Critical Care

Critical Care

Edited by

John M. Oropello, MD, FACP, FCCP, FCCM

Professor of Surgery & Medicine
Program Director, Critical Care Medicine
Co-Director, Surgical ICU
Icahn School of Medicine at Mount Sinai
New York, New York

Stephen M. Pastores, MD, FACP, FCCP, FCCM

Professor of Medicine and Anesthesiology
Weill Cornell Medical College of Cornell University
Program Director, Critical Care Medicine
Department of Anesthesiology and Critical Care Medicine
Memorial Sloan Kettering Cancer Center
New York, New York

Vladimir Kvetan, MD

Director
Jay B. Langner Critical Care System
Professor of Anesthesiology & Clinical Medicine
Associate Professor of Surgery
Montefiore Medical Center
Albert Einstein College of Medicine
Bronx, New York

Mc
Graw
Hill
Education

New York   Chicago   San Francisco   Athens   London   Madrid   Mexico City
Milan   New Delhi   Singapore   Sydney   Toronto

Critical Care

Cover image © 2016, Memorial Sloan Kettering Cancer Center.

2 3 4 5 6 7   QVS   23 22 21 20 19

ISBN 978-0-07-182081-3
MHID 0-07-182081-7

This book was set in Minion Pro by Cenveo® Publisher Services.
The editors were Brian Belval and Christie Naglieri.
The production supervisor was Catherine Saggese.
Project Management was provided by Srishti Malasi, Cenveo Publisher Services.
Quad/Graphics was printer and binder.

This book is printed on acid-free paper.

Library of Congress Cataloging-in-Publication Data

Names: Oropello, John M., editor. | Pastores, Stephen M., editor. | Kvetan,
   Vladimir, editor.
Title: Current diagnosis and treatment. Critical Care / [edited by]
   John M. Oropello, Stephen M. Pastores, Vladimir Kvetan.
Other titles: Critical Care
Description: First edition. | New York : McGraw-Hill, [2016] | Includes
   bibliographical references and index.
Identifiers: LCCN 2016003118| ISBN 9780071820813 (pbk.) | ISBN 0071820817
   (pbk.)
Subjects: | MESH: Critical Care—methods | Emergency Medical
   Services—methods | Critical Illness—therapy | Diagnostic Techniques and
   Procedures
Classification: LCC RC86.7 | NLM WX 218 | DDC 616.02/8—dc23
LC record available at http://lccn.loc.gov/2016003118

McGraw-Hill Education books are available at special quantity discounts to use as premiums and
sales promotions or for use in corporate training programs. To contact a representative, please visit the
Contact Us pages at www.mhprofessional.com.

We dedicate this 1st edition of Lange Critical Care to:
Our families:
Hiromi, Adrianna, and Luke Oropello
Cindy Conley and Henry Kvetan
Maria Teresa DeSancho, MD, MSc, Steven Michael, and Monica Cristina Pastores
For their love and understanding
and
To Our Critical Care Fellows, past, present, and future
and
To the generations of intensivists whose selfless clinical and academic work will change
the face of our chosen specialty for our patients, as well as advance the governance of
critical care with the leadership of our institutions.

Contents

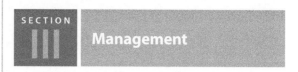

SECTION III   Management

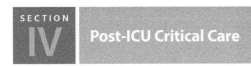

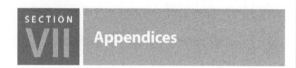

Contributors

Jason Adelman, MD, MS
Chief Patient Safety Officer
Associate Chief Quality Officer
New York Presbyterian/Columbia University
    Medical Center
New York, New York

Muhammad Adrish, MD, FCCP
Attending, Pulmonary and Critical Care
Bronx-Lebanon Hospital Center
Affiliated with Icahn School of Medicine at Mount Sinai
Bronx, New York

Ylaine Rose T. Aldeguer, MD
Intensivist
Regional Medical Center of San Jose
San Jose, California

Mark Ault
Department of Medicine
Cedars-Sinai Medical Center
Los Angeles, California

Elie Azoulay, MD
Medical ICU, Saint Louis Hospital AP-HP
Faculté de Médecine Paris-Diderot
Sorbonne Paris-Cité
Paris, France

Jan Bakker, MD, PhD, FCCP
Department of Intensive Care Adults
Erasmus MC University Medical Centre
Rotterdam, The Netherlands

Erica Bang, MD
Assistant Professor of Emergency Medicine
Mount Sinai Beth Israel Medical Center
New York, New York

Maneesha D. Bangar, MD
Attending Physician
Department of Critical Care Medicine
Jay B. Langner Critical Care System
Assistant Professor of Clinical Medicine
Montefiore Medical Center
Albert Einstein College of Medicine
Bronx, New York

Philip S. Barie, MD, MBA, FIDSA, FCCM, FACS
Professor of Surgery
Professor of Public Health in Medicine
Weill Cornell Medical College
Attending Surgeon
NewYork-Presbyterian Hospital-Weill Cornell
    Medical Center
New York, New York

Adel Bassily-Marcus, MD
Associate Professor, Surgery
Icahn School of Medicine at Mount Sinai
New York, New York

Tara T. Bellamkonda, DO
Assistant Professor of Medicine
Division of Critical Care Medicine
Albert Einstein College of Medicine of Yeshiva University
Bronx, New York

Jay Berger, MD, PhD
Assistant Professor, Department of Anesthesiology
Department of Medicine, Division of Critical
    Care Medicine
Montefiore Medical Center
Bronx, New York

Samarth Beri, MD
Attending Critical Care Physician
Department of Medicine
New York Presbyerian Hospital Queens
Flushing, New York

Saad Bhatti, MD
Clinical Instructor, Surgical/Trauma Intensive Care Unit
Elmhurst Hospital Center
Elmhurst, New York

Leon Boudourakis, MD, MHS
Assistant Professor, Surgery
SUNY Downstate College of Medicine
Kings County Hospital
Brooklyn, New York

Daniel Caplivski, MD
Medical Director
Travel Medicine Program
Assistant Professor of Medicine
Division of Infectious Diseases
Icahn School of Medicine at Mount Sinai
New York, New York

Anthony Carlese, DO, FCCP
Medical Director
Cardiothoracic Intensive Care Unit
Jay B. Langner Critical Care System
Montefiore Medical Center
Bronx, New York
Assistant Professor of Clinical Medicine and Neurology
Albert Einstein College of Medicine
Bronx, New York

John Cavagnaro, PA
Department Critical Care
Montefiore Medical Center
Bronx, New York

Subani Chandra, MD
Division of Pulmonary, Allergy and Critical
    Care Medicine
Columbia University College of Physicians and Surgeons
New York, New York

Alfredo Lee Chang, MD
Division of Pulmonary Medicine
Department of Medicine
Albert Einstein College of Medicine
Bronx, New York

John C. Chapin, MD
Assistant Professor of Medicine
Weill Cornell Medical College
New York, New York

Mohit Chawla, MD, FCCP
Assistant Attending Director Interventional
    Pulmonology Program
Pulmonary Service
Department of Medicine
Memorial Sloan Kettering Cancer Center
New York, New York

Sanjay Chawla, MD, FACP, FCCP
Critical Care Medicine Service
Department of Anesthesiology and Critical
    Care Medicine
Memorial Sloan Kettering Cancer Center
New York, New York

Julie Chen, PharmD, BCPS
Department of Pharmacy
Montefiore Medical Center
Bronx, New York

Leon Chen, MSc, AGACNP-BC, CCRN, CEN
Nurse Practitioner
Critical Care Medicine Service
Department of Anesthesiology and Critical
    Care Medicine
Memorial Sloan Kettering Cancer Center
New York, New York
Clinical Faculty
Graduate and Undergraduate Program
NYU Rory Meyers College of Nursing
New York, New York

Ko Eun Choi, MD
Department of Neurology
Cedars-Sinai Medical Center
Advanced Health Sciences Pavilion—Neurosciences
Los Angeles, California

David Chong, MD
Division of Pulmonary, Allergy and Critical
    Care Medicine
Columbia University College of Physicians and Surgeons
New York, New York

Mabel Chung, MD
Assistant Professor, Department of Anesthesiology
Department of Medicine, Division of Critical
    Care Medicine
Montefiore Medical Center
Bronx, New York

Mai O. Colvin, MD
Department of Internal Medicine
Montefiore Medical Center
Bronx, New York

George Coritsidis, MD
Associate Professor
Icahn School of Medicine at Mount Sinai
New York, New York
Director, Surgical/Trauma Intensive Care Unit; Chief,
    Division of Nephrology
Elmhurst Hospital Center
Elmhurst, New York

Wilma Correa-Lopez, MD
Montefiore Medical Center
Bronx, New York

Annette Czernik, MD
Department of Dermatology
Icahn School of Medicine at Mount Sinai
New York, New York

Rhonda D'Agostino, RN, ACNP-BC, CCRN, FCCM
ICU/PACU NP Coordinator
Department of Anesthesiology and Critical Care
Memorial Sloan Kettering Cancer Center
New York, New York

Alexandre Demoule, MD
Sorbonne Universités, UPMC Univ Paris 06
INSERM, UMRS1158 Neurophysiologie respiratoire
    expérimentale et Clinique
Paris, France
AP-HP, Groupe Hospitalier Pitié-Salpêtrière Charles
    Foix, Service de Pneumologie et Réanimation
    Médicale (Département "R3S")
Paris, France

Maria T. Desancho, MD, MSc
Associate Professor of Clinical Medicine
Clinical Director of Benign Hematology
Division of Hematology and Medical Oncology
Department of Medicine
Weill Cornell Medical College
New York, New York

Vikram Dhawan, MD
Assistant Professor, Medicine/Neurology
Critical Care Medicine
Mount Sinai Beth Israel, Mount Sinai Hospital
New York, New York

Fred DiBlasio, MD
Director, Critical Care
Huntington Hospital
Hofstra School of Medicine
Northshore University
New York, New York

Kevin C. Doerschug MD, MS, FCCP
Professor of Medicine
Division of Pulmonary Diseases, Critical Care, and
    Occupational Medicine
University of Iowa Carver College of Medicine
Iowa City, Iowa

John T. Doucette, PhD
Associate Professor
Department of Environmental Medicine and
    Public Health
Icahn School of Medicine at Mount Sinai
New York, New York

Michael Duff, MD
Intensivist, Advanced ICU Care
St. Louis, Missouri

Alina Dulu, MD
Assistant Professor, Department of Medicine
    Critical Care
Assistant Professor, The Saul R. Korey Department
    of Neurology
Montefiore Medical Center
Albert Einstein College of Medicine
Bronx, New York

Lewis Ari Eisen, MD
Division of Critical Care Medicine
Department of Medicine
Albert Einstein College of Medicine
Bronx, New York

Michael Elias, MD
Fellow, Critical Care Medicine
Icahn School of Medicine at Mount Sinai
New York, New York

Adebayo Esan, MBBS, FCCP, FACP
Director, Pulmonary Hypertension Center
Associate Director, Medical Intensive Care Unit
New York Methodist Hospital
New York, New York

Eddy Fan, MD, PhD
Assistant Professor of Medicine
Interdepartmental Division of Critical Care
    Medicine and Institute of Health Policy, Management
    and Evaluation
University of Toronto
Ontario, Canada
Director, Critical Care Research
University Health Network and Mount Sinai Hospital
Ontario, Canada

Emily Fish, MD
Harvard Medical School
Boston, Massachusetts

Robert Foronjy, MD
Department of Medicine
Division of Pulmonary, Critical Care and Sleep Medicine
St. Luke's Roosevelt Hospital of the Mount Sinai
    Health System
New York, New York
Department of Critical Care Medicine, Montefiore
    Medical Center
Albert Einstein College of Medicine
Bronx, New York

Oren A. Friedman, MD
Associate Director, Cardiac Surgery ICU
Cedars Sinai Medical Center
New York, New York

Patrick Geraghty, PhD
Department of Medicine
Division of Pulmonary, Critical Care and Sleep Medicine
St. Luke's Roosevelt Hospital
Mount Sinai Health System
New York, New York

Hayley B. Gershengorn, MD
Division of Critical Care Medicine
Albert Einstein College of Medicine
Montefiore Medical Center
Bronx, New York

Carmine Gianatiempo, MD
Director of Critical Care
Englewood Hospital and Medical Center
Englewood, New Jersey

Umesh K. Gidwani, MD
Chief, Cardiac Critical Care
Associate Professor, Cardiology, Pulmonary, Critical Care, and Sleep Medicine
Icahn School of Medicine at Mount Sinai
New York, New York

Mark Gillespie, PA-C, MS
Icahn School of Medicine at Mount Sinai
New York, New York

Dena Goffman, MD
Associate Professor
Department of Obstetrics and Gynecology and Women's Health
Columbia University Medical Center
New York, New York

Martin E. Goldman, MD
Professor of Cardiology & Medicine
Program Director, Academic Track Cardiology
Icahn School of Medicine at Mount Sinai
New York, New York

Baruch Goldstein, MD
Banner iCare/Banner Health
Mesa, Arizona

Lawrence T. Goodnough, MD
Professor
Departments of Pathology and Medicine
Stanford University School of Medicine
Stanford, California

Yonatan Y. Greenstein, MD
Division of Pulmonary, Critical Care, and Sleep Medicine
Hofstra North Shore-LIJ School of Medicine
New Hyde Park, New York

Michael A. Gropper, MD, PhD
Professor and Acting Chairman
Department of Anesthesia and Perioperative Care
University of California
San Francisco, California

Jay N. Gross, MD
Montefiore Medical Center
Bronx, New York

Michael J. Grushko, MD
Attending, Arrhythmia and Electrophysiology
Jacobi Medical Center/North Central Bronx Hospital
Montefiore Einstein Heart and Vascular Care Center
Assistant Professor of Medicine
Albert Einstein College of Medicine
Bronx, New York

Perminder Gulani, MD
Department of Medicine
Division of Critical Care Medicine
Montefiore Medical Center
Bronx, New York

Dipti Gupta, MD, MPH
Assistant Attending Physician
Cardiology Service, Department of Medicine
Memorial Sloan Kettering Cancer Center
New York, New York

Rohit R. Gupta, MD
Fellow, Critical Care Medicine
Icahn School of Medicine at Mount Sinai
New York, New York

Cristina Gutierrez, MD
Assistant Professor of Critical Care
Department of Critical Care Medicine
The University of Texas MD Anderson Cancer Center
Houston, Texas

Edward Pellerano Guzman, MD
Fellow, Critical Care Medicine
Icahn School of Medicine at Mount Sinai
New York, New York

Negin Hajizadeh, MD, MPH
Intensivist, Critical Care Medicine
North Shore-LIJ Health System
Manhasset, New York

Kaye Hale, MD
Assistant Attending
Department of Anesthesiology and Critical Care Medicine
Memorial Sloan Kettering Cancer Center
New York, New York

Zaffar K. Haque
Division of Pulmonary Medicine
Montefiore Medical Center—Moses Campus
Bronx, New York

Renzo H. Hidalgo, MD
Fellow, Critical Care Medicine
Icahn School of Medicine at Mount Sinai
New York, New York

Vanessa P. Ho, MD, MPH
Assistant Professor of Surgery
Department of Surgery
Case Western Reserve University
Cleveland, Ohio
Attending Surgeon
University Hospitals of Cleveland
Cleveland, Ohio

Carol Hodgson PhD, FACP
ANZIC Research Centre and the Department of
    Epidemiology and Preventive Medicine (CH)
School of Public Health and Preventive Medicine
Monash University, Melbourne, Australia
Interdepartmental Division of Critical Care
    Medicine (EF), University of Toronto
Ontario, Canada

Aluko A. Hope, MD, MSCE
Department of Medicine, Division of Critical Care
    Medicine, Montefiore Medical Center
Albert Einstein College of Medicine of Yeshiva University
Bronx, New York

Leila Hosseinian, MD
Assistant Professor
Department of Anesthesiology
Icahn School of Medicine at Mount Sinai
New York, New York

S. Jean Hsieh, MD
Associate Professor of Medicine
Division of Critical Care Medicine
Department of Medicine
Montefiore Medical Center
Albert Einstein College of Medicine
Bronx, New York

Ella Illuzzi, RN, ANP-BC
Icahn School of Medicine
Mount Sinai Hospital
New York, New York

William Jakobleff, MD
Assistant professor
Montefiore medical center
Bronx, New York
Albert Einstein College of Medicine
Bronx, New York

Aaron Joffe, DO, FCCM
Department of Anesthesiology and Pain Medicine
Harborview Medical Center
University of Washington Medical School
Seattle, Washington

Jeremy M. Kahn, MD MSc
Professor of Critical Care, Medicine, and Health Policy
Department of Critical Care
Department of Medicine
University of Pittsburgh School of Medicine
Pittsburgh, Pennsylvania
Department of Health Policy and Management
University of Pittsburgh Graduate School of
    Public Health
Pittsburgh, Pennsylvania

Satish Kalanjeri, MD
Assistant Professor of Clinical Medicine
Interventional Pulmonology
Louisiana State University Health Sciences Center
Shreveport, Louisiana

Pankaj Kapadia, MD
Fellow, Critical Care Medicine
Icahn School of Medicine at Mount Sinai
New York, New York

Massoud G. Kazzi, MD
Intensivist
Bronx, New York

Adam Keene, MD
Associate Professor of Clinical Medicine and Neurology
Fellowship Director
Division of Critical Care Medicine
Department of Medicine
Montefiore Medical Center
Bronx, New York

David Keith, PA-C, MS
Critical Care Medicine Service
Montefiore Medical Center
Bronx, New York

Inga Khachaturova, MD
Critical Care Fellow
Icahn School of Medicine at Mount Sinai
New York, New York

Felix Khusid, RRT-ACCS, NPS, RPFT, FAARC
Administrative Director of Respiratory Therapy and
    Pulmonary Physiology Center
New York Methodist Hospital
New York, New York

Claude Killu, MD
Cardiac Surgery Intensive Care, Kaiser Permanente
Los Angeles Medical Center
Los Angeles, California

Brian Kim, MD
Assistant Professor of Clinical Medicine
Division of Gastrointestinal and Liver Diseases
    Transplant Hepatology Keck School of Medicine
University of Southern California
Los Angeles, California

Min Jung Kim, MD
Intensivist, Cardiopulmonary Intensive Care Unit
CAMC Memorial Hospital
Charleston, West Virginia

Leona Kim-Schluger, MD
Professor of Medicine
Associate Director of the Recanati/Miller
    Transplantation Institute
Icahn School of Medicine at Mount Sinai
New York, New York

Roopa Kohli-Seth, MD
Professor, Surgery
Director Surgical ICU
Icahn School of Medicine at Mount Sinai
New York, New York

Bonnie Koo, MD
Assistant Professor & Director, Hospital-Based
    Dermatology
Department of Dermatology
Hofstra Northwell School of Medicine
Lake Success, New York

Natalie Kostelecky, RN, BSN
Clinical Research Nurse Coordinator, Critical
    Care Medicine
Department of Anesthesiology and Critical
    Care Medicine
Memorial Sloan Kettering Cancer Center
New York, New York

Steven Krasnica, MD
Attending Physician
Tristar Cenennial Medical Center
Nashville, Tennessee

James A. Kruse, MD
Professor, Columbia University College of Physicians
    and Surgeons
Chief, Critical Care
Bassett Medical Center
Cooperstown, New York

Vladimir Kvetan, MD
Director
Jay B. Langner Critical Care System
Professor of Anesthesiology & Clinical Medicine
Associate Professor of Surgery
Montefiore Medical Center
Albert Einstein College of Medicine
Bronx, New York

Sheron Latcha, MD, FASN
Associate Attending Physician
Memorial Sloan Kettering Cancer Center
New York, New York
Assistant Professor of Clinical Medicine
Weill Cornell Medical College
New York, New York

Ilde Manuel Lee, MD
Clinical Faculty
Department of Critical Care Medicine
Kendall Regional Medical Center
Miami, Florida

Robert Lee, MD
Assistant Attending
Interventional Pulmonology Program
Pulmonary Service
Department of Medicine
Memorial Sloan Kettering Cancer Center
New York, New York

Andrew Leibowitz, MD
Chairman of Anesthesiology
Icahn School of Medicine at Mount Sinai
New York, New York

Sharon Leung, MD, MS, MHA, FCCP
Director of Clinical Operations
Director of Quality and Safety
Jay B. Langner Critical Care System
Montefiore Medical Center
Bronx, New York
Associate Professor of Clinical Medicine
Department of Medicine
Albert Einstein College of Medicine
Bronx, New York

Leonard Lim, MD
Montefiore Medical Center
Bronx, New York

Angela K. M. Lipshutz, MD, MPH
Assistant Professor
Department of Anesthesia and Perioperative Care
University of California
San Francisco, California

George Lominadze, MD
Staff Intensivist
Assistant Clinical Professor of Medicine
Columbia University
New York-Presbyterian/Lawrence Hospital
Bronxville, New York

Dana Lustbader MD, FCCM, FCCP
Section Head, Palliative Medicine
Intensivist, Critical Care Medicine
North Shore-LIJ Health System
Manhasset, New York

Nagendra Y. Madisi, MD
Fellow, Critical Care Medicine
Icahn School of Medicine at Mount Sinai
New York, New York

Jibran Majeed, ACNP-BC, CCRN
Critical Care Medicine Service
Memorial Sloan Kettering Cancer Center
New York, New York

Jun Makino, MD
Fellow, Critical Care Medicine
Icahn School of Medicine at Mount Sinai
New York, New York

Anthony Manasia, MD, FCCP
Associate Professor, Surgery and Medicine
Icahn School of Medicine at Mount Sinai
New York, New York

Halinder S. Mangat, MD
Assistant Professor
Department of Neurology and Neurosurgery
Division of Stroke and Critical Care
Weill Cornell Medical Center
New York, New York

Paul Marik, MD, FCCP, FCCM
Chief, Pulmonary and Critical Care Medicine
Professor of Medicine
Eastern Virginia Medical School
Norfolk, Virginia

Roshen Mathew, MD
Montefiore Medical Center
Bronx, New York

Paul H. Mayo, MD, FCCP
Division of Pulmonary, Critical Care, and Sleep Medicine
Hofstra North Shore-LIJ School of Medicine
New Hyde Park, New York

Russell J. McCulloh, MD
Assistant Professor
University of Missouri-Kansas City SOM
Pediatric Infectious Diseases
Children's Mercy Hospital
Kansas City, Missouri

Jeffrey I. Mechanick, MD
Clinical Professor of Medicine
Director, Metabolic Support
Division of Endocrinology, Diabetes, and Bone Disease
Icahn School of Medicine at Mount Sinai
New York, New York

Daniel Miller, MD
Critical Care Medicine Physician
Westchester Medical Center
Valhalla, New York

Edward Mossop, MD
Cardiac Surgery Intensive Care
Kaiser Permanente
Los Angeles Medical Center
Los Angeles, California

Nelson Moussazadeh, MD
Department of Neurological Surgery
New York-Presbyterian Hospital/Weill Cornell
    Medical Center
New York, New York

Victor Murgolo, CCRN
Nurse Clinician, Surgical ICU
Mount Sinai Hospital
New York, New York

Jon Narimasu, MD
Fellow, Critical Care Anesthesiology
Icahn School of Medicine at Mount Sinai
New York, New York

Tzvi Neuman, DO
Montefiore Medical Center
Albert Einstein College of Medicine
Bronx, New York

John K. Nia, MD
New York Medical College
New York, New York

Steven M. Opal, MD, FIDSA
Professor of Medicine
Infectious Disease Division
Alpert Medical School of Brown University
Providence, Rhode Island
Co-Director of the Ocean State Clinical
    Coordinating Center
Rhode Island Hospital
Providence, Rhode Island

John M. Oropello, MD, FACP, FCCP, FCCM
Professor of Surgery and Medicine
Program Director, Critical Care Medicine
Co-Director, Surgical ICU
Icahn School of Medicine at Mount Sinai
New York, New York

Deborah Orsi, MD
Montefiore Medical Center
Bronx, New York

Amit Pandit, MD
Department of Emergency Medicine
University of Mississippi Medical Center
Jackson, Mississippi

Stephen M. Pastores, MD, FACP, FCCP, FCCM
Professor of Medicine and Anesthesiology
Weill Cornell Medical College of Cornell University
New York, New York
Program Director, Critical Care Medicine
Department of Anesthesiology and Critical
    Care Medicine
Memorial Sloan Kettering Cancer Center
New York, New York

Pritul Patel, MD
Assistant Clinical Professor
Division of Critical Care
Division of Cardiothoracic Anesthesiology
Department of Anesthesiology and
    Perioperative Medicine
Ronald Reagan-UCLA Medical Center
Los Angeles, California

Annie Lynn Penaco, MD
Resident
Department of Anesthesiology
Montefiore Medical Center
Albert Einstein College of Medicine
Bronx, New York

Anuja Pradhan, MD
Critical Care Medicine
Hackensack University Medical Center
Hackensack, New Jersey
Infectious Disease
St. Barnabas Medical Center
Livingston, New Jersey

Nida Qadir, MD
Assistant Professor of Medicine
Assistant Professor of Neurology
Montefiore Medical Center
Bronx, New York
Albert Einstein College of Medicine
Bronx, New York

Ellie S. Ragsdale, MD
Instructor
Department of Obstetrics and Gynecology and
    Women's Health
Cleveland, Ohio

Marjan Rahmanian, MD
Division of Critical Care Medicine
Department of Medicine
Albert Einstein College of Medicine
Bronx, New York

Preethi Rajan, MD
Critical Care Medicine Service
Department of Anesthesiology and Critical
    Care Medicine
Memorial Sloan Kettering Cancer Center
New York, New York

Meenakshi M. Rana, MD
Assistant Professor
Division of Infectious Disease
Department of Medicine
Icahn School of Medicine at Mount Sinai
New York, New York

Jamie M. Rand, MD, FACS
Assistant Professor of Surgery
Trauma/Surgical Critical Care
St. Louis University Hospital
St Louis, Missouri

Suhail Raoof, MD, FCCP, MACP, FCCM
Professor of Medicine
Hofstra Northwell School of Medicine Chief
Pulmonary Service
Lenox Hill Hospital
New York, New York

J. David Roccaforte, MD
Associate Professor of Anesthesiology and Surgery
Department of Anesthesiology
New York University School of Medicine
Surgical Intensive Care Unit
Bellevue Hospital Center
New York, New York

Nancy Roistacher, MD
Attending Physician
Memorial Sloan Kettering Cancer Center
New York, New York

Axel Rosengart, MD, PhD, MPH
Professor, Departments of Neurology, Neurosurgery and
    Biomedical Sciences
Director, Neurocritical Care
Cedars-Sinai Medical Center, Advanced Health Sciences
    Pavilion—Neurosciences
Los Angeles, California

Katerina Rusinova, MD
Department of Anaesthesia and Intensive Care
Institute for Medical Humanities
1st Medical Faculty, Charles University
General University Hospital
Prague, Czech Republic

Omar Saeed, MD
Montefiore Medical Center
Bronx, New York

Tarang Safi, MD
Resident, Department of Anesthesiology
Montefiore Medical Center
Bronx, New York

Venketraman Sahasranaman, MD
Fellow, Department of Medicine
Division of Critical Care Medicine
Montefiore Medical Center
Bronx, New York

Amar Anantdeep Singh Sarao, MD, RCPSC, D.ABIM
Intensivist, Division of Critical Care Medicine
The University Hospital of Northern BC
British Columbia, Canada

Mark Schattner, MD
Gastroenterology and Nutrition Service
Department of Medicine
Memorial Sloan Kettering Cancer Center
New York, New York

Bradley A. Schiff
Associate Professor
Department of Otorhinolaryngology—Head and
    Neck Surgery
Montefiore Medical Center
Albert Einstein College of Medicine
Bronx, New York

Gregory A. Schmidt, MD, FCCP
Professor of Medicine
Division of Pulmonary Diseases, Critical Care, and
    Occupational Medicine
University of Iowa Carver College of Medicine
Iowa City, Iowa

Christopher W. Seymour, MD MSc
Department of Critical Care
Department of Emergency Medicine
University of Pittsburgh School of Medicine
Pittsburgh, Pennsylvania

Pari Shah, MD, MSCE
Gastroenterology and Nutrition Service
Department of Medicine
Memorial Sloan Kettering Cancer Center
New York, New York

Aryeh Shander, MD
Chair, Department of Anesthesiology, Critical Care
    Medicine, Pain Management and Hyperbaric
    Medicine, Englewood Hospital and Medical Center
Englewood, New Jersey
Clinical Professor Anesthesiology, Medicine and Surgery
Icahn School of Medicine at Mount Sinai
New York, New York

Ariel L. Shiloh, MD
Director, Critical Care Consult Service
Assistant Professor of Clinical Medicine and Neurology
Jay B. Langner Critical Care Service
Department of Medicine
Montefiore Medical Center
Albert Einstein College of Medicine
Bronx, New York

Shant Shirvanian, MD
Pulmonary Fellow
Cedars-Sinai Medical Center
Los Angeles, California

Effie Singas MD, FACP, FCCP
Division of Pulmonary, Critical Care and Sleep Medicine
North Shore-LIJ Hofstra School of Medicine
Manhasset, New York

Daniel J. Singer, MD
Associate Director Emergency Department Intensive
    Care Unit
Lincoln Medical Center
Bronx, New York

Anil Singh, MD
Pulmonary Fellow
University of Tennessee
Knoxville, Tennessee

Charanya Sivaramakrishnan, MD
Fellow, Critical Care Medicine
Icahn School of Medicine at Mount Sinai
New York, New York

Isaac Soo, MD
Gastroenterology Service
Department of Medicine
University of Alberta
Calgary, Alberta

Graciela J. Soto, MD, MS
Montefiore Medical Center
Bronx, New York

Tihomir Stefanec
Assistant Professor of Medicine and Neurology
Albert Einstein College of Medicine
Bronx, New York
Attending Physician
Critical Care Medicine
Department of Medicine
Montefiore Medical Center
Bronx, New York

Philip E. Stieg, PhD, MD
Chairman and Neurosurgeon-in-chief
Department of Neurological Surgery
Weill Cornell Brain and Spine Center
Weill Cornell Medical Center
New York, New York

Erik Stoltenberg, MD
Department of Anesthesiology and Pain Medicine
Veterans Administration Puget Sound Health Care
    System University of Washington Medical School
Seattle, Washington

Reuben J. Strayer, MD, FRCPC, FAAEM
Department of Emergency Medicine
Icahn School of Medicine at Mount Sinai
NYU School of Medicine
New York, New York

Samantha Strickler, DO
Fellow, Critical Care Medicine
Icahn School of Medicine at Mount Sinai
New York, New York

Rami Tadros, MD
Associate Program Director
Assistant Professor of Surgery and Radiology, Icahn
    School of Medicine at Mount Sinai
New York, New York
Division of Vascular Surgery, Department of Surgery,
    The Mount Sinai Hospital
New York, New York

Daniel Talmor, MD, MPH
Edward Lowenstein Professor and Chair
Department of Anesthesia, Critical Care, and
    Pain Medicine
Beth Israel Deaconess Medical Center and Harvard
    Medical School
Boston, Massachusetts

Victor F. Tapson, MD
Director, Venous Thromboembolism and Pulmonary
    Vascular Disease Research
Director, Clinical Research, Women's Guild
    Lung Institute
Associate Director, Division of Pulmonary and
    Critical Care
Cedars-Sinai Medical Center
Los Angeles, California

James M. Tauras, MD, FACC
Assistant Professor of Medicine
Albert Einstein Medical College
Medical Director, CCU
Montefiore Medical Center/Einstein Division
Bronx, New York

Rafael Tolentino, MD
Research Fellow
Department of Critical Care Medicine
Cedimat
Santo Domingo, Dominican Republic

Matthew I. Tomey, MD, FACC
Assistant Professor of Medicine (Cardiology), Icahn
    School of Medicine at Mount Sinai
New York, New York
Attending Physician, Cardiac Care Unit
Attending Physician, Cardiothoracic Intensive Care Unit
Attending Interventional Cardiologist, Cardiac
    Catheterization Laboratory
The Institute for Critical Care Medicine
The Zena and Michael A. Wiener Cardiovascular Institute
Mount Sinai Health System
New York, New York

Jamie S. Ullman, MD, FACS, FAANS
Associate Professor of Neurosurgery
Hofstra North Shore-LIJ School of Medicine
Manhasset, New York

Elvis Umanzor, MD
Assistant Professor of Anesthesiology
Elmhurst Hospital Center
Elmhurst, New York

Aditya Uppalapati, MD
Assistant Professor of Clinical Medicine
Weill Cornell Medical College and Institute of Academic
    Medicine at Houston Methodist Hospital
Houston, Texas

Carla Venegas-Borsellino, MD
Montefiore Medical Center
Bronx, New York

Michael A. Via, MD
Assistant Professor of Medicine
Division of Endocrinology and Metabolism
Beth Israel Medical Center
Albert Einstein College of Medicine
Bronx, New York

Louis P. Voigt, MD
Associate Professor of Medicine and Anesthesiology
Weill Cornell Medical College of Cornell University
New York, New York
Attending Physician
Department of Anesthesiology and Critical
    Care Medicine
Memorial Sloan Kettering Cancer Center
New York, New York

Jennifer Wang, DO
Fellow, Critical Care Medicine
Icahn School of Medicine at Mount Sinai
New York, New York

Richard Weiner, MSN, RN, ANP-BC
Memorial Sloan Kettering Cancer Center
New York, New York

Scott Weingart, MD FCCM
Associate Professor
Chief, Division of Emergency Critical Care
Department of Emergency Medicine
Stony Brook Medicine
Director, Resuscitation and Acute Critical Care Unit
Stony Brook Hospital
New York, New York

Sara Wilson, MS, RD, CNSC
Senior Director Clinical Nutrition
The Mount Sinai Hospital
Mount Sinai Beth Israel
New York, New York

Hannah Wunsch, MD, MSc
Department of Anesthesiology, College of Physicians and
    Surgeons, Columbia University
Department of Epidemiology, Mailman School of Public
    Health, Columbia University
New York, New York

Mekeleya Yimen, MD
Intensivist
Lenox Hill Hospital
New York, New York

Joanna Yohannes-Tomicich, MSN, RN, NP-C
Memorial Sloan Kettering Cancer Center
New York, New York

Jose R. Yunen, MD
Assistant Professor
Department of Critical Care Medicine
Montefiore Medical Center
Bronx, New York

Rafael Alba Yunen, MD
Fellow, Critical Care Medicine
Icahn School of Medicine at Mount Sinai
New York, New York

Christopher Zammit, MD
Assistant Professor of Emergency Medicine, Neurology,
    Neurosurgery, and Internal Medicine
Attending Neurointensivist and Emergency Physician
School of Medicine & Dentistry
University of Rochester Medical Center
Rochester, New York

Ronald Zolty, MD, PhD
Professor
Division of Cardiology
University of Nebraska Medical Center (UNMC)
Heart Failure Fellowship Program Director
Advanced Heart Failure and Pulmonary
    Hypertension Program
Omaha, Nebraska

Preface

We present *Lange Critical Care* in the spirit of our philosophy that the distinctions between critical care medicine, critical care surgery, and critical care anesthesiology are artificial; more the result of politics than medicine. All intensivists, regardless of primary discipline, must possess a core set of critical care skills that allow them to manage the sickest of patients. Surgical, medical, anesthesia, or neurological problems can arise in any patient, particularly in the critically ill. Furthermore, most hospitals today contain intensive care units (ICUs) that are mixed by intention or by overflow and multidisciplinary trained intensivists are best equipped to both recognize and manage the wide range of acute care problems.

The chapters reflect the growing scope of critical care provided outside of the ICU and the increasing importance and recognition of critical care services within the hospital structure. The Pre-ICU Critical Care section focuses on triage, transport, resuscitation, and stabilization, and includes forward-looking chapters on pre-ICU syndromes, hypothermia, military-related injuries, regionalization of critical care, and biomarkers in decision making. The second and largest section, ICU Critical Care, contains over 74 chapters and subchapters on multidisciplinary critical care that includes comprehensive coverage of medical, surgical, anesthetic, and neurological issues involving multiple organ systems. The third section, Management, includes chapters on education and simulation, bed utilization, the ICU's role in the global hospital environment, ICU staffing models, telemedicine issues, ethics, palliative care, and ICU governance. The fourth section, Post-ICU

Critical Care, contains chapters on postintensive care syndrome and outcomes research. The fifth section, Genomics of Critical Care, contains one chapter, Critical Care Medicine in the Era of Omics, written to provide a basic understanding of the potential applications of genomics unique to tackling critical illnesses. An integral part of critical care practice is addressed in the sixth section, Critical Care Procedures, that includes guidance in maintaining patient safety and extracting accurate information from monitors. The seventh section, Appendices, contains reference material and formulas, including a chapter on bedside statistics, an essential skillset for the modern intensivist. Sprinkled throughout each section are "Controversies" chapters provided to address some of the more ambiguous aspects of critical care.

In keeping with the team approach and multiprofessional nature of critical care delivery, several chapters are authored or coauthored with critical care fellows, ICU nurses, physician assistants, nurse practitioners, and pharmacists.

In addition to practicing critical care physicians and fellows in training, this edition is designed to be a valuable resource for all critical care providers-hospitalists, subspecialty physicians, residents, nurses, physician assistants, nurse practitioners, nutritionists, pharmacists, respiratory therapists, and medical students.

We are grateful to the publishing editors at McGraw-Hill (Brian Belval, Christie Naglieri, and Kathryn Schell) for their tireless efforts and guidance in the production of this textbook.

Triage and Transport in the Field for the Critically Ill Patient

Carla Venegas-Borsellino, MD

KEY POINTS

1 The combination of an increasing patient population and diminished funding for hospital services is creating a need for optimized distribution of medical resources. Efficient management of major incidents involves triage, treatment and transport.

2 Triaging tools would benefit initial allocation and future allocation of resources over time to support ongoing needs of survivors of critical illness. Over triage might overburden the local health care systems, have a negative impact on patient outcomes, and decrease cost effectiveness.

3 This is a review of the most common triage protocols used for illness scoring as methods to identify the severity of the

injury, and the most often recommended guidelines for field triage of injured patients.

4 Critical care regionalization is becoming more common and studies have supported that the transport of critically ill patients to a tertiary care center leads to better patient outcomes.

5 Patients' and providers' safety, as well as the benefits and cost-effectiveness of the mode of transport are key considerations when assessing whether to transport a critically ill patient. Current standards for interfacility transport dictate that the decision on transport mode and team composition is based on individual patient requirements, considering minimization of transport time and anticipated treatment requirements during transport.

INTRODUCTION

The word "triage" originates from the French "trier" (to choose from among several) and was originally applied around 1792 by Baron Dominique Jean Larrey, surgeon-in-chief to Napoleon's Imperial Guard, in reference to the process of sorting wounded soldiers. Its aim was to optimize the use of available medical resources to maximize efficacy; patients with the greatest chance of survival and the least

resource use are treated first.[1] Currently, the combination of an increasing patient population and diminished funding for hospital services is creating a need for optimized distribution of medical resources. Efficient management of major incidents involves triage, treatment, and transport. Useful triage tools would predict which patients have the greatest chance of survival, which patients are likely to die, and which will benefit most from advanced medical care such as mechanical ventilation. These are important issues not only for initial allocation of resources but also for future allocation of resources over time to support the ongoing needs of survivors of critical illness.

The challenges associated with the triaging process have caused health systems to initiate a number of adaptational strategies, including regionalization of care, specialization of critical care facilities, and better allocation of available personnel and equipment; the triaging process impacts multiple practices such as pre-hospital care, emergency department services, intensive care, surgical intervention, and the process of determining the order of rank for patients to receive advanced therapeutic treatments (including renal replacement therapy and organ transplantation). In the field, emergency medical services (EMS) providers must ensure that patients receive prompt and appropriate emergency care and are transported in a timely manner to a health care facility for further evaluation and treatment. Identifying the severity of the injury or illness, prioritizing medical management, and determining the appropriate facility to which a patient should be transported can have a profound impact on subsequent morbidity and mortality.[2]

It is well described that overtriage might overburden the local health care systems, have a negative impact on patient outcomes, and decrease cost-effectiveness. Frykberg and Tepas[3] in their published experience with terrorist bombings found a mean over triage rate of 59% and identified a linear relationship between overtriage rate and critical mortality. However, being too selective might lead to unacceptably high rates of undertriage and also increased morbidity and mortality.[4] Because poor triage quality may lead to adverse consequences and bring multiple ethical and legal questions, the process should be based on recommended (research-based) protocols and guidelines, and be clear, transparent, and consistent. Unfortunately, an extensive literature review published in 2013[5] reported that even though there are some scoring systems available to evaluate the severity of injury, algorithms to guide the initial clinical management, and recommendations about where to transport injured patients, there is little documentation about the effectiveness of these strategies on clinical outcomes.

In this chapter, we review the most common triage protocols used for illness scoring as methods to identify the severity of the injury, and the most often recommended guidelines for field triage of injured patients, along with accompanying recommendations regarding transport of critically ill patients in the field.[6]

It is important to emphasize that these guidelines are based on anatomic, physiologic, and/or situational factors intended to be applicable to patients with major risk of injury and/or significant negative outcomes; however, in light of a relative dearth of evidence-based medicine support, such scores must be used with full appreciation of their limitations. Though the guidelines are useful for comparing institutional performances and outcomes in studies of certain groups of patients, great caution must be exercised when applying these protocols to individual patients.

EVIDENCE-BASED TRIAGE AND TRANSPORT OF THE CRITICALLY ILL PATIENT

In general, evidence-based guidelines focused on pre-hospital care are lacking. Beate Lidal et al[5] conducted a systematic review of 120 publications to identify available research on the effects on health outcomes of validated triage systems used in the pre-hospital EMS, and found that none of the identified articles fulfilled their inclusion criteria or answered their scientific questions. They concluded that there is a lack of scientific documentation evaluating whether pre-hospital triage systems are effective, whether one triage system is more effective than others, and whether it is effective to use the same triage system in 2 or more settings of an EMS. This lack of validated efficacy was related to a gamut of important aspects of care: health outcomes, patient safety, patient satisfaction, user friendliness, resource use, goal achievement, and the quality of the information flow between the different settings of the EMS.

For medical transportation studies, the HEMS Manuscript[7] is a draft in progress, developed by a multidisciplinary panel of experts on trauma funded by the National Highway Traffic Safety Administration, which attempts to develop guidelines recommending an evidence-based strategy for the triage and transportation of all pre-hospital trauma patients who use 911 services. After an extensive literature review considering mortality, morbidity, and undertriage of critically ill patients as critical outcomes, the panel concluded 2 strong and 3 weak recommendations for (1) the mode of transport (Helicopter Emergency Medical Services [HEMS] vs Ground Emergency Medical Services [GEMS]), (2) the use of online medical control, and (3) considerations for local adaptation. All recommendations were supported only by low- or very-low-quality evidence. In their manuscript they recommend:

1. Triage criteria for all trauma patients should include anatomic, physiologic, and situational components to risk-stratify injury severity and guide decisions as to destination and transport modality. (Strong recommendation, low-quality evidence.)

2. EMS providers should not be required to consult with online medical direction (OLMD) before activating HEMS for trauma patients meeting appropriate physiologic and anatomic criteria for serious injury (Strong recommendation, low-quality evidence); for all other trauma patients, OLMD may be used to determine transportation method as long as it does not result in a significant delay. (Weak recommendation, very-low-quality evidence.)

3. HEMS should be used to transport patients meeting appropriate physiologic and anatomic criteria for serious injury to an appropriate trauma center if there will be a significant time savings over GEMS. (Weak recommendation, very-low-quality evidence.)

4. GEMS should be used to transport all other patients to an appropriate hospital, so long as system factors do not preclude safe and timely transportation. (Weak recommendation, very low-quality evidence.)

In general, these recommendations consider the most seriously injured patients and their families to serve them with the most expedient transport possible to the hospital. Although none of the HEMS activation variables has been prospectively validated in multicenter trials, and while the time and cost-effectiveness of HEMS remain disputable, the panel recommends that the most seriously injured patients should be transported by HEMS over GEMS.

TRIAGE SCORING SYSTEM

Triage protocols should only be initiated when it is apparent that resource deficits will occur across a broad geographical area despite efforts to expand or acquire additional capacity. Different triaging scorings have been developed to help providers in making the critical decisions necessary to increase the likelihood of favorable outcomes for patients. However, there is insufficient scientific documentation to decide whether triage scales are reproducible, and also whether the current triage scales differ concerning safety, reliability, and reproducibility, especially in the pre-hospital setting.[8] Some of the most used triage scales are discussed as follows.

Field Triage Decision Scheme

In 1986, the American College of Surgeons developed the Field Triage Decision Scheme (called "Decision Scheme"),[6] which serves as the basis for triage protocols for state and local EMS systems across the United States. The Decision Scheme is the most often recommended algorithm that guides EMS providers through a 4-step decision-making process to determine the most appropriate destination facility within the local trauma care system. Since its initial publication, the Decision Scheme has been revised multiple times, updated last in 2011.

The recommendations are based on physiologic, anatomic, mechanism of injury, or situational factors, where each of these categories includes at least some variables that are associated with risk of major injury and more severe outcomes. The algorithm is divided into a step-by-step approach as described in Table 1–1.

Although decisions might be dictated by standing protocols, for patients meeting the criteria in step 4, OLMD should be consulted to determine the most appropriate facility to treat patients requiring special consideration. If patients do not meet criteria for triage to a trauma center in steps 1 through 4 of the Decision Scheme, EMS providers should use local protocols for transport without the need to

TABLE 1-1 The field triage decision scheme.

Step	Criteria	Recommendations
Step One-Physiologic Criteria: Identify critically injured patients measuring vital signs and assessing level of consciousness. (Sen 65%, ppv 42%, Spe 85%)	Any patient with: • Glasgow ComaScale of < 14 • Systolic blood pressure < 90 mm Hg • Respiratory rate of < 10 or > 29 bxm (< 20 in infant aged < 1 year)	These patients have potentially serious injuries and should be transported to the highest level trauma center (Level I, if available).
Step Two-Anatomic Criteria: Recognition of patients who might have a severe injury but do no meet physiologic parameters. Anatomic criteria alone has Sen 50% and PPV of 22%. Combining anatomic and physiologic criteria have Sen 80% and PPV of 27%	Patients with: • Any penetrating injuries to head, neck, torso, and extremities proximal to elbow and knee • Two or more proximal long-bone fractures • Flail chest or pelvic fractures • Crushed, degloved, or mangled extremity • Amputation proximal to wrist and ankle • Open or depressed skull fracture • Paralysis	These patients might have a severe injury and need care at a high-level trauma center but do not meet physiologic criteria. They should be transported to the highest level trauma center available in the system, typically Level I or II.
Step Three-Mechanism of injury Criteria: A patient who does not meet Step One or Step Two criteria might still have severe, but occult injury. The mechanism of injury should be evaluated next to determine whether the injured person should be transported to a trauma center.	Transport to a trauma center if: • Adults: fall > 20 feet, children aged < 15 years: fall > 10 feet or two to three times child's height • High-risk auto crash; intrusion > 12" to the occupant site or > 18" to any site ejection from automobile, death in same passenger compartment; vehicle telemetry data consistent with high risk of injury; autoversus pedestrian/bicyclist thrown: run over, or with significant (> 20 mph) impact • Motorcycle crash > 20 mph.	These patients whose injuries meet mechanism-of-injury criteria but not physiologic or anatomic criteria should be transported to the closest appropriate trauma center, not necessarily to a center offering the highest level of trauma care available.
Step Four-Special Considerations: Determining whether a patient who has not met the previous criteria has underlying conditions or comorbid factors that place him/her at higher risk for severe injury.	Include: • Aged > 55 or < 15 years • On anticoagulation or bleeding disorders • Burns with trauma mechanism should be triage to trauma center; without other trauma mechanism should go to burn facility • Time-sensitive extremity injury • End-stage renal disease on HD • Pregnancy > 20 weeks • EMS provider judgment	These patients might require trauma-center care.

Data from Sasser SM, Hunt RC, Faul M, et al: Guidelines for field triage of injured patients: recommendations of the National Expert Panel on Field Triage, 2011, MMWR Recomm Rep. 2012 Jan 13;61(RR-1):1-20.

contact medical control. Owing to the complexity of traumatic injury and its evaluation, the last line of the Decision Scheme, essentially unchanged from previous versions, is "When in doubt, transport to a trauma center."

The Sequential Organ Failure Assessment and Modified SOFA

The Sequential Organ Failure Assessment (SOFA) score is a validated measure of organ failure over time

and a predictor of mortality in critically ill patients[9] that has been incorporated into triage protocols for critical care in the event of an influenza pandemic or a mass influx of patients during a disaster.[10] The SOFA score combines a clinical assessment of 2 organ systems (cardiovascular and central nervous) with laboratory measurements for evaluation of 4 other organ systems: respiratory, hematologic, liver, and renal. The SOFA score has been shown to reliably evaluate and quantify the degree of organ dysfunction present on admission to the intensive care unit (ICU) (initial score) or developing during ICU stay. The maximum SOFA score reflects cumulative organ dysfunction that develops and correlates with mortality, whereas the mean score is a good prognostic indicator-predicting outcome throughout an ICU stay.[9]

As the SOFA score requires laboratory measurement of 4 parameters (creatinine, platelet count, partial pressure of arterial oxygen, and serum bilirubin), this scoring system may be impractical with constrained resources. Looking for an alternative, Grissom et al[11] proposed a modified SOFA (MSOFA) score that requires only 1 laboratory measurement (creatinine, which can be measured using a bedside point-of-care testing device), eliminates the platelet count, and replaces the other laboratory test results with clinical measurements: saturation of oxygen and jaundice. They evaluated the accuracy of both scores in 2 key areas: (1) ability to predict mortality and (2) ability to predict need for mechanical ventilation in critically ill patients after admission to the ICU. Findings were that for predicting mortality on days 1 and 3, the MSOFA and SOFA scores are equally accurate, but for predicting mortality at day 5 of ICU stay, the predictive accuracy for both was diminished.

Both scores are equivalent in predicting ongoing requirements for mechanical ventilation, but because both scores exclude the patients with more than 11 points, the system excluded about 94% of total patients in their cohort, but up to 40% of these excluded patients would survive in a setting where ample critical care resources were available. This illustrates that these scoring systems can only be 1 part of an overall system of triage.[10] The overall triage process should be based on a consideration of scoring systems and the analysis of preexisting comorbidities; to successfully use limited resources to save lives, strategically excluding patients with high risk of mortality must be considered.

Simple Triage Scoring System

Initially during the influenza pandemic in 2009, the UK Department of Health recommended the SOFA score as part of a staged triage and treatment prioritization tool during the initial weeks of an overwhelming influenza pandemic and to prioritize admission to critical care beds.[12] Further

data analysis suggests that SOFA score may not be a good predictor of outcome in this cohort of patients, and had surge capacity been overwhelmed, it may have led to inappropriate limitation of therapy. Before the pandemic, in 2007 Talmor et al[13] proposed the Simple Triage Scoring System (STSS) as a potential alternative tool in predicting mortality and optimizing the utilization of critical care resources during epidemics. It uses only vital signs and patient characteristics that are readily available at initial presentation (age, shock index [heart rate > blood pressure], respiratory rate, oxygen saturation, and altered mental state). In 2011 Adeniji and Cusack[12] reviewed the performance of the admission STSS and SOFA scoring systems as indicators of optimal utilization of hospital resources, and of mortality during the H1N1 infection; they found that the STSS accurately risk-stratified patients with this viral illness with regard to the need for admission to the ICU and for mechanical ventilation, suggesting that the STSS performs better in this population and overall would be a more appropriate early assessment triage rule.

Abbreviated Injury Scale, Injury Severity Score, and the New Injury Severity Score

The Abbreviated Injury Scale (AIS) ranks different injuries with a numerical score from 1 for minor injury to 6 for probably lethal/maximum injury. In 1974, the Injury Severity Score (ISS) was derived from AIS scores and it uses an ordinal scale (range: 1-75) that summarizes and takes account of the effect of multiple injuries.[14] The ISS is calculated by assigning AIS scores to injuries in each of 6 body regions (head/neck, face, thorax, abdomen/visceral pelvis, bony pelvis/extremities, and external structures) and then adds the squares of the highest AIS scores in each of the 3 most severely injured body regions. Only the most severe injury in each body region is used in the score. If an AIS score of 6 is assigned to any body region, the maximal ISS of 75 is assigned. The ISS is an accepted method of determining the overall severity of injury and correlates with mortality, morbidity, and length of hospital stay, and it has been used to predict mortality and risk for postinjury multiple organ failure.[14]

In a more recent study developed in a level 1 university trauma center, the New Injury Severity Score (NISS) showed that 7.5% patients with discrepant scores (NISS > ISS) had longer hospital and ICU stay and higher mortality rate (all $P < .01$), suggesting that the NISS has better predictive power related with these outcomes.[15]

Trauma Score and Revised Trauma Score

Because of the increasing number of trauma patients admitted to critical care facilities, familiarity with trauma scales is important. The Trauma Score (TS) is based on the Glasgow Coma Scale (GCS), and on the status of the cardiovascular and respiratory systems, it assigns values to each parameter and the scores are summed to obtain the total TS, which ranges from 1 to 16. Mortality risk varies inversely with the TS.[16]

After an evaluation of the TS by the same author, it was found that it underestimates the importance of head injuries, so the Revised Trauma Score (RTS)[17] was proposed. The RTS demonstrated substantially improved reliability in outcome predictions compared to the TS and yielded more accurate outcome predictions for patients with serious head injuries than the TS. Currently, the RTS is the most widely used physiologic trauma scoring tool.

CRAMS Scale

The Circulation, Respiration, Abdomen, Motor, Speech (CRAMS) scale is another trauma triage scale that is frequently used to decide which patients require triage to a trauma center. Patients with lower CRAMS scale scores would be expected to require critical care unit admission.[18]

TRANSPORT OF THE CRITICALLY ILL PATIENT

Critical care regionalization is becoming more common and studies have supported that the transport of critically ill patients to a tertiary care center leads to better patient outcomes.[19] As a result, there is increased interfacility transport of critically ill patients and the need to develop methods for transport of these patients using practices based on the best scientific and management evidence.

Composition of the Transport Team

There are no national data on overall transport volumes or team composition within transport systems. Published guidelines recommend that a minimum of 2 medically qualified people in addition to vehicle operators accompany a critically ill patient, but there are no standard recommendations regarding which patients may be transferred solely with paramedics, which patients require a nurse in attendance, and which patients require a physician in attendance.[20]

While in urban areas ground transport is most common, in rural areas air transport is more often required because of the distances involved and the difficulties of road travel. In most settings, the emergency medical technician (EMT) is the highest-level care provider on the interfacility transport team, but for critical care transports, it is most often a physician, nurse, or paramedic; many critical care transport programs are using physicians who are still in training on board transport vehicles. However, again, there is little information speaking to how the level of experience of the physicians affects outcome. Therefore, current standards for interfacility transport dictate that the decision on transport mode and team composition is based on individual patient requirements, considering minimization of transport time and anticipated treatment requirements during transport.

Medical Management during the Transport

After a literature review concerning medical management in the pre-hospital setting, Ryynänen et al[21] concluded that cardiopulmonary resuscitation and early defibrillation are essential for survival, but providing these interventions in the pre-hospital setting has not shown improved survival, so the data regarding their effectiveness are contradictory. Better documentation is available supporting a reduction in mortality in patients with myocardial infarction when pre-hospital thrombolytic treatment is provided. Regarding the trauma patient, it is accepted to provide basic life support (BLS) in the case of penetrating trauma and in cases of short distance to a hospital, but in patients with severe head injuries, advance life support (ALS) provided by paramedics and intubation without anesthesia can even be harmful. There is also some evidence supporting use of ALS among patients with epileptic seizures as well as those with respiratory distress.

Managing Airway

Critical care transport often involves advanced airway management that includes establishment of an advanced airway with standard endotracheal tube or backup tools such as laryngeal mask, pharyngotracheal lumen tube, or needle cricothyrotomy with emergency transtracheal jet ventilation. In addition to advanced airway management, ALS transport crews should have equipment available for decompression of tension pneumothorax (ie, either needle or chest tube thoracostomy).[20]

Mechanical ventilation of intubated patients during transport has been shown to be optimal in comparison with manual ventilation; therefore, several types of ventilators are available for the transport environment. Transport ventilators must be monitored continuously during transport as they are subject to problems such as power failure and disconnection. Pressure-controlled ventilators are used most commonly during transport, and in aircraft they must be adjusted for altitude changes. While providing mechanical ventilation, patients need continuous oximetry and end-tidal carbon dioxide monitoring, to identify clinically unrecognized hypoxia.[22]

Hemodynamic Monitoring

Interfacility critical care transport requires continuous monitoring and clinical management of the patient throughout the transport environment.[22] The transporting vehicle should have the necessary power converters for all equipment that could be needed, battery backup in case of electrical failure, and backup oxygen supply in case of vehicle breakdown. In cold climates, provision must be made for maintenance of a warm environment in case of vehicle failure. Transport monitor devices include devices for measuring electrocardiography (ECG), blood pressure, oxygen saturation, and, if necessary, end-tidal carbon dioxide level, pulmonary artery pressure, intra-arterial pressure, and intracranial pressure.[20]

Defibrillation has been performed safely during flight, and its use does not interfere with other systems on helicopters and fixed-wing aircraft. Medications should be administered by an infusion pump throughout transport to ensure accurate dosing. Many small infusion pumps are available and can be reprogrammed rapidly to manage unstable patients. In addition, new portable intra-aortic balloon pumps and left-ventricular assist devices are available, and can be transported on most ambulances, helicopters, and airplanes.[22]

Medication

Medication lists have been published for the management of the obstetric, neonatal, pediatric, and adult patients during transport.[20] Special medications may be required according to patient needs, and protocols should be prepared beforehand for the use of these medications on route. Some common pharmacologic practices include the use of paralytic agents to facilitate endotracheal intubation, and thrombolytic agents for acute cardiac and stroke patients, but in general their use is still controversial.

Intravascular Access

Intraosseous (IO) access is an accepted method for providing vascular access in the out-of-hospital critically ill patients when traditional intravenous access is difficult or impossible. Different IO techniques have been used showing overall success rates of 50% using the manual needle, 55% using the bone injection gun, and 96% using the EZ-IO.[23]

Controversies in Management

Blood product transfusion during interfacility transport is controversial. It has been shown that in HEMS using flight nurses, the transfusion of blood can be performed safely and is feasible during transport,[24] but the use of blood product transfusions is still limited to the length of the transport during which crystalloid infusion alone will not stabilize a patient. Use of blood products during transport requires adherence to strict standard blood transfusion protocols, with blood administered by properly trained transport personnel.

Modes of Transport

Current options for mode of transport are the ground ambulance, either a helicopter or a fixed-wing aircraft, and watercraft.[20] In many urban centers, all options are available, and in more remote rural areas the airplane is essential. Factors that will influence the mode of transport include the distance and duration of transport, the diagnosis and complications that may arise during transport, the level of training and techniques the transporting personnel can provide, the urgency of access to tertiary care, and local weather conditions and geography. In the United States, helicopters are used frequently for the transportation of trauma patients; a 2007 overview estimated that 753 helicopters and 150 dedicated fixed-wing aircraft are in EMS.[25]

Ground Ambulance

Ground ambulances have the advantage of rapid deployment, high mobility, and lower cost. However, patients and equipment are subject to significant deceleration and vibration forces.[20] Ground ambulance vehicles are usually most readily available and should be considered for transport distances of 30 miles or less. They are categorized as vehicles for BLS or ALS. BLS ambulances are most often staffed with 2 EMTs whereas ALS ambulances are staffed with a paramedic, nurse, or physician as the highest-level provider. Ground ambulances are limited by surface conditions or traffic congestion. All of them should have a backup equipment supply (ie, batteries or oxygen tanks), and ALS ambulances, particularly, must have the necessary outlets for managing ventilators or balloon pumps for interfacility critical transfers. The US Department of Transportation (DOT) has published standards that have been adopted by most states that relate to minimum ambulance configuration and equipment requirements.[26] Communication between the ground ambulance and the receiving facility or designated medical control center can be considered during transport.

Helicopter

Fixed-wing or rotary aeromedical transport may be necessary during disasters to extricate victims via air.[20] Helicopters should be considered for transports over distances of 30 to 150 miles. They travel at ground speeds of 120 to 180 miles/h and often are dispatched from the receiving tertiary facility or urban area emergency service providers. The physical location of the helicopter at the time of dispatch is important to consider because an inflight round trip to transport a patient may not offer advantages over a 1-way trip by an available ground vehicle. Helicopters usually require a warm-up time of 2 to 3 minutes before liftoff and, allowing for communication time, can be launched within 5 to 6 minutes of receipt of the flight request. Medical transport helicopters are usually staffed by critical care crews, and the number of patients who can be transported is determined by aircraft capacity. Under normal weather conditions, helicopters can fly point to point and land at accident scenes or sending facilities; the liftoff capability depends on the type of helicopter used. Helicopter transports are limited by adverse weather conditions and available landing sites (often a problem in densely populated areas).

Fixed-Wing Aircraft

Fixed-wing aircraft should be considered for transport over distances exceeding 100 to 150 miles. Being faster, they have the advantage of having a greater range and the ability to fly in difficult weather conditions, but they are limited by the need for ground transportation at both ends.[20] Though there is reduced noise, significant forces (fore/aft) are exerted on the patient and may affect critically ill patients who have a decreased physiologic reserve. Aircraft cabins are normally pressurized at altitudes between 6000 and 8000 ft, and this may have effects not only on the patient's clinical condition but also on medical devices.

Watercraft

Watercrafts are rarely used for interfacility critical care transport. However, in special environments, such as offshore islands and oil platforms, watercrafts play a role in medical transport.[20] Their use usually comes into play in situations where inclement weather does not allow for helicopter transport. Because of problems with water damage to electric equipment and dangers of staff electric shock from defibrillators, the monitoring and ALS activities that can be supported on watercraft are limited.

NEW CHALLENGES IN TRIAGE AND TRANSPORT OF CRITICALLY ILL PATIENTS

Critical care triage and transport are not uncommon practices; yet there is a relative lack of available comparative research studies that address (sometimes controversial) practices in this area of medicine because of the ethical implications of such studies, the nature of urgent and intensive care, and the large number of variables to consider.

Ethical Impact

When resource scarcities occur, ethical and international laws dictate that triage protocols should be used to guide resource allocation, and that they should equitably provide every person the "opportunity" to survive.[27] As this law does not guarantee either treatment or survival, performing triage of critical care services introduces several ethical challenges. To conscientiously meet these challenges, it is important to be familiar with the 4 principles of biomedical ethics developed by Beauchamp and Childress[28] and to understand their application to the critically ill patient.

Autonomy: Respect for autonomy is a fundamental criterion for decision making in health care and provides that competent persons have the right to make choices regarding their own health care.[28] In the critical care setting, autonomy is very difficult to assess due to the urgency of the situations, lack of privacy, and lack of an established medical relationship. For the health care provider, it is important to focus on good and clear communication, even when the informed consent is not part of triage procedure.

Beneficence: Beneficence is the moral obligation of contributing to the benefit or well-being of people, and thus is a positive action done for the benefit of others, rather than merely refraining from harmful acts.[28] By applying a system of triage, the health care provider strives to improve the quality of care by using the available resources as effectively and efficiently as possible. The ultimate goal of triage is to preserve and protect endangered human lives as much as possible by assigning priority to patients with an immediate need for life-sustaining treatment. In triage, the tendency of overtriage, particularly in patients with trauma, may be a tendency for beneficence, to "err on the side of caution." However, overtriage not only increases the cost of medical care but also may result in worse outcome.[29]

Nonmaleficence: The principle of nonmaleficence can be described as "do no harm" and it is part of The Hippocratic Oath every health care provider commits to. Harm is not directly inflicted by triage except, perhaps when hopelessly injured patients are considered in the dead category.[28] Even during disasters, health care professionals are always obligated to reasonably provide the best care. So the aim of triage is to secure fair and equitable resources and protections for vulnerable groups. Triage guidelines aim to avoid harm to the patient by sorting the patients as quickly and efficiently as possible. However, in emergency care, especially in situations of overcrowding, treating one patient might indirectly threaten the welfare of another patient; any delay in treatment can potentially be harmful, but may be unavoidable if resources are limited. Our best efforts to use good communication skills and maximize allocation of resources can help us preserve principle of nonharming by reducing as much as possible any delay in treatment.

Justice: Distributive justice requires that, given limited resources, allocation decisions must be made fairly, and that the benefits and burdens are distributed in a just and fair way.[28] Triage schemes are designed to allocate the benefits of receiving health care among the injured persons, but it does not mean than each person will receive equality if there are scarce resources; this aspect makes the triage of critically ill patients especially challenging. The triage equity perspective should be based on 3 principles: (1) Principle of equality: Based on the idea that each person's life is of equal worth and everyone should have an equal chance to receive necessary care. But this does not imply that the triage system can simply operate on a first-come first-service basis, because in an emergency care scenario this is a suboptimal strategy. (2) Principle of utility: It considers providing the greatest good for the greatest number. To respect this principle, the triage system should allocate scarce medical resources as efficiently as possible, seeking to achieve survival, restoration or preservation of function, and minimize suffering. To maximize benefit at the macro level, bad consequences for some (at micro level) may be justified if an action produces the greatest overall benefit. (3) The principle of worst-off: This principle depends on how worst-off is defined; most likely in critical care it means the severely ill or injured patient with greatest risk of death. To consider this principle, triage systems would give priority to treat this sickest group, but when resources are scattered, this approach can be inefficient if maximizing the benefits for the close-to-death group of patients who are not likely to survive consumed resources that could have saved lives of those not as sick, but more likely to survive. Triage systems should focus on minimizing the number of avoidable deaths, directing resources to salvageable patients.

Most of the available literature related to triage focuses just on a medical perspective (clinically based guidelines recommendations) or an ethical perspective (with its conflicting principles). Aacharya et al[28] conducted a literature review, in an attempt to bring together these 2 strands of thought. They consolidated the results from the analysis, using the 4 principles of biomedical ethics, proposing a clinically integrated and ethically based framework of emergency department triage planning. After their review they concluded that emergency triage is a dynamic process that takes relevant ethical principles into account; as triage involves significant moral implications, public representatives and ethics scholars should participate in the development of ethically sound institutional policies on triage planning. As a dynamic process, triage planning is a process susceptible to change and should be reviewed by multidisciplinary task forces and hospital ethics committees.

Safety

Safety of patients and EMS providers as well as the benefits and cost-effectiveness of the mode of transport are key considerations when assessing whether to transport a critically ill patient by ground or air, but the support regarding this topic is still controversial: One study has found no difference in transport times for HEMS versus GEMS[30]; one found a positive, but not statistically significant, point estimate for the association between HEMS transport and scene trauma mortality[31]; and another, focused only on patients with severe injury as defined by ISS, found that transport by helicopter was associated with improved hospital-to-discharge outcomes, compared to ground transport.[32] Methodologically, it is very difficult to evaluate the different transport modalities due to the influence of multiple variables such as local weather, traffic congestion, and EMS crew training. In general, the data indicate that the risks of aeromedical transport are very low, and the risk of ground transportation cannot be ignored.

Medical Legal Issues

Interfacility transport of patients has received increased legal attention especially regarding topics such as transfers of unstable patients, transfers of uninsured patients, and "antidumping legislation."[20] Legally the sending facility is responsible for initiating the transfer, selecting the mode of transportation and the equipment on the transporting vehicle (including the level of expertise of transferring personnel), and ensuring that the receiving facility has space and personnel available for care of the patient. The sending physician is responsible for the risks of transfer and for deciding that the benefits to the patient following successful transfer outweigh the risks. A receiving facility that has specialized units shall not refuse to accept an appropriate transfer if that hospital has the capability to treat the individual. This is a nondiscrimination clause and is designed to prevent receiving facilities from accepting only funded patients.

In addition, owing to the high degree of acuteness of these patients and potential for adverse outcomes, the resultant liability implications make it mandatory that transferring personnel have medical malpractice coverage.

Education and Training

A study has showed that training on triage skills using standardized simulated cases can decrease undertriage by 12%.[33] Training modules for all transporting personnel should be developed in such a way that it is consistent with the policies and practices of the local emergency medical services and critical care community. The facilities and the crew should be subjected to ongoing curriculum development and quality assurance by the medical director.

CONCLUSION

Triage, treatment, and transport of injured patients require careful attention to priorities, prevention of further injuries, and delivering reassurance and compassion to those who are injured. As mentioned by Pepe and Kvetan,[34] early treatment in the field should be focused on seriously injured persons who require immediate care but with a chance of survival. And most importantly, beyond the pre-hospital injury "management" or "treatment," we should always provide the best possible pre-hospital care.

Critically ill patients generally require a high level of care during transport. Recommendations regarding transport of critically ill patients are supported by data that show that the critically ill patient has better outcomes in tertiary centers than in other facilities and that transport of the critically ill patient does not adversely affect the patient during transport and improves outcome when compared with national norms. Established systems of care (encompassing critical transport as a component) have societal outcomes better than those of comparable communities without such a system and better than those in the same community before the system was in place; regionalization of specialized care is cost-effective and improves utilization of community resources.

Even though conducting research in the pre-hospital environment and in EMS presents multiple challenges, there is a real need for more research specifically related to field triage recommendations, cost-effectiveness recommendations, how to improve trauma surveillance, and data systems able to analyze the impact of various policies and procedures affecting the care of acutely injured persons.

REFERENCES

1. Robertson-Steel I. Evolution of triage systems. *Emerg Med J.* 2006;23:154-155.
2. Sasser S, Varghese M, Joshipura M, et al. *Preventing Death and Disability Through the Timely Provision of Prehospital Trauma Care.* Geneva, Switzerland: World Health Organization; 2006. http://www.who.int/bulletin/volumes/84/7/editorial20706html/en/print.html.
3. Frykberg ER, Tepas JJ. Terrorist bombings. Lessons learned from Belfast to Beirut. *Ann Surg.* 1988;208:569-576.
4. Mackersie RC. Field triage, and the fragile supply of "optimal resources" for the care of the injured patient. *Prehosp Emerg Care.* 2006;10:347-350.
5. Beate Lidal I, Holte HH, Vist GE. Triage systems for pre-hospital emergency medical services—a systematic review. *Scand J Trauma Resus Emerg Med.* 2013;21:28.
6. Centers for Disease Control. Guidelines for field triage of injured patients: recommendations of the national expert panel on field triage, 2011. *MMWR Recomm Rep.* 2012;61:1-20.
7. Thomas S, Brown K, Oliver Z, et al. *An Evidence-Based Guideline for the Transportation of Prehospital Trauma Patients.* HEMS Manuscript—Draft 3. 23.
8. Harding KE, Taylor NF, Leggat SG. Do triage systems in healthcare improve patient flow? A systematic review of the literature. *Aust Health Rev.* 2011;35(3):371-383.
9. Ferreira FL, Bota DP, Bross A, Mélot C, Vincent JL. Serial evaluation of the SOFA score to predict outcome in critically ill patients. *JAMA.* 2001;286(14):1754-1758.
10. Devereaux AV, Dichter JR, Christian MD, et al. Definitive care for the critically ill during a disaster: a framework for allocation of scarce resources in mass critical care: from a Task Force for Mass Critical Care summit meeting, 2007, Chicago, IL. *Chest.* 2008:51S-66S.

11. Grissom CK, Brown SM, Kuttler KG, et al. A modified sequential organ failure assessment score for critical care triage. *Disaster Med Public Health Prep*. 2010;4(4):277-284.

12. Adeniji KA, Cusack R. The Simple Triage Scoring System (STSS) successfully predicts mortality and critical care resource utilization in H1N1 pandemic flu: a retrospective analysis. *Crit Care*. 2011;15(1):R39.

13. Talmor D, Jones AE, Rubinson L, et al. Simple triage scoring system predicting death and the need for critical care resources for use during epidemics. *Crit Care Med*. 2007;35:1251-1256.

14. Baker SP, O'Neill B, Haddon W Jr, et al: The Injury Severity Score: a method for describing patients with multiple injuries and evaluating emergency care. *J Trauma*. 1974;14:187-196.

15. Balogh Z, Offner PJ, Moore EE, et al. NISS predicts postinjury multiple organ failure better than the ISS. *J Trauma*. 2000;48:624-628.

16. Champion HR, Sacco WJ, Carnazzo AJ, et al. Trauma score. *Crit Care Med*. 1981;(9):672-676.

17. Champion HR, Sacco WJ, Copes WS, et al. A revision of the trauma score. *J Trauma*. 1989;29:623-629

18. Gormican SP. CRAMS scale: field triage of trauma victims. *Ann Emerg Med*. 1982;11(3):132-135.

19. Frankema SP, Ringburg AN, Steyerberg EW, Edwards MJ, Schipper IB, van Vugt AB. Beneficial effect of helicopter emergency medical services on survival of severely injured patients. *Br J Surg*. 2004;91:1502-1506.

20. Stratton S. Transport. In: *Current Diagnosis & Treatment Critical Care*. 3rd ed. New York, NY: McGraw-Hill; 2008:208-214.

21. Ryynänen OP, Iirola T, Reitala J, et al. Is advanced life support better than basic life support in prehospital care? A systematic review. *Scand J Trauma Resus Emerg Med*. 2010;18:62.

22. Warren J, Fromm RE, Jr, Orr RA, Rotello LC, Horst HM; American College of Critical Care Medicine. Guidelines for the inter- and intrahospital transport of critically ill patients. *Crit Care Med*. 2004;32:256-262.

23. Sunde G, Heradstveit BE, Vikenes BH, et al. Emergency intraosseous access in a helicopter emergency medical service: a retrospective study. *Scand J Trauma Resus Emerg Med*. 2010;18:52.

24. Sumida MP, Quinn K, Lewis PL, et al. Prehospital blood transfusion versus crystalloid alone in the air medical transport of trauma patients. *Air Med J*. 2000;19:104.

25. McGinnis KK, Judge T, Nemitz B, et al. Air medical services: future development as an integrated component of the Emergency Medical Services (EMS) System: a guidance document by the Air Medical Task Force of the National Association of State EMS Officials, National Association of EMS Physicians, Association of Air Medical Services. *Prehosp Emerg Care*. 2007;11:353-368.

26. Document Number DOT HS 808 721. Rev. June 1995, by the National Highway Traffic Safety Administration, an operating administration of the U.S. Department of Transportation.

27. Domres B, Koch M, Manger A. Ethics and triage. *Prehospital Disaster Med*. 2001;16:53-58.

28. Aacharya RP, Gastmans C, Denier Y. Emergency department triage: an ethical analysis. *BMC Emerg Med* 2011;11:16.

29. Armstrong JH, Hammond J, Hirshberg A, et al. Is overtriage associated with increased mortality? The evidence says "yes." *Disaster Med Public Health Prep*. 2008;2(1):4-5.

30. Lerner EB, Billittier AS. Delay in ED arrival resulting from a remote helipad at a trauma center. *Air Med J*. 2000;19:134-136.

31. Bulger EM, Guffey D, Guyette FX, et al. Impact of prehospital mode of transport after severe injury: a multicenter evaluation from the Resuscitation Outcomes Consortium. *J Trauma Acute Care Surg*. 2012;72:567-573.

32. Galvagno SM, Jr, Haut ER, Zafar SN, et al. Association between helicopter vs ground emergency medical services and survival for adults with major trauma. *JAMA*. 2012;307:1602-1610.

33. Rehn M, Andersen JE, Vigerust T, et al: A concept for major incident triage: full-scaled simulation feasibility study. *BMC Emerg Med*. 2010;10:17.

34. Pepe PE, Kvetan V. Field management and critical care in mass disasters. *Crit Care Clin*. 1991;7(2):401-420.

Resuscitation and Stabilization

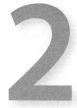

Daniel J. Singer, MD; Scott Weingart, MD, FCCM and
Reuben J. Strayer, MD, FRCPC, FAAEM

KEY POINTS

1. The goal of the first 5 minutes of resuscitation is to establish conditions in which resuscitation can be effectively carried out, identify immediate life threats, and initiate stabilizing therapies.

2. Cardiac arrest must be recognized immediately, and may be missed in unresponsive or intubated patients unless specifically sought.

3. The four signs of airway embarrassment are change in voice, stridor, mishandling of secretions, and airway posturing.

4. Point-of-care sonography is indicated early in the management of all patients.

5. Blood pressure is the most basic proxy for tissue perfusion; however, a more reliable indicator of successful resuscitation is end-organ function.

Resuscitation—*reanimation* in many languages—is the restoration of life where it is absent or diminished. Resuscitation is the simultaneous identification and treatment of threats to life, limb, or function and is initiated by any qualified person whenever and wherever such a threat is recognized.

The need for resuscitation may announce itself with obvious signs such as a patient struggling to breathe or speak, by dramatic alterations in mental status, or by abnormal vital signs, but may also be manifested by more subtle markers of serious illness such as singed nasal hair, muffled voice, or a mottled extremity.

We will first describe a stepwise approach to the initial phase of resuscitation of the undifferentiated, critically ill patient—the *primary survey*—and then more comprehensively discuss the basic assessments, maneuvers, and strategies central to any resuscitation paradigm.

THE PRIMARY SURVEY

The goal of the first 5 minutes of resuscitation is to establish the conditions in which resuscitation can be effectively carried out, identify the most immediate life threats, and initiate stabilizing therapies (Table 2–1). The acronym used here is DC3A-J:

D: Danger

The first priority in resuscitation is to determine that it is safe to approach the patient; the first D stands for Danger—danger *to the provider and the treatment team*. This preliminary step assumes much greater importance in the prehospital environment than the operating theater, but all patients pose a potential threat to their treating clinicians. Scene security (from fire, armed aggressors, etc) is a clear priority in the field. In all settings, appropriate personal protective

TABLE 2–1 The primary survey.

Danger
Call for help
Calm
Cardiac arrest
Airway
Breathing
Circulation
Neurologic **D**isability
Exposure
Family and friends
Anal**G**esia
Hcg
Infection
Ultrasound **J**el

equipment to shield against bloodborne or airborne infectious disease is essential. Occasional patients will have a dangerous substance on their skin or clothes and require decontamination.

The agitated patient deserves special consideration. In addition to the potential for violence against providers, which by itself would indicate appropriate chemical and physical restraint as an early priority, agitated patients can be broadly divided into two groups. In many cases, agitation can be confidently attributed to benign etiologies such as psychiatric disease or safe intoxicants; these patients can be managed in a measured, methodical fashion using de-escalation techniques or titrated chemical or physical restraints. Agitation, however, can either accompany or be caused by life-threatening disease, and in these cases the patient interfering with their care becomes an additional threat to their own safety. When sufficient concern for a dangerous condition exists, agitated patients must be immediately controlled using assertive doses of powerful

sedatives; we prefer ketamine, droperidol, and/or midazolam.[1]

C: Call for help

Verify at the outset of care that the patient is in the appropriate location, and that the appropriate personnel and equipment are either at bedside or summoned. This may mean activating emergency medical service (EMS), activating an in-house critical patient alert, or pushing the patient to another area in the department.

C: Calm

An important impediment to optimal patient care is apprehension and the resuscitationist's own anxiety level should be actively managed. An early step to take in this regard is to make a loud room quiet. This can be accomplished with a forceful *quiet please* and by requesting that observers not directly participating in patient care move to the perimeter or out of the room altogether. This maneuver also establishes the resuscitation leader, which if not apparent should be done at this point.

In medical resuscitation, operator catecholamines generally rise in response to anxiety around the patient deteriorating despite efforts, or in anticipation of an infrequently performed procedure. An effective technique to combat this anxiety and lower catecholamines is to consider how the patient could deteriorate and decide, in as much detail as achievable, how to respond. *Invisible simulation* of this sort can be augmented if necessary by tactical breathing,[1] where relaxation physiology is harnessed to effect calm, which allows optimal decision making.

C: Cardiac arrest

Cardiac arrest must be recognized immediately, and may be missed in unresponsive or intubated patients unless specifically sought. In patients who are unresponsive to a painful stimulus and not certainly breathing (gasping can occur in arrest or just prior to arrest) or intubated patients, the first consideration is

---

[1] One tactical breathing technique has the operator breathe in through the nose for 4 seconds, hold the breath for 4 seconds, exhale through the mouth for 4 seconds, then hold for 4 seconds. This sequence is repeated 4 times.[2]

to establish the presence or absence of a pulse. This can be accomplished by palpation, a pulse oximetry waveform, or cardiac ultrasound.

As soon as pulselessness is detected, chest compressions are initiated, then the rhythm is established so that ventricular fibrillation and ventricular tachycardia may be defibrillated. While the search for the cause of arrest is ongoing, supportive therapies such as vasopressors and empiric treatment of relevant reversible causes of cardiac arrest are often provided; the establishment of vascular access is therefore an early priority in most scenarios, using an intraosseous cannula if venous access is not quickly obtained. This is the time to consider placing large-bore femoral cannulae if intra-arrest extracorporeal membrane oxygenation (ECMO) is available.

A: Airway

The goal of the airway assessment in the primary survey is to determine if an airway intervention is needed now or in the near term. Patients with dynamic airway lesions such as neck trauma, anaphylaxis, angioedema, and thermal or caustic inhalational injury demand a high level of vigilance and preparation for definitive airway management, even without signs of airway compromise. These *bullets, bites and burns* lesions can cause rapid deterioration of airway patency and escalation of difficulty in airway management. Otherwise, a patient who is able to speak comfortably with a clear voice is unlikely to require an immediate airway intervention.

The four signs of airway embarrassment are change in voice, stridor, mishandling of secretions, and airway posturing. Many patients who require resuscitation have decreased level of consciousness and demonstrate a patent, defended airway by handling their secretions: Drooling, gurgling, coughing, gagging, or sonorous respirations indicate the potential for an unprotected airway.

The airway interventions to consider in the primary survey include head and neck positioning (including jaw thrust), suctioning of oral secretions, removal of a foreign body, placement of oral or nasal airways, placement of a laryngeal mask airway, or endotracheal intubation.

B: Breathing

The primary breathing assessment focuses on the adequacy of oxygenation and the provision of therapies to augment oxygenation when needed. In an alert patient, breathing competence is best assessed by respiratory effort; distress is indicated by high respiratory rate, recruitment of accessory muscles, and speaking in less than complete sentences. Pulse oximetry—especially room air pulse oximetry—is a reliable indicator of respiratory status in awake or obtunded patients, provided a good waveform is present. Auscultation of the lungs should be performed briefly, with the intent of identifying bilateral breath sounds, wheezes, and crackles.

Supplemental oxygen is the cardinal empiric therapy for breathing disorders. All critically ill patients should be placed on nasal cannula oxygen, which can be augmented with face mask oxygen or noninvasive ventilation (continuous positive airway pressure [CPAP]/bilevel positive airway pressure [BiPAP]) depending on the oxygenation deficit and its suspected etiology.

Other therapies to consider in the primary survey include nebulized albuterol for reactive airway disease, nitroglycerine for pulmonary edema, and thoracostomy (with needle, chest tube, or finger) for an unstable patient with pneumothorax. A portable chest radiograph may be called for when indicated.

C: Circulation

The initial assessment of circulation centers on the adequacy of organ perfusion, as evidenced by mentation and warm, dry skin with brisk capillary refill. Heart rate and blood pressure are measured, usually by placing the patient on a telemetry monitor. The presence of gross jugular venous distention should be sought, as it indicates heart failure/volume overload or circulatory obstruction.

Resuscitative vascular access is an early, crucial priority. In the non-exsanguinating critically ill patient, prompt placement of a short, large-gauge catheter into a peripheral vein is usually sufficient for initiating the first phase of treatment. The patient with life-threatening hemorrhage requires an additional high-flow cannula—either a 16-gauge or larger angiocath or a 7-Fr or larger introducer placed in a large peripheral or central vein—to facilitate transfusion at the outset of care. If intravenous access is unable to be obtained immediately, an intraosseous catheter should be inserted without delay.

The most important therapies to support circulation to consider in the primary survey are crystalloid and blood. Epinephrine is indicated in the primary survey when anaphylaxis is a high concern.

An electrocardiogram (ECG) may be obtained in the primary survey when the patient is suspected to be critically ill from an arrhythmia or acute coronary syndrome. Unstable tachycardias are shocked and unstable bradycardias are paced at this juncture unless an immediately reversible cause is identified. Perhaps the most important of these is hyperkalemia, which is common and dangerous enough that calcium therapy should be specifically considered in the primary survey, especially in renal failure patients.

D: neurologic Disability

The initial evaluation of neurologic disability is four maneuvers: assessment of level of consciousness and mentation; pupillary size, symmetry, and reactivity; movement at four extremities; and capillary glucose measurement.

Level of consciousness is adequately described in the primary survey as either agitated, alert, responsive to verbal stimuli, responsive to painful stimuli, or unresponsive to painful stimuli. Agitation or confusion can be as ominous as obtundation as a marker of serious disease.

All patients with neurologic signs should have hypoglycemia either excluded or empirically treated. Signs of brain herniation may be treated straightaway with mannitol or hypertonic saline. Early brain imaging is appropriate in patients thought to be critically ill from a structural brain lesion.

E: Exposure

Patients who require resuscitation should have all clothing removed and every inch of skin examined as early as can be done safely. Evidence of trauma, rashes, medication patches, medical alert tags, scars, and medical devices often direct care and are easily missed unless sought. If the history is incomplete, clothing and possessions should be inspected for clues.

A rectal temperature can be taken at this time, and active warming or cooling is initiated in the primary survey when indicated.

F: Family and friends

Many patients who require resuscitation cannot provide a complete history, making the collateral history offered by EMS, family, companions, or other providers crucial. Goals of care should be clarified or established early, when appropriate. In cardiac arrest, offer family the opportunity to be present during the resuscitation. Otherwise, provide an early report to the family, erring on the side of cautious prognosis. Language like *I'm very concerned* usually appropriately sets expectations and conveys a suitable degree of uncertainty.

G: analGesia

Pain should be rapidly, aggressively treated as a primary goal of care but also to reduce catecholamine release. Intravenous opiates are first line in most cases: Fentanyl offers rapid onset of action and is an excellent initial choice, followed by longer-acting agents such as morphine or hydromorphone. Analgesic-dose ketamine (0.15 mg/kg) is an effective alternative or addition when opiates are ineffective or not desired.[3] Intramuscular or subcutaneous dosing should be provided to the patient in severe pain if intravascular access is not immediately available.

H: Human chorionic gonadotropin

Pregnancy may be occult and usually changes the trajectory of resuscitation; it must be specifically considered early in the care of any ill woman of childbearing age. This is most easily accomplished by placing two drops of blood on a standard urine human chorionic gonadotropin (hCG) cassette assay.[4]

The uterus of the hypotensive late trimester patient should be manually displaced to the left. A woman who presents arrested or nearly arrested with a gravid abdomen should be considered for perimortem caesarean section.

I: Infection

Isolation of patients who may have dangerous communicable illness is an essential step when indicated. Patients thought to be critically ill from an infection should have appropriate cultures drawn and promptly treated with broad-spectrum antibiotics. Early source control, such as the removal of an infected catheter or surgical debridement of infected tissue, may be lifesaving and should be initiated as rapidly as practicable.

J: ultrasound Jel

Point-of-care sonography is indicated early in the management of all patients with hypotension of uncertain etiology to narrow the differential diagnosis, guide procedures such as vascular access, and direct fluid resuscitation. Specific ultrasound techniques will be highlighted in the following sections.

Emergency Airway Management

The Decision to Intubate

Endotracheal intubation (ETI) is the most dangerous procedure that most resuscitationists routinely perform. While performing ETI on a patient who would have done well without it is suboptimal, delaying or omitting ETI when it is required is much more likely to result in patient harm. Understanding the indications for intubation is therefore a cardinal skill for providers who care for the critically ill; these are summarized in Table 2–2.

Anatomic airway lesions—especially dynamic airway lesions mentioned earlier—can progress rapidly and demand a particularly aggressive, early airway strategy that also accounts for their expected difficulty. Disorders of breathing are the most common reason for ETI in most environments but are also the most treatable with noninvasive ventilation, as discussed later. Failure to protect the airway from neurologic disability is classically confirmed by the

TABLE 2–2 Indications for intubation.

Anatomic **airway** compromise: neck trauma, angioedema/anaphylaxis, thermal or caustic exposures, mouth and neck infections, tumor, oral bleeding.

Failure of oxygenation or ventilation (**breathing**): asthma/COPD, pulmonary edema, pneumonia.

Support tissue oxygen delivery (**circulation**) by unloading the muscles of respiration: sepsis, multiple organ dysfunction syndrome.

Neurologic failure to protect the airway (**disability**): intracranial catastrophes (stroke, trauma), profound central nervous system (CNS) depression, status epilepticus. Neuromuscular weakness syndromes (myasthenia gravis, amyotrophic lateral sclerosis (ALS), Guillain-Barré syndrome) may cause critical airway or breathing embarrassment depending on whether they primarily insult airway reflexes or the muscles of respiration.

Expected clinical deterioration, especially if the patient is to be moved away from a resuscitation bay (to radiology or another institution).

A **fighting** patient—especially with high concern for an associated dangerous condition—too agitated to properly manage without aggressive sedation.

absence of a gag reflex, but this is no longer considered good practice because a significant portion of the population has a poor gag reflex, and performing an emetogenic stimulus on a patient with compromised airway defenses is dangerous.[5]

Preparation for Endotracheal Intubation

In optimal airway management technique, preparation is deliberate and meticulous, while the procedure itself is brief and anticlimactic. Preparation is divided into preoxygenation, cognitive readiness, and material readiness. In addition to complex decision making, ETI requires many simple steps that, when accidentally omitted, can bring disaster; we therefore strongly recommend using a checklist (Figure 2–1).

Preoxygenation should start as soon as the decision to intubate is made. In addition to large-volume oxygenation techniques, all patients should be oxygenated with a nasal cannula, which augments conventional maneuvers and provides positive pressure oxygenation during the airway attempt, prolonging safe apnea time.[6] Most patients can be fully preoxygenated with a reservoir face mask. Patients who do

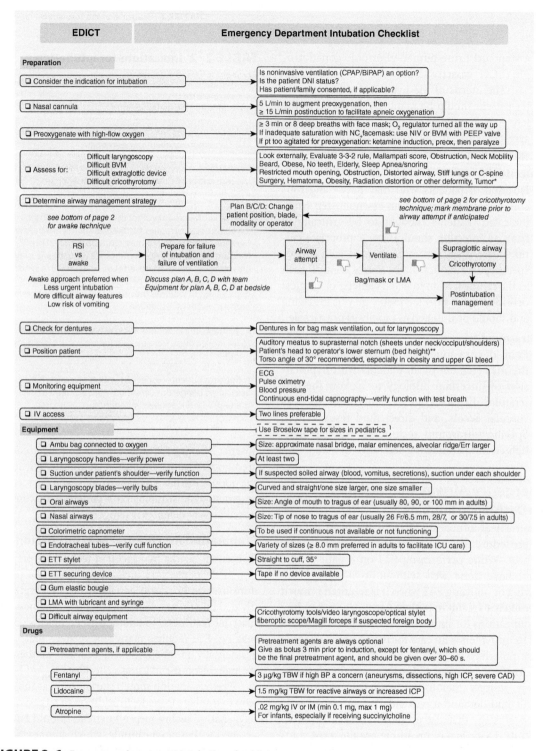

EDICT   **Emergency Department Intubation Checklist**

Preparation

☐ Consider the indication for intubation
> Is noninvasive ventilation (CPAP/BiPAP) an option?
> Is the patient DNI status?
> Has patient/family consented, if applicable?

☐ Nasal cannula
> 5 L/min to augment preoxygenation, then
> ≥ 15 L/min postinduction to facilitate apneic oxygenation

☐ Preoxygenate with high-flow oxygen
> ≥ 3 min or 8 deep breaths with face mask; O₂ regulator turned all the way up
> If inadequate saturation with NC facemask: use NIV or BVM with PEEP valve
> If pt too agitated for preoxygenation: ketamine induction, preox, then paralyze

☐ Assess for:
Difficult laryngoscopy
Difficult BVM
Difficult extraglottic device
Difficult cricothyrotomy
> Look externally, Evaluate 3-3-2 rule, Mallampati score, Obstruction, Neck Mobility
> Beard, Obese, No teeth, Elderly, Sleep Apnea/snoring
> Restricted mouth opening, Obstruction, Distorted airway, Stiff lungs or C-spine
> Surgery, Hematoma, Obesity, Radiation distortion or other deformity, Tumor*

☐ Determine airway management strategy

see bottom of page 2 for awake technique

Plan B/C/D: Change patient position, blade, modality or operator

see bottom of page 2 for cricothyrotomy technique; mark membrane prior to airway attempt if anticipated

RSI vs awake → Prepare for failure of intubation and failure of ventilation → Airway attempt → Ventilate → Supraglottic airway / Cricothyrotomy

Bag/mask or LMA → Postintubation management

Awake approach preferred when
Less urgent intubation
More difficult airway features
Low risk of vomiting

Discuss plan A, B, C, D with team
Equipment for plan A, B, C, D at bedside

☐ Check for dentures
> Dentures in for bag mask ventilation, out for laryngoscopy

☐ Position patient
> Auditory meatus to suprasternal notch (sheets under neck/occiput/shoulders)
> Patient's head to operator's lower sternum (bed height)**
> Torso angle of 30° recommended, especially in obesity and upper GI bleed

☐ Monitoring equipment
> ECG
> Pulse oximetry
> Blood pressure
> Continuous end-tidal capnography—verify function with test breath

☐ IV access
> Two lines preferable

Equipment
> Use Broselow tape for sizes in pediatrics

☐ Ambu bag connected to oxygen
> Size: approximate nasal bridge, malar eminences, alveolar ridge/Err larger

☐ Laryngoscopy handles—verify power
> At least two

☐ Suction under patient's shoulder—verify function
> If suspected soiled airway (blood, vomitus, secretions), suction under each shoulder

☐ Laryngoscopy blades—verify bulbs
> Curved and straight/one size larger, one size smaller

☐ Oral airways
> Size: Angle of mouth to tragus of ear (usually 80, 90, or 100 mm in adults)

☐ Nasal airways
> Size: Tip of nose to tragus of ear (usually 26 Fr/6.5 mm, 28/7, or 30/7.5 in adults)

☐ Colorimetric capnometer
> To be used if continuous not available or not functioning

☐ Endotracheal tubes—verify cuff function
> Variety of sizes (≥ 8.0 mm preferred in adults to facilitate ICU care)

☐ ETT stylet
> Straight to cuff, 35°

☐ ETT securing device
> Tape if no device available

☐ Gum elastic bougie

☐ LMA with lubricant and syringe

☐ Difficult airway equipment
> Cricothyrotomy tools/video laryngoscope/optical stylet
> fiberoptic scope/Magill forceps if suspected foreign body

Drugs

☐ Pretreatment agents, if applicable
> Pretreatment agents are always optional
> Give as bolus 3 min prior to induction, except for fentanyl, which should
> be the final pretreatment agent, and should be given over 30–60 s.

Fentanyl
> 3 µg/kg TBW if high BP a concern (aneurysms, dissections, high ICP, severe CAD)

Lidocaine
> 1.5 mg/kg TBW for reactive airways or increased ICP

Atropine
> .02 mg/kg IV or IM (min 0.1 mg, max 1 mg)
> For infants, especially if receiving succinylcholine

FIGURE 2–1 Emergency department intubation checklist.
R. Strayer/S. Weingart/P. Andrus/R. Arntfield Mount Sinai School of Medicine/v13/7.8.2012.
*From Walls RM and Murphy MF: *Manual of Emergency Airway Management*. Philadelphia, Lippincott, Williams and Wilkins, 3rd edition, 2008; with permission.
**From Levitan RM: Airway•Cam Pocket Guide to Intubation. Exton, PA, Apple Press, 2005; with permission.

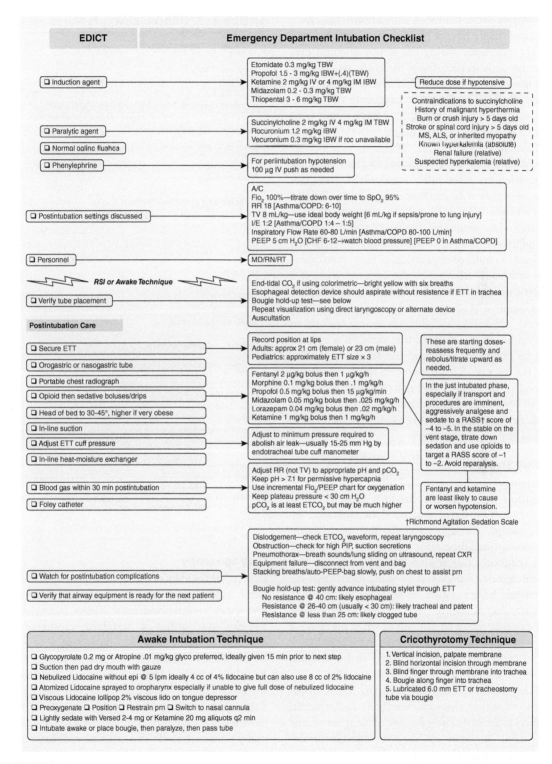

| EDICT | Emergency Department Intubation Checklist |

☐ Induction agent → Etomidate 0.3 mg/kg TBW / Propofol 1.5 - 3 mg/kg IBW+(.4)(TBW) / Ketamine 2 mg/kg IV or 4 mg/kg IM IBW / Midazolam 0.2 - 0.3 mg/kg TBW / Thiopental 3 - 6 mg/kg TBW → Reduce dose if hypotensive

Contraindications to succinylcholine
History of malignant hyperthermia
Burn or crush injury > 5 days old
Stroke or spinal cord injury > 5 days old
MS, ALS, or inherited myopathy
Known hyperkalemia (absolute)
Renal failure (relative)
Suspected hyperkalemia (relative)

☐ Paralytic agent → Succinylcholine 2 mg/kg IV 4 mg/kg IM TBW / Rocuronium 1.2 mg/kg IBW / Vecuronium 0.3 mg/kg IBW if roc unavailable

☐ Normal saline flushes

☐ Phenylephrine → For periintubation hypotension 100 µg IV push as needed

☐ Postintubation settings discussed → A/C / Fio$_2$ 100%—titrate down over time to SpO$_2$ 95% / RR 18 [Asthma/COPD: 6-10] / TV 8 mL/kg—use ideal body weight [6 mL/kg if sepsis/prone to lung injury] / I/E 1:2 [Asthma/COPD 1:4 – 1:5] / Inspiratory Flow Rate 60-80 L/min [Asthma/COPD 80-100 L/min] / PEEP 5 cm H$_2$O [CHF 6-12→watch blood pressure] [PEEP 0 in Asthma/COPD]

☐ Personnel → MD/RN/RT

RSI or Awake Technique

☐ Verify tube placement → End-tidal CO$_2$ if using colorimetric—bright yellow with six breaths / Esophageal detection device should aspirate without resistence if ETT in trachea / Bougie hold-up test—see below / Repeat visualization using direct laryngoscopy or alternate device / Auscultation

Postintubation Care

☐ Secure ETT → Record position at lips / Adults: approx 21 cm (female) or 23 cm (male) / Pediatrics: approximately ETT size × 3

☐ Orogastric or nasogastric tube

☐ Portable chest radiograph

☐ Opioid then sedative boluses/drips → Fentanyl 2 µg/kg bolus then 1 µg/kg/h / Morphine 0.1 mg/kg bolus then .1 mg/kg/h / Propofol 0.5 mg/kg bolus then 15 µg/kg/min / Midazolam 0.05 mg/kg bolus then .025 mg/kg/h / Lorazepam 0.04 mg/kg bolus then .02 mg/kg/h / Ketamine 1 mg/kg bolus then 1 mg/kg/h

☐ Head of bed to 30-45°, higher if very obese

☐ In-line suction

☐ Adjust ETT cuff pressure → Adjust to minimum pressure required to abolish air leak—usually 15-25 mm Hg by endotracheal tube cuff manometer

☐ In-line heat-moisture exchanger

☐ Blood gas within 30 min postintubation → Adjust RR (not TV) to appropriate pH and pCO$_2$ / Keep pH > 7.1 for permissive hypercapnia / Use incremental Fio$_2$/PEEP chart for oxygenation / Keep plateau pressure < 30 cm H$_2$O / pCO$_2$ is at least ETCO$_2$ but may be much higher

☐ Foley catheter

These are starting doses-reassess frequently and rebolus/titrate upward as needed.

In the just intubated phase, especially if transport and procedures are imminent, aggressively analgese and sedate to a RASS† score of −4 to −5. In the stable on the vent stage, titrate down sedation and use opioids to target a RASS score of −1 to −2. Avoid reparalysis.

Fentanyl and ketamine are least likely to cause or worsen hypotension.

†Richmond Agitation Sedation Scale

☐ Watch for postintubation complications → Dislodgement—check ETCO$_2$ waveform, repeat laryngoscopy / Obstruction—check for high PIP, suction secretions / Pneumothorax—breath sounds/lung sliding on ultrasound, repeat CXR / Equipment failure—disconnect from vent and bag / Stacking breaths/auto-PEEP-bag slowly, push on chest to assist prn

Bougie hold-up test: gently advance intubating stylet through ETT
No resistance @ 40 cm: likely esophageal
Resistance @ 26-40 cm (usually < 30 cm): likely tracheal and patent
Resistance @ less than 25 cm: likely clogged tube

☐ Verify that airway equipment is ready for the next patient

Awake Intubation Technique

☐ Glycopyrolate 0.2 mg or Atropine .01 mg/kg glyco preferred, ideally given 15 min prior to next step
☐ Suction then pad dry mouth with gauze
☐ Nebulized Lidocaine without epi @ 5 lpm ideally 4 cc of 4% lidocaine but can also use 8 cc of 2% lidocaine
☐ Atomized Lidocaine sprayed to oropharynx especially if unable to give full dose of nebulized lidocaine
☐ Viscous Lidocaine lollipop 2% viscous lido on tongue depressor
☐ Preoxygenate ☐ Position ☐ Restrain prn ☐ Switch to nasal cannula
☐ Lightly sedate with Versed 2-4 mg or Ketamine 20 mg aliquots q2 min
☐ Intubate awake or place bougie, then paralyze, then pass tube

Cricothyrotomy Technique

1. Vertical incision, palpate membrane
2. Blind horizontal incision through membrane
3. Blind finger through membrane into trachea
4. Bougie along finger into trachea
5. Lubricated 6.0 mm ETT or tracheostomy tube via bougie

FIGURE 2–1 *(Continued)*

not saturate better than 95% with a non-rebreathing face mask likely have a physiologic shunt and will quickly desaturate during the airway attempt; pre-oxygenation is in these cases therefore ideally done with noninvasive ventilation.[7] Patients whose respiratory effort is insufficient to oxygenate with high-flow supplemental oxygen should have respirations assisted by bagging across a face mask or via a supra-glottic airway device.

Patients who are too agitated to allow adequate oxygenation are more safely managed by using dissociative sedation to facilitate oxygenation. *Delayed sequence intubation* calls for the administration of induction-dose ketamine (1 mg/kg IV over 30 seconds with additional doses of 0.5 mg/kg as needed), followed by closely monitored application of usual preoxygenation technique, followed by the administration of a paralytic and commencement of the airway attempt.[8]

Cognitive readiness entails assessment of the patient's physiology and difficult airway features to develop an airway strategy that includes a specific plan for failure of intubation and failure of ventilation; the roles of all team members should be clearly defined at this stage. Material readiness stipulates that all equipment that may be needed for initial and failed airway management is either at bedside or is located and quickly available.

Airway Strategy

Most patients are best intubated using rapid sequence intubation (RSI), the simultaneous administration of an induction agent and paralytic, followed by laryngoscopy. Through paralysis, RSI immediately provides optimal intubating conditions and reduces the likelihood of aspiration. RSI also renders the patient apneic, however, and ventilation must be established before critical desaturation occurs. RSI therefore may not be the best choice when laryngoscopy is predicted to be difficult or when maneuvers to rescue failed laryngoscopy—bag mask ventilation and cricothyrotomy—are expected to be difficult (Table 2–3).

The most important alternative to RSI is *awake intubation*, which uses local anesthesia and systemic sedation to facilitate laryngoscopy while spontaneous respirations are preserved. The more difficult the airway features and the less procedural urgency, the more likely awake intubation should be used instead of RSI.

TABLE 2–3 Difficult airway features.

Difficult laryngoscopy
Look externally for gestalt
Evaluate 3-3-2: 3 fingers in between incisors, 3 fingers from mentum to hyoid, 2 fingers from hyoid to thyroid
Mallampati classification
Obstructed airway
Neck mobility
Difficult bag mask ventilation
Beard
Obese
No teeth
Elderly
Sleep apnea/snoring
Difficult cricothyrotomy
Surgery
Hematoma
Obesity
Radiation
Tumor

Data from Walls RM, Murphy MF. *Manual of Emergency Airway Management.* 3rd ed. Philadelphia, PA: Lippincott Williams & Wilkins; 2008.

Laryngoscopy

Direct and video-assisted laryngoscopy are the chief airway management techniques in most resuscitation environments. Video laryngoscope devices that utilize a standard geometry (eg, Macintosh) blade offer the advantages of video laryngoscopy (better view of the glottis, viewable by others who can thus advise or assist) as well as the advantages of direct laryngoscopy (easier tube delivery, no soiling of camera). For either direct or video laryngoscopy, the patient should be optimally positioned with the external auditory meatus parallel to the suprasternal notch; in obese patients this often means building a "ramp" of sheets under upper back, shoulders, neck, and head. Inclining the torso 15° to 45°, either by raising the head of the bed or using reverse Trendelenburg position, improves glottic view and oxygenation as well as reducing the likelihood of regurgitation or emesis, and should be used routinely but especially in obese or vomiting/hematemesis patients.[9,10]

The laryngoscope of either a direct or video device should be inserted into the mouth under direct vision. Once the blade has controlled the tongue, gaze may be shifted to the video monitor. The first goal is to visualize the epiglottis; once identified, the blade is positioned to lift the epiglottis and expose the vocal cords. If an adequate view of the glottis is obtained, the endotracheal tube may be delivered at this point—if using video, advance the tube under direct vision until the tip of the tube approaches the end of the blade, then return gaze to the screen. Inadequate views may be enhanced by an assistant performing jaw thrust, repositioning of the head, or external manipulation of the larynx.[11] Poor glottic views may be intubated using a gum elastic bougie; we recommend using the bougie routinely so that its advantages may be skillfully leveraged in difficult airway scenarios.

As soon as these maneuvers have failed to produce an intubatable view of the glottis, or significant desaturation has occurred, laryngoscopy should be aborted and ventilation established. Bag mask ventilation is more likely to be effective and less likely to dangerously insufflate the stomach if nasal and oral airways are placed and the mask is applied to the face with two hands, the Ambu bag compressed by an assistant. Alternatively, when laryngoscopy has failed, immediate ventilation through a supraglottic airway device is both easier and more effective than bag mask ventilation.

Once ventilation is established and the patient is reoxygenated, the equipment, modality, patient position, or operator is changed and another airway attempt is undertaken. If after failed intubation ventilation and oxygenation also fail, it is imperative that a surgical airway be initiated early, before critical desaturation.

Postintubation Management

After tracheal position is confirmed by capnography, supracarinal position is confirmed by auscultation of both lungs. The tube is secured and postintubation analgesia and sedation are initiated. In the just-intubated patient, it is appropriate to provide aggressive sedation, as the patient may still be paralyzed and require invasive procedures or transport. Once the patient has settled and is stable on the ventilator, sedation should be lightened to a more physiologic level of arousal.

Noninvasive Ventilation

Noninvasive ventilation (NIV, variously referred to as noninvasive positive pressure ventilation [NIPPV], CPAP or BiPAP) uses a ventilator attached to a tight-fitting mask that covers the nose or both the mouth and nose to deliver oxygen at positive pressure. NIV has emerged as a valuable therapy in the management of various types of respiratory failure. In particular, the care of patients with pulmonary edema, decompensated chronic obstructive pulmonary disease (COPD), and severe asthma has been transformed by the application of NIV in resuscitation environments. To realize the potential of NIV to reduce the incidence of ETI and its attendant morbidity, all equipment and expertise needed to initiate NIV must be present at the point of care, that is, clinicians are able (and encouraged) to initiate NIV without summoning assistance or materials from outside the department.

Arrested patients require invasive ventilation techniques, and full face mask NIV should not be used if vomiting is a high concern, however most other patients with respiratory failure of any type deserve a trial of NIV, if only as preoxygenation while preparations are being made for ETI. NIV is appropriate for use in patients with noncurative goals of care,[12] and has an emerging role in supporting ventilation during procedures that require deep sedation or analgesia.[13]

Hypotension

Along with airway and breathing embarrassment, the management of patients with circulatory compromise, as evidenced by hypotension and/or hypoperfusion, is a foundational charge of the resuscitationist. Empiric therapies to support circulation are instituted in the primary survey as the differential diagnosis—perhaps the most important in resuscitation medicine—is considered (Table 2–4).

TABLE 2–4 Hypotension differential diagnosis.

Vasodilatory
Sepsis
Anaphylaxis
Neurogenic

Obstructive
Tension pneumothorax
Cardiac tamponade
Pulmonary embolism
Auto-PEEP (if intubated)
Abdominal compartment syndrome

Cardiogenic
Arrhythmia
Ischemia
Valvulopathy
Myopathy

Hypovolemic (hemorrhagic)
Chest
Abdomen
Retroperitoneum
GI tract
Thigh
External (street)

Hypovolemic (ahemorrhagic)
Vomiting, diarrhea
Inadequate fluid intake
Diuresis, hyperglycemia
Diaphoresis, hyperthermia
Cirrhosis, pancreatitis, burn

Toxicologic
Calcium channel blocker
Beta blocker
Clonidine
Digoxin
Opiates
Sedatives
Valproic acid
Heterocyclic antidepressants
Phenothiazines
Carbon monoxide, cyanide

Metabolic
Hypoadrenalism
Hypo/hyperthyroidism
Hypocalcemia

Spurious
Equipment or technique failure

Bedside Sonography for Hypotension

Goal-directed point-of-care ultrasound has assumed a central role in the management of patients with undifferentiated hypoperfusion states. Bedside sonography can be quickly performed in the resuscitation bay simultaneously with other maneuvers, is noninvasive, repeatable, and powerfully enhances the diagnostic power of the history and physical examination.[14]

The evaluation of traumatic hypotension was among the earliest indications for nonradiologist-performed ultrasound.[15] Focused Assessment with Sonography for Trauma (FAST) entails a series of targeted ultrasound windows (Table 2–5) to rule in common causes of hypotension in blunt or penetrating trauma. FAST has reduced computed tomography (CT) use, marginalized invasive diagnostic peritoneal lavage (DPL), and improved patient-oriented outcomes in the management of trauma.[16]

Bedside sonography is of high utility in both the diagnosis and management of atraumatic hypotension. The Rapid Ultrasound for Shock and Hypotension (RUSH) examination outlines a goal-directed algorithm[17] which has been supplemented with additional assessments since its inception to produce a comprehensive evaluation of the hypoperfused patient.[18]

Focused echocardiography is often of great value in hypotension. The parasternal long-axis view is generally used to identify pericardial effusion and, if present, to assess for diastolic collapse of the right atrium and ventricle, suggesting tamponade physiology. The apical four-chamber view can be used to assess for right ventricular dilation and paradoxical motion of the interventricular septum; this is evidence of pulmonary hypertension, raising the specter of pulmonary embolism as the etiology of hypotension.[19] Left ventricular contractility, qualitatively assessed in parasternal long or short axis,

TABLE 2–5 Focused assessment with sonography for trauma.

Subxiphoid view of the heart: Is there a pericardial effusion?
Hepatorenal space: Is there fluid in the right upper quadrant?
Splenorenal space: Is there fluid in the left upper quadrant?
Rectovesical space: Is there fluid in pouch of Douglas?
Lung apices: Is there a pneumothorax?

is classified as hyperdynamic (as seen in hypovolemia), normal, or depressed (seen in coronary ischemia, cardiomyopathy, or myocardial depression from sepsis). Left ventricle (LV) function may also be used to guide the administration of IV fluids and vasoactive drugs.

Respirophasic variation in diameter of the inferior vena cava (IVC), as measured by bedside sonography, has been shown to correlate with central venous pressure and intravascular volume, and may predict fluid responsiveness.[20] The IVC is readily assessed in its longitudinal axis and measured 2 cm from its entrance into the right atrium; the greater the variation in the diameter of the IVC with respiration, the more likely the patient is to benefit from fluid administration.

Lung ultrasound is used to exclude pneumothorax, as in trauma, by visualizing sliding of the visceral pleura on the parietal pleura with the linear array probe positioned at the third intercostal space, midclavicular line. Pulmonary edema

is identified sonographically by the prevalence of hyperechoic vertical beam artifacts, *B-lines*, that arise at the interface of water and air. The presence of three or more B-lines per field indicates interstitial fluid and, together with LV and IVC assessment, can be used to predict fluid responsiveness (Figure 2–2).[21]

In appropriate circumstances, the abdomen is assessed for free fluid, as in the FAST examination, which in medical resuscitation could indicate bleeding or ascites. The aorta is imaged for aneurysm from its origin inferior to the xiphoid process to its iliac artery bifurcation point; diameter greater than 3 cm is abnormal with higher likelihood of rupture greater than 5 cm.

If pulmonary embolism is in the differential, bedside two-point compression sonography of the femoral and saphenous veins accurately detects deep vein thrombosis (DVT).[22]

Lastly, ultrasound is used to guide resuscitative venous access, pericardiocentesis, paracentesis,

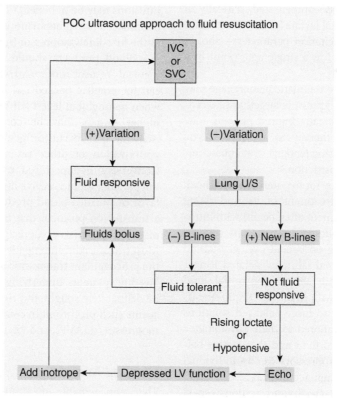

FIGURE 2–2 Point-of-care (POC) ultrasound approach to fluid resuscitation.

chest drainage, and lumbar puncture, as well as determine endotracheal tube position.[23]

Resuscitation Goals and Therapies in Hypotension

Blood pressure is the most basic proxy for tissue perfusion, and remains a valuable guide to therapy, with a mean arterial pressure (MAP) of 65 mm Hg often used as a target.[24] A more reliable indicator of successful resuscitation, however, is end-organ function. Normal mentation, urine output, and skin quality demonstrate adequate perfusion, though young, healthy patients have high physiologic reserve and may not manifest hypotension and organ failure despite significant perfusion deficit.

Serum lactic acid clearance has emerged as a powerful resuscitation barometer and predictor of patient outcome in a variety of shock states[25,26] and is recommended as a resuscitation goal by the Surviving Sepsis Campaign.[27] While treatment-resistant hyperlactatemia is an ominous sign demanding a diagnostic and therapeutic reevaluation, a significant proportion of decompensated, critically ill patients will have normal lactate levels.[28] Serum lactic acid—like all resuscitation parameters—should therefore be interpreted as a single data point in a larger clinical context.

Patients shocked by traumatic hemorrhage may benefit from lower blood pressure targets until bleeding is controlled.[29] Critically injured patients may benefit from titrating therapy to a sympatholytic blood pressure target, using fentanyl to attenuate catecholaminergic vasoconstriction.[30]

The cardinal therapy for hypotension and shock is identification and treatment of its underlying cause. Empiric management often begins with intravenous fluids, with colloidal preparations such as albumin demonstrating no benefit over crystalloid in most studies.[31] Normal saline or lactated Ringer solution are appropriate choices for initial fluid resuscitation; patients with high fluid requirements should be transitioned to more balanced solutions or fluid preparations tailored to their physiology.[32] The utility of additional fluid and the relative balance of fluids and vasopressors in the individual hypotensive patient remains a central resuscitation challenge. The ideal test of fluid responsiveness demonstrates an augmentation of cardiac output

TABLE 2–6 Tests of fluid responsiveness.

Central venous pressure (CVP)
Right atrial pressure
Pulmonary artery occlusion pressure
Stroke volume variation
Pulse pressure variation
Inferior vena cava diameter variation
Superior vena cava diameter variation
Passive leg raise

with fluid challenge. When direct measurement of cardiac output is not feasible, a variety of surrogates have been used to predict and evaluate the benefit of volume (Table 2–6). Vasopressors are traditionally added when the patient is thought to be volume replete or fluid unresponsive; however, especially in distributive shock, earlier use of low-dose pressor infusions may be of benefit.[33] Although data are not definitive,[34] norepinephrine is often recommended as the first-line vasopressor in many shock states.[27]

Blood products should be used sparingly in medical resuscitation. Current recommendations call for empiric packed red blood cell transfusion when hemoglobin levels fall below 7 g/dL,[35] though higher targets may be considered in coronary ischemia or if perfusion goals are not met despite optimization of other resuscitation parameters.[36] Conversely, hypoperfused trauma or hemorrhaging patients should receive little if any crystalloid in favor of warmed blood products, ideally as part of a transfusion protocol that balances red cells with platelets, plasma, cryoprecipitate, and calcium.[30] Most transfused trauma patients should also receive the procoagulant tranexamic acid,[37] and in critically bleeding patients underlying coagulopathy should be deliberately sought and treated with appropriate agents such prothrombin complex concentrate, desmopressin (ddAVP), and vitamin K.

Cardiac Arrest

The management of atraumatic cardiac arrest starts with the immediate provision of supportive therapies, followed by consideration of specific therapies to address the precipitating cause. After cardiac arrest has been identified, if resuscitation is consistent with the goals of care, the earliest priority is the initiation of chest compressions at a rate of at least 100 per minute, a depth of approximately 2 in, and allowing full recoil between compressions. If a chest compression device is not used, the compressor should be switched at regular, brief intervals to maintain quality. Chest compressions should proceed with minimal interruption until return of spontaneous circulation, implementation of extracorporeal life support, or pronouncement.

The determination of the cardiac rhythm and defibrillation of pulseless ventricular tachycardia or ventricular fibrillation should occur as early as feasible and at regular intervals thereafter. Vascular access is established with large-bore peripheral venous catheters or an intraosseous catheter. Ventilation may be initiated using a supraglottic device such as an laryngeal mask airway (LMA), to be replaced with an endotracheal tube if needed for gas exchange or definitive airway control. Most arrested patients should be ventilated with an explicitly low rate and volume, preferably using a mechanical ventilator. The empiric use of vasopressors and antidysrhythmics in cardiac arrest is recommended by widely adopted guidelines[38] and is routine in most environments. The use of specific intra-arrest therapies is guided by history, physical examination, and ultrasound (Table 2–7).

Continuous capnography should be initiated at the outset of cardiac arrest care to verify the efficacy of ventilation (through bag mask, supraglottic device, or endotracheal tube) and monitor intra-arrest care. End-tidal CO_2 ($ETCO_2$)reflects cardiac output and a drop in $ETCO_2$ often indicates chest compressor fatigue.[39] Return of spontaneous circulation is detected by a sudden rise in $ETCO_2$ and an $ETCO_2$ value persistently less than 10 mm Hg predicts failure of resuscitation.[40] When supportive therapies have been provided and reversible causes of cardiac arrest are considered and addressed, ongoing cardiac arrest predicts a poor likelihood of successful reanimation (in the absence of extracorporeal oxygenation).[41] A low $ETCO_2$ value and the absence of sonographic cardiac contractility are often used as further evidence of poor recoverability

TABLE 2–7 Causes of cardiac arrest.

Acute coronary syndrome, dysrhythmia, pump failure
Airway obstruction, hypoxia, respiratory failure
Massive pulmonary embolism
Tension pneumothorax
Pericardial tamponade
Hypoglycemia
Hyperkalemia or hypokalemia
Hemorrhage, trauma
Ahemorrhagic hypovolemia
Hyperthermia, hypothermia
Poisons (recreational, medicinal, environmental)
Sepsis
Anaphylaxis
Aortic catastrophe
Intracranial catastrophe (CVA, SAH)

CVA, cardiovascular accident; SAH, subarachnoid hemorrhage.

and an appropriate point to terminate efforts and pronounce the patient as deceased.[42]

Emerging therapies in intra-arrest care include extracorporeal oxygenation and transesophageal echocardiography (TEE). In capable centers, selected patients in cardiac arrest are stabilized with emergency department–based ECMO, which replaces cardiac and pulmonary function while the underlying lesion is addressed. Extracorporeal cardiopulmonary resuscitation requires specialized equipment, training, and a multidisciplinary protocol, but can produce remarkable rates of neurologically intact cardiac arrest survival.[43,44] Intra-arrest TEE provides anatomic windows to the heart and surrounding anatomy in detail not degraded by body habitus or lung disease, while allowing access to the chest for compressions and other procedures. TEE is more likely to identify the precipitant of arrest than TTE, provides real-time feedback on the adequacy of chest compressions, reveals electrocardiographically occult ventricular fibrillation, and distinguishes pulseless electrical activity from pseudo–pulseless electrical activity (PEA) (myocardial contractions too weak to generate a pulse).[45]

When return of spontaneous circulation (ROSC) is achieved, patients who do not have return of mentation should be maintained at 36°C.[46] Further efforts to determine the arrest precipitant should be undertaken if uncertain and the patient considered for immediate coronary angiography.[47] Priorities in postarrest care include lung-protective ventilation with normoxia, inotropic and vasopressor agents to address hypocontractility and hypotension, careful attention to glucose and electrolytes, and optimization of end-organ perfusion.

External chest compressions and vasoactive medications do not benefit patients who arrest following trauma.[48,49] The management of traumatic arrest centers on prognostication based on mechanism, signs of life, and duration of cardiac arrest.[50] Appropriate patients should receive bilateral chest decompression and consideration for resuscitative thoracotomy, where pericardial tamponade is relieved and penetrating injuries to the heart or pulmonary vessels temporarily controlled, the aorta cross-clamped, and internal cardiac massage performed.[51]

REFERENCES

1. Roberts JR, Geeting GK. Intramuscular ketamine for the rapid tranquilization of the uncontrollable, violent, and dangerous adult patient. *J Trauma.* 2001;51(5):1008-1010; Nov. 2014.
2. Grossman D, Christensen LW. *On Combat: The Psychology and Physiology of Deadly Conflict in War and Peace.* 3rd ed. Millstadt, IL: Warrior Science Publications; 2008.
3. Beaudoin FL, Lin C, Guan W, Merchant RC. Low-dose ketamine improves pain relief in patients receiving intravenous opioids for acute pain in the emergency department: results of a randomized, double-blind, clinical trial. *Acad Emerg Med.* 2014;21(11):1193-1202.
4. Fromm C, Likourezos A, Haines L, Khan AN, Williams J, Berezow J. Substituting whole blood for urine in a bedside pregnancy test. *J Emerg Med.* 2012;43(3):478-482.
5. Mackway-Jones K, Moulton C. Towards evidence based emergency medicine: best bets from the manchester royal infirmary. Gag reflex and intubation. *J Accid Emerg Med.* 1999;16(6):444-445.
6. Weingart SD. Preoxygenation, reoxygenation, and delayed sequence intubation in the emergency department. *J Emerg Med.* 2011;40(6):661-667.
7. Baillard C, Fosse JP, Sebbane M, et al. Noninvasive ventilation improves preoxygenation before intubation of hypoxic patients. *Am J Respir Crit Care Med.* 2006;174(2):171-177.
8. Weingart SD, Trueger S, Wong N, Scofi J, Singh N, Rudolph SS. Delayed sequence intubation: a prospective observational study. *Ann Emerg Med.* 2015;65(4):349-355.
9. Levitan RM, Mechem CC, Ochroch EA, Shofer FS, Hollander JE. Head-elevated laryngoscopy position: improving laryngeal exposure during laryngoscopy by increasing head elevation. *Ann Emerg Med.* 2003;41(3):322-330.
10. Ramkumar V, Umesh G, Philip FA. Preoxygenation with 20° head-up tilt provides longer duration of non-hypoxic apnea than conventional preoxygenation in non-obese healthy adults. *J Anesth.* 2011;25(2):189-194.
11. Levitan RM, Kinkle WC, Levin WJ, Everett WW. Laryngeal view during laryngoscopy: a randomized trial comparing cricoid pressure, backward-upward-rightward pressure, and bimanual laryngoscopy. *Ann Emerg Med.* 2006;47(6):548-555.
12. Azoulay E, Demoule A, Jaber S, et al. Palliative noninvasive ventilation in patients with acute respiratory failure. *Intensive Care Med.* 2011;37(8):1250-1257.
13. Cabrini L, Nobile L, Cama E, et al. Non-invasive ventilation during upper endoscopies in adult patients. A systematic review. *Minerva Anesthesiol.* 2013;79(6):683-694.
14. Volpicelli G, Lamorte A, Tullio M, et al. Point-of-care multiorgan ultrasonography for the evaluation of undifferentiated hypotension in the emergency department. *Intensive Care Med.* 2013;39(7):1290-1298.
15. Scalea TM, Rodriguez A, Chiu WC, et al. Focused assessment with sonography for trauma (fast): results from an international consensus conference. *J Trauma.* 1999;46(3):466-472.
16. Moore CL, Copel JA. Point-of-care ultrasonography. *N Engl J Med.* 2011;364(8):749-757.
17. Weingart SD, Duque D, Nelson B. Rapid ultrasound for shock and hypotension (rush-himapp). 2009. http://emedhome.com/.
18. Seif D, Perera P, Mailhot T, Riley D, Mandavia D. Bedside ultrasound in resuscitation and the rapid

ultrasound in shock protocol. *Crit Care Res Pract.* 2012;2012:503254.

19. Dresden S, Mitchell P, Rahimi L, et al. Right ventricular dilatation on bedside echocardiography performed by emergency physicians aids in the diagnosis of pulmonary embolism. *Ann Emerg Med.* 2014;63(1):16-24.

20. Barbier C, Loubieres Y, Schmit C, et al. Respiratory changes in inferior vena cava diameter are helpful in predicting fluid responsiveness in ventilated septic patients. *Intensive Care Med.* 2004;30(9):1740-1746.

21. Lichtenstein DA. Lung ultrasound in the critically ill. *Ann Intensive Care.* 2014;4(1):1.

22. Crisp JG, Lovato LM, Jang TB. Compression ultrasonography of the lower extremity with portable vascular ultrasonography can accurately detect deep venous thrombosis in the emergency department. *Ann Emerg Med.* 2010;56(6):601-610.

23. Chou HC, Tseng WP, Wang CH, et al. Tracheal rapid ultrasound exam (t.R.U.E.) for confirming endotracheal tube placement during emergency intubation. *Resuscitation.* 2011;82(10):1279-1284.

24. Asfar P, Meziani F, Hamel JF, et al. High versus low blood-pressure target in patients with septic shock. *N Engl J Med.* 2014;370(17):1583-1593.

25. Abramson D, Scalea TM, Hitchcock R, Trooskin SZ, Henry SM, Greenspan J. Lactate clearance and survival following injury. *J Trauma.* 1993;35(4):584-588; discussion 588-589.

26. Nguyen HB, Loomba M, Yang JJ, et al. Early lactate clearance is associated with biomarkers of inflammation, coagulation, apoptosis, organ dysfunction and mortality in severe sepsis and septic shock. *J Inflamm (Lond).* 2010;7:6.

27. Vassalos A, Rooney K. Surviving sepsis guidelines 2012. *Crit Care Med.* 2013;41(12):e485-e486.

28. Rivers EP, Elkin R, Cannon CM. Counterpoint: should lactate clearance be substituted for central venous oxygen saturation as goals of early severe sepsis and septic shock therapy? No. *Chest.* 2011;140(6):1408-1413; discussion 1413-1409.

29. Bickell WH, Wall MJ, Jr., Pepe PE, et al. Immediate versus delayed fluid resuscitation for hypotensive patients with penetrating torso injuries. *N Engl J Med.* 1994;331(17):1105-1109.

30. Dutton RP. Haemostatic resuscitation. *Br J Anaesth.* 2012;109(suppl 1):i39-i46.

31. Perel P, Roberts I, Ker K. Colloids versus crystalloids for fluid resuscitation in critically ill patients. *Cochrane Database Syst Rev.* 2013;2:CD000567.

32. Raghunathan K, Shaw A, Nathanson B, et al. Association between the choice of IV crystalloid and in-hospital mortality among critically ill adults with sepsis*. *Crit Care Med.* 2014;42(7):1585-1591.

33. Beck V, Chateau D, Bryson GL, et al. Timing of vasopressor initiation and mortality in septic shock: a cohort study. *Crit Care.* 2014;18(3):R97.

34. Havel C, Arrich J, Losert H, Gamper G, Mullner M, Herkner H. Vasopressors for hypotensive shock. *Cochrane Database Syst Rev.* 2011(5):CD003709.

35. Carson JL, Carless PA, Hebert PC. Transfusion thresholds and other strategies for guiding allogeneic red blood cell transfusion. *Cochrane Database Syst Rev.* 2012;4:CD002042.

36. Carson JL, Brooks MM, Abbott JD, et al. Liberal versus restrictive transfusion thresholds for patients with symptomatic coronary artery disease. *Am Heart J.* 2013;165(6):964-971; e961.

37. Shakur H, Roberts I, Bautista R, et al. Effects of tranexamic acid on death, vascular occlusive events, and blood transfusion in trauma patients with significant haemorrhage (crash-2): a randomised, placebo-controlled trial. *Lancet.* 2010;376(9734):23-32.

38. Neumar RW, Otto CW, Link MS, et al. Part 8: adult advanced cardiovascular life support: 2010 American Heart Association Guidelines for Cardiopulmonary Resuscitation and Emergency Cardiovascular Care. *Circulation.* 2010;122(18 suppl 3):S729-S767.

39. Santos LJ, Varon J, Pic-Aluas L, Combs AH. Practical uses of end-tidal carbon dioxide monitoring in the emergency department. *J Emerg Med.* 1994;12(5):633-644.

40. Levine RL, Wayne MA, Miller CC. End-tidal carbon dioxide and outcome of out-of-hospital cardiac arrest. *N Engl J Med.* 1997;337(5):301-306.

41. Cooper S, Janghorbani M, Cooper G. A decade of in-hospital resuscitation: outcomes and prediction of survival? *Resuscitation.* 2006;68(2):231-237.

42. Blaivas M, Fox JC. Outcome in cardiac arrest patients found to have cardiac standstill on the bedside emergency department echocardiogram. *Acad Emerg Med.* 2001;8(6):616-621.

43. Maekawa K, Tanno K, Hase M, Mori K, Asai Y. Extracorporeal cardiopulmonary resuscitation for patients with out-of-hospital cardiac arrest of cardiac origin: a propensity-matched study and predictor analysis. *Crit Care Med.* 2013;41(5):1186-1196.

44. Shin TG, Choi JH, Jo IJ, et al. Extracorporeal cardiopulmonary resuscitation in patients with inhospital cardiac arrest: a comparison with conventional cardiopulmonary resuscitation. *Crit Care Med.* 2011;39(1):1-7.

45. Blaivas M. Transesophageal echocardiography during cardiopulmonary arrest in the emergency department. *Resuscitation*. 2008;78(2):135-140.

46. Nielsen N, Wetterslev J, Cronberg T, et al. Targeted temperature management at 33 degrees c versus 36 degrees c after cardiac arrest. *N Engl J Med*. 2013;369(23):2197-2206.

47. Peberdy MA, Callaway CW, Neumar RW, et al. Part 9: post-cardiac arrest care: 2010 American Heart Association Guidelines for Cardiopulmonary Resuscitation and Emergency Cardiovascular Care. *Circulation*. 2010;122(18 suppl 3):S768-S786.

48. Luna GK, Pavlin EG, Kirkman T, Copass MK, Rice CL. Hemodynamic effects of external cardiac massage in trauma shock. *J Trauma*. 1989;29(10):1430-1433.

49. Sperry JL, Minei JP, Frankel HL, et al. Early use of vasopressors after injury: caution before constriction. *J Trauma*. 2008;64(1):9-14.

50. Hunt PA, Greaves I, Owens WA. Emergency thoracotomy in thoracic trauma—a review. *Injury*. 2006;37(1):1-19.

51. Burlew CC, Moore EE, Moore FA, et al. Western trauma association critical decisions in trauma: resuscitative thoracotomy. *J Trauma Acute Care Surg*. 2012;73(6):1359-1363.

Targeted Temperature Management After Cardiac Arrest

Oren A. Friedman, MD

KEY POINTS

1 Targeted temperature management (TTM) refers to the global practice of controlling temperature after cardiac arrest. Mild therapeutic hypothermia refers to a temperature between 32°C and 34°C.

2 The positive effects of TTM postarrest are believed to be related to its effects in suppressing the whole body reperfusion injury, and preventing exacerbation of that injury by hyperthermia.

3 Device therapy for TTM can be divided into surface cooling and invasive technology.

4 The three phases of TTM are induction, maintenance, and rewarming.

5 There is no consensus on the optimal rate of rewarming although it is recognized that uncontrolled or rapid rewarming can lead to vasodilation, hemodynamic instability, and dangerous electrolyte shifts.

6 The lack of pupillary reflexes 3 days postcardiac arrest, the presence of myoclonic status epilepticus (MSE), and the absence of somatosensory-evoked potentials (SSEPs) all very likely portend an extremely poor prognosis.

The implementation of therapeutic hypothermia (TH) and targeted temperature management postcardiac arrest has arguably been one of the most significant contributions to resuscitation care. It should be viewed as the most important intervention in the postresuscitation period.

HISTORY OF HYPOTHERMIA

The modern application of TH had its origins in the 1950s. In 1956, Bigelow pioneered the use of hypothermia for neurologic protection during cardiac surgeries, a practice that has since become standard.[1] In 1964 Peter Safar's historic paper "the first ABC's of resuscitation" recommended the use of hypothermia after cardiac arrest in patients who do not regain consciousness after return of spontaneous circulation.[2] Physicians hypothesized that hypothermia's ability to suppress metabolic activity would translate into a tissue preservative capacity. Low target temperatures were used to accentuate the reduction in metabolism. However, a core body temperature below 30°C which we now refer to as "deep hypothermia," exposes patients to the dangers of cardiac instability. Presumably whatever beneficial effects existed at these temperatures were outweighed by harm, and the therapy was abandoned. Then the 1980s and 1990s saw the emergence of animal research on the beneficial effects of "mild hypothermia." Mild TH, that is a temperature between

32°C and 34°C, has profound effects on stemming reperfusion injury, without the deleterious consequences of cardiac instability.

INTRODUCTION INTO MODERN PRACTICE

The modern framework of TH postcardiac arrest stems from two landmark trials in the *New England Journal of Medicine* in 2002. The larger study known as the "Hypothermia after Cardiac Arrest (HACA) trial" was a multicenter randomized controlled trial (RCT) in Europe involving 273 postventricular fibrillation (VF)/ventricular tachycardia (VT) cardiac arrest patients who were randomized to either cooling to 32°C to 34°C for 24 hours, or "normothermia." The normothermia control group did not have any temperature management. The neurologic outcome at 6 months was favorable in 55% of the hypothermia patients versus 39% of the control group.[3] The second major trial enrolled 77 patients in Australia with out-of-hospital arrest from VF. At hospital discharge 49% of patients who were cooled went home or to rehabilitation, versus only 26% in the control group.[4] The odds ratio for a favorable neurologic outcome with TH was 5.25 (95% confidence interval [CI], 1.47-18.76; P = 0.01), after adjustment for age and duration of the arrest.

It is important to note that two studies investigated patients with out-of-hospital electrical arrests who remained unconscious. The International Liaison Committee on Resuscitation (ILCOR) published a recommendation to use TH after electrical arrests in 2003. The most recent recommendations from the American Heart Association (AHA) in 2010 gave hypothermia after VF/VT a class I recommendation and a class IIb for pulseless electrical activity (PEA)/asystole.[5]

Since the two initial RCTs targeted a temperature range between 32°C and 34°C, the majority of centers began targeting a temperature of 33°C. In late 2013, the large multicenter trial known as the Targeted Temperature Management (TTM) trial randomized 950 postarrest patients to a temperature target of 33°C versus 36°C for 28 hours, and demonstrated equivalent mortality and neurologic outcome.[6] It is emphasized that temperature was tightly controlled in both arms, as opposed to the earlier two trials in which the control group was allowed to become hyperthermic. The study included all rhythms, but a prespecified subgroup analysis of VF/VT also failed to show a difference between the two temperatures. Given how recent this important article was published, it remains to be seen how this will impact provision of TH. Most of the knowledge surrounding the practice of temperature management after cardiac arrest derives from studies and experience targeting a temperature of 33°C. One option many will take is to change to a target of 36°C in all patients. There could also be more variability in targeted temperatures going forward. While it is reasonable to continue to cool to 33°C in many patients with VF or VT as the presenting rhythm, for those with higher cooling risk (ie, more hemodynamically unstable, more bleeding concerns) and/or less clear clinical benefit (PEA, asystole), a temperature target of 36°C may be a better alternative (Table 3–1).

TABLE 3-1 Landmark trials of therapeutic hypothermia.

Trial	Study Group	Intervention	Outcome
HACA 2002 (*n* = 253)	Out of hospital VF/VT	32°C-34°C for 24 h vs normothermia[a]	Improved neurologic outcome and mortality at 6 mo
Bernard 2002 (*n* = 77)	Out of hospital VF	32°C-34°C for 12 h vs normothermia[a]	Improved good outcome at discharge[b]
TTM 2013 (*n* = 950)	Out of hospital all rhythms	33°C versus 36°C for 28 h	Equivalent neurologic outcome and mortality at 6 mo

[a]Normothermia groups were allowed to be hyperthermic.
[b]Good outcome was defined as discharge to home or rehabilitation center.

To clarify terminology, TTM will refer to the global practice of controlling temperature after cardiac arrest and the "TTM trial" will refer to this above study. TH will refer to a target temperature of 33°C, and minimal hypothermia (MH) will refer to a target temperature of 36°C.

WHY HYPOTHERMIA IS BENEFICIAL

The therapeutic value of TH is believed to lie mainly in its ability to decrease reperfusion injury. Cells subject to ischemia become injured and stunned, but do not necessarily undergo cell death immediately. A large proportion of the cytotoxicity from broad ischemic injury occurs in the period of time following tissue reperfusion. Ischemic cells have lost normal oxidative and metabolic function and an immediate burst of oxygenated free radicals and mitochondrial damage occurs on reperfusion. A second phase of injury involves inflammation, apoptosis and necrosis, which can play out over hours to days. Numerous complicated pathways of reperfusion injury include but are not limited to intracellular calcium and glutamate dysregulation, proinflammatory cytokines, and complement activation.[1] Hypothermia impacts this cascade at multiple steps, stemming calcium and glutamate imbalance, reducing oxidative damage, and ultimately decreasing apoptosis.[7] The brain is particularly susceptible to ischemia-reperfusion injury, and particularly sensitive to temperature. However, in cardiac arrest, the ischemia is global, and damage is widespread. There is reason to believe that systemic cooling as opposed to local brain cooling accounts for some of the impact of TH in reducing mortality. It is not clear how low of a temperature is required to have clinical benefit, and the TTM trial suggests minimal hypothermia may be enough. Hyperthermia (fever) exacerbates the reperfusion injury, and may explain why its prevention alone has therapeutic potential. The TTM trial also raises the question of whether simply preventing hyperthermia has enough therapeutic power as to negate any beneficial effects of lower temperature.

In summary the positive effects of TTM postarrest are believed to be related to its effects in suppressing the whole body reperfusion injury, and preventing exacerbation of that injury by hyperthermia.

WHO TO COOL
Neurologic Status After Arrest

TTM is not recommended for patients who have clear return to baseline neurologic status after their arrest. Criteria for enrollment in the HACA trial was the inability to follow verbal commands; the Australian study used the more vague description of "unconscious," and the recent TTM trial specified a Glasgow Coma Scale (GCS) less than 8. It is not known whether there is any benefit to TTM in patients who have less severe neurological examinations postreturn of spontaneous circulation (ROSC). The 2010 AHA guidelines recommend TH for patients who have a lack of meaningful response to verbal commands,[5] and it is reasonable to apply this criteria to TTM in general. As for patients who may have received sedatives thereby confounding their presenting examination, it may be prudent to wait a reasonable period to see if they regain the ability to follow commands before deciding to cool. It is suggested not to provide TTM in patients who are severely neurologically impaired at baseline, terminally ill, those for whom intensive care does not seem appropriate, or in whom they or their surrogates have indicated that they would not want intensive care.[7]

Location and Other Rhythms

In terms of location, the core studies were limited to out-of-hospital arrests. Accumulating evidence however supports TH for in-hospital arrests, and aside from the higher proportion of nonarrhythmic arrests there is no reason to believe the difference in physical location would have any detrimental impact on the therapy. Although TH is best established in VF and VT arrests, there has always been interest in its application to nonshockable rhythms. Irrespective of the dominant rhythm during cardiac arrest, ischemia and reperfusion injury occurs and may therefore be responsive to TH. The 2015 AHA guidelines gave a class I recommendation that all comatose patients post ROSC irrespective of rhythm receive TTM in the range between 32°C and 36°C.[6] A large retrospective study in 2011 showed that TH was associated with improved outcomes in out-of-hospital nonshockable rhythms.[8] However, a recent prospective review of a French registry from 2000 to 2009, did not find improved outcomes of TH in PEA/asystole patients.[9] The authors raised the possibility that the anoxic/hypoxic insult in nonarrhythmic arrests is likely much greater and therefore may require deeper or longer periods of hypothermia to address. On the other hand, it is also possible that the risk-benefit ratio may simply be altered in this high-risk population and that PEA and asystole are better served by targeting a (potentially safer) temperature of 36°C. In conclusion, data supporting TH (33°C) in PEA/asystole are lacking and the benefit of TTM in general in this population is not clear. However, given the physiologic rationale for benefit of TH, it is arguable to target a potentially safer goal of 36°C.

Physiologic Effects of Cooling

The following sections on the physiologic effects of cooling refer mainly to a temperature of 33°C. The effects of minimal hypothermia (36°C) are less well characterized, but presumably milder.

Cardiovascular Effects

Hypothermia raises systemic vascular resistance (SVR) but its effects on blood pressure are variable as are its effects on cardiac output. The hypothermic heart develops diastolic dysfunction and there is an expected and physiologically adaptive bradycardia. It is not uncommon to see heart rates (HRs) in the low 40s (occasionally high 30s) with core temperatures of 33°C. Artificially elevating the HR could result in worsening contractility and cardiac output.[10] Therefore, it is not recommended to treat bradycardia (with catecholamine infusions or pacing) unless evidence suggests it is directly responsible for poor perfusion. Mild TH has an antiarrhythmic effect and suppresses the development of ventricular arrhythmias. But overcooling should be avoided because a core temperature under 30°C frequently results in cardiac arrhythmias including spontaneous VF.[11]

Although initial studies excluded hemodynamically unstable patients, increasing experience shows the safety in TH even in very unstable patients. A case series of patients in cardiogenic shock post-cardiac arrest from acute coronary syndrome (ACS) on multiple vasopressors/inotropes including a large percentage requiring intra-aortic balloon pumps reported the safety of TH.[12] Another study of cardiac arrest patients from ACS suggests that TH may have a favorable impact on the hemodynamics of cardiogenic shock. Hypothermic patients had a higher SVR and HR. But more surprisingly, they also had improved cardiac output and index[13] (as measured by a minimally invasive cardiac output monitoring device and echocardiography).

Neurologic

The brain is particularly sensitive to ischemic injury and temperature. For every decrease in 1°C, brain metabolism decreases by 6% to 7%.[1] There is abundant evidence that hyperthermia is associated with poor outcomes after many different brain injured states (stroke, traumatic brain injury). Postcardiac arrest cerebral edema may be more common than readily recognized and hypothermia is very effective in lowering intracranial pressure (ICP). Lastly, TH may provide an anti-antiepileptic effect.[14]

Hematologic

It has been long recognized that hypothermia potentiates coagulopathy during trauma and surgery. Accidental hypothermia is widely considered a marker of mortality in trauma victims, as well as a marker of morbidity during surgery. The oft-repeated bloody vicious triad of trauma "hypothermia, coagulopathy, and acidosis," is thought critical to avoid. Studies of TH effects on coagulation demonstrate a prolongation of prothrombin time (PT) and activated partial thromboplastin time (aPTT), as well as reversible thrombocytopenia and platelet dysfunction.[15] A mild prolongation of time to clot formation, but not clot propagation or clot firmness using more sophisticated clotting testing (ROTEM) has also been found.[16] However, while unintentional hypothermia may be important to avoid during massive resuscitation of a bleeding patient, the clinical relevance of its effects on coagulopathy in controlled hypothermic conditions however is less clear. Importantly, major clinical studies have not shown a significant increase in bleeding. There is accumulated experience of TH safely being applied concurrent with heparinization for pulmonary embolism, as well as in extremely anticoagulated patients with ACS (who may receive aspirin, clopidogrel, or heparin). Routine intensive care unit (ICU) procedures such as arterial and venous catheterization should not be affected by TH. In summary, the coagulopathy of TH is well tolerated, and safe with concurrent anticoagulation, but should be considered contraindicated in patients who arrest secondary to bleeding, especially those with ongoing uncontrolled bleeding. TH at 36°C is expected to have trivial effects on coagulation.

Renal/Electrolytes

A major concern is the effect of TH on potassium. Induction of hypothermia drives intracellular flux of potassium and the reverse occurs upon rewarming. Hypokalemia on induction is usually not a huge problem, but caution and possibly intervention should be taken in the hyperkalemic patient before rewarming. Magnesium levels mimic potassium, falling on cooling and rising again on rewarming. Hypophosphatemia is also common but rarely a problem. Hypothermia also inhibits insulin sensitivity and release leading to hyperglycemia.[15] TH may lead to an increase in urine output, dubbed the "cold diuresis." Whether this is related to a more centrally distributed circulation or a direct tubular effect is not clear.

Immune Suppression

TH is thought to be immunosuppressive but the degree is not well characterized, and may do not have clinical relevance. Pneumonia is common after cardiac arrest in general, and it is unclear if TH increases that risk. It is possible that TH can indirectly lead to an increase in infections by requiring sedation, paralysis, and mechanical ventilation.

Acid Base

As temperature falls the solubility of gases in the blood decreases. Temperature uncorrected arterial blood gases (ABGs) therefore overestimate both Pco_2 and Po_2. The patient therefore may have a slight respiratory alkalosis and be slightly more hypoxemic. The significance of this effect is unknown, and it is controversial whether to aim for a normal pH (pH stat) or normal CO_2 (alpha stat) level during TH. It is likely that the impact is more important at deeper levels of hypothermia used during cardiopulmonary bypass. This author recommends addressing the pH/Pco_2 on the uncorrected ABG as you would any other critically ill patient, but aim for a slightly higher Po_2 than normal (ie, 70 mm Hg) to give buffer room.

In summary, TH routinely leads to well-tolerated bradycardia and electrolyte shifts. Other effects such as coagulopathy, immune suppression, and acid-base imbalances, are uncommon severe problems. TH effects on any of these conditions are expected to be minimal.

PRACTICAL CONSIDERATIONS OF TTM

1. Measuring temperature
2. Device therapy
3. Controlling shivering

Measuring Temperature

Surface or tympanic temperature measurements are not accurate enough for implementation of TTM. Core temperature monitoring via bladder or esophagus is recommended. Esophageal temperature rapidly reflects changes to core temperature, whereas bladder temperature may lag by 15 to 30 minutes as it equilibrates. Concern is raised in using bladder temperature probes with low or absent urine output, and therefore in a dialysis patient for example, esophageal monitoring is recommended.

Device Therapy

Good outcomes are possible with simple surface methods (ice packs, blankets); however the practice is very labor-intensive, messy, and less precise. Simple surface methods frequently lead to both over- and undershooting in temperature.[17] Device therapy is recommended, as it provides strict control of temperature during the maintenance phase, while also allowing for a very steadily controlled rewarming rate. It is not clear that TH is easier (less deep temperature) to achieve without device therapy, and therefore device therapy is still recommended.

Device therapy can easily be divided into surface cooling and invasive technology. Surface cooling devices typically circulate water through a cooling pad or blanket which relies on heat dissipation through the skin. Modern sophisticated devices work off feedback from a continuous core temperature monitor. Popular options include the Arctic Sun by Medivance and Medi-Therm by Gaymar. There is also a cooling pad by EMCOOLS that is studded with multiple square-shaped conductors containing a proprietary water graphite mixture called hydrocarbon.

Invasive devices require the insertion of a cooling catheter into a central vein (internal jugular femoral or subclavian). The device circulates cold fluid through the catheter cooling the blood by contact. Popular models include the CoolGuard and Thermogard systems made by Zoll, and the InnerCool systems by Philips.

Studies directly comparing simple surface cooling methods to intravascular cooling showed equivalent outcomes but better temperature control with device therapy.[18,19] But when compared against sophisticated surface devices there is no evidence that invasive cooling results in either faster cooling or decreased shivering. More important than the choice of device is being familiar with operating the device that you choose.

Extracorporeal cooling is very effective and convenient if the patient is already being placed on extracorporeal membrane oxygenation (ECMO) as part of their resuscitation, but this is not routine.

Controlling Shivering

If a patient is not achieving goal temperature target, the first consideration should be uncontrolled shivering. Shivering is not only counterproductive to cooling efforts but also detrimental to the critically ill patient who is unable to tolerate the high metabolic energy expenditure required to generate heat. This author has seen shivering lead to a drop in saturation of the central venous oxygenation ($S_{CV}O_2$) to the 50s only to see it normalize after the shivering was addressed with paralysis. Shivering can occur in very obvious gross myoclonic form, or may be so subtle as to not be visible to the eye. Sometimes

shivering can only be recognized by looking for baseline vibration artifact on the cardiac monitor tracing, or with electroencephalogram (EEG) monitoring (if present). Nonpharmacologic methods of shivering control such as skin counter warming have been explored, but virtually every patient undergoing TH will need pharmacologic control of shivering. Many medications have been successfully used to control shivering including opiates, benzodiazepines, propofol, and dexmedetomidine. Although there are subtle differences in response to one medication over another, there is no proof of a superior drug. Neuromuscular blockade (NMB) will definitely stop shivering and was used routinely in both of the 2002 trials and widely in the 2013 TTM trial. Although many have argued against using NMB during TTM, there is no proof of a deleterious effect, and this author believes that the downside of uncontrolled shivering far outweighs the potential of critical illness neuropathy. Many have reported an ability to stop paralytics or decrease sedatives once at 33°C, presumably due to suppression of the shivering reflex at a lower core temperature. Notably, in the TTM trial there was no difference in shivering between the 33°C and 36°C groups. It remains to be seen whether real-world practice will see less shivering at 36°C (because it is closer to normothermia) or more (because there will no longer be suppression of the shivering reflex). As always, the use of NMB should be accompanied by continuous sedation. For TH, this author favors starting continuous sedation and NMB on induction and continuing up through the rewarming phase.

THREE PHASES OF TTM (INDUCTION, MAINTENANCE, AND REWARMING)

Induction

Induction Techniques

Hypothermia devices can certainly be used for the induction phase of cooling. If cooling to 33°C, the only potential disadvantage of device therapy is a slow cooling rate (1°C-1.5°C per hour on average). A faster induction can be achieved with chilled IV saline. Kim et al showed that infusion of intravenous saline by emergency medical service (EMS) shortly after ROSC was a safe and effective way to lower core body temperature by on average 1.5°C.[20] There was no evidence that cold saline led to recurrent arrests or significant pulmonary edema. Another small series of the use of intra-arrest cold saline showed that this could safely be done with the effect of lowering temperature by 2°C,[21] with a median time to reach 33°C of only 16 minutes. There is no evidence that mild TH inhibits ROSC and in fact one study showed that TH improves defibrillation success.[22] Years of experience since the initial studies also supports the safety of IV chilled saline.

Chilled saline can either be kept ready in a refrigerator or can be made by placing a saline bag in ice water for 15 minutes. Induction can also be enhanced by placing ice packs over superficial vascular points including the neck, axilla, and groin.

Safety and Efficacy of Early Cooling

How early to start cooling, how fast to bring down the temperature, and how long to cool are areas of ongoing academic study. There is a multitude of animal data suggesting that earlier cooling is beneficial. One mouse study showed that intra-arrest cooling had better neurologic effects when compared with cooling initiated postarrest.[23] Certainly there is physiologic rationale to slow and prevent the reperfusion injury earlier on in the process, and like most interventions in resuscitation, the earlier the better.

In one recent trial, out-of-hospital arrest patients were randomized to prehospital cooling with IV saline versus cooling initiated in the emergency department (ED). There was no difference found in outcome, but due to the fast EMS response time and aggressive cooling in the ED, within 1 hour of arrival to the ED both groups were at the same temperature. The study, however, bolsters the safety of early IV cooling, and draws attention to the need for more trials addressing the topic.[24]

The normal physiologic response to maintain thermostasis appears to be disturbed in sicker patients. Patients who are passively cooler post-ROSC, and who are less resistant to the induction of cooling tend to do worse overall. This phenomenon has complicated efforts to study time to goal temperature and outcome. Studies that have emerged seemingly linking earlier cooling to worse outcomes may reflect a selection bias toward sicker patients.[25]

Most patients will have a significant drop in body temperature upon ROSC presumably due to heat loss, low metabolism, and low-flow state during the arrest. Rather than allowing the body to rewarm, the clinician can take advantage of the lower temperature and build upon it by either rapidly inducing TH, or maintaining the temperature at 36°C. The Fire Department of New York began intra-arrest cold saline administration in 2010.

How Late After Cardiac Arrest is too Late to Start Treating?

In the HACA trial it is important to note that target temperature was not reached for an average of 6 to 8 hours postarrest, a very long induction time compared to modern practice. There is animal research suggesting loss of benefit of hypothermia when started beyond 4 to 6 hours of ROSC.[25] However reperfusion injury postarrest occurs over hours to days, so if there is a delay in therapy for whatever reason, an impact may still be possible. Although it is reasonable to consider not treating if the patient is 8 hours post-ROSC, it is also important to emphasize that the upper limit of delay to implementation is not known.

Maintenance

Once at goal temperature, patients tend to stabilize. Temperature is continually monitored and controlled. Similarly, shivering is monitored and addressed. Aggressive critical care including ventilator management, replacing nonsterile lines, fluid resuscitation, and vasopressor agent titration is crucial. In the HACA trial patients were maintained at goal for 24 hours after arrival to the ED, whereas in the Australian trial induction of TH was earlier but maintenance was only for 12 hours. In the TTM trial patients were rewarmed 28 hours after randomization (which roughly corresponded to 24 hours at target temperature). The luxury of having RCTs with different intervals is that it provides a basis for modifying the treatment interval. There has been experience of using longer cooling intervals (up to 72 hours) in conjunction with extracorporeal life support in Japan.[27] A case report also details a good outcome in a patient cooled to 33°C for 48 hours postarrest.[28] It is possible that like many critical care therapies, the maintenance interval of TTM should be adjusted on a sliding scale tailored to the particular injury of the patient. However, until more data are available, the consensus opinion is to maintain 24 hours at target temperature.

Rewarming

Although there is no consensus on the optimal rate of rewarming it is recognized that uncontrolled or rapid rewarming can lead to vasodilation, hemodynamic instability, and dangerous electrolyte shifts. There is also limited evidence that rapid rewarming may trigger deleterious cellular injury, obviating the potential benefits of the initial cooling.[15] Herein lies a major advantage in using a TH device, as rewarming can be extremely difficult to control otherwise. Studies have shown that you can safely rewarm between 0.1°C and 0.5°C per hour although the latter may be too rapid for less stable patients. Seizures which are common in the postarrest period tend to occur during rewarming. This author will frequently pause or decrease the rate of rewarming if the patient shows hemodynamic instability or develops seizures until these problems can be addressed. It is likely that the principles of practice listed above are more important when rewarming from a target of 33°C as opposed to 36°C.

Normothermia After Rewarming

It is a common practice to maintain 24 to 48 hours of normothermia (37°C) after rewarming. Rebound hyperthermia is common and the injured brain may be susceptible to further damage. However, despite the logic, there is currently little clinical evidence to support its benefit.[27] The only potential harm of normothermia maintenance is that some patients require ongoing sedation to prevent shivering which could delay extubation and neurologic prognostication.

NEUROLOGIC PROGNOSIS

Neurologic prognostication is arguably the most complicated and least well-understood aspect of care revolving around the application of TTM. The medical world is still in its infancies in understanding how temperature management affects healing of the injured brain. Much of what is known about anoxic encephalopathy originated from studies published prior to

the era of TTM. It is crucial to avoid an errant negative prognosis that might lead to withdrawal of care in a patient who could go on to have a good outcome. On the other hand, many individuals would not opt for ongoing care if they were in a persistent vegetative state. Additionally, ongoing care for neurologically devastated patients leads to undue burden on the medical system. Tests should ideally have a zero false-positive rate for determining a poor prognosis, and most of the research has thus been focused on prediction of poor outcomes. Unfortunately, many studies of neurologic tests after TH suffer from the "self-fulfilling prophecy bias." It is hard to draw conclusions regarding the predictive value of tests that were in turn used as criteria to withdraw care (Table 3–2).

Neurologic Examination: The basic neurologic examination arguably remains the centerpiece for prognostication. Rosetti et al showed that motor response (ability to withdraw from pain and follow motor commands) is often delayed by TH. Absence of motor response on day 3 had a high false-positive rate (24%), and should not be used alone as criteria to withdraw care.[30] However, several studies support that the absence of either pupillary or corneal reflexes

TABLE 3-2 Neurologic prognosis.

Reliable Tests (Good Data)	
Examination	Absence of pupil or corneal response at 72 h = bad outcome
SSEP	If bilateral absence = bad outcome
Indeterminate Tests (Limited Data or Less Reliability)	
EEG reactivity	If present associated with good outcome
NSE	Levels > 33 associated with bad outcome
Imaging	Severely abnormal imaging associated with bad outcome
Treatment Refractory Status Epilepticus	If present associated with bad outcome
MSE	If present = bad outcome

at 72 hours postcardiac arrest consistently portends a very poor neurologic prognosis irrespective of the use of TH.[31,32] A recent meta-analysis suggested that absence of pupillary reflex was a better negative predictor than absence of corneal reflex, and reinforced the lack of reliability of the motor examination.[33]

Advanced Testing and Monitoring

EEG

Although there is no RCT showing mortality or neurologic benefit to routine (continuous or spot) EEG monitoring during TTM, EEG helps in the identification and treatment of seizures and also in neurologic prognostication. Seizures are common postcardiac arrest, occurring in 30% to 50% of patients, and may contribute to further brain damage and prolong coma.[15] They are often difficult to detect, due to the high percentage of nonconvulsive status epilepticus as well as the use of sedatives and NMB during TH. However, the abnormal EEG patterns seen after severe brain injury may be difficult to interpret and can be very refractory to treatment. Some believe that treatment refractory nonconvulsive status on rewarming may in fact be "electrical chaos" from a severely injured dying brain and not seizures in the conventional sense. In terms of prognosis, a flat EEG, nonpharmacologic burst suppression, and electrographic status, are all patterns associated with a poor outcome. MSE, bilaterally synchronous twitches of limb, trunk or facial muscles jerks associated with EEG correlate has a well-established association with poor outcome in many forms of anoxic brain injury including cardiac arrest.[34] Although this association still largely holds, some reports have suggested that MSE may not be as dismal as a marker in a patient treated with TH.[35] The presence of EEG reactivity (an electrographic response to visual, auditory, or painful stimuli) during TH, portends a good outcome while the lack of reactivity portends a bad outcome.

Somatosensory-evoked Potentials

SSEPs are particularly helpful as negative prognostic markers. The median nerve is stimulated electrically at the wrist and a cranial electrode records a response wave called the N20 which reflects stimulation of the somatosensory cortex. The bilateral absence of N20 response on SSEP is possibly the most accurate

predictor of a poor neurologic prognosis, with many early studies showing nearly a 0% false-positive response.[36] The 2006 American Academy of Neurology guidelines recommended withdrawing care if there is an absent bilateral N20 response.[37] The accuracy of SSEP was again supported by a meta-analysis of over 1000 patients.[32] However, there does exist a very small false-positive rate, and there is still a need for caution in interpreting SSEPs in isolation.[38]

Brain Imaging

There is not enough information to support neurologic prognostication based on head computed tomography (CT) or magnetic resonance imaging (MRI) alone. There are situations in which the imaging is dramatically abnormal and shows for example diffuse cerebral edema, loss of gray-white differentiation, or herniation. However in these cases usually the examination also reflects the extent of injury, so imaging ends up playing a supportive role.

Biomarkers

Neuron-specific enolase is a biomarker of neuronal injury, and there is accumulating evidence of its predictive value during TH. Levels above 33 generally correlate with poor outcome but there have been exceptions.[39,40]

When to Prognosticate

Caution needs to be exercised against holding to rigid time frames postcardiac arrest. There is wide variability in time to awakening post-TH. In one study the median time to awakening post-TH was 3.2 days but the variability was wide and patients often awaken after 3 days. In this study, 15% of the patients woke more than 72 hours after their arrest.[41] Sedative choices, accumulative doses, and renal function all potentially can impact time to awakening.

SUMMARY OF NEUROLOGIC PROGNOSIS

The TTM trial used a combination of different criteria for prognostication, and this is a well-advised approach. The following were used as criteria to recommend withdrawal of care: MSE plus negative SSEP at 24 hours, GCS motor score 1 to 2 at 72 hours plus negative SSEP, or GCS motor score

1 to 2 at 72 hours plus treatment refractory status epilepticus.[6] An important general premise is that it is easier to predict who will do very well (eg, the patient who is waking and following commands soon after TH), and easy to predict who will do very poorly (those with lack of brainstem reflexes at 3 days, absent SSEPs). Nevertheless, it is hard to predict long-term outcomes for those who fall in between. It is strongly recommended to take precautions that sedatives are not negatively influencing the neurologic examination post-TH. The lack of pupillary reflexes 3 days postcardiac arrest, the presence of MSE, and the absence of SSEPs all very likely portend an extremely poor prognosis. However, caution should be exercised in using any one test in isolation. Information from imaging, EEG, and neuron-specific enolase levels may be helpful adjuncts, especially in those patients who fall into the gray zone.

REFERENCES

1. Bernard SA, Buist M. Induced hypothermia in critical care medicine: a review. *Crit Care Med.* 2003;31:2041-2051.
2. Kochanek P. The brain, the heart, and therapeutic hypothermia. *Cleveland Clin J Med.* 2009;76:S8-S12.
3. Hypothermia after Cardiac Arrest Study Group: mild therapeutic hypothermia to improve the neurologic outcome after cardiac arrest. *N Engl J Med.* 2002;346:549-556.
4. Bernard SA, Gray TW, Buist MD, et al. Treatment of comatose survivors of out-of-hospital cardiac arrest with induced hypothermia. *N Engl J Med.* 2002;346:557-563.
5. Nielsen N, Wetterslev J, Cronberg T, et al. Targeted temperature management at 33°C versus 36°C after cardiac arrest. *N Engl J Med.* 2013;369:2197-2206.
6. Callaway CW, Donnino MW, Fink EL, et al. Part 8: Post-Cardiac Arrest Care: 2015 American Heart Association Guidelines for Cardiopulmonary Resuscitation and Emergency Cardiovascular Care. Circulation.2015; 132 (18 suppl 2): S465-S476.
7. Holzer M. Targeted temperature management for comatose survivors of cardiac arrest. *N Engl J Med.* 2010;363(13):1256-1264.
8. Testori C, Sterz F, Behringer W, et al. Mild therapeutic hypothermia is associated with favourable outcome in patients after cardiac arrest with non-shockable rhythms. *Resuscitation.* 2011;82(9):1162-1167.
9. Dumas F, Grimaldi D, Zuber B, et al. Is hypothermia after cardiac arrest effective in both shockable and nonshockable patients: insights from a large registry. *Circulation.* 2011;123(8):877-886.
10. Lewis ME, Al-Khalidi AH, Townend JN, Coote J, Bonser RS. The effects of hypothermia on human left ventricular contractile function during cardiac surgery. *J Am Coll Cardiol.* 2002;39(1):102-108.
11. Danzl DF, Pozos RS. Accidental hypothermia. *N Engl J Med.* 1994;331(26):1756-1760.
12. Hovdenes J, Laake JH, Aaberge L, Haugaa H, Bugge JF. Therapeutic hypothermia after out-of-hospital cardiac arrest: experiences with patients treated with percutaneous coronary intervention and cardiogenic shock. *Acta Anaesthesiol Scand.* 2007;51(2):137-142.
13. Zobel C, Adler C, Kranz A, et al. Mild therapeutic hypothermia in cardiogenic shock syndrome. *Crit Care Med.* 2012;40(6):1715-1723.
14. Orlowski JP, Erenberg G, Lueders H, et al. Hypothermia and barbiturate coma for refractory status epilepticus. *Crit Care Med.* 1984;12:367-372.
15. Polderman KH. Application of therapeutic hypothermia in the intensive care unit. Opportunities and pitfalls of a promising treatment modality. *Intensive Care Med.* 2004;30:757-769.
16. Spiel AO, Kliegel A, Janata A. Hemostasis in cardiac arrest patients treated with mild hypothermia initiated by cold fluids. *Resuscitation.* 2009;80:762-765.
17. Merchant RM, Abella BS, Peberdy MA, et al. Therapeutic hypothermia after cardiac arrest: unintentional overcooling is common using ice packs and conventional cooling blankets. *Crit Care Med.* 2006;34(12):S490-S494.
18. Tømte Ø, Draegni T, Mangschau A, et al. A comparison of intravascular and surface cooling techniques in comatose cardiac arrest survivors. *Crit Care Med.* 2011;39(3):443-449.
19. Gillies MA, Pratt R, Whiteley C, et al. Therapeutic hypothermia after cardiac arrest: a retrospective comparison of surface and endovascular cooling techniques. *Resuscitation.* 2010;81(9):1117-1122.
20. Kim F, Olsufka M, Longstreth WT, Jr, et al. Pilot randomized clinical trial of prehospital induction of mild hypothermia in out-of-hospital cardiac arrest patients with a rapid infusion of 4 degrees C normal saline. *Circulation.* 2007;115:3064-3070.

21. Bruel C, Parienti JJ, Marie W, et al. Mild hypothermia during advanced life support: a preliminary study in out-of-hospital cardiac arrest. *Crit Care.* 2008;12(1):R31.

22. Boddicker KA, Zhang Y, Zimmerman MB, Davies LR, Kerber RE. Hypothermia improves defibrillation success and resuscitation outcomes *Circulation.* 2005;111:3195-3201.

23. Abella BS, Zhao D, Alvarado J, Hamann K, Vanden Hoek TL, Becker LB. Intra-arrest cooling improves outcomes in a murine cardiac arrest model. *Circulation.* 2004;109:2786-2791.

24. Bernard SA, Smith K, Cameron P, et al. Induction of therapeutic hypothermia by paramedics after resuscitation from out-of-hospital ventricular fibrillation cardiac arrest: a randomized controlled trial. *Circulation.* 2010;122(7):737-742.

25. Italian Cooling Experience (ICE) Study Group. Early-versus late-initiation of therapeutic hypothermia after cardiac arrest: preliminary observations from the experience of 17 Italian intensive care units. *Resuscitation.* 2012;83(7):823-828.

26. Che D, Li L, Kopil CM, et al. Impact of therapeutic hypothermia onset and duration on survival, neurologic function, and neurodegeneration after cardiac arrest. *Crit Care Med.* 2011;39(6):1423-1430.

27. Nagao K, Hayashi N, Kanmatsuse K, et al. Cardiopulmonary cerebral resuscitation using emergency cardiopulmonary bypass, coronary reperfusion therapy and mild hypothermia in patients with cardiac arrest outside the hospital. *J Am Coll Cardiol.* 2000;36(3):776-783.

28. Kung DH, Friedman OA. Prolonged hypothermia for neurological protection. *Ther Hypothermia Temp Manag.* 2013;3(2):88-91.

29. Leary M, Grossestreuer AV, Iannacone S, et al. Pyrexia and neurologic outcomes after therapeutic hypothermia for cardiac arrest. *Resuscitation.* 2013;84:1056-1061.

30. Rossetti AO, Oddo M, Logroscino G, Kaplan PW. Prognostication after cardiac arrest and hypothermia: a prospective study. *Ann Neurology.* 2010;67(3):301-307.

31. Greer D, Jingun Y, Patricia DS, Sims J, et al. Clinical examination for prognostication in comatose cardiac arrest patients. *Resuscitation.* 2013;84:1546-1551.

32. Rittenberger JC, Sangl J, Wheeler M, Guyette FX, Callaway CW. Association between clinical examination and outcome after cardiac arrest. *Resuscitation.* 2010;81:1128-1132.

33. Kamps M, Horn J, Oddo M, Fugate J, et al. Prognostication of neurologic outcome in cardiac arrest patients after mild therapeutic hypothermia: a meta-analysis of the current literature. *Intensive Care Med.* 2013;39:1671-1682.

34. Zandbergen EG, HIjdra A, Koelman JH, et al. Prediction of poor outcomes within the first 3 days of postanoxic coma. *Neurology.* 2006;66:62-68.

35. Dattta S, Hart GK, Opdam H, Gutteridge G, Archer J. Post-hypoxic myoclonic status: the prognosis is not always hopeless. *Crit Care Resusc.* 2009;11:39-41.

36. Chen R, Bolton CF, Young B. Prediction of outcome in patients with anoxic coma: a clinical and electrophysiologic study. *Crit Care Med.* 1996;24(4):672-678.

37. Wijdicks EF, Hijdra A, Young GB, et al. Practice parameter: prediction of outcome in comatose survivors after cardiopulmonary resuscitation (an evidence-based review): report of the Quality Standards Subcommittee of the American Academy of Neurology. *Neurology.* 2006;67(2):203-210.

38. Tiainen M, Kovala TT, Takkunen OS, Roine RO. Somatosensory and brainstem auditory evoked potentials in cardiac arrest patients treated with hypothermia. *Crit Care Med.* 2005;33:1736-1740.

39. Daubin C, Quentin C, Allouche S, et al. Serum neuron-specific enolase as predictor of outcome in comatose cardiac-arrest survivors: a prospective cohort study. *BMC Cardiovasc Disord.* 2011;42:985-992.

40. Tiainen M, Roine RO, Pettial V, Takkunen OS. Serum neuron-specific enolase and S-100B protein in cardiac arrest patients treated with hypothermia. *Stroke.* 2003;34:2881-2886.

41. Grossestreuer AV, Abella BS, Leary M, et al. Time to awakening and neurologic outcome in therapeutic hypothermia-treated cardiac arrest patients. *Resuscitation.* 2013;84(12):1741-1746.

Military-Related Injuries

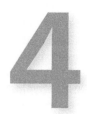

Jamie M. Rand, MD, FACS and Aditya Uppalapati, MD

KEY POINTS

1. Military personnel treat injuries which are similar to the civilian population as well as those specific to war and combat.

2. Multiple factors influence the five levels of aeromedical evacuation. Patients are moved through the system as quickly and safely as possible with consideration for combat activities and terrain.

3. It is important to understand the mechanism of injury. Projectile injuries are influenced by kinetic energy (KE), depth of penetration, and yaw.

4. Explosive trauma, resulting in thermal, blast and/or ballistic injury, is the most common mechanism of military-related injury in current conflicts.

5. In patients with significant hemorrhage, massive transfusion protocols and viscoelastic coagulation testing guided resuscitation may be helpful. Fresh whole blood transfusion can be an important component in austere conditions.

6. Nuclear, biological, and chemical warfare can affect a massive number of individuals. Exposure prevention and decontamination are paramount. Supportive care and exposure-specific management then follow based on patient-specific presentation and factors.

Conflicts in far-reaching and diverse areas of the world have resulted in a myriad of traumatic injuries which health care providers are tasked to treat. Some military injuries are comparable to civilian traumatic injuries, while others are unique to wartime/conflict operations. Unfortunately, with the current state of terrorism, the line between the two is becoming more blurred, making it all the more important for all providers to be aware of what classically have been thought of as "military-related injuries." In addition to the severity and pattern of injuries, the conflict environment itself adds an additional complexity to providing medical care in these situations. This chapter will provide an overview of the injuries traditionally associated with military operations, as well as highlight operational considerations.

"Lessons learned" from our military colleagues can be lifesaving when applied to disaster situations no matter the location or specific circumstance.

While many surgical advances have been, and are being made, because of the vast experiences of military wartime trauma, many civilian injuries are treated in a similar fashion as military their counterparts. The sheer number of seriously injured in recent conflicts has allowed the military to further evidence-based transfusion practices. For example, the numerous multiple-injured military personnel have allowed for improved mortality in massive transfusion with the creation of 1:1:1 ratio protocols[1] and the addition of tranexamic acid.[2] In the end, however, these strategies are not significantly different from the massive transfusion protocols in place in civilian institutions. Similarly, splenic lacerations, whether sustained from a car crash in Missouri or an improvised explosive device (IED) detonating under a tank in Afghanistan, are treated the same. Furthermore, while traumatic brain injury (TBI) may be seen in an increased frequency in current military conflicts, its management is also comparable to its stateside counterpart. The military may be more in tune to the effects of repeat concussions, but the underlying management is the same. This chapter will highlight instances where military trauma varies from civilian trauma.

AEROMEDICAL EVACUATION: FROM THE BATTLEFIELD TO HOME

Before specific injuries are addressed, it is important to understand the basics of how a military member goes from being injured on the battlefield to eventual admission to a hospital in the United States. There are five levels of care described in the military aeromedical evacuation system.[3] Unlike the American College of Surgery levels of trauma care, an increase in the military level represents an increase in medical capability.

Level I care is provided by the injured member themselves, other members of their unit, or a medic. This "Self-Aid/Buddy Care" allows for quick control of hemorrhage via pressure dressings, tourniquets, and topical hemostatic agents to stave off early hemorrhagic death. At this level, medical care is frequently complicated by the combat environment. Moving the injured to safety prior to providing medical care can be lifesaving for both the injured as well as the provider.

Level II is the first time a military member will encounter an advanced health care provider. Each branch of service has a slightly different medical team at this level, but it typically either consists of an area support facility staffed with a nonsurgeon advanced health care provider, or a mobile surgical unit which has basic general and orthopedic surgical capabilities. Units at this level typically have a holding capacity of 24 to 72 hours with supplies to support up to 10 operations each day for those 1 to 3 days without being resupplied, with specifics

being dependent on the branch of service. Most of these units are modular in nature and can be supplemented with additional personnel and equipment to further enhance the medical care provided in the tactical environment.

Level III, the theater hospital, is approximately equivalent to a stateside Level III trauma center. This facility is still within the combat zone but has an increased capability, both in terms of the medical/surgical care and holding capacity. For example, Craig Joint Theater Hospital (CJTH), one of the Level III hospitals in support of Operation Enduring Freedom in Afghanistan, has advanced radiology support with computed tomography (CT), magnetic resonance imaging (MRI), and interventional radiology, as well as numerous subspecialty surgical services and 5 to 6 operating room tables. Holding capacity is increased to 44 to 248 beds and to 30 days.

Level IV is a major medical facility, still within the theater of war but outside the combat zone. **Level V** is a major medical center in the United States. These upper echelons have capabilities and staffing similar to civilian hospitals.

Where a patient enters the aeromedical evacuation chain depends on multiple factors, primarily proximity to medical facilities and severity of injury. While most point-of-injury care is provided by Level II facilities, if a member is injured near a Level III facility, then that is where they will receive their initial evaluation. Keep in mind that prior to entering any facility, all patients must be cleared—inspected for unexploded ordinance, booby-traps, or bombs. Safety is paramount while still trying to quickly evacuate the wounded out of the combat zone. For the Afghanistan theater the g oal is for patients to reach Level II within 1 hour from time of injury and to be transported to Level III within 24 hours. Transport from the point of injury to Level II is typically by ground or by tactical rotor aircraft. Transport between Levels II and III is also usually via tactical rotor aircraft under the medical supervision of Critical Care Air Transport (CCAT) teams given the smaller and more temporary nature of where these units are located. Transport between Levels III, IV, and V facilities is via fixed-wing aircraft. The goal is to have patients evacuated out to a Level IV facility within 48 to 72 hours from the time of injury. In all cases, the philosophy is to "get the right patient to the right hospital in the right amount of time," while preserving the safety and security of all involved.[3,4]

Spectrum of Injuries

Military-related injuries are comprised of battle and nonbattle injuries, with all possible mechanisms of traumatic injury being represented. In the military setting, these mechanisms of injury are not usually mutually exclusive; one patient may have penetrating wounds, blunt injuries, and blast trauma as well as burns, all from a single incident. Penetrating injury can be from gunshot wounds of varying caliber, knives, or flying projectiles from a myriad of explosive ordinance. Blunt mechanisms include falls, motor vehicle crashes, as well as assaults and sports-related injuries. Burns can occur from accidental or intentional household exposures, fires, explosions, or nuclear/radiation or chemical sources. The most common injury in recent conflicts is a result of explosive trauma, namely IEDs.

Distribution of Injuries

Since the advent of modern warfare, patterns of injury have remained remarkably constant. From World War I to the present, the anatomic distribution of wounds has remained approximately 60% to 70% to the extremities, 15% to the head, and 10% to each the thorax and the abdomen.[5] Body armor is improving, becoming lighter and more flexible than in previous conflicts. The enhanced capability of body armor likely has contributed to the improved casualty to mortality ratio of 16:1 in Iraq and Afghanistan compared to 2.6:1 in Vietnam.[6] Furthermore, the most common mechanism of injury is explosive trauma, with IED blasts being more common than gunshot wounds.

Projectiles

Projectiles cause injury through the creation of a permanent cavity as well as a temporary cavity. The permanent cavity is a result of the physical crush injury created by the projectile moving through tissue. The temporary cavity is created by a stretch injury from energy imparted to the tissues as the projectile travels. The permanent cavity is readily apparent at the time of injury, while the temporary cavity may not be as obvious at the initial evaluation. This tissue may initially look viable, but will ultimately become necrotic over time.

The specific characteristics of each type of projectile contribute to the overall damage that is caused. The most important of these characteristics are mass, velocity, depth of tissue penetration, yaw within the tissue, deformation, and fragmentation. KE is directly proportional to the mass and the square of the velocity of the projectile: $KE = \frac{1}{2} \text{ mass} \times \text{velocity}^2$. Thus, for two projectiles with the same kinetic energy, a large slow projectile will directly crush more tissue resulting in a larger permanent cavity, whereas a small fast projectile will impart more of its energy to the surrounding tissues causing more stretch and a larger temporary cavity.[7]

Yaw is defined as the angle between the projectile's long axis and its line of flight. A bullet can yaw during flight prior to encountering a target, or within the target tissue itself. The amount of yaw during flight is relatively inconsequential to the degree of tissue damage, affecting mainly the angle of entry, while the amount of yaw within the tissue contributes significantly to the amount of destruction caused. For example, Figures 4–1 to 4–3 compare the 7.62-mm AK-47 round, 5.6-mm M-16A1 round, and 7.62-mm M-14 or M-60 round with respect to anticipated permanent and temporary cavities.

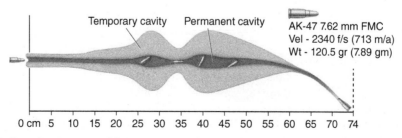

Temporary cavity   Permanent cavity

AK-47 7.62 mm FMC
Vel - 2340 f/s (713 m/a)
Wt - 120.5 gr (7.89 gm)

0 cm 5   10   15   20   25   30   35   40   45   50   55   60   65   70 74

FIGURE 4–1 Ballistic characteristics of the 7.62-mm round, typical ammunition of the AK-47. (*Reproduced with permission from Borden Institute Army Medical Center: Emergency War Surgery, 4th edition. Washington, DC: Department of the Army; 2013.*)

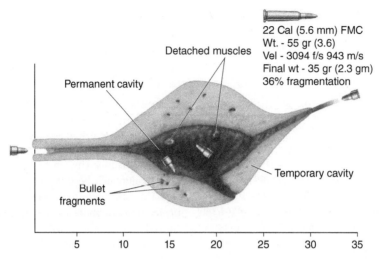

FIGURE 4–2 Ballistic characteristics of the 5.6-mm round, typical ammunition of the M-16A1. (*Reproduced with permission from Borden Institute Army Medical Center: Emergency War Surgery, 4th edition. Washington, DC: Department of the Army; 2013.*)

The M-16A1 round is lighter and faster than the AK-47 or M-14 rounds, with a much higher percentage of fragmentation. It also begins to yaw within a shorter distance, 10 to 15 cm, compared with 15 to 20 cm for the M-14 bullet and 25 cm for the AK-47. The characteristics of the M-16A1 lend to a greater amount of injury compared to the AK-47 or M-14, despite its being a smaller projectile.[5]

Explosive Ordinance

Explosive trauma is currently the most common cause of military-related injury. Depending on proximity to the explosion's epicenter, three distinct types of injuries are encountered: thermal, blast, and ballistic (Figure 4–4).[5] Those closest to the explosion can be affected by the heat and flames of the explosion resulting in thermal or chemical burns of varying severity. Blast injury can present in three different classes of injury. Primary blast injury is a result of overpressure from the blast wave itself. All air-containing body structures are at risk of rupture when a victim experiences this sonic shock wave. A ruptured tympanic membrane is the most common injury sustained in blast trauma, followed by pneumothorax and gastrointestinal (GI) perforation. GI perforation can take up to 48 hours to manifest clinical symptoms, so a high index of suspicions is necessary to limit morbidity and mortality from a delayed diagnosis. Ballistic trauma, also classified as secondary blast trauma, is due to flying fragments. These fragments cause injury in a similar manner as projectiles, with permanent and temporary cavities. However, they are typically smaller, less uniform in shape, and impart lower amounts of energy. Ballistic trauma is classified both as secondary blast injury, for projectiles in the environment being thrown

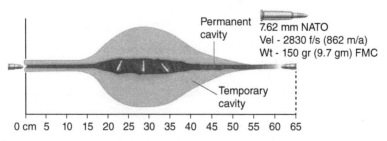

FIGURE 4–3 Ballistic characteristics of the 7.62 NATO round, typical ammunition of the M-14 and M-60. (*Reproduced with permission from Borden Institute Army Medical Center: Emergency War Surgery, 4th edition. Washington, DC: Department of the Army; 2013.*)

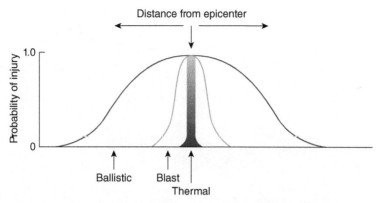

FIGURE 4–4 Type of injury relative to proximity to explosion. (*Reproduced with permission from Borden Institute Army Medical Center: Emergency War Surgery, 3rd edition. Washington, DC: Department of the Army; 2004.*)

by the blast wind, or ballistic injury from fragments of the explosive device itself—either pieces of the explosive's casing or other objects deliberately placed in the explosive with the intent of causing injury as projectiles. The subtle difference between intentional and unintentional flying pieces of debris allows for ballistic trauma to be classified both with the category of blast trauma and is mentioned separately. Tertiary blast trauma is a result of the explosive force propelling the casualty into surrounding objects. This blunt force trauma results in injuries comparable with other types of blunt trauma, such as motor vehicle crashes or falls. Thus, a patient involved in a significant explosion can sustain burns, overpressure perforations, penetrating trauma, and blunt trauma simultaneously. A detailed thorough systematic evaluation is required to properly identify and address all injuries.

Not only does the type of explosive ordnance influence the injuries sustained, but also where that explosion occurs is of great importance. If the explosion occurs with the patient in a vehicle, it is termed a "mounted" IED event. An explosion triggered by a person outside of an armored vehicle is termed a "dismounted" detonation. In a mounted IED event, an IED or landmine explodes under an armored vehicle (Figure 4–5).[5] The three forms of blast trauma can still affect the occupants, even though they may still be protected from the outside environment.[5] Primary blast trauma exists from the blast wave overpressure. Secondary blast trauma exists from objects inside the vehicle becoming projectiles. Tertiary blast trauma exists as occupants collide with

other occupants or portions of the vehicle. Furthermore, toxic gases can be released from the explosive device or the vehicle itself.

In a "dismounted" detonation, the person experiences significant explosive force directly beneath them, with the pressure wave driving debris upwards along fascial planes (Figure 4–6).[5] Tissue far remote from the most distal site of injury can be damaged from the explosive force, much in the same way as the temporary cavity of a projectile is remote from the permanent cavity.

Given their prevalence worldwide and potential to cause devastating injuries, landmines and other explosive ordnance deserve further consideration. Landmines can be either antipersonnel or antivehicle depending on the intended trigger. Antipersonnel mines can be static, bounding, or horizontal spray.[5] Static mines explode where they lie once pressure is applied to them, that is, stepped upon. Bounding mines have a separate explosive charge which causes the mine to "pop up" approximately 1 to 2 m prior to exploding. Horizontal spray mines expel fragments in a specific direction. This type of mine can be triggered via tripwire or command detonation. The location of the injuries inflicted depends greatly on the type of antipersonnel mine that is encountered. Static mines cause mainly lower extremity injuries, while bounding and horizontal spray mines can also cause torso injuries.

Another category of explosive ordnance is termed "explosive remnants of war" (ERW). This category is comprised of "unexploded ordnance" (UXO) and "abandoned explosive ordnance" (AXO).

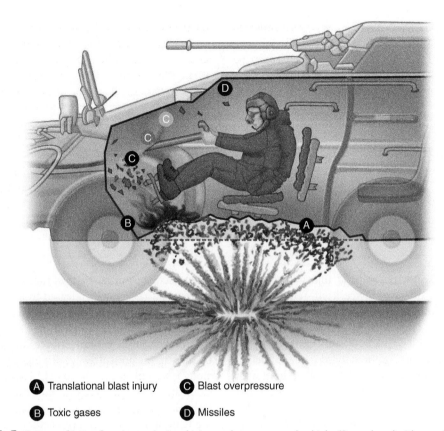

A Translational blast injury   C Blast overpressure

B Toxic gases   D Missiles

FIGURE 4-5 Pattern of injury from an explosive device under an armored vehicle. (*Reproduced with permission from Borden Institute Army Medical Center: Emergency War Surgery, 4th edition. Washington, DC: Department of the Army; 2013.*)

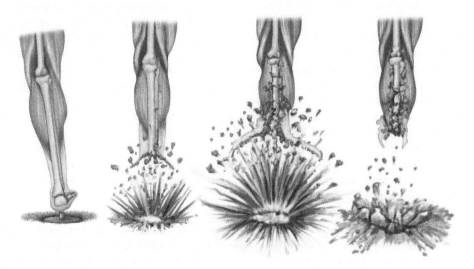

FIGURE 4-6 Pattern of injury from a static landmine explosion. (*Reproduced with permission from Borden Institute Army Medical Center: Emergency War Surgery, 4th edition. Washington, DC: Department of the Army; 2013.*)

Both are unexploded devices. UXOs were deployed as weapons but did not properly explode whereas AXOs were left in an area of conflict without being attempted to be used. While UXO and AXO differ as to why they exist as unattended explosive ordnance in an area of current or former conflict, both types result in similar explosive injuries if detonated. Landmines and ERW are indiscriminant weapons. Personnel or vehicle—man, woman, or child—military or civilian—during an ongoing war or long after the conflict has been resolved—these ordinances affect all the same with devastating results.

According to figures reported by the International Campaign to Ban Landmines, in 2012 there were 3628 casualties of landmines and ERWs.[8] These casualties were located in 62 countries. Approximately 78% of victims were civilians, with 47% of the civilians being children. While the total number of victims is decreased from 4474 reported in 2011, it is likely that these figures are an underrepresentation of the true morbidity and mortality sustained by these explosive devices. The emotional, physical, and financial toll of these injuries cannot be overestimated.

BLEEDING: WHAT TO GIVE AND HOW MUCH?

As mentioned earlier, combat operations in Iraq and Afghanistan have provided copious amounts of data to help develop improved transfusion strategies. From the analysis of these two wars, as well as large amounts of civilian data, massive transfusion protocols have been developed which provide for earlier transfusion of fresh frozen plasma and platelets, with improved mortality.[9] The military continues with its civilian colleagues to determine the optimum transfusion strategy. Is it ratio driven? Is it guided by viscoelastic testing—thromboelastography (TEG) or rotational thromboelastometry (ROTEM)—in which whole blood clotting is examined?[10] Military and civilian doctors alike are trying to create rational transfusion strategies which maximally benefit our patients while limiting the inherent risk associated with blood transfusion.

One area where the military differs from its civilian counterparts is the potential use of fresh whole blood. The military often operates in austere environments in which fractional blood components are not readily available, where supply lines are long, and where the limited supply of blood products, if existent at all, may not be adequate to correct the hemorrhagic shock and associated coagulopathy in the casualties present. In these dire circumstances, fresh whole blood (FWB) is an option.[11]

FWB provides red blood cells (RBCs), clotting factors, platelets, and fibrinogen—all the components which are required to reestablish hemostasis. The blood is warm, thus not contributing to hypothermia, and is more functional, as clotting is not hampered by the loss of factor or platelet activity through cold storage. Additionally, the RBCs in FWB do not have the lessened oxygen delivery capacity from acquired storage lesions.

However, FWB does have disadvantages. Even with rapid testing for malaria, HIV, hepatitis B, hepatitis C, and syphilis, bloodborne transmission is possible. There is a theoretical increased risk of bacterial contamination given the decreased sanitary conditions inherent to most field conditions. Furthermore, given the chaotic situation in which FWB would be required, the chance of clerical error is increased, compounded by the fact that FWB must be type specific. If more than one person requires FWB, this increased risk for clerical error and a transfusion of incompatible blood is increased even more. Another strictly military consideration is that the donor, also a military member, will have a decreased exercise tolerance for a period of time while the body adjusts to the acute, albeit voluntary, blood loss. It must be remembered that in all situations, the success of the fight trumps any individual. Weakening the remaining fighting force is not a decision to be made lightly.

Nuclear Warfare

Another facet of military-related injuries involves nonconventional weapons. Unfortunately, with the increased activity of terrorist organizations these attacks have been seen in the civilian sector as well. A strong suspicion and good working relationship with the public health sector can greatly assist in determining if a nonconventional attack has taken place and how best to treat those already affected and prevent others from becoming affected.

A nuclear explosion has all the same explosive causes of injury as a conventional explosive—thermal, blast, and ballistic—with the addition of radiation. Radiation exposure requires decontamination prior to being brought into the medical facility, in the same manner as the safety clearance is performed. Triage is first based on a patient's conventional injuries, and then modified based on radiation exposure.[12]

Radioactive particles are classified as alpha, beta, gamma, and neutron. Alpha particles can be shielded by a sheet of paper and are harmful if internalized. Beta particles require a thicker material for shielding such as a layer of clothing or a few millimeters of aluminum. These can cause skin burns and are also harmful if ingested. Gamma particles and neutrons destroy living cells and are only shielded by a few feet of concrete or inches of lead. Radiosenstivity is directly correlated with mitotic rate, as only replicating cells are vulnerable to radiation's effects. Less mitotically active cells are affected only when larger doses of radiation are absorbed. Thus, a patient's symptoms can be used to estimate the amount of exposure incurred. Furthermore, these symptoms and their time-to-onset can be used to predict mortality as the adverse effects of radiation following a fairly consistent pattern.

Radiation exposure is expressed in gray (Gy) or rad. One Gy is equivalent to 100 rad which is equal to 1 J of energy per kilogram.[13] LD_{50} is defined as the dose which results in death of half of the people exposed. Exposure of 0.35 Gy can cause transient nausea or headache but is not classified as acute radiation syndrome (ARS). At least 2 Gy are required for ARS to develop.

The hematologic system is affected first with a decline in all cell lines. Radiation exposure affecting only the patient's bone marrow could be latent for 2 to 6 weeks, with the main symptom being fatigue. If there aren't other injuries prompting a medical evaluation, it is possible that medical attention would not be sought, even though it is direly needed. The GI system is affected next. At doses of 6 to 10 Gy, within 2 hours of exposure the patient will have acute-onset cramping abdominal pain, nausea, vomiting, and diarrhea as cells of the GI tract slough. Paradoxically, at doses greater than 10 Gy, nausea is suppressed. Early-onset diarrhea, especially without

nausea, is a particularly poor prognostic sign. Neurologic symptoms, mainly ataxia, seizures, dizziness, and disorientation, suggest an exposure of greater than 10 Gy. Cardiovascular collapse occurs with doses of greater than 35 Gy.[13]

Without supportive care, the LD_{50} is only 3.5 Gy. Death typically occurs within 60 days as a result of the patient's impaired immunity.[13] With supportive care, namely fluids, antimicrobials, cytokines, and transfusion, the LD_{50} increases to approximately 6 Gy. However, these LD_{50}s are based on radiation injury alone. If a patient sustains additional trauma, the LD_{50} will decrease in accordance with the morbidity and mortality of the other injuries. Furthermore, while some conventional wounds are allowed to heal by secondary intention after repeated debridement, it is important for wounds in irradiated tissue to be closed primarily within 36 to 48 hours. Wounds in irradiated tissue left open for longer than this time frame serve as a source of infection.[12]

Treatment of radiation injury is primarily decontamination to prevent continuing exposure and symptomatic relief. Intravenous fluids are provided for hypotension and increased fluid losses from damaged skin and gastrointestinal cells. Antiemetics provide relief from nausea and vomiting, limiting further fluid losses. Lymphocyte counts can be very useful in determining if a lethal dose of radiation was experienced as well as for directing cytokine therapy. If lymphocyte counts are greater than $1.7 \times 10^3/\mu L$, a fatal dose is unlikely. Patients with lymphocyte counts less than 300 to 500/μL can be considered for cytokine supplementation to counteract the radiation's effect on bone marrow. Given these suppressive effects, surgical procedures need to be delayed for weeks if possible, or completed within the first 36 hours. Other supportive measures include potassium iodide to prevent thyroid uptake of radioactive isotopes, chelating agents to bind absorbed metals, and Prussian blue to prevent gastrointestinal absorption of radionuclides.[12]

The evaluation of patients exposed to radiation needs to involve an accurate assessment of those who have a potential for survival. As a general rule, in any military mass casualty situation, if a patient presents with GI symptoms after radiation exposure their chance of survival is low enough and the anticipated utilization of resources is high enough that they will be triaged to "expectant," and provided with comfort care measures.

Biological Warfare

Biological warfare also requires close communication between the medical care providers and public health officials. An attack should be suspected in scenarios with an unusual number of illnesses, unusual presentations, or simultaneous outbreaks, especially of diseases not endemic to the area. Weaponized biological agents can be difficult to identify, treat and isolate if a high index of suspicion is not maintained.

Prevention, protection, decontamination, and infection control are key while treating those suspected to be involved in a biological attack. Primary protection through vaccination is one of the most effective ways of minimizing the impact of a biological agent. Vaccination is possible for anthrax, plague, and smallpox. Postexposure chemoprophylaxis is available for anthrax, plague, Q fever, and tularemia. Decontamination, either mechanical via physical removal of the agent or chemical via destruction of the agent, helps to limit spread of the agent from people or clothing. Dilute bleach solutions are also effective for decontamination—either a 0.5% solution for skin or a 5% solution for equipment. Furthermore, ultraviolet (UV) light or heat can be utilized to effectively kill biological agents on inanimate objects.

The type of infection control precautions that are utilized depend on how the biological agent is transmitted. Universal precautions, consisting of hand washing, gloves, gown, eye protection, and masks, are always recommended when it is likely that body fluids may be encountered. When there is concern about transmission via droplets the patient should also be wearing a mask to limit the transmission of these larger particles. Droplet precautions should be instituted for *Bordetella pertussis*, influenza virus, adenovirus, rhinovirus, *Neisseria meningitidis*, and group A *Streptococcus*. Airborne precautions for particles less than 5 μm in size require special surgical masks/respirators. Agents which require airborne precautions include measles, varicella zoster, *Legionella*, disseminated herpes zoster, and tuberculosis. When possible, patients should be kept in private rooms or cohorted with others experiencing similar symptoms.

Table 4–1 lists known potential biological agents, likely symptoms, and appropriate medical management.[14]

Chemical Warfare

Toxic chemicals can be used intentionally as weapons, or released unintentionally from industrial accidents. Personal protective gear is required when there is a known threat or attack. Preventing exposure is key. Safe decontamination is paramount when exposure has already occurred. Specific antidotes should be provided as quickly as possible to limit morbidity and mortality. Table 4–2 lists many of the known chemical agents, mechanisms of action, symptoms, and treatments.[15,16] Surgical procedures can be safely performed after decontamination, but precautions must still be maintained. Double gloves should be worn, instruments should be cleaned with 5% bleach, and removed objects or tissue should be placed in bleach for disposal. Debridement should be performed with a no-touch technique as much as possible.

TRIAGE PRINCIPLES: MILITARY VERSUS CIVILIAN MINDSET

In most scenarios in the US civilian sector, resources are unlimited, personnel are plentiful, and the facility cannot be easily overwhelmed. In the military, the opposite is frequently true. In a mass casualty situation, resource and personnel limitations can force a change in triage principles that can be difficult to enact. As health care providers, we are usually trained to treat patients in a vacuum. Each patient's viability is based solely on the extent of their injuries. The sickest patient is treated first, but heroic measures will be available to all.

On the battlefield, the goals change. The battle itself remains the overarching goal. "Return the greatest number of soldiers to the fight" is the mantra. The sickest are not always treated first. "Limited resources" literally means that what is used for one patient is not available for the next. "Saving the greatest number of lives" equates to a patient who is deemed expectant in one situation may have been treated further in a less dire situation. Resources may need to be withheld from one so that multiple

TABLE 4-1 Biological agents, signs/symptoms, and treatments.

Biological Toxin	Signs/Symptoms	Medical Management
Botulinum	Cranial nerve palsies, paralysis, respiratory failure	Antitoxin, supportive care
Ricin	Fever, cough, dyspnea, arthralgias, pulmonary edema	Supportive care
Bacteria	**Signs/Symptoms**	**Medical Management**
Anthrax (*Bacillus anthracis*)	Fever, malaise, cough, dyspnea, cyanosis	Ciprofloxacin
Plague (*Yersinia pestis*)	High fever, chills, headache, cough, dyspnea, cyanosis	Streptomycin
Brucellosis (*Brucella sp.*)	Fever, headache, myalgias, sweats, chills	Doxycycline
Cholera (*Vibrio cholerae*)	Massive watery diarrhea	Fluids; tetracycline, doxycycline, or ciprofloxacin
Tularemia (*Francisella tularensis*)	Local ulcer, lymphadenopathy, fever, chills, headache, malaise	Streptomycin
Q-fever (*Coxiella burnetii*)	Fever, cough, pleuritic chest pain	Tetracycline
Virus	**Signs/Symptoms**	**Medical Management**
Venezuelan equine encephalitis (VEE)	Fever, encephalitis	Supportive care
Smallpox	Malaise, fever, rigors, vomiting, headache, pustular vesicles	Investigational antiviral
Viral hemorrhagic fever (VHF)	Facial flushing, petechiae, bleeding, fever, myalgias, vomiting, diarrhea	Supportive care

Reproduced with permission from Borden Institute Army Medical Center: Emergency War Surgery, 4th edition. Washington, DC: Department of the Army; 2013.

others may live. Mass casualty situations test not only medical skill, but emotional fortitude and resiliency as well.

Triage systems exist to prioritize patients for treatment. One common system utilizes 4 categories: immediate, delayed, minimal, and expectant.[17] The immediate group requires lifesaving surgery or other intervention provided without delay. The delayed group also is likely to require lifesaving surgery; however for this group, surgery can be delayed for a short time without adversely affecting mortality as long as temporizing measures are provided. The minimal group is comprised of minor injuries, the care of which can be provided by nonmedical personnel or be delayed hours to days without adverse effect. Expectant patients are those who have injuries so extensive that the time or resources required

to treat them with the goal of survival exceed that which are available. Expectant patients are provided with necessary pain control and other reasonable comfort measures but lifesaving measures are not pursued.

Another system divides patients into only 3 categories: emergent, nonemergent, and expectant. The emergent group can be thought of as those requiring immediate (within minutes) and urgent (within hours) intervention. Nonemergent patients still require care but do not currently have a threat to life, limb, or eyesight. Expectant patients are again those who, given the circumstances, have nonsurvivable injuries. No matter which system is utilized, the goal remains the same—to quickly identify which patients need attention first. It is important to remember that triage needs to be repeated.

TABLE 4–2 Chemical agents: mechanism, signs/symptoms, and treatment.

	Mechanism of Action	Signs/Symptoms	Treatment
Nerve agents			
Organophosphates (GA, GB, GD, GF, VX)	Bind acetylcholinesterase	Miosis, rhinorrhea, dyspnea, loss of consciousness, apnea, seizures, paralysis, copious secretions	Atropine, pralidoxime chloride
Vesicants	**(blister agents)**		
Sulfur mustard (HD), nitrogen mustard (HN), Lewisite (L), phosgene oxime (CX)	Alkylating agent, denatures DNA	Skin blisters, airway irritation, conjunctivitis, mucus membrane burns	Decontamination (M291 kit), dimercaprol
Inhalation injury	**(choking agents)**		
Phosgene (CG) (smells like freshly mown grass/hay)	Oxidative stress, neutrophil influx	Throat irritation, pulmonary edema	N-acetylcysteine, ibuprofen, aminophylline, isoproterenol, colchicine, steroids
Chlorine (Cl)	Inhalation burn	Small airway and alveolar irritation, dyspnea	Nebulized steroids, sodium bicarbonate, and beta agonists; mechanical ventilation
Diphosgene (DP)	Airway irritation	Dyspnea	Supportive care, mechanical ventilation
Chloropicrin (PS)	Airway irritation	Dyspnea	Supportive care, mechanical ventilation
Cyanogens	**(blood agents)**		
Hydrogen cyanide (AC) Cyanogen chloride (CK)	Binds to cytochrome oxidase	Seizures, cardiac arrest, respiratory arrest	100% oxygen, activated charcoal, sodium nitrite, sodium thiosulfate
Hydrogen sulfide (smells like rotten eggs)	Binds to cytochrome oxidase	Loss of consciousness, seizures, myocardial ischemia, pulmonary edema, keratoconjunctivitis	Sodium nitrite
Incapacitation agents			
BZ and indoles: atropine, scopolamine, hyoscyamine	CNS effects	Mydriasis, dry mouth, dry skin, increased reflexes, hallucination, impaired memory	Physostigmine

Data from Borden Institute: Emergency War Surgery, 4th edition. Washington, DC: Department of the Army; 2013.

A patient's condition over time can change, requiring either an elevation in priority if they become more critical or perhaps even a change to expectant if their condition severely deteriorates or the overall situation becomes more dire with an influx of additional casualties. A successful medical operation in a mass casualty situation requires swift, accurate, and repeated triage.

CONCLUSION

In many ways, military-related injuries are treated in very much the same way as their civilian counterparts. However, some differences do exist. The injuries themselves can differ as military-related trauma can be caused by ordinances not typically encountered in the civilian environment. The priorities of treatment may vary as the strength of the remaining fighting force must be maintained. Returning members to the fight is a real consideration. What isn't different is the goal of "getting the right patient to the right hospital in the right amount of time."

REFERENCES

1. Holcomb JB, del Junco DJ, Fox EE, et al. The prospective, observational, multicenter, major trauma transfusion (PROMMTT) study: comparative effectiveness of a time-varying treatment with competing risks. *JAMA Surg.* 2013;148(2):127-136.
2. CRASH-2 trial collaborators, Shakur H, Robert I, et al. Effects of tranexamic acid on death, vascular occlusive events and blood transfusion in trauma patients with significant haemorrhage (CRASH-2): a randomized placebo-controlled trial. *Lancet.* 2010;376(9734):23-32.
3. Nessen SC, Lounsbury DE, Hetz SP. Prologue: trauma system development and medical evacuation in the combat theater. In: Nessen SC, Lounsbury DE, Hetz SP, eds. *War Surgery in Afghanistan and Iraq.* 1st ed. Washington DC: Department of the Army; 2008:1-10.
4. Szul AC, Davis LB, Walter Reed Army Medical Center Borden Institute. Levels of medical care. In: Szul AC, Davis LB, eds. *Emergency War Surgery.* 3rd ed. Washington, DC: Department of the Army; 2004:2.1-2.11.
5. Szul AC, Davis LB, Walter Reed Army Medical Center Borden Institute. Effects and parachute injuries. In: Szul AC, Davis LB, eds. *Emergency War Surgery.* 3rd ed. Washington, DC: Department of the Army; 2004:1.1-1.15.
6. Glasser RJ. *Broken Bodies Shattered Minds: A Medical Odyssey from Vietnam to Afghanistan.* Palisades, NY: History Publishing Company; 2011:33-34, 83-84.
7. Hollerman JJ, Fackler ML, Coldwell DM, Ben-Menachem Y. Gunshot wounds: 1. Bullets, ballistics, and mechanisms of injury. *AJR Am J Roentgenol.* 1990;155(4):685-690.
8. International Campaign to Ban Landmines. Landmine Monitor 2013, 2013. www.the-monitor. org. Accessed December 2013.
9. Spinella PC, Holcomb JB. Resuscitation and transfusion principles for traumatic hemorrhagic shock. *Blood Rev.* 2009;23(6):231-240.
10. Wegner J, Popovsky MA. Clinical utility of thromboelastography: one size does not fit all. *Semin Thromb Hemost.* 2010;36(7):699-706.
11. Joint Theater Trauma System. Clinical practice guideline: Fresh whole blood (FWB) transfusion. Department of the Army, 2012. http://www.usaisr. amedd.army.mil/clinical_practice_guidelines.html. Accessed December 2013.
12. Szul AC, Davis LB, Walter Reed Army Medical Center Borden Institute. Radiological injuries. In: Szul AC, Davis LB, eds. *Emergency War Surgery.* 3rd ed. Washington, DC: Department of the Army; 2004:30.1-30.7.
13. Donnelly EH, Nemhauser JB, Smith MJ, et al. Acute radiation syndrome: assessment and management. *South Med J.* 2010;103(6):541-544.
14. Szul AC, Davis LB, Walter Reed Army Medical Center Borden Institute. Biological warfare. In: Szul AC, Davis LB, eds. *Emergency War Surgery.* 3rd ed. Washington, DC: Department of the Army; 2004:31.1-31.6.
15. Szul AC, Davis LB, Walter Reed Army Medical Center Borden Institute. Chemical injuries. In: Szul AC, Davis LB, eds. *Emergency War Surgery.* 3rd ed. Washington, DC: Department of the Army; 2004:32.1-32.7.
16. Joint Theater Trauma System. Clinical practice guideline: inhalation injury and toxic industrial chemicals. Department of the Army, 2012. http:// www.usaisr.amedd.army.mil/clinical_practice_ guidelines.html. Accessed December 2013.
17. Szul AC, Davis LB, Walter Reed Army Medical Center Borden Institute. Mass casualty and triage. In: Szul AC, Davis LB, eds. *Emergency War Surgery.* 3rd ed. Washington, DC: Department of the Army; 2004:3.1-3.17.

Regionalization

*Christopher W. Seymour, MD, MSc and
Jeremy M. Kahn, MD, MSc*

5

KEY POINTS

1 Regionalization refers to the systematic transfer of high-risk critically ill patients to regional referral centers where intensivists provide high-intensity care.

2 Regionalization has several unrealized benefits including the potential to increase survival for critically ill patients through greater use of evidence-based practices and clinical experience with performing of advanced interventions, and shorter time to definitive therapy. Concentrating high-risk, high-cost care for the critically ill also has the potential to reduce overall costs for the health system.

3 Potential unintended consequences include the downscaling of critical care capacity at smaller hospitals resulting in reduced ability to provide advanced care in emergencies due to an erosion of clinical skills, inadequate equipment, or familiarity of clinicians with best practice.

4 Regionalization may increase intensive care unit (ICU) occupancy or census beyond the capabilities of high-volume referral centers and may also strain the capacity for interhospital transport.

5 Barriers to implementation of regionalization include the lack of a strong centralized authority to regulate and enforce the regionalized system; strain on families due to the longer distances to travel for care at referral hospitals, lack of familiarity with physicians/care team at new hospitals, and risks of interfacility transport to new hospital; capacity constraints at large-volume hospitals; and both hospitals' and physicians' potential unwillingness to sacrifice income when patients are transferred to other hospitals for care.

6 Special challenges include the need to educate new clinicians in understanding when patients should or should not be treated at referral hospitals, balancing stakeholder needs, and maintaining patient centeredness.

Critical care is usually perceived as a local activity within one hospital—nurses and physicians providing high-intensity care to seriously ill patients within a defined geographic space, without considering the larger health care system outside the hospital. More recently, however, critical care has evolved into a regional activity, one in which intensivists across many hospitals collaborate to provide high-intensity care to all individuals in an entire geographic area. Large hospitals functioning as "regional referral centers" now routinely provide specialty critical care to the sickest patients,[1] often after long distance interhospital transfers,[2] while the threats of pandemics and natural disasters are forcing hospitals to align within regions in a state of critical care preparedness.[3] Moreover, governmental agencies will soon require that regional critical care services not only be coordinated but also be accountable—that is, hospitals and regions will have to show that they are capable of effectively providing high-quality critical care to all patients in need.[4] Such is the mandate of the United States Patient Protection and Affordable Care Act—which seeks to link payment to quality, coordinated care, and more efficient health care delivery at the level of the system, not just the individual provider.

Many factors might explain the shifting paradigm in the delivery of critical care. First, critical care is expanding and now accounts for more than $80 billion per year in US health care costs, almost 1% of the gross domestic product (GDP).[5] These extreme financial burdens and the increasing volume of patients demand attention to more efficient care strategies in critical illness. Second, an expanding information technology system allows hospitals to share clinical information rapidly and securely, enabling more effective cross-hospital care coordination.[6] Third, interfacility transport is increasingly safe over long distances, even for the critically ill.[7,8] Fourth, a limited supply of trained intensivist physicians in the United States makes it difficult to match intensivist supply with the increasing demand for critical care, necessitating system-level approaches to matching supply and demand.[9]

Additionally, and perhaps most importantly, health care stakeholders increasingly recognize that hospitals vary widely in their capabilities and overall quality of critical care.[10] Not all hospitals are capable of providing 24-hour trauma care, emergency stroke assessments and treatment, emergency surgery, advanced interventional cardiology, or specialty medical services like continuous renal replacement therapy or extracorporeal membrane oxygenation (ECMO), as there are substantial fixed costs to keep these critical care services "at the ready." The few hospitals that do provide these services are not readily accessible to the general US population.[11]

This chapter will review the concept of *regionalization*, a regional care coordination strategy designed to address these problems. Under critical care regionalization, high-risk patients would be systematically transferred to regional referral centers. The chapter will outline conceptual models for regionalization, review the existing evidence, and provide practical guidance for clinicians who will increasingly be required to develop, manage, and practice regionalization in their health care system. Of note, regionalization is only one of several approaches to regional critical care coordination.[12] Others include ICU telemedicine and community-based education. These topics are discussed elsewhere in this textbook. Regionalization should be viewed as complementary to these other approaches, to be undertaken in concert as part of a holistic, regional approach to critical care.[13]

WHAT IS MEANT BY "REGIONALIZATION"?

Regionalization is the systematic transfer of high-risk critically ill patients to regional referral centers. A regionalized critical care system requires the following four components:

a. A method to define regions, either by geography or by political boundaries

b. A method to identify hospitals by their critical care capability

c. A strategy to triage patients to designated referral hospitals

d. A regulatory body to manage and provide oversight for the system

Each of these individual components are important for different reasons. Without a consensus-based definition for regions, it will be impossible to hold providers accountable for their coordinator efforts or to enact local legislation to support the process. Without an objective method to stratify hospitals based on capability, it will be impossible to identify regional critical care centers. Without a valid approach to triage, it will be impossible to get the right patients to the right hospitals. And without a regulatory body to oversee the system, it will be impossible to effect meaningful change.

The care for many diseases and syndromes in the US health care system is already organized in regionalized systems based on these four components. These include time-sensitive conditions that are similar to those commonly cared for ICUs. Most notably, patients with traumatic injury are cared for in a mature regional system. Early trauma systems grew out of advances in emergency medicine and triage made during the Vietnam conflict. This was followed by extensive advocacy by professional societies that recognized the potential for improved outcomes by centralizing care for seriously injured patients.[14] In addition, a broad evidence base establishes that injured patients receiving care in a trauma center are more likely to experience improved outcomes as a result of their injury than similar patients receiving care in a nontrauma center.[15] These systems continue to be evaluated for their ability to improve patient-centered outcomes.

Other syndromes or diseases that are considered for regionalization include ST-segment elevation myocardial infarction (STEMI),[16] neonatology,[17] stroke,[18] and cardiac arrest, although formal regionalization for these areas is far less prevalent than for trauma. Many features of these conditions make them amenable to centralized care, including the following:

a. The high risk for an adverse outcome

b. The time-sensitive nature of the conditions

c. The extensive infrastructure and stand-ready costs for effective 24-hour care

d. Established volume-outcome relationships that suggest that outcomes might be improved by centralizing care at high-volume centers[19]

Based on these examples in comparable syndromes and a broad conceptual foundation, critical care regionalization is supported by several multidisciplinary stakeholder groups.[20] In fact, there are calls for the implementation of regionalized care for critical care in general as well as for the specific disease states with a high-likelihood of critical illness (eg, acute myocardial infarction [MI], acute stroke, high-risk surgeries, and out-of-hospital cardiac arrest).[21] In the United States, these calls were followed on by proposed legislation in the US Congress that seeks novel methods of critical care delivery for highest-risk patients.[22]

POTENTIAL BENEFITS

Regionalization has several unrealized benefits, including the potential to increase survival for critically ill patients. If sickest patients are rapidly triaged to centers of excellence, several time-sensitive evidence-based practices could be provided, including thrombolysis for stroke,[23] targeted temperature management after cardiac arrest,[24] or quantitative fluid resuscitation for septic shock.[25,26] High-volume centers may also facilitate evidence-based practices, which although not time sensitive, may be more thoroughly delivered at referral centers with regular use. These might include low-tidal volume ventilation for acute lung injury,[27] daily interruption of continuous sedative infusions,[28] and ECMO for severe acute respiratory failure.[29] Improved outcomes at higher-volume centers (ie, volume outcome relationship) may derive from a variety of factors. These could include on-call resources for advanced procedures (eg, ECMO), greater clinical experience with performing and management of advanced interventions, or shorter time to definitive therapy. Although untested in a randomized trial, the concentration of these critically ill patients at centers of excellence may improve critical care outcomes.

Regionalization could also have financial implications for critical care. ICUs exhibit economies of scale. In other words, the greater the throughput of patients in an ICU is accompanied by lower per unit costs.[30] Because most hospital costs are fixed, higher-volume hospitals share those fixed costs over more patients, improving overall efficiency. For example, high-cost equipment and personnel like the oxygenator and perfusionists for an ECMO machine may be too expensive for a small community hospital if only used occasionally each year. However, if a referral center uses ECMO every day, the costs of that machine and personnel are spread over many patients, reducing the per patient costs. In this way, concentrating high-risk, high-cost care for the critically ill has the potential to reduce overall costs for the health system.

In addition, regionalization may have subtle benefits to the prevalent disparities in the delivery of critical care. Recent evidence suggests that certain critical care services are unequally distributed across racial and ethnic groups, as well as ability to pay, and these differences may impact patient outcomes like 30-day mortality.[31] In fact, transfers of patients for common critical illnesses like sepsis or complaints like chest pain may be less common among the uninsured.[32] Such disparities by race, ethnicity, or insurance status could be mitigated through structured regionalization in which transfers to regional referral centers are determined by explicit criteria based on illness severity, rather than on implicit criteria that are more subject to bias.

POTENTIAL UNINTENDED CONSEQUENCES

The potential clinical and economic benefits of regionalization may be offset by a number of potential unintended consequences.[33] First, the upscaling of critical care capacity at referral hospitals may require the downscaling capacity at others. Downscaling may result in a reduced ability of small hospitals to provide advanced care in emergencies due to an erosion of clinical skills, inadequate equipment, or familiarity of clinicians with best practice. For example, under a regionalized scenario smaller hospitals may see fewer cases of septic shock. Septic patients receiving care in these hospitals may be subject to increased morbidity as a result.[34] Although regionalization may benefit patients up-triaged to regional referral centers, it may harm patients who remain at smaller community hospitals. Regionalization may also extend harm to other patients, as many high-margin medical services such as oncology and cardiac surgery require high-quality ICUs. The downscaling of critical care may force these hospitals to abandon other profitable programs that require intensivists to care for their patients, limiting access to these services in rural communities.

Second, regionalization of the critically ill may increase ICU occupancy or census beyond the capabilities of high-volume referral centers. Many large academic medical centers are operating at high capacity, and are under pressure to expand with rising number of critically ill patients. If ICU occupancy is at capacity limits, access to ICU beds may be reduced for other patients—potentially worsening their outcomes. Indeed, boarding critically ill patients in the emergency department or in ICUs unequipped to care for specialty cases is associated with higher mortality,[35,36] a situation that may increase under regionalization. As well, Gabler et al found that across 155 US ICUs in more than 200,000 patients, small increases in ICU strain were associated with 2% to 7% increase in the odds of mortality.[37]

Regionalization may also strain our capacity for interhospital transport, or the ability to move patients from small hospitals to referral centers. Multiple studies demonstrate that long-distance transfer of critically ill patients by both ground or aeromedical transport is both feasible and safe.[38] However, these observations occur under the existing system, which likely limits transfers only to those most likely to survive. The capacity of this system to accommodate a larger volume of patients, sicker patients, and patients earlier in their hospital course in the setting of predefined transfer criteria, has not been empirically tested.

Despite the economy-of-scale rationale for regionalization, regionalization may increase health care utilization in some scenarios, leading to higher costs. Unforeseen costs may include flight or transport costs to a new facility, and added fixed costs to oversee and regulate the coordinated system. Many trauma systems struggle with issues of costs and cost-effectiveness, in particular how to manage stand-ready costs for unpredictable and unscheduled, high-priced patients. With even more general critically ill patients than trauma, it is likely that a regionalized critical care system will have multiple competing financial implications at both the referral and referring hospitals.

CLINICAL EVIDENCE

Little empiric data support regionalization for critical care. As previously mentioned, regionalization is indirectly supported by the existence of volume-outcome relationships and successful implementation of regionalized systems in trauma and neonatal care.[33]

Additional indirect evidence for regionalization of the critically ill derives from the conventional ventilatory support versus extracorporeal membrane oxygenation for severe adult respiratory failure (CESAR) trial. In this United Kingdom–based, multicenter trial, 180 patients with severe but potential reversible acute respiratory failure were randomized to receive conventional management or referral to a specialty center for consideration for ECMO. Because of the intent-to-treat analysis and that only 75% (N = 57 of 90) assigned to ECMO centers actually received ECMO, the study has findings that speak toward referral center care as opposed to just ECMO. In fact, those referred experienced a 16% increase in months without disability, and 0.03 increase in quality-adjusted life-years (QALYs) at 6-month follow-up.

An additional study during the 2009 H1N1 influenza pandemic revealed differences in outcome among acute respiratory distress syndrome (ARDS) patients who were and were not referred for ECMO at 4 adult ECMO centers in the United Kingdom.[39] Using multiple strategies to account for patient differences, this observational study found between 22% and 29% reduction in mortality for H1N1-related ARDS patients referred to ECMO centers. Randomized trials of this regionalization strategy are particularly challenging from ethical, logistic, and practical barriers—and even more so during pandemics. Yet this observational study provides strong observational evidence of the power of transfer to a regional referral center to save lives in critical illness.

Finally, indirect support derives from simulated data which evaluated the impact of regionalization for nonsurgical patients in the United States receiving mechanical ventilation.[40] Therein, the authors analyzed hospital discharge data from 8 US states in which 50% of mechanically ventilated patients received care in ICUs with very low admission volumes. By simulating the transfer or those patients to high-volume centers and assuming a mortality benefit similar to prior volume-outcome studies, the authors found that transferring 16 patients would prevent one death. Trade-offs were small for patients, and transfer distances were relatively small for most patients in urban areas. The study concluded that regionalizing care was feasible and might result in a significant mortality benefit for many who are critically ill.

This study has many limitations. The authors assumed that patients transferred to regional referral centers would receive the same mortality benefit as patients originally admitted to those centers. Additionally, the study assumed a perfect triage model whereby all eligible patients were successfully triaged to a regional referral center. In reality, triage of critically ill patients is a complex decision informed by severity of illness, insurance status, distance, and preexisting relationships between clinicians (both referring and receiving) and patients. And as shown in trauma, where triage criteria are relatively standardized and objective,[41] optimal triage that is adherent to guidelines is difficult to achieve. In critical care, triaging patients to referral centers may be more challenging, as there are no commonly accepted strategies to assess who would benefit most at referral centers, nor agreement among providers. Several strategies are under development that may inform critical illness triage, both at the beginning of critical care in the ambulance and after initial stabilization at referring hospitals.[42]

BARRIERS TO IMPLEMENTATION

The implementation of regionalized critical care faces several key barriers (Table 5-1). As identified in a 2009 survey of ICU physicians, one such barrier is the lack of a strong centralized authority to regulate and enforce the regionalized system.[43] No central health authority exists in the United States to oversee a regionalized system—and even trauma regionalization pieces together multiple authorities across many regions. Central oversight has been proposed for cardiac arrest centers but has been difficult to adopt and implement.[44] Competition among

TABLE 5-1 Barriers for stakeholders in the development of regionalized care systems for critical care.

Barriers for hospitals
   Potential to decrease quality of care at smaller hospitals
   Financial implications for hospitals and physicians
   Potential to overwhelm census and capacity at large hospitals

Barriers for patients
   Long(er) distances to travel for care at referral hospitals
   Lack of familiarity with physicians/care team at new hospitals
   Risks of interfacility transport to new hospital

Barriers for the system
   Absence of criteria to determine if patients should be transferred
   No standardized consensus criteria to designate referral center
   No central authority to oversee and regulate the system

US hospitals may lead to additional barriers for criterion-based categorization of hospitals as critical care "centers of excellence." Some countries such as the United Kingdom, Canada, and Australia have public health systems and regional health authorities capable of regulating a regionalized critical care system, however even in these countries hospitals may resist efforts to dictate the services they can provide.

Families may also be strained by regionalized critical care. Some families may be forced to travel long distances to receive critical care, often by unfamiliar clinicians in new hospitals. In a simulation study of regionalized mechanically ventilated patients,[40] the increase in distance from moving patients to referral centers was 8.5 mi. As such, the regionalized system may therefore place undo burden on families and compromise the patient-physician relationship, leading to adverse consequences such as cognitive and emotional dysfunction among family members.[45] As shown in other conditions like pancreatic cancer,[46] patients and families may be willing to accept a higher risk of death if it means receiving care closer to home. This may be more prevalent in patients less likely to survive the hospitalization.

Many other barriers limit regionalization. These include capacity constraints at large-volume hospitals, the difficulty in accurately identifying patients in triaging patients for transfer in a consistent, reliable manner, and both hospitals' and physicians' potential unwillingness to sacrifice income when patients are transferred to other hospitals for care. And crucial to any regionalized system is the efficient ability to move patients between hospitals. This requires both aeromedical and ground emergency medical services personnel to be trained, available, and compensated for participation in critical care transport.[47]

STRATEGIES FOR IMPLEMENTATION

The effective implementation of regionalized critical care will require both intelligent system design and coordination among stakeholders. First, regional systems can be designed around either a traditional hub-and-spoke model or a model with multiple disease-specific referral centers (Figure 5–1). The relative merits of each of these approaches are unknown. Second, policy makers must explicitly define the methods to identify regional referral centers. In cardiac arrest, proposed criteria include (1) capability and timeliness of advanced

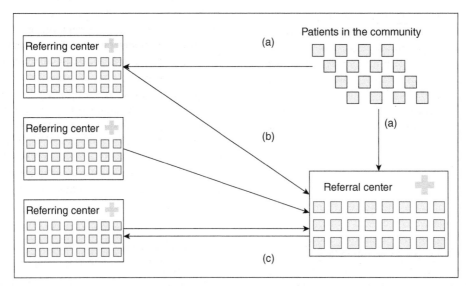

FIGURE 5-1 Schematic of regionalized critical care system where patients can be routed on a variety of paths: (**A**) admission to referring or referral hospitals from the community, (**B**) Up-triage of higher acuity patients from referring to referral hospitals, or (**C**) Down-triage of lower-acuity patients to referring hospitals.

procedures, (2) monitoring and reporting of outcomes, (3) aligned with others in the system of care (eg, emergency medical service [EMS] and emergency department [ED]), and (4) participation in certification programs. Potential structural criteria for referral center certification include intensivist physician staffing and the availability of definitive surgical, coronary, and cardiac care, among others (Table 5–2).[15,29,48-53] Certification as a regional referral centers should be voluntary to ensure maximal buy-in, yet certification should be regulated by existing governmental bodies in order to ensure that the number and location of regional referral centers best meet population needs.

In addition, stakeholders need to standardize the method to identify patients in need to transfer to a regional care center. Transfer criteria are more objective and reliable among ST-elevation MI patients, but may be more difficult to establish for the medical critically ill. It is essential that these criteria be objective to avoid subjective and arbitrary decisions that impact hospital economies or facilitate gaming of the system. The overall goals include improving access to best care but also delivering best care in an equitable fashion. Such equity may be harmed if some regions are overserved by regional centers and other regions are underserved.

In practical terms, the implementation of a regionalized system requires dedicated, coordinated efforts by participating clinicians and critical care policy makers. Such broad stakeholder support is essential, with leadership needed from professional societies to develop evidence-based standards for hospital certification, and governmental accreditation bodies those are in the best position to enforce those standards. Regionalization will also require demonstration products supporting both feasibility and effectiveness. Given the large-scale system change that is mandated through regionalization, it is unlikely that we can proceed until initial studies demonstrate improvements in patient-centered outcomes.

THE ROLE OF INTENSIVISTS

Intensivists will play a major role in a regionalized system. In fact, many intensivists in large health systems participate in *ad hoc* regionalization already. If critical care is further regionalized in a systematic fashion, it will occur as an *inclusive* system, whereby many hospitals are capable of providing some level of critical care but the sickest patients are transferred to higher levels. In contrast, an *exclusive* system occurs when only some hospitals provide critical care, and initial triage is performed by emergency department and EMS personnel prior to hospital admissions. Such a distinction has great implications for emergency care clinicians who may not be positioned or available to perform this triage. In addition, intensivists will also be called upon to inform overall system design, including the outcomes by which integrated critical care systems will be evaluated for quality and outcomes. Thus, intensivists will take an active role in the development of these regional systems, and challenged to maintain a patient-centered view during the process.

SPECIAL CHALLENGES FOR REGIONALIZATION

The gap between evidence and critical care practice, substantial variation in critical care across hospitals, and the growing intensivist workforce crisis in the

TABLE 5–2 Candidate structural characteristics and services of a regional referral center for critical care.

Personnel availability
  Perfusionists for extracorporeal membrane oxygenation (ECMO)
  24-h neurosurgeons
  24-h percutaneous transluminal coronary angioplasty

Certifications in other specialties
  Stroke center
  Level I trauma center

Advanced procedures
  Percutaneous transluminal coronary angioplasty for diagnosis and treatment
  Renal replacement therapy
  Extracorporeal membrane oxygenation

Structural characteristics
  Multidisciplinary rounds for all intensive care patients
  All ICUs staffed by trained intensivists under closed or mandatory consult model

United States are unlikely to go away soon. As such, the need for studying more efficient, cheaper critical care strategies is likely to expand. Consequently, there are special challenges we must face in the reorganization of critical care.

Educating New Clinicians

Traditional medical education emphasizes individual patient care at the bedside, with lessons on the pathophysiology of disease tightly linked to the patient history and physical examination, a focus on communication with the patients, ethics, and professionalism in response to new challenges faced by doctors. Yet, this multidisciplinary curriculum does not prepare trainees to practice in the fully integrated health system of the future. This health system provides care across regions using a combination of technological, physical approaches, and shared resources. The Accreditation Council for Graduate Medical Education has been proactive in this regard by incorporating "systems-based practice" as a core competency critical care fellowship education. To ensure a prepared workforce we must continue to emphasize a system's view in the education of our future intensivists. This will include an understanding of when patients should or should not be treated at referral hospitals.

Balancing Stakeholder Needs

If critical care is organized into a regionalized system, competing stakeholder needs will require careful balancing. The relevant stakeholders in critical care include community physicians, academic physicians, other clinicians, hospitals, governmental agencies, EMS personnel who transport patients, and health care purchasers. All these stakeholders have different needs and incentives that do not always align. For example, regionalization may require community physicians to sacrifice autonomy, patients, and procedures in order to achieve greater health care quality. Conversely, hospitals that receive patients from smaller centers may operate with high census, straining staff, and resources. A balance of stakeholder views and appropriate "buy-in" is a major practical hurdle to future implementation studies.

Maintaining Patient Centeredness

Most importantly, the patient should be at the center of future proposals for regionalized care. Patients have shown that they will not always choose longer distances for specialized care,[46] and we must not forget to consider patient and family wishes when we suggest transferring critically ill patients. In fact, many important components of multidisciplinary critical care, including pastoral services, end-of-life care, and family presence may be more challenging when far from home.

In the end, we face a growing challenge to maximize health care value, whereby the greatest benefit is achieved for the greatest number of people in the most efficient manner. Mindful of the importance of the patient, regionalization is one strategy to accomplish this goal.

REFERENCES

1. Angus DC, Linde-Zwirble WT, Lidicker J, et al. Epidemiology of severe sepsis in the United States: analysis of incidence, outcome, and associated costs of care. *Crit Care Med.* 2001;29:1303-1310.
2. Iwashyna TJ, Christie JD, Moody J, et al. The structure of critical care transfer networks. *Med Care.* 2009;47:787-793.
3. Rubinson L, Hick JL, Hanfling DG, et al. Definitive care for the critically ill during a disaster: a framework for optimizing critical care surge capacity: from a Task Force for Mass Critical Care summit meeting, January 26-27, 2007, Chicago, IL. *Chest.* 2008;133(suppl 5):S18-S31.
4. Institute of Medicine. *Hospital-Based Emergency Care: at the Breaking Point.* Washington, DC: National Academies Press; 2007.
5. Halpern NA, Pastores SM. Critical care medicine in the United States 2000-2005: an analysis of bed numbers, occupancy rates, payer mix, and costs*. *Crit Care Med.* 2010;38:65-71.
6. Jha AK, DesRoches CM, Campbell EG, et al. Use of electronic health records in U.S. hospitals. *N Engl J Med.* 2009;360:1628-1638.
7. Seymour CW, Kahn JM, Schwab CW, Fuchs BD. Adverse events during interhospital, aeromedical transport of mechanically ventilated patients. *Crit Care.* 2008;12(3): R71.
8. Fan E, MacDonald RD, Adhikari NK, et al. Outcomes of interfacility critical care adult patient transport: a systematic review. *Crit Care.* 2006;10:R6.

9. Angus DC, Kelley MA, Schmitz RJ, et al. Current and projected workforce requirements for care of the critically ill and patients with pulmonary disease: can we meet the requirements of an aging population? *JAMA*. 2000;284:2762-2770.

10. Knaus WA, Wagner DP, Zimmerman JE, et al. Variations in mortality and length of stay in intensive care units. *Ann Intern Med*. 1993;118:753-761.

11. Wallace DJ, Angus DC, Seymour CW, et al. Geographic access to high capability severe acute respiratory failure centers in the United States. *PLoS One*. 2014;9:e94057.

12. Nguyen YL, Kahn JM, Angus DC. Reorganizing adult critical care delivery: the role of regionalization, telemedicine, and community outreach. *Am J Respir Crit Care Med*. 2010;181:1164-1169.

13. Carr B, Martinez R. Executive summary—2010 consensus conference. *Acad Emerg Med*. 2010;17:1269-1273.

14. Mullins RJ. A historical perspective of trauma system development in the United States. *J Trauma*. 1999;47(suppl 3):S8-S14.

15. MacKenzie EJ, Rivara FP, Jurkovich GJ, et al. A national evaluation of the effect of trauma-center care on mortality. *N Engl J Med*. 2006;354:366-378.

16. Jollis JG, Roettig ML, Aluko AO, et al. Implementation of a statewide system for coronary reperfusion for ST-segment elevation myocardial infarction. *JAMA*. 2007;298:2371-2380.

17. Cifuentes J, Bronstein J, Phibbs CS, et al. Mortality in low birth weight infants according to level of neonatal care at hospital of birth. *Pediatrics*. 2002;109:745-751.

18. Rymer MM, Thrutchley DE. Organizing regional networks to increase acute stroke intervention. *Neurol Res*. 2005;27(suppl 1):S9-S16.

19. Halm EA, Lee C, Chassin MR. Is volume related to outcome in health care? A systematic review and methodologic critique of the literature. *Ann Intern Med*. 2002;137:511-520.

20. Barnato AE, Kahn JM, Rubenfeld GD, et al. Prioritizing the organization and management of intensive care services in the United States: the PrOMIS Conference. *Crit Care Med*. 2007;35:1003-1011.

21. Carr BG, Matthew Edwards J, Martinez R. Regionalized care for time-critical conditions: lessons learned from existing networks. *Acad Emerg Med*. 2010;17:1354-1358.

22. Schakowsky J. H.R. 3886 (110th): Patient Focused Critical Care Enhancement Act, 2007.

23. Lees KR, Bluhmki E, von Kummer R, et al. Time to treatment with intravenous alteplase and outcome in stroke: an updated pooled analysis of ECASS, ATLANTIS, NINDS, and EPITHET trials. *Lancet*. 2010;375:1695-1703.

24. Bernard SA, Gray TW, Buist MD, et al. Treatment of comatose survivors of out-of-hospital cardiac arrest with induced hypothermia. *N Engl J Med*. 2002;346:557-563.

25. Rivers E, Nguyen B, Havstad S, et al. Early goal-directed therapy in the treatment of severe sepsis and septic shock. *N Engl J Med*. 2001;345:1368-1377.

26. Lilly C. The ProCESS Trial—a new era of sepsis management. *N Engl J Med*. 2014;370:1750-1751.

27. Cooke CR, Watkins TR, Kahn JM, et al. The effect of an intensive care unit staffing model on tidal volume in patients with acute lung injury. *Crit Care*. 2008;12:R134.

28. Kress JP, Pohlman AS, O'Connor MF, et al. Daily interruption of sedative infusions in critically ill patients undergoing mechanical ventilation. *N Engl J Med*. 2000;342:1471-1477.

29. Peek GJ, Mugford M, Tiruvoipati R, et al. Efficacy and economic assessment of conventional ventilatory support versus extracorporeal membrane oxygenation for severe adult respiratory failure (CESAR): a multicentre randomised controlled trial. *Lancet*. 2009;374:1351-1363.

30. Jacobs P, Rapoport J, Edbrooke D. Economies of scale in British intensive care units and combined intensive care/high dependency units. *Intensive Care Med*. 2004;30:660-664.

31. Lyon SM, Benson NM, Cooke CR, et al. The effect of insurance status on mortality and procedural utilization in critically ill patients. *Am J Respir Crit Care Med*. 2011;184:809-815.

32. Hanmer J, Lu X, Rosenthal GE, et al. Insurance status and the transfer of hospitalized patients: an observational study. *Ann Intern Med*. 2014;160:81-90.

33. Kahn JM, Branas CC, Schwab CW, et al. Regionalization of medical critical care: what can we learn from the trauma experience? *Crit Care Med*. 2008;36:3085-3088.

34. Walkey AJ, Wiener RS. Hospital case volume and outcomes among patients hospitalized with severe sepsis. *Am J Resp Crit Care Med*. 2014;189:548-555.

35. Chalfin DB, Trzeciak S, Likourezos A, et al. Impact of delayed transfer of critically ill patients from the emergency department to the intensive care unit. *Crit Care Med*. 2007;35:1477-1483.

36. Lott JP, Iwashyna TJ, Christie JD, et al. Critical illness outcomes in specialty versus general intensive care units. *Am J Respir Crit Care Med.* 2009;179:676-683.
37. Gabler NB, Ratcliffe SJ, Wagner J, et al. Mortality among patients admitted to strained intensive care units. *Am J Resp Crit Care Med.* 2013;188:800-806.
38. Seymour CW, Kahn JM, Schwab CW, et al. Adverse events during rotary-wing transport of mechanically ventilated patients: a retrospective cohort study. *Crit Care.* 2008;12:R71.
39. Noah MA, Peek GJ, Finney SJ, et al. Referral to an extracorporeal membrane oxygenation center and mortality among patients with severe 2009 influenza A (H1N1). *JAMA.* 2011;306:1659-1668.
40. Kahn JM, Linde-Zwirble WT, Wunsch H, et al. Potential value of regionalized intensive care for mechanically ventilated medical patients. *Am J Respir Crit Care Med.* 2008;177:285-291.
41. Ma MH, MacKenzie EJ, Alcorta R, et al. Compliance with prehospital triage protocols for major trauma patients. *J Trauma.* 1999;46:168-175.
42. Seymour CW, Kahn JM, Cooke CR, et al. Prediction of critical illness during out-of-hospital emergency care. *JAMA.* 2010;304:747-754.
43. Kahn JM, Asch RJ, Iwashyna TJ, et al. Physician attitudes toward regionalization of adult critical care: a national survey. *Crit Care Med.* 2009;37:2149-2154.
44. Nichol G, Aufderheide TP, Eigel B, et al. Regional systems of care for out-of-hospital cardiac arrest: a policy statement from the American Heart Association. *Circulation.* 2010;121:709-729.
45. Kentish-Barnes N, Lemiale V, Chaize M, et al. Assessing burden in families of critical care patients. *Crit Care Med.* 2009;37(suppl 10):S448-S456.
46. Finlayson SR, Birkmeyer JD, Tosteson AN, et al. Patient preferences for location of care: implications for regionalization. *Med Care.* 1999;37:204-209.
47. Munjal K, Carr B. Realigning reimbursement policy and financial incentives to support patient-centered out-of-hospital care. *JAMA.* 2013;309:667-668.
48. Pronovost PJ, Angus DC, Dorman T, et al. Physician staffing patterns and clinical outcomes in critically ill patients: a systematic review. *JAMA.* 2002;288:2151-2162.
49. Kim MM, Barnato AE, Angus DC, et al. The effect of multidisciplinary care teams on intensive care unit mortality. *Arch Intern Med.* 2010;170:369-376.
50. Ferrer R, Artigas A, Levy MM, et al. Improvement in process of care and outcome after a multicenter severe sepsis educational program in Spain. *JAMA.* 2008;299:2294-2303.
51. Alberts MJ, Latchaw RE, Selman WR, et al. Recommendations for comprehensive stroke centers: a consensus statement from the Brain Attack Coalition. *Stroke.* 2005;36:1597-1616.
52. Vogt A, Niederer W, Pfafferott C, et al. Direct percutaneous transluminal coronary angioplasty in acute myocardial infarction. Predictors of short-term outcome and the impact of coronary stenting. Study Group of The Arbeitsgemeinschaft Leitender Kardiologischer Krankenhausarzte (ALKK). *Eur Heart J.* 1998;19:917-921.
53. Pannu N, Klarenbach S, Wiebe N, et al. Renal replacement therapy in patients with acute renal failure: a systematic review. *JAMA.* 2008;299:793-805.

Pre-ICU Syndromes

George Lominadze, MD; Massoud G. Kazzi, MD and Ariel L. Shiloh, MD

KEY POINTS

1. A demand on the limited number of ICU beds requires more acute and complex patient care to be delivered on the general wards, outside of the ICU.

2. Rapid response systems are designed to address this goal and rapid response teams (RRTs) or medical emergency teams (METs) have become increasingly prevalent in the US hospital systems as the means to intervene in the care of hospitalized patients with acute clinical deterioration.

3. The identification of prearrest physiology such as abnormal vital signs, or a sudden change in vital signs, can help identify

clinical deterioration minutes to hours before a serious adverse event, often providing sufficient time to deliver an intervention.

4. The Society of Critical Care Medicine has identified the 5 principal admitting ICU diagnoses as respiratory failure or insufficiency, the need for postoperative management, ischemic heart disorders, sepsis, and decompensated heart failure. The correlating rapid response triggers for these conditions are often identified as hypotension, altered mental status, and respiratory distress.

PRE-ICU SYNDROMES: RECOGNITION AND RAPID RESPONSE

Rapid Response Teams

The Joint Commission's National Patient Safety Goals, directs health care providers to improve the identification of clinical deterioration in hospitalized patients and select "a suitable method that enables health care staff members to directly request additional assistance from a specially trained individual(s) when the patient's condition appears to be worsening."[1]

Rapid response systems are designed to address this goal and RRTs or METs have become increasingly prevalent in the US hospital systems

as the means to intervene in the care of hospitalized patients with acute clinical deterioration.[2,3] RRTs are called to evaluate and treat not only the patients who had a cardiorespiratory arrest (for which traditional code teams exist), but also to assess patients who are having symptoms indicative of an impending cardiorespiratory or neurologic deterioration, thus supplementing traditional code teams in scope and frequency of response.[2-5] RRTs may be called for signs of clinical deterioration, such as vital sign abnormalities, arrhythmias, dyspnea, and altered consciousness. A demand on the limited number of intensive care unit (ICU) beds requires more acute and complex patient care to be delivered on the general wards, outside of the ICU.[6]

Rapid Response Activation

The RRT team is activated in instances of perceived patient deterioration and recognition of clinical deterioration. RRT calls are most commonly prompted by cardiorespiratory and neurologic symptoms identified by hospital staff (clinical and nonclinical) or even family members.

The identification of prearrest physiology such as abnormal vital signs, or a sudden change in vital signs, can help identify clinical deterioration minutes to hours before a serious adverse event, often providing sufficient time to deliver an intervention.[7-9] Indeed, diurnal variation of RRT activation rates generally correlate with the timing of caregiver visits.[10] Delays in provider notification and failure to seek help in a timely manner by ward personnel can also contribute to suboptimal outcomes and increased mortality even when RRT systems

are in place.[11,12] Providing objective criteria as a guide for the activation of RRT improves utilization of the RRT systems.

Studies have searched for the minimal criteria for RRT activation. Universally, vital signs monitoring and evaluation of mental status is reproducible and effective.[13] Trigger systems that rely on these parameters alone are known as single and multiple parameter systems based on the number of physiologic criteria included (Figure 6–1). Continuous vital sign monitoring is not feasible for non-ICU patients; so the optimal frequency of vital sign monitoring is patient dependent and difficult to generalize to all patient populations.[14]

In a review of current early warning systems for recognizing and responding to clinically deteriorating patients, relevant policies were examined to determine the vital sign parameters and trigger

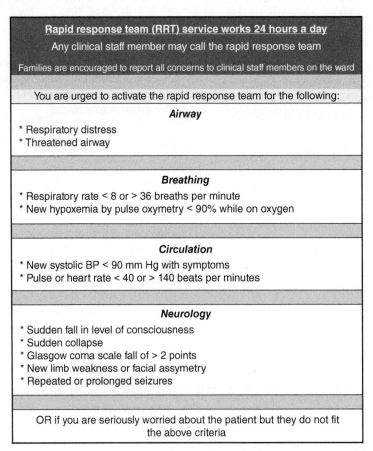

FIGURE 6–1 Example of a rapid response activation care based on single-parameter system. Cards can be distributed, or posted, to instruct clinical staff about activating the rapid response team.

---

thresholds that activate RRT. Most hospitals scored respiratory rate, heart rate, systolic blood pressure, and consciousness level as triggers, and some additionally scored urine output, oxygen saturation, and need for oxygen administration. The thresholds for classifying the values as abnormal varied between the hospitals and were chosen seemingly arbitrarily based on local preferences and expertise.[15] A study of 400 rapid response calls at a large Australian teaching hospital found the most common reasons for RRT activation to be hypoxia (41%), hypotension (28%), altered consciousness (23%), tachycardia (19%), increased respiratory rate (14%), and oliguria (8%). Infection, pulmonary edema, and arrhythmias featured prominently as underlying morbidities and were thought to be responsible for 53% of all triggers for RRT calls.[16]

Traditional ICU scoring systems, such as the sequential organ failure assessment (SOFA) score or the multiple organ dysfunction score (MODS) which are used to predict ICU mortality have been adopted by some institutions as markers for clinical deterioration of non-ICU patients.

The National Early Warning Score Design and Implementation Group (NEWSDIG) in the United Kingdom developed the VitalPac Early Warning Score (ViEWS), a validated scoring system for the early detection of clinical deterioration and prediction for cardiac arrest or need for ICU transfer. The aggregate weighted system scores physiologic parameters to determine the need for more frequent monitoring or ICU-level care. The parameters include respiratory rate, oxygen saturation, supplemental oxygen use, temperature, systolic blood pressure, heart rate, and level of consciousness. Higher scores indicate the need for more frequent reassessment and higher level of care (Figure 6–2A-C). Similar scoring systems such as the cardiac arrest risk triage (CART) have been

National early warning score (NEWS)

Physiological parameters	3	2	1	0	1	2	3
Respiration rate	≤ 8		9-11	12-20		21-24	≥ 25
Oxygen saturations	≤ 91	92-93	94-95	≥ 96			
Any supplemental oxygen		Yes		No			
Temperature	≤ 35.0		35.1-36.0	36.1-38.0	38.1-39.0	≥ 39.1	
Systolic BP	≤ 90	91-100	101-110	111-219			≥ 220
Heart rate	≤ 40		41-50	51-90	91-110	111-130	≥ 131
Level of consciousness				A			V, P, or U

The NEWS Score Initiative flowed from the Royal College of Physicians' NEWS Development and Implementation Group (NEWSDIG) report, and was jointly developed and funded in collaboration with: The Royal College of Physicians, The Royal College of Nursing, The National Outreach Forum, and NHS Training for Innovation

NHS
Training for Innovation

FIGURE 6–2A The National Early Warning Score physiologic parameters scoring chart. A, alert; P, any response to pain; V, any response to voice; U, unresponsive/unconscious. (*Reproduced with permission from Royal College of Physicians. National Early Warning Score (NEWS): Standardising the assessment of acute illness severity in the NHS. Report of a working party. London: RCP, 2012.*)

The national early warning score (NEWS) thresholds and triggers

New scores	Clinical risk
0	Low
Aggregate 1-4	
RED score* (Individual parameter scoring 3)	Medium
Aggregate 5-6	
Aggregate 7 or more	High

Royal College of Physicians

NHS Training for Innovation

The NEWS trigger system aligned to the scale of clinical risk

*RED score refers to an extreme variation in a single physiological parameter (ie a score of 3 on the NEWS chart, coloured RED to aid identification and represents an extreme variation in a single physiological parameter). The consensus of the NEWS Development and Implementation Group (NEWSDIG) was that extreme values in one physiological parameter (eg heart rate ≤ 40 beats per minute, or a respiratory rate of ≤ 8 per minute or a temperature of ≤ 35°C) could not be ignored and on its own required urgent clinical evaluation.

Reproducing this chart: please note that this chart must be reproduced in colour, and should not be modified or amended.

The NEWS initiative: the NEWS initiative flowed from the Royal College of Physicians' NEWSDIG report, and was jointly developed and funded in collaboration with the Royal College of Physicians, Royal College of Nursing, National Outreach Forum and NHS Training for Innovation.

FIGURE 6–2B The National Early Warning Score threshold and triggers. (*Reproduced with permission from Royal College of Physicians. National Early Warning Score (NEWS): Standardising the assessment of acuteillness severity in the NHS. Report of a working party. London: RCP, 2012.*)

developed using logistic regression. The CART score has been validated for in-hospital cardiac arrest (AUC 0.84) and the need for ICU transfer (AUC 0.71).[17] Over 100 track and trigger systems have been developed in recent years, making it extremely difficult to accurately compare and validate them with each other.

More recently, prediction models using vital sign, demographic, location, and laboratory data in electronic health records have been developed as early warning systems for adverse outcomes on the wards. The models are able to calculate a risk score based on computerized data to alert caregivers with automated, real-time, information regarding patient deterioration. Compared to manually calculated systems, automated systems are the least error prone to calculation errors and are the least labor intensive. Although potentially quite useful, these automated scoring systems should not be regarded as the sole solution for detecting patient deterioration; the systems are highly sensitive and may overestimate clinical deterioration or need for higher level of care. Rather, their use could be an adjunct to alert staff to the need to further clinically assesses patients.[18]

A large systematic review demonstrated that implementation of single parameter triggering systems alone are unlikely to improve hospital survival, and that there was only weak evidence in the reduction of cardiac arrest. In contrast, aggregate weighted scoring systems improved hospital survival and reduced both unexpected ICU admission and cardiac arrest rates.[19]

Outcomes

Typical call rates are 20 to 40 per 1000 admissions and the in-hospital mortality of such patients is 24% to 34%.[3,20] Although the MERIT study, a multicenter, cluster-randomized, controlled trial of RRT systems

Outline clinical response to NEWS triggers

News score	Frequency of monitoring	Clinical response
0	Minimum 12 hourly	• Continue routine NEWS monitoring with every set of observations
Total: 1-4	Minimum 4-6 hourly	• Inform registered nurse who must assess the patient; • Registered nurse to decide if increased frequency of monitoring and/or escalation of clinical care is required;
Total: 5 or more or 3 in one parameter	Increased frequency to a minimum of 1 hourly	• Registered nurse to urgently inform the medical team caring for the patient; • Urgent assessment by a clinician with core competencies to assess acutely ill patients; • Clinical care in an environment with monitoring facilities;
Total: 7 or more	Continuous monitoring of vital signs	• Registered nurse to immediately inform the medical team caring for the patient—this should be at least at specialist registrar level; • Emergency assessment by a clinical team with critical care competencies, which also includes a practitioner/s with advanced airway skills; • Consider transfer of clinical care to a level 2 or 3 care facility, i.e. higher dependency or ITU;

Royal College of Physicians · NHS *Training for Innovation*

FIGURE 6-2C The National Early Warning Score outline for recommended frequency of monitoring and clinical response. (*Reproduced with permission from Royal College of Physicians. National Early Warning Score (NEWS): Standardising the assessment of acuteillness severity in the NHS. Report of a working party. London: RCP, 2012.*)

failed to demonstrate that implementation of RRTs led to a decrease in cardiac arrests, ICU admissions, or unexpected deaths;[21] post hoc analysis showed a significant improvement in outcomes when the data were analyzed in an as-treated model rather than an intention-to-treat model.[22] Further single-center trials also point to improved outcomes in hospitals that implemented RRTs.[20] A meta-analysis of 18 studies reviewing the effectiveness of RRT systems in acute care settings demonstrated that the implementation of RRTs is associated with reduced rates of cardiorespiratory arrests outside of the ICU with relative risk reduction of 33%.[23] In addition, a retrospective study of nearly 6 million admissions over a 10-year period showed the presence of a hospital RRT system for more than 2 years was associated with 0.14% absolute risk reduction of in-hospital mortality across a major metropolitan health network, which translated to 56 lives saved per year in a hospital with 40,000 admissions per year.[24] Mortality benefits after the introduction of RRTs are not always immediate and may take time to become apparent.

In general, triage decisions based on rapid response evaluation regarding transfer of patients to the ICU or general ward care seem to be appropriate. In a large study, 12.7% of patients that had RRT activation required repeat RRT activation and of those around 80% were transferred to the ICU. A total of 0.4% died within 24 hours of the index RRT activation, with half of the mortalities occurring as unexpected cardiac arrests on the wards, while the other half occurred in the setting of ICU care, or palliative care, after the repeat RRT call.[25]

Inappropriate triage and disposition of unrecognized critical illness at the time of initial admission are contributing factors to unfavorable patient outcomes. Indeed, RRTs occurring early in hospitalizations (hospital days 0 and 1) constitute approximately 27% of all calls and partially reflect suboptimal triage decisions.[10]

Team Composition

The composition of the RRT can vary significantly based on the hospital system and available resources.[26] Teams are often comprised of multidisciplinary staff that may include critical care medicine fellows or attendings, internal medicine housestaff or hospitalists, respiratory therapists, physician assistants, nurse practitioners or an ICU nurse. Studies evaluating ideal team composition are sparse.[27] It is difficult to assess the optimal team composition and subsequent outcomes due to the amount of variation that exists. While it has been shown that response teams led by attending intensivists and senior medical residents had similar outcomes, teams led by nurses alone had equivocal outcomes.[19]

PRE-ICU SYNDROMES: ASSESSMENT AND TREATMENT

The Society of Critical Care Medicine has identified the five primary ICU admission diagnoses as: respiratory system diagnosis with ventilator support, acute myocardial infarction, intracranial hemorrhage or cerebral infarction, percutaneous cardiovascular procedure with drug-eluting stent, and septicemia or severe sepsis. Additional diagnoses that often require ICU admission include: toxins, heart failure, arrhythmias, renal failure, and gastrointestinal hemorrhage.[28]

The correlating rapid response triggers for these conditions are often identified as hypotension, altered mental status, and respiratory distress.

Hypotension and Shock

Hypotension is not defined by a fixed number, but often precedes or is the manifestation of shock. Classically shock has been divided into four categories: hypovolemic, obstructive, cardiogenic, and distributive.[29] Hypovolemic shock is explained by hemorrhage or fluid losses. Obstructive shock indicates a structural impediment to the circulatory apparatus as seen with pericardial tamponade, tension pneumothorax, or pulmonary embolism. Cardiogenic shock occurs secondary to valvular dysfunction, arrhythmia, or ventricular compromise. Distributive shock is often a marker of an inflammatory process disrupting the integrity of small vessels that can be seen in sepsis or anaphylaxis. The classification may be overly simplistic as septic patients in distributive shock may also present with relative hypovolemia and cardiomyopathy contributing to their shock state. Still, the classification provides a useful framework through which to approach a difficult problem.

Shock is the clinical diagnosis that represents the imbalance between oxygen delivery and demand. Physiologically it is based on the principle of oxygen delivery to end organs, accomplished by adequate circulating blood volume and red blood cells, vascular tone, and cardiac function. These physiologic principles are the backbone for the early goal-directed therapy in the treatment of severe sepsis and septic shock.[30] Clinical signs of end-organ damage such as decreased urine output and encephalopathy as well as biomarkers (increased lactate, creatinine, troponins, and liver enzymes) are indicative of hypoperfusion and shock.

Altered Mental Status and Neurologic Deterioration

Altered mental status is a broad term encompassing a spectrum of alterations of an individual's normal mental facilities. The differential diagnosis of altered mental status can be more succinctly divided into four categories: primary intracranial processes, systemic or metabolic diseases secondarily affecting the central nervous system, exogenous toxins, and drug withdrawal.[31] Differential diagnosis may be difficult upon initial evaluation. Focal neurologic symptoms often indicate an intracranial process such as a stroke or seizure. Encephalopathy and delirium are more often associated with systemic illness, toxins, and withdrawal. Furthermore, toxidromes have been described with specific drug exposures and poisonings.

Deterioration in mental status can be measured serially with the Glasgow Coma Scale (GCS). A GCS of 8 or less is associated with the inability to protect one's airway and the risk of aspiration, prompting emergent transfer to a monitored setting, or intubation.[32]

Respiratory Distress and Failure

Acute respiratory failure and the need for mechanical ventilation are among the most common causes of ICU admission. The cause for respiratory failure can be of a primary pulmonary pathology or secondary to cardiac, infectious, metabolic, neurologic, and overall systemic illness. An increased work of breathing, low oxygen saturation, or depressed respiratory status should all prompt an ICU evaluation as such patients rapidly deteriorate into cardiopulmonary collapse. Pulse oximetry and blood gases are readily available and can be repeated serially to determine the degree of oxygenation and ventilation deficit. When appropriate, the need for mechanical ventilation should not be delayed. In select cases, such as exacerbation of heart failure or obstructive pulmonary disease, a trial of noninvasive positive pressure ventilation (NIPPV) while implementing targeted therapies has been shown to be effective and may alleviate the need for mechanical ventilation.[33]

APPROACH TO THE PRE-ICU PATIENT

Implementation of RRT is meant for the early identification of pre-ICU syndromes and prevention of cardiac arrests. While the causes for shock, neurologic deterioration, or respiratory failure may not be initially evident, the "Hs and Ts" (Table 6–1), described in Advanced Cardiac Life Support guidelines, provide a framework for diagnostics and treatment.[35] They are major contributing factors to developing cardiac arrest that can be identified and

TABLE 6–1 The "Hs and Ts" of advanced cardiac life support guideline.

Hs	Ts
Hypoxia	Toxins—drug overdose
Hypovolemia	Tamponade
Hypoglycemia and other metabolic disorders	Tension pneumothorax
Hypothermia	Thrombosis—coronary
Hydrogen ion—acidosis	Thrombosis—pulmonary
Hypokalemia and hyperkalemia	Trauma

potentially treated at the bedside, before transfer to the ICU. The rapid identification of these factors helps guide therapy in the crucial moments leading up to a cardiac arrest. These findings are present, or are the presenting symptoms, in many patients requiring ICU-level care.

First steps when evaluating the critically ill patient include cardiac monitoring, vital signs, pulse oximetry, and establishing intravenous access. The advanced cardiac life support and advanced trauma life support algorithms have popularized an "ABCD" approach to critically ill patients: irway, breathing, circulation, and neurological disability and differential diagnosis (Table 6–2).[34] A rapid primary survey evaluating for and intervening upon life-threatening conditions is a fundamental underpinning of effective resuscitation and is a useful model to follow in critical care. Clinically experienced physicians will proceed in an order dictated by their experience—often delegating tasks to team members. For the less experienced physician the framework is a reminder of the critical elements that must be assessed and intervened upon with immediacy.

Equipment and Medications

Equipment and medications are limited on general wards. When responding to a rapid response, the appropriate equipment should be brought to the bedside. The following are examples of equipment and medications that supplement standard intubation supplies and cardiac arrest medications required for the ACLS algorithm.

TABLE 6-2 An example of the ABCD approach to the pre-ICU Patient.

	Clinical Examination	Analysis	Imaging	Initial Rapid Response Interventions
Airway/ Breathing	Respiratory rate Accessory muscle use Airway patency Auscultation	Pulse oximetry Arterial blood gas Electrocardiogram	Thoracic and pleural ultrasound Vascular ultrasound Chest radiography	Jaw thrust Removal of foreign bodies Supplemental oxygen Bag valve mask ventilation Noninvasive positive pressure ventilation Intubation and mechanical ventilation Thrombolytics (myocardial infarction, pulmonary embolism) Relief of pneumothorax or plural effusion
Circulation	Blood pressure Pulse rate and quality Capillary refill Urine output Extremity temperature Pulses: faint or bounding Auscultation	Arterial blood gas Lactate Creatinine Troponin Liver function tests Central and mixed venous oxygenation Electrocardiogram	Echocardiography Abdominal ultrasound Thoracic and pleural ultrasound Vascular ultrasound	Vascular access (peripheral, central, intraosseous) Volume administration Vasopressors Inotropes Thrombolytics (myocardial infarction, pulmonary embolism) Relief of pneumothorax or pericardial effusion
Neurologic Disability	Neurologic Examination Glasgow Coma Scale Respiratory rate and patterns Toxidromes	Glucose Ammonia level Arterial blood gas	Brain computed tomography Brain magnetic resonance imaging Electroencephalogram	Antiepileptics and benzodiazepines (seizures) Naloxone (opiate overdose) Glucose (hypoglycemia) Supplemental oxygen (hypoxemia) Mechanical ventilation (hypercarbia) Thrombolytics (ischemic stroke)

- Airway/equipment bag: The contents of the bag should include equipment for intubation of the difficult airway. This includes laryngeal mask airways, a bougie or endotracheal tube introducer, video laryngoscopes, peep valves, and a cricothyroidotomy kit. The addition of an intraosseous infusion kit allows for rapid circulatory access when appropriate intravenous access is lacking.
- Medication bag: The contents of the bag should include medications for appropriate induction of anesthesia prior to intubation and blood pressure support. This includes propofol, etomidate, short-acting paralytics and vasoactive medications such as phenylephrine or norepinephrine.

- Portable ultrasound: Goal-directed ultrasonography during a rapid response assists in formulating a diagnosis, focusing therapy, and guiding procedures without having to transport critically ill patients to imaging suites.

The medications and equipment listed above are used as an example. Local hospital practice, protocols, equipment availability, and expertise should dictate the contents of RRT equipment.

Postoperative, Postprocedure, and Specialized Care

Often admissions to the ICU are not related to the above-described, unexpected, syndromes. Rather, they are admissions that require postoperative, postprocedural, or specialized care. These are planned or protocoled admissions that are based on local hospital policy and procedure and the need for additional monitoring. Specialized units include, but are not limited to, surgical, cardiothoracic, neurologic, neurosurgical, burn, trauma, respiratory, and cardiac units. Unplanned, or unexpected, postoperative or postprocedural admissions are often related to the previously described syndromes.

SUMMARY

The majority of ICU admissions can be characterized by the presence of respiratory failure, a shock state, neurologic deterioration, or a combination of the three. While often times the need for ICU care is evident on initial presentation to the hospital, it is not always possible to predict the need. Pre-ICU syndromes develop rapidly, unexpectedly, and have the potential for detrimental outcomes. It is imperative to have functional rapid response systems, in terms of both triggering and response, to expedite care to such patients in a ward setting.

REFERENCES

1. The Joint Commission. National Patient Safety Goals. Available at: http://www.jointcommission.org/patientsafety/nationalpatientsafetygoals. Accessed August 1, 2016.
2. Devita M, Bellomo R, Hillman K, et al. Findings of the first consensus conference on medical emergency teams. *Crit Care Med.* 2006;34(9):2463-2478.
3. Jones DA, DeVita MA, Bellomo R. Rapid-response teams. *N Engl J Med.* 2011;365(2):139-146.
4. Winters BD, Pham J, Pronovost PJ. Rapid response teams—walk, don't run. *JAMA.* 2006;296(13):1645-1647.
5. Litvak E, Pronovost PJ. Rethinking rapid response teams. *JAMA.* 2010;304(12):1375-1376.
6. Jaderling G, Bell M, Martling CR, et al. ICU admittance by a rapid response team versus conventional admittance, characteristics, and outcome. *Crit Care Med.* 2013;41(3):725-731.
7. Buist M, Jarmolowski E, Burton P, Bernard SA, Waxman BP, Anderson J. Recognising clinical instability in hospital patients before cardiac arrest or unplanned admission to intensive care. A pilot study in a tertiary-care hospital. *Med J Aust.* 1999;171(1):22-25.
8. DeVita M. Medical emergency teams: deciphering clues to crises in hospitals. *Crit Care.* 2005;9(4):325-326.
9. Franklin C, Mathew J. Developing strategies to prevent in hospital cardiac arrest: analyzing responses of physicians and nurses in the hours before the event. *Crit Care Med.* 1994;22(2):244-247.
10. Investigators METE-o-LC. The timing of rapid-response team activations: a multicentre international study. *Crit Care Resusc.* 2013;15(1):15-20.
11. Downey AW, Quach JL, Haase M, et al. Characteristics and outcomes of patients receiving a medical emergency team review for acute change in conscious state or arrhythmias*. *Crit Care Med.* 2008;36(2):477-481.
12. Wilson R, Harrison B, Gibberd R, Hamilton JD. An analysis of the causes of adverse events from the Quality in Australian Health Care Study. *Med J Aust.* 1999;170(9):411-415.
13. Harrison GA, Jacques TC, Kilborn G, et al. The prevalence of recordings of the signs of critical conditions and emergency responses in hospital wards—the SOCCER study. *Resuscitation.* 2005;65(2):149-157.
14. DeVita MA, Smith GB, Adam SK, et al. "Identifying the hospitalised patient in crisis"—a consensus conference on the afferent limb of rapid response systems. *Resuscitation.* 2010;81(4):375-382.
15. Psirides A, Hill J, Hurford S. A review of rapid response team activation parameters in New Zealand hospitals. *Resuscitation.* 2013;84(8):1040-1044.
16. Jones D, Duke G, Green J, et al. Medical emergency team syndromes and an approach to their management. *Crit Care.* 2006;10(1):R30.
17. Churpek MM, Yuen TC, Edelson DP. Risk stratification of hospitalized patients on the wards. *Chest.* 2013;143(6):1758-1765.
18. Churpek MM, Yuen TC, Park SY, Gibbons R, Edelson DP. Using electronic health record data to develop and validate a prediction model for adverse outcomes in the wards. *Crit Care Med.* 2014;42:841-848.
19. McNeill G, Bryden D. Do either early warning systems or emergency response teams improve hospital patient survival? A systematic review. *Resuscitation.* 2013;84(12):1652-1667.
20. Jones D, Opdam H, Egi M, et al. Long-term effect of a Medical Emergency Team on mortality in a teaching hospital. *Resuscitation.* 2007;74(2):235-241.
21. Hillman K, Chen J, Cretikos M, et al. Introduction of the medical emergency team (MET) system:

a cluster-randomised controlled trial. *Lancet.* 2005;365(9477):2091-2097.

22. Chen J, Bellomo R, Flabouris A, et al. The relationship between early emergency team calls and serious adverse events*. *Crit Care Med.* 2009;37(1):148-153.

23. Winters BD, Weaver SJ, Pfoh ER, et al. Rapid-response systems as a patient safety strategy: a systematic review. *Ann Intern Med.* 2013;158(5 pt 2):417-425.

24. Tobin A, Santamaria J. Medical emergency teams are associated with reduced mortality across a major metropolitan health network after two years service: a retrospective study using government administrative data. *Crit Care.* 2012;16(5):R210.

25. Schneider AG, Warrillow S, Robbins R, et al. An assessment of the triage performance of the efferent arm of the rapid response system. *Resuscitation.* 2013;84(4):477-482.

26. Jones D, Drennan K, Hart GK, et al. Rapid response team composition, resourcing and calling criteria in Australia. *Resuscitation.* 2012;83(5):563-567.

27. Morris DS, Schweickert W, Holena D, et al. Differences in outcomes between ICU attending and senior resident physician led medical emergency team responses. *Resuscitation.* 2012;83(12):1434-1437.

28. Society of Critical Care Medicine. Critical Care Statistics. Available at: http://www.sccm.org/ Communications/Pages/CriticalCareStats.aspx, Accessed August 1, 2016.

29. Herget-Rosenthal S, Saner F, Chawla LS. Approach to hemodynamic shock and vasopressors. *Clin J Am Soc Nephrol.* 2008;3(2):546-553.

30. Rivers E, Nguyen B, Havstad S, et al. Early goal-directed therapy in the treatment of severe sepsis and septic shock. *N Engl J Med.* 2001;345(19):1368-1377.

31. Lipowski ZJ. Delirium in the elderly patient. *N Engl J Med.* 1989;320(9):578-582.

32. Duncan R, Thakore S. Decreased Glasgow Coma Scale score does not mandate endotracheal intubation in the emergency department. *J Emerg Med.* 2009;37(4):451-455.

33. Garpestad E, Brennan J, Hill NS. Noninvasive ventilation for critical care. *Chest.* 2007;132(2):711-720.

34. Neumar RW, Otto CW, Link MS, et al. Part 8: adult advanced cardiovascular life support: 2010 American Heart Association guidelines for cardiopulmonary resuscitation and emergency cardiovascular care. *Circulation.* 2010;122(18 suppl 3):S729-S767.

35. Part 7: Adult Advanced Cardiovascular Life Support: 2015 American Heart Association Guidelines Update for Cardiopulmonary Resuscitation and Emergency Cardiovascular Care. Link MS, Berkow LC, Kudenchuk PJ, Halperin HR, Hess EP, Moitra VK, Neumar RW, O'Neil BJ, Paxton JH, Silvers SM, White RD, Yannopoulos D, Donnino MW. Circulation. 2015 Nov 3;132(18 Suppl 2):S444-64

Biomarkers in Decision Making

Anthony Manasia, MD and Jon Narimasu, MD

1 An ideal biomarker has a high sensitivity and allows for clinical applications in the diagnosis, staging, prognosis, and treatment of disease.

2 Early identification of ischemia after the rupture or erosion of an atherosclerotic coronary plaque and before myonecrosis occurs is currently under investigation. Biomarkers of myocardial ischemia include choline, a chemical released during membrane damage; unbound free fatty acids, a chemical released by ischemic myocytes and ischemia-modified albumin.

3 The cardiac biomarkers B-type natriuretic peptide (BNP) and N-terminal proBNP (NT-proBNP) are elevated in 80% of patients who present to the emergency department (ED) with chronic heart failure (CHF).

4 Neutrophil gelatinase-associated lipocalin (NGAL) is a novel serum biomarker that can identify acute kidney injury (AKI) early after the initial renal insult and can be reliably measured in the plasma by point-of-care immunoassay. NGAL levels were elevated up to 48 hours prior to the diagnosis of AKI based on the *r*isk or renal dysfunction, *i*njury to the kidney, *f*ailure of kidney function, *l*oss of kidney function, and *e*nd-stage kidney disease (RIFLE) criteria in a recent study.

5 The use of procalcitonin (PCT) in the diagnosis and discrimination of bacterial infection, sepsis, and response to antibiotic therapy from noninfectious causes of systemic inflammatory response syndrome (SIRS) (ie, pancreatitis) is currently in use by some institutions.

INTRODUCTION

A biological marker (biomarker) is a characteristic that is objectively measured and evaluated as an indicator of normal biological processes, pathogenic processes, or pharmacologic responses to a therapeutic intervention.[1] An ideal biomarker enables sensitivity and allows for clinical applications in the diagnosis, staging, prognosis, and treatment of disease. The utility of biomarkers in clinical decision making can be organized into a multitude of categories (Figure 7–1). Diagnostic biomarkers may afford rapid screening and stratification of patients into specific groups that may respond to a particular intervention or treatment. Prognostic biomarkers may predict the course or trajectory of disease allowing for early determination of disposition (ie, floor vs ICU) and goals of care. Surrogate biomarkers are those, which are substituted for a clinical end point (ie, response to therapy).

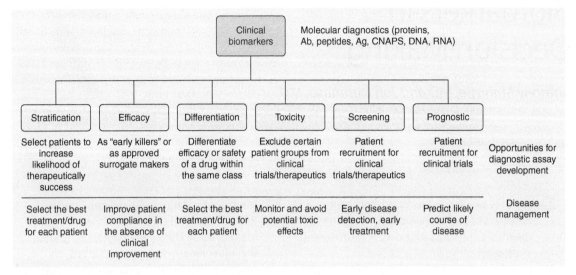

FIGURE 7-1 Clinical biomarkers: categories/types.
Currently, only a handful of serum biomarkers are used in clinical practice. This chapter will highlight these biomarkers, and provide a systematic review by organ. (*Reproduced with permission from Drucker E, Krapfenbauer K: Pitfalls and limitations in translation from biomarker discovery to clinical utility in predictive and personalised medicine, EPMA J. 2013 Feb 25;4(1):7.*)

CARDIAC MARKERS

Myocardial Injury

Since 1900 (with exception of 1918), cardiovascular disease has been the leading cause of mortality in the United States.[2] In 2009, statistics indicated that cardiovascular disease accounted for approximately 800,000 or 32% of deaths annually. Coronary heart disease also remains the number one cause of morbidity in the United States, accounting for an estimated 7.6 million myocardial infarctions (MIs), 7.8 million cases of angina pectoris, and 5.1 million occurrences of heart failure. Due to the tremendous health and economic burdens of cardiovascular disease, the search for diagnostic, prognostic, and therapeutic cardiac biomarkers continues.

Early identification of ischemia after the rupture or erosion of an atherosclerotic coronary plaque and before myonecrosis occurs is an appealing concept.[3] Biomarkers of myocardial ischemia include choline, a chemical released during membrane damage; unbound free fatty acids, a chemical released by ischemic myocytes; and ischemia-modified albumin, a form of albumin that is unable to bind cobalt during myocardial ischemia. While the identification of these novel biomarkers initially showed promise, they have not been validated in clinical studies.

The World Health Organization, American College of Cardiology and European Society of Cardiology consider cardiac troponins (cTn), biomarkers of myocardial injury, as the "gold standard" for the diagnosis of MI. cTn are cardiospecific and released as an intact molecule from injured myocytes. Further specification of cTn T or I (cTnT or cTnI, respectively) is analogous to the discovery and utility of creatinine kinase myocardial band (CK-MB) after CK was identified.

In clinical use, cTn levels stratify risk in patients presenting with angina and in the determination of acute coronary syndrome (ACS). In patients with electrocardiogram (ECG) changes consistent with ST-segment elevation myocardial infarction (STEMI), the presence of cTn is primarily used to confirm the diagnosis. However, biomarker confirmation with cTn should not delay early intervention to reestablish coronary blood flow via primary percutaneous coronary intervention or thrombolysis. In addition, there is also some evidence that the level of cTn may quantify the degree and extent of myocyte injury and perhaps predict impairment of the ejection fraction.

In patients who present with angina, but without classic ST-segment elevation, cTn levels indicate those at low risk for ACS and those with non-ST-segment elevation myocardial infarction (NSTEMI). Patients with normal cTn levels have low risk for ACS, and can undergo observation and potentially outpatient evaluation with cardiac stress testing or a myocardial perfusion scan. In contrast, patients with NSTEMI should be admitted to the hospital and should receive antiplatelet and antithrombotic therapy with or without percutaneous coronary intervention.

Although cTn remains the gold standard to determine myocardial infarction, both ischemic and nonischemic conditions can cause elevated levels. It is important to recognize these secondary causes (Table 7–1). Prognostic application of cTn in medical intensive care unit (ICU) patients has also been studied retrospectively to identify short-term and long-term survival. Elevated cTn levels were independently associated with mortality at 1-month, 1 year, 2 years, and 3 years.[4]

Heart Failure

Heart failure affects 5.1 million Americans each year, but identifying cardiac dysfunction remains a challenge in the acute care setting. Acute dyspnea caused by cardiac dysfunction (ie, heart failure) needs to be discriminated from pulmonary disease (ie, pneumonia, chronic obstructive pulmonary disease [COPD] exacerbation, acute respiratory distress syndrome [ARDS]) because management and therapeutic strategies differ. The cardiac biomarkers BNP and NT-proBNP were found to be elevated in up to 80% of patients who present to the ED with CHF.[5]

BNP is a hormone secreted by ventricular myocytes in response to increased ventricular volume and pressure, which results in wall stretch. BNP is actually a cleaved byproduct of proBNP, which is a prohormone that is upregulated within the cardiac myocyte after stimulus. As proBNP traverses the cardiac myocyte membrane into the plasma, it is cleaved into two products: BNP (active; $T_{1/2}$ 20 minutes) and NT-proBNP (inactive; $T_{1/2}$ 1.5-2 hours). The physiologic actions of BNP results in diuresis, natriuresis, vasodilation (causing decreased systemic vascular resistance and preload), anti-inflammatory, antiplatelet, and antihypertrophic effects.[6]

Diagnostic cutoff values for patients without renal failure provide the best sensitivity and specificity for BNP and NT-proBNP, and should be stratified

into ranges instead of a single value. Levels of BNP less than 100 ng/L make the diagnosis of heart failure unlikely, and a level greater than 500 ng/L favors the diagnosis.[5] For NT-proBNP, the proposed diagnostic cutoff levels are affected by age. NT-proBNP less than 300 ng/L make the diagnosis of heart failure unlikely, and levels greater than 450 ng/L (age < 50), greater than 900 ng/L (50-75 years), and greater than 1800 ng/L (> 75 years) favor a heart failure diagnosis. Although NT-proBNP is the inactive portion of the proBNP hormone, it has a longer half-life relative to BNP, which could offer better diagnostic sensitivity. Measurements that fall in between the proposed cutoff values for BNP and NT-proBNP require additional information obtained from echocardiography for diagnosis of heart failure.

Patients with renal failure and obesity warrant special consideration because their cutoff levels for BNP and NT-proBNP are different. Further, morbidly obese patients (body mass index [BMI] > 35 kg/m²) will have a cutoff level of BNP less than 55 ng/L to rule out heart failure. For patients with stage 3 chronic kidney disease (glomerular filtration rate [GFR] 30-59 mL/min/1.073 m²), the cutoff levels that likely rule out heart failure are BNP less than 200 to 225 ng/L, and NT-proBNP less than 1200 ng/L.

In ICU patients, the role of cardiac biomarkers is limited by multisystem organ pathology. In critically ill patients, without renal disease who develop acute dyspnea, a cutoff level for BNP less than 250 ng/L may favor the diagnosis of ARDS over cardiogenic pulmonary edema.

RENAL
Acute Kidney Injury

AKI is one of the most common diagnoses encountered in acute care in the United States. It affects more than 20% of hospitalized patients,[7] and more than 30% of critically ill patients.[8] The development of AKI is independently associated with increased mortality. In noncritically ill hospitalized patients, the presence of AKI was associated with an overall mortality rate of 10% compared to 1.5% in patients without AKI. The mortality rate increases with the severity of AKI. In critically ill patients, mortality rates are based on the severity of AKI: stage I AKI

TABLE 7–1 Secondary ischemic and non-ischemic causes of cardiac injury.

Primary ischemic cardiac injury (PICI)		
Thrombotic coronary artery occlusion due to platelets/fibrin	ST elevation MI	
	Non-ST elevation ML (non Q wave MI plus cTn plus cTn-positive unstable angina)	
Secondary ischemic cardiac injury (SICI)		
Coronary intervention	Primary PTCA	Distal embolization from atheroma or debris Side branch occlusion
	Elective PTCA	Distal embolization or debris Side branch occlusion
	CABG	Global ischemia form inadequate perfusion, myocardial cell production of anoxia
Sympathomimetics	Cocaine abuse	
	Catecholamine storm	Head injury, stroke, intracerebral bleeding
Pulmonary embolus	Presumed right heart strain or hypoxia	
Coronary artery spasm	In Japan—up to 10% of admissions for chest pain	
Coronary artery embolization	Clot Air CABG	
Coronary artery inflammation with microvasular occlussion	Vasculitidies	
	Connective tissue damage (eg, Pompe's disease) Systemic lupus erythematosus (SLE)	
End-stage renal failure	More severe coronary artery disease, but 50% ESRD patients have normal coronaries	
Rhythm disorders	Prolonged tachycardia or bradycardia with IHD	
Acute heart failure	Only if due to IHD	
Direct coronary trauma		
Extreme endurance exercise	Extreme marathons	Wall motion abnormalities
	Extreme training	cTn positive deaths presumed due to extreme oxygen debt producing ischemia
Non-ischemic cardiac injury (NICI)		
Known causes of myocarditis	Infection	Bacterial or viral Rheumatic myocarditis Septic shock Acute pericarditis
	Inflammation	
	Autoimmune	Polymyositis Scleroderma Sarcoidosis
	Drug-induced	Alcohol Cocaine abuse Chemotherapy
	Toxins	Snake, puffer fish envenomation
Cardiac Trauma	Direct	Motor Vehicle Accident (MVA) Stabbing
	Cardiac surgery	
Metabolic/toxic	Renal failure Multiple organ failure (MOF)	

Reproduced with permission from Collinson PO, Gaze DC. Biomarkers of cardiovascular damage and dysfunction- an overview, *Heart Lung Circ.* 2007;16 Suppl 3:S71-S82.

is associated with a mortality rate of 13.9%; stage II AKI of 16.4%; and stage III AKI of 33.8%.[9]

The current diagnostic criteria used to define AKI are based primarily on increases in serum creatinine (SCr) levels relative to baseline, with high associated morbidity and mortality. The search for novel serum biomarkers identifying AKI earlier after the initial renal insult, has led to the recognition of neutrophil gelatinase-associated lipocalin (NGAL). NGAL is a protein that is transcribed early in the process of renal injury, and can be reliably measured in the plasma by point-of-care immunoassay.[10] In a prospective, observational study of 301 patients, investigators evaluated the utility of NGAL as an early serum biomarker of AKI compared to the commonly used RIFLE criteria.[10] The RIFLE criterion, which utilizes SCr and GFR, was defined by the Acute Dialysis Quality Initiative (ADQI) group in 2004.[11] Results demonstrated that NGAL levels were elevated up to 48 hours prior to the diagnosis of AKI based on the RIFLE criteria (Figure 7–2). Plasma NGAL levels greater than 150 ng/mL were associated with an increased incidence of AKI of 11.8 (95% confidence interval [CI], 3.5-39.2). In addition, NGAL levels greater than 150 ng/mL were also a good predictor of renal replacement therapy. Further evaluation is required to determine if plasma NGAL will ultimately translate into the renal "troponin" in clinical practice.

While NGAL has been demonstrated as a renal biomarker, there are others under investigation including kidney injury molecule 1 (KIM-1), cystatin-C, interleukin (IL)-6, IL-18, urinary N-acetyl-beta-(D) glucosaminidase activity (NAG), and matrix metalloproteinase 9 (MMP-9).[10]

Infectious Disease
Sepsis and Shock

In the United States, sepsis-related health care costs remain the number one economic burden accounting for more than $20 billion as of 2011.[12] Even more alarming are the number of reported cases (> 1,000,000), and the incidence of hospital admissions due to sepsis continues to rise each year from 266,895 in 2005 to 353,516 in 2011.[13] However, mortality rates related to sepsis remain high (25%-50%), and account for greater than 200,000 deaths each year.[14]

Studies have evaluated numerous biomarkers involved in the sepsis cascade as potential targets for therapy. Unfortunately, immunotherapy trials (ie, recombinant activated protein C, eritoran tetrasodium—E5564, a toll-like receptor 4 antagonist, and talactoferrin alpha) have failed to demonstrate mortality benefit.[15] Focus may need to be

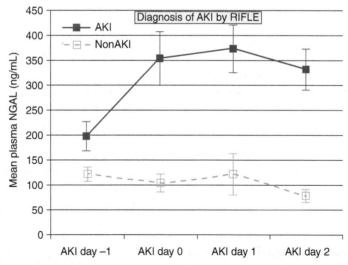

FIGURE 7–2 Mean plasma NGAL concentrations at various timepoints in patients with acute kidney injury. (*Reproduced with permission from Cruz DN, de Cal M, Garzotto F, et al. Plasma neutrophil gelatinase-associated lipocalin is an early biomarker for acute kidney injury in an adult ICU population,* ntensive Care Med. *2010 Mar;36(3):444-451.*)

on when to target each biomarker with immunotherapy, instead of just inhibiting or augmenting an ongoing process in the sepsis cascade. In a study of patients with severe sepsis and septic shock, levels of serum biomarkers (ie, IL-1 beta, 1ra, 6, 8, and 10; intercellular adhesion molecule, tumor necrosis factor alpha, caspase 3, D-dimer, high-mobility group protein 1, vascular endothelial growth factor, matrix metalloproteinase, and myeloperoxidase) known to be involved in the pathogenesis of sepsis were measured at various times (0, 3, 6, 12, 24, 48, 60, and 72 hours).[15] The results demonstrated various times to peak levels of each biomarker ranging from 3 to 48 hours, and different patterns (ie, bimodal) of peak and nadir levels. These results indicate a 3-hour window for appropriate intervention from peak levels of some of the above biomarkers and development of sepsis. In contrast, for other biomarkers, successful immunotherapy may require multiple time-sensitive interventions based on changing levels. Further understanding of biomarkers and sepsis will lead to a new paradigm of early and "time-sensitive" goal-directed therapies.

During shock, anaerobic glycolysis produces lactate, which is converted to glucose via the Cori cycle in the liver as a source of energy. Approximately 1300 to 1500 mmol of lactate is produced each day under normal physiologic conditions by various organs including the brain, skeletal muscle, intestine, skin, and red blood cells.[16] Normal serum lactate levels are less than 2 mmol/L.

Hyperlactatemia (> 2 mmol/L) is caused by excess production (ie, anaerobic glycolysis), reduced clearance, or a combination of both states. Hyperlactatemia occurs in patients with tissue dysoxia, or in other conditions where hypoxia is not the primary etiology such as SIRS and sepsis. Lactate clearance (ie, decrease of 10% from baseline levels within 2 hours and up to 12 hours), or normalization of lactate levels within 24 hours is associated with decreased mortality, organ failure, and ICU days.[16-18]

Lactate Clearance

A randomized, multicenter trial evaluated the mortality outcomes of a protocol-driven treatment plan, comparing the use of the $ScvO_2$ greater than 70% versus lactate clearance of 10% within 2 hours of initiating resuscitation.[19] Patients with severe sepsis or septic shock were treated with a protocol consistent with the SSC guidelines. The two treatment groups utilized resuscitation to sequentially achieve a central venous pressure (CVP) greater than or equal to 8 mm Hg, then a mean arterial pressure greater than or equal to 65 mm Hg, followed by either an $ScvO_2$ greater than 70% or lactate clearance greater than 10% (within 2 hours of initiating the protocol). The mortality rate in the $ScvO_2$ group was 23%, versus 17% in the lactate clearance group, demonstrating a mortality benefit of 6% when using lactate clearance as a primary goal of initial resuscitation.

Other studies have also supported the concept of lactate normalization, as it is known that hyperlactatemia is independently associated with increased morbidity and mortality regardless of the etiology.[16,20]

Procalcitonin: Diagnosis of Bacterial Infections/Sepsis & Guidance of Antibiotic Therapy

Discrimination of sepsis (defined as probable or documented infection) from noninfectious causes of SIRS remains a challenge. The difficulty in diagnosing bacterial infection is a reflection of the nonspecific symptoms and signs of SIRS. Studies have revealed promise with the use of procalcitonin in the diagnosis of bacterial infection, sepsis, and response to antibiotic therapy.[21] However, there is no single biomarker of sepsis that has 100% sensitivity or specificity.

PCT is a prohormone of calcitonin, which is synthesized in the parafollicular C cells of the thyroid gland.[22] In response to inflammatory and noninflammatory mediators released by bacterial infection, procalcitonin is upregulated and produced by C cells of the thyroid and other organs (ie, liver, lung, small intestine, kidney) throughout the body. Upregulation and plasma levels increase within 6 to 12 hours of bacterial infection. PCT is specific for bacterial infection since interferon gamma is released in response to viral infection and inhibits the upregulation of PCT. Once appropriate antibiotic therapy has been administered, the levels of endotoxin and cytokines fall resulting in the decline of serum PCT levels by 50% each day. PCT has a plasma half-life of 25 to 30 hours. Plasma PCT levels correlate with the severity of infection, prognosis, allow for monitoring response to antibiotic therapy, and guide duration of treatment. The implementation of algorithms using PCT in clinical practice have been studied and validated. Different patient populations and care settings have led to the development of practical algorithms (see Figure 7–1) with specific cutoff values of PCT.[21,23] In low-acuity (ie, outpatient) and moderate acuity (ie, emergency department and inpatient) settings, antibiotic therapy is encouraged if the PCT level is greater than or equal to 0.25 µg/L, and strongly encouraged if the level is greater than or equal to 0.5 µg/L. In high-acuity settings (ie, ICU) or with septic patients, PCT levels should not be used to determine when to initiate antibiotic therapy but rather to guide early discontinuation of treatment.

PULMONARY

Chronic Obstructive Pulmonary Disease and Asthma

Severe exacerbations of COPD and asthma account for a significant number of hospitalizations, but the decision for ICU admission is based on clinical presentation and empiric therapy. Biomarkers evaluated include interleukins, interferons, and leukotrienes; tumor necrosis factor alpha; myeloperoxidase; eosinophil cationic protein; eosinophil peroxidase; and exhaled nitric oxide.[24] Unfortunately, biomarkers in COPD and asthma lack sensitivity, specificity, and have not translated into clinical medicine.

Pulmonary Embolism

The development and widespread application of computed tomography pulmonary angiography (CTPA) to diagnosis pulmonary embolism (PE) has led to a significant rise in the incidence of reported cases from 62 to 112 per 100,000.[25] The downside of the high-sensitivity of CTPA has led to increased diagnosis of chronic and clinically insignificant cases of PE. Mortality rates have remained steady around 12%, but complications related to the treatment of PE with thrombolysis and anticoagulation increased from 3 to 5 cases per 100,000. The challenge in the management of PE is to stratify patients into risk categories to determine which patients will benefit the most from treatment. The highest mortality (25%-50%) is associated with patients who develop hemodynamic instability and right ventricular dysfunction.[26] Biomarkers have been evaluated alone,

and compared to conventional scoring systems (ie, pulmonary embolism severity index [PESI]) and imaging (CTPA and echocardiography) to identify high-risk patients. proBNP greater than 600 pg/mL and BNP greater than 75 pg/mL are associated with right ventricular dysfunction and increased mortality (> 6-fold). In addition, acute right ventricular pressure overload may lead to myocardial injury and elevated cTn levels. cTnI greater than 0.1 ng/mL and cTnT greater than 0.01 ng/mL have been associated with increased mortality (> 5-fold).

D-Dimers

Fibrin degradation products (FDPs) are released when fibrin is cleaved by plasmin. D-Dimer is one of the major FDPs. D-Dimer is generated from cross-linked fibrin and an increase in D-dimer is an indication of intravascular coagulation. D-Dimer levels are helpful but not sufficient on their own to diagnose PE. However, patients with a low clinical suspicion of PE and normal D-dimer level, less than 500 ng/mL, PE can be excluded and no further testing is warranted.[27] In patients with a low clinical suspicion of PE, elevated levels of D-dimer (> 500 ng/mL) should prompt further testing with computed tomography (CT) angiogram. Patients with a moderate or high suspected PE should undergo imaging studies without the need of D-dimer testing. D-Dimer is best tested using quantitative and semiquantitative enzyme-linked immunosorbent assay (ELISA).

GASTROINTESTINAL

Acute Mesenteric Ischemia

Acute mesenteric ischemia is a surgical emergency with a 50% mortality rate.[28] Early diagnosis remains a challenge with clinicians relying heavily on a patient's clinical history, nonspecific symptoms and signs on physical examination, and laboratory studies (ie, leukocytosis, amylase, lipase, lactate) for diagnosis. CT angiography has increased the diagnostic sensitivity and specificity, but not enough to change overall mortality. Serum lactate has been used as a primary biomarker in the diagnosis of acute mesenteric ischemia, and studies have demonstrated that levels vary even in severe cases with complete arterial occlusion.[29]

In an attempt to improve diagnostic utility, investigators have evaluated two stereoisomers of lactate: L-lactate and D-lactate. L-Lactate is produced by anaerobic glycolysis by many cells in the body and is metabolized by the liver. D-Lactate is a specific byproduct of bacterial metabolism in the lumen of the intestine that is absorbed into the bloodstream. During periods of intestinal hypoperfusion, it was proposed that bacterial overgrowth would lead to increased production of D-lactate, absorption, and plasma levels. Most laboratories measure both stereoisomers of lactate but do not distinguish between the two forms. However, when D-lactate and L-lactate were measured individually, there was no diagnostic sensitivity or specificity for acute mesenteric ischemia. Currently, studies are evaluating intestinal fatty acid–binding protein (i-FABP), which is released into the blood by injured enterocytes. Future research is needed to determine the significance of i-FABP as a biomarker in the diagnosis of acute mesenteric ischemia.

Acute Pancreatitis

Acute pancreatitis regardless of the etiology leads to a prolonged clinical course in 20% of patients, which can be complicated by multisystem organ failure and death.[30] Of the subset of patients who develop severe pancreatitis, the risk of death approaches 60%. In the first 2 weeks of developing acute severe pancreatitis, deaths are primarily attributed to SIRS and multiorgan dysfunction syndrome. In contrast, after 2 weeks, mortality is mostly due to sepsis-related complications.[31] Research has focused on identifying risk factors for the development of severe acute pancreatitis. In practice, a multitude of clinical scoring systems (ie, Ranson, APACHE II, BISAP, CTSI) involving patient characteristics, radiologic findings, and biomarkers are used to predict the severity and clinical course of acute pancreatitis. Comparisons of these various scoring systems revealed that the biomarkers, IL-6, and C-reactive protein (CRP) are useful in predicting disease severity and the development of pancreatic necrosis. IL-6 is a proinflammatory cytokine released by leukocytes activated by SIRS. IL-6 and other cytokines then stimulate the production of acute-phase reactants such as CRP by the liver. For severe pancreatitis, the diagnostic timing and cutoff levels are IL-6 greater than or equal to 50 pg/mL within 24 hours, and CRP greater than or equal to 150 mg/L at 48 hours. The use of IL-6 and CRP to identify patients at risk of developing severe, acute pancreatitis may create a window for early intervention.

NEUROLOGIC

Ischemic Stroke

Ischemic stroke affects approximately 700,000 people in the United States each year. Diagnosis is based on clinical history, physical examination, and initial imaging with computed tomography. In the last decade, there has been limited success in evaluating potential stroke biomarkers.[32] The inability to identify a single reliable diagnostic biomarker for ischemic stroke is likely due to various underlying mechanisms and the blood-brain barrier. Other studies have evaluated biomarker panels (ie, matrix metalloproteinase 9, BNP, D-dimer, S-100β) but clinical utility has not been demonstrated.

Traumatic Brain Injury

In the United States, traumatic brain injury (TBI) affects 1.7 million people and accounts for approximately 50,000 deaths.[33] Diagnosis of TBI is based on clinical findings and reliance on imaging with CT and magnetic resonance imaging (MRI). Imaging modalities have limitations with regard to time sensitivity, ability to predict the evolution or extent of injury, and detection of intracranial hypertension, all of which may ultimately delay surgical intervention. Ideally, brain biomarkers would help clinicians triage patients with TBI through the early diagnosis of diffuse and focal injury, and intracranial hypertension. Research has evaluated numerous brain biomarkers, which are mainly proteins released into the bloodstream after TBI. Some of the brain biomarkers which have been studied include neurofilament, tau protein, microtubule-associated protein 2, myelin basic protein, neuron-specific enolase, S-100β, glial fibrillary acidic protein, ubiquitin c-terminal hydrolase-L1, alpha-II spectrin breakdown product, and microRNA. Unfortunately, the diagnosis of TBI and intracranial hypertension utilizing brain biomarkers is in the early phase of discovery.

CONCLUSION

The use of biomarkers in current clinical practice is limited. However, with the exponential growth in biomarker research, there is enthusiasm that our expanding knowledge will translate into improved decision making and outcomes. Continuous evaluation of our practice and incorporation of these new ideas and studies has the potential to improve patient care. The future development and adoption of guidelines and protocols using biomarkers has potential to minimize variability and maximize benefit. Through thoughtful study design and collaboration, the biomarker era will surely transform and shape the future of medicine.

REFERENCES

1. Atkinson AJ, Colburn WA, Degruttola VG, et al. Biomarkers and surrogate endpoints: preferred definitions and conceptual framework. *Clin Pharmacol Ther*. 2001;69(3):89-95.
2. Go AS, Mozaffarian D, Roger VL, et al. Heart disease and stroke statistics—2013 update: a report from the American Heart Association. *Circulation*. 2013;127:e6-e245.
3. Collinson PO, Gaze DC. Biomarkers of cardiovascular damage and dysfunction—an overview. *Heart, Lung Circ*. 2007;16:S71-S82.
4. Babuin L, Vasile VC, Rio Perez JA, et al. Elevated cardiac troponin is an independent risk factor for short- and long-term mortality in medical intensive care unit patients. *Crit Care Med*. 2008;36(3):759-765.
5. Thygesen K, Mair J, Mueller C, et al. Recommendations for the use of natriuretic peptides in acute cardiac care: a position statement from the study group on biomarkers in cardiology of the ESC working group on acute cardiac care. *Eur Heart J*. 2012;33(16):2001-2006.
6. Clerico A, Recchia FA, Passino C, Emdin M. Cardiac endocrine function is an essential component of the homeostatic regulation network: physiological and clinical implications. *Am J Physiol Heart Circ Physiol*. 2006;290(1):H17-H29.
7. Wang HE, Muntner P, Chertow GM, Warnock DG. Acute kidney injury and mortality in hospitalized patients. *Am J Nephrol*. 2012;35(4):349-355.
8. Clec'h C, Gonzalez F, Lautrette A, et al. Multiple-center evaluation of mortality associated with acute kidney injury in critically ill patients: a competing risks analysis. *Crit Care*. 2011;15(3):R128.
9. Mandelbaum T, Scott DJ, Lee J, et al. Outcome of critically ill patients with acute kidney injury using the acute kidney injury network criteria. *Crit Care Med*. 2011;39(12):2659-2664.
10. Cruz DN, de Cal M, Garzotto F, et al. Plasma neutrophil gelatinase-associated lipocalin is an early biomarker for acute kidney injury in an adult ICU population. *Intensive Care Med*. 2010;36:444-451.
11. Bellomo R, Ronco C, Kellum JA, Mehta RL, Palevsky P. Acute renal failure—definition, outcome measures, animal models, fluid therapy and information technology needs: the second international consensus conference of the acute dialysis quality initiative (ADQI) group. *Crit Care*. 2004;8(4):R204-R212.
12. Torio CM, Andrews RM. National inpatient hospital costs: the most expensive conditions by payer, 2011: statistical brief #160. *Healthcare Cost and Utilization Project (HCUP) Statistical Briefs [Internet]*. Rockville, MD: Agency for Health Care Policy and Research (US); 2006.
13. Sutton JP, Friedman B. Trends in septicemia hospitalizations and readmissions in selected HCUP states, 2005 and 2010: statistical brief #161. *Healthcare Cost and Utilization Project (HCUP) Statistical Briefs [Internet]*. Rockville, MD: Agency for Health Care Policy and Research (US); 2006.
14. Murphy SL, Xu J, Kochanek KD. Deaths: final data for 2010. *Natl Vital Stat Rep*. 2013;61(4):1-118.
15. Rivers EP, Jaehne AK, Nguyen HB, et al. Early biomarker activity in severe sepsis and septic shock and a contemporary review of immunotherapy trials: not a time to give up, but to give it earlier. *Shock*. 2013;39(2):127-137.
16. Attana P, Lazzeri C, Picariello C, et al. Lactate and lactate clearance in acute cardiac patients. *Eur Heart J Acute Cardiovasc Care*. 2012;1(2):115-121.
17. Fuller BM, Dellinger RP. Lactate as a hemodynamic marker in the critically ill. *Curr Opin Crit Care*. 2012;18(3):267-272.
18. Marty P, Roquilly A, Vallee F, et al. Lactate clearance for death prediction in severe sepsis or septic shock patients during the first 24 hours in intensive care unit: an observational study. *Ann Intensive Care*. 2013;3(1):3.
19. Jones AE, Shapiro NI, Trzeciak S, et al. Lactate clearance versus central venous oxygenation saturation as goals of early sepsis therapy: a randomized clinical trial. *JAMA*. 2010;303(8):739-746.
21. Andersen LW, Mackenhauer J, Roberts JC, et al. Etiology and therapeutic approach to elevated lactate levels. *Mayo Clin Proc*. 2013;88(10):1127-1140.

22. Schuetz P, Litke A, Albrich WC, Mueller B. Blood biomarkers for personalized treatment and patient management decisions in community-acquired pneumonia. *Curr Opin Infect Dis.* 2013;26(2):159-167.

23. Meisner M. Pathobiochemistry and clinical use of procalcitonin. *Clin Chim Acta.* 2002;323(1-2):17-29.

24. Matthaiou DK, Ntani G, Kontogiorgi M, et al. An ESICM systematic review and meta-analysis of procalcitonin-guided antibiotic therapy algorithms in adult critically ill patients. *Intensive Care Med.* 2012;38(6):940-949.

25. Snell N, Newbold P. The clinical utility of biomarkers in asthma and COPD. *Curr Opin Pharmacol.* 2008;8:222-235.

26. Wiener RS, Schwartz LM, Woloshin S. Time trends in pulmonary embolism in the United States: evidence of over diagnosis. *Arch Intern Med.* 2011;171(9):831-837.

27. Stamm JA. Risk stratification for acute pulmonary embolism. *Crit Care Clin.* 2012;28(2):301-321.

28. Perrier A, Sylvie D, Catherine G, et al. D-dimer testing for suspected pulmonary embolism in outpatients. *Am J Respir Crit Care Med.* 1997;156(2):492-496.

29. Sise MJ. Acute mesenteric ischemia. *Surg Clin North Am.* 2014;94(1):165-181.

30. Demir IE, Ceyhan GO, Friess H. Beyond lactate: is there a role for serum lactate measurement in diagnosing acute mesenteric ischemia? *Dig Surg.* 2012;29:226-235.

31. Cardoso FS, Ricardo LB, Oliveira AM, et al. C-reactive protein prognostic accuracy in acute pancreatitis: timing of measurement and cutoff points. *Eur J Gastroenterol Hepatol.* 2013;25(7):784-789.

32. Khanna AK, Meher S, Prakash S, et al. Comparison of Ranson, Glasgow, MOSS, SIRS, BISAP, APACHE-II, CTSI Scores, IL-6, CRP, and procalcitonin in predicting severity, organ failure, pancreatic necrosis, and mortality in acute pancreatitis. *HPB Surg.* 2013;2013:367581.

33. Kim SJ, Moon GJ, Bang OY. Biomarkers for stroke. *J Stroke.* 2013;15(1):27-37.

34. Yokobori S, Hosein K, Burks S, et al. Biomarkers for the clinical differential diagnosis in traumatic brain injury—a systematic review. *CNS Neurosci Ther.* 2013;19:556-565.

Controversies in Therapeutic Hypothermia

Jose R. Yunen, MD and Rafael Tolentino, MD

8

Induced TH is currently used in several medical conditions. However, it is by far more commonly employed in today's clinical practice to prevent or diminish hypoxic-ischemic encephalopathy (HIE) and its deleterious outcomes in postcardiac arrest patients.

OVERVIEW OF HIE

HIE is a syndrome of acute global brain injury resulting from critical reduction or loss of blood flow and supply of oxygen and nutrients. Some of the terms used to describe this clinical syndrome include anoxic encephalopathy, postcardiac arrest brain injury, and other terms denoting a diminution of blood or oxygen to the whole brain. The pathologic injury to the brain results in cell injury and death from an intracellular energetic crisis that selectively affects vulnerable areas such as CA-1 of the hippocampus, caudate, putamen and neocortex, and relative sparing of brain stem. High-quality cardiopulmonary resuscitation (CPR) with prompt restoration of spontaneous circulation is crucial to survival. The mainstay of postresuscitation care is TH. ICU management also includes optimizing hemodynamic status, diagnosing and treating seizures, and other supportive care.

The most common cause of HIE is cardiac arrest, which is commonly secondary to cardiac etiologies (infarction or arrhythmia). Each year over half a million cardiac arrests occur in the United States. Approximately 380,000 of these occur outside of health care facilities, and another 210,000 occur in hospital every year.

Outcomes of Postanoxic Brain Injury After Cardiac Arrest

The outcome of patients experiencing SCA is poor. The primary cause of mortality after SCA is primarily related to the effects of anoxic brain injury and not necessarily from cardiac complications.

Outcomes differ based on initial rhythm found at scene of SCA. For example, outcomes are poorer with so-called "nonshockable" rhythms (asystole, pulseless electrical activity [PEA]) compared to "shockable" rhythms (ventricular tachycardia [VT] or ventricular fibrillation [VF]). Improved survival may be best when initial rhythm is VF, but still dependent on prompt delivery of effective CPR. Clinical factors identified as predictors of greater likelihood of survival to hospital discharge are witnessed arrest, VT or VF as initial rhythm, return to spontaneous circulation (ROSC) during first 10 minutes, and longer duration of overall resuscitation efforts.[1]

The Controversies

Since the development of modern CPR techniques in the 1950s, numerous pharmacologic trials with putative neuroprotective effects have failed to improve survival and quality of life of patients resuscitated from cardiac arrest. Mild TH has become a standard component of postcardiac arrest to prevent or mitigate various types of neurologic injury. The ultimate goal of resuscitation is to improve survival with good neurologic outcome. The evidence supporting this practice came from two randomized trials published consecutively in 2002—one small-sized Australian study done by Bernard et al that showed good neurologic outcome in 49% survivors in the hypothermia to 33°C group versus 26% of normothermic patients, among 77 patients with out-of-hospital cardiac arrest due to VT.[2] The other, a medium-sized randomized controlled multicenter trial was done in 9 European centers by the Hypothermia After Cardiac Arrest (HACA) group wherein among 273 patients with out-of-hospital arrest due to shockable initial rhythms (VF or VT), hypothermia to 34°C led to improved neurologic outcome 55% versus 39% with usual care.[3]

TH (also called targeted temperature management) had demonstrated a robust benefit with a number needed to treat (NNT) of 6. While these 2 landmark studies focused on out-of-hospital cardiac arrest with VT/VF as initial rhythms, subsequent studies showed likely survival and quality-of-life benefits for victims of cardiac arrest with initial rhythms of asystole or PEA with hypothermia (TH).[4] While no prospective randomized controlled trial has been undertaken to show the benefit of TH in patients with PEA and asystole,[5-8] existing studies have also shown that TH is not harmful either. Current recommendations strongly favor cooling all comatose cardiac arrest victims regardless of presenting ECG rhythm in accordance to the International Liaison Committee on Resuscitation (ILCOR) guidelines (American Heart Association [AHA] class I recommendation for out-of-hospital arrest with VT/VF as the initial rhythm, and IIB for those with PEA and asystole as initial rhythm), and the European Resuscitation Council.[9]

This approach was recommended despite arguments by some investigators that the evidence was weak, owing to the risk of bias and small samples.[10,11] Furthermore, its use has been extended to cardiac arrest of other causes and with other presenting rhythms as well as to the in-hospital setting.[12] Although a Cochrane review supports these guidelines,[13] some investigators have suggested a need for additional trials to confirm or refute the current treatment strategy.[14-16] In addition, one trial showed that fever developed in many patients in the standard treatment group.[17] It is therefore unclear whether the reported treatment effect was due to hypothermia or to the prevention of fever, which is associated with a poor outcome.[18-20]

The subsequent debate has focused on 2 issues. The first issue is whether TH should be extended to patients outside the originally described populations.[21-23] It may be reasoned that the potential benefits of temperature management on brain injury due to circulatory arrest would be the same irrespective of the cause of arrest. However, whole body hypothermia influences all organ systems and any potential benefit should be balanced against

possible side effects.[24] The population of patients with cardiac arrest is heterogeneous, and the potential risks and benefits of temperature intervention may not be the same across subgroups. The second issue is the most beneficial target temperature for therapeutic hypothermia.[25] The recommended temperature of 32°C to 34°C has been extrapolated from experiments in animals[26,27]; however, similar results have been observed with milder cooling.[28]

AREAS OF UNCERTAINTY

Therapeutic Hypothermia in Nonshockable Cardiac Arrest

There are less robust recommendations with the use of mild TH in cardiac arrest with nonshockable initial rhythm (PEA or asystole). Only few studies have been published to evaluate the potential benefit of therapeutic hypothermia in comatose subjects presenting with nonshockable initial rhythm with conflicting results. The meta-analysis of studies by Kim et al done before 2010 using mild therapeutic hypothermia in survivors of nonshockable cardiac arrest found that TH is associated with reduced in-hospital mortality but no significant neurologic benefit.[29] Three retrospective analyses of out-of-hospital nonshockable cardiac arrest found possible improvement of neurologic outcomes using TH.[30-32] A large cohort study by Dumas et al found no benefit for therapeutic hypothermia in nonshockable cardiac arrest.[33]

It is not clear whether other factors influence the outcome in nonshockable cardiac arrest. It would be logical to think that neurologic injury whether shockable or nonshockable cardiac arrest could have the same mechanism. Adult patients with PEA or asystole cardiac arrest are usually sicker, with ongoing hypoxemia and circulatory shock that often result in bradycardia or hypotension before progressing to pulseless cardiac arrest.[34] Additional brain insult may have been incurred during prearrest asphyxia and circulatory shock.

Cooling and Rewarming

The optimal time to initiate TH, the optimal method of cooling, the optimal rate of induction, level and duration of hypothermia, and the optimal rate of rewarming are still unknown. In animal models of cardiac arrest, the benefit of hypothermia declines when it is started more than 15 minutes after Reperfusion.[35] Bernard et al[36,37] hypothesized that early initiation of cooling in the field after ROSC would improve both survival and neurologic outcome. Rapid cooling after resuscitation from cardiac arrest with an intravenous infusion of cold saline appears feasible and safe.[38] Infusion of cold intravenous fluid is an attractive strategy to achieve early cooling because of its portability, ease in administration, and potential widespread availability in the prehospital setting. However, no benefit was observed among 234 patients resuscitated from prehospital VF and then randomized to early field cooling.[39]

This large randomized trial[40] found that prehospital, rapid infusion of up to 2 L of 4°C normal saline did induce mild hypothermia faster than standard care but did not improve survival or neurologic status at discharge after resuscitation from prehospital shockable (VF) or nonshockable (without VF) cardiac arrest. The resuscitation and intervention were performed by paramedics from emergency medical service (EMS) agencies with a high overall rate of resuscitation. The intervention reduced core body temperature by hospital arrival, and patients reached the goal temperature about 1 hour sooner than in the control group. The intervention was associated with significantly increased incidence of rearrest during transport, time in the prehospital setting, pulmonary edema, and early diuretic use in the emergency department (ED). Mortality in the out-of-hospital setting or ED and hospital length of stay did not differ significantly between the treatment groups.

Clinical evidence in humans undergoing intra-arrest therapeutic hypothermia (IATH) is limited, but has been shown to be both safe and feasible, and in one study it showed improvements in ROSC, survival to hospital discharge, and neurologic outcomes.[41-43]

In the pivotal clinical trials,[2-3] therapeutic hypothermia was achieved with use of noninvasive surface cooling methods by application of ice packs in the Australian trial and with the use cold air mattress covering the entire body in the European trial. Other studies made use of invasive core cooling via intravascular catheters, ice-cold fluid infusion, peritoneal lavage, and use of extracorporeal circulation. Each method has their advantages and disadvantages. It is important however that the chosen method could rapidly induce cooling as well as maintain the target temperature within a narrow range.

Temperature Modulation

After maintaining a TH of 32°C to 34°C for 24 hours, active, controlled rewarming at a rate of 0.25°C to 0.5°C per hour is recommended until a core temperature of 36°C to 37°C is achieved. Upon rewarming, the therapeutic temperature management system should remain in place for a further 48 to 72 hours to ensure normothermia, protecting the brain from the detrimental effects of hyperthermia. Rebound pyrexia is a common phenomenon occurring in about 40% of patients posttherapeutic hypothermia. Only temperatures greater than 38.7°C appear to be associated with worse neurologic outcomes in patients who survive to discharge.[44] The mechanism for this common presentation of fever after therapeutic hypothermia is not well understood, however several factors are thought to contribute to its presence: altered thermoregulation from damage to thalamic structures, rebound hyperthermia, infection, and proinflammatory states all are likely contributors.

Shivering

Another important consideration when treating with hypothermia is the management and prevention of shivering. Shivering is a centrally mediated thermoregulatory response that normally sets in at 35.5°C, and is usually overcome below 34°C. However, these reference temperatures apply to healthy individuals, and may not be the same in all cardiac arrest patients. The absence of shivering after induction of hypothermia, or spontaneous hypothermia prior to induction of hypothermia has been associated with worse outcomes[45]; it is possible that damage to the hypothalamus impairing thermoregulation may be a marker for more severe injury. On the other hand, the presence of shivering is known to increase body temperature which has been shown to worsen brain injury and negatively impact outcome.[44]

Does It Really Work?

To make things more uncertain, in the largest randomized trial yet published in 2013, Nielsen et al probe further whether TH is effective in cardiac arrest with and without shockable rhythms, if fever is also prevented as standard of care. This study included 939 patients after out-of-hospital cardiac arrest of presumed cardiac cause between 2010 and 2013 in 36 centers in Europe and Australia, regardless of the initial rhythm (80% had a shockable initial rhythm, 12% had asystole, and 8% had PEA). They were randomized to receive targeted temperature management using any cooling method to either 33°C or a near-normal temperature of 36°C, induced as soon as possible, for 28 hours, followed by rewarming, followed by fever-reduction methods for 72 hours postarrest. This trial showed that hypothermia at a targeted temperature of 33°C did not confer a benefit as compared with a targeted temperature of 36°C regardless of initial rhythm. There were no differences between groups in the rate of death (50% with hypothermia, 48% without), or in the composite outcome of poor neurologic outcome or death after 6 months (risk ratios were almost exactly 1). When the analysis was restricted only to the 80% of subjects with shockable cardiac arrest, there was still no benefit from TH: The relative risk for death among the cooled patients was 1.06.

The investigators did not find any harm with a targeted temperature of 33°C as compared with 36°C. However, it is worth recognizing that for all outcomes, none of the point estimates were in the direction of a benefit for the 33°C group. On the basis of these results, decisions about which temperature to target after out-of-hospital cardiac arrest require careful consideration.

There are multiple possible explanations for the absence of benefit from lower temperatures in patients with cardiac arrest.[46] The population was less select than in previous trials, including patients with shockable rhythms and those with nonshockable rhythms. There has been evolution of intensive care over the past decade, and improvements in patient care may have reduced the potential incremental benefits of a single intervention. In addition, illness severity varies greatly among patients with cardiac arrest, and there may be subgroups of patients who do benefit from induced hypothermia but who were not designated in advance. Particularly if the degree or duration of hypothermia must be adjusted to

match the severity of brain injury, the benefits to a subgroup may be missed in a trial of one regimen of hypothermia for all comers.

One interpretation of these results is that they reinforce the importance of controlling temperature, even while they question whether 33°C is the best temperature. For example, many patients in the "normothermia" group of the older trials actually became hyperthermic,[47,48] which is deleterious.[49,50] The exceptional rates of good outcomes in both the 33°C and 36°C groups in the present trial may reflect the active prevention of hyperthermia.

Further investigation is needed to address and define the population of cardiac arrest patients for whom the costly and intensive method of therapeutic hypothermia should be applied to or withheld.

Other Applications

Hypothermia is utilized in the management of severe traumatic brain injury (TBI) to lower cerebral metabolic rate of oxygen ($CMRO_2$) despite the lack of unequivocal evidence supporting its use. Most single-center studies suggest that induced hypothermia is associated with improved outcome. However, 2 large randomized multicenter studies in adults with severe TBI (National Acute Brain Injury Study: Hypothermia I and II) failed to show benefit,[51,52] and a randomized study of hypothermia in children with TBI suggested harm.[53] While mild-to-moderate hypothermia has not been shown to improve outcome, the preponderance of literature suggests it is effective in lowering intracranial pressure (ICP).

In laboratory investigations of traumatic spinal cord injury, no treatment appears as promising as therapeutic hypothermia. The current issue remains translating this putative success into an approved human clinical therapy. The issue began to receive copious public interest after the case of football player whose recovery was widely credited to TH. He was said to be complete (ASIA A) below the clavicles. Of note, he received methylprednisolone infusion in the ambulance as well as IV chilled saline and ice packs to the groin. In the ED, he was hemodynamically stable with a temperature of 36°C. His C3-C4 facet dislocation was operatively reduced about 3 hours after injury. The following day, he was cooled for several days at 33°C, recovering strength about 15 hours postinjury.[54] Was this the effect of hypothermia, or of the combination of steroids and early open reduction with adjunctive hypothermia? Such is the potential confounding where steroids and other aspects of care have varied in the setting of varied hypothermia protocols. For now, the use of TH after spinal cord injury (SCI) is considered experimental.

A recently published multicenter randomized controlled clinical trial[55] by Mourvillier et al showed that moderate hypothermia did not improve outcome in patients with severe bacterial meningitis and may even be harmful. After inclusion of 98 comatose patients, the trial was stopped early at the request of the DSMB because of concerns over excess mortality in the hypothermia group (25 of 49 patients [51%]) versus the control group (15 of 49 patients [31%]; relative risk [RR], 1.99; 95% confidence interval [CI], 1.05-3.77; $P = 0.04$).

The use of therapeutic hypothermia poses some potential risks, and some considerations need to be noted for its possible adverse effects. The clinical trials showed nonsignificant occurrence of adverse events between TH and control groups. Nonetheless, the more common adverse conditions to be vigilant for include pneumonia, sepsis, bleeding, electrolyte abnormalities, cardiac arrhythmias, and dysglycemia.[56] Establishing treatment protocols of care for induction and maintenance of hypothermia and rewarming, as well as tracking and correction of potential adverse events have enhance the delivery of care and contributed to the success of the TH.

REFERENCES

1. Bunch TJ, White RD, Gersh BJ, et al. Outcomes and in-hospital treatment of out-of-hospital cardiac arrest patients resuscitated from ventricular fibrillation by early defibrillation. *Mayo Clinic Proc.* 2004;79:613.
2. Bernard SA, Gray TW, Buist MD, et al. Treatment of comatose survivors of out-of-hospital cardiac arrest with induced hypothermia. *N Engl J Med.* 2002;346:557-563.
3. Hypothermia after Cardiac Arrest Group. Mild therapeutic hypothermia to improve neurologic outcome after cardiac arrest. *N Engl J Med.* 2002;346(8):549-556.
4. Nolan JP, Morley PT, Vanden Hoek TL, et al. Therapeutic hypothermia after cardiac arrest: an advisory statement by the advanced life support task force of the International Liaison Committee on Resuscitation. *Circulation.* 2003;108:118-121.
5. Dumas F, Grimaldi D, Zuber B, et al. Is hypothermia after cardiac arrest effective in both shockable and nonshockable patients?: insights from a large registry. *Circulation.* 2011;123(8):877-886.
6. Oddo M, Ribordy V, Feihl F, et al. Early predictors of outcome in comatose survivors of ventricular fibrillation and non-ventricular fibrillation cardiac arrest treated with hypothermia: a prospective study. *Crit Care Med.* 2008;36(8):2296-2301.
7. Don CW, Longstreth WT, Maynard C, et al. Active surface cooling protocol to induce mild therapeutic hypothermia after out-of-hospital cardiac arrest: a retrospective before-and-after comparison in a single hospital. *Crit Care Med.* 2009;37(12):3062-3069.
8. Kory P, Fukunaga M, Mathew JP, et al. Outcomes of mild therapeutic hypothermia after in-hospital cardiac arrest. *Neurocrit Care.* 2012;16(3):406-412.
9. Peberdy MA, Callaway CW, Neumar RW, et al. Part 9: post-cardiac arrest care: 2010 American Heart Association Guidelines for Cardiopulmonary Resuscitation and Emergency Cardiovascular Care. *Circulation.* 2010;122(18 suppl 3):S768-S786.
10. Nielsen N, Friberg H, Gluud C, Herlitz J, Wetterslev J. Hypothermia after cardiac arrest should be further evaluated—a systematic review of randomised trials with meta-analysis and trial sequential analysis. *Int J Cardiol.* 2011;151(3):333-341.
11. Gibson A, Andrews PJ. Therapeutic hypothermia, still "too cool to be true?" *F1000Prime Rep.* 2013;5:26-29.
12. Peberdy MA, Callaway CW, Neumar RW, et al. Post-cardiac arrest care: 2010 American Heart Association Guidelines for Cardiopulmonary Resuscitation and Emergency Cardiovascular Care. *Circulation.* 2010;122(suppl 3):S768-S786. [Errata, *Circulation.* 2011;123(6):e237, 124(15):e403.]
13. Arrich J, Holzer M, Havel C, Müllner M, Herkner H. Hypothermia for neuroprotection in adults after cardiopulmonary resuscitation. *Cochrane Database Syst Rev.* 2012;9:CD004128.
14. Nielsen N, Friberg H, Gluud C, Herlitz J, Wetterslev J. Hypothermia after cardiac arrest should be further evaluated—a systematic review of randomised trials with meta-analysis and trial sequential analysis. *Int J Cardiol.* 2011;151(3):333-341.
15. Fisher GC. Hypothermia after cardiac arrest: feasible but is it therapeutic? *Anaesthesia.* 2008;63:885-886.
16. Moran JL, Solomon PJ. Therapeutic hypothermia after cardiac arrest—once again. *Crit Care Resusc.* 2006;8:151-154.

17. Hypothermia after Cardiac Arrest Study Group. Mild therapeutic hypothermia to improve the neurologic outcome after cardiac arrest. *N Engl J Med*. 2002;346:549-556. [Erratum, *N Engl J Med*. 2002;346:1756.]

18. Zeiner A, Holzer M, Sterz F, et al. Hyperthermia after cardiac arrest is associated with an unfavorable neurologic outcome. *Arch Intern Med*. 2001;161:2007-2012.

19. Bro-Jeppesen J, Hassager C, Wanscher M, et al. Post-hypothermia fever is associated with increased mortality after out-of-hospital cardiac arrest. *Resuscitation*. 2013;84(12):1734-1740.

20. Leary M, Grossestreuer AV, Iannacone S, et al. Pyrexia and neurologic outcomes after therapeutic hypothermia for cardiac arrest. *Resuscitation*. 2013;84:1056-1061.

21. Dumas F, Rea TD. Long-term prognosis following resuscitation from out-ofhospital cardiac arrest: role of aetiology and presenting arrest rhythm. *Resuscitation*. 2012;83:1001-1005.

22. Nichol G, Huszti E, Kim F, et al. Does induction of hypothermia improve outcomes after in-hospital cardiac arrest? *Resuscitation*. 2013;84:620-625.

23. Dumas F, Grimaldi D, Zuber B, et al. Is hypothermia after cardiac arrest effective in both shockable and nonshockable patients? Insights from a large registry. *Circulation*. 2011;123:877-886.

24. Nielsen N, Sunde K, Hovdenes J, et al. Adverse events and their relation to mortality in out-of-hospital cardiac arrest patients treated with therapeutic hypothermia. *Crit Care Med*. 2011;39:57-64.

25. Holzer M. Targeted temperature management for comatose survivors of cardiac arrest. *N Engl J Med*. 2010;363:1256-1264.

26. Colbourne F, Corbett D. Delayed and prolonged post-ischemic hypothermia is neuroprotective in the gerbil. *Brain Res*. 1994;654:265-272.

27. Sterz F, Safar P, Tisherman S, Radovsky A, Kuboyama K, Oku K. Mild hypothermic cardiopulmonary resuscitation improves outcome after prolonged cardiac arrest in dogs. *Crit Care Med*. 1991;19:379-389.

28. Logue ES, McMichael MJ, Callaway CW. Comparison of the effects of hypothermia at 33 degrees C or 35 degrees C after cardiac arrest in rats. *Acad Emerg Med*. 2007;14:293-300.

29. Kim YM, Yim HW, Jeong SH, Klem ML, Callaway CW. Does therapeutic hypothermia benefit adult cardiac arrest patients presenting with nonshockable initial rhythms?: a systematic review and meta-analysis of randomized and non-randomize studies. *Resuscitation*. 2012;83(2):188-196.

30. Soga T, Nagao K, Sawano H, et al. Neurological benefit of therapeutic hypothermia following return of spontaneous circulation for out-of-hospital nonshockable cardiac arrest. *Circ J*. 2012;76(11):2579-2585.

31. Testori C, Sterz F, Behringer B, et al. Mild therapeutic hypothermia is associated with favourable outcome in patients after cardiac arrest with nonshockable rhythms. *Resuscitation*. 2011;82(9):1162-1167.

32. Lundbye JB, Rai M, Ramu B, et al. Therapeutic hypothermia is associated with improved neurological outcome and survival in cardiac arrest survivors of nonshockable rhythms. *Resuscitation*. 2012;83(2):202-207.

33. Dumas F, Grimaldi D, Zuber B, et al. Is hypothermia after cardiac arrest effective in both shockable and nonshockable patients?: insights from a large registry. *Circulation*. 2011;123:877-886.

34. Nadkarni VM, Larkin GL, Peberdy MA, et al. First documented rhythm and clinical outcome from in hospital cardiac arrest among children and adults. *JAMA*. 2006;295(1):50-57.

35. Kuboyama K, Safar P, Radovsky A, et al. Delay in cooling negates the beneficial effect of mild resuscitative cerebral hypothermia after cardiac arrest in dogs. *Crit Care Med*. 1993;21(9):1348-1358.

36. Bernard S. Hypothermia after cardiac arrest. *Crit Care Med*. 2004;32(3):897-899.

37. Bernard S, Buist M, Monteiro O, Smith K. Induced hypothermia using large volume, ice-cold intravenous fluid in comatose survivors of out-of-hospital cardiac arrest: a preliminary report. *Resuscitation*. 2003;56(1):9-13.

38. Kim F, Olsufka M, Longstreth WT, Jr, et al. Pilot randomized clinical trial of prehospital induction of mild hypothermia in out-of-hospital cardiac arrest patients with a rapid infusion of 4 degrees C normal saline. *Circulation*. 2007;115(24):3064-3070.

39. Bernard SA, Smith K, Cameron P, et al; Rapid Infusion of Cold Hartmanns (RICH) Investigators. Induction of therapeutic hypothermia by paramedics after resuscitation from out-of-hospital ventricular fibrillation cardiac arrest: a randomized controlled trial. *Circulation*. 2010;122(7):737-742.

40. Kim F, Nichol G, Maynard C, et al. Effect of prehospital induction of mild hypothermia on survival and neurological status among adults with cardiac arrest a randomized clinical trial. *JAMA*. 2014;311(1):45-52.

41. Castrén M, Nordberg P, Svensson L, et al. Intra-arrest transnasal evaporative cooling: a randomized, prehospital, multicenter study (PRINCE: Pre-ROSC IntraNasal Cooling Effectiveness). *Circulation.* 2010;122(7):729-736.

42. Deasy C, Bernard S, Cameron P, et al. Design of the RINSE trial: the rapid infusion of cold normal saline by paramedics during CPR. *BMC Emerg Med.* 2011;11(1):17.

43. Garrett JS, Studnek JR, Blackwell T, et al. The association between intra-arrest therapeutic hypothermia and return of spontaneous circulation among individuals experiencing out of hospital cardiac arrest. *Resuscitation.* 2011;82(1):21-25.

44. Leary M, Grossestreuer AV, Iannacone S, et al. Pyrexia and neurologic outcomes after therapeutic hypothermia for cardiac arrest. *Resuscitation.* 2013;84(8):1056-1061.

45. Benz-Woerner J, Delodder F, Benz R, et al. Body temperature regulation and outcome after cardiac arrest and therapeutic hypothermia. *Resuscitation.* 2012;83(3):338-342.

46. Rittenberger JC, Callaway CW. Temperature management and modern ost-cardiac arrest care. *N Engl J Med.* 2013;369:23.

47. Hypothermia after Cardiac Arrest Study Group. Mild therapeutic hypothermia to improve the neurologic outcome after cardiac arrest. *N Engl J Med.* 2002;346:549-556. [Erratum, *N Engl J Med.* 2002;346:1756.]

48. Bernard SA, Gray TW, Buist MD, et al. Treatment of comatose survivors of out-of-hospital cardiac arrest with induced hypothermia. *N Engl J Med.* 2002;346:557-563.

49. Zeiner A, Holzer M, Sterz F, et al. Hyperthermia after cardiac arrest is associated with an unfavorable neurologic outcome. *Arch Intern Med.* 2001;161:2007-2012.

50. Gebhardt K, Guyette FX, Doshi AA, Callaway CW, Rittenberger JC. Prevalence and effect of fever on outcome following resuscitation from cardiac arrest. *Resuscitation.* 2013;84:1062-1067.

51. Clifton GL, Miller ER, Choi SC, et al. Lack of effect of induction of hypothermia after acute brain injury. *N Engl J Med.* 2001;344:556.

52. Clifton GL, Valadka A, Zygun D, et al. Very early hypothermia induction in patients with severe brain injury (the National Acute Brain Injury Study: Hypothermia II): a randomized trial. *Lancet Neurol.* 2011;10:131.

53. Hutchison JS, Ward RE, Lacroix J, et al. Hypothermia therapy after traumatic brain injury in children. *N Engl J Med.* 2008;258(23):2447-2456.

54. Cappuccino A, Bisson LJ, Carpenter B, et al. The use of systemic hypothermia for the treatment of an acute cervical spinal cord injury in a professional football player. *Spine.* 2010;35:E57-E62.

55. Mourvillier B, Tubach F, Beek D, et al. Induced hypothermia in severe bacterial meningitis: a randomized clinical trial. *JAMA.* 2013;310(20):2174-2183.

56. Neumar RW, Nolan JP, Adrie C, et al. Post-cardiac arrest syndrome: epidemiology, pathophysiology, treatment, and prognostication. A consensus statement from the International Liaison Committee on Resuscitation. *Circulation.* 2008;118(23):2452-2483.

C H A P T E R

Bedside Technology

Tara T. Bellamkonda, DO; Victor Murgolo, CCRN and John M. Oropello, MD, FACP, FCCP, FCCM

9

KEY POINTS

1. Physicians, advanced care practitioners, and nurses all share the responsibility of having basic knowledge about bedside technology to properly manage patients as well as to ensure patient safety and reduce complications due to user error.

2. Standard pulse oximeters use transmittance spectrophotometry, that is, the light source and photodetector regions of the sensor should be directly opposite each other; they are completely unreliable if placed on the forehead or in any configuration that does not allow the transmitter and receiver to be opposite each other.

3. Medical air is 21% oxygen from a yellow-coded outlet that is used to power air-driven medical equipment; 100% oxygen supplied by a green-coded outlet is for oxygen delivery to the patient. Make sure they are connected properly.

4. Patients on positive end-expiratory pressure (PEEP) to maintain oxygenation, and require bag-valve-mask (BVM) ventilation during disconnection from mechanical ventilation, should be ventilated with a BVM containing a built-in PEEP valve or with a PEEP valve added to the exhalation port of the BVM.

The critically ill patient is in constant flux and both monitoring and therapeutic equipment are essential for managing these patients in the intensive care unit (ICU). Physicians, advanced care practitioners, and nurses all share the responsibility of having basic knowledge about bedside technology to properly manage patients as well as to ensure patient safety and reduce complications due to user error.

BEDSIDE MONITORING SYSTEM

The bedside monitor is the most prominent device garnering the most attention for both medical staff and patients and their families. Bedside monitoring is designed to display, store, and trend the patient's heart rate, respiratory rate, blood pressure reading (noninvasive and invasive), oxygen saturation, electrocardiographic (ECG) tracing, and pressure waveforms generated from arterial, venous, or bladder catheters. The individual bedside monitor is connected to a computerized central monitoring system outside of the patient's room that will sound an alarm when abnormal measurements are recorded prompting immediate notification of the ICU staff and evaluation of the patient.

Alarm limits and scales are set by the nursing staff depending on the patient's clinical status (Figure 9–1). For instance, the ECG scale may be

91

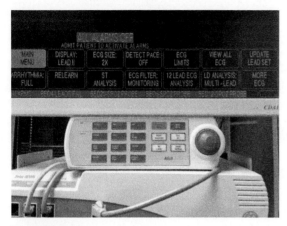

FIGURE 9–1 Monitor settings.

TABLE 9–1 Electrode placement for 5-lead system.

Electrode	Placement
Right arm (RA)	Apply to the right shoulder near the junction of the right arm and torso
Left arm (LA)	Apply to the left shoulder near the junction of the left arm and torso
Right leg (RL)	Apply at the level of the lowest right rib, on the right abdominal region, or right hip
Left leg (LL)	Apply at the level of the lowest left rib, on the left abdominal region, or left hip
Precordial (choose either V_1 or V_6)	V_1 Apply to fourth intercostal space on right sternal border V_6 Apply to fifth intercostal space on midaxillary line

Data from AACN, Wiegand DJ: ACCN Procedure Manual for Critical Care. 6th ed. St. Louis, MO: Elsevier; 2011.

set to amplify the tracing 2- to 4-fold in a low-voltage state. Pressure waveform scales can vary based on the patient's pressure range; generally, the right atrial pressure is set at 20 mm Hg, pulmonary artery systolic pressure is set at 40 mm Hg, and systolic arterial blood pressure is set at 180 mm Hg.[1]

Electrophysiologic Monitor

Cardiac monitoring is indicated for all critically ill patients and is used for the assessment of hemodynamics, rhythm diagnosis, and detection of ischemic changes. Monitors can employ 3-lead or 5-lead wire systems to depict the electrical activity of the heart; however, 5-lead systems are most common for continuous monitoring and provide a readout of 2 or more leads simultaneously.[1]

Lead placement must be standardized in order to maintain precise and accurate results and interpretation (Table 9–1). In order for the monitor's heart rate counter to detect the correct heart rate, the height of the R wave should be twice the height of the other electrocardiographic waves. The alarm mechanism relies on R-wave height for proper detection; false alarms can occur if T-wave height is equivalent to R-wave height, which causes double counting.[1] Most monitors have the capability of taking a 12-lead ECG. In terms of lead placement, when only monitoring, the lower limb leads should be placed on the abdomen to pick up the breaths, when taking a 12-lead ECG they should be placed on the thigh.

Electrode resistance changes as the gel dries; if a problem occurs with one electrode, it is recommended that all electrodes be changed to prevent discordance in resistance between electrodes.[1] Other key elements needed to ensure proper cardiac monitoring include adequately preparing the skin by cleaning and drying the sites of lead placement, testing the center of the pregelled electrode to make sure it is not dry, and reducing tension on wires. If these measures are not performed, interference and incorrect recordings can result.

Pulse Oximetry

Hemoglobin oxygen saturation is measured by pulse oximetry and is expressed as the percentage of oxygen (O_2) that hemoglobin carries relative to the total amount of hemoglobin that is capable of carrying oxygen and is noted as "Spo_2," to differentiate it from "Sao_2" obtained from arterial blood gas analysis. Pulse oximetry employs the technologies of spectrophotometry and optical plethysmography. Spectrophotometry estimates the hemoglobin oxygen saturation by using a light source with 2 light-emitting diodes (LEDs) that emit light at red (660 nm) and infrared (940 nm) wavelengths. Deoxyhemoglobin absorbs red light and oxyhemoglobin absorbs infrared light; absorbed light is transmitted to a photodetector and converted to a digital value. Optical plethysmography detects pulsatile arterial changes at the pulse oximeter sensor site as the path length of light through the sensor site alternately increases or decreases with each pulsation.[2] The plethysmography component of the pulse oximeter differentiates light absorption by hemoglobin from light absorption by surrounding tissue.

Pulse oximeter sensor probes should be placed on the best pulsatile vascular bed available; potential sites include fingers, great toe, and earlobe. Sensor probes should not be used on sites that are near indwelling arterial catheters, blood pressure cuffs, or areas of venous engorgement such as arteriovenous fistulas and blood transfusions. Standard pulse oximeters use transmittance spectrophotometry, that is, the light source and photodetector regions of the sensor should be directly opposite each other on the vascular bed and should be positioned so that all light from the sensor makes contact with perfused tissue beds. This minimizes ambient light interference and optical shunting which occurs when light bypasses the vascular bed.[1] If the these probes are placed on the forehead or nasal bridge (as is sometimes erroneously done if there is difficulty detecting an adequate pulse waveform on the digits or earlobe) or in any configuration that does not allow the transmitter and receiver to be opposite each other, the SpO_2 is completely unreliable. Specialized pulse oximeters that use reflectance spectrophotometry can be placed on the forehead and give reliable SpO_2 readings. Make sure you know the capabilities of the device used in your ICU.

Two-wavelength pulse oximetry as described above is standard, but is inaccurate in the presence of dyshemoglobins such as carboxyhemoglobin and methemoglobin. Other causes of spurious readings (usually erroneously decreased SpO_2) include low perfusion states, clinical motion, venous pulsation at sensor site, dark skin, intense ambient light, nail polish, artificial nails, and intravenously administered dyes such as methylene blue, indigo carmine, and indocyanine green.[2]

Transducer System

The function of the transducer system is to convert a biophysical event into an electrical signal that is

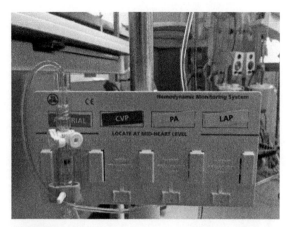

FIGURE 9–2   Multiple-pressure transducer system.

transmitted as a waveform to the bedside monitor. The transducer system can be a single-pressure unit for arterial or right atrial monitoring or a multiple-pressure unit for arterial, right atrial, and pulmonary artery monitoring (Figure 9–2). The system consists of a catheter, pressure tubing, stopcocks, and a flushing device.

To ensure accuracy, the system must be zeroed against atmospheric pressure and then leveled with the phlebostatic axis which approximates the right atrium. The phlebostatic axis is located at the intersection of an imaginary line from the fourth intercostal space at the sternal border extending laterally to the right chest and the midaxillary line with the patient in supine position with the head of the bed between 0° to 45°s.

The pressure bag (Figure 9–3) should encase a bag of normal saline and be inflated to 300 mm Hg. If blood is noted to be flowing back into the system, the pressure is inadequate. Inadequate pressure may be due to an empty bag of normal saline, initially inadequate inflation of the pressure bag or later deflation of the pressure bag from leaks; or the tubing connected to the catheter might be disconnected from the circuit.

Gas Delivery Systems

Flowmeters (Figure 9–4) measure the flow rate of the gas (usually medical air or oxygen) attached to the meter. Medical air or compressed air is filtered atmospheric air (ie, 21% oxygen, yellow-coded

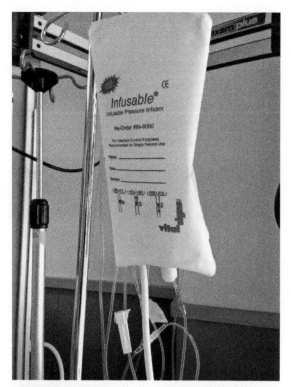

FIGURE 9–3 Pressure bag.

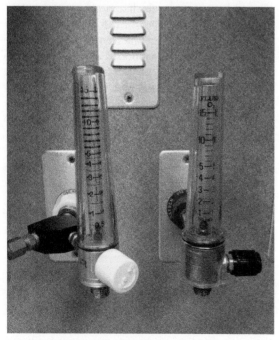

FIGURE 9–4 Flowmeters. Compressed air (color-coded yellow) on the left; oxygen (color-coded green) on the right.

outlet) and its clinical uses include nebulizer treatments, providing clean air in ventilators, and powering air-driven medical equipment. Oxygen is 100% oxygen (green-coded outlet).

Nasal cannulae deliver oxygen at flow rates of 0.5 to 6 L/min and are generally more comfortable for patients than face masks, making talking and eating easier. Although it can be approximated that the fraction of inspired oxygen (FIO_2) increases by 0.03 to 0.04 per increase of 1 L/min in oxygen flow rate, this estimate is usually inaccurate as FIO_2 also depends on the patient's tidal volume, inspiratory flow rate, respiratory rate, and the volume of the nasopharynx.[3] Nasal cannulae are effective in the setting of mouth breathing since inspiratory air flow occurs while breathing through the mouth which causes entrainment of oxygen from the nose via the posterior pharynx.[3] A bubble canister (Figure 9–5) for humidification should be used when patients require more than 4 L of oxygen to minimize irritation of nasal and oropharyngeal mucosa.

A simple face mask or variable performance mask delivers oxygen at flow rates of 5 to 8 L/min with a corresponding FIO_2 of 0.40 and 0.60, respectively.[4] The mask has holes on either side for entrainment of air and venting of exhaled gas but rebreathing may occur if the expiratory pause is absent. The FIO_2

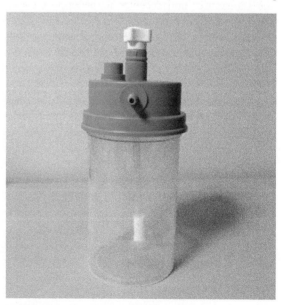

FIGURE 9–5 Bubble canister for delivery of humidified oxygen therapy or nebulizer treatments.

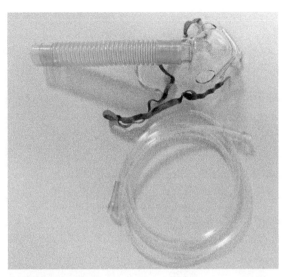

FIGURE 9-6A Venturi-style face mask.

delivered is variable according to flow rate, pattern and rate of ventilation, inspiratory flow rate, and fit of mask and should not be used in patients who require a fixed oxygen concentration.[3]

The air-entrainment or Venturi mask (Figure 9–6A) delivers a predetermined and fixed oxygen concentration mechanistically by the Bernoulli principle. The mask comes with color-coded concentration dials or dilator jets labeled with the corresponding oxygen flow rate required for the desired fixed delivery of oxygen concentration ranging from 24% to 60%. The differently colored dilator nozzles (Figure 9–6B) have apertures of varying

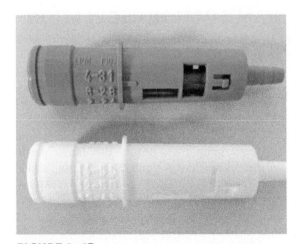

FIGURE 9-6B Color-coded concentration nozzles.

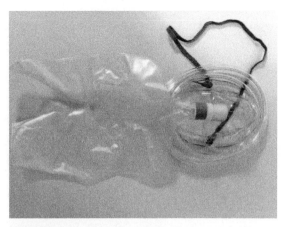

FIGURE 9-7 Non-rebreather face mask.

size that control the amount of atmospheric air entrained (a smaller nozzle entrains more room air and delivers lower F_{IO_2}) and subsequently the amount of inspired oxygen delivered to the patient. Expired gas rapidly exits the mask due to high flow rates and rebreathing does not occur.[3]

A non-rebreather mask (Figure 9–7) has 3 one-way valves in order to provide an inspired oxygen concentration of 100% and to allow venting of exhaled gas and prohibit entrainment of room air.[4] However they usually deliver less than 100% (eg, ~60%-80%) F_{IO_2} due to entrainment of room air since a completely sealed face mask could result in asphyxiation. Non-rebreather masks should not be used for extended periods of time given risk of absorption atelectasis and oxygen toxicity.

The bag valve mask (BVM) (often called an Ambu bag) is a portable device that provides intermittent positive-pressure ventilation with a self-inflating bag and one-way valve (Figure 9–8). The valve has 3 distinct ports: an inspiratory inlet which permits the entry of fresh gas during inspiration, an expiratory outlet for the exit of exhaled gas, and a connection to the face mask or endotracheal tube.[3]

While specifications may vary according to the manufacturer, the volume of an adult-sized BVM is 2100 mL. The average stroke volume delivered with one hand is 600 mL and using two hands yields 900 mL. A reservoir bag or corrugated tube is attached to the tubing and should be fully extended to its maximum length for maximum concentration of oxygen (90%

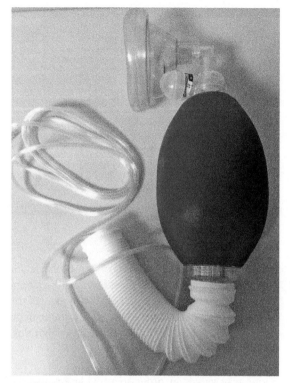

FIGURE 9–8 Bag valve mask (Ambu bag).

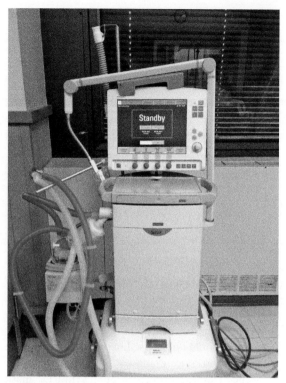

FIGURE 9–9 Ventilator with humidifier on the left and gas tubing on the right.

for reservoir bag and 100% for corrugated tube). The recommended oxygen flow rate is 15 L/min. Patients that need PEEP to maintain oxygenation (eg, adult respiratory distress syndrome [ARDS]) and require BVM ventilation during disconnection from mechanical ventilation (eg, for transport, ventilator troubleshooting) should be ventilated with a BVM containing a built-in PEEP valve or with a PEEP valve added to the exhalation port of the BVM. This PEEP valve is adjusted to provide the current level of PEEP set on the ventilator and maintain oxygenation during BVM.

BASIC VENTILATOR SETUP

The mechanical ventilator circuit includes a conventional humidifier or disposable heat and moisture exchangers to minimize the drying effect of gases that flow from the ventilator since the natural humidification of gas that occurs in the upper airways is circumvented by endotracheal intubation.

The yellow tubing for compressed air and the green tubing for oxygen delivery that exit the back of the ventilator should be attached to the appropriate wall outlets (Figures 9–9 and 9–10).

WALL SUCTION REGULATION

Disposable wall suction (Figure 9–11) is most commonly used in the ICU setting and can be attached to orogastric (OG) or nasogastric (NG) tubes, abdominal sump drains, or chest drainage systems. Low intermittent suction is used for small-bore OG and NG tubes to minimize damage to the gastric mucosa. Low continuous suction is used with OG or NG Salem sump drains because they have an additional air vent which prevents the drain from adhering to the gastric mucosa due to force of suction.

The suction regulator displays the degrees of suction (low, medium, high, and full vacuum) and dials to select the degree of suction and intermittent versus continuous suction (Figure 9–12). If the

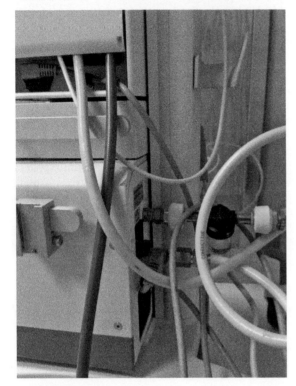

FIGURE 9–10 Compressed air (yellow) and oxygen (green) outlets from the wall (right) and entering the back of the ventilator (left).

suction is not working, disconnect from the drainage canister and feel for suction flow; make sure that caps and lids are secured tightly on the collection canister.

INFUSION DEVICES

Smart pumps are the standard of care for administering intravenous therapy in order to maximize patient safety. The device incorporates computerized dose error reduction software with a library of intravenous drugs and fluids and their administration rate limits.[5] Patient data is first entered

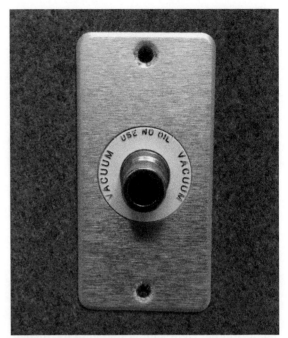

FIGURE 9–11 Vacuum outlet.

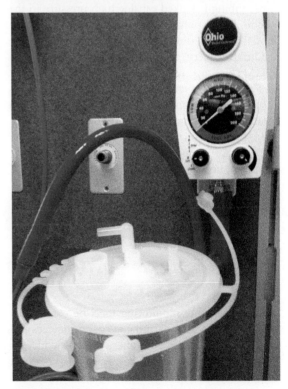

FIGURE 9–12 Wall suction setup displaying the suction regulator attached to the collection canister below.

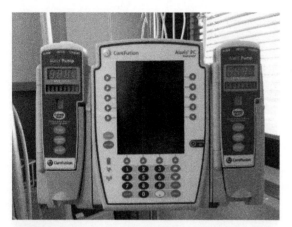

FIGURE 9–13 Smart pumps attached to a central module.

into the computer module followed by selection of the drug or fluid and its concentration and rate; if the rate selected is predetermined to be unsafe, the pump will not allow administration of the therapy. Pumps may alarm if air is detected in the tubing or if the tubing is kinked causing high pressure in the circuit. Smart pumps are capable of many infusion modalities including large-volume pump, syringe or epidural delivery, and patient-controlled analgesia (PCA) (Figure 9–13).

PCA can be ordered as a basal or continuous infusion, patient-initiated boluses only, or both an established basal rate with intermittent boluses. The PCA prescription is entered into the smart pump and should include whether the patient is opiate naive, normal, or tolerant, the concentration of medication, basal rate, loading dose, demand dose, lockout interval, and cumulative dose limit over 1 or more hours.

EXTERNAL TEMPERATURE CONTROL DEVICES

Core temperature monitoring must be continuous when using external warming or cooling devices and can be obtained from pulmonary artery, bladder, or esophageal temperature probes. The Bair Hugger is a forced-air warming blanket that can raise a patient's core temperature 2°C to 3°C an hour by delivering warm airstreams onto the patient's skin.[1]

Traditional cooling or hypothermic blankets utilize a reservoir filled with distilled water that is cooled to the targeted temperature that flows to the blanket through hoses. The device can be turned off manually or automatically once the desired body temperature is reached; however, the patient's temperature probe must be connected to the cooling blanket in order for the unit to function in automatic mode.[1]

SEQUENTIAL COMPRESSION DECOMPRESSION DEVICES

Sequential compression decompression devices (SCDs) are used to reduce the risk of deep venous thrombosis and consist of garments or bladders applied to the calves and a pump system (Figure 9–14). The garments come in 3 sizes—small, medium, and extra large. Foot pumps are available for patients who require a size beyond extra large.

The compression cycle entails 40 mm Hg of pressure applied for 12 seconds followed by deflation for 48 seconds. The alternate leg then undergoes a compression/decompression cycle 30 seconds after deflation is completed for the preceding leg. The skin under the bladder should be cleaned each nursing shift, as excess moisture can be associated with skin damage.

Contraindications to pneumatic compression include severe vascular disease, active wounds involving the lower extremities, conditions that could deteriorate due to augmented preload, and known or suspected (eg, after acute pulmonary embolism) deep venous thrombosis.

BED ELECTRONICS

Modern critical care beds have many capabilities including measuring patient weight, providing chest physiotherapy, promoting patient mobility, and reducing the incidence of pressure ulcers and ventilator-associated pneumonia (Figures 9–15 through 9–17).

Weights are determined after zeroing the bed and are stored in the electronic interface. The bed should be kept at the lowest height to maximize patient safety and reduce the risk of falls and can be

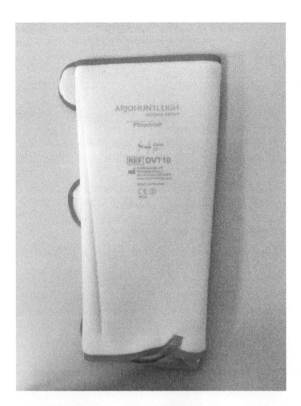

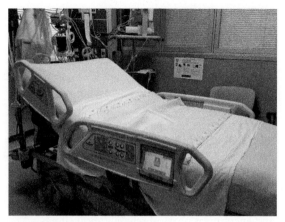

FIGURE 9–15 Critical care bed.

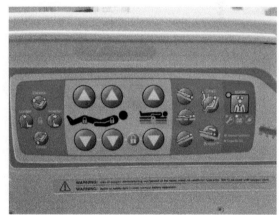

FIGURE 9–16 Bed positions.

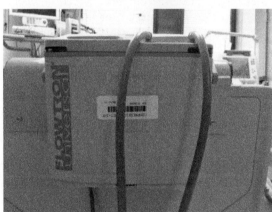

FIGURE 9–14 Sequential compression decompression (SCD) device. Bladder (top) and pump (bottom).

locked so that patients are unable to modify the bed position. Patients who are spontaneously breathing should be in the sitting position to optimize their respiratory status. Mechanically ventilated patients should have the head of bed elevated to 30° to enhance diaphragmatic excursion, decrease

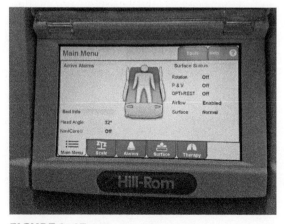

FIGURE 9–17 Bed control panel.

intrathoracic pressure, and aid in preventing aspiration and ventilator-associated pneumonia.

Continuous lateral rotation therapy causes rotation of the bed by an arc of 30° to 50° in increments of 8 cycles/h with the dual goal of decreasing pooled secretions that may lead to pneumonia and possibly preventing pressure ulcers. The pressure redistribution mattress also functions to reduce pressure-related skin damage. Percussion and vibration is denoted as "P&V" on the main menu and can be selected to improve pulmonary hygiene.

Removing the foot of the bed and placing the bed in a chair position can facilitate exiting the bed and encourages physical rehabilitation efforts.

REFERENCES

1. Lynn-McHale Wiegand DJ, ed. *AACN Procedure Manual for Critical Care*. 6th ed. St. Louis, MO: Elsevier; 2011.
2. Reich DL, ed. *Monitoring in Anesthesia and Perioperative Care*. 1st ed. New York, NY: Cambridge University Press; 2011.
3. Al-Shaikh B, Stacey S. *Essentials of Anaesthetic Equipment*. 2nd ed. London, UK: Churchill Livingstone; 2002.
4. O'Donnell JM, Nacul FE, eds. *Surgical Intensive Care Medicine*. 2nd ed. New York, NY: Springer; 2010.
5. Harding AD. Intravenous smart pumps. *J Infus Nurs*. 2013;36(3):191-194.

Physical Examination in the ICU

10

Ella Illuzzi, RN, ANP-BC and Mark Gillespie, PA-C, MS

KEY POINTS

1 The key to a good physical exam in critically ill patients is the ability to interface medical technology with the patient's clinical presentation.

2 Performing both planned and quick focused (ie, unplanned or emergent) exams can make the difference in timely diagnosis and

treatment, thus having a positive impact on patient outcome.

3 Acute and life-threatening situations in the intensive care unit are inevitable and timely examination is imperative. The initial visual assessment should take no more than 10 seconds.

The presence of advanced medical technology and sophisticated laboratory tests allow healthcare practitioners to provide the highest standard of care to patients particularly in the acute care setting. However, the importance of the physical examination should not be underestimated. The key to a good physical exam in the intensive care unit (ICU) setting is the ability to interface this medical technology with the patient's clinical presentation. Performing both planned and quick focused (ie, unplanned or emergent) exams can make the difference in timely diagnosis and treatment, thus having a positive impact on patient outcome.

Performing a physical exam in the ICU is often difficult. The bedside examination in an ICU may be hindered by various conditions. These include noisy alarms (eg, monitor, ventilator, IV pumps, etc), limited assessment due to sedation or analgesia, inability to easily change the patient's position, wounds, dressings and multiple invasive lines or tubes. Amid these obstacles, this exam should be performed quickly and efficiently. This chapter will demonstrate how to perform a physical examination on routine

assessment and in certain critical situations in the acute care setting.

PLANNED PHYSICAL EXAMINATION

Physical examination on daily rounds is a vital part of ICU management. Before performing a physical exam, review the patient's chart; obtain a history and gather information from the patient, relatives, medical staff, or review of notes. For all patients whether awake or unresponsive, it is best to begin the exam by introducing yourself and explaining what you intend to do. In the ICU, it is easy to divert attention from the patient and focus on the alarming monitors and machines. The main focus should remain on the patient's clinical presentation while integrating information from the monitors and diagnostic tests. The patient's current illness and status will prioritize the exam. Use a structured method to the examination by reviewing all major organ systems; this will avoid omitting important information. Accurate documentation of physical exam findings will identify trends or any change in a patient's clinical status.

Central Nervous System

Frequent evaluation of pain, sedation and delirium in the ICU is generally underestimated. There are various scales to assess level of sedation and pain and choosing 2 reliable scales, for example the Sedation-Agitation Scale (SAS)[1] (Table 10-1) to assess the level of sedation and the Wong-Baker FACES Pain Rating Scale[2] to communicate how much pain the patient is experiencing. In the ICU, most patients are unable to self-report pain or communicate, which makes this exam more challenging. If the patient cannot participate in this exam then look for signs of pain such as facial cues, restlessness/positioning, and/or physiological changes (rise in heart rate and blood pressure). However, vital signs are not used solely to assess for pain. Make note of the analgesic or sedative agent the patient is receiving, titrate and taper to maintain goal. In an adult ICU, light levels of sedation are recommended and daily interruptions can reduce the amount of time on a ventilator and the ICU stay.[3]

Critically ill patients may be obtunded, agitated, or delirious. For patients who are not sedated, assess whether they are alert and oriented. For critically ill patients, the cause in cognitive impairment can be variable and include, but is not limited to, metabolic disturbances or medications such as analgesics and sedatives. According to the 2013 clinical practice guidelines for Pain, Agitation, and Delirium (PAD), delirium should be assessed daily in mechanically ventilated patients.[4] Delirium can occur in nearly 60% to 80% of mechanically ventilated patients and is associated with increased mortality in the ICU and long-term cognitive impairment.[4] Adult ICU patients can be assessed for delirium by using The Confusion Assessment Method for the ICU (CAM-ICU)[5] (Figure 10-1).

Patients admitted to the ICU with intracranial pathology should have a more focused and detailed neurological assessment adjusted to their diagnosis and presentation. For all patients, pupils should be checked for size, equality, and reaction to light.

Respiratory System

Routine examination of the respiratory includes examining the airway and auscultating the lungs. Further evaluation includes inspecting the patient's overall appearance, work of breathing, accessory muscle use, bilateral chest rise, oxygen saturation, and arterial blood gas findings. The patient may require supplemental oxygen and the decision for such support (nasal cannula, nonrebreathing mask, noninvasive, and invasive ventilation) should be based on clinical presentation and laboratory findings.

TABLE 10-1 Riker sedation-agitation scale.

Score	Term	Descriptor
7	Dangerous agitation	Pulling at ET tube, trying to remove catheters, climbing over bedrail, striking at staff, thrashing side-to-side
6	Very agitated	Requiring restraint and frquent verbal reminding of limits, biting ETT
5	Agitated	Anxious or physically agitated, calms to verbal instructions
4	Calm and cooperative	Calm, easily arousable, follows commands
3	Sedated	Difficult to arouse but awakens to verbal stimuli or gentle shaking, follows simple commands but drifts off again
2	Very sedated	Arouses to physical stimuli but does not communicate or follow commands, may move spontaneously
1	Unarousable	Minimal or no response to noxious stimuli, does not communicate or follow commands

Reproduced with pemission from Riker RR, Picard JT, Fraser GL: Prospective evaluation of the Sedation-Agitation Scale for adult critically ill patients, *Crit Care Med* 1999 Jul;27(7):1325-1329.

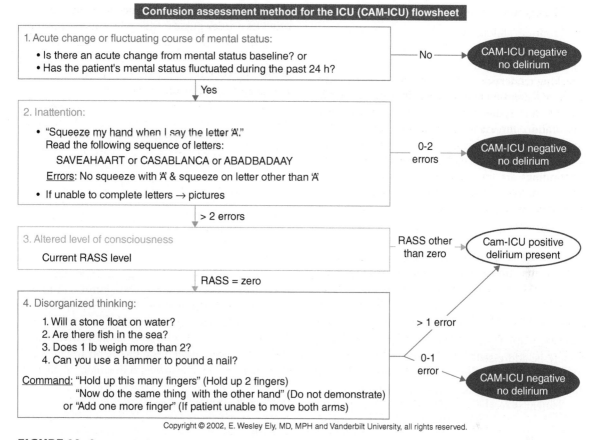

FIGURE 10-1 CAM-ICU.[5]

For intubated and mechanically ventilated patients, examine the endotracheal tube (ETT) position both on exam (eg, 21 cm at the lips) and on chest x-ray (CXR) (eg, ETT tip 5 cm above the carina) and review the ventilator settings and the output information. Basic ventilator settings include the ventilator mode, respiratory rate, tidal volume, fraction of inspired oxygen (FiO_2) and positive end expiratory pressure (PEEP). Make note of the measured or output tidal volumes, minute volumes, flow rate and peak, and plateau pressures. Other parameters to include during respiratory examination are correlating the patient's current condition with their chest x-ray, lung sonogram (if available), and any chest tubes or drains. Most importantly, take this opportunity to assess the readiness of the patient's ability to wean off the ventilator, which should be the ultimate daily goal.

Cardiovascular System

An assessment of the cardiovascular system should be obtained which includes auscultation of heart sounds, evaluation of pulses, capillary refill, and edema. Most ICU patients are continuously monitored with beat-by-beat measurements via the electrocardiogram (ECG) and blood pressure (via noninvasive cuff or invasive arterial catheter monitor). Use this information and integrate it with the patient's clinical status. Observe the medications, especially continuous infusions that the patient is receiving such as inotropic agents, vasopressors and antiarrhythmic medications. A bedside transthoracic echocardiogram is relatively quick and useful in the evaluation of the right and left ventricular function and can guide the use of intravenous fluids, vasopressors, or other cardiac agents.

Abdomen

The routine abdominal exam is very important, owing to the fact that it tends to mask infection. The abdomen should be thoroughly examined by checking tenderness, distention, and bowel sounds. Pay close attention to any surgical incisional sites or wounds for erythema or other signs of infection or perforation, for example, purulent, enteric, or bilious drainage. Make note of any drains or stomas and trend the output volumes and color. If clinical findings are consistent with abdominal hypertension or compartment syndrome, then perhaps intraabdominal pressure measurements may be further warranted.

The patient's nutritional status should be addressed including daily weights and whether the patient's nutritional needs are being met. Bowel function should also be noted and the output recorded.

Renal

The necessity for an indwelling urinary catheter should be addressed daily. A patient on strict input and output measurements should have recorded urine output hourly. Note the type of fluid therapy the patient is receiving and whether the amount or rate is accurate or appropriate based on the patient's clinical status, weight, cardiac status, and sensible and insensible fluid losses. Daily laboratory trends in renal function should be monitored and if indicated, assess the need for renal replacement therapy.

Skin

Points of particular interest during this exam are the color of the skin (cyanosis or pallor), temperature, and presence of any rash. In patients that have indwelling catheters (ventriculostomy or lumbar drains) and vascular access (central or arterial catheters), examine these sites routinely for signs of infection and determine whether the catheter is still indicated based on the patient's clinical status. Check common sites such as bony prominences and the sacrum for decubiti ulcers or evidence of skin break down.

In addition to the physical exam, recent laboratory tests, microbiology findings, imaging results, and current medications should be reviewed frequently for appropriate management of the critical care patient. Table 10–2, modified from Runcie et al[6] provides a quick guide for the physical examination.

UNPLANNED PHYSICAL EXAMINATION

Almost all ICU patients are continuously observed on cardiac and hemodynamic monitors, which is cornerstone of management in critically ill patients. Continuous observation of vital parameters such as heart rate, blood pressure, respiratory rate, and oxygen saturation allows the medical staff to stay apprised of any acute changes and the general condition of the patient.

Acute situations in the ICU are inevitable. In most instances, there are a plethora of possible diagnoses for a patient's presenting symptoms and time is of the essence. Therefore, thoughtful and timely examination is imperative. The following circumstances are frequent life-threatening conditions that may arise in the ICU that warrant immediate attention. A stepwise guide to follow upon reaching the bedside is provided below with the intent of offering a template that the reader may customize to their practice environment.

You Are Called to the Bedside for...

Acute Bradycardia

Visual examination—The first thing you do as you walk into the room is observe the patient, their overall condition (eg, level of distress) and whether or not they are on oxygen or mechanical ventilation. Glance at the monitor to assess the ECG rate and rhythm, arterial blood pressure, and waveform or the noninvasive blood pressure (NBP) reading (may need to be cycled), the pulse oximetry reading/waveform, and respiratory rate. This assessment should take less than 10 seconds.

Physical examination—Then look more closely at the patient and note the level of alertness and distress. Is the patient awake or unresponsive? Is the patient in no acute distress (NAD) or in distress? Quickly glance at the patient's skin and lips for signs of cyanosis. Manually check for a pulse. Does the monitor accurately reflect the patient's pulse and clinical condition? Is the patient showing signs and symptoms of hypoxia? Quickly auscultate the chest

TABLE 10–2 ICU guide for physical assessment.

System	Primary Variable	Interrelated or Secondary Variable
General	Overall appearance Acute distress Level of consciousness	Sedation
Central nervous system	Level of consciousness (SAS) Pain level (Wong-Baker Pain Scale) Neurologic function examination Focal neurologic examination CAM-ICU	Sedation Analgesia
Respiratory system	Physical examination Oxygen saturation Arterial blood gas (ABG) Ventilator settings Chest imaging (x-ray, CT scan, lung ultrasound)	Signs of respiratory distress Breath sounds Cyanosis (skin, lips) Chest drains/tubes FiO_2, PEEP, tidal volume, minute volumes, peak and plateau pressures, flow
Cardiovascular system	Physical examination EKG Echocardiogram Direct parameters	Assess tissue perfusion (mental status, skin temperature, capillary refill time, and urine output) Heart rate, arterial/noninvasive blood pressure
Abdomen	Abdominal examination GI function Nutrition	Tenderness, distention, bowel sounds Wounds/drains/stomas Nasogastric/orogastric tube output Bowel movements Enteral or parenteral feeding
Renal	Urine output and fluid status	Peripheral edema
Skin	Physical examination Color Temperature	Edema, rashes, pressure ulcers, vascular access sites, indwelling catheter sites Cyanosis, hemoglobin level, oxygen saturation Signs of infection
Catheters	Peripheral, central and arterial catheters, Foley catheter	
Tubes/drains	ETT, nasogastric/orogastric tube, chest tube, pigtail drain, Jackson-Pratt drain, Penrose drain, negative pressure wound therapy	
Laboratory/diagnostic tests		
Medications		

Data from Runcie CJ, Dougall JR. Assessment of the critically ill patient, *Br J Hosp Med* 1990;43(1):74-76.

for bilateral breath sounds and verify that the patient is receiving adequate oxygenation and ventilation. Is the patient on a ventilator or breathing spontaneously? If the patient is on a ventilator look for the following: What are the settings? Do the ventilator inputs (ie, tidal volume) match the outputs? Are the alarms going off? If so, which alarms- high pressure, low pressure, and/or low tidal volume? What is the breathing pattern and are the ventilator waveforms synchronous or dyssynchronous? Also, is the patient receiving the set tidal volume? Does the patient's ETT or tracheostomy need to be suctioned?

Acute management—If the patient is awake and in NAD, spontaneously breathing, not hypotensive and no complaints, obtain a 12 lead ECG and analyze rhythm, perform further testing if necessary, assess for drug-induced causes, and discontinue the offending medication depending on the diagnosis and clinical scenario. If the patient is stable continue to monitor and observe closely. However, if the patient is unstable and symptomatic with a change in mental status, hypotension, and complaints of chest pain, then treatment should focus on optimizing the patient's hemodynamic status by initiation of the Advanced Cardiovascular Life Support (ACLS) protocol for bradyarrhythmia and treat the underlying cause.

If the underlying cause is hypoxia and the pulse oximeter shows desaturation, patient-ventilator dyssynchrony and/or the ventilator is alarming, refer to the section on *Acute Respiratory Distress*.

Acute Tachycardia

Visual exam—The first thing you do as you walk into the room is observe the patient and their overall condition. Observe the oxygen-ventilator-patient interface (are they connected to oxygen or the ventilator?). Glance at the monitor to assess the ECG rate and rhythm, the arterial blood pressure, and waveform or NBP reading and the pulse oximetry reading. This assessment should take less than 10 seconds.

Physical examination—Connect the oxygen or ventilator if disconnected. At the same time observe the patient and note the level of alertness and distress. Is the patient awake or unresponsive? Is the patient in NAD or in distress? Manually check the pulse. Does the monitor accurately reflect the patient's pulse and clinical condition? Simultaneously, assess the skin: hypothermic/hyperthermic, poor skin turgor, cold, and clammy. Is the patient febrile and/or in shock (hypovolemic, cardiogenic, obstructive, or distributive)?

Acute management—Obtain a 12-lead ECG and analyze rhythm. Your management will depend on the rhythm and whether the patient is stable or unstable. If the patient is stable then proceed with further testing if necessary, discontinue, and/or adjust medications depending on the diagnosis and clinical scenario and treat the underlying cause. If the patient is unstable, initiate the ACLS protocol, prepare for synchronized cardioversion and further pharmacologic treatment.

Acute Hypotension

Visual examination—The first thing you do as you walk into the room is observe the patient, the oxygen-ventilator-patient interface (are they connected to oxygen or the ventilator?) and glance at the monitor to assess the ECG rate and rhythm, the arterial blood pressure and waveform or the NBP reading, and the pulse oximetry reading. This assessment should take less than 10 seconds.

Physical examination—Connect the oxygen or ventilator if disconnected. Assess for accuracy of the blood pressure reading by checking cuff or arterial catheter placement. Note the mean arterial pressure and quickly check for signs of organ perfusion. At the same time, look at the patient and note their level of alertness and distress. Is the patient awake or unresponsive? Is the patient in NAD or in distress? Is there an arrhythmia associated with hypotension? Is the patient in shock (hypovolemic, cardiogenic, obstructive, or distributive)? Has the patient received any medications that can cause hypotension?

Acute management—If there is an arrhythmia associated with hypotension, obtain an ECG and analyze rhythm, perform further testing if necessary, assess for drug-induced causes, and discontinue the offending medication depending on the diagnosis and clinical scenario. If the patient is in truly in shock, begin resuscitation and treatment of the underlying cause. Perform a bedside echocardiogram to evaluate right and left ventricular function and volume status to direct treatment.

Acute Chest Pain

Visual examination—The first thing you do as you walk into the room is observe the patient and glance at the monitor to assess the ECG rate and rhythm, the arterial blood pressure and waveform or NBP reading, and the pulse oximetry reading. This assessment should take less than 10 seconds.

Physical examination—At the same time, look at the patient and note the level of alertness and distress. Is the patient awake or unresponsive? Is the patient in NAD or in distress?

If the patient can participate in the exam: Follow OPQRST algorithm: Onset of the event, provocation or palliation, quality of pain, region and radiation, severity, and time.

Acute management—Obtain 12-lead ECG for rhythm assessment specifically to rule out ST-changes, new onset left bundle branch block, or any arrhythmia. If EKG is noted for ST-elevation myocardial infarction, obtain an immediate cardiology consultation for possible need of emergent percutaneous catheter intervention. Make note of any arrhythmia (stable or unstable rhythm). If the patient is unstable and presumed cardiac ischemic etiology, start necessary pharmacologic treatment and initiate the ACLS protocol if needed. If the cause of chest pain is less likely due to cardiac etiology then rule out chest etiology. Auscultate bilateral breath sounds, assess for bilateral chest rise and perform an ultrasound of the chest to evaluate lung sliding or B-lines. Other unstable etiologies of acute chest pain that need to be considered include thoracic aneurysm, pulmonary embolus, pneumothorax, and mediastinitis. If the patient is stable, consider ultrasound, computed tomography (CT) scan and/or ventilation perfusion scan of the chest. If a pneumothorax is present, determine if the patient is stable or unstable. If the patient is unstable and experiencing signs of obstructive shock, immediate intervention for decompression is warranted.

Acute Respiratory Distress (Not on a Ventilator)

Visual examination—The first thing you do as you walk into the room is observe the patient, are they connected to supplemental oxygen, if so what type? Then glance at the monitor to assess the ECG rate and rhythm, the arterial blood pressure and waveform or the NBP reading, respiratory rate, and the pulse oximetry reading. This assessment should take less than 10 seconds.

Physical examination—Apply supplemental oxygen as needed. At the same time, look at the patient and note their overall appearance, level of consciousness, skin color (cyanosis), work of breathing, accessory muscle use, airway resistance, airflow, and ability to speak in full sentences or not. Auscultate the lungs for any adventitious sounds, which may include the following: wheezing (asthma, bronchospasm), rales, or stridor. Has the patient been recently extubated and not tolerating it well? Has the patient had any recent intervention that may have caused a pneumothorax? Is the patient high risk for

pulmonary embolism and experiencing any associated symptoms? Is the patient exhibiting signs of anxiety and agitation? Is there any known previous pertinent medical history that could be attributing to this distress?

Acute management—If there are no signs of imminent respiratory failure, you have some time to retrieve an arterial blood gas sample, review valuable laboratory results and diagnostic findings (CXR or CT Chest) and bedside lung ultrasonography to assess for lung sliding to rule out pneumothorax, B-lines to rule out fluid overload and pleural effusion. This will help provide a list of differential diagnoses for the patient's respiratory status.

There are multiple strategies to treating a patient in respiratory distress whether it is close observation, medication, supplemental oxygenation, the need for an advanced airway, or an emergent intervention (chest tube thoracostomy). The patient's clinical status and arterial blood gas findings will help guide the management decisions.

Acute Respiratory Distress (on a Ventilator)

Visual examination—The first thing you do as you walk into the room is observe the patient and glance at the ETT or tracheostomy tube making sure it is connected and not dislodged. Then look at the monitor to assess the ECG rate and rhythm, the arterial blood pressure waveform or the NBP reading, and the pulse oximetry reading. Quickly look at the ventilator, its waveforms (tidal volume, pressure, and flow) and make note of which ventilator alarms are being triggered. This exam should take less than 10 seconds.

Physical examination—At the same time, look at the patient and note the overall appearance, level of consciousness, skin color (cyanosis), work of breathing, accessory muscle use, airway resistance, and airflow, and if there is ventilator synchrony versus dyssynchrony. Auscultate the lungs for bilateral and any adventitious sounds.

The main focus should always be on the patient rather than solely the ventilator. If the patient is rapidly deteriorating or abruptly unstable, disconnect the patient from the ventilator and hand ventilate with a bag valve mask providing 100% oxygen and use a PEEP valve if the patient was receiving PEEP. If the patient is orally intubated with an ETT, note the position of tube at lips or teeth. Check the cuff of the ETT and listen for a leak, if there is a leak, inflate air using an empty syringe to assess for adequate filling. Determine if the patient needs suctioning of their ETT from possible obstruction or mucous plug. If the patient has a tracheostomy, assess for adequate placement in airway, adequate cuff volume, and inner cannula for patency.

If there is enough time to troubleshoot the ventilator, observe the ventilator waveforms, settings and alarming parameters. The ventilator alarms that are being triggered will give insight to why the patient may be in respiratory distress. Common ventilator alarms are high pressure, low pressure, high/low minute volume, apnea, disconnection in the circuit, and high-exhaled tidal volume. Check the current settings: ventilator mode, tidal volume, respiratory rate, FiO_2, PEEP, and inspiratory to expiratory ratio. Make note of the measured tidal volumes, minute volumes, and peak and plateau pressures.

High-pressure alarms may indicate the following: mucus plug, pneumothorax, mainstream intubation, obstructed ETT (patient biting or mucus plug), asynchrony, or abdominal compartment syndrome affecting ability of adequate ventilation.

Low-pressure alarms may indicate the following: air leak, extubation, tube, or ventilator disconnection; note that there are many areas on the ventilator circuit tubing that can allow for a disconnection and the tubing must be examined carefully fully along its path.

Acute Lethargy/Unresponsiveness

Visual examination—The first thing you do as you walk into the room is observe the patient and glance at the monitor to assess the ECG rate and rhythm, the arterial blood pressure and waveform or the NBP reading, and the pulse oximetry reading. This assessment should take less than 10 seconds.

Physical examination—At the same time, look at the patient and note the level of consciousness and/or distress. If there is no contradiction, gently rub the patient's sternum with a closed fist to stimulate the patient. This will help assess whether they are awake, alert, and able to move extremities. Quickly assess the patient's pulses, extremities, and respiratory status. If the patient is receiving any sedative or analgesic, discontinue the offending agent and consider a pharmacologic reversal agent if indicated (flumazenil or naloxone).

Is there concern for hepatic encephalopathy or metabolic encephalopathy?

Is the patient in acute respiratory distress? Is the patient obtunded or experiencing signs of herniation?

Is the patient having a seizure? Assess pupillary response, eye movement, nystagmus, or spontaneous movement of bilateral eyes?

Is the patient exhibiting any signs or symptoms of a stroke (cerebral vascular accident/transient ischemic attack)? If the patient can cooperate with a neurological exam, assess for facial drooping, arm drift, and slurred speech.

Acute management—If the patient is unresponsive, unstable, or experiencing signs of a stroke, initiate the ACLS protocol. If the patient is obtunded or unable to protect their airway, then consider intubation and initiation of mechanical ventilation. If the patient is in respiratory distress, refer to the section above on *acute respiratory distress*. Support the patient and treat the underlying cause.

Seizure

Visual examination—The first thing you do as you walk into the room is observe the patient and glance at the monitor to assess the ECG rate and rhythm, the arterial blood pressure and waveform or the NBP reading, and the pulse oximetry reading. This assessment should take less than 10 seconds.

Physical examination—At the same time, look at the patient for abnormal movements or shaking and note the level of consciousness and/or distress. Perform a quick assessment of the patient's respiratory status. Some patients need an advanced airway for airway protection. Observe the type of seizure activity: partial seizure, tonic clonic seizure, grand mal seizure, or status epilepticus.

Acute management—Provide a safe environment and administer a first line agent, such as an intravenous benzodiazepine (lorazepam, midazolam, or diazepam). Do not place anything in the patient's mouth. Review current medications and possible side effects that may have precipitated the seizure. Obtain a neurology consultation. For ongoing status epilepticus, continue further seizure treatment and consider airway protection with intubation and mechanical ventilation.

Acute Extremity Symptom or Coolness

Visual examination—The first thing you do as you walk into the room is observe the patient and glance at the monitor to assess whether the vital signs are stable.

Physical examination—Is the patient in distress and experiencing severe pain, weakness, numbness, or paresthesias of the extremity? Is the patient at risk for ischemic limb or compartment syndrome? Does the patient have a history of vascular disease or recent vascular surgery in the affected extremity? Check for indwelling catheters (peripheral intravenous catheter and arterial catheters) that may cause vascular compromise. Has the patient any recent surgery or trauma to the affected extremity? Assess any surgical or nonsurgical dressings that may be compressing the area.

Perform a thorough assessment of the affected extremity's proximal and distal pulses, coolness and capillary refill. Consider using a doppler if the pulse is unable to be palpated.

Acute management—Remove any invasive catheter, dressing, cast or splint that may be compromising the extremity. For concerns of ischemia or compartment syndrome call the appropriate consult.

Acute Abdominal Distention

Visual examination—The first thing you do as you walk into the room is observe the patient and glance at the monitor to assess the ECG rate and rhythm, the arterial blood pressure and waveform or the NBP reading, and the pulse oximetry reading.

Physical examination—At the same time, look at the patient and note the level of alertness and distress. Is the patient awake or unresponsive, in NAD or in distress? Pay close attention to the patient's general appearance, examine for pain, and note any recent fevers. A patient with peritoneal irritation is likely to remain still, contrary to a patient with obstruction, who usually presents with restlessness. Assess the abdomen and skin. Has the patient had recent abdominal surgery? Recent large volume resuscitation? Risk for intra-abdominal bleeding? Recent anticoagulation and possible skin ecchymosis? Be sure to ask about the patient's last bowel movement or recent vomiting. Has the urine output abruptly decreased or was there a change in color? Does the patient have any intraabdominal surgical drains in

place and is there any fluid output? Are you having any difficulty ventilating the patient with oxygen? If the patient is on mechanical ventilation and experiencing respiratory distress and desaturation from inadequate ventilation, are the peak inspiratory pressures elevated? Is the patient experiencing signs of obstructive hypotension and shock?

Acute Management

If the patient is stable, consider an abdominal x-ray, CT scan, or surgical consult. Review medications that could be further potentiating an obstructive process or gastroparesis. Obtain an intra-abdominal pressure via bladder pressure measurement. If the etiology is primary abdominal compartment syndrome, immediate surgical intervention is required for abdominal decompression. For unstable patients, especially those experiencing signs of obstructive shock, provide adequate oxygenation, ventilation, and cardiovascular support.

Acute Anuria

Visual examination—The first thing you do as you walk into the room is observe the patient and glance at the monitor to assess the ECG rate and rhythm, the arterial blood pressure and waveform or the NBP reading, and the pulse oximetry reading.

Physical examination—At the same time, look at the patient and note their level of consciousness and/or distress. Check the Foley catheter for kinks and hand irrigate to assess patency. Evaluate the patient's volume status; is the patient volume depleted, hypoperfused, or has a low cardiac output? Is the patient hypotensive or in shock? Is there an obstruction? Is the patient exhibiting signs of acute renal failure?

Assess abdomen for distention, tenderness, rigidity, or a possible complication or failure of drains, such as an ileal conduit or nephrostomy tube. Obtain intra-abdominal pressures to rule out compartment syndrome. Review laboratory and chemistry information.

Acute management—If there in an indwelling urinary catheter, consider mechanical obstruction and frequently administer saline flushes to assure patency. Administer a fluid bolus challenge to assess the response to fluid. If the patient has oliguric or anuric acute renal failure further testing is required. Obtain a bedside renal ultrasound to assess for signs of obstruction, for example, bladder distension and hydronephrosis. If a patient's clinical status is deteriorating, consider a nephrology consultation and possible initiation of renal-replacement therapy.

REFERENCES

1. Riker RR, Picard JT, Fraser GL. Prospective evaluation of the Sedation-Agitation Scale for adult critically ill patients. *Crit Care Med.* 1999;27(7):1325-1329.
2. Foundation W-BF. Wong-Baker FACES® Pain Rating Scale. 2015; http://www.WongBakerFACES.org. Accessed October, 2015.
3. Girard TD, Kress JP, Fuchs BD, et al. Efficacy and safety of a paired sedation and ventilator weaning protocol for mechanically ventilated patients in intensive care (Awakening and Breathing Controlled trial): a randomised controlled trial. *Lancet.* 2008;371(9607):126-134.
4. Barr J, Fraser GL, Puntillo K, et al. Clinical practice guidelines for the management of pain, agitation, and delirium in adult patients in the intensive care unit. *Crit Care Med.* 2013;41(1):263-306.
5. Ely EW, Margolin R, Francis J, et al. Evaluation of delirium in critically ill patients: validation of the Confusion Assessment Method for the Intensive Care Unit (CAM-ICU). *Crit Care Med.* 2001;29(7):1370-1379.
6. Runcie CJ, Dougall JR. Assessment of the critically ill patient. *Br J Hosp Med.* 1990;43(1):74-76.

Imaging of the Critically Ill Patient: Radiology

11

Nida Qadir, MD and Roshen Mathew, MD

KEY POINTS

1 Chest radiography is particularly useful in the initial placement, positioning of invasive hardware, and for monitoring of complications postprocedure in critically ill patients.

2 Contrast imaging should be used judiciously in critically ill patients. Computed tomography (CT) with contrast helps further evaluation of lung parenchyma and pulmonary vascular lesions.

3 Atelectasis and pneumonia are common causes of respiratory failure in the intensive care unit (ICU). Unrecognized it can progresses to cavitation and abscess formation.

4 High probability ventilation perfusion scans have good positive predictive value for Pulmonary Embolism, and is in par with CT Pulmonary Angiography which show intraluminal filling defects for the same.

5 Pulmonary edema and acute respiratory distress syndrome (ARDS) may have similar radiologic features but have a different time of onset, presentation, and its ensuing clinical progression.

6 Bedside ultrasound is a convenient option for the evaluation and drainage of the pleural space.

IMAGING PROCEDURES

Imaging is an essential tool in the clinical assessment and management of critically ill patients. Although bedside ultrasound and chest radiography are the mainstays of initial assessment, an extensive variety of imaging options are available to the physician in the ICU, including CT, magnetic resonance imaging (MRI), and nuclear medicine studies. Interventional procedures, either at the bedside or in the radiology suite, are also playing an increasingly important role in the management of critical illness.

The choice of a particular imaging modality is occasionally difficult and should be based on recommendations in the literature, local expertise, type of equipment available, and the experience of the radiologists. Given the increasing emphasis on cost-effective practice, clinicians and radiologists must maximize the diagnostic and therapeutic yield of procedures while minimizing costs. The main indications, strengths, and weaknesses of imaging modalities used in common ICU scenarios are reviewed in this chapter. Although abdominal, neurologic, and musculoskeletal imaging studies play an important role in the care of the critically ill patient, this chapter will focus primarily on imaging of the chest and devices used in the ICU.

IMAGING TECHNIQUES
Plain Radiography

Portable chest radiographs are the most commonly requested imaging examination in the ICU. Despite their limitations, these films play an important role in the management of ICU patients. Chest radiographs are used to identify and follow pulmonary and cardiac disorders as well as evaluate the positions of and complications from catheters and support devices used in the care of critically ill patients.

Imaging of the abdomen can also often begin with plain radiographs, which provide a readily accessible means of diagnosing perforation, bowel obstruction, and ileus. However, because the overall sensitivity of plain radiographs remains low, further imaging with CT is frequently necessary to confirm suspected pathology and to inspect the features of the bowel walls and surrounding fat. Supine radiographs are appropriate for verifying nasogastric or feeding tube placement and for initial investigation of renal stones and ileus or bowel obstruction. Additional views obtained with the patient in a semiupright or lateral decubitus position are used to show air-fluid levels in the gastrointestinal tract or free intraperitoneal gas and may be helpful in patients with suspected bowel perforation or obstruction.

Ultrasound

Ultrasound examination at the bedside in the ICU is relatively inexpensive and does not use ionizing radiation. In the thorax, ultrasound is useful in imaging lung consolidation, pleural-based masses and effusions, pneumothorax, and diaphragmatic dysfunction. It can identify complex or loculated effusions and be used as a guide to thoracentesis or thoracostomy tube insertion.

In the abdomen, ultrasound provides for rapid evaluation of hepatobiliary and genitourinary disease, as well as assessment of vascular structures such as the aorta and the inferior vena cava. Similar to its use in the thorax, ultrasound can be used for identification and qualitative assessment of intraperitoneal fluid, as well as a guide for paracentesis.

In addition to its use in pleural and peritoneal fluid aspiration, ultrasound can be used as a tool in a multitude of bedside procedures such as central line placement, pulmonary artery catheterization, biopsies, and drainage of fluid collections. Its use in cardiac and hemodynamic assessment is becoming increasingly important in critical care.

Computed Tomography

By virtue of multiplanar imaging capabilities and improved contrast resolution, multidetector CT (MDCT) has been shown to be very valuable in increasing diagnostic accuracy and guiding therapeutic procedures for critically ill patients. MDCT allows for more rapid scanning of patients, with imaging of the entire chest, abdomen, and pelvis with thin sections during a single breath-hold. Such short acquisition times have facilitated the use of CT for evaluation of vascular disorders such as aortic dissection and pulmonary embolism. CT is a critical diagnostic tool for the evaluation of an acute abdomen and also allows for improved characterization of pulmonary diseases.

Transportation of the ICU patient to the CT scanner poses significant risks and requires a coordinated effort from hospital personnel, including ICU physicians and nurses, respiratory therapists, radiology technologists, and radiologists. Careful monitoring during transport and throughout the procedure is essential and should be performed by a dedicated team skilled in airway management and resuscitation.

Nuclear Scintigraphy

Nuclear scintigraphy has a number of applications in the critically ill patient. Myocardial perfusion and infarct scanning in cardiac disease, ventilation-perfusion scanning in patients with suspected pulmonary embolism, evaluation of gastrointestinal hemorrhage and acute cholecystitis, and localization of occult infection are among the most common indications for radionuclide imaging in the ICU patient.

Magnetic Resonance Imaging

MRI provides excellent differentiation of vascular and nonvascular structures without the use of intravenous contrast material or ionizing radiation and provides cross-sectional images in multiple planes. It is generally considered the single best imaging method for evaluation of the central nervous system (CNS), head and neck, liver, and musculoskeletal system. However, in many cases, MRI is not feasible in the evaluation of the critically ill patient because of interference caused by ferromagnetic monitoring devices, the difficulty of adequately ventilating and monitoring patients within the narrow MRI gantry, and long scan times. MRI may be appropriate in selected diagnostic dilemmas if MR-compatible equipment and coordinated effort among caregivers can be arranged.

IODINATED CONTRAST AGENTS

Peripheral venous access, particularly in an antecubital or large forearm vein is the preferred route of contrast agent administration in imaging. The flow rate should be appropriate for the gauge of the catheter used; a 20-gauge or larger catheter is preferable for flow rates of 3 mL/s or higher. When peripheral access is difficult, existing central venous catheters (CVCs) may be considered, provided that certain precautions are followed. First, catheter placement should be confirmed prior to its use, and its integrity and patency should be checked before and after injection. Additionally, flow rates greater than 2.5 mL/s should be avoided in order to keep intraluminal pressures below most manufacturers' specified limits; this flow rate limitation may in turn produce a suboptimal study. Finally, contrast media should not be administered by a power injector unless permitted by the manufacturer's specifications because of the risk of catheter breakage. Hospital personnel should be knowledgeable about the specific catheters used at their institution and adapt their practice accordingly.

Adverse reactions to iodinated contrast agents occur at low rates but are encountered not infrequently given their widespread use. Idiosyncratic reactions range from benign urticaria to, very rarely, life-threatening hypotension, laryngeal edema, and bronchospasm. These events are not considered truly allergic in nature because they are not antibody mediated and are inconsistently reproducible with subsequent administrations. Prior allergy-like reaction to contrast media is associated with an up to 5-fold increased likelihood of the patient experiencing a subsequent reaction. A history of asthma or other allergic diatheses may also predispose individuals to reactions. The predictive value of allergy to shellfish, previously thought to be helpful, is now recognized to be unreliable.

In high-risk patients, pretreatment with steroids should be given beginning at least 6 hours prior to the injection of contrast media whenever possible. Supplemental administration of an H_1 antihistamine

(eg, diphenhydramine) may reduce the frequency of urticaria, angioedema, and respiratory symptoms. Although pretreatment with corticosteroids appears to be effective for mild events, no randomized controlled clinical trials have demonstrated premedication protection against severe life-threatening adverse reactions. In the latter situation, an alternative imaging modality such as MRI should be considered.

Contrast-induced nephropathy (CIN) is another important complication of intravascular iodinated contrast use. The most important risk factor for CIN is preexisting renal insufficiency. Multiple other predisposing factors have been proposed, including diabetes mellitus, dehydration, cardiovascular disease, advanced age, and exposure to multiple doses of iodinated contrast in a short time interval (< 24 hours), but these have not been rigorously confirmed as independent risk factors. There is no specific creatinine or estimated glomerular filtration rate (eGFR) level that absolutely precludes the use of contrast agents; the decision to use contrast must be made on a case-by-case basis, carefully weighing the need for the study in high-risk patients. The major preventive action against CIN is to ensure adequate hydration with isotonic fluid. Substitution of sodium bicarbonate for 0.9% saline or addition of N-acetylcysteine to intravenous hydration is controversial. Multiple studies and a number of meta-analyses have had disparate results and neither strategy can be definitively recommended.

If CIN does develop, its clinical course depends on a number of variables, including baseline renal function, coexisting risk factors, and degree of hydration. Serum creatinine usually begins to rise within 24 hours of intravascular iodinated contrast medium administration, peaks within 4 days, and often returns to baseline within 7 to 10 days. Progression to end-stage renal disease is exceptionally rare and usually develops in the setting of multiple risk factors.

IMAGING OF SUPPORT AND MONITORING DEVICES

Endotracheal and Tracheostomy Tubes

Both endotracheal intubation and tracheostomy may cause potentially serious complications. Malpositioning of the endotracheal tube (ETT) occurs in approximately 15% of endotracheal intubations. The clinical assessment of tube location is frequently inaccurate, and a chest radiograph should be obtained immediately following intubation. With the neck in neutral position, the ideal position of the tube tip is 5 to 7 cm above the carina; flexion of the head and neck causes a 2-cm descent of the tip of the tube, whereas extension of the head and neck causes a 2-cm ascent of the tip. In 90% of patients, the carina projects between the fifth and seventh thoracic vertebrae on the portable radiograph; when the carina cannot be clearly seen, the ideal positioning of the ETT is at the T2-T4 level. The aortic arch also may be used to estimate tube location because the carina is typically at the level of the undersurface of the aortic arch. If the ETT is too high, there is a risk of either inadvertent extubation or hypopharyngeal intubation, which can cause ineffective ventilation, gastric distention, or vocal cord injury. If the ETT is too low, selective intubation of the right mainstem bronchus may occur, resulting in segmental or complete collapse of the left lung,

hyperinflation of the right lung, and possible pneumothorax (Figure 11–1). The balloon cuff should fill but not dilate the trachea. Cuff overinflation can cause tracheal injury, including tracheomalacia, tracheal stenosis, or acute tracheal rupture.

Inadvertent placement of the ETT into the esophagus is uncommon but may be catastrophic when it does occur. Esophageal intubation may be difficult to diagnose on the portable chest film because the esophagus frequently projects over the tracheal air column. Gastric or distal esophageal distention, location of the tube lateral to the tracheal air column, and deviation of the trachea secondary to an overinflated intraesophageal balloon cuff are radiographic signs of esophageal intubation. The right posterior oblique view with the patient's head turned to the right allows ease of separation of the esophagus and trachea and can be obtained in equivocal cases.

Tracheostomy is typically performed in the patient who requires relatively long-term ventilatory support. The tip of the tracheostomy tube should be

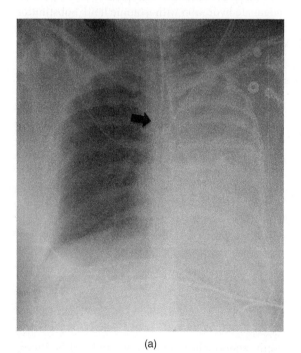

(a)

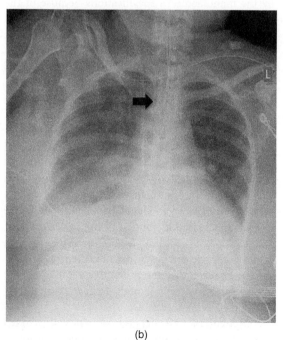

(b)

FIGURE 11–1 Right mainstem intubation. **A.** Placement of the endotracheal tube (*arrow*) into the right mainstem bronchus with resulting collapse of the left lung. **B.** Reexpansion of the left lung after retraction of the endotracheal tube.

located at approximately one-half to two-thirds of the distance from the stoma to the carina, and unlike the ETT's position, the tracheostomy tube's position is not changed by extension or flexion of the patient's head. Although small amounts of subcutaneous emphysema and pneumomediastinum may be seen after an uncomplicated tracheostomy tube placement, significant emphysema may be a sign of tracheal perforation. Pneumothorax can occur after tracheostomy tube placement and may also be a sign of tracheal perforation. Late complications include tracheal stenosis, stomal infection, aspiration, tube occlusion, and development of a fistula between the trachea and esophagus, pleura, or mediastinum. The fistula is caused by erosion through the posterior tracheal membrane and usually occurs at the level of the tracheal cuff. If the fistula develops below the level of the cuff, gastric contents may be aspirated into the lungs. If the fistula develops above the level of the cuff, gastric contents may collect in the upper trachea.

Central Venous Catheters

CVCs are used frequently in the ICU patient for venous access, monitoring central venous pressure, and hemodialysis. The subclavian, internal jugular, and femoral veins are the sites of venous access used most commonly; smaller-caliber central catheters can also be peripherally inserted via antecubital veins. CVCs inserted via a thoracic vein are visible on the chest radiograph, and knowledge of normal thoracic venous anatomy is required to assess catheter location. The subclavian vein originates by the lateral aspect of the first rib and courses posterior to the clavicle, and anterior to the first rib. The internal jugular vein courses vertically in the neck; its convergence with the subclavian vein to form the brachiocephalic vein usually occurs behind the sternal end of the corresponding clavicle. Whereas the right brachiocephalic vein has a vertical course as it forms the superior vena cava, the left brachiocephalic vein crosses the mediastinum from left to right in a retrosternal position to enter the superior vena cava. The superior vena cava is formed by the junction of the right and left brachiocephalic veins at the level of the first anterior intercostal space, with its upper border usually just superior to the angle of the right mainstem bronchus and the trachea. On a chest radiograph, the junction of the superior vena cava and right atrium lies approximately 4 cm below the carina, or 1 to 2 cm below the superior right heart border. CVCs are optimally positioned when the tip within the superior vena cava, ideally slightly above the right atrium.

Appropriate catheter position must be verified radiographically, as malposition has been described in up to 40% of CVCs. Positioning of the catheter tip within the right atrium is common and may result in cardiac perforation and tamponade. Placement into the right ventricle may result in arrhythmias secondary to irritation of the endocardium or interventricular septum. A misplaced CVC may have its tip terminating in central systemic veins, which can result in inaccurate venous pressure readings as well as venous thrombosis or venous wall perforation. The most common location for a misplaced catheter entering the subclavian vein is the ipsilateral internal jugular vein. Less frequently, thoracic CVCs may enter the azygous, internal mammary, superior intercostal (Figure 11–2), thymic, left pericardiophrenic, or inferior thyroid veins. Looping, knotting, and kinking of the catheter may also occur (Figure 11–3), which can place mechanical stress on the vein and occasionally require removal by surgical or interventional radiology techniques.

Other complications of central venous catheterization include pneumothorax, hemothorax,

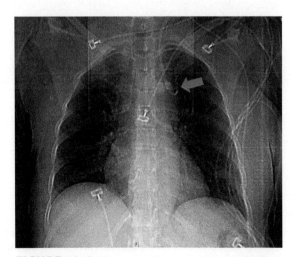

FIGURE 11–2 Placement of central venous catheter in the left superior intercostal vein (*red arrow*).

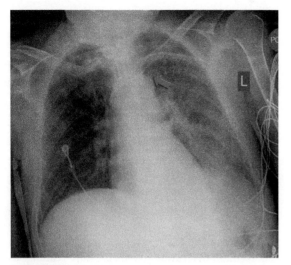

FIGURE 11–3 Chest radiograph showing a central venous catheter forming a loop in the left brachiocephalic vein and terminating in the subclavian vein (*arrow*).

and perforation, which may result in pericardial effusion, hydrothorax, mediastinal hemorrhage, or ectopic infusion of intravenous solutions (Figure 11–4). Less common complications include

air embolism and catheter fracture or embolism. Pneumothorax occurs in up to 5% of CVC insertions; the incidence of is higher with a subclavian approach than with an internal jugular approach. Pneumothorax may be clinically occult, and a chest radiograph should be obtained to exclude a pneumothorax following line placement. A radiograph should be obtained even following an unsuccessful attempted line placement.

Venous air embolism is an uncommon complication of central venous catheterization. Radiographically, air in the main pulmonary artery is diagnostic, but other features include focal oligemia, pulmonary edema, and atelectasis. Intracardiac air or air within the pulmonary artery is seen easily on CT.

Long-term complications of venous access devices include delayed perforation, pinch-off syndrome, thrombosis, catheter knotting, and catheter fragmentation. Left-sided catheters have a greater risk for perforation, with increased risk in catheters abutting the right lateral wall of the superior vena cava. In pinch-off syndrome, the catheter lumen is compromised by compression between the clavicle

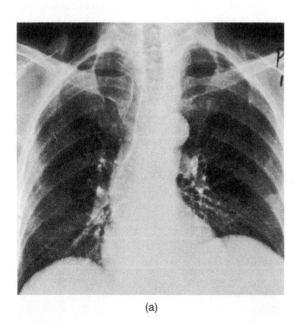

(a)

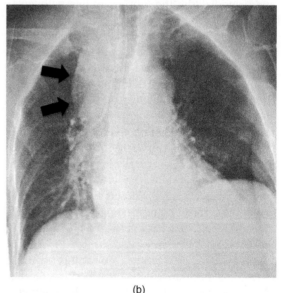

(b)

FIGURE 11–4 Mediastinal hematoma following attempted central venous catheterization. **A.** Mediastinum appears unremarkable prior to catheter placement. **B.** Following attempted central line placement, there is widening of the superior mediastinum (*arrows*) secondary to mediastinal hemorrhage due to a lacerated subclavian artery. (*Reproduced with permission from Bongard FS, Sue D, Vintch J: Current Diagnosis and Treatment Critical Care, 3rd edition. New York: McGraw-Hill Education; 2008.*)

and the first rib, leading to catheter malfunction and possible catheter fracture. This is frequently first observed as subtle focal narrowing of the catheter as it crosses the intersection of clavicle and rib.

Pulmonary Artery Catheters

The pulmonary artery catheter (PAC) plays an important role in the hemodynamic monitoring of the critically ill patient. The catheter is inserted via the subclavian or internal jugular vein and its tip should lie within the right or left main pulmonary artery. The catheter tip should remain within 2 cm of the hilum so that it does not extend beyond the proximal interlobar arteries. Complications related to CVC insertion, such as pneumothorax, vascular injury, infection, and knotting, kinking, or coiling of the catheter may also occur with PAC insertion. Ventricular arrhythmias are also common during PAC insertion, though usually self-limited. Another major complication is pulmonary infarction (Figure 11–5), usually caused by peripheral migration and occlusion of the vascular lumen by the catheter, or by continuous wedging of the inflated balloon in a central pulmonary artery. The radiographic appearance of pulmonary infarction secondary to a PAC is similar to that of infarction from other causes and consists of a wedge-shaped

parenchymal opacity seen in the distribution of the vessel distal to the catheter. Management consists of removal of the catheter. Anticoagulation is generally not required, and resolution of consolidation usually occurs in 2 to 4 weeks.

Pulmonary artery rupture is a catastrophic complication of pulmonary artery catheterization, with a reported mortality rate of 46%. The incidence is low—no more than 0.2% of catheter placements. Risk factors include pulmonary hypertension, advanced age, and improper balloon location or inflation. The mortality rate increases in anticoagulated patients. Pseudoaneurysm formation has been reported secondary to rupture or dissection by the balloon catheter tip. This appears radiographically as a well-defined nodule at the site of the aneurysm, but it may be obscured initially by extravasation of blood into the adjacent air spaces. Chest radiographic findings often precede clinical manifestations, and death due to rupture of pseudoaneurysm may occur weeks following catheterization. The CT appearance of a pulmonary artery pseudoaneurysm has been described as a sharply defined nodule with a surrounding halo of faint parenchymal density. Pulmonary artery pseudoaneurysm now may be treated in some patients with transcatheter embolization rather than surgical resection.

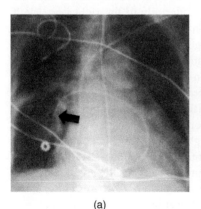 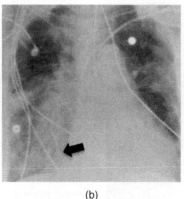 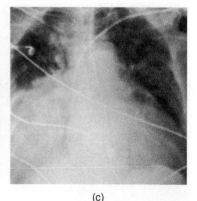

(a)   (b)   (c)

FIGURE 11–5 Lung infarction secondary to pulmonary artery catheterization. **A.** Initial radiograph after catheterization shows the tip of the catheter at the level of the right interlobar pulmonary artery (*arrows*). Mild redundancy of the catheter is present within the dilated heart. **B.** At 24 hours, the patient developed hemoptysis. Radiograph now shows migration of the catheter into a segmental arterial branch (*arrows*) with increased density in the right lower lobe. **C.** Follow-up film demonstrates dense consolidation of the right middle and lower lobes secondary to infarction. (*Reproduced with permission from Aberle DA, Brown K: Radiologic considerations in the adult respiratory distress syndrome,* Clin Chest Med. *1990 Dec;11(4):737-754.*)

Intra-Aortic Balloon Counterpulsation

Intra-aortic balloon counterpulsation is used to improve cardiac function in patients with cardiogenic shock and in the perioperative period in cardiac surgery patients. The device consists of a fusiform inflatable balloon surrounding the distal portion of a catheter that is placed percutaneously from a femoral artery into the proximal descending thoracic aorta. The balloon is inflated during diastole, thereby increasing diastolic pressure in the proximal aorta and increasing coronary artery perfusion. During systole, the balloon is forcibly deflated, allowing aortic blood to move distally and decreasing the afterload against which the left ventricle must contract, thus decreasing left ventricular workload. The tip of the balloon ideally should be positioned just distal to the origin of the left subclavian artery at the level of the aortic knob (Figure 11–6). Complications occur in 8% to 36% of intra-aortic balloon pump (IABP) placements and are most often secondary to malpositioning of the catheter. Overadvancement of the catheter may cause occlusion of the left subclavian artery, resulting in arm ischemia, or obstruction of the left common carotid or left vertebral arteries, causing cerebral ischemia. Caudal placement of the catheter

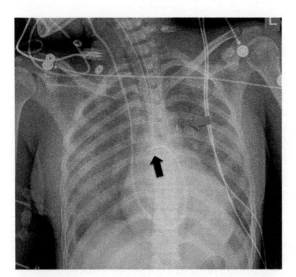

FIGURE 11–6 Intra-aortic balloon pump positioned in the proximal descending thoracic aorta (*red arrow*). A pulmonary artery catheter is also seen with its tip located in the right main pulmonary artery (*black arrow*).

can obstruct renal or mesenteric arterial flow. Aortic dissection has been reported in 1% to 4% of IABP catheter insertions, and an indistinct aorta on chest radiographs has been suggested as an early clue to intramural location, requiring confirmation by angiography. Balloon leak or rupture with gas embolization has also been described as an extremely rare but potentially fatal complication.

Cardiac Pacemakers and Automatic Implantable Cardioverter-Defibrillators

Cardiac pacemakers can be inserted by 3 approaches: transvenous, epicardial, and subxiphoid. Most often the transvenous approach is used, whereby an introducer sheath is used to establish central venous access and allow for insertion of the pacing wire, which is then guided into the right ventricle under electrocardiogram (ECG), ultrasound, or fluoroscopic guidance. The right internal jugular and the left subclavian veins are often preferred, as these routes take advantage of the natural curve of the pacing catheter, allowing for smoother, more direct placement of the wire.

When viewed on a chest radiograph, the pacemaker lead should terminate in the right ventricular apex, slightly to the left of the thoracic spine and at the anterior-inferior aspect of the cardiac shadow. A lateral view can be obtained to confirm that the catheter courses anteriorly to the right ventricle if proper placement is in question. The pacemaker lead should curve gently throughout its course, as regions of sharp angulation will have increased mechanical stress and enhance the likelihood of lead fracture. Excessive lead length can result in myocardial perforation, causing hemopericardium and cardiac tamponade. Shorter leads can become dislodged and enter the right atrium. Leads also may become displaced and enter the pulmonary artery, coronary sinus, or inferior vena cava. Other complications include venous thrombosis or infection, either at the pulse generator pocket or within the vein.

Nasogastric Tubes

Nasogastric tubes are used frequently to provide nutrition and administer oral medications as well as for suctioning gastric contents. Ideally, the tip of the tube should be positioned at least 10 cm beyond the gastroesophageal junction. This ensures that all side holes are located within the stomach and decreases the risk of aspiration.

Small-bore flexible feeding tubes have been developed to facilitate insertion and improve patient comfort. However, inadvertent passage of the nasogastric tube into the tracheobronchial tree is not uncommon, most often occurring in the sedated or neurologically impaired patient. In patients with endotracheal tubes in place, low-pressure, high-volume balloon cuffs do not prevent passage of a feeding tube into the lower airway. If sufficient feeding tube length is inserted, the tube actually may traverse the lung and penetrate the visceral pleura (Figure 11–7). Removal of the tube from an intrapleural location may result in tension pneumothorax, and preparations should be made for potential emergent thoracostomy tube placement at the time of removal. Other complications of nasogastric intubation include esophagitis, stricture, and, rarely, rupture of the pharynx, esophagus, or stomach.

In addition to feeding tubes, balloon tamponade tubes occasionally are used for nasogastric

intubation in the treatment of bleeding esophageal and gastric varices. The balloon can be easily recognized when distended, and correct positioning can be evaluated radiographically (Figure 11–8). Esophageal rupture complicates approximately 5% of cases in which balloon tamponade tubes are used.

Thoracostomy Tubes

Thoracostomy tubes ("chest tubes") are used for the evacuation of air or fluid from the pleural space. When chest tubes are used for relief of pneumothorax (Figure 11–9), apical location of the tip of the tube is most effective, whereas a tube inserted to drain free-flowing effusions should be placed in the dependent portion of the thorax. Chest radiographs, ultrasound, or CT should be used to guide correct placement of the tube for adequate drainage of a loculated effusion. Failure of the chest tube to decrease the pneumothorax or the effusion within several hours should arouse suspicion of a malpositioned tube. Tubes located within the pleural fissures are usually less effective in evacuating air or fluid collections. An interfissural location is suggested by

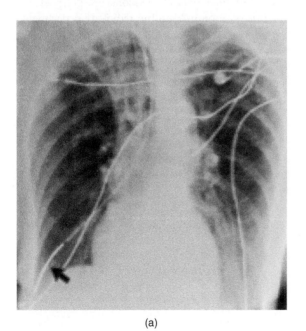 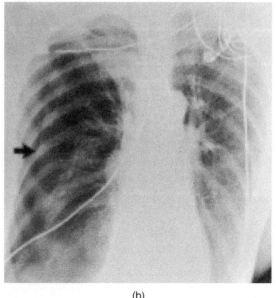

(a)   (b)

FIGURE 11–7 Malpositioned feeding tube. **A.** Feeding tube courses via the right mainstem bronchus with the tip (*arrow*) overlying the right costophrenic angle. An endotracheal tube is present. **B.** Following removal of the feeding tube, a pneumothorax is seen (*arrow*). (*Reproduced with permission from Bongard FS, Sue D, Vintch J:urrent Diagnosis and Treatment Critical Care, 3rd edition. New York: McGraw-Hill Education; 2008.*)

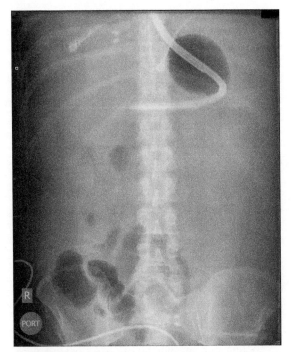

FIGURE 11–8 An abdominal radiograph showing placement of a Blakemore tube. The distal (gastric) balloon has been inflated.

orientation of the tube along the plane of the fissure on frontal radiographs and by lack of a gentle curvature near the site of penetration of the pleura, indicating failure of the tube to be deflected anteriorly or posteriorly in the pleural space. The lateral view may be confirmatory. Uncommonly, thoracostomy tubes may penetrate the lung, resulting in pulmonary laceration and bronchopleural fistula. Unilateral pulmonary edema may occur following rapid evacuation of a pneumothorax or pleural effusion that is of long standing or has produced significant compression atelectasis of lung.

CHEST RADIOGRAPHS IN THE INTENSIVE CARE UNIT: TECHNICAL CONSIDERATIONS AND UTILITY

Portable chest radiographs are frequently obtained in ICU patients. Almost all portable chest radiographs are taken with the patient supine and with the film placed behind the back of the patient (anteroposterior) rather than in the conventional upright, posteroanterior position used in the radiology department.

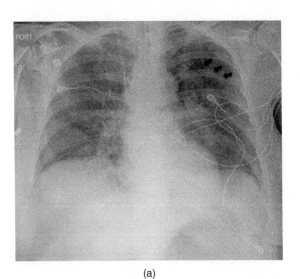

(a)

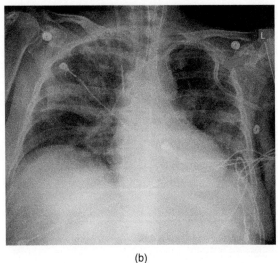

(b)

FIGURE 11–9 Pneumothorax. **A.** Development of a right-sided pneumothorax (*black arrows*) after placement of a subclavian central venous catheter (CVC). **B.** Reexpansion of the right lung after placement of a chest tube (*red arrow*).

Supine chest radiographs result in decreases in lung volume and can alter the size and appearance of the lungs, the pulmonary vasculature, and the mediastinum. Anteroposterior chest radiographs cause cardiac magnification, making evaluation of true cardiac size more difficult. Inspiratory films may be difficult to obtain because of respiratory distress, pain, sedation, or alterations in mental status. These technical limitations complicate diagnostic interpretation. Nonetheless, portable radiography continues to be a primary method of imaging critically ill patients.

Traditionally, routine daily chest radiographs have been performed on ICU patients, particularly those requiring mechanical ventilation. However, the benefit of this practice has recently been questioned. Multiple recent studies have found a low incidence of significant findings in routine radiographs, and no significant difference in mortality, length of stay, or ventilator days in patients receiving chest radiographs on a daily basis compared with those receiving chest radiographs for specific clinical indications. The American College of Radiology Thoracic Expert Panel concluded that chest radiographs should be obtained if there is a change in the clinical condition of the patient, or after placement of an ETT, central venous pressure or pulmonary artery catheter, chest tube, or nasogastric tube. Routine daily chest radiographs are not indicated.

ATELECTASIS

Atelectasis is one of the most common pulmonary parenchymal abnormalities seen in the ICU. It refers to collapse of previously inflated lung and results in diminished lung volume. The spectrum can be subtle, with only segmental or subsegmental involvement and minimal clinical significance, or extensive, with lobar involvement and ventilation-perfusion defects. Distinguishing atelectasis from pneumonia can be a challenge as the signs and symptoms often coexist. Atelectasis has a basilar predominance, particularly in the left lower lobe, and can be influenced by gravity. It also has a more rapid resolution than pneumonia.

Multiple factors contribute to the development of atelectasis. Hypoventilation results in atelectasis of the dependent lung in the bedridden patient. Bronchial obstruction from retained secretions cause

mucous plugging and may result in postobstructive collapse of the distal lung. A right mainstem bronchial intubation can cause atelectasis of the nonventilated left lung (see Figure 11–1). In postcardiac surgery patients, left lower lobe collapse occurs frequently due in part to the weight of the heart unsupported by pericardium, which compresses the left lower lobe bronchus. Central neurogenic depression, anesthesia, or splinting may decrease alveolar volume, reducing surfactant and promoting diffuse microatelectasis. Pleural processes, including pneumothorax and pleural effusion, may also result in compressive atelectasis.

Radiographic Features

The radiographic appearance of atelectasis depends largely on the degree and cause of lung collapse. Dependent (gravity-related) atelectasis occurring in supine patients may be demonstrated on thoracic CT even in healthy individuals but is usually not appreciated on plain chest radiography. Linear bands of opacity may be seen in "discoid" or "platelike" atelectasis on a subsegmental level. Focal patchy opacities can be seen with atelectasis of lung subtended by a segmental bronchus. Lobar or lung collapse (Figure 11–10) results in a dense homogenous opacity of the involved lobes and radiologic signs of volume loss. These signs include displacement of fissures and the hila, mediastinal shift, deviation of the trachea, elevation of hemidiaphragm, and sometimes hyperexpansion of the uninvolved lung.

The left lower lobe is the most frequent location of lobar atelectasis, followed by the right lower lobe and right upper lobe. The radiographic features of left and right lower lobe collapse are similar and involve triangular opacities and silhouetting of the corresponding hemidiaphragm (Figure 11–10A). The right upper lobe also collapses into a triangular density, with superior and medial migration of the horizontal fissure, anterior migration of the oblique fissure, and silhouetting of the right superior mediastinum. Due to the lack of a horizontal fissure in the left lung, the left upper lobe collapses anteriorly; atelectasis in this region presents as a hazy opacification in the left upper lung zone that gradually fades inferiorly. Collapse of the lingula or right middle lobe usually results

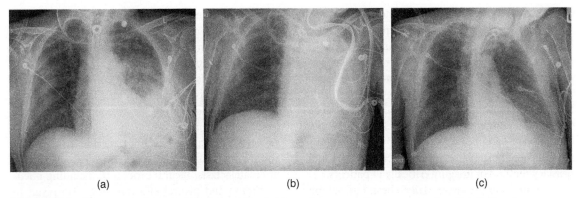

(a)   (b)   (c)

FIGURE 11–10 Lobar atelectasis. **A.** Collapse of the left lower lobe secondary to mucus plugging. **B.** Ongoing mucus plugging in the same patient resulting in collapse of the entire left lung. **C.** Reexpansion of the left lung after bronchopulmonary toileting.

in obscuring of the corresponding heart border but causes minimal signs of volume loss.

PNEUMONIA

Patients with severe pneumonia complicated by sepsis, respiratory failure, hypotension, or shock are seen frequently in the ICU. While many patients will have acquired pneumonia outside of the hospital, a substantial number will have nosocomial pneumonia, defined as lower respiratory tract infection occurring more than 48 hours after admission. Nosocomial pneumonia is the second most common nosocomial infection in the United States and is associated with high morbidity and mortality. Factors contributing to the high incidence of nosocomial pneumonias include endotracheal intubation or tracheostomy, prolonged mechanical ventilation, aspiration, and impaired host defenses. Inappropriate use of antimicrobials and emerging patterns of resistance has created additional treatment challenges.

Most radiologists sort the radiographic appearance of pneumonia into 3 categories that may aid in differentiation: lobar (alveolar or air space) pneumonia, lobular pneumonia (bronchopneumonia), and interstitial pneumonia. *Lobar pneumonia* is characterized on x-ray by relatively homogeneous regions of increased lung opacity and air bronchograms. The entire lobe does not need to be involved, and since the airways are not primarily involved, volume loss is not a frequent finding. *Streptococcus pneumonia* is the classic lobar pneumonia, although other organisms produce a similar pattern. *Lobular*

pneumonia (bronchopneumonia) results from inflammation involving the terminal and respiratory bronchioles. The distribution is more segmental and patchy-appearing, affecting some lobules while sparing others. Mild volume loss may also be present. The most common organisms producing typical bronchopneumonia are *Staphylococcus aureus* and *Pseudomonas* species. *Interstitial pneumonia* is typically caused by viruses, *Mycoplasma pneumoniae* or, in immunocompromised patients, *Pneumocystis jiroveci*. Chest radiographs demonstrate an increase in linear or reticular markings in the lung parenchyma with peribronchial thickening.

Radiographic Features
Plain Films

The chest radiograph assesses for the presence and extent of pneumonia, as well as the existence of associated complications such as parapneumonic effusions, pneumatoceles, cavitation, and abscess formation. It also helps to gauge response to antibiotic therapy. A persistent pneumonia on the radiograph despite adequate therapy may raise suspicion for mimics of infectious pneumonia, including cryptogenic organizing pneumonia or bronchioalveolar carcinoma, or the presence of an obstructing mass.

The silhouette sign on the chest radiograph is useful for determining the site of pneumonia. When consolidation is adjacent to a structure of soft tissue density (eg, the heart or the diaphragm), the margin of the soft tissue structure will be obscured by the opaque lung. Thus, a right middle lobe consolidation may cause loss of the margin of the right heart border, lingular consolidation may cause loss of the left heart border, and lower lobe pneumonia may obliterate the diaphragmatic contour.

Cavitation and abscess formation are also important complications of pneumonia caused by necrosis of the pulmonary parenchyma. Typical causative agents include anaerobes and gram-negative organisms, but cavitation can also be caused by staphylococci, *Mycobacterium tuberculosis*, atypical mycobacteria, and fungi. Lung abscesses may also be polymicrobial. Complications of lung abscess include sepsis, cerebral abscess, hemorrhage, and spillage of contents of the cavity into uninfected lung or pleural space. A lung abscess usually appears as a rounded, focal mass with a thickened (5-15 mm), irregular wall and an air-fluid level. An air crescent sign (crescentic radiolucency around lung parenchyma) or a halo sign (pulmonary opacity surrounded by a zone of ground-glass attenuation) may also be present (Figure 11–11). Abscesses may be surrounded by adjacent parenchymal consolidation (Figure 11–12) or appear as areas of lucency within an area of consolidation.

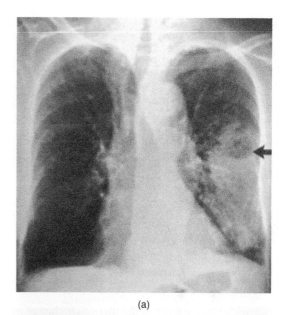

(a)

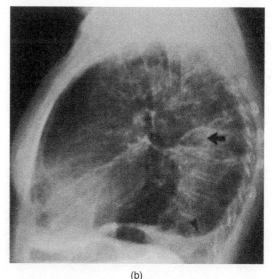

(b)

FIGURE 11–12 Cavitary pneumonia. Posteroanterior (**A**) and lateral (**B**) chest radiographs demonstrate consolidation with cavitation (*arrows*) in the superior segment of the left lower lobe. (*Reproduced with permission from Bongard FS, Sue D, Vintch J:* Current Diagnosis and Treatment Critical Care, *3rd edition. New York: McGraw-Hill Education; 2008.*)

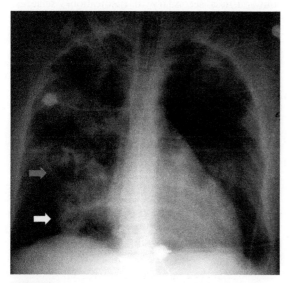

FIGURE 11–11 Pulmonary aspergillosis with cavitation. Chest radiograph demonstrates a pulmonary opacity surrounded by a zone of ground-glass attenuation (*halo sign, white arrow*) and a crescent-shaped air density surrounding a parenchymal opacity (*crescent sign, red arrow*).

Pneumatoceles (Figure 11–13) are associated with pneumonia and are caused by alveolar rupture and resulting formation of subpleural air collections. Radiographically, they appear as single or multiple

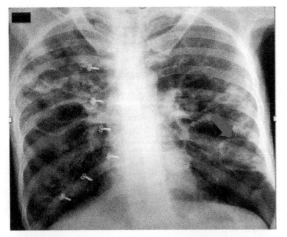

FIGURE 11–13 Pneumatocele in *Staphylococcus* pneumonia.

cysts with thin, smooth walls that often change in size and location on serial imaging. The most common causative agent is *S aureus*. Complications include pneumothorax and secondary infection.

Computed Tomography

The cross-sectional imaging plane and superior contrast resolution make CT useful in the evaluation of complicated inflammatory diseases. Cavitation,

which may be obscured on plain films, is easily identified on CT.

Localization of parenchymal diseases facilitates the direction of invasive studies such as bronchoscopy or open lung biopsy. Superimposed pleural and parenchymal processes are more easily differentiated on CT than on plain films (Figure 11–14). The administration of intravenous contrast material can further facilitate the differentiation of pleural and parenchymal disease; pleural lesions will exhibit little to no enhancement with contrast, whereas parenchyma will demonstrate enhancement as well as the presence of blood vessels.

ASPIRATION

Aspiration results from inhalation of oropharyngeal or gastric secretions into the larynx or lower respiratory tract. Aspiration can result in multiple pulmonary syndromes, including aspiration pneumonitis, a chemical injury caused by the inhalation of gastric contents, or aspiration pneumonia, an infectious process in which oropharyngeal secretions colonized by pathogenic bacteria are inhaled, resulting in lower respiratory tract infection. Several clinical conditions predispose patients to aspiration. Depressed levels of consciousness secondary to medications, seizures,

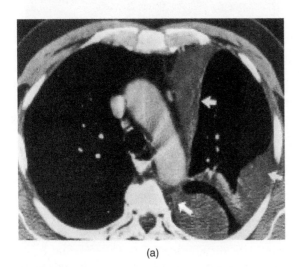

(a)

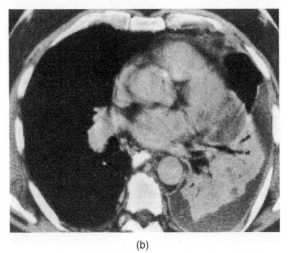

(b)

FIGURE 11–14 Pneumonia with loculated empyema. **A.** CT shows a loculated pleural effusion in the left hemithorax (*arrows*). **B.** Dense consolidation with air bronchograms in the left lower lobe. The consolidated lung enhances with contrast and is easily distinguished from the surrounding pleural effusion. (*Reproduced with permission from Bongard FS, Sue D, Vintch J: Current Diagnosis and Treatment Critical Care, 3rd edition. New York: McGraw-Hill Education; 2008.*)

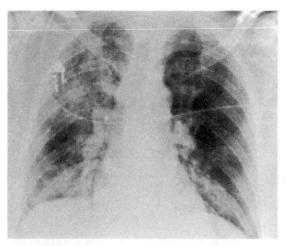

FIGURE 11–15 Aspiration following drug overdose. Multiple areas of pulmonary opacification are present bilaterally. (*Reproduced with permission from Bongard FS, Sue D, Vintch J:* Current Diagnosis and Treatment Critical Care, *3rd edition. New York: McGraw-Hill Education; 2008.*)

drug overdose, anesthesia, or neurologic disease result in impaired upper airway reflexes (Figure 11–15). Mechanical factors predisposing patients to aspiration include endotracheal intubation, enteral feeding tubes, gastric distention, vomiting, gastroesophageal reflux, and decreased esophageal and gastrointestinal motility. Pneumonia can develop when oral or gastric secretions contaminated with bacteria are aspirated. Poor oral care may result in bacterial colonization of oropharyngeal secretions. Although gastric acidity maintains sterility of stomach contents in normal circumstances, antacid therapy for stress ulcers prophylaxis increases gastric pH, which may result in gastric colonization with pathogenic bacteria. Enteral feedings, small bowel obstruction, and gastroparesis may also result in bacterial colonization of gastric contents.

Radiographic Features

The radiographic pattern seen in aspiration depends on the position of the patient, as well as the volume and the nature of aspirated contents. In a supine patient, the posterior segments of the upper lobes and superior segments of the lower lobes are typically affected. In a semirecumbent or upright patient, the basilar segments of the lower lobes are usually involved. The right lung is more frequently involved than the left due to the larger caliber and straighter course of the right mainstem bronchus.

Aspiration of small amounts of water or neutralized gastric content may produce minimal airspace opacities that rapidly resolve. If acidic gastric contents are aspirated (*Mendelson syndrome*), airspace disease rapidly develops, and can resemble pulmonary edema if the amount of aspirate is massive. Aspiration of bacteria resulting in pneumonia will produce infiltrates in characteristic bronchopulmonary segments; bilateral and multilobar consolidation may occur. Complications result from parenchymal necrosis and include the development of cavitary disease, empyema, or lung abscess.

PULMONARY EMBOLISM

Pulmonary embolism (PE) is a common, life-threatening disorder that results from venous thrombosis, usually arising in the deep veins of the lower extremities. The signs and symptoms of pulmonary embolism are nonspecific, and can be seen in a variety of pulmonary and cardiovascular diseases. The clinician must stay alert to the possibility of pulmonary embolism in any patient at risk for Virchow triad of venous stasis, intimal injury, and hypercoagulable state. A variety of imaging resources, including chest radiography, ventilation-perfusion scans, pulmonary angiography, and spiral or helical CT, play a role in the diagnosis of pulmonary embolism.

Radiographic Features
Chest Radiograph

The chest radiograph is often abnormal but rarely, if ever, diagnostic of PE. Common findings can include cardiomegaly, pulmonary artery enlargement, atelectasis, and pleural effusion. Less frequently, Westermark sign (focal oligemia distal to the site of PE), or Hampton hump (wedge-shaped peripheral consolidation resulting from infarction, Figure 11–16A) may be seen, but these are also poor predictors of PE. Consequently, the role of the chest radiograph in PE is mainly limited to ruling out other diagnoses and aiding in the interpretation of the ventilation-perfusion radionuclide scan.

Ventilation-Perfusion Lung Scan

Ventilation-perfusion scans are based on the premise that pulmonary thromboembolism results in a region of lung that is ventilated but not perfused. The study consists of two scans—the perfusion scan and the ventilation scan—that are compared for interpretation. The perfusion scan involves injection of technetium-99m-labeled macroaggregated albumin. This agent is trapped via the precapillary arterioles and identifies areas of normal lung perfusion; regions of the lung with absent perfusion will appear photon deficient. The ventilation scan is performed by obtaining images after having the patient inhale a radioactive gas (xenon) or radioaerosol (technetium-99m diethylenetriamine penta-acetic acid). Perfusion and ventilation images are compared; perfusion defects in areas of normal ventilation are suggestive of pulmonary embolism.

Although the concept behind V/Q scanning is simple, image interpretation is complex and has several limitations in ICU patients. V/Q scanning must be done in conjunction with a chest radiograph, as perfusion abnormalities may have many etiologies other than PE, including chronic obstructive pulmonary diseae (COPD), pulmonary edema, lung mass, pneumonia, and atelectasis, all frequently seen in ICU patients. Additionally, the reliability of radionuclide inhalation in intubated patients is unclear. Finally, while normal and high-probability V/Q scans have high negative and positive predictive values for PE, respectively, many V/Q scans are interpreted as intermediate- or low-probability and require further diagnostic testing.

CT Pulmonary Angiography

Ventilation-perfusion imaging has been largely replaced by multidetector computed tomography pulmonary angiography (CTPA), which is the current standard of care for detecting PE. Based on data obtained from the prospective investigation of pulmonary embolism diagnosis (PIOPED) II study, CTPA has a sensitivity of 83% and specificity of 96% in the diagnosis of pulmonary embolism. When CTPA was combined with CT venography (CTV), the sensitivity increased to 90% without significant changes in specificity. Data from PIOPED II also demonstrated high concordance between lower limb compression ultrasonography (CUS) and CTV

in the detection of lower extremity deep venous thrombosis (DVT); use of CUS obviates the additional radiation exposure associated with CTV.

CT findings of pulmonary embolism (Figure 11–16B) include the following:

- Intraluminal filling defects that sharply interface with intravascular contrast material.

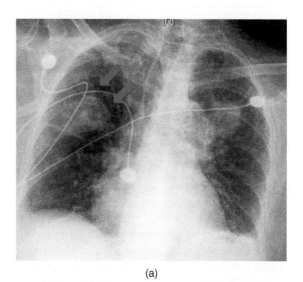

(a)

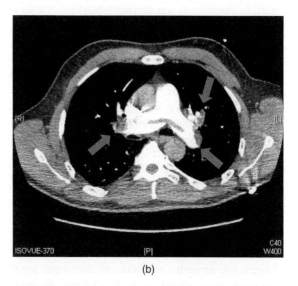

(b)

FIGURE 11–16 Pulmonary embolism. **A.** Chest radiograph shows a wedge-shaped, peripheral consolidation, known as Hampton hump. **B.** CT scan revealing bilateral intraluminal filling defects.

- Complete arterial occlusion resulting in dilation of the artery in comparison with the adjacent bronchus.
- Partial filling defects surrounded by contrast. These may manifest as the "rim sign" in the axial plane or the "railway track sign" in the long axis of a vessel.
- Partial eccentric intraluminal filling defects making an acute angle with the arterial wall.

Of note, small subsegmental filling defects must be seen definitively in more than one axial image in order to be considered consistent with PE. Other nonspecific CT findings include ground-glass opacities consistent with pulmonary hemorrhage, wedge-shaped consolidations resulting from pulmonary infarction and pleural effusions. Oligemia of lung parenchyma distal to the occluded vessel may be present. Signs of right ventricular dysfunction, such as right ventricular dilatation or leftward deviation of the interventricular septum, may also be present.

Pitfalls in the interpretation of CTPA include breathing artifact, inadequate contrast opacification of the pulmonary arteries, and suboptimal visualization of obliquely oriented vessels (eg, segmental branches of the right middle lobe and lingula). Partially opacified veins may be confused with thrombosed arteries; hilar lymph nodes and mucus-filled bronchi may be misinterpreted as thrombi. Flow- and motion-related artifacts can also result in false-positive findings.

Pulmonary Angiography

Pulmonary angiography is an invasive test and is considered the gold standard for the diagnosis of pulmonary embolism. Angiography is indicated when the pretest probability for PE is high and the results of CT angiography and V/Q show conflicting or indeterminate results. It also may be useful when therapy involves more complicated treatment such as an inferior vena cava filter, surgical embolectomy, or thrombolytic therapy.

Pulmonary angiography requires the percutaneous placement of an intravascular catheter through the femoral vein, past the right ventricle and into the pulmonary artery. Contrast is then injected at a rapid rate and images are acquired. A filling defect or abrupt cutoff of a small vessel is indicative of an

embolus in this study. Other nonspecific findings may include decreased perfusion, delayed venous return, abnormal parenchymal stain, and crowded vessels. Complications of pulmonary angiography are frequently related to catheter insertion and manipulation and include arrhythmias, heart block, cardiac perforation, right-sided heart failure, and cardiac arrest.

Magnetic Resonance Angiography

The PIOPED III study investigated the diagnostic accuracy of gadolinium-enhanced magnetic resonance angiography (MRA) alone or in combination with venous phase magnetic resonance venogram (MRV) for the diagnosis of PE. The sensitivity and specificity of MRA was 78% and 99%, respectively; combined MRA/MRV had a sensitivity of 92% and specificity of 96%. However, due to an unacceptably high percentage of patients with technically inadequate examinations, the investigators recommended that MRA only be performed in centers with significant pulmonary MRA experience and in patients with contraindications to all other standard tests.

SEPTIC PULMONARY EMBOLISM
General Considerations

Septic pulmonary emboli occur as a result of infections of the right side of the heart or of the peripheral veins. Major risk factors include intravenous drug use, indwelling catheters, and skin and soft tissue infections. Oropharyngeal infections can result in infectious thrombophlebitis of the internal jugular vein (Lemierres syndrome), a rare but significant cause of septic pulmonary emboli. Most patients with septic pulmonary emboli have positive blood cultures at the time of imaging, with S aureus being the most commonly isolated organism.

Radiographic Features

The radiographic features of septic pulmonary emboli include multiple wedge-shaped or rounded peripheral opacities of varying size and lower lobe predominance, reflecting increased blood flow to dependent portions of lung. Cavitation is common, with necrotic debris often present within cavities.

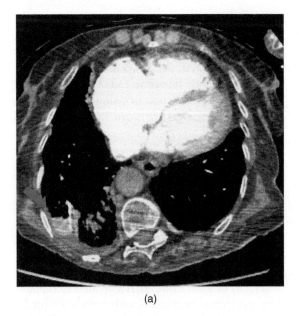
(a)

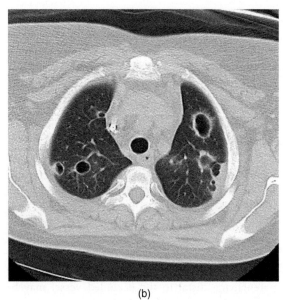
(b)

FIGURE 11–17 Septic pulmonary embolism. **A.** CT scan demonstrating a feeding vessel leading to a peripheral nodule (*arrow*). **B.** Multiple cavitary lesions varying in size.

Hilar and mediastinal lymphadenopathy can occur, as can empyema.

CT imaging may detect disease earlier than the plain radiograph and better characterize its extent. In addition to the above findings, CT may also reveal peripheral nodules with feeding vessels and contrast enhancement of wedge-shaped lesions (Figure 11–17).

PULMONARY EDEMA

General Considerations

Pulmonary edema—an excess of water in the extravascular lung space—is a frequent cause of respiratory distress in the critically ill patient. According to Starling law, fluid accumulates in the extravascular space in one of two ways:

- Increased hydrostatic pressure within the lung capillaries (cardiogenic pulmonary edema), resulting from fluid overload or cardiac dysfunction.
- Increased capillary membrane permeability (noncardiogenic pulmonary edema), which

can be caused by a variety of insults to the microvasculature of the lung.

In the ICU patient, more than one mechanism may contribute to the formation of edema, increasing the difficulty of diagnostic interpretation on radiographs.

Radiographic Features

The earliest sign of cardiogenic pulmonary edema is vascular redistribution, manifested as hyperperfusion of the upper lobes, or cephalization. This finding is best seen in an upright film and may be difficult to see in the supine or semiupright films obtained in critically ill patients. As hydrostatic pressure increases, fluid accumulates in the interstitium; corresponding radiographic signs may be present prior to the onset of symptoms and include Kerley lines, peribronchial cuffing, loss of vascular definition, thickening of the fissures, and pleural effusions (Figure 11–18). Kerley A lines represent distension of anastomotic channels between lymphatics and appear as long, irregular linear opacities extending from the hila to the periphery. Kerley B lines are caused by edematous interlobular septa and are short, horizontal lines

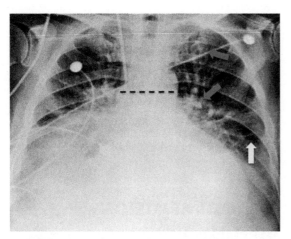

FIGURE 11–18 Chest radiograph displaying multiple signs of cardiogenic pulmonary edema, including pleural effusions, cardiomegaly, prominent pulmonary vasculature (*red arrow*), Kerley B lines extending to periphery (*yellow arrow*), and peribronchial cuffing (*blue arrow*). A widened vascular pedicle is marked by the dotted line. (*Reproduced with permission from Bongard FS, Sue D, Vintch J*: Current Diagnosis and Treatment Critical Care, *3rd edition. New York: McGraw-Hill Education; 2008.*)

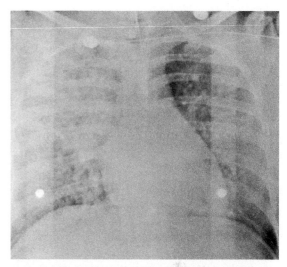

FIGURE 11–19 Noncardiogenic pulmonary edema. The chest radiograph displays bilateral asymmetric air space opacities. There are no pleural effusions. The heart and vascular pedicle are of normal size. (*Reproduced with permission from Bongard FS, Sue D, Vintch J*: Current Diagnosis and Treatment Critical Care, *3rd edition. New York: McGraw-Hill Education; 2008.*)

found predominantly at the lung bases. Kerley C lines are reticular opacities primarily seen at the lung bases and signify thickened interlobular septa in transverse orientation. Kerley B lines are seen more frequently than Kerley A or C lines. Peribronchial cuffing results when fluid-thickened bronchial walls become visible producing rounded, "doughnut-like" densities in the lung parenchyma.

As extravascular fluid continues to accumulate, alveolar edema develops. Clinical signs and symptoms of heart failure are generally apparent at this point, and the chest radiograph will reveal airspace opacities that can coalesce into diffuse consolidations, frequently with a perihilar or basilar distribution. Air bronchograms are usually absent, and the lung periphery is often spared, sometimes resulting in a "batwing" appearance. In general, cardiogenic pulmonary edema is bilateral and symmetric, but atypical edema patterns may be seen in patients with underlying lung disease or as a consequence of gravitational forces related to patient positioning. Destruction of the lung due to emphysema may cause a patchy, asymmetric distribution of edema that spares regions of bullous disease.

Widening of the vascular pedicle is also seen in cardiogenic pulmonary edema. The vascular pedicle width extends from the superior vena cava on the right side of the mediastinum to the proximal descending aorta on the left. Vascular pedicle width greater than 7 cm is consistent with volume overload.

Distinguishing cardiogenic from noncardiogenic pulmonary edema is not always possible radiographically, and the 2 processes may be seen concurrently in ICU patients. In noncardiogenic pulmonary edema (Figure 11–19), the vascular pedicle width tends to be normal, and pleural effusions, septal thickening, and peribronchial cuffing are absent. Edema is more likely to be patchy and peripheral in distribution, in contrast to the central or basilar distribution seen in cardiogenic pulmonary edema.

ACUTE RESPIRATORY DISTRESS SYNDROME
General Considerations

ARDS is a diffuse, acute, inflammatory lung injury manifested by severe hypoxia and bilateral radiographic infiltrates of noncardiogenic etiology. It can result from either direct pulmonary injury or in response to a systemic insult. Imaging plays an important role in the diagnosis of ARDS and may help determine its underlying etiology.

Radiographic Features

The radiographic manifestations correlate with the pathologic changes seen in the lung parenchyma and vary with the stage of lung injury. There are 3 phases of ARDS as described below:

- **Exudative phase (days 1-7):** This phase is characterized by endothelial and epithelial injury and an influx of protein-rich fluid, first into the interstitium and subsequently into the alveoli. Alveolar atelectasis and hyaline membrane formation are seen. Radiographically, interstitial edema is initially seen, followed by alveolar consolidation; both patterns may be present concurrently (Figure 11–20A). Additionally, if a direct lung injury such as pneumonia was the trigger for ARDS, its presence may be evident.

- **Proliferative phase (days 8-14):** Infiltration with fibroblasts and type II pneumocytes occurs in this phase as a response to injury and coarse reticular opacities may develop on the chest radiograph. Imaging will otherwise remain relatively static, as alveolar and interstitial edema will persist. The development of additional airspace opacities should generate concern for new infection or other complications.

- **Fibrotic phase (day 15 onward):** This late phase of ARDS may overlap with the proliferative phase and is characterized by collagen deposition and fibrosis. The degree of fibrosis is variable and the radiographic findings can range from complete resolution to the development of widespread reticular markings, cysts, airway distortion, and persistent ground-glass opacities (Figure 11–20B).

PLEURAL EFFUSION

General Considerations

Pleural fluid is primarily formed on the parietal pleural surface and absorbed on the visceral pleural surface. Approximately 25 mL of fluid is normally present in the pleural space. When there is an imbalance between production and absorption of pleural fluid, excess intrapleural fluid accumulates and pleural effusions form. While the plain chest radiograph can be useful for detecting and estimating the amount of pleural effusion, pleural fluid is more easily visualized and distinguished from lung parenchyma with CT or bedside ultrasound. The role of ultrasound in visualizing pleural effusions is detailed in Chapter 12.

Radiographic Features

The appearance and distribution of fluid within the pleural space is greatly affected by lung elastic recoil

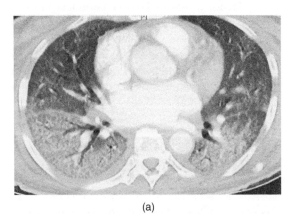

(a)

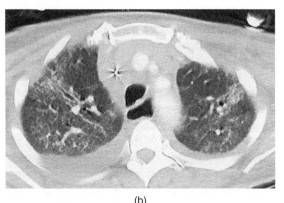

(b)

FIGURE 11–20 ARDS. **A.** Exudative phase of ARDS. CT demonstrates bilateral consolidations with air bronchograms and interstitial edema. **B.** Fibrotic phase of ARDS. CT reveals traction bronchiectasis and honeycombing.

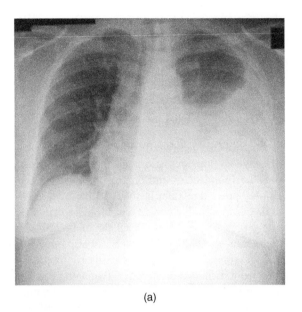

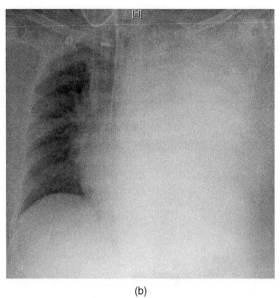

(a)   (b)

FIGURE 11–21 Pleural effusion. **A.** Chest radiograph displaying a left-sided pleural effusion with a meniscus sign. **B.** Massive left pleural effusion with rightward tracheal deviation.

and gravity. On erect frontal and lateral radiographs, free pleural effusions typically have a concave, upward-sloping interface with the lung (the meniscus sign) and result in blunting of the costophrenic angle (Figure 11–21A). Blunting of the costophrenic angle may occur with as little as 175 mL of fluid on an erect frontal radiograph; smaller amounts of fluid can be detected on a lateral upright or lateral decubitus view but these views are logistically difficult to obtain in the ICU patient. A massive pleural effusion can produce near-complete opacification of the involved hemithorax, accompanied by contralateral mediastinal shift (Figure 11–21B).

Multiple diagnostic challenges exist when visualizing pleural effusions with a chest radiograph. Atelectasis and lung consolidation may be difficult to distinguish from pleural effusion because they too may obscure the hemidiaphragm. Pleural fluid can accumulate along the pleural fissures and result in a mass-like appearance, or pseudotumor. However, unlike a true mass, a pseudotumor will change in shape and size as the patient is repositioned. Pleural effusions may also be found in a subpulmonary location between the lung base and diaphragm without causing blunting of the lateral costophrenic sulcus.

The chest radiograph will reveal what appears to be an elevated hemidiaphragm, which is actually the displaced pleural-visceral interface simulating a "pseudodiaphragm." Signs that can help distinguish subpulmonic effusion from diaphragmatic elevation include the flatter shape of the pseudodiaphragm in comparison with a true hemidiaphragm, and increased distance between the gastric bubble and the pseudodiaphragm (Figure 11–22).

An additional challenge specific to ICU patients is that many radiographs are performed with the patient in the supine position, making the diagnosis of pleural effusion more difficult, particularly with smaller effusions. When a patient is supine, the most dependent regions of the pleural space are the posterior aspects of the bases and the lung apex. Free pleural effusions layer posteriorly, resulting in a homogeneous increased density of the lower involved hemithorax. Fluid also may accumulate at the apex of the thorax, resulting in apical capping.

Given the limitations of chest radiography in visualizing pleural effusions, ultrasound and CT are frequently utilized. Ultrasound imaging is detailed in Chapter 12. Pleural effusions on CT typically appear as sickle-shaped, posterior opacities (Figure 11–23).

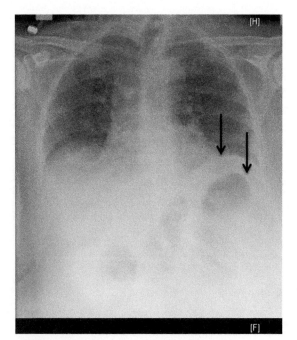

FIGURE 11–22 Separation of the left "hemidiaphragm" (*arrows*) from the stomach bubble suggesting a subpulmonic pleural effusion.

CT is extremely sensitive in the detection of small effusions, demonstrating loculations, and distinguishing pleural and parenchymal processes. In complicated cases, intravenous contrast administration can help differentiate parenchyma from pleura, as consolidated lung will enhanced, whereas pleural processes will not. While the attenuation of the effusion cannot help distinguish all transudates from exudates, very high attenuation may suggest the presence of a hemorrhagic or proteinaceous collection.

One typically high-attenuation collection is an empyema. Empyema is defined as pus in the pleural space and warrants additional radiographic considerations. While empyemas may initially appear as free-flowing pleural effusions, they often subsequently develop loculations as they pass through their fibrinopurulent and organizing phases. Loculations appear lenticular in shape with obtuse angles to the chest wall. If a concurrent bronchopleural fistula is present, an air-fluid level can be identified in the pleural space. Air-fluid levels can also be seen in lung abscesses, making the 2 difficult to distinguish on a frontal chest radiograph; CT imaging can better distinguish the 2 given its cross-sectional nature. The visceral and parietal pleura frequently enhance due to increased blood supply to the inflamed pleural surfaces during the organizing phase with resultant uptake of intravenous contrast. The "split pleura" sign results from this enhancement as well as separation of the visceral and parietal pleura. Surrounding edema and a local increase in extrapleural fat are also often seen, suggesting the chronic nature of the empyema (Figure 11–24).

PNEUMOTHORAX
General Considerations

Pneumothorax is a frequent and serious complication in the ICU. Iatrogenic pneumothorax frequently develops as a sequela of invasive diagnostic or therapeutic procedures, or barotrauma from mechanical ventilation. Other etiologies of pneumothorax include chest trauma and complications of pulmonary diseases such as COPD, asthma, interstitial lung disease, and cavitary pneumonia. Recognition of even small pneumothoraces is crucial for the prevention of progressive accumulation of pleural air collections, particularly in patients being maintained on mechanical ventilation.

Radiographic Features

As with fluid in the pleural space, the distribution of a pneumothorax is influenced by gravity, lung elastic

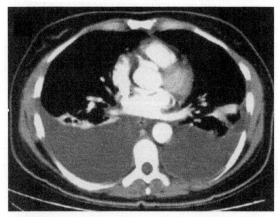

FIGURE 11–23 Large bilateral pleural effusions demonstrated on CT scan.

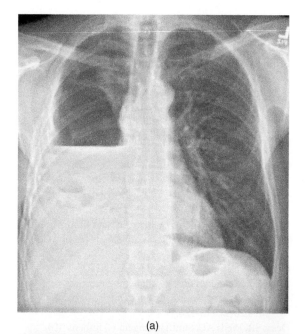

(a)

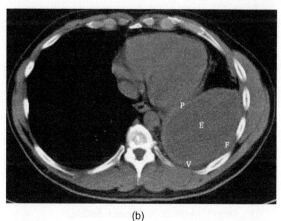

(b)

FIGURE 11–24 **A.** Air-fluid level in an empyema with a bronchopleural fistula. **B.** Split pleura sign: large empyema (E) with separated, enhanced visceral (V) and parietal (P) pleura as well as thickening of extrapleural fat (F).

recoil, potential adhesions in the pleural space, and the anatomy of the pleural recesses. Radiographically, a pneumothorax is identified by separation of the visceral pleural surface from the chest wall and the absence of pulmonary vessels peripheral to the pleural line. A pneumothorax is typically better seen on expiratory images because of a relative decrease in lung volumes compared with the air in the pleural

space. In the upright patient, air accumulates in the nondependent region of the pleural space, the apex.

Expiratory, upright radiographs are generally unattainable in ICU patients; images are usually obtained in the supine position, altering the radiographic appearance of pneumothorax. In this position, the least dependent regions of the pleural space are the anteromedial and subpulmonary regions. Pleural air in the anteromedial space results in sharp delineation of mediastinal contours, including the superior vena cava, the azygos vein, the heart border, the inferior vena cava, and the left subclavian artery. The accumulation of air in the subpulmonary region results in a hyperlucent upper quadrant of the abdomen, a deep, hyperlucent lateral costophrenic sulcus ("deep sulcus sign"), sharp delineation of the ipsilateral diaphragm, and visualization of the inferior surface of the lung (Figure 11–25). Air can accumulate in the apicolateral pleural space in the supine patient just as in the erect patient, especially when a large pneumothorax is present. In the presence of lower lobe pneumothorax, air can accumulate in the posteromedial pleural recess, resulting in sharp delineation of the posterior mediastinal structures, including the descending aorta and the costovertebral sulcus.

Tension pneumothorax occurs when the pressure of air in the pleural space exceeds ambient

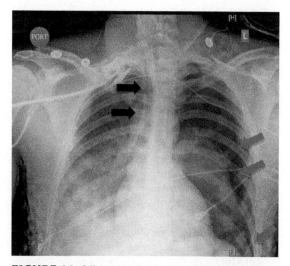

FIGURE 11–25 Large left-sided pneumothorax (*red arrows*) as a complication of subclavian line placement. Rightward tracheal shift (*black arrows*) and sharp delineation of the left hemidiaphragm (*blue arrow*) can be seen.

pressure during the respiratory cycle. With this pressure gradient, air enters the pleural space on inspiration but is prevented from exiting the pleural space during expiration. A tension pneumothorax may result in acute respiratory distress and, if untreated, cardiopulmonary arrest. Radiographic signs include displacement of the mediastinum toward the contralateral thorax, inferior displacement or inversion of the diaphragm, and total lung collapse. Adhesions may prevent mediastinal shift, and lung collapse may not occur in patients with stiff lungs such as those with ARDS.

Bedside ultrasound is a reliable tool for the diagnosis of pneumothorax and is further described in Chapter 12. CT may be particularly useful in the diagnosis of loculated pneumothorax and in guiding appropriate chest tube placement.

Several conditions may be confused with a pneumothorax. Pneumoperitoneum may result in a hyperlucent upper abdomen, mimicking pneumothorax. Skin folds can be confused with apicolateral pneumothorax but should be recognized when they extend outside the bony thorax or are traced bilaterally. Pneumomediastinum may simulate medial pneumothorax; however, pneumomediastinum will often cross the midline and extend into the retroperitoneum.

REFERENCES

Abramowitz Y, Simanovsky N, Goldstein MS, Hiller N. Pleural effusion: characterization with CT attenuation values and CT appearance. *AJR Am J Roentgenol.* 2009;192:618-623.

ACR Manual on Contrast Media. Version 9. Reston: American College of Radiology, ACR Committee on Drugs and Contrast Media; 2013.

American Thoracic Society; Infectious Diseases Society of America. Guidelines for the management of adults with hospital-acquired, ventilator-associated, and healthcare-associated pneumonia. *Am J Respir Crit Care Med.* 2005;171(4):388-416.

Amorosa JK, Bramwit MP, Mohammed TL, et al. ACR appropriateness criteria routine chest radiographs in intensive care unit patients. *J Am Coll Radiol.* 2013;10(3):170-174.

Aronchick JM, Miller WT, Jr. Tubes and lines in the intensive care setting. *Semin Roentgenol.* 1997;32(2):102-116.

Ashizawa K, Hayashi K, Aso N, Minami K. Lobar atelectasis: diagnostic pitfalls on chest radiography. *Br J Radiol.* 2001;74(877):89-97.

Bellingan GJ. The pulmonary physician in critical care * 6: the pathogenesis of ALI/ARDS. *Thorax.* 2002;57(6):540-546.

Bettmann MA, Baginski SG, White RD, et al. ACR Appropriateness Criteria® acute chest pain—suspected pulmonary embolism. *J Thorac Imaging.* 2012;27:W28-W31.

Caironi P, Carlesso E, Gattinoni L. Radiological imaging in acute lung injury and acute respiratory distress syndrome. *Semin Respir Crit Care Med.* 2006;27:404-415.

Chen KY, Jerng JS, Liao WY, et al. Pneumothorax in the ICU: patient outcomes and prognostic factors. *Chest.* 2002;122:678-683.

Cullu N, Kalemci S, Karakaş Ö, et al. Efficacy of CT in diagnosis of transudates and exudates in patients with pleural effusion. *Diagn Interv Radiol.* 2014;20(2):116-120.

Desai SR, Wells AU, Suntharalingam G, Rubens MB, Evans TW, Hansell DM. Acute respiratory distress syndrome caused by pulmonary and extrapulmonary injury: a comparative CT study. *Radiology.* 2001;218(3):689-693.

Dodd JD, Souza CA, Müller NL. High-resolution MDCT of pulmonary septic embolism: evaluation of the feeding vessel sign. *AJR Am J Roentgenol.* 2006;187(3):623-629.

Ely EW, Haponik EF. Using the chest radiograph to determine intravascular volume status: the role of vascular pedicle width. *Chest.* 2002;121(3):942-950.

Franquest T. Imaging of pneumonia: trends and algorithms. *Eur Respir J.* 2001;18(1):196-208.

Franquet T, Giménez A, Rosón N, Torrubia S, Sabaté JM, Pérez C. Aspiration diseases: findings, pitfalls, and differential diagnosis. *Radiographics.* 2000;20:673-685.

Gluecker T, Capasso P, Schnyder P, et al. Clinical and radiologic features of pulmonary edema. *Radiographics.* 1999;19:1507-1531.

Godoy MC, Leitman BS, de Groot PM, Vlahos I, Naidich DP. Chest radiography in the ICU: part 1, evaluation of airway, enteric, and pleural tubes. *AJR Am J Roentgenol.* 2012;198(3):563-571.

Godoy MC, Leitman BS, de Groot PM, Vlahos I, Naidich DP. Chest radiography in the ICU: part 2, evaluation of cardiovascular lines and other devices. *AJR Am J Roentgenol.* 2012;198(3):572-581.

Hejblum G, Chalumeau-Lemoine L, Ioos V, et al. Comparison of routine and on-demand prescription of chest radiographs in mechanically ventilated adults: a multicentre, cluster-randomised, two-period crossover study. *Lancet*. 2009;374(9702):1687-1693.

Hill JR, Horner PE, Primack SL. ICU imaging. *Clin Chest Med*. 2008;29(1):59-76.

Ichikado K, Suga M, Muranaka H, et al. Prediction of prognosis for acute respiratory distress syndrome with thin-section CT: validation in 44 cases. *Radiology*. 2006;238(1):321-329.

Iwasaki Y, Nagata K, Nakanishi M, et al. Spiral CT findings in septic pulmonary emboli. *Eur J Radiol*. 2001;37(3):190-194.

Jang JS, Jin HY, Seo JS, et al. Sodium bicarbonate therapy for the prevention of contrast-induced acute kidney injury: a systematic review and meta-analysis. *Circ J*. 2012;76(9):2255-2265.

Kearney SE, Davies CW, Davies RJ, Gleeson FV. Computed tomography and ultrasound in parapneumonic effusions and empyema. *Clin Radiol*. 2000;55(7):542-547.

Kong A. The deep sulcus sign. *Radiology*. 2003;228:415-416.

Kwon WJ, Jeong YJ, Kim KI, et al. Computed tomographic features of pulmonary septic emboli: comparison of causative microorganisms. *J Comput Assist Tomogr*. 2007;31(3):390-394.

Lewin S, Goldberg L, Dec GW. The spectrum of pulmonary abnormalities on computed chest tomographic imaging in patients with advanced heart failure. *Am J Cardiol*. 2000;86:98-100.

Marik PE. Aspiration pneumonitis and aspiration pneumonia. *N Engl J Med*. 2001;344(9):665-671.

Martin GS, Ely EW, Carroll FE, Bernard GR. Findings on the portable chest radiograph correlate with fluid balance in critically ill patients. *Chest*. 2002;122:2087-2095.

Moss HA, Roe PG, Flower CDR. Clinical deterioration in ARDS: an unchanged chest radiograph and functioning chest drains do not exclude an acute tension pneumothorax. *Clin Radiol*. 2000;55:637-651.

Mullett R, Jain A, Kotugodella S, Curtis J. Lobar collapse demystified: the chest radiograph with CT correlation. *Postgrad Med J*. 2012;88(1040):335-347.

Nicolaou S, Talsky A, Khashoggi K, Venu V, et al. Ultrasound-guided interventional radiology in critical care. *Crit Care Med*. 2007;35(suppl 5):S186-S197.

Oba Y, Zaza T. Abandoning daily routine chest radiography in the intensive care unit: meta-analysis. *Radiology*. 2010;255(2):386-395.

Qureshi NR, Gleeson FV. Imaging of pleural disease. *Clin Chest Med*. 2006;27:193-213.

Rankine JJ, Thomas AN, Fluechter D. Diagnosis of pneumothorax in critically ill adults. *Postgrad Med J*. 2000;76:399-404.

Rubinowitz AN, Siegel MD, Tocino I. Thoracic imaging in the ICU. *Crit Care Clin*. 2007;23(3):539-573.

Ruskin JA, Gurney JW, Thorsen MK, Goodman LR. Detection of pleural effusions on supine chest radiographs. *AJR Am J Roentgenol*. 1987;148:681-683.

Sharma S, Maycher B, Eschun G. Radiological imaging in pneumonia: recent innovations. *Curr Opin Pulm Med*. 2007;13(3):159-169.

Sheard S, Rao P, Devaraj A. Imaging of acute respiratory distress syndrome. *Respir Care*. 2012;57(4):607-612.

Stathopoulos GT, Karamessini MT, Sotiriadi AE, Pastromas VG. Rounded atelectasis of the lung. *Respir Med*. 2005;99(5):615-623.

Stein PD, Chenevert TL, Fowler SE, et al. Gadolinium-enhanced magnetic resonance angiography for pulmonary embolism: a multicenter prospective study (PIOPED III). *Ann Intern Med*. 2010;152:434-443.

Stein PD, Fowler SE, Goodman LR, et al. Multidetector computed tomography for acute pulmonary embolism. *N Engl J Med*. 2006;354:2317-2327.

Stein PD, Woodard PK, Weg JG, et al. Diagnostic pathways in acute pulmonary embolism: recommendations of the PIOPED II Investigators. *Radiology*. 2007;242:15-21.

Sun Z, Fu Q, Cao L, Jin W, Cheng L, Li Z. Intravenous N-acetylcysteine for prevention of contrast-induced nephropathy: a meta-analysis of randomized, controlled trials. *PLoS One*. 2013;8(1):e55124.

The PIOPED Investigators. Value of the ventilation-perfusion scan in acute pulmonary embolism. *JAMA*. 1990;263:2753-2759.

Thomason JW, Ely EW, Chiles C, Ferretti G, Freimanis RI, Haponik EF. Appraising pulmonary edema using supine chest roentgenograms in ventilated patients. *Am J Respir Crit Care Med*. 1998;157:1600-1608.

Trotman-Dickenson B. Radiology in the intensive care unit (part 1). *J Intensive Care Med*. 2003;18:198-210.

Vilar J, Domingo ML, Soto C, Cogollos J. Radiology of bacterial pneumonia. *Eur J Radiol*. 2004;51(2):102-113.

Woodside KJ, vanSonnenberg E, Chon KS, et al. Pneumothorax in patients with acute respiratory distress syndrome: pathophysiology, detection, and treatment. *J Intensive Care Med*. 2003;18:9-20.

Ye R, Zhao L, Wang C, Wu X, Yan H. Clinical characteristics of septic pulmonary embolism in adults: a systematic review. *Respir Med*. 2014;108(1):1-8.

Imaging The Critically Ill: Bedside Ultrasound

Alfredo Lee Chang, MD; Lewis Ari Eisen, MD and Marjan Rahmanian, MD

KEY POINTS

1. Focused critical care ultrasound (CCU) answers specific clinical questions and is an extension of the physical examination.

2. Bedside ultrasound can benefit patients by decreasing ionizing radiation exposure and improving patient safety by decreasing the need for transport out of the intensive care unit (ICU).

3. Bedside ultrasound is better for ruling in diagnoses than ruling out diagnoses.

4. If the diagnosis is unclear after a focused ultrasound, expert consultation or additional imaging is advised.

5. Bedside ultrasound is shown to decrease complications and improve success rates for many common critical care procedures.

INTRODUCTION TO BEDSIDE ULTRASOUND

Ultrasound technology was introduced to the medical field in the early 1950s. It was not until 1970s that multiple specialties in medicine adopted ultrasound as a useful diagnostic tool. Slasky et al mentioned the importance of ultrasound in the ICU. He reported a 2-year retrospective study of ultrasound indications in the ICU and found that 64.4% of patients had abnormal findings and 52% of these patients' clinical course and therapy were modified by ultrasonography.[1] Other authors reported similar findings.[2-4]

Bedside ultrasonography differs from the ultrasound studies done by consult services (ie, cardiology, radiology, etc). The intensivist uses real-time (image acquisition and interpretation are done at the same time) point-of-care ultrasonography (POC-US) to answer simple clinical questions that will change patient's management. One clear example of POC-US frequently used by emergency physicians and trauma surgeons is the focused assessment by sonography for trauma (FAST). This became standard of care and it is fully integrated into advanced trauma life support teaching. For intensivists, POC-US helps diagnose, evaluate response to treatment and guide procedures safely.

In this chapter we will cover the basics of image acquisition and clinical applications of POC-US.

BASICS OF ULTRASONOGRAPHY

Understanding the basic physics of how ultrasound images are generated will help interpreting images and identifying artifacts. The ultrasound frequency ranges within millions of Hertz (MHz). It is generated when electric current is applied to a piezo-electric crystal. These mechanical vibrations are transmitted through tissues; each tissue will have

TABLE 12-1 Important artifacts in ultrasonography.

Artifacts	Mechanism	Description
Acoustic enhancement	Attenuation of sound	Usually seen after an anechoic structure that does not attenuate the ultrasound wave and generates a brighter image than we would expect.
Acoustic shadows	Attenuation of sound	Usually seen after a hyperechoic structure that obliterate the ultrasound wave and creates a dark shadow.
Side lobe artifacts	Propagation	Consist of low-intensity ultrasound beams located outside of the main beam, generating a "sludge" appearance.
Refraction "edge artifact"	Propagation assumption	Seen when ultrasound waves encounter a curved surface at a tangential angle, these waves are scattered and refracted, thus creating a linear shadow.
Refraction "ghosting"	Propagation assumption	Seen when ultrasound waves travel through materials with different acoustic transmission speeds causing a shadow.
Reverberation artifacts	Propagation assumption	Seen when ultrasound waves are reflected back and forth at close intervals, eg, A-line and B-lines.

different impedance, generating echoes throughout. The same transducer, then receives and transduces into a grayscale image that is generated at 20 to 40 frames per second. This is perceived as continuous images on the screen. For deeper structures, low-frequency waves such as 1 to 5 MHz are preferred and for superficial structures, high-frequency waves such as 5 to 15 MHz are preferred. By convention, tissues like the liver and kidneys are isoechoic. Bone, stones, and other tissues that reflect more echoes are hyperechoic and fat, fluid, and blood have low impedance generating hypoechoic or anechoic images.

Basic understanding of acoustic artifacts can help with image interpretation; these are described in Table 12-1.

GUIDELINES AND INTERNATIONAL STATEMENTS

Training and Competency

Despite the potential benefit of POC-US, the use of ultrasound is not universal in critical care medicine. Benefits will only be appreciated if the operator is capable of acquiring and interpreting ultrasound images. Multiple international critical care societies had partnered to establish guidelines to provide competency in POC-US.[5,6] These guidelines are intended to create a framework toward an universal standard. For those intensivists interested in POC-US, the World Interactive Network Focused on Critical Ultrasound (WINFOCUS) and the American College of Chest Physician (ACCP) have well-developed training programs that consist of basic concepts of ultrasonography, hands-on image acquisition, and interpretation.

Competency for general critical care ultrasound (GCCU) and critical care echocardiography (CCE) are different, CCE competency is described in chapter 95 of this book.

It is a consensus that courses designed to teach GCCU and CCE should be at least 10 hours divided into lectures and didactic image-acquisition training. The numbers of examination to achieve competency is controversial.[6]

The basic requirements needed to achieve competency as per the ACCP allows the operator to foster self-directed learning (Table 12-2.)

INTERNATIONAL EVIDENCE-BASED RECOMMENDATIONS

To date, the only evidence-based recommendation for POC-US is for lung ultrasonography (LUS).[7] A panel of experts voted for the level of evidence in each condition where lung ultrasonography is used.

TABLE 12–2 American College of Chest physician requirements to achieve critical care ultrasonography competency.

Areas of Study	Required Images for Competency
Lung/pleural study	1. Three pleural effusions of any size 2. Three lung sliding 3. Three alveolar consolidation
Abdominal study	1. Four longitudinal view of the left kidney with splenorenal space 2. Four longitudinal view of the right kidney with hepatorenal recess 3. Four transverse bladder views
Vascular diagnostic study	1. Three right common femoral vein with compression 2. Three left common femoral vein with compression 3. Three right common femoral vein at saphenous intake with compression 4. Three left common femoral vein at saphenous intake with compression 5. Three right superficial femoral vein with compression 6. Three left superficial femoral vein with compression 7. Three right popliteal vein with compression 8. Three left popliteal vein with compression

The level of evidence was classified as following: Level A: high-quality evidence and further research is very unlikely to change the estimated effect or accuracy of evidence. Level B: Moderate quality and further research is likely to have an important impact on estimated effect or accuracy and may change level of evidence. Level C: Low quality of evidence and further research is likely to change the estimated effect or accuracy of evidence (Table 12–3).

Lung Ultrasonography

Ultrasound Probe Selection and Orientation

The preferred probe to evaluate the thorax is a 3.5 to 5 MHz with a small footprint and the cursor pointing cephalad. If more superficial structures of the thorax are being investigated, a 7.5- to 10-MHz linear probe can be used.

The classical views of the chest are in the midclavicular line, midaxillary line, and posterior axillary line or mid scapular line. However, scanning other parts of the chest may be indicated as long as good images are obtained for interpretation.

Clinical Implications and Description of Syndromes

In the hands of an experienced operator, LUS in the critically ill is superior to chest roentgenogram (CXR) and comparable to computerized tomography of the chest (CT-Chest) in several conditions.[8,9] It is important to understand the air-fluid ratio in the lung to understand and interpret LUS. The air-fluid ratio in pneumothorax (PTX) is pure air, no fluid; normal lung has air and very little fluid, the interstitial syndrome has air with more fluid; alveolar consolidation has little air but a lot of fluid and pleural effusion consists of pure fluid, no air. (Figure 12–1).

The only way to image the lung is in between the ribs (Figure 12–2). The lung has to be centered in the screen and the two rib shadows are seen on the side; this is referred to as the *bat sign*. The pleural line can be identified as a bright structure. Standard ultrasound probes cannot separate the visceral from the parietal pleura so only one line is seen. In a healthy lung, the pleural surfaces move against each other during the respiratory cycle causing a shimmering line, this is called *lung sliding*. *Lung pulse* is referred to the pleural line moving synchronously with each cardiac cycle. A normal aerated lung will show reverberations artifact from ultrasound reflection between the pleural line and the skin surface, these are called A-lines. In the presence of lung sliding, A-lines indicate normally aerated lung. In the absence of lung sliding, A-lines do not necessarily indicate normal lung and pneumothorax could be present.

The Interstitial Syndrome—B-lines represents thickened subpleural interlobular septa and/or ground-glass opacity,[10] either of cardiogenic or noncardiogenic etiology. They are described as comet-tail artifact and must fulfill all of these requirements: (1) Starts from the pleural surface, (2) moves with lung sliding, (3) erases A-lines (4) reaches the bottom of the screen. If any one of the requirements is not met, it is not a B-line.

B-line artifact can be seen in interstitial syndromes (Table 12–4). A few B-lines in the bases of

TABLE 12-3 Evidence bases recommendations for lung ultrasonography.

Level of Evidence	Clinical Syndromes and Recommendations

A (High quality) Further research is very unlikely to change estimates	1. Pneumothorax (PTX)
	  • Signs suggesting PTX: presence of lung point, B-lines, lung pulse, or absence of lung sliding.
	  • Ultrasound rules out PTX more accurately than supine anterior chest radiography (CXR).
	2. Interstitial syndrome
	  • Diffuse B-lines indicate interstitial syndrome.
	  • A positive sign is defined by the presence of 3 or more B-lines between 2 ribs.
	3. Alveolar consolidation
	  • Lung ultrasound for detection of lung consolidation can differentiate consolidation due to pulmonary embolism, pneumonia, or atelectasis.
	  • Lung ultrasound is an alternative diagnostic tool to computerized tomography (CT) in diagnosis of pulmonary embolism when it is contraindicated or unavailable.
	  • In mechanically ventilated patients, lung ultrasonography is more accurate than CXR in detecting and distinguishing various types of consolidations.
	4. Pleural effusions
	  • A hypoechoic space between the parietal and visceral pleura with respiratory movement of the lung within the effusion is very specific for such condition.
	  • Internal echoes in the effusion suggest that fluid is an exudate or hemorrhagic.
	  • Lung ultrasound is more accurate that supine radiography and nearly as accurate as CT.
	  • Lung ultrasound is more accurate in distinguishing effusion from consolidation than CXR.
	5. Monitoring lung disease
	  • In cardiogenic pulmonary edema, severity of congestion is proportional to number of B-lines.
	  • B-lines can be used to monitor response to therapy in patients with cardiogenic pulmonary edema.
	  • In patients with increased extravascular lung water, assessment of lung reaeration can be assessed by a decrease in the number of B-lines.
	  • In acute lung injury or acute respiratory distress syndrome (ARDS), tracking changes in sonographic findings may quantitatively assess lung reaeration.

B (Moderate quality) Further research is likely to have an important impact in changing	1. Pneumothorax
	  • Ultrasound rules in PTX more accurately than supine anterior CXR.
	2. Interstitial syndrome
	  • Diffuse bilateral B-lines indicate interstitial syndrome of various causes, ie, pulmonary edema/ interstitial pneumonia/diffuse parenchymal lung disease.
	  • Localized B-lines are seen in pneumonia/pneumonitis/atelectasis/pulmonary contusions/ pulmonary infarctions/pleural disease/neoplasia.
	  • Pulmonary fibrosis can be evaluated with ultrasound, diffuse multiple B-lines with pleural abnormalities are seen often.
	  • Sonographic findings of ARDS include anterior subpleural consolidations/absence or reduction of lung sliding/pleural line abnormalities/nonhomogeneous B-lines.
	3. Alveolar consolidation
	  • Ultrasound is a useful tool to rule in pneumonia provided consolidation reaches the pleura.
	  • Ultrasound should be considered for the evaluation of pulmonary conditions in patients with pleuritic pain.
	4. Pleural effusions
	  • The optimal site to detect a nonloculated pleural effusion is at the posterior axillary line above the diaphragm.
	5. Monitoring lung disease
	  • Serial evaluation of B-lines in hemodialyzed patients with pulmonary congestion may be of clinical utility.
	  • In cardiogenic pulmonary edema, semi-quantitative B-line assessment is a prognostic indicator of adverse outcomes and mortality.

(Continued)

TABLE 12–3 Evidence bases recommendations for lung ultrasonography. (*Continued*)

Level of Evidence	Clinical Syndromes and Recommendations

C (Low Quality) Further research is very likely to have an important impact as the evidence is currently very uncertain	1. Pneumothorax
	  • Ultrasound is a better initial study compared to chest radiography and may lead to better patient outcomes.
	  • Ultrasound compares well to computerized tomography in assessment for PTX.
	  • Lung point ultrasound is a useful tool to differentiate large and small PTX.
	2. Interstitial syndrome
	  • Lung ultrasound used as first-line diagnostic approach in the evaluation of suspected interstitial syndromes compared to CXR may lead to better outcomes.
	3. Alveolar consolidation
	  • Low-frequency ultrasound scanning may allow for better evaluation of the extent of a consolidation.
	  • Lung ultrasound used as an initial diagnostic strategy in consolidations improves outcomes compared to CXR.
	4. Monitoring lung disease
	  • Semiquantitative techniques of B-line evaluation are useful as a prognostic indicator of outcomes or mortality in patients with left-sided heart failure.

Data from Volpicelli G, Elbarbary M, Blaivas M, et al: International evidence-based recommendations for point-of-care lung ultrasound, *Intensive Care Med.* 2012 Apr;38(4):577-591.

the lung are considered normal but more than three B-lines in a single field should be considered abnormal (Figure 12–3).

Diffuse bilateral B-line pattern with smooth pleura is consistent with cardiogenic interstitial edema.[11] Diffuse bilateral B-line pattern with an irregular pleura is usually seen in adult respiratory distress syndrome. Focal irregular pleura with B-lines can be interpreted as early or atypical pneumonia in an appropriate clinical setting.

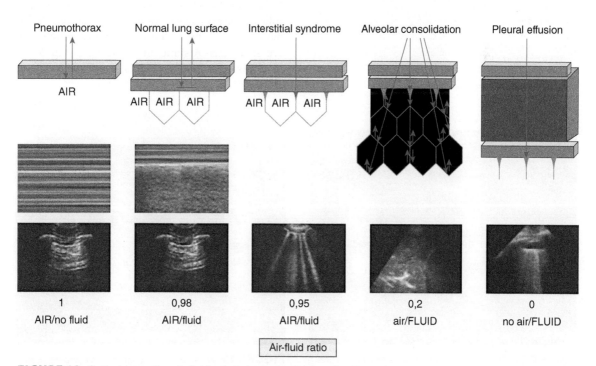

FIGURE 12–1 Understanding air-fluid ratio in lung ultrasonography. (*Reproduced with permission from Lichtenstein DA: Lung Ultrasound in the Critically Ill: The BLUE Protocol. Switzerland: Springer; 2016*).

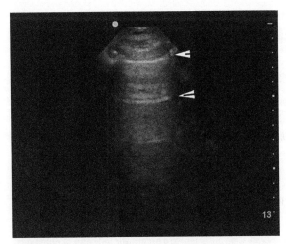

FIGURE 12–2 This is the bat sign representing normal lung. Arrowheads are pointing the A-lines.

TABLE 12–4 Causes of interstitial syndrome.

Pathophysiology	Etiologies
Cardiogenic	Acute hemodynamic pulmonary edema
Noncardiogenic	Adult respiratory distress syndrome Pneumonias Interstitial lung disease Lung contusion Pneumonitis Alveolar hemorrhage

Used with permission from Sahar Ahmad, MD.

TABLE 12–5 Causes of consolidation.

Etiology
Bacterial infection Mycobacterial infection Fungal infection Viral infection Malignancies Lung infarction Absorptive atelectasis

The Alveolar Consolidation Syndrome—The alveolar consolidation syndrome refers to any condition that can fill the alveoli with fluid (Table 12–5). About 98.5% of alveolar consolidations reach the pleura, enabling ultrasound examination. In a supine patient, 90% of consolidations can be found in the most dependent area of the thorax.[8] The *tissue-like sign* is an echoic pattern, with regular trabeculation reminiscent of an ill-defined liver (Figure 12–4). Ultrasound has a 90% and 98% sensitivity and specificity, respectively.[8] In alveolar consolidation syndromes 2 types of air bronchograms can be seen, static and dynamic. Dynamic air bronchograms indicate the presence of air moving within the bronchus with each breathing cycle, ruling out absorptive atelectasis. A static air bronchogram indicates obstruction of the bronchus causing absorptive atelectasis.

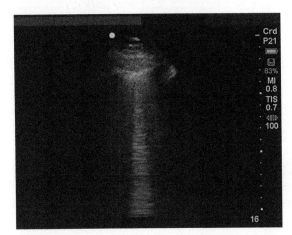

FIGURE 12–3 B-lines are comet-tail artifacts that are seen in interstitial lung syndrome.

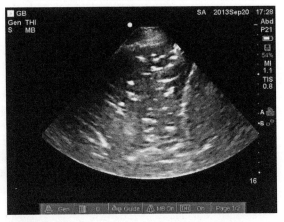

FIGURE 12–4 Alveolar consolidation syndrome seen in pneumonia. *(Image courtesy of Sahar Ahmad, MD).*

Pleural Ultrasonography

PTX occurs in 6% of the ICU patients[12] and up to 30% of those can be misdiagnosed on conventional CXR owing to the supine position of the critically ill patient.[13] The gold standard to diagnose PTX is CT-Chest; this involves transferring the patient with all the risks associated with it. Luckily ultrasound can help us identify PTX by scanning the anterior chest. Once the bat sign is identified, the absence of lung sliding plus a diffuse A-line pattern should prompt us to consider the diagnosis of PTX (Figure 12–5). Lung point indicates the point where the lung is touching the chest wall and moves with each respiratory cycle, this is 100% specific for PTX. The sensitivity of lung point for PTX detection is not 100% since this is usually absent in large PTX. It is important to mention that the presence of lung pulse or B-lines rule out PTX in 100% of the cases.

Another phenomenon described in left side PTX is the flickering image in the parasternal long axis view of the heart. The heart is seen in mid-diastole and disappears in midsystole. This is explained by the transient interposition of air between the chest wall and the heart, making it hard to visualize when it is empty and not in contact with the chest wall. This is called *heart point* (Figure 12–6).[14]

Pleural effusion is a very common finding in ICU patients.[15] It collects in dependent areas unless

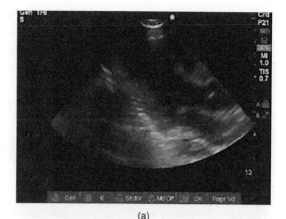

(a)

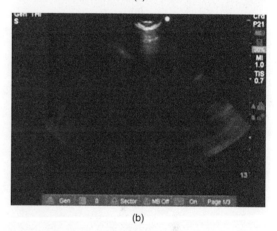

(b)

FIGURE 12–6 Heart point. In a parasternal long axis view of the heart Image A represents the heart in diastole, when it is fully seen, Image B represents the heart in systole, contact of the heart with the chest wall has disappeared as well as the image. (*Reprinted with permission of the American Thoracic Society. Copyright © 2016 American Thoracic Society. Khan R, Rahmanian M, Kaufman M, et al: The Heart Point Sign: An Ultrasonographic Confirmation Of Pneumothorax, 2013.*)

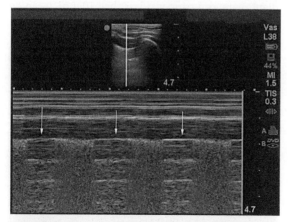

FIGURE 12–5 This image shows pneumothorax, note the absence of lung sliding that is represented as stratosphere sign (*arrows*) and sliding lung represented by seashore sign (*in between arrows*) in M-mode. Intermittent seashore and stratosphere sign is seen in the lung point.

loculated. By using the signs described below, ultrasound can achieve a sensitivity and specificity of 93%.[9]

A big pleural effusion is easily identified and must be distinguished from ascites. Using simple static and dynamic signs, we can tell them apart. The lung can be identified as a consolidated mass usually with air bronchograms, floating in fluid. This is called the *jellyfish sign*. The diaphragm should be identified above the liver and the spleen, if there is no *jellyfish sign* in a big effusion; the structure is likely to be the liver (or spleen), not the lung (Figure 12–7).

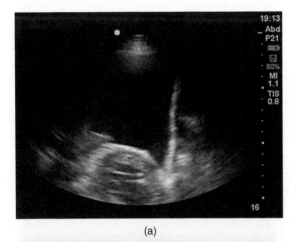

(a)

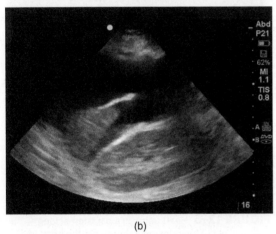

(b)

FIGURE 12-7   Image A represents a pleural effusion; look at the similarities with ascites in Image B. It is important to determine static and dynamic signs to differentiate between pleural effusions from ascites.

Ultrasound can also help identify the nature of the pleural effusion. A complex anechoic or hypoechoic space with septations most likely represents an exudative effusion (Figure 12–8).[16] Sometimes this effusion can be seen as a "thick effusion" meaning a tissue-like echogenicity but with particles swirling around. This is called the *plankton sign*, which is seen in empyema and hemothorax (Figure 12–9).

Diaphragm Evaluation

This structure usually is easily visualized above the liver or spleen. There have been studies examining diaphragm thickness and strength. It is well

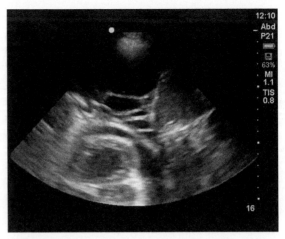

FIGURE 12-8   Septated pleural effusion usually seen in an exudative effusion. These strands resembling spider webs are floating in the pleural effusion.

known that thinning of the diaphragm starts within 18 hours of muscle inactivity.[17] This was demonstrated by ultrasonography in 7 patients measuring the diaphragm using the 7.5- to 10-MHz linear probe placed in the midaxillary line to measure the apposition area (Figure 12–10).[18] The utility of this should be further studied. Another promising use for ultrasonography of the diaphragm includes evaluation of its excursion during weaning from mechanical ventilation. Kim et al found that in patients with diaphragm dysfunction, defined when diaphragm excursion was less than 10 mm, weaning

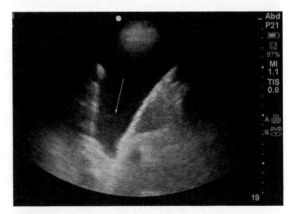

FIGURE 12-9   Plankton sign is usually seen when debris exist within the pleural effusion; it can be pus or blood (see *arrow*).

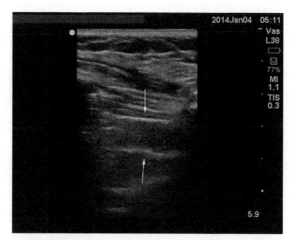

FIGURE 12-10 Diaphragm thickness (*in between arrows*). Image acquired in the apposition area.

failure rate was higher when compared to patients with diaphragm excursion of more than 10 mm.[19]

Critical Care Echocardiography

Echocardiography, either transthoracic echocardiography or transesophageal is a very helpful tool in the critically ill patient. This will be discussed in detail in Chapter 94 of this book.

Abdominal Ultrasonography

Ultrasound Probe Selection and Orientation

The preferred ultrasound probe to evaluate the abdominal area will be a 3.5 to 5 MHz with a small footprint with the cursor pointing cephalad.

Clinical Implications of Abdominal Ultrasonography and Recognition of Important Structures

The intensivist should be capable of performing and interpreting simple abdominal ultrasonography. Detailed ultrasound examination of the abdominal organs is out of the scope of this book. It is our practice to perform abdominal POC-US paying attention to liver, spleen, kidney, bladder, gallbladder, aorta, and intestines.

Recognition of the Peritoneal Space

The parietal and visceral layers are in touch with each other and slide with each respiratory cycle; this is called *gut sliding*.

It is imperative to look for free fluid in an unstable patient. We have found FAST very useful in different situations outside the classic trauma population.

The peritoneal fluid can range from anechoic to hyperechoic, depending on the etiology. Transudates will have an anechoic nature, an hemoperitoneum can be visualized depending on the amount and time elapsed since bleeding started; it could be mildly hyperechoic with plankton sign or more hyperechoic if the blood had already organized. An exudative effusion causing infectious peritonitis could have septations. Ultrasound is more sensitive for detecting septations than CT scan.

Pneumoperitoneum (Figure 12–11) can be detected with ultrasound using the same concepts we have learned in pneumothorax. There are a couple of signs that will help us identify this condition: (a) Gut sliding: as described above, can rule out pneumoperitoneum. (b) Splanchnogram: it is when an abdominal organ can be seen with ultrasound, thus, ruling out pneumoperitoneum between the probe and the organ.

The presence of these 2 signs can rule out pneumoperitoneum accurately.

Kidney and Bladder

The probe should be oriented with the pointer cephalad and placed in the posterior axillary line under the costal border; once the liver or the spleen is identified, the kidney is easier to find.

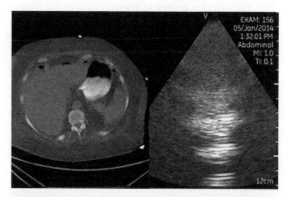

FIGURE 12-11 Pneumoperitoneum detected through ultrasonography. Please note the reverberation artifact resembling the lung A-line. There is no splagnogram. Used with permission from Sahar Ahmad, MD.

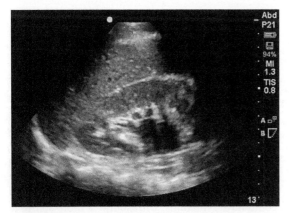

FIGURE 12-12 Acute hydronephrosis of the right kidney.

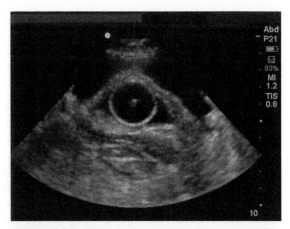

FIGURE 12-13 Urinary catheter balloon inside the bladder.

Acute renal failure (ARF) is frequently encountered in the critically ill patient. The etiologies are classified into prerenal, renal, and postrenal. Ultrasound is useful as an initial screening tool.

The evaluation of the renal parenchyma by ultrasound is complex but we can briefly mention some concepts. ARF can be differentiated from chronic renal failure (CRF) because in the latter small kidneys with thin parenchyma and irregular borders are seen. Corticomedullary dedifferentiation can be seen in multiple conditions. In acute medical renal disease the renal parenchyma becomes more echogenic. The renal pelvises are well visualized under ultrasound. Chronic dilatation causes rounded renal calyces and the acute dilatation causes flatter renal calyces (Figure 12–12).

The bladder is very well visualized in the suprapubic area with the probe held transversely. A full bladder can be identified as an anechoic structure, if the patient has an urinary catheter, this can be easily visualized (Figure 12–13). Furthermore, ultrasound of the bladder can be used to check for urinary retention without using a catheter.

Ultrasound of the Abdominal Aorta

This is a very important structure to evaluate in an unstable patient and in someone who has been complaining of abdominal or flank pain. Abdominal aortic aneurysm (AAA) rupture has a high mortality rate (around 50%) and ultrasound has been shown to be a reliable method of evaluating AAA.

The thoracic aorta is better evaluated with a transesophageal echocardiogram or contrast computerized tomography. The abdominal aorta is easily visualized by transabdominal ultrasound.

The aorta is evaluated with the ultrasound probe placed in the midline of the abdomen and the cursor pointing toward the patient's right when a transverse view is desired and pointing toward the head when a longitudinal view is desired. The aorta should be studied from the epigastrium until the bifurcation to the iliac arteries (Figure 12–14). A diameter greater than 3 cm is considered aneurysmal. Ultrasound is not very sensitive to evaluate for aortic dissections but if a false lumen is seen, it is highly specific for such disease.

Gastrointestinal Tract

The esophagus is usually very difficult to visualize under ultrasound. It becomes visible and feasible for ultrasound assessment once it enters the abdomen to join the stomach. Ultrasound evaluation of the abdominal part of the gastrointestinal (GI) tract is very useful in the critically ill patient.

One observational study showed the utility of identifying gastric contents with ultrasound and performing suctioning prior to emergent endotracheal intubation.[20] It is thought that this can potentially decrease the chances of aspiration during intubation. The use of ultrasound had also been described for confirmation of

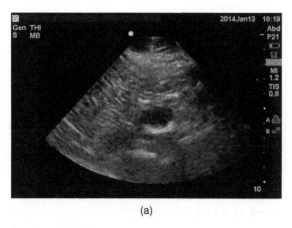

(a)

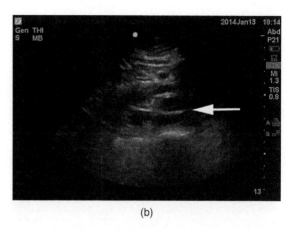

(b)

FIGURE 12–14 Image A shows a normal abdominal aorta with the inferior vena cava located on the left. Image B shows a dissection flap (*arrow*) inside the abdominal aorta.

nasogastric tube and Sengstaken-Blakemore tube positioning.[21-23]

When evaluating the GI tract, it is important to observe the wall thickness that usually ranges around 2 to 4 mm. It is also very important to observe for gut sliding and peristalsis; the latter are permanent dynamic crawling contractions seen from the antrum of the stomach until the terminal ileus. The presence of peristalsis is rare in a true surgical abdomen.

Liver, Gallbladder, and Spleen

The liver is rarely a target in a critically ill patient despite its size. It acts as an acoustic window to access the heart, Morrison pouch and inferior vena cava analysis. However in some occasions, gross abnormalities can arise such as the following: (a) Liver abscess: yields a round heterogenous hypoechoic image within the regular hepatic echostructure easily identifiable. A highly hyperechoic image can represent microbial gas. (b) Portal gas: as a result of mesenteric infarction. Hyperechoic images disseminated within the liver parenchyma mainly in the periphery and resembling alveolar consolidation with air bronchograms. (c) Liver cirrhosis: yields a coarse and nodular pattern with atrophy (Figure 12–15). (d) Hepatic tumors: Metastatic tumors are usually multiple iso- or hypoechoic masses. However an echoic heterogeneous mass within a cirrhotic parenchyma suggests hepatoma.

A simple biliary cyst is usually described as a simple anechoic structure with thin walls (Figure 12–16).

The gallbladder can be viewed during ultrasound of the right upper quadrant. The following findings are suggestive of acute cholecystitis: (1) Enlarged gallbladder over 90 mm in long axis and over 50 mm in short axis. (2) Thickening of the wall greater than 3 mm. (3) Sludge or stones seen within gallbladder. (4) Perivesicular fluid collection. (5) Murphy sign. The sensitivity drops if all the criteria are used but specificity increases.

Cardiogenic or noncardiogenic gallbladder wall edema can confound the diagnosis of acute cholecystitis.

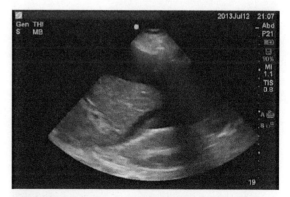

FIGURE 12–15 A small liver compatible with liver cirrhosis, the similarity with a consolidated lung can confuse the nonexperienced operator between ascites and pleural effusion.

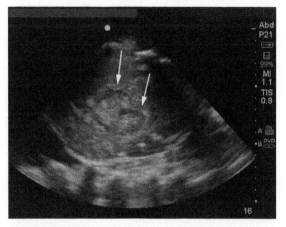

FIGURE 12–16 Liver tumor with metastasis (*arrows*).

Spleen analysis in the critically ill is seldom revealing. It acts as an acoustic window for different organs and also to localize the diaphragm while planning for thoracentesis. In a trauma patient, splenic laceration can be detected and in rare instances a splenic abscess is seen.

Deep Venous Thrombosis Assessment
Ultrasound Probe Selection and Orientation
The high-frequency 7.5 to 10 MHz linear probe is preferred in our institution with the cursor pointing toward the right of the patient.

Introduction of Venous Ultrasonography of the Lower Extremities
Deep vein thrombosis (DVT) and pulmonary embolism (PE) are a spectrum of the same disease. In a rapidly decompensating patient, either in the hospital ward or in the ICU, DVT and PE should always be in the differential diagnosis. Blood test such as D-dimer is nonspecific in the hospitalized patient. Ultrasound of the lower extremities can successfully diagnose DVT. When done by a trained intensivist, the sensitivity and specificity are very similar to examinations done by the radiology technician and interpreted by a radiologist.[24] A DVT can be found in the upper and lower extremities. We will focus on lower extremity anatomy here.

The patient should be positioned in the decubitus position with the leg slightly flexed and externally rotated (Figure 12–17). The leg should be examined by performing gentle and firm compression, enough to collapse (Figure 12–18) the vein but not the artery. A vein with DVT will not collapse. (Figures 12–19 and 12–20).

The operator should be familiar with the lower extremity venous anatomy (see Figure 12–20). The ultrasound probe should be placed at the level of the inguinal ligament to localize the femoral vein, which is medial to the femoral artery. Once this is identified, a compression movement is performed to check for collapsibility, a collapsible vein rules out DVT. A noncollapsible vein, rules in DVT. Color

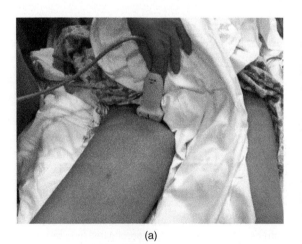

(a)

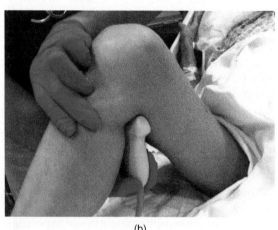

(b)

FIGURE 12–17 Position of deep venous thrombosis (DVT) study for femoral and popliteal vein.

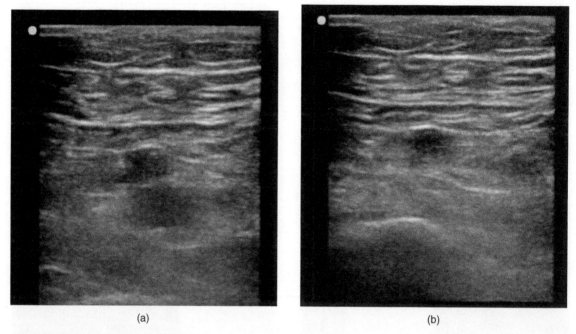

(a)   (b)

FIGURE 12–18 Femoral vein in a patient with suspected deep venous thrombosis. Image A without compression and Image B showing vein completely collapsible.

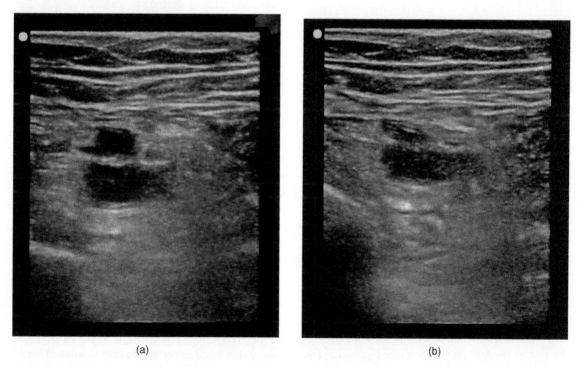

(a)   (b)

FIGURE 12–19 Femoral vein in a patient with suspected deep venous thrombosis. Image A without compression and Image B showing the vein is not collapsible.

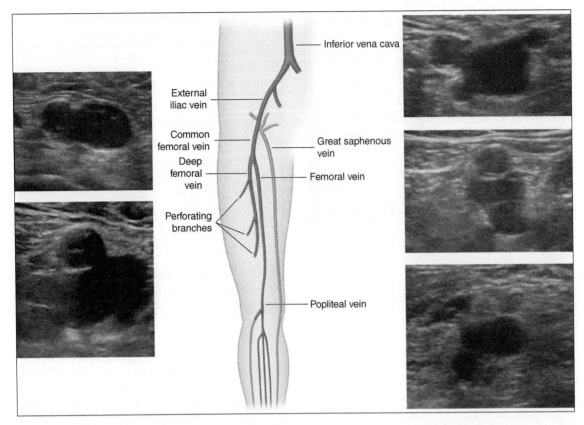

FIGURE 12–20 Important veins of the lower extremity, it is important to be familiar with the anatomy in order to interpret where the DVT is located. Dark blue: Deep vein. Light Blue: superficial vein.

Doppler can be used but will increase study time without adding much information. Unfortunately, the external iliac veins are not visualized fully but can be partially visualized if the probe is tilted and pointing the ultrasound beam "under" the inguinal ligament. Once the common femoral vein (CFV) is studied, the drainage of the greater saphenous vein can be seen medially. A couple of centimeters below, the CFV bifurcates in deep femoral vein and superficial femoral vein (SFV). It is important to recall that the SFV is still part of the deep venous system. Compression should be done every 2 to 3 cm while identifying the perforating branches until the vein enters the adductor canal if visibility allows. The popliteal vein should also be studied with the leg bent and the sole of the foot on the bed (see Figure 12–17). The popliteal vein should be located superficially to

the artery. Again, firm pressure is applied to evaluate compressibility.

How can we integrate these findings in our clinical assessment? A hypoxic patient with positive DVT and bilateral A-line pattern in the lung, PE should be suspected. Furthermore, a quick echocardiogram should be done and if there are signs of right ventricle overload, submassive or massive PE is highly suspected.

Optic Nerve Ultrasonography
Probe Selection and Orientation
It is usually performed with the high-frequency 7.5 to 10 MHz linear probe and it is placed over the eyelid. The optic nerve sheath (ONS) will be identified and then measured (Figure 12–21).

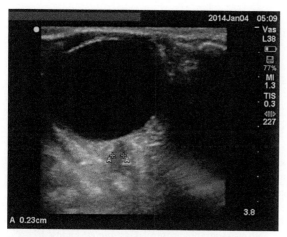

FIGURE 12–21 Optic nerve sheet measurement. In this particular case, it was not enlarged.

Competency Requirements

It is estimated that 10 studies could be sufficient in experienced US operators and 25 studies for inexperienced US operators to achieve competency.[25]

Clinical Implications

The gold standard for detection of an elevated intracranial pressure (ICP) is invasive measurement. These methods can lead to complications such as infection or bleeding. Other methods are described but we found US measurement of the optic nerve sheath diameter (ONSD) an excellent screening test for elevated ICP.

When ONSD is compared to the gold standard, a pooled analysis using cutoff value range from 5.2 to 5.9 mm showed a sensitivity and specificity of 74% to 95% and 74% to 100%, respectively.[26] In another meta-analysis[27] the pooled sensitivity and specificity was 90% and 85%, respectively. One study using 5 mm as a cutoff[28] yielded 100% and 95% sensitivity and specificity, respectively.

PROCEDURAL GUIDANCE

Several procedures can be done in the intensive care unit (Table 12–6). These procedures will be described in details in subsequent chapters. When possible, the dynamic technique, which involves direct visualization of the needle tip, is highly

TABLE 12–6 Procedures done under ultrasound guidance in critical care.

- Paracentesis
- Thoracentesis
- Pericardiocentesis
- Central venous line placement
- Arterial line placement
- Transthoracic-guided biopsy, for microbiological sampling or malignancy
- Lung abscess drainage
- Liver or spleen abscess drainage
- Lumbar puncture
- Peritoneal collection drainage
- Pacemaker placement
- Percutaneous gallbladder drainage
- Percutaneous bladder drainage

recommended for nearly all procedures. Continuous vision of the needle tip will ensure low complication rates.

CONCLUSION

POC-US is a helpful noninvasive tool that benefits the critically ill patient. It is easy to perform and learn but requires practice to master. POC-US should be incorporated in the skills of every intensivist.

REFERENCES

1. Slasky BS, Auerbach D, Skolnick ML. Value of portable real-time ultrasound in the ICU. *Crit Care Med.* 1983;11(3):160-164.
2. Harris RD, Simeone JF, Mueller PR, Butch RJ. Portable ultrasound examinations in intensive care units. *J Ultrasound Med.* 1985;4(9):463-465.
3. Schunk K, Pohan D, Schild H. The clinical relevance of sonography in intensive care units. *Aktuelle Radiol.* 1992;2(5):309-314.
4. Lichtenstein DA, Axler O. Intensive use of general ultrasound in the intensive care unit. *Intensive Care Med.* 1993;19:353-355.
5. Mayo PH, Beaulieu Y, Doelken P, et al. American College of Chest Physicians/La Societe de Reanimation de Langue Francaise statement on competence in critical care ultrasonography. *Chest.* 2009;135(4):1050-1060.
6. Expert Round Table on Ultrasound in ICU. International expert statement on training standards

for critical care ultrasonography. *Intensive Care Med.* 2011;37(7):1077-1083.

7. Volpicelli G, Elbarbary M, Blaivas M, et al. International evidence-based recommendations for point-of-care lung ultrasound. *Intensive Care Med.* 2012;38(4):577-591.

8. Litchteinstein DA, Lascols N, Mezière G, Gepner A. Ultrasound diagnosis of alveolar consolidation in the critically ill. *Intensive Care Med.* 2004;30(2):276-281.

9. Litchteinstein DA, Goldstein I, Mourgeon E, Cluzel P, Grenier P, Rouby. Comparative diagnostic performances of auscultation, chest radiography and lung ultrasonography in acute respiratory distress syndrome. *Anesthesiology.* 2004;100(1):9-15.

10. Lichtenstein D, Mézière G, Biderman P, Gepner A, Barré O. The comet-tail artifact. An ultrasound sing of alveolar-interstitial syndrome. *Am J Respir Crit Care Med.* 1997;156:1640-1646.

11. Lichtenstein DA, Mézière GA, Lagoueyte JF, Biderman P, Goldstein I, Gepner A. A-lines and B-lines: lung ultrasound as a bedside tool for predicting pulmonary artery occlusion pressure in the critically ill. *Chest.* 2009;136(4):1014-1020.

12. Kollef MH. Risk factors for the misdiagnosis of pneumothorax in the intensive care unit. *Crit Care Med.* 1991;19(7):906-910.

13. Tocino IM, Miller MH, Fairfax WR. Distribution of pneumothorax in the supine and semirecumbent critically ill adult. *AJR Am J Roentgenol.* 1985;144(5):901-905.

14. Stone MB, Chilstrom M, Chase K, Lichtenstein D. The heart point sign: description of a new ultrasound finding suggesting pneumothorax. *Acad Emerg Med.* 2010;17(11):e149-e150.

15. Mattison LE, Coppage L, Alderman DF, Herlong JO, Sahn SA. Pleural effusions in the medical ICU. Prevalance, causes and clinical implications. *Chest.* 1997;111(4):1018-1023.

16. Yang PC, Luh KT, Chang DB, Wu HD, Yu CJ, Kuo SH. Value of sonography in determining the nature of pleural effusion: analysis of 320 cases. *AJR Am J Roentgenol.* 1992;159(1):29-33.

17. Levine S, Nguyen T, Taylor N, et al. Rapid disuse atrophy of diaphragm fibers in mechanically ventilated humans. *N Engl J Med.* 2008;358(13):1327-1335.

18. Grosu HB, Lee YI, Lee J, Eden E, Eikermann M, Rose KM. Diaphragm muscle thinning in patients who are mechanically ventilated. *Chest.* 2012;142(6):1455-1460.

19. Kim WY, Suh HJ, Hong SB, Koh Y, Lim CM. Diaphragm dysfunction assessed by ultrasonography: influence on weaning from mechanical ventilation. *Crit Care Med.* 2011;39(12):2627-2630.

20. Koenig SJ, Lakticova V, Mayo PH. Utility of ultrasonography for detection of gastric fluid during urgent endotracheal intubation. *Intensive Care Med.* 2011;37(4):627-631.

21. Lock G, Reng M, Messman H, Grüne S, Schölmerich J, Holstege A. Inflation and positioning of the gastric balloon of a Sengstaken-Blakemore tube under ultrasonographic control. *Gastrointest Endosc.* 1997;45(6):538.

22. Lin AC, Hsu YH, Wang TL, Chong CF. Placement confirmation of Sengstaken-Blakemore tube by ultrasound. *Emerg Med J.* 2006;23(6):487.

23. Kim HM, So BH, Jeong WJ, Choi SM, Park KN. The effectiveness of ultrasonography in verifying the placement of a nasograstric tube in patients with low consciousness at an emergency center. *Scand J Trauma Resusc Emerg Med.* 2012;20:38.

24. Kory PD, Pellecchia CM, Shiloh AL, Mayo PH, DiBello C, Koenig S. Accuracy of ultrasonography performed by critical care physicians for the diagnosis of DVT. *Chest.* 2011;139(3):538-542.

25. Tayal VS, Neulander M, Norton HJ, Foster T, Saunders T, Blaivas M. Emergency department sonographic measurement of optic nerve sheath diameter to detect findings of increased intracranial pressure in adult head injury patients. *Ann Emerg Med.* 2007;49(4):508-514.

26. Rosenberg JB, Shiloh AL, Savel RH, Eisen LA. Non-invasive methods of estimating intracranial pressure. *Neurocrit Care.* 2011;15(3):599-608.

27. Dubourg J, Javouhey E, Geeraerts T Messerer M, Kassai B. Ultrasonography of optic nerve sheath diameter for detection of raised intracranial pressure: a systematic review and meta-analysis. *Intensive Care Med.* 2011;37(7):1059-1068.

28. Blaivas M, Theodoro D, Sierzenski PR. Elevated intracranial pressure detected by bedside emergency ultrasonography of the optic nerve sheath. *Aca Emerg Med.* 2001;10(4):376-381.

Patient Safety in the ICU

Jason Adelman, MD, MS

---

1 The intensive care unit (ICU) is particularly prone to medical errors as patients are very ill and require continuous monitoring.

2 A patient safety program that drives improvement for critical care patients can be categorized into 4 general domains: (1) ensuring compliance with patient safety regulations; (2) responding to adverse events by performing root cause analyses and implementing targeted corrective actions; (3) applying evidence-based risk reduction strategies that are not required by regulations, but are considered best practices; and (4) implementing strategies to meet and exceed patient safety metrics that are publicly reported or tied to pay-for-performance programs.

3 To prevent wrong patient errors, the Joint Commission requires the use of at least 2 patient identifiers when administering medications and blood products, when collecting laboratory specimens and taking imaging tests, and when providing any type of treatment.

4 The majority of adverse events are never reported and therefore cannot be addressed.

5 When a serious adverse event happens to a critical care patient, a systematic investigation of the event, called a root cause analysis, should be completed by an interdisciplinary team that has expertise in the areas involved in the event.

6 According to the Just Culture concept, the major focus of an adverse event investigation should be on potential system failures that led to the error as opposed to simply attributing blame to the providers involved in the error.

7 Team training is a well-established approach for preventing errors in high-risk industries such as the military and the airline industry, and is now being applied to the medical industry.

8 Simulation is a promising new strategy for improving patient safety. Similar to flight simulators used by the airline industry, health care simulators allow providers to learn a procedure or protocol using high-tech mannequins instead of live patients.

9 Pay-for-performance is a new approach for driving improvement in medical care by using financial incentives to reward hospitals that perform well on preestablished safety and quality measures.

10 Those who want to lead in patient safety should innovate new approaches for preventing errors, and study these approaches using rigorous research methodology.

PATIENT SAFETY IN THE INTENSIVE CARE UNIT

The modern patient safety movement began with the release of the 1999 Institute of Medicine (IOM) report "To Err Is Human," which estimated that up to 98,000 patients die each year from medical errors. This high number of deaths exceeded the number attributed to the eighth leading cause of death at the time, and helped refocus the health care community on the importance of patient safety. The ICU is particularly prone to medical errors as patients are very ill and require continuous monitoring. The care of ICU patients can be complex, involving multiple consultants and many medications, where life-and-death decisions often need to be made quickly. A 2006 international study of 205 ICUs found an average of 38.8 events that compromised patient safety per every 100 patient critical care days, highlighting the need for risk reduction and complication avoidance strategies in ICUs.

The Four Domains of a Patient Safety Program

A patient safety program that drives improvement for critical care patients can be categorized into 4 general domains (Figure 13-1): (1) ensuring compliance with patient safety regulations (eg, The Joint Commission National Patient Safety Goals [NPSGs]); (2) responding to adverse events by performing root cause analyses and implementing targeted corrective actions (eg, delayed response to a ventilator alarm); (3) applying evidence-based risk reduction strategies that are not required by regulations, but are considered best practices (eg, checklists); and (4) implementing strategies to meet and exceed patient safety metrics that are publicly reported or tied to pay-for-performance programs (eg, hospital-associated infections reported on public report cards). Hospitals that are leaders in patient safety excel in each of these 4 domains, and also contribute to the science of patient safety by developing new strategies for preventing errors, conducting research, and publishing their findings.

Patient Safety Regulations

The Joint Commission NPSGs are the predominant patient safety regulations that guide hospitals'

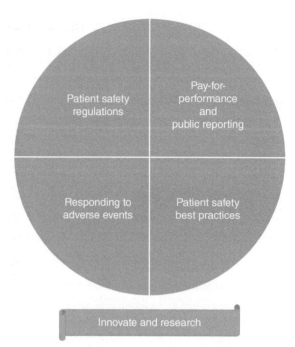

FIGURE 13-1 Four domains of a patient safety program.

medical error reduction strategies. Established in 2002, the NPSGs require organizations to address specific areas of concern in regard to patient safety. Many of these goals target important patient safety issues in critical care units including proper patient identification, timely response to critical tests, and appropriate use of clinical alarms. Table 13-1 has a complete list of the 2016 Joint Commission NPSGs.

Patient Identification

Wrong patient errors occur in virtually all stages of diagnosis and treatment. On critical care units, patients are often in close proximity, elderly and encumbered with tubes and cannulas. Under these conditions patients can look alike and be confused with one another. To prevent wrong patient errors, the Joint Commission requires the use of at least 2 patient identifiers when administering medications and blood products, when collecting laboratory specimens and taking imaging tests, and when providing any type of treatment.

Critical Test Results

Critical test results that fall significantly outside the normal range and indicate potentially

TABLE 13–1 2016 Joint commission patient safety goals.

Identify patients correctly	• Use at least 2 ways to identify patients. For example, use the patient's name and date of birth. This is done to make sure that each patient gets the correct medicine and treatment. • Make sure that the correct patient gets the correct blood when they get a blood transfusion.
Improve staff communication	• Get important test results to the right staff person on time.
Use medicines safely	• Before a procedure, label medicines that are not labeled. For example, medicines in syringes, cups, and basins. Do this in the area where medicines and supplies are set up. • Take extra care with patients who take medicines to thin their blood. • Record and pass along correct information about a patient's medicines. Find out what medicines the patient is taking. Compare those medicines to new medicines given to the patient. Make sure the patient knows which medicines to take when they are at home. Tell the patient it is important to bring their up-to-date list of medicines every time they visit a doctor.
Use alarms safely	• Make improvements to ensure that alarms on medical equipment are heard and responded to on time.
Prevent infection	• Use the hand cleaning guidelines from the Centers for Disease Control and Prevention or the World Health Organization. Set goals for improving hand cleaning. Use the goals to improve hand cleaning. • Use proven guidelines to prevent infections that are difficult to treat. • Use proven guidelines to prevent infection of the blood from central lines. • Use proven guidelines to prevent infection after surgery. • Use proven guidelines to prevent infections of the urinary tract that are caused by catheters.
Identify patient safety risks	• Find out which patients are most likely to try to commit suicide.
Prevent mistakes in surgery	• Make sure that the correct surgery is done on the correct patient and at the correct place on the patient's body. • Mark the correct place on the patient's body where the surgery is to be done. • Pause before the surgery to make sure that a mistake is not being made.

life-threatening conditions are common in intensive care patients. The Joint Commission requires these critical test results be reported within reasonable time frames that are established by the hospital. The intent is for patients to receive appropriate treatment as soon as possible. The Joint Commission also requires that procedures are put in place for tracking these reporting times, and that performance improvement programs are used when reporting times are not within acceptable time frames.

Clinical Alarms

A newly added Joint Commission regulation addresses the safety of improperly managed clinical alarm systems, which are an important part of the care and monitoring of critically ill patients. Clinical alarm systems are intended to alert caregivers of potential patient emergencies, but when improperly configured they can compromise patient safety. Critical care units have numerous clinical alarms,

and the resulting noise and visual warnings can desensitize staff and cause them to miss or ignore these alarms. In some instances critical care staff will disable alarms or set alarm limits to inappropriate thresholds to decrease distractions. This new Joint Commission regulation requires that leaders establish alarm system safety as a hospital priority, establish policies addressing critical issues in alarm management (Table 13–2), and educate staff about the proper operation of alarm systems for which they are responsible.

Failure Mode and Effects Analysis

In addition to the NPSGs, the Joint Commission requires hospitals to perform yearly proactive risk assessments of a high-risk process called a Failure Mode and Effects Analysis (FMEA). When doing an FMEA, an interdisciplinary team of experts create a detailed flow diagram of the high-risk process being evaluated. After this is completed, each step of the

TABLE 13-2 Critical issues in alarm management.

- Establish clinically appropriate settings for alarm signals and who has the authority to set or change alarm parameters.
- Determine when alarm signals can be disabled and who has the authority to set alarm parameters to "off."
- Develop a system for monitoring and responding to alarm signals.
- Create a process for checking individual alarm signals for accurate settings, proper operation, and detectability.

process is assigned 3 scores: (1) the risk of failure (1-10, with 10 representing the highest risk of failure); (2) the likelihood that the failure will be intercepted before reaching the patient (1-10, with 10 representing the least likelihood of interception); (3) the risk that the failure will cause harm (1-10, with 10 representing the highest risk for harm). The product of these three numbers is the hazard score. The steps in the workflow with the highest hazard score should be the first to be evaluated for performance improvement. In a critical care setting, some high-risk practices that may benefit from an FMEA include responding to clinical alarms, preventing hospital-acquired infections from catheters and central lines, and handoffs between clinicians.

State Regulations

Many states also issue patient safety regulations. Often these regulations pertain to the reporting of adverse events. For example, New York State requires serious adverse events to be reported along with a detailed analysis of what happened and proposed corrective actions. In Pennsylvania, all errors are reported, ranging from near-miss errors that do not cause harm to the most serious errors that lead to death. Other examples of state regulations concern surgical safety, sepsis, and perinatal safety. State regulations that address patient safety continue to evolve, requiring hospital leadership to pay close attention to new state-led initiatives aimed at preventing medical errors.

Responding to Adverse Events

While patient safety regulations address hazards that are believed to be universal in health care

(eg, requiring confirmation of patient identification prior to administering medications), investigating adverse events and implementing corrective actions are opportunities to address issues that may be organization specific. When a serious adverse event happens to a critical care patient, a systematic investigation of the event, called a root cause analysis, should be completed by an interdisciplinary team that has expertise in the areas involved in the event. After a detailed analysis, corrective actions aimed at preventing similar events should be implemented, which can involve rethinking a poorly functioning workflow, purchasing new technology, updating a policy, and/or reeducating staff.

Reporting Adverse Events

Unfortunately, the majority of adverse events are never reported and therefore cannot be addressed. A 2011 study by Classen et al found that among 393 adverse events detected by various mechanisms, only 4 (1%) were identified through voluntary reporting. Several strategies are being implemented to increase the reporting of adverse events. For example, many institutions are moving to electronic adverse event reporting systems that make reporting easier. These systems allow for the reporting of incidents that cause harm (eg, a patient who falls and fractures a hip), near-miss errors that do not cause harm but still provide information about hidden hazards (eg, a patient who trips over a loose wire but catches himself before falling), and unsafe conditions which can potentially lead to adverse events (eg, a loose wire). Reports of incidents, near misses, and unsafe conditions are collectively called "patient safety work product."

Just Culture

In addition to implementing electronic reporting systems, some hospitals are embracing a concept called Just Culture. According to the Just Culture concept, the major focus of an adverse event investigation should be on potential system failures that led to the error as opposed to simply attributing blame to the providers involved in the error. The need to focus on system failures was highlighted in the IOM report "To Err Is Human" (Figure 13–2), and has become an important staple of modern patient safety programs. Based on this IOM report, a hospital that

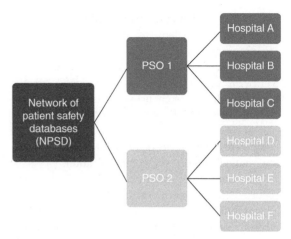

Why Do Errors Happen?

"The common initial reaction when an error occurs is to find and blame someone. However, even apparently single events or errors are due most often to the convergence of multiple contributing factors. Blaming an individual does not change these factors and the same error is likely to recur. Preventing errors and improving safety for patients require a systems approach in order to modify the conditions that contribute to errors. People working in health care are among the most educated and dedicated workforce in any industry. The problem is not bad people; the problem is that the system needs to be made safer."

FIGURE 13–2 Excerpt from the Institute of Medicine Report "To Err Is Human".

FIGURE 13–3 The network of patient safety databases.

implements Just Culture policies can expect to see an increase in reporting of adverse events as providers come to believe that leadership is committed to improving systems instead of punishing human errors.

Patient Safety Organizations

To optimize lessons learned from adverse events, the federal government enacted the Patient Safety and Quality Improvement Act of 2005 which authorized the creation of patient safety organizations (PSOs) to collect and analyze patient safety work product from health care facilities, and provide feedback and assistance to effectively minimize patient risk. The Patient Safety and Quality Improvement Act also provides federal protections that prohibit the use of patient safety work product in criminal, civil, or disciplinary proceedings in order to encourage providers to report medical errors without fear of repercussions and lawsuits. In addition, the federal Agency for Healthcare Quality and Research (AHRQ) produced a set of common definitions and reporting formats, known as "common formats," which allow health care facilities to exchange data with PSOs in a standardized manner. PSOs, in turn, transmit deidentified patient safety work product to the national network of patient safety databases (NPSD), which is maintained by AHRQ. The NPSD has been aggregating patient safety data from across the United States, analyzing the data, and eventually will make recommendations for improving patient safety (Figure 13–3).

Patient Safety Best Practices

There are many approaches to improving patient safety that are not required by regulation, and not implemented as a direct response to an adverse event. They are good ideas, with strong evidence to support their effectiveness in preventing errors and avoiding complications. Many of these best practices are appropriate in a critical care setting.

Teamwork

Team training is a well-established approach for preventing errors in high-risk industries such as the military and the airline industry, and is now being applied to the medical industry. The underlying theory behind medical team training is that highly trained individuals (eg, physicians, nurses, and technicians) acting together as a cohesive team are more effective and in the best interest of their patients. This includes strong leadership, where the team leader articulates clear goals and makes decisions using input from team members. Effective team work also requires clear communication with briefs and debriefs before and after procedures and complex patient encounters, and ad hoc huddles when unexpected urgent situations arise. It is important that team members "cross-check" each other, offering assistance when needed, and that team members are respectful of each other, so that all team members feel comfortable speaking up.

AHRQ collaborated with the United States Department of Defense to develop a team training program called Team Strategies and Tools to Enhance Performance and Patient Safety (TeamSTEPPS), which is specifically designed for the medical industry. Many hospitals are now using the AHRQ TeamSTEPPS program to teach the principles of medical team work, with a focus on 4 core competencies: team leadership, situation monitoring, mutual support, and communication.

In one study, an academic medical center reported on the implementation of the TeamSTEPPS program in their pediatric and surgical ICUs, where all pediatric ICU (PICU), surgical ICU (SICU), and respiratory therapy staff received TeamSTEPPS training. The staff felt the implementation was effective and improved teamwork on the unit and objective patient safety measures significantly improved after the TeamSTEPPS program was implemented. Another study examined the relationship between the level of self-identified teamwork and their mortality rates in 17 ICUs. This study found that the units with lower mortality rates had teams with a deeper understanding of how well their teams functioned, were more trusting of other team members, and perceived themselves as more organized when compared to the units with the higher mortality rates.

Simulation

Simulation is a promising new strategy for improving patient safety. Similar to flight simulators used by the airline industry, health care simulators allow providers to learn a procedure or protocol using high-tech mannequins instead of live patients. The old adage, "see one, do one, teach one" is being replaced by continuous practice in a simulation laboratory. Simulation allows providers to learn new technical skills, practice their responsiveness to high-stress clinical emergencies, and practice working as a team. It is being incorporated into medical school curricula, as well as the continuing education classes of nurses, residents, and attending physicians.

Health care simulation is usually conducted in replicate clinical settings with the same equipment used to treat real patients. It is common for simulation centers to have mock inpatient rooms, emergency bays, and operating suites, each equipped with sophisticated video equipment that captures multiple angles. Outside the simulation room, often behind a one-way mirror, is a trained technician controlling the faux clinical scenario by manipulating the simulated patient's vital signs, clinical alarms, and even their verbal responses through a microphone.

The most important part of health care simulation is the debriefing which occurs once the simulated clinical scenario is completed. A video of the simulation is played back, and all participants review their actions with a trained specialist who facilitates the conversation, making sure to highlight what went right and where there are potential areas for improvement. In the ICU, simulation is an ideal tool for teaching residents, fellows, and nurses many aspects of critical care medicine, ranging from the technical skills of placing a central catheter with ultrasound guidance to the essential cultural skill of working effectively together as a team.

Critical Care Staffing and Telemedicine

Patients in critical care units often have life-threatening illnesses which require complicated care plans, rapid decision making, close monitoring, and constant support from highly trained doctors and nurses who specialize in caring for the sickest of patients. Several studies have demonstrated improved outcomes when these patients are cared for in closed units, and when their care is supervised by critical care attending physicians. The Leapfrog Group, which is a consortium of Fortune 500 companies and other large health care purchasers that work together to drive improvements in patient safety, have made appropriate ICU staffing a major pillar in their patient safety program. To meet the Leapfrog Group's standard on ICU staffing, a hospital must (1) have an intensivist present during daytime hours and provide clinical care exclusively in the ICU, (2) ensure that the intensivists return pages at least 95% of the time when they are not present on site, and (3) arrange for a Fundamental Critical Care Support (FCCS) certified physician or physician extender to reach ICU patients within 5 minutes of being called or paged. When an intensivist is not available on site, it is acceptable if they are available via telemedicine.

The telemedicine model was initially envisioned as a tool for providing specialty medical expertise to rural communities that do not have ready access to tertiary care; today it is used by critical care medicine as a means of expanding the geographic range of critical care physicians. The critical care physician is often physically located in a room offsite, with access to patient monitors and electronic health records. He or she remotely keeps a watchful eye on the vital signs, laboratory results, and overall well-being of dozens of critically ill patients, sometimes from several different units across a health system. The critical care physician has direct communication with the local ICU team, and is available to them 24 hours a day, 7 days a week.

Pay-for-Performance and Public Reporting

Pay-for-performance is a new approach for driving improvement in medical care by using financial incentives to reward hospitals that perform well on preestablished safety and quality measures. The broad categories of measures used by these programs include surveys of patients' experiences and timeliness and effectiveness of care, as well as readmissions, complications, and deaths. For example, the Center for Medicare and Medicaid Services (CMS) has implemented the 2014 Hospital Value-Based Purchasing (Hospital VBP) Program which adjusts hospitals' payments based on their performance on several safety and quality metrics, some of which are directly affected by the care patients receive in ICUs (eg, pneumonia 30-day mortality rate).

In addition to financial incentives, safety and quality measures are used in publicly displayed hospital report cards that inform patients of each hospitals strengths and weaknesses (eg, Medicare's Hospital Compare website hospitalcompare.gov), thus motivating hospitals to implement programs for improving their performance on these measures and ultimately improving patient safety. Many of the quality and safety measures used in these programs are collected in the ICUs (eg, infection control surveillance data reported for both central line-associated bloodstream infections [CLABSIs] and catheter-associated urinary tract infections historically have been collected exclusively from ICUs).

Pneumonia 30-Day Mortality Rate

In the United States, pneumonia results in more than a million admissions each year, and is the second leading cause of hospitalization among patients over 65 years. As a result, pneumonia has been a focus of quality improvement programs for a decade. The CMS has attempted to accelerate the improvement in the care of patients with pneumonia by publically reporting the 30-day mortality rate for pneumonia patients on Hospital Compare, and have included this same metric in their pay-for-performance value-based purchasing program.

Central Line-Associated Bloodstream Infections

An estimated 80,000 CLABSIs occur in United States' hospitals each year, causing up to 28,000 deaths in ICUs. The majority of patients in an ICU have a central venous catheter to ensure reliable intravenous access. However, the presence of these devices places the patients at risk for developing a CLABSI. These hospital-acquired infections are an important measure on Medicare's Hospital Compare report card portal which compares the quality of care at over 4000 Medicare-certified hospitals across the country. Hospital Compare uses the CLABSI data that the Centers for Disease Control and Prevention (CDC) collect from hospitals' ICUs via the National Healthcare Safety Network (NHSN) tool.

As CLABSIs have become an important and often-used publicly reported metric, they have received much attention from quality improvement and patient safety researchers. One noteworthy study, led by Dr. Peter Pronovost and widely known as the "Keystone Project," measured the effectiveness of decreasing the rate of CLABSIs by implementing various interventions across 103 ICUs. The study interventions included 5 procedures recommended by the CDC, including hand washing, using full-barrier precautions during the insertion of central venous catheters, cleaning the skin with chlorhexidine, avoiding the femoral site if possible, and removing unnecessary catheters. At the start of the study clinicians were educated about practices to control infection and harm resulting from CLABSIs: a central-line cart with necessary supplies was created; a checklist was used to ensure adherence to infection-control practices; providers were stopped (in nonemergency situations) if these practices were not being followed; the removal of catheters was discussed at daily rounds; and the teams received feedback regarding the number and rates of CLABSIs. The study lasted 18 months, and demonstrated a large and sustained reduction (up to 66%) in rates of CLABSIs that was maintained throughout the study period. The success of this initiative has led to the adoption of many of the best practices used in the study by ICUs across the country, particularly the use of the checklist.

Innovate and Research

When "To Err Is Human" was first released by the IOM in 1999, many of the recommendations for improving patient safety were based on anecdotal accountings of errors and expert opinion. Now, 15 years later, there is increasingly more evidence defining best practices. Critical care leaders who are committed to providing safe care for their patients should exert effort to implement these evidence-based practices. Those who want to lead in patient safety should innovate new approaches for preventing errors, and study these approaches using rigorous research methodology.

REFERENCES

Agency for Healthcare Research and Quality (AHRQ) Patient Safety Organizations. http://www.pso.ahrq.gov/.

Classen DC, Resar R, Griffin F, et al. "Global trigger tool" shows that adverse events in hospitals may be ten times greater than previously measured. *Health Aff (Millwood)*. 2011;30:581-589.

Groves RH, Jr, Holcomb BW, Jr, Smith ML. Intensive care telemedicine: evaluating a model for proactive remote monitoring and intervention in the critical care setting. *Stud Health Technol Inform*. 2008;131:131-146.

Kohn LT, Corrigan JM, Donaldson MS (Institute of Medicine). *To Err Is Human: Building A Safer Health System*. Washington, DC: National Academy Press; 2000.

Lindenauer PK, Bernheim SM, Grady JN, et al. The performance of US hospitals as reflected in risk-standardized 30-day mortality and readmission rates for Medicare beneficiaries with pneumonia. *J Hosp Med*. 2010;5(6):E12-E18.

Mayer C, Lin W, Willis T, et al. Evaluating efforts to optimize TeamSTEPPS implementation in surgical and pediatric intensive care units. *Jt Comm J Qual Patient Saf*. 2011;37(8):365-374.

Nishisaki A, Keren R, Nadkarni V. Does simulation improve patient safety? Self-efficacy, competence, operational performance, and patient safety. *Anesthesiol Clin*. 2007;25:225-236.

Piquette D, Tarshis J, Regehr G, Fowler RA, Pinto R, LeBlanc VR. Effects of clinical supervision on resident learning and patient care during simulated ICU scenarios. *Crit Care Med*. 2013;41(12):2705-2711.

Pronovost P, Needham D, Berenholtz S, et al. An intervention to decrease catheter-related bloodstream infections in the ICU. *N Engl J Med*. 2006;355:2725-2732.

Pronovost PJ, Angus DC, Dorman T, et al. Physician staffing patterns and clinical outcomes in critically ill patients: a systematic review. *JAMA*. 2002;288:2151-2162.

The Joint Commission 2016 National Patient Safety Goals. http://www.jointcommission.org/standards_information/npsgs.aspx.

The Leapfrog Group ICU Physician Staffing Fact Sheet. http://www.leapfroggroup.org/ratings-reports/icu-physician-staffing.

Valentin A, Capuzzo M, Guidet B, et al. Patient safety in intensive care: results from the multinational Sentinel Events Evaluation (SEE) study. *Intensive Care Med*. 2006;32:1591-1598.

Wheelan SA, Burchill CN, Tilin F. The link between teamwork and patients' outcomes in intensive care. *Am J Crit Care*. 2003;12:527-534.

ICU-Acquired Weakness and Early Mobilization in the Intensive Care Unit

14

Carol Hodgson, PhD, FACP and Eddy Fan, MD, PhD

KEY POINTS

1 ICU-acquired weakness is common and occurs early during the ICU stay.

2 Bed rest is a contributing factor and may be modifiable.

3 Early mobilization is a promising intervention to prevent ICU-acquired weakness.

4 Early mobilization requires a coordinated, multidisciplinary approach.

INTRODUCTION

The decreasing mortality from critical illness over recent decades has led to an increasing number of intensive care unit (ICU) survivors.[1-3] As a result, there has been a shift in focus from short-term mortality to longer-term morbidities within the field of critical care. Neuromuscular complications, leading to ICU-acquired weakness (ICUAW) and impaired physical function, are common in survivors of critical illness, with a prevalence ranging from 9% to 87%.[4] Furthermore, these complications are frequently severe and persistent, contributing to functional decline and significant decrements in health-related quality of life.[5-11]

Reasons for muscle weakness following critical illness are multifactorial, including premorbid weakness associated with chronic diseases. Recently, there has been growing recognition that both critical illness and its associated treatments are toxic to muscles and nerves and contribute to the development of ICUAW.[1,2] Unfortunately, there are limited interventions to prevent or treat ICUAW. There is currently evidence from observational studies and small randomized controlled trials that establishes proof-of-principle that early mobilization (EM) may improve patient outcomes. This chapter will focus on the development, detection, and outcomes of ICUAW, with a particular emphasis on the role of EM in the critically ill. We will also discuss the barriers to EM in the ICU, the safety considerations for EM, strategies for measuring outcomes, and setting goals that include both the patient and their families.

ETIOLOGY AND PATHOPHYSIOLOGY OF WEAKNESS IN THE ICU

Bed Rest, Immobilization, and Disuse Muscle Atrophy

Prolonged bed rest and immobilization is common in many ICU patients and may contribute to the development of ICUAW.[3] A meta-analysis of 39 randomized trials examining the effects of bed rest on 15 different medical conditions and procedures demonstrated that bed rest was not beneficial, and may be associated with harm.[4]

Prolonged bed rest leads to decreased muscle protein synthesis, increased muscle catabolism, and decreased muscle mass, especially in the lower extremities.[5,6] In healthy volunteers, muscle atrophy can begin within hours of immobility,[7] resulting in a 4% to 5% loss of muscle strength for each week of bed rest.[8] Immobility results in the activation of specific biochemical pathways that lead to enhanced proteolysis and decreased protein synthesis, resulting in a net loss in muscle mass, cross-sectional muscle area, and contractile strength.[9-12] Moreover, there is a general shift from slow twitch (type I) to fast twitch (type II) muscle fibers, with reduced muscle endurance due to fewer fatigue-resistant (type I) fibers.[13-15] Consequently, disuse atrophy results in deleterious effects on muscle strength, with nearly 2% of quadriceps' strength lost for each day of bed rest in healthy individuals.[16,17] In a multisite study of patients with acute respiratory distress syndrome (ARDS), the duration of bed rest during critical illness was the only risk factor consistently associated with weakness throughout the entire follow-up, with each additional day of bed rest having up to an 11% relative decrease in muscle strength at 24-months post-ARDS.[18] In addition, the interaction of bed rest and critical illness appears to result in more significant muscle loss than bed rest alone.[19-21] Furthermore, short-term immobility may impair microvascular function and induce insulin resistance, both of which may further potentiate injuries to muscle and nerves in the critically ill.[22]

In addition to its direct effects on muscle, immobility can lead to a proinflammatory state via increased proinflammatory cytokines.[23,24] This cytokine shift may potentiate the systemic inflammatory milieu commonly observed during critical illness leading to further muscle damage and loss.[25] The proinflammatory state associated with bed rest also may cause increased production of reactive oxygen species (ROS), with a concomitant decrease in antioxidative defenses.[26,27] ROS play a role in oxidization of myofilaments, resulting in contractile dysfunction and atrophy.[28,29] This concomitant increase in ROS and imbalance in the cytokine profile can further disrupt the balance between muscle synthesis and proteolysis, with a net loss of muscle protein and subsequent muscle weakness.

Finally, bed rest may produce indirect consequences that lead to further intolerance of physical activity. Immobility may lead to increased postural hypotension and tachycardia due to alterations in baroreceptor function.[30,31] Furthermore, prolonged physical inactivity can result in generalized pain and changes in mood which may limit physical function.[32] Even in healthy adults, the effects of prolonged immobilization and disuse atrophy alone are often persistent, and require extensive physical reconditioning to allow a return to their baseline level of functioning.[30,31]

Critical Illness Polyneuropathy and Critical Illness Myopathy

Critical illness polyneuropathy (CIP) is a diffuse and symmetric sensorimotor axonal neuropathy that was first described in 1984.[33] Electrophysiologic changes, detected with nerve conduction studies (NCS) and electromyography (EMG), can occur within 24 hours after the onset of critical illness.[34] The development of primary axonal degeneration in CIP is likely multifactorial, but a number of mechanistic hypotheses have been posited.[35-37] Critical illness myopathy (CIM) represents metabolic, inflammatory, and bioenergetic derangements in muscle similar to those seen in CIP.[38] These changes result in early and rapid skeletal muscle wasting during the first week of critical illness.[39] Functional inactivation of the remaining muscle may occur due to membrane inexcitability from acquired ion-channel dysfunction.[40-42] CIP and CIM share many pathologic mechanisms, often coexist, and may represent a form of neuromuscular organ dysfunction from systemic critical illness.[1] As such, similar emphasis should be placed on prevention and recovery as would be for ICU patients that develop acute kidney injury or lung injury.[43]

Although immobilization and the effects of critical illness traditionally have been considered to predominantly affect peripheral muscles groups, recent preclinical and clinical studies have suggested diaphragmatic involvement, including reduced muscle force and increased muscle atrophy.[44-46] A preliminary study in humans suggests that even short-term diaphragmatic inactivity and controlled mechanical ventilation (with effective functional denervation) can result in marked diaphragmatic atrophy.[47] A "two-hit" combination of immobilization and the early development of subclinical CIP/CIM may contribute to the rapid development of muscle atrophy.[48]

RISK FACTORS FOR ICU-ACQUIRED WEAKNESS

Although many studies have investigated risk factors for ICUAW, most have been limited by small sample size, retrospective design, and single-center experiences.[49] Furthermore, lack of comparable patient populations and standard definitions for ICUAW makes comparisons across studies difficult.[43,49] Thus, although there are a number of commonly cited risk factors for ICUAW, many lack support from rigorous clinical investigations.[43]

Hyperglycemia

A recent systematic review found that hyperglycemia is the most consistently identified risk factor for ICUAW.[49] Two large randomized controlled trials (RCTs) of intensive insulin therapy for tight glycemic control in the ICU[50,51] and associated subanalyses,[37,52] demonstrated a substantial decrease in the incidence of ICUAW in patients randomized to intensive insulin therapy. However, the overall safety and efficacy of intensive insulin therapy and tight glycemic control in a heterogeneous population of critically ill patients remains controversial,[53-55] and clinicians should be cautious in using the results of these secondary analysis to support the use of tight glycemic control for the prevention of ICUAW.

Sepsis and Systemic Inflammation

Given the potential mechanistic relationship between systemic inflammation (ie, the systemic inflammatory response syndrome [SIRS]), with or without concomitant infection (ie, sepsis), and the development of ICUAW, several studies have examined this issue.[56-58] Two prospective studies reported a significant association of ICUAW with the presence of SIRS[57] and the duration of SIRS (odds ratio [OR] 1.05; 95% confidence interval [CI] 1.01-1.15 for each day in the first week).[56] However, another prospective study demonstrated no association between the presence of sepsis and ICUAW.[58]

Corticosteroids and Neuromuscular Blocking Agents

There has been substantial controversy regarding the role of systemic corticosteroids in the development of ICUAW. A prospective study reported that exposure to corticosteroids was the single largest risk factor for the development of weakness (OR 14.9; 95% CI 3.2-69.8).[59] However, this study revealed no relationship between the dose or duration of corticosteroid therapy and the development of weakness. A number of other clinical studies, including a systematic review, have failed to demonstrate a consistent association between corticosteroids and ICUAW.[18,37,49,56-58,60-64] Conversely, a recent study demonstrated decreased ICUAW in patients randomized to intensive insulin therapy who also received corticosteroids in the ICU (OR 0.91; 95% CI 0.86-0.97).[52] The investigators suggested that the deleterious effects of corticosteroids on the neuromuscular system may be mediated through hyperglycemia, such that when blood glucose is strictly controlled, the anti-inflammatory effects of corticosteroids may be protective against ICUAW.

Despite early reports of persistent weakness following prolonged administration of neuromuscular blockade, 5 prospective trials,[18,37,49,56,57] an RCT (which demonstrated at significant reduction in 28-day mortality)[65] and a systematic review[66] did not find a significant association between their use and the development of ICUAW. However, 2 other studies did find a significant association, possibly due to larger doses and longer duration of neuromuscular blockade use.[52,61] Thus, clinicians should consider the use of corticosteroids or neuromuscular blocking agents on a case-by-case basis, weighing the potential risks and benefits based on the individual patient characteristics.[67]

CLINICAL MANIFESTATION AND DIAGNOSIS OF ICU-ACQUIRED WEAKNESS

ICUAW is often difficult to diagnose in critically ill patients during the acute phase of their illness due to the frequent use of deep sedation. As a result, ICUAW is usually recognized in 2 distinct contexts: (1) prolonged or failed weaning from mechanical ventilation, despite otherwise global improvement in other organ systems; or (2) profound bilateral weakness in an awake patient recovering from critical illness.[68] In either scenario, neuromuscular dysfunction is usually detected after the recovery of other organ systems as the patient wakes.

Typically, symmetric motor weakness is observed in all limbs, ranging from mild paresis to frank quadriplegia. In noncooperative patients, noxious stimuli may be applied to each extremity in order to grossly evaluate the strength of patient withdrawal. Since facial muscles are typically spared in patients with ICUAW, patients may have normal facial grimacing with application of noxious stimuli.

Physical Examination

The bedside physical examination of the neuromuscular system in a critically ill patient is often difficult due to deep sedation or delirium. The standard physical examination of individual muscle groups is typically done using the Medical Research Council (MRC) Manual Muscle Test scale,[69] which is dependent on patient effort and cooperation. This scale evaluates muscle strength with a score ranging from 0 (no muscle contraction) to 5 (normal strength). Physical examination of 3 muscle groups in each limb, yielding a composite MRC score, has demonstrated excellent inter-rater reliability within specific non-ICU patient populations,[70] with very good inter-rater reliability in ICU patients and survivors.[71] Clinically detectable muscle weakness has been arbitrarily defined as a composite MRC score less than 80% of normal (eg, composite MRC score less than 48 out of a maximum score of 60 for 3 muscle groups in each limb).[59,70,72] Other methods of volitional muscle testing that could be employed in these patients include handheld or handgrip dynamometry.

Similar to the motor examination, a sensory examination is often limited by sedation, altered sensorium, as well as peripheral edema. Deep tendon reflexes may be diminished or absent, but normal reflexes do not rule out ICUAW. Hyperreflexia and/or associated spasticity should suggest an alternative diagnosis (eg, central nervous system etiology), and further investigations (eg, brain and spinal cord imaging) should be obtained.

Electrophysiology and Muscle Biopsy

Given the limitations of physical examination, there has been growing interest in the use of electrodiagnostic testing (ie, motor/sensory NCS and needle EMG) for the diagnosis of ICUAW. In patients with CIP, NCS often reveal a mixed sensorimotor axonopathy manifested by a reduced amplitude of the compound muscle action potential (CMAP) and sensory nerve action potential (SNAP) with relative preservation of the nerve conduction velocity.[36] The electrophysiologic changes seen in CIP can be detected as early as 24 to 48 hours following the onset of critical illness, and often precede clinical findings in these patients.[73-75] Despite their potential utility in sedated or comatose patients, there are still certain technical factors, including local edema and limb temperature, which can interfere with NCS.[2]

In patients with CIM, prolongation of CMAP duration on NCS can be seen and suggests the presence of a myopathic process (ie, not due to muscle denervation). On needle EMG, CIM will manifest as short-duration, low-amplitude motor unit action potentials (MUAP) with early recruitment of MUAPs on volitional contraction. Furthermore, abnormal spontaneous activity, including fibrillation potentials and positive sharp waves, may be present.[76] Therefore, diagnosis of CIM with EMG requires a cooperative patient that can perform voluntary contraction, and an experienced clinician to interpret the results.

Definitive diagnosis of an underlying myopathy requires histologic confirmation with a muscle biopsy. Histopathologic findings consistent with CIM include muscle fiber atrophy (with preferential loss of type II fibers), occasional fiber necrosis and regeneration, and selective loss of myosin filaments (pathognomonic for CIM).[38]

Diagnostic Strategy

Despite its limitations, routine bedside physical examination should be the starting point for the identification of ICUAW. Given the relative cost, invasiveness, and need for specialist physicians and technicians, comprehensive electrophysiology studies and muscle biopsy should be reserved for weak patients with slower-than-expected improvement on serial clinical examination.[68]

OUTCOMES IN PATIENTS WITH ICU-ACQUIRED WEAKNESS

Weaning From Mechanical Ventilation

Prolonged or failed weaning from mechanical ventilation is a common manifestation of ICUAW in patients recovering from critical illness. Involvement of both chest wall muscles and the diaphragm in ICUAW likely contribute to the difficulty with weaning from mechanical ventilation. In a recent systematic review, 12 of 13 studies that evaluated ICUAW and the duration of mechanical ventilation revealed that ICUAW was associated with prolonged mechanical ventilation in patients with ICUAW.[49] In one study, the presence of ICUAW was the only significant predictor of failure to wean from mechanical ventilation (OR 15.4; 95% CI 4.6-52.3).[77]

Patient Outcomes After ICU Discharge

A recent systematic review was inconclusive regarding differences in patient outcomes with CIP versus CIM.[49] Existing evidence is also inconclusive regarding whether ICUAW is associated with increased hospital mortality.[49,61,78] In survivors of critical illness, recovery from ICUAW is possible, with a majority (94%) of patients in one cohort demonstrating meaningful clinical recovery of muscle strength at 9 months.[59] However, in some patients, ICUAW may persist and result in severe and prolonged functional deficits,[18,79-81] with concomitant decrements in health-related quality of life.[18,82,83]

STRATEGIES FOR THE PREVENTION AND TREATMENT OF ICU-ACQUIRED WEAKNESS

There are currently few options for the prevention and/or treatment of ICUAW. During critical illness, exposure to hyperglycemia and certain medications (eg, corticosteroids and neuromuscular blocking agents) may be associated with the development of ICUAW. At present, the strongest evidence for the prevention of ICUAW is tight glycemic control with intensive insulin therapy, which may decrease neuromuscular abnormalities in critically ill patients who are mechanically ventilated for more than or equal to 7 days. However, the potential benefits of intensive insulin therapy should be carefully weighed against the possibility of serious hypoglycemia, as demonstrated in recent clinical trials.[55,84] Finally, despite a strong evidence base, maintenance of electrolyte homeostasis (eg, phosphate, magnesium) and adequate nutrition to ameliorate muscle catabolism may be reasonable clinical recommendations for minimizing ICUAW.[85]

Beneficial Effects of Exercise in ICU

A potential therapeutic option to reduce ICUAW is avoidance of bed rest via EM in the ICU setting. EM in the ICU is a candidate intervention to improve muscle strength, physical function, and quality of survival.[86] EM is the intensification and acceleration of the usual physical therapy (PT) that is administered to critically ill patients, along with additional novel concepts that include the mobilization of patients requiring mechanical ventilation and the use of novel techniques such as cycle ergometry and electrical muscle stimulation.[86] EM is applied with the intention of maintaining or restoring musculoskeletal strength and function and thereby, potentially, improving functional, patient-centered outcomes.[87]

Usual Physical Therapy in ICU

The management of critically ill patients appears to vary widely within countries and internationally.[88,89] This is partly due to cultural differences, funding differences (eg, staffing ratios of nurses to patient), and partly due to differences in medical management as a result of local practice. To date there is no published data comparing the practice of early mobilization in ICUs internationally. However, there are 2 multicenter point prevalence studies of EM in ICU that may be informative. The first studied all patients from 38 ICUs in Australia and New Zealand at a single time on a single day in 2009 and 2010.[88] Of the 514 patients included, 45% were mechanically ventilated. Overall, mobilization activities were classified into 5 categories that were not mutually exclusive: 140 patients (28%) completed an in-bed exercise regimen, 93 (19%)

sat over the side of the bed, 182 (37%) sat out of bed, 124 (25%) stood and 89 (18%) walked. Adverse events occurred on 24 occasions (5%). Importantly, none of the mechanically ventilated patients sat out of bed or walked on the day of the study. The main barrier to mobilization was that the patient was unconscious (20%) or deeply sedated (17%).

A similar study was conducted in 116 German ICUs including 783 mechanically ventilated patients.[89] Overall, 185 patients (24%) were mobilized out of bed which was defined as sitting on the edge of the bed or a higher level of mobilization. Among patients with an endotracheal tube, tracheostomy, and noninvasive ventilation, 8%, 39%, and 53% were mobilized out of bed, respectively. This study identified cardiovascular instability (17%) and deep sedation (15%) as the main barrier to mobilization, however mobilization out of bed was not associated with a higher frequency of complications.

Safety

Clinical practice guidelines endorsed by the European Society of Intensive Care Medicine (ESICM) on the safety of EM have been published and serve as a guide to clinicians working in the ICU.[90] Active mobilization of a critically ill patient, particularly if they require mechanical ventilation, involves a complex assessment that has not been standardized and may differ between ICUs and individual patients. In part this may be due to the heterogeneity of critical illness, the changing stability of the patient and the cointerventions; however it is also affected by the individual response to EM.[91]

The decision to actively mobilize a patient, both in bed and out of bed, should be made by the multidisciplinary ICU team, preferably during the morning rounds. The decision should include the individual assessment of the patient's past medical history and exercise tolerance, respiratory and cardiovascular stability over the previous 24-hour period, management of lines and tubes, consideration of orthopedic and neurologic conditions, medications that may affect the patients' safety during mobilization, and the available staff and equipment to ensure patient safety. Occasionally medical staff outside the ICU may need to be consulted about the safety of mobilization, for example in a polytrauma patient with lower leg injuries, an orthopedic surgeon may need

to be contacted regarding the lower limb weight-bearing status if it is not clearly documented in the patient history.

Ideally, each ICU would formulate a protocol to guide EM, where decisions are predetermined about the safety criteria acceptable within that ICU to commence mobilization and the safety criteria to cease if the patient deteriorates during mobilization.

Cardiovascular Reserve

Cardiovascular stability is determined by assessing the heart rate and rhythm, blood pressure, requirement and dose of vasoactive or antiarrhythmic drugs, and other major cardiac conditions or support (eg, intra-aortic balloon pump, extracorporeal membrane oxygenation [ECMO]).[90] The blood pressure and heart rate should be considered stable by the medical staff, with minimal variability (< 20%) over the preceding hours and stable requirements of vasoactive drugs. If there is any doubt about cardiovascular stability, the medical team should be consulted prior to mobilization.

Respiratory Reserve

Respiratory stability is determined by the respiratory rate and pattern, the fraction of inspired oxygen and the arterial oxygen concentration measured either with blood gases or a pulse oximeter and the ventilator settings if the patient is on mechanical ventilation, including the rate, pressure, volume, and requirement for positive end-expiratory pressure (PEEP). In general, the respiratory rate and oxygen requirements should not have increased in the preceding hours prior to mobilization and the patient should have a clear airway with minimal work of breathing.[90] The oxygen saturation should be greater than 90% and the fraction of inspired oxygen 0.6 with PEEP less than 15 cm H_2O. The respiratory rate should be less than 30 breaths/min.

Prior to each episode of mobilization, an appropriate ICU staff member should check the position of the artificial airway and ensure that the artificial airway is secure (ie, an orotracheal, nasotracheal, or tracheostomy tube). Additionally, if the plan is to move away from the bed, any supplementary gas supply required by the patient during mobilization should be available and there should be adequate reserve for the expected duration of the mobility session, and a little extra reserved for any unexpected additional requirements.

Neurologic Stability

Ideally, prior to mobilization, the patient is awake, calm, and able to follow instructions. This can be assessed with standardized tools, such as the Richmond Agitation and Sedation Scale (RASS), where a score of –1 to +1 is ideal. Delirium is common in the ICU and can also be assessed using the Confusion Assessment Method for the ICU (CAM-ICU). Other neurologic precautions for EM include active treatment for intracranial hypertension, craniectomy, open lumbar drains, spinal precautions, or the presence of an acute spinal injury.

Other Considerations

Medical Conditions—Patients should also be assessed with regards to oxygen carrying capacity (Hb > 7 g/dL and stable), white cell and platelet count, deep vein thrombosis or pulmonary embolus, body temperature, unstable fractures, skin grafting, and open surgical wounds. If there is any doubt about the safety of mobilization, the senior consultant or surgeon should be asked to make a final decision prior to commencing EM.

Staffing—There must be adequate trained staff and equipment to ensure safe mobilization of an ICU patient. In the case of a mechanically ventilated patient, one person should always be designated to ensure the security of the airway during mobilization. The patient should be assessed for strength prior to mobilizing out of bed, for example using the MRC manual muscle test, and if there is significant weakness the patient may not be strong enough to mobilize against gravity or they may require specific equipment designed to assist with EM. This may include a hoist, standing lifter or a walking frame designed to include a pole (to attach intravenous fluids), and a stand for the mechanical ventilator and oxygen tank (Figure 14–1).

Other Lines, Drains, and Attachments—Each ICU may differ in its policy regarding attachments that are safe for mobilization, or attachments that are contraindicated for mobilisation. Discussion about the safety of various patient lines and attachments must be considered on an individual basis. There is some evidence that femoral catheters,

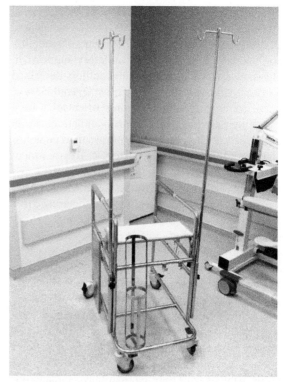

FIGURE 14–1 A custom made walking frame on wheels, including 2 poles for intravenous fluids, a stand for the mechanical ventilator, and a frame to hold the oxygen cylinder.

including femoral catheterization for hemofiltration, should not be a contraindication to EM in the ICU.[92] Similarly, some extracorporeal devices are considered safe for EM with adequately trained staff conducting the activities.[93]

In a recent systematic review of physiotherapy in intensive care, 17 observational studies of EM reported outcomes regarding feasibility, safety, and physiologic effects.[91] Mobilization activities were reported as both safe and feasible, with the frequency of serious adverse events reported to be less than or equal to 1%. There were occasional short-term physiologic changes associated with EM that requires careful assessment throughout the mobilization activity.

Clinical Evidence—Early mobilization in ICU is an emerging new focus of intensive critical care research, representing a potentially lower-cost, high-impact intervention. However, there are few RCTs evaluating its efficacy.

Three RCTs[94-96] and a number of observational studies[97-102] have provided data on the safety and preliminary efficacy of the concept of mobilizing patients dependent on ventilatory support. In the first observational study, the authors described 1449 activity events in 103 patients. Overall, 53% of these events included ambulating patients that were dependent on positive pressure ventilation via an endotracheal tube or tracheostomy; there was less than 1% adverse events related to EM. This treatment was resourced from within the existing ICU staff structure, including ICU nurses, technicians, physical therapists (PTs), and respiratory therapists. In a further study, the same authors describe a before-and-after cohort study in 104 patients with respiratory failure who were transferred from another ICU to their respiratory ICU. Transfer to the study respiratory ICU with a culture of EM increased the probability of ambulation ($P < 0.0001$) during ICU stay.

Schweikert and colleagues reported findings from a prospective, outcome assessor-blinded, randomized trial of early physical therapy (PT) and occupational therapy (OT) from two centers in the USA.[95] In this study, patients who were mechanically ventilated for less than 72 hours and expected to stay ventilated in the next 24 hours were randomized either to an EM protocol which progressed from passive range of motion (PROM), active range of motion (AROM), bed mobility, sitting balance, standing, standing transfers, and gait reeducation during sedation interruption, or a control group which underwent PT and OT as prescribed by standard care. This trial demonstrated safety and feasibility for EM, as well as improved functional outcomes with early intervention.

COMMON BARRIERS TO EARLY MOBILIZATION IN THE ICU

Sedation

The aim of sedation management in ICU is to keep patients awake and comfortable where appropriate[103] and to use sedation when medically indicated in the following manner:

1. Target therapy to a desired sedation score (eg, RASS)

2. Use analgesic therapy over sedative/hypnotic therapy

3. Limit excessive doses of sedative and analgesic medications

4. Reduce the incidence of medication-induced delirium

5. Promote daily sedation interruption to facilitate early mobilization

Analgesic and sedative infusions are routinely used in the ICU in patients requiring mechanical ventilation.[104] Although these infusions are often required for patient comfort, to facilitate procedures and for patient-ventilator synchrony, heavy sedation (RASS $\leq$ –3) is commonly used. There are some circumstances when heavy sedation is required (eg, to control raised intracranial pressure [ICP]). However, it is now understood that excessive sedation may result in delayed extubation and prolonged ICU length of stay, as well as a decrease in sleep quality, an increase in delirium, and even an increase in mortality.[104]

Targeted sedation protocols involve the use of a validated sedation scale. Treating teams determine a required level of sedation and then titration algorithms are used to maintain the patient's level of sedation within the target range. Targeted sedation protocols have been shown to reduce time to arousal and decrease the duration of mechanical ventilation, as well as limiting exposure to benzodiazepines without an increase in self-extubation rates. A recent survey of Australian and New Zealand ICUs found that although 74% of ICUs used continuous infusions as the primary means of sedation and 70% used a sedation scale, only 48% of units had a written sedation policy.[104]

Delirium

Assessment for delirium is recommended using either the CAM-ICU or the Intensive Care Delirium Screening Checklist (ICDSC). Delirium is known to be associated with the use of sedative medications and there is evidence that the use of a sedation protocol can decrease the number of days with delirium. The CAM-ICU tool should be used daily if the RASS score is greater than or equal to –2. A delirious patient may be unsafe when mobilized out of bed, and particular caution is required as their behavior may be unpredictable.

Pre-ICU Level of Function

It is important to set realistic goals for mobilization based on previous levels of physical function. Communication with the family and caregivers of the patient is essential to determine premorbid level of physical function, including whether the patient could transfer from bed to chair independently prior to the critical illness. For instance, it is essential to determine if the patient previously walked independently or with a gait aid, whether they could walk outside, on uneven surfaces, to the mailbox, around the shops, or further? Patients who were unable to walk independently or transfer independently prior to ICU admission will require increased supervision and increased staff numbers when attempting mobilization. This reduces the risk of injury to both patients and staff.

MEASURING EARLY MOBILIZATION IN ICU

Mobility milestones are the most commonly reported outcome measure in ICU research projects of early mobilization.[105] Several studies have reported mobility milestones, such as sitting, standing, or walking, as an important indication of patient physical function in ICU.[97,99,101] They have not reported the level of assistance required to achieve the mobility milestone and they have not reported the same milestones. A recent systematic review described measures of physical function used in studies investigating EM in the ICU.[105] The ability to perform activities of mobility, or mobility milestones, was the most common end point reported in these studies. However, between these studies there was no consensus on the functional activities that should be included in measures of mobility in the ICU, or reports of the feasibility or inter-rater reliability of such measures.[105]

ICU Mobility Scale

The IMS is an 11-point ICU mobility scale (Table 14–1).[106] The IMS was based on functional patient activities that can reasonably be achieved across the spectrum of recovery while in the ICU. Moreover the reliability assessment was conducted at 2 large ICUs with a varied clinical case mix, including surgical, medical, and trauma patients, and included nurses and junior and senior PTs.

Despite the busy ICU environment, the IMS was administered with ease. The inter-rater agreement in the scale was excellent between PTs and good between nursing staff and PTs. This simple scale of mobility milestones will not replace other tests of physical function, but may assist as a daily record of mobility for both clinical and research purposes in order to allow greater standardization and comparability across time and between ICUs.

Other measures of mobilization have been developed for specific patient groups. For example, the Surgical Intensive Care Unit Optimal Mobility Score (SOMS) consists of a simple numeric scale that describes patients' mobilization capacity in a surgical ICU. A SOMS of 0 indicates that no mobilization should be considered. This score was assigned to patients who were either moribund or had an unstable head or spinal cord injury; those in whom any change in position led to profound respiratory or hemodynamic changes; and those with elevated ICPs (> 20 cm H_2O). A SOMS of 1 was used to describe patients receiving PROM exercises while in bed, and SOMS 2 was given to patients who were able to sit up in bed greater than 45° or in a chair. A SOMS 3 described patients who were able to stand with or without assistance, and a SOMS of 4 was assigned to patients able to ambulate. The SOMS demonstrated that in surgical critically ill patients presenting without preexisting impairment of functional mobility, it is a reliable and valid tool to predict mortality and ICU and hospital length of stay.[107]

Protocols

Several types of protocols have been suggested to allow mobilization in the ICU to occur as early as possible.[99,107] All protocols include a stepwise prescription of mobilization activity based on the physical capacity of the patient (Figure 14–2). Protocols such as these have been safely and effectively introduced into clinical practice. Further to this, a protocol that considers both the cognitive and the physical capacity of the patient has been implemented in one center in the United States, and resulted in patients walking at least 3 days sooner, an adverse event occurrence of less than 1% and an increase in mobility of up to 2-fold.[108] In another US center, an increase in routine mobilization occurred.[95]

TABLE 14-1 ICU mobility scale.[27]

	Classification	Definition
0	Nothing (lying in bed)	Passively rolled or passively exercised by staff, but not actively moving.
1	Sitting in bed, exercises in bed	Any activity in bed, including rolling, bridging, active exercises, cycle ergometry, and active assisted exercises; not moving out of bed or over the edge of the bed.
2	Passively moved to chair (no standing)	Hoist, passive lift or slide transfer to the chair, with no standing or sitting on the edge of the bed.
3	Sitting over edge of bed	May be assisted by staff, but involves actively sitting over the side of the bed with some trunk control.
4	Standing	Weight bearing through the feet in the standing position, with or without assistance. This may include use of a standing lifter device or tilt table.
5	Transferring bed to chair	Able to step or shuffle through standing to the chair. This involves actively transferring weight from one leg to another to move to the chair. If the patient has been stood with the assistance of a medical device, they must step to the chair (*not* included if the patient is wheeled in a standing lifter device).
6	Marching on spot (at bedside)	Able to walk on the spot by lifting alternate feet (must be able to step at least 4 times, twice on each foot), with or without assistance.
7	Walking with assistance of 2 or more people	Walking away from the bed/chair by at least 5 m (5 yd) assisted by 2 or more people.
8	Walking with assistance of 1 person	Walking away from the bed/chair by at least 5 m (5 yd) assisted by 1 person.
9	Walking independently with a gait aid	Walking away from the bed/chair by at least 5 m (5 yd) with a gait aid, but no assistance from another person. In a wheelchair-bound person, this activity level includes wheeling the chair independently 5 m (5 yd) away from the bed/chair.
10	Walking independently without a gait aid	Walking away from the bed/chair by at least 5 m (5 y) without a gait aid or assistance from another person.

Goal Setting

Setting goals for rehabilitation, particularly EM, is important to patients, family, and the staff in ICU. Functional rehabilitation can be progressed based on the clinical assessment discussed previously in this chapter and may be an important motivation for critically ill patients to recover. Family and friends often express delight at finding the patient out of bed, standing, or walking, even while attached to mechanical ventilation. Concerns about safety of early mobilization may arise from visitors to the ICU and it is important for clinicians prescribing and delivering exercise to explain the physiologic response expected in these circumstances and the safety precautions utilized by ICU staff.

Goals of EM should be clearly documented and progress reported. This is required both for hospital records and for patients and their families to celebrate progress. Diaries, journals, photographs, and documentation of progress made available to the patients and their families may be beneficial for physical and psychological recovery.[106,109,110]

PRACTICAL TIPS FOR STAFF PERFORMING EM

The S.T.A.N.D. Principle

Safety and stability: Assess the respiratory, hemodynamic and neurologic stability, muscle strength, and cooperation of the patient. Most

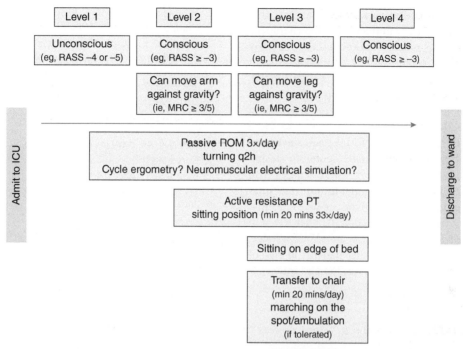

FIGURE 14-2 An example of a graded early mobilization protocol for ICU patients. Patients are initially assessed for their level of consciousness and motor strength to determine the highest level of activity they can start at. It is important to note that patients can skip directly to any level, as long as it is safe and feasible to do so, and they do not need to progress through the levels sequentially if they are capable of a higher level of activity. ICU, intensive care unit; MRC, Medical Research Council; PT, physical therapy; RASS, Richmond Agitation-Sedation Scale; ROM, range of motion.

importantly, discuss this with the ICU team if any concerns are raised prior to mobilization.

Teamwork: Early mobilization requires a team of people to work together with clear communication and an understanding of the safety requirements of the ICU. One person should be appointed as the leader of the team to direct the mobilization activity. The leader ensures that everyone in the team knows their role, including one person to be dedicated to protecting the airway.

Airway management: Airway management is the main priority during mobilization. One person is dedicated to maintaining the airway. Emergency equipment and portable oxygen supplies are checked and should remain easily accessible at all times. The patient should be suctioned prior to mobilizing and suction equipment should be available during EM.

Number of lines/tubes/attachments and equipment: Prepare the environment by double checking that all lines and tubes are secure, the area is clear of hazards, and the equipment required for mobilization is prepared.

Determine an alternate plan: If the patient does not tolerate the mobilization activity, have an alternative plan for repositioning the patient into sitting or supine. Be prepared for bowel movements and ensure there is adequate staff around to assist if the patient becomes unstable.

FUTURE DIRECTIONS

ICU survivors recovering from a prolonged critical illness often have severe muscle weakness and functional impairment. Future studies are needed to further elucidate the various mechanisms that lead to ICUAW, and to find and develop therapeutic targets for this morbid ICU complication. Early mobilization is a promising intervention to prevent or attenuate ICUAW and requires a coordinated, interprofessional team approach to assess readiness to mobilize and to optimize the progression of patient activity. Observational studies and small randomized trials evaluating EM suggest safety and feasibility, but are mostly single center in design with limited external validity. These studies also suggest that EM has the potential to improve functional outcomes in these survivors, reduce readmissions, and reduce health care costs. Further research is warranted to define baseline standard practice, identify risk factors that predict patients at risk of weakness, and define an intervention and intervention dose for EM.

TAKE HOME POINTS

- ICUAW is common, occurs early in critical illness, and is associated with significant long-term morbidity, and potentially mortality.

- Despite its limitations, routine bedside physical examination should be the starting point for the identification of ICUAW. Given the relative cost, invasiveness, and need for specialist physicians and technicians, comprehensive electrophysiology studies and muscle biopsy should be reserved for weak patients with slower-than-expected improvement on serial clinical examination.

- Early mobilization is a promising intervention to prevent or attenuate ICUAW.

- Early mobilization requires a coordinated, interprofessional team approach to assess readiness to mobilize and to optimize the progression of patient activity.

REFERNCES

1. Fan E, Zanni JM, Dennison CR, Lepre SJ, Needham DM. Critical illness neuromyopathy and muscle weakness in patients in the intensive care unit. *AACN Adv Crit Care*. 2009;20(3):243-253.

2. Hermans G, de Jonghe B, Bruyninckx F, Berghe G. Clinical review: critical illness polyneuropathy and myopathy. *Crit Care*. 2008;12(6):238.

3. Puthucheary Z, Harridge S, Hart N. Skeletal muscle dysfunction in critical care: wasting, weakness, and rehabilitation strategies. *Crit Care Med*. 2010;38(suppl 10):S676-S682.

4. Allen C, Glasziou P, Del Mar C. Bed rest: a potentially harmful treatment needing more careful evaluation. *Lancet*. 1999;354(9186):1229-1233.

5. Kortebein P, Ferrando A, Lombeida J, Wolfe R, Evans WJ. Effect of 10 days of bed rest on skeletal muscle in healthy older adults. *JAMA*. 2007;297(16):1772-1774.

6. Ferrando AA, Lane HW, Stuart CA, Davis-Street J, Wolfe RR. Prolonged bed rest decreases skeletal muscle and whole body protein synthesis. *Am J Physiol*. 1996;270(4 pt 1):E627-E633.

7. Kasper CE, Talbot LA, Gaines JM. Skeletal muscle damage and recovery. *AACN Clin Issues*. 2002;13(2):237-247.

8. Berg HE, Larsson L, Tesch PA. Lower limb skeletal muscle function after 6 wk of bed rest. *J Appl Physiol*. 1997;82(1):182-188.

9. Reid MB. Response of the ubiquitin-proteasome pathway to changes in muscle activity. *Am J Physiol Regul Integr Comp Physiol*. 2005;288(6):R1423-R1431.

10. Bodine SC, Stitt TN, Gonzalez M, et al. Akt/mTOR pathway is a crucial regulator of skeletal muscle hypertrophy and can prevent muscle atrophy in vivo. *Nat Cell Biol*. 2001;3(11):1014-1019.

11. Stevenson EJ, Giresi PG, Koncarevic A, Kandarian SC. Global analysis of gene expression patterns during disuse atrophy in rat skeletal muscle. *J Physiol*. 2003;551(pt 1):33-48.

12. Batt J, Santos dos CC, Cameron JI, Herridge MS. Intensive care unit-acquired weakness: clinical phenotypes and molecular mechanisms. *Am J Respir Crit Care Med*. 2013;187(3):238-246.

13. Giger JM, Haddad F, Qin AX, Zeng M, Baldwin KM. Effect of unloading on type I myosin heavy chain gene regulation in rat soleus muscle. *J Appl Physiol*. 2005;98(4):1185-1194.

14. Jones SW, Hill RJ, Krasney PA, O'Conner B, Peirce N, Greenhaff PL. Disuse atrophy and exercise rehabilitation in humans profoundly affects the expression of genes associated with the regulation of skeletal muscle mass. *FASEB J*. 2004;18(9):1025-1027.

15. Krawiec BJ, Frost RA, Vary TC, Jefferson LS, Lang CH. Hindlimb casting decreases muscle mass in

part by proteasome-dependent proteolysis but independent of protein synthesis. *Am J Physiol Endocrinol Metab*. 2005;289(6):E969-E980.

16. Honkonen SE, Kannus P, Natri A, Latvala K, Järvinen MJ. Isokinetic performance of the thigh muscles after tibial plateau fractures. *Int Orthop*. 1997;21(5):323-326.

17. Muller EA. Influence of training and of inactivity on muscle strength. *Arch Phys Med Rehabil*. 1970,51.449-462.

18. Fan E, Dowdy DW, Colantuoni E, et al. Physical complications in acute lung injury survivors: a 2-year longitudinal prospective study. *Crit Care Med*. 2014;42:849-859.

19. Ferrando AA, Paddon-Jones D, Wolfe RR. Bed rest and myopathies. *Curr Opin Clin Nutr Metab Care*. 2006;9(4):410-415.

20. Finn PJ, Plank LD, Clark MA, Connolly AB, Hill GL. Progressive cellular dehydration and proteolysis in critically ill patients. *Lancet*. 1996;347(9002):654-656.

21. Paddon-Jones D, Sheffield-Moore M, Cree MG, et al. Atrophy and impaired muscle protein synthesis during prolonged inactivity and stress. *J Clin Endocrinol Metab*. 2006;91(12):4836-4841.

22. Hamburg NM, McMackin CJ, Huang AL, et al. Physical inactivity rapidly induces insulin resistance and microvascular dysfunction in healthy volunteers. *Arterioscler Thromb Vasc Biol*. 2007;27(12):2650-2656.

23. Bruunsgaard H. Physical activity and modulation of systemic low-level inflammation. *J Leukoc Biol*. 2005;78(4):819-835.

24. Winkelman C. Inactivity and inflammation in the critically ill patient. *Crit Care Clin*. 2007;23(1):21-34.

25. Bozza FA, Salluh JI, Japiassu AM, et al. Cytokine profiles as markers of disease severity in sepsis: a multiplex analysis. *Crit Care*. 2007;11(2):R49.

26. Pawlak W, Kedziora J, Zolynski K, Kedziora-Kornatowska K, Blaszczyk J, Witkowski P. Free radical generation by granulocytes from men during bed rest. *J Gravit Physiol*. 1998;5:P131-P132.

27. Pawlak W, Kedziora J, Zolynski K, et al. Effect of long term bed rest in men on enzymatic antioxidative defense and lipid peroxidation in erythrocytes. *J Gravit Physiol*. 1998;5(1):P163-P164.

28. Andrade FH, Reid MB, Allen DG, Westerblad H. Effect of hydrogen peroxide and dithiothreitol on contractile function of single skeletal muscle fibres from the mouse. *J Physiol*. 1998;509(pt 2):565-575.

29. Buck M, Chojkier M. Muscle wasting and dedifferentiation induced by oxidative stress in a murine model of cachexia is prevented by inhibitors of nitric oxide synthesis and antioxidants. *EMBO J*. 1996;15(8):1753-1765.

30. Convertino VA, Bloomfield SA, Greenleaf JE. An overview of the issues: physiological effects of bed rest and restricted physical activity. *Med Sci Sports Exerc*. 1997;29(2):187-190.

31. Fortney SM, Schneider VS, Greenleaf JE. The physiology of bed rest. In: Fregly MJ, Blatteis CM, eds. *Handbook of Physiology*. New York, NY: Oxford University Press; 1996.

32. Hough CL, Needham DM. The role of future longitudinal studies in ICU survivors: understanding determinants and pathophysiology of weakness and neuromuscular dysfunction. *Curr Opin Crit Care*. 2007;13(5):489-496.

33. Bolton CF, Gilbert JJ, Hahn AF, Sibbald WJ. Polyneuropathy in critically ill patients. *J Neurol Neurosurg Psychiatr*. 1984;47(11):1223-1231.

34. Latronico N, Bertolini G, Guarneri B, et al. Simplified electrophysiological evaluation of peripheral nerves in critically ill patients: the Italian multi-centre CRIMYNE study. *Crit Care*. 2007;11(1):R11.

35. Witt NJ, Zochodne DW, Bolton CF, et al. Peripheral nerve function in sepsis and multiple organ failure. *Chest*. 1991;99(1):176-184.

36. Bolton CF. Neuromuscular manifestations of critical illness. *Muscle Nerve*. 2005;32(2):140-163.

37. van den Berghe G, Schoonheydt K, Becx P, Bruyninckx F, Wouters PJ. Insulin therapy protects the central and peripheral nervous system of intensive care patients. *Neurology*. 2005;64(8):1348-1353.

38. Puthucheary Z, Montgomery H, Moxham J, Harridge S, Hart N. Structure to function: muscle failure in critically ill patients. *J Physiol*. 2010;588(pt 23):4641-4648.

39. Puthucheary ZA, Rawal J, McPhail M, et al. Acute skeletal muscle wasting in critical illness. *JAMA*. 2013;310(15):1591-1600.

40. Rich MM, Pinter MJ. Crucial role of sodium channel fast inactivation in muscle fibre inexcitability in a rat model of critical illness myopathy. *J Physiol*. 2003;547(pt 2):555-566.

41. Rossignol B, Gueret G, Pennec JP, et al. Effects of chronic sepsis on contractile properties of fast twitch muscle in an experimental model of critical illness neuromyopathy in the rat. *Crit Care Med*. 2008;36(6):1855-1863.

42. Allen DC, Arunachalam R, Mills KR. Critical illness myopathy: further evidence from muscle-fiber excitability studies of an acquired channelopathy. *Muscle Nerve.* 2008;37(1):14-22.

43. Lee CM, Fan E. ICU-acquired weakness: what is preventing its rehabilitation in critically ill patients? *BMC Med.* 2012;10(1):115.

44. Fujimura N, Sumita S, Narimatsu E, Nakayama Y, Shitinohe Y, Namiki A. Effects of isoproterenol on diaphragmatic contractility in septic peritonitis. *Am J Respir Crit Care Med.* 2000;161(2 pt 1):440-446.

45. Shanely RA, Zergeroglu MA, Lennon SL, et al. Mechanical ventilation-induced diaphragmatic atrophy is associated with oxidative injury and increased proteolytic activity. *Am J Respir Crit Care Med.* 2002;166(10):1369-1374.

46. Maes K, Testelmans D, Powers S, Decramer M, Gayan-Ramirez G. Leupeptin inhibits ventilator-induced diaphragm dysfunction in rats. *Am J Respir Crit Care Med.* 2007;175(11):1134-1138.

47. Levine S, Nguyen T, Taylor N, et al. Rapid disuse atrophy of diaphragm fibers in mechanically ventilated humans. *N Engl J Med.* 2008;358(13):1327-1335.

48. Fan E, Needham DM. Mechanical ventilation and disuse atrophy of the diaphragm. *N Engl J Med.* 2008;359(1):90-91; author reply 91-92.

49. Stevens RD, Dowdy DW, Michaels RK, Mendez-Tellez PA, Pronovost PJ, Needham DM. Neuromuscular dysfunction acquired in critical illness: a systematic review. *Intensive Care Med.* 2007;33(11):1876-1891.

50. van den Berghe G, Wouters P, Weekers F, et al. Intensive insulin therapy in the critically ill patients. *N Engl J Med.* 2001;345(19):1359-1367.

51. van den Berghe G, Wilmer A, Hermans G, et al. Intensive insulin therapy in the medical ICU. *N Engl J Med.* 2006;354(5):449-461.

52. Hermans G, Wilmer A, Meersseman W, et al. Impact of intensive insulin therapy on neuromuscular complications and ventilator dependency in the medical intensive care unit. *Am J Respir Crit Care Med.* 2007;175(5):480-489.

53. Brunkhorst FM, Engel C, Bloos F, et al. Intensive insulin therapy and pentastarch resuscitation in severe sepsis. *N Engl J Med.* 2008;358(2):125-139.

54. Preiser JC, Devos P, Ruiz-Santana S, et al. A prospective randomised multi-centre controlled trial on tight glucose control by intensive insulin therapy in adult intensive care units: the Glucontrol study. *Intensive Care Med.* 2009;35(10):1738-1748.

55. NICE-SUGAR Study Investigators, Finfer S, Chittock DR, et al. Intensive versus conventional glucose control in critically ill patients. *N Engl J Med.* 2009;360(13):1283-1297.

56. Bednarík J, Vondracek P, Dusek L, Moravcova E, Cundrle I. Risk factors for critical illness polyneuromyopathy. *J Neurol.* 2005;252(3):343-351.

57. de Letter MA, Schmitz PI, Visser LH, et al. Risk factors for the development of polyneuropathy and myopathy in critically ill patients. *Crit Care Med.* 2001;29(12):2281-2286.

58. Coakley JH, Nagendran K, Yarwood GD, Honavar M, Hinds CJ. Patterns of neurophysiological abnormality in prolonged critical illness. *Intensive Care Med.* 1998;24(8):801-807.

59. de Jonghe B, Sharshar T, Lefaucheur JP, et al. Paresis acquired in the intensive care unit: a prospective multicenter study. *JAMA.* 2002;288(22):2859-2867.

60. Bercker S, Weber-Carstens S, Deja M, et al. Critical illness polyneuropathy and myopathy in patients with acute respiratory distress syndrome. *Crit Care Med.* 2005;33(4):711-715.

61. Garnacho-Montero J, Madrazo-Osuna J, García-Garmendia JL, et al. Critical illness polyneuropathy: risk factors and clinical consequences. A cohort study in septic patients. *Intensive Care Med.* 2001;27(8):1288-1296.

62. Hough CL, Steinberg KP, Thompson BT, Rubenfeld GD, Hudson LD. Intensive care unit-acquired neuromyopathy and corticosteroids in survivors of persistent ARDS. *Intensive Care Med.* 2009;35(1):63-68.

63. Tang B, Craig J, Eslick G, Seppelt I, McLean A. Use of corticosteroids in acute lung injury and acute respiratory distress syndrome: a systematic review and meta-analysis. *Crit Care Med.* 2009;37:1594-1603.

64. Peter JV, John P, Graham PL, Moran JL, George IA, Bersten A. Corticosteroids in the prevention and treatment of acute respiratory distress syndrome (ARDS) in adults: meta-analysis. *BMJ.* 2008;336(7651):1006-1009.

65. Papazian L, Forel JM, Gacouin A, et al. Neuromuscular blockers in early acute respiratory distress syndrome. *N Engl J Med.* 2010;363(12):1107-1116.

66. Alhazzani W, Alshahrani M, Jaeschke R, et al. Neuromuscular blocking agents in acute respiratory distress syndrome: a systematic review and meta-analysis of randomized controlled trials. *Crit Care.* 2013;17(2):R43.

67. Puthucheary Z, Rawal J, Ratnayake G, Harridge S, Montgomery H, Hart N. Neuromuscular blockade

and skeletal muscle weakness in critically ill patients: time to rethink the evidence? *Am J Respir Crit Care Med*. 2012;185(9):911-917.

68. Koo K, Fan E. ICU-acquired weakness and early rehabilitation in the critically ill. *J Clin Outcomes Manag*. 2013;20(5):223-231.

69. Medical RCGOB. *Aids to the Examination of the Peripheral Nervous System*. London, UK: Bailliere Tindall; 1986.

70. Kleyweg RP, van der Meché FG, Schmitz PI. Interobserver agreement in the assessment of muscle strength and functional abilities in Guillain-Barré syndrome. *Muscle Nerve*. 1991;14(11):1103-1109.

71. Vanpee G, Hermans G, Segers J, Gosselink R. Assessment of limb muscle strength in critically ill patients: a systematic review. *Crit Care Med*. 2014;42(3):701-711.

72. Fan E, Ciesla ND, Truong AD, Bhoopathi V, Zeger SL, Needham DM. Inter-rater reliability of manual muscle strength testing in ICU survivors and simulated patients. *Intensive Care Med*. 2010;36(6):1038-1043.

73. Tennilä A, Salmi T, Pettilä V, Roine RO, Varpula T, Takkunen O. Early signs of critical illness polyneuropathy in ICU patients with systemic inflammatory response syndrome or sepsis. *Intensive Care Med*. 2000;26(9):1360-1363.

74. Bednarik J, Lukas Z, Vondracek P. Critical illness polyneuromyopathy: the electrophysiological components of a complex entity. *Intensive Care Med*. 2003;29(9):1505-1514.

75. Khan J, Harrison TB, Rich MM, Moss M. Early development of critical illness myopathy and neuropathy in patients with severe sepsis. *Neurology*. 2006;67(8):1421-1425.

76. Goodman BP, Boon AJ. Critical illness neuromyopathy. *Phys Med Rehabil Clin N Am*. 2008;19(1):97-110, vii.

77. Garnacho-Montero J, Amaya-Villar R, García-Garmendía JL, Madrazo-Osuna J, Ortiz-Leyba C. Effect of critical illness polyneuropathy on the withdrawal from mechanical ventilation and the length of stay in septic patients. *Crit Care Med*. 2005;33(2):349-354.

78. Ali NA, O'Brien JM, Hoffmann SP, et al. Acquired weakness, handgrip strength, and mortality in critically ill patients. *Am J Respir Crit Care Med*. 2008;178(3):261-268.

79. Berek K, Margreiter J, Willeit J, Berek A, Schmutzhard E, Mutz NJ. Polyneuropathies in critically ill patients: a prospective evaluation. *Intensive Care Med*. 1996;22(9):849-855.

80. Herridge MS, Tansey CM, Matté A, et al. Functional disability 5 years after acute respiratory distress syndrome. *N Engl J Med*. 2011;364(14):1293-1304.

81. Herridge MS, Cheung AM, Tansey CM, et al. One-year outcomes in survivors of the acute respiratory distress syndrome. *N Engl J Med*. 2003;348(8):683-693.

82. Dowdy DW, Eid MP, Dennison CR, et al. Quality of life after acute respiratory distress syndrome: a meta-analysis. *Intensive Care Med*. 2006;32(8):1115-1124.

83. Dowdy DW, Eid MP, Sedrakyan A, et al. Quality of life in adult survivors of critical illness: a systematic review of the literature. *Intensive Care Med*. 2005;31(5):611-620.

84. Griesdale DEG, de Souza RJ, van Dam RM, et al. Intensive insulin therapy and mortality among critically ill patients: a meta-analysis including NICE-SUGAR study data. *CMAJ*. 2009;180(8):821-827; discussion 799-800.

85. Schweickert WD, Hall J. ICU-acquired weakness. *Chest*. 2007;131(5):1541-1549.

86. Hodgson CL, Berney S, Harrold M, Saxena M, Bellomo R. Clinical review: early patient mobilization in the ICU. *Crit Care*. 2013;17(1):207.

87. Needham DM. Mobilizing patients in the intensive care unit: improving neuromuscular weakness and physical function. *JAMA*. 2008;300(14):1685-1690.

88. Berney S, Harrold M, Webb SA, et al. Intensive care unit mobility practices in Australia and New Zealand: a point prevalence study. *Crit Care Resusc*. 2013;15(4):260-265.

89. Nydahl P, Ruhl AP, Bartoszek G, et al. Early mobilization of mechanically ventilated patients: a 1-day point-prevalence study in Germany. *Crit Care Med*. 2014;42:1178-1186.

90. Stiller K. Safety issues that should be considered when mobilizing critically ill patients. *Crit Care Clin*. 2007;23(1):35-53.

91. Stiller K. Physiotherapy in intensive care: an updated systematic review. *Chest*. 2013;144(3):825-847.

92. Winkelman C. Ambulating with pulmonary artery or femoral catheters in place. *Crit Care Nurse*. 2011;31(5):70-73.

93. Hodgson CL, Fan E. A step up for extracorporeal membrane oxygenation: active rehabilitation. *Respir Care*. 2013;58(8):1388-1390.

94. Burtin C, Clerckx B, Robbeets C, et al. Early exercise in critically ill patients enhances short-term functional recovery. *Crit Care Med*. 2009;37(9):2499-2505.

95. Schweickert WD, Pohlman MC, Pohlman AS, et al. Early physical and occupational therapy in mechanically ventilated, critically ill patients: a randomised controlled trial. *Lancet.* 2009;373(9678):1874-1882.

96. Denehy L, Skinner EH, Edbrooke L, et al. Exercise rehabilitation for patients with critical illness: a randomized controlled trial with 12 months of follow-up. *Crit Care.* 2013;17(4):R156.

97. Bailey P, Thomsen GE, Spuhler VJ, et al. Early activity is feasible and safe in respiratory failure patients. *Crit Care Med.* 2007;35(1):139-145.

98. Bourdin G, Barbier J, Burle JF, et al. The feasibility of early physical activity in intensive care unit patients: a prospective observational one-center study. *Respir Care.* 2010;55(4):400-407.

99. Morris PE, Goad A, Thompson C, et al. Early intensive care unit mobility therapy in the treatment of acute respiratory failure. *Crit Care Med.* 2008;36(8):2238-2243.

100. Needham DM, Korupolu R, Zanni JM, et al. Early physical medicine and rehabilitation for patients with acute respiratory failure: a quality improvement project. *Arch Phys Med Rehabil.* 2010;91(4):536-542.

101. Thomsen GE, Snow GL, Rodriguez L, Hopkins RO. Patients with respiratory failure increase ambulation after transfer to an intensive care unit where early activity is a priority. *Crit Care Med.* 2008;36(4):1119-1124.

102. Zanni JM, Korupolu R, Fan E, et al. Rehabilitation therapy and outcomes in acute respiratory failure: an observational pilot project. *J Crit Care.* 2010;25(2):254-262.

103. Barr J, Fraser GL, Puntillo K, et al. Clinical practice guidelines for the management of pain, agitation, and delirium in adult patients in the intensive care unit. *Crit Care Med.* 2013;41(1):263-306.

104. Shehabi Y, Bellomo R, Reade MC, et al. Early intensive care sedation predicts long-term mortality in ventilated critically ill patients. *Am J Respir Crit Care Med.* 2012;186(8):724-731.

105. Tipping CJ, Young PJ, Romero L, Saxena MK, Dulhunty J, Hodgson CL. A systematic review of measurements of physical function in critically ill adults. *Crit Care Resusc.* 2012;14(4):302-311.

106. Hodgson C, Needham D, Haines K, et al. Feasibility and inter-rater reliability of the ICU Mobility Scale. *Heart Lung.* 2014;43(1):19-24.

107. Kasotakis G, Schmidt U, Perry D, et al. The surgical intensive care unit optimal mobility score predicts mortality and length of stay. *Crit Care Med.* 2012;40(4):1122-1128.

108. Morris PE, Griffin L, Berry M, et al. Receiving early mobility during an intensive care unit admission is a predictor of improved outcomes in acute respiratory failure. *Am J Med Sci.* 2011;341(5):373-377.

109. Roulin MJ, Hurst S, Spirig R. Diaries written for ICU patients. *Qual Health Res.* 2007;17(7):893-901.

110. Egerod I, Christensen D. A comparative study of ICU patient diaries vs. hospital charts. *Qual Health Res.* 2010;20(10):1446-1456.

Pharmacology in Critical Illness

15

Julie Chen, PharmD, BCPS and Adam Keene, MD

KEY POINTS

1 Complex pharmacokinetic and pharmacodynamic variations occur in critically ill patients secondary to underlying illness and acute organ failures as well as the multiple supportive modalities employed.

2 Failure to appreciate variabilities in pharmacokinetic and pharmacodynamic characteristics may contribute to suboptimal dosing, adverse outcome, increased risk of medication errors and adverse drug reactions.

3 Altered drug absorption, plasma protein binding, volume of distribution, renal and hepatic clearance, and affinity of binding to target receptors in critically-ill patients can all affect the therapeutic response and clinical outcome.

4 For medications with monitoring parameters available and a fairly rapid onset of action, careful dose titration based on clinical observation is appropriate; many of the cardiovascular active agents fall into this category.

5 For medications with slower onset of action and dose-dependent pharmacology, proper loading and maintenance doses should be determined; changes in drug volume

of distribution and clearance observed or measured in individual patients should be taken into consideration.

6 Therapeutic drug monitoring (TDM) is recommended for certain medications, including some antimicrobials, antiepileptics and cardiovascular agents. These tests are widely available with quick turnaround time for the results to assist in dose adjustment.

7 Different renal replacement regimens may have different impacts on the volume of distribution and clearance of each medication. Dosing need to be tailored to the dialysis modality utilized and delivered. In general, higher doses and more frequent dosing are necessary with continuous renal replacement therapy as compared to intermittent HD.

8 Other supportive modaltites, such as ECMO and plasmaphoresis, can also affect the pharmacology of some medications.

9 Polypharmacy is inevitable in critically ill and may contribute to adverse outcome secondary to drug interactions or toxicity; careful monitoring and patient assessment remains the key for optimal therapeutic outcome.

INTRODUCTION

Medication errors and adverse drug reactions (ADRs) occur more frequently in critically ill patients due to complex polypharmacy, frequent off-label drug use and multiorgan dysfunction. Requests to provide "STAT" doses during emergent situations further complicate this issue. Clinicians require an adequate knowledge of drug pharmacokinetics (PK) and pharmacodynamics (PD) to ensure safe and effective drug use in intensive care units (ICUs).

PK describes the movement of a drug through the body including the processes of absorption, distribution, metabolism, and elimination. PD describes the physiologic effects once the drug reaches the site of action. Most PK data are derived from healthy volunteers or from stable patients with specific disease states and may not be applicable to critically ill patients. Failure to anticipate significant changes in PK and PD in critical illness may contribute to suboptimal patient management.

PHARMACOKINETIC CONSIDERATIONS

Volume of distribution (Vd) and clearance (CL) are the 2 most important PK parameters for appropriate drug dosing. Initial loading dose (LD) is determined by Vd whereas maintenance dosing (MD) is determined by CL. Alterations of Vd and CL can occur during critical illness. These changes may result in an increased pharmacologic effect and/or undesired toxicity. The following provides a brief review focusing on general principles related to drug PK and changes that can occur during critical illness. All discussion is based on a one-compartment model using first-order PK principles.[1-6]

Absorption of medications from the gastrointestinal (GI) tract during critical illness is frequently low due to shunting of blood flow to support vital organs. Poor peripheral perfusion also impairs systemic absorption from muscles and subcutaneous tissues. Thus, intravenous (IV) administration is usually preferred for patients in shock. However, oral administration may be considered once patient is hemodynamically stable and enteral feeding is tolerated. Medications such as antihypertensive agents can be titrated to the

effect and provide smooth blood pressure coverage when given orally as compared to the intravenous alternatives. Some antimicrobial agents, such as cotrimoxazole, quinolones, linezolid, fluconazole, and voriconazole, have excellent oral bioavailability and can safely be given enterally once the infection is under control.

Vd is calculated by dividing the amount of drug in the body by the plasma concentration. Drug distribution in the body depends on blood flow, body composition, and plasma protein binding (PPB). In general, drugs that have high PPB stay mainly in the intravascular space and have a small Vd (Table 15–1). Lipophilic drugs have a large Vd because they tend to diffuse into the tissue and have a low plasma concentration. Vd can be used to determine the LD required to achieve a desired serum drug concentration ($Cp_{desired}$) by using the following equation (Equation 15–1):

$$LD~(mg) = Cp_{desired}~(mg/L) \times Vd~(L/kg) \times weight~(kg)$$
$$(15\text{–}1)$$

After appropriate fluid resuscitation, patients in septic shock and other forms of multiorgan dysfunction tend to have both greatly increased intra- and extravascular fluid volume. This can increase the Vd for hydrophilic medications significantly. Thus, much higher initial dose (LD) is required to achieve a desired therapeutic effect for a hydrophilic drug such as vancomycin and aminoglycosides. Lipophilic drugs have larger Vd and their Vd is usually not affected by the fluid shift.

PPB may affect the Vd and the therapeutic effect of a drug. Only free or unbound drugs can be readily distributed into tissues and thus have pharmacologic effect. Albumin and alpha 1-acid glycoprotein (AAG) are 2 primary proteins. Acidic drugs, such as phenytoin, bind to albumin whereas basic drugs, such as lidocaine, bind to AAG. The increased vascular permeability and protein catabolism seen in critically ill patients can result in decreased albumin concentrations. Thus, increased free plasma concentration for acidic drugs. AAG, an acute phase reactant, is increased in critically ill patients, thus, decreasing the free plasma concentration of basic drugs. Metabolic abnormalities, uremia, and drug interactions may further displace a drug from PPB. Warfarin, a drug frequently avoided in ICU patients, is 99% PPB with only 1% free drug responsible for its

TABLE 15–1 Medications with high plasma protein binding.

Drug	PPB (%)
Antiepileptics	
Phenytoin	88-93
Valproic acid	90
Anticoagulants	
Apixaban	87
Rivaroxaban	92-95
Warfarin	99
Antifungals	
Amphotericin B	> 90
Echinocandins	
Anidulafungin	98
Caspofungin	97
Micafungin	99
Posaconazole	98
Antimicrobials	
Ceftriaxone	83-96
Clindamycin	60-95
Daptomycin	84-93
Nafcillin	87-90
Oxacillin	94
Tigecycline	71-89
Benzodiazepines	
Chlordiazepoxide	90-98
Diazepam	94-99
Lorazepam	85-91
Midazolam	95
Calcium channel blockers	
Diltiazem	77-93
Nicardipine	> 95
Nifedipine	90-96
Nimodipine	> 95
Nitrendipine	97-99
Verapamil	88-94
Diuretics	
Bumetanide	90-99
Ethacrynic acid	90
Furosemide	91-99
Torsemide	> 99
Endothelin receptor antagonists	
Ambrisentan	99
Bosentan	> 98
Macitentan	>99
Other	
Amiodarone	96
Dexmedetomidine	94
Haloperidol	> 90
Hydralazine	88-90

therapeutic effect. A displace of 1% PPB can double its free drug in the plasma and cause excessive anticoagulation. Meanwhile, phenytoin is approximately 90% bound to albumin and can be displaced in uremia. It is important to recognize that these patients frequently have a low measured total phenytoin level with adequate free phenytoin level (1-2 µg/mL) for therapeutic effect. Equations have been proposed to account for increased free plasma phenytoin in patients with hypoalbuminemia (Equation 15–2) and uremia (Equation 15–3).

$$C_{adjusted} = \frac{C_{measued}}{0.2 \times Alb + 0.1} \qquad (15\text{–}2)$$

$$C_{adjusted} = \frac{C_{measued}}{0.1 \times Alb + 0.1} \qquad (15\text{–}3)$$

$C_{measured}$ and $C_{adjusted}$: measured and adjusted phenytoin concentrations.
Alb: patient's albumin levels in g/dL.

As explained above, a patient with a serum albumin of 2 g/dL will only need a measured phenytoin level between 5 and 10 µg/mL to maintain a therapeutic effect. In the presence of uremia, a measured level between 3 and 6 µg/mL may be adequate. Although only supported by limited data, these equations are useful in ICU setting to guide dosage adjustment. Monitoring free phenytoin concentration may be impractical due to rapid changes in serum albumin levels and slow laboratory turnaround times.

CL measures drug removal from the body by all elimination pathways, including metabolism and excretion. To maintain therapeutic effect, the amount of drug removed during the dosing interval should be replaced as maintenance dose. In critically ill patients, both hepatic and renal CL is usually reduced. However, in early stage of septic shock, a compensatory hyperdynamic phase accompanied by an increase in cardiac output and organ perfusion may result in increased drug clearance. Appropriate dosage adjustment is critical to provide the desired effect while minimizing toxicity. Serum creatinine (SCr) and urine output are frequently monitored to estimate the extent of renal dysfunction. However, changes in SCr lag behind changes in actual renal function during acute kidney injury and recovery. Also, extensive muscle injury or drug interactions (ie, concurrent trimethoprim) may cause elevated SCr unrelated to renal dysfunction. Monitoring the trend of organ dysfunction for proactive dosing adjustments is recommended. Maintenance dose for medications mainly cleared renally should be reduced in patients with oliguria or anuria, while prompt dosing increase is imperative with renal recovery. Various dosing guidelines are available based on the estimated creatinine clearance (CrCl) using Cockroft-Gault equation (Equation 15–4):

Estimated CrCl (mL/min) for males =

$$\frac{(140-age)\times weight*(kg)}{72\times SCr} \qquad (15\text{--}4)$$

($\times 0.85$ for females—adjust for smaller muscle mass)

*Ideal body weight (IBW) should be used for obese patients:

IBW (kg) for females = 45 + 2.3 ×
(height in inches − 60)
IBW (kg) for males = 50 + 2.3 ×
(height in inches − 60)

It is important to know that this estimate is not reliable in patients with acute changes in SCr or very low SCr. In addition to estimated CrCl, extent of dose reduction should be based on the trend in renal function, and the indication for therapy. This is especially important to avoid inadequate dosing of antibiotic therapy. MD adjustment can be done by either dose reduction or interval extension. Dosing for many cardiovascular drugs (ie, antihypertensive and inotrope agents), analgesics and central nervous system (CNS) depressants can be initiated conservatively and titrated to desired effect based on clinical assessment. It is also important to remember that toxic or active metabolites (ie, of opiates and benzodiazepines) may also accumulate in patients with renal dysfunction; close monitoring is required when an extended duration of therapy is indicated. Goal-directed sedation and sedation vacations are probably the most useful approaches to avoid excessive sedation in ICU patients with multiorgan failure.

Metabolism may be affected by decreased hepatic blood flow, altered PPB, decreased hepatic enzyme activity, and other metabolic abnormalities

seen in critically ill patients. Concurrent renal and cardiac dysfunction further complicates this issue. Acute hepatic dysfunction usually does not affect drug metabolism significantly. Extent of hepatic dysfunction cannot be quantified for dosage adjustment in acute or chronic liver failure. Dosing for medications that require hepatic metabolism should be initiated conservatively and titrated to the effect based on risk and benefit assessment. Concurrent or excessive use of hepatotoxic agents such as acetaminophen should be avoided whenever possible.

Half-life ($T_{1/2}$), the time required for plasma drug concentration (Cp) to reduce by 50%, is determined by Vd and CL as shown in Equation 15–5:

$$T_{1/2} = 0.693 \times \frac{Vd}{CL} \qquad (15\text{--}5)$$

$T_{1/2}$ is increased with a decrease in CL, or an increase in Vd. Under normal circumstance, 4 to 5 half-lives are required for serum drug concentrations to reach steady state after a therapy is started. It may take much longer for an ICU patient to reach steady state due to rapid changes in CL and Vd. When a drug regimen is discontinued, it also takes 4 to 5 half-lives for a drug to be cleared from the plasma compartment. Dosing strategy is frequently determined by the $T_{1/2}$. For drugs with long $T_{1/2}$ (such as amiodarone with a $T_{1/2}$ of 1 month or longer with chronic use) initial LDs are required to achieve a more rapid therapeutic response. On the other hand, aminoglycosides (AGs) have a short $T_{1/2}$ of 1 to 2 hours in patients with normal renal function. Serum concentration would approach 0 before the next dose for once-a-day AG regimen. This dosing approach utilizes the concentration-dependent killing effect of AG to enhance bactericidal action while lowering the risk of nephrotoxicity. The postantibiotic effect of AGs allows for continued bacterial killing even when trough concentrations of 0 are reached.

Specific PD considerations Medications with long $T_{1/2}$ do not always have a long duration of action. This is especially true for CNS depressants including opioids, benzodiazepines, and barbiturates. These agents are highly lipid soluble and have a rapid onset of action after an IV dose. However, disproportion to the relatively long $T_{1/2}$, the duration of action is frequently short lived secondary to a rapid decline of CNS concentration after a rapid redistributed into peripheral "lipid-rich" tissues. Clinical experience has shown that the effect and duration of these medications also depends heavily on the past exposure history of the patient. Patients with chronic use of alcohol, opioids, and benzodiazepines tend to develop tolerance to these agents and require much higher doses and more frequent dosing for the required sedative or analgesic effect. Receptor desensitization and/or downregulation may be responsible for this observation. In these patients, medications with long $T_{1/2}$, such as diazepam and chlordiazepoxide may still accumulate after repeated doses. This is the rationale of repeating the doses of benzodiazepines until the patient is calm in the acute management of alcohol withdrawal. At this stage, enough benzodiazepine accumulates in the tissue (adipose) to sustain adequate concentration in the CNS. Further doses may be used less frequently and as needed for recurrent symptoms of delirium tremens (DT). The amount accumulated in the tissue will serve as a drug depot to support a slow benzodiazepine taper and complete DT management. It is also important to recognize that all benzodiazepines will have longer duration of action and longer half-lives once the agent is accumulated in the tissue. Thus, a short-acting agent, such as midazolam, may have a long-lasting sedative effect with prolonged use.

Because of increased multiple-drug resistance infections, some specific PD-based antibiotic dosing approaches have been advocated. Aminoglycoside antibiotics have concentration-dependent killing and a pronounced postantibiotic effect. Once-daily AG regimens (gentamicin and tobramycin: up to 7 mg/kg; amikacin: up to 20 mg/kg) can achieve high peak serum concentrations with better bactericidal effect than the same dose divided into multiple doses per day. Beta-lactam antibiotics, such as piperacillin/tazobactam, have time-dependent killing. Maintaining serum beta-lactam concentrations above the minimum inhibitory concentration (MIC) during the dosing interval can achieve better antibacterial activity. When piperacillin/tazobactam is administered as an extended infusion over 4 hours, compared to a 30-minute bolus infusion, serum concentration can be maintained above the MIC for a greater proportion of time during the dosing interval.

EXTRACORPOREAL DRUG CLEARANCE

Renal Replacement Therapy

In addition to intermittent hemodialysis (IHD), continuous renal replacement therapy (CRRT),[7-9] especially continuous venovenous hemofiltration (CVVH) and continuous venovenous hemodiafiltration (CVVHDF), is often provided to ICU patients with acute and chronic kidney injury. Removal of solutes and fluid from blood through semipermeable membranes occurs by means of either diffusion and/or convection during RRT. While IHD utilizes diffusion for clearance, CVVH utilizes convection and CVVHDF utilizes a combination of both. Small molecules (MW < 1000 Da) are removed effectively by IHD with conventional hemofilters (small pores). Modern high-flux membranes (large pores) utilized in CRRT are permeable to large molecules (30,000-50,000 Da) and therefore, most drug molecules. The characteristics of high-flux hemofilters and the continuous, prolonged nature of CRRT result in efficient solute removal and enhanced drug clearance. In general, the relative extent of drug removal in CRRT is CVVHDF greater than CVVH greater than IHD. However, the extent of CRRT clearance still depends on specific physiochemical properties of the drug and how CRRT is prescribed and delivered. Compared to IHD or patients with renal failure, drugs that are normally cleared by the kidney may require a much higher dose during CRRT. Drugs with a high Vd (> 1 L/kg), high PPB (> 80%), and predominant nonrenal clearance may need no dose adjustment due to poor CRRT removal.

Only unbound and water-soluble drug molecules are removed effectively during CRRT. It is evident that an increase in unbound fraction secondary to changes in systemic pH, plasma protein concentrations, organ function, and drug interactions can contribute to increased CRRT elimination. Another potential mechanism for solute removal during CRRT is "adsorption." The clinical significance of drug adsorption to the dialysis circuitry and membrane is unclear. Many published data are available to guide proper drug dosing in CRRT. However, these dosing recommendations have been derived from diverse patient populations in which different modes of CRRT were prescribed. Other clinical and patient variables, such as interruptions or inconsistency of CRRT delivery, fluid overload, and residual renal function, may also affect drug clearance. Thus, dosing in patients requiring CRRT needs to be individualized. Drugs such as analgesics, sedatives, and cardiovascular agents can be dosed based on clinical response. Therapeutic drug monitoring (TDM) is available for some antiepileptics, antimicrobials, and cardiovascular agents. The turnaround time for TDM should be short enough for the monitoring to be clinically relevant.

As a general rule, a proper LD is usually required for an agent with a long $T_{1/2}$ to achieve therapeutic plasma levels rapidly. This initial dose is determined largely by the Vd of the drug and need not be adjusted in CRRT. However, Vd might be increased significantly in ICU patients as described in the PK section. Using vancomycin as an example, a regular or even higher LD (25 mg/kg or more) should be administered initially. Subsequent MDs require modification based on the PK and PD characteristics, and CRRT clearance. For medications such as most beta-lactam antibiotics that are renally cleared, 50% to 100% of the regular MD has been recommended for patients undergoing CRRT. It is important to recognize that aggressive antibiotic dosing during CRRT along with proper monitoring is always preferred to underdosing in patients with septic shock, especially within the first few days of therapy. The nurse in charge of the CRRT delivery should also document the actual delivery of CRRT and must inform the physicians and pharmacists if any significant interruptions of CRRT occur. This information should be communicated every 6 to 8 hours, if not more often, to ensure timely dosing adjustment. This rule should also be followed when CRRT is discontinued or a different CRRT mode is prescribed.

Plasmapheresis and Therapeutic Plasma Exchange

These are automated extracorporeal apheresis techniques designed to remove or reduce the concentration of large-molecular-weight substances such as immunoglobulins and autoantibodies from the plasma. This treatment may increase drug CL.

During the process, plasma proteins are removed. Drugs with a small Vd and/or high PPB, such as basiliximab, ceftriaxone, and propranolol, may be removed significantly and supplemental doses may be required at the completion of plasmapheresis. Another approach to retain drug efficacy is to schedule the plasmapheresis toward the end of the dosing interval, allowing the regular dose to be administered at the completion of the session.[10]

Extracorporeal Membrane Oxygenation

Extracorporeal membrane oxygenation (ECMO)[11,12] is an advanced life support system to provide support for patients with respiratory and/or or cardiac failure who have failed conventional management. ECMO may influence PK through hemodilution (increased Vd) as well as by binding or sequestration of drugs in the ECMO circuit. Significant sequestration of opioids (fentanyl, morphine), benzodiazepines (diazepam, lorazepam, midazolam), nitroglycerin, propofol, and antimicrobials (ampicillin, cefazolin, voriconazole) has been reported. This sequestration can lower serum drug concentrations and potentially reduced the therapeutic effect. There is limited data available to guide dosing adjustment in adult patients. Most of the data have been derived from pediatric populations. Decreased serum levels of gentamicin, heparin, phenobarbital, phenytoin, and vancomycin have been reported in neonates maintained on ECMO. It is important to note that children supported by ECMO require a relative larger volume (compared to their body size) to prime the circuit and blood transfusion is frequently utilized to maintain acceptable hemoglobin levels. Although pediatric data may not be applicable to adults, higher LD and MD may be needed to maintain therapeutic levels in adult ICU patients requiring ECMO support. Proper monitoring to guide dose adjustment is essential. Serum drug monitoring is not possible for many drugs used in ICU. Tailoring therapy to the individual clinical response is often a more practical approach.

Dosing Adjustment in Obese Patients

Most recent reports indicate that 12% to 37% of ICU patients are obese. Obesity presents unique challenge because only limited PK data are available to guide dosing. Many drug investigations either exclude or do not include enough obese patients for data extrapolation. In general, both Vd and CL of drugs are altered by obesity. Lipophilic medications are distributed to adipose tissue and a larger dose is required to achieve therapeutic serum or tissue levels. Loading doses of lipophilic agents, such as phenytoin, should be based on the actual body weight followed with MD adjusted based on serum concentrations. Also, higher doses of sedatives and opioids (most are lipophilic) are usually required initially for the desired sedative or analgesic effect. However, obese patients are also at increased risk for drug accumulation after prolonged infusion or frequent dosing. Thus, proper dose titration to goal or patient response is essential. More hydrophilic medications with smaller Vd and limited distribution to adipose tissue may be dosed based on adjusted weight as per Equation 15–6.[13]

Adjusted body weight = ideal body weight +
40% (actual body weight –
ideal body weight*)

(15–6)

*See Equation 15–4 for ideal body weight.

Since most antimicrobial agents are hydrophilic, adequate blood concentrations may be achieved at the usual recommended doses. However, more aggressive antibiotic dosing approaches may be indicated based on the severity of the infection and the safety profile of the agent chosen. Again, with limited data to support dosing, seeking assistance from an experienced clinical pharmacist is recommended. Close monitoring for drug efficacy and toxicity is essential in the management of obese ICU patients.

Therapeutic Drug Monitoring

Serum drug concentrations of some medications may need to be monitored to ensure therapeutic effect without excessive toxicity (Table 15–2). Timing of a blood sample in relation to previous dose influences the interpretation of a drug concentration measurement. As a general rule, TDM should be done when steady state has been reached (after 4-5 half-lives). Check a peak level "immediately" after a LD is rarely justified. To confirm if a LD is adequate

TABLE 15–2 Therapeutic ranges for drugs commonly used in ICU.

Drugs	Therapeutic Range[a]
Amikacin	Peak: depends on dosing strategy and severity/site of infection Trough < 5 µg/mL
Carbamazepine	4-12 µg/mL
Gentamicin	Peak: depends on dosing strategy and severity/site of infection Trough < 2 µg/mL
Digoxin	0.5-1.2 µg/L
Phenobarbital	15-40 µg/mL
Phenytoin	Total: 10-20 µg/mL Free[b]: 1-2 µg/mL
Theophylline (in COPD)	5-10 µg/mL
Tobramycin	Peak: depends on dosing strategy and severity/site of infection Trough < 2 µg/mL
Valproic acid	50-140 µg/mL
Vancomycin	15-20 µg/mL (10-15 is acceptable for less severe infections)

[a]Trough level is preferred unless otherwise specified.
[b]Although free phenytoin levels are occasionally indicated or recommended, they are not practical in critically ill patients secondary to slow test turnaround times and rapid changes in serum albumin (see text for details).

or further LD is needed, the level should be checked after the completion of the distribution phase. Most drugs, such as vancomycin and aminoglycosides, have a distribution phase of 30 to 60 minutes after IV administration. Digoxin is an exception to this rule. The distribution phase of digoxin is prolonged and a level (if indicated) should be drawn at least 4 to 6 hours after an IV dose or 6 to 8 hours after an oral dose. Otherwise, the measured serum digoxin level will be falsely high and misleading. Although a peak level may be required for some medications (ie, AGs), most drug levels should be checked as steady-state troughs just before the next dose is due. These trough levels represent the lowest level in the blood which can be used to guide dose adjustment based on clinical assessment. If trough monitoring is not feasible, another approach is sampling blood for drug levels consistently during a dosing interval after the completion of distribution phase. This means drawing a level at the same time of the day when such monitoring is indicated. The trend of serum drug concentration changes can then be used to guide MD adjustment. After a target level is achieved, drug levels only need to be rechecked as clinically indicated such as in patients with acute changes in organ function, suspected toxicity, or clinical failure. Also, it is important to allow at least 2 to 4 hours to elapse after any form of renal replacement therapy before sampling blood if a drug level is indicated. This is to allow redistribution of the drug from other tissues into the intravascular space. Otherwise, a falsely low level may lead to unnecessary dosing increase. The extent of this rebound of serum concentration after dialysis is more significant for a drug with a larger Vd and/or after prolonged therapy secondary to increased tissue drug accumulation.

Adverse Drug Events

Adverse drug events (ADEs)[14-17] are defined as harm or injury caused by the use of a drug. These events can occur at any stage in treatment. Approximately 25% of ADEs are either unpredictable or caused by an allergic reaction. The rest ADRS (> 70%) are dose related or predictable based on pharmacologic characteristics. Critically ill patients are at high risk for ADEs because of their organ dysfunctions as well as the complexity of the medications they are prescribed. Acute renal failure in ICU patients has been linked to increased morbidity/mortality, length of stay, and cost. Up to 20% of all cases of renal failure in ICUs may be associated with drug toxicity. The benefit of using any nephrotoxic agent (Table 15–3) in ICU patients needs to be weighed against the risk. Patients should be monitored carefully and evidence-based preventive measures should be provided whenever possible. Efforts should also be directed to minimize the exposure to other potential causes of renal injury. Adequate hydration with isotonic fluid and maintenance of renal perfusion are crucial for reducing renal toxicity associated with many agents including acyclovir, amphotericin B, radiocontrasts, and sulfonamides. Aggressive diuretic therapy should be used with caution when a patient is maintained on a therapy with known nephrotoxicity. If drug-induced renal failure is suspected,

TABLE 15–3 Medications frequently associated with nephrotoxicity in ICUs (not all inclusive).

Angiotensin-converting enzyme inhibitors/angiotensin receptor antagonists
Captopril
Lisinopril
Losartan, etc
Antimicrobials
Aminoglycosides—amikacin, gentamicin, tobramycin, etc
Amphotericin B—including all lipid complex formulations
Antivirals—acyclovir, foscarnet, cidofovir, pentamidine
Beta-lactams—penicillins and cephalosporins may cause interstitial nephritis in rare cases
Sulfonamides—sulfadiazine, sulfamethoxazole, etc
Calcineurin inhibitors
Cyclosporine
Tacrolimus
Diuretics—secondary to intravascular volume depletion
Bumetanide
Furosemide
Torsemide
Nonsteroidal anti-inflammatory agents (include cyclooxygenase-2 inhibitors)
Ketorolac
Ibuprofen
Naprosyn, etc
Miscellaneous
Allopurinol
Immunoglobulins
Mannitol
Radiocontrasts
Starches—hetastarch, etc

the therapy should be discontinued whenever possible. Medication profiles should be reviewed for proper dose adjustment while renal supportive care is provided. Many drugs used in ICU have been associated with prolongation of the QT interval (Table 15–4). Amiodarone and methadone are the 2 most frequently reported drugs to cause prolonged QT interval and torsades de pointes based on the data from the Food and Drug Administration (FDA) Adverse Event Reporting System (January 2004 to December 2007). Patients receive concurrent medications with QT prolongation potential should be

TABLE 15–4 Medications associated with prolonged QT interval[a] in ICUs (not all inclusive).

Analgesics—Methadone

Antiarrhythmic agents
Amiodarone
Dofetilide
Ibutilide
Procainamide
Quinidine
Sotalol

Anesthetics
Inhaled—Halothane, Enflurane, Isoflurane, Sevoflurane
Intravenous—Thiopental

Antidepressants
Tricyclics—Imipramine, etc
SSRIs[b]—Citalopram, Fluoxetine, Venlafaxine

Antimicrobial agents
Fluoroquinolones—Levofloxacin > Moxifloxacin > Ciprofloxacin
Macrolides—Erythromycin (esp. high-dose IV) > Clarithromycin > Azithromycin
Azole antifungals[c]—(Ketoconazole, Itraconazole) > voriconazole > Fluconazole

Antipsychotics
Butyrophenones—Droperidol, Haloperidol
Clozapine
Olanzapine
Phenothiazines—Thioridazine, etc
Quetiapine
Risperidone
Ziprasidone

Antiemetics
5-HT3 antagonists—Dolasetron > Ondansetron
Droperidol

Neuromuscular blocking and reversal agents
Succinylcholine
Atropine, Glycopyrrolate, Neostigmine

[a]Risk is increased with higher dose or repeated doses in short period of time; risk is also increased in drug overdose.
[b]SSRIs: selectiveserotonin reuptake inhibitors.
[c]Azoles usually cause prolonged QT interval through interaction with another agent with QT prolongation potential.

monitored properly. Clinical decisions about drug discontinuation should be made based on the extent of QT prolongation. The risk of developing torsades de points is significantly increased in patients with QT intervals of greater than 500 msec.

Drug-Drug Interactions

Drug-drug interactions (DDIs) are major contributors to ADEs but can easily be prevented or managed when identified in advance. It has been estimated that at least 11% of patients admitted to a general ICU may experience DDIs. Polypharmacy, altered organ function, and advanced age are risk factors identified. DDIs may contribute to adverse events and compromise patient care with increased morbidity, mortality, and health care cost. Most DDIs can be classified as PK or PD interactions. A PK interaction occurs when one drug alters the absorption, distribution, metabolism, or elimination of another agent. A PD interaction occurs when one agent enhances or antagonizes the pharmacologic action of another agent. Antibiotics and antithrombotic agents have frequently been implicated in DDIs. Drugs that are potent inhibitors or inducers of liver cytochrome P-450 enzyme system should be used with caution. Among many of the P-450 isoenzmes identified, CYP3A4 is involved in liver metabolism of up to 50% of medications. Protease inhibitors (ie, ritonavir), macrolides (ie, erythromycin), and triazoles (ie, fluconazole, posaconazole, voriconazole) are potent CYP3A4 inhibitors. Serious DDIs with significant toxicity may develop if any of these agents is initiated concurrently with a drug that is also a CYP3A4 substrate (ie, amiodarone, cyclosporine, tacrolimus, HMG-CoA reductase inhibitors). Warfarin, an agent with narrow therapeutic index, is metabolized by several CYP enzymes, especially CYP1A2, 2C9, 2C19, and 3A4. Rifampin, a potent inducer of CYP2C9, can result in decreased warfarin effect while CYP2C9 inhibitors (ie, amiodarone, sulfonamides, voriconazole, and metronidazole) can increase the effect of warfarin. Alternative medications with minimal or no DDI should always be considered. If this approach is not possible, most of the DDIs encountered clinically can be monitored with careful dosing adjustment. A multidisciplinary team approach, especially with the presence of a clinical pharmacist on rounds, may facilitate the detection, prevention, and resolution of potential DDIs. Potential DDIs should be evaluated at the time a medication is initiated or discontinued, especially if a high-risk medication (Table 15–5) is involved.

TABLE 15–5 High-risk medications for potential drug-drug interactions in ICUs (not all inclusive).

Medications	Comments

Antiepileptics
  Barbiturates
  Carbamazepine
  Phenytoin*
  Valproic acid
	Valproic acid is a P-450 enzyme system inhibitor, barbiturates, carbamazepine and phenytoin are P-450 enzyme system inducers; *Decrease GI absorption of phenytoin with concurrent enteral nutrition—may be overcome by using higher dose.

Antithrombotic agents
  Heparin, unfractionated
  Low-molecular-weight heparins
  Warfarin*
	Interact with any agent that can affect hematologic system and hemostasis, such as antibiotics, antiplatelets. *Warfarin is highly plasma protein bound (PPB—99%) and can be displaced by other high PPB agents.

Cardiac medications
  Amiodarone
  Calcium channel blockers
    Diltiazem
    Nicardipine
    Verapamil
  Digoxin
	Amiodarone and calcium channel blockers interact with each other and many drugs that rely on P-450 enzyme system for clearance. Serum digoxin level may be doubled or tripled with concurrent amiodarone, Cardizem, and verapamil administration—if combination is crucial, reduce digoxin maintenance dose by 35%-50% after regular loading dose.

CNS depressants **Benzodiazepines, opioids, propofol**	Synergistic sedative effect, goal-directed sedation with daily wake-up assessment if feasible to avoid excessive sedation.

Fluoroquinolones
  Ciprofloxacin
  Levofloxacin
  Moxifloxacin
	GI absorption is impaired by concurrent polyvalent cations, such as Zn, Fe, Al, Mg; cause prolonged QT interval—potentiate other drugs that cause prolonged QT.

GI medications
  Proton pump inhibitors
  H$_2$-blockers
	Increased gastric pH results in decreased GI absorption of certain HIV regimens, itraconazole, ketoconazole, and iron supplement.

HIV antiretroviral regimens	Ritonavir-boosted regimens: many inhibit P-450 enzyme system. Atazanavir, nelfinavir, and rilpivirine: GI absorption is reduced with stress ulcer prophylaxis.

Immunosuppresive regimens
  Cyclosporine
  Tacrolimus
  Sirolimus
	Many interactions with medications that inhibit or induce P-450 enzyme system.

Triazole antifungals
  Itraconazole*
  Ketoconazole*
  Voriconazole
	Many Interactions via potent inhibition of P-450 enzyme system; cause prolonged QT interval—potentiate other drugs that cause prolonged QT. *GI absorption is gastric pH dependent.

Macrolides:
  Azithromycin
  Clarithromycin
  Erythromycin
	Cause prolonged QT interval—potentiate other drugs that cause prolonged QT; inhibit P-450 enzyme system; erythromycin is the most potent inhibitor.

Nephrotoxic agents **Acyclovir, Aminoglycosides, Amphotericin b, Cidofovir, Cotrimoxazole, Foscarnet, Tenofovir, etc**	Close monitoring of renal function is essential—concurrent administration of these drugs need clear risk and benefit assessment; acute renal failure can also lead to excessive dosing or toxicity from other renally eliminated medications.

Medication Errors and Prevention

Medication errors (MEs) are a reality of medicine.[18-20] Harmful MEs are reported more frequently in the ICU than in the non-ICU setting. Although ME data are generally underreported, it has been estimated, that critically ill patients experience an average of 1.7 MEs per day, and many patients suffer a potential life-threatening ME during their ICU stay. Reduction of MEs is the focus of many hospital quality improvement programs. Several interventions have been shown to decrease MEs in the ICU. Improved medication safety can be accomplished by medication standardization (prophylaxis for venous thromboembolism and stress ulcer, standardized IV concentrations, etc.) computerized physician order entry, barcode technology, smart intravenous infusion devices, and medication reconciliation programs. "Medication reconciliation" has been incorporated into National Patient Safety Goal #3 as of July 2011. Patient's complete medication regimen should be reviewed at the time of ICU admission and transfer, and should be compared with the regimen being considered for the new setting of care. This process is to ensure consistencies in medication regimens and prevent possible harms from unintentional medication omissions or therapeutic duplicates. Elimination of situational risk factors, such as inadequate trainee supervision, excessive nurse and physician work hours or work load, and distractions from the work flow, can prevent MEs. In addition, multidisciplinary team approach with physicians, physician assistants, nurses, and pharmacists is essential to medication oversight and error interception.

CLINICAL PEARLS FOR CRITICAL CARE PHARMACOLOGY

1) Apply pharmacokinetic and pharmacodynamic knowledge to determine the best dosing approach for critically ill patients with rapidly changing multiorgan dysfunction.

2) Loading dose is required to achieve desired therapeutic response timely, especially for drugs with long $T_{1/2}$. Critically ill patients must receive adequate loading dose as indicated.

3) Loading (initial) dose is determined mainly by the volume of distribution – no dose adjustment is required in the presence of organ dysfunction.

4) Maintenance doses should be adjusted based on the extent and trend of organ dysfunction, as well as the clinical indication for the therapy— lower doses may be needed if organ function continues to deteriorate whereas higher doses may be indicated in the recovery phase of organ dysfunction.

5) Be proactive to avoid improper dosing for patients with rapidly changing organ function—look at the trend to maximize therapeutic effect while minimizing toxicity.

6) Prevent medication errors and adverse drug-drug interactions—review medication profiles when high-risk drugs with known toxicity or drug-drug interactions are initiated or discontinued.

7) Multidisciplinary team work is the key for safe and effective pharmacologic management.

REFERENCES

1. Smith BS, Yagaratnam D, Levasseur-Franklin KE, Forni A, Fong J. Introduction to drug pharmacokinetics in the critically ill patients. *Chest.* 2012;141(5):1327-1336.

2. Quintiliani R, Sr, Quintiliani R, Jr. Pharmacokinetics/pharmacodynamics for critical care clinicians. *Crit Care Clin.* 2008;24:335-348.

3. Lodise TP, Drusano GL. Pharmacokinetics and pharmacodynamics: optimal antimicrobial therapy in the intensive care unit. *Crit Care Clin.* 2011;27:1-18.

4. Varghese JM, Roberts JA, Lipman J. Antimicrobial pharmacokinetic and pharmacodynamic issues in the critically ill with severe sepsis and septic shock. *Crit Care Clin.* 2011;27:19-34.

5. Winter ME. *Basic Principles in Basic Clinical Pharmacokinetics.* 5th ed. Lippincott Williams & Wilkins; 2010:2-133.

6. Peppard WJ, Peppard SR, Somberg L. Optimizing drug therapy in the surgical intensive care unit. *Surg Clin N Am.* 2012;92:1573-1620.

7. Choi G, Gomersall CD, Tian Q, Joynt GM, Freebairn R, Lipman J. Principles of antibacterial dosing in

continuous renal replacement therapy. *Crit Care Med*. 2009;37(7):2268-2282.

8. Heintz BH, Matzke GR, Dager WE. Antimicrobial dosing concepts and recommendations for critically ill adult patients receiving continuous renal replacement therapy or intermittent hemodialysis. *Pharmacotherapy*. 2009;29(5):562-577.

9. Pea F, Viale P, Pavan F, Furlanut M. Pharmacokinetic consideration for antimicrobial therapy in patients receiving renal replacement therapy. *Clin Pharmacokinet*. 2007;46(12):997-1038.

10. Ibrahim RB, Liu C, Cronin SM, et al. Drug removal by plasmapheresis: an evidence-based review. *Pharmacotherapy*. 2007;27(11):1529-1549.

11. Mousavi S, Levcovich B, Mojtahedzadeh M. A systemic review on pharmacokinetic changes in critically ill patients: role of extracorporeal membrane oxygenation. *Drug*. 2011;19(5):312-321.

12. Watt K, Li JS, Benjamin DK, Cohen-Wolkowiez M. Pediatric cardiovascular drug dosing in critically ill children and extracorporeal membrane oxygenation. *J Cardiovasc Pharmacol*. 2011;58(2):126-132.

13. The impact of obesity on critical care resource use and outcomes. *Crit Care Nurs Clin N Am*. 2009;21:403-422.

14. Askari M. Frequency and nature of drug-drug interactions in the intensive care unit. *Pharmacoepidemiol Drug Saf*. 2013;22(4):430-437.

15. Smithburger PI, Seybert AL, Armahizer MJ, Kane-Gill SL. QT prolongation in the intensive care unit: commonly used medications and the impact of rug-drug interactions. *Expert Opin Drug Saf*. 2010;9(5):699-712.

16. Papadopoulos J, Smithburger PL. Common drug interactions leading to adverse drug events in the intensive care unit: management and pharmacokinetic considerations. *Crit Care Med*. 2010;38(suppl 6);S126-S135.

17. Kane-Gill SL, Jacobi J, Rothschild JM. Adverse drug events in intensive care units: risk factors, impact, and the role of team care. *Crit Care Med*. 2010;38(suppl 6);S83-S89.

18. Camire E, Moyen E, Stelfox HT. Medication errors in critical care: risk factors, prevention and disclosure. *CMAJ*. 2009;180(9):936-943.

19. Latif A, Rawat N, Pustavoitau A, Pronovost PJ, Pham JC. National study on the distribution, causes, and consequences of voluntarily reported medication errors between the ICU and non-ICU settings. *Crit Care Med*. 2013;41(2):389-398.

20. Patient Safety Primer, Medication Reconciliation. Agency for Healthcare Research and Quality PSNet. https://psnet.ahrq.gov/primers/primer/1/medication-reconciliation. Accessed March 2015.

Analgesia, Sedation, and Neuromuscular Blockade

Erik Stoltenberg, MD and Aaron M Joffe, DO, FCCM

KEY POINTS

1. Older paradigms of analgesia and sedation in the intensive care unit (ICU) have evolved to incorporate patient-centered outcomes, such as quality of life and functional status after ICU discharge in survivors.

2. Techniques for appropriate pain management must be individualized to each patient, starting with an appropriate assessment of its severity. Based upon their psychometric properties (reliability and validity), the Critical Care Pain Observation Tool and Behavioral Pain Scale are currently recommended for use in adults over other reported scales.

3. Systemic opioids (fentanyl, morphine, and hydromorphone) are traditionally the cornerstone of postoperative and critical care pain management. The ideal method of opioid administration will vary considerably with the clinical context and include opioids by mouth or parenteral administration either via intermittent intravenous or via patient-controlled infusion pumps.

4. Regional analgesia should be considered in certain ICU scenarios: (1) thoracic epidural analgesia in open abdominal aortic aneurysm surgery and (2) thoracic epidural analgesia in traumatic rib fractures, especially in the elderly.

5. Compared with propofol and dexmedetomidine, benzodiazepines (midazolam and lorazepam) have significantly longer context-sensitive half-times at both short- and long-duration infusions. Caution should be used when using benzodiazepines in the elderly, both because these agents can cause paradoxical agitation and because altered pharmacokinetic factors, such as increased volume of distribution and decreased elimination half-life often increase time to awakening.

6. The depth of sedation should be routinely monitored and quantified using a validated assessment tool. Sedative medications should be titrated to keep patients continuously lightly sedated unless a contraindication exists (severe acute respiratory distress syndrome [ARDS], refractory intracranial hypertension, status asthmaticus, or epilepticus) appears noninferior to standard therapy with daily sedative interruptions.

7. Neuromuscular blocking agents (cisatracurium) may still play an important role in management of critically ill patients in well-defined situations including to facilitate tracheal intubation, minimize systemic oxygen consumption in the setting of severe and refractory hypoxemia, improve outcomes in moderate and severe ARDS, treat shivering in patients undergoing targeted temperature management therapy, or treat refractory intracranial hypertension.

In addition to providing vital organ support and treatment of the underlying condition responsible for admission to the intensive care unit (ICU), the health care team must assure patient comfort and limitation of further stress on the patient. Failure in this regard may result in physiologic derangement and unwanted cognitive side effects. In order to attain these goals, a thorough knowledge of the pharmacokinetics (what the body does to the drug) and pharmacodynamics (what the drug does to the body) of a variety of medications is necessary; many of these agents are used exclusively in the ICU or by anesthesiologists in the operating room.

Over the past decade, an expanding body of basic science and clinical research has changed the way intensivists think about the treatment of pain and the management of sedation in the ICU. The use of newer drugs, such as dexmedetomidine as well as newfound indications for older drugs (eg, ketamine and lidocaine), have improved our ability to provide appropriate analgesia and sedation in the ICU. Recent trial results have provided high-quality evidence for use of neuromuscular blockade, despite its side-effect profile, in specific clinical circumstances (eg, severe acute respiratory distress syndrome [ARDS]). Older paradigms of analgesia and sedation in the ICU have evolved to incorporate patient-centered outcomes, such as quality of life and functional status after ICU discharge in survivors. This has been accomplished by aggressive assessment and treatment of patient discomfort and focusing on maintaining the ability of the patient to interact with caregivers and their environment through lighter sedation. The goals of this chapter are to underscore the necessity of analgesia and sedation in the ICU; describe pharmacologic properties of important analgesics, sedatives, and neuromuscular blocking drugs (NMBDs); and describe clinical strategies that improve patient outcomes.

ANALGESIA

Epidemiology of Pain in the ICU

Pain is common in the ICU, but is more difficult to assess than in acute care patients because of a common inability for critically ill patients to subjectively express pain. The inherent subjective nature of pain is well described by the International Association for the Study of Pain, which defines pain as an "unpleasant sensory and emotional experience associated with actual or potential tissue damage, or described in terms of such damage."[1] However, the inability to communicate pain does not mean it is not being experienced by the patient. In fact, it has been reported that the majority of critically ill patients (both medical and surgical) do experience pain[1,2]—which patients describe as a significant source of stress, if not *the most* significant source of stress during their ICU stay, even when asked 6 months later.[3]

In addition to an unpleasant experience, undertreated pain may have negative somatic and long-term consequences. The pain response increases plasma catecholamine levels, causing vasoconstriction, impaired tissue oxygenation, and increased myocardial oxygen demand. Pain can cause neuroendocrine activation resulting in a catabolism state, breakdown of muscle tissue, and impaired immune function, which can increase susceptibility to infection. In addition to acute anxiety and fear, acute pain is associated with chronic pain, posttraumatic stress disorder, and lower health-adjusted quality of life after ICU discharge.

Physiology and Anatomy of Pain

The pleiotropic effects of pain are due to the complicated processing of pain from stimulus to cerebral cortex. There are four described elements of pain processing:

1) *Transduction*. Noxious stimuli are converted to an action potential.

2) *Transmission*. Action potentials are conducted via afferent neurons.

3) *Modulation*. Afferent pain signals are altered by efferent neural inhibition via neurotransmitters, especially in the dorsal horn of the spinal cord or by augmentation via neuronal plasticity (eg, central sensitization).

4) *Perception*. Integration of afferent pain signals in the cerebral cortex.

Specific analgesic drugs and drug classes, which act at each of these four pathways, are presented in Table 16–1. Multimodal analgesic strategies are those

TABLE 16–1 Specific analgesic drug classes and how pain signals are modulated.

Transduction	Transmission	Modulation	Perception
NSAIDs	Local anesthetics:	Spinal opioids	Parenteral opioids
Antihistamines	Peripheral nerve blocks	α_2-Agonists	α_2-Agonists
Membrane stabilizing agents	Epidural analgesia	NMDA receptor antagonists (ketamine)	Inhaled anesthetics
Opioids		NSAIDs	
Bradykinin and serotonin antagonists		CCK antagonists	
Topical anesthetics		K+ channel openers	
		NO inhibitors	

NSAIDs, nonsteroid anti-inflammatory drugs; NMDA, *N*-methyl-D-aspartate; CCK, cholecystokinin.

considered to target more than one pathway simultaneously. Pain chronicization—a transition from acute pain to chronic pain—is a feared consequence of painful critical illness, and much research has addressed neuronal plasticity in this pathophysiology. Fortunately, therapeutic options have been developed to decrease the risk of this transition, and will be discussed further as follows (see Nonopioid Analgesics).

Strategies for Pain Management
Assessment of Pain

Techniques for appropriate pain management must be individualized to each patient, starting with an appropriate assessment of its severity. This assessment should be more detailed than a simple visual analog scale (VAS). If the patient is able to adequately communicate pain, the following should be assessed: site, onset and timing, quality, severity, exacerbating and relieving factors, response to analgesics, and assessment of pain with movement, breathing, and cough.

As mentioned earlier, critically ill patients may not be able to self-report, so behavioral assessments should be used. Based upon their psychometric properties (ie, reliability and validity), the Critical Care Pain Observation Tool and Behavioral Pain Scale are currently recommended for use in adults over other reported scales. It should also be noted that the use of vital signs as the sole surrogate for pain is strongly discouraged. Although more

validation testing in certain patient populations who may fail to exhibit typical pain behaviors (eg, neurologically injured) is warranted, implementation of behavioral scales is associated with lower resource consumption—such as days of mechanical ventilation—and ICU length of stay (LOS).[3]

Opioids—Systemic opioids are traditionally the cornerstone of postoperative and critical care pain management. As shown in Table 16–1, opioids' sites of action affect 3 of 4 pain-processing pathways. Opioids act as ligands at G protein-coupled opioid receptors, namely, the μ (mu), δ (delta), and κ (kappa) receptors. These receptors are located peripherally, in the spinal cord dorsal horn as well as at various locations in the brain. Opioid receptors are located on primary afferent neurons and inhibit release of nociceptive substances, decrease neurotransmitter release in the spinal cord, and activate descending inhibitory neurons. The μ-receptor is thought to be responsible for much of the peripheral analgesia caused by opioid agonists. There are a number of opioid receptor subtypes that have been discovered and are expressed on a variety of different cells, some unrelated to the central nervous system (CNS) and peripheral nervous system (such as on leukocytes and vascular tissue). This broad expression of opioid receptors is likely because there are number of endogenous opioids. The complicated interaction and broad expression of opioid receptors has led to opioids being implicated in such diverse pathophysiology as increased rates of

TABLE 16-2A Opioid analgesics (adapted from Joffe et al[6]).

Opioid	IV Dose (mg)	PO Dose (mg)	Time to Onset	Time to Peak Effect	Duration of Effect	Infusion Rate
Morphine	5	15	< 5 min (IV), 30 min (PO)	30 min (IV)	3-4 h	2-30 mg/h
Hydromorphone	0.7	4	< 5 min (IV), 30 min (PO)	30 min (IV)	4-5 h	0.5-3 mg/h
Fentanyl	0.05	N/A	Immediate	< 5 min	30-60 min	25-300+ mcg/h
Remifentanil	N/A	N/A	Immediate	< 3 min	< 10 min	0.05-0.3 mcg/kg/h
Oxycodone	N/A	10	20-30 min	< 1h	3-4 h	N/A
Methadone		(variable)	10-20 min (IV), 30 min (PO)	10-20 min (IV), 30-60 min (PO)	3-6 h (longer with repeat dosing)	N/A

cancer recurrence and modulation of inflammation. Intensivists should, therefore, have an appreciation not only for the acute adverse effects of opioids (respiratory depression and sedation), but also more subtle, long-term effects of opioid therapy. For more information regarding specific opioids, see Table 16-2a and 16-2b.

The ideal method of opioid administration will vary considerably with the clinical context and include opioids by mouth or parenteral administration either via intermittent intravenous or via patient-controlled infusion pumps (PCA, patient-controlled analgesia). For patients requiring mechanical ventilation, bolus or continuous infusion of opioids can treat both pain and ventilator-associated anxiety.

PCA—For awake, alert patients with moderate to severe pain—most commonly postoperative patients—PCA is an appropriate choice. Before initiating a PCA order, the patient must be able to

TABLE 16-2B Opioid analgesics (adapted from Joffe et al[6]).

Opioid	Elimination Half-Life	Metabolic Pathway	Active Metabolites	Notes
Morphine	1.5-2 h	Liver: glucuronidation	Morphine 6- and 3-glucuronide	Histamine release may be important from a cardiovascular and pulmonary perspective. Caution in renal failure.
Hydromorphone	2-3 h	Liver: glucuronidation	None	Accumulation with hepatic dysfunction.
Fentanyl	3-4 h	Liver: N-dealkylation CYP3A4/5	None	Significant increase in context-sensitive half-time with infusions >12 h.
Remifentanil	10-20 min	Plasma esterase hydrolysis	None	Abrupt discontinuation of analgesia.
Oxycodone	3-4 h	Liver: CYP2D6	Noroxycodone and oxymorphone	
Methadone	8-59 h	Liver: N-methylation CYP3A4, 2D6	none	NMDA receptor-antagonist, unpredictable pharmacokinetics (risk for accumulation). Multiple drug–drug interactions. Can prolong QTc.

NMDA, *N*-methyl-D-aspartate.

understand how to appropriately use the PCA apparatus. To determine the PCA prescription, the following parameters must be specified: (1) opioid, (2) incremental (or demand) dose, (3) lockout interval, (4) background infusion rate (if any), (5) 1- and 4-hour dose limits, and (6) bolus dose administration (for breakthrough pain). A reasonable starting prescription in an opioid-naïve patient would be morphine with an incremental dose of 1 to 2 mg, a lockout of 6 to 10 min, no continuous infusion rate, a 4-hour maximum dose of 30 mg, and a bolus dose of 2 to 4 mg every 5 min for 5 doses.

Although PCA has gained significant popularity for its ease of use, when compared to intermittent bolus opioids, outcome studies show mixed results. There is some evidence that patient satisfaction is improved, possibly because of the patients' increased sense of control over pain.[4] In general, there seems to be little change in analgesic efficacy, with patients reporting similar VAS pain scores with PCA and intermittent IV bolus analgesia. For patients that are taking chronic opioids when treated with a PCA, total dose of opioid was thrice higher than patients not taking opioids previously.[5] Interestingly, patients with opioid tolerance had increased rates of sedation compared with opioid-naïve patients, which suggests the therapeutic index for opioid-tolerant patients may be narrower than opioid-naïve patients.

Nonopioid Analgesics

Acetaminophen and Nonsteroidal Anti-inflammatory Drugs

Acetaminophen is a ubiquitous centrally acting cyclooxygenase inhibitor with a long history of use outside the ICU, but very little research has been applied to critically ill patients. Much of the research in non-ICU patients showed modest (but statistically significant) reductions in mild and moderate pain. The notable exception regards research studying the IV formulation of acetaminophen, which became available in the United States in early 2011. Pharmacokinetic studies showed increased plasma and cerebrospinal fluid levels of acetaminophen after IV administration compared with oral or rectal administration. Although studies results are mixed, decreased VAS pain scores, opioid side effects, and early extubation following major surgery have all been demonstrated with IV

acetaminophen.[6] Given the common scenario of treating patients in the ICU with moderate to severe pain and concern for impaired absorption from the gastrointestinal tract or when side effects of opioids are particularly harmful, IV acetaminophen may play an important role, but attention should be paid to the increased cost of the IV formulation.

Many acetaminophen and nonsteroidal anti-inflammatory drugs (NSAIDs) are used in acute postoperative pain and pain associated with critical illness; these drugs work primarily though cyclooxygenase and prostaglandin synthesis inhibition. All are generally effective in decreasing moderate and severe pain in equal-analgesic doses, but their utility is limited by their side effect profiles. NSAIDs can indirectly cause constriction of the afferent renal arterioles and inhibit platelet function (both in clinically significant ways), so their use is relatively contraindicated in patients at risk for renal injury and significant bleeding.

Ketamine

Ketamine, historically used as an IV dissociative general anesthetic with hypnotic and analgesic properties, has been the subject of much research in the treatment of acute pain. Ketamine acts primarily though N-methyl-D-aspartate (NMDA) receptor antagonism, which plays an important role in pain modulation and prevention of the transition of acute pain to chronic pain. Prevention of pain chronicization is a particularly useful characteristic of ketamine, especially in those patients that are opioid tolerant, as evidenced by a randomized controlled trial (RCT) of patients undergoing spine surgery that showed reductions in pain scores at 48 hours and 6 weeks after ketamine versus placebo infusion intraoperatively.[7] Ketamine also may reduce opioid-related side effects, including nausea and vomiting. Because analgesic adjunct doses of ketamine (0.05-0.4 mg/kg/h) are significantly smaller than anesthetic doses (1-3 mg/kg/h), psychomimetic reactions from ketamine are significantly less common at these doses, and only slightly more common than placebo. Other side effects of ketamine (sympathetic stimulation and salivation) are not usually observed with analgesic doses.

Lidocaine

Lidocaine is a well-known sodium channel antagonist local anesthetic that also has antiarrhythmic, general anesthetic, and analgesic (both antinociceptive and antineuropathic) properties. It has been studied extensively in the perioperative setting as an IV infusion, with mainly mixed results. Cytokine levels decrease after lidocaine infusion, suggesting that inflammation causing nociceptive pain may be decreased. Lidocaine has also been shown to modestly decrease VAS scores, opioid requirements, and duration of postoperative ileus postoperatively.[6] A recent study enrolling patients with complex spine surgery showed a significant improvement in subjective physical health months after surgery with lidocaine infusion versus placebo (a secondary outcome measure).[8] Lidocaine has significant cardiac toxicity and his cleared by the liver, and therefore, should be used with caution in critically ill patients with hepatic dysfunction.

Gabapentin and Pregabalin

As with lidocaine and ketamine, the calcium channel blockers gabapentin and pregabalin have been useful in treating neuropathic pain. There is considerable research demonstrating increased analgesic

efficacy of gabapentin as part of a regimen that also includes opioids in patients with chronic pain. There is also evidence for effectiveness in reducing opioid requirements and opioid-related side effects in patients with acute postoperative pain. Data supporting use of gabapentin and pregabalin in the ICU is limited, but a study evaluating patients with pain related to Guillain-Barre demonstrated decreased pain scores and opioid consumption in the ICU compared with placebo. In a meta-analysis of postoperative patients (not necessarily in the ICU) the number-needed-to-treat-to-benefit (NNT) to achieve 50% reduction in pain for gabapentin (NNT 11) is higher than that of naproxen (2.7), ibuprofen (2.5-2.7), or oral oxycodone 15 mg (4.6).[1,9-12] The most common side effect of gabapentin is sedation, but this effect is relatively rare— number needed to harm was 35.[7,13] Taken together, these data suggest gabapentin and pregabalin are safe and effective adjuncts in the treatment of pain in the ICU.

A summary of nonopioid analgesics is provided in Table 16–3.

TABLE 16–3 Nonopioid analgesics.

Drug	IV or PO Dose	Half-Life	Metabolism	Notes
Ketamine	IV: 0.1-0.5 mg/kg bolus, then 0.05-0.4 mg/kg/h	2-3 h	CYP450: 2B6, 2C9, 3A4, urinary excretion	Attenuates opioid-induced hyperalgesia, may decrease persistent postoperative pain
Acetaminophen	IV/PO: 650-1000 mg q4-6 h (<4000 mg per day)	2-4 h	CYP450: 1A2, 2E1, urinary excretion	Use caution in hepatic impairment
Ketorolac	IV: 15-30 mg q6 h up to 5 days	2.4-8.6 h	CYP450. Less than 50% metabolized. 90% excreted in the urine, 6% in bile/feces	Avoid use in patients with aspirin allergy. Caution with renal dysfunction, patients at high risk for bleeding, and in elderly patients.
Ibuprofen	PO: 400 mg q 4 h	1.8-2.5 h	CYP450: 2C9, urinary excretion	Same caution as with ketorolac, IV formulation also available.
Gabapentin	PO: 100 mg TID, can titrate up to maximum dose 1800 mg/day	5-7 h	Minimal. Excreted intact in urine.	May cause sedation. Abrupt discontinuation may cause seizures.
Pregabalin	PO: 50 mg TID, may increase to 100 mg TID	5.5-6.7 h	Minimal metabolism (2%). Renally excreted.	
Lidocaine	IV: 1.5 mg/kg loading dose, 1-2 mg/kg/h	1.5-2 h	Hepatic CYP450 (1A2 and 3A4), 10% unchanged in the urine	Active metabolites may accumulate in hepatic or renal failure

Adapted with permission from Joffe A, Hallman M, Gélinas C, et al: *Evaluation and Treatment of Pain in Critically Ill Adults. Semin Respir Crit Care Med.* 2013 Apr;34(2):189-200.

Regional Analgesia and Nonpharmacologic Techniques

Regional analgesia—targeted administration of local anesthetics and analgesics to certain anatomic locations—may have considerable advantage in the management in acute postsurgical and traumatic pain. Lower doses of medication can be delivered in a targeted fashion to decrease the risk of side effects of systemic delivery of medication, and analgesia is often significantly improved compared to IV opioids. In certain ICU scenarios regional analgesia should be considered: (1) thoracic epidural analgesia in open abdominal aortic aneurysm surgery and (2) thoracic epidural analgesia in traumatic rib fractures, especially in the elderly. Using thoracic epidural analgesia in both these scenarios is supported by clinical practice guidelines from the Society of Critical Care Medicine,[3] and have improved clinical outcomes—mainly by decreasing respiratory complications.

Although data supporting regional analgesia as a means to reduce morbidity is limited, in a broader array of scenarios regional analgesia decreases VAS pain scores, decreases systemic opioid requirements, decreases opioid side effects (postoperative ileus and urinary retention), and it may improve patient satisfaction.[6] In a recent meta-analysis, regional anesthesia decreased the incidence of persistent postoperative pain 6 months postsurgery after thoracotomy and breast surgery by two-thirds (odds ratio = 0.33, 95% confidence interval [CI]: 0.2-0.66).[14]

In addition to pharmacologic analgesic therapy, there are a variety of nonpharmacological analgesic techniques that may be helpful to patients. These techniques include music therapy, relaxation, therapy, family presence, distraction, massage, and deep breathing. Although empiric evidence of their efficacy is mixed and precludes high-level recommendations, their low cost and safety make them a valuable consideration within the context of a multimodal analgesia strategy in the ICU.

SEDATION

Sedation Pharmacology

Once determining that sedation is necessary for a critically ill patient, the selection of sedative should be based on the predicted length of required sedation, the reason sedation is necessary (eg, agitation, increased intracranial pressure, or alcohol withdrawal) as well as the pharmacodynamics and pharmacokinetics of the drug (Table 16–4). This strategy should involve patient factors, such as hepatic and renal dysfunction, hemodynamic stability, and inferred changes in drug volume of distribution (V_D).

Critical illness can significantly alter sedative pharmacokinetics in a variety of ways. Most sedatives undergo hepatic metabolism, many with a high hepatic extraction ratio, and therefore, decrease in hepatic blood flow that occur commonly in patients with shock, after abdominal surgery, or with increased intra-abdominal pressure can significant decrease drug clearance. Sedatives are often significantly bound to plasma proteins, and therefore, decrease in plasma protein concentration can increase the concentration of drug in the CNS. Perhaps the most important pharmacokinetic principle with respect to sedative infusions is the context-sensitive half-time, which is a calculated multicompartment model-derived graph of the time required for a 50% reduction in drug concentration at the effect site versus infusion duration for a constant-rate infusion. Some drugs (propofol) have a short half-time if the infusion is relatively short-lived (hours), but the half-time may increase significantly if the infusion is continued for days. The main difference in context-sensitive half-times between sedatives is the rate at which the half-times increase with infusion time. Compared with propofol and dexmedetomidine, benzodiazepines have significantly longer context-sensitive half-times at both short and long duration infusions—an important fact to consider when choosing a sedative.

Propofol

Propofol is a commonly used IV anesthetic induction agent that has excellent effectiveness in the ICU for varying levels of sedation. It works on a variety of CNS receptors to block neural transmission, including gamma-aminobutyric acid (GABA), and not only cause sedation, hypnosis, and amnesia, but also has anticonvulsant and antiemetic properties. It has no analgesic properties. It is highly lipid soluble and therefore crosses the blood-brain barrier and redistributes to vessel-poor compartments quickly,

TABLE 16-4 Sedating medications.

Drug	IV Loading Dose	Infusion Rate	Time to Onset	Elimination Half-Life*	Active Metabolites	Notes
Midazolam	0.01-0.05 mg/kg	0.02-0.1 mg/kg/h	2-5 min	1.7-2.6 h	Yes (α-hydroxy-midazolam and conjugated α-hydroxy-midazolam)	Active metabolites especially important in renal failure; adverse effects—hypotension, respiratory depression
Lorazepam	0.02-0.04 mg/kg	0.01-0.1 mg/kg/h	15-20 min	11-22 h	No	Propylene glycol (carrier solution) can cause acidosis; adverse effects—hypotension, respiratory depression
Propofol	0.1-0.3 mg/kg	5-50 μg/kg/min	1-3 min	4-23 h	No	Soybean oil and lecithin carrier (avoid with egg allergy) Adverse effects: hypotension, respiratory depression, propofol-related infusion syndrome, pain on injection, hypertriglyceridemia, pancreatitis
Dexmedetomidine	1 μg/kg over 10 min	0.2-0.7 μg/kg/**h**	5-10 min	1.8-3.1 h	No	Adverse effects—bradycardia and hypotension, hypertension with loading dose; difficult to achieve deep sedation

*For short-term infusions. Half-lives can be significantly longer after longer infusions given context-sensitive half-time (see text).
Adapted with permission from Barr J, Fraser GL, Puntillo K, et al: Clinical practice guidelines for the management of pain, agitation, and delirium in adult patients in the intensive care unit, *Crit Care Med* 2013 Jan;41(1):263-306.

resulting in a fast-onset, fast-recovery when given in bolus doses and short infusions. It is, therefore, useful in spontaneous awakening trial (SAT) protocols (see "the case of lighter sedation" later) and in patients that require frequent neurological assessments. Given the context-sensitive half time, delayed awakening after prolonged infusions still occurs.

The most common adverse effect with propofol is hypotension caused by arterial and venous vasodilation in addition to direct myocardial depression. The hemodynamic effects are dose dependent, and are less profound with infusion rates targeted to moderate sedation than with bolus induction doses. The carrier solution (lipid solution containing egg lecithin and soybean oil) is potentially allergenic and has been implicated in the rare propofol infusion syndrome—a potentially devastating severe metabolic acidosis associated with hypotension, hypertriglyceridemia, rhabdomyolysis, ECG changes, and multiorgan dysfunction.

Dexmedetomidine

Dexmedetomidine is a potent α_2-adrenergic receptor agonist with a potency several fold higher than clonidine (α_2: α_1 activity = 1,620:1 and 220:1 for dexmedetomidine and clonidine, respectively). The relative densities of these receptors in the CNS account for the sedative, sympatholytic, and analgesic properties of the drug. Dexmedetomidine usually results in a lightly sedated, interactive, cooperative patient. Because of minimal respiratory depression, it is particularly useful in facilitation of liberation from mechanical ventilation and extubation, as an infusion can be safely continued during a spontaneous breathing trial through extubation. Although it is only Food and

Drug Administration (FDA)-approved for ICU sedation at doses up to 0.7 µg/kg/h for 24 hours, there is empiric evidence to support safety at higher doses (1.5 µg/kg/h) for longer durations (up to 28 days).

Concerns with dexmedetomidine are primarily hemodynamic, as it can cause hypotension at rates similar to that of propofol. Loading doses of dexmedetomidine delivered too rapidly can cause severe life-threatening hypertension and bradycardia. Hypertension is likely caused by agonism of the peripheral α_1 or α_{2B} receptor subtype in the periphery resulting in vasoconstriction. Because of sympatholysis seen with continuous infusion, attempts to achieve deeper levels of sedation may be limited by bradycardia and hypotension. Lastly, it should be noted that the dosing of dexmedetomidine is unique among standard critical care infusions owing to its potency—µg/kg/*h* and not µg/kg/*min*.

Benzodiazepines

Benzodiazepines provide anxiolysis, sedation, hypnosis, and anticonvulsant effects through activation of $GABA_A$ receptors in the brain. The most common benzodiazepines used in the ICU are midazolam and lorazepam, because they can be used effectively both as intermittent boluses and as infusions. However, the context-sensitive half-times of benzodiazepines are significantly longer than that of propofol or dexmedetomidine, and therefore, benzodiazepines may cause residual sedation hours to days after infusions are stopped. Because of hepatic metabolism, benzodiazepine clearance may be reduced in patients with hepatic dysfunction or when coadministered with cytochrome P_{450} inhibitors.

Although midazolam has a shorter elimination half-life than other benzodiazepines, there is greater variability and potentially longer time to awakening with midazolam, likely secondary to accumulation of an active metabolite (conjugated and unconjugated α-hydroxymidazolam). This accumulation is especially important with concomitant renal dysfunction. Caution should be used in the elderly, both because benzodiazepines can cause paradoxical agitation and because altered pharmacokinetic factors such as increased volume of distribution and decreased elimination half-life often increase time to awakening.

Historical Context of Sedation for Mechanical Ventilation

Because the widespread implementation of positive pressure ventilation, use of sedatives to ensure patient-ventilator synchrony has been a mainstay of the practice of critical care. In the early days of mechanical ventilation, synchronized patient-ventilator interaction was very difficult or impossible, and was thought to require deep sedation to ensure optimal respiratory physiology. The patient experience of ICU care was considered to be inhumane and the provision of deep sedation was felt to provide comfort and amnesia to the experience. Treatment of ARDS involved normalizing respiratory physiology and gas exchange, which often involved deep sedation and comatose patients. In general, protocols to systematically assess the depth of sedation were not used. High infusion rates of intermediate-acting benzodiazepines and opioids were common, and patients were often unresponsive for days at a time. Although it is now apparent that this sedation paradigm directly contributes to worse outcomes, change in clinical practice has been slow. Even after a number of studies suggested that deep sedation may be harmful, 40% to 50% of patients were observed to be deeply sedated.[15] Finally, strategies of ICU sedation have changed considerably; the evidence for these changes will be discussed here. As follows, the reader will find summaries of seminal works that have greatly informed current sedation paradigms, but are strongly encouraged to perform a more in-depth reading of the primary source material.

The Case for Lighter Sedation

Observations from more than 20 years ago noted that mechanically ventilated ICU patients sedated by continuous infusion had significantly longer duration of mechanical ventilation, ICU, and hospital lengths of stay than those who were sedated by intermittent intravenous boluses.[16] Likely as a result, rates of documented ventilator-associated pneumonia (VAP) were also higher. In response, Kress and colleagues performed a trial comparing a protocol of daily sedative interruption (DSI, now referred to as SAT) to sedation as directed by the physician.[17] About 150 patients were enrolled in the study at a single center, and the duration of mechanical ventilation, hospital LOS and ICU LOS were the primary endpoints. Duration of mechanical ventilation and ICU LOS were both decreased in the DSI group by 2.4 days (4.9 days, 95% CI: 2.5-8.6 vs 7.3 days, 95% CI: 3.4-16.1, $P = 0.004$) and 3.5 days (6.4 days, 95% CI: 3.9-12 vs 9.9 days 95% CI: 4.7-17.9, $P = 0.02$), respectively. There was no difference in rates of self-extubation or mortality. The authors concluded, "daily interruption of sedation is a safe and practical approach to treating patients who are receiving mechanical ventilation."

Recognizing the results of this trial and appreciating the intertwined nature of mechanical ventilation and sedation, Girard et al published a multicenter study combining protocols of SATs (after a SAT safety screen) with spontaneous breathing trials (SBTs) and compared the protocol with usual care.[18] The so-called "Awakening and Breathing Controlled Trial" (ABC trial) enrolled 336 patients in 4 centers with a primary outcome of time breathing without assistance during the first 28 days after enrollment. Not only did the protocol patients have an increased mean/median number of ventilator-free days of 14.7/20 versus 11.6/8.1 ($P = 0.02$ for mean), but secondary outcomes of 1 year mortality were significantly decreased in the protocol patients (44% vs 58%, $P = 0.01$). It is important to note that the rate of self-extubation was higher in the intervention group, but the rate of reintubation was not different.

Both the Kress et al trial and ABC trial had a control group with usual care, which usually consisted of sedation that was not interrupted. Although the Kress et al trial targeted sedation depth in both groups to achieve a score of 3 or 4 on the Ramsay sedation scale (3—*responsive to commands* and 4—*asleep with a brisk response to a light glabellar tap or loud sound*), patients in the control arm were only "awake" (responsive to commands) on 9% of patient-days. In the ABC trial, both control and intervention group had sedation that was titrated to different institution-specific endpoints. However, the control group had an increased duration of coma during the study period (3 days, IQR 1-7 vs 2 days, IQR 0-4, $P = 0.002$). Given these data, both control group patients were comatose for a significantly greater amount of time than the intervention group patients. An important question remained—would

a SAT/SBT be superior to a strategy that simply titrated sedation to a lighter, noncomatose, level?

A multicenter trial attempted to answer this question by randomizing 430 patients to one of two protocols: (1) protocoled sedation targeting a RASS of –3 to 0 (sedated but opening eyes to voice [–3] to alert and calm [0]) plus daily sedation interruption or 2) protocoled sedation (RASS –3 to 0) alone without interruption of sedating medications.[19] The primary outcome measure was time to successful extubation. There was no difference in time to successful extubation in the groups. Interestingly, secondary outcome measures showed an increase in the dose of sedating medications and the self-perceived nurse workload in the *interruption* group. There were no differences in self-extubation or delirium.

Given that sedation interruptions and perhaps lighter sedation improves outcomes, some ICUs have adopted a practice of no sedation for mechanical ventilation. In one such mixed medical-surgical ICU in Denmark where the nurse: patient ratio is 1:1 and extra staff are available to "verbally comfort and reassure the patient," a RCT was performed to compare the intervention group (no sedatives) to the control group (sedation with goal Ramsay score 3-4 and daily sedation interruption).[20] Analgesia with as needed IV morphine was administered in both groups. The primary outcome measure was the number of days without mechanical ventilation in a 28-day period, with secondary endpoints being brain imaging (MRI or CT), accidental extubation, and VAP. The no sedation group had 4.2 days (95% CI: 0.3-8.1) more without mechanical ventilation in the 28 days after randomization (corrected for baseline variables). The secondary outcomes were not different between the groups. As assessed by the gold standard criteria, the DSM IV, more patients in the no sedation group experienced agitated delirium than in the control group (20% vs 7%, $P = 0.04$); these patients were treated with higher average doses of haloperidol, although the dose was small in both groups. This trial addressed the frequent appeals for a RCT comparing strategies of sedation versus no sedation and showed that, in carefully selected patients within a particular staffing model, sedation may contribute to prolonged mechanical ventilation and may be unnecessary. A large multicenter trial in

Denmark and Norway (NONSEDA Study Group) is attempting to confirm these findings by enrolling 700 patients using the same protocol.

From currently available data, it is now apparent that (1) depth of sedation should be routinely monitored and quantified using a validated assessment tool, (2) titrating medications to keep patients continuously lightly sedated unless a contraindication exists (severe ARDS, refractory intracranial hypertension, status asthmaticus, or epilepticus) appears noninferior to standard therapy with DSIs, (3) titration of sedation and SBTs should be closely coordinated in a multidisciplinary team that involves respiratory therapists, nurses, and the medical team.

NEUROMUSCULAR BLOCKADE

As the paradigm of ICU sedation continues to shift away from deep sedation and immobility, the list of accepted indications for use of NMBDs in mechanically ventilated patients has diminished considerably. However, NMBDs may still play an important role in management of critically ill patients in well-defined situations. These may include use to facilitate tracheal intubation, minimize systemic oxygen consumption in the setting of severe and refractory hypoxemia, improve outcomes in moderate and severe ARDS, treat shivering in patients undergoing targeted temperature management therapy, or treat refractory intracranial hypertension. Other "relative" indications, such as in protection of important vascular anastomoses (free flaps), taut wound closures and tracheal anastomoses, are dubious in nature and should be questioned. It is also important to note that administration of a NMBD excludes the use of subjective assessments of pain and sedation depth. In this setting, use of objective measures of brain function, such as bispectral index monitoring (BIS) or formal electroencephalography (EEG) to monitor depth of sedation should be considered.

NMBD Pharmacology

NMBDs have unique pharmacology that necessitates knowledge of the biochemistry of nicotinic acetylcholine receptors at the neuromuscular junction (NMJ). NMBDs are classified as either depolarizing or nondepolarizing based on their action at the postsynaptic nicotinic acetylcholine receptor.

Succinylcholine is the only depolarizing NMBD available in the United States—it depolarizes nicotinic acetylcholine receptors and either desensitizes the receptor, inactivates sodium channels and prevents propagation of an action potential, or a combination of both. It acts similarly to acetylcholine at the receptor, but binds significantly longer, and therefore, can cause significant hyperkalemia by the resulting efflux of potassium from muscle cells, especially in the setting of extrajunctional acetylcholine receptors. These extrajunctional receptors are expressed more frequently on muscle cells that have been denervated by neurologic disease (stroke, Guillian–Barre, spinal cord injury, severe burns, and prolonged immobility), and therefore, fatal hyperkalemia can result in these cases. Succinylcholine has other important adverse effects including hypertension, tachycardia, bradycardia, ventricular arrhythmias, and less commonly, increased intracranial pressure and malignant hyperthermia.

Nondepolarizing NMBDs are competitive inhibitors of acetylcholine, and inhibit depolarization at the NMJ. Therefore, the presence of extrajunctional acetylcholine receptors is not a concern with this class of NMBDs. These NMBDs are subclassified by duration of action (short, intermediate, and long) and chemical structure (benzylisoquinoline or aminosteroid). All commonly used nondepolarizing NMBDs are intermediate acting. A summary of the pharmacology of NMBDs commonly used in the ICU is presented in Table 16–5.

Neuromuscular Blockade for Facilitation of Mechanical Ventilation

NMBDs have been used to avoid patient-ventilator dyssynchrony in the setting of severe and/or refractory gas exchange abnormalities, particularly hypoxemia, but a number of case series suggest that they are associated with prolonged neuromuscular weakness. Although some of these cases were ascribed to decreased drug clearance in the setting of renal and hepatic dysfunction, some were thought to result from pathologic myopathy.[21] This myopathy has also been demonstrated in rats after prolonged exposure to vecuronium. Many of the cases with

TABLE 16-5 Neuromuscular blocking drugs.

Drug	Use	Category	Duration of Action	Intubating Dose (RSI) (mg/kg)	Notable Pharmacology
Succinylcholine	RSI	Depolarizing	Short	1-1.5	Contraindications: denervated muscle, hyperkalemia, increased intraocular pressure, susceptibility to MH
Rocuronium	RSI	Nondepolarizing, aminosteroid	Intermediate	1.2	Variable recovery with repeated dosing, renal and hepatic clearance
Vecuronium	Induction, infusion	Nondepolarizing, aminosteroid	Intermediate	N/A	Renal and hepatic clearance
Cisatracurium	Induction, infusion, ARDS	Nondepolarizing, benzylisoquinoline	Intermediate	N/A	Hoffman degradation

potential myopathy involved aminosteroid NMBDs (see Table 16–5). Although there have been case reports of prolonged weakness after infusion of benzylisoquinoline, it is thought to be less of a concern than with aminosteroid compounds. The most commonly used benzylisoquinoline NMBD, cisatracurium, also has the advantage of being degraded by Hoffman elimination and ester hydrolysis in the plasma, and is therefore, not dependent on renal or hepatic function for clearance.

Infusion with cisatracurium for 48 hours for treatment of moderately severe and severe ARDS was recently studied in a double-blind RCT in France in 340 patients.[22] The primary outcome measure (adjusted hazard ratio for death at 90 days) was 0.68 (95% CI: 0.48-0.98, $P = 0.04$) for the cisatracurium group, with no difference in ICU-acquired paresis. In both groups, a large number of patients were receiving corticosteroids for septic shock, which may contribute to ICU myopathy. A meta-analysis including this trial as well as two smaller studies also supports the notion that short-trem use of cisatracurium reduces hospital mortality and barotrauma without an increased risk of ICU-acquired weakness. Thus, current evidence supports the short-term use of cisatracurium for severe ARDS, and should be in any intensivist's armamentarium for treatment of severe ARDS. As mentioned previously, depth of sedation monitoring with BIS or EEG should be considered if

NMBDs are used. However, NMBD use to facilitate mechanical ventilation in patients without moderately severe to severe ARDS is strongly discouraged.

REFERENCES

1. Bonica JJ. The need of a taxonomy. *Pain.* 1979;6:247-248.
2. Erstad BL, Puntillo K, Gilbert HC, et al. Pain management principles in the critically ill. *Chest.* 2009;135:1075-1086.
3. Barr J, Fraser GL, Puntillo K, et al. Clinical practice guidelines for the management of pain, agitation, and delirium in adult patients in the intensive care unit. *Crit Care Med.* 2013;41:263-306.
4. Macintyre PE. Safety and efficacy of patient-controlled analgesia. *Br J Anaesth.* 2001;87:36-46.
5. Rapp SE, Ready LB, Nessly ML. Acute pain management in patients with prior opioid consumption: a case-controlled retrospective review. *Pain.* 1995;61:195-201.
6. Joffe A, Hallman M, Gélinas C, Herr D, Puntillo K. Evaluation and treatment of pain in critically ill adults. *Semin Respir Crit Care Med.* 2013;34:189-200.
7. Loftus RW, Yeager MP, Clark JA, et al. Intraoperative ketamine reduces perioperative opiate consumption in opiate-dependent patients with chronic back pain undergoing back surgery. *Anesthesiology.* 2010;113:639-646.

8. Farag E, Ghobrial M, Sessler DI, et al. Effect of perioperative intravenous lidocaine administration on pain, opioid consumption, and quality of life after complex spine surgery. *Anesthesiology.* 2013;119:932-940.

9. Straube S, Derry S, Moore RA, Wiffen PJ, McQuay HJ. Single dose oral gabapentin for established acute postoperative pain in adults. *Cochrane Database Syst Rev.* 2010:CD008183.

10. Derry C, Derry S, Moore RA, McQuay HJ. Single dose oral naproxen and naproxen sodium for acute postoperative pain in adults. *Cochrane Database Syst Rev.* 2009:CD004234.

11. Derry C, Derry S, Moore RA, McQuay HJ. Single dose oral ibuprofen for acute postoperative pain in adults. *Cochrane Database Syst Rev.* 2009:CD001548.

12. Gaskell H, Derry S, Moore RA, McQuay HJ. Single dose oral oxycodone and oxycodone plus paracetamol (acetaminophen) for acute postoperative pain in adults. *Cochrane Database Syst Rev.* 2009:CD002763.

13. Tiippana EM, Hamunen K, Kontinen VK, Kalso E. Do surgical patients benefit from perioperative gabapentin/pregabalin? A systematic review of efficacy and safety. *Anesth Analg.* 2007;104:1545-1556.

14. Andreae MH, Andreae DA. Regional anaesthesia to prevent chronic pain after surgery: a Cochrane systematic review and meta-analysis. *Br J Anaesth.* 2013;111:711-720.

15. Payen J-F, Chanques G, Mantz J, et al. Current practices in sedation and analgesia for mechanically ventilated critically ill patients: a prospective multicenter patient-based study. *Anesthesiology.* 2007;106:687-695—quiz 891-892.

16. Kollef MH, Levy NT, Ahrens TS, Schaiff R, Prentice D, Sherman G. The use of continuous i.v. sedation is associated with prolongation of mechanical ventilation. *Chest.* 1998;114:541-548.

17. Kress JP, Pohlman AS, O'Connor MF, Hall JB. Daily interruption of sedative infusions in critically ill patients undergoing mechanical ventilation. *N Engl J Med.* 2000;342:1471-1477.

18. Girard TD, Kress JP, Fuchs BD, et al. Efficacy and safety of a paired sedation and ventilator weaning protocol for mechanically ventilated patients in intensive care (Awakening and Breathing Controlled trial): a randomised controlled trial. *Lancet.* 2008;371:126-134.

19. Mehta S, Burry L, Cook D, et al. Daily sedation interruption in mechanically ventilated critically ill patients cared for with a sedation protocol: a randomized controlled trial. *JAMA.* 2012;308:1985-1992.

20. Strøm T, Martinussen T, Toft P. A protocol of no sedation for critically ill patients receiving mechanical ventilation: a randomised trial. *Lancet.* 2010;375:475-480.

21. Watling SM, Dasta JF. Prolonged paralysis in intensive care unit patients after the use of neuromuscular blocking agents: a review of the literature. *Critical Care Medicine.* 1994;22:884-893.

22. Papazian L, Forel J-M, Gacouin A, et al. Neuromuscular blockers in early acute respiratory distress syndrome. *N Engl J Med.* 2010;363:1107-1116

23. Alhazzani W, Alshahrani M, Jaeschke R, et al. Neuromuscular blocking agents in acute respiratory distress syndrome: a systematic review and meta-analysis of randomized controlled trials. *Crit Care.* 2013;17(2):R43. Review.

Airway Management/ The Difficult Airway

Venketraman Sahasranaman, MD; Tarang Safi, MD; Mabel Chung, MD and Jay Berger, MD/PhD

KEY POINTS

1. The anatomy of the airway starts at either the nasopharynx or oropharynx, and continues inferiorly past the larynx into the trachea.

2. In an emergency when the patient cannot be intubated or ventilated, the airway can be surgically entered via the cricothyroid membrane.

3. Difficult ventilation is a situation in which adequate ventilation cannot be achieved.

4. Identifying patients with potentially difficult airways is essential due to the increased incidence of complications associated with difficult intubations.

5. Preoxygenation increases the safety buffer time available during the peri-intubation period.

6. In order to insure amnesia, analgesia, and muscle relaxation during intubation, a balanced approach utilizing multiple medications are required.

7. Confirmation of correct placement of the endotracheal tube can be accomplished directly by visualizing the tube passing through the vocal cords or indirectly by auscultating bilateral breath sounds, observing rise and fall of the chest wall, and by capnography.

8. The risk of aspiration in patients with suspected or known full stomachs can be decreased by utilizing a rapid sequence intubation technique.

INTRODUCTION

The majority of patients admitted to the intensive care unit have varying degrees of respiratory failure. The intensivist must decide whether these patients would benefit from supplemental oxygen, noninvasive positive pressure ventilation (NIPPV), or endotracheal intubation with mechanical ventilation. The ability to secure an airway with a tracheal tube is therefore a necessity for all intensivists. As can be seen in Table 17–1, there are multiple indications for intubation. In this chapter, the airway management of critically ill patients will be discussed, including the preintubation assessment, the process of intubation, and weaning to extubation.

TABLE 17-1 Indications for endotracheal intubation in critical care.

Hypoxemic respiratory failure	ARDS Cardiogenic pulmonary edema Pneumonia Status asthmaticus
Hypercapnic respiratory failure	COPD exacerbation
Circulatory failure	Shock/cardiac arrest Anticipated hemodynamic instability
Neurologic emergency	Treatment of increased ICP
Airway protection	Airway edema Airway obstruction (secretions/blood) Altered mental status Surgical procedures

FUNCTIONAL ANATOMY OF THE AIRWAY

The upper airway (Figure 17–1) includes all of the structures externally from the nares and mouth to the vocal cords. The nasal passage way is highly vascular; disruption of Kiesselbach's plexus, located in the anterior aspect of the nasal septum, is the most common cause of epistaxis. The floor of the nasal passage way slopes very gently downward. As such, nasal airways, nasogastric tubes, and endotracheal tubes (ETTs) should be directed perpendicularly or with a slightly caudad tilt in the supine patient. The nasal passages open into the nasopharynx. Laceration of the mucosa and creation of a false passage during nasotracheal intubation most commonly occurs in the region of the eustachian tubes.

The larynx is continuous with the trachea inferiorly. The thyroid cartilage, cricoid cartilage, and the hyoid bone are the main components of the laryngeal skeleton. The epiglottis and arytenoids contribute to this structure. The piriform recesses, which reside on each side of the larynx, function to divert the food bolus laterally and away from the glottic opening. The thyroid cartilage supports most of the soft tissue structures in the larynx. The cricoid cartilage is the only complete ring in the larynx and serves to support the posterior laryngeal structures. During an emergent intubation in which the patient cannot be ventilated or intubated, the cricothyroid membrane, which is located between the thyroid

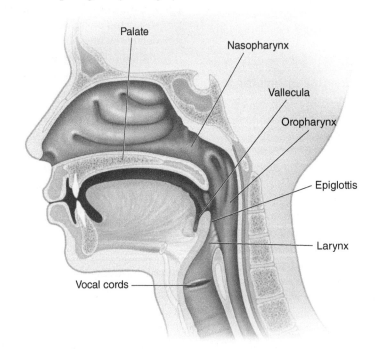

FIGURE 17-1 Normal anatomy of the upper airway.

and cricoid cartilages, may be surgically accessed to obtain an airway. The epiglottis projects posteriorly from the tongue and aids in airway protection during deglutition. Arytenoid cartilages articulate with the posterior parts of the cricoid cartilage. The muscles of voice control are attached to the two arytenoid cartilages, and the vocal cords project anteriorly from the arytenoid cartilages to the thyroid cartilage. Movement of the cricoarytenoid joints from the action of the laryngeal muscles causes a change in size of the opening between the vocal cords. The larynx is heavily innervated by the vagus nerve.[1]

The trachea starts at the inferior border of the cricoid cartilage and extends 12 to 15 cm distally to the carina, the first branch point marking the start of the right and left main bronchus. The anterior portion of the trachea is composed of structured cartilaginous rings, while the posterior portion is membranous. The average internal diameter is 9 to 15 mm. Typically, an ETT with an internal diameter of 7 to 7.5 and 7.5 to 8.5 mm is used for intubation of adult female and male patients, respectively. If bronchoscopy is anticipated, the minimum ETT size is 7.5 mm to allow passage of the bronchoscope. In some circumstances, such as pregnancy, a smaller ETT could be required due to swelling and edema of the airway.[2]

AIRWAY EVALUATION

Predictors of Difficult Ventilation

Bag valve mask (BVM) ventilation is a fundamental skill in airway management. Adequate ventilation is essential to provide oxygenation and removal of carbon dioxide. The American Society of Anesthesiologists (ASA) Task Force on Management of the Difficult Airway described difficult mask ventilation as a situation where a conventionally trained anesthesiologist experiences difficulty with ventilation due to one or more of the following problems: inadequate mask or supraglottic airway seal, excessive gas leak, or excessive resistance to the ingress or egress of gas.[3] Fortunately, the incidence of difficult ventilation in the operating room is relatively low at 1.4% to 5%, with the incidence of impossible ventilation at 0.006% to 0.15%.[4-6] Likely, the incidence of both situations is higher outside of the controlled setting of the operating room.

The predictors of difficult mask ventilation include factors that prevent proper seal of the mask and that obstruct air flow to and from the lungs. Identified risk factors for difficult ventilation are of age greater than 55, body mass index greater than 26, edentulous, history of snoring, and the presence of a beard.[7] The risk factors associated with impossible ventilation include a history of neck radiation, male sex, history of sleep apnea, Mallampati III or IV score, and the presence of a beard.[4]

Predictors of Difficult Tracheal Intubation

Tracheal intubation is the process by which the airway is secured by placing an ETT past the vocal cords and into the trachea to facilitate ventilation and oxygenation. The difficulty of intubation and the difficulty of ventilation should be considered as two distinct issues. In some instances, they may be concordant, such as with Ludwig's angina, where swelling of the posterior aspect of the tongue can interfere with both intubation and ventilation. However, in other situations, the ability to intubate and ventilate may be mutually exclusive. A male patient with a large bushy beard may be difficult to ventilate with a BVM, but easy to intubate. Conversely, a thin patient with severe rheumatoid arthritis affecting the cervical spine may be easy to ventilate, but extremely difficult to intubate due to limited range of motion of the neck.

The ASA has defined the difficult intubation as a situation involving "three or more laryngoscopic attempts to place the ETT into the trachea" or a situation where the attempts last for more than 10 minutes using conventional laryngoscopy.[8] In the operating room, the incidence of difficult intubation is around 5.8%. In the nonoperative emergent setting, the incidence varies from 10% to 24%.[8-10] Patients who were difficult to intubate had a 51% incidence of life threatening complications defined by death, cardiac arrest, cardiovascular collapse, shock, or hypoxic injury.[8] A difficult intubation increased the incidence of esophageal intubation, aspiration, pneumothorax, dental injury, and death in those requiring emergent intubation.[12] Identifying patients who may be a difficult intubation is essential. By anticipating a difficult intubation, advance airway equipment can be procured and additional personnel, such as a more experienced laryngoscopist or a surgeon experienced in emergent surgical airways can be assembled for help.

The probability of a difficult airway may be predicted by a thorough upper airway exam. "LEMON" is a mnemonic tool that can be used in assessing and predicting the difficult airway. The mnemonic stands for: L = look externally, E = evaluate using the 3-3-2 rule (a minimum of 3 finger breadths for the mouth opening measured as the distance between the top and bottom incisors, 3 finger breadths for the thyromental distance, and 2 finger breadths for the distance between the hyoid and thyroid), M = Mallampati score (Figure 17–2), O = obstruction (anything that might interfere with intubation, such as a foreign body), and N = neck mobility. Numerous prediction models and scores have been devised and validated for the prediction of a difficult intubation.[11] Most of these scores are comprised of a mix of patient characteristics, disease characteristics, and operator characteristics, and have been validated in the operating room. One multicenter study evaluated the usefulness of the MACOCHA score, which consists of several risk factors that can be easily evaluated in the intensive care unit (ICU), to predict difficult intubations (Table 17–2). A score of 0-3 is associated with a low incidence of difficult intubation, while a score of 10-12 is associated with a very

TABLE 17–2 Derivation of the MACOCHA score.

	Variables	Score
Patient-related factors	Mallampati score of 3 or 4	5
	Obstructive sleep apnea	2
	Reduced cervical spine mobility	1
	Limited mouth opening < 3 cm	1
Pathology-related factors	Coma	1
	Severe hypoxemia	1
Operator-related factors	Nonanesthesiologist	1
Total score		12

high incidence of difficult intubation.[8] An easy intubation is predicted by a large mouth opening, lack of top teeth, adequate thyromental distance, and adequate range of motion of the neck. A small mouth opening, protruding top teeth, short thyromental distance, and decreased range of motion of the neck conspire to prevent adequate alignment of the oral and pharyngeal axes during laryngoscopy and decreases the probability of visualization of the glottis (see "Visualizing the Larynx"). A normal airway

Mallampati classification

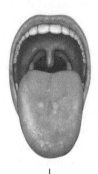 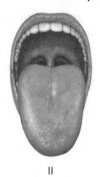 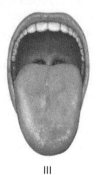 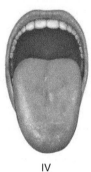

I   II   III   IV

FIGURE 17–2 Mallampati score.
Class 1: Complete visualization of the soft palate
Class 2: Complete visualization of the uvula
Class 3: Partial visualization of the uvula
Class 4: Soft palate cannot be visualized (*Reproduced with permission from Manabe Y, Iwamoto S, Miyawaki H, et al: Mallampati classification without tongue protrusion can predict difficult tracheal intubation more accurately than the traditional Mallampati classification*, Oral Science International *2014;11(2):52-55.*)

can subsequently become difficult due to processes, such as angioedema.

History of a prior difficult intubation appears to be strongly predictive of a difficult airway.[13] The association between obesity and difficult airway has been studied. Though a link between the two would be expected, Brodsky et al showed in their study that obesity as an isolated factor does not increase chance of difficult intubation.[14] Ultrasound has been proposed as a method of identifying patients with difficult airway. The recommended technique is to image and measure the soft tissue thickness over the vocal cords. These studies have had variable outcomes; at this time, ultrasound cannot be recommended as a definite tool to identify a difficult airway.[15,16]

PREOXYGENATION

A key step in securing an airway is to maintain adequate oxygenation in the peri-intubation period. Prolonged periods of hypoxia can result in significant hemodynamic instability and hypoxic brain injury. Preoxygenation increases the safety buffer time available during the process of intubation. The terms safe period of apnea and duration of apnea without desaturation (DAWD) have been defined as the peri-intubation period where the patient is apneic and still able to maintain saturation more than 90%.[17]

During an elective intubation for general anesthesia in the operating room, the patient is preoxygenated prior to induction of anesthesia. Following induction, the patient is ventilated until the optimal intubation conditions are achieved. For the period of time required for the actual intubation, the patient remains apneic; however, the aforementioned maneuvers typically prevent desaturation. Emergent intubations are not as slow and controlled as elective intubations. In addition, patients undergoing emergent intubations are typically presumed to be full stomachs, where the benefit of ventilation prior to intubation must be weighed against the risk of insufflating the stomach and increasing the risk of aspiration.

Oxygen can be delivered by a simple face mask providing a FiO_2 of 60% to 70% or a nonrebreather (NRB) face mask with a reservoir bag providing a FiO_2 of greater than 90%. A BVM may be required for preoxygenation prior to intubation; however, its use increases the risk of gastric insufflation and aspiration even if used properly.[18] Irrespective of how the oxygen is delivered, the flow rate must be high enough to wash out all nitrogen from the circuit prior to delivery to the patient. This is typically accomplished by using high flow rates of 10 to 15 L/min. In patients who have failed a trial of NIPPV, preoxygenation may be more efficient using the NIPPV circuit than switching to NRB mask. NIPPV may also be considered for preoxygenation in morbidly obese patients and in those patients that cannot support a SaO_2 of greater than 95% by other means of oxygen delivery.[19] Preoxygenation can be improved by having the patient in a sitting up or reverse Trendelenburg position so to increase their total respiratory system compliance and subsequently their functional residual capacity (FRC) and DAWD.[20] Failure of preoxygenation most commonly occurs due to low oxygen flow rates, inadequate preoxygenation time, air leak, and rebreathing.[17]

INTRAVENOUS ANESTHETICS

Intravenous anesthetics play an important role in airway management. They permit rapid induction of anesthesia and facilitate securing of the airway with an ETT with minimal stress to the patient. The ideal medication would provide amnesia, analgesia, and muscle relaxation. In addition, the ideal medication would have minimal effect on the patient's hemodynamics, preventing both hypotension due to sedation and analgesia and hypertension from the stimulation of laryngoscopy. Unfortunately, no one medication encompasses all of these properties. Instead, a balanced approach with a combination of medications is utilized. In elective intubations, the availability of time and the presence of an empty stomach allow for premedication; this is followed by an induction agent, which provides unconsciousness, and then a paralytic to help facilitate intubation. In emergent intubations, premedication may not be possible due to the lack of time or a contraindication to its use such as a full stomach. The hemodynamics of the patient may limit the amount of induction agent utilized; those who are particularly tenuous may not tolerate any induction agent. If paralysis is required, only fast acting paralytics will be of benefit

TABLE 17–3 Common endotracheal intubation medication indications and dosages.

Indication	Medication Class	IV dose	Onset
Premedications			
Midazolam	Benzodiazepine	1-2 mg	60-90 s
Fentanyl	Opioid	1-3 mcg/kg	< 30 s
Lidocaine	Local anesthetic	1.5 mg/kg	45-90 s
Induction agents			
Propofol	GABA receptor agonist	1-2 mg/kg	15-45 s
Etomidate	Imidazole	0.3 mg/kg	15-45 s
Ketamine	NMDA receptor antagonist	1-2 mg/kg	30 s
Paralytics			
Succinylcholine	Depolarizing	1.5 mg/kg	60-90 s
Rocuronium	Nondepolarizing	0.6-1.2 mg/kg	60-120 s

during an emergent intubation. Common medication dosages are listed in Table 17–3.

Premedication

Midazolam

Midazolam is a fast-acting intravenous benzodiazepine that allows for anxiolysis and anterograde amnesia by crossing the brain blood barrier and activating the gamma-butyric acid (GABA) receptor complex. The acidic nature of the intravenous preparation keeps midazolam in solution; however, exposure to the pH of the blood causes a structural change making midazolam extremely lipophilic. Hepatic metabolism results in formation of an active metabolite (1-hydroxymidazolam), which is renally cleared and may contribute to prolonged sedation with extended infusions. The short duration of action is aided by its lipophilicity, which promotes rapid redistribution from the brain to inactive tissue sites, such as fat and skeletal muscle. Side effects include respiratory depression, especially when given in conjunction with an opioid.[21]

Fentanyl

Fentanyl is a synthetic centrally acting opioid agonist that is structurally related to meperidine. It is approximately 100 times more potent than morphine. The rapid onset of action is attributed to its high lipophilicity, which also leads to its short duration of action by redistribution. Hepatic metabolism results in an inactive metabolite. Side effects include respiratory depression, especially when given with a benzodiazepine, and chest wall rigidity at high doses.[21]

Lidocaine

Lidocaine is an amide local anesthetic that is capable of suppressing the sympathetic response to intubation by inhibiting the gag and cough reflex. Blunting the sympathetic response can limit the rise in blood pressure due to manipulation of the airway during intubation and can prevent an increase in intracranial pressure (ICP) in a patient with known or presumed head injury.[21]

Induction Agents

Propofol

Propofol is an alkylphenol compound that is insoluble in water, and therefore, must be administered as an emulsion, containing soybean oil, glycerol, and egg lecithin. The rapid onset of action is attributed to its high lipophilicity. The short duration of action is primarily due to redistribution from highly perfused compartments such as the brain to the poorly perfused compartments such as skeletal muscle. In addition to its hypnotic properties, propofol is both a respiratory and cardiac depressant. Hypotension following induction is primarily due to vasodilation; however, the baroreceptor response is also attenuated preventing an adequate increase in heart rate to compensate for the decrease in blood pressure.[22] Hypotension following emergent intubation in critically ill patients is a strong predictor of mortality.[23] As a result, propofol should be used with caution if at all in hypotensive patients requiring emergent intubation. Hypotension should be immediately treated with a vasopressor, such as phenylephrine (IV dose 50-200 mcg).

Etomidate

Etomidate is a carboxylated imidazole that acts as a hypnotic by inhibiting the GABA receptors of the reticular activating system. Etomidate is poorly soluble in water and therefore is administered in a 35% propylene glycol solution. Onset of action is similar to propofol with a duration of effect of 3 to 12 minutes. Unlike propofol, etomidate has minimal effects on myocardial contractility and cardiac output resulting in less hypotension.[21] Myoclonus caused by a disinhibitory effect on the central nervous system is characteristic. A single induction dose of etomidate causes adrenal suppression by inhibiting the activity of 11-β-hydroxylase, an enzyme required for cortisol and aldosterone synthesis.[24,25] Subgroup analysis in the Corticus trial indicated a decreased responsiveness to cortisol and increased mortality in septic patients who received etomidate.[26] In summary, etomidate is an attractive induction agent in hemodynamically unstable patients; however, recent studies demonstrating adrenal suppression and increased mortality in septic patients has called its use into question.

Ketamine

Ketamine is a phencyclidine derivative that causes a dose-dependent state of "dissociative anesthesia" that produces both amnesia and analgesia. Ketamine interacts with a variety of receptors. Its amnestic property is likely due to the inhibition of the N-methyl-D-aspartate (NMDA) complex. Stimulation of the sympathetic nervous system causes an increase in heart rate, myocardial contractility, and mean arterial blood pressure, making it an ideal agent in hemodynamically compromised patients.[27] The mechanism of this indirect stimulatory effect is via inhibition of norepinephrine reuptake. The direct myocardial depressant effect of ketamine may be unmasked in patients with poor catecholamine stores such as the chronically or severely critically ill patient. Stimulation of the sympathetic nervous system will also result in increased cerebral oxygen consumption, cerebral blood flow, and ICP making it a poor choice in patients with suspected head injury and elevated ICP. Ketamine is infamous for its ability to cause hallucinations; however, the coadministration of a benzodiazepine can usually attenuate this effect.[28]

Paralytics

Succinylcholine

Succinylcholine (SCh) is a depolarizing neuromuscular blocking drug (NMBD) that has a fast onset time and short duration of action, making it ideal for rapid sequence induction (RSI). Structurally, SCh is related to acetylcholine (ACh) and functions by binding to the ACh receptor on the motor end plate, resulting in continued depolarization of the receptor and subsequent skeletal muscle paralysis. The onset of paralysis is typically preceded by fasciculations, which are caused by transient generalized skeletal muscle contractions. Normal muscle function does not return until the receptor is allowed to repolarize to its resting state, which occurs after metabolism of SCh by pseudocholinesterase. Pseudocholinesterase metabolizes SCh at such a high rate that only a small portion of the injected dose reaches the motor end plate. Altered pseudocholinesterase function can result in paralysis lasting 6 to 8 hours after a single dose. A relative decrease in pseudocholinesterase levels in patients with liver disease, kidney disease, anemia, pregnancy, and cocaine and amphetamine abuse has a minimal clinical effect and no alteration in the dose of SCh is required.[29]

Certain adverse effects may prevent SCh from being utilized as a RSI paralytic. On average, the serum potassium level increases 0.5 mEq/L following administration of SCh. If a paralytic is required in a patient with symptomatic hyperkalemia, an alternative medication should be considered; however, renal failure in a patient with normal potassium levels is not a contraindication to the administration of SCh.[30] Severe hyperkalemia causing cardiac arrest has been documented in patients with disorders of the nervous system (eg, spinal cord transection, amyotrophic lateral sclerosis, Guillain-Barre, etc) or extensive burn injury. Approximately 5 to 15 days after an acute injury, the body produces extrajunctional ACh receptors (ie, outside of the motor end plate) that may cause excessive potassium release following administration of SCh. This phenomenon puts patients at increased risk of hyperkalemic cardiac arrest. Nonetheless, it is generally considered safe to administer SCh within 24 hours of the acute injury nerve injury or stroke.[31] Hyperkalemia may also occur in patients with disorders of the musculoskeletal system, such as Duchenne muscular dystrophy, and SCh should be avoided in such patients. The increase in potassium level after SCh administration has been associated with length of stay in the ICU, which acts a surrogate marker for immobility. The risk of acute hyperkalemia ($\geq$ 6.5 mEq/L) is highly significant after 16 days in the ICU.[32]

The administration of SCh increases intraocular pressure (IOP) by 5 to 10 mm Hg for 2 to 6 minutes.[33] In patients with open eye injuries, the concern that increased IOP will cause extrusion of intraocular contents has limited the use of SCh in these patients. Nonetheless, there has never been a reported case of this occurring in the literature. The effect of SCh on ICP is controversial. Studies demonstrating a modest increase in ICP after SCh administration are inconsistent.[34] SCh may act as a trigger for malignant hyperthermia, a life-threatening complication resulting in high fever, muscle rigidity, rhabdomyolysis, and renal failure, which requires immediate treatment with dantrolene. Fortunately, the incidence of malignant hyperthermia after administration of SCh is rare. While SCh may cause a number of potential adverse side effects, no medication has been able to match its fast onset time and short duration to replace it as the paralytic of choice during an emergent intubation.

Rocuronium

Rocuronium is a nondepolarizing NMBD that causes paralysis by antagonism of the ACh receptor. The onset of action is slightly slower than that of SCh at a rapid sequence intubating dose of 1.2 mg/kg (normal intubating dose 0.6 mg/kg), but faster than the other nondepolarizing NMBDs. The major concern with rocuronium is its prolonged duration of action of approximately 1 hour. If a patient needs to be woken up due to difficulty in intubating or ventilating, they will not be able to regain spontaneous respiration for a prolonged period of time. Sugammadex is a specific reversal agent for rocuronium, preventing its interaction with the ACh receptor, and reverses paralysis within 3 minutes of administraion.[35] Sugammadex is currently not available in the United States due to Food and Drug Administration concerns regarding hypersensitivity and allergic reactions.

BAG MASK VENTILATION

The ability to oxygenate and ventilate a patient is an essential skill for anyone involved in airway management. While much emphasis is often placed on the ability to intubate, the morbidity associated with emergent intubations is in fact more closely correlated to the inability to ventilate and provide gas exchange. When an unanticipated difficult airway is encountered, the ability to ventilate the patient allows the practitioner to breathe for the patient, allowing time to obtain help in the form of additional equipment or personnel. Many practitioners insist that the ability to ventilate a patient be demonstrated prior to the administration of a paralytic. Paradoxically, ventilation can be made easier by paralysis due to loss of muscular tone. In addition, the administration of a paralytic can be crucial in increasing the intubatability of a patient assessed to be a moderately difficult airway. Ventilation with a BVM is relatively contraindicated during rapid sequence intubation (RSI) as it can lead to insufflation of the stomach and increase the risk of aspiration.

Facemasks for BVM are available in multiple sizes. Clear masks have the benefit of allowing visualization of vapor condensation, skin color, and signs of regurgitation. The last three digits of the practitioner's left hand are utilized to open the patient's airway with either a chin lift or jaw thrust. Compression of the soft tissue below the mandible should be avoided to prevent obstruction of the airway. The thumb and index finger are utilized to hold the facemask in place. The bag mask ventilation is a self-inflating resuscitation bag with reservoir connected to a high-flow oxygen source.[36]

Maintaining an open airway is one of the first steps required to insure adequate ventilation. Typically, a head tilt chin lift position is used. However, in patients with suspected spinal injuries, a jaw thrust maneuver is performed. Adjuncts, such as oral and nasal airways can be used to improve ventilation by moving an obstructing tongue from the posterior pharyngeal wall. In lightly anesthetized patients, an oral airway may trigger the gag reflex with a nasal airway being better tolerated. Nasal airways are relatively contraindicated in patient on blood thinners and antiplatelet therapy due to the risk of epistaxis and in any patient with a suspected basilar skull fracture. In a patient who is difficult to ventilate despite these maneuvers and adjuncts, a two person technique may be required. One person opens the airway using two hands and the other ventilates the patient.[37-39] The adequacy of BVM ventilation may be assessed by looking for chest rise and condensation on the mask due to the return of humidified exhaled air.

SUPRAGLOTTIC DEVICES

Laryngeal Mask Airways

The first supraglottic device was the laryngeal mask airway (LMA) classic invented by Dr Archie Brain in 1981. This first-generation LMA device was a reusable device, but a disposable version was soon developed. The LMA consists of a ventilation tube and an elliptical mask with a cuff, pilot tube, and balloon. Aperture bars in the mask prevent the epiglottis from obstructing ventilation. When inserted, the LMA moves along the hard then soft palate to the hypopharynx and then resides in the proximal esophagus, ultimately acting as a "mask" for the glottic opening with the distal tip located posterior to the cricoid cartilage and the proximal portion against the base of the tongue. Advantages of LMA use during general anesthesia include less irritation to the vocal cords and decreased hemodynamic changes upon awakening. Since its introduction, the use of LMAs has been extended from purely elective use to rescue situations where a patient cannot be ventilated. Other variations in the LMA have evolved and include the flexible LMA, ProSealLMA, LMA supreme, and LMA Excel. The Fastrach LMA was designed to aid with intubation as well as ventilation. Other supraglottic devices such as the Ambu laryngeal mask, Air Q intubating laryngeal airway, Cobra perilaryngeal airway, and others are based on the same concept as the LMA.

Combitube

The Combitube was developed for patients that could not be intubated by traditional laryngoscopy. The device is designed to be inserted blindly. Ventilation can be supported regardless of whether the distal portion of the tube is placed in the esophagus or trachea. The tube is a disposable, double lumen, and double cuffed device with separate pilot balloons for the proximal and distal cuffs. Approximately 95% of the time the distal tip of the tube enters the esophagus allowing the lungs to be ventilated via the proximal lumen. Less than 5% of the time, the tip of the tube enters the trachea and ventilation occurs via the distal lumen. Disadvantages of the Combitube include the inability to suction the trachea when the distal tip of the tube is in the esophagus. Contraindications for the use of the Combitube include patients with esophageal disease, suspected caustic substance ingestion, and history of esophageal varices.[41,42]

TRACHEAL INTUBATION

Tracheal intubation consists of three steps: visualization of the larynx, placement of the ETT proximal to the larynx, and then advancement of the ETT distal to the glottis.

Visualizing the Larynx

Laryngoscopic visualization of the vocal cords is made easier when the patient is placed in the sniffing position. The sniffing position, which is defined as flexion of the neck on the body and extension of the head on the neck, may be achieved by elevating the head in the extended position.[43] In the sniffing position, the oral and pharyngeal are placed into greater alignment facilitating direct visualization of the glottis (Figure 17–3). Modifications to patient positioning such as ramping up of the morbidly obese patient can lead to improved visualization as well (Figure 17–4).

Direct laryngoscopy involves using a laryngoscope, which contains a handle, blade and light source. Laryngoscope blades come in a variety of shapes and sizes. The most commonly used blades include the Macintosh and Miller blades. The curved Macintosh blade requires insertion in the right corner of the mouth, sweeping the tongue to the left with concurrent insertion, and placement of the tip into the vallecula, which indirectly elevates the epiglottis. The Miller, or straight blade, is inserted under and directly lifts the epiglottis. The choice of the blade is typically operator dependent; however, a straight blade that directly lifts the epiglottis may work better in certain situations such as with a patient with a large floppy epiglottis.[44]

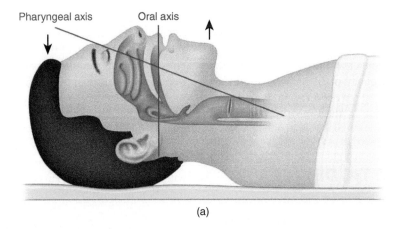

Pharyngeal axis   Oral axis

(a)

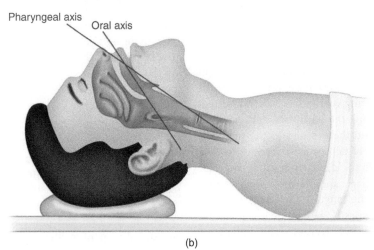

Pharyngeal axis
Oral axis

(b)

FIGURE 17–3   Sniffing position for endotracheal intubation—head extended and neck flexed.

Confirmation of Endotracheal Placement of ETT

The best confirmation of tracheal placement of an ETT is by directly visualizing the tube passing through the vocal cords. Other confirmatory measures may be utilized including bilateral breath sounds, rise and fall of the chest wall, and condensation on the ETT. Capnography detects the presence of carbon dioxide in the exhaled air and is another positive indicator of tracheal intubation. False negatives may occur in the presence of decreased pulmonary blood flow, such as with a cardiac arrest or with airflow limiting processes, such as bronchospasm.

Rapid Sequence Intubation

RSI is typically utilized in situations where the risk of aspiration is deemed to be high due to known or suspected full stomach, physiological conditions, such as late-term pregnancy, and pathological conditions, such as bowel obstruction or severe ascites. The goal of RSI is to decrease the risk of aspiration by minimizing the time between loss of airway reflexes, which occurs upon induction of anesthesia, and protection of the airway by ETT placement. RSI is accomplished by preoxygenation, application of cricoid pressure, administration of an induction agent and paralytic, and then intubation when the paralytic has come into full effect.

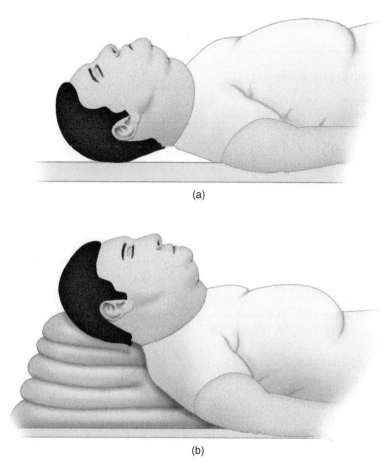

(a)

(b)

FIGURE 17–4 Improved Cormack–Lehane view with head elevation.

The goal of applying downward pressure at the cricoid cartilage is to prevent regurgitation of stomach contents by collapsing the esophagus between the trachea and spine. The utility of this maneuver has recently been called into question and may in the future be removed from the algorithm.[40] If cricoid pressure obscures the view of the vocal cords, it should be stopped immediately. In order to lessen the time between induction and intubation, only fast acting induction agent and paralytic should be chosen, and the two agents should be administered in rapid succession. As discussed in "Intravenous Anesthetics," SCh provides paralysis with a fast onset and short duration. When a contraindication to SCh exists, "double-dose" rocuronium (twice the usual intubating dose of 0.6 mg/kg, ie, 1.2 mg/kg)

provides an onset of paralysis nearly as fast as SCh, but with a prolonged duration of action. Ventilation with a BVM is typically avoided in order to prevent insufflation of the stomach with air, which increases the risk of aspiration. However, if the risk of injury from hypoxemia is judged to be greater than the risk of aspiration, manual ventilation should be utilized. In addition, injury from hypercarbia may also necessitate ventilation if the intubation is not immediately successful. Table 17–4 outlines various conditions where ventilation during RSI may need to be utilized. RSI is contraindicated in the setting of a known difficult airway. In this circumstance, an awake intubation will maintain protective airway reflexes while the airway is being secured.

TABLE 17–4 Indications for ventilation during RSI.

Severe hypoxemia
Conditions where worsening hypercapnia would be deleterious:
Cerebral edema or high ICP
Severe pulmonary hypertension
Right heart failure
Severe metabolic acidosis
Hyperkalemia

INDIRECT LARYNGOSCOPY

Videolaryngoscopy

Recently, a number of devices that utilize a high-resolution camera and a small monitor screen have been developed to improve the view and the success rate of intubation over that of direct laryngoscopy. All of these devices allow a view of the glottis without requiring alignment of the oral and pharyngeal axes (Figure 17–3). The learning curve of these newer devices appears to be less than that of direct laryngoscopy, especially for novice laryngoscopists.[45]

Fiberoptic Intubation

The gold standard for management of an anticipated difficult airway is fiberoptic intubation. Fiberoptic intubation via the nasopharynx as compared to the oropharynx is technically easier because of the gentler curve toward the glottis, but the high vascularity of the nasal passage increases the incidence of bleeding which can interfere with fiberoptic visualization of the glottis. Subsequently, an inherent weakness of the fiberoptic bronchoscope is that the camera view can easily be obscured by any contamination of the larynx. In addition, fiberoptic bronchoscopy is a modality that is not easily utilized during a truly emergent intubation.

In an awake, nonemergent fiberoptic intubation the patient is instructed about the procedure. The upper airway is topicalized with local anesthetic such as 4% lidocaine. Mild sedation typically aids in the patient tolerating the intubation; however, care must be taken not to over-sedate the patient, causing respiratory depression. Pretreatment with glycopyrrolate, a potent antisialagogue, decreases secretions. If time allows, a topical vasoconstrictor to the nares can help prevent bleeding. If the oral approach is attempted, a bite block will prevent damage to the fiberoptic scope. Once the tip of the scope is advanced past the glottis the ETT is advanced. Frequently, full advancement of the tip of the ETT into the trachea is hindered by the arytenoids. Gentle pressure and a clockwise rotation usually allow passage into the trachea. The correct position of the tube can then be confirmed by bronchoscopy.[46]

Other Techniques

In patients that are spontaneously breathing and cannot be intubated orally or have failed traditional oral intubation, a blind nasal intubation can be utilized to secure the airway. This procedure became popular during pre-hospital intubations when the use of paralytics was restricted. Typically the ETT is lubricated to aid in insertion. If time allows, the nasal passage way can be pretreated with a vasoconstricting agent to minimize bleeding. As the ETT is advanced from the nasopharynx to the oropharynx, the transmission of breath sounds via the tube are used to guide advancement through the glottis. Complications of this procedure include epistaxis, sinusitis, turbinate injury, perforation of the pharynx, and failed intubation and loss of airway. Contraindications include patients who are not spontaneously breathing and suspected basilar skull[47,48] or neck injuries.

LMAs have officially been identified as a rescue device during difficult intubation as well as ventilation. The Fastrach LMA was specifically designed to allow ventilation as well as to facilitate intubation. It differs from the classic LMA by having an anatomically curved rigid airway tube, integrated guiding handle, epiglottic elevating bar, and a guiding ramp. A Fastrach LMA with an internal diameter of 13 mm can accommodate up to an 8.0 sized lubricated ETT. The insertion technique of the Fastrach LMA is similar to other LMAs; however, after insertion, it is recommended to first rotate the Fastrach LMA in the sagittal plane to align with the glottis opening and then to move the metal handle vertically to prevent pressure on the arytenoids. Once in place with the cuff inflated, this LMA can be used to ventilate the patient. The ETT is inserted blindly through the LMA, although this method can be modified by use of the fiberoptic bronchoscope if blind insertion is not successful. After insertion, the LMA must be removed very carefully with an obturator holding the tube in place. In certain circumstances, the LMA may be deflated and left in place if risk of tube displacement is high. Complications of the intubating LMA include esophageal intubation, injury to the larynx and teeth, and aspiration of gastric contents.[49,50]

SURGICAL AIRWAY

If a patient cannot be intubated, one of two options remains. The first is to continue ventilating the patient and to allow them to awaken from sedation. The second option is to proceed to a surgical airway, which may need to be performed emergently if the patient cannot be ventilated or intubated. Cricothyroidotomy involves placement of an airway device by piercing the cricothyroid membrane. The prevalence of out-of-hospital cricothyroidotomy placement by emergency services varies based on location—from 4/100,000 overall up to 10% in a single center study.[51,52] The cricothyroid membrane is located above the cricoid cartilage and 1 to 1.5 fingerbreadths below the thyroid cartilage in the midline of the neck. The airway can be entered by a surgical technique that involves a vertical skin incision, blunt dissection down to the trachea, and a horizontal incision in the trachea. Otherwise, the airway is entered by a percutaneous puncture technique. Confirmation of successful placement of the airway into the trachea involves capnography, chest auscultation and a confirmatory chest x-ray. Generally, the cricothyroidotomy is converted to a regular tracheostomy within 24 hours, provided the patient has stabilized.[53]

ENDOTRACHEAL TUBE EXCHANGE

Despite proper care and suctioning, an ETT may need to be exchanged for a host of reasons such as development of a pilot balloon leak or tube obstruction. One method to exchange the tube is to induce anesthesia with or without a paralytic, remove the ETT, and reintubate the patient. Even if the patient was originally an easy intubation, it is not uncommon for airway swelling and edema to make a subsequent

reintubation more difficult. If the patient was originally a difficult airway or the patient's condition has changed and a difficult airway is now anticipated, a safer method of changing the ETT may involve using an airway exchange catheter (AEC). These catheters are thin, elongated, hollow tubes. Various sizes and diameters are available ranging from the Cook AEC (8-11 Fr) to the Aintree intubating catheter (14Fr). These tubes come with a ventilation port that can be used to oxygenate the patient if reintubation becomes prolonged.[54] The AEC is inserted through the ETT until resistance is encountered, usually between 30 and 40 cm. Some studies now suggest that the AEC should not be inserted more than 23 cm to prevent injury to the lung.[55] The indwelling ETT is removed and a new ETT is advanced over the catheter. Advancement of the tip of the ETT can be impeded by the posterior arytenoids. Gentle rotation in a clock-wise fashion will typically allow passage. The first pass success rate of reintubation over an AEC is 80% to 90%. If unable to pass the tube into the trachea, direct or indirect laryngoscopy may be required for reintubation. If that fails, a surgical airway may be emergently required. Complications associated with AEC use are direct injury to the airway by the catheter, which can on rare occasion lead to a pneumothorax.[56,57]

EXTUBATION

Critically ill patients are intubated for a host of different reasons that range from respiratory failure to prophylactically securing the airway. Objective clinical criteria and weaning predictors help predict if a patient is ready to be extubated. The required and optional criteria are listed in Table 17–5.[58] The rapid shallow breathing index (RSBI), which compares the respiratory frequency to the tidal volume (f/V_T), is the most commonly used and best studied weaning parameter. A RSBI of more than 105 breaths/min/L suggests that that patient is not ready to be liberated from the ventilator. As a patient is being weaned from support on the ventilator, they can be placed on a spontaneous breathing trial (SBT) either with a progressive pressure support wean with or without PEEP or with a T-piece trial. The rationale for performing a SBT with decreasing/minimal pressure support rather than no support with a T-piece trial is that the

TABLE 17–5 Required and optional criteria for tracheal extubation.

Required criteria
1. Cause of respiratory failure has improved
2. Adequate oxygenation
   $PaO_2/FiO_2 \geq 150$
   $SpO_2 > 90\%$ on minimal vent settings
3. Arterial pH > 7.35
4. Hemodynamic stability
5. Adequate ventilation with a spontaneous respiratory rate and adequate tidal volume
6. Airway protective reflexes: cough, gag, swallow
7. Awake and alert or easily arousable

Optional criteria
1. Hemoglobin ≥ 7-10 mg/dL
2. Afebrile with core temp ≤ 38°C

lumen of the ETT tends to become occluded over time, and this occlusion can cause resistance to air flow movement that is equivalent to a tube that is 1 to 4 times smaller.[59] Additional support for using low-level pressure support comes from a study that took patients who were failing a T-piece trial; after being placed immediately on pressure support ventilation at 7 cm of H_2O for 30 minutes, 21 of 31 patients were successfully weaned.[60] Common causes of weaning failures are volume overload, cardiac dysfunction, neuromuscular weakness, delirium, anxiety, metabolic disturbances, and adrenal insufficiency, in addition to unresolved lung pathology.

Following a successful weaning trial and the achievement of minimal ventilator settings, the patient's ability to protect their airway and the patency of the airway must be assessed. The ability to protect the airway is dependent on the strength of the patient's cough and inversely correlated with the required frequency of suctioning.[61] Airway patency is commonly demonstrated with a positive cuff leak prior to extubation. A cuff leak refers to airflow around the ETT after the cuff balloon has been deflated. The absence of a leak suggests that the space between the ETT and larynx is reduced, which places the patient at risk for postextubation stridor. A cuff leak can be quantitatively determined by placing the patient on full mechanical support and measuring the difference between the inspired tidal volume and the expired tidal volume. A difference less than 110 mL or 12% to 24% of delivered tidal volume suggests that airway patency is diminished.[62]

Once the decision to extubate the patient has been made, the patient should be seated in an upright position. The oral cavity and ETT should be suctioned. The patient is instructed to inhale deeply and during exhalation the cuff balloon is deflated and the tube is removed. Typically, an orogastric tube is removed simultaneously with the ETT. The oral cavity is again suctioned after extubation and the patient is placed on supplemental oxygen. If the concern for postextubation failure/complication is high and the airway was not easily secured, an AEC can be left in place after extubation. Early aggressive management with bronchodilators, suctioning, diuresis, and/or NIPPV can prevent reintubation. The caveat is that NIPPV applied after the onset of postextubation complications appears to be ineffective and may be harmful; therefore, patients who are anticipated to need NIPPV after extubation should be extubated directly to NIPPV.[63]

SPECIAL SITUATIONS
Severe Sepsis and Septic Shock

Indications for intubating patients with severe sepsis and septic shock are to reduce the work of breathing, treat hypoxic respiratory failure, and for airway protection in patients with septic encephalopathy. Typically, these patients must be assumed to be a full stomach with a RSI as the preferred method of intubation. Etomidate is typically used as the induction in hypotensive patients because it causes less vasodilation than propofol. However, a growing amount of evidence argues against its use in this patient population.[64-66]

Head Injury

Head-injured patients are specifically at a higher risk of worsening neurologic injury with increasing ICP. The act of laryngoscopy, intubation, and tracheal suctioning has been shown to induce a sympathetic response,[67] which causes an increase in the systemic blood pressure and subsequently can lead to increased ICP. A balance must be obtained between RSI, which tends to elicit more hemodynamic lability, but may protect against aspiration, versus a slower and gentler induction and intubation, which may mitigate increases in blood pressure and ICP, but may increase the risk of aspiration. A complicating aspect is the fact that hypotension is also detrimental to these patients. Increasing the amount of narcotic administered during induction can block the sympathetic response with minimal effect on systemic blood pressure; however, the sedative effects will last longer than with propofol or etomidate and may interfere with the postintubation neurological exam. Esmolol is an ultrashort acting β-blocker that can block sympathetic simulation; however, care must be taken to not cause hypotension.[67]

Lidocaine is a local anesthetic that can also block the sympathetic response to intubation for a few minutes with minimal effect on blood pressure and effect on the postintubation neurological exam.[68,69] Muscle relaxation with SCh might cause a temporary rise in ICP.[67] Pretreatment with a low dose of nondepolarizing neuromuscular blocker (NDMB) can attenuate this effect; however, this technique should not be used in an anticipated difficult airway because even that small dose of a NDMB can interfere with waking a patient up after a failed intubation attempt and may drive the algorithm toward a surgical airway. The patient with suspected head injury should be positioned with the head up at least 30° to facilitate venous drainage and mitigation of the ICP.[70] Hyperventilation should only be utilized for the emergent treatment of impending cerebral herniation.

Cervical Spine Injury

All trauma patients are assumed to have a cervical spine injury unless proven otherwise. Studies have estimated that all airway devices cause some degree of extension of the cervical spine. In a cadaver study, the McCoy laryngoscope caused maximal extension at the C_0-C_1 level and the Macintosh caused maximal extension at the C_2-C_3 level.[71] While the least amount of cervical manipulation occurs with fiberoptic intubation, direct laryngoscopy may still be required in the patient with an unstable C-spine if the airway must be secured emergently.[72] In order to secure the airway without causing movement at the C-spine, manual inline stabilization is mandatory. The C-collar is removed and an assistant stands at the head of the stretcher and gently, but firmly maintains the head in a neutral position during laryngoscopy.[73]

Cardiac Arrest

The latest ACLS guidelines from the American Medical Association emphasize good chest compressions and ventilation with end-tidal carbon dioxide ($EtCO_2$) monitoring over placement of an advanced airway.[74] If BVM ventilation is ineffective, then a supraglottic devices, such as a LMA can be placed fairly quickly. If endotracheal intubation is to be attempted, it is usually done without any sedation or paralysis. Tube placement is confirmed by visualizing the ETT going through the vocal cords as well as with auscultation and positive capnography. The positivity of capnography may be diminished due to decreased pulmonary blood flow.

SUMMARY

Airway management is the process by which differing degrees of respiratory failure are treated. Mild respiratory failure may only require supplemental oxygen via a nasal cannula, while more severe forms of respiratory failure may require endotracheal intubation. The intensivist must be facile with all aspects of securing the airway including assessment of the anticipated ease or difficulty of ventilation and intubation, the role of RSI, the anesthetic agents to be utilized, and the advanced equipment available for placing an ETT in the trachea. Of even greater importance is the ability to recognize the unanticipated difficult airway and to call for help immediately when difficulty with intubation or especially ventilation is encountered. In addition to securing the airway, the intensivist must be able to evaluate the safety and appropriateness of removing an ETT. These basic principles of airway management are frequently utilized in the intensive care and are foundational to the care of those critically ill with respiratory processes or in need of airway protection.

REFERENCES

1. Murphy MF. Applied functional anatomy of the airway. In: Walls RM, ed. *Manual of Emergency Airway Management*. Wolters Kluwer/Lippincott Williams & Wilkins Heath; 2012:36-44.
2. Richard SI. Anatomy and physiology of the upper airway. *Anesthesiol Clin North America*. 2002;20(4):733-745.

3. Apfelbaum JL, Hagberg CA, Caplan RA, et al. American Society of Anesthesiologists Task Force on Management of the Difficult Airway. Practice guidelines for management of the difficult airway: an updated report by the American Society of Anesthesiologists Task Force on Management of the Difficult Airway. *Anesthesiology*. 2013;118(2):251-270.

4. Kheterpal S, Han R, Tremper KK, et al. Incidence and predictors of difficult and impossible mask ventilation. *Anesthesiology*. 2006;105(5):885-891.

5. Langeron O, Masso E, Huraux C, et al. Prediction of difficult mask ventilation. *Anesthesiology*. 2000;92(5):1229-1236.

6. Kheterpal S, Martin L, Shanks AM, Tremper KK. Prediction and outcomes of impossible mask ventilation: a review of 50,000 anesthetics. *Anesthesiology*. 2009;110(4):891-897.

7. El-Orbany M, Woehlck HJ. Difficult mask ventilation. *Anesth Analg*. 2009;109(6):1870-1880.

8. De Jong A, Molinari N, Terzi N, et al. AzuRéa Network for the Frida-Réa Study Group. Early identification of patients at risk for difficult intubation in the intensive care unit: development and validation of the MACOCHA score in a multicenter cohort study. *Am J Respir Crit Care Med*. 2013;187(8):832-839.

9. Heuer JF, Barwing TA, Barwing J, et al. Incidence of difficult intubation in intensive care patients: analysis of contributing factors. *Anaesth Intensive Care*. 2012;40(1):120-127.

10. Martin LD, Mhyre JM, Shanks AM, et al. 3,423 emergency tracheal intubations at a university hospital: airway outcomes and complications. *Anesthesiology*. 2011;114(1):42-48.

11. Arné J, Descoins P, Fusciardi J, et al. Preoperative assessment for difficult intubation in general and ENT surgery: predictive value of a clinical multivariate risk index. *Br J Anaesth*. 1998;80(2):140-146.

12. Schwartz DE, Matthay MA, Cohen NH. Death and other complications of emergency airway management in critically ill adults. A prospective investigation of 297 tracheal intubations. *Anesthesiology*. 1995;82(2):367-376.

13. Lundstrøm LH, Møller AM, Rosenstock C, et al. Danish Anaesthesia Database. A documented previous difficult tracheal intubation as a prognostic test for a subsequent difficult tracheal intubation in adults. *Anaesthesia*. 2009;64(10):1081-1088.

14. Brodsky JB, Lemmens HJ, Brock-Utne JG, et al. Morbid obesity and tracheal intubation. *Anesth Analg*. 2002;94(3):732-736.

15. Komatsu R, Sengupta P, Wadhwa A, et al. Ultrasound quantification of anterior soft tissue thickness fails to predict difficult laryngoscopy in obese patients. *Anaesth Intensive Care*. 2007;35(1):32-37.

16. Ezri T, Gewürtz G, Sessler DI, et al. Prediction of difficult laryngoscopy in obese patients by ultrasound quantification of anterior neck soft tissue. *Anaesthesia*. 2003;58(11):1111-1114.

17. Tanoubi I, Drolet P, Donati F. Optimizing preoxygenation in adults. *Can J Anaesth*. 2009;56(6):449-466.

18. Weingart SD, Levitan RM. Preoxygenation and prevention of desaturation during emergency airway management. *Ann Emerg Med*. 2012;59(3): 165-175.e1.

19. Baillard C, Fosse JP, Sebbane M, et al. Noninvasive ventilation improves preoxygenation before intubation of hypoxic patients. *Am J Respir Crit Care Med*. 2006;174(2):171-177.

20. Dixon BJ, Dixon JB, Carden JR. Preoxygenation is more effective in the 25 degrees head-up position than in the supine position in severely obese patients: a randomized controlled study. *Anesthesiology*. 2005;102(6):1110-1115.

21. Stollings JL, Diedrich DA, Oyen LJ, et al. Rapid-sequence intubation: a review of the process and considerations when choosing medications. *Ann Pharmacother*. 2014;48(1):62-76.

22. Smith I, White PF, Nathanson M, et al. Propofol. An update on its clinical use. *Anesthesiology*. 1984;81(4):1005-1043.

23. Reich DL, Hossain S, Krol M, et al. Predictors of hypotension after induction of general anesthesia. *Anesthesia and Analgesia*. 2005;101(3):622-628.

24. Wagner RL, White PF, Kan PB, et al. Inhibition of adrenal steroidogenesis by the anesthetic etomidate. *New England J Med*. 1984;310(22):1415-1421.

25. Hildreth AN, Mejia VA, Maxwell RA, et al. Adrenal suppression following a single dose of etomidate for rapid sequence induction: a prospective randomized study. *J Trauma*. 2008;65(3):573-579.

26. Cuthbertson BH, Sprung CL, Annane D, et al. The effects of etomidate on adrenal responsiveness and mortality in patients with septic shock. *Inten Care Med*. 2009;35(11):1868-1876.

27. Morris C, Perris A, Klein J, et al. Anaesthesia in haemodynamically compromised emergency patients: does ketamine represent the best choice of induction agent? *Anaesthesia*. 2009;64(5):532-539.

28. White PF, Way WL, Trevor AJ. Ketamine – its pharmacology and therapeutic uses. *Anesthesiology*. 1982;56(2):119-136.

29. Vissers RJ. Tracheal intubation and mechanical ventilation. In: Tintinalli JE, Stapcynski JS, Cline DM, Ma OJ, Cydulka RK, eds. *Tintinalli's Emergency Medicine: A Comprehensive Study Guide.* 7th ed. New York, NY: McGraw-Hill; 2011:S4.

30. Thapa S, Brull SJ. Succinylcholine-induced hyperkalemia in patients with renal failure: an old question revisited. *Anesth Analg.* 2009;91:1237-1241.

31. Saunders DB. Lambert-Eaton myasthenic syndrome: clinical diagnosis, immune-medicated mechanisms and update on therapeutics. *Ann Neurol.* 1995;37:S63-S73.

32. Blaine A, Ract C, Leblanc PE, et al. The limits of succinylcholine for critically ill patients. *Anesth Analg.* 2012;155(4):873-879.

33. Cunningham AJ, Barr P. Intraocular pressure-physiology and implications for anesthetic management. *Canadian J Anaesth.* 1986;33:195-208.

34. Mace SA. Challenges and advances in intubation: rapid sequence intubation. *Emerg Med Clin North America.* 2008;26:10436-10468.

35. Schaller SJ, Fink H. Sugammadex as a reversal agent for neuromuscular block: an evidence-based review. *Core Evid.* 2013;8:57-67.

36. Na JU, Han SK, Choi PC, et al. Influence of face mask design on bag-valve-mask ventilation performance: a randomized simulation study. *Acta Anaesth Scand.* 2013;57:1192.

37. Hart D, Reardon R, Ward C, et al. Face mask ventilation: a comparison of three techniques. *J Emerg Med.* 2013;44(5):1028-1033.

38. Joffe AM, Hetzel S, Liew EC. A two-handed jaw-thrust technique is superior to the one-handed "EC-clamp" technique for mask ventilation in the apneic unconscious person. *Anesthesiology.* 2010;113(4):873-879.

39. Otten D, Liao MM, Wolken R, et al. Comparison of bag-valve-mask hand-sealing techniques in a simulated model. *Ann Emerg Med.* 2014;63(1):6-12.e3.

40. Ellis DY, Harris T, Zideman D. Cricoid pressure in emergency department rapid sequence tracheal intubations: a risk-benefit analysis. *Ann Emerg Med.* 2007;50(6):653-665.

41. Ostermayer DG, Gausche-Hill M. Supraglottic airways: the history and current state of prehospital airway adjuncts. *Prehosp Emerg Care.* 2014;18(1):106-115.

42. Hernandez MR, Klock PA, Jr, Ovassapian A. Evolution of the extraglottic airway: a review of its history, applications, and practical tips for success. *Anesth Analg.* 2012;114(2):349-368.

43. El-Orbany M, Woehlck H, Salem MR. Head and neck position for direct laryngoscopy. *Anesth Analg.* 2011;113(1):103-109.

44. Arino JJ, Velasco JM, Gasco C, et al. Straight blades improve visualization of the larynx while curved blades increase ease of intubation: a comparison of the Macintosh, Miller, McCoy, Belscope and Lee-Fiberview blades. *Can J Anaesth.* 2003;50(5):501-506.

45. Malik MA, Hassett P, Carney J, Higgins BD, et al. A comparison of the Glidescope, Pentax AWS, and Macintosh laryngoscopes when used by novice personnel: a manikin study. *Can J Anaesth.* 2009;56(11):802-811.

46. Koerner IP, Brambrink AM. Fiberoptic techniques. *Best Pract Res Clin Anaesthesiol.* 2005;19(4):611-621.

47. Hall CE, Shutt LE. Nasotracheal intubation for head and neck surgery. *Anaesthesia.* 2003;58(3):249-256.

48. Dong Y, Li G, Wu W, et al. Lightwand-guided nasotracheal intubation in oromaxillofacial surgery patients with anticipated difficult airways: a comparison with blind nasal intubation. *Int J Oral Maxillofac Surg.* 2013;42(9):1049-1053.

49. Gerstein NS, Braude DA, Hung O, Sanders JC, Murphy MF. The Fastrach Intubating Laryngeal Mask Airway: an overview and update. *Can J Anaesth.* 2010;57(6):588-601.

50. Niforopoulou P, Pantazopoulos I, Demestiha T, et al. Video-laryngoscopes in the adult airway management: a topical review of the literature. *Acta Anaesthesiol Scand.* 2010;54(9):1050-1061.

51. Wang HE, Mann NC, Mears G, Jacobson K, Yealy DM. Out-of-hospital airway management in the United States. *Resuscitation.* 2011;82(4):378-385.

52. Bair AE, Panacek EA, Wisner DH, et al. Cricothyrotomy: a 5-year experience at one institution. *J Emerg Med.* 2003;24(2):151-156.

53. Helm M, Gries A, Mutzbauer T. Surgical approach in difficult airway management. *Best Pract Res Clin Anaesthesiol.* 2005;19(4):623-640.

54. Duggan LV, Law JA, Murphy MF. Brief review: supplementing oxygen through an airway exchange catheter: efficacy, complications, and recommendations. *Can J Anaesth.* 2011;58(6):560-568.

55. deLima LG, Bishop MJ. Lung laceration after tracheal extubation over a plastic tube changer. *Anesth Analg.* 1991;73(3):350-351.

56. Rashid AM, Williams C, Noble J, et al. Pneumothorax, an underappreciated complication

with an airway exchange catheter. *J Thorac Dis.* 2012;4(6):659-662.

57. McLean S, Lanam CR, Benedict W, et al. Airway exchange failure and complications with the use of the cook airway exchange catheter®: a single center cohort study of 1177 patients. *Anesth Analg.* 2013;117(6):1325-1327.

58. MacIntyre NR, Cook DJ, Ely EW, Jr, et al. American College of Chest Physicians; American Association for Respiratory Care; American College of Critical Care Medicine. Evidence-based guidelines for weaning and discontinuing ventilatory support: a collective task force facilitated by the American College of Chest Physicians; the American Association for Respiratory Care; and the American College of Critical Care Medicine. *Chest.* 2001;120(6 Suppl):375S-395S.

59. Wilson AM, Gray DM, Thomas JG. Increases in endotracheal tube resistance are unpredictable relative to duration of intubation. *Chest.* 2009;136(4):1006-1013.

60. Ezingeard E, Diconne E, Guyomarc'h S, et al. Weaning from mechanical ventilation with pressure support in patients failing a T-tube trial of spontaneous breathing. *Intens Care Med.* 2006;32(1):165-169.

61. Khamiees M, Raju P, DeGirolamo A, et al. Predictors of extubation outcome in patients who have successfully completed a spontaneous breathing trial. *Chest.* 2001;120(4):1262-1270.

62. Jaber S, Chanques G, Matecki S, et al. Post-extubation stridor in intensive care unit patients. Risk factors evaluation and importance of the cuff-leak test. *Intens Care Med.* 2003;29(1):69-74.

63. Esteban A, Frutos-Vivar F, Ferguson ND, et al. Noninvasive positive-pressure ventilation for respiratory failure after extubation. *N Engl J Med.* 2004;350(24):2452-2460.

64. Sprung CL, Annane D, Keh D, et al. CORTICUS Study Group. Hydrocortisone therapy for patients with septic shock. *N Engl J Med.* 2008;358(2):111-124.

65. McPhee LC, Badawi O, Fraser GL, et al. Single-dose etomidate is not associated with increased mortality in ICU patients with sepsis: analysis of a large electronic ICU database. *Crit Care Med.* 2013;41(3):774-783.

66. Chan CM, Mitchell AL, Shorr AF. Etomidate is associated with mortality and adrenal insufficiency in sepsis: a meta-analysis. *Crit Care Med.* 2012;40(11):2945-2953.

67. Walls RM. Rapid-sequence intubation in head trauma. *Ann Emerg Med.* 1993 Jun;22(6):1008-1013.

68. Lev R, Rosen P. Prophylactic lidocaine use preintubation: a review. *J Emerg Med.* 1994;12(4):499-506.

69. Kuzak N, Harrison DW, Zed PJ. Use of lidocaine and fentanyl premedication for neuroprotective rapid sequence intubation in the emergency department. *CJEM.* 2006;8(2):80-84.

70. Ampel L, Hott KA, Sielaff GW, et al. An approach to airway management in the acutely head-injured patient. *J Emerg Med.* 1988;6(1):1-7.

71. Kiliç T, Goksu E, Durmaz D, et al. Upper cervical spine movement during intubation with different airway devices. *Am J Emerg Med.* 2013;31(7):1034-1036.

72. Crosby ET. Airway management in adults after cervical spine trauma. *Anesthesiology.* 2006;104(6):1293-1318.

73. Robitaille A. Airway management in the patient with potential cervical spine instability: continuing professional development. *Can J Anaesth.* 2011;58(12):1125-1139.

74. Field JM, Hazinski MF, Sayre MR, et al. Part 1: executive summary: 2010 American Heart Association Guidelines for Cardiopulmonary Resuscitation and Emergency Cardiovascular Care. *Circulation.* 2010;122(18 Suppl 3):S640-S656.

Ventilator Technology and Management

18

Adebayo Esan, MBBS, FCCP, FACP; Felix Khusid RRT- ACCS, NPS, RPFT, FAARC, FCCM, FCCP and Suhail Raoof, MD, FCCP, MACP, CCM

KEY POINTS

1 The goals of mechanical ventilation are to provide safe gas exchange, decrease the work of breathing, improve patient–ventilator interactions, minimize iatrogenic injury, and promote liberation from mechanical ventilation in a timely manner.

2 Mechanical ventilation is indicated in individuals who are unable to sustain normal gas exchange as a result of established or impending respiratory failure from hypoxemia, hypercapnia, or both; airway problems, and to provide support to individuals undergoing general anesthesia.

3 A ventilator mode can be classified by specifying the control variable, breath sequence, and targeting scheme.

4 Conventional modes of ventilatory support include continuous mandatory ventilation, assist-control ventilation, intermittent mandatory ventilation and synchronized intermittent mandatory ventilation, and pressure support ventilation.

5 Alternative modes of ventilatory support include dual control modes, such as volume-assured pressure support or pressure augmentation, volume support ventilation or variable pressure support ventilation, pressure-regulated volume control and auto mode ventilation.

6 Nonconventional modes of ventilatory support include airway pressure release ventilation, proportional assist ventilation, adaptive support ventilation, neurally adjusted ventilatory assist, and high-frequency ventilation including high-frequency oscillatory ventilation and high-frequency percussive ventilation.

7 Monitoring during mechanical ventilation includes measurement of peak and plateau pressures, intrinsic positive end-expiratory pressure, and work of breathing.

8 Prerequisites prior to conducting a spontaneous breathing trial include partial or complete recovery of conditions that resulted in respiratory failure; adequate oxygenation with low PEEP, that is, PaO_2/FIO_2 more than 200, PEEP ≤ 8 cm H_2O, and $FIO_2 \leq 0.5$; absence of severe acidosis (pH ≥ 7.25); hemodynamic stability with minimal or no vasopressor support; and presence of spontaneous inspiratory effort.

9 Noninvasive positive pressure ventilation avoids complications of invasive ventilation (eg, trauma, cardiac arrhythmias, hypotension, volutrauma, and ventilator-associated pneumonia).

10 Indications for noninvasive positive pressure ventilation include acute hypercapnic respiratory failure in the setting of chronic obstructive pulmonary disease (COPD) and cardiogenic pulmonary edema and immunosuppressed patients with pulmonary infiltrates, fever, and acute respiratory failure.

INTRODUCTION

Mechanical ventilation may prove to be life-saving in patients with acute respiratory failure. The use of mechanical ventilation has evolved over the years from the application of positive pressure with bellows to negative-pressure deployment with devices like the tank respirator to the modern day complex microprocessor-controlled positive-pressure devices. In recent years, new modes of mechanical ventilation have been devised for the purpose of enhancing patient comfort, minimizing patient-ventilator dyssynchrony, reducing lung injury, and automatically escalating or deescalating ventilatory support as needed. Regardless of these advancements, the goals of mechanical ventilation remain the same: providing safe gas exchange; decreasing the work of breathing (WOB); improving patient–ventilator interactions; minimizing iatrogenic injury; improving patient-ventilator interactions; and promoting liberation from mechanical ventilation in a timely manner.[1-3] Nonetheless, it must be pointed out that there is limited data to show that newer modes of mechanical ventilation reduce morbidity and mortality over conventional modes of mechanical ventilation.[4]

INDICATIONS OF MECHANICAL VENTILATION

Mechanical ventilation is indicated in individuals who are unable to sustain normal gas exchange as a result of established or impending respiratory failure from hypoxemia, hypercapnia, or both; airway problems, and for providing support to individuals undergoing general anesthesia. The decision to institute mechanical ventilation must take into account both the clinical circumstances (eg, clinical signs of respiratory distress, cardiovascular compromise, impaired mentation, reversibility of underlying disease, or presence of multiorgan dysfunction) as well as the patient's acceptance of the treatment. The indications for mechanical ventilation are shown in Table 18–1.[5,6]

TABLE 18–1 Indications for mechanical ventilation.

Type of Respiratory Failure	Area of Involvement	Common Examples
Ventilatory failure	Central nervous system (respiratory center)	Drug overdose, narcotics or sedatives, brain injury, brain tumors, hemorrhage, infection, edema, infarction, trauma, hypothyroidism
	Spinal cord	Cervical or thoracic spinal cord injury, poliomyelitis, amyotrophic lateral sclerosis
	Peripheral nervous system	Phrenic nerve paralysis, polyneuritis, Guillain-Barre syndrome
	Neuromuscular junction	Myasthenia gravis, Lambert-Eaton disease, botulism, tick paralysis, neuromuscular blocking drugs
	Respiratory muscles	Diaphragmatic weakness, endocrine disorders, electrolytes impairment, corticosteroid usage, critical care myopathy
	Bony rib cage	Flail chest
	Airway	Laryngeal edema, airways obstruction, acute bronchospasm, profuse airway secretions
Oxygenation failure	Diffusion abnormality	Pulmonary edema, interstitial lung disease
	Shunt	Atelectasis, pneumonia, acute respiratory distress syndrome
	Cellular extraction impairment	Sepsis, carbon monoxide poisoning
	Perioperative care	Routine anesthesia, major or prolonged surgery

BASIC PRINCIPLES OF VENTILATORY SUPPORT

Ventilators are either powered electrically or pneumatically. Ventilator classification schemes serve to elucidate the mechanism by which a ventilator operates.[7,8] Technological advancements with complex (microprocessor-controlled), dual modes with built-in intra- or interbreath feedback mechanisms have made the classification schemas more difficult. This is further compounded by the absence of a universally established classification system for ventilators.[1,9] To add to the increasing complexity, various ventilator manufacturers have given different proprietary names for the same mode of ventilation.[1,10,11] An example of this is adaptive pressure control (PC), which depending on the ventilator brand, is also called pressure-regulated volume control, adaptive pressure ventilation, autoflow, volume control plus, volume-targeted PC, and pressure-controlled volume guaranteed.[10] Table 18–2 outlines the essential components of a ventilator delivered breath, which gives a better understanding of how these modes work.

Equation of Motion

The equation of motion is a mathematical expression of the interaction between a patient and a ventilator, and elucidates the events within a breath.[9] It is expressed as

$$P = V_T/C_{RS} + \dot{V} \times R$$

where P is the sum of the pressures generated by the patient and the ventilator, V_T is the tidal volume that the patient receives (ventilator driven) or generates (intrinsic inspiratory effort), C_{RS} is the compliance of the respiratory system, $\dot{V}$ is the flow, and R is the resistance of the respiratory system (airway tubing, endotracheal tube, and airways). Thus, V_T/C_{RS} is the elastic load and $\dot{V} \times R$ the resistive load that has to be overcome to deliver volume and flow to the patient.

Control Variables

A ventilator regulates inspiration of a mechanical breath by manipulating control variables such as pressure, volume, flow, or time as feedback signals.[7-9,11] The control variable is based on the equation of motion expressed earlier. During inspiration, a ventilator controls one variable at a time; that is, pressure, volume, or flow. The control variable remains constant as the ventilatory load imposed by the patient's respiratory system (ie, lung compliance and airway resistance) changes.[7-9,11] In some ventilators, neither pressure, nor volume nor flow can be kept constant with changes in the ventilatory load resulting from the patient's lung mechanics. In such ventilators, only inspiratory and expiratory times are the variables being controlled, such as is seen in high-frequency ventilation.[8,9,11]

Phase Variables

Further description of a mechanical breath can be made by identifying what triggers (initiates), limits (sustains) and cycles (ends) a breath. These aforementioned events that initiate different phases of the ventilatory cycle (Figure 18–1) are referred to as phase variables.[8,11] The *trigger variable* initiates inspiration

TABLE 18–2 Terminology used to define components of a ventilator-delivered breath.

Variable	Definitions	Parameter Used
Control	The parameter that the ventilator controls	Pressure, volume, flow, or time
Phase	Trigger—initiates inspiration	Pressure, flow, or time
	Limit—maximum level that can be reached and sustained during inspiration	Pressure, volume, or flow
	Cycle—terminates inspiration	Pressure, volume, flow, or time
	Baseline—sustains functional residual capacity	Pressure
Conditional	Determines whether change in breath pattern is needed	Pressure, volume, flow, minute ventilation, or time

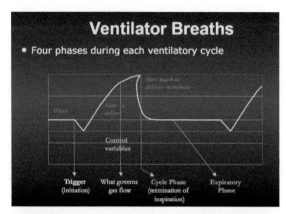

FIGURE 18–1 Different components of a ventilatory breath cycle.

and could either be machine-triggered (usually timed) or patient-triggered (usually pressure or flow).[8,11] Flow triggering has become standard in most modern ventilators and has been shown to reduce the inspiratory WOB in comparison to pressure triggering as well as enhance the patient-ventilator synchrony.[12,13] The *limit variable* is the maximum preset value of pressure, volume, or flow that can be reached and sustained before inspiration ends. The preset limit value being reached does not end the inspiratory phase.[7,8,11] The *cycle variable* is the preset value of pressure, volume, flow, or time that ends inspiration. In pressure, volume, or flow cycling, a ventilator delivers inspiratory flow until a preset pressure, volume, or flow is attained, after which inspiration ends and exhalation begins. With time cycling, inspiration ends once a preset inspiratory period has elapsed.[7,8,11] Exhalation begins once inspiration ends. The *baseline variable* is the parameter that is controlled during exhalation. Even though pressure, volume, or flow can function as baseline variables, modern ventilators utilize pressure because it is the most practical to implement. This is done by employing the positive end-expiratory pressure (PEEP) setting such that if baseline pressure is to be equal to or exceed atmospheric pressure, PEEP is set at 0 or a positive value, respectively.[7,8,11]

CONDITIONAL VARIABLES

A ventilator creates specific patterns of control from each breath and decides at preset intervals if that

pattern of breathing should be altered. An example of this is when a ventilator switches from a patient-triggered (spontaneous) breath to a machined-triggered (mandatory) breath in synchronized intermittent mandatory ventilation (SIMV), delivers sighs at regular intervals, or switches to mandatory minute ventilation mode.[8,11]

BREATH SEQUENCE

The breath sequence describes the manner in which spontaneous and mandatory breaths are delivered by a ventilator. A spontaneous breath is one in which inspiration is both triggered (initiated) and cycled (terminated) by the patient, while a mandatory breath is one in which inspiration is either triggered and/or cycled by the ventilator.[7,8,11] A mandatory breath is described as assisted if it is patient triggered.[11] In addition, a spontaneous breath is described as supported if the airway pressure during inspiration rises above baseline pressure. This is commonly seen in the pressure support mode where airway pressure rises to a preselected level above PEEP.[7,11] Alternatively, a spontaneous breath is described as unassisted if the airway pressure during inspiration does not rise above baseline as is seen in the continuous positive airway pressure (CPAP) setting.[7]

Three breath sequences have been described in the literature and they include the following:[7,10,11,14]

a. *Continuous spontaneous ventilation* in which all breaths are spontaneous.

b. *Intermittent mandatory ventilation (IMV)* in which mandatory (machine-triggered) breaths are delivered with spontaneous breaths permitted in between. If the mandatory breath is patient triggered, it is referred to as SIMV.

c. *Continuous mandatory ventilation (CMV)* in which all breaths are mandatory, but may be patient or machine triggered. No spontaneous breaths are permitted between mandatory breaths. This is also referred to as controlled mechanical ventilation.

Targeting Schemes

Targeting schemes are the feedback control system by which a ventilator delivers a specific ventilatory pattern, that is, it represents the relationship between operator inputs and ventilator outputs to obtain a specific ventilator pattern.[1,15] Output (eg, airway pressure generated) is used as a feedback signal that is compared to operator-set input (eg, preset inspiratory pressure) to change the characteristics of the delivered breath.[7] It comprises the ventilator settings and programming that determine the ventilator's response to the patient's lung compliance, airway resistance, and respiratory effort.[10]

There are two types of control systems, namely, *open-loop control* and *closed-loop control*.[16] The open-loop control scheme is the simplest type of control. It is unable to correct for variations such as changes in the patient's ventilatory drive, respiratory system mechanics, or leaks. The information available from the ventilator is not utilized to the advantage of the patient in a meaningful way.[16] The closed-loop control is used in all modern ventilators. It is also called the feedback control. The closed-loop control is used to keep pressure and flow waveforms consistent in the midst of altering patient/system conditions.[7,16]

There are, at present, seven fundamental targeting schemes used as feedback control loops (ie, closed-loop systems) to create a varying number of ventilator modes.[1,7,15] With *set-point targeting*, specific target parameters are set such as V_T or inspiratory flow in volume-control (VC) mode or inspiratory pressure in PC, and the ventilator attempts to deliver them. The goal is to perpetuate a constant output to match a constant input. Set-point targeting is the least complex of the targeting schemes and assumes constant respiratory system mechanics. This is seen in assist-control (AC) modes.[1,7,15,16] *Dual targeting* occurs when a ventilator can automatically switch between VC and PC (or vice versa) during a single inspiration based on attaining certain preset parameters such as V_T. It can adapt to changing patient conditions and guarantees either a preset V_T or peak inspiratory pressure (PIP).[1] This is seen in volume-assured pressure support (VAPS).[1,7,15,16] *Servo control* is a targeting scheme in which the output of the ventilator, such as pressure, volume or flow, automatically follows a varying input. The ventilator support is proportional to the patient's inspiratory effort. Examples include proportional assist ventilation (PAV), automatic tube compensation, and neurally

adjusted ventilatory assist (NAVA).[1,7,15,16] *Biovariable targeting* occurs when a ventilator automatically modifies the inspiratory pressure or V_T in a random manner thereby simulating the biologically variable ventilation seen during normal breathing.[1] This is seen with variable pressure support.[1] *Adaptive targeting* occurs when a ventilator automatically sets one or more targets between breaths to adjust to varying patient conditions.[1,7,15] This automatic adjustment of one set point is to perpetuate a different operator-selected set point, such as adjusting the pressure limit of a breath so as to meet an operator-set V_T target over several breaths.[16] This is seen with pressure-regulated volume control (PRVC).[1,7,15,16] *Optimal targeting* is a form of adaptive targeting schemes that enables a ventilator to set both volume and pressure set points, thereby enabling adjustment to varying patient conditions.[7,15,16] It occurs when a ventilator automatically modifies the targets of the ventilatory pattern to either minimize or maximize some overall performance characteristic. Once an operator has set a target percentage minute volume, it enables the ventilator to make all subsequent adjustments in response to respiratory-system mechanics and patient effort.[15,16] An example of this is the adaptive support ventilation (ASV).[1,7,15] *Intelligent targeting* is another form of adaptive targeting schemes that uses artificial-intelligence techniques, such as rule-based expert systems, fuzzy logic, and artificial neural networks, and is also able to adjust to varying patient conditions.[1,7] There are limited randomized control trials evaluating the use of advanced targeting schemes, and superiority has not been clearly demonstrated. A myriad of commercially available ventilator mode names exist, majority of which are not particularly different modes. Understanding this is essential in appropriately utilizing the right ventilator mode for optimal patient care that would promote safety, comfort, and eventually liberation.

CLASSIFICATION OF MECHANICAL VENTILATION
Modes of Mechanical Ventilation

A ventilator mode describes the manner in which a breath is delivered to a patient in order to meet physiological demands.[7] It has been proposed that a ventilator mode can be classified by specifying the control variable, breath sequence, and targeting scheme.[7,10] It incorporates variables that control, initiate, sustain, and terminate the breath (phase variables) as well as determine if a change in breath pattern is needed (conditional variables). The emergence of a new generation of microprocessor-based ventilators has resulted in advancements in triggering, monitoring, and safety at the cost of added complexity and expense.[4,17,18] None of these newer modes of have been shown to reduce morbidity or mortality.[4,17,18] Following are some of the common conventional and alternative modes of ventilatory support utilized in clinical practice (Table 18–3).

Conventional Modes of Ventilatory Support

Continuous Mandatory Ventilation

In the CMV mode, all breaths are mandatory and delivered by the ventilator at a predetermined frequency and inspiratory time (Figure 18–2). The breaths could either be volume or pressure targeted (or controlled), triggered by the ventilator (ie, time triggered), pressure, volume or flow limited, and time, flow, pressure, or volume cycled by the ventilator.[19,20] Patients receiving this mode usually require deep sedation or paralysis, or do not have ventilatory drive.[19] Most modern ventilators do not prevent patients from triggering a breath; therefore, this mode has been replaced by the A/C mode.[19] In some ventilator brands, CMV and A/C modes are the same.

Assist-Control Ventilation

In assist-control ventilation (ACV) mode, breaths are mandatory and delivered by the ventilator at a predetermined minimum frequency. The breaths could be volume or pressure targeted (A/C VC or A/C PC), and are either ventilator, that is, time triggered based on a set rate, or patient triggered (using flow or pressure) depending on patient effort and set sensitivity (Figure 18–3). In this mode, assisted breaths (mandatory breaths that are patient triggered) can be delivered at the predetermined pressure or volume in between the ventilator triggered breaths. Similar to CMV, the breaths are also pressure, volume or flow limited and flow, volume, pressure, or time cycled by the ventilator.[20] ACV is the preferred mode in most clinical settings, but common problems encountered include respiratory

alkalosis in patients with a high respiratory drive, increased WOB by patients if the sensitivity and flow rates are inadequately set and dyssynchrony in awake patients.[19,21]

Intermittent Mandatory Ventilation and Synchronized Intermittent Mandatory Ventilation

In the IMV mode, breaths are mandatory and delivered by the ventilator at a set frequency, and are either volume or pressure targeted. Furthermore, the mandatory breaths are triggered and cycled by the ventilator. In between the mandatory breaths delivered, a patient can breathe spontaneously at a frequency and V_T determined by the patient, irrespective of the set ventilator frequency. These spontaneous breaths are patient triggered and patient cycled, and may be augmented by pressure support.[22-26] Nevertheless, the lack of coordination between spontaneous and mandatory breaths can result in breath stacking if a mandatory breath is triggered before the patient completely exhales a spontaneous breath. The SIMV mode (Figure 18–4) is a form of IMV in which mandatory breaths are delivered at a preset frequency with the patient taking spontaneous breaths in between. However, if the ventilator detects patient effort at the time a mandatory breath is to be triggered, the mandatory breath is delivered in coordination (ie, synchronized) with the patient's effort, that is, it becomes patient triggered instead of ventilator triggered.[19] If no inspiratory effort is detected from the patient within a set interval (ie, synchronization window) at the time scheduled for a mandatory breath, then the ventilator will deliver a time triggered mandatory breath. Modern day ventilators provide SIMV rather than IMV. This mode of ventilation has been used for both primary support as well as weaning from mechanical ventilation, though there is evidence suggesting that its use as a weaning mode may contribute to prolonged weaning time.[17] Additionally, the premise that mandatory breaths of SIMV allow respiratory muscles to rest has been questioned.[27,28] It is felt that since the respiratory center does not anticipate when the ventilator will deliver the next breath, it continues to provide its output and stimulate respiratory muscle activity even during mechanically generated or supported

TABLE 18–3 Commonly used ventilator modes.

Ventilator Modes	Description	Proprietary Name
Conventional Modes of Ventilation		
CMV	All breaths are mandatory and delivered at a predetermined frequency and inspiratory time. Ventilator triggers all breaths. Patients usually require deep sedation or paralysis, or do not have ventilatory drive. This mode has been replaced by the assist-control mode.	CMV-VC, CMV-PC
ACV	All breaths are mandatory and delivered at a predetermined minimum frequency. Breaths could be triggered by ventilator or patient. Preferred mode for primary support in most clinical settings.	A/C VC, A/C PC
IMV	Breaths are mandatory and delivered by the ventilator at a preset frequency. Mandatory breaths are triggered by the ventilator. In between mandatory breaths, patient can breathe spontaneously.	IMV-VC, IMV-PC
SIMV	Is a form of IMV but differs by ventilator's ability to detect patient effort during preset intervals and delivering a mandatory breath is in coordination with (ie, synchronized) patient's effort. If no effort detected, ventilator will deliver a mandatory breath at the scheduled time (ie, time triggered). SIMV has replaced IMV in clinical practice. Used for primary support and weaning.	SIMV-VC, SIMV-PC
PSV	All breaths are spontaneous. Patient determines the respiratory rate, inspiratory time, and V_T. Patient-ventilator synchrony is enhanced. Used commonly as a weaning mode but can also be used for primary support or in combination with other modes such as SIMV.	Pressure support
Dual-Control Modes of Ventilation		
Dual control	Pressure or volume delivered is controlled by the ventilator via a feedback loop. Ventilator regulation of the pressure or volume occurs within a breath, ie, intrabreath. V_T is guaranteed by switching between PSV and VC. Breaths may be triggered by patient or ventilator.	VAPS or PA
	Pressure or volume delivered is controlled by the ventilator via a feedback loop. Ventilator regulation of the pressure or volume occurs breath to breath, ie, *interbreath*. V_T is guaranteed by adjusting PS level. Breaths are all patient-triggered.	VS or VPS
	Pressure or volume delivered is controlled by the ventilator via a feedback loop. Ventilator regulation of the pressure or volume occurs breath to breath, ie, *interbreath*. V_T is guaranteed by adjusting PC. Breaths may be triggered by patient or ventilator.	PRVC, APV, Autoflow, VPC or VCV+
	Combines dual-control, breath-to-breath, time-cycled (mandatory), and flow-cycled (spontaneous) breaths into a single mode. Can switch between PRVC and VS, or PC and PS, or VC and VS. Breaths may be triggered by patient or ventilator.	AutoMode
	Combines dual-control, breath-to-breath, time-cycled (mandatory), and flow-cycled (spontaneous) breaths into a single mode. Ventilator chooses ventilator parameter based on clinician input of IBW and percent minute volume to meet minute ventilation target while minimizing WOB. Can switch between APC and PS, and SIMV-PC and PS. Breaths may be triggered by patient or ventilator.	ASV

(Continued)

TABLE 18–3 Commonly used ventilator modes. (*Continued*)

Ventilator Modes	Description	Proprietary Name
Nonconventional Modes of Ventilation		
APRV	Uses 2 levels of continuous airway pressure, high and low, with intermittent release to the lower level. Patients are able to take spontaneous breaths during any phase of the respiratory cycle. It is commonly used as an alternative modality in ARDS patients.	APRV
PAV	Continuous spontaneous ventilation in which pressure generated is proportional to patient's inspiratory effort (volume and flow). It enhances patient-ventilator synchrony.	PAV
NAVA	Continuous spontaneous ventilation in which pressure generated is proportional to the electrical activity of the diaphragm. It enhances patient-ventilator synchrony.	NAVA
HFV	Generates very small tidal volumes with respiratory rates > 100/min. Has been used in patients with ARDS.	HFOV
	Generates very small tidal volumes with respiratory rates > 100/min. Has been used in patients with ARDS, bronchopleural fistulas, burns with significant airway secretions, and patients with raised ICP.	HFPV

A/C, assist control; ACV, assist control ventilation; APV, adaptive pressure ventilation; ARDS, acute respiratory distress syndrome; APRV, airway pressure release ventilation; ASV, adaptive support ventilation; CMV, continuous mandatory ventilation; HFOV, high-frequency oscillatory ventilation; HFPV, high-frequency percussive ventilation; HFV, high-frequency ventilation; ICP, intracranial pressure; IMV, intermittent mandatory ventilation; NAVA, neurally adjusted ventilatory assist; PA, pressure augmentation; PAV, proportional assist ventilation; PC, pressure control; PS, pressure support; PSV, pressure support ventilation; SIMV, synchronized intermittent mandatory ventilation; VAPS, volume assured pressure support; VC, volume control; VCV, volume control ventilation; VPC, variable pressure control; VPS, variable pressure support; VS, volume support; V_T, tidal volume.

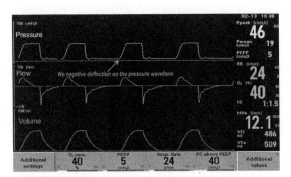

FIGURE 18–2 Continuous mechanical ventilation (CMV) using pressure-controlled breaths. All the breaths are triggered by the ventilator as depicted by the absence of a negative deflection on the pressure waveform (top waveform), flow limited (middle waveform), and time cycled. The bottom waveform shows the tidal volume that is being generated, which can be variable based on changes in the patient's compliance and resistance.

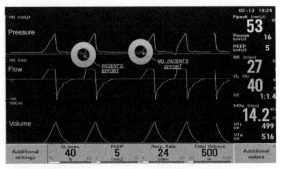

FIGURE 18–3 Assist control ventilation (ACV) using volume-controlled breaths. Some breaths are patient-triggered (depicted by the negative deflection on the pressure waveform [top waveform]), that is, assisted, and some breaths are ventilator-triggered (depicted by the absence of a negative deflection on the pressure waveform [top waveform]), that is, mandatory. The pressure generated can be variable based on changes in the patient's compliance and resistance, while the flow (middle waveform) and volume (bottom waveform) remain constant.

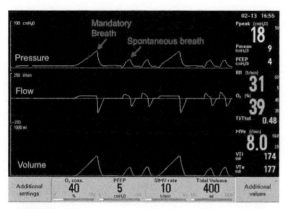

FIGURE 18–4 Synchronized intermittent mechanical ventilation (SIMV) showing both volume-controlled mandatory breaths triggered by the ventilator at a set frequency and spontaneous pressure supported breaths triggered by the patient in between the mandatory breaths.

breaths. Hence, the patient ends up performing as much WOB in spontaneous as in ventilator generated or supported breaths.

Pressure Support Ventilation

Pressure support ventilation (PSV; Figure 18–5) is a spontaneous ventilatory mode in which a patient's inspiratory effort is assisted by the ventilator up to a predetermined inspiratory pressure level. Each breath is patient triggered, pressure limited, and flow cycled, thus the patient determines the frequency, inspiratory time and V_T and thereby

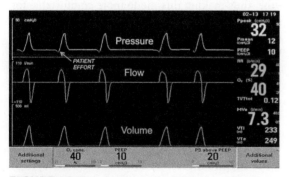

FIGURE 18–5 Pressure support ventilation (PSV) in which all breaths are spontaneous and the patient's inspiratory effort is assisted by the ventilator up to a predetermined inspiratory pressure level. Each breath is patient triggered, pressure limited, and flow cycled; thus the patient determines the respiratory frequency, inspiratory time, and tidal volume.

patient-ventilator synchrony is enhanced.[26,29,30] This mode is often confused with PC ventilation which is patient or ventilator triggered, pressure limited, and time cycled (Figure 18–2). Inspiration in PSV ceases when the peak inspiratory flow rate decreases to a predetermined minimum level (eg, 5 L/min) or a percentage of the initial inspiratory flow (eg, 25%).[19,31] The WOB related to this mode is a function of the selected pressure level, such that higher levels provide more ventilatory support and decrease the workload of the respiratory muscles.[19] This is used commonly as a weaning mode, but can also be used for primary support or in combination with other modes, such as SIMV.[29,31] It should not be used in patients with unstable respiratory drive.

Alternative Modes of Ventilatory Support

Changes in ventilatory support continue to occur as a result of microprocessor control of mechanical ventilators. This has led to the production of devices that are increasingly more complex. Some of the more common alternative modes are described below briefly.

Dual Control Modes

Dual control is a mode of ventilation in which the pressure or volume delivered is controlled by the ventilator via a feedback loop.[32] Ventilator regulation of the pressure or volume could occur within a breath, that is, *intrabreath* or from breath-to-breath, that is, *interbreath*. In the former, the ventilator switches from PC to VC during the breath, while in the latter the ventilator functions in either the PS or PC mode, adjusting the pressure limit to automatically maintain a predetermined V_T.[32]

VAPS or pressure augmentation uses dual control within a single breath. The breath may be patient triggered or ventilator triggered. After a breath is triggered, the ventilator attempts to reach the predetermined pressure target, that is, the PS setting. This portion of the breath is the pressure-limited portion. As the pressure level is attained, the ventilator determines the adequacy of the V_T delivered to the patient by comparing the volume delivered with the predetermined V_T. If the ventilator senses that the desired V_T will not be reached, inspiration continues (ie, increase in inspiratory time $[T_I]$) according to the set peak flow, whereby the breath

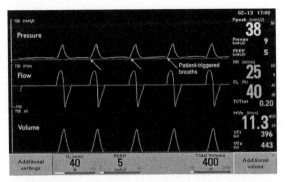

FIGURE 18–6 Volume support (VS) ventilation in which all breaths are triggered by the patient and are pressure supported. A constant tidal volume is maintained by the ventilator by adjusting the pressure support level, that is, variable pressure support.

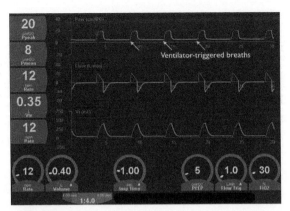

FIGURE 18–7 Pressure-regulated volume control (PRVC) (ie, adaptive pressure ventilation) in which the breaths are currently being triggered by the ventilator and not the patient. The ventilator adjusts the pressure limit based on the patient's respiratory mechanics to guarantee the targeted tidal volume.

changes from a pressure limited to a volume limited mode. This assures the predetermined volume is delivered to the patient.[19,32] However, if the delivered V_T and predetermined V_T are the same, the breath remains in the PS mode and is flow cycled. Consequently, VAPS combines the high initial flow of a pressure-limited breath with the constant volume delivery of a volume-limited breath.

Volume support ventilation (VS) or variable pressure support ventilation uses dual control from breath-to-breath (Figure 18–6). The breaths are pressure-limited and flow-cycled and are all triggered by the patient.[19] The ventilator maintains V_T by adjusting the PS, that is, V_T is used as a feedback control for continuously adjusting the pressure support level for the next breath.[33] Because all breaths are PS breaths, cycling occurs when the flow falls less than 25% of peak value.[33] It is a combination of the positive attributes of PSV with the constant minute volume and V_T seen with volume-controlled ventilation (VCV).

PRVC uses dual control from breath-to-breath (Figure 18–7). It has also been described as adaptive pressure ventilation, autoflow, VCV+, variable pressure control, though small technical differences exist.[10,33] The breaths are ventilator or patient triggered, pressure limited, and time cycled. In this mode of ventilation, the V_T is used as the feedback control mechanism (conditional variable) for continuously adjusting the pressure limit.[10,32] Initially, a series of test breaths are delivered to determine the inspiratory pressure required, based on the patient's

respiratory mechanics, to deliver the desired V_T within the chosen T_I.[29] This mode maintains a minimum peak pressure which provides a constant predetermined V_T and an automatic reduction of inspiratory pressure as the patient's efforts increase or lung mechanics improve. Conversely, an increase in inspiratory pressure will occur on the next breath if a change in lung mechanics or patient effort causes the V_T delivered to below the target V_T.[29,32] A major benefit of this mode is that the ventilator can adjust inspiratory flow according to the patient's demand while maintaining a constant minimum minute volume, thus making this mode more comfortable for the patient. Conversely, the fixed minute ventilation may result in alveolar overdistention in the face of varying compliance of the lung.[34]

AutoMode ventilation combines dual control breath-to-breath time cycled breaths (PRVC) with dual control breath-to-breath flow-cycled breaths (VS) into a single mode. In this mode, the ventilator is able to switch from either PRVC to VS or vice versa based on whether the breaths are mandatory (time triggered, pressure limited, and time cycled) or spontaneous (patient triggered, pressure limited, and flow cycled). In a similar fashion, this mode can also switch from PS to PC (Figure 18–8) or from VS to VC if the patient is unable to sustain spontaneous breathing and requires mandatory breaths to be delivered.[32,35]

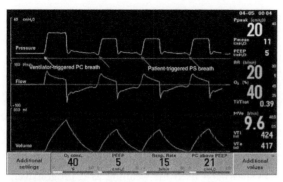

FIGURE 18-8 AutoMode ventilation combining pressure control and pressure support into a single mode. The ventilator is able to switch from either pressure control to pressure support or vice versa based on whether the breaths are mandatory (time triggered, pressure limited and time cycled) or spontaneous (patient triggered, pressure limited, and flow cycled). If the patient is unable to sustain spontaneous breathing, mandatory breaths are delivered.

Nonconventional Modes of Ventilatory Support
Airway Pressure Release Ventilation

Airway pressure release ventilation (APRV) is a pressure limited, time cycled (flow cycled in some ventilator brands) mode (Figure 18–9) that uses a high continuous airway pressure level (P_{high}) with a periodic release to a low continuous airway pressure level (P_{low}).[36,37] Patients are able to spontaneously breathe in both phases of the ventilator cycle, that is, during P_{high} and P_{low}.[36] Time spent at P_{high} (T_{high}) is usually longer than T_I in conventional ventilation, thereby promoting adequate alveolar recruitment and oxygenation. However, the brief periodic expiratory release to P_{low} in addition to the patient's ability to breathe spontaneously allow for adequate ventilation. The V_T generated is a function of the lung compliance, airway resistance, periodicity, and duration of the release phase.[38] Recently, several studies and editorials have questioned the usefulness and safety of spontaneous breathing in the setting of ARDS.[39]

Proportional Assist Ventilation

PAV is a ventilatory mode that amplifies a patient's effort without imposing predetermined targets such as flow or volume.[40,41] The ventilator applies pressure in proportion to the patient's inspiratory effort.[42-44]

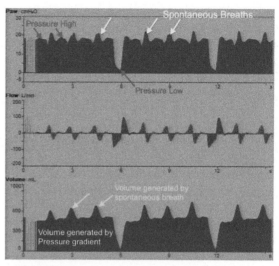

FIGURE 18-9 Airway pressure release ventilation (APRV) that is a pressure-limited and time-cycled mode that uses high and low levels of continuous airway pressure with a periodic release between the two. As is seen in this figure, patients are able to spontaneously breathe in both phases of the ventilator cycle that enhances oxygenation and further lung recruitment. However, this capability also increases the risk of producing higher tidal volumes than would be conventionally recommended.

Unlike in PSV where the inspiratory pressure provided by the ventilator is constant, with PAV, the ventilator provides dynamic inspiratory pressure assistance in linear proportion to the patient-generated flow and volume as a result of the pressure generated by the respiratory muscles. The ventilator-applied pressure increases and decreases according to the proportion of the patient's effort and this results in better patient-ventilator synchrony.[19] The ventilator amplifies the patient's instantaneous effort while leaving complete autonomy over the breathing pattern (such as tidal volume, inspiratory and expiratory duration, and flow) to the patient. The proportion of assist provided is determined by the continuous calculation of the resistive and elastic loads and this is amplified to assist the patient.[19] Hence, the system functions by positive feedback (ie, mechanical unloading). In this mode, the proportionality between applied pressure and both flow and volume is selected, and this determines the magnitude of the decrease in both the resistive and elastic loads faced by the inspiratory muscles.

The necessity of the accurate measurements of airway resistance and respiratory system elastance are limitations to the use of PAV. However, the development of PAV with load adjustable gain (PAV+) may have solved this, thereby facilitating broader clinical use.[45,46]

Adaptive Support Ventilation

ASV is a pressure-targeted closed loop mode of ventilation with optimal targeting schemes for V_T, respiratory rate and $\dot{V}_E$, in response to changes in respiratory mechanics and spontaneous breathing (Figure 18–10).[47] The ventilator determines the predicted $\dot{V}_E$ (ie, 0.1 L/kg/min) based on the patient's ideal body weight (IBW) and estimated dead space (ie, 2.2 mL/kg), which represents 100% minute ventilation.[10,48] The clinician then inputs the target percent of minute ventilation (%MinVol) that the ventilator will support. Subsequently, the ventilator automatically utilizes the Otis' equation to predict a V_T and optimal frequency (f) combination that minimizes the WOB.[49] The target V_T is calculated as $\dot{V}_E/f$. If the patient is making respiratory efforts, ASV delivers

PS breaths (patient triggered, pressure targeted, and flow cycled), and can only adjust the inspiratory pressure level and thereby V_T in order to maintain target $\dot{V}_E$. However, in the absence of respiratory efforts, ASV delivers adaptive pressure controlled breaths (ventilator triggered, pressure targeted, and time cycled) while still maintaining the target $\dot{V}_E$ by being able to adjust both V_T and f.[10,47,50] The ventilator will continuously monitor WOB relative to selected %MinVol, by adjusting peak pressure, V_T, and f accordingly. ASV has been used for weaning as it progressively and automatically decreases inspiratory pressure as the patient's respiratory mechanics improve and all breaths remain spontaneous.[51]

Neurally Adjusted Ventilatory Assist

NAVA is a ventilator mode whereby positive pressure is applied to the airway opening in proportion to the electrical activity of the diaphragm (EAdi).[52,53] This diaphragmatic activity is directly related to phrenic nerve impulse. A specially designed esophageal catheter with multiple electrodes is inserted to collect the EAdi.[54] The use of EAdi to estimate respiratory center output needs the integrity of the respiratory center, phrenic nerve, and neuromuscular junction to be intact, and assumes the diaphragm to be the primary inspiratory muscle. This diaphragmatic electrical activity is picked up by the electrode, and acts as a trigger for a pressure support breath to be delivered by the ventilator (Figure 18–11). The pressure delivered by the ventilator is calculated by multiplying the EAdi by a proportionality factor called "NAVA level" (expressed as cm $H_2O/\mu V$). Ultimately, the pressure delivered by the ventilator is cycled-off as the EAdi falls to 40% to 70% of the peak EAdi reached during inspiration.[52,53] NAVA is said to represent the first form of assisted ventilation in which the patient's respiratory center can assume full control of the magnitude and timing of the mechanical support provided, in spite of changes in respiratory drive, mechanics, and muscle function. This results in a better patient-ventilator synchrony, reduction in the risk of iatrogenic hyperinflation, respiratory alkalosis, and hemodynamic impairment.[52,53]

High-Frequency Ventilation

High-frequency ventilation (HFV) is a mechanical ventilatory technique that uses respiratory rates

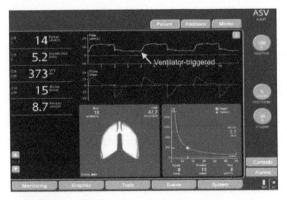

FIGURE 18–10 Adaptive support ventilation (ASV). The ventilator determines the predicted minute ventilation (V_E) based on the patient's ideal body weight (IBW) that represents 100% minute ventilation and the clinician decides on the target percent of minute ventilation (%MinVol) that the ventilator will support. If the patient makes respiratory efforts, ASV delivers pressure support breaths (patient triggered, pressure targeted, and flow cycled). However, in the absence of respiratory efforts, as in this figure, ASV delivers adaptive pressure-controlled (APC) breaths (ventilator triggered, pressure targeted, and time cycled) so as to maintain the target V_E.

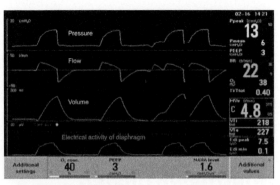

FIGURE 18-11   Neurally adjusted ventilatory assist (NAVA) in which positive pressure is delivered in proportion to the electrical activation of the diaphragm (EAdi). Ventilatory support begins when the neural drive to the diaphragm starts to increase, such that as the EAdi progressively rises, inspiratory airway pressure also rises proportionally. The pressure delivered is reached by multiplying the EAdi by a proportionality factor called "NAVA level" (in this patient: 1.6 cm $H_2O/\mu V$). The pressure delivered by the ventilator is cycled-off as the EAdi is terminated by the respiratory centers.

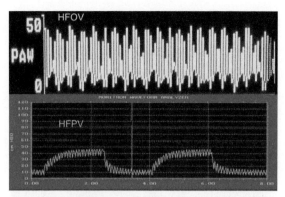

FIGURE 18-12   The waveforms that can be generated in high-frequency oscillatory ventilation (HFOV) versus high-frequency percussive ventilation (HFPV). With HFPV, small volumes are delivered in a stepwise manner with scheduled interruptions that result in the formation of high- and low-frequency cycles. It has crudely been described as an amalgam of HFOV and pressure-controlled breaths into one.

greater than 100 breaths/min along with the generation of small V_T, that are smaller than traditional estimations of both anatomic and physiologic dead space and range from approximately 1 to 5 mL/kg.[55,56] Three types of HFV exist, but the two types discussed are high-frequency oscillatory ventilation (HFOV) and high-frequency percussive ventilation (HFPV) whose waveforms are shown in Figure 18-12. In contrast to conventional ventilation where gas transport takes place by bulk delivery of gas, further theoretical mechanisms believed to enhance gas exchange in these forms of HFV have been described in the literature and include asymmetric velocity profiles, longitudinal (Taylor) dispersion, pendelluft, cardiogenic mixing, and molecular diffusion.[55,57,58] There has been interest in the use of HFV in severe hypoxemic respiratory failure, however, studies have failed to demonstrate mortality benefit in adult patients.

HFOV is characterized by the generation of small V_T as a result of the oscillation of a bias gas flow that result in pressure swings within the airway at frequencies ranging from 3 to 15 Hz (usually 3–6 Hz in adults). These pressure swings may be significant proximally, but become attenuated as they reach the distal airways and alveoli resulting

in the low V_T. The oscillations are produced by an oscillatory diaphragm/piston pump, and result in an active inspiratory and expiratory phase. The rapid oscillations of gas are delivered at pressures above and below a constant mean airway pressure (mPaw), which in addition to the fraction of inspired oxygen (FIO_2), determine the level of oxygenation. Ventilation, on the other hand, is directly related to the pressure amplitude of oscillation (ΔP); that is, degree of displacement by the oscillatory diaphragm/piston pump, but inversely related to the set frequency.[59] The combined effects of a high mPaw and small V_T potentially result in improved recruitment of alveoli and gas exchange with an associated reduced risk of overdistention.[60-62] Because of the low V_T generated, it is considered to be lung protective. It has been used primarily in patients with ARDS in whom conventional ventilatory strategies have failed. However, recent trials have demonstrated that it has limited benefit for the treatment of these patients.[63,64]

HFPV is a pressure-limited, flow-regulated, and time-cycled ventilator mode that delivers a series of high-frequency (200-900 cycles/min) small volumes in a consecutive stepwise stacking manner resulting in the formation of low-frequency (4–30 cycles/min) convective pressure-limited breathing cycles (Figure 18-13).[62,65-67] Gas exchange is a function of the

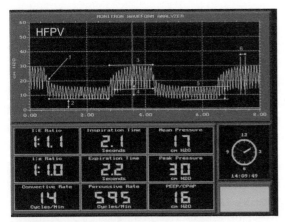

FIGURE 18–13 High-frequency percussive ventilation in which the breaths are pressure-limited, flow-regulated, and time-cycled, but are delivered at a high frequency (in this case 655 cycles/min) with very small volumes. These volumes are delivered in a consecutive stepwise stacking manner resulting in the formation of low-frequency (in this case 14 cycles/min) convective pressure-limited breathing cycles. Gas exchange is a function of the percussion frequency. The interplay of its control variables plays a role in determining the mPaw and degree of gas exchange. 1. Periodic scheduled interruptions signifying end of inspiration and onset of expiration. 2. Demand continuous positive airway pressure (CPAP). 3. Pulsatile flow during inspiration at 595 cycles/min. 4. Convective pressure-limited breath with low-frequency-cycle at 14 cycles/min. 5. Oscillatory CPAP. 6. Single percussive breath.

percussion frequency, such that at average percussion frequencies (500-600 cycles/min) oxygenation and ventilation are augmented, while low percussion frequencies less than 500 cycles/min may be utilized in patients with deep-seated secretions so as to enhance clearance.[62,67-69] The interplay of its control variables (ie, inspiratory and expiratory time, percussion frequency, PIP, pulsatile flow rate, and PEEP) either individually or in combination, play a role in determining the mPaw and degree of gas exchange.[62,67,69] HFPV has been used as a rescue modality in patients with severe hypoxemic respiratory failure, such as those with ARDS in whom conventional ventilatory strategies have failed. It has also been used in patients who tend to have a significant amount of airway secretions and debris because of its pulsatile flow mechanism. There is a paucity of literature with regards to its use and it has not been demonstrated to bring about a reduction in mortality.

Adjuncts to Mechanical Ventilation

Nonventilatory strategies that have been used in conjunction with mechanical ventilation either to enhance oxygenation, patient comfort or maintain other goals of mechanical ventilation, include prone positioning, extracorporeal membrane oxygenation also called extracorporeal life support, use of neuromuscular blocking agents or inhaled vasodilators.[70-75]

MONITORING DURING MECHANICAL VENTILATION

Pulmonary mechanics are usually assessed during mechanical ventilation. This is essential for monitoring the course of the pulmonary disease, providing adequate ventilatory support while minimizing iatrogenic effects, and determining time of discontinuation from mechanical ventilation.[76] The rapid airway occlusion technique is the most commonly used method for measuring pulmonary mechanics.[77,78]

Measurement of Peak and Plateau Pressures

Measurement of peak (PIP) and plateau (Pplat) pressures (Figure 18–14) can give valuable information regarding the patient's airways (resistance) and the respiratory system compliance. It is recommended that these pressures be measured regularly, especially when there is a change in the patient's condition. In a mechanically ventilated patient, the ventilator tubing is connected via the endotracheal tube to the patient's airways. These components are responsible for the resistive properties of the respiratory system. The lungs and chest wall are responsible for the elastic properties of the respiratory system (Figure 18–15a).[79] When a breath is delivered to the patient, the patient and the ventilator have to overcome the airways resistance and the respiratory system elastance. At the end of delivery of the V_T, the maximum pressure is recorded. This is the PIP (Figure 18–15b),[79] and it reflects the pressure that has to be developed to overcome the airway resistance and to expand the lungs and chest wall, that is, PIP reflects airways resistance + respiratory system compliance. At the end of inspiration, when an end-inspiratory pause is introduced, a newer lower pressure is reached. This is called the Pplat (Figure 15c).[79] The plat is measured in a no flow state. Since airways

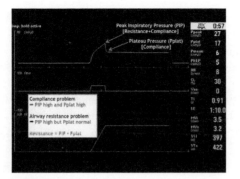

FIGURE 18–14 Graphical representation of the peak inspiratory pressure (PIP) and the plateau pressure (Pplat). The PIP is the maximum airway pressure measured at the end of inspiration and it represents the pressure required to overcome the elastic and resistive forces of the respiratory system. The application of a rapid end-inspiratory occlusion in a passively ventilated patient results in the interruption of constant gas flow with a subsequent rapid drop from PIP to Pplat, which represents the compliance of the lung. The difference between PIP and Pplat represents the pressure lost in overcoming the resistance to the flow of gas within the airways. Elevations in PIP or both PIP and Pplat assists in determining whether the patient is having primarily an airway problem versus a compliance problem.

resistance is flow dependent, it (airways resistance) will be 0 cm H_2O/L/s in a no flow state. Thus, the Pplat reflects only the state of respiratory system compliance (C_{RS}), that is, Pplat is proportional to C_{RS} and is expressed as[76]:

$$C_{RS} = V_T/(\text{Pplat} - \text{Total PEEP})$$

Furthermore, PIP – Pplat reflects airway resistance. Airway resistance (R_I) during inspiration can be expressed as[76,80]:

$$R_I = (\text{PIP} - \text{Pplat})/\dot{V}_I$$

where $\dot{V}_I$ is inspiratory flow.

The clinical applications of these pressure measurements are tabulated in Table 18–4.

With the placement of an esophageal balloon manometer in a passively ventilated patient, the direct measurement of esophageal pressure (P_{ES}; Figure 18–16) can occur and this is used as a surrogate for pleural pressure (P_{PL}). As a result, the true distending pressure across the lungs, that is, the transpulmonary pressure (P_{TP}), expressed as the difference between the alveolar pressure and pleural

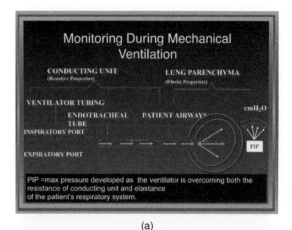

(a)

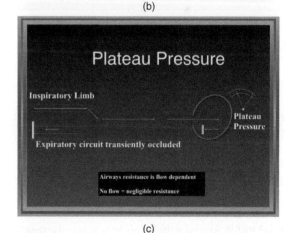

(c)

FIGURES 18–15 Parts a to c respectively show how peak inspiratory pressure (PIP) is generated to overcome both the resistive and elastic loads, features that can cause an elevation in PIP and how plateau pressure is obtained by performing an inspiratory hold maneuver. (*Reproduced with permission from Raoof S, Khan F: Mechanical Ventilation Manual. Philadelphia: American College of Physicians; 1998.*)

TABLE 18–4 Applications of peak and plateau pressures.

Clinical Condition	PIP	Pplat	Finding
Deterioration of respiratory status	High	Normal	Airway resistance problem
Deterioration of respiratory status	High	Elevated	Respiratory system elastance problem from the lung (pulmonary edema, pneumothorax, ARDS, lung contusion), chest wall or abdominal compartment (obesity, ascites, chest wall deformities) or both
Deterioration of respiratory status	High	Elevated	Determination of the pleural pressure may assist in determining the transpulmonary pressure in cases where Pplat may be falsely elevated
Determination of pressure support level	—	—	Equal to PIP-Pplat to overcome airways resistance
ARDS patients	—	< 30 cm	Keep Pplat pressures below 30 cm H$_2$O

ARDS, acute respiratory distress syndrome; PIP, peak inspiratory pressure; Pplat, plateau pressure.

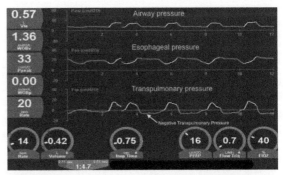

FIGURE 18–16 This figure shows how placing an esophageal probe to determine esophageal pressure (surrogate for pleural pressure) can provide accurate measurements of the transpulmonary pressure, that is, the distending pressure within the lungs. This assists in managing patients who may have conditions causing elevated pleural pressures, for example, pleural effusion, morbid obesity, ascites, etc, that would result in an elevated plateau pressure and thereby limit the amount of PEEP that may be administered to enhance their oxygenation or recruit the lungs.

pressure ($P_{ALV} - P_{PL}$), may be obtained. This is useful in cases where elevated abdominal pressures such as in obesity, ascites, or abdominal compartment syndrome, may falsely elevate the Pplat.

Intrinsic PEEP

It is important to clarify the following terms with regards to PEEP, namely, intrinsic PEEP (PEEP*i* or auto-PEEP), extrinsic PEEP (or set PEEP) and total PEEP. At end exhalation in a passively ventilated patient, airway pressure (P_{AW}) may be equal to atmospheric pressure (P_{ATM}) or may be raised to a level commensurate with the applied PEEP.[81] When an end-expiratory pause maneuver is performed causing airflow to cease and equilibration to occur

between end-expiratory pressure and proximal P_{AW}, the pressure measured is referred to as total PEEP.[82] Intrinsic PEEP is the difference between the total PEEP and extrinsic PEEP. Common features that suggest the presence of PEEP$_i$ include the presence of flow at end expiration (Figure 18–17), if end-expiratory pause pressure exceeds the externally applied PEEP (ie, extrinsic PEEP), and if the addition of extrinsic PEEP does not raise the PIP. This is commonly seen in situations of dynamic hyperinflation and active breathing efforts in which hemodynamic compromise, increased WOB (Figure 18–18), and barotrauma can result.[82]

Work of Breathing

Work is performed by the ventilator to overcome the elastic and frictional resistances of the lungs and chest wall during mechanical ventilation. Factors that may affect the WOB in mechanically ventilated patients include compliance, resistance, PEEP$_i$ (Figure 18–18), endotracheal tube diameter, V_T, and minute ventilation.[78] WOB is not commonly calculated in clinical practice, and its use has not been shown to be superior to simpler and more commonly used measurements such as PIP, Pplat, or PEEP$_i$.[78]

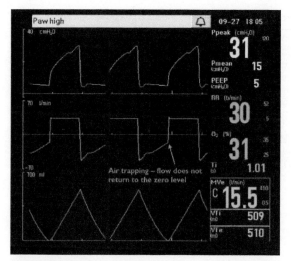

FIGURE 18–17 This figure shows how intrinsic positive end-expiratory pressure (PEEP$_i$) can be revealed on the flow waveform as a result of air trapping. This is seen as the expiratory limb does not return back to baseline at the end of exhalation. This can be further confirmed by performing an end-expiratory pause maneuver. It is seen in situations of dynamic hyperinflation and active breathing efforts, resulting in hemodynamic compromise, increased work of breathing, and barotrauma.

MECHANICAL VENTILATION IN SPECIFIC CONDITIONS

The choice of which ventilator mode and what settings to be used may be influenced by the patient's underlying condition. Nevertheless, the goals of mechanical ventilation in such situations must be maintained.[1-3] Ventilatory management in some common conditions are presented in Table 18–5.[83-88]

Ventilatory Support in Severe Hypoxemic Respiratory Failure

It is imperative to institute the Acute Respiratory Management in ARDS (ARMA) guidelines in all patients with ARDS.[83] After instituting a lung protective strategy (low V_T, low stretch), the patient should receive a V_T of 6 mL/kg IBW. After ensuring that the patient is breathing synchronously with the ventilator, the Pplat is checked. If the Pplat is more than 30 cm H$_2$O, the V_T is lowered gradually to 4 mL/kg IBW. After stabilizing the patient more than 12 to 24 hours and instituting PEEP, the

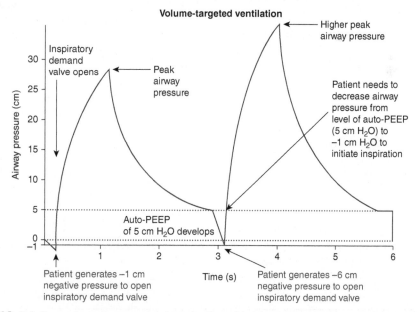

FIGURE 18–18 This figure shows how a patient's work of breathing can increase as a result of the development of intrinsic positive end-expiratory pressure (PEEP$_i$). The patient now has to generate 6 cm H$_2$O instead of 1 cm H$_2$O of negative pressure to open the inspiratory demand valve as a result of the development of 5 cm H$_2$O of PEEP$_i$. (*Reproduced with permission from Raoof S, Khan F:* Mechanical Ventilation Manual. *Philadelphia: American College of Physicians; 1998.*)

TABLE 18–5   Ventilatory management in specific conditions.

Clinical Condition	Initial Ventilator Setting	Monitoring
ARDS	• Mode: A/C VC • Low V_T: 4-8 mL/kg IBW • Pplat: < 30 cm H_2O • RR: up to 35/min • F_{IO_2}: 1 (initially) • PEEP is set according to F_{IO_2}/PEEP combinations to achieve oxygenation goals	• Avoid $PEEP_i$ • Spo_2 goal 88%-95% • Pao_2 goal 55-80 mm Hg • pH goal 7.30-7.45 • Permissive hypercapnia may be needed • Patient-ventilator synchrony • Hemodynamic status
COPD	• NIPPV should be considered in COPD patients prior to invasive ventilation • Mode: A/C VC or PC • Low V_T: 6-8 mL/kg IBW • Pplat: < 30 cm H_2O • RR: 8-12/min • F_{IO_2}: ≤ 0.5 (or to meet Spo_2 goal) • PEEP: ≤ 5 cm H_2O or as needed to offset $PEEP_i$ (80% of $PEEP_i$) • T_i: 0.6-1.25 s • Peak flow: ≥ 80 L/min (decelerating flow) in VC	• Avoid $PEEP_i$ • Spo_2 goal > 88% • Avoid hyperventilation • $Paco_2$ goal is patient's baseline in COPD • Permissive hypercapnia may initially be required in asthmatic patients • Patient-ventilator synchrony • Hemodynamic status • Airway pressure assessment and flow-volume patterns can be used to monitor bronchodilator effectiveness
Asthma	• Mode: A/C VC or PC • Low V_T: 6-8 mL/kg IBW • Pplat: < 30 cm H_2O • RR: 10-15/min • F_{IO_2}: ≤ 0.5 (or to meet Spo_2 goal) • PEEP: 0-≤ 5 cm H_2O or as needed to offset $PEEP_i$ (80% of $PEEP_i$) • T_i: 0.6-1.25 s • Peak flow: 60 L/min (constant flow) or 80-100 L/min (decelerating flow) in VC	• Avoid $PEEP_i$ • Spo_2 goal > 90% • Permissive hypercapnia may initially be required in asthmatic patients • Patient-ventilator synchrony • Hemodynamics • Use of helium-oxygen mixtures should be considered • Airway pressure assessment and flow-volume patterns can be used to monitor bronchodilator effectiveness
Chronic Restrictive Disease	• Mode: A/C VC or PC • Low V_T: 4-8 mL/kg IBW • Pplat: < 30 cm H_2O • RR: 15-30/min • F_{IO_2}: ≤ 0.5 • PEEP: 5 cm H_2O • T_i: < 1 s • Peak flow: ≥ 60 L/min in VC	• Spo_2 goal 88%-95% • Pao_2 goal 55-80 mm Hg • Patient-ventilator synchrony • Hemodynamic status

Neuromuscular Disease	• NIPPV should be considered early
	• Mode: A/C VC or PC
	• Low V_T: 6-8 mL/kg IBW
	• Pplat: < 30 cm H_2O
	• RR: 10-15/min
	• F_{IO_2}: ≤ 0.5 (or to meet Spo_2 goal)
	• PEEP: 5 cm H_2O
	• T_i: 1 s
		• Spontaneous V_T and RR
		• Vital capacity
		  • Intubate if < 10 mL/kg
		  • Wean if = 10 mL/kg
		  • Extubate if > 15 mL/kg post-SBT
		• PImax
		  • Intubate if < –20 cm H_2O
		  • Wean if = –20 cm H_2O
		  • Extubated if > –30 cm H_2O post-SBT

(Continued)

TABLE 18–5 **Ventilatory management in specific conditions. (*Continued*)**

Clinical Condition	Initial Ventilator Setting	Monitoring
Head Trauma	Mode: A/C VC or PC Low V_T: 6-8 mL/kg IBW Pplat: < 30 cm H_2O RR: 15-20/min F_{IO_2}: ≤ 0.5 (or to meet Spo_2 goal) PEEP: 5 cm H_2O T_i: 1 s	• Monitor ICP or signs of raised ICP • Avoid hypoxia or hypercapnia; can raise ICP • Pao_2 goal 70-100 mm Hg • $Paco_2$ goal 35-40 mm Hg • Ensure PEEP level does not raise ICP • Avoid $PEEP_i$

A/C, assist control; F_{IO_2}, fraction of inspired oxygen; IBW, ideal body weight; PC, pressure control; Pao_2, partial pressure of arterial oxygen; PEEP, positive end-expiratory pressure; $PEEP_i$, intrinsic PEEP; PImax, maximal inspiratory pressure; Pao_2, plateau pressure; RR, respiratory rate; SBT, spontaneous breathing trial; Spo_2, oxygen saturation by pulse oximetry; T_i, inspiratory time; VC, volume control; V_T, tidal volume.

PaO_2/FIO_2 (P/F) ratio is checked. If the P/F ratio is 100 or less, the patient falls into the severe ARDS category, as defined by the Berlin criteria.[89] The mortality in these patients is an average of 52% (range 36-68%). This is in contrast to those who show an improvement in their P/F ratio (> 200) within 24 hours after institution of lung protective strategies. Their mortality ranges from 12.5% to 23%.[90,91] Other variables that define severe ARDS include[62] high ventilatory requirements as demonstrated by FIO_2 ≥ 0.7 or PEEP >15 cm H_2O or inability to maintain Pplat less than 30 cm H_2O on V_T 4 mL/kg IBW or oxygenation index more than 30. In these individuals, rescue therapy may be considered. A review of the published literature regarding rescue therapies indicates the following: (a) there is very limited data to show that these rescue therapies reduce mortality; (b) most of these therapies result in improvement in oxygenation, especially in the subset of patients who show recruitment with the application of higher PEEP; (c) improvement of oxygenation does not translate to reduction in mortality; (d) the window period to use these rescue therapies is limited to 72 to 96 hours; (e) if instituted late, conventional mechanical ventilation has inflicted ventilator-induced lung injury leaving very little recruitable lung; and (f) the choice of recruitment strategies is based upon their availability, and the familiarity of the treating team with these modes.

The data regarding individual modalities used as rescue therapy are shown in Table 18–6.

COMPLICATIONS OF MECHANICAL VENTILATION

Although in many clinical situations mechanical ventilatory support can be life-saving, it is commonly associated with many complications. The goal is always to prevent iatrogenic injury; however, avoiding these untoward events may not always be achievable. It is, therefore, important to promptly recognize and address these complications as it may be life-saving. Table 18–7 lists the common pulmonary and extra-pulmonary complications that have been associated with mechanical ventilation.[19,92-99]

DISCONTINUATION OF MECHANICAL VENTILATION

As stated earlier, one of the goals of mechanical ventilation is to promote liberation from it as quickly and as safely as possible. Once the inciting event or condition that resulted in mechanical ventilation begins to resolve, the focus should be on discontinuation so as not to expose the patient to potential complications (Table 18–7). Weaning has been used synonymously with discontinuation from mechanical ventilation; however, weaning is the systematic method of gradually decreasing the ventilatory support level as tolerated.[100] This can result in unnecessary prolongation of ventilatory support in those who no longer require it.

Current evidence-based guidelines focus attention on establishing readiness for a spontaneous

TABLE 18–6 Strategies used in rescue therapy.

Modality	Data Supporting Use
Higher levels of PEEP than used in ARMA trial[113-115]	No reduction in mortality based on 3 articles listed. However, if recruiters are identified by recruitment trials, it is possible that this subgroup may experience greater benefit than harm.
Lung recruitment maneuvers[112]	Not routinely recommended. Desaturation and hypotension are seen in 22% of patients, although serious complications such as air leak are uncommon.
Prone position[75]	Recent data indicate that patients with P/F ratio < 100, who are proned early in the course of ARDS, kept proned approximately 75% of the time, in centers that are well versed with proning patients, there is a reduction in 28- and 90-d mortality.
HFOV[63,64]	Based on 2 recent trials (OSCILLATE study and OSCAR trial), HFOV cannot be recommended as first mode of therapy for ARDS. It is one of the rescue therapies that have not shown reduced mortality when compared with conventional lung protective strategies. In fact, in the OSCILLATE study, using an aggressive strategy with high mean airway pressures, more hemodynamic compromise, larger number of organ failure, and higher mortality was noted.
APRV[111]	Should be used with caution. Very few studies have shown survival benefits.
ECMO/ECLS[73,74,110]	May be considered in patients at hospitals with this technology available.

APRV, airway pressure release ventilation; ARDS, acute respiratory distress syndrome; ARMA, acute respiratory management in ARDS; ECLS, extracorporeal life support; ECMO, extracorporeal membrane oxygenation; HFOV, high-frequency oscillatory ventilation; OSCAR trial, high-frequency OSCillation in ARDS; OSCILLATE trial, oscillation for acute respiratory distress syndrome (ARDS) treated early trial; PEEP, positive end-expiratory pressure.

breathing trial (SBT) by clinical assessment of stability or recovery, then carrying out a SBT to determine the potential for ventilator discontinuation, and finally identifying the causes of a failed SBT if it occurs.[101] It is essential to properly time the performance of a SBT as premature discontinuation is fraught with its own complications such as airway compromise, muscle overload and fatigue, cardiovascular stress, and impaired gas exchange. Discontinuation of mechanical ventilation is a process that must, therefore, be carried out with proper caution and monitoring.

Contemplating Mechanical Ventilation Discontinuation

A patient should be considered daily for ventilator withdrawal if the following prerequisites are present prior to conducting a SBT[101]: partial or complete recovery of conditions that resulted in respiratory failure; adequate oxygenation with low PEEP, that is, PaO_2/FIO_2 more than 200, PEEP 8 cm H_2O or less, and FIO_2 0.5 or less; absence of severe acidosis, that is, pH 7.25 or more; hemodynamic stability with minimal or no vasopressor support; and presence of spontaneous inspiratory effort. Multiple physiological parameters have been investigated as predictors

for successful discontinuation of mechanical ventilation. However, these indices have demonstrated limited value in doing so.[102]

Mechanical Ventilation Discontinuation Assessment

Patients who fulfill the aforementioned prerequisites should undergo a SBT. Regardless of the SBT method used (ie, CPAP of 5 cm H_2O, PSV of 5-7 cm H_2O, or T-piece breathing trial), an initial screening phase of a SBT lasting a few minutes should be performed to assess tolerance of the trial. Tolerance is determined by assessing objective parameters, such as adequacy of gas exchange, hemodynamic stability, ventilatory pattern, and subjective parameters, such as mental status changes, patient discomfort, diaphoresis, and signs of increased WOB. Based on a successful outcome of the initial screen, the SBT should continue for a total duration of 30 to 120 min. To determine SBT success, an integrated assessment of the following parameters should take place[101]:

- Respiratory pattern—RR less than 35 per minute

- Gas exchange—oxygen saturation more than 90%

TABLE 18-7 Complications associated with mechanical ventilation.

Complication	Clinical Presentation
Upper airway and tracheobronchial tree problems related to intubation	• Early problems: trauma, right main stem intubation • Late problems: ulcerations, tracheomalacia, tracheoesophageal fistula, tracheoinnominate fistula
Pulmonary barotrauma resulting from high peak airway pressures and/or underlying disease process	• Subcutaneous emphysema, pneumothorax, pneumomediastinum, pneumopericardium, bronchopleural fistula resulting from the placement of a chest tube
Ventilator-induced lung injury	• Exposure to high transpulmonary pressures (barotrauma), alveolar overdistension (volutrauma), and/or repetitive opening and closing of the alveoli (atelectrauma) resulting in lung damage, as well as triggering an inflammatory response (biotrauma) that leads to injury to nonpulmonary organs and possible organ failure
Ventilator-associated event	• Development of worsening oxygenation after a baseline period of stability or improvement, subsequent development of signs of infection (ie, fever, purulent respiratory secretions, positive cultures), and pneumonia
Ventilator-induced diaphragm dysfunction	• Disuse muscle atrophy particularly from prolonged mechanical ventilation, use of ventilation modes that minimize patient effort and overuse of sedative and analgesic agents that decrease respiratory drive, thereby decreasing patient work during assisted breaths
Patient-ventilator dyssynchrony	• Can result in hypoxemia, increased work of breathing, hemodynamic compromise, discomfort, and agitation
Oxygen toxicity	• Prolonged use of high F_{IO_2} can trigger the release of oxygen-free radicals that can further cause lung damage
Cardiovascular effects	• Hemodynamic compromise
Gastrointestinal effects	• Stress-related mucosal disease that can lead to gastrointestinal bleeding, motility disturbances, pneumoperitoneum
Renal effects	• Renal hypoperfusion leading to decreased urine output and risk of developing renal failure
Neuromuscular effects	• Critical illness polyneuropathy and myopathy resulting in limb weakness and flaccidity, respiratory muscle weakness, difficulty in weaning from ventilator

F_{IO_2}, fraction of inspired oxygen.

• Hemodynamic status—systolic blood pressure less than 180 mm Hg, heart rate less than 140 per minute or heart rate change less than 20% from baseline

• Patient comfort—absence of development of anxiety or diaphoresis

Extubation Assessment

Following a successful SBT, there is a high likelihood that a patient may tolerate permanent discontinuation of mechanical ventilation.[101] In removing the artificial airway, the following considerations need to be made prior to extubation[101]:

• Airway patency—the presence of an air leak of less than 110 mL (cuff leak test) when the endotracheal tube balloon is deflated may identify patients who may be at risk for postextubation upper airway obstruction, for example, prolonged mechanical ventilation, female gender, trauma, and repeated or traumatic intubation.

• Ability to protect airway—patient must be able to expel secretions with an effective cough, lack excessive secretions, or require infrequent airway suctioning (less than every 2 hours).

Extubation failure occurs if there is a need to reinstitute ventilatory support within 24 to 72 hours of a planned extubation. About 4% to 23% of patients who pass a SBT may fail extubation.[101,103] Nevertheless, a successful SBT coupled with a patent upper airway and ability to protect the airway remains the best predictor of extubation success.

Failure of SBT

If a patient fails the SBT, they are placed back on a comfortable form of ventilatory support and the reason for the SBT failure is determined. Once the reversible causes are corrected and the patient again meets the previously mentioned prerequisites, subsequent SBTs can be performed every 24 hours.[17,101] In patients who persistently fail, in spite of clinical stability or reversal of their clinical condition, a tracheostomy may be required for prolonged mechanical ventilation during which a gradual ventilatory support reduction strategy is implemented in conjunction with rehabilitative interventions.[101]

NONINVASIVE POSITIVE PRESSURE VENTILATION

Noninvasive ventilation implies the provision of mechanical ventilatory assistance without the need of an invasive airway. Noninvasive ventilatory techniques can be either negative pressure (eg, tank respirator) or positive pressure ventilation (eg, CPAP and bilevel NIPPV). It is important to distinguish the usage of NIPPV in the setting of acute respiratory failure (hospital setting usually) versus chronic respiratory failure (home setting). The ICU ventilators may combine CPAP with pressure support to provide two separate levels of pressure in the two phases of the breathing cycle. Other modes of ventilation may be utilized to administer NIPPV. These include noninvasive NAVA, proportional pressure ventilation + (PPV+) and average volume assured pressure support. It should be pointed out that PAV does not exist in the noninvasive form commercially.

Advantages of NIPPV

NIPPV avoids complications of invasive ventilation, such as aspiration, trauma, cardiac arrhythmias or hypotension, and volutrauma (early complications) as well as ventilator associated pneumonia, sinusitis, stress gastritis, airways injury, and problems associated with tracheostomy (late complications). It is more comfortable, requires less sedation, and in the long run proves to be less costly.

Physiological Rationale for Using NIPPV

- Acute exacerbation of COPD: application of NIPPV counterbalances PEEP$_i$ and reduces the WOB.

- Pulmonary edema: NIPPV increases the lung compliance via the application of PEEP or CPAP, thereby preventing alveolar collapse, redistributing intra-alveolar fluid, and improving oxygenation. Additionally, it allows muscle rest by the application of pressure support ventilation.

Indications of NIPPV

It is important to select patients who are likely to benefit from NIPPV. The strong (level A) indications for NIPPV include the following:

1. *Acute hypercapnic respiratory failure in the setting of COPD*
    In a Cochrane systemic review of 14 studies, bilevel NIPPV decreased the risk of intubation [number needed to treat (NNT) = 4] and lowered the mortality (NNT = 10).[104]

2. *Cardiogenic pulmonary edema*
    Both CPAP or bilevel NIPPV may be utilized in this setting. A Cochrane systemic review of 32 studies comparing NIPPV plus standard medical care (SMC) with SMC alone demonstrated that the institution of NIPPV (CPAP and bilevel NIPPV) reduced the need for intubation (NNT = 8) and mortality (NNT = 14).[105] Furthermore, there did not appear to be any significant different between CPAP and bilevel NIPPV with regards to the reduction in intubation or mortality. In addition, there was no increased incidence of acute myocardial infarction either during or after the usage of CPAP or bilevel NIPPV.[105]

3. *Immunosuppressed patients with pulmonary infiltrates, fever, and acute respiratory failure*

In a study of 52 immunosuppressed patients with pulmonary opacities and fever with early hypoxemic respiratory failure, NIPPV delivered by face mask every 3 hours for at least 45 minutes, was administered to 26 patients. An equal number of patients were used as control and given standard treatment without NIPPV. There were fewer patients in the NIPPV group as compared to the standard treatment group who required endotracheal intubation (12 [46%] vs 20 [77%]; $P = 0.03$), fewer who died in the ICU (10 [38%] vs 18 [69%]; $P = 0.02$) and fewer who died in the hospital (13 [50%] vs 21 [81%]; $P = 0.02$). Each of these values was considered significant.[106]

A weaker level B indication for the use of NIPPV in acute respiratory failure includes the following conditions:

1. Asthma

2. Extubation failure in COPD patients

3. All other causes of hypoxemic respiratory failure (except cardiogenic pulmonary edema)

4. Postoperative respiratory failure

5. Do not intubate (DNI) patients especially those with COPD and left ventricular failure

Practical Aspects and Institution of NIPPV

Step 1: Indications for use
NIPPV should be considered when dyspnea is at least moderate, that is, respiratory rate more than 24 per minute in the setting of COPD and more than 30 per minute in hypoxemic respiratory failure. Usually there is recruitment of accessory muscle usage. Gas exchange abnormalities generally indicate the development of hypercapnia in COPD exacerbations with falling pH or a drop in the PaO_2/FIO_2 to less than 300 in the setting of pulmonary edema. In assessing these patients, the likelihood of needing intubation should be approximately 50% or higher.

Step 2: Exclude contraindications to using NIPPV
These include: imminent risk of having respiratory arrest; medical instability (acute shock, upper

gastrointestinal bleeding, etc); agitated or uncooperative patient; profuse secretions which require frequent suctioning; facial trauma; severe hypoxemic respiratory failure with PaO_2/FIO_2 less than 200; and multisystem organ failure.

Step 3: Selection of appropriate interfaces
It is imperative that appropriate time and resources be utilized to select the mask that is most comfortable to the patient. This should take into consideration patient preferences, nasal or mouth breathing patterns, risk of vomiting, and degree of respiratory failure. In a controlled trial of oronasal versus nasal mask ventilation in the treatment of acute respiratory failure, 35 patients received oronasal masks and a similar number received nasal masks.[107] Sixty-six percent of those receiving oronasal masks were successfully managed versus 49% with the nasal mask although this did not reach statistical significance. However, intolerance to the oronasal mask was 11% versus 34% who were on the nasal mask ($P = 0.02$).

Step 4: Selection of ventilatory modes
Noninvasive ventilatory modes available on critical care ventilators allow for leak compensation, have an adjustable rise time, allow an inspiratory time limit to be set, and have the provision to silence alarms. Usually CPAP with pressure support is instituted to apply pressures to both exhalation and inspiration phases of the breath. However, other modes mentioned previously can also be applied. It is imperative to observe the patient's breathing patterns on these modes rather than just empirically selecting the mode.

Step 5: Settings
Usual practice is to start with low inspiratory positive pressures at about 8 to 10 cm H_2O as well as expiratory positive pressures at about 4 to 5 cm H_2O and readjust relatively soon to achieve adequate V_T of about 5 to 7 mL/kg IBW. More importantly, observing an improvement in respiratory distress with a lowering of the respiratory rate and unloading of accessory muscles must be actively sought. Usually inspiratory positive pressures of up to 20 cm H_2O

and expiratory positive pressures of up to 8 to 10 cm H_2O are utilized. Oxygen is blended to achieve SpO_2 of more than 90% to 92%.

Step 6: Monitoring

Depending upon the clinical acuity, patients may be monitored in an ICU or on a step-down facility. Clinical parameters that are commonly monitored are the level of dyspnea, synchrony with the ventilator, air leaks, mask acceptability, and oxygen saturation. Occasional blood gases are performed within the first 1 to 2 hours after institution of NIPPV. It is also important to stand at the patient's bedside and observe the patient frequently in the first 1 to 2 hours of institution of NIPPV. Those who will fail NIPV will generally do so in the first 2 hours. It is important to ascertain that the patient is breathing synchronously with the ventilator as indicated by the following signs[108,109]: air leak is minimal (< 24 L/min); desaturation dips less than 3%; and tidal volumes more than 7 mL/kg IBW.

Step 7: When to decide NIPPV is unsuccessful

It is important to assess when NIPPV should be stopped. If there is lack of improvement within 1 to 2 hours, if the patient is intolerant to therapy, if adverse side effects, such as hypotension develop, or if the patient wishes to stop this therapy, NIPPV should be terminated.

SUMMARY

Mechanical ventilation can be life-saving in patients with acute respiratory failure. The goals of mechanical ventilation include providing safe gas exchange; decreasing the WOB; minimizing iatrogenic injury; improving patient–ventilator interactions; and promoting liberation from mechanical ventilation in a timely manner. Technological advancements with complex (microprocessor controlled) modes have made the classification schemas more difficult. None of the new complex modes have been shown to improve morbidity or mortality, although patient–ventilator synchrony is enhanced in some. The choice of the ventilator mode to use and parameters to set may be influenced by the patient's underlying condition, that is, one glove does not fit all. There

is a higher likelihood of permanent discontinuation of mechanical ventilation if a properly timed SBT is utilized to evaluate readiness. The use of NIPPV avoids the complications associated with invasive mechanical ventilation. However, it is important to select the appropriate group of patients who would benefit from its use.

REFERENCES

1. Mireles-Cabodevila E, Hatipoglu U, Chatburn RL. A rational framework for selecting modes of ventilation. *Resp Care.* 2013;58(2):348-366.
2. Marini JJ. Mechanical ventilation: past lessons and the near future. *Crit Care.* 2013;17(Suppl 1):S1.
3. Tobin MJ. Advances in mechanical ventilation. *N Engl J Med.* 2001;344(26):1986-1996.
4. Branson RD, Johannigman JA. What is the evidence base for the newer ventilation modes? *Resp Care.* 2004;49(7):742-760.
5. Ponte J. Assisted ventilation. 2. Indications for mechanical ventilation. *Thorax.* 1990;45(11):885-890.
6. Tobin MJ, Laghi F, Jubran A. Ventilatory failure, ventilator support, and ventilator weaning. *Compr Physiol.* 2012;2(4):2871-2921.
7. Chatburn RL. Classification of mechanical ventilators and modes of ventilation. In: Tobin MJ, ed. *Principles and Practice of Mechanical Ventilation.* 3rd ed. New York: McGraw-Hill; 2013:45-64.
8. Hess DR, Kacmarek RM. Overview of the mechanical ventilator system and classification. *Essentials of Mechanical Ventilation.* 2nd ed. New York: McGraw-Hill; 2002:26-33.
9. Chatburn RL. Classification of ventilator modes: update and proposal for implementation. *Resp Care.* 2007;52(3):301-323.
10. Mireles-Cabodevila E, Diaz-Guzman E, Heresi GA, Chatburn RL. Alternative modes of mechanical ventilation: a review for the hospitalist. *Cleveland Clin J Med.* 2009;76(7):417-430.
11. Chatburn RL, Branson RD. Classification of mechanical ventilators. In: MacIntyre NR, Branson RD, eds. *Mechanical Ventilation.* 2nd ed. St. Louis, MO: Saunders Elsevier; 2009:1-48.
12. Branson RD, Campbell RS, Davis K, Jr, Johnson DJ, 2nd. Comparison of pressure and flow triggering systems during continuous positive airway pressure. *Chest.* 1994;106(2):540-544.
13. Sassoon CS, Giron AE, Ely EA, Light RW. Inspiratory work of breathing on flow-by and

demand-flow continuous positive airway pressure. *Crit Care Med.* 1989;17(11):1108-1114.

14. Hess DR, Kacmarek RM. Traditional modes of mechanical ventilation. *Essentials of Mechanical Ventilation.* 2nd ed. New York: McGraw-Hill; 2002:34-42.

15. Chatburn RL, Mireles-Cabodevila E. Closed-loop control of mechanical ventilation: description and classification of targeting schemes. *Resp Care.* 2011;56(1):85-102.

16. Chatburn RL. Computer control of mechanical ventilation. *Resp Care.* 2004;49(5):507-517.

17. Esteban A, Alia I, Ibanez J, Benito S, Tobin MJ. Modes of mechanical ventilation and weaning. A national survey of Spanish hospitals. The Spanish Lung Failure Collaborative Group. *Chest.* 1994;106(4):1188-1193.

18. Branson RD. Dual control modes, closed loop ventilation, handguns, and tequila. *Resp Care.* 2001;46(3):232-233.

19. George L, Khusid F, Raoof S. Basic and advanced mechanical ventilation modalities. In: Fein A, Kamholz S, Ost D, eds. *Respiratory Emergencies.* 1st ed. Florida: CRC Press; 2006:57-82.

20. Branson RD. Modes of ventilator operation. In: MacIntyre NR, Branson RD, eds. *Mechanical Ventilation.* 2nd ed. St. Loius, MO: Saunders Elsevier; 2009:49-88.

21. Koh SO. Mode of mechanical ventilation: volume controlled mode. *Crit Care Clin.* 2007;23(2): 161-167, viii.

22. Luce JM, Pierson DJ, Hudson LD. Intermittent mandatory ventilation. *Chest.* 1981;79(6):678-685.

23. Downs JB, Block AJ, Vennum KB. Intermittent mandatory ventilation in the treatment of patients with chronic obstructive pulmonary disease. *Anesth Analg.* 1974;53(3):437-443.

24. Downs JB, Klein EF, Jr, Desautels D, Modell JH, Kirby RR. Intermittent mandatory ventilation: a new approach to weaning patients from mechanical ventilators. *Chest.* 1973;64(3):331-335.

25. Downs JB, Stock MC, Tabeling B. Intermittent mandatory ventilation (IMV): a primary ventilatory support mode. *Annales chirurgiae et gynaecologiae. Supplementum.* 1982;196:57-63.

26. Sassoon CS, Mahutte CK, Light RW. Ventilator modes: old and new. *Crit Care Clin.* 1990;6(3):605-634.

27. Imsand C, Feihl F, Perret C, Fitting JW. Regulation of inspiratory neuromuscular output during synchronized intermittent mechanical ventilation. *Anesthesiology.* 1994;80(1):13-22.

28. Marini JJ, Smith TC, Lamb VJ. External work output and force generation during synchronized intermittent mechanical ventilation. Effect of machine assistance on breathing effort. *Am Rev Respir Dis.* 1988;138(5):1169-1179.

29. Singer BD, Corbridge TC. Pressure modes of invasive mechanical ventilation. *Southern Med J.* 2011;104(10):701-709.

30. Sassoon CS. Positive pressure ventilation. Alternate modes. *Chest.* 1991;100(5):1421-1429.

31. Burns SM. Pressure modes of mechanical ventilation: the good, the bad, and the ugly. *AACN Advan Crit Care.* 2008;19(4):399-411.

32. Branson RD, Davis K, Jr. Dual control modes: combining volume and pressure breaths. *Resp Care Clin North Am.* 2001;7(3):397-408, viii.

33. Branson RD, Johannigman JA. The role of ventilator graphics when setting dual-control modes. *Respir Care.* 2005;50(2):187-201.

34. Guldager H, Nielsen SL, Carl P, Soerensen MB. A comparison of volume control and pressure-regulated volume control ventilation in acute respiratory failure. *Crit Care.* 1997;1(2):75-77.

35. Holt SJ, Sanders RC, Thurman TL, Heulitt MJ. An evaluation of Automode, a computer-controlled ventilator mode, with the Siemens Servo 300A ventilator, using a porcine model. *Respir Care.* 2001;46(1):26-36.

36. Downs JB, Stock MC. Airway pressure release ventilation: a new concept in ventilatory support. *Crit Care Med.* 1987;15(5):459-461.

37. Stock MC, Downs JB, Frolicher DA. Airway pressure release ventilation. *Crit Care Med.* 1987;15(5):462-466.

38. Habashi NM. Other approaches to open-lung ventilation: airway pressure release ventilation. *Crit Care Med.* 2005;33(3 Suppl):S228-S240.

39. Hess DR, Thompson BT, Slutsky AS. Update in acute respiratory distress syndrome and mechanical ventilation 2012. *Am J Respir Crit Care Med.* 2013;188(3):285-292.

40. Grasso S, Ranieri VM. Proportional assist ventilation. *Resp Care Clin North Am.* 2001;7(3):465-473, ix-x.

41. Ambrosino N, Rossi A. Proportional assist ventilation (PAV): a significant advance or a futile struggle between logic and practice? *Thorax.* 2002;57(3):272-276.

42. Younes M. Proportional assist ventilation, a new approach to ventilatory support. Theory. *Am Rev Respir Dis.* 1992;145(1):114-120.

43. Sinderby C, Beck J. Proportional assist ventilation and neurally adjusted ventilatory assist—better

approaches to patient ventilator synchrony? *Clin Chest Med.* 2008;29(2):329-342, vii.

44. Turner DA, Rehder KJ, Cheifetz IM. Nontraditional modes of mechanical ventilation: progress or distraction? *Expert Rev Respir Med.* 2012;6(3):277-284.

45. Xirouchaki N, Kondili E, Vaporidi K, et al. Proportional assist ventilation with load-adjustable gain factors in critically ill patients: comparison with pressure support. *Intens Care Med.* 2008;34(11):2026-2034.

46. Costa R, Spinazzola G, Cipriani F, et al. A physiologic comparison of proportional assist ventilation with load-adjustable gain factors (PAV+) versus pressure support ventilation (PSV). *Intens Care Med.* 2011;37(9):1494-1500.

47. Chen CW, Wu CP, Dai YL, et al. Effects of implementing adaptive support ventilation in a medical intensive care unit. *Resp Care.* 2011;56(7):976-983.

48. Wu CP, Lin HI, Perng WC, et al. Correlation between the %MinVol setting and work of breathing during adaptive support ventilation in patients with respiratory failure. *Resp Care.* 2010;55(3):334-341.

49. Otis AB. The work of breathing. *Physiol Reviews.* 1954;34(3):449-458.

50. Brunner JX, Iotti GA. Adaptive Support Ventilation (ASV). *Minerva Anestesiologica.* 2002;68(5):365-368.

51. Burns KE, Lellouche F, Lessard MR. Automating the weaning process with advanced closed-loop systems. *Intens Care Med.* 2008;34(10):1757-1765.

52. Sinderby C, Beck J, Spahija J, et al. Inspiratory muscle unloading by neurally adjusted ventilatory assist during maximal inspiratory efforts in healthy subjects. *Chest.* 2007;131(3):711-717.

53. Sinderby C, Navalesi P, Beck J, et al. Neural control of mechanical ventilation in respiratory failure. *Nat Med.* 1999;5(12):1433-1436.

54. Wysocki M, Brunner JX. Closed-loop ventilation: an emerging standard of care? *Crit Care Clin.* 2007;23(2):223-240, ix.

55. Krishnan JA, Brower RG. High-frequency ventilation for acute lung injury and ARDS. *Chest.* 2000;118(3):795-807.

56. Fessler HE, Hess DR. Respiratory controversies in the critical care setting. Does high-frequency ventilation offer benefits over conventional ventilation in adult patients with acute respiratory distress syndrome? *Resp Care.* 2007;52(5):595-605; discussion 606-598.

57. dos Santos CC, Slutsky AS. Overview of high-frequency ventilation modes, clinical rationale, and gas transport mechanisms. *Resp Care Clin North Am.* 2001;7(4):549-575.

58. Chang HK. Mechanisms of gas transport during ventilation by high-frequency oscillation. *J Appl Physiol: Resp, Environ Exer Physiol.* 1984;56(3):553-563.

59. Chan KP, Stewart TE, Mehta S. High-frequency oscillatory ventilation for adult patients with ARDS. *Chest.* 2007;131(6):1907-1916.

60. Ferguson ND, Chiche JD, Kacmarek RM, et al. Combining high-frequency oscillatory ventilation and recruitment maneuvers in adults with early acute respiratory distress syndrome: the Treatment with Oscillation and an Open Lung Strategy (TOOLS) Trial pilot study. *Crit Care Med.* 2005;33(3):479-486.

61. Mehta S, Granton J, MacDonald RJ, et al. High-frequency oscillatory ventilation in adults: the Toronto experience. *Chest.* 2004;126(2):518-527.

62. Esan A, Hess DR, Raoof S, George L, Sessler CN. Severe hypoxemic respiratory failure: part 1— ventilatory strategies. *Chest.* 2010;137(5):1203-1216.

63. Ferguson ND, Cook DJ, Guyatt GH, et al. High-frequency oscillation in early acute respiratory distress syndrome. *N Engl J Med.* 2013;368(9):795-805.

64. Young D, Lamb SE, Shah S, et al. High-frequency oscillation for acute respiratory distress syndrome. *N Engl J Med.* 2013;368(9):806-813.

65. Allan PF, Osborn EC, Chung KK, Wanek SM. High-frequency percussive ventilation revisited. *J Burn Care Res.* 2010;31(4):510-520.

66. Chung KK, Wolf SE, Renz EM, et al. High-frequency percussive ventilation and low tidal volume ventilation in burns: a randomized controlled trial. *Crit Care Med.* 2010;38(10):1970-1977.

67. Lucangelo U, Fontanesi L, Antonaglia V, et al. High frequency percussive ventilation (HFPV). Principles and technique. *Minerva Anestesiol.* 2003;69(11): 841-848, 848-851.

68. Lucangelo U, Zin WA, Antonaglia V, et al. High-frequency percussive ventilation during surgical bronchial repair in a patient with one lung. *British J Anaesth.* 2006;96(4):533-536.

69. Salim A, Martin M. High-frequency percussive ventilation. *Crit Care Med.* 2005;33(3 Suppl): S241-S245.

70. Raoof S, Goulet K, Esan A, Hess DR, Sessler CN. Severe hypoxemic respiratory failure:

part 2—nonventilatory strategies. *Chest.* 2010;137(6):1437-1448.

71. Davies A, Jones D, Bailey M, et al. Extracorporeal membrane oxygenation for 2009 influenza A(H1N1) acute respiratory distress syndrome. *JAMA.* 2009;302(17):1888-1895.

72. Peek GJ, Clemens F, Elbourne D, et al. CESAR: conventional ventilatory support vs extracorporeal membrane oxygenation for severe adult respiratory failure. *BMC Health Serv Res.* 2006;6:163.

73. Peek GJ, Mugford M, Tiruvoipati R, et al. Efficacy and economic assessment of conventional ventilatory support versus extracorporeal membrane oxygenation for severe adult respiratory failure (CESAR): a multicentre randomised controlled trial. *Lancet.* 2009;374(9698):1351-1363.

74. Marasco SF, Lukas G, McDonald M, McMillan J, Ihle B. Review of ECMO (extra corporeal membrane oxygenation) support in critically ill adult patients. *Heart, Lung Circ.* 2008;17(Suppl 4):S41-S47.

75. Guerin C, Reignier J, Richard JC, et al. Prone positioning in severe acute respiratory distress syndrome. *N Engl J Med.* 2013;368(23):2159-2168.

76. Grinnan DC, Truwit JD. Clinical review: respiratory mechanics in spontaneous and assisted ventilation. *Crit Care.* 2005;9(5):472-484.

77. Lucangelo U, Bernabe F, Blanch L. Lung mechanics at the bedside: make it simple. *Curr Opin Crit Care.* 2007;13(1):64-72.

78. Polese G, Serra A, Rossi A. Respiratory mechanics in the intensive care unit. In: Gosselink R, Stam H, eds. *European Respiratory Monograph.* Vol. 31. United Kingdom: European Respiratory Society; 2005:195-206.

79. Raoof S. Monitoring during mechanical ventilation. In: Raoof S, Khan F, eds. *Mechanical Ventilation Manual.* Philadelphia, Pennsylvania: American College of Physicians; 1998:56-68.

80. Henderson WR, Sheel AW. Pulmonary mechanics during mechanical ventilation. *Respir Physiol Neurobiol.* 2012;180(2-3):162-172.

81. MacIntyre NR. Respiratory system mechanics. In: MacIntyre NR, Branson RD, eds. *Mechanical Ventilation.* 2nd ed. St. Loius, MO: Saunder Elsevier; 2009:159-170.

82. Bekos V, Marini JJ. Monitoring the mechanically ventilated patient. *Crit Care Clin.* 2007;23(3):575-611.

83. Ventilation with lower tidal volumes as compared with traditional tidal volumes for acute lung injury and the acute respiratory distress syndrome. *N Engl J Med.* 2000;342(18):1301-1308.

84. Peigang Y, Marini JJ. Ventilation of patients with asthma and chronic obstructive pulmonary disease. *Curr Opin Crit Care.* 2002;8(1):70-76.

85. Koh Y. Ventilatory management in patients with chronic airflow obstruction. *Crit Care Clin.* 2007;23(2):169-181, viii.

86. Mannam P, Siegel MD. Analytic review: management of life-threatening asthma in adults. *J Intens Care Med.* 2010;25(1):3-15.

87. Oddo M, Feihl F, Schaller MD, Perret C. Management of mechanical ventilation in acute severe asthma: practical aspects. *Intens Care Med.* 2006;32(4):501-510.

88. Johnson VE, Huang JH, Pilcher WH. Special cases: mechanical ventilation of neurosurgical patients. *Crit Care Clin.* 2007;23(2):275-290, x.

89. Ranieri VM, Rubenfeld GD, Thompson BT, et al. Acute respiratory distress syndrome: the Berlin Definition. *JAMA.* 2012;307(23):2526-2533.

90. Villar J, Perez-Mendez L, Kacmarek RM. Current definitions of acute lung injury and the acute respiratory distress syndrome do not reflect their true severity and outcome. *Intens Care Med.* 1999;25(9):930-935.

91. Ferguson ND, Kacmarek RM, Chiche JD, et al. Screening of ARDS patients using standardized ventilator settings: influence on enrollment in a clinical trial. *Intens Care Med.* 2004;30(6):1111-1116.

92. Slutsky AS. Ventilator-induced lung injury: from barotrauma to biotrauma. *Resp Care.* 2005;50(5):646-659.

93. Slutsky AS, Ranieri VM. Ventilator-induced lung injury. *N Engl J Med.* 2013;369(22):2126-2136.

94. Anzueto A, Frutos-Vivar F, Esteban A, et al. Incidence, risk factors and outcome of barotrauma in mechanically ventilated patients. *Intens Care Med.* 2004;30(4):612-619.

95. Haitsma JJ. Diaphragmatic dysfunction in mechanical ventilation. *Curr Opin Anaesthesiol.* 2011;24(2):214-218.

96. Tobin MJ, Laghi F, Jubran A. Narrative review: ventilator-induced respiratory muscle weakness. *Ann Intern Med.* 2010;153(4):240-245.

97. Kollef MH. Ventilator-associated complications, including infection-related complications: the way forward. *Crit Care Clin.* 2013;29(1):33-50.

98. Provost KA, El-Solh AA. Complications associated with mechanical ventilation. In: Tobin MJ, ed. *Principles and Practice of Mechanical Ventilation.* 3rd ed. New York: McGraw-Hill; 2013:973-993.

99. Magill SS, Klompas M, Balk R, et al. Executive summary: developing a new, national approach to

surveillance for ventilator-associated events. *Ann Am Thorac Soc.* 2013;10(6):S220-S223.

100. Hess DR, MacIntyre NR. Ventilator discontinuation: why are we still weaning? *Am J Respir Crit Care Med.* 2011;184(4):392-394.

101. MacIntyre NR, Cook DJ, Ely EW, Jr, et al. Evidence-based guidelines for weaning and discontinuing ventilatory support: a collective task force facilitated by the American College of Chest Physicians; the American Association for Respiratory Care; and the American College of Critical Care Medicine. *Chest.* 2001;120(6 Suppl):375S-395S.

102. Meade M, Guyatt G, Cook D, et al. Predicting success in weaning from mechanical ventilation. *Chest.* 2001;120(6 Suppl):400S-424S.

103. Rothaar RC, Epstein SK. Extubation failure: magnitude of the problem, impact on outcomes, and prevention. *Curr Opin Crit Care.* 2003;9(1):59-66.

104. Ram FS, Picot J, Lightowler J, Wedzicha JA. Non-invasive positive pressure ventilation for treatment of respiratory failure due to exacerbations of chronic obstructive pulmonary disease. *Coch Database System Rev.* 2004;(3):CD004104.

105. Vital FM, Ladeira MT, Atallah AN. Non-invasive positive pressure ventilation (CPAP or bilevel NPPV) for cardiogenic pulmonary oedema. *Coch Database System Rev.* 2013;5:CD005351.

106. Hilbert G, Gruson D, Vargas F, et al. Noninvasive ventilation in immunosuppressed patients with pulmonary infiltrates, fever, and acute respiratory failure. *N Engl J Med.* 2001;344(7):481-487.

107. Kwok H, McCormack J, Cece R, Houtchens J, Hill NS. Controlled trial of oronasal versus nasal mask ventilation in the treatment of acute respiratory failure. *Crit Care Med.* 2003;31(2):468-473.

108. Rabec C, Georges M, Kabeya NK, et al. Evaluating noninvasive ventilation using a monitoring system coupled to a ventilator: a bench-to-bedside study. *Eur Respir J.* 2009;34(4):902-913.

109. Storre JH, Magnet FS, Dreher M, Windisch W. Transcutaneous monitoring as a replacement for arterial PCO(2) monitoring during nocturnal non-invasive ventilation. *Resp Med.* 2011;105(1):143-150.

110. Brodie D, Bacchetta M. Extracorporeal membrane oxygenation for ARDS in adults. *N Engl J Med.* 2011;365(20):1905-1914.

111. Neumann P, Golisch W, Strohmeyer A, Buscher H, Burchardi H, Sydow M. Influence of different release times on spontaneous breathing pattern during airway pressure release ventilation. *Intens Care Med.* 2002;28(12):1742-1749.

112. Fan E, Checkley W, Stewart TE, et al. Complications from recruitment maneuvers in patients with acute lung injury: secondary analysis from the lung open ventilation study. *Resp Care.* 2012;57(11):1842-1849.

113. Brower RG, Lanken PN, MacIntyre N, et al. Higher versus lower positive end-expiratory pressures in patients with the acute respiratory distress syndrome. *N Engl J Med.* 2004;351(4):327-336.

114. Meade MO, Cook DJ, Guyatt GH, et al. Ventilation strategy using low tidal volumes, recruitment maneuvers, and high positive end-expiratory pressure for acute lung injury and acute respiratory distress syndrome: a randomized controlled trial. *JAMA.* 2008;299(6):637-645.

115. Mercat A, Richard JC, Vielle B, et al. Positive end-expiratory pressure setting in adults with acute lung injury and acute respiratory distress syndrome: a randomized controlled trial. *JAMA.* 2008;299(6):646-655.

The Acute Respiratory Distress Syndrome

19

Emily Fish, MD, MPH and Daniel Talmor, MD, MPH

KEY POINTS

1 Acute respiratory distress syndrome (ARDS) is characterized by a severe inflammatory process, which causes diffuse alveolar epithelial and capillary damage.

2 A number of medical and surgical conditions have been associated with the development of ARDS, with pneumonia and sepsis being the two most common predisposing conditions.

3 The Berlin definition of ARDS includes four diagnostic criteria: (1) bilateral opacities on chest radiograph or computed tomography, (2) P_aO_2/F_iO_2 300 mm Hg or less with 5 cm or more H_2O PEEP, (3) respiratory failure not fully explained by cardiogenic edema or volume overload, and (4) 7 days or less from predisposing clinical insult.

4 Severity of ARDS is classified by the Berlin definition according to P_aO_2/F_iO_2: mild (201-300), moderate (101-200), and severe (< 100).

5 Management strategies for ARDS are centered on treatment of the underlying clinical disorder while providing supportive care that minimizes ventilator-induced lung injury.

6 Current clinical practice guidelines for reducing lung injury include low tidal-volume ventilation, application of PEEP (while maintaining plateau pressures < 30 cm H_2O), and reduction of FiO_2 to lowest necessary value to maintain a goal oxygen saturation of 88% to 95%.

7 A number of novel therapies and ventilation strategies are currently under investigation.

8 Despite significant advancements in the diagnosis and management of ARDS over the last two decades, mortality estimates remain more than 30% with significant morbidity among survivors.

INTRODUCTION

The acute respiratory distress syndrome (ARDS) was first described in 1967 by Dr David Ashbaugh and colleagues.[1] ARDS is a life-threatening lung condition characterized by acute onset and rapidly progressive dyspnea, tachypnea, and hypoxemia. Several clinical precipitants are associated with the development of ARDS, including sepsis, pneumonia, aspiration, and transfusion of blood products. Pathogenesis is through a severe inflammatory process, which causes diffuse alveolar damage and alveolar capillary leakage, resulting in a ventilation-perfusion mismatch and poor lung compliance. A significant amount of basic and clinical research has resulted in a greater understanding of ARDS and subsequent improvement in outcomes through improved ventilatory strategies and supportive care of other organ systems. Morbidity and mortality, however, remain high. This chapter discusses the current understanding of the epidemiology, pathophysiology, management approaches, and prevention of ARDS.

Epidemiology

Accurate estimation of the incidence of ARDS is limited due to variations in diagnostic criteria over the last two decades. In 2005, a prospective cohort study estimated the incidence of acute lung injury (ALI) and ARDS to be approximately 190,600 cases annually in the United States.[2] Additional cross-sectional studies demonstrated that patients with ARDS represent approximately 5% of hospitalized, mechanically ventilated patients.[3] Over the last decade, there has been a decrease in the incidence of hospital-acquired ARDS, which has been attributed to overall improvements in the care of critically ill patients. However, it appears the incidence of community-acquired ARDS is unchanged.[4]

Prior literature has suggested that mortality from ARDS differs by sex and race, with males and African Americans suffering disproportionately lower survival rates.[5] This sex-related mortality difference may be partially explained by recent data suggesting sex differences exist in patient presentation and likelihood of development of ALI with males more likely than females to develop ALI. The same explanation was not true for race-related differences, as White patients were found more likely than Black patients to develop ALI.[6]

PATHOPHYSIOLOGY

Predisposing Conditions

A number of medical and surgical conditions have been associated with the development of ARDS. Traditionally, these disorders have been categorized into direct (pulmonary) lung injury or indirect (extrapulmonary) lung injury resulting from inflammatory disease states. Direct/pulmonary injuries account for the majority of cases, while pneumonia and sepsis are the two most common causes overall.[7] Table 19-1 summarizes pulmonary and extrapulmonary predisposing conditions.

TABLE 19-1 Predisposing conditions associated with development of ARDS.

Direct Lung Injury	Indirect Lung Injury
Pneumonia	Sepsis
Aspiration	Acute pancreatitis
Inhalation injury	Burns
Pulmonary contusion	Severe trauma
Near-drowning	Drug or alcohol overdose
Fat embolus	Cardiopulmonary bypass
Amniotic fluid embolus	Transfusion-related lung injury

Mechanism of Injury

ARDS is characterized by a severe inflammatory process, which causes diffuse alveolar epithelial and capillary damage, resulting in three distinct pathologic stages. During the acute exudative stage, increased alveolar capillary permeability leads to alveolar flooding with protein-rich fluid. A release of proinflammatory cytokines coupled with neutrophil extravasation into the alveoli leads to diffuse alveolar injury. Damage to type I and II alveolar cells results in exposition of the underlying basement membrane and impaired surfactant synthesis, respectively. Alveolar collapse ensues and is accompanied by alveolar hemorrhage and hyaline membrane formation. Approximately 7 to 14 days following the initial insult the second fibroproliferative stage begins, represented by varying degrees of neovascularization and fibrosis. From here, most patients enter into a subsequent resolution and repair phase. Few individuals, however, progress to a fibrotic stage resulting in obliteration of the normal lung architecture.[8]

CLINICAL FEATURES AND DIAGNOSIS

Clinical Presentation

The clinical features of ARDS typically manifest within 72 hours of the predisposing event and worsen rapidly. In addition to clinical findings related to the precipitating condition, patients typically present in

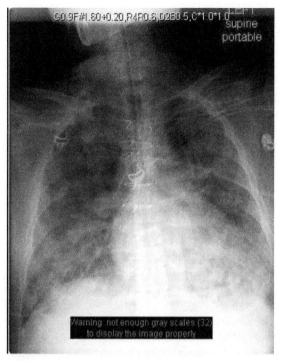

FIGURE 19–1 Chest radiograph of ARDS.

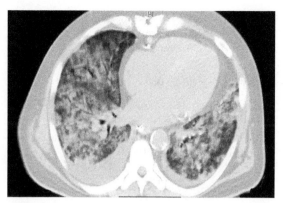

FIGURE 19–2 Chest computed tomography of ARDS.

respiratory distress with tachypnea, dyspnea, and hypoxemia. Laboratory evaluation reveals hypoxemia with an elevated alveolar-arterial gradient. Supplemental oxygenation is generally inadequate, and endotracheal intubation is often required. Imaging exhibits bilateral alveolar infiltrates on chest radiograph (CXR; Figure 19–1) and generalized airspace opacities on computed tomography (CT) with predominance in the dependent lung zones (Figure 19–2).

Diagnosis

In 1994, the American-European Consensus Conference (AECC) defined diagnostic criteria for ALI and ARDS which included four components: appropriate clinical setting, acute severe hypoxemia (defined as a ratio of $P_aO_2/F_iO_2 \leq 200$ mm Hg for ARDS), bilateral infiltrates on CXR, and unelevated pulmonary capillary wedge pressure (PCWP $\leq$ 18 mm Hg) or no clinical evidence of left atrial hypertension. The AECC used a P_aO_2/F_iO_2 threshold of 200 to differentiate ALI (P_aO_2/F_iO_2 201-300 mm Hg) from ARDS ($P_aO_2/F_iO_2 \leq 200$ mm Hg).[9]

Due to AECC definition limitations in sensitivity and reproducibility,[10] these criteria were reevaluated and eventually superseded by the Berlin definition of ARDS in 2012. Important modifications to the AECC definition include (1) specification of "acute" as 7 days or less from the predisposing event, (2) elimination of the use of PCWP to rule out cardiogenic edema, and (3) elimination of ALI as a diagnostic category and instead implementing a mild, moderate, and severe grading system.[11] Table 19–2 outlines the Berlin definition, which is the current standard for diagnosis.

There is ongoing research into the predictive value of plasma biomarkers for the diagnosis of ARDS. Several ARDS-associated biomarkers have been identified, such as Krebs von den Lungen-6, lactate dehydrogenase, receptor for advanced glycation end products, von Willebrand factor, and interleukin-8.[12] Definitive validation of the use of these biomarkers for

TABLE 19–2   2012 Berlin definition of ARDS.

1. Bilateral opacities on CXR or CT not fully explained by effusion, lung collapse, or nodules
2. P_aO_2/F_iO_2 300 mm Hg or less with 5 cm H_2O or more PEEP
3. Respiratory failure not fully explained by cardiogenic pulmonary edema or volume overload
4. About 7 or less days from predisposing clinical insult, or new/worsening symptoms within prior week
5. Severity classification
   Mild ARDS: P_aO_2/F_iO_2 201-300
   Moderate ARDS: P_aO_2/F_iO_2 101-200
   Severe ARDS: $P_aO_2/F_iO_2 < 100$

Data from ARDS Definition Task Force, Ranieri VM, Rubenfeld GD, et al: Acute respiratory distress syndrome: the Berlin Definition, *JAMA* 2012 Jun 20;307(23):2526-2533.

diagnosis has not been accomplished, however, and the diagnosis of ARDS remains a clinical one.

MANAGEMENT

Management strategies for ARDS are centered on treatment of the underlying clinical disorder while providing supportive care that minimizes ventilator-induced lung injury (VILI).

Mechanical Ventilation

The majority of patients with ARDS develop respiratory failure severe enough to necessitate mechanical ventilation. While positive-pressure ventilation helps to ensure adequate oxygenation, our understanding of the potential harms of mechanical ventilation has evolved over the last decade. There are four potential mechanisms of alveolar damage in ventilated patients with ARDS: (1) barotrauma caused by excessive airway pressures, (2) volutrauma caused by over distension of alveoli from high tidal-volume ventilation, (3) atelectrauma caused by shearing forces on alveoli from inspiratory opening and expiratory collapse, and (4) biotrauma caused by the release of proinflammatory cytokines from excessive mechanical forces on the lung.[13]

A substantial amount of basic and clinical research has been devoted to understanding optimal ventilator strategies to reduce VILI, which are summarized as follows.

Low Tidal-Volume Ventilation

One strategy for reducing lung injury during mechanical ventilation is the use of low tidal-volume (V_t) ventilation. This became the standard of care following the landmark National Heart, Lung, and Blood Institute's ARDS Network (ARDSNet) trial in 2000, in which a lower V_t (goal 6 mL/kg ideal body weight) with lower plateau-pressure (< 30 cm H_2O) was compared to a higher V_t and plateau-pressure (12 mL/kg ideal body weight and < 50 cm H_2O). Patients randomized to the low V_t/low plateau-pressure group had a reduced 28-day mortality and developed fewer instances of organ failure.[14] These findings have been confirmed by additional work showing increased intensive care unit and hospital mortality in patients ventilated with higher V_t.[15]

Positive End-Expiratory Pressure

Another strategy used to reduce injury during mechanical ventilation is the application of positive end-expiratory pressure (PEEP) to reduce cyclical alveolar opening/collapse. However, the optimal level of PEEP in ventilated patients with ARDS remains controversial given the opposing risks of alveolar overdistension and hemodynamic compromise. In a meta-analysis of trials comparing high-PEEP and low-PEEP strategies (14 cm H_2O vs ~8 cm H_2O), patients with moderate to severe ARDS ($P_aO_2/F_iO_2 \leq 200$) showed a small but significant improvement in survival among the higher PEEP group. However, this mortality benefit did not exist when all ARDS patients ($P_aO_2/F_iO_2 \leq 300$) were included in the analysis.[16] One possible explanation for these findings is that patients with moderate to severe ARDS (with more significant edema and potentially recruitable lung) may respond favorably to higher PEEP, whereas patients with mild ARDS (and less proportion of recruitable lung) may experience alveolar distension of their healthy, already-aerated lung tissue. At this time, clinical practice guidelines recommends titrating PEEP to maintain an oxygen saturation of 88% to 95% and a plateau pressure of 30 cm H_2O or less to avoid barotrauma.

Fraction of Inspired Oxygen

While the use of high concentrations of inspired oxygen (FiO_2) is commonly necessary, at least temporarily, for patients with severe ARDS, excessive use of high FiO_2 can cause a spectrum of lung injury. Cellular injury appears to be related to increased production of reactive oxygen species, which impair intracellular molecule function and cause cell death.[17] This can lead to damage of the airways and pulmonary parenchyma. Reducing the FiO_2 to the lowest tolerable level is desirable for all critically ill patients and particularly in patients with ARDS who have already sustained some form of lung injury.

Novel Ventilation Strategies

Transpulmonary pressure-guided ventilation— Transpulmonary pressure-guided ventilation uses an esophageal balloon-catheter to estimate pleural pressure and titrate PEEP to each individual's lung and chest wall mechanics. This approach targets a positive transpulmonary pressure (P_{TP}) to deliver enough PEEP to prevent repetitive airspace collapse yet avoiding alveolar overdistension. A preliminary single-centered trial showed that optimizing P_{TP} significantly improved oxygenation and lung mechanics compared to a conventional ventilation strategy.[18] Further investigations are being conducted to examine potential survival benefit.

High-frequency oscillation ventilation—High-frequency oscillation ventilation (HFOV) delivers very small tidal volumes at a high frequency (180-1800 per minute) in an effort to maintain a high mean airway pressure. The supporting theory is that sustaining a constant mean airway pressure during inspiration and expiration will prevent end-expiratory collapse. An initial randomized, controlled trial showed an early, transient improvement in oxygenation among patients ventilated with HFOV versus conventional ventilation.[19] However, a subsequent trial showed no significant differences between both groups and was stopped prematurely due to low inclusion.[20]

Airway pressure release ventilation—Airway pressure release ventilation is a mode of pressure-controlled mechanical ventilation, which applies continuous positive airway pressure for a prolonged time, followed by a release phase to a lower pressure for a shorter period of time. The prolonged high-pressure phase allows for maintenance of adequate lung volume and alveolar recruitment while the shorter low-pressure phase provides the majority of ventilation and carbon dioxide removal.[21] APRV was developed to provide lung recruitment while minimizing VILI. Several studies have shown APRV to improve clinical outcomes, such as oxygenation, lung recruitment, respiratory mechanics, and sedation requirement. However, thus far it has not been shown to improve mortality as compared to other lung protective ventilation strategies.[22]

Supportive Care

Patients with ARDS require diligent supportive care, including judicious use of sedatives, appropriate fluid management, and adequate nutritional support.

Sedation

The use of sedatives and analgesia in patients with ARDS improves ventilator tolerance[23] and decreases

oxygen consumption.[24] However, given the significant morbidity associated with excessive sedation, judicious use of agents is recommended. Moreover, improved outcomes have been demonstrated through the application of strategies for frequent sedation liberation and awakening as well as early mobilization.[25]

Fluid Management

Although the ARDS definition excludes patients with pulmonary edema exclusively due to volume overload or cardiogenic etiologies, an estimated 30% of patients with ARDS have an elevated pulmonary artery occlusion pressure less than 18 mm Hg. Even in patients without elevated filling pressures, a positive fluid balance is associated with poorer outcomes.[26] Thus, conservative fluid management for patients with hemodynamic stability and adequate urine output may be beneficial in patients with ARDS.

Nutritional Support

Given the tremendously catabolic state present among patients with ARDS, nutritional support is advantageous. Enteral feedings are preferable if the gastrointestinal tract is acceptable for intake. Theoretically, enteral feeds with increased fat and decreased carbohydrates should result in less carbon dioxide production, thereby decreasing the degree of respiratory acidosis. The ARDSNet EDEN trial showed no difference in physical function, survival, or cognitive performance among patients receiving trophic versus full enteral feedings.[27]

Novel Therapies

Paralysis

Neuromuscular blocking agents are used to achieve paralysis and decrease ventilator dyssynchrony. Improved patient–ventilator synchrony is thought to reduce VILI by improving control of low tidal-volume ventilation and decreasing the inflammatory response.[28] In patients with ARDS, early, short-term paralysis has been shown to improve mortality without a significant increase in development of muscle weakness.[29]

Prone Positioning

Prone positioning results in improved oxygenation through three primary mechanisms. First, redistribution of blood flow to healthier lung regions results in a decreased ventilation perfusion mismatch and recruitment of dependent lung units.[30] Mechanically, lung tissue relieved of compression from anterior mediastinal and abdominal structures. Lastly, clearance of respiratory secretions is improved with an associated reduction in ventilator-associated pneumonia.[31] For patients with severe ARDS ($P_aO_2/F_iO_2 \leq 100$ mm Hg), early application of prone positioning has been shown to confer a survival benefit at 28 and 90 days.[32]

Extracorporeal Membrane Oxygenation

During extracorporeal membrane oxygenation (ECMO) blood is rerouted outside the body to an external membrane oxygenator, which acts as an artificial lung to facilitate adequate gas exchange. Major risks include bleeding due to anticoagulation (in particular, intracranial hemorrhage) and complications of large bore vascular access. While initial studies showed no improvement in mortality, a more recent trial suggested a potential survival benefit for patients put on ECMO,[33] though other studies have not reproduced this benefit. Currently, ECMO is reserved as an option for rescue therapy for patients with severe ARDS and refractory hypoxemia.

Pulmonary Vasodilator Pharmacotherapy

Inhaled vasodilators, such as nitric oxide (NO) have been used in ARDS to improve oxygenation by selectively dilating pulmonary arterial vasculature and decreasing ventilation/perfusion mismatching. While inhaled NO has been shown to improve oxygenation in some ARDS patients with refractory hypoxemia, it has not shown a reduction in mortality.[34] Thus, inhaled NO has not used routinely and is instead reserved for patients with intractable hypoxemia.

PROGNOSIS AND OUTCOMES

Despite significant advancements in the diagnosis and management of ARDS over the last two decades, recent mortality estimates remain more than 40%.[35] Recent studies have suggested an improvement in survival over time; however, this appears to instead reflect a shift in clinical trials to enroll patients with less severe ARDS.[37]

Among patients who survive ARDS, there is frequently appreciable morbidity that persists years later. Decreased functionality, impaired exercise intolerance, negative psychosocial sequelae, and decreased quality of life have been shown to persist up to 5 years following discharge.[38]

REFERENCES

1. Ashbaugh DG, Bigelow DB, Petty TL, Levine BE. Acute respiratory distress in adults. *Lancet.* 1967;2(7511):319-323.
2. Rubenfeld GD, Caldwell E, Peabody E, et al. Incidence and outcomes of acute lung injury. *N Engl J Med.* 2005;353(16):1685-1693.
3. Esteban A, Ferguson ND, Meade MO, et al. Evolution of mechanical ventilation in response to clinical research. *Am J Respir Crit Care Med.* 2008;177(2):170-177.
4. Li G, Malinchoc M, Cartin Ccba R, et al. Eight-year trend of acute respiratory distress syndrome: a population-based study in Olmsted County, Minnesota. *Am J Respir Crit Care Med.* 2011;183(1):59-66.
5. Erickson SE, Shlipak MG, Martin GS, et al. Racial and ethnic disparities in mortality from acute lung injury. *Crit Care Med.* 2009;37(1):1-6.
6. Lemos-Filho LB, Mikkelsen ME, Martin GS, Artigas A, Brigham KL, et al. Sex, race, and the development of acute lung injury. *Chest.* 2013;143(4):901-909.
7. Ware LB and MA Matthay. The acute respiratory distress syndrome. *N Engl J Med.* 2000;342(18):1334-1349.
8. Matthay MA and Zemans RL. The acute respiratory distress syndrome: pathogenesis and treatment. *Annu Rev Pathol.* 2011;6:147-163.
9. Bernard GR, et al. Report of the American-European consensus conference on ARDS: definitions, mechanisms, relevant outcomes and clinical trial coordination. The Consensus Committee. *Intensive Care Med.* 1994;20(3):225-232.
10. Esteban A, Fernandez-Segoviano P, Frutas-Vivar F, et al. Comparison of clinical criteria for the acute respiratory distress syndrome with autopsy findings. *Ann Intern Med.* 2004;141(6):440-445.
11. Ranieri VM, Rubenfeld GD, Thompson BT, et al. Acute respiratory distress syndrome: the Berlin Definition. *JAMA.* 2012;307(23):2526-2533.
12. Terpstra ML, Aman J, van Nieuw Amerongen GP, Groeneveld AB. Plasma biomarkers for acute respiratory distress syndrome: a systematic review and meta-analysis*. *Crit Care Med.* 2014;42(3):691-700.

13. Slutsky AS, Ranieri VM. Ventilator-induced lung injury. *N Engl J Med*. 2013;369(22):2126-2136.

14. The Acute Respiratory Distress Syndrome Network. Ventilation with lower tidal volumes as compared with traditional tidal volumes for acute lung injury and the acute respiratory distress syndrome. *N Engl J Med*. 2000;342(18):1301-1318.

15. Determann RM, Royakkers A, Wolthuis EK, et al. Ventilation with lower tidal volumes as compared with conventional tidal volumes for patients without acute lung injury: a preventive randomized controlled trial. *Crit Care*. 2010;14(1):R1.

16. Briel M, Meade M, Mercat A, et al. Higher vs lower positive end-expiratory pressure in patients with acute lung injury and acute respiratory distress syndrome: systematic review and meta-analysis. *JAMA*. 2010;303(9):865-873.

17. Fridovich I. Oxygen toxicity: a radical explanation. *J Exp Biol*. 1998;201(Pt 8):1203-1209.

18. Talmor D, Sarge T, Malhotra A, et al. Mechanical ventilation guided by esophageal pressure in acute lung injury. *N Engl J Med*. 2008;359(20):2095-2104.

19. Derdak S, Mehta S, Stewart TE, et al. High-frequency oscillatory ventilation for acute respiratory distress syndrome in adults: a randomized, controlled trial. *Am J Respir Crit Care Med*. 2002;166(6):801-808.

20. Ferguson ND, Cook DJ, Guyatt GH, et al. High-frequency oscillation in early acute respiratory distress syndrome. *N Engl J Med*. 2013;368(9):795-805.

21. Daoud EG Airway pressure release ventilation. *Ann Thorac Med*. 2007;2(4):176-179.

22. Maung AA, Kaplan LJ. Airway pressure release ventilation in acute respiratory distress syndrome. *Crit Care Clin*. 2011;27(3):501-509.

23. Hansen-Flaschen J. Improving patient tolerance of mechanical ventilation. Challenges ahead. *Crit Care Clin*. 1994;10(4):659-671.

24. Swinamer DL, Phang PT, Jones RL, Grace M, King EG. Effect of routine administration of analgesia on energy expenditure in critically ill patients. *Chest*. 1988;93(1):4-10.

25. Pandharipande P, Banaerjee A, McGrane, S, Ely EW. Liberation and animation for ventilated ICU patients: the ABCDE bundle for the back-end of critical care. *Crit Care*. 2010;14(3):157.

26. Wiedemann HP, Wheeler AP, Bernard GR, et al. Comparison of two fluid-management strategies in acute lung injury. *N Engl J Med*. 2006;354(24):2564-2575.

27. Rice TW, Wheeler AP, Thompson BT, et al. Initial trophic vs full enteral feeding in patients with acute lung injury: the EDEN randomized trial. *JAMA*. 2012;307(8):795-803.

28. Forel JM, Roch A, Marin V, et al. Neuromuscular blocking agents decrease inflammatory response in patients presenting with acute respiratory distress syndrome. *Crit Care Med*. 2006;34(11):2749-2757.

29. Papazian L, Forel JM, Gacouin A, et al. Neuromuscular blockers in early acute respiratory distress syndrome. *N Engl J Med*. 2010;363(12):1107-1116.

30. Pelosi P, Brazzi L, Gattinoni L. Prone position in acute respiratory distress syndrome. *Eur Respir J*. 2002;20(4):1017-1028.

31. Sud S, Friedrich JO, Taccone P, et al. Prone ventilation reduces mortality in patients with acute respiratory failure and severe hypoxemia: systematic review and meta-analysis. *Intensive Care Med*. 2010;36(4):585-599.

32. Guerin C, Reignier J, Richard JC, et al. Prone positioning in severe acute respiratory distress syndrome. *N Engl J Med*. 2013;368(23):2159-2168.

33. Peek GJ, Mugford M, Tiruvoipati R, et al. Efficacy and economic assessment of conventional ventilatory support versus extracorporeal membrane oxygenation for severe adult respiratory failure (CESAR): a multicentre randomised controlled trial. *Lancet*. 2009;374(9698):1351-1363.

34. Adhikari NK, Dellinger RP, Lundin S, et al. Inhaled nitric oxide does not reduce mortality in patients with acute respiratory distress syndrome regardless of severity: systematic review and meta-analysis. *Crit Care Med*. 2014;42(2):404-412.

35. Villar J, Blanco J, Anon JM, et al. The ALIEN study: incidence and outcome of acute respiratory distress syndrome in the era of lung protective ventilation. *Intensive Care Med*. 2011;37(12):1932-1941.

36. Erickson SE, Martin GS, Davis JL, Matthay MA, Eisner MD. Recent trends in acute lung injury mortality: 1996-2005. *Crit Care Med*. 2009;37(5):1574-1579.

37. Phua J, Badia JR, Adhikari NK, et al. Has mortality from acute respiratory distress syndrome decreased over time?: A systematic review. *Am J Respir Crit Care Med*. 2009;179(3):220-227.

38. Herridge MS, Tansey CM, Matte A, et al. Functional disability 5 years after acute respiratory distress syndrome. *N Engl J Med*. 2011;364(14):1293-1304.

Venous Thromboembolism

Erica Bang, MD and
Stephen M. Pastores, MD, FACP, FCCP, FCCM

KEY POINTS

1. Venous thromboembolism (VTE) continues to elude diagnosis due to its diverse presentations and etiologies.

2. Proximal deep vein thromboses (DVT) have a 90% likelihood of progressing to pulmonary embolism (PE).

3. Although DVT and PE have similar risk factors and many overlapping features, the risk of death within 1 month is far higher in patients with PE than with DVT; thus, aggressive management for PE is recommended compared to isolated DVT.

4. Risk stratification based on pretest probability results in a cost-effective and practical diagnostic evaluation of VTE.

5. The major complications of anticoagulant therapy for VTE are hemorrhage and heparin-induced thrombocytopenia.

6. Focus must lie in the diagnosis, treatment, and prevention in order to improve survival of the critically ill patient with VTE.

INTRODUCTION

Venous thromboembolism (VTE), manifested as either deep venous thrombosis (DVT) or pulmonary embolism (PE), is a leading cause of morbidity and mortality in the critically ill patient. Standardizing for age and race, the incidence of VTE in the United States is approximately 70 to 120 cases per 100,000 individuals. The incidence of VTE increases exponentially as the population ages although no difference is apparent between genders. The high incidence of VTE is mainly dominated by PE diagnosed at autopsy and as a contributory factor in 4% to 11% of deaths. Despite appropriate therapy, 1% to 8% of patients with PE will not survive and others will experience long-term complications including postphlebitic syndrome (40%) and chronic thromboembolic pulmonary hypertension (4%). In the International Cooperative Pulmonary Embolism Registry, the death rate was 58% in patients who were hemodynamically unstable at the time of presentation and 15% among those who were hemodynamically stable.

VTE often eludes diagnosis due to its wide variety of presentations and diverse pathophysiological mechanisms. The diagnosis of PE is confirmed by objective testing in only about 20% of patients. Accurate diagnosis of VTE can minimize the risk of thromboembolic events and complications related to unnecessary anticoagulation and treatment. Consequently, the Agency for Healthcare Research and Quality ranks prevention of VTE as the first priority out of 79 preventive initiatives that can improve patient safety in healthcare settings.

Because DVT and PE have a spectrum of presentations, they have been approached by many clinicians in an algorithmic manner to address diagnosis, treatment, and prevention. The clinical presentation of VTE ranges from asymptomatic tachycardia to respiratory failure and hemodynamic instability. Additionally, VTE can occur spontaneously or from predisposing risk factors, catheter related, and may arise from genetic predisposition. In more than half of the cases, VTE is provoked by surgery, immobilization, advanced age, pregnancy, the use of oral contraceptives, or hormone-replacement therapy. The difficulty for clinicians lies in the early recognition and prompt treatment of VTE because of these widely diverse presentations. Prevention of DVT/PE in the ICU patient also poses many difficulties in choosing the appropriate regimen for prevention based on the risk-benefit ratios. The goal is to prevent recurrence because this can be fatal in approximately 5% of patients and prolonged therapy with anticoagulants in itself carries bleeding risks.

RISK FACTORS AND PATHOPHYSIOLOGY

Risk factors for VTE include increased age (≥ 40 years), obesity, prior VTE, malignancy, prolonged immobilization, major surgery, trauma, cardiac failure, pregnancy, hormone replacement therapy, and oral contraceptive therapy. Critically ill patients are especially at high risk for VTE due to severe underlying disease, immobility, and central venous catheterization.

According to Virchow's triad, the pathophysiology of thrombosis lies in three mechanisms: vessel wall injury, stasis, and hypercoagulability. A failure of one of these components leads to clot formation and DVT/PE. Hypercoagulable states may be inherited or acquired. The inherited type should be expected in patients with recurrent or life-threatening VTE, family history of thromboembolism, those younger than 45 years old, no acquired risk factors, and females with multiple miscarriages. Inherited risk factors for VTE include factor V Leiden (activated protein C resistance), protein C and S deficiency, antithrombin III deficiency, prothrombin gene mutation, dysfibrinogenemia, and disorders of plasminogen. Acquired hypercoagulable states include antiphospholipid antibody syndrome (anticardiolipin antibodies, lupus anticoagulant) and hyperhomocysteinemia.

The location of the VTE is another factor in risk evaluation and treatment with anticoagulation. The most common site of DVT is the calf vein but only 15% to 20% will extend proximally into the deep proximal veins. The deep vein thromboses that are of significance are those that occur more proximally, which typically is in the posterior tibial vein and the common femoral vein. Those with proximal vein thromboses have a 90% likelihood of developing PE. Identifying high-risk thrombi in the proximal veins is imperative to prevent the progression to PE; superficial veins thromboses rarely are associated with PE. Hypercoagulable states can also lead to venous thromboses in the superior and inferior vena cava (IVC), renal veins, and hepatic veins.

Upper extremity DVT can occur and involve the brachial, axillary, and subclavian veins and can extend proximally to the brachiocephalic vein, internal jugular vein, or superior vena cava. They account for less than 10% of all DVTs and approximately 75% are provoked by the placement of pacemakers and central venous catheters either in the internal jugular or in subclavian vein. In addition, right atrial thrombi can occur due to venous catheters or cardiac disease, such as atrial fibrillation, cardiomyopathy, ventricular aneurysms, and malignancy. About 5% of patients with arm DVT will have a PE, 20% will have postthrombotic syndrome, and 8% will have recurrence if untreated.

The hypoxemia that is observed in patients with PE is caused by the ventilation-perfusion mismatch resulting from increased physiologic dead space and intrapulmonary shunting. This is commonly associated with increases in minute ventilation and airways resistance, decreased vital and diffusion capacities, and in patients with a potentially patent foramen ovale, progressive pulmonary hypertension may lead to intra-arterial right-to-left shunting and severe refractory hypoxemia. Hemodynamic instability may result from the obstruction of the pulmonary circulation and increase in pulmonary vascular resistance, which impedes right ventricular outflow leading to reduced left ventricular preload and ultimately, a decreased cardiac output. Patients with underlying cardiopulmonary disease are more likely not to tolerate increases in pulmonary artery pressures and thus are more susceptible to developing right heart failure.

CLINICAL PRESENTATION

The clinical presentation of VTE can extend to a wide spectrum of signs and symptoms which present a multitude of diagnostic challenges. Both DVT and PE can present with nonspecific signs and symptoms, such as shortness of breath, fever, tachycardia, pain, and even no symptoms at presentation. However, both can have specific presentations, such as patients with DVT can present with erythema, leg swelling, tenderness, or pain, whereas those with acute PE can present with chest pain, dyspnea, unexplained sustained hypotension, hemoptysis, syncope, increased P_2 on physical exam, right heart failure, respiratory failure, and death. It is important to note that many of the signs and symptoms of PE may frequently be seen in patients with concomitant cardiac and pulmonary disease, and that these manifestations may be a result of a coexisting disease or a superimposed acute PE.

Acute PE can be massive or massive. Massive PE is characterized by hypotension (defined as a systolic blood pressure < 90 mm Hg) or shock and accounts for 5% of all cases of PE. Submassive PE is variably defined on the basis of right ventricular (RV) enlargement, dysfunction, ischemia, or strain on echocardiography, computed tomography (CT), or with cardiac biomarkers (troponins or B-type natriuretic peptide, BNP) with no associated hemodynamic instability.

DIAGNOSTIC WORKUP

The diagnostic workup for VTE should be tailored to the severity of the clinical presentation and depends on whether the patient is hemodynamically stable or hemodynamically unstable. Clinical judgment and clinical prediction rules are useful in establishing a pretest probability of DVT and PE in which patients are typically classified into low-, moderate-, or high-risk categories. These clinical prediction rules should drive the diagnostic workup and facilitates the interpretation of diagnostic tests.

IMAGING STUDIES

Acute DVT

Several imaging modalities are available to detect acute DVT, including venous ultrasonography, impedance plethysmography, computed tomography (CT) venography, magnetic resonance imaging (MRI), and contrast venography. Venous ultrasonography of the lower extremities is the preferred noninvasive test for the diagnosis of symptomatic proximal DVT. Failure to demonstrate collapsibility or flow indicates a DVT. Venous ultrasonography has a very high sensitivity and specificity of 95% and 98%, respectively. Additionally, both compression and Doppler ultrasonography can be used to diagnose upper extremity DVT.

Impedance plethysmography uses electrical current to estimate venous outflow obstruction when blood flows out of the leg venous system after release of a thigh pressure cuff. Failure to change impedance is presumptive evidence of a proximal DVT. However, other forms of venous obstruction and congestive heart failure can provide false-positive results.

MRI and CT venography can be highly accurate and have the advantage of evaluating both PE and DVT in a single study. However, MRI is expensive, time consuming, and restricted in patients with metallic devices and the additional irradiation associated with CT venography may not be desirable. Contrast venography is invasive and also requires radiocontrast material and should only be considered if noninvasive testing is nondiagnostic or impossible to obtain.

Pulmonary Embolism

Initial evaluation of a patient with suspected PE with nonspecific symptoms should include examination of the electrocardiogram for tachycardia, T-wave and ST-segment changes, and right- or left-axis deviation, arrhythmias, and less commonly for the classic pattern of $S_1Q_3T_3$, right ventricular strain, and new, incomplete right bundle branch block. Chest radiography is usually abnormal in more than 80% of patients with PE and helps to rule out and identify other conditions, such as pneumothorax, rib fracture, pneumonia, and pulmonary edema. Classic radiographic signs suggestive of PE include Westermark's sign (focal decrease in vascularity or oligemia distal to the pulmonary artery occlusion) and Hampton's hump (wedge-shaped opacity at the costophrenic angle indicating pulmonary infarction).

CT angiography has essentially replaced ventilation/perfusion (V/Q) scan and pulmonary angiography as the diagnostic imaging modality of choice in patients with suspected PE. In the Prospective Investigation of Pulmonary Embolism Diagnosis II (PIOPED II) trial, CT angiography had sensitivity and specificity rates of 83% and 96%, respectively. Limitations of CT angiography include the risk of adverse reactions to contrast (nephrotoxicity or anaphylaxis) and lack of portability.

Ventilation-perfusion scans are generally reserved for patients with renal failure or allergy to contrast dye. A normal V/Q scan essentially rules out PE. However, V/Q scanning is diagnostic in only 30% to 50% of patients with suspected PE. In PIOPED II with the exclusion of patients with intermediate or low probability scans, the sensitivity of a high probability (PE present) scan finding was 77%, whereas the specificity of very low probability or normal (PE absent) scan finding was 98%. Contrast-enhanced magnetic resonance angiography may also be useful in patients with suspected PE in whom radiographic contrast material or ionizing radiation are relatively contraindicated (eg, renal failure and pregnancy).

Echocardiography (transthoracic or transesophageal) is particularly useful in patients suspected of acute PE who may not be stable for transport for CT angiography or V/Q scanning and may also help to guide management. Classic echocardiography signs of PE on echocardiography include dilatation and hypokinesis of the right ventricle, McConnell's sign (free wall RV hypokinesis that spares the apex), paradoxical motion of the interventricular septum, tricuspid regurgitation, and lack of collapse of the IVC during inspiration. Transesophageal echocardiography can confirm the diagnosis of PE by showing emboli in the main pulmonary arteries. Right ventricular dysfunction defined as RV dilation (apical 4-chamber RV diameter divided by LV diameter > 0.9) or RV systolic dysfunction is associated with increased mortality in patients with acute PE. Additionally, among hemodynamically stable patients with PE, the association between an increased troponin level and RV dysfunction on echocardiography identifies a subgroup of patients at particularly high risk for an adverse outcome.

Pulmonary angiography remains the gold standard for diagnosis of PE. However, it is invasive and associated with several complications including renal failure, respiratory failure and bleeding and thus is now rarely utilized for diagnosis of PE.

LABORATORY FINDINGS

D-Dimer

D-dimer is a specific fibrin degradation product that has been widely studied in patients with acute DVT and PE. The rapid enzyme-linked immunosorbent assay is the most commonly used method for measurement of D-dimer. When used in conjunction with a low clinical pretest probability for VTE, D-dimer testing is very sensitive and has a high negative predictive value in excluding the presence of DVT. Several studies have shown that D-dimer testing can decrease the need for further testing such as repeat venous ultrasonography. However, the specificity rates of D-dimer testing are low particularly in patients with cancer, pregnant women, and hospitalized and elderly patients.

Arterial Blood Gas

Arterial blood gases (ABG) have a limited role in diagnosing acute PE. In those with PE associated with hemodynamic instability, the ABG typically shows hypoxemia with an increased alveolar-arterial (A-a) gradient. However, in the PIOPED study, 7% of patients with angiographically documented PE had completely normal ABG measurements. Due to the increase in minute ventilation, patients with PE can demonstrate normal or decreased pCO_2 and respiratory alkalosis.

Cardiac Biomarkers

Elevated levels of serum troponin I or T are noted in 30% to 50% of patients with a moderate or large PE and can indicate RV strain, ischemia, or impending myocardial infarction and are predictive of a poor outcome. One meta-analysis showed that elevated levels of troponin were associated with an increase in the short-term risk of death by a factor of 5.2 (95% confidence interval [CI], 3.3-8.4) and an increase in the risk of death from PE by a factor of 9.4 (95% CI, 4.1-21.5).

BNP (and its precursor, N-terminal pro-BNP) are released in response to increased cardiac filling pressure and are frequently elevated in patients with significant PE. Similar to patients with PE who have elevated troponins, patients with elevated levels of BNP and pro-BNP have an increased risk of an adverse in-hospital outcome as compared with patients with normal levels.

Algorithms for DVT and PE

Validated algorithms are important to evaluate patients with suspected DVT along with objective testing to confirm the diagnosis. Risk factors for DVT should be identified including malignancy, recent surgery, history of prolonged bed rest or immobilization, obesity, lower extremity trauma, pregnancy, and use of oral contraceptives or hormone replacement therapy. The 2012 American College of Chest Physicians (ACCP) consensus guidelines recommend the following goals for nonpregnant patients with a suspected first DVT of the lower extremity: reduce overall false negatives to 2% or less as defined by symptomatic DVT or PE within 3 to 6 months after a negative test; reduce the risk of fatal PE after testing less than 0.1%, and reduce the risk of fatal hemorrhage due to anticoagulation to less than 0.1%. The guidelines endorse using the Wells score for risk stratification of patients for likelihood of DVT into low-, moderate-, and high-risk categories. The Wells criteria for DVT include risk factors, such as active cancer, bedridden recently more than 3 days or major surgery within 4 weeks, calf swelling more than 3 cm compared to the other leg, collateral superficial veins present, entire leg swollen leg, localized tenderness along the deep venous system, pitting edema greater in the symptomatic leg, previously documented DVT and alternative diagnosis to DVT as likely or more likely. Wells score of 4 or less is consistent with a low (5%) pretest probability for DVT; 4.5 to 6 is consistent with a moderate (17%) pretest probability, and more 6 with a high (53%) pretest probability of DVT (Table 20–1).

TABLE 20–1 Wells criteria and pretest probability of DVT.

Wells Score	Probability of DVT
Low	5%
Moderate	17%
High	53%

In patients with a low pretest probability for DVT in the leg, the guidelines recommend checking either a moderately or highly sensitive D-dimer and compression ultrasound of the proximal leg veins rather than whole leg ultrasound. D-dimer testing is preferred over compression ultrasound of the proximal veins as the initial test. If D-dimer is negative, no further testing is necessary; if D-dimer is positive, compression ultrasound of the proximal leg veins should be performed, and if this is positive, then the patient should be treated without further testing.

In patients with a moderate pretest probability for DVT in the leg, the guidelines recommend checking either a highly sensitive D-dimer (unless the patient has a comorbid condition that would likely elevate the D-dimer level, such as cancer or recent surgery or trauma), compression ultrasound of the proximal leg veins, or whole leg ultrasound. If the highly sensitive D-dimer is negative, then no further testing is needed. If the highly sensitive D-dimer is positive, then compression ultrasound of the proximal leg veins or the whole leg is recommended. A negative ultrasound should lead to a repeat compression ultrasound in 1 week and checking a moderate/high sensitivity D-dimer. If the compression ultrasound is negative, no further testing is warranted. If the D-dimer test is negative, no further testing is needed. If whole leg ultrasound is chosen and is negative, no further testing is also recommended. If compression ultrasound of the proximal leg veins or whole leg ultrasound is positive, the patient should be treated without further testing. If whole leg ultrasound is only positive for isolated distal (calf vein) DVT, serial ultrasounds are recommended to ensure the DVT does not propagate proximally rather than treating with anticoagulation. Approximately 15% to 20% of calf vein thrombi can extend into the proximal veins especially within the first 7 days; thus the need for serial ultrasound examinations.

In patients with a high pretest probability for DVT in the leg, the guidelines recommend either compression ultrasound of proximal leg veins or whole leg ultrasound. If either ultrasound examination is positive, the patient should be treated without further testing. If the whole leg ultrasound is negative for DVT, no further testing is recommended. If the compression ultrasound of the proximal leg veins is negative, one can either repeat the ultrasound in 1 week and if negative no further testing is recommended, or check a high sensitivity D-dimer and if negative, no further testing is needed. If D-dimer is positive, repeat compression ultrasound in one week is recommended and if negative, no further testing. D-dimer should not be used as a stand-alone test to rule out DVT in patients with a high pretest probability for DVT.

A diagnostic algorithm (Figure 20–1) with a dichotomized version of the Wells clinical decision rule, D-dimer testing, and CT has been shown to be useful in guiding management decisions in almost 98% of patients with clinically suspected PE.

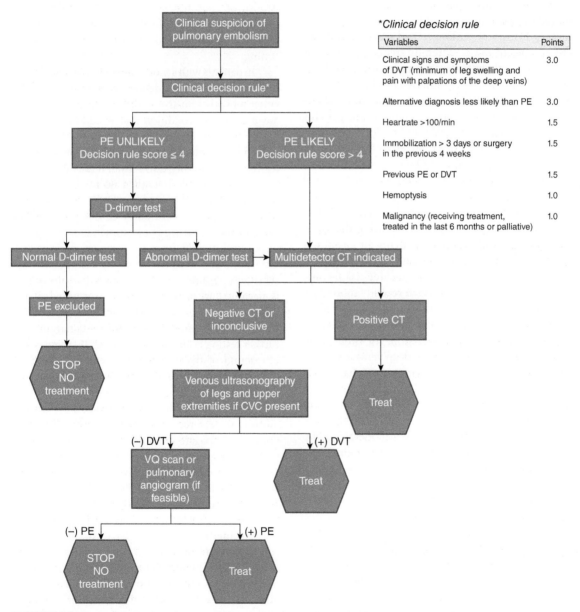

FIGURE 20–1 Diagnostic algorithm in patients with clinically suspected PE. (*Reproduced with permission from Pastores SM: Management of venous thromboembolism in the intensive care unit, J Crit Care. 2009 Jun;24(2):185-191.*)

TREATMENT

Anticoagulation

In patients with a high clinical suspicion of acute DVT, treatment with parenteral anticoagulants is recommended while awaiting the results of diagnostic tests. For those with documented DVT and PE, anticoagulation is the mainstay of treatment if no contraindications exist. The recently released 2016 ACCP guidelines suggest the use of direct oral anticoagulants (DOACs) such as dabigatran, rivaroxaban, apixaban, or edoxaban over vitamin K antagonist (VKA) in patients with DVT of the leg or PE and no cancer. For patients with DVT of the leg or PE and no cancer who are not treated with DOACs, the guidelines suggest the use of VKA therapy over low-molecular weight heparin (LMWH). Initial parenteral anticoagulation with unfractionated heparin or LMWH is given before dabigatran and edoxaban, is not given before rivaroxaban and apixaban, and is overlapped with VKA therapy. In patients with DVT of the leg or PE and cancer, LMWH is favored over VKA therapy and DOACs for the first 3 months. Routine use of compression stockings to prevent postthrombotic syndrome is not recommended in patients with acute DVT or PE who are treated with anticoagulants.

With regards to duration of therapy, at least 3 months of anticoagulation is recommended in patients with a proximal DVT of the leg or PE provoked by surgery or by a nonsurgical transient risk factor. After 3 months of treatment, patients with unprovoked DVT of the leg or PE should be evaluated for the risk-benefit ratio of extended therapy. Extended anticoagulant therapy is recommended in patients with a first VTE that is an unprovoked proximal DVT of the leg or PE and who have a low or moderate bleeding risk.

Administration of IV heparin is usually undertaken using the weight-based heparin dosing nomogram where patients receive a loading bolus dose of 80 units/kg followed by an 18 units/kg/h per hour infusion. The heparin dose is adjusted to maintain an activated partial thromboplastin time of 1.5 to 2.3 times control. IV heparin is favored in LMWH have greater bioavailability when given by SC injection, do not require strict laboratory monitoring, and have a lower risk of heparin-induced thrombocytopenia (HIT) compared with UFH. Enoxaparin, dalteparin, and tinzaparin are approved for use in the United States. Enoxaparin is typically given at 1 mg/kg SC twice daily or 1.5 mg/kg SC daily, while tinzaparin is given at 175 units/kg SC once daily. Monitoring antifactor Xa levels typically 4 hours after injection may be considered in patients who are morbidly obese, pregnant patients, and patients with renal insufficiency. Fondaparinux is given at a dose of 5 mg SC once daily for patients weighing less than 50 kg, 7.5 mg SC once daily for patients weighing 50 to 100 kg, and 10 mg SC once daily for patients weighing more than 100 kg. Caution should be observed in patients with renal impairment as both LMWH and fondaparinux are retained in these patients.

UFH is suggested for patients with renal impairment (creatinine clearance < 30 mL/min). Warfarin for the treatment of VTE is not ideal in ICU patients given the many drug and food interactions associated with its use and genetic variations in drug metabolism.

Complications of Anticoagulation

The major complications of anticoagulant therapy are hemorrhage and HIT. The frequency of major bleeding was reported at 1.9% and a fatal hemorrhage rate of 0.2% in a large meta-analysis involving over 15,000 patients treated with either UFH or LMWH. HIT is an immune-mediated adverse reaction to heparin that is associated with thrombocytopenia and can lead to venous and arterial thrombosis. Commonly, there is an otherwise unexplained fall in platelet count (absolute thrombocytopenia or > 50% decrease if the platelet nadir remains in the normal range) 5 to 10 days following exposure to heparin. In patients who develop HIT, the heparin should be immediately discontinued and direct thrombin inhibitors such as argatroban or lepirudin should be administered if anticoagulation continues to be required.

In patients receiving UFH or LMWH who develop clinically significant or devastating hemorrhage, protamine sulfate can be administered although the anticoagulant effect of LMWH is only partially reversed. Allergic reactions and bradycardia are side effects of protamine.

Thrombolytic Therapy

The guidelines recommend the use of systemically administered thrombolytic agents (alteplase, streptokinase, and alteplase) in patients with acute PE associated with hypotension (systolic BP < 90 mm Hg) who do not have a high bleeding risk. Thrombolysis may also be considered in selected patients with acute PE not associated with hypotension and with low bleeding risk whose initial clinical presentation or clinical course suggests a high risk of developing hypotension. In the Pulmonary Embolism Thrombolysis (PEITHO) trial published in 2014, the administration of tenecteplase plus heparin was associated a significant reduction in all-cause mortality or hemodynamic decompensation within 7 days, when compared to placebo plus heparin in patients with intermediate-risk PE (acute PE associated with RV dysfunction on echocardiography and myocardial injury as evidenced by a positive troponin I or T test). However, thrombolytic treatment with tenecteplase was associated with a 2% incidence of hemorrhagic stroke. Short-term infusion times (eg, 2-hour infusion of 100 mg of alteplase) through a peripheral vein are suggested over prolonged infusion times and over a pulmonary artery catheter, respectively. Urokinase and streptokinase are given as a loading dose (streptokinase 250,000 units over 30 minutes) followed by continuous infusion of 100,000 units/hour for 24 hours; urokinase 4400 units/kg over 10 minutes followed by a continuous infusion of 4400 units/kg/h for 12 to 24 hours. Heparin infusion is typically continued after thrombolytic therapy. Contraindications to thrombolysis include surgery in the past 10 days, recent puncture or invasion of noncompressible vessels, recent intracerebral hemorrhage or stroke, uncontrolled hypertension, recent trauma, pregnancy, hemorrhagic retinopathy, other sites of potential bleeding, and infective endocarditis. Thrombolytic therapy should be tailored to the complicated ICU patient and risks and benefits heavily weighed prior to administration.

Inferior Vena Cava Filter

The guidelines recommend the use of an IVC filter in patients with acute PE and contraindications to anticoagulation. No randomized clinical trial (RCT) has evaluated IVC filters as sole therapy in patients with DVT. IVC filters may increase the risk of recurrent DVT and do not reduce the risk of PE or alter mortality. If an IVC filter is indicated in a patient with acute DVT or PE because anticoagulant therapy is temporarily contraindicated (eg, active bleeding), a retrievable filter may be inserted and subsequently removed when it is safe to start anticoagulant therapy. Patients who have an IVC filter inserted should receive a conventional course of anticoagulation (eg, parenteral and long-term anticoagulation) if the contraindication to anticoagulation resolves and should be treated for the same length of time similar to patients who had not had an IVC filter placed. For upper extremity DVT, some institutions can place superior vena cava filters although these are associated with high complication rates than IVC filters; thus, their use should be confined to exceptional circumstances in specialized centers. The risk of recurrent pulmonary emboli after IVC filter placement is 2% to 3%. Complications of IVC filter placement include venous thrombosis at the site of filter insertion, procedural complications, filter malposition and migration, caval occlusion, and sepsis due to device infection. Permanent IVC filters may also predispose to postthrombotic syndrome.

Other Modalities

Surgical pulmonary embolectomy is recommended only in patients with acute PE who have contraindications to thrombolysis, have failed thrombolysis or catheter-assisted embolectomy, or shock that is likely to cause death before thrombolysis can take effect (eg, within hours), provided surgical expertise and resources are available. Mortality from emergency pulmonary embolectomy can be as high as 30% and should be performed only in highly specialized centers.

Other modalities that have investigated include interventional catheterization techniques for massive such as mechanical fragmentation of thrombus with a standard pulmonary artery catheter, clot pulverization with a rotating basket catheter, percutaneous rheolytic thrombectomy, or pigtail rotational catheter embolectomy. Pharmacologic thrombolysis and mechanical interventions are usually combined unless bleeding risk is high.

PREVENTION

Due to the significant morbidity and mortality associated with VTE, prevention is pivotal particularly in high-risk patients, such as those admitted to the ICU. Prevention lies in risk stratification and focusing on identifying preventable or predisposing conditions, such as hypercoagulability and immobility. The Padua Risk Assessment Model (RAM) is the best available validated predictor for DVT/PE risk. Patients scored as low risk (RAM < 4) have a 0.3% risk of developing a DVT and do not require prophylaxis, while those scored as high-risk (RAM score ≥ 4) have a 2.2% risk of developing a DVT and require prophylaxis. The guidelines recommend against the use of pharmacologic prophylaxis or mechanical prophylaxis for acutely ill-hospitalized medical patients at low risk of thrombosis. However, the Padua prediction score should not be utilized in critically ill patients who already have an elevated risk for DVT/PE. Patients at moderate or high risk of developing DVT/PE by the Padua prediction score including all critically ill patients who are not bleeding or at high risk for bleeding should receive anticoagulant thromboprophylaxis with either LMWH, UFH, or fondaparinux. Screening for asymptomatic DVT with routine ultrasounds in critically ill patients is not recommended.

Intermittent pneumatic compression devices or graduated compression stockings should be used for patients who are bleeding or at high risk for bleeding. These patients should be switch to anticoagulant prophylaxis as soon as bleeding resolves or once the bleeding risk is considered to be low. Patients considered to be high risk for bleeding and warrant compression devices over anticoagulant prophylaxis include patients with active gastroduodenal ulcer, bleeding in 3 months prior to admission and platelets less than 50,000 mm³.

REFERENCES

1. Goldhaber SZ, Visani L, De Rosa M. Acute pulmonary embolism: clinical outcomes in the International Cooperative Pulmonary Embolism Registry (ICOPER). *Lancet.* 1999;353:1386-1389.
2. Seligsohn Uri, Lubetsky A. Genetic susceptibility to venous thrombosis. *N Engl J Med.* 2001;344:1222-1231.
3. Scarvelis D, Wells PS. Diagnosis and treatment of deep-vein thrombosis. *CMAJ.* 2006;175(9):1087-1092.
4. Dentali F, Douketis JD, Gianni M, et al. Meta-analysis: anticoagulant prophylaxis to prevent symptomatic venous thromboembolism in hospitalized medical patients. *Ann Intern Med.* 2007;146(4):278-288.
5. White RH. The epidemiology of venous thromboembolism. *Circulation.* 2003;107(23 Suppl 1): I4-I8.
6. Agnelli G, Becattini C. Acute pulmonary embolism. *N Engl J Med.* 2010;363:266-274.
7. Samama MM. An epidemiologic study of risk factors for deep vein thrombosis in medical outpatients: the Sirius study. *Arch Intern Med.* 2000;160(22):3415-3420.
8. Heit JA, Silverstein MD, Mohr DN, et al. Risk factors for deep vein thrombosis and pulmonary embolism: a population-based case-control study. *Arch Intern Med.* 2000;160(6):809-815.
9. Bates SM, Jaeschke R, Stevens SM, et al. Diagnosis of DVT. *Chest.* 2012;141:e351S-e418S.
10. Kearon C, Akl EA, Comerota AJ, et al. Antithrombotic therapy for VTE disease: Antithrombotic Therapy and Prevention of Thrombosis, 9th ed: American College of Chest Physicians Evidence-Based Clinical Practice Guidelines. *Chest.* 2012;141(2 suppl):e419-e494S.
11. Guyatt GH, Akl EA, Crowther M, et al. Executive summary: Antithrombotic Therapy and Prevention of Thrombosis, 9th ed: American College of Chest Physicians Evidence-Based Clinical Practice Guidelines. *Chest.* 2012;141(2 suppl):7S-47S.
12. Jaff MR, McMurthy MS, Archer SL, et al. Management of massive and submassive pulmonary embolism, iliofemoral deep vein thrombosis, and chronic thromboembolic pulmonary hypertension: a scientific statement from the American Heart Association. *Circulation.* 2011;123(16):1788-1830.
13. Klok FA., Inge CM Mos, Huisman MV. Brain-type natriuretic peptide levels in the prediction of adverse outcome in patients with pulmonary embolism: a systematic review and meta-analysis. *Am J Respir Crit Care Med.* 2008;178:425-430.
14. Bates SM, Greer IA, Hirsh J, Ginsberg JS. Use of antithrombotic agents during pregnancy: the Seventh ACCP Conference on Antithrombotic and Thrombolytic Therapy. *Chest.* 2004;126(3 Suppl): 627S-644S.
15. Wells P, Anderson DR, Rodger M, et al. Evaluation of D-dimer in the diagnosis of suspected deep-vein thrombosis. *N Engl J Med.* 2003;349(13):1227-1235.

16. Schulman S, Kearon C, Kakkar AK, et al. Dabigatran versus warfarin in the treatment of acute venous thromboembolism. *N Engl J Med.* 2009;361:2342-2352.

17. Stein P, Fowler SE, Goodman LR, et al. Multidetector computed tomography for acute pulmonary embolism. *N Engl J Med.* 2006;354(22):2317-2327.

18. Kuo WT, Gould MK, Louie JD, et al. Catheter-directed therapy for the treatment of massive pulmonary embolism: systematic review and meta-analysis of modern techniques. *J Vasc Interv Radiol.* 2009;20:1431-1440.

19. Pastores SM. Management of venous thromboembolism in the intensive care unit. *J Crit Care.* 2009;24:185-191.

20. Stein PD, Woodard PK, Weg JG, et al. Diagnostic pathways in acute pulmonary embolism: recommendations of the PIOPED II investigators. *Am J Med.* 2006;119(12):1048-1055.

21. Wells PS, Owen C, Doucette S, Fergusson D, Tran H. Does this patient have deep vein thrombosis? *JAMA.* 2006;295(2):199-207.

22. Tapson VF. Acute pulmonary embolism. *N Engl J Med.* 2008;358(10):1037-1052.

23. Meyer G, Vicaut E, Danays T, et al. Fibrinolysis for patients with intermediate-risk pulmonary embolism. *N Engl J Med.* 2014;370(15):1402-1411.

24. Konstantinides SV, Torbicki A, Agnelli G, et al. 2014 ESC guidelines on the diagnosis and management of acute pulmonary embolism. *Eur Heart J.* 2014;35(43):3033-3069.

25. Kearon C, Akl EA, Ornelas J, et al. Antithrombotic therapy for VTE Disease: CHEST Guideline and Expert Panel Report. *Chest.* 2016;149(2):315-352.

Shock: Diagnosis and Management

*Kevin C. Doerschug MD, MS, FCCP and
Gregory A. Schmidt, MD, FCCP*

KEY POINTS

1. Shock is acute circulatory failure threatening multiple organ systems and demands prompt diagnosis and urgent resuscitation.

2. The main types of shock are hypovolemic, cardiogenic, and distributive shock.

3. Shock must be managed rapidly by identifying and treating acute, reversible causes; restoring intravascular volume; infusing vasoactive drugs; using mechanical adjuncts, when applicable; and supporting vital functions until recovery.

4. Bedside goal-directed echocardiography should be performed to clarify or confirm the etiology of shock; identify readily treatable contributors (such as tension pneumothorax or cardiac tamponade); and seek clues to fluid responsiveness.

5. A comprehensive assessment of the adequacy of perfusion is useful to guide resuscitation, rather than merely aiming for an arbitrary mean arterial pressure.

INTRODUCTION

Shock is acute circulatory failure threatening multiple organ systems and producing a grave threat to survival. Most patients will be hypotensive (mean arterial blood pressure [MAP] < 60 mm Hg) and are often tachycardic, tachypneic, and exhibit overt end-organ dysfunction, such as oliguria, encephalopathy, or lactic acidosis (Table 21–1). The basis for shock may be readily evident from the presentation, such as following trauma, or when symptoms or signs of hemorrhage, fluid loss, or sepsis are evident. A subset of shock patients will have normal blood pressure (even hypertension is possible); many will also lack tachycardia. In such patients, the diagnosis may be challenging, especially since there is such interindividual variance in normal values for blood pressure. Subtle or atypical presentations of shock may require a high index of clinical suspicion. Initially, shock is reversible, but rapidly progresses to cellular injury, cell death, failure of critical organ systems, and an irreversible state that terminates in death. Timely resuscitation blunts inflammation and mitochondrial damage, potentially reducing the burden of early and late morbidity. Because delays in

TABLE 21–1 Recognizing shock.

Hypotension
Tachycardia
Tachypnea, respiratory failure, or respiratory alkalosis
Encephalopathy, anxiety, or agitation
Oliguria or AKI
Lactic acidosis
Skin mottling, cool extremities, cyanosis, livedo reticularis
Low mixed venous or central venous oxyhemoglobin saturation values

resuscitation may be lethal, shock demands prompt diagnosis and urgent resuscitation.

DIFFERENTIAL DIAGNOSIS OF SHOCK

Shock is divided into three types: hypovolemic, cardiogenic, or distributive. In a patient with new-onset shock, it is usually possible to categorize the type of shock within minutes based on a concise history and targeted examination. In a patient with shock, a wide pulse pressure accompanied by warm extremities and brisk capillary refill is evidence of high cardiac output (CO; distributive shock). Alternatively, a narrow pulse pressure, cool extremities, and delayed capillary refill suggest low CO. Low CO shock is comprised of hypovolemia and pump failure. In the subset of low output shock, an assessment of intravascular volume can further differentiate hypovolemia from cardiogenic causes of shock. Bedside goal-directed echocardiography[1] (GDE) should be performed to clarify or confirm the etiology of shock (Table 21–2); identify readily treatable contributors (such as tension pneumothorax or cardiac tamponade); and seek clues to fluid-responsiveness.

Certainly, there may be overlapping causes, as in the patient with septic shock who has both hypovolemic (before resuscitation) and distributive components; or following calcium channel blocker overdose when there may be both cardiogenic and distributive contributors. These more complex cases can generally be recognized by a systematic approach of performing GDE; identifying fluid responsiveness; estimating global perfusion through venous oximetry, lactate clearance, or measures of stroke volume; and repeating these measures until shock remits or a diagnosis is established. For patients already critically ill who progress to new shock, discerning the type may rely on more invasive measurements or diagnostic steps.

TOOLS FOR DIAGNOSIS AND MONITORING OF RESPONSE

Lactic Acid Levels and Clearance

Shock often produces significantly elevated blood levels of lactic acid; sometimes this precedes hypotension and serves as an early indicator.[2] In a similar vein, successful resuscitation typically produces

TABLE 21–2 Manifestations of the types of shock.

	Hypovolemic	Cardiogenic	Distributive
Symptoms	Overt blood or other fluid loss	Those of acute cardiovascular disease	Those of infection, inflammation, intoxication, or other
Signs	Cool, clammy extremities	Cool, clammy extremities	Warm extremities, bounding or normal pulses
Pulse pressure	Low	Low	Normal or high
Cardiac output or stroke volume	Low	Low	Normal or high
Venous oxyhemoglobin saturation	Low	Low	Normal or high
Lactic acid concentration	High	High	High
Goal-directed echo findings	IVC small, varying with respiration	IVC full; RV, LV, or valve dysfunction; pericardial effusion	Normal or hyperdynamic
Central venous pressure (or pulmonary wedge pressure)	Low	High	Any

rapidly falling values. In a trial of early goal-directed therapy, targeting a lactate clearance of 10% was as good as aiming for normal central venous oxyhemoglobin saturation.[3] Moreover, normalization of lactate values is strongly associated with survival.[4] For patients with low CO shock (hypovolemic or cardiogenic), the genesis of hyperlactatemia is easy to understand: limited oxygen delivery to tissues cripples oxidative metabolism, causing tissues to shift to anaerobic production of ATP, and increases the generation and release of lactic acid. The lactic acidosis of sepsis (and perhaps some other forms of distributive shock) is more complex. In some patients, tissues may be deprived of oxygen, especially before resuscitation or perhaps in the mesenteric circulation, and produce lactic acid anaerobically. Yet many resuscitated septic patients have high CO, total body oxygen delivery, venous saturations, and tissue oxygen saturations,[5] along with oxidation-reduction ratios that do not support a theory of anaerobic metabolism. These findings cannot exclude oxygen lack, since microvascular dysfunction[6] and maldistribution of blood flow[7] may create hidden zones of hypoxia. Nevertheless, other mechanisms are likely, including enhanced aerobic glycolysis through activation of Na+/K ATPase, perhaps mediated by catecholamines.[8] This may be one reason that treatments for shock directed at augmenting oxygen delivery fail to lower lactic acid values or improve outcomes.[9,10]

Venous Oximetry

Venous oximetry entails measuring the oxyhemoglobin saturation of central or mixed venous blood. Although central and mixed venous values are not identical, they are closely related and usually change in the same direction. Venous oximetry relies on the Fick Principle for oxygen, stating that the difference between arterial and venous oxygen contents is related inversely to the CO as long as oxygen consumption is constant. Because clinicians defend the arterial content value by maintaining minimum values for arterial saturation, low CO tends to be matched by a low venous saturation value. Some support for the importance of venous oximetry derives from the trial of Early Goal-Directed Therapy in which resuscitation based on central venous oximetry during the first 6 hours of septic shock

led to improved survival.[11] Similarly, in trauma patients, low venous saturation was a better harbinger of blood loss than conventional hemodynamic parameters.[12] On the other hand, resuscitation of a broad population of critically ill subjects according to mixed venous oxyhemoglobin saturation had no impact on outcome.[13]

Pulmonary Artery Catheter

The pulmonary artery catheter (PAC) has been widely used to assess CO; mixed venous oxygen saturation; and intrapulmonary and intra-cardiac pressures, and provides a wealth of derived information on the systemic and pulmonary circulation. However its use in the ICU, once considered the standard of care for hemodynamic monitoring, has declined in the last decade due to lack of mortality benefit in critically ill patients,[14] and even in congestive heart failure.[15] Newer, less invasive technologies have largely supplanted the PAC for most critical care monitoring and are considered as follows.

Near-Infrared Spectroscopy

The continuous measurement of oxyhemoglobin saturation in thenar capillaries by near-infrared spectroscopy (NIRS) has the promise of directly monitoring the microvasculature. This technique has provided an early warning of shock progression during acute hemorrhage following trauma.[16] Moreover, the microvascular dysfunction of septic shock is related to organ failures,[6] while increased microcirculatory flow during resuscitation is associated with reduced subsequent organ dysfunction.[17] Static NIRS measures generally normalize, however, presumably due to shunting and cellular dysoxia, and so may be less useful during prolonged shock states.

Stroke Volume Estimation

Stroke volume can be estimated through a variety of techniques, such as arterial pulse contour analysis, bioreactance, bioimpedance, CO_2 rebreathing, and pulse-wave Doppler analysis of the left ventricular outflow tract. These methods all demonstrate reasonable correlations with invasive measures of stroke volume, with the advantage of minimally or noninvasive technology. None has been shown to improve outcomes in patients with shock so their potential value remains inconclusive. Further, since large studies of hemodynamic optimization using the PAC failed to demonstrate improved outcomes, it seems unlikely that gathering similar information noninvasively will produce major advances in care.

Goal-Directed Echocardiography

Bedside GDE is now commonplace for the assessment of shock in the ICU, emergency department, and on rapid-response teams. Typically, an intensivist acquires four standard chest views to evaluate ventricular size and function, along with a subcostal view of the inferior vena cava. It allows for rapid assessment, often serially in a patient with rapidly changing conditions, and can prove to be crucial in cases of unsuspected ventricular dysfunction, hypovolemia, cardiac tamponade, or severe acute valve failure. The subcostal view is especially helpful in assessing the inferior vena cava, showing significant cyclic variation with respiration in hypovolemic states, as discussed as follows.[18]

MANAGEMENT OF SHOCK

Shock is managed (1) at an urgent tempo; and by (2) identifying and treating acute, reversible causes; (3) restoring intravascular volume; (4) infusing vasoactive drugs; (5) using mechanical adjuncts, when applicable; and (6) supporting vital functions until recovery.

Tempo of Management

Minutes matter when recognizing and resuscitating shock. This principle is emphasized in speaking of the "golden hour" in which the circulation and tissue perfusion are restored before progressive tissue injury and organ failures that rapidly become refractory to subsequent attempts at resuscitation. This golden hour is a time-honored tenet in trauma, and more recently recognized to be also pertinent in septic shock. The initial Early Goal Directed Therapy (EGDT) trial demonstrated that rapid resuscitation to endpoints of central venous pressure, mean arterial pressure, and central venous oxyhemoglobin saturation within 6 hours of presentation improved outcomes compared to a less-aggressive resuscitation.[11] Three subsequent trials of

septic shock did not confirm the utility of the original EGDT protocol.[19-21] However, the mortality rates reported in these later trials, performed in an era when aggressive early resuscitation was the norm, were significantly lower than in previous reports. One interpretation of these results is that, while the appropriate endpoints of resuscitation remain unclear, an environment that favors early, aggressive resuscitation improves outcomes in septic shock.

The appropriate endpoints of shock resuscitation remain elusive. Importantly, resuscitation to an arbitrarily set MAP of at least 65 mm Hg is not sufficient and possibly not necessary. As an example, treatment with a nitric oxide synthase inhibitor leads to increased blood pressures and lower catecholamine use, but also increased mortality.[22] These seemingly contradictory effects of therapy may be explained by discrepancies between systemic hemodynamics and the microcirculation; lack of validity of the targets of macrovascular resuscitation (perhaps MAP is less important than believed); or to unrecognized adverse effects of the drug. Several studies have compared specific blood pressure targets finding that achieving a MAP of higher than 65 mm Hg (such as 75 or 85 mm Hg) does not improve outcomes. Targeting microvascular resuscitation is attractive in theory, but real-time assessments of microvascular function are not readily available for clinical use, and effective methods to safely and reliably increase microvascular function have not been found. We advocate a comprehensive assessment of the adequacy of perfusion to guide resuscitation, rather than merely aiming for an arbitrary mean arterial pressure. Serial assessments are likely to be valuable since shock and its resuscitation can produce dramatic changes within hours.

Identify and Treat Reversible Causes

Several causes of shock require specific identification and treatment because general supportive measures will surely fail. Good examples include tension pneumothorax, cardiac tamponade, and ruptured abdominal aortic aneurysm (Table 21–3). These can be subtle at times, requiring a careful, systematic approach to shock. Intensivist-conducted ultrasound has changed fundamentally the initial examination of the shock patient. Its ability to quickly signal cardiac dysfunction, pericardial

TABLE 21-3 Differential diagnosis of shock.

Hypovolemic shock
  Intravascular hypovolemia
    Hemorrhagic shock (GI, trauma, aortic rupture, etc)
    Renal loss (diuresis, osmotic loss, diabetes insipidus)
    Gastrointestinal loss (diarrhea, vomiting)
    "Third space" loss (pancreatitis, postsurgical, sepsis, anaphylaxis, trauma, toxin, idiopathic systemic capillary leak syndrome)
  Venodilation
    Anaphylaxis
    Neurogenic shock
    Drugs (sedatives, analgesics, nitrates, Ca-channel blockers)
  Impaired cardiac filling
    Cardiac tamponade
    High pleural pressure (PEEP, autoPEEP, tension pneumothorax, massive effusion, abdominal compartment syndrome)
    Other obstruction to cardiac filling (tumor, thrombus)

Cardiogenic shock
  Arrhythmia (fast or slow)
  Systolic LV or RV dysfunction
    Ischemia
    Cardiomyopathy
    Metabolic derangement
    Drugs (Ca-channel blockers, beta-blockers, other)
    Sepsis
    Myocardial contusion
    Toxins
  Diastolic dysfunction
    Ischemia
    Hypertrophy
    Restrictive cardiomyopathy
    Tamponade (as above)
  Excessive afterload
    Pulmonary embolism
    Aortic stenosis; hypertrophic obstructive cardiomyopathy
    ARDS and its treatment (elevated alveolar pressure)
    Malignant hypertension
  Valve dysfunction
    Aortic insufficiency
    Papillary muscle rupture
    Endocarditis
    Mitral stenosis
  Device malfunction (ECMO, VAD, IABP)

Distributive (high cardiac output) shock
  Sepsis
  Hepatic failure (acute and chronic)
  Adrenal insufficiency
  Thiamine deficiency
  Toxins (salicylate, cyanide, carbon monoxide)
  Thyroid storm
  Arteriovenous shunts
  Cellular dysoxia (prolonged shock states)

effusion, hypovolemia, deep vein thrombosis, pulmonary embolism-in-transit, pneumothorax, aortic rupture, free peritoneal blood, traumatic injuries, sources of sepsis, and other crucial findings makes ultrasound an essential skill for early diagnosis.[23] Moreover, the intensivist can repeat the ultrasound examination at will to judge the response to interventions or identify complications.

The timing of antibiotics in confirmed or suspected septic shock deserves specific mention in relation to the tempo of shock resuscitation. Appropriate antibiotics must be given within the first hour following the recognition of septic shock. Antibiotic therapy is frequently delayed and often ineffective for the final microbiologic diagnosis. Orders may be delayed due to diagnostic confusion and caregiver attention toward invasive procedures and hemodynamic resuscitation. Systems issues between ordering and administering antibiotics also contribute to these delays. Regardless of cause, delays in appropriate antibiotic administration worsen mortality by approximately 8% per hour of delay.[24] For these reasons, broad-spectrum antibiotics should be ordered and administered promptly after a diagnosis of shock when sepsis is in the differential, preferably guided by preplanned order sets. Antibiotics should then be tailored to microbial susceptibilities, as these data are available, or discontinued promptly if an alternative etiology of shock is identified.

Restoring Intravascular Volume

Rapid restoration of intravascular volume is an essential principle of shock resuscitation since fluids may promptly restore perfusion and prevent organ failures. Fluids should be infused at a rapid pace (usually much faster than typical ICU infusion pumps will allow), and in sufficient volume (which can be many liters). This practice allows for periodic reevaluation for clinical response: slower infusions of small volumes may confound the perception of response. Although colloid-containing fluids have some theoretical advantages over crystalloids, clinical trials generally show equivalence. Some colloids, especially synthetic starches, are clearly detrimental and should not be used.[25] Because crystalloids are more widely available, cheaper, and at least as effective, they are preferred for shock resuscitation. Although vasomotor function and vasopressors are both less active in acidemic environments, attempts to correct a metabolic acidosis with bicarbonate infusions do not speed resuscitation nor reduce vasopressor requirements, and may lead to worsening intracellular acidosis. Accordingly, bicarbonate infusions should be avoided.

In the setting of acute traumatic shock, questions have been raised about the targets of early fluid resuscitation. Potential downsides of restoring blood pressure to normal before surgical exploration include dilution of clotting factors, hypothermia, and an increased rate of hemorrhage as arterial pressure rises. Several studies suggest that delayed fluid resuscitation for victims of penetrating trauma (aiming for a systolic blood pressure of 70 mm Hg) might improve outcomes.[26] Concerns about the risks of persisting hypotension and doubts about whether these data can be generalized to the broad group of patients with traumatic shock have limited its appeal.

While the importance of urgent fluid resuscitation is undeniable, many patients with shock fail to respond, especially following initial resuscitation when shock is due to sepsis.[27] Indiscriminant fluid may produce harm by causing pulmonary edema or other organ failures so, especially in the sickest patients with lung and renal failure, an effort should be made to predict fluid responsiveness. In this regard, static measures of the central venous and pulmonary artery occlusion pressures have been shown invalid[28] and have been supplanted by dynamic indicators. High-volume positive-pressure ventilation produces pleural pressure changes that affect stroke volume in a cyclical fashion (largely by varying right atrial filling), giving rise to larger fluctuations in stroke volume; vascular flow; and vena caval diameter in preload-dependent individuals. A 13% variation in pulse pressure with breathing is highly sensitive and specific for predicting fluid responders.[29] Similarly, useful cutoff values have been determined for variations in vena caval diameter (superior and inferior); aortic and brachial artery flow velocity; left ventricular outflow tract velocity-time integral; and cardiac volumes derived from bioimpedance and bioreactance. Prerequisites for validity include tidal volume of 8 to 12 mL/kg; a fully passive patient; regular cardiac rhythm; and the absence of acute cor pulmonale. Since this tidal volume is larger than generally appropriate, the ventilator should be adjusted before the measurement of variation in order to produce the conditions for validity but then returned to lung-protective volumes. Passive leg raising is a reliable indicator of fluid-responsiveness irrespective of ventilation mode and cardiac rhythm,[30] but is not reliable when there is severe intra-abdominal hypertension. By returning blood held in the capacitance veins to the circulation and thereby raising stroke volume in patients who are on the ascending limb of the Starling curve, it avoids potentially harmful fluid boluses in patients who will not benefit. This method is particularly useful for patients who cannot easily be made passive on the ventilator.

Infusing Vasoactive Drugs

In addition to careful assessment and restoration of circulatory volume, many patients in shock require vasoactive infusions. Norepinephrine is the preferred initial agent given its potency, relatively low propensity to induce arrhythmias, and association with improved mortality compared to dopamine.[31] To avoid injury caused by accidental infiltration of vasoconstrictors into peripheral tissues, norepinephrine and other vasopressors should be infused through central venous or intraosseous catheters. However, in keeping with the urgent tempo of shock resuscitation, vasoactive infusions into severely ill patients should not be delayed merely because central access is not yet available. Similarly, vasopressors should not be initiated without attempts to restore circulating volume, yet severely ill patients should be resuscitated simultaneously with vasopressors and fluids, with titration of the vasopressors as circulating volume is restored.

The initiation of vasoactive infusions may also provide additional important clues to the underlying physiology. For example, norepinephrine consistently increases blood pressure. However, a concomitant increase in lactic acidosis and fall in venous oxyhemoglobin should prompt reevaluation for inadequate fluid loading or for cardiogenic shock.

When cardiogenic shock is identified or suspected, inotropic agents, such as dobutamine are useful. Like norepinephrine, careful examination during dobutamine initiation may identify additional physiologic perturbations. A rise in arterial pressure (or decrease in norepinephrine requirements) after initiating inotropic agents supports cardiogenic shock physiology. Because dobutamine also causes some arteriolar dilation, if arterial pressure falls with dobutamine one may suspect inadequate

preload or, alternatively, a severely dysfunctional myocardium.

Mechanical Adjuncts for Circulatory Support

When ventricular dysfunction is so extensive that it is refractory to vasoactive infusions (or when valvular incompetence contributes to cardiogenic shock), mechanical adjuncts to aid circulation may be employed. Ideally, these devices are employed as a bridge to definitive correction of the cardiac dysfunction. Intra-aortic balloon counterpulsation has been used extensively in this fashion for decades, although more recent evidence show that it does not improve outcomes in patients with acute myocardial infarction or cardiogenic shock.[32,33] Veno-arterial extracorporeal membrane oxygenation (ECMO) also provides circulatory support and can be employed rapidly, even during cardiopulmonary resuscitation. The practice of E-CPR (initiation of ECMO within 15 minutes of cardiac arrest) may lead to improved patient outcomes. Ventricular assist devices (VADs) also provide circulatory support: while slower to employ than ECMO, VADs may be more appropriate for medium- and even long-term support.

General Supportive Care

Patients in shock often have deranged cerebral perfusion and metabolic encephalopathy that would benefit from endotracheal intubation and mechanical ventilation. In severe shock states, lactic acidosis leads to increased respiratory effort, which subsequently increases lactate production, diverts blood flow to respiratory muscles, and draws CO from other vital organs. Mechanical ventilation (either invasive or noninvasive) may decrease oxygen consumption and increase vital organ blood flow and should be considered even in the absence of encephalopathy.

Because shock is usually characterized by inadequate oxygen delivery, increasing arterial oxygen content through transfused red blood cells may be helpful, particularly when shock results from massive hemorrhage. However, this theoretical benefit of transfusions must be balanced with its negative effects, including circulatory overload, inflammatory effects, and immune suppression as well as recognition that transfused red cells may exhibit impaired oxygen carrying capacity. Studies in patients with acute gastrointestinal hemorrhage and in those with septic shock show that liberal transfusion strategies (to keep the [Hgb] > 9 g/dL) are no better and may be inferior to restrictive targets ([Hgb] > 7 g/dL).[34,35] While there may be some patients in whom higher targets for hemoglobin may be appropriate (eg, acute coronary syndrome, low central venous oxyhemoglobin saturation despite resuscitation, and other overt manifestation of anemia), we recommend that transfusion be avoided in most patients with shock until the hemoglobin falls lower than 7 g/dL. It is even possible that lower targets could be beneficial for some patients, but these have not been tested.

Critically ill patients with shock have historically been considered fragile, leading to orders for strict bed rest and minimization of physical interventions. More recently, early physical and occupational therapy has been shown safe for critically ill patients and effective in preserving functional independence.[36] Many of the subjects in this and similar studies have been in shock, on vasoactive infusions, suggesting that shock is not a contraindication to mobilization. Some patients experience a decrease in vasoactive infusion requirements following mobility sessions suggesting a previously unrecognized, but important intervention for the management of shock.

REFERENCES

1. Schmidt GA, Koenig S, Mayo PH. Shock: ultrasound to guide diagnosis and therapy. *Chest.* 2012;142:1042-1048.
2. Howell MD, Donnino M, Clardy P, et al. Occult hypoperfusion and mortality in patients with suspected infection. *Intensive Care Med.* 2007;33:1892-1899.
3. Jones AE, Shapiro NI, Trzeciak S, et al. Lactate clearance vs central venous oxygen saturation as goals of early sepsis therapy: a randomized clinical trial. *JAMA.* 2010;303:739-746.
4. Puskarich MA, Trzeciak S, Shapiro NI, et al. Whole blood lactate kinetics in patients undergoing quantitative resuscitation for severe sepsis and septic shock. *Chest.* 2013;143:1548-1553.
5. Boekstegers P, Weidenhofer S, Kapsner T, et al. Skeletal muscle partial pressure of oxygen in patients with sepsis. *Critical Care Med.* 1994;22:640-650.
6. Doerschug KC, Delsing AS, Schmidt GA, et al. Impairments in microvascular reactivity are related to organ failure in human sepsis. *Am J Physiol Heart Circ Physiol.* 2007;293:H1065-H1071.
7. Walley KR. Heterogeneity of oxygen delivery impairs oxygen extraction by peripheral tissues: theory. *J Appl Physiol.* 1996;81:885-894.
8. Levy B, Gibot S, Franck P, et al. Relation between muscle Na+K+ ATPase activity and raised lactate concentrations in septic shock: a prospective study. *Lancet.* 2005;365:871-875.
9. Silverman HJ. Lack of a relationship between induced changes in oxygen consumption and changes in lactate levels. *Chest.* 1991;100:1012-1015.
10. Heyland DK, Cook DJ, King D, et al. Maximizing oxygen delivery in critically ill patients: a methodologic appraisal of the evidence. *Critical Care Med.* 1996;24:517-524.
11. Rivers E, Nguyen B, Havstad S, et al. Early goal-directed therapy in the treatment of severe sepsis and septic shock. *N Engl J Med.* 2001;345:1368-1377.
12. Scalea TM, Hartnett RW, Duncan AO, et al. Central venous oxygen saturation: a useful clinical tool in trauma patients. *J Trauma.* 1990;30:1539-1543.
13. Gattinoni L, Brazzi L, Pelosi P, et al. A trial of goal-oriented hemodynamic therapy in critically ill patients. SvO2 Collaborative Group. *N Engl J Med.* 1995;333:1025-1032.
14. Harvey S, Harrison DA, Singer M, et al. Assessment of the clinical effectiveness of pulmonary artery catheters in management of patients in intensive care (PAC-Man): a randomised controlled trial. *Lancet.* 2005;366:472-477.
15. Binanay C, Califf RM, Hasselblad V, et al. Evaluation study of congestive heart failure and pulmonary artery catheterization effectiveness: the ESCAPE trial. *JAMA.* 2005;294:1625-1633.
16. Cohn SM, Nathens AB, Moore FA, et al. Tissue oxygen saturation predicts the development of organ dysfunction during traumatic shock resuscitation. *J Trauma.* 2007;62:44-54; discussion 54-45.
17. Trzeciak S, McCoy JV, Phillip Dellinger R, et al. Early increases in microcirculatory perfusion during protocol-directed resuscitation are associated with reduced multi-organ failure at 24 h in patients with sepsis. *Intensive Care Med.* 2008;34:2210-2217.
18. Barbier C, Loubieres Y, Schmit C, et al. Respiratory changes in inferior vena cava diameter are helpful in

predicting fluid responsiveness in ventilated septic patients. *Intensive Care Med.* 2004;30:1740-1746.

19. Yealy DM, Kellum JA, Huang DT, et al. A randomized trial of protocol-based care for early septic shock. *N Engl J Med.* 2014;370:1683-1693.

20. Peake SL, Delaney A, Bailey M, et al. Goal-directed resuscitation for patients with early septic shock. *N Engl J Med.* 2014;372:1301-1311.

21. Mouncey PR, Osborn TM, Power GS, et al. Trial of early, goal-directed resuscitation for septic shock. *N Engl J Med.* 2015.

22. Watson D, Grover R, Anzueto A, et al. Cardiovascular effects of the nitric oxide synthase inhibitor NG-methyl-L-arginine hydrochloride (546C88) in patients with septic shock: results of a randomized, double-blind, placebo-controlled multicenter study (study no. 144-002). *Critical Care Med.* 2004;32:13-20.

23. Schmidt GA. ICU ultrasound. The coming boom. *Chest.* 2009;135:1407-1408.

24. Kumar A, Roberts D, Wood KE, et al. Duration of hypotension before initiation of effective antimicrobial therapy is the critical determinant of survival in human septic shock. *Critical Care Med.* 2006;34:1589-1596.

25. Brunkhorst FM, Engel C, Bloos F, et al. Intensive insulin therapy and pentastarch resuscitation in severe sepsis. *N Engl J Med.* 2008;358:125-139.

26. Bickell WH, Wall MJ, Jr, Pepe PE, et al. Immediate versus delayed fluid resuscitation for hypotensive patients with penetrating torso injuries. *N Engl J Med.* 1994;331:1105-1109.

27. Durairaj L, Schmidt GA. Fluid therapy in resuscitated sepsis: less is more. *Chest.* 2008;133:252-263.

28. Osman D, Ridel C, Ray P, et al. Cardiac filling pressures are not appropriate to predict hemodynamic response to volume challenge. *Critical Care Med.* 2007;35:64-68.

29. Michard F, Boussat S, Chemla D, et al. Relation between respiratory changes in arterial pulse pressure and fluid responsiveness in septic patients with acute circulatory failure. *Am J Respir Critical Care Med.* 2000;162:134-138.

30. Cavallaro F, Sandroni C, Marano C, et al. Diagnostic accuracy of passive leg raising for prediction of fluid responsiveness in adults: systematic review and meta-analysis of clinical studies. *Intensive Care Med.* 2010;36:1475-1483.

31. De Backer D, Biston P, Devriendt J, et al. Comparison of dopamine and norepinephrine in the treatment of shock. *N Engl J Med.* 2010;362:779-789.

32. Patel MR, Smalling RW, Thiele H, et al. Intra-aortic balloon counterpulsation and infarct size in patients with acute anterior myocardial infarction without shock: the CRISP AMI randomized trial. *JAMA.* 2011;306:1329-1337.

33. Thiele H, Zeymer U, Neumann FJ, et al. Intra-aortic balloon counterpulsation in acute myocardial infarction complicated by cardiogenic shock (IABP-SHOCK II): final 12 month results of a randomised, open-label trial. *Lancet.* 2013;382:1638-1645.

34. Villanueva C, Colomo A, Bosch A, et al. Transfusion strategies for acute upper gastrointestinal bleeding. *N Engl J Med.* 2013;368:11-21.

35. Holst LB, Haase N, Wetterslev J, et al. Lower versus higher hemoglobin threshold for transfusion in septic shock. *N Engl J Med.* 2014;371:1381-1391.

36. Schweickert WD, Pohlman MC, Pohlman AS, et al. Early physical and occupational therapy in mechanically ventilated, critically ill patients: a randomised controlled trial. *Lancet.* 2009;373:1874-1882.

CPR and ACLS Updates

Carla Venegas-Borsellino, MD and
Maneesha D. Bangar, MD

KEY POINTS

1 In- and out-of-the-hospital cardiac arrest remains a substantial public health problem and a leading cause of death in many parts of the world. There is a dramatic variation in the survival rates across various systems of care.

2 Major changes were made in the 2010 American Heart Association (AHA) guidelines for cardiopulmonary resuscitation (CPR) and emergency cardiovascular care. We will review the studies behind these recommendations.

3 Identifying the most accurate and relevant post–cardiac arrest outcomes to measure is a major challenge. The most used measurements are survival to hospital discharge, or neurologically intact survival to discharge.

4 Five main components of high-performance CPR have been identified: chest compression fraction, chest compression rate, chest compression depth, chest recoil, and ventilation. Minimizing the interval between stopping chest compressions and delivering a shock improves the chances of shock success and patient survival.

4 The 2010 AHA guidelines recommend education to improve the effectiveness of resuscitation. Recommended educational tools include high-quality medical simulators, videos, and written tests accompanied with a performance assessment.

INTRODUCTION

Cardiac arrest is the abrupt cessation of cardiac pump function which leads to death, but in some cases can be reversible by a prompt intervention in the form of cardiopulmonary resuscitation (CPR).[1] In- and out-of-the-hospital cardiac arrest remains a substantial public health problem and a leading cause of death in many parts of the world.[2] In the United States and Canada, approximately 350,000 people/year suffer a cardiac arrest (approximately half of them in-hospital) and receive attempted resuscitation; approximately 25% of these present with pulseless ventricular arrhythmias.[3,4] Cardiac-arrest victims who present with ventricular fibrillation (VF) or pulseless ventricular tachycardia (VT) have a substantially better outcome compared with those who present with asystole or pulseless electrical activity (PEA).[4] Emergency systems that can immediately and effectively implement life support measurement can achieve witnessed VF cardiac arrest survival of almost 50%.[5] However, there is a dramatic variation in the survival rates across various systems of care, with the most successful systems reporting survival rates five times higher than the least successful.[3]

The survival rate and the quality of life (specially measured as a neurological performance) after a cardiac arrest have also changed over time; for example, the US survival rates for hospitalized patients with cardiac arrest improved from 30.4% in 2001 to 42.2% in 2009 as per the US National In-Patient Sample, a national hospital discharge database.[6] It is important to understand that CPR outcomes are significantly influenced by the underlying pathology and the initial cardiac rhythm at the time of the cardiac arrest. In a nutshell, survival is best for patients with VT or VF.

It is an integrated and coordinated system, starting from initial responders (including both medical professionals and bystanders) to in-hospital caregivers, functioning as a comprehensive whole that will produce the highest likelihood of achieving the desired survival to discharge from hospital outcome. However, research has shown that several factors prevent bystanders from taking action; including fear that they will perform CPR incorrectly, fear of legal liability, and fear of infection from performing mouth-to-mouth.[7] But a hospital setting does not have these inhibitory factors; hence, hospital personnel have tools in the form of the knowledge about CPR guidelines and resources to fight against cardiac arrest.

Resuscitation is one of the most widely studied topics in medicine. It has been known and practiced since 1740 when performance of mouth-to-mouth resuscitation for drowning victims was recommended by the Paris Academy of Science.[8] As of December 2013, there were close to 19,000 related references cited in PubMed, with new changes being recommended every few years in how CPR should be administered; so it is important to keep ourselves updated with the latest knowledge and practice of the art of CPR. The American Heart Association (AHA), in cooperation with the International Liaison Committee on Resuscitation, leads the research and management guidelines for CPR. The latest guidelines available for CPR were established in 2010[7] after an extensive evidence evaluation process that included 356 resuscitation experts from 29 countries who reviewed and analyzed the available literature during the 36-month period before the 2010 Consensus Conference. The experts produced 411 scientific evidence reviews on 277 topics in resuscitation and emergency cardiovascular care. The purpose of this chapter is to review the fundamentals of these

recommendations, to emphasize the new changes made in 2010, and review the evidence-base literature that support these guidelines.

HISTORY OF CPR

Upon review of the history of CPR, the earliest recorded reference to artificial breathing is in the Old Testament, in the book of Kings, where the prophet Elisha restored the life of a boy through a technique that included placing his mouth on the mouth of the child.[8] Around the 1700s, there was a large number of drowning deaths in the Rhine river near Paris, and even though there were case reports and references to mouth to mouth resuscitation for many years before this, it was not until the 1740s that the technique became well known after the Paris Academy of Science's official recommendation of mouth-to-mouth resuscitation for drowning victims.[8] In 1891, Dr Friedrich Maass performed the first equivocally documented chest compression on a human.[8] This resuscitation technique was rediscovered in the 1940s during the polio epidemic in Minneapolis by the anesthesiologist James Elam.[9]

The three most important contributors to modern CPR are Doctors Zoll, Safar, and Kouwenhoven.[10] Safar in the 1950s investigated techniques for airway management and showed that the optimal position for CPR was with the patients' neck extended, mandible supported, in order to insert the oropharyngeal tube to deliver oxygen; Zoll performed and recorded the first successful closed chest human defibrillation in a man with syncope and VF; and Kouwenhoven in 1950s to 1960s developed a closed chest cardiac massage and external defibrillation. Later in the 1960s, Safar et al[11] published a paper showing circulatory efficacy of closed-chest cardiac massage and postulated that rhythmic sternal pressure must be accompanied by intermittent positive-pressure ventilation.

In 1960, Dr Kouwenhoven, in association with Drs Knickerbocker and Jude, documented 14 patients who survived cardiac arrest with the application of closed chest cardiac massage[12]; that same year, at the meeting of the Maryland Medical Society in Ocean City, the combination of chest compressions and rescue breathing was introduced.[13] Two years later, in 1962, direct-current, monophasic waveform defibrillation was described, and in 1966, the AHA developed the first CPR guidelines, which have been followed by periodic updates.[14] Since then, the AHA has maintained a program to acquaint physicians with closed chest cardiac resuscitation; this program is the forerunner of CPR training for the general public.

In 1979, the concept of Advanced Cardiovascular Life Support (ACLS) was introduced during the Third National Conference on CPR, and in the 1990s, Early Public Access Defibrillation programs were developed with goal in mind of providing training, resources, and the ability of the general public to become proactive and integral in the successful resuscitation of sudden cardiac arrest victims.[15] It was not until 2005 that the International Consensus on Emergency Cardiovascular Care (ECC) and CPR Science with Treatment Recommendations (CoSTR) Conference produced the 2005 AHA guidelines for CPR and ECC.[7]

Two studies published just before the 2005 International Consensus Conference documented the poor quality of CPR performed in both out-of- and in-hospital resuscitations;[16,17] addressing this, changes in the compression-ventilation ratio and in the defibrillation sequence (from 3 stacked shocks to 1 shock followed by immediate CPR) were recommended to minimize interruptions in chest compressions.[7] Since 2005, as mentioned earlier, it is more clear that after CPR with early, noninterrupted chest compressions and early defibrillation and ACLS, the best survival chance is for patients with VT or VF. To follow, we will review the major changes from 2010 AHA guidelines for CPR and ECC,[7] and some of the studies behind these recommendations.

NEW RECOMMENDATIONS FROM 2010 AHA GUIDELINES FOR BASIC LIFE SUPPORT

Traditionally, basic life support (BLS) has three components: achieving a patent airway, delivering lung inflations via mouth to mouth or bag-mask to mouth, and promoting circulation with chest compressions. Studies have demonstrated improved outcomes after out-of-hospital cardiac arrest (OHCA), particularly from shockable rhythms when there are minimal interruptions in compressions without excessive ventilation.[5,18,19] In order to prevent wasting time on potentially improper airway maneuvers, the most recent AHA guidelines recommend a significant change in BLS sequence.

CHANGE IN BLS SEQUENCE OF STEPS FOR TRAINED RESCUER FROM A-B-C TO C-A-B

Reasoning: High-quality CPR is the cornerstone of a system of care that can optimize outcomes beyond return of spontaneous circulation (ROSC), where return to a prior quality of life and functional state of health is the ultimate goal. The newest development in the 2010 AHA Guidelines for CPR and ECC is a change in the BLS sequence of steps from "A-B-C" (Airway, Breathing, Chest compressions) to "C-A-B" (Chest compressions, Airway, Breathing) for adult patients. As explained in the AHA guidelines, the A-B-C sequence could be reason why fewer people in cardiac arrest received bystander CPR. A-B-C starts with the most difficult and time consuming set of tasks: positioning the patient's head correctly, opening the airway, achieving a mouth to mouth seal, and delivering rescue breaths. Also there may be hesitancy on part of a rescuer's willingness to provide mouth-to-mouth resuscitation. By changing to C-A-B sequence, chest compressions will be initiated sooner and ventilation only minimally delayed until the first cycle of chest compressions is completed. The only exception to this sequence is in drowning victims and newborn patients where conventional CPR must be done.

In a prospective, population-based, observational study involving patients with emergency responder resuscitation attempts from 1998 through 2003, Iwami et al[18] found that 1 year survival with favorable neurologic outcome was similar for bystander-initiated cardiac-only resuscitation (4.3%; odds ratio [OR], 1.72; 95% confidence interval [CI], 1.01-2.95) and conventional CPR for most adult OHCAs.

Olasveengen et al[20] did a retrospective, observational study between 2003 and 2006 in all nontraumatic cardiac arrest adult patients treated by the community-run emergency medical service (EMS) in Oslo, Norway in which they measured outcomes for patients receiving Standard basic life support (S-BLS), compared with patients receiving only continuous chest compression (CCC). They found that there were no differences in outcomes between the two patient groups, with 13% discharged with a favorable outcome for the S-BLS group and 10% in the CCC group ($P = 0.85$). Similarly, there was no difference in survival subgroup analysis of patients presenting with initial VF/VT after witnessed arrest, with 29% and 28% patients discharged from hospital in the S-BLS and CCC groups, respectively ($P = 0.97$).

"LOOK, LISTEN, AND FEEL" HAS BEEN REMOVED FROM THE BLS ALGORITHM

Reasoning: "Look, listen, and feel" is an inconsistent and time-consuming practice. In a study by Rupert et al[21] four different populations were tested for their ability to assess breathlessness: EMS personnel, physicians, medical students, and laypersons. Only 55.6% of all participants showed correct diagnostic skills. They concluded that this diagnostic procedure takes more time than recommended in international guidelines and checking for breathing was shown to be mostly inaccurate and unreliable. Professional as well as lay rescuers may be unable to accurately determine the presence or absence of adequate or normal breathing in unresponsive victims because the airway is not open or because the victim has occasional gasps.

1. A "chest compression rate of at least 100/min" is now recommended, different from the "approximately 100/min" recommended in 2005.

    Reasoning: The number of chest compressions per minute is an important factor for attaining ROSC. Studies show that delivery of more frequent compressions is associated with better survival. A prospective observational study by Abella[17] showed that in-hospital chest-compression rates were below published resuscitation recommendations; suboptimal compression rates were correlated with poor ROSC.

2. "Chest compression depth of at least 2 in (5 cm)," different from the "approximately 2 in" recommended in 2005.

    Reasoning: Chest compression delivers blood flow and oxygen to heart and brain. Studies show that rescuers often do not push hard enough. Steil et al[22] found suboptimal compression depth in half of patients by 2005 guideline standards and in almost all patients by 2010 standards; a strong association between increased compression depth and higher survival outcomes was found.

3. If a bystander is not trained in CPR, it is recommended he/she perform hands-only CPR with the emphasis to push fast and hard at the center of the chest. AHA 2005 guidelines did not provide different recommendations for trained versus untrained rescuers. However, according to the N2010 AHA recommendations, the trained rescuer should perform cardiac compression and give breaths.

    Reasoning: During the past 5 years, there has been an effort to simplify CPR recommendations and emphasize the fundamental importance of high-quality CPR. For most adults with OHCA, bystander CPR with chest compression only (Hands-Only CPR) appears to achieve outcomes similar to those of conventional CPR (compressions with rescue breathing).[18,19] However, for children, conventional CPR is superior. Hands only CPR is easier for an untrained person. Studies written above[19,20] show hands only CPR to be as effective as conventional CPR.

4. The new guidelines do not recommend routine use of cricoid pressure.

    Reasoning: Cricoid pressure may impede ventilation and it can delay or prevent placement of an advanced airway, and some aspiration can still occur despite cricoid pressure. It is also difficult to train rescuers in using this maneuver. A study by Li et al[23] showed that cricoid pressure impedes insertion of, and ventilation through the ProSeal laryngeal mask airway in anesthetized, paralyzed patients.

NEW RECOMMENDATIONS FROM 2010 AHA GUIDELINES FOR ADVANCE CARDIAC LIFE SUPPORT

ACLS is an extension of BLS and is implemented by a team which can provide advanced therapeutic care. At the time of the 2010 International Consensus Conference, there was still insufficient data to demonstrate that any drugs or mechanical CPR devices improve long-term outcomes after cardiac arrest. So the 2010 AHA Guidelines for CPR and ECC continue to emphasize that the foundation of successful ACLS is good BLS, beginning with prompt high-quality CPR with minimal interruptions, and for VF/pulseless VT, attempted defibrillation within minutes of collapse.[7] The new recommendations focus on the Post–Cardiac Arrest Care, as comprehensive multidisciplinary care that begins with recognition of cardiac arrest and continues after ROSC, through hospital discharge and beyond.

1. Continuous quantitative waveform capnography is a major new Class I recommendation for intubated adults throughout the periarrest period. It should be used for confirming tracheal tube placement and for monitoring CPR quality and detecting return of spontaneous circulation, based on end-tidal carbon dioxide values.

    Reasoning: Blood has to circulate through the lungs for carbon dioxide to be exhaled and measured, so capnography can be used for monitoring the effectiveness of chest compressions. Inadequate chest compressions, failing cardiac output, or rearrest causes decreased end tidal carbon dioxide. Grmec[24] studied adult patients intubated by an emergency physician in the field, with tube position confirmed by auscultation, infrared capnometry, and infrared capnography. He concluded that capnography is the most reliable method to confirm endotracheal tube placement in

    emergency conditions in the prehospital setting

2. Atropine is not recommended for Pulseless electrical activity (asystole) while adenosine is recommended in the initial diagnosis and treatment of stable, undifferentiated, monomorphic tachycardia.

    Reasoning: Evidence suggests that routine use of Atropine for PEA/Asystole is unlikely to have therapeutic benefit.[7] Adenosine is safe and efficient and so recommended for aforementioned tachycardia.[25] The effects of atropine were assessed in 7448 adults with nonshockable rhythm from the SOS-KANTO study; they found that administration of atropine had no long-term neurological benefit in adults with OHCA due to nonshockable rhythm and concluded that atropine is not useful for adults with PEA.[26]

3. Post–Cardiac arrest care to improve survival for victims of cardiac arrest admitted to hospital after return of spontaneous circulation. It should include cardiopulmonary and neurologic support, therapeutic hypothermia, and percutaneous coronary interventions when indicated; EEG for the diagnosis of seizures, monitored frequently in a comatose patient after ROSC; optimizing cardiopulmonary function and vital organ perfusion after ROSC; transportation to an appropriate hospital or critical-care unit with a comprehensive post–cardiac arrest treatment system of care; identification of and intervention for acute coronary syndromes; anticipation, treatment, and prevention of multiple organ dysfunction.

    Reasoning: Systematically organized multidisciplinary treatment programs for post–cardiac arrest (in- or out-of-hospital) patients may improve survival to hospital discharge outcomes among victims who attain ROSC.[27] Coordinated programs focusing on optimizing neurologic, metabolic, and hemodynamic function have shown some promise when deployed in an integrated system of care. As of now, the individual effects of such therapies have not been conclusively studied, but there is emerging evidence that use of such therapies may effectively improve outcomes. Studies have shown possible benefit of therapeutic hypothermia after cardiac arrest and that organized post–cardiac arrest care may improve survival to hospital discharge. Study done by hypothermia study group[28] found that therapeutic mild hypothermia increased the rate of a favorable neurologic outcome and reduced mortality for in-hospital patients who had been successfully resuscitated after cardiac arrest due to VF. It is recommended that post–cardiac arrest patient treated with therapeutic hypothermia be monitored for clinical neurologic signs using electrophysiological studies, biomarkers, and imaging where available, at 3 days after cardiac arrest, to be used for prognostication.

The steps in BLS (shown in Figure 22–1) and ACLS (shown in Figure 22–2) are shown as algorithms to be followed.

EVIDENCE-BASED MEDICINE: RECENT AND CONTROVERSIAL TOPICS

Evidence-based medicine is the conscientious, explicit, and judicious use of current best evidence in making decisions about the care of individual patients; the practice of evidence-based medicine means integrating individual clinical expertise with the best available external clinical evidence from systematic research.[29] Resuscitation research is particularly challenging because it must be scientifically

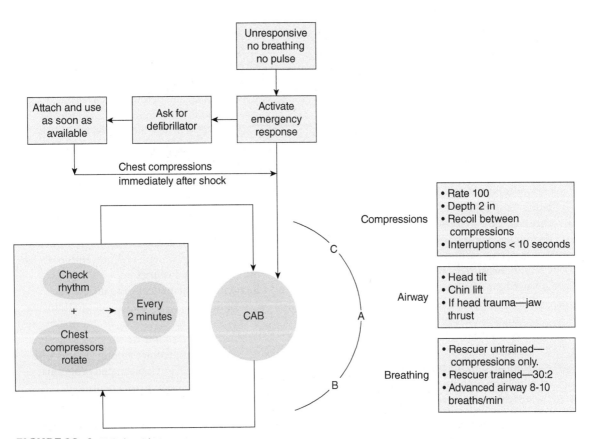

FIGURE 22–1 BLS algorithm.

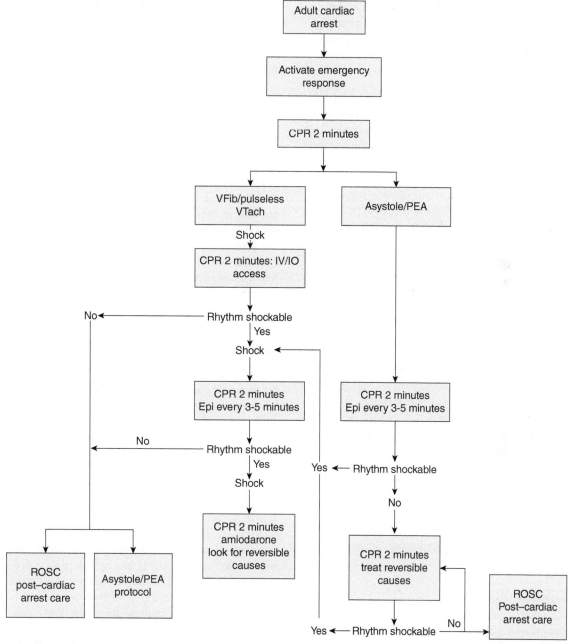

FIGURE 22–2 ACLS algorithm.

rigorous, while confronting ethical, regulatory, and public relations concerns that arise; life or death scenarios presented by the need for CPR make it impossible to receive informed consent from the patient. Regulatory requirements, community notification, and consultation requirements often impose expensive and time-consuming demands that may not only delay important research, but also render it cost prohibitive, with little significant evidence that these measures effectively address the concerns about research.[30] The following are some more recent and perhaps controversial topics/studies that arise when discussing evidence base CPR recommendations.

CPR OUTCOMES

Identifying the most accurate and relevant post–cardiac arrest outcomes to measure is a major challenge that requires further research. The most used measurements are survival to hospital discharge, or neurologically intact survival to discharge. Caution is advised, for example, when considering limiting care or withdrawing life-sustaining therapy because the predictors of neurological recovery currently in use have not been validated for patients who are treated with therapeutic hypothermia.

Hollenberg et al[19] conducted a study during a 14 year time period (1992-2005) in Sweden describing changes in 1-month survival in patients given CPR after OHCA. He found improved survival rates over that time period; factors that potentially contributed to the improved survival rate were an increase in emergency medical crew-witnessed cases (from 9% in 1992 to 15% in 2005 [$P < 0.01$]) and, to a lesser degree, an increase in bystander CPR (from 31% in 1992 to 50% in 2005 [$P < 0.01$]).

Hinchey et al[5] did an observational multiphase before-after cohort study to assess survival from OHCA in adult patients with cardiac arrest managed by emergency responders. They concluded that in the context of a community-wide focus on resuscitation, the sequential implementation of 2005 AHA guidelines for compressions, ventilations, and induced hypothermia significantly improved survival after cardiac arrest.

CPR Quality

Minimizing the interval between stopping chest compressions and delivering a shock (ie, minimizing the preshock pause) improves the chances of shock success and patient survival.[31]

Edelson et al[32] did a study on internal medicine residents at a university hospital who attended weekly debriefing sessions of the prior week's resuscitations, reviewing CPR performance transcripts obtained from a CPR-sensing and feedback-enabled defibrillator. Compared with the control period, the mean (SD) ventilation rate decreased (13 [7]/min vs 18 [8]/min; $P < 0.01$) and compression depth increased (50 [10] vs 44 [10] mm; $P < 0.01$), among other CPR improvements. These changes correlated with an increase in the rate of ROSC in the RAPID (Resuscitation with Actual Performance Integrated Debriefing) group (59.4% vs 44.6%; $P < 0.05$). They concluded that the combination of RAPID and real-time audiovisual feedback improved CPR quality compared with the use of feedback alone and was associated with an increased rate of ROSC. Survival from cardiac arrest depends on early recognition of the event and immediate activation of emergency response system, but equally critical is the quality of CPR delivered.

Five main components of high performance CPR have been identified: chest compression fraction (proportion of time chest compressions are administered in each minute of CPR), chest compression rate, chest compression depth, chest recoil, and ventilation.[33]

CPR Devices

Several devices to provide effective CPR have been the focus of recent clinical trials. To date, no adjunct has consistently been shown to be superior to standard conventional (manual) CPR for out-of-hospital BLS, and no device other than a defibrillator has consistently improved long-term survival from OHCA.

Integration of AEDs into a system of care is critical in the Chain of Survival in public places outside of hospitals. To give the victim the best chance of survival, 3 actions must occur within the first moments of a cardiac arrest: activation of the EMS system, provision of CPR, and operation of a defibrillator.[7] An area of continued interest is whether delivering a longer period of CPR before defibrillation improves outcomes in cardiac arrest. Early studies showed improved survival when 1.5 to 3 minutes of CPR preceded defibrillation for patients with cardiac arrest for more than 5 minutes duration prior to EMS arrival, but more recent trials did not improved outcomes.[7]

Transcutaneous pacing has also been the focus of several recent trials. In the current 2010 AHA recommendations, pacing is not generally recommended for patients in asystolic cardiac arrest since randomized controlled trials indicate no improvement in rate of admission to hospital or survival to hospital discharge when pacing was attempted in patients with cardiac arrest in the prehospital or in-hospital (ED) setting.[7]

Medications Used During CPR

A meta-analysis of 5 randomized trials[34] showed no statistically significant differences between vasopressin and epinephrine for ROSC, 24-hour survival, or survival to hospital discharge.

It is appropriate to administer a 1-mg dose of epinephrine IV/IO every 3 to 5 minutes during adult cardiac arrest or one dose of vasopressin 40 U IV/IO may replace either the first or second dose of epinephrine in the treatment of pulseless arrest.[7]

Hypothermia

Therapeutic hypothermia is one intervention that has been shown to improve outcome for comatose adult victims of witnessed OHCA when the presenting rhythm was VF.[28] Since 2005, nonrandomized studies with concurrent controls or historic controls have indicated the possible benefit of hypothermia following in- and out-of-hospital cardiac arrest from all other initial rhythms in adults. Holzer's study found 53% survival with favorable neurological outcome in the endovascular cooling group, compared to 34% in the control group (OR 2.15, 95% CI, 1.38 to 3.35; $P < 0.05$).[35] Therapeutic hypothermia is a "game changer," changing the specificity of neurological prognostication decision rules that were previously established from studies of post–cardiac arrest patients not treated with hypothermia.

Extracorporeal Membrane Oxygenation

Extracorporeal membrane oxygenation (ECMO) is a form of external cardiopulmonary life support (ECLS). Its goal is supporting the body's circulation in the absence of an adequately functioning cardiac pump. The initiation of ECLS and the management of a patient on ECLS require highly trained personnel and specialized equipment. ECLS has been associated with improved survival rates when compared with conventional CPR in patients less than 75 years old with potentially correctable conditions in case

series and observational studies for in-hospital and OHCA sufferers. Although there are no randomized studies that compare ECLS with conventional CPR for patients in cardiac arrest, there are data from several case series that demonstrate the feasibility and safety of ECLS in highly specialized centers,[36] but, as of this writing, there is not enough evidence to recommend the routine use of ECLS in this population.

Study by Thiagarajan[37] showed that ECMO used to support CPR rescued one third of patients in whom death was otherwise certain; improved survival was found in association with patient diagnosis, absence of severe metabolic acidosis before ECMO support, and uncomplicated ECMO course.

In a study by Lamhaut L et al[38] published in 2013, prehospital ECMO (PH-ECLS) was implemented by a PH-ECLS team for refractory cardiac arrest in 7 patients with a witnessed cardiac arrest, with CPR initiated within the first 5 minutes, and absence of severe comorbidities. This pilot study suggests that PH-ECLS performed by nonsurgeons is potentially safe and feasible. Further studies are needed to confirm the time saved by this strategy and its potential effect on survival.

Ethical Issues

1. Should resuscitative efforts be started? Ethical issues associated with CPR start with the question as to whether or not to initiate resuscitation as some patients might prefer palliative care without heroic measures to prolong life; advance directives play a very important role in these matters, and if an advance directive in the form of a living will is not available then a health care proxy or surrogate decision maker is helpful. Acknowledgment of a verbal or written do-not-attempt-resuscitation order may decrease the number of futile resuscitation attempts; however, there is insufficient evidence to support this without further validation.

2. When should resuscitative efforts stop? The final decision to stop resuscitative efforts often is not simple; clinical judgment and respect for patients' and their families' wishes must enter into decision making. Research addressing issues related to the appropriate termination

of resuscitative efforts is limited. Goto et al[39] performed a study with Japanese database on patients with OHCA. The main outcome measures were specificity, positive predictive value (PPV), and area under the receiver operating characteristic curve for the new developed termination of resuscitation (TOR) rule for emergency department physicians. They validated that the TOR rule consisting of 3 prehospital variables (no prehospital ROSC, unshockable initial rhythm, and unwitnessed by bystanders) had a more than 99% PPV of very poor outcome. However, the implementation of this new rule in other countries or EMS systems requires further validation studies.

3. Should family be present during CPR? Jabre P et al[40] enrolled 570 relatives of patients who were in cardiac arrest and were given CPR by 15 pre-hospital EMS units that were randomly assigned either to systematically offer the family member the opportunity to observe CPR (intervention group) or to follow standard practice regarding family presence (control group). The primary end point was the proportion of relatives with post-traumatic stress disorder-related symptoms on day 90; secondary end points included the presence of anxiety and depression symptoms, the effect of family presence on medical efforts at resuscitation, the well-being of the health care team, and the occurrence of medico-legal claims. They concluded that family presence during CPR was associated with positive results on psychological variables and did not interfere with medical efforts, increase stress in the health care team, or result in medico-legal conflicts. Some other studies indicate that no clear conclusion is derived from studies done so far and more studies have to be done in this area.

4. *Organ donation.* Because of the growing need for transplant tissue and organs, all provider teams who treat postarrest patients should also plan and implement a system of tissue and organ donation that is timely, effective, and supportive of family members for that subset of patients in whom brain death is confirmed or for organ donation after cardiac arrest.

EDUCATION AND IMPLEMENTATION

The 2010 AHA guidelines recommend education to improve the effectiveness of resuscitation.[7] The recommendations include frequent practicing of skills; training of teamwork and leadership skills; formal training in CPR techniques, including compression-only (Hands-Only) in CPR to potential bystander rescuers; training in dispatcher instructions over the telephone by EMS providers. Recommended educational tools include high-quality medical simulators, videos, and written tests accompanied with a performance assessment.

CONCLUSION

The art of resuscitation has developed over thousands of years. The guidelines for resuscitation have had significant updates and as strong evidence-based studies continually provide the medical community with more information, methods used in resuscitative efforts may likely evolve further to improve patient outcomes. Extensive training and education of nonmedical staff in BLS and medical staff in BLS and ACLS is necessary so that we properly implement them. Simulation training on mannequins, for example, is one tool that can aid in the application of these guidelines effectively. Extensive studies have been done on CPR techniques but more research has to be done on the ethical and other aspects of CPR. We have come a long way in our understanding of what life-saving measures work best, and further understanding and evolution of CPR practices most likely will improve our ability to effectively save lives through CPR.

REFERENCES

1. Fauci A, Braunwald E, Isselbacher K, et al. *Harrison's Principles of Internal Medicine.* 14th international ed. Chap. 39, P. 222.
2. Lloyd-Jones D, Adams RJ, Brown TM, et al. American Heart Association Statistics Committee and Stroke Statistics Subcommittee. Heart disease and stroke statistics–2010 Update: a report from the American Heart Association. *Circulation.* 2010;121:e46-e215.

3. Nichol G, Thomas E, Callaway CW, et al. Regional variation in out-of-hospital cardiac arrest incidence and outcome. *JAMA*. 2008;300:1423-1431.

4. Nadkarni VM, Larkin GL, Peberdy MA, et al. First documented rhythm and clinical outcome from in-hospital cardiac arrest among children and adults. *JAMA*. 2006;295:50-57.

5. Hinchey PR, Myers JB, Lewis R, et al. Improved out-of-hospital cardiac arrest survival after the sequential implementation of 2005 AHA guidelines for compressions, ventilations, and induced hypothermia: the Wake County experience. *Ann Emerg Med*. 2010;56(4):348-357.

6. Fugate JE, Brinjikji W, Mandrekar JN, et al. Post-cardiac arrest mortality is declining: a study of the US National Inpatient Sample 2001 to 2009. *Circulation*. 2012;126(5):546-550.

7. Field J, Hazinski MF, Sayre M, et al. 2010 American Heart Association Guidelines for Cardiopulmonary Resuscitation and Emergency Cardiovascular Care Science. *Circulation*. 2010;122:S639.

8. Taw RL, Jr. Dr. Friedrich Maass: 100th anniversary of "new" CPR. *Clin Cardiol*. 1991;14(12):1000-1002.

9. Ornato J, Peberdy MA. *Cardiopulmonary Resuscitation 2005*. History of the science of cardiopulmonary resuscitation. Mickey Eisenberg. Chap. 1. P. 2. ISBN 978-1-59259-814-4.

10. Hollenberg J. *Thesis: Out of Hospital Cardiac Arrest*. Elanders; 2008:9-10. ISBN: 978-91-7409-027-7.

11. Safar P, Brown TC, Holtey WJ. Ventilation and circulation with closed-chest cardiac massage in man. *JAMA*. 1961;176(7):574-576.

12. Kouwenhoven WB, Jude JR, Knickerbocker GG. Closed-chest cardiac massage. *JAMA*. 1960;173:1064-1067.

13. Eisenberg M. *Resuscitate! How Your Community Can Improve Survival from Sudden Cardiac Arrest*. Seattle, WA: University of Washington Press; 2009.

14. Cardiopulmonary resuscitation: statement by the Ad Hoc Committee on Cardiopulmonary Resuscitation, of the Division of Medical Sciences, National Academy of Sciences, National Research Council. *JAMA*. 1966;198:372-379.

15. Chan P, Krumholz H, Nichol G, et al. Delayed time to defibrillation after in-hospital cardiac arrest. *N Engl J Med*. 2008;358:9-17.

16. Wik L, Kramer-Johansen J, Myklebust H, et al. Quality of cardiopulmonary resuscitation during out-of-hospital cardiac arrest. *JAMA*. 2005;293:299-304.

17. Abella BS, Sandbo N, Vassilatos P, et al. Chest compression rates during cardiopulmonary resuscitation are suboptimal: a prospective study during in-hospital cardiac arrest. *Circulation*. 2005;111(4):428-434.

18. Iwami T, Kawamura T, Hiraide A, et al. Effectiveness of bystander-initiated cardiac-only resuscitation for patients with out-of-hospital cardiac arrest. *Circulation*. 2007;116:2900-2907.

19. Hollenberg J, Herlitz J, Linqvist J. Improved survival after out-of-hospital cardiac arrest is associated with an increase in proportion of emergency crew-witnessed cases and bystander cardiopulmonary resuscitation. *Circulation*. 2008;118(4):389-396.

20. Olasveegen TM, Wik L, Steen PA. Standard basic life support vs. continuous chest compressions only in out-of-hospital cardiac arrest. *Acta Anaesthesiol Scand*. 2008;52(7):914-919.

21. Ruppert M, Reith MW, Widmann JH, et al. Checking for breathing: evaluation of the diagnostic capability of emergency medical services personnel, physicians, medical students, and medical laypersons. *Ann Emerg Med*. 1999;34(6):720-729.

22. Stiell IG, Brown SP, Christenson J, et al. What is the role of chest compression depth during out-of-hospital cardiac arrest resuscitation? *Crit Care Med*. 2012;40(4):1192-1198.

23. Li CW, Xue FS, Xu YC, et al. Cricoid pressure impedes insertion of, and ventilation through, the ProSeal laryngeal mask airway in anesthetized, paralyzed patients. *Anesth Analg*. 2007;104(5):1195-1198.

24. Grmec S. Comparison of three different methods to confirm tracheal tube placement in emergency intubation. *Intensive Care Med*. 2002;28(6):701-704.

25. Herbert ME, Votey SR. Adenosine in wide-complex tachycardia. *Ann Emerg Med*. 1997;29(1):172-174.

26. Survey of Survivors After Out-of-hospital Cardiac Arrest in KANTO Area, Japan (SOS-KANTO) Study Group Atropine sulfate for patients with out-of-hospital cardiac arrest due to asystole and pulseless electrical activity. *Circ J*. 2011;75(3):580-588.

27. Gaieski DF, Band RA, Abella BS, et al. Early goal-directed hemodynamic optimization combined with therapeutic hypothermia in comatose survivors of out-of-hospital cardiac arrest. *Resuscitation*. 2009;80:418-424.

28. The Hypothermia after Cardiac Arrest Study Group. Mild therapeutic hypothermia to improve the neurologic outcome after cardiac arrest. *N Engl J Med*. 2002;346:549-556.

29. Sackett DL, Rosenberg W, Muir Gray JA, et al. Evidence based medicine: what it is and what it isn't. *BMJ*. 1996;312:71.

30. Dickert NW, Sugarman J. Getting the ethics right regarding research in the emergency setting: lessons from the PolyHeme study. *Kennedy Inst Ethics J.* 2007;17:153-169.
31. Christenson J, Andrusiek D, Everson-Stewart S, et al. Chest compression fraction determines survival in patients with out-of-hospital ventricular fibrillation. *Circulation.* 2009;120:1241-1247.
32. Edelson DP, Litzinger B, Arora V, et al. Improving in-hospital cardiac arrest process and outcomes with performance debriefing. *Arch Intern Med.* 2008;168(10):1063-1069.
33. Meaney PA, Bobrow BJ, Mancini ME, et al. CPR Quality: improving cardiac resuscitation outcomes both inside and outside the hospital: a consensus statement from American Heart Association. *Circulation.* 2013;128:417-435.
34. Aung K, Htay T. Vasopressin for cardiac arrest: a systematic review and meta-analysis. *Arch Intern Med.* 2005;165:17-24.
35. Holzer M, Müllner M, Sterz F, et al. Efficacy and safety of endovascular cooling after cardiac arrest: cohort study and Bayesian approach. *Stroke.* 2006;37(7):1792-1797.
36. Chen YS, Yu HY, Huang SC, et al. Extracorporeal membrane oxygenation support can extend the duration of cardiopulmonary resuscitation. *Crit Care Med.* 2008;36:2529-2535.
37. Thiagarajan R, Laussen PC, Rycis PT, et al. Extracorporeal membrane oxygenation to aid cardiopulmonary resuscitation in infants and children. Pediatric cardiology. *Circulation.* 2007;116:1693-1700.
38. Lamhauta L, Jouffroya R, Soldana M, et al. Safety and feasibility of prehospital extra corporeal life support implementation by non-surgeons for out-of-hospital refractory cardiac arrest. *Resuscitation.* 2013;84:1525-1529.
39. Goto Y, Maeda T, Goto YN. Termination-of-resuscitation rule for emergency department physicians treating out-of-hospital cardiac arrest patients: an observational cohort study. *Crit Care.* 2013;17(5):R235.
40. Jabre P, Belpomme V, Azoulay E, et al. Family presence during cardiopulmonary resuscitation. *N Engl J Med.* 2013;368(11):1008-1018.

Arrhythmia Diagnosis and Management

Dipti Gupta, MD, MPH and Nancy Roistacher, MD

KEY POINTS

1 Between 12% and 19% of patients in intensive care unit (ICU) settings have sustained arrhythmias.

2 In the ICU, the most common causes of arrhythmias are infection, electrolyte abnormalities, medications, ischemia, anemia, hypoxia, and changes in volume status and hemodynamics.

3 Tachycardias are more common than bradycardias and atrial arrhythmias are more common than ventricular arrhythmias.

4 Common causes of bradycardia include beta-blockers, calcium channel blockers, digoxin, narcotics, and antiemetics.

5 Patients are less likely to remain hemodynamically stable with higher degrees of atrioventricular (AV) block and usually require temporary pacing (transthoracic or transvenous), and ultimately permanent pacing if the heart block persists.

6 AV dissociation occurs when there is loss of the usual pattern of atrial and ventricular synchrony and there is no association between P waves and the QRS complexes.

7 The majority of atrial tachyarrhythmias in the critically ill patient are due to atrial fibrillation, atrial flutter, AV nodal reentry tachycardia, ectopic atrial tachycardia with rapid ventricular rates, and underlying preexcitation with an atrial arrhythmia.

8 For the hemodynamically unstable or symptomatic patient with AV nodal reentrant tachycardia, initial choices include adenosine or direct current cardioversion to restore sinus rhythm and hemodynamic stability.

9 Multifocal atrial tachycardia is usually associated with underlying pulmonary disease especially severe chronic obstructive lung disease or respiratory failure in older, acutely ill individuals.

10 Atrial fibrillation is the most common dysrhythmia in the critically ill. Recent clinical trials have demonstrated similar outcomes with rate and rhythm control strategies for atrial fibrillation.

11 Indications for urgent cardioversion in atrial fibrillation include hypotension/shock, acute or ongoing myocardial ischemia, congestive heart failure and/or acute pulmonary edema, and underlying preexcitation with rapid ventricular rates and/or hemodynamic instability.

12 Torsade de pointes and other forms of polymorphic tachycardia are rapid ventricular rhythms associated with hemodynamic instability and

—Continued next page

Continued—

a predisposition to degenerate into ventricular fibrillation.

13 Patients with nonsustained ventricular tachycardias and ischemic heart disease in ICU settings should be given beta-blockers to control heart rate, blood pressure

and rhythm disturbances, electrolyte replacement, and control of stimulatory factors, such as anemia, pain, and fever.

14 Ventricular fibrillation requires emergency defibrillation.

INTRODUCTION

Acutely ill patients frequently have significant arrhythmias. By some estimates between 12% and 19% of patients in critical care unit settings have sustained arrhythmias.[1,2] Patients following cardiac and thoracic surgery have a significant incidence of postoperative arrhythmias, specifically atrial fibrillation. Tachycardias are more common than bradycardias and atrial arrhythmias are more common than ventricular arrhythmias. Patients with underlying heart disease are more likely to have clinically significant arrhythmias. In the intensive care unit (ICU), multiple stimuli and associated elevated catecholamine levels contribute to arrhythmias. These include infection, electrolyte abnormalities, medications, ischemia, anemia, hypoxia, and changes in volume status and hemodynamics. Majority of these arrhythmias are secondary to at least one of these factors and usually respond to treatment of the primary medical or surgical processes.

Cardiac arrhythmias prolong the ICU length of stay of patients even if they are not the primary cause of their admissions and contribute to the morbidity and mortality of these patients. It is important to differentiate between those arrhythmias that need to be treated and those that are more benign so that a proper treatment plan can be instituted.

Tachycardias can be due to increased automaticity, reentry, or triggered activity. The stress seen in ICU patients can bring out or exacerbate underlying genetic or congenital predispositions, such as accessory pathways like Wolff-Parkinson-White Syndrome, Brugada syndrome, reentry arrhythmias, and congenital long QT syndromes. When assessing 12-lead electrocardiograms (EKG), monitor strips and a careful physical examination are important in addition to looking for structural heart disease.

Myocardial dysfunction, valvular abnormities, pericardial disease, congenital heart disease, and conduction abnormalities may be present. Acute cardiac dysfunction due to sepsis or related to high catecholamine states (Takotsubo syndrome) should also be considered in these critically ill patients.

The hemodynamic stability of the patient also needs to be assessed in addition to blood test analysis, medication lists, and EKG and telemetry analysis. Electrolyte abnormalities and renal or hepatic failure can be contributory. The presence of hemodynamic compromise or associated ischemia indicates the need for acute intervention. Reversible factors should be identified and treated. Significant prolongation of the QT interval is likely due to electrolyte abnormalities, such as hypomagnesemia and hypokalemia or to medications. The use of inotropes and vasopressor agents can increase heart rate (HR) and induce tachyarrhythmias. Fever, respiratory failure and severe anemia can also be contributing factors.

BRADYARRHYTHMIAS

Increased vagal tone can slow HR and sometimes can cause delays in cardiac conduction. Medications used to control blood pressure and tachyarrhythmias can cause further delays in conduction and heart block in patients with underlying conduction system disease. Beta-blockers, calcium channel blockers, digoxin, narcotics, and antiemetics can cause bradycardia and sometimes higher degree atrioventricular (AV) block. Bradycardia rarely needs to be treated unless there is associated hemodynamic instability.

Progressive delay in conduction of intracardiac electrical impulses can occur. Isolated first-degree AV block with prolongation of the PR interval to more than 200 ms does not need treatment although it can be associated with other conduction abnormalities. Second-degree AV block occurs when not all sinus impulses are transmitted to the ventricle. In Mobitz type I (Wenckebach) second-degree AV block there is progressive lengthening of the PR interval with constant P-P intervals eventually

leading to nonconducted P waves in a pattern of group beating (ratio of P waves to QRS complexes). This is usually due to a reversible delay of conduction in the AV node and is likely due to increased vagal tone or medications. It rarely needs treatment unless there is severe bradycardia and associated hypotension. Mobitz type II second-degree AV block, high-degree block, and complete heart block involve varying degrees of delay in the infranodal conduction system and are usually due to intrinsic conduction system disease. A lower ventricular escape rhythm with a rate of 25 to 40 beats/min is often present in complete heart block in an attempt to maintain cardiac output but may not provide an adequate HR (Figure 23–1a). Patients are less likely

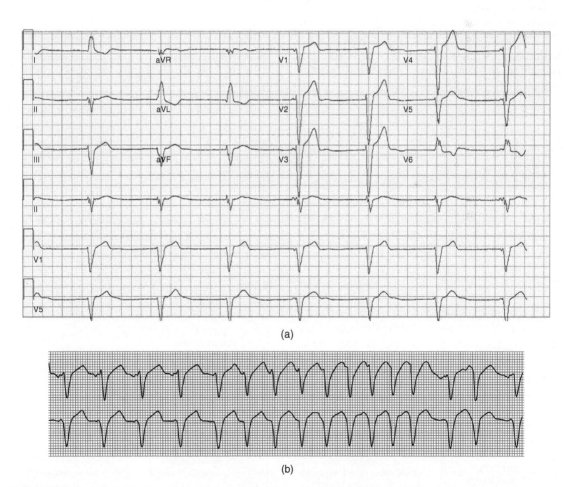

(a)

(b)

FIGURE 23–1 (a) A 12-lead electrocardiogram with atrioventricular dissociation with severe sinus bradycardia and an idioventricular escape rhythm of 43 beats/min with left bundle branch conduction. (b) Monitor strip showing atrioventricular dissociation with an underlying sinus rhythm of 70 beats/min and a monomorphic ventricular tachycardia.

to remain hemodynamically stable with higher degrees of AV block and usually require temporary pacing with either a transthoracic or transvenous pacemaker and ultimately permanent pacing if the heart block persists. While atropine increases HR by decreasing vagal tone and the degree of AV block with type I AV block, it is usually ineffective in increasing HR with infranodal conduction delays and may actually increase the degree of block by increasing sinus rate without the ability to increase ventricular rate. Another common cause of bradycardia in the ICU occurs in patients with alternating bradycardia and tachyarrhythmias (Tachy–Brady syndrome) or paroxysmal atrial fibrillation, who have delayed sinus node recovery times either due to intrinsic conduction system disease or to the medications used to control the tachycardia. They can have prolonged pauses when they convert to sinus rhythm and may require pacing to allow adequate medication to control their arrhythmia without periods of symptomatic bradycardia.

AV dissociation occurs when there is loss of the usual pattern of atrial and ventricular synchrony and there is no association between P waves and the QRS complexes. This can be caused by heart block as discussed earlier where impulses cannot be transmitted through the AV node and a lower focus (escape rhythm) takes over (Figure 23–1a). Persistent heart block usually leads to permanent pacemaker implantation. A benign form of AV dissociation is called isoarrhythmic AV dissociation (Figure 23–2), which occurs when the sinus rate is slower than or approximately the same as a lower intrinsic cardiac rhythm so the rhythms alternate. This is commonly a junctional rhythm of 50 to 60 beats/min and does not need treatment unless there is associated hemodynamic instability. Isoarrhythmic AV dissociation resolves with an increase in the sinus rate. Acceleration of a lower focus such as a junctional or ventricular tachycardia can also cause AV dissociation. These rhythms usually require treatment if sustained or symptomatic.

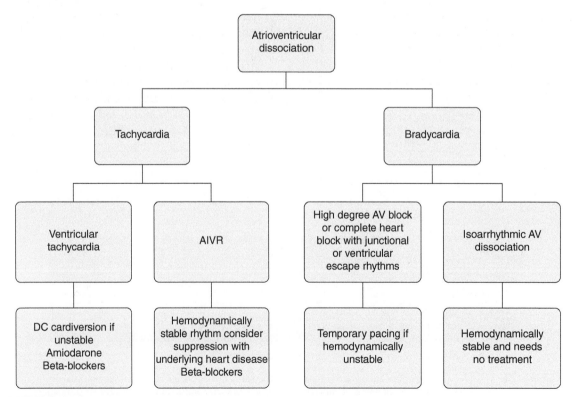

FIGURE 23–2 Differential diagnosis and treatment of atrioventricular dissociation.

TACHYARRHYTHMIAS

ICU patients frequently have atrial and ventricular beats, which rarely need to be treated unless there is a sustained arrhythmia. Even frequent ventricular premature contractions (VPCs) with couplets, periods of bigeminy, and short runs do not need treatment unless the cardiac output is compromised. Underlying provocative causes, such as ischemia, left ventricular dysfunction, medication toxicity (eg, digoxin), or electrolyte abnormalities should be identified and addressed.

Sustained arrhythmias are less frequent but not uncommon. It is usually possible to differentiate between atrial and ventricular arrhythmias, but one of the biggest challenges in critically ill patients is to define the etiology of a wide complex tachycardia. Knowledge of the baseline EKG is important to help differentiate these arrhythmias. Patients with baseline right or left bundle branch blocks (LBBBs) have wide complex tachycardias, which are supraventricular with a QRS morphology that is the same as their baseline EKGs and are usually preceded by P waves. Some patients develop rate-related bundle branch blocks usually with an increase in HR that can cause confusion, but similarly are supraventricular, usually sinus in origin and due to variable delay in the conduction system and refractory periods of the bundle branches. Another form of wide complex supraventricular tachycardia can occur in patients with preexcitation syndromes when there is orthodromic conduction down the accessory pathway. These forms of supraventricular tachycardias need to be differentiated from ventricular rhythms.

The morphology of the QRS complexes can help differentiate supraventricular from ventricular rhythms. Ventricular tachycardias, while more likely to have LBBB configurations, have varying conduction patterns, have longer QRS durations (> 0.14-0.16 ms) and have greater leftward axis deviation. Evidence of AV dissociation with fusion or capture beats usually indicates a lower origin of the arrhythmia such as ventricular tachycardia.

SUPRAVENTRICULAR TACHYCARDIAS

Atrial fibrillation, atrial flutter, AV nodal reentry tachycardia, ectopic atrial tachycardia with rapid ventricular rates, and underlying preexcitation with an atrial arrhythmia form the majority of atrial tachyarrhythmias that manifest in the critically ill patient. Figure 23–3 lays out a classification scheme for narrow complex supraventricular tachycardias based on the regularity of the rhythm.

Initial evaluation is directed toward assessing hemodynamic stability. In the setting of hemodynamic compromise (eg, symptomatic hypotension, angina, heart failure, or myocardial ischemia) urgent

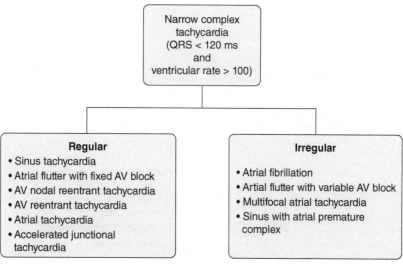

FIGURE 23–3 Classification of narrow complex tachycardias.

electrical cardioversion is indicated. The major goal of acute treatment is to slow the ventricular rate so as to restore hemodynamic stability by improving cardiac output and blood pressure. For patients that are hemodynamically stable, initial rate control strategy should be considered. Further treatment is directed toward eliminating or reversing the precipitating or exacerbating causes. Correction of alkalosis, hypokalemia, hypomagnesemia, and hypoxemia will increase the likelihood of rate control and eventual conversion to or maintenance of sinus rhythm.

ATRIOVENTRICULAR NODAL REENTRANT TACHYCARDIA

About 65% of regular supraventricular tachycardias are due to atrioventricular nodal reentrant tachycardia (AVNRT).[3] AV nodal reentrant tachycardias are rhythm disturbances that depend on the properties of the AV node for initiation and propagation. In a typical circuit, activation proceeds down the anterograde "slow" pathway and returns via the retrograde "fast" pathway. The arrhythmia results from an endless circle of electrical impulses conducted down one pathway and up another with slow and fast pathways cooperating to facilitate and maintain the circuit. The atypical form of AVNRT involves antegrade conduction down the "fast" perinodal pathway and retrograde conduction via the "slow" perinodal pathway. AV nodal reentrant tachycardias usually have ventricular rates of 150 to 220 beats/min, but can be as fast as 250 beats/min. AV conduction is usually 1:1, but rarely 2:1. It usually begins with a premature atrial depolarization. There can be a pseudo R' in lead V1, a pseudo-S wave in the inferior leads and retrograde P wave can be seen in other leads. If the initial diagnosis is unclear, adenosine (6-12-12 mg intravenously) usually will break the reentry circuit and restore sinus rhythm (Figure 23–4). A brief intervening period of sinus bradycardia or complete heart block may occur. With atrial tachycardia, atrial flutter, or atrial fibrillation, increasing AV block with adenosine will usually make the diagnosis apparent while with sinus tachycardia the heart will slow gradually in response to adenosine and then return to the pretreatment rate.

For the hemodynamically unstable or symptomatic patient with AVNRT, initial choices include

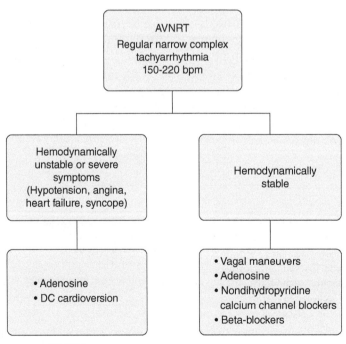

FIGURE 23–4 Management of AVNRT.

adenosine or direct current (DC) cardioversion to restore sinus rhythm and hemodynamic stability. Adenosine has a rapid onset and an extremely short half-life, making it the drug of choice for acute treatment of narrow complex tachyarrhythmias, but it is not useful in preventing recurrences.

For the hemodynamically stable patient, treatment approaches include vagal maneuvers (eg, Valsalva maneuver or carotid sinus massage), adenosine, nondihydropyridine calcium channel blockers (eg, verapamil 5 mg IV bolus or diltiazem 0.25 mg/kg infusion given over 2 minutes) and beta-blockers (eg, metoprolol with 5 mg boluses or esmolol, 0.5-1.0 mg/m² bolus). These drugs alter conduction velocity through the AV node (see Figure 23–4). Calcium channel blockers and beta-blockers decrease the likelihood of recurrence and should be considered in patients with early recurrent arrhythmia after administration of adenosine. Continued intravenous (IV) infusions may be needed to prevent early recurrences. For long-term management of patients with symptomatic episodes of this tachyarrhythmia, options include pharmacologic therapy and radiofrequency catheter ablation with the latter providing high curative success rates.

ATRIAL TACHYCARDIA

Atrial tachycardia is a narrow complex tachyarrhythmia with impulse generation outside of the sinus node that does not rely on accessory pathways, AV node, or ventricular tissue for generation and propagation.[3] Atrial tachycardia is usually focal in origin and can arise from any ectopic focus in the left atrium, right atrium, vena cava, or pulmonary veins. The underlying mechanism can involve reentry, enhanced automaticity, or triggered activity. Atrial tachycardia may occur from atrial stretch, digitalis toxicity, electrolyte imbalance, and catecholamine excess with or without underlying cardiac disease. On the EKG, the P wave generally precedes the QRS complex; however, it has a morphology that is distinct from the sinus P wave. The P wave axis is usually abnormal and may help in localizing the site of origin of the tachycardia. AV nodal blockers and digoxin do not terminate this arrhythmia, but can be used to slow down the ventricular rate and improve hemodynamics. In select cases, there may

be a role for class Ia, Ic, or III antiarrhythmic agents. Electrical cardioversion plays a limited role in the management of atrial tachycardia as the underlying pathophysiology is usually enhanced automaticity, which in most cases renders cardioversion ineffective with a high rate of arrhythmia recurrence.

MULTIFOCAL ATRIAL TACHYCARDIA

Multifocal atrial tachycardia is usually associated with underlying pulmonary disease especially severe chronic obstructive lung disease or respiratory failure in older, acutely ill individuals.[3] It can also occur in patients with other forms of pulmonary or cardiac disease. Electrolyte imbalance, hypoxia, acidosis, and drugs, such as isoproterenol and theophylline are also associated with this arrhythmia. It is characterized by an irregularly irregular rhythm with a ventricular rate greater than 100 beats/min and at least 3 unique P-wave morphologies each felt to indicate multiple atrial activation sites. Treatment is aimed at the underlying disease. Verapamil may be effective and sometimes slows ventricular response, but is not effective in all patients.

ATRIAL FLUTTER

Atrial flutter is a macroreentrant atrial tachycardia typically involving the right atrium. It usually coexists with atrial fibrillation and is uncommon in a structurally normal heart.[3] The atrial flutter rate is usually 300 beats/min, but can be slower (240-440 beats/min) especially in patients on antiarrhythmic therapy. The ventricular rate which is determined by the AV conduction ratio is usually a 2:1 with the resultant ventricular rate of approximately 150 beats/min (Figure 23–5). Higher degrees of AV block and variable HRs can be seen in patients due to underlying cardiac disease or AV nodal conduction disease and those on antiarrhythmic agents. Atrial flutter with 1:1 AV conduction and ventricular rates as high as 300 beats/min is poorly tolerated and can be seen in cases of sympathetic stimulation or in the presence of an accessory pathway. Flutter waves are best identified in the inferior leads and demonstrate a typical "sawtooth pattern" with

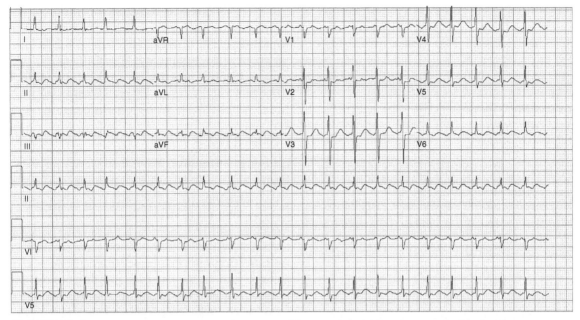

FIGURE 23-5 A 12-lead electrocardiogram showing atrial flutter with variable atrioventricular block with a ventricular rate of 128 beats/min. Note the presence of "saw tooth" waves in the inferior leads indicative of a typical or counterclockwise reentry circuit.

absence of an isoelectric baseline. The flutter waves are negative in the inferior leads if the reentry circuit is anticlockwise and positive if the reentry circuit is clockwise (uncommon variant). The rhythm while usually regularly can be irregular in the presence of variable AV block.

In patients with acute hemodynamic collapse or severe symptoms due to atrial flutter, DC synchronized cardioversion is indicated. Atrial flutter can be converted using relatively small amounts of electrical energy, usually less than 50 joules. Alternatively, if pharmacologic conversion is deemed necessary, ibutilide is considered the drug of choice, but carries a risk of QT prolongation and torsade de pointes mandating close monitoring with aggressive repletion of magnesium and potassium.

Atrial flutter also can be converted to sinus rhythm with overdrive pacing. Atrial flutter is amenable to radiofrequency ablation, with success rates approaching those for other supraventricular tachycardias and provides effective long-term treatment. AV nodal blockers can be used to slow down the ventricular rate in hemodynamically stable patients; however, rate control is more difficult to achieve in

atrial flutter. Digoxin can be considered for ventricular rate control in patients with congestive heart failure or hypotension.

Regardless of whether a rate or rhythm control method is employed, anticoagulation strategies to prevent systemic embolization must be considered in patients with atrial flutter. The risk assessment and therapeutic recommendations follow the same principal as atrial fibrillation.

ATRIAL FIBRILLATION

Atrial fibrillation is the most common dysrhythmia in the general population and is highly prevalent in the critically ill.[4] Affected patients are at increased risk of cardiovascular morbidity and mortality.[5] It is characterized by disorganized atrial electrical activity probably owing to multiple reentry circuits within the atria that results in loss of atrial contraction and irregular and often times rapid ventricular rates. It is easily recognized on the surface EKG as a narrow complex, irregularly irregular, supraventricular rhythm with a loss of clear P waves, and/or the presence of fibrillatory waves (Figure 23-6).

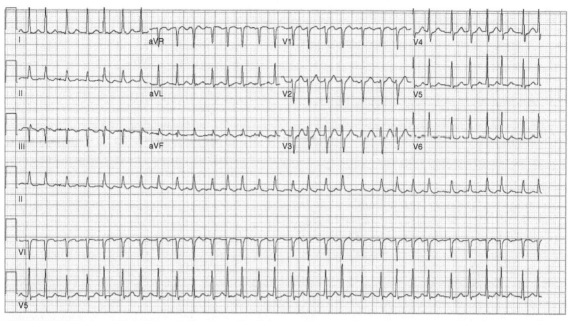

FIGURE 23-6 A 12-lead electrocardiogram showing atrial fibrillation with a rapid ventricular rate of 179 beats/min. Note the absence of clear P waves and an irregularly irregular rhythm.

This feature distinguishes atrial fibrillation from the other organized atrial arrhythmias.

Atrial fibrillation increases with age and is greater in men compared to women. Most forms of structural heart disease are associated with atrial fibrillation; most commonly hypertensive heart disease, underlying coronary artery disease, and rheumatic heart disease. Other cardiopulmonary and systemic diseases including obstructive sleep apnea, diabetes, obesity, metabolic syndrome, hyperthyroidism, chronic kidney disease, and postsurgical states have also been associated with atrial fibrillation. Premature atrial contractions are a trigger for atrial fibrillation. In addition, transition between atrial fibrillation and other supraventricular arrhythmias, especially typical atrial flutter is noted frequently. Initial diagnostic workup should include a careful history and physical examination(focusing on the duration and symptoms associated with the arrhythmia, identifiable exacerbating factors, and underlying cardiopulmonary or systemic disease processes), pertinent labs (including serum electrolytes and thyroid function tests), and specific cardiovascular workup (transthoracic and in select cases transesophageal echocardiogram).

As with other arrhythmias, initial assessment should focus on hemodynamic stability as well as identification and correction of underlying causes. Therapeutic considerations in atrial fibrillation include the three nonmutually exclusive strategies of rate control, rhythm control, and systemic thromboembolism prevention.[6-9] Recent clinical trials have demonstrated similar outcomes with rate and rhythm control strategies; however, there may be crossover from one to another strategy due to the natural history of the disease, failure of the initial strategy, or patient preference.[10]

Rhythm control strategies include synchronized DC cardioversion, pharmacologic conversion using antiarrhythmic drugs, radiofrequency catheter ablation, and/or surgical procedures (eg, Maze procedure). Urgent cardioversion should be considered for hemodynamically unstable, severely symptomatic patients, and in the presence of underlying preexcitation. Indications have been summarized in Table 23-1. Several antiarrhythmic agents can be used for pharmacologic rhythm control; however, careful attention should be paid to appropriate patient selection and the side-effect profile and proarrhythmic potential of these medications.

TABLE 23–1 Indications for urgent cardioversion in atrial fibrillation.

Hypotension/shock
Acute or ongoing myocardial ischemia
Congestive heart failure and/or acute pulmonary edema
Underlying preexcitation with rapid ventricular rates and/or hemodynamic instability

For patients without evidence of structural heart disease or coronary artery disease, class Ic agents like propafenone or flecainide can be considered. Patients should be monitored for QRS widening after initiation of these drugs. For patients with evidence of structural heart disease, amiodarone, sotalol, dronedarone, ibutilide, and dofetilide are the most commonly recommended antiarrhythmic agents. In patients with coronary artery disease without left ventricular dysfunction sotalol, dofetilide, amiodarone, and dronedarone are reasonable choices. In patients with left ventricular (LV) dysfunction and clinical heart failure, antiarrhythmic choices include amiodarone and dofetilide. QT interval should be monitored with class III antiarrhythmics. Sotalol and dofetilide are both affected by renal insufficiency and may require dose adjustment or discontinuation. Amiodarone requires dose adjustment in hepatic dysfunction and has significant systemic side effects with a propensity to cause pulmonary, cardiac, thyroid, ocular, dermatologic, hepatic, and gastrointestinal side effects which must be carefully considered prior to initiating treatment.

Most patients will require slowing of the ventricular rate associated with atrial fibrillation. Pharmacologic approach includes AV nodal blocking agents, namely, nondihydropyridine calcium channel blockers and beta-blockers. In patients with congestive heart failure or hypotension, digoxin can be considered. In select patients, combination therapy may be necessary, but excessive AV nodal blockade should be avoided. A-V node ablation with ventricular pacing is an alternative nonpharmacologic rate control approach, but rarely an acute treatment.

An important aspect of atrial fibrillation management includes prevention of thromboembolism. Patients with atrial fibrillation are at risk for systemic embolization and stroke. The noncontracting atria are a potential nidus for thrombus formation, which usually occurs in the left atrium and left atrial appendage. Multivariate risk models are available to aid in estimation of the thromboembolic risk in patients with nonvalvular atrial fibrillation so that appropriate antithrombotic prevention strategies can be recommended. The most commonly used and well validated being the CHADS2 point score (Congestive heart failure, Hypertension, Age ≥ 75 years, Diabetes mellitus, and prior Stroke or transient ischemic attack) index.[11] Patients without any of these risk factors have a CHADS2 score of 0 are at low risk of thromboembolic events and do not require long-term antithrombotic therapy. Patients with a score of 1 are at intermediate risk and can be treated with oral anticoagulant therapy or aspirin. Patients with a score of 2 or higher on the CHADS2 index are considered to be at high risk for thromboembolic events and anticoagulant therapy is recommended unless there are contraindications. Choices include the conventionally used vitamin K antagonist warfarin or newer direct thrombin inhibitor such as dabigatran and factor Xa inhibitors, such as rivaroxaban or apixaban. The new agents should not be used in the presence of severe renal insufficiency, prosthetic heart valves, and in cases of valvular atrial fibrillation. Initial therapy in critically ill patients may be unfractionated or fractionated heparin in the acute period of care prior to conversion to one of these agents.

Hemodynamically stable patients with atrial fibrillation of unknown duration or those with atrial fibrillation for more than 48 hours should be therapeutically anticoagulated for 3 to 4 weeks before elective conversion is attempted. Alternatively, the patient can be started on anticoagulation and if a transesophageal echocardiogram rules out existing thrombi, elective cardioversion can be performed safely. Anticoagulation should be continued for 4 weeks after cardioversion.

The differences in the pathophysiology and management of patients that present with atrial fibrillation with an underlying accessory pathway are noteworthy. A rapid ventricular rate (usually greater than 200 beats/min) and evidence of preexcitation are clues to this diagnosis. For hemodynamically unstable patients urgent cardioversion should be considered. AV nodal blockers should be avoided as they can promote conduction down the accessory pathway resulting in rapid ventricular rates and ventricular fibrillation. Digoxin and adenosine should also be avoided. Antiarrhythmic choices for rhythm control include procainamide, amiodarone, ibutilide, flecainide, and propafenone. Transvenous radiofrequency catheter ablation of bypass tracts obviates the need for long-term pharmacologic therapy and has largely replaced surgical ablation due to its high curative success rates in patients with bypass tracts.

VENTRICULAR TACHYCARDIAS

Ventricular tachycardia is defined as 3 or more consecutive VPCs at a rate of at least 100 beats/min, but is not considered sustained unless it is persists for at least 30 seconds. It is usually monomorphic and is a reentry arrhythmia (Figure 1b). This is easily differentiated from an accelerated idioventricular rhythm (AIVR) which is a wide complex rhythm at 40 to 60 beats/min that is usually due to increased automaticity or is an escape rhythm due to bradycardia (Figure 1a). AIVR is usually transient and does not require treatment other than addressing the underlying cause. Rapid ventricular tachyarrhythmias, especially in patients with structural heart disease and ischemia are more likely to cause hemodynamic compromise and to degenerate into ventricular fibrillation. Ventricular fibrillation requires emergency defibrillation as per Advanced Cardiac Life Support recommendations and protocols.[12] Unstable patients such as those with hypotension, exacerbation of heart failure, obtundation, or unstable ischemic chest pain who develop ventricular tachycardia should be treated by emergency electrical cardioversion starting with 100 to 200 J and increasing up to 360 J to restore sinus rhythm. Pharmacologic treatment may be needed in addition, but can be used alone in patients who have sustained ventricular tachycardia and remain hemodynamically stable.[13] These drugs need to be used carefully as many antiarrhythmic agents have significant proarrhythmic side effects and potassium and magnesium replacement should be given. Initial treatment with amiodarone is recommended as a first-line agent. IV infusion of 150 mg of amiodarone over 10 minutes can be given. The full loading dose of amiodarone is given over 24 hours at 1 mg/min over the first 6 hours followed by 0.5 mg/min over the next 18 hours for a total of 1050 mg. Subsequent maintenance doses can be given orally or intravenously as tolerated. Beta-blockers and procainamide are alternatives. Lidocaine can be used in patients with acute cardiac syndromes and other drugs, such as sotalol, propafenone, and flecainide are second-line agents due to their high incidence of proarrhythmic effects. Overdrive pacing can be considered in patients with sustained ventricular arrhythmias that are refractory to antiarrhythmic agents.

Torsade de pointes and other forms of polymorphic tachycardia are rapid ventricular rhythms associated with hemodynamic instability and a predisposition to degenerate into ventricular fibrillation.[14] Polymorphic ventricular tachycardia is commonly associated with ischemia and is likely to require cardioversion and consideration of rapid myocardial revascularization. In Torsades de pointes, the morphology of the QRS complexes varies in a pattern of twisting points and changes of axis associated with marked QT prolongation of greater than 500 ms (Figure 23–7). It can be caused by electrolyte abnormalities, ischemia, and proarrhythmic effects of antiarrhythmic agents such as flecainide, propafenone, quinidine, and sotalol and by other agents and drug interactions that increase the QT interval. Common causative agents include antibiotics, antihistamines, antifungal agents, tricyclic antidepressants, and phenothiazines. Although less common than acquired QT prolongation are patients with congenital QT prolongation (Romano–Ward Syndrome and Lange–Jervell–Neilson Syndrome) who are at risk for polymorphic ventricular tachycardia. Treatment is directed to reversing the inciting causes of the arrhythmia and to shortening the QT interval. IV magnesium should be given and potassium level repleted to 4.5 to 5 mmol/L. The stimulating factors should be removed or corrected as much as possible. The absolute QT interval should be shortened by increasing the HR with atropine, isoproterenol infusion, or overdrive pacing. As with any unstable patient with ventricular tachycardia, electrical cardioversion may be needed.

Other less common causes of ventricular tachycardia/ventricular fibrillation can sometimes be

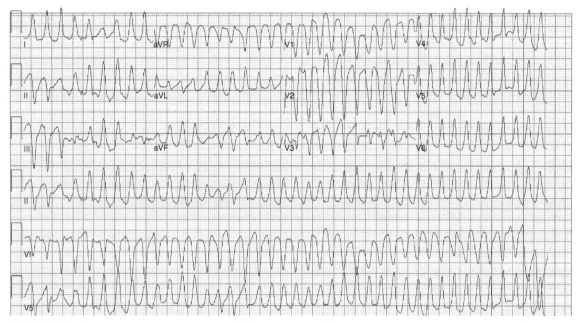

FIGURE 23–7 A 12-lead electrocardiogram of Torsade de pointes. Unstable rapid polymorphic ventricular tachycardia demonstrating the shifting heights and constantly changing axes of the ventricular complexes.

found in patients in the ICU and need to be recognized. Patients with Brugada syndrome may be predisposed to polymorphic ventricular tachycardia and ventricular fibrillation. EKGs show varying degrees of right bundle branch block and right precordial ST elevations, which may not always be present at baseline, but can be induced during periods of stress and by medications. These patients with life threatening arrhythmias will require automatic implantable cardioverter defibrillator (AICD) implantation in addition to the acute treatment described earlier. Another variant of stress or exercise-induced ventricular tachycardia usually arises from the right ventricular outflow tract and less commonly from a site in the left ventricular outflow tract. This is usually a more benign arrhythmia that presents with paroxysmal ventricular tachycardia with a LBBB pattern that responds to adenosine or beta-blockers. This rhythm can eventually be treated with radiofrequency catheter ablation of the initiating site in the outflow tract although long-term treatment with beta-blockers can be effective.

All ventricular arrhythmias can be markers for poorer long-term prognosis and sudden death in patients associated with left ventricular dysfunction and ischemic heart disease.[13] Patients with nonsustained ventricular tachycardias and ischemic heart disease in ICU settings, especially those with acute cardiac syndromes should be given beta-blockers to control HR, blood pressure, and rhythm disturbances in addition to electrolyte replacement and control of other stimulatory factors such as anemia, pain, and fever. Long-term treatment strategies for these patients may include AICDs and biventricular pacing especially if there is persistent left ventricular dysfunction with no reversible inciting factors for the ventricular arrhythmia. While these devices have improved outcome in some patients, they are rarely indicated acutely in the treatment of patients in the ICU. Patients should eventually be referred for cardiac evaluation to see if they qualify for device implantation under the current guidelines.[13,15,16] Patients with ventricular arrhythmias and structural heart disease, such as hypertrophic cardiomyopathies and congenital syndromes, such as Brugada syndrome may benefit from earlier electrophysiologic referral for secondary prevention of ventricular arrhythmias and sudden death.

REFERENCES

1. Reinelt P, Karth GD, Geppert A, et al. Incidence and type of cardiac arrhythmias in critically ill patients: a single center experience in a medical-cardiological ICU. *Intensive Care Med.* 2001;27(9):1466-1473.
2. Annane D, Sebille V, Duboc D, et al. Incidence and prognosis of sustained arrhythmias in critically ill patients. *Am J Respir Crit Care Med.* 2008;178(1):20-25.
3. Blomström-Lundqvist C, Scheinman MM, Aliot EM, et al. ACC/AHA/ESC guidelines for the management of patients with supraventricular arrhythmias—executive summary: a report of the American College of Cardiology/American Heart Association Task Force on Practice Guidelines and the European Society of Cardiology Committee for Practice Guidelines (Writing Committee to Develop Guidelines for the Management of Patients With Supraventricular Arrhythmias). *Circulation.* 2003;108:1871-1909.
4. Go AS, Hylek EM, Phillips KA, et al. Prevalence of diagnosed atrial fibrillation in adults: national implications for rhythm management and stroke prevention: the Anticoagulation and Risk Factors in Atrial Fibrillation (ATRIA) study. *JAMA.* 2001;285:2370-2375.
5. Benjamin EJ, Wolf PA, D'Agostino RB, et al. Impact of atrial fibrillation on the risk of death: the Framingham Heart Study. *Circulation.* 1998;98:946-952.
6. Fuster V, Ryden LE, Cannom DS, et al. ACC/AHA/ESC 2006 guidelines for the management of patients with atrial fibrillation—Executive Summary: a report of the American College of Cardiology/American Heart Association Task Force on Practice Guidelines and the European Society of Cardiology Committee for Practice Guidelines (Writing Committee to Revise the 2001 Guidelines for the Management of Patients with Atrial Fibrillation). *J Am Coll Cardiol.* 2006;48:854-906.
7. Fuster V, Ryden LE, Cannom DS, et al. 2011 ACCF/AHA/HRS focused updates incorporated into the ACC/AHA/ESC 2006 guidelines for the management of patients with atrial fibrillation: a report of the American College of Cardiology Foundation/American Heart Association Task Force on practice guidelines. *Circulation.* 2011;123:e269-e367.
8. Wann LS, Curtis AB, January CT, et al. 2011 ACCF/AHA/HRS focused update on the management of patients with atrial fibrillation (Updating the 2006 Guideline): a report of the American College of Cardiology Foundation/American Heart Association Task Force on Practice Guidelines. *J Am Coll Cardiol.* 2011;57:223.
9. American College of Cardiology Foundation, American Heart Association, European Society of Cardiology, et al. Management of patients with atrial fibrillation (compilation of 2006 ACCF/AHA/ESC and 2011 ACCF/AHA/HRS recommendations): a report of the American College of Cardiology/American Heart Association Task Force on practice guidelines. *Circulation.* 2013;127:1916.
10. Wyse DG, Waldo AL, DiMarco JP, et al. A comparison of rate control and rhythm control in patients with atrial fibrillation. *N Engl J Med.* 2002;347:1825-1833.
11. Gage BF, Waterman AD, Shannon W, et al. Validation of clinical classification schemes for predicting stroke: results from the National Registry of Atrial Fibrillation. *JAMA.* 2001;285:2864-2870.
12. Neumar RW, Otto CW, Link MS, et al. Part 8: Adult advanced cardiovascular life support: 2010. American Heart Association Guidelines for Cardiopulmonary resuscitation and emergency cardiovascular care. *Circulation.* 2010;122:S729.
13. European Heart Rhythm Association, Heart Rhythm Society, Zipes DP, et al. ACC/AHA/ESC 2006 guidelines for management of patients with ventricular arrhythmias and the prevention of sudden cardiac death. *J Am Coll Cardiol.* 2006;48:e247.
14. Drew BJ, Ackerman MJ, Funk M, et al. Prevention of Torsade de Pointes in Hospital settings: A scientific statement from the American Heart Association and the American College of Cardiology Foundation endorsed by the America Association of Critical-Care Nurses and the International Society for Computerized Electrocardiology. *J Am Coll Cardiol.* 2010;55(9):934-947.
15. Epstein AD, DiMarco JP, Ellenbogen KA, et al. ADD/AHA/HRS 2008 Guidelines for Device—Based Therapy of Cardiac Rhythm abnormalities; A Report of the American College of Cardiology/American Heart Association task force on Practice Guidelines(Writing Committee to revise the ADD/AHA/NASPE 2002 guideline update for implantation of cardiac pacemakers and antiarrhythmia devices). *Circulation.* 2008;117:e350.
16. Russo AM, Stainback RF, Bailey SR, et al. ACCF/HRS/AHA/ASE/HFSA/SCCT/SCMR 2013. Appropriate Use criteria for implantable Cardioverter-Defibrillators and Cardiac Resynchronization Therapy: A report of the America

College of Cardiology Foundation, Appropriate Use Criteria Task Force, Heart Rhythm Society, American Heart Association, American Society of Echocardiography, Heart Failure Society of America, Society for Cardiovascular Angiography and Interventions, Society of Cardiovascular Computed Tomography and Society for Cardiovascular Magnetic Resonance. *J Am Coll Cardiol.* 2013;61(12):1318-1368.

Acute Cardiac Ischemia

Matthew I. Tomey, MD and Umesh K. Gidwani, MD

KEY POINTS

1. Any acute imbalance between myocardial oxygen supply and demand may result in a syndrome of acute cardiac ischemia. Potential mechanisms include acute changes in coronary anatomy, as in plaque rupture and thrombosis, and acute changes in physiology as in sepsis and hemorrhage.

2. Acute cardiac ischemia progresses in a typical cascade through perfusion abnormality, metabolic disturbances, diastolic and systolic dysfunction, electrocardiographic changes, symptoms, and ultimately myocardial necrosis, with associated rise in serum biomarkers of myocardial infarction. Therapy to interrupt this cascade is time sensitive in order to prevent irreversible loss of myocytes.

3. Key elements of initial evaluation of suspected acute cardiac ischemia include a chest pain history, focused examination to exclude alternate diagnoses and assess hemodynamic stability, and a 12-lead electrocardiogram to identify ST-segment elevations. Serum biomarkers of myocardial infarction including troponin

creatine kinase and its MB fraction should be measured for diagnostic and prognostic purposes, but should not delay urgent management.

4. Directed therapy for acute cardiac ischemia should target the suspected mechanism of ischemia. When plaque rupture, thrombosis, and acute obstruction to coronary blood flow are suspected, appropriate treatment includes dual antiplatelet therapy with aspirin and an adenosine diphosphate receptor antagonist, anticoagulation, statin therapy, and consideration of reperfusion therapy. When stable coronary anatomy and an acute change in physiology are suspected, treatment should prioritize correction of the offending physiologic derangements.

5. Acute cardiac ischemia with ST-segment elevations is a medical emergency requiring immediate cardiology consultation and consideration of reperfusion therapy, including potential primary percutaneous coronary intervention or fibrinolytic therapy.

INTRODUCTION

Acute cardiac ischemia is defined by new or worsening imbalance between myocardial oxygen supply and demand, most commonly in the setting of coronary artery disease. Despite improvements in medical therapy, the burden of coronary artery disease remains high, affecting over 15 million United States adults.[1] Acute cardiac ischemia describes a physiologic disturbance underlying a spectrum of disorders encountered in critical care, from so-called "demand ischemia" in the setting of an acute physiologic insult and stable ischemic heart disease, to acute coronary syndromes (ACS), including unstable angina (UA), non-ST segment elevation myocardial infarction (NSTEMI), and ST-segment elevation myocardial infarction (STEMI).

Whereas certain physiologic principles of acute cardiac ischemia are common across this spectrum, providing the basis for understanding its natural history and therapy, appropriate management varies importantly with the mechanism of disease. As such, the ability to both identify and discriminate acute cardiac ischemia is fundamental to timely selection and implementation of appropriate therapy. In this chapter, we aim to provide a practical, intuitive review of the spectrum of acute cardiac ischemia for the critical care provider.

ANATOMIC AND PHYSIOLOGIC CONSIDERATIONS

Cardiac ischemia results from an imbalance between myocardial oxygen supply and demand. Acute disturbances in supply, demand, or both can precipitate a syndrome of acute cardiac ischemia. Major determinants of myocardial oxygen supply and demand are presented in Table 24–1.

Determinants of Myocardial Oxygen Supply

Oxygen uptake by tissue is governed by oxygen delivery and oxygen extraction. Because myocardial oxygen extraction is near-maximal, at 70% to 80%, variation in myocardial oxygen supply is primarily driven by delivery of oxygen. Delivery of oxygen is directly related to cardiac output, or blood flow, and the content of oxygen in arterial blood (**Equation 24–1**). Cardiac output is the product of heart rate and left ventricular stroke volume (**Equation 24–2**). Arterial oxygen content is determined by the hemoglobin concentration, arterial oxygen saturation, and partial pressure of oxygen in arterial blood (**Equation 24–3**).

$$DO_2 \; \alpha \; CO \times CaO_2 \qquad (24\text{–}1)$$

$$CO = HR \times SV \qquad (24\text{–}2)$$

$$CaO_2 = (Hb \times 1.39 \times SaO_2) + (PaO_2 \times 0.003) \qquad (24\text{–}3)$$

Oxygenated blood is delivered to the myocardium via branches of the coronary arteries. Normal coronary anatomy consists of a right coronary artery (RCA) arising from the right sinus of Valsalva and a left main coronary artery arising from the left sinus of Valsalva, which in turn bifurcates into the left anterior descending and left circumflex arteries (Figure 24–1). The coronary arteries and their branches develop as anatomical "end arteries," providing all or most of the blood supply to specific areas of subtended myocardium. Typically, the RCA supplies blood to the right ventricle and inferior wall of the left ventricle, the left circumflex supplies blood to the lateral and inferior walls of the left ventricle, and the left anterior descending supplies blood to the anterior wall of the left ventricle. Anatomic variations are common. Furthermore, collateral circulation can develop over time as an adaptation to chronic ischemia.

Myocardial blood flow is driven by the pressure gradient from the aortic root to the myocardial capillaries, the coronary perfusion pressure, and inversely related to coronary arterial resistance.

Coronary perfusion pressure is equal to the difference between aortic diastolic pressure and left ventricular end-diastolic pressure. Blood flow to the left ventricular myocardium occurs primarily during diastole, when aortic pressure exceeds left ventricular

TABLE 24–1 Key factors influencing myocardial oxygen supply and demand.

Supply	Demand
Cardiac output	Contractility
Hemoglobin concentration and oxygen saturation	Systolic blood pressure/afterload
Diastolic blood pressure	Preload
Left ventricular end-diastolic pressure	Heart rate
Coronary vasomotor tone	
Heart rate	

Right coronary artery

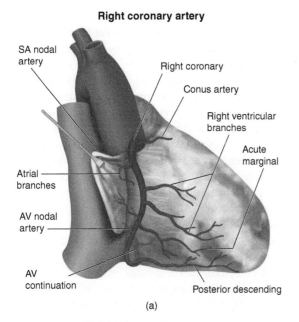

(a)

Left coronary artery

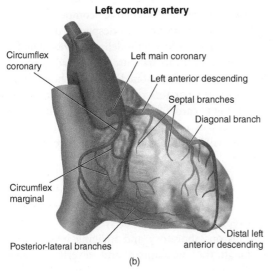

(b)

FIGURE 24–1 Normal coronary anatomy. (*Reproduced with permission from Doherty GM:* Current Diagnosis and Treatment: Surgery, *14th edition. New York: McGraw-Hill, Inc; 2015.*)

pressure due to closure of the aortic valve. During systole, in contrast, left ventricular pressure equals or exceeds (in the case of any left ventricular outflow tract obstruction) aortic pressure. Accordingly, decreases in aortic diastolic pressure and increases

in left ventricular end-diastolic pressure will tend to decrease myocardial blood flow. In a given coronary artery, anatomic obstruction (such as by atherosclerotic plaque, thrombus or embolus) may cause limitation or complete interruption of blood flow. Clinically important obstruction may occur at the macrovascular or microvascular level. Whereas the duration of systole is fairly fixed, the duration of diastole is variable and dependent on heart rate. As such, myocardial blood flow is also heart rate dependent; other things being equal, increases in heart rate decrease diastolic filling time and tend to reduce myocardial blood flow.

Resistance to coronary arterial blood flow is dynamic. A complex array of paracrine, endocrine, neural, and mechanical factors mediate local and global increases or decreases in coronary arterial resistance, in large part through modulation of coronary vasomotor tone. The capacity for localized changes in coronary vasomotor tone permits heterogeneity in coronary arterial resistance and local adaptation to physiologic circumstances, including ischemia. Decreases in local or global coronary arterial resistance tend to increase myocardial blood flow and, in turn, myocardial oxygen delivery.

DETERMINANTS OF MYOCARDIAL OXYGEN DEMAND

Oxygen is used by cells, including cardiac myocytes, as the ultimate electron acceptor in a series of redox reactions that culminate in generation of adenosine triphosphate (ATP) by oxidative phosphorylation. ATP is required to power energy-dependent cellular processes; in cardiac myocytes, this includes regulation of membrane potential, regulation of sarcoplasmic reticulum calcium concentration, and both cross-bridge formation and dissociation of actin and myosin (required for contraction and relaxation, respectively). Demand for ATP and, in turn, demand for oxygen, relates to the magnitude of this cellular work.

Accordingly, beyond myocardial basal energy expenditure, myocardial oxygen demand is driven by the work of each cardiac cycle and the number of cardiac cycles per minute (the heart rate). The work of a given cardiac cycle relates closely to wall stress—the force applied to a unit area of myocardium. As expressed by the Law of Laplace (**Equation 24–4**), *wall stress* is directly proportional to pressure and radius and inversely proportional to wall thickness. As such, wall stress and, in turn, myocardial oxygen demand will tend to increase in association with increases in contractility and systolic blood pressure (increasing left ventricular systolic pressure), obstruction to left ventricular outflow (increasing left ventricular systolic pressure), volume overload (increasing left ventricular radius and end-diastolic pressure), and decreased compliance (increasing left ventricular end-diastolic pressure).

$$\text{Wall stress} = \frac{P \times r}{2h} \qquad (24\text{--}4)$$

The Ischemic Cascade

Following onset of acute cardiac ischemia, a typical sequence of events ensues, referred to as the ischemic cascade (Figure 24–2). The earliest detectable change is a local abnormality in myocardial perfusion. This is followed in course by tissue-level metabolic disturbances, regional diastolic dysfunction, regional systolic dysfunction, electrocardiographic changes, symptoms, and finally irreversible cellular injury progressing to cell death (myocardial infarction).

The pace of this cascade depends on the severity of myocardial ischemia. With acute thrombotic total occlusion of an epicardial coronary artery, contractile changes are evident within 1 to 2 minutes; within 10 minutes, alterations in membrane potential increase predisposition to malignant ventricular arrhythmias; by 20 minutes, cellular injury becomes irreversible, beginning the process of myocardial infarction.[2] This rapid progression to risk of life-threatening arrhythmia and irreversible myocardial injury underscores the urgency of evaluation and management of suspected acute cardiac ischemia.

Myofibrillar changes are followed within hours by acute inflammation and coagulation necrosis, which proceeds over several days, followed by removal of dead myocytes by infiltrating macrophages. During this phase of phagocytosis, cardiac tissue is particularly friable and at risk of rupture. After 1 week, granulation tissue begins to form and mature, with progressive removal of cellular tissue and deposition of collagen. The process of scarring completes over 2 months. In parallel, the healing ventricle undergoes a process of remodeling, including changes in ventricular geometry and size. Although an increase in left ventricular end-diastolic volume allows hemodynamic compensation by maintaining stroke volume despite a decrease in systolic function, this remodeling proves maladaptive, contributing to increased myocardial oxygen demand (as aforementioned), chronic heart failure and mortality. For this reason, therapies to prevent such adverse cardiac remodeling are an important component of management of acute cardiac ischemia, as will be discussed in sections to follow.

CLINICAL PRESENTATION

Onset of acute cardiac ischemia is accompanied by a typical constellation of symptoms, signs, and findings on laboratory and imaging investigation. Although the mechanism and severity of acute cardiac ischemia may vary across the spectrum of responsible disorders, elements of the clinical presentation are conserved, which we review here.

HISTORY

The cardinal symptom of acute cardiac ischemia is chest pain. Chest pain typical of cardiac ischemia (*angina pectoris*) is characterized by provocation by exertion or emotional upset and alleviation by rest or nitrates. Pain is typically retrosternal in location and may radiate to the jaw, throat, or arms. The quality of

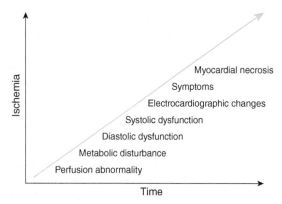

FIGURE 24–2 The ischemic cascade.

TABLE 24-2 Differential diagnosis of acute chest pain in the intensive care unit.

Diagnosis	Historical Features
Pulmonary embolism	Pleuritic Venous thromboembolism risk factors may be present
Pneumonia	Fever Productive cough
Aortic dissection	Tearing quality Sudden onset Radiation to back
Gastritis/esophageal reflux	May vary with meals or antacids
Esophageal spasm	May improve with nitrates
Pericarditis	Positional Pleuritic
Musculoskeletal	Localized May be elicited with palpation, motion or sometimes respiration

pain may be described as pressure-like or squeezing, and patients may even demonstrate this as a clenched fist in front of the chest (the Levine sign). Accompanying symptoms may include dyspnea, diaphoresis, and nausea. Importantly, the chest discomfort of acute cardiac ischemia may be a typical or absent, notoriously in women and patients with diabetes mellitus as well as postoperative or critically ill patients. A high index of suspicion is therefore mandatory. The angina of acute cardiac ischemia is *unstable*, being of new onset, occurring with rest or minimal exertion, or worsening in intensity, frequency, or duration (typically longer than 20 minutes).

Features on history may suggest a noncardiac source of chest pain. Pain that is pleuritic, positional, sharp, or reproducible with palpation is less likely to represent acute cardiac ischemia. A differential diagnosis is presented in Table 24–2.

Physical Examination

Abnormalities on physical examination are insufficient to rule in or rule out acute cardiac ischemia. Careful physical diagnosis is nonetheless necessary in the setting of suspected acute cardiac ischemia to identify signs of alternative diagnoses; to assess disease severity; and to identify systemic precipitants of worsening imbalance in myocardial oxygen supply and demand.

A focused investigation for alternative diagnoses should include simultaneous palpation of the bilateral radial pulses and measurement of bilateral brachial blood pressures to look for discrepancy, as might be seen in acute aortic dissection; palpation of the locus of chest discomfort to elicit tenderness, as would be suggestive of a musculoskeletal origin of pain; and auscultation of the chest and precordium to listen for a friction rub, as might be heard in pleuritis or pericarditis, or adventitious lung sounds, as might be heard in pneumonia. It should be noted that fever, while raising the question of alternate diagnoses, does not exclude acute cardiac ischemia, as indeed fever (along with leukocytosis) may be observed during acute myocardial infarction in conjunction with a robust systemic inflammatory response, with adverse prognostic implications.

When acute cardiac ischemia is the most likely diagnosis, physical examination is useful to identify evidence of acute heart failure, hemodynamic instability, and mechanical complications of ischemia and infarction. Manifestations of acute heart failure may include a third heart sound and signs of decreased cardiac output (such as sinus tachycardia, narrow pulse pressure, hypotension, decreased alertness, cool extremities, and thready pulses) or congestion (such as jugular venous distension, tachypnea, hypoxemia, labored breathing, rales, and frank pink, frothy sputum). A new systolic murmur may represent acute mitral regurgitation, resulting from acute ischemic dysfunction of a papillary muscle or, in the setting of acute myocardial infarction, papillary muscle rupture, or formation of a ventricular septal defect. The clinical triad of hypotension, jugular venous distension, and muffled heart sounds mandates investigation for pericardial tamponade, which may result from ventricular free wall rupture.

Electrocardiogram

The surface 12-lead electrocardiogram is the *sine qua non* of diagnosis and triage of acute cardiac ischemia, and should be performed within 10 minutes of medical contact. While the electrocardiogram should be approached systematically, including analysis of the rhythm, rate, axis, intervals, and evidence of chamber enlargement, particular attention is paid to the ST segments, T waves, and presence or absence of pathologic Q waves.

ST-segment elevation is the defining feature of STEMI, and a red flag that emergent action may be required. When caused by acute cardiac ischemia, ST-segment elevation is indicative of severe and often transmural ischemia, most commonly secondary to an acute total obstruction to coronary blood flow. Several conditions may explain ST-segment elevations (Table 24–3). To be diagnostic of STEMI, ST-segment elevations of sufficient magnitude (at least 0.1 mV and higher in leads V2-V3) must be present in at least two contiguous leads. The ST-segment elevations of acute cardiac ischemia are characterized by a territorial distribution; elevations in leads V2-V4; V5-V6, I, aVL; and II, III, aVF reflect ischemia in the anterior, lateral and inferior walls, respectively. Ischemic ST-segment elevations are typically characterized by a convex morphology, in contrast to the concave ST-segment elevations observed in pericarditis and early repolarization.

Clinical syndromes consistent with acute cardiac ischemia with no ST-segment elevations on the surface electrocardiogram are considered non-ST elevation ACS, and comprise UA and NSTEMI. The

acute cardiac ischemia of non-ST elevation ACS is typically nontransmural, but may still be extensive, often associated with multivessel coronary artery disease. ST-segment depressions or T wave inversions may be present, but these findings are not required for the diagnosis of UA or NSTEMI.

Of note, in certain syndromes of myocardial infarction, ST-segment elevations may be absent from the standard electrocardiogram despite presence of acute total occlusion of a coronary artery. True lateral, posterior, and right ventricular myocardial infarctions may be occult on the standard electrocardiogram due to their peripheral locations, requiring special placement of posterior (V7-V9) or right-sided (V3R-V5R) leads to reveal the diagnostic ST-segment elevations. These myocardial infarctions are pathophysiologically indistinguishable from those with overt ST-segment elevations and require the same urgency in management. It is of particular importance to recognize right ventricular infarction when it occurs—occasionally in isolation, but most frequently in conjunction with an inferior wall myocardial infarction due to occlusion of the RCA—as acute ischemia of the right ventricle causes exquisite preload dependence and susceptibility to severe hypotension with nitroglycerin.

Serum Biomarkers

Acute cardiac ischemia associated with myocardial infarction is characterized by a typical rise and fall of serum biomarkers of cardiac injury. The most sensitive and specific of these markers are the MB-fraction of creatine kinase (*CK-MB*), which tends to peak in the first day and fall over the next two, and *troponin I* or *T*, which also peaks in the first day but falls more slowly over several days (Figure 24–3). Less-specific serum markers which also rise and fall with acute myocardial infarction include *myoglobin*, total *creatine kinase, aspartate aminotransferase*, and *lactate dehydrogenase*.

Improvements in the sensitivity of laboratory measurements of serum troponin have not only permitted superior recognition of myocardial injury in the setting of acute cardiac ischemia, but also identification of troponin elevations in the setting of other acute illnesses. This is particularly relevant in the critical care setting. Troponin elevations

TABLE 24–3 Differential diagnosis of ST-segment elevations.

Acute myocardial infarction
Early repolarization
Left ventricular hypertrophy
Left bundle branch block
Acute myopericarditis
Hyperkalemia
Brugada syndrome
Pulmonary embolism
Vasospasm
Ventricular aneurysm
Apical ballooning syndrome (Takotsubo cardiomyopathy)

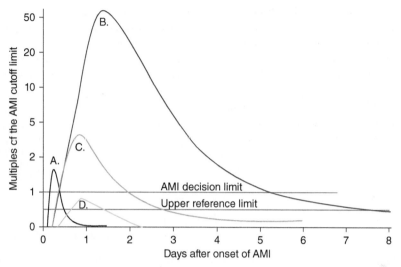

FIGURE 24–3 Kinetics of cardiac-specific biomarkers in myocardial infarction. A, myoglobin after MI; B, troponin after MI; C, CK-MB after MI; D, troponin in UA. (*Reproduced with permission from Wu AH, Apple FS, Gibler WB, et al: National Academy of Clinical Biochemistry Standards of Laboratory Practice: recommendations for the use of cardiac markers in coronary artery diseases, Clin Chem 1999 Jul;45(7):1104-1121.*)

can be seen with nonischemic myocardial injury, as in myocarditis, toxic insults, rhabdomyolysis, defibrillator shocks, and cardiac contusion as well as severe systemic illnesses, such as sepsis, stroke, and renal failure.[3] In isolation, an elevation in serum troponin is insufficient for diagnosis of acute cardiac ischemia.

Adjunctive Imaging

When laboratory studies, clinical examination, and the electrocardiogram are indeterminate for the diagnosis of cardiac ischemia, adjunctive imaging modalities with increased sensitivity to detect ischemia may be useful. The role of these tools is intuitive in the context of the ischemic cascade (see Figure 24–2). *Echocardiography* may detect new regional or global abnormalities in systolic or diastolic function as well as potential complications of acute cardiac ischemia, such as new onset mitral regurgitation. The transthoracic echocardiogram is a particularly useful tool in the intensive care unit as it can readily be performed portably at the bedside without requirement for radiation or nephrotoxic contrast media. For patients sufficiently stable to undergo stress testing, vasodilator testing with

myocardial perfusion imaging can be used to identify regional abnormalities in myocardial perfusion.

Coronary angiography, performed either noninvasively via computed tomography or invasively via cardiac catheterization, provides an anatomic depiction of coronary arterial patency. Although a 70% or greater diameter stenosis of the lumen of a coronary artery tends to connote a hemodynamically important obstruction to blood flow, it is important to recognize that angiography, by itself, is not a physiologic test of ischemia. For lesions of uncertain hemodynamic significance in the catheterization laboratory (and soon, the computed tomography suite), *fractional flow reserve* may be used to verify obstruction.

Universal Definition and Classification of Myocardial Infarction

Acute myocardial infarction is defined by clinical evidence of acute cardiac ischemia and a rise and/or fall in troponin, exceeding the 99th percentile of the normal reference population for a given laboratory.[3] Based on the clinical scenario, myocardial infarction may be classified into one of 6 types (1, 2, 3, 4a, 4b, or 5; see Table 24–4).

TABLE 24–4 Universal classification of myocardial infarction.

Type	Description
1	Spontaneous
2	Secondary to an ischemic imbalance
3	Resulting in death when biomarkers are unavailable
4a	Related to percutaneous coronary intervention
4b	Related to stent thrombosis
5	Related to coronary artery bypass grafting

Data from Thygesen K, Alpert JS, Jaffe AS, et al: Third universal definition of myocardial infarction, *J Am Coll Cardiol* 2012 Oct 16; 60(16):1581-1598.

THERAPEUTIC APPROACH

Critical care pathways differ importantly across the spectrum of acute cardiac ischemia. However, the core principle of therapy is shared: to restore balance between myocardial oxygen supply and demand. In this respect, it is fruitful to first undertake a general review of therapies used in the acute management of acute cardiac ischemia (Table 24-5) from a physiologic perspective.

Antithrombotic Therapy

Antithrombotic therapies, including antiplatelet and anticoagulant drugs, are useful in the acute setting when acute cardiac ischemia results from an acute coronary anatomic change (eg, atherosclerotic plaque rupture) associated with a tendency to thrombosis. This is to be contrasted with the scenario of "demand ischemia," in which coronary anatomy is stable, but an acute physiologic change has occurred resulting in increased myocardial oxygen demand. (Initiation of dual antiplatelet therapy is *not* the treatment of choice for acute cardiac ischemia secondary to a gastrointestinal hemorrhage!)

Aspirin is the cornerstone of antiplatelet therapy for patients with ACS. Aspirin inhibits platelets via inhibition of cyclooxygenase and, in turn, down regulation of thromboxane A2. In the setting of ACS, aspirin should be administered as soon as possible as a chewable loading dose (162-325 mg) followed by a daily oral maintenance dose of 75 to 100 mg.

TABLE 24–5 Evidence-based pharmacotherapies in the management of ACS.

Therapy	Examples
Aspirin	Aspirin
Platelet P2Y$_{12}$ adenosine diphosphate receptor antagonist	Clopidogrel Prasugrel Ticagrelor
Anticoagulation	Unfractionated heparin Enoxaparin Fondaparinux
High-potency statin	Atorvastatin 80 mg Rosuvastatin 40 mg
Beta-adrenergic blockade	Metoprolol
Angiotensin converting enzyme inhibitor *or* Angiotensin receptor blocker	Lisinopril Valsartan

Dual antiplatelet therapy using aspirin and an antagonist of the platelet adenosine diphosphate receptor has been shown to be superior to aspirin alone in the setting of ACS with or without ST-segment elevation for the prevention of recurrent ischemic events.[4,5] Originally documented with clopidogrel, this benefit has since been extended to the newer agents prasugrel and ticagrelor.[6,7] Clopidogrel is administered as an oral loading dose (300 or 600 mg) followed by a daily oral maintenance dose of 75 mg. Prasugrel should only be initiated at the time of coronary angiography, and never in patients with active bleeding or a history of stroke; when used, it is administered as an oral loading dose (30 or 60 mg) followed by a daily oral maintenance dose of 5 or 10 mg. Ticagrelor is administered as an oral loading dose (180 mg) followed by a twice daily oral maintenance dose of 90 mg.

Anticoagulation in the setting of ACS is typically accomplished using an inhibitor of the intrinsic coagulation cascade. Options include unfractionated heparin, administered as an intravenous bolus of 60 units/kg followed by an infusion of 12 units/kg/h, titrated to an activated partial thromboplastin time of 50 to 70 seconds; the low molecular weight heparin enoxaparin, administered as a subcutaneous injection 1 mg/kg twice daily; and fondaparinux.

Glycoprotein IIb/IIIa inhibitors are potent antiplatelet agents still used, in select cases, with cardiology guidance, typically in association with invasive management. Due to an increased risk of bleeding without clear benefit, routine early use of glycoprotein IIb/IIIa inhibitors upstream of invasive angiography is not recommended.[8]

Anti-ischemic Therapy

Multimodal therapies directed at improving balance between myocardial oxygen supply and demand are useful in all forms of acute cardiac ischemia, but must be tailored carefully to an individual patient.

Beta-adrenergic blockers increase myocardial oxygen supply by increasing diastolic filling time and decrease myocardial oxygen demand by reducing heart rate, contractility, and systolic blood pressure. This mechanism explains the utility of uninterrupted beta-adrenergic blockade during the perioperative setting of patients with known coronary artery disease. When feasible, as tolerated by blood pressure, beta-adrenergic blockade should be uptitrated to achieve a resting heart rate of 60 to 80 bpm. When acute cardiac ischemia is accompanied by signs of reduced cardiac output, and in particular tachycardia and hypotension, however, caution should be taken beta-blockade may inhibit the heart's compensatory response to acute systolic dysfunction, precipitating worsening heart failure or cardiogenic shock.

Nitrates, available in transdermal, sublingual, oral, and intravenous formulations, increase myocardial oxygen supply by reducing coronary vasomotor tone and left ventricular end-diastolic pressure and reduce myocardial oxygen demand by decreasing preload and systolic blood pressure. In the setting of ACS, nitrates are useful for the treatment of refractory angina or hypertension, and should be uptitrated as tolerated by blood pressure to achieve chest pain resolution.

Nitrates should be used only with caution in patients with suspected right ventricular infarction or recent use of phosphodiesterase type 5 inhibitors, as this combination may result in hypotension.

Angiotensin converting enzyme inhibitors and *angiotensin receptor blockers* serve multiple purposes in the setting of ACS, among which is a reduction in myocardial oxygen demand via reduction in systolic blood pressure. As tolerated by blood pressure and renal function, an agent should be started within 24 to 48 hours of presentation with ACS.

In patients with diminished content of arterial oxygen due to anemia or hypoxemia, *red blood cell transfusion* or *supplemental oxygen* may be warranted. Liberal transfusion and superoxygenation, however, are not helpful in the setting of acute cardiac ischemia, and may be harmful.

Analgesic therapy with *morphine* may indirectly decrease myocardial oxygen demand via reduction in pain and, in turn, heart rate. As morphine may also mask ongoing ischemia, however, it is reserved as a second-line to more direct anti-ischemic therapies. Nonsteroidal anti-inflammatory therapies should be avoided in the setting of ACS.

In select cases of acute cardiac ischemia refractory to medical therapies, mechanical support may be warranted to optimize balance of myocardial oxygen supply and demand. *Positive pressure ventilation* may reduce myocardial oxygen demand via reduction in work of breathing and preload. *Intra-aortic balloon counterpulsation* improves myocardial oxygen supply by augmenting coronary perfusion pressure during diastole and reduces myocardial oxygen demand by reducing afterload during systole.

REPERFUSION THERAPY

When acute cardiac ischemia results from acute interruption of blood flow in a coronary artery, reperfusion therapy restores myocardial oxygen supply via restoration of myocardial blood flow. Reperfusion therapy may be accomplished via fibrinolytic therapy, percutaneous coronary intervention, or coronary artery bypass graft surgery. Whereas fibrinolytic therapy is appropriate only for STEMI, percutaneous coronary intervention or bypass grafting may be used in cases of ACS with or without ST-segment elevation.

STATINS

While not strictly an anti-ischemic therapy, inhibitors of 3-hydroxy-3-methyl-glutaryl-coenzyme A reductase (statins) are a fundamental component of management of ACS. Through not only lipid lowering, but also pleiotropic effects, statins stabilize atherosclerotic plaque and reduce risk of recurrent ischemic events in patients with ACS. As soon as possible upon diagnosis of ACS, in the absence of contraindications, patients should be treated with a high-potency statin, examples of which include atorvastatin 80 mg and rosuvastatin 40 mg.

SPECIFIC CLINICAL SYNDROMES

In patients with suspected acute cardiac ischemia, prompt evaluation and triage is mandatory to permit assignment to syndrome-specific critical care

pathways (Figure 24–4). For detailed, up-to-date discussion of management considerations particular to UA/NSTEMI and STEMI, readers are encouraged to refer directly to current American College of Cardiology/American Heart Association guidelines.[9,10]

Acute Cardiac Ischemia in the Setting of Stable Coronary Artery Disease

Myocardial infarction "type 2" may result from anatomically stable coronary artery disease when physiologic derangements result in an acute imbalance

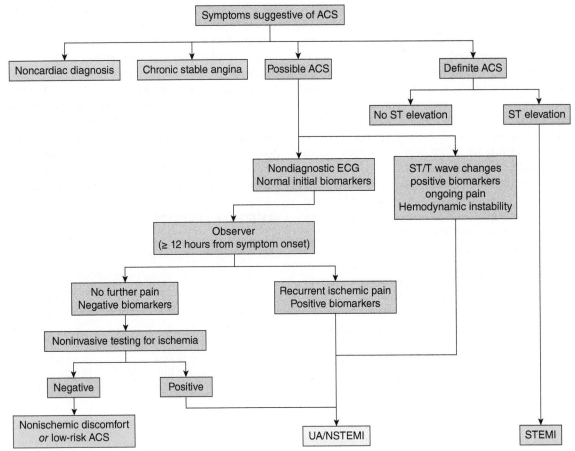

FIGURE 24–4 Diagnostic algorithm for patients with suspected acute cardiac ischemia. ACS, acute coronary syndrome; ECG, electrocardiogram; NSTEMI, non-ST elevation myocardial infarction; STEMI, ST elevation myocardial infarction; UA, unstable angina. (*Adapted with permission from Anderson JL, Adams CD, Antman EM, et al. 2012 ACCF/AHA focused update incorporated into the ACCF/AHA 2007 guidelines for the management of patients with unstable angina/non-ST-elevation myocardial infarction: a report of the American College of Cardiology Foundation/American Heart Association Task Force on Practice Guidelines, J Am Coll Cardiol 2013;61(23):e179-347.*)

TABLE 24–6 Common sources of myocardial infarction type 2 and management.

Illness	Potential Management
Acute blood loss/anemia	Transfusion Source control
Decompensated heart failure	Diuresis Inotropes
Tachyarrhythmia *or* bradyarrhythmia	Rate control Pacing
Sepsis	Antibiotics Volume resuscitation Source control
Hypertensive emergency	Blood pressure reduction
Hypotension	Volume resuscitation Pressors
Aortic stenosis	Valvuloplasty Valve replacement

between myocardial oxygen supply and demand and elevation in serum biomarkers of myocardial injury. The key to management of this syndrome is identification and correction of the underlying cause of increased myocardial oxygen demand. Potential etiologies of myocardial infarction type 2 are listed in Table 24–6. In conjunction with this disease-directed approach, supportive measures to mitigate cardiac ischemia include use of anti-ischemic therapies, as discussed earlier.

Of note, demand-mediated acute ischemia in the intensive care unit may not present with classical angina. Symptoms may be atypical or absent ("silent ischemia"). Among patients with known coronary artery disease or coronary risk factors, such silent ischemia is common in the intensive care unit, often unrecognized, and linked with increased morbidity and mortality.[11] Reported incidence has varied in series studying different settings and using test modalities with different sensitivities, with ischemic ST changes observed in 11% to 21% and troponin elevations noted in 15% to 38% of patients in published series.[11-13] Continuous electrocardiographic monitoring using 5 electrodes and 2 leads (typically

II and V5) has a low sensitivity in comparison with a standard 12-lead electrocardiogram and may miss clinically important ischemia.[13] It is important to recognize, however, that elevation in serum biomarkers of myocardial infarction may occur in the absence of epicardial coronary artery disease, deriving instead from direct effects of catecholamines or other circulating toxins on myocardial cells.

NSTE-ACS (UA/NSTEMI)

UA and NSTEMI account for the majority of ACS. When a diagnosis of UA/NSTEMI is suspected, the early priority of management is risk stratification. High-risk cases of UA/NSTEMI benefit from an early invasive management strategy, whereas lower-risk cases may be managed with an initial conservative strategy and provisional invasive angiography. Clinical features indicating high risk include refractory angina, hemodynamic or electrical instability, left ventricular systolic dysfunction, elevated serum biomarkers of cardiac injury, and ST-segment deviation. Global risk scores are also useful for risk stratification; commonly used scores include the TIMI, GRACE, and PURSUIT risk scores.

Regardless of risk profile, all patients diagnosed with UA/NSTEMI should be managed with dual antiplatelet therapy, anticoagulation, a high-potency statin, and optimal anti-ischemic therapy, as discussed earlier. Useful markers of therapeutic efficacy include resolution of chest pain and ST-segment deviations and a downward trend in serum CK-MB. Patients judged to be at high-risk and assigned to an early invasive strategy should undergo invasive angiography to define coronary anatomy and facilitate triage to an appropriate revascularization strategy. Patients deemed to be at low risk may be evaluated first using noninvasive stress testing, with subsequent triage to invasive angiography as warranted.

STEMI

STEMI is a medical emergency. Most commonly resulting from acute thrombotic occlusion of a coronary artery in the setting of coronary atherosclerosis, STEMI reflects severe, acute often transmural cardiac ischemia. "Time is muscle": reperfusion therapy is time-sensitive to save jeopardized myocardium. As such, management algorithms for

STEMI, including interhospital systems of care, are designed to minimize time to reperfusion therapy, for which primary percutaneous coronary intervention is preferred. Reperfusion therapy is indicated in all eligible patients within 12 hours of symptom onset; between 12 and 24 hours after symptom onset, reperfusion therapy may still be indicated for patients with clinical or electrocardiographic evidence of ongoing ischemia. Current time to reperfusion therapy systems goals include a door-to-needle time of 30 minutes (for fibrinolytic therapy) and a door-to-device time of 90 minutes (for primary percutaneous coronary intervention). In conjunction with expeditious reperfusion therapy, patients diagnosed with STEMI should receive dual antiplatelet therapy, anticoagulation, a high-potency statin, and optimal anti-ischemic therapy, as discussed above. In a limited proportion of cases, patients ineligible for reperfusion therapy will be managed with these medical therapies alone.

Complications of STEMI are of particular concern, and become the focus of critical care following reperfusion therapy. These may be grouped in terms of ischemic, electrical, and mechanical complications.

Ischemic complications include reinfarction and, following percutaneous coronary intervention with stent implantation, acute or subacute stent thrombosis. Symptoms and signs may include recurrent ischemic chest discomfort, ST-segment deviations, and a new rise in serum biomarkers of cardiac injury. Management may require intensification of antithrombotic and anti-ischemic therapy and may include repeat invasive angiography.

Electrical complications may include new onset bradyarrhythmias (including conduction blocks) and tachyarrhythmias, and in particular within the first 24 to 48 hours, ventricular tachycardia. Continuous electrocardiographic monitoring is mandatory to permit prompt identification and acute management of dysrhythmia; indeed, facilitation of prompt defibrillation was a primary motivating factor in the creation of coronary care units.

Mechanical complications include pump failure and cardiogenic shock; acute mitral regurgitation; ventricular septal defect formation; and free wall rupture with pericardial tamponade. Clinicians must maintain a high index of suspicion for these mechanical complications, which may manifest as fulminant clinical deterioration and which, importantly, may present late, 3 to 7 days following myocardial infarction.

In addition to these complications of STEMI itself, attention must be paid to the complications of our therapy. In particular, patients with both STEMI and UA/NSTEMI are exposed to risk of bleeding as a consequence of the acute provision of antiplatelet, anticoagulant, and invasive vascular therapies. Bleeding complications of ACS are important, with adverse prognostic implications. Patients who bleed are at risk for morbidity and mortality related to bleeding itself as well as heightened risk of recurrent ischemic events, which may relate to withholding of antithrombotic therapies or adverse effects of transfusion.

TRANSITION FROM ACUTE CARE TO SECONDARY PREVENTION

While the emphasis of critical care for acute cardiac ischemia is expeditious restoration of balance between myocardial oxygen supply and demand, also of critical importance is the transition from this acute phase to the work of preventing recurrent ischemic events. The critical care provider has a unique chance to "set the ship on course," seizing the episode of acute cardiac ischemia as an opportunity to educate the patient about therapeutic lifestyle changes (such as smoking cessation), identify and correct modifiable risk factors for coronary artery disease, arrange for cardiac rehabilitation, and emphasize the importance of medication adherence.

REFERENCES

1. Go AS, Mozaffarian D, Roger VL, et al. Heart disease and stroke statistics—2014 update: a report from the American Heart Association. *Circulation.* 2014;129(3):e28-e292.
2. Schoen FJ, Mitchell RN. The Heart. In: Kumar V, Abbas AK, Fausto N, Aster JC, eds. *Robbins and Cotran Pathologic Basis of Disease.* 8th ed. Philadelphia, PA: Saunders Elsevier; 2009.

3. Thygesen K, Alpert JS, Jaffe AS, et al. Third universal definition of myocardial infarction. *J Am Coll Cardiol*. 2012;60(16):1581-1598.

4. Yusuf S, Zhao F, Mehta SR, et al. Effects of clopidogrel in addition to aspirin in patients with acute coronary syndromes without ST-segment elevation. *N Engl J Med*. 2001;345(7):494-502.

5. Sabatine MS, Cannon CP, Gibson CM, et al. Addition of clopidogrel to aspirin and fibrinolytic therapy for myocardial infarction with ST-segment elevation. *N Engl J Med*. 2005;352(12):1179-1189.

6. Wiviott SD, Braunwald E, McCabe CH, et al. Prasugrel versus clopidogrel in patients with acute coronary syndromes. *N Engl J Med*. 2007;357(20):2001-2015.

7. Wallentin L, Becker RC, Budaj A, et al. Ticagrelor versus clopidogrel in patients with acute coronary syndromes. *N Engl J Med*. 2009;361(11):1045-1057.

8. Giugliano RP, White JA, Bode C, et al. Early versus delayed, provisional eptifibatide in acute coronary syndromes. *N Engl J Med*. 2009;360(21):2176-2190.

9. Anderson JL, Adams CD, Antman EM, et al. 2012 ACCF/AHA focused update incorporated into the ACCF/AHA 2007 guidelines for the management of patients with unstable angina/non-ST-elevation myocardial infarction: a report of the American College of Cardiology Foundation/American Heart Association Task Force on Practice Guidelines. *J Am Coll Cardiol*. 2013;61(23):e179-e347.

10. O'Gara PT, Kushner FG, Ascheim DD, et al. 2013 ACCF/AHA guideline for the management of ST-elevation myocardial infarction: a report of the American College of Cardiology Foundation/American Heart Association Task Force on Practice Guidelines. *J Am Coll Cardiol*. 2013;61(4):e78-e140.

11. Guest TM, Ramanathan AV, Tuteur PG, et al. Myocardial injury in critically ill patients. A frequently unrecognized complication. *JAMA*. 1995;273(24):1945-1949.

12. Landesberg G, Vesselov Y, Einav S, et al. Myocardial ischemia, cardiac troponin, and long-term survival of high-cardiac risk critically ill intensive care unit patients. *Crit Care Med*. 2005;33(6):1281-1287.

13. Martinez EA, Kim LJ, Faraday N, et al. Sensitivity of routine intensive care unit surveillance for detecting myocardial ischemia. *Crit Care Med*. 2003;31(9):2302-2308.

14. Wu AH, Apple FS, Gibler WB, et al. National Academy of Clinical Biochemistry Standards of Laboratory Practice: recommendations for the use of cardiac markers in coronary artery diseases. *Clin Chem*. 1999;45(7):1104-1121.

Heart Failure Syndromes in the Critical Care Setting

Omar Saeed, MD and James M. Tauras, MD

KEY POINTS

1 The incidence of heart failure (HF) is increasing significantly due to the aging population, improved drug, and device therapies for myocardial infarction as well as heart failure.

2 Categorizing HF patients based on volume status ("wet/dry") and perfusion status ("cold/warm") can guide treatment as well as risk stratify patients.

3 Routine use of inotropic agents in HF patients without a definitive low output state and end organ failure is generally not indicated, since these medications can increase myocardial oxygen demand and can promote arrhythmias, and outcomes data from randomized trials and registry data typically demonstrate worse outcomes with inotropic therapy compared to vasodilator therapy.

4 Pulmonary artery catheterization is typically reserved for HF patients with respiratory distress or evidence of hypoperfusion in whom intracardiac filling pressures cannot be determined from bedside assessment as well as patient who are doing poorly with empiric treatment based on clinical assessment.

4 Mechanical circulatory support (intra-aortic balloon pump, Impella device, tandem heart, and extracorporeal membrane oxygenation) can be extremely effective therapy in select patients.

HEART FAILURE SYNDROME

Heart failure (HF) is a global clinical syndrome which occurs when the metabolic demands of the body are not met by the circulation due to impairment of cardiac structure and function. Patients typically present with symptoms of progressive dyspnea, decreased exercise tolerance, and may or may not have signs of volume overload and congestion. The final diagnosis of HF must be made by a comprehensive clinical assessment and is not determined by a solitary laboratory value or radiological test.[1-5]

HF WITH REDUCED OR PRESERVED LEFT VENTRICULAR EJECTION FRACTION

HF may occur with or without the presence of left ventricular (LV) systolic dysfunction and thus it is widely categorized into 2 separate entities, namely, HF with reduced ejection fraction (HFrEF) and HF with preserved ejection fraction (HFpEF). Though different investigators and societies have used different definition of HFrEF and HFpEF, the current

American College of Cardiology Foundation/ American Heart Association (ACCF/AHA) Heart Failure Guidelines define HFrEF as patients with an LV ejection fraction of 40% or lower; these patients often have varying degrees of diastolic dysfunction as well. Oral HF therapies (beta-blockers, angiotensin converting enzyme inhibitors, mineralocorticoid receptor antagonists, hydralazine, and nitrates) have been extensively validated to provide a quality of life and mortality benefit by many randomized-control trials in patients with chronic HFrEF.

HFpEF includes patients with a left ventricular ejection fraction (LVEF) of 50% or higher and such patients may comprise up to 50% of the entire HF population. HFpEF is described by clinical signs of volume overload, preserved or normal LVEF, and diastolic dysfunction, typically demonstrated by Doppler echocardiography or cardiac catheterization. Patients with HFpEF tend to be older women with hypertension, and other prevalent comorbidities in this group include coronary artery disease, obesity, diabetes mellitus, and atrial fibrillation. To date, no oral HF therapies are proven to demonstrate mortality benefit in this heterogeneous category.

HEART FAILURE DEMOGRAPHICS

Acute heart failure (AHF) is the most common cause of hospitalization in patients more than 65 years old. The relative incidence of heart failure in women is lower than that of men, however, due to their longer life expectancy woman represent half the cases of heart failure. The incidence of heart failure increases dramatically with population age. Additionally, the incidence of heart failure admissions to US hospitals has been increasing significantly due to the aging population, improved therapies, and survival for acute myocardial infarction as well as improved drug and device therapies for chronic heart failure. Hospitalization is a key prognostic event in patients with heart failure with reduced ejection fraction as it is predictive of a 30% mortality rate in 1 year and a 50% risk of recurrent hospitalization in 6 months.

ASSESSMENT ACUTE HEART FAILURE SYNDROMES

History

Obtaining and performing a thorough history and physical examination are critical in reaching an accurate diagnosis of AHF and determining the cause of acute decompensation. The major elements of history that should be queried included changes in exercise tolerance, increase in baseline body weight, symptoms of ongoing cardiac ischemia, adherence to, and recent changes in heart failure medications, and signs or symptoms of infection. It is well known that signs and symptoms of heart failure (ie, weight gain, development of peripheral edema, dyspnea, and on exertion) can begin days to even weeks prior to hospital admission. Specific historical information can estimate if AHF involves right- or left-sided cardiac failure. Symptoms of left-sided AHF include dyspnea, orthopnea, and paroxysmal nocturnal dyspnea, while symptoms of right-sided failure may include early satiety and leg edema.

Physical Examination

Although patients with AHF often have a reduced cardiac output, hypotension may not be present. According to the ADHERE registry (a national registry of AHF admissions at 263 hospitals in the United States) the majority of patients with AHF present with a systolic blood pressure (SBP) of greater than 140 mm Hg. This maintenance of blood pressure is due to a catecholamine-mediated increase in systemic vascular resistance. Narrow pulse pressure may be a marker of severe LV dysfunction and tachycardia may be present as a compensatory response or due to ongoing cardiac ischemia. The level of the jugular venous pulsation (JVP) can be used to estimate the central venous pressure and serves as an important bedside measure of intravascular volume. Cardiac auscultation is critical as it can point toward structural and arrhythmic causes of AHF and signs of congestion can be confirmed by pulmonary examination. It is important to note that patients with chronic HF may not have signs of pulmonary congestion due to compensatory lymphatic drainage. Extremities should be examined for warmth or coolness as an indirect measure of perfusion.

Chest X-Ray and Electrocardiogram

Chest radiography is crucial as it cannot only confirm the presence and severity of pulmonary edema, but may also reveal other characteristics of cardiac disease. The cardiac silhouette should be examined for enlargement, size of the pulmonary artery may indicate elevated pulmonary arterial pressures, increased mediastinum width can point to aortic pathology, and the presence of any cardiovascular implantable electronic devices or prosthetic heart valves would indicate preexisting disease. The electrocardiogram is essential to determine if AHF is related to ischemia and arrhythmia and should be serially monitored in patients admitted with acute coronary syndromes.

Laboratory Analysis

Laboratory data can provide more clues in determining the causes of AHF including anemia, thyroid disease, infection, and biomarkers, such as sodium and brain natriuretic peptides cannot only assist in determining volume status, but may also have prognostic value. Renal function is a sensitive marker of perfusion and intravascular volume, but it should be used in conjunction with the overall clinical assessment, since a decrease in creatinine clearance may occur from reduced cardiac output from either a drop or rise in intravascular volume, direct renal toxicity, or postrenal obstruction. Liver function test abnormalities may be related to congestive hepatopathy or ischemia from severely reduced cardiac output.

Clinical Assessment

The overall clinical assessment is aimed toward placing patients with AHF into one of 4 categories (Figure 25–1) based on their volume and perfusion status, and determining the acute precipitants of AHF. For patients with evidence of intravascular volume overload described as "wet" (elevated JVP, pulmonary rales, and peripheral edema) decongestive therapies such as diuretics or ultrafiltration can be administered to reduce intracardiac filling pressures and reduce dyspnea. If there are signs of reduced perfusion (such as decreased urine output, worsening renal function, and cool extremities)

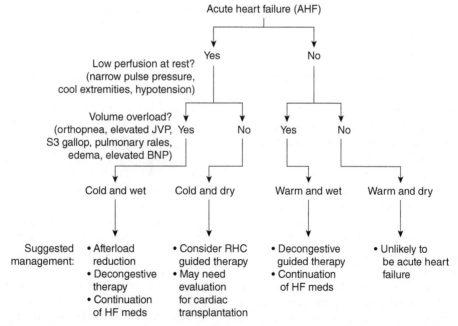

FIGURE 25–1 The overall clinical assessment is aimed toward placing patients with AHF into one of 4 categories.

patients are considered "cool" and in the absence of hypotension, therapies are geared toward augmenting cardiac output by reducing afterload (oftentimes with nitrates and hydralazine). Routine use of inotropic agents without a definitive low output state and end organ failure is generally not indicated, since these medications can increase myocardial oxygen demand and can promote arrhythmias, and outcomes data from randomized trials and registry data typically demonstrate worse outcomes with inotropic therapy compared to vasodilator therapy.

RIGHT HEART CATHETERIZATION

The appropriate use of right heart catheterization in patients with AHF is a subject of considerable controversy. The ESCAPE trial, in which AHF patients were randomized to management with a pulmonary artery catheter (PAC) or careful clinical assessment, demonstrated no mortality benefit or decrease in length of hospitalization with PAC; the trial also demonstrated increased adverse events in the PAC arm driven principally by catheter related infections. Based on these results routine use of PAC in stable AHF patients is not recommended. The

2013 ACCF/AHA Heart Failure Guidelines recommend PAC monitoring for patients in respiratory distress or with clinical evidence of impaired perfusion in whom intracardiac filling pressures cannot be determined from clinical assessment, as well as in patients who are failing (ie, still symptomatic, worsening renal function, and hypotensive) initial empiric therapy based on best clinical assessment. Figure 25–2 shows the typical intravascular and intracardiac pressure profiles of common AHF syndromes.

NONINVASIVE TESTING

Echocardiography is indicated to confirm a new diagnosis of AHF and in those with a significant clinical change from baseline. However, there is limited value in obtaining serial echocardiograms without a significant clinical alteration. This noninvasive modality is a cornerstone for diagnosing pathology involving the pericardium, heart valves, ventricular function, cardiac masses, and congenital defects. In cases of valvular pathology, valve area, valvular gradient, and regurgitant severity can be calculated to determine lesion severity, prognosis and drive further clinical management. Echocardiography can also provide

Clinical scenerio	Systemic blood pressure nL: 120/80 mm Hg	Right atrial pressure nL: 2-6 mm Hg	Pulmonary artery pressure nL: 15-25/ 8–15 mm Hg	Pulmonary capillary wedge pressure nL: 6-12 mm Hg	Cardiac Index nL: 2.5-4 L/min/m²	Systemic vascular resistance nL: 800-1200 Dynes-s/cm⁵
Decompensated systolic heart failure (LV dysfunction)	↑ ↔	↑	↑	↑	↓	↑
Cardiogenic shock	↓↓	↑	↑	↑	↓↓	↑
Septic shock	↓↓	↓	↔	↑ ↔	↑	↓
Right heart failure	↓↓	↑↑	↑ ↔	↑ ↔	↓↓	↑
Pericardial tamponade	↓↓	↑	↑ ↔	↑	↓↓	↔
Severe mitral regurgitation	↓	↑	↑	↑↑	↑	↑

FIGURE 25–2 Typical intravascular and intracardiac pressure profiles of common AHF syndromes.

supplementary information about intracardiac pressures in specific cardiac chambers to assist in determination of intravascular volume. For example, in a nonintubated patient if the inferior vena cava is noted to be dilated (> 2 cm) and not collapsing with respiration, the CVP is generally elevated beyond 10 mm Hg. Moreover, pulmonary artery and left sided pressures can be estimated by Doppler echocardiography of tricuspid regurgitation (TR) and mitral inflow, respectively. TR velocities greater than 3 m/s may indicate pulmonary hypertension and diastolic mitral inflow E wave velocities greater 0.12 m/s coupled with a prolonged deceleration time are present with elevated left atrial pressure. Diastolic dysfunction can also be graded by echocardiography.

COMMON PRECIPITANTS OF AHF AND THEIR MANAGEMENT

In addition to improving loading conditions, it is paramount to address the underlying cause of AHF. In cases of acute coronary syndrome, cardiac catheterization is usually indicated to define coronary anatomy and determine either a percutaneous or surgical revascularization strategy. Management of regurgitant valvulopathy typically involves reduction of loading conditions, while stenotic lesions may need surgical intervention. Infections can raise metabolic demand to leading to AHF, especially in patients with reduced LV function and should be promptly treated with antibiotics. Another common scenario is uncontrolled hypertension leading to acute LV diastolic dysfunction and pulmonary edema. Intravenous agents, such as nitroprusside or nitroglycerin, can be administered to reduce blood pressure and diuretics can be given to reduce congestive symptoms. If AHF is caused by persistent tachyarrhythmias, that is, tachycardia-induced cardiomyopathy, then cardioversion may be indicated and an electrophysiologic consultation may be sought to determine optimal pharmacologic or ablative strategies for maintaining sinus rhythm. Dietary and pharmacologic nonadherence are common and recurrent causes of AHF in patients with preexisting chronic HF. In such cases, it is critical to educate patients on appropriate dietary modifications and address any psychosocial or financial

TABLE 25-1 Common precipitating causes of Acute Heart Failure.

Dietary and medication nonadherence
Myocardial ischemia
Uncontrolled hypertension
Arrhythmia
Pulmonary embolism
Medication induced salt retention (NSAIDS, steroids)
Excessive alcohol consumption or illicit drug use
Uncontrolled thyroid disease
Infection
Valvular heart disease
Aortic dissection
Pericardial disease
Chemotherapy
Anemia

problems that may preclude further compliance with HF medications. Please see Table 25-1 for additional precipitants of AHF.

SEPSIS CARDIOMYOPATHY

Myocardial dysfunction can occur in patients with severe sepsis and is characterized by a reduction in ejection fraction and stroke volume. Cardiac output may be reduced or even normal due to a significant reduction in SVR. Cardiovascular dysfunction during sepsis can increase mortality up to 70% to 90%, in comparison to a 20% mortality in patients with sepsis without cardiovascular involvement. Although several biochemical mechanisms, such as upregulation of endothelin-1, higher expression of inducible nitric oxide synthase leading to free radical toxicity, activation of coagulation pathways and monocyte infiltration have been associated with sepsis cardiomyopathy, the precise mechanism of cardiac dysfunction remains elusive. Management rests upon treating the underlying infectious source and supporting the cardiovascular system.

BRAIN NATRIURETIC PEPTIDE

BNP is a biomarker which has had an increasingly important role in the management of acute as well as chronic heart failure. Originally described in porcine brain extract (and hence "brain natriuretic peptide" or BNP), in human biology it is principally secreted by ventricular myocytes in response to increased ventricular filling pressures and ventricular stretch. The molecule is secreted as an inactive peptide pro-BNP, and is then lysed into the biologically active BNP as well as the biologically inert amino terminal BNP (NT-BNP). The biologically active BNP acts as a balanced veno- and arteriolar vasodilator and also has direct renal effects, which promote natriuresis and diuresis. Both of the cleaved molecules are used in modern chemistry laboratories for BNP levels.

BNP testing was well validated in emergency room settings in the Breathing Not Properly trial, where BNP testing was demonstrated to be useful in establishing the diagnosis of heart failure in the acutely dyspneic patient. Use of BNP in the critical care setting can be more complicated, as in addition to heart failure, there are many cardiac and noncardiac causes of elevated BNP in hospitalized patients, including but not limited to myocarditis, acute coronary syndrome, pulmonary embolism and sepsis (Table 25–2). BNP levels can be falsely low in very obese patients, and are also lower in HFpEF patients compared to HFrEF patients. Additionally, BNP

levels are elevated in those with renal insufficiency compared to those without renal insufficiency. Finally, higher BNP levels are associated with a higher risk of mortality in both acute and chronic heart failure populations.

MEDICATIONS IN ACUTE HEART FAILURE SYNDROMES

Sodium Nitroprusside

Sodium nitroprusside (SNP) is a potent vasodilator, with balanced action in the arteriolar and venous beds. It has a very short (seconds to minutes) half-life, and produces a dramatic increase in cardiac output, decrease in pulmonary capillary wedge pressure (PCWP), and decrease in mitral regurgitant fraction; this is typically associated with a decrease in mean arterial pressure. The initial dose is 10 mcg/min, with up titration to as high as 350 mcg/min. Since the coronary vasodilatory properties of SNP can promote coronary steal and ischemia in those with significant unrevascularized coronary artery disease, it is not recommend in patient with active ischemia. The metabolism of SNP leads to the release of nitric oxide and cyanide. The symptoms of cyanide toxicity include nausea, abdominal discomfort and dysphoria. As there can be accumulation of cyanide and thiocyanate, caution must be used in patients with renal and hepatic dysfunction.

Nitroglycerin

Nitroglycerin is a potent venodilator, producing rapid decreases in pulmonary congestion, left ventricular end diastolic pressure, LV wall stress, and myocardial oxygen consumption. It has coronary vasodilatory effects as well, making it a good option for patient with ongoing ischemia. Initial intravenous dose is typically 20 mcg/min, with a doubling of the dose every 5 to 15 minutes. Other options for administration include sublingual tablets and sprays as well as topical pastes. Major side effects include hypotension and headache.

Nesiritide

Nesiritide is recombinant B-type natriuretic peptide. It has balanced venous and arteriolar actions,

TABLE 25–2 Causes of elevated natriuretic peptide concentrations.

Cardiac
- Heart failure, including RV syndromes
- Acute coronary syndrome
- Heart muscle disease, including LVH
- Valvular heart disease
- Pericardial disease
- Atrial fibrillation
- Myocarditis
- Cardiac surgery
- Cardioversion

Noncardiac
- Advancing age
- Anemia
- Renal failure
- Obstructive sleep apnea, severe pneumonia, pulmonary hypertension
- Critical illness
- Bacterial sepsis
- Severe burns
- Toxic-metabolic insults, including cancer chemotherapy and envenomation

and modestly enhances diuresis through direct renal effects. The dose starts at 0.01 mcg/kg/min. Major side effects include headache and hypotension. The ASCEND trial randomized 7141 patients with ADHF to either standard care or nesiritide plus standard of care. Nesiritide demonstrated a modest, statistically nonsignificant improvement in dyspnea; however, there was a higher rate of hypotension in the nesiritide arm of the trial. Importantly, there was no significant change in the rate of death, rehospitalization, or renal function in the nesiritide arm. Though there may be a role for nesiritide in some special populations (ie, diuretic resistant patients), the results of the ASCEND trial do not support the routine use of nesiritide in acute decompensate heart failure.

Milrinone

Milrinone is a positive inotropic agent as well as a vasodilator. It is a phosphodiesterase 3 inhibitor, and its mechanism of action is the inhibition of the breakdown of cyclic adenosine monophosphate (cAMP) in cardiac myocytes, leading to the increase of cAMP-mediated Ca++ in the myocyte and hence enhanced myocyte contractility. Similarly, in the vascular smooth muscle, its action is that of increasing cAMP-mediated contractile protein phosphorylation, leading to vascular relaxation. The hemodynamic changes seen with milrinone include an increased cardiac output, decreased SVR, reduced PCWP, and typically a mild decrease in mean arterial pressure. The half-life is approximately 2.4 hours, and it is renally cleared. The largest randomized clinical trial involving milrinone was the OPTIME-CHF trial, which randomized ADHF patients to either milrinone or placebo. Milrinone did not significantly decrease hospitalization length of stay, and did lead to significantly more hypotension and atrial arrhythmias. Use of milrinone is typically reserved patient with evidence of severely reduced cardiac output and end organ damage.

Dobutamine

Dobutamine is a direct beta-1 agonist, which produces positive inotropic and chronotropic effects. The mechanism of action is the binding of the beta-1 receptor, leading to phosphorylation of protein kinase A, which ultimately leads to an increase in intracellular cAMP and Ca++, leading to enhanced myocardial contractility. There is also a modest alpha and beta-2 effect, which causes mild peripheral vasodilation; in the context of increasing cardiac output, this can cause a variable effect on mean arterial pressure. The major side effects of dobutamine are atrial and ventricular tachyarrhythmias. There is no equivalent large, randomized trial experience with dobutamine in AHF as there is with milrinone, however registry data of AHF patients suggest worse outcomes with dobutamine and hence its use is limited to patients with poor response to diuretics and vasodilators and patients in overt cardiogenic shock.

Dopamine

Dopamine is a naturally occurring compound that plays an important role in many aspects of human body homeostasis, including major roles in neural, cardiovascular, and renal physiology. Dopamine has variable effects on different receptors at different doses; conventionally at low doses (0-2 mcg/kg/min), there is preferential dopamine receptor activation leading to enhanced renal artery vasodilation and enhanced renal perfusion; at 2 to 10 mcg/kg/min, there is enhanced norepinephrine release, leading to enhanced myocardial contractility and mild peripheral vasoconstriction; at doses above 10 mcg/kg/min, there is preferential alpha adrenergic receptor activation causing peripheral vasoconstriction and an increase in mean arterial pressure. In the context of treatment of AHF, dopamine is often used at low or "renal" dose in diuretic resistant patients, or at higher doses in those with frank cardiogenic shock. The limited clinical trial data evaluating the use of "renally dosed" dopamine in heart failure has been mixed. The most recent trial examining this issue (ROSE trial) randomized 360 AHF patients with renal dysfunction to either usual care or renally dosed dopamine (there was an additional low-dose nesiritide arm of the trial); the trial did not demonstrate a significant benefit of dopamine infusion in terms of urine output or change in renal function. Based on prior trial data, renally dosed dopamine is currently given a IIb recommendation by the ACC/AHA Heart Failure guidelines to help enhance urine output and renal perfusion in AHF patients.

Ultrafiltration

Ultrafiltration is a decongestive therapy in which water and small solutes are moved across a semipermeable membrane to reduce volume overload. Potential benefits of ultrafiltration over intravenous diuretics include more effective removal of sodium, minimal effects on serum electrolytes, decreased neurohormonal activation, and adjustable and potentially very rapid fluid removal rates. The outcomes in prospective heart failure trials in which patients were randomized to ultrafiltration versus diuretic therapy have varied. In the UNLOAD trial, 200 AHF patients were randomized to diuretics versus ultrafiltration; the ultrafiltration arm demonstrated greater fluid loss at 48 hours and a decrease in heart failure admissions in 90 days, with similar safety profile as diuretics. The CARESS-HF trial randomized AHF patients with cardiorenal syndrome to ultrafiltration or diuretics and failed to demonstrate a benefit with ultrafiltration. The cost, need for vascular access, need for nursing training and support are all potential barriers to ultrafiltration in clinical practice. Identifying the most appropriate patients for ultrafiltration therapy is an area of controversy and active clinical research.

Mechanical Circulatory Support

In cases of severe AHF, which is refractory to medical therapy, temporary circulatory support (TCS) can be utilized to improve end organ perfusion. TCS ranges from percutaneously inserted devices, such as intra-aortic balloon pump, tandem heart, and Impella which are able to augment cardiac output by up to 5 L/min. In cases of complete hemodynamic collapse or severe right ventricular failure, venoarterial extracorporeal membrane oxygenation can be placed to completely bypass the cardiopulmonary

circulation. Additional surgically placed TCS includes semidurable continuous-flow ventricular assist devices, such as CentriMag. TCS can serve as a "bridge to recovery" or as a "bridge to decision" in patients who may need implantation of permanent LV assist devices or cardiac transplantation.

REFERENCES

1. Binanay C, Califf RM, Hasselblad V, et al. Evaluation study of congestive heart failure and pulmonary artery catheterization effectiveness: the ESCAPE trial. *JAMA.* 2005;294(13):1625-1633.
2. Fanarow G, Adams KF, Jr, Abraham WT, Yancy CW, Boscardin WJ; ADHERE Scientific Advisory Committee, Study Group, and Investigators. Risk stratification for in-hospital mortality in acutely decompensated heart failure: classification and regression tree analysis. *JAMA.* 2005;293(5):572-580.
3. Merx MW, Weber C. Sepsis and the Heart. *Circulation.* 2007;116:793-802.
3a. O'Conner CM, Starling RC, Hernandez AF. Effect of nesiritide in patients with acute decompensated heart failure. *N Engl J Med.* 2011;365(1):32-43.
4. Quinones MA, Otto CM, Stoddard M, Waggoner A, Zoghbi WA; Doppler Quantification Task Force of the Nomenclature and Standards Committee of the American Society of Echocardiography. Recommendations for quantification of Doppler echocardiography: a report from the Doppler Quantification Task Force of the Nomenclature and Standards Committee of the American Society of Echocardiography. *J Am Soc Echocardiogr.* 2002;15(2):167-184.
5. Yancy C, Jessup M, Bozkurt B. ACCF/AHA guideline for the management of heart failure: a report of the American College of Cardiology Foundation/American Heart Association Task Force on practice guidelines. *Circulation.* 2013;128(16):e240-e319.

Pulmonary Arterial Hypertension in the ICU

Noam Broder, MD and Ronald Zolty, MD, PhD

26

KEY POINTS

1. Pulmonary arterial hypertension is a chronic, progressive disease affecting pulmonary arteries that results in increased pulmonary vascular resistance and pulmonary arterial pressures. As the disease progresses, chronic or acute increases in pulmonary arterial pressures result in right ventricular failure (RVF) which is the most common cause of death in this patient population. RVF is clinically defined as a reduced cardiac output and an increase in right ventricular filling pressure.

2. Pulmonary arterial hypertension is diagnosed with a right heart catheterization or Swan–Ganz catheter showing pulmonary arterial mean pressure greater than 25 mm Hg and not by echocardiogram.

3. Given the lack of physiologic reserve of patients with pulmonary hypertension, any further physiologic imbalance, such as infection, arrhythmia, or pulmonary embolism can trigger hemodynamic collapse, RVF and result in an ICU admission.

4. Patients with pulmonary hypertension are at risk for developing sepsis, pulmonary embolism, and arrhythmia.

5. Treatment of patients in the ICU with evidence of right heart failure due to pulmonary hypertension involves supportive care, correcting the underlying cause of the hemodynamic instability and supporting hemodynamic function of the right heart.

6. Intubation of patients with pulmonary hypertension and RVF should be avoided.

7. Pulmonary vasodilators are used to reduce RV afterload by reducing pulmonary arterial pressures. Medications effective at reducing RV afterload, such as IV Prostanoids, Inhaled Nitric oxide cause improvements in cardiac output and oxygenation.

8. Inotropes, such as Dobutamine and Milrinone are used to maintain cardiac output in the presence of cardiogenic shock from right heart failure due to pulmonary hypertension.

9. In extreme cases atrial septostomy can be used to reduce RV pressures by shunting blood from the right atrium to left atrium.

10. Pressure support medications, such as norepinephrine and vasopressin should be used to maintain systemic blood pressure as well as right coronary artery perfusion of the right ventricle.

11. For patients with end stage PAH and RVF refractory to optimized medical treatment, lung transplantation with bridging via extracorporeal life support should be considered.

INTRODUCTION

Pulmonary arterial hypertension (PAH) is a chronic, progressive disease affecting small pulmonary arteries that results in increased pulmonary arterial pressures and eventual right ventricular failure (RVF). PAH can be caused by idiopathic or heritable sources, induced by drugs and toxins, has associations with connective tissue disease, HIV infection, portal hypertension, congenital heart disease, schistosomiasis, chronic hemolytic anemia, and can also result from persistent pulmonary hypertension (PHTN) of the newborn.[1] Clinically, PHTN is diagnosed with a right heart catheterization showing pulmonary arterial pressure greater than 25 mm Hg. As the disease progresses, chronic or acute increases in pulmonary arterial pressures result in RVF which is the most common cause of death in this patient population.[2] RVF is clinically defined as a reduced cardiac output and an increase in RV filling pressure.[3] Due to their delicate hemodynamic states and advanced disease, PAH patients in the ICU have mortality rates reported as high as 41%.[4]

Chronic destruction of pulmonary vasculature as well as increases in pulmonary vascular resistance (PVR) and pulmonary arterial pressures cause RVF.[5] The right ventricle responds to increased pulmonary pressures with compensatory structural changes that compromise the heart's ability to maintain sufficient cardiac output. As such, an understanding of the underlying physiology of PHTN and the right heart is required in order to treat this complex and dangerous disorder in the ICU.

PHYSIOLOGY OF THE RIGHT HEART

The normal structure and function of the right ventricle reflects the low resistance and high compliance and capacitance of the pulmonary vasculature system to which it delivers blood. The thin-walled structure of the right ventricle implies the low resistance of the pulmonary vasculature. Functionally, the right ventricle spends little time in isovolumic contraction or relaxation and as a result is able to generate cardiac output with only a fifth of the energy demanded by the left ventricle (LV).[6] The right ventricle receives a continuous flow of coronary blood via the RCA during both systole and diastole.[6] This blood supply is possible given the thin-walled structure of the RV as well as its relatively small isovolumic activity. Given this physiology adapted specifically for the low resistance pulmonary vasculature, the right ventricle has difficulty responding to the increased resistance of PHTN.[6] The adaptive changes that the RV undergoes cause structural changes that compromise its ability to maintain cardiac output.

PATHOPHYSIOLOGY OF PAH AND RVF

In order to reduce wall tension caused by the increased afterload of PHTN, hypertrophy of the right ventricle occurs. As a result, coronary flow no longer occurs in diastole despite the increased demand of the hypertrophied right ventricle. Also, the right ventricle spends more time in isovolumic contraction and relaxation in order to overcome increased pulmonary pressures, which results in a reduction of right heart output and greater energy demand.[6] RV hypertrophy also interferes with the normal motion of the tricuspid valve and together with increased pulmonary pressures results in tricuspid regurgitation.[6] The growth of the right ventricle also impedes on the function of the LV as the interventricular septum bulges into the LV.[6] These changes in the right ventricle all contribute to the reduction of cardiac output, which in turn decreases coronary flow to the RV and causes ischemic damage. Finally, this hypertrophy of the right ventricle accompanied by ischemic damage eventually leads to ventricular dilatation and total right heart failure.

CAUSES FOR ICU ADMISSION IN PATIENTS WITH PAH

Given the lack of physiologic reserve of patients with PHTN, any further physiologic imbalance can trigger hemodynamic collapse and result in an ICU admission. The differential diagnosis for patients with PHTN presenting with acute RVF should include the pathologies unique to PHTN discussed later. It is also important to note that advanced treatments for PHTN work to slow progress of the disease, and do not cure the disease. As such, RVF occurs when the compensatory mechanisms of the RV are overwhelmed by progressive destruction of the pulmonary vasculature even with use of advanced therapies.

Patients with PHTN are at risk for developing sepsis. Patients with low cardiac output may poorly perfuse the bowel, leading to a leaky endothelial barrier that allows bacteria and their toxins to invade, which can result in sepsis.[7] Prostacyclin, one of the advanced medications for the treatment of PHTN has an immunosuppressive effect.[8] Additionally, prostacyclin is delivered via an indwelling catheter, which has its own infection risk.[8] As such, sepsis was found to be the most common identifiable trigger for ICU admission in a study of 46 patients with PAH or inoperable chronic thromboembolic pulmonary hypertension (CTEPH) admitted to the ICU.[4]

The effects of sepsis on the patient with PHTN can be devastating. Sepsis-induced drops in systemic vascular resistance (SVR) can severely compromise patients with reduced cardiac output from PHTN. Furthermore, sepsis has been shown to cause pulmonary vasoconstriction and dysfunction as well as produce cytokines that reduce right heart contractility.[9,10] Clinically, sepsis was found to be a leading cause of patient mortality in the ICU for patients with PHTN exacerbations.[4]

Iatrogenic causes can also trigger hemodynamic instability leading to an ICU admission in a patient with PHTN. Negative inotropes, such as beta-blockers and calcium channel blockers can depress the contractile ability of the right ventricle and cause an acute decrease in cardiac output. Abrupt cessation of pulmonary vasodilator medications can cause rebound pulmonary vasoconstriction.

PAH also provides a setting for pulmonary emboli to form. Patients with PAH often live sedentary lifestyles due to poor exercise capacity resulting in venous stasis.[6] Also, pulmonary blood travels slowly through the pulmonary vasculature in PHTN with RVF. A PE with a resulting loss of oxygenation, shunting of blood, and increased pulmonary arterial pressures can severely destabilize the hemodynamics of a patient with PHTN.

As the heart remodels in response to PAH, patients become susceptible to atrial arrhythmias. The remodeling process predisposes patients with PAH to arrhythmias by modulating autonomic activity and delaying cardiac repolarization.[11] Also, ischemic myocardial damage to the RV itself can predispose patients to developing an arrhythmia.[11] One study of 231 patients with PAH or CTEPH showed a yearly incidence of 2.8% for new onset supraventricular tachycardia, most commonly atrial fibrillation or flutter.[12] Any loss of the ability of the LA to fill the LV can further reduce CO in addition to the already decreased RV CO. Also, the poorly compliant RV is dependent on the atrial kick of the RA to fill and produce adequate output. As such, onset of arrhythmias was related to clinical deterioration in patients with PHTN and patients with sustained atrial fibrillation had a cumulative mortality rate of 82%, emphasizing the need for conversion to sinus rhythm.[12]

Atrial arrhythmias are challenging to manage in the ICU given the potential negative inotropic effects of beta-blockers and high doses of calcium channel blockers on the right heart. Therefore, rhythm control may be a better management choice than rate control, with amiodarone, cardioversion, or ablation as potential therapies.[11]

MONITORING IN THE ICU

Careful monitoring of patients with PAH and RVF is necessary given their fragile hemodynamic state.

Hypoxia causes selective pulmonary vessel vasoconstriction as the body attempts to shunt blood to areas of the lung with better oxygenation. However, this process will increase pulmonary arterial pressures and exacerbate PHTN, so pulse oximetry or more invasive methods of monitoring can be valuable tools in the prevention of desaturation.

Troponins should be checked to identify if myocardial infarction was the trigger event for the ongoing PHTN/RVF episode. Trending troponins may also give insight into any ongoing ischemia occurring in the right ventricle due to the PHTN exacerbation.

BNP can be used to confirm dilation of the right ventricle and to trend the function of the right ventricle over time. High admission BNP levels in patients with PAH or inoperable CTEPH were found to be predictive of mortality.[4]

Hemoglobin levels should be monitored and maintained at a level above 10 mg to avoid compensatory cardiac reaction to anemia as per expert opinion.[3]

Due to the delicate hemodynamic state of the right heart in PAH, electrolyte disturbances have potential to be very harmful and should be carefully monitored. BUN and creatinine should be followed as measures of kidney function and cardiogenic shock. AST, ALT, and bilirubin should be monitored as markers for liver damage caused by cardiogenic shock. Finally, lactate is a useful marker for ischemia and RV insufficiency.

Echocardiography is a valuable noninvasive monitoring modality used to observe the function and structure of the right ventricle. Echocardiographic signs of right heart failure include RV dilation and loss of the RV's normal, triangular shape.[13] Systolic paradoxical motion of the interventricular septum is another sign of RVF as it represents RV systolic overload.[13] An echocardiogram can also help identify possible causes of the PHTN associated right heart failure exacerbation such as left heart failure, RV ischemia, new valvular abnormalities, or pericardial effusions.[13] Furthermore, right atrial enlargement, septal displacement, pericardial effusion, and low tricuspid annual plane systolic excursion are echocardiographic signs associated with poor outcomes in patients with chronic right heart failure.[14] However, these associations were identified in chronic right heart failure patients only, and the value of these signs in an acutely ill patient is unclear. For patients with poor transthoracic echocardiographic imaging, a transesophageal echocardiogram is a valuable option, although it is more invasive and, therefore, carries greater risks.

Outcomes of invasive monitoring with pulmonary artery (PA) catheters have not been specifically studied in patients with PAH. Studies of PA catheterization (PAC) in the ICU patient population have shown no mortality benefit and possibly increased mortality with PAC.[15] Furthermore, PAC involves risks including PA rupture and tachyarrhythmia and one study of patients with PHTN receiving nonacute PAC in an expert center showed an incident rate of 1.1% for adverse events.[16] However, information on PA pressures and RVF can be directly obtained from PAC. As such, the decision to monitor patients with RVF/PAH should be made based on individual patient presentation and course, as hemodynamic

information obtained from PAC may give valuable physiologic information only hinted at by indirect biomarkers such as lactate.

ICU MANAGEMENT OF PAH AND RVF

Treatment of patients in the ICU with evidence of right heart failure due to PHTN involves supportive care, correcting the underlying cause of the hemodynamic instability and supporting hemodynamic function of the right heart. Specifically, the goals of supportive cardiac care for PHTN in the ICU focus on maintaining aortic root pressure, systemic blood pressure, and cardiac output as well as reducing pulmonary arterial pressures. If these treatments are ineffective, invasive strategies, such as extracorporeal support and ultimately lung transplantation should be considered. Unfortunately, PAH in the ICU has not been studied extensively, and much of the following information is based on animal studies and studies of other classes of PHTN.

Supportive Care

As discussed earlier, hypoxia can exacerbate elevated pulmonary pressures, so supplemental oxygenation should be used to maintain hemoglobin oxygen saturation to at least 90% to prevent or reverse any hypoxia induced pulmonary vasoconstriction. Also, there is evidence showing the efficacy of oxygen as a selective pulmonary vasodilator in patients with PAH, as treatment with 100% O_2 for 5 minutes in patients undergoing PAC increased cardiac index and reduced PVR.[17]

PAH patients should be anticoagulated as they are at high risk for new DVT or PE given their limited mobility and altered pulmonary hemodynamics as discussed above.

Diuresis helps reduce the pressure of fluid overload on a failing right ventricle that is on the far right of the Frank Starling curve. Dialysis should be considered if the patient fails to respond to diuresis. Patients should be followed clinically with regards to fluid management, as over diuresis can reduce cardiac output. As such, input and outputs for the patient should be carefully monitored to ensure diuresis is proceeding appropriately. In the case of pure diastolic failure of the RV with signs of fluid overload and normal CO, diuresis alone would be the appropriate choice for management.

Intubation of patients with PHTN and RVF should be avoided as sedatives can depress cardiac function and lower SVR and increased transpulmonary pressures can further lower CO. If mechanical ventilation is necessary, pretreatment with catecholamines to avoid a drop in BP may be necessary. Etomidate is a preferred induction agent, as it has relatively fewer effects on vascular tone or cardiac contractility than propofol.[6] In general, ventilator strategies should avoid high intrathoracic pressures in order to prevent PVR increases or RV preload decrease. Also, ventilation strategies should attempt to prevent compression of pulmonary vasculature by avoiding high lung volumes and should also avoid hypercapnia, hypoxia, and atelectasis, which can increase PVR.[18]

Pulmonary Vasodilators

Pulmonary vasodilators are used to reduce RV afterload by reducing pulmonary arterial pressures. Medications effective at reducing RV afterload cause improvements in CO and oxygenation.

Intravenous (IV) prostanoids are short acting pulmonary vasodilators and platelet aggregation inhibitors delivered by continuous IV infusion or implanted perfusion devices. IV prostanoids are potent pulmonary vasodilators and have been used in the treatment of acute RVF in patients after cardiac surgery where they significantly reduced PVR and increased RV function.[19,20] IV prostanoids should specifically be avoided in patients with PHTN due to left heart failure, as increased volume delivered to the LV can result in pulmonary edema. Hypotension is a significant adverse effect of IV prostanoids and must be watched for as prostanoids are up titrated. Also, IV prostanoids can cause nonselective pulmonary vasodilation resulting in V/Q mismatch and worsening of cardiac and pulmonary function. Other systemic side effects of IV prostanoids include nausea, diarrhea, flushing, and headache.

In order to avoid hypotension V/Q mismatch from IV prostanoids, inhaled prostanoids, which are only approved for chronic treatment of PAH, should be strongly considered in the care of the acutely ill patient. One study of 35 patients with PAH undergoing right heart catheterization showed greater efficacy of inhaled iloprost versus NO as an inhaled pulmonary vasodilator.[21] The ultrasonic nebulizer is being used as a delivery device for inhaled prostanoids in the postsurgical setting to treat RVF.[6]

Inhaled NO directly vasodilates the pulmonary vasculature and may be especially useful in patients who cannot tolerate IV prostanoids due to hypotension and v/q mismatch. NO has a short half-life given its rapid deactivation by hemoglobin in pulmonary capillaries. A study of 26 patients with acute RVF admitted to the ICU and treated with inhaled NO showed in half of all patients a significant decrease more than 20% in PVR and pressure.[22] Additionally, in a study comparing NO to IV prostanoids in patients with RVF following cardiac surgery, NO was shown to increase CI and reduce PVR with similar efficacy to IV prostanoids.[20] However, prolonged use of high concentration inhaled NO can cause methemoglobinemia so cyanosis should be watched for and periodic methemoglobin levels should be drawn. Withdrawal of NO therapy should be carefully monitored as rebound increases in PA pressure can result from abrupt withdrawal.

Although unstudied in an acute setting, IV PDE5 inhibitors, such as Sildenafil may be a possible therapy for patients with PAH and acute RVF. IV sildenafil does have risks of systemic hypotension and V/Q mismatch from nonselective pulmonary vasodilation.

After patients are stabilized with IV or inhaled medications, endothelin receptor blockers and PDE5 antagonists can be added as oral medications for discharge. These oral medications should be bridged carefully over the ICU medication, as abrupt withdrawal of IV prostanoids, inhaled NO or inhaled prostanoids can cause rebound PHTN.

Inotropes

Inotropes are used to maintain cardiac output in the presence of cardiogenic shock from right heart failure due to PHTN.

Dobutamine is a beta-1 receptor agonist that augments cardiac contractility and reduces RV and LV afterload. Animal models of RVF and PHTN had increased CO and RV-PA coupling with little effects on the PA after dobutamine treatment.[23]

Dobutamine significantly improved hemodynamics and cardiac function of patients with PH after RV infarction[24] as well as increasing RV contractility and decreasing afterload in patients with PH at liver transplantation.[25] However, dobutamine is a direct adrenergic agonist and also has an agonistic effect at beta-2 receptors, which can cause vasodilation resulting in hypotension and tachycardia. This vasodilation and tachycardia can be especially harmful as it reduces diastolic filling time on an already volume deprived LV. Dobutamine-induced hypotension should be anticipated at higher doses and may be treated with vasopressors should the need arise.

Another inotrope used in the ICU treatment of patients with PHTN is Milrinone, a PDE3 inhibitor. Milrinone directly increases cAMP which causes increased contractility and reduced afterload. Animal models of chronic PAH treated with Milrinone showed significant increases in RV function, pulmonary blood flow and LV filling.[26] One example of Milrinone's efficacy in human RVF can be seen in a study of patients with RVF after LVAD placement who received Milrinone and had a resulting significant reduction in PVR and an increase in LVAD flow.[27] As with any systemic inotrope, there is a risk of systemic hypotension with milrinone usage and vasopressors should be used as necessary to prevent hypotension.

Inhaled milrinone has been used as salvage therapy when other PAH therapies could not be increased due to hypotension.[28] Also, in a study of patients with PHTN undergoing mitral valve surgery inhaled milrinone decreased mean PA pressure and PVR in a similar range as IV milrinone.[29] As such, inhaled milrinone should be considered in the patient with hypotension and for any patient in which V/Q mismatching and shunting is a major concern.

Vasopressors

Pressure support medications should be used to maintain aortic root pressure and RCA perfusion of the RV. These medications are especially important given the loss of CO in RVF as well as the hypotensive side effects of advanced PAH therapies and inotropes. Also, by increasing the afterload, vasopressors have an additional benefit of normalizing the shape of the LV against an enlarged RV.

Norepinephrine causes vasoconstriction and improves SVR via alpha-1 receptor agonist activity as well as exerting inotropic effect by beta-1 receptor agonist activity. In a study comparing mortality and adverse event outcomes of norepinephrine versus dopamine treatment in patients with shock in the ICU, the subset of patients with cardiogenic shock treated with norepinephrine had a decreased rate of 28-days mortality and arrhythmias as compared to patients treated with dopamine.[30] However, in a small study of 10 patients with septic shock, PH and RVF treated with norepinephrine showed an increase in PVR and no improvement in RV EF.[31] This increase in PVR was thought to be from a dose-dependent beta-1 effect of norepinephrine on the pulmonary vasculature.

Vasopressin acts at V1 receptors on vascular smooth muscle cells to cause vasoconstriction. Vasopressin also potentiates the vascular effects of catecholamines. Vasopressin has been shown to cause pulmonary vasodilation in animal models via endothelial NO production[32] and a reduction in PVR and PVR/SVR ratio in humans,[18] making it a theoretically better choice than norepinephrine for patients with PHTN. Vasopressin has been used effectively to treat sepsis induced hypotension, RVF and PHTN after cardiac surgery and chronic PHTN.[18] However, vasopressin does have dose related toxicities such as coronary vasoconstriction and depressed myocardial function at higher doses and has not been studied as well as norepinephrine in the ICU setting.[18] As such, for patients with pulmonary vascular dysfunction and vasodilatory shock, vasopressin can be used at low doses in those not responding to norepinephrine and other conventional treatments.

ATRIAL SEPTOSTOMY, EXTRACORPOREAL LIFE SUPPORT, AND END OF LIFE IN THE ICU

Atrial septostomy (AS) can be used to reduce RV pressures by shunting blood from the RA to LA. This shunting decompresses the dilated RV, improves LV function and RV contractility, and reduces deforming pressure on the LV from the enlarged RV. Paradoxically, this procedure does not result in decreased oxygenation as the increased cardiac function resulting from AS outweighs the loss of hemoglobin oxygenation from the atrial shunt. However, this procedure is not appropriate for the end stages of the disease or hemodynamically unstable patients, as patients with RA pressures greater than 20 mm Hg or O_2 sat less than 80% on room air or low CI who underwent this procedure had a significantly higher risk of fatal complications.[33,34]

For patients with end stage PAH and RVF refractory to optimized medical treatment, lung transplantation with bridging via extracorporeal life support (ECLS) should be considered. ECLS unloads the RV, increases organ perfusion and can even remove the need for catecholamine medications. As such, ECLS as a bridge to transplantation is a good choice of therapy for patients with PAH refractory to treatment exhibited by persistent hypoperfusion and continuous end organ dysfunction.

Venoarterial ECMO draws blood from the RA via a femoral venous cannula, oxygenates the blood externally to the patient, and returns the newly oxygenated blood into the lower abdominal aorta. A series of 5 patients in Germany with PH and RVF showed rapid improvement in end organ function and reversal of cardiovascular failure with V/A ECMO treatment while awake and breathing spontaneously without intubation.[35] Of these 5 patients, 4 survived to transplantation and 3 of these patients survived for one additional year.[35] A follow-up retrospective study comparing awake V/A ECMO to patients receiving traditional intubated V/A ECMO showed a significant increase in 6 months survival after lung transplantation and shortened postoperative stay in patients receiving awake V/A ECMO.[36] As such, awake V/A ECMO seems to be a promising bridging strategy to lung transplant for patients with PHTN. However, bleeding complications are a risk given the anticoagulation required to use V/A ECMO and 2 weeks may be the maximum time patients can remain on ECMO before other complications such as hemolysis, organ failure, sepsis, renal failure, and cerebral vascular accidents begin to occur with greater frequency.[37]

Pumpless lung assist devices have been used in hemodynamically unstable patients with PAH and veno-occlusive disease as a bridge to lung transplantation.[37] Pumpless lung assist devices are low-resistance membrane oxygenators, which are connected between the PA and the left atrium. This device effectively offloads the RV in the same way as BAS, but instead allows for oxygenation of the shunted blood over the membrane device.

If a patient does have cardiac arrest during their ICU stay, CPR has very little efficacy. One study of 132 patients with PAH who had CPR performed after circulatory arrest showed that only 8 patients survived for more than 90 days and 7 of these patients had identifiable causes of circulatory arrest.[38] Given the high PVR present in patients with PAH in the ICU, it is not surprising that chest compressions are unable to generate forward flow of blood from the RV through the constricted pulmonary vasculature. Timely discussions of goals of care and DNR orders are, therefore, appropriate for patients with PAH and RVF in the ICU.

REFERENCES

1. Simonneau G, Robbins IM, Beghetti M, et al. Updated clinical classification of pulmonary hypertension. *J Am Coll Cardiol*. 2009; 54(1 Suppl):S43-S54.
2. D'Alonzo GE, Barst RJ, Ayres SM, et al. Survival in patients with primary pulmonary hypertension. Results from a national prospective registry. *Ann Intern Med*. 1991;115(5):343-349.
3. Hoeper MM, Granton J. Intensive care unit management of patients with severe pulmonary hypertension and right heart failure. *Am J Respir Crit Care Med*. 2011;184(10):1114-1124.
4. Sztrymf B, Souza R, Bertoletti L, et al. Prognostic factors of acute heart failure in patients with pulmonary arterial hypertension. *Eur Resp J*. 2010;35(6):1286-1293.
5. Bogaard HJ, Natarajan R, Henderson SC, et al. Chronic pulmonary artery pressure elevation is insufficient to explain right heart failure. *Circulation*. 2009;120(20):1951-1960.
6. Poor HD, Ventetuolo CE. Pulmonary hypertension in the intensive care unit. *Prog Cardiovasc Dis*. 2012;55(2):187-198.
7. Krack A, Sharma R, Figulla HR, Anker SD. The importance of the gastrointestinal system in the pathogenesis of heart failure. *Eur Heart J*. 2005;26(22):2368-2374.
8. Papierniak ES, Lowenthal DT, Mubarak K. Pulmonary arterial hypertension: classification

and therapy with a focus on prostaglandin analogs. *Am J Ther.* 2012;19(4):300-314.

9. Bull TM, Clark B, McFann K, Moss M; National Institutes of Health/National Heart, Lung, and Blood Institute ARDS Network. Pulmonary vascular dysfunction is associated with poor outcomes in patients with acute lung injury. *Am J Respir Crit Care Med.* 2010;182(9):1123-1129.

10. Court O, Kumar A, Parrillo JE, Kumar A. Clinical review: myocardial depression in sepsis and septic shock. *Crit Care.* 2002;6(6):500-508.

11. Rajdev A, Garan H, Biviano A. Arrhythmias in pulmonary arterial hypertension. *Prog Cardiovasc Dis.* 2012;55(2):180-186.

12. Tongers J, Schwerdtfeger B, Klein G, et al. Incidence and clinical relevance of supraventricular tachyarrhythmias in pulmonary hypertension. *Am Heart J.* 2007;153(1):127-132.

13. Gayat E, Mebazaa A. Pulmonary hypertension in critical care. *Curr Opin Crit Care.* 2011;17(5):439-448.

14. Ghio S, Klersy C, Magrini G, et al. Prognostic relevance of the echocardiographic assessment of right ventricular function in patients with idiopathic pulmonary arterial hypertension. *Int J Cardiol.* 2010;140(3):272-278.

15. Harvey S, Harrison DA, Singer M, et al. Assessment of the clinical effectiveness of pulmonary artery catheters in management of patients in intensive care (PAC-Man): a randomized controlled trial. *Lancet.* 2005;366(9484):472-477.

16. Hoeper MM, Lee SH, Voswinckel R, et al. Complications of right heart catheterization procedures in patients with pulmonary hypertension in experienced centers. *J Am Coll Cardiol.* 2006;48(12):2546-2552.

17. Roberts DH, Lepore JJ, Maroo A, Semigran MJ, Ginns LC. Oxygen therapy improves cardiac index and pulmonary vascular resistance in patients with pulmonary hypertension. *Chest.* 2001;120(5):1547-1555.

18. Price LC, Wort SJ, Finney SJ, Marino PS, Brett SJ. Pulmonary vascular and right ventricular dysfunction in adult critical care: current and emerging options for management: a systematic literature review. *Crit Care.* 2010;14(5):R169.

19. Ocal A, Kiriş I, Erdinç M, Peker O, Yavuz T, Ibrişim E. Efficiency of prostacyclin in the treatment of protamine-mediated right ventricular failure and acute pulmonary hypertension. *Tohoku J Exp Med.* 2005;207(1):51-58.

20. Schmid ER, Bürki C, Engel MH, Schmidlin D, Tornic M, Seifert B. Inhaled nitric oxide versus intravenous vasodilators in severe pulmonary hypertension after cardiac surgery. *Anesth Analg.* 1999;89(5):1108-1108.

21. Hoeper MM, Olschewski H, Ghofrani HA, et al. A comparison of the acute hemodynamic effects of inhaled nitric oxide and aerosolized iloprost in primary pulmonary hypertension. *J Am Coll Cardiol.* 2000;35(1):176-182.

22. Bhorade S, Christenson J, O'connor M, Lavoie A, Pohlman A, Hall JB. Response to inhaled nitric oxide in patients with acute right heart syndrome. *Am J Respir Crit Care Med.* 1999;159(2):571-579.

23. Kerbaul F, Rondelet B, Motte S, et al. Effects of norepinephrine and dobutamine on pressure load-induced right ventricular failure. *Crit Care Med.* 2004;32(4):1035-1040.

24. Ferrario M, Poli A, Previtali M, et al. Hemodynamics of volume loading compared with dobutamine in severe right ventricular infarction. *Am J Cardiol.* 1994;74(4):329-333.

25. Acosta F, Sansano T, Palenciano CG, et al. Effects of dobutamine on right ventricular function and pulmonary circulation in pulmonary hypertension during liver transplantation. *Transplant Proc.* 2005;37(9):3869-3870.

26. Chen EP, Bittner HB, Davis RD, Jr, Van Trigt P 3rd. Milrinone improves pulmonary hemodynamics and right ventricular function in chronic pulmonary hypertension. *Ann Thorac Surg.* 1997;63(3):814-821.

27. Kihara S, Kawai A, Fukuda T, et al. Effects of milrinone for right ventricular failure after left ventricular assist device implantation. *Heart Vessels.* 2002;16(2):69-71.

28. Buckley MS, Feldman JP. Nebulized milrinone use in a pulmonary hypertensive crisis. *Pharmacotherapy.* 2007;27(12):1763-1766.

29. Wang H, Gong M, Zhou B, Dai A. Comparison of inhaled and intravenous milrinone in patients with pulmonary hypertension undergoing mitral valve surgery. *Adv Ther.* 2009;26(4):462-468.

30. De Backer D, Biston P, Devriendt J, et al. Comparison of dopamine and norepinephrine in the treatment of shock. *N Engl J Med.* 2010;362(9):779-789.

31. Schreuder WO, Schneider AJ, Groeneveld AB, Thijs LG. Effect of dopamine vs norepinephrine on hemodynamics in septic shock. Emphasis on right ventricular performance. *Chest.* 1989;95(6):1282-1288.

32. Evora PR, Pearson PJ, Schaff HV. Arginine vasopressin induces endothelium-dependent

vasodilatation of the pulmonary artery. V1-receptor-mediated production of nitric oxide. *Chest.* 1993;103(4):1241-1245.

33. Rich S, Dodin E, McLaughlin VV. Usefulness of atrial septostomy as a treatment for primary pulmonary hypertension and guidelines for its application. *Am J Cardiol.* 1997;80(3):369-371.

34. Galie N, et al. Guidelines for the diagnosis and treatment of pulmonary hypertension. *Eur Respir J.* 2009;34(6):1219-1263.

35. Fuehner T, Kuehn C, Hadem J, et al. Extracorporeal membrane oxygenation in awake patients as bridge to lung transplantation. *Am J Respir Crit Care Med.* 2012;185(7):763-768.

36. Olsson KM, Simon A, Strueber M, et al. Extracorporeal membrane oxygenation in nonintubated patients as bridge to lung transplantation. *Am J Transplant.* 2010;10(9):2173-2178.

37. Strueber M, Hoeper MM, Fischer S, et al. Bridge to thoracic organ transplantation in patients with pulmonary arterial hypertension using a pumpless lung assist device. *Am J Transplant.* 2009;9(4):853-857.

38. Hoeper MM, Galié N, Murali S, et al. Outcome after cardiopulmonary resuscitation in patients with pulmonary arterial hypertension. *Am J Respir Crit Care Med.* 2002;165(3):341-344.

Electrolyte Disorders in Critically Ill Patients

27

Sheron Latcha, MD, FASN

1 A careful assessment of the patient's osmolality and volume status are vital to appropriately evaluate the patient with either hypernatremia or hyponatremia.

2 The syndrome of inappropriate antidiuretic hormone is characterized by inappropriately concentrated urine in the setting of a low serum osmolality and a normal plasma volume.

3 Treatment strategies for syndrome of inappropriate antidiuretic hormone include fluid restriction to 1 to 1.5 L of free water per day, sodium chloride tablets, isotonic saline along with furosemide or hypertonic saline (2% or 3%) alone, and vasopressin-2 (V2) receptor antagonists (conivaptan and tolvaptan).

4 For patients with symptomatic and/or severe hyponatremia (mental status changes, seizures, coma, sodium < 115mEq/L), 3% normal saline should be used to correct the sodium deficit with close monitoring of their neurologic status and serum sodium values.

5 The goals in treating hypernatremia include identifying correcting any reversible factors (hypercalcemia, hypokalemia, and hypertonic solutions); correcting volume depletion if present; and replacing the calculated free water deficit.

6 The clinical signs and symptoms of hyperkalemia are predominantly neuromuscular (weakness, and muscle paralysis) and cardiac (electrocardiographic [EKG] changes—peaked T waves, prolonged PR interval, widened QRS, arrhythmias, and asystole).

7 The most rapid way to lower serum potassium is with the use of inhaled beta agonists (nebulized albuterol 10-20 mg over 15 minutes) and insulin (50 s of D50W and 10U regular insulin over 15-30 minutes). Other treatments include IV sodium bicarbonate, isotonic saline infusion, loop diuretics alone or in combination with saline infusion, and sodium polystyrene given as a rectal suppository or orally in combination with sorbitol for faster delivery to its site of action at the colonic mucosa.

8 Clinical manifestations of hypokalemia are predominantly cardiac (arrhythmias, EKG changes [flattening of the T wave, and U wave]) and neuromuscular (muscle weakness, paralysis, ileus, and constipation).

9 Symptoms of severe hypocalcemia include tetany, seizures, a prolonged QT interval, and ventricular arrhythmias. For acute correction of symptomatic hypocalcemia, IV calcium gluconate, or calcium chloride

—Continued next page

Continued—

(10 mL of a 10% solution) can be administered over 10 minutes.

(10) For patients with symptomatic hypercalcemia, aggressive volume expansion with 0.9% normal saline at rates needed to promote a urine output of 100 to 150 cc/h is recommended. Other treatments include furosemide after adequate volume resuscitation is achieved, calcitonin, bisphosphonates (pamidronate and zoledronate), and dialysis.

(11) Hypophosphatemia may be associated with decreased myocardial contractility, respiratory failure due to diaphragmatic paralysis, dysphagia, ileus, paresthesias, seizures, rhabdomyolysis, and myopathy.

(12) Hyperphosphatemia may result from tumor lysis syndrome, massive blood transfusions, rhabdomyolysis, acute extracellular shifts of phosphorus (lactic and diabetic ketoacidosis), ingestion of large amounts of phosphorus containing laxatives, hypoparathyroidism, and vitamin D toxicity.

(13) Clinically important manifestations of hypomagnesemia include EKG changes (arrhythmias and torsades de pointes), neuromuscular problems (tetany and seizures), electrolyte disorders (hypokalemia and hypocalcemia) and impaired parathyroid hormone release and action.

INTRODUCTION

Fluid and electrolyte disorders are ubiquitous in the intensive care unit (ICU) setting. This text will focus on common clinical scenarios in the ICU and assumes a basic fund of knowledge about fluid and electrolyte disorders.

SODIUM DISORDERS

Sodium is the most copious extracellular (EC) cation and is the most important osmotically active constituent of the EC fluid. Changes in serum sodium represent changes in salt and water balance. Therefore, a careful assessment of the patient's osmolality and volume status are vital to appropriately evaluate the patient with either hypernatremia or hyponatremia.

Hyponatremia

Hyponatremia is one of the most common electrolyte disorders in hospitalized patients, with a reported prevalence of 30% to 40%. It has been observed in 14% of patients upon admission to the ICU and in 30% of patients in the critical care setting.[1,2] This diagnosis is associated with statistically significantly increased mortality, length of hospital stay, admission to the ICU, and cost for hospitalization.[3] An algorithm for evaluating the patient with hyponatremia is proposed in Figure 27–1.

Pseudohyponatremia and Hyperosmolar Hyponatremia

The first step in the evaluation of a hyponatremic patient is to obtain a serum osmolality in order to identify those patients with pseudohyponatremia and those who have hyperosmolar hyponatremia. As its name implies, pseudohyponatremia refers to a spuriously low-measured serum sodium value. In the presence of severe hyperlipidemia and paraproteinemia, the water phase of serum becomes displaced by these particles, and when flame photometry or indirect potentiometry is used to the measure sodium, the values are reported as spuriously low. Measuring serum sodium by direct potentiometry should remove this problem. Patients with pseudohyponatremia require no further treatment.

The presence of exogenously or endogenously derived osmotically active particles in serum will cause hyperosmolar hyponatremia. In normal

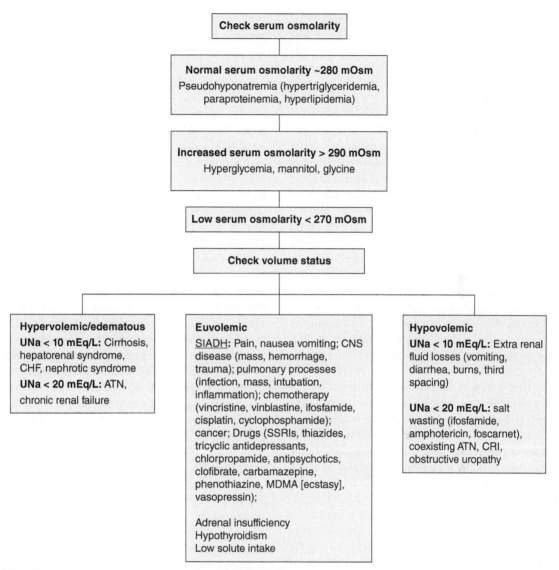

FIGURE 27–1 Clinical approach to the patient with hyponatremia.

homeostasis, water will shift across the cell membrane to equalize the osmolality between the intracellular (IC) and EC spaces. When there are osmotically active particles in the EC space, large volumes of water can transfer from the IC, causing a true dilutional hyponatremia. Patients who undergo procedures, such as hysteroscopies or transurethral resections of bladder tumor (TURBTs) are exposed to glycine containing fluids. Glycine is an osmotically active particle. Because large volumes of these solutions are instilled into the body cavity during surgical procedures, the high intravesical pressures can cause glycine to be absorbed into the venous circulation. Subsequent translocation of free water from the IC to the EC space will cause a dilutional hyponatremia. A similar process occurs in the presence of other osmotically active particles, such as mannitol and in the setting of hyperglycemia.[4] Importantly, the patient with hyperosmolar hypernatremia should never receive hypertonic saline as part of the management of hyponatremia, even if they have mental status changes associated with hypernatremia, since hypertonic saline will only exacerbate the hyperosmolar state. A renal consultation should be obtained since these patients may require hemodialysis (HD).

Hypo-Osmolar Hyponatremia

Most patients will fall into the remaining category of hypo-osmolar hyponatremia. Since disorders of serum sodium are best approached as disorders of relative concentrations of salt and water, all hyponatremic patients, whether they are volume overloaded, euvolemic or hypervolemic, have an excess of total body water relative to total body sodium. Therefore, an assessment of the patient's volume status helps to define the primary disorder in this category of patients. Be mindful that the presence of edema does not accurately identify a patient as hypervolemic. Deep venous thrombosis, inferior vena cava (IVC) clots, and lymphatic or venous obstruction from pelvic masses can all produce lower extremity edema. However, these patients may have a state of diminished effective intravascular volume due to diminished venous return to the right atrium from the primary disease process. Since patients in the ICU can have nonvolume mediated causes of tachycardia and dry mucous membranes, whenever possible, it can be very helpful to check orthostatic vital signs at the bedside to assess the volume status in patients who is not frankly hypotensive. A patient is considered to be orthostatic if the heart rate increases more than 20 beats/min or the systolic blood pressure drops more than 10 mm Hg from the supine to upright position. Patients should be allowed spend 2 to 3 minutes in the sitting and standing position before the vitals are checked to allow for appropriate autoregulation.

Hypovolemic hyponatremia—This scenario can be observed in patients on diuretics, or who have diarrhea, excessive sweating (marathon runners), or insensible losses from the skin (burn victims). A similar scenario can be observed in the intubated ICU patient because the positive intrathoracic pressures generated by mechanical ventilation will impair cardiac filling. The volume deficit in these patients will cause activation of the baroreceptors, the release of antidiuretic hormone (ADH), and activation of the renin angiotensin aldosterone system and the sympathetic nervous system. The end result of triggering these pathways is the retention of free water and salt. ADH and angiotensin are also dipsogens and will stimulate thirst. Consequently, there will be net retention of free water and salt, but a relative excess of free water retention. These patients typically have "prerenal" indices—a urine sodium less than 20 mEq/L, urine osmolarity more than 500 mOsm and a fractional excretion of sodium (FENa) less than 1%. Since diuretics can affect urine sodium excretion, for patients who have received diuretics within the preceding 24 hours, the fractional excretion of urea (FEurea) can be checked instead. A FEurea of <15% suggests volume contraction.

A more complex presentation of hypovolemic hypovolemia occurs with renal salt wasting and cerebral salt wasting. Renal salt wasting has been described following exposure to chemotherapeutic agents (cisplatin and ifosfamide) and anti-infectives (amphotericin, trimethoprim-sulfamethoxazole, and amikacin).[5] Cerebral salt wasting has been described following CNS trauma, neurosurgery, and traumatic brain injury. In contrast to the previously described group of hypovolemic patients, those individuals with salt wasting syndromes tend to have polyuria and will have inappropriately high urine sodium and osmolality values and the FENa can be more than 1%. Similar urine values can be observed in patients with the syndrome of inappropriate ADH release (SIADH) which is discussed in the section on normovolemic hyponatremia. However, the patient with SIADH, by definition, is euvolemic.

Appropriate treatment for salt wasting syndromes is isotonic normal saline (0.9% NS), which can be delivered as a bolus or infusion, depending on the severity of the volume depletion. Some patients with severe salt wasting may require hypertonic saline solutions (2% or 3% NS) to replace the amount of salt being lost in the urine.

There is a subset of critically ill patients who appear volume overloaded on exam, but have diminished effective arterial blood flow and who are hypotensive or orthostatic on exam. Patients with hepatorenal syndrome, systemic inflammatory response syndrome, and those who are "third spacing" (rhabdomyolysis and pancreatitis) will have prerenal indices. In hepatorenal syndrome, increased nitric oxide levels results in preferential pooling of blood in the splanchnic circulation, resulting in diminished effective intraarterial blood volume (EABV) to other vital organs, including the kidneys.[6] These patients can be frankly hypotensive in the presence of substantial edema on exam. In systemic inflammatory response syndrome, although the pathophysiology is not well delineated, several cytokines pathways, which include tumor necrosis factor, nitric oxide, and interleukins appear to be responsible for the substantial capillary leak and diminished EABV. These patients may require significant amounts of crystalloid and/or colloid fluids to expand their intravascular volume.

Hypervolemic hyponatremia—This group of visibly volume overloaded patients have excessive amounts of total body free water and sodium, with relatively more free water than sodium in the EC space. Classically, patients with congestive heart failure, cirrhosis, nephrotic syndrome (NS), and pregnancy fall into this category. In the case of a normal pregnancy, serum sodium declines up to 5 mEq/L below normal values because ADH is released at a lower set point. Hyponatremia in pregnancy is physiologic and does not require correction.[7] On the other hand, the hyponatremia associated with congestive heart failure and cirrhosis is best treated with the use of loop diuretics. Thiazide diuretics should be avoided in the setting of hyponatremia because they can actually cause hyponatremia. This is because thiazides impeded the ability of the collecting tubules to maximally concentrate urine and will, therefore, cause overall retention of free water.

Normovolemic hyponatremia—The 2 physiologic stimuli for ADH release are an elevated serum osmolality and a diminished plasma volume. Therefore, in the setting of a low-serum osmolarity and a normal plasma volume, there is no physiologic stimulus for ADH release. There are, however, numerous nonphysiologic stimuli for ADH, and these stimuli are prevalent in the ICU. Pain, nausea, drugs (catecholamines, chemotherapy, antidepressants, and diuretics), and any lung or CNS disease can cause inappropriate release of ADH. The postoperative state is also associated with inappropriate ADH release, and potentially severe hyponatremia can develop in patients receiving hypotonic intravenous (IV) solutions in the perioperative period.

Death and permanent neurologic deficits in the setting of postoperative hyponatremia is more commonly observed in menstruating women and pre pubertal children.[8] Adrenal and thyroid deficient states are also associated with SIADH. Figure 27–1 lists some causes of SIADH that can be encountered in the ICU setting.

The defining feature of the SIADH state is the presence of inappropriately concentrated urine in the setting of a low-serum osmolality and a normal plasma volume. The urine sodium is > 20 mEq/L and the FENa is more than 1%.

Importantly, administering 0.9% NS to a patient with SIADH will actually worsen the hyponatremia. Because these patients have a normal plasma volume, there is no stimulus for the kidney to retain the 9 g of sodium contained in each liter of 0.9% NS. However, the presence of ADH will cause the renal tubules to retain the IL of water. This free water retention will dilute and further lower the serum sodium. Inappropriately administering 0.9% NS to patients with SIADH who have a very low serum sodium values or abruptly lowing the sodium significant amounts can precipitate hyponatremic seizures. Therefore, 0.9% NS without furosemide or any hypotonic fluids (D5W, 1/2NS) are all contraindicated in the setting of SIADH.

Several approaches can be employed to correct the imbalance between sodium and water concentration in the setting of SIADH. Patients can be asked to restrict their fluid intake to 1 to 1.5 L of free water per day and can be given NaCl tablets. These interventions may be limited in the ICU patient since the often require IV medications and cannot tolerate oral medications. In this case, 0.9% NS given along with furosemide or hypertonic saline (2% or 3%) alone can be used to increase the serum sodium concentration. Usual doses of furosemide in patients with normal renal function are 10 to 20 mg/d and can be give IV or orally. Higher doses of furosemide may be required in patients with renal function. Vasopressin-2 (V2) receptor antagonists are the newest class of agents which can be used in the management of hypervolemic and euvolemic hyponatremia. V2 receptor antagonists will block ADH-mediated insertion of aquaporin channels at the apical membrane of the renal collecting duct cells and will ultimately result in free water losses in the urine. Conivaptan is an IV formulation (20 mg infused over 30 minutes as a loading dose, followed by a continuous infusion of 20 mg over 24 hours) and tolvaptan can be given to patients who are able to take oral medications (initial dose is 15 mg once daily can increase to 30 mg once daily after 24 hours). Any combination of fluid restriction, NaCl tablets, furosemide, and/or a V2 receptor antagonist can be used to achieve a normal serum sodium value. Conivaptan and tolvaptan have been shown to reliably increase serum sodium by 6 to 8 mEq/L with a 48 hours period and have the advantage of not producing the hypokalemia and metabolic alkalosis that can result from treatment with diuretics.[9]

If nausea, vomiting and pain are inappropriately stimulating ADH, then appropriate use of antiemetics and pain medications can diminish these nonphysiologic stimuli for ADH release. Any of the culprit medications that have been implicated as a cause of hyponatremia (see Figure 27–1) should be discontinued if it is safe to do so. For patients with adrenal or thyroid deficient states, hormone replacement therapy will be necessary to correct the hyponatremia.

Clinical Manifestations and Management of Severe Hyponatremia

The clinical signs and symptoms of hyponatremia are in large part manifestations of increased intracerebral pressure due to brain edema. When the serum sodium and serum osmolality are lower than that within the brain cells, water will shift into the brain cells. Since the skull is a fixed cavity, it cannot expand to accommodate this increase in brain volume. Some clinical signs of increased intracranial pressure include nausea, confusion vomiting, a decline in mental status, ataxia, and seizures. When hyponatremic encephalopathy develops, the associated mortality rate is as high as 20%.[8] If the brain volume markedly exceeds the skull volume, frank herniation of the brainstem and death can occur. There are adaptive mechanisms in place to mitigate brain edema in the setting of hyponatremia. However, when the serum sodium drops too rapidly relative to the ability of the brain to adapt to the change in osmolality, clinical signs, and symptoms will develop. This explains why one patient can present

with seizures and another can appear asymptomatic at equivalent serum sodium values.

The brain's adaptive mechanisms are essentially aimed at decreasing its water content back to normal by extruding solute. In rat models, Na^{2+} and Cl^- are extruded via the Na^{2+} and Cl^- channels present in the cell membrane within 30 minutes of induction of hyponatremia. These electrolyte losses are maximal at around 3 hours. After longer periods of persistent hyponatremia, organic osmolytes such as glutamate, creatine, and taurine exit the brain cell.[10] These compensatory adaptations explain why rapid correction of chronic hyponatremia leads to rapid egress of water from the brain cell. In mild cases, dehydration of the brain tissue occurs, and in severe cases, osmotic demyelination can occur. The current recommendation for correcting chronic hyponatremia or hyponatremia of unknown duration is to correct the serum sodium no more than 10-12 mEq/L within the first 24 hours, and at a rate of no more than 10 to 12 mEq/L within the first 24 hours, and generally, at a rate of no more than 0.5 mEq/L/h.[11]

Treatment for mild hyponatremia is discussed in the aforementioned sections. When symptomatic hyponatremic develops (mental status changes, seizures, and coma), and when serum sodium levels are very low (less than 115 mEq/L), patients needs to be closely monitored with repeated neurologic evaluations and frequent monitoring of their serum sodium values while they receive 3% NS to correct the sodium deficit. One of the numerous online resources available to calculate the sodium deficit is http://www.mdcalc.com/sodium-deficit-in-hyponatremia/, or the sodium deficit can be calculated using the equation: Sodium deficit = total body water × (desired serum Na − actual serum Na), where total body water is total body weight (kg) × 0.5. Each IL of 3% NS contains 512 mEq of sodium. Importantly, the severely symptomatic patient with hyperosmolar hyponatremia should not receive 3% NS. Administration of a hypertonic solution in this setting is contraindicated as it will worsen the hyperosmolar state. This category of patients may require urgent dialysis. Patients with significant hypovolemia should be treated with boluses of NS until a euvolemic state is achieved. Thereafter, the rate of correction of the serum sodium should not exceed 10 to 12 mEq/L in a 24 hours period.

Hypernatremia

The incidence of hypernatremia in the general hospital population is only 1%. The reported incidence in the ICU population ranges from 10% to 26%, and it is most commonly hospital acquired.[12] When hypernatremia is acquired in the ICU, the adjusted hazard ratio for ICU mortality increased twofold in patients with mild hypernatremia (> 145 mEq/L) and 2.67-fold in patients with moderate to severe hypernatremia (> 150 mEq/L).[13]

Hypernatremia arises when there is a relative or absolute free water deficit so patients are either hypervolemic or hypovolemic, respectively. Normally, a rise in serum sodium, and consequent rise in serum osmolarity causes ADH release, which is a potent stimulus for thirst. Patients with an intact thirst mechanism and access to free water are able to maintain normal serum sodium levels notwithstanding considerable urine outputs in hyperosmolar states from hyperglycemia or diabetes insipidus. By contrast, ICU patients oftentimes have an impaired thirst response, impaired access to free water or restricted fluid intake.

Hypervolemia Hypernatremia

Administration of sodium bicarbonate, trisodium citrate, hypertonic saline, or other fluids containing an excess of solute relative to free water results in hypervolemic hypernatremia.

Hypovolemic Hypernatremia

Conditions that cause excessive amounts of free water losses via the kidneys include central and nephrogenic diabetes insipidus (CDI and NDI, respectively). Acquired causes of NDI include amphotericin, foscarnet, lithium, hypokalemia, and hypercalcemia. Hyperglycemia and mannitol cause an osmotic diuresis and hyperalimentation solutions can also produce diuresis due to urea generation. Nonrenal free water losses can occur via the gastrointestinal (GI) tract (nasogastric suction, diarrhea, and vomiting), skin (burns, hyperthermia, open wounds, and drains), and from the respiratory tract in intubated patients.

Clinical Manifestations and Management

The clinical signs of hypernatremia are the result of shrinkage of the brain away from the skull and the mechanical stress that this causes on blood vessels, which can lead to ischemia and hemorrhage. Symptoms include agitation, lethargy, seizures, and coma. When hypernatremia develops rapidly, osmotic demyelination can occur.

The goals in treating hypernatremia include (1) identifying correcting any reversible factors (hypercalcemia, hypokalemia hypertonic solutions); (2) correcting volume depletion if present; and (3) replacing the calculated free water deficit. Additionally, if compatible, all IV medications should be administered in hypotonic solutions (1/2 NS or D5W). In hypervolemic patients, thiazides can be used to decrease edema as well as the serum sodium. In patients with polyuria due to partial NDI or CDI, arginine vasopressin administration will permit free water retention in the kidneys and correction of the sodium to a normal value permitting free water retention in the kidneys. In the hypovolemic patient with hemodynamic compromise, isotonic NS can be given to first correct the volume deficit and to ward off hemodynamic collapse. Thereafter, hypotonic solutions (1/2 NS or D5W) can be used with the goal of correcting 1/2 the free water deficit in the initial 24 hours period, and the remaining deficit over the ensuing 48 to 72 hours. The free water deficit can be calculated using the formula: Water deficit = 0.5 Wt (kg) [Serum Na/140-1]. Ongoing losses should be considered when replacing the water deficit. The serum sodium should not decrease by more than 0.5 mEq/L/h. Overly rapid correction of hypernatremia can cause increased intracranial pressure and the signs associated with hyponatremia (see section on hyponatremia).

POTASSIUM

Approximately 98% of the body's potassium is found in the IC space. Normally, when potassium enters the circulation acutely, it is rapidly shifted to the IC space by the action of insulin and catecholamines. The kidneys are the major site for excretion of potassium and chronic potassium homeostasis. Eighty percent of potassium is excreted from the kidneys, and 90% is reabsorbed via the renal tubules. Aldosterone is the major hormone governing renal potassium excretion.[14] About 15% of potassium is eliminated from the GI tract and 5% is lost in sweat.[15] The major clinical manifestations potassium disorders are cardiac and neuromuscular abnormalities.

Hyperkalemia

Keeping in mind the key regulators of potassium homeostasis mentioned in the previous paragraph, a simple and effective approach to evaluating hyperkalemia is to make the following inquiries: (1) Is there is too much exogenous potassium being delivered to the patient? (2) Is there is a problem with the usual mechanism for shifting potassium into the IC space? (3) Is there is a problem with eliminating potassium via the kidneys or GI tract? A number of conditions can predispose ICU patient to developing hyperkalemia, including insulin deficiency or resistance, renal dysfunction, adrenal insufficiency, and exposures to medications that are known to derange normal potassium homeostasis.

Acute potassium loads from cell destruction in the setting tumor lysis syndrome, massive blood transfusions and rhabdomyolysis can overwhelm the normal mechanisms available to acutely shift potassium into the IC space. In patients with hyperglycemia, insulin deficiency will cause diminished influx of potassium to the IC space. Moreover, when hyperglycemia is present, in response to the osmotic gradient generated across the cell membrane by the hyperglycemia, water will shift from teh IC to the EC space to equalize the gradient across the cell membrane. By the process of solvent drag, potassium will move with the water to the EC space, further increasing serum potassium levels.

A host of medications commonly used in the ICU can (1) impair the kidney's ability to appropriately excrete potassium (triamterene, trimethoprim, pentamidine, and spironolactone); (2) inhibit the ATPase driven movement of potassium into cells (beta-blockers and digoxin; (3) inhibit aldosterone synthesis (angiotensin converting enzyme inhibitors, angiotensin 2 receptor blockers, heparin, and azole antifungals); (4) inhibit prostaglandin (nonsteroidal anti-inflammatory medications); and (5) suppress the release of low renin and consequently low aldosterone levels (cyclosporine and tacrolimus).[16]

Patients who are volume-depleted patient are unable to properly excrete potassium, since the delivery of sodium to the distal renal tubule is necessary for urinary potassium secretion. Patients with obstructive uropathy also have an impaired ability to excrete potassium properly. Potential sources of exogenous potassium that can go unnoticed in the ICU patient include the administration of inappropriate enteral or parenteral nutrition, and chronic absorption of potassium from degenerated RBCs from a retroperitoneal hematoma or GI bleed.

Clinical Manifestations and Management

The clinical signs and symptoms of hyperkalemia are predominantly neuromuscular (muscle weakness, paralysis) and cardiac (electrocardiographic [EKG] changes—peaked T waves, prolonged PR interval, widened QRS, arrhythmias, and asystole).

The patient with hyperkalemia is best approached with following principles in mind: (1) identify and discontinue all medications that may be deranging normal potassium homeostasis; (2) discontinue all potassium containing IV fluids; (3) shift potassium into the IC space; and (4) increase potassium elimination through the kidneys and the GI tract.

For patients who have EKG changes associated with hyperkalemia, IV calcium (10% calcium chloride or calcium gluconate 500-1000 mg over 2-5 minutes) is needed to stabilize the cardiac cells and lower the risk of fatal arrhythmias. Patients with muscle weakness or paralysis and those who have acute renal failure may require urgent dialysis. An early renal consultation is recommended for these patients.

The most rapid way to lower serum potassium is with the use of inhaled beta agonists (nebulized albuterol 10-20 mg over 15 minutes) and insulin (50 mL of D50W + 10U regular insulin over 15-30 minutes). These agents will acutely shift potassium into the IC space. In the hyperglycemic patient, insulin therapy will dissipate the gradient for solvent drag across the cell membrane in addition to pushing potassium back into the IC space. If a patient is acidemic, neutralizing the serum pH with IV sodium bicarbonate (50 mEq intravenous push (IVP)) will facilitate potassium entry back into cells. While beta agonists and insulin acutely shift potassium into cells, these measures are short lived and rebound hyperkalemia can occur if additional steps are not taken at the same time to permanently remove potassium from the body. Infusion with 0.9% NS will promote a kaliuresis by increasing delivery of sodium to the distal tubule. If clinically appropriate, a loop diuretic can be used alone or in combination with IV 0.9% NS to promote renal potassium elimination. Potassium losses can also be affected via the GI tract. Sodium polystyrene (15-30 g) will exchange potassium for sodium across the colonic mucosa. However, it may take several days to appreciably lower the serum potassium since delivery to the colon is dependent on GI transit time. Sodium polystyrene can be given as a rectal suppository or orally in combination with sorbitol for faster delivery to its site of action at the colonic mucosa. Care should be taken when prescribing this medication to patients in the post-operative period following abdominal surgery and in patients who are hypotensive or have decreased GI motility. These patients may be at increased risk of bowel necrosis with this therapy.[17] Sodium polystyrene and sodium bicarbonate can both worsen fluid retention in patients with volume overload and should be used with caution in this setting.

Hypokalemia

The frequency of hypokalemia in the adult ICU population has not been well documented, but it is encountered fairly commonly. In the pediatric ICU population, the reported frequency is 40%.[18] The same principles apply when approaching hypokalemia as is the case with hyperkalemia. That is to say, it is necessary to systematically identify factors that will (1) shift potassium into the IC space (beta agonists, epinephrine, insulin, dobutamine, respiratory alkalosis, and refeeding); (2) increase GI losses of potassium (nasogastric tube (NGT) suction; vomiting, diarrhea, and sodium polystyrene sulfonate); (3) increase renal potassium losses (diuretics, hypomagnesemia, aminoglycosides, amphotericin, cisplatin, ifosfamide, fludrocortisone, postobstructive diuresis, and post-acute tubular necrosis (ATN) diuresis); and (4) diminish oral potassium intake. In the setting of a post-ATN and a postobstructive diuresis, renal tubular resorptive function is impaired so patients can excrete large amounts of isosthenuric urine containing significant amounts of electrolytes. In the refeeding syndrome, the introduction of carbohydrates and subsequent increase in insulin release will shift potassium to the IC compartment.

Clinical Manifestations and Treatment

The clinical manifestations of hypokalemia are predominantly cardiac (arrhythmias, EKG changes [flattening of the T wave, U wave]) and neuromuscular (muscle weakness, cramping and ileus, and constipation). Fairly small decrements in serum potassium values can actually represent significant potassium deficits since most of the potassium stores are in the IC space. For example, mild hypokalemia with a serum K of 3.0 mEq/L can actually reflect up to a 300 mEq total body deficit.[19] There is no reliable way to measure the total body potassium deficit.

In general, ICU patients receive potassium replacement intravenously, but oral administration of potassium is preferable if possible. Potassium infusions can be caustic to peripheral veins, so for doses exceeding 10 mEq/h, a central line should be used. Continuous EKG monitoring is appropriate in those patients with an abnormal EKG for whom it may be necessary to infuse potassium at rates exceeding 20 mEq/h. In all patients, especially those with renal impairment, serum potassium levels should be repeated after electrolyte replacement to ensure adequate correction and to avoid over correction. In patients with concomitant hypomagnesemia, the hypomagnesemia needs to corrected first because hypomagnesemia will cause efflux of potassium from the renal tubules and can result in resistance to potassium supplementation. For ICU patients with diuretic-induced hypokalemia who require further diuretic therapy, in addition to correcting the hypokalemia, consideration should be given to adding to or replacing the loop diuretic with a potassium sparing diuretic such as spironolactone, triamterene, or amiloride.

CALCIUM

Serum calcium reflects less than 1% of total body calcium, as 99% of total body calcium resides in the bones. Of the remaining 1% of serum calcium, 50% is bound to albumin and 50% is unbound or biologically active calcium. Common conditions in ICU patients can affect the amount of unbound (free) calcium. For example, in the setting of metabolic alkalosis, there is increased calcium binding to albumin and in the setting of metabolic acidosis, decreased calcium binding to albumin. Because ICU patients are often hypoalbuminemic and have derangements in their acid base status, measuring ionized serum calcium levels is the best method for determining an individual's true serum calcium status.[20]

The chief regulators of serum calcium levels are parathyroid hormone (PTH), vitamin D levels, and calcitonin. Calcium acts as a key IC regulator and messenger. As a result, some clinically important manifestations of disordered calcium homeostasis in the ICU patient include neuromuscular and cardiac dysfunction. Symptoms of severe hypocalcemia include tetany, seizures, a prolonged QT interval, and ventricular arrhythmias.

Hypocalcemia

Hypocalcemia is ubiquitous in the ICU, affecting 80% to 90% of all patients,[16] and when present, is associated with longer ICU stays, increased mortality and higher rates of bacteremia.[21] It can be the result of low vitamin D levels and abnormalities in the release or effect of PTH. Hypoparathyroidism and hypomagnesemia can both decrease PTH secretion and hypomagnesemia additionally diminishes the effect of PTH on skeletal tissue and so will decrease calcium release from bone.

The patients who come to the ICU following a parathyroidectomy can have severe and abrupt hypocalcemia. Following resection of the parathyroid gland for secondary or tertiary hypoparathyroidism, the tonic release of high levels of PTH suddenly dramatically decreases. Serum calcium rushes into the skeletal compartment and can result in severe symptomatic hypocalcemia. This is referred to as the "hungry bone syndrome."

In cancer patients, tumor lysis syndrome can occur spontaneously or following chemotherapy. As the tumor cells release their IC contents, the resultant acute hyperphosphatemia becomes the source for calcium phosphate precipitates and this will abruptly lower the serum calcium. A similar scenario of acute calcium phosphorus precipitate formation occurs in the setting of rhabdomyolysis and following exposure to phosphorus containing laxatives and enemas which are commonly used prior to colonoscopies. Hyperphosphatemia will further lower serum calcium levels by causing decreased levels of $1,25(OH)_2$ vitamin D.

In patients who transfused with large amounts of blood products, and in those patients receiving citrate anticoagulation during plasmapheresis or continuous renal replacement therapy (CRRT), hypocalcemia can result from citrate acting as a chelator of ionized calcium. Gadolinium contrast interferes with calcium assays and can cause spurious hypocalcemia. However, the ionized serum calcium measurements are not affected.[22]

Clinical Manifestations and Treatment

For acute correction of symptomatic hypocalcemia, IV calcium gluconate or calcium chloride (10 mL of a 10% solution) can be administered over 10 minutes. For patients with hungry bone syndrome, in addition to IV pushes of calcium chloride or calcium gluconate, a continuous IV calcium infusion, with frequent monitoring of serum calcium, may be necessary to maintain normal serum calcium levels. When hypocalcemia is accompanied by hypomagnesemia, the hypomagnesemia will need to be corrected first or the hypocalcemia can become resistant to calcium supplementation due to the effect of hypomagnesemia on PTH release and action on its end organs. When hypocalcemia is accompanied by metabolic acidosis, the hypocalcemia should be corrected before the acidosis because correcting the acidosis first will further lower the serum calcium and possibly precipitate symptomatic hypocalcemia. In patients with hypocalcemia due to formation of calcium phosphorus complexes (pancreatitis, tumor lysis syndrome), hypocalcemia should only be corrected if patients become symptomatic. If the calcium phosphorus product exceeds 60, then dialysis should be considered to lower the calcium phosphorus product prior to calcium repletion.

Hypercalcemia

Hypercalcemia occurs less often than hypocalcemia in the ICU. When present, the level of hypercalcemia can be an important clue to its pathogenesis. Serum calcium values above 13 mg/dL should raise suspicion for hypercalcemia of malignancy in the appropriate clinical setting. Hypercalcemia of malignancy is most often attributable to PTH related protein and, less frequently, to osteolytic cytokines and exogenous calcitriol production. Less severe levels of hypercalcemia can be seen in association diseases that increase bone resorption (immobility, thyrotoxicosis, and Paget's and hypervitaminosis A); diseases that increase intestinal absorption of calcium (milk alkali syndrome and hypervitaminosis D); any cause of increased PTH levels (primary, secondary, or tertiary hyperparathyroidism); elevated Vitamin D levels (from oral supplements, or granulomatous diseases, such as tuberculosis or sarcoidosis); and medications (thiazide diuretics, lithium, theophylline, and teriparatide). Adrenal insufficiency causes hypercalcemia via several mechanisms (volume contraction, increased bone resorption, and increased tubular absorption of calcium).

Clinical Manifestations and Treatment

Some neurologic manifestations of hypercalcemia include anorexia, confusion, and obtundation. Cardiac manifestations include arrhythmias and EKG changes (shortened QT). Importantly, hypercalcemia can cause a NDI. Free water losses in the urine from the NDI, in addition to diminished oral intake due to decrease mental acuity and anorexia in these patients, results in significant volume depletion in hypercalcemic patients. Therefore, aggressive volume resuscitation is a cornerstones of therapy for hypercalcemia.

The primary goals in the management of hypercalcemia are to (1) increase urinary excretion of calcium and (2) inhibit bone resorption. To this end, in the absence of edema, aggressive volume expansion with 0.9% NS at rates needed to promote a urine output of 100 o 150 cc/h is recommended. These patients often may require a 1 to 2 L bolus of 0.9% NS to replace the fluid deficit and then require an infusion rate of 150 to 200 mL/h. Once the patient is adequately volume replete, furosemide can be used to promote a calciuresis. It is recommended that furosemide not be given prior to adequate volume resuscitation since the diuretic can further compromise the hemodynamic status of these dehydrated patients. Calcitonin (4 units/kg every SQ every 12 hours for 4-6 doses) will begin to lower serum calcium within 4 to 6 hours of administration, with a maximum effect of 1 to 2 mg/dL (0.3-0.5 mmol/L). It does so by inhibiting bone resorption and by increasing urinary calcium excretion. Unfortunately, tachyphylaxis due to downregulation of it receptors occurs after repeated

dosing so the medication loses efficacy after 48 hours. In patients who are volume overloaded or anuric, dialysis with a low calcium dialysate (2.5 mEq/L) may be necessary to treat hypercalcemia.

Bisphosphonates (BPs) have become another cornerstone for management of hypercalcemia. Pamidronate and zoledronate currently have Food and Drug Administration (FDA) approval for the management of hypercalcemia, but pamidronate should be preferentially used in patients with renal insufficiency and a creatine clearance less than 30 mL/min. Please consult dosing guidelines for zoledronic acid for patients with mildly impaired renal function. Since the onset of action of BPs is 2 to 4 days, it is recommended that they be administered at the time that hypercalcemia is first diagnosed.

PHOSPHORUS

Phosphorus is another anion which is primarily contained in the bones and soft tissue, with only 1% circulating in the EC space. Phosphorus is the building block for adenosine triphosphate, which is required for all energy requiring physiologic and metabolic functions. Therefore, IC phosphate depletion can produce multiorgan dysfunction due to decrease oxygen release to the cardiac (decreased myocardial contractility), pulmonary (respiratory failure due to diaphragmatic paralysis), GI (dysphagia and ileus), neurologic (parasthesias and seizures) and skeletal systems (rhabdomyolysis and myopathy).

Hypophosphatemia

In the general hospital wards, about 5% of patients have serum phosphorus levels less than 2.5 mg/dL, while the prevalence of hypophosphatemia in patients with severe sepsis and trauma is reported to be 30% to 50%.[23] Patients in the ICU have conditions which predispose them to developing hypophosphatemia via the three major mechanisms: (1) redistribution of phosphorus to the IC space (due to respiratory alkalosis, glucose, and insulin release during carbohydrate refeeding in malnourished patients); (2) redistribution of phosphorus into the bone (hungry bone syndrome [see section on hypocalcemia] and bisphosphonate therapy); (3) decreased intestinal absorption of phosphorus (steatorrhea, chronic diarrhea, or prolonged starvation, phosphate binding in the gut by aluminum or magnesium containing antacids); and (4) increased phosphaturia (any cause of increased PTH, vitamin D deficiency, acetazolamide, thiazide diuretics, or Fanconi syndrome [multiple myeloma and ifosfamide]). Patients on continuous CRRT will also lose phosphorus to the dialysate.

Treatment

Phosphorus replacement is available as potassium phosphate and sodium phosphate. Keep in mind that each mmol of potassium phosphate contains 1.47 mEq of potassium. Therefore, 15 mmol of potassium phosphate will deliver 22.5 mEq of potassium to the patient. For patients with symptomatic hypophosphatemia, phosphorus can be given at a rate of up to 7 mmol/h.[24] Serum phosphorus levels should be checked 2 to 4 hours after IV repletion since phosphorus can quickly shift into the IC space. Whenever possible, oral phosphorus is preferred for the correction of asymptomatic hypophosphatemia and when the serum phosphorus level is more than 2 mg/dL.

Hyperphosphatemia

Since the kidneys are very efficient at maintaining normal phosphorus balance, there has to be some element of renal dysfunction present for hyperphosphatemia to develop. Most of the total body phosphorus is contained within cells and the skeletal tissue. Therefore, release massive amounts of IC phosphorus from cell lysis (tumor lysis syndrome and massive blood transfusions), muscle injury (rhabdomyolysis), and acute EC shifts of phosphorus (lactic and diabetic ketoacidosis) will acutely increase serum phosphorus. Acute elevations in the levels of serum phosphorus have been also been reported following ingestion of large amounts of phosphorus containing laxatives used for colonoscopy bowel preparation. Hypoparathyroidism and vitamin D toxicity are also causes of hyperphosphatemia.

When there is an acute increase in serum phosphorus levels, phosphorus will complex with calcium to form calcium phosphate crystals, which in turn can cause obstructive uropathy and acute kidney injury. The acute kidney injury will in turn further compromise renal clearance of phosphorus.

Treatment

In addition to identifying and correcting underlying causes of hyperphosphatemia and infusion of NS to promote phosphaturia is central in the management of this disorder. In those patients with oral intake, oral phosphate binders can be used to bind phosphorus in the gut. However, oral phosphate binders have no benefit to those patients who are not being fed orally. HD may be required to lower the serum phosphorus in patients who are anuric or oliguria AND for those with a calcium phosphorus product more than 55-60; and in the patient with symptomatic hypocalcemia. Continuous dialysis (CRRT) will lower the phosphorus more continuously that intermittent HD and there may be rebound hyperphosphatemia in between treatments when intermittent HD is used.

MAGNESIUM

Magnesium is principally an IC cation, with only 1% of the total body content contained in the EC space. Magnesium homeostasis is predominantly handled by the kidneys with important contributions from the GI tract and parathyroid hormone. Importantly, the cation serves as a cofactor for reactions involving adenosine triphosphate. Hypomagnesemia can result from renal losses (aminoglycosides, thiazide and loop diuretics, amphotericin, cisplatin, epithelial growth factor inhibitors [cetuximab] alcoholism, and cyclosporine), GI losses (proton pump inhibitors, short bowel syndrome, malabsorption, and steatorrhea), and diminished intake (malnutrition). Magnesium can also be chelated in circulation by citrate (massive blood transfusions) and foscarnet. Hypokalemia and hypocalcemia frequently coexist with hypomagnesemia. The hypokalemia may be due to impaired function of the sodium potassium pump and the hypocalcemia is due to impaired PTH secretion and activity. Hypermagnesemia is often the result of iatrogenesis and oftentimes occurs in the setting of impaired renal function.

Hypomagnesemia

Hypomagnesemia is frequently found in critically ill patients, with a reported prevalence of 60% to 65%.[25] When it is present, it is associated with greater morbidity and mortality.[26] Clinically important manifestations of hypomagnesemia include EKG changes (arrhythmias and torsades de pointes), neuromuscular problems (tetany and seizures), electrolyte disorders (hypokalemia and hypocalcemia), and impaired PTH release and action.

Treatment

In patients with cardiac and neuromuscular manifestations of hypomagnesemia, 1 to 2 g of magnesium sulfate can be given as a IV bolus or over 60 minutes, followed by an IV infusion to keep the serum magnesium more than 1.5 mEq/L.[27] When repleting magnesium, it is important to keep in mind that magnesium distributes into the tissue space very slowly, and that acute increases in serum magnesium inhibits magnesium reabsorption in the renal tubules. Therefore, when magnesium is given rapidly, up to 50% of the IV dose is lost in the urine. Therefore, the best way to supplement magnesium intravenously is to do so very slowly, at a rate not exceeding 1 g/h. It is best to allow several hours to elapse before checking the postrepletion serum magnesium levels since levels drawn immediately after supplementation may be spuriously elevated. In ICU patients with asymptomatic hypomagnesemia who are able to tolerate oral magnesium, the oral route for magnesium repletion is preferable. Unfortunately, oral magnesium supplements can cause diarrhea.

Hypermagnesemia

Since the kidneys are rapidly able to excrete magnesium when serum magnesium increases acutely, hypermagnesemia most frequently occurs when patients with underlying renal insufficiency are given a large dose of magnesium. For example, when ICU patients are given magnesium containing laxatives or antacids.

Clinical manifestations of hyperkalemia include neurologic (loss of deep tendon reflexes), cardiac (bradycardia, hypotension, heart block, and cardiac arrest), neuromuscular disturbances (respiratory paralysis), and death.

Treatment

In all cases of hypermagnesemia, the exogenous magnesium needs to be discontinued. In patients with asymptomatic hypomagnesemia, loop diuretics can be used in nonoliguric patients and dialysis may be required in oliguric and anuric patients. When the patient is symptomatic, IV calcium chloride 500 to 1000 mg (via a central line), or IV calcium gluconate 1 to 3 g (if a central line is not available) can be rapidly infused until the neuromuscular and cardiac disturbances are reversed. HD may be required as well.

REFERENCES

1. DeVita MV, Gardenswartz MH, Konecky A, Zabetakis PM. Incidence and etiology of hyponatremia in an intensive care unit. *Clin nephrol.* 1990;34(4):163-166.
2. Upadhyay A, Jaber BL, Madias NE. Incidence and prevalence of hyponatremia. *Am J Med.* 2006; 119(7 Suppl 1):S30-S35.
3. Callahan MA, Do HT, Caplan DW, Yoon-Flannery K. Economic impact of hyponatremia in hospitalized patients: a retrospective cohort study. *Postgrad Med.* 2009;121(2):186-191.
4. Adrogue HJ, Madias NE. Hyponatremia. *N Engl J Med.* 2000;342(21):1581-1589.
5. Kaufman AM, Hellman G, Abramson RG. Renal salt wasting and metabolic acidosis with trimethoprim-sulfamethoxazole therapy. *Mt Sinai J Med.* 1983; 50(3):238-239.
6. Martin PY, Gines P, Schrier RW. Nitric oxide as a mediator of hemodynamic abnormalities and sodium and water retention in cirrhosis. *N Engl J Med.* 1998;339(8):533-541.
7. Lindheimer MD, Barron WM, Davison JM. Osmoregulation of thirst and vasopressin release in pregnancy. *Am J Physiol.* 1989;257(2 Pt 2):F159-F169.
8. Ayus JC, Wheeler JM, Arieff AI. Postoperative hyponatremic encephalopathy in menstruant women. *Ann Intern Med.* 1992;117(11):891-897.
9. Schrier RW, Gross P, Gheorghiade M, Berl T, Verbalis JG, Czerwiec FS, et al. Tolvaptan, a selective oral vasopressin V2-receptor antagonist, for hyponatremia. *N Engl J Med.* 2006;355(20):2099-2112.
10. Gullans SR, Verbalis JG. Control of brain volume during hyperosmolar and hypoosmolar conditions. *Annu Rev Med.* 1993;44:289-301.
11. Verbalis JG, Goldsmith SR, Greenberg A, Schrier RW, Sterns RH. Hyponatremia treatment guidelines 2007: expert panel recommendations. *Am J Med.* 2007;120(11 Suppl 1):S1-S21.
12. Pokaharel M, Block CA. Dysnatremia in the ICU. *Curr Opin Crit Care.* 2011;17(6):581-593.

13. Darmon M, Timsit JF, Francais A, Nguile-Makao M, Adrie C, Cohen Y, et al. Association between hypernatraemia acquired in the ICU and mortality: a cohort study. *Nephrol Dial Transplant.* 2010;25(8):2510-2515.

14. Halperin ML, Kamel KS. Potassium. *Lancet.* 1998;352(9122):135-140.

15. Mandal AK. Hypokalemia and hyperkalemia. *Med Clin North Am.* 1997;81(3):611-639.

16. Sedlacek M, Schoolwerth AC, Remillard BD. Electrolyte disturbances in the intensive care unit. *Semin Dial.* 2006;19(6):496-501.

17. McGowan CE, Saha S, Chu G, Resnick MB, Moss SF. Intestinal necrosis due to sodium polystyrene sulfonate (Kayexalate) in sorbitol. *South Med J.* 2009;102(5):493-497.

18. Cummings BM, Macklin EA, Yager PH, Sharma A, Noviski N. Potassium abnormalities in a pediatric intensive care unit: frequency and severity. *J Intensive Care Med.* 2014;29(5):269-274.

19. Weiner ID, Wingo CS. Hypokalemia—consequences, causes, and correction. *J Am Soc Nephrol.* 1997;8(7):1179-1188.

20. Kelly A, Levine MA. Hypocalcemia in the critically ill patient. *J Intensive Care Med.* 2013;28(3):166-177.

21. Desai TK, Carlson RW, Geheb MA. Prevalence and clinical implications of hypocalcemia in acutely ill patients in a medical intensive care setting. *Am J Meds.* 1988;84(2):209-214.

22. Williams SF, Meek SE, Moraghan TJ. Spurious hypocalcemia after gadodiamide administration. *Mayo Clin Proc.* 2005;80(12):1655-1657.

23. King AL, Sica DA, Miller G, Pierpaoli S. Severe hypophosphatemia in a general hospital population. *South Med J.* 1987;80(7):831-835.

24. Rosen GH, Boullata JI, O'Rangers EA, Enow NB, Shin B. Intravenous phosphate repletion regimen for critically ill patients with moderate hypophosphatemia. *Crit Care Med.* 1995;23(7):1204-1210.

25. Ryzen E. Magnesium homeostasis in critically ill patients. *Magnesium.* 1989;8(3-4):201-212.

26. Tong GM, Rude RK. Magnesium deficiency in critical illness. *J Intensive Care Med.* 2005;20(1):3-17.

27. Kraft MD, Btaiche IF, Sacks GS, Kudsk KA. Treatment of electrolyte disorders in adult patients in the intensive care unit. *Am J Health Syst Pharm.* 2005;62(16):1663-1682.

Acid-Base Disorders

James A. Kruse, MD

1. Recognition of acid-base disturbances through interpretation of arterial blood gases is of fundamental importance to the daily clinical practice of critical care.

2. The carbonic acid-bicarbonate buffer is the most important buffer system. The relation of pH to this buffering system is defined by the Henderson–Hasselbalch equation.

3. There are four cardinal acid-base disorders: metabolic acidosis, metabolic alkalosis, respiratory acidosis, and respiratory alkalosis.

4. The etiologies of metabolic acidosis can be classified by the typical serum anion gap association (elevated or normal anion gap acidosis).

5. The serum osmole gap is often used as a screening test when methanol or ethylene glycol intoxication is suspected.

6. Gastric fluid loss, diuretic use, and extracellular volume contraction are among the most common causes of metabolic alkalosis.

7. The etiologies of metabolic alkalosis can be classified by the expected urine chloride concentration or excretion (normal, high, or low urine chloride).

8. Common causes of respiratory acidosis are pulmonary disorders (eg, chronic obstructive lung disease, severe pneumonia, aspiration pneumonitis, and smoke inhalation), neurologic injury, neuromuscular and metabolic disorders, and narcotic and sedative agents.

9. Respiratory alkalosis is common with severe sepsis, hepatic failure, mechanical ventilation, and with drugs such as salicylates and illicit stimulants (eg, cocaine and amphetamine).

10. Mixed acid-base disorders are not uncommon in critically ill patients and frequently complicate interpretation of arterial blood gases in the intensive care unit setting.

INTRODUCTION

Recognition of acid-base disturbances through interpretation of arterial blood gases is of fundamental importance to the day-to-day clinical practice of critical care. Knowledge of the underlying basic chemical relationships and established nomenclature is prerequisite to this understanding. Several different paradigms of acid-base relationships have been proposed and are in current clinical use for framing the results of blood gas and related laboratory measurements. These paradigms include the base excess method, the Stewart or physicochemical method, and the bicarbonate-pH-Pco_2 method, and they all basically arrive at common endpoints of interpretation.[1,2] The bicarbonate-pH-Pco_2 method, also known as the physiological method, will be described herein. It is based on the carbonic acid-bicarbonate buffer system, is well established, has an empiric basis, and is in wide clinical use. Starting with a review of acid-base terminology and basic chemical relationships, this chapter will describe the basis of the physiological method for arriving at a diagnosis of simple and mixed acid-base disorders, and show how readily available laboratory testing, in conjunction with clinical information from the history and physical examination, can narrow the differential diagnosis with the goal of pin-pointing the underlying causative process or disease.

CHEMICAL RELATIONSHIPS

One definition for an acid is a chemical compound capable of donating a hydrogen ion (ie, a proton). The degree of acidity of a solution can thus be quantified as the hydrogen ion activity, which is closely related to the molar concentration of hydrogen ions. Normal hydrogen ion concentration of plasma averages about 40 nmol/L, which is considerably less than other plasma cations commonly assayed in the clinical setting. For example, plasma sodium concentration normally averages about 140 mmol/L, which is 3.5 million-fold higher than normal H^+ concentration. To avoid using small numbers and to allow simple expression of H^+ activity or concentration over a wide range of values, the pH scale was developed. The relationship between pH and hydrogen ion concentration is defined by

$$pH = -\log_{10}[H^+] \qquad (28\text{-}1)$$

where the square brackets here signify molar concentration units.

A buffer is a solution containing a weak acid (HA) and its conjugate base (A^-), which can coexist in an equilibrated reversible chemical reaction represented generically as

$$HA \leftrightharpoons H^+ + A^- \qquad (28\text{-}2)$$

The molar proportions of the substances represented in this chemical equation assume definite proportional relationships to one another at equilibrium, dependent on the chemical nature of the specific acid, temperature, and certain other variables. These proportions are expressible numerically by the modified equilibrium constant (K′) as

$$K' = \frac{[H^+] \times [A^-]}{[HA]} \qquad (28\text{-}3)$$

The prime symbol is added to signify that molar concentrations are employed rather than thermodynamic activities.[3] Buffers resist changes in pH when additional acid or base is introduced into the solution because the added acid reacts with the conjugate base, while added base reacts with the existing acid or the acid's dissociated protons. Bodily fluids contain multiple buffers, but the proportions of their acid form to their conjugate base form are all related by way of the shared hydrogen ion concentration of the fluid as

$$[H^+] = K_1' \times \frac{[HA_1]}{[A_1^-]} = K_2' \times \frac{[HA_2]}{[A_2^-]} = K_3' \times \frac{[HA_3]}{[A_3^-]}$$

$$= \cdots K_n' \times \frac{[HA_n]}{[A_n^-]} \qquad (28\text{-}4)$$

Thus, only one buffer pair needs to be considered to describe the system in terms of $[H^+]$ or pH. Carbonic acid and its conjugate base (bicarbonate) are selected as the representative buffer pair because of the ability of carbonic acid to dissociate to form carbon dioxide, the body's ability to excrete large amounts of carbon dioxide by way of the lungs, and ready availability of suitable assay methods.

In the presence of carbonic anhydrase, the reversible dissociation of carbonic acid to carbon dioxide occurs rapidly and in accordance with the principle of chemical mass action as

$$H_2CO_3 \leftrightharpoons CO_2 + H_2O \qquad (28\text{-}5)$$

Following the general form of equation (28-2), carbonic acid can also form ionic dissociation products, a hydrogen cation and bicarbonate anion, as

$$H_2CO_3 \leftrightharpoons H^+ + HCO_3^- \qquad (28\text{-}6)$$

Combining equations (28-5) and (28-6) yields[2]

$$H^+ + HCO_3^- \leftrightharpoons H_2CO_3 \leftrightharpoons CO_2 + H_2O \qquad (28\text{-}7)$$

Assuming equilibrium conditions, and substituting the carbonic acid dissociation reaction in equation (28-6) into the general form given in equation (28-3), yields[3]

$$K' = \frac{[H^+] \times [HCO_3^-]}{[H_2CO_3]} \text{ or, by re-arrangement:}$$

$$[H^+] = K' \times \frac{[H_2CO_3]}{[HCO_3^-]} \quad (28\text{-}8)$$

K' for this reaction can be empirically demonstrated to be 7.9×10^{-7}. Applying the negative logarithm function, and using analogous symbolism as employed by equation (28-1), yields a more convenient form for the constant, pK', equal to approximately 6.1.[4] The stoichiometric relationship shown in equation (28-5) allows substitution of CO_2 for carbonic acid as

$$[H^+] = K' \times \frac{[CO_2]}{[HCO_3^-]} \quad (28\text{-}9)$$

Molar concentration units of carbon dioxide are related to clinically familiar gas tension units by way of the gas's solubility coefficient, α (0.03 mmol/L per torr at 37°C), as

$$[CO_2] = \alpha \times P_{CO_2} \quad (28\text{-}10)$$

Substituting equation (28-10) into equation (28-9), supplying numerical approximations for the equilibrium and solubility constants, and using units of nanomoles per liter for $[H^+]$, millimoles per liter for $[HCO_3^-]$, and torr (equivalent to millimeters of mercury) for P_{CO_2}, yields

$$H^+ = 24 \times \frac{P_{CO_2}}{HCO_3^-} \quad (28\text{-}11)$$

which is known as the Henderson equation. Taking the negative logarithm of both sides of equation (28-9), and performing substitutions allowed by equations (28-1) and (28-10), yields[2,4]

$$pH = pK' - \log \times \frac{\alpha \times P_{CO_2}}{[HCO_3^-]} \text{ or, by re-arrangement:}$$

$$pH = pK' + \log \frac{[HCO_3^-]}{\alpha \times P_{CO_2}} \quad (28\text{-}12)$$

which is known as the Henderson–Hasselbalch equation, basically a logarithmic form of the Henderson equation. Note that the K' term has been replaced by the symbol pK', the negative logarithm of the modified equilibrium constant. Although equation (28-12) is based on equilibrium conditions, the relationship between the three acid-base variables pH, bicarbonate concentration, and carbon dioxide tension empirically prevail, even in unstable critically ill patients.[4] This relationship also provides the basis for determining bicarbonate concentration in virtually all commercial blood gas analyzers, which utilize a hydrogen ion-selective glass electrode to determine pH and a Severinghaus electrode to determine P_{CO_2}, and then solve equation (28-12) for bicarbonate concentration. Either the Henderson equation or the Henderson–Hasselbalch equation can also be used in the clinical setting to check the internal consistency of the three acid-base variables obtained by blood gas analysis. This is accomplished by selecting any two of the reported variables, calculating the third variable, and comparing the calculated value to that reported. A significant discrepancy (after accounting for rounding to significant digits) signifies that one or more of the reported values is faulty, usually due to transcription error.

Multiphasic plasma or serum electrolyte profiles usually include measurements of sodium, potassium, chloride, and total carbon dioxide content (tCO_2). The latter analyte is often used interchangeably with bicarbonate concentration in clinical parlance. However, tCO_2 actually represents the combined molar concentrations of CO_2 and various acid-labile precursor forms of carbon dioxide. These include bicarbonate and several other chemical entities. Thus,

$$tCO_2 = HCO_3^- + CO_2 + CO_3^{2-} + H_2CO_3 \\ + R - NH - COO \quad (28\text{-}13)$$

where $R - NH - COO^-$ represents labile carbamino compounds formed by combination of carbon dioxide with amine moieties of plasma proteins by

$$R - NH_2 + CO_2 \rightleftharpoons R - NH - COO^- + H^+ \quad (28\text{-}14)$$

Quantitatively, however, the main constituents of tCO_2 are bicarbonate and dissolved CO_2 gas.

Thus, equation (28-13) can be closely approximated by eliminating the negligible terms, and substituting from equation (28-10), as[3]

$$tCO_2 = HCO_3^- + 0.03 \times P_{CO_2} \qquad (28\text{-}15)$$

where total CO_2 content and bicarbonate concentration are given in millimoles per liter and P_{CO_2} is given in torr. Substituting average normal values for bicarbonate concentration (24.0 mmol/L) and arterial P_{CO_2} (Pa_{CO_2}), 40 torr, yields a tCO_2 level of 25.2 mmol/L, which is only marginally higher than the bicarbonate concentration. However, in patients with marked hypercapnia, more significant discrepancies may be seen. For example, at a Pa_{CO_2} of 100 torr and bicarbonate concentration of 28.0 mmol/L, tCO_2 would equal 31.0 mmol/L.

SIMPLE ACID-BASE DISORDERS

A simple acid-base disorder is one in which there is either acidosis or alkalosis (Table 28-1), but not

TABLE 28–1 Basic nomenclature for describing primary acid-base disorders.

Acidemia	A state of abnormally low blood pH (< 7.36)
Alkalemia	A state of abnormally high blood pH (> 7.44)
Acidosis	A pathological process tending to acidify body fluids
Alkalosis	A pathological process tending to alkalinize body fluids
Metabolic	In describing an acid-base disorder, a disturbance caused by pathological gain or loss of acid (other than carbonic acid) or bicarbonate from the body
Respiratory	In describing an acid-base disorder, a disturbance caused by pathological gain or loss of carbonic acid (or CO_2) from the body
Acute	In describing a primary respiratory acid-base disorder, a disturbance present from minutes to hours
Chronic	In describing a primary respiratory acid-base disorder, a disturbance present for more than about 2 days

both simultaneously, and this primary pathologic process is either of metabolic or respiratory origin, but not both. If sufficiently severe, a simple acid-base disturbance will always result in an abnormality in blood pH, that is, either alkalemia or acidemia. Thus, there are four cardinal acid-base disorders: metabolic acidosis, metabolic alkalosis, respiratory acidosis, and respiratory alkalosis. The patterns of pH, Pa_{CO_2}, and bicarbonate concentration representing these cardinal disturbances, uncomplicated by any superimposed acid-base disorder, have been observed in animal models in which the cardinal disturbance is imposed by an experimental procedure (eg, infusing an acid, such as HCl or lactic acid intravascularly, or manipulating minute ventilation in mechanically ventilated animals). These patterns have also been observed clinically in patients by independently surmising the particular acid-base process present and then examining the associated arterial blood gas assay results. Limited studies have also been performed in healthy human volunteers. The next four sections explain the patterns observed in these simple cardinal disorders, delineate the associated quantitative relationship between blood gas variables, list the differential diagnosis (ie, the underlying causes) of each cardinal disorder, and provide some simple methods for narrowing the differential diagnosis.

Metabolic Acidosis

From equation (28-7), it can be seen that loss of bicarbonate from the body, for example, from diarrhea, will result in formation of excessive hydrogen ion concentration by the principle of chemical mass action. On the other hand, addition of acid, either exogenous or generated by pathophysiologic metabolic processes, can directly increase hydrogen ion concentration and therefore lower pH. Also, equation (28-7) shows that addition of acid (H^+) to body fluids generates carbon dioxide above and beyond the amount would be produced by normal physiologic mechanisms. Blood pH is expected to decrease from the added hydrogen ions that have not reacted with bicarbonate, and bicarbonate concentration will decrease from the hydrogen ions that combine with bicarbonate to form carbon dioxide. To prevent hypercapnia, the body has a built-in reflexive mechanism for dealing with this increased

CO_2 generation, namely, hyperventilation mediated through the brainstem at the level of the medulla. The afferent limb of this physiologic reflex reacts to the fall in pH to neurogenically effect hyperventilation. The increase in ventilation does not simply suffice to maintain baseline $Paco_2$, but rather it lowers $Paco_2$ below the normal range to a degree that is proportional to the extent of the metabolic acidosis. Empiric analysis of this proportionality in humans has been found to be linear, and can be represented by[5]

$$\text{Expected } Paco_2 = 1.5 \times HCO_3^- + 8 \pm 2 \quad (28\text{-}16)$$

where HCO_3^- is the patient's observed bicarbonate concentration (in millimoles per liter), and expected $Paco_2$ is the arterial carbon dioxide gas tension (in torr) that occurs statistically (ie, on average) in uncomplicated metabolic acidosis of a severity level corresponding to the observed bicarbonate concentration in the patient at hand.

Equation (28-16) follows the general form of a linear equation: $y = mx + b$, where m represents the slope of the linear equation when graphed on Cartesian coordinates with the X-axis representing HCO_3^- concentration and the Y-axis representing $Paco_2$, and b represents the point of interception of the line along the Y-axis. The slope, given above by the factor 1.5 in equation (28-16), has been shown in some studies to be closer to 1.2.[6] The term ± 2 is appended to represent the 95% confidence interval derived from empiric data. If simple (ie, uncomplicated by another primary acid-base disorder) metabolic acidosis is present, substituting the patient's bicarbonate concentration into equation (28-16) and finding the patient's $Paco_2$ to be within the expected range derived from solving the equation, would signify that the patient's arterial blood gas findings are consistent with metabolic acidosis. A $Paco_2$ value lying outside this range implies that metabolic acidosis either is not present, is incompletely developed, or is present in combination with some other cardinal acid-base disturbance. The latter situation would constitute a mixed acid-base disturbance.

Table 28–2 provides a differential diagnosis for metabolic acidosis. A classic method for narrowing this differential diagnosis is to use the results of a basic multiphasic serum (or plasma) electrolyte panel to arrive at the anion gap by[7-9]

$$\text{Serum anion gap} = Na^+ - Cl^- - tCO_2 \quad (28\text{-}17)$$

where each analyte concentration is expressed in units of millimoles (or milliequivalents) per liter. The normal range for the serum anion gap varies among clinical chemistry laboratories, and has declined somewhat following the adoption of contemporary assay methods, but for some laboratories, it is 12 ± 4 mEq/L. Values exceeding the upper normal limit imply that an anion, other than chloride or bicarbonate, is present at pathological concentrations. The cause of abnormally high anion gap values, particularly if the degree of elevation is not subtle, often can be confirmed, in whole or in part, by measurement of the culpable anion; for example, lactate if the cause is lactic acidosis, or β-hydroxybutyrate if the cause is ketoacidosis. Assays for some organic anions that can increase the anion gap, for example, glycolate in ethylene glycol poisoning as well as some inorganic anions, for example, sulfate accumulation in chronic renal failure, are not commonly available; however, information from the patient's medical history, physical examination, and ancillary laboratory assays can often corroborate the specific diagnosis in these cases.

If the anion gap is normal, the cause of the metabolic acidosis is basically either loss of bicarbonate from the body or an etiology that does not involve excessive production of an organic acid. In cases of metabolic acidosis where the serum anion gap is not elevated, clinical information coupled with other simple laboratory tests can often facilitate delineation of the cause.[10,11] In cases of mild metabolic acidosis due to organic anion accumulation, the corresponding mild perturbation in the anion gap may not be sufficient to increase the gap above the upper normal limit. Similarly, a low baseline serum anion gap, as can occur in marked hypoalbuminemia, can have the same effect.[8] The latter phenomenon can be taken into account by measuring serum albumin and recognizing that for every 1 g/dL decrease in serum albumin concentration, the serum anion gap decreases by about 2.4 mEq/L, on average.[12]

The serum osmole gap, often used as a screening test when methanol or ethylene glycol intoxication

TABLE 28-2 Etiologies of metabolic acidosis classified by typical serum anion gap association.

Elevated Serum Anion Gap	Normal Serum Anion Gap
Chronic Renal Failure	**Gastrointestinal Related**
Lactic Acidosis	Diarrhea (some forms, especially small bowel secretory
Type A: due to tissue hypoxia or shock	causes)
Type B1: due to certain disease states, but ostensibly not	Ileostomy drainage
due to tissue hypoxia or hypoperfusion (eg, thiamine	Enterocutaneous fistula
deficiency and some neoplasms)	Pancreatic or biliary drainage
Type B2: due to certain drugs of toxins (eg, cyanide,	Some rectal villous adenomas
metformin, propylene glycol, and nucleoside reverse	**Kidney Related**
transcriptase inhibitors)	Acute kidney injury
Type B3: congenital forms* (eg, glycogen storage disease	Renal tubular acidosis (types I, II, and IV)
type I and hereditary fructose intolerance)	Other tubulointerstitial renal disorders
Ketoacidosis	Ureterosigmoidostomy
Diabetic ketoacidosis	Ileal loop bladder
Starvation ketoacidosis	**Endocrine Related**
Alcoholic ketoacidosis	Diabetic ketoacidosis (mainly in recovery phase)
Infantile forms* (eg, succinyl CoA:3-ke-toacid CoA	Adrenal insufficiency
transferase deficiency)	Primary hypoaldosteronism
Intoxications	Pseudohypoaldosteronism (types I and II)
Methanol or ethylene glycol poisoning	Hyporeninemic hypoaldosteronism
Salicylate overdose	**Respiratory Related**
Drug-induced pyroglutamic acidosis (eg, secondary to	Posthypocapnia
acetaminophen)	Toluene-containing glue inhalation
Paraldehyde intoxication	**Pharmacotherapy Related**
Other Congenital Organic Acidoses*	Excessive volumes of normal saline (ie, dilutional acidosis)
including those which do not necessarily	Carbonic anhydrase inhibitors (eg, acetazolamide)
manifest as ketoacidosis or lactic acidosis (eg,	Cationic amino acids (total parenteral nutrition infusions with
3-hydroxy-3-methylglutaryl-CoA lyase deficiency and	insufficient organic anion additive)
maple syrup urine disease)	Hydrochloric acid administration
	NH_4Cl administration
	Arginine HCl administration

*Infantile organic acidosis due to inborn errors of metabolism.

is suspected, is another simple derived laboratory-based expression that can be helpful in the differential diagnosis of metabolic acidosis when either of these poisonings is suspected.[13] The osmole gap can be elevated after methanol or ethylene glycol ingestion even before the metabolic acidosis develops. As methanol is metabolized to formate, or ethylene glycol is metabolized to glycolate, both of which are acid anions, the serum osmole gap declines, the serum anion gap rises, and metabolic acidosis evolves.[14] The osmole gap is the difference between serum osmolality determined by freezing point depression osmometry (Osm_{fp}) and serum osmolality estimated from routinely available clinical chemistry testing (Osm_{est}), expressed as

$$\text{Serum osmole gap} = Osm_{fp} - Osm_{est} \quad (28\text{-}18)$$

Osm_{est} is calculated from simultaneous measurements of the main osmotically active constituents of normal plasma: sodium, urea nitrogen (BUN), and glucose, along with ethanol, if applicable, by:

$$Osm_{est} = 2 \times Na^+ + BUN/2.8 + Glucose/18$$
$$+ \, Ethanol/4.6 \quad (28\text{-}19)$$

where Na^+ is expressed in millimoles per liter and the other serum assay results are expressed in milligrams per deciliter. The sodium concentration is doubled to account for osmotically active attendant anions that balance the positive charges of the sodium ions. The divisors in the other terms are derived from their respective molecular weights and convert their concentration units to millimoles (equivalent to milliosmoles) per liter. An elevated osmole gap (>15 mOsm/kg H_2O or so) suggests the presence of occult osmoles, such as methanol or ethylene glycol molecules present in the sample and contributing to total osmolality.[13] Other potential causes of an elevated serum osmole gap include ethanol intoxication (if the ethanol term is deleted from equation [28-19]), ketoacidosis, and severe degrees of circulatory shock.[9,13]

Metabolic Alkalosis

Addition of bicarbonate or loss of hydrogen ions from the body elevates extracellular bicarbonate concentration, decreases hydrogen ion concentration, and correspondingly increases pH. As in metabolic acidosis, there is normally an associated reflexive change in pulmonary minute ventilation, but in this case manifesting as hypoventilation and resulting in CO_2 retention. The resulting hypercapnia does not represent respiratory dysfunction, but is an expected physiologic response to the metabolic alkalosis. The proportional change in ventilation, as manifested by $Paco_2$, is related to the degree of metabolic alkalosis as expressed by the plasma bicarbonate concentration. One empirically derived equation describing this relationship is

$$\text{Expected PaCO}_2 = 0.9 \times \text{HCO}_3^- + 15 \qquad (28\text{-}20)$$

The slope, given above as 0.9, has been shown in some studies to be closer to 0.7.[6] Greater variability in this relationship has been observed compared to that seen in metabolic acidosis. Nevertheless, arterial blood gas values that approximate this relationship are consistent with simple metabolic alkalosis.

Once the diagnosis of metabolic alkalosis is established, the range of possible mechanisms or etiologies is considered (Table 28–3). As with metabolic acidosis, the applicable etiology is often apparent from information available through the medical history and physical examination.[11,15] Gastric fluid loss, diuretic use, and extracellular volume contraction are among the most common causes. Excess alkali intake (< 10 mEq/kg) is excreted rapidly in most patients with normal renal function. However, exogenous alkali administration can lead to alkalosis in patients with compromised renal function, low chloride intake, or mineralocorticoid excess.[16] Sources of exogenous alkali include oral or

TABLE 28–3 Etiologies of metabolic alkalosis classified by expected urine chloride concentration or excretion.

High (or normal) Urine Chloride (> 20 m Eq/L)
Active diuretic use or abuse
Severe potassium depletion
Severe magnesium depletion
Chronic diarrhea (colonic origin, chiefly)
Chronic laxative abuse
Primary aldosteronism
Cushing syndrome
Apparent mineralocorticoid excess syndrome
Renal artery stenosis
Accelerated hypertension
Bartter syndrome
Gitelman syndrome
Liddle syndrome
Therapeutic corticosteroid use
Renin-secreting tumor
Licorice abuse
Carbenoxolone use
Refeeding alkalosis (normal NaCl intake)
Alkali ingestion or treatment (normal Cl⁻ intake and normal circulating volume, or nonoliguric renal failure)
Nonabsorbable antacids plus sodium polystyrene sulfonate
Milk-alkali syndrome
Low Urine Chloride (< 20 mEq/L)
Vomiting or nasogastric suction
Some colonic villous adenomas
Congenital chloridorrhea
Cystic fibrosis
Recently discontinued diuretic treatment
Extracellular volume depletion in general (ie, contraction alkalosis)
Chloride-deficient diet (eg, soybean and protein-based infant formula diet)
Alkali ingestion or treatment (low Cl⁻ intake and low circulating volume)
Acute correction of chronic hypercapnia
Refeeding alkalosis (in the face of low NaCl intake)
Nonreabsorbable anion (eg, high-dose penicillin or carbenicillin) in the face of extracellular volume contraction

parenteral bicarbonate (including oral baking soda or overtreatment with intravenous $NaHCO_3$), acetate (eg, in parenteral nutrition formulas or dialysate solutions), citrate (including secondary to multiple blood transfusions), lactate (including Ringer's lactate solutions), and gluconate salts (found, eg, in certain proprietary intravenous balanced salt solutions), or $CaCO_3$ (eg, in oral calcium supplements).

In cases when the etiology is not straightforward, a simple laboratory test, urine chloride measurement, can sometimes be helpful. Low urine chloride concentration (< 20 mmol/L), commonly points to gastric fluid losses (by vomiting or gastric suction), recently discontinued diuretic therapy, or a posthypercapnic state. The latter occurs commonly in patients with chronic carbon dioxide retention due to chronic obstructive pulmonary disease who are placed on mechanical ventilation with resultant rapid lowering of $Paco_2$. High urine chloride concentration (> 20 mmol/L), on the other hand, points to a renal mechanism that involves chloride wasting with retention of the alternative anion bicarbonate. Common causes of chloride wasting in the intensive care unit setting are active diuretic administration and corticosteroid therapy. The urine chloride concentration also has therapeutic implications. Low urine chloride concentrations in the face of metabolic alkalosis are often readily corrected by simply supplying chloride in the form of ample sodium chloride-containing intravenous fluids. Patients with high urine chloride levels, for example, mediated by excessive mineralocorticoid activity, are resistant to therapy with chloride-containing parenteral fluid administration because the administrated chloride load is excreted without correction of the alkalosis. Note that some patients with chloride-resistant forms of metabolic alkalosis may not manifest high urine chloride levels if they have been deprived of dietary or parenteral chloride.

Respiratory Acidosis

Acute hypoventilation in an otherwise normal subject results in decreased elimination of carbon dioxide, with a resultant rise in $Paco_2$. Accompanying this rise is an immediate concomitant rise in the plasma bicarbonate level. This rapid rise in bicarbonate concentration is not mediated by renal mechanisms, but rather by the principle of chemical mass action affecting equation (28-7), shifting accumulated CO_2 leftward to form bicarbonate. Controlled and observational studies have demonstrated that the average rise in bicarbonate concentration (here measured in millimoles per liter) is approximately one-tenth the increase in arterial CO_2 tension (measured in torr), that is,[2,6,17]

$$\text{Expected } \Delta HCO_3^- \approx 0.1 \times \Delta Paco_2 \quad (28\text{-}21)$$

When a hypercapnic patient's arterial blood gas values ($Paco_2$ tension and bicarbonate concentration) conform to equation (28-21) by comparison to known or assumed baseline (prehypercapnic) values, the results are consistent with simple acute respiratory acidosis.

The kidney normally reclaims bicarbonate filtered at the glomerulus by secreting hydrogen ions into the renal tubular lumen. The reaction between bicarbonate and hydrogen ions forms CO_2 by equation (28-7), and the CO_2 is readily absorbed from the tubules into the bloodstream where equation (28-7) then can operate in reverse, thus effectively resulting in bicarbonate reabsorption.[2] In sustained hypercapnia, the kidney normally responds by gradually increasing tubular hydrogen ion secretion, thereby enhancing bicarbonate reabsorption, adding to the bicarbonate-elevation effect given by equation (28-21). This renal effect on plasma bicarbonate concentration takes several days to fully evolve and is proportional to the degree of prevailing hypercapnia. Although the relationship is not precisely linear, the combined mass action and renal effects of chronic hypercapnia on bicarbonate concentration can be approximated by[2,6]:

$$\text{Expected } \Delta HCO_3^- \approx 0.35 \times \Delta Paco_2 \quad (28\text{-}22)$$

When the patient's arterial blood gas values yield a plasma bicarbonate concentration that approximately conforms to that given by equation (28-22), the results are consistent with simple chronic respiratory acidosis. Patients having a bicarbonate concentration intermediate between the values obtained using equations (28-21) and (28-22) either have an intermediate degree of chronicity with respect to their hypercapnia, or have a mixed acid-base disturbance (see the final section).

Etiologies of hypercapnia can be divided into primary pulmonary derangements, primary neurological abnormalities, and metabolically mediated causes, with the latter potentially including drug or toxin-mediated causes (Table 28–4). The patient's medical history, physical examination, chest imaging studies and, where necessary, other investigations will assist in narrowing the differential diagnosis and arriving at the reason for respiratory acidosis.

TABLE 28–4 Etiologies of respiratory acidosis.

Pulmonary Disorders
Chronic obstructive lung disease
Status asthmaticus
Severe pneumonia
Aspiration pneumonitis
Acute respiratory distress syndrome
Cardiogenic pulmonary edema (severe)
Smoke inhalation
Pneumothorax or hemothorax
Thoracic skeletal disorders (eg, kyphoscoliosis, rib fractures, and flail chest)
Extrathoracic restrictive processes (eg, obesity, ascites, and abdominal compartment syndrome)
Mechanical ventilation with excessive deadspace
Incorrect mechanical ventilation settings or ventilator malfunction
Upper airway obstruction (eg, laryngospasm, airway tumor or foreign body, and obstructive sleep apnea)

Neurologic Illness or Injury
Traumatic brain injury
Spinal cord injury
Cerebrovascular accident
Intracranial hemorrhage
Brain tumor
Intracranial hypertension
Central nervous system infection
Guillain–Barré syndrome
Poliomyelitis
Amyotrophic lateral sclerosis
Obesity hypoventilation syndrome

Muscle and Neuromuscular Disorders
Myasthenia gravis
Muscular dystrophy
Polymyositis

Metabolic Disorders
Myxedema coma
Severe hypokalemia
Thyrotoxic hypokalemic periodic paralysis
Familial hypokalemic periodic paralysis
Severe hyperkalemia (rare)

Drug and Toxin Related
Sedative hypnotic drugs (eg, benzodiazepines, barbiturates, and propofol)
General anesthetic (eg, halothane and other volatile anesthetics; nitrous oxide)
Opioids (eg, morphine, heroin, hydromorphone, oxycodone, and fentanyl)
Succinylcholine
Nondepolarizing neuromuscular blocking drugs (eg, pancuronium, vecuronium, and atracurium)
Reversible carbamate cholinesterase inhibitor overdose (eg, physostigmine and pyridostigmine)
Organophosphate insecticide poisoning (eg, malathion and diazinon)
Military nerve agents (eg, sarin, soman, and VX)
Sodium bicarbonate administration in the face of ventilatory limitation
Botulism
Tetrodotoxin poisoning (eg, from puffer fish ingestion)

Respiratory Alkalosis

Acute hyperventilation in an otherwise normal subject results in increased elimination of carbon dioxide and therefore a fall in Pa_{CO_2}. Accompanying this fall is an immediate concomitant decrease in plasma bicarbonate concentration. This rapid fall in bicarbonate is not mediated by renal mechanisms, but rather by the principle of chemical mass action affecting equation (28-7), causing a rightward shift in the reaction sequence to partially fill the void left by the expired CO_2. Human observational studies have shown that the fall in bicarbonate concentration (measured in millimoles per liter) is approximately two-tenths the decrease in arterial CO_2 tension (measured in torr), that is,[6]

$$\text{Expected } \Delta HCO_3^- \approx 0.2 \times \Delta Pa_{CO_2} \qquad (28\text{-}23)$$

Arterial blood gas values showing hypocapnia and decreased plasma bicarbonate concentrations that approximate those given by equation (28-23) are consistent with simple acute respiratory alkalosis.

As described earlier, the kidney normally regulates bicarbonate reabsorption by adjusting hydrogen ion secretion into the renal tubular lumen. Sustained hypocapnia downregulates this hydrogen ion secretion, resulting in less reclaimed bicarbonate and thus enhancing bicarbonate excretion, adding to the bicarbonate lowering effect accounted for by equation (28-23). This added renal effect on bicarbonate concentration takes several days to fully evolve and is proportional to the degree of prevailing hypocapnia, as given by[6,18]

$$\text{Expected } \Delta HCO_3^- \approx 0.4 \times \Delta Pa_{CO_2} \qquad (28\text{-}24)$$

However, this proportionality, representing the combined mass action and renal bicarbonate wasting effects of hypocapnia on plasma bicarbonate concentration, eventually reaches a limit such that further degrees of hypocapnia have little additional effect on the plasma bicarbonate level. Thus, plasma HCO_3^- concentrations much less than 17 mmol/L are not commonly observed in simple chronic respiratory alkalosis. Within this limit, arterial blood gas results that show hypocapnia and plasma bicarbonate concentrations that conform to that given by equation (28-24) are consistent with simple chronic respiratory alkalosis. Patients having a bicarbonate concentration intermediate between the values obtained by equations (28-23) and (28-24) either have an intermediate degree of chronicity to their hypocapnia, or have a mixed acid-base disturbance (see the following section).

Etiologies of hypocapnia can be classified according to whether the primary disorder is pulmonary, neurological, metabolic, or a drug or toxin-mediated cause (Table 28–5). The patient's medical history, physical examination, chest imaging studies and, where necessary, other investigations will assist in narrowing the differential diagnosis and arriving at the reason for respiratory acidosis.

TABLE 28–5 Etiologies of respiratory alkalosis.

Pulmonary Disorders
  Asthma
  Pneumonia
  Pulmonary edema (mild to moderate)
  Interstitial lung disease
  Pulmonary embolism
  Mechanical ventilation
  High-altitude hypoxemia
  Ventilation-perfusion mismatch
  Intrapulmonary shunting
  Other causes of hypoxemia
Neurological Disorders
  Traumatic brain injury
  Central nervous system infection
  Brain tumors
  Cerebrovascular accident
  Hyperventilation syndrome
  Anxiety
  Pain
Metabolic Causes
  Pyrexia
  Severe sepsis
  Pregnancy
  Hepatic failure
  Burn injury or trauma
  Recovery phase of metabolic acidosis
Drug Related
  Salicylate overdose
  Caffeine overdose
  Nicotine intoxication
  Progesterone administration
  Exogenous catecholamines
  Stimulant drug overdose (eg, cocaine, amphetamine)

MIXED ACID-BASE DISORDERS

Whereas simple acid-base disturbances involve a single primary underlying causative mechanism, either metabolic or respiratory, mixed acid-base disorders involve more than one cardinal acid-base derangement simultaneously. Co-occurrence of two or three of the cardinal acid-base disorders is not uncommon in critically ill patients and frequently complicates interpretation of arterial blood gas determinations in the intensive care unit setting.

The data used to derive the empiric formulas given for the cardinal acid-base disorder in the preceding sections have also been used to generate statistical confidence limits for each disorder. These confidence bands are approximated graphically in Figure 28–1, a plot of $Paco_2$ versus bicarbonate concentration.[2,5,6,17,19] According to equation (28-12), a given $Paco_2$ and bicarbonate concentration defines a specific pH; therefore, lines of equal pH can be superimposed on the graph (the diagonal lines in Figure 28–1). The elliptical area near the center of the graph represents the 95% confidence area for the combined normal ranges for $Paco_2$ and bicarbonate concentration. The normal range for arterial blood pH (7.36-7.44) can be indirectly appreciated on the graph by interpolating between the diagonal lines. The dark bands represent confidence areas defining patterns of blood gas values that have been observed when the depicted cardinal acid-base disorder is present and is not complicated by another cardinal acid-base disturbance. For the respiratory disorders, both acute and chronic confidence bands are given. The overlap in the confidence bands near the center of the graph (at the outskirts of the normal confidence ellipse) illustrates that mild blood gas abnormalities can present greater diagnostic uncertainty compared to more severe abnormalities. Figure 28–1 also highlights the quantitative relationship between the three blood gas variables and shows that merely examining the directional changes in one or two of the variables, without considering the quantitative relationship between them, may not allow accurate identification of the cardinal disturbance. For example, finding that a patient has a low bicarbonate concentration does not allow one to distinguish whether the patient has metabolic acidosis or respiratory alkalosis. Similarly, knowing

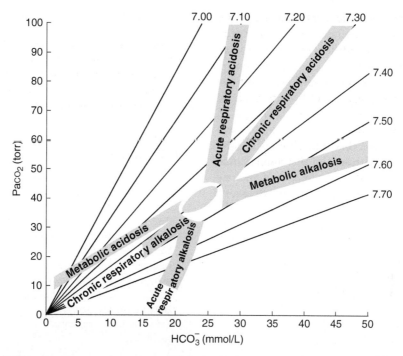

FIGURE 28–1 Acid-base nomogram showing confidence bands for simple acid-base disturbances. Conversion factor: 1 torr = 0.13 kPa. (*Adapted from Kruse JA. Acid-base interpretations. In: Prough DS, Traystman RJ, eds.* Critical Care. State of the Art. *Vol. 14. Mt. Prospect, Ill: Society of Critical Care Medicine: 1993:275-297. Used with permission.*)

that a patient has a low bicarbonate level and low $Paco_2$ does not discriminate between these two disturbances. Quantifying the relationship between the acid-base variables, however, often identifies which disorder is present.

When one of the cardinal respiratory disturbances is present, and the time course of the disorder is intermediate between an acute and a fully developed chronic disturbance, the blood gas values will lie between the acute and chronic respiratory bands. Analogously, when two cardinal disturbances are present simultaneously (eg, metabolic acidosis and respiratory alkalosis), the range of possible arterial blood gas values can lie anywhere between the confidence areas given for the two cardinal disorders in Figure 28–1. Thus, abnormal blood gas findings that do not fall within any of the confidence bands imply that a mixed disturbance is present. If there are two cardinal disorders present, the point representing the blood gas values will usually lie between the two bands representing the disorders.

Note that although blood gas results lying within a confidence band are consistent with the disorder represented by the band, it is still possible that a mixed disorder could be present. For example, a patient with simultaneous development of severe metabolic alkalosis (say, from protracted vomiting) and severe metabolic acidosis (say, from concomitant diabetic ketoacidosis) could present with arterial blood gas values that are within normal limits.[8] Similarly, if metabolic acidosis and metabolic alkalosis are simultaneously present, but one of the disorders is more severe, the blood gas results may lie squarely within the confidence band of the more severe disorder, concealing the presence of the opposing metabolic disorder. Although this is a limitation of the method, consideration of information from the history and screening laboratory testing, particularly the serum anion gap in this case, will usually overcome the diagnostic challenge. As another example, a patient with metabolic acidosis and simultaneous chronic respiratory alkalosis

(Figure 28–1) may have blood gas values that are consistent with acute respiratory alkalosis. Again, the medical history and ancillary testing commonly surmount these limitations.

Each of the descriptive cardinal acid-base disturbances directly depicted in Figure 28–1 can be considered an acid-base diagnosis. Arriving at an acid-base diagnosis, however, is not an end in itself. Rather, the purpose of this identification process is to characterize the disorder so that a differential diagnosis can be formulated and the specific etiology then discerned. Pin-pointing the specific diagnosis requires additional information, available from the clinical context of the case, including the patient's medical, surgical, and medication use history, physical examination, and sometimes simple laboratory test results such as the serum potassium level, serum anion gap, or urine chloride concentration. Once the specific underlying diagnosis is ascertained, appropriate treatment can be implemented.

REFERENCES

1. Adrogué HJ, Gennari FJ, Galla JH, et al. Assessing acid-base disorders. *Kidney Int.* 2009;76(12):1239-1247.
2. Bruno CM, Valenti M. Acid-base disorders in patients with chronic obstructive pulmonary disease: a pathophysiological review. *J Biomed Biotechnol.* 2012;2012:915150.
3. Kruse JA. Calculation of plasma bicarbonate concentration *versus* measurement of serum CO_2 content. pK' revisited. *Clin Intensive Care.* 1995;6(1):15-20.
4. Kruse JA, Hukku P, Carlson RW. Relationship between the apparent dissociation constant of blood carbonic acid and severity of illness. *J Lab Clin Med.* 1989;114(5):568-574.
5. Albert MS, Dell RB, Winters RW. Quantitative displacement of acid-base equilibrium in metabolic acidosis. *Ann Intern Med.* 1967;66(2):312-322.
6. Adrogué HJ, Madias NE. Secondary responses to altered acid-base status: the rules of engagement. *J Am Soc Nephrol.* 2010;21(6):920-923.
7. Kraut JA, Nagami GT. The serum anion gap in the evaluation of acid-base disorders: what are its limitations and can its effectiveness be improved? *Clin J Am Soc Nephrol.* 2013;8(11):2018-2024.
8. Kruse JA. Clinical utility and limitations of the anion gap. *Int J Intensive Care.* 1997;4(2):51-66.
9. Holstege CP, Borek HA. Toxidromes. *Crit Care Clin.* 2012;28(4):479-498.
10. Kraut JA, Madias NE. Differential diagnosis of nongap metabolic acidosis: value of a systematic approach. *Clin J Am Soc Nephrol.* 2012;7(4):671-679.
11. Perez GO, Oster JR, Rogers A. Acid-base disturbances in gastrointestinal disease. *Digest Dis Sci.* 1987;32(9):1033-1043.
12. Feldman M, Soni N, Dickson B. Influence of hypoalbuminemia or hyperalbuminemia on the serum anion gap. *J Lab Clin Med.* 2005;146(6):317-320.
13. Kruse JA, Cadnapaphornchai P. The serum osmole gap. *J Crit Care.* 1994;9(3):185-197.
14. Kruse JA. Methanol and ethylene glycol intoxication. *Crit Care Clin.* 2012;28(4):661-711.
15. Melvin E, Laski ME, Sabatini S. Metabolic alkalosis, bedside and bench. *Semin Nephrol.* 2006;26(6):404-421.
16. Gennari FJ. Pathophysiology of metabolic alkalosis: a new classification based on the centrality of stimulated collecting duct ion transport. *Am J Kidney Dis.* 2011;58(4):626-636.
17. Brackett NC, Jr, Cohen JJ, Schwartz WB. Carbon dioxide titration curve of normal man: effect of increasing degrees of acute hypercapnia on acid-base equilibrium. *N Engl J Med.* 1965;272(1):6-12.
18. Krapf R, Beeler I, Hertner D, et al. Chronic respiratory alkalosis. The effect of sustained hyperventilation on renal regulation of acid-base equilibrium. *N Engl J Med.* 1991;324(20):1394-1401.
19. Kruse JA. Acid-base interpretations. In: Prough DS, Traystman RJ, eds. *Critical Care. State of the Art.* Vol. 14. Mt. Prospect, Ill: Society of Critical Care Medicine; 1993:275-297.

Nutrition Support

Ylaine Rose T Aldeguer, MD; Sara Wilson, MS, RD, CNSC and Roopa Kohli-Seth, MD

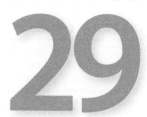

KEY POINTS

1. Malnutrition is associated with increased mortality and remains an underdiagnosed condition affecting critically ill patients. Timely and adequate screening is important to identify patients who are at risk.

2. Early enteral nutrition has been proven to be beneficial in ICU patients. Every effort should be made to initiate enteral nutrition within 48 hours of ICU admission unless clinically contraindicated.

3. Developing feeding protocols has been shown to increase nutrient administration and utilization of enteral nutrition in critically ill patients. Identifying procedures that focus on the use of promotility agents and avoiding unnecessary feeding interruptions is essential.

4. Inappropriate parenteral nutrition use has been associated with increased risk of infectious and metabolic complications. Delaying initiation of parenteral nutrition for at least 7 days may be prudent.

MALNUTRITION AND CRITICAL ILLNESS

An estimated 40% to 50% of patients admitted to the ICU are undernourished or at risk for malnutrition.[1] Malnutrition is known to impair tissue function, delay wound healing, prolong ventilator dependence, and increase length of hospital stay.[2,3] During critical illness, metabolic changes can lead to hyperglycemia, increased energy expenditure, and protein catabolism. This cytokine-driven and hormone-mediated response to stress is not only vital in stabilizing organ function and preserving immune competency, but it may also contribute to the loss of body mass and development of malnutrition. Therefore, adequate nutrition should aim to reduce severity and duration of the catabolic phase and optimize nutritional status for recovery.

CLASSIFICATION AND SEVERITY OF ADULT MALNUTRITION

Adult malnutrition is poorly defined and frequently unrecognized, hence the incidence and prevalence are difficult to determine. Clinical terms, such as marasmus, kwashiorkor, and protein-calorie malnutrition have previously been used to identify malnutrition; however, the use of some of these terms is confusing and antiquated. They were originally meant to distinguish the different clinical features of acute malnutrition in children (Table 29–1).

While numerous tools for identifying and classifying malnutrition have been developed, their application has often led to further confusion and

TABLE 29–1 Malnutrition definitions.

Protein-calorie malnutrition: Malnutrition usually seen in infants and young children whose diets are deficient in both proteins and calories. Clinically, the condition may be precipitated by other factors, such as infection of intestinal parasites.

Kwashiorkor: A severe protein-deficiency type of malnutrition in children. It occurs after the child is weaned. The clinical signs are, at first, a vague type of lethargy, apathy, or irritability and later, failure to grow, mental deficiency, inanition, increased susceptibility to infections, edema, dermatitis, and liver enlargement. The hairs may have reddish color.

Marasmus: Emaciation and wasting in an infant due to malnutrition. Causes include caloric deficiency secondary to acute diseases, esp. diarrheal diseases of infancy, deficiency in nutritional composition, inadequate food intake, malabsorption, child abuse, failure-to-thrive syndrome, deficiency of vitamin D, or scurvy.

Reproduced with permission from *Taber's Cyclopedic Medical Dictionary* ©1997.

misdiagnoses. More recently, focus has shifted away from using prognostic indicators, such as protein stores, as they are not an accurate indicator of nutritional status. The Academy of Nutrition and Dietetics and the American Society for Parenteral and Enteral Nutrition (ASPEN) have developed standardized diagnostic criteria for defining and documenting adult malnutrition in the clinical setting. The consensus defined adult malnutrition in the context of acute illness or injury, chronic diseases or conditions, and starvation-related malnutrition. Since there is no single parameter for identifying malnutrition, presence of 2 or more of the following characteristics is recommended for the diagnosis: insufficient energy intake, weight loss, loss of muscle mass, loss of subcutaneous fat, localized or generalized fluid accumulation, and diminished functional status as measured by hand grip (Table 29–2).[4]

TABLE 29–2 Diagnostic criteria for malnutrition. Patient must meet 2 or more characteristics for the diagnosis of malnutrition.

Characteristic	Acute Illness/Injury-Related Malnutrition		Chronic Disease-Related Malnutrition		Social/Environmental-Related Malnutrition	
	Nonsevere	Severe	Nonsevere	Severe	Nonsevere	Severe
Energy intake	< 75% for > 7 days	≤ 50% for ≥ 5 days	< 75% for ≥ 1 month	≤ 75%/ ≥ 1 month	< 75% for ≥ 3 months	≤ 50% for ≥ 1 month
Weight loss	1%-2%/1 week 5%/1 month 7.5%/3 months	> 2%/1 week > 5%/1 week > 7.5%/3 months	5%/1 month 7.5%/3 months 10%/6 months 20%/1 year	> 5%/1 month > 7.5%/3 months > 10%/6 months > 20%/1 year	5%/1 month 7.5%/3 months 10%/6 months 20%/1 year	> 5%/1 month > 7.5%/3 months > 10%/6 months > 20%/1 year
Physical Findings						
Body fat	Mild depletion	Moderate depletion	Mild depletion	Severe depletion	Mild depletion	Severe depletion
Muscle mass	Mild depletion	Moderate depletion	Mild depletion	Severe depletion	Mild depletion	Severe depletion
Fluid accumulation	Mild	Moderate to severe	Mild	Severe	Mild	Severe
Grip strength	Not applicable	Not recommended in ICU	Not applicable	Reduced for age/gender	Not applicable	Reduced for age/gender

Adapted with permission from White JV, Guenter P, Jensen G, et al: Consensus statement: Academy of Nutrition and Dietetics and American Society for Parenteral and Enteral Nutrition: characteristics recommended for the identification and documentation of adult malnutrition (undernutrition), JPEN *J Parenter Enteral Nutr.* 2012 May;36(3):275-283.

NUTRITION ASSESSMENT

The application of conventional risk and assessment tools is generally not practical in critically ill patients. Use of body weight (BW) as a marker of nutritional status can be problematic because of fluids shifts associated with critical illness. Markers of protein status, such as albumin and prealbumin levels are also of limited use, as they tend to be more reflective of acute phase response than a patient's nutritional status.[5]

A review of weight, caloric intake prior to ICU admission, and gastrointestinal tract function should be conducted prior to initiating any form of nutrition support.[6,7] Risk assessment in critically ill patients should include evaluation of clinical status, length of time on mechanical ventilation, and severity and duration of stress response. Early and adequate nutrition support is important to avoid large cumulative energy deficits, which can lead to increased ventilator days and increased ICU length of stay (LOS).[7] Avoiding overfeeding in critically ill patients is equally important, as excessive calories can result in hyperglycemia and increased carbon dioxide production, thus exacerbating respiratory insufficiency and prolonged weaning from the ventilator.

CALCULATING NEEDS

Measuring nutrient requirements is the first step in providing adequate nutrition. The use of an established amount of calories per kilogram has historically been applied when calculating energy needs. The most frequently used amount is 25 kcal/kg/day. When using calories per kilogram to determine energy needs, it is important to identify the appropriate weight. The patient's height should first be obtained, followed by calculation of an ideal BW (IBW) (Table 29–3). Once calculated, the IBW should then be compared to the admission dry weight. In patients who weigh less than 90% of their IBW, practitioners should consider using the actual BW to calculate needs and avoid overfeeding, particularly in the early stages of critical illness.

Indirect calorimetry, which measures oxygen consumption and carbon dioxide production to calculate resting energy expenditure, remains the gold standard for estimating needs in the critically ill patient. However, its use is often not practical, due to the expense of the machines, lack of reimbursement, shortage of personnel trained in its use, and length of actual testing. Predictive equations offer another method for estimating calorie needs by using measurable data, including anthropometrics, to calculate estimated energy expenditure. Table 29–4 outlines equations developed for critically ill patients.

Identifying the appropriate method for estimating needs in critically ill overweight and obese patients can be challenging. Table 29–5 outlines the interpretations for BMI classifications. In patients defined with class I to III obesity (BMI > 30), calculating 22 to 25 kcal/kg of IBW has been recommended.[6,7] Adjusted BW calculations should be used with caution as they may be unreliable. In 2013, the ASPEN published guidelines for hospitalized adult patients with obesity, recommending the Penn State University 2010 equation and the modified Penn State University equation for obese patients over 60 years of age. A 70% or greater accuracy was found using Penn State compared to other predictive equations.[8]

Valdation studies have demonstrated improved accuracy with predictive equations, even though they are less accurate than indirect calorimetry. In the absence of indirect calorimetry, Gguidelines suggest using predictive equations or simple weight based equations (kcal/kg) for estimating calorie needs in critically ill patients.[7] However, the use of predictive equations can be time consuming, and therefore, less appealing in the clinical setting.

TABLE 29–3 Formulas for determining IBW.

Females: IBW = 100 lbs for the first 5 ft of height, and an additional 5 lbs for each inch above
Males: IBW = 106 lbs for the first 5 ft of height, and an additional 6 lbs for each additional inch above

NUTRITION SUPPORT AND THERAPY

Enteral Nutrition

Enteral feeding is physiologic and the preferred route of providing nutrition in the ICU. In patients

TABLE 29–4 Summary of predictive equations for calculating energy needs.

Penn–State equation (2003)	$RMR = Mifflin(0.96) + V_E(31) + T_{max}(167) - 6212$
	V_E = minute ventilation (L/min) T_{max} = maximum temperature (°C) Mifflin = Mifflin–St. Joer equation
Modified Penn (2010)	$RMR = Mifflin(0.71) + V_E(64) + T_{max}(85) - 3085$
	V_E = minute ventilation (L/min) T_{max} = maximum temperature (°C) Mifflin = Mifflin–St. Joer equation
Ireton Jones (1992)	$IJEE$ (ventilator dependent) $= 1925 - 10(A) + 5(W) + 281(S) + 851(B)$ $IJEE$ (spontaneous breathing) $= 629 - 11(A) + 25(W) - 609(O)$
	$IJEE$ = estimated energy expenditure (kcal/day)
	A = age (years); T = trauma (present = 1, absent = 0) W = weight (kg); B = burns (present = 1, absent = 0) S = sex (male = 1, female = 0); O = BMI > 27 kcal/m² (present = 1, absent = 0)
Mifflin–St. Jeor equation (1990)	Female = $(10 \times Wt) + (6.25 \times Ht) - (5 \times Age) - 161$ Male = $(10 \times Wt) + (6.25 \times Ht) - (5 \times Age) + 5$
	W (kg): use actual weight/Ht (cm)/age (years)

who are unable to start oral diet, nutrition support should be initiated, preferably enteral feeding, if the gut is functional. In conditions where enteral nutrition is contraindicated, such as in the case of intestinal obstruction, severe ileus, high-output ileostomy, active gastrointestinal bleeding, or hemodynamic instability, and the patient requires non–per-orem

TABLE 29–5 BMI classifications.

BMI [Weight (kg)/Height (m²)]	Classification
< 18.5	Underweight
18.5-24.9	Normal weight
25-29.9	Overweight
30-34.9	Obesity class I
35-39.9	Obesity class II
> 40	Obesity class III

status for more than 7 days, parenteral nutrition (PN) should be considered. However, once these conditions resolve, enteral feeding should be started or resumed.

Enteral feeding maintains gut integrity and function, helps attenuate inflammatory responses, maintains gastrointestinal blood flow and peristalsis, and prevents bacterial translocation. Enteral nutrition should be initiated within the first 24 to 48 hours of ICU admission. In hemodynamically stable patients, providing enteral nutrition may reduce the incidence of infectious complications, reduce ICU and hospital mortality, and may be cost effective.[9,10] ASPEN/SCCM guidelines support the early initiation of enteral feeds with advancement toward goal over the next 48 to 72 hours.[6,7]

Enteral feeding is commonly provided via a nasogastric tube, orogastric tube, nasojejunal tube, or endoscopically or surgically inserted gastrostomy (G-tube) or jejunostomy (J-tube) tubes. In practice, gastric feeding is the preferred method for providing nutrition in the ICU because it is more physiological and easier to place than more distal enteral access devices. Intragastric feeds can be given either as a bolus or continuously via pump infusion. Impaired gastric emptying, which is a relatively common problem, may preclude the use of intragastric feeding. Known factors that predispose patients to develop impaired gastric emptying include drugs (sedatives, opioids, anticholinergics, and neuromuscular blocking agents), the presence of metabolic abnormalities (hypokalemia, acidosis, hypothyroidism, and long-standing diabetes), and the presence of anatomic abnormalities, infections, or muscle disease. Symptomatic patients with gastroparesis may benefit from decreasing doses of sedatives and opioid analgesics, or by adding prokinetic drugs, such as metoclopramide, erythromycin, or domperidone, which may help facilitate gastric motility. In severe cases of impaired gastric emptying, such as recurrent vomiting, persistently elevated gastric residual volumes, presence of gastric reflux refractory to medical treatment, or in the presence of severe acute pancreatitis,

postpyloric feeding may be favorable and should be considered.

Enteral Formulas

There are several enteral formulas designed for use in the ICU.[11] Generally, these formulas differ in their protein and fat content and are classified as standard (polymeric), specialized (disease-specific and immune-enhancing), semielemental (oligomeric), or elemental (monomeric).[11,12] Standard or polymeric enteral formulas contain intact protein, complex carbohydrates, long-chain triglycerides, a balanced amount of micronutrients, and are usually less expensive than specialized formulas. The caloric density of a standard enteral formula can range from 1.0 to 2.0 kcal/mL. Calorie dense products are formulas that contain higher amounts of calories per milliliter and are intended for patients that require less volume of free water, such as in congestive heart failure or renal failure. They can also be used in patients who require nocturnal or bolus feedings to avoid large volumes of feeding being infused at higher rates. Table 29–6 outlines various enteral formulas commonly used in the ICU. Some enteral

TABLE 29–6 Enteral formulas commonly used in the ICU.

Description	Concentration (kcal/mL)	Carbohydrate (%)	Protein (%)	Fat (%)	Free H$_2$O (%)
Semielemental, isotonic eg, Peptamen 1.0, Vital 1.0	1.0	51	16	33	84
Semielemental low CHO, high protein eg, Peptamen AF, Vital 1.2	1.2	35-36	25	39-40	81
Semielemental, concentrated eg, Peptamen 1.5, Vital 1.5	1.5	49	18	33	77
Elemental, low fat eg, Vivonex RTF	1	70	20	10	85
Intact, electrolyte restricted eg, Nepro, Novasource Renal	1.8-2.0	34-37	18	45-48	72-73
Intact, high fiber eg, Jevity 1.2, Fibersource	1.2	53	19	29	81
Intact, low carbohydrate eg, DiabetiSource AC, Glucerna 1.2	1.2	35-36	20	44-45	81-82

formulas contain fiber, which may help improve diarrhea; however, studies have revealed conflicting results.[13,14] Guidelines suggest formulas free of soluble and insoluble fiber be used in critically ill patients that are at high risk for bowel ischemia or obstruction.[7]

Specialized enteral formulas are designed for patients with existing medical conditions that may require adjustment of calories, carbohydrate, protein, electrolytes, vitamins, and minerals. Formula selection in patients with renal disease can vary depending on the degree of renal function, the presence or absence of renal replacement therapy, and the patient's nutrient requirement. These patients require formulas that are low in water content, potassium, phosphorus, and magnesium. Patients receiving renal replacement therapy, hemodialysis, or continuous veno-venous hemofiltration have higher protein requirements of up to 2.5 g/kg/day and do not necessarily require fluid restriction from enteral feedings. In the absence of hyperkalemia, hyperphosphatemia, or hypermagnesemia, a standard, high-protein enteral formula should be used.

Enteral formulas that contain a lower amount of carbohydrates and higher fat content are intended for use in patients with diabetes mellitus. There is no significant difference in glycemic control, mortality, ICU LOS, or ventilator days when using diabetic formulas compared to standard formulas.[15-18] However, some studies showed a trend toward lower infection rate and lower daily insulin requirements in patients receiving the diabetic formula.[18]

Hepatic formulas contain increased amounts of branched-chain amino acids, for example, valine, leucine, isoleucine, and reduced amounts of aromatic amino acids, such as phenylephrine, tyrosine, and tryptophan, purposely designed to reduce the neurological symptoms of hepatic encephalopathy. Evidence supporting the use of these formulas is limited and routine use of these branched-chain amino acid–enriched enteral formulas in patients with advanced liver disease, with or without hepatic encephalopathy, are currently not recommended.[19,20]

Conflicting evidence limits the routine use of specialized formulas for patients with chronic obstructive pulmonary disease and acute respiratory distress syndrome (ARDS). The enteral formulas for patients with chronic obstructive pulmonary disease, generally, have lower carbohydrate content which theoretically were created to limit carbon dioxide production and reduce ventilatory load. An enteral formula with modified lipid component containing borage and fish oils as well as high amounts of antioxidants, believed to modulate inflammatory response, is also available for use in patients with ARDS. Although previous studies have revealed some evidence of improvement in gas exchange, fewer ventilator days, and lower ICU LOS in patients receiving specialized ARDS formulas, a recent multicenter RCT found that the use of omega 3 fatty acids, linolenic acid, and antioxidant in patients with acute lung injury did not improve clinical outcome (ventilator-free days) and may be harmful.[21-23] Therefore, the routine use of these formulas in patients with ARDS should be discouraged.

Although known to be 4 times as costly compared to standard formulas, the use of semielemental and elemental enteral formulas has gained popularity in patients with severe uncontrolled diarrhea and malabsorptive states. Elemental formulas contain amino acids, glucose polymers, and lower amounts of long-chain triglycerides, and were developed mainly for better absorption in patients suffering from malabsorption. They are preferentially used in patients with pancreatitis to avoid exocrine pancreatic stimulation. Semielemental formulas contain hydrolyzed proteins, such as oligopeptides, dipeptides, and tripeptides, simple sugars, glucose polymers, starch, and medium chain triglycerides absorbed directly across the small intestinal mucosa into the portal vein in the absence of lipase or bile salts.[11] In clinical studies, both formulas were found to be nonsuperior to standard formulas in providing nutrition and nitrogen balance in patients with malabsorption, and therefore, should be reserved for patients who have failed previous attempts at providing enteral feeding with a standard formula.[24-26]

Determining Goal Rates

Once the patient's caloric requirement and appropriate enteral formula are chosen, it is important to determine the daily duration of feeding. In the ICU, a 24-hour continuous pump infusion of gastric feeding is commonly employed. Table 29–7 shows an example for calculating the enteral goal rate.

TABLE 29–7 Enteral nutrition formula sample.

1. Use caloric estimate (predictive equations vs kcal/kg) to figure total calorie goal
2. Choose a tube feed (TF) formula
3. Divide goal calories by kcal/mL of formula to determine daily volume of formula (= 1200 mL)
4. Divide daily volume by number of hours TF to infuse to determine goal rate

Example:

1. **Caloric estimate: 1440 kcal**
2.

Description	Concentration (kcal/mL)	CHO (%)	Protein (%)	Fat (%)	Free H₂O (%)
Semielemental low CHO, high protein	1.2	36	25	39	81

5. 1600 kcal/1.2 kcal/mL = 1200 mL
6. 1200 mL/24 h = 50 mL/h

Risks and Complications of Enteral Nutrition

Commonly encountered problems with enteral feeding in the ICU include gastrointestinal complications, mechanical problems, and metabolic derangements. In a multicenter, prospective cohort study of 400 patients evaluating 3700 feeding days, gastrointestinal complications associated with enteral nutrition were found to occur in about 62.8% of cases. These complications included high gastric residuals (39%), constipation (15.7%), diarrhea (14.7%), abdominal distention (13.2%), vomiting (12.2%), and regurgitation (5.5%).[27] The occurrence of diarrhea in the ICU is very rarely related to enteral nutrition use alone. Once diarrhea occurs, the investigation should first focus on ruling out pathologic causes as a result of infection, inflammation, or secretory or osmotic mechanisms, which occur in many states of malabsorption. More commonly, diarrhea can be caused by various medications and so obtaining a good drug history is very important to avoid sending unnecessary tests. Drugs that are well known to cause diarrhea include laxatives, magnesium-containing antacids, antibiotics, colchicine, lactose or sorbitol based products, non-steroidal anti-inflammatory drugs, and prostaglandins. A common infectious cause of diarrhea in the ICU is pseudomembranous colitis caused by Clostridium difficile from prolonged use of antibiotics. Addressing the underlying cause is the first step in the management of diarrhea in the ICU, and once diarrhea is proven to be nonpathologic, adding medications such as bismuth salicylate, loperamide, diphenoxylate/atropine, octreotide, or opium tincture may be practical. Changing the enteral feeds to a more elemental form may also be of potential benefit.

Feeding intolerance often results in withdrawal of enteral nutrition which translates into decreased nutrient intake, longer ICU LOS and higher mortality.[28] An association between 12-day caloric adequacy and 60-day hospital mortality found that as the amount of calories delivered increases and reaches at least 80% to 85% of prescribed calories, mortality decreases.[7,29] Essentially, the fewer calories the patient is able to receive, the greater the mortality. These findings validate the importance of receiving adequate nutrition during critical illness and the importance of developing strategies that maximize the benefits and minimize the risk of enteral nutrition. Some strategies developed to optimize delivery of enteral nutrition in the ICU include elevating head of bed at least 30°, proactive use of prokinetic agents, use of small bowel feeding, and implementation of feeding protocols.[30]

The occurrence of hyperglycemia in patients fed enterally is relatively rare as compared to patients receiving PN. In the ICU, hyperglycemia is mostly multifactorial, a result of a combination of factors commonly seen in the critical setting, eg, use of steroids, insulin resistance during critical illness, and presence of preexisting diabetes mellitus. Evaluating appropriate caloric requirements and correct administration rates as well as reducing inciting medications, and adding insulin, may be necessary in addressing hyperglycemia. Currently, aiming at moderate glycemic control with a blood glucose (BG) target between 140 and 180 mg/dL in critically ill patients is beneficial over strict BG control of 81 to 108 mg/dL.[31] Electrolytes should also be monitored as imbalances in sodium, potassium, and phosphorus may also occur in patients receiving enteral feedings.

Though relatively rare in commercially available enteral formulas, microbial contamination of enteral feeding decanted in feeding bags occurs and is usually related to poor hand-hygiene of health care providers.[32,33] Commercially prepared enteral formulas are considered sterile until opened. In most clinical settings, implementing strict hand washing and routine change of feeding bags (every 24 hours) are practices employed to reduce the risks of contamination.

Mechanical problems associated with enteral nutrition are generally related to placement and maintenance of enteral access. Difficulties during initial placement of nasogastric tube or nasojejunal tube may result in nasopharyngeal irritation, esophageal irritation and bleeding, tube misplacement, or perforation of the esophagus, stomach, or lungs. At particular risk are patients who are agitated and fail to cooperate during the insertion process. The use of stiffer feeding tubes and stylets may also contribute to these problems. Previously placed temporary feeding tubes should also be monitored for possible migration, kinking, and occlusion, and replaced as needed. Long-term enteral access is also associated with formidable risk that occurs either during initial placement or maintenance of these feeding tubes. Commonly associated complications are abdominal pain, tube leakage, irritation, or infection around the insertion site, peritonitis, fistulas, tube clogging or occlusion, and dislodgment of the tube, collar, or button. Regular use of water flushes may reduce incidence of clogging or occlusion of feeding tubes.

Feeding Protocols in the ICU

Clinical evidence has shown that the use of enteral feeding protocols in the ICU may lead to an overall increase in the utilization of enteral nutrition and improvement in the delivery of enteral feedings to critically ill patients.[34,35] Additionally, the use of protocols and algorithms in enteral feeding increases

use of promotility agents and decreases unnecessary feeding interruptions related to intolerance from high gastric residual volume.[35]

Parenteral Nutrition

PN is intravenous nutrition designed to meet the needs of patients with a compromised GI tract or other conditions that preclude the delivery of enteral nutrition. While the appropriate use of PN may improve patient outcomes, inappropriate use has been associated with infectious complications, increased metabolic abnormalities, and higher medical costs.[36] Efforts to reduce the inappropriate use of PN highlight the importance of developing guidelines for initiating PN support, which are carried out by multidisciplinary nutrition support teams who specialize in its provision. Indications for PN include short bowel syndrome, high output enteric fistula, small bowel obstruction, paralytic ileus and intractable vomiting, diarrhea, or high ostomy output.[37] Additionally, patients undergoing major upper GI surgery, who are unable to be fed enterally, and are identified as being severely malnourished, have been shown to benefit from perioperative PN. Timing of PN initiation is a controversial topic, specifically in patients who are well nourished prior to ICU admission. In well-nourished patients, delaying PN initiation has been shown to improve outcomes.[6,7,38] In patients identified as having poor nutritional status or severe malnutrition, early PN use should be considered if enteral nutrition is unable to meet a patient's needs.

PN can be administered via central or peripheral venous access. Total PN (TPN) requires central venous access, where the tip of the catheter lies in or close to the superior vena cava allowing for infusion of hypertonic formulations. TPN is intended for patients who require PN support for greater than 7 to 14 days; however, patients can be maintained on PN for extended periods of time, years in some cases.[5]

In patients who require long-term TPN, a peripherally inserted central catheter or a tunneled cuffed catheter is placed for long-term access. Peripheral PN utilizes a peripheral vessel for administration. It is generally designed for short-term use, as the osmolarity of the solution must be less than 800 to 900 mOsm/L to prevent thrombophlebitis.[5] In the critically ill patient, peripheral PN is generally not practical, as large fluid volumes (2.4-3.0 L) are often required to provide significant calories and protein.

Calculating Needs

Calculating nutrient needs for patients on PN support is similar to that of patients being fed enterally. Providing less than 30 kcal/kg is recommended to avoid overfeeding. As previously stated, 25 kcal/kg is frequently used.

Once the appropriate weight and calories per kilogram are determined, energy needs can be calculated. and divided among carbohydrate and lipids (non-protein calories). The use of nonprotein calories, particularly in PN, is designed to spare protein in order to preserve lean body mass. When dividing estimated energy needs among carbohydrate (dextrose), protein (AA) and fat (lipids), a 60%/40% or 70%/30% 50%/25%/25% ratio is often employed (Table 29-8). However, adjusting protein requirements may result in altered distributions.

The amount of protein provided is calculated according to the underlying condition. In the case of critical illness, 1.5 g protein/kg BW is generally appropriate. In patients with large wounds or pressure ulcers, additional protein is required. Obese patients may require more than 2 g protein/kg. Standard recommendations for estimating protein should be followed for patients with renal failure. Patients on mechanical renal replacement therapy, such as hemodialysis or continuous venovenous hemofiltration, have higher requirements ($\geq$ 1.5 g/kg BW) due to losses, and protein needs should be adjusted accordingly.

If an institution is equipped with an on-site PN pharmacy, there is greater opportunity for customizing the formulations to meet individualized patient needs. Hospitals without a PN pharmacy on site rely on outside vendors to mix and deliver the formulas to the institution. Turnaround time may be extended in this case; however, more companies are providing these services and meeting the needs of institutions by customizing bags and making timely deliveries.

Fluid and electrolyte requirements in critically ill patients can vary depending on a number of factors, including preexisting medical conditions, presence of renal dysfunction, and overall clinical status. Communication with the ICU team on the addition of fluids and electrolytes is imperative to ensure that PN solutions are consistent with the therapies being provided by the ICU team. No more than 154 mEq/L of sodium is generally provided. Infusing more than 10 mEq/h of potassium should be avoided, unless the patient is severely hypokalemic. Prescribers should proceed with caution when increasing amounts of calcium and phosphorus in the PN solution, and are encouraged to work closely with pharmacy to ensure that formulations are not at risk for developing precipitates. Daily review of lab values is recommended to ensure PN is addressing the constantly changing needs of the patient.[39]

The inclusion of micronutrients in PN solutions is important to avoid the complications that can result from deficiencies. Standard additions of multivitamins and trace elements are generally included. If serum total bilirubin is more than 4 mg/dL, trace elements can be eliminated to avoid accumulating copper and manganese, which are excreted in bile. Other additives included in PN formulas are H2 blockers, vitamin K, heparin, regular insulin, and carnitine which plays a role in the transport and metabolism of fat.[40]

Risks and Complications of Parenteral Nutrition

The complications associated with PN infusion are generally divided into 3 categories: mechanical, infectious, and metabolic. The most common mechanical complication is catheter occlusion, which can be related to thrombotic and nonthrombotic sources. While catheter-related infections are not common, their occurrence can significantly affect morbidity, mortality, and LOS. Instituting guidelines and following the appropriate standards of care to reduce infectious complications improve outcomes and ensure safe delivery of PN support.[5,40]

Hyperglycemia is among the most common metabolic complications of PN infusion. Considerable controversy surrounding optimal BG levels for ICU patients exist. In postoperative cardiac patients, improved outcomes have been observed when implementing measures to maintain tight glycemic control (80-110 mg/dL). However, in most critically ill populations, the complications that result from hypoglycemia can have far more significant consequences. Moderate glycemic control (BG between

TABLE 29-8 Parenteral nutrition formula sample.

Calculate macronutrients:
Use caloric estimate (predictive equations v. kcal/kg) to estimate total calories:
1. Calculate Protein (AA) needs:
   - .8-1.0 g/kg for adult maintenance
   - 1.2- 2.0 kg for stress, s/p surgery, wound healing
   - **1.5g/kg for critical illness**
     - ≥ 2g/kg IBW for Class I, II obesity (BMI 30-40)
     - ≥ 2.5g/kg IBW for Class III obesity (BMI ≥ 40)
     - ≥ 1.5 g/kg (hemodialysis, continuous veno-venous hemofiltration)

   Multiply weight (kg) × desired protein (g/kg; see above) = _____ g AA
   AA g × 4 kcal/g = _____ kcals from AA

2. Calculate Carbohydrates (CHO) needs:
   Total kcal × 50% = _____ kcals from CHO
   CHO kcals / 3.4 kcals/g = _____ g CHO
3. Calculate Fat (Lipid) needs; remaining calories after AA and CHO are calculated
   Total kcals – AA kcals – CHO kcals = Lipid kcals
   Lipid kcals / 10 kcals/g = _____ g Lipid
(CHO and fat ratio can be adjusted per medical condition, for example in patients with rising worsening liver failure and rising LFTs can consider higher %CHO and lower% Lipid)

Example (using 60 kg BW):
Total Calories: 1500 kcal
1. **Protein (AA):**
   60 kg x 1.5 g/kg = 90 g
   90 g x 4 kcal/g = 360 kcal

2. **Carbohydrate (Dextrose):**
   1500 kcal × .5 = 750 kcal
   750 kcal/3.4 kcal/g = 220 g

3. **Fat (Lipid):**
   1500 kcal – 750 kcal (from CHO) – 360 kcal (from Protein) = 390 kcal
   390 kcal/10 kcal/g = 39 g (can be rounded to 40 g)

Calculate fluid requirements:
Grams AA/CHO/Lipid divided by [concentration of solutions] = minimum volume (ml)

   Protein (AA): 10 - 15% concentration
   Carbohydrate (CHO): standard dextrose solution- 70% concentration
   Fat: (Intralipid): 30% concentration
   Add 150 ml for additives (vitamins, minerals, trace elements, etc)

Example
90 g AA / 0.1 = 900 ml
+ 220 g dextrose / 0.7 = 314.2 ml
+ 40 g lipid / 0.3 = 133.3 ml
+ 150 ml (for additives)

Total = 1497.5 ml

140 and 180 mg/dL) helps avoid hypoglycemia and appears to be safer than strict control.[6,7,31,36,41] Steps to avoid hyperglycemia in patients receiving PN support include avoiding glucose infusion rates that exceed 5 mg/kg/min, close monitoring of BG levels, and providing insulin coverage as indicated. The addition of chromium in TPN, for presumed deficiency, may also be considered in patients with unexplained hyperglycemia. When initiating PN a reduced concentration (half-strength) is recommended to observe glycemic response and determine whether insulin therapy is required.

Hypoglycemia is often a result of excess insulin provided either directly in the PN formulation or subcutaneously. A patient who experiences hypoglycemic episodes during PN infusion can be treated with ampules of 50% dextrose or continuous infusion of 10% dextrose. The PN solution may also be discontinued until a reformulation is available. In patients receiving large doses of insulin, who no longer require PN infusion, a 1 to 2 hours taper of PN at half the prescribed rate is helpful in reducing the occurrence of rebound hypoglycemia.[6]

Hypertriglyceridemia results from excessive dextrose infusion or rapid infusion of intravenous fat emulsions (IVFE). It is recommended that IVFE in PN formulations should not exceed 1 g/kg/day. Serum triglycerides should also be obtained prior to advancing IVFE to goal, and monitored weekly for changes. An acceptable serum triglyceride level for patients on PN support is less than 400 mg/dL. Intravenous lipids are considered acceptable for patients with pancreatitis whose serum triglyceride levels are within normal limits.[6,39]

PN-associated liver dysfunction (PNALD) refers to liver and biliary dysfunction associated with the initiation of PN support. The 3 hepatobiliary disorders associated with PN infusion are steatosis, cholestasis, and gallbladder sludge/stones. Steatosis generally occurs within 2 weeks of initiation of PN support and may be the result of excessive infusion of calories. Biliary obstruction or impaired biliary secretion can cause cholestasis. In patients who require long-term PN support, cholestasis can progress to cirrhosis and liver failure.

Decreased enteral stimulation and suppression of cholecystokinin as a result of PN infusion can increase the risk for gallbladder sludge/stones.[42] Patients who are more at risk for developing PNALD include those with intestinal failure, or extensive bowel resection. In patients with suspected PNALD, it is important to avoid overfeeding, particularly of nonprotein calories, which can promote lipogenesis and inhibit lipolysis. Trials of enteral nutrition and ultimate discontinuation of PN should also be explored.[6,7,43]

Patients who are PN dependent generally receive IVFE as their source of essential fatty acids. Essential fatty acid deficiency (EFAD) can present within 1 to 3 weeks of receiving IVFE-free formulations, and include dermatitis, alopecia,

thrombocytopenia, fatty liver, and anemia. To prevent EFAD, 50 g weekly, eg, 250 mL of 20% IVFE or 500 mL of 10% IVFE should be provided.[5]

REFEEDING SYNDROME

Refeeding syndrome occurs when nutrition is reintroduced following a period of severe nutritional deprivation. The rapid delivery of nutrients can lead to glycogen and protein synthesis and quick uptake of glucose and amino acids, resulting in hypokalemia, hypophosphatemia, hypomagnesemia, and symptoms of acute thiamine deficiency. If left untreated, consequences include cardiac failure and neurological complications. Refeeding syndrome occurs in roughly 50% of severely malnourished patients fed orally, enterally, or parenterally. For severely malnourished patients, nutrition should be initiated and steadily increased with close monitoring and aggressive repletion of electrolytes as indicated.[44]

IMMUNONUTRITION

The practical use of immune enhancing products in critically ill patients is controversial. Conflicting results on the variable effects of pharmaconutrients, such as glutamine, arginine, omega 3 fatty acids, and selenium make it difficult to implement routine guidelines for their use. As more data emerge on the potential benefits of these immune modulating agents, more specific guidelines and recommendations for the appropriate dosing, timing, and duration may emerge.[45]

REFERENCES

1. Souba WW. Nutritional support. *N Engl J Med*. 1997;336:41-48.
2. Correia MI, Waitzberg DL. The impact of malnutrition on morbidity, mortality, length of stay and costs evaluated through a multivariate model analysis. *Clin Nutr*. 2003;22(3):235-239.
3. Goiburu ME, Goiburu MM, Bianco H, et al. The Impact of malnutrition on morbidity, mortality, and length of hospital stay in trauma patients. *Nutr Hosp*. 2006;21(5):604-610.
4. JV White, Guenter P, Jensen G, Malone A, Schofield M. Academy Malnutrition Work

Group, A.S.P.E.N. Malnutrition Task Force, and A.S.P.E.N. Board of Directors. Consensus statement: Academy of Nutrition and Dietetics and American Society for Parenteral and Enteral Nutrition: characteristics recommended for the identification and documentation of adult malnutrition (undernutrition). *J Parenter Enteral Nutr*. 2012;36(3):275-283.

5. Mueller C. *The A.S.P.E.N. Adult Nutrition Support Core Curriculum*, 2nd ed. Silver Spring, MD: American Society for Parenteral and Enteral Nutrition; 2012:155-169, 234-244 and 377-391.

6. McClave SA, Martindale RG, Vanek VW, et al. A.S.P.E.N. Board of Directors; American College of Critical Care Medicine; Society of Critical Care Medicine. Guidelines for the Provision and Assessment of Nutrition Support Therapy in the Adult Critically Ill Patient: Society of Critical Care Medicine (SCCM) and American Society for Parenteral and Enteral Nutrition (A.S.P.E.N.). *JPEN J Parenter Enteral Nutr*. 2009;33(3):277-316.

7. McClave SA, Taylor BE, Martindale RG, et al. Guidelines for the Provision and Assessment of Nutrition Support Therapy in the Adult Critically Ill Patient: Society of Critical Care Medicine (SCCM) and American Society for Parenteral and Enteral Nutrition (A.S.P.E.N.). *J Parenter Enteral Nutr*. 2016;40(2):159-211.

8. Alberda C, Gramlich L, Jones N, et al. The relationship between nutritional intake and clinical outcomes in critically ill patients: results of an international multicenter observational study. *Intensive Care Med*. 2009;35:1728-1737.

9. Choban P, Dickerson R, Malone A, Worthington P, Compher C, and the American Society for Parenteral and Enteral Nutrition. A.S.P.E.N. Clinical guidelines: nutrition support of hospitalized adult patients with obesity. *J Parenter Enteral Nutr*. 2013;37(6):714-744.

10. Khalid I, Doshi P, DiGiovine B. Early enteral nutrition and outcomes of critically ill patients treated with vasopressors and mechanical ventilation. *Am J Crit Care*. 2010;19(3):261-268.

11. Doig GS, Chevrou-Séverac H, Simpson F. Early enteral nutrition in critical illness: a full economic analysis using US costs. *Clinicoecon Outcomes Res*. 2013;5:429-436.

12. Malone A. Enteral formula selection: a review of selected product categories. *Nutrition Issues in Gastroenterology, Series #28. Practical Gastroenterology*, 2005.

13. Makola D. Elemental and semielemental formulas: are they superior to polymeric formulas? *Nutrition Issues in Gastroenterology, Series #34. Practical Gastroenterology*, 2005.

14. Dobb GJ, Towler SC. Diarrhea during enteral feeding in the critically ill: a comparison of feeds with and without fiber. *Intensive Care Med*. 1990;16(4):252-255.

15. Belknap D, Davidson LJ, Smith CR. The effects of psyllium hydrophilic mucilloid on diarrhea in enterally fed patients. *Heart Lung*. 1997;26(3):229-237.

16. Peters AL, Davidson MB. Lack of glucose elevation after simulated tube feeding with a low-carbohydrate, high-fat enteral formula in patients with type I diabetes. *Am J Med*. 1989;87(2):178-182.

17. Peters AL, Davidson MB. Effects of various enteral feeding products on postprandial blood glucose response in patients with type I diabetes. *JPEN J Parenter Enteral Nutr*. 1992;16(1):69-74.

18. Leon-Sanz M, Garcia-Luna PP, Planas M, et al. Glycemic and lipid control in hospitalized type 2 diabetic patients: evaluation of 2 enteral nutrition formulas (low carbohydrate-high monounsaturated fat vs high carbohydrate). *JPEN J Parenter Enteral Nutr*. 2005;29(1):21-29.

19. Craig LD, Nicholson S, Silverstone FA, Kennedy RD. Use of a reduced-carbohydrate, modified-fat enteral formula for improving metabolic control and clinical outcomes in long-term care residents with type 2 diabetes: results of a pilot trial. *Nutrition*. 1998;14(6):529-534.

20. Cerra FB, Cheung NK, Fischer JF. Disease-specific amino acid infusion in hepatic encephalopathy: a prospective, randomized, double-blind, controlled trial. *JPEN J Parenter Enteral Nutr*. 1985;9(3):288-295.

21. Michel H, Bories P, Aubin JP, Pomier-Layrargues G, Bauret P, Bellet-Herman H. Treatment of acute hepatic encephalopathy in cirrhotics with a branched-chain amino acids enriched versus a conventional amino acids mixture. A controlled study of 70 patients. *Liver*. 1985 Oct;5:282-289. PMID: 4079669.

22. Gadek JE, DeMichele SJ, Karlstad MD, et al. Effect of enteral with eicosapentanoic acid, gamma-linolenic acid, and antioxidants in patients with acute respiratory distress syndrome. *Crit Care Med*. 1999;27(8):1409-1420.

23. Tehila M, Gibstein L, Gordgi D, Cohen JD, Shapira M, Singer P. Enteral fish oil, borage oil and antioxidants in patients with acute lung injury (ALI). *Clin Nutr*. 2003;22(S1):S20.

24. Rice TW, Wheeler AP, Taylor Thompson BT, et al. Enteral omega 3-fatty acid, gamma-linolenic acid, and antioxidant supplementation in acute lung injury. *JAMA*. 2011;306(14):1574-1581.

25. Viall C, Porcelli K, Teran JC, Varma RN, Steffee WP. A double-blind clinical trial comparing the gastrointestinal side effects of two enteral feeding formulas. *JPEN J Parenter Enteral Nutr*. 1990;14(3):265-269.

26. Mowatt-Larssen CA, Brown RO, Wojtysiak SL, Kudsk KA. Comparison of tolerance and nutritional outcome between a peptide and a standard enteral formula in critically ill, hypoalbuminemic patients. *JPEN J Parenter Enteral Nutr*. 1992;16(1):20-24.

27. Heimburger DC, Geels VJ, Bilbrey J, Redden DT, Keeney C. Effects of small-peptide and whole-protein enteral feedings on serum proteins and diarrhea in critically ill patients: a randomized trial. *JPEN J Parenter Enteral Nutr*. 1997;21(3):162-167.

28. Montejo, JC. Enteral nutrition-related gastrointestinal complications in critically ill patients: a multicenter study. The Nutritional and Metabolic Working Group of the Spanish Society of Intensive Care Medicine and Coronary Units. *Crit Care Med*. 1999;27(8):1447-1453.

29. Heyland DK, Cahill N, Day AG. Optimal amount of calories for critically ill patients: depends on how you slice the cake! *Crit Care Med*. 2011;39(12):2619-2626.

30. Heyland DK, Stephens KE, Day AG, McClave SA. The success of enteral nutrition and ICU-acquired infections: a multicenter observational study. *Clin Nutr*. 2011;30(2):148-155.

31. Heyland, DK. Strategies to Optimize Enteral Nutrition in the ICU; PENSA 2011 Highlights; NNI Luncheon Symposium Proceedings from the 14th Congress of PENSA; Taipei, October 15, 2011.

32. The NICE-SUGAR Study Investigators, Finfer S, Chittock DR, et al. Intensive versus conventional glucose control in critically ill patients. *N Engl J Med*. 2009;360(13):1283-1297.

33. Bussy V, Marechal F, Masca S. Microbial contamination of enteral feeding tubes occurring during nutritional treatment. *JPEN J Parenter Enteral Nutr*. 1992;16(6):552-557.

34. Beyer, P. Complication of enteral feedings. In: Matarese LE, Gottschlich MM (eds). *Contemporary Nutrition Support Practice*. Philadelphia: WB Saunders Company; 1998.

35. Heyland, DK, Cahill, N, Dhaliwal, R, Sun X, Day AG, McClave SA. Impact of enteral feeding protocols on enteral nutrition delivery: results of a multicenter observational study. *JPEN J Parenter Enteral Nutr*. 2010;34(6):675-684.

36. Racco, M. An enteral nutrition protocol to improve efficiency in achieving nutritional goals. *Crit Care Nurse*. 2012;32(4):72-75.

37. Van den Berghe G, Wilmer A, Hermans G, et al. Intensive insulin therapy in the critically ill patients. *N Engl J Med*. 2001;345:449-461.

38. Kohli-Seth R, Sinha R, Wilson S, Bassily-Marcus A, Benjamin E. Adult parenteral nutrition utilization at a tertiary care hospital. *Nutr Clin Pract*. 2009;24(6):728-732.

39. Casaer MP, Mesotten D. Hermans G, et al. Early versus late parenteral nutrition in critically ill adults. *N Engl J Med*. 2011. Aug 11; 365 (6): 506-517. PMID: 21714640.

40. Neuman T, Kohli-Seth R, Wilson S, Bassily-Marcus A. Total parenteral nutrition in the ICU. *ICU Director*. 2010;1:203-209.

41. Deshpande KS. Total parenteral nutrition and infections associated with use of central venous catheters. *Am J Crit Care*. 2003;12(4):326-327.

42. Devos P, Preiser JC. Current controversies around tight glucose control in critically ill patients. *Curr Opin Clin Nutr Metab Care*. 2007;10(2):206-209.

43. Kumpf VJ. Parenteral nutrition-associated liver disease in adult and pediatric patients. *Nutri Clin Pract*. 2006;21(3):279-290.

44. A.S.P.E.N. Board of Directors and the Clinical Guidelines Task Force. Guidelines for the use of parenteral and enteral nutrition in adult and pediatric patients. *JPEN J Parenter Enteral Nutr*. 2002;26(1 Suppl):1SA-138SA.

45. Stanga Z, Brunner A, Leuenberger M, et al. Nutrition in clinical practice-the refeeding syndrome: illustrative cases and guidelines for prevention and treatment. *Eur J Clin Nutr*. 2008 Jun;62(6):687-694. PMID: 17700652.

46. Pierre J, Heneghan A, Lawson C, Wischmeyer P, Kozar R, Kidsk K. Pharmaconutrition review: physiological mechanisms. *JPEN J Parenter Enteral Nutr*. 2013;37(1):51S-65S.

Acute Kidney Injury and Failure

Pritul Patel, MD and Leila Hosseinian, MD

KEY POINTS

1. Current concepts of AKI in sepsis indicate that systemic inflammation, microvascular dysregulation, and mitochondrial alteration, leading to cell death may be more important than global renal hypoperfusion.

2. Urine output and SCr are at best surrogate markers of renal function, but can be "normal" in the presence of renal dysfunction.

3. Recent studies have identified new biomarkers of renal injury that can diagnose AKI earlier than SCr, but these are still in the primary stages of clinical adoption.

4. Prevention of contrast-induced AKI focuses on the use of noniodinated contrast media, minimizing contrast-media volume, avoiding repeat exposure to contrast media, and expanding plasma volume before administration of contrast media.

5. The published literature suggests that periprocedural dialysis has no protective effect against CI-AKI.

INTRODUCTION

Acute kidney injury (AKI) is the sudden decline of renal function resulting in the retention of nitrogenous waste products and the inability to regulate electrolytes and extracellular volume. The development of AKI is associated with increased morbidity and mortality. These patients have an increased hospital length of stay and hospital readmissions, all of which translate into increasing resource utilization. The number of deaths resulting from AKI continues to increase even though the treatment of AKI and care of critically ill patients has improved. The reason for this increase in absolute mortality from AKI is twofold: the incidence of AKI is increasing and patients with AKI are older, with a greater number and severity of comorbid conditions.[1] Furthermore, we are pushing the boundaries in medicine; sicker patients who once were untreatable are now undergoing more complex and invasive diagnostic and surgical procedures.

PATHOPHYSIOLOGY

Although the kidneys receive approximately 20% of the total cardiac output, they are still at very high risk for ischemic injury. This dichotomy is explained by the fact that most renal blood flow (80%-90%) is directed toward the renal cortex, where it passes through the glomerulus and is filtered.[2] The most metabolically active portion of the kidney, however, is not the cortex but the medulla, which is responsible for creating the osmotic gradient that serves to reabsorb water and concentrate urine. In order to maintain this osmotic gradient, blood flow to the medulla is kept low. In fact, the oxygen tension in the medulla is only approximately 10 mm Hg.[2] This lack of luxury perfusion to a metabolically active portion of the kidney predisposes it to ischemic injury. Furthermore, the kidney concentrates toxins that the body is exposed to, thereby amplifying the exposure of renal cells to toxic substances.

The etiology of AKI is traditionally divided into prerenal, intrinsic renal, and postrenal. Prerenal azotemia occurs as a complication of decreased renal perfusion with preservation of the cellular architecture of the renal parenchyma. Direct injury to the kidneys results in renal azotemia, or intrinsic renal injury. Postrenal azotemia occurs as a result of obstruction of the urinary outflow tract. The overwhelming majority of AKI in critically ill patients is caused by sepsis, whose mechanism does not quite fit within any of the traditional categories of AKI. It was traditionally thought that sepsis-induced AKI was caused by renal hypoperfusion due to systemic hypotension and renal vasoconstriction, along with reperfusion injury to the kidneys. However, this theory has recently come into question. It is now thought that while ischemia may play a role, there are many other pathophysiologic mechanisms at work. Recent human and animal studies have shown that renal blood flow is preserved in sepsis. Current concepts of AKI in sepsis indicate that systemic inflammation, microvascular dysregulation, and mitochondrial alteration, leading to cell death may be more important than global renal hypoperfusion.[3] This theory claims that sepsis induces an "inflammatory danger signal" that is initially adaptive and later becomes maladaptive, leading ultimately to, metabolic reprioritization of renal cells which favors cell adaptive processes (like maintenance of cell membrane potential and cell cycle arrest) at the expense of actual filtration of blood.[3]

Renal hypoperfusion is the hallmark of prerenal AKI. Renal hypoperfusion (resulting from prolonged hypotension, hemorrhage, abdominal compartment syndrome, low cardiac output states, or cirrhosis) is a common cause of prerenal AKI in the ICU. Medications that interfere with normal renal autoregulation (nonsteroidal anti-inflammatory drugs, angiotensin converting enzyme inhibitors, angiotensin receptor blockers, cyclosporine, and tacrolimus) can precipitate AKI in patients with marginal renal perfusion. Prerenal azotemia

presents with decreased glomerular filtration rate (GFR) and little evidence of cellular damage in most cases. Therefore, the condition is usually completely reversible. Prolonged prerenal azotemia, however, can lead to evidence of cellular damage, usually in the form of acute tubular necrosis.

Intrarenal AKI has many causes and is best understood when classified by the location of the lesion: glomerulus, tubule, vasculature, or interstitium. Most intrarenal AKI in the ICU setting is due to acute tubular necrosis from prolonged hypotension, nephrotoxic medications, recent exposure to radiographic contrast agents; or interstitial nephritis from nephrotoxic medications, such as antibiotics. Glomerular and vascular causes of intrarenal AKI are more commonly causes of renal failure outside of the ICU.

Urinary indices can be helpful in distinguishing prerenal and renal azotemia in non-ICU settings. A fractional excretion of sodium (FE_{Na}) less than 1% is commonly used in the non-ICU setting to identify patients with prerenal AKI. However, in the ICU, where many patients receive diuretics, the FE_{Na} becomes unreliable and should not be routinely used as a diagnostic test. An elevated blood urea nitrogen (BUN)/creatinine ratio is also not necessarily indicative of prerenal AKI in ICU patients due to the lengthy list of comorbidities that may elevate the BUN/creatinine ratio in a euvolemic ICU patient (gastrointestinal hemorrhage, total parenteral nutrition, steroids, catabolic stress). Analysis of urinary sediment can be used to distinguish prerenal and intrarenal AKI, but these tests have limited use in an ICU setting. Generally, the microscopic examination of urine in patients with prerenal or postrenal AKI is normal. Red blood cell casts, protein, white blood cells or leukocyte casts, or hematuria suggest intrarenal causes of AKI.

Postrenal AKI occurs when there is bilateral or unilateral obstruction in urinary flow. This leads to an increase in intratubular pressure, eventually leading to a decrease in glomerular filtration pressure. Postrenal AKI is a very rare cause of AKI in the ICU, since most patients in the ICU have a urinary catheter. Obstruction of the urinary tract can be extrarenal or renal. Extrarenal causes include prostatic hypertrophy, and abdominal/retroperitoneal masses compressing the ureters. Intrarenal obstruction can be caused by deposition of stones, crystals, clots, or tumors.

DEFINITION

The RIFLE (acronym stands for: risk, injury, failure, loss, and end-stage renal disease) criteria established a universal definition of AKI, facilitating communication among clinicians and researchers. The criteria include three severity grades (risk, injury, and failure), which are based on changes in serum creatinine and urine output, using the worst of each measure.[4] The criteria also include two outcome criteria (loss and end-stage renal disease), which are based on the duration of the loss of kidney function.[4] The RIFLE criteria have been validated with multiple trials showing that the severity of AKI, as defined by the RIFLE criteria, is associated with increased mortality.

The Acute Kidney Injury Network (AKIN) made modifications to the RIFLE criteria in order to take into account the importance of timing in kidney injury. Their diagnostic criteria for AKI include an abrupt (within 48 hours) reduction in kidney function defined by an absolute increase in SCr of more than or equal to 0.3 mg/dL, a percentage increase in SCr of more than or equal to 50% (1.5-fold from baseline) or a reduction in urine output (less than 0.5 mL/kg/h for more than 6 hours).[4] Their classification system involves a numbered system where stage 1 corresponds with RIFLE R, stage 2 with RIFLE I, and stage 3 with RIFLE F. Loss and end stage kidney disease were removed from the staging system (Table 30–1).

The AKIN and RIFLE criteria are useful measures of AKI, but are also fraught with limitations. Urine output and SCr are at best surrogate markers of renal function, but can be "normal" in the presence of renal dysfunction. The use of SCr can delay the diagnosis of renal injury and increases in SCr are only detected after a substantial reduction in GFR. In this sense, creatinine reflects renal injury that has already occurred. Creatinine is also affected by many factors other than renal dysfunction including muscle mass, catabolic state, rhabdomyolysis, dilutional effects, and drugs. Recent studies have identified new biomarkers of renal injury that can diagnose AKI earlier than SCr,

TABLE 30–1 Comparison of AKI staging criteria versus RIFLE staging criteria.[4]

AKI Staging		RIFLE	
Serum Creatinine	**Urine Output (Common to Both)**	**Class**	**Serum Creatinine of GFR**
Stage 1 Increase of more than or equal to 0.3 mg/dl (≥ 26.5 µmol/l) or increase to more than or equal to 150% to 200% (1.5- to 2-fold) from baseline	Less than 0.5 ml/kg/h for more than 6 hours	Risk	Increase in serum creatinine × 1.5 or GFR decrease > 25%
Stage 2 Increased to more than 200% to 300% (> 2- to 3-fold) from baseline	Less than 0.5 ml/kg/h for more than 12 hours	Injury	Serum creatinine × 2 or GFR decreased > 50%
Stage 3 Increased to more than 300% (> 3-fold) from baseline, or more than or equal to 4.0 mg/dl (≥ 354 µmol/l) with an acute increase of at least 0.5 mg/dl (44 µmol/l) or on RRT	Less than 0.3 ml/kg/h for 24 hours or anuria for 12 hours	Failure	Serum creatinine × 3, or serum creatinine > 4 mg/dl (> 354 µmol/l) with an acute rise > 0.5 mg/dl (> 44 µmol/l) or GFR decreased > 75%
		Loss	Persistent acute renal failure=complete loss of kidney function > 4 weeks
		End-stage kidney disease	ESRD > 3 months

Reproduced with permission from KDIGO Clinical Practice Guideline for Acute Kidney Injury. Section 2: AKI Definition, *Kidney Int Suppl.* 2012 Mar;2(1):19-36).

but these are still in the primary stages of clinical adoption.

AKI RISK FACTORS

The risk of developing AKI is dependent on the interplay between a patient's preexisting susceptibility to kidney injury combined with the duration of exposure to insults that result in AKI.[4] Table 30–2 summarizes the most common risk factors and exposures leading to AKI.

AKI MANAGEMENT

There are some general underlying management strategies that are common to all types of AKI. The mainstay of AKI management relies on early diagnosis and prompt intervention to minimize injury to the kidneys. In addition, adjusting to renal doses of renally metabolized medications is crucial as is avoiding any additional exposure to nephrotoxic drugs.[5]

In general, hemodynamic management, assessment of volume status, and management of fluid administration become even more important once

TABLE 30–2 Causes of AKI.[4]

Exposures	Susceptibilities
Sepsis	Dehydration or volume depletion
Critical illness	Advanced age
Circulatory shock	Female gender
Burns	Black race
Trauma	CKD
Cardiac surgery (especially with CPB)	Chronic diseases (heart, lung, liver)
Major noncardiac surgery	Diabetes mellitus
Nephrotoxic drugs	Cancer
Radiocontrast agents	Anemia
Poisonous plants and animals	

Reproduced with permission from KDIGO Clinical Practice Guideline for Acute Kidney Injury. Section 2: AKI Definition, *Kidney Int Suppl.* 2012 Mar;2(1):19-36.)

renal function has deteriorated. Hypotension and decreased circulating volume can lead to hypoperfusion and ischemia of the kidneys; especially since injured kidneys lose the ability to autoregulate blood flow and become dependent on the mean arterial pressure to maintain perfusion. Conversely, overaggressive fluid resuscitation can lead to tissue edema, hypoxia, and heart failure, exacerbating poor perfusion to the kidneys. Positive fluid balance in AKI has been correlated with increased 60 days mortality in large multicenter studies.[6] Strict hemodynamic monitoring and control of volume status in patients with AKI is critical and sometimes requires invasive cardiac monitoring or frequent bedside echocardiographic monitoring.

The type of fluid used for resuscitation in AKI and critically ill patients remains controversial. The Saline versus albumin fluid evaluation (SAFE) trial showed that albumin and crystalloids were equivalent in terms of renal outcomes.[7] It is probably prudent to avoid volume resuscitation with hetastarch in patients with AKI as recent evidence points to increased renal injury and increased incidence of renal replacement therapy with the use of hetastarches.[8] It is generally accepted that buffered salt solutions (such as lactated ringers, or Plasmalyte) may be the best agents for intravascular fluid resuscitation.[4] Some studies indicate that normal saline administered in large quantities can cause hyperchloremia, leading to decreased renal perfusion and increased incidence of AKI and need for renal replacement therapy. There is also a trend towards a hyperchloremic metabolic acidosis, leading to hyperkalemia.[9]

Frequently, patients in the ICU have shock of various etiologies, and after adequate fluid resuscitation, the use of vasopressors is often necessary to maintain an adequate arterial blood pressure. A large randomized study comparing the use of dopamine to norepinephrine infusions in patients with septic shock found that there was no difference in mortality or renal function, but dopamine was associated with more adverse events.[10] Both norepinephrine and vasopressin are suitable agents for the treatment of septic shock in patients that have been adequately volume resuscitated. Vasopressin has been gaining popularity because of some evidence that it may be superior to norepinephrine at reducing the progression of AKI, leading to less patients requiring RRT.[11] Finally, inotropes in conjunction with vasopressors also have a place in the treatment of hypotension due to cardiogenic shock as they help improve overall perfusion to all organs.

GLUCOSE MANAGEMENT IN AKI

Glycemic control among the critically ill is a controversial topic. Hyperglycemia and insulin resistance seem to be natural physiologic responses to critical illness, which occur in response to inflammatory mediators that are released during critical illness. Multiple studies have not shown any benefits of intensive insulin therapy and instead have shown an increased risk of hypoglycemia. The largest randomized trial of intensive glucose control in the ICU (NICE-SUGAR trial) failed to show a benefit in prevention of organ dysfunction, mortality, or bacteremia in patients with tight glucose control (81-108 mg/dL) compared to standard glucose control (140-180 mg/dL).[12] The KDINGO guidelines for the management of AKI suggest that critically ill patients should be treated with insulin for the prevention of severe hyperglycemia. Currently the blood glucose target supported by the majority of medical associations is 110 to 180 mg/dL.[4]

DOPAMINE, FENOLDOPAM, ATRIAL NATRIURETIC PEPTIDE, NESIRITIDE

Dopamine has been used in the past as prophylaxis against and treatment of renal failure in critically ill patients. Low-dose dopamine (1-3 mcg/kg/min) administered to healthy individuals results in renal afferent arteriole vasodilation, natriuresis, and increased GFR.[13] However, in patients with AKI, low-dose dopamine has in fact been shown to increase renal vascular resistance.[13] A large, randomized, placebo controlled, double-blinded study showed that dopamine had no renal protective effects.[13] There is some evidence that shows that the use of dopamine in AKI can even cause harm. It has been linked with tachy-dysrhythmias, myocardial ischemia, decreased intestinal blood flow, and can suppress immune function. Therefore, the use of dopamine to prevent or treat AKI has been abandoned.[4]

A promising agent for the prevention and treatment of AKI involves the use of fenoldopam. Fenoldopam is a pure dopamine 1-type receptor agonist with no alpha- or beta-receptor properties that is currently only indicated for treatment of hypertension. It reduces systemic vascular resistance and increases renal blood flow. Fenoldopam has been shown in small trials to have a renal protective effect, preventing the development of AKI.[14] While the data is promising, there are still no multicenter, highly powered, randomized controlled trials showing a clinically significant benefit of using fenoldopam in AKI. Furthermore, the hypotension that it causes is a significant side effect particularly in critically ill patients.

Atrial natriuretic peptide (ANP) is another potential therapy for the prevention and treatment of AKI. ANP is an amino acid that is released from the atrium in response to atrial stretch. It has diuretic, natriuretic, and renal vasodilatory activity, and can potentially increase GFR. There have been several negative studies concerning the use of ANP as prophylaxis against AKI.[15] Therefore, until further research proves a benefit, ANP should not be used for treatment of prevention of AKI.

Nesiritide is a recombinant form of brain natriuretic peptide that has been approved by the Food and Drug Administration for use in decompensated heart failure.[4] It may improve GFR, decrease rise in SCr, and improve urine output in patients, especially those with baseline renal insufficiency. In a pilot trial, nesiritide infusion started during and after cardiopulmonary bypass was shown to improve SCr values in patients with left ventricular dysfunction undergoing cardiac surgery.[4] Nesiritide is not FDA approved for this indication.

DIURETICS

Patients with AKI are frequently administered diuretics, either before or after being diagnosed with AKI. According to one observational study, approximately 59% to 70% of patients with AKI were shown to have been administered a diuretic before the onset of RRT.[16] There are multiple reasons for administering diuretics to a patient with AKI. Nonoliguric renal failure has a better prognosis than oliguric renal failure; therefore, many clinicians administer diuretics to convert oliguric renal failure into nonoliguric renal failure. Diuretics can sometimes ameliorate fluid overload, commonly seen with AKI. Furthermore, some diuretics are thought to have renoprotective effects. However, improper diuretic use can lead to a decrease in intravascular volume, exacerbating prerenal insult to the kidneys.

Loop diuretics, such as furosemide, have a potentially renoprotective profile that may serve to protect the kidneys from AKI. They inhibit the Na^{2+}-K-2Cl$^-$ transporter in the ascending limb of the Loop of Henle. Inhibition of this active sodium transporter may decrease the oxygen demand of the renal tubule and protect the kidney against ischemia.[17] Furosemide also increases the flow of urine in the renal tubules, helping to wash out ischemia-related necrotic debris blocking the tubules.[17]

A meta-analysis by Ho et al examined the effect of loop diuretics in AKI. They found that furosemide had no impact on hospital mortality, the requirement for RRT, number of dialysis sessions, or the incidence of oliguria. Furosemide was not effective for the prevention of AKI; it did not improve mortality in AKI and did not reduce the severity of AKI. Furosemide also did not decrease the duration of CRRT therapy and did not facilitate the return of renal function.[18] However, furosemide does have a role for the management of hypervolemia, hyperkalemia, and hypercalcemia in AKI.[4]

Mannitol has been used to prevent AKI, however, most of the studies showing a beneficial effect of mannitol are underpowered, retrospective, and of poor quality.[4] Mannitol may be beneficial when administered just prior to the arterial clamp removal in renal transplantation. In this setting, mannitol has been shown to decrease posttransplant AKI, but has not been shown to have a positive impact on renal graft function after 3 months.[19] There is some underwhelming evidence that mannitol may be beneficial in treating rhabdomyolysis by stimulating osmotic diuresis. But again, the studies were not randomized and are underpowered.[20]

NUTRITION

Protein-calorie malnutrition is an independent risk factor for in-hospital mortality for patients with AKI. The nutritional considerations in patients with AKI must take into account a multitude of patient factors, including metabolic and inflammatory derangements, renal replacement therapy–induced nutrient imbalance, the underlying etiology of AKI, and patient comorbidities.

AKI is associated with hyperglycemia from peripheral insulin resistance, and increased hepatic gluconeogenesis. Hypertriglyceridemia is another consequence of AKI and occurs due to decreased lipolysis and impaired ability to metabolize exogenous lipids.[21] When considering nutritional supplementation, it should be noted that patients with AKI do not manifest increased energy consumption. The optimal energy to nitrogen ratio is not known. One study of AKI patients on CVVH showed that there was a less negative/weakly positive nitrogen balance with energy intake of 25 kcal/kg/d.[22] Another randomized study of AKI patients provided 30 or 40 kcal/kg/d of energy. The higher caloric intake did not improve the nitrogen balance of these patients and instead was associated with worsening hyperglycemia, and hypertriglyceridemia.[23] Therefore, it is reasonable to suggest that patients with AKI be provided with at least 20 kcal/kg/d, but not more than 30 kcal/kg/d.[4]

Protein catabolism is a common finding in critically ill patients, including those with AKI. Consequently, protein intake should not be withheld in order to attenuate the rise in BUN and SCr in order to stave off RRT.[4] However, administration of high doses of protein have not been proven to improve the nitrogen balance of patients with AKI, and may in fact be associated with increased acidosis, azotemia, and increasing dialysis dose requirements.[24] Patients on RRT lose extra protein during therapy in addition to the protein catabolism occurring as a result of their critical illness. Patients on CRRT lose 0.2 g of amino acids per liter of filtrate (5-10 g/d)[4]; patients on intermittent HD may lose less protein per day. The KDINGO guidelines suggest administering 0.8 to 1.0 g/kg/d of protein in AKI patients not on RRT; 1.0 to 1.5 g/kg/d in AKI patients on RRT; and a maximum of 1.7 g/kg/d in patients on CRRT.[4]

Enteral nutrition should be used whenever possible in all critically ill patients, including those with AKI. Critically ill patients may not tolerate enteral nutrition due to delayed gastric emptying and decreased nutritional uptake from bowel wall edema. The use of enteral nutrition has been shown to improve outcome and survival in ICU patients. The provision of nutrients via the gut helps maintain gut integrity, decreases gut atrophy, and decreases bacterial translocation.

ANTIBIOTIC-RELATED AKI

Aminoglycoside

Aminoglycosides are very potent bactericidal agents that are being used with increasing frequency because of growing antibiotic resistance. The advantages of aminoglycosides include: predictable pharmacokinetics, and lack of hematologic and hepatic toxicity. However, they are also fraught with considerable side effects, including: nephrotoxicity and ototoxicity.[4] The risk of aminoglycoside induced AKI can be as high as 25%.[26] When used appropriately, with proper dosing and monitoring of levels, the risk of AKI with aminoglycosides can be minimized.

Repeated dosing of aminoglycosides results in the accumulation of aminoglycosides in the renal tubular epithelial cells, leading to a higher incidence of nephrotoxicity with repeated exposure.[27] Single daily dosing or extended interval dosing can potentially decrease the amount of aminoglycoside that is taken up in the renal tubules and may limit the potential for nephrotoxicity without sacrificing the therapeutic effect.[27] Monitoring of aminoglycoside levels during therapy is essential in critically ill patients with frequent fluctuations in GFR.

Amphotericin B

Amphotericin B is a widely used antifungal drug with many systemic side effects including chills, hypotension, cytokine release, thrombophlebitis, electrolyte disturbances, and hypoplastic anemia. Nephrotoxicity is commonly seen with amphotericin B and is the primary dose-limiting side effect.[28]

Prevention of amphotericin toxicity relies on judicious use of amphotericin. Amphotericin should be avoided, and azole antifungal agents should be used whenever feasible. One major advance in the avoidance of amphotericin nephrotoxicity has been the advent of lipid formulations of amphotericin. The original formulation of amphotericin used deoxycholate as the solvent.[28] Clinical trials have shown that the lipid formulations of amphotericin are less nephrotoxic, while preserving the potent antifungal effect of amphotericin.[28]

CONTRAST-INDUCED AKI

Many critically ill patients receive diagnostic or therapeutic procedures that require exposure to intravenous (IV) contrast medium. The nephrotoxic potential of contrast media is well known and not inconsequential. Diabetes mellitus, Chronic kidney disease (CKD), and advanced age have been identified as the three risk factors that are common amongst patients that develop contrast induced (CI)-AKI. Preexisting renal disease is the most important risk factor, with the incidence of CI-AKI approaching 25% in this setting.[30] Precautions to reduce the risk of CI-AKI should be taken in patients whose baseline creatinine is greater than 1.8 mg/dL.[29]

Prevention of CI-AKI focuses on the use of non-iodinated contrast media[29], minimizing contrast-media volume, avoiding repeat exposure to contrast media, and expanding plasma volume before administration of contrast media. Using iso-osmolar or low-osmolar iodinated contrast media should be used whenever feasible. In general, repeated exposure to contrast should be delayed for 48 hours in patients without risk factors, and for 72 hours in those with diabetes mellitus or previous AKD/AKI. The risk of AKI seems to be highest after inter arterial injection of iodinated contrast media.[29] The published literature suggests that periprocedural dialysis has no protective effect against CI-AKI.

Extracellular volume expansion may serve to prevent CI-AKI by a variety of mechanisms. Exposure of the kidneys to radiocontrast agents causes renal damage via a direct nephrotoxic effect, secretion of vasopressin and stimulation of the renin-angiotensin axis (stimulates renal afferent artery vasoconstriction resulting in renal hypoperfusion).[29] Extracellular volume expansion causes decreased secretion of vasopressin and also attenuates the renin-angiotensin axis stimulation. Furthermore, by directly diluting the radiocontrast agent, volume expansion may attenuate the direct nephrotoxicity from the contrast. The type of IV fluid used for extracellular volume expansion plays a role in averting CI-AKI. The two solutions that have shown to help prevent CI-AKI are isotonic normal saline and sodium bicarbonate solutions. The REINFORCE trial, however, found no difference in the incidence of CI-AKI in patients receiving sodium bicarbonate when compared to normal saline.[30]

There have been many trials examining the use of N-acetyl cysteine (NAC) before contrast exposure in order to decrease the incidence of CI-AKI. Although the evidence supporting the use of NAC in preventing CI-AKI is not particularly strong, considering its negligible side effects, some clinicians include oral NAC along with IV fluid resuscitation as a strategy to prevent CI-AKI.[31]

REFERENCES

1. Bagshaw SM, Bellomo R, Prasad D. Review article: acute kidney injury in critical illness. *J Can Anesth.* 2010;57:985-998.
2. Vincent JL, Abraham E, Moore F, Kochanek P, Fink M (eds). *Textbook of Critical Care*, 6th ed. Philadelphia, PA: Saunders Elsevier; 2011:885-891.
3. Gomez H, Ince C, DeBacker D, et al. A unified theory of sepsis-induced acute kidney injury: inflammation, microcirculatory dysfunction, bioenergetics, and the tubular cell adaption to injury. *Shock.* 2014;41:3-11.
4. Kidney Disease: Improving Global Outcomes (KDIGO) Acute Kidney Injury Work Group. KDIGO clinical practice guideline for acute kidney injury. *Kidney Int.* 2012;2:1-138.
5. Himmelfarb J, Sayegh MH (eds.). *Chronic Kidney Disease, Dialysis, and Transplantation: A Companion to Brenner and Rector's The Kidney*, 3rd ed. London, UK: Saunders Elsevier; 2011:654-667.
6. Payen D, de Pont AC, Sakr Y, et al. A positive fluid balance is associated with a worse outcome in patients with acute renal failure. *Crit Care.* 2008;12:R74.
7. Finfer S, Bellomo R, Boyce N, et al. A comparison of albumin and saline for fluid resuscitation in the intensive care unit. *N Engl J Med.* 2004;350(22):2247-2256.
8. Perner A, Haase N, Guttormsen AB, et al. Hydroxyethyl starch 130/0.42 versus Ringer's acetate in severe sepsis. *N Engl J Med.* 2012;367(2):124-134.
9. Lobo D, Awad S. Should chloride-rich crystalloids remain the mainstay of fluid resuscitation to prevent "pre-renal" acute kidney injury?: con. *Kidney Int.* 2014;86(6):1096-1105.
10. De Backer D, Biston P, Devriendt J, et al. Comparison of dopamine and norepinephrine in the treatment of shock. *N Engl J Med.* 2010;362(9):779-789.
11. Gordon AC, Russell JA, Walley KR, et al. The effects of vasopressin on acute kidney injury in septic shock. *Intensive Care Med.* 2010;36(1):83-91.
12. Finfer S, Chittock DR, Su SY, et al. Intensive versus conventional glucose control in critically ill patients. *N Eng J Med.* 2009;360(13):1283-1297.
13. Lauschke A, Teichgraber UK, Frei U, Eckardt KU. "Low-dose" dopamine worsens renal perfusion in patients with acute renal failure. *Kidney Int.* 2006;69(9):1669-1674.
14. Cogliati AA, Vellutini R, Nardini A, et al. Fenoldopam infusion for renal protection in high-risk cardiac surgery patients: a randomized clinical study. *J Cardiothorac Vasc Anesth.* 2007;21(6):847-850.
15. Ricksten SE, Sward K. Atrial natriuretic peptide in acute renal failure. In: Ronco C, Bellomo R, Kellum J (eds). *Critical Care Nephrology*, 2nd ed. Philadelphia, PA: Saundners Elsevier; 2009:429-433.
16. Mehta RL, Pascual MT, Soroko S, Chertow GM; PICARD Study Group. Diuretics, mortality, and nonrecovery of renal function in acute renal failure. *JAMA.* 2002;288(20):2547-2553.
17. Ludens JH, Hook JB, Brody MJ, Williamson HE. Enhancement of renal blood flow by furosemide. *J Pharmacol Exp Ther.* 1968;163(2):456-460.
18. Ho KM, Sheridan DJ. Meta-analysis of frusemide to prevent or treat acute renal failure. *BMJ.* 2006;333(7565):420.
19. Weimar W, Geerlings W, Bijnen AB, et al. A controlled study on the effect of mannitol on immediate renal function after cadaver donor kidney transplantation. *Transplantation.* 1987;44:784-788.
20. Vanholder R, Sever MS, Erek E, Lameire N. Rhabdomyolysis. *J Am Soc Nephrol.* 2000;11(8):1553-1561.
21. Druml W, Mitch WE. Metabolic abnormalities in acute renal failure. *Semin Dial.* 1996;9:484-490.
22. Macias WL, Alaka KJ, Murphy MH, Miller ME, Clark WR, Mueller BA. Impact of the nutritional regimen on protein catabolism and nitrogen balance in patients with acute renal failure. *JPEN J Parenter Enteral Nutr.* 1996;20(1):56-62.
23. Fiaccadori E, Maggiore U, Rotelli C, et al. Effects of different energy intakes on nitrogen balance in patients with acute renal failure: a pilot study. *Nephrol Dial Transplant.* 2005;20(9):1976-1980.
24. Scheinkestel CD, Adams F, Mahony L, et al. Impact of increasing parenteral protein loads on amino acid

levels and balance in critically ill anuric patients on continuous renal replacement therapy. *Nutrition.* 2003;19(9):733-740.

25. English WP, Williams MD. Should aminoglycoside antibiotics be abandoned? *Am J Surg.* 2000;180(6): 512-515; discussion 515-516.

26. Falagas ME, Kopterides P. Old antibiotics for infections in critically ill patients. *Curr Opin Crit Care.* 2007;13:592-597.

27. Harbarth S, Burke JP, Lloyd JF, Evans RS, Pestotnik SL, Samore MH. Clinical and economic outcomes of conventional amphotericin B-associated nephrotoxicity. *Clin Infect Dis.* 2002;35(12):e120-127.

28. Johansen HK, Gotzsche PC. Amphotericin B lipid soluble formulations vs. amphotericin B in cancer patients with neutropenia. *Cochrane Database Sys Rev.* 2000;3:CD000969.

29. Mehran R, Nikolsky E. Contrast-induced nephropathy: definition, epidemiology, and patients at risk. *Kidney Int Suppl.* 2006;100:S11-15.

30. Adolph E, Holdt-Lehmann B, Chatterjee T, et al. Renal Insufficiency Following Radiocontrast Exposure Trial (REINFORCE): a randomized comparison of sodium bicarbonate versus sodium chloride hydration for the prevention of contrast-induced nephropathy. *Coron Artery Dis.* 2008;19:413-419.

31. Fishbane S. N-acetylcysteine in the prevention of contrast-induced nephropathy. *Clin J Am Soc Nephrol* 2008;3:281-297.

Renal Replacement Therapy

George Coritsidis, MD and Saad Bhatti, MD

KEY POINTS

1. Renal replacement therapy (RRT) is one of the most expensive interventions used in an already cost burdensome intensive care unit (ICU) setting. Prescribing RRT in the critically ill is complex and ideally should involve clear communication between nephrologist and intensivist.

2. RRT modalities include peritoneal dialysis, intermittent hemodialysis, continuous renal replacement therapies, and sustained low-efficiency daily dialysis.

3. These modalities utilize 2 transport mechanisms in providing renal replacement: *diffusion* and *convection*. These forces result in solute **clearance** and plasma water removal or **ultrafiltration (UF)**.

4. RRT is initiated early in patients whose renal function is not expected to quickly improve due to severity of illness and is unresponsive to resuscitation: multiorgan failure, high fractional excretion of sodium (FENa), rising azotemia (without plateau of urea or creatinine levels), and oliguria all suggestive of acute tubular necrosis (ATN).

5. At present, randomized trials and meta-analyses, do not support a mortality benefit for one modality over another. However, a gradual clearance rate may be wise in hemodynamic instability, acute coronary syndromes, elevated intracranial pressures (ICPs), or hypo/hypernatremia.

INTRODUCTION

Almost 60 years ago, RRT was first used to treat acute kidney injury (AKI) during the Korean War.[1] Within 25 years, continuous therapies were first attempted in Germany.[2] RRT modalities have since expanded, becoming commonplace in most hospitals of the developed world. In AKI, when preventative and supportive management fails we turn to RRT.

In the past decade, admissions for AKI increased with a doubling in the incidence of severe AKI (Figure 31–1).[3] In parallel, approximately 200,000 patients required RRT in 2012.[3] The incidence of RRT-requiring AKI now surpasses that of end-stage renal disease (ESRD).[4] What's more, the morbidity

and mortality of AKI requiring RRT extends beyond hospitalization.[3,5]

The necessity for RRT in the ICU arises in 1 of 3 clinical situations: AKI, critically ill ESRD patients,[6] and drug or toxic overdoses. RRT for AKI is dramatic but less common than most think. The incidence of AKI in the ICU is relatively low between 6% and 19%, but can be higher depending on population studied and risk, injury, failure loss, and end-stage kidney disease (RIFLE) criteria.[7,8] RRT needs occur in up to 5% of AKI.[8,9] Unfortunately, mortality continues to remain high, between 24% and 50%.[3,8,10] AKI incrementally adds to short- and long-term mortality, and especially when RRT is

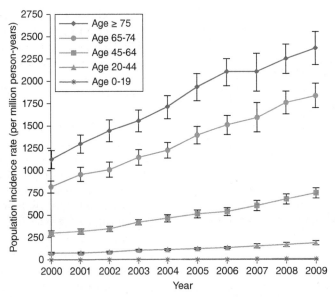

FIGURE 31-1 Population incidence of dialysis-requiring acute kidney injury (AKI) in the United States from 2000 to 2009 (count and incidence rate per million person-years). I bars represent 95% confidence intervals (CIs). The number of cases of dialysis-requiring AKI increased from 63,000 (2000) to almost 164,000 (2009); population incidence increased 10% per year from 222 to 533 cases/million person-years.[3] (*Reproduced with permission from Hsu RK, McCulloch CE, Dudley RA, et al: Temporal Changes in Incidence of Dialysis-Requiring AKI,* J Am Soc Nephrol *2013 Jan: 24(1):37-42.*)

required,[6,9] with up to 14% requiring chronic dialysis on discharge.[5,8,11]

Prescribing RRT in the critically ill is complex and ideally should involve clear communication between nephrologist and intensivist.[12] The choice of modality, the goals, its timing, as well as patient-specific findings, are collectively crucial in the decision for RRT.[12] Understanding the shortcomings and function of the modalities must also be a part of the process. In centers where selection is limited to intermittent hemodialysis (IHD), adaptations are not only viable but presently adequate.[13]

RRT: PHYSIOLOGY

Clearance of any substance depends on modality characteristics, (convection vs diffusion), size, time on RRT, flow rates (both blood and dialysate), and dialyzer membrane characteristics (Figure 31–2).[14] This coupled with patient acuity, hemodynamics, nutritional status, volume status, and diagnosis determines eventual success.

RRT attempts to support the kidneys' responsibilities in maintaining homeostasis. To some extent it

succeeds in volume control and to a lesser extent in solute and acid/base homeostasis. The various modalities, whether peritoneal or hemodialysis, utilize 2 transport mechanisms in providing renal replacement: *diffusion* and *convection*. These forces result in solute **clearance** and plasma water removal or **UF**. Other renal responsibilities such as calcium/phosphate balance and anemia control are not provided with RRT.

Clearance, removal of solute from plasma, is most efficiently accomplished by diffusion. Namely plasma is cleared of certain solutes across a semipermeable membrane (the dialyzer), as it travels down a concentration gradient. Each fluid medium (plasma and dialysate), flows in a direction counter current to the other, maintaining the concentration gradient between plasma and dialysate. Hence a plasma potassium of 7 mEq/L approaches that of the dialysate's 2 mEq/L over time. Dialysate can be adjusted to approximate the desired goal of net solute change. Clearance is determined by the solutes' serum concentration, molecular weight, and dialysis membrane characteristics (pore size and surface area). Diffusion becomes relatively inefficient as solute molecular weight increases, while with convection

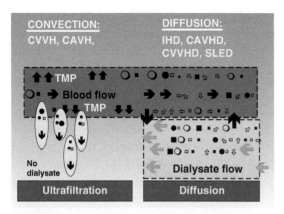

FIGURE 31-2 Mechanisms of solute clearance in various modalities of Renal Replacement. TMP, transmembrane pressure, or hydrostatic pressure; UF, ultrafiltration; •□*■ = solutes.

large-molecular-weight solute clearance is more effective.[15] Diffusion is a key mechanism of clearance in RRT using dialysate such as IHD.

Convection, which is preferred in treating the critically ill, is capable of removing large quantities of "plasma" water or UF. Blood hydrostatic pressure in the dialyzer supports a transmembrane pressure, through which UF is generated. Accompanying UF is the clearance of solute via **solvent drag**, signifying that this fluid is not pure water but

laden with solute. In fact, convection plays a significant role in providing clearance in continuous RRTs. UF rate is what determines clearance and is dependent on blood flow rate. Though inefficient in providing clearance, convention by adding the luxury of 24 hours surpasses what IHD can do in 4 (Figure 31–3).

An added benefit with convection is the enhanced clearance of larger molecules or middle molecules (500-5000 Da), felt to include uremic toxins. There are over 115 compounds identified as toxins that correlate more closely with uremic symptoms such as encephalopathy.[16] Since middle molecule clearance depends on the duration of a plasma-dialysate interface, continuous RRTs are more effective. Though at present conjectural, middle molecule clearance may in time provide for an important element of treatment in AKI due to sepsis. For instance, evidence indicates that continuous modalities may enhance clearance of various mediators of inflammation (see later).

RRT: INDICATIONS

RRT indications include the critically ill ESRD patient, the critically ill AKI patient, and the toxic overloaded patient. Only the first 2 are actual renal replacement.

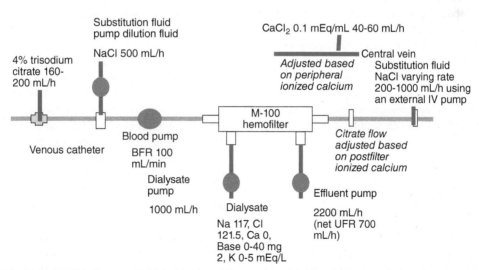

FIGURE 31-3 Continuous renal replacement therapy (CRRT) circuit (Gambro PRISMA and M-100 filter). Regional citrate is infused for anticoagulation; CaCl₂ adjusts peripheral ionized Ca levels; substitution fluid (replacement fluid [RF]) can be either pre- or postfilter and determines net fluid balance; effluent represents spent dialysate and/or UF. (*Reproduced with permission from Mehta RL, et al. Continuous renal replacement therapy in the critically ill patient,* Kidney Int 2005 *Feb; 67(2):781-795.*)

The Critically Ill Esrd Patient: Maintenance Dialysis

RRT for ESRD patients may be the most common reason (up to 40% of all patients receiving RRT) for its use in the ICU.[6,17] The etiology is most often related to ESRD comorbidities, primarily cardiovascular problems (31% of ICU ESRD cases) and most commonly arrhythmias and congestive heart failure.[6] Admissions may result from missed dialysis and/or compliance issues resulting in volume or electrolyte imbalances. ICU monitoring provides ventilator support, or if hyperkalemic, telemetry for possible arrhythmias, or cardiogenic shock. After prompt RRT the patient is stabilized, often resulting in relatively short admissions.

ICU care may also be required for acute events unrelated to ESRD, such as sepsis (15% of ICU ESRD cases), trauma, or complications from surgery. They have twice the rate of sepsis and higher readmission rates than nonrenal failure patients.[6,17] Mortality is lower than AKI patients requiring RRT, but higher than the general population.

The Critically Ill AKI Patient: Bridge RRT

In treating AKI, RRT is supportive, bridging the patient while treating the initiating event. About 7.5% of hospitalized patients with AKI require RRT.[5] In the ICU, AKI is most often due to sepsis thought to be from ATN, though glomerular hemodynamics play a significant role.[8,18] The need for RRT is relatively uncommon in AKI when all RIFLE classes are included. It requires a process of involved decision making between nephrologist and intensivist: recognizing the patient's needs; weighing issues of hypotension and anticoagulation; selecting the proper RRT; and balancing them with realistic capabilities. This includes possibly avoiding RRT, waiting for renal recovery, or not even considering it due to futility.

Emergent RRT

Clear indications for immediate RRT include life-threatening hyperkalemia, severe metabolic acidosis, and volume overload; overt symptomatic manifestations of uremia such as pericarditis and encephalopathy; and intoxications (lithium, aspirin, ethylene glycol, methanol, metformin, amanita).

Adequate treatment of uremia through the clearance of uremic toxins is unclear since such toxins are not clinically measured.[16] Since, for every small increment of creatinine there is a significant rise in mortality,[19] uremic toxins may be clinically more important than realized. Unfortunately, we are limited to assuming uremia in the azotemic patient with a pericardial rub, or encephalopathy. Given the multiple reasons for mental status changes in the ICU, the encephalopathy is particularly difficult to discern and ideally RRT should be initiated well before uremic symptoms occur.

In uremic pericarditis, treatment is daily, continued RRT. When entertaining the diagnosis, it is important to evaluate and rule out, cardiac tamponade. Aggressive RRT without initial decompression may decrease preload and result in shock.

Early or Urgent RRT

RRT is initiated early in patients whose renal function is not expected to quickly improve due to severity of illness: multiorgan failure, AKI unresponsive to resuscitation, high FENa, rising azotemia (without plateau of creatinine or urea levels), and oliguria all suggestive of ATN. In such "extreme" conditions the concept of early RRT to replace renal function and/or support multiorgan dysfunction may make most sense and benefit.[20] RRT maintains volume despite hemodynamic, nutritional, antibiotic, and other infusion needs, while providing balance of electrolytes and pH.

The decision for early RRT remains a difficult one especially since the benefits to mortality or otherwise is not clear.[21] A meta-analysis of 30 RCTs and 8 prospective cohort studies was inconclusive,[9] while a recent meta-analysis of 23 studies (1960-2006), suggested some benefit.[22] Importantly, these trials differed considerably in clinical settings and definitions of early RRT. Many excluded patients that recovered or died without starting RRT, rendering a recommendation for early RRT difficult.

The question becomes more complicated prompting clinical discussion in less dramatic presentations, such as nonoliguric AKI,[23] and/or slow rising azotemia (risk or injury on the RIFLE scale). Since there is no key single marker to use as a starting point for RRT, the decision is based on the multiple facets of the presentation.

Traditional markers of AKI, serum creatinine and blood urea nitrogen (BUN) are limited in this regard, though, a lower mortality risk has been reported when starting RRT at lower BUN levels.[26,27] Urea generation (BUN levels) varies depending upon on protein intake and catabolism[26]. Its highly variable volume of distribution (Vd) is exemplified by the BUN rebound seen in sepsis after RRT. What's more, dialysis efficacy using urea kinetics has not been assessed in either AKI or in the critically ill.[14]

Pursuing this question, the BEST study[28] separated azotemic patients by BUN, creatinine, and time in ICU. The answers were mixed. In the BUN-based analysis, there was no outcome difference in timing of RRT.[28] "Late" initiation based on creatinine had lower mortality while those initiated early based on ICU duration prior to RRT had lower mortality. These observations were confounded due to some having chronic kidney disease (CKD) and variability in patient presentations. However, the study did suggest that early RRT in patients with preexisting CKD may impart a higher survival advantage.[28]

Another reported reason in delaying RRT is the perception of impending renal recovery.[25] RRT is invasive and can result in complications from access placement, hypotension, electrolyte abnormalities, and arrhythmias.[13,29] Hemodynamic instability is common in the ICU and the intensivist needs to balance RRT safety with its need. Hypotension during RRT, along with issues of dialyzer bioincompatibility may delay renal recovery.[30] Dialyzer membranes induce monocyte-derived proinflammatory cytokines (interleukin [IL] 1, 6, 8, tumor necrosis factor alpha [TNF-α]), which can increase renal toxicity. So-called biocompatible membranes may lessen these responses. Therefore when taken into account a prudent decision may be to wait and monitor volume, potassium, protein intake, and supplement bicarbonate as needed, selecting extended or continuous RRTs if condition worsens. Recently published AKIKI trial with early vs late initiations of RRT in critically ill patients suggest delaying initiation based on clinical indications may avoid the need for RRT. ELAIN trial suggests reduced 90 days mortality with early RRT initiation.[25,26]

Finally, delays can also arise from issues of logistic support involving nursing and staff availability as well as their timeliness.[25]

Fluid Overload

In severe sepsis and AKI, positive fluid balance is independently associated with increased mortality.[31,32] Recent studies suggest fluid overload to be more critical indication for initiating RRT earlier. In both the pediatric and adult literature, fluid overloaded patients had better outcomes with early RRT even after severity of illness adjustments.[31,33] Furthermore, survivors had lower fluid accumulation at RRT initiation compared to nonsurvivors even with RRT modality and severity adjustments. Always influential, volume status may now provide a greater urgency for *early* RRT.

Fluid overload is also associated with more days on dialysis, and greater ICU and hospital length of stay.[28,34] Though adjusted for severity, it is not clear the difference in volumes suggest hemodynamically dissimilar patients or that volume should be applied more conservatively and/or ultrafiltrated more aggressively.

Cessation

Similar to commencement, no prespecified single finding or estimated glomerular filtration rate (eGFR) exists to trigger cessation. Actually, attempting to assess GFR is inaccurate when renal function is not in steady state. As patient acuity improves, the first decision is to transfer to IHD. In deciding, it is important to consider if IHD can support present and daily volume load. Moreover, drug dosing must be adjusted to IHD or level of renal function.

In general, RRT is terminated when urine output increases and creatinine is stable or decreases. The return of renal function is often preceded by an improvement in the patient's overall condition. Continuing may not only be unnecessary but any RRT, and possibly more so IHD, may delay renal recovery from hypotension and/or continued inflammation. Conversely, continued RRT may be of benefit for maximizing uremic toxin clearance.[35] The answer is not known.

RRT: MODALITIES

The coupling of adequate solute and UF control with satisfactory patient outcomes are the goals of RRT. Practical issues that include nursing scheduling and

TABLE 31–1 Comparison of the RRT modalities.

Modality	1° Mode of Clearance	BFR cc/min	Dialysate	RF	Anticoagulation	Time
IHD	Diffusion	250-400	Yes	No	Short heparin	3-4 h
SLEDD	Diffusion	100-200	Yes	No	Long heparin	8-24 h
CVVH	Convection	200-300	No	Yes	Continuous heparin/citrate	24 h
CVVHD	Both	200-300	Yes	Yes	Continuous Heparin/citrate	24 h
SCUF	Convection	100-200	No	No	Long heparin/citrate	Variable

BFR, blood flow rate; CVVH, continuous venovenous hemofiltration; CVVHD, continuous venovenous hemodiafiltration; IHD, intermittent hemodialysis; RF, replacement fluid; SCUF, sustained continuous ultrafiltration; SLEDD, sustained low-efficiency daily dialysis. Data from Schortgen F, Soubrier N, Delclaux C, et al: Hemodynamic tolerance of intermittent hemodialysis in critically ill patients: usefulness of practice guidelines, *Am J Respir Crit Care Med* 2000 Jul;162(1):197-202.

cost are coupled to the patient's presentation when selecting the RRT modality (Table 31–1).

Peritoneal dialysis

In North America, peritoneal dialysis (PD) was extensively used into the 1990s to treat AKI in the ICU.[36] PD requires placement of an intra-abdominal catheter, with continuous exchanges of high dextrose dialysate into the abdominal cavity. PD, therefore, is a continuous RRT. The high osmolarity dextrose generates UF, and hemodynamically it tends to fare better than IHD. Catheters were temporarily placed at the bedside by nephrologists, or Tenckhoff catheters were placed by surgeons. In the following decades, acute PD was largely abandoned due to inefficient solute clearance, infection concerns, and its contraindication in patients with abdominal problems or recent surgery. PD may also be difficult in ventilated patients or in severe obstructive lung disease.

Recently, the modality has been reassessed in the ICU setting, where the use of high-volume PD was examined.[37] One study which excluded severely hypercatabolic patients, had few complications (7.5%) and 12% had peritonitis. In certain critically ill patients, PD may be a viable alternative,[37] where its characteristic continuous slow clearance may better suit patients with elevated ICP.[38]

Intermittent Hemodialysis

This is essentially conventional outpatient dialysis averaging 4 hours, 3 times per week, with blood flow rates (BFR) up to 400 cc/min. Due to the higher BFR

and dialysate flow rates (DFRs) it is more likely to induce hypotension than other modalities. Therefore, the traditional arguments against using IHD in the ICU have been relatively less hemodynamic stability and clearance compared to continuous RRT. Furthermore, IHD is also a concern in situations where rapid changes in solute (sodium or potassium) or osmoles (elevated ICP) can be detrimental (see below). Financially, the use of roller blood pumps and rapid clearance requires skilled dialysis nursing, increasing costs.

Earlier studies demonstrated IHD a hemodynamic risk compared to continuous RRT (CRRT). Since then, advancements such as in-line bicarbonate baths and biocompatible membranes have improved IHD stability.[30,39] Presently, IHD is the most commonly selected RRT in American ICUs, utilized in 57% of cases.[40]

Furthermore, in the severely ill, nephrologists can improvise IHD by slowing BFR, increasing hours and/or increasing its use to 6 d/wk. This increases net clearance while maintaining hemodynamic stability, essentially becoming sustained low-efficiency daily dialysis (SLEDD) (see later). What's more, adding a separate UF procedure (blood through the dialyzer without counter current dialysate, excising diffusion), facilitates volume removal with less hypotension. UF is better tolerated when solute and osmole clearance is not concomitant.

In the critically ill requiring the use of vasopressor agents, IHD may still be attempted by increasing the dose of the vasopressor as needed. The suggested guidelines in Table 31–2 can largely be met by most institutions.

TABLE 31–2 Guidelines for IHD in critically ill patients.[a]

- Biocompatible, modified cellulosic membranes (not cuprophane)
- Connect both sides of circuit simultaneously with .9% saline at start
- Adjust dialysate sodium at 145, calcium 1.5 mmol/L
- Limit maximum blood flow to 150 mL/min
- Increase time on dialysis and/or days per week (6 days per week)
- Dialysate temperature ≤ 37°C
- Stop vasodilators; increase vasopressors as needed
- Start with dialysis and then continue with ultrafiltration alone
- Ultrapure water

[a]Adapted from Schortgen F, Soubrier N, Delclaux C, et al. Hemodynamic tolerance of intermittent hemodialysis in critically ill patients: usefulness of practice guidelines. *Am J Respir Crit Care Med.* 2000;162:197-202.

Continuous Renal Replacement Therapy

Continuous modalities (see Table 31–1) are considered in hemodynamically unstable patients less likely to tolerate abrupt fluid shifts associated with IHD. CRRT is distinguished by lower BFR, allowing for greater stability in treating fluid overload. Indeed, fluid accumulation is more likely seen with IHD than CRRT.[33] Also, acidosis and volume control are more consistent with CRRT. Both convective and diffusion modes of solute clearance can be utilized depending on CRRT type. Surprisingly, outcome benefits of CRRT over IHD have not been demonstrated.

Patients for which CRRT is preferred include those with hypotension as in severe sepsis, cirrhosis, liver transplant, and congestive heart failure (CHF). It also benefits patients with markedly elevated BUN and/or ICP due to gradual solute removal avoiding disequilibrium.

As implied, CRRT is administered continuously for as long as required. In actuality, due to interruptions for diagnostic and/or therapeutic interventions treatment time is closer to 18 hours. The long duration on the CRRT circuit cools the blood, resulting in reflexive vasoconstriction supporting hemodynamics.[41] CRRT can be used in operating rooms during prolonged procedures such as liver transplantation, and requires frequent hemodynamic, laboratory and electrolyte assessments.

Continuous Arteriovenous Hemofiltration

Arteriovenous modalities (continuous arteriovenous hemofiltration [CAVH] and continuous arteriovenous hemodialysis [CAVHD]) required placement of catheters in an artery and central vein. This system utilized the patient's arterial pressure rather than a rolling pump for blood flow. CAVH is rarely used since the advent of continuous venovenous hemofiltration (CVVH) due to more invasive arterial access, variable BFR, and increased filter clotting issues.

CVVH

Essentially through convection, clearance is dependent on large UF rates. To maintain hemodynamic and electrolyte stability large volumes (between 1 and 3 L/h) of electrolyte solutions are necessary. Frequent close attention to volume and electrolyte status is essential. Effluent flow is reported as mL/kg/h. The difference between infused volume and UF generated is the net fluid balance. Recent studies have not demonstrated superiority of a particular flow over another.[29]

REPLACEMENT FLUIDS:—Replacement fluids (RFs) are provided as prefilled sterilized bags by the equipment manufacturer. They have varying concentrations of sodium, magnesium, calcium, and potassium, and allow for modification. Either bicarbonate or lactate is the alkali source. Ideally, lactate-based RF should be avoided in liver failure and/or lactic acidosis, and periodic lactate measurements are needed with bicarbonate replacement when higher than 5 mmol/L.[42] Bicarbonate has become the buffer of choice despite issues with storage and preparation.

The RF with the added clearance of solute has effects on blood composition and requires periodic monitoring of blood chemistries. It is added either before the dialyzer (predilution/inflow) or after blood has passed through the dialyzer (postdilution/outflow).

Predilution RF lowers (dilutes) solute concentration and theoretically decreases CVVH clearance efficiency. The UF is not 100% saturated with urea having been diluted by RF prior to passage through the dialyzer/filter. Advantages lie in requirements of low BFR and less clotting of circuit also due to the dilutional effect of the RF.

In *postdilution* outflow mode, UF rate should not be more than 20% of BFR to avoid excess hemoconcentration and clotting of the circuit. This requires higher BFR of 150 to 200 mL/min to achieve adequate fluid removal in excess of 25 L/d. Predilution inflow overcomes this problem at the expense of clearance efficiency but overall better treatment due to less clotting and more fluid processed for UF generation.[43] As an example, 35 L of daily replacement fluid addition in predilution/inflow mode dilutes the blood by 15% at a BFR of 140 mL/min. (35 L/d = 24 mL/min; 24/140 + 24 = 15%).

Continuous Venovenous Hemodiafiltration

Diffusion is now introduced enhancing clearance, by running dialysate countercurrent to blood flow in the extracorporeal circuit. As a combined modality, it requires large volumes of RF in maintaining hemodynamic and electrolyte stability. Again, close attention to the volume and electrolyte status is essential. Comparing CVVH to continuous venovenous hemodiafiltration (CVVHDF) meta-analysis has failed to show any benefit in mortality, renal recovery, vasopressor use, or organ failure.[44]

Anticoagulation

All RRT requires anticoagulation to avoid circuit clotting that can result in blood loss, fluid administration to flush the circuit, and minimize blood loss. Treatment disruption to replace the circuit, associated costs for dialyzer and line changes, and resource utilization of personnel, since many institutions mandate dialysis staff to replace circuits. Due to lower BFRs, CRRT have higher clotting risks than IHD.

As in IHD, heparin is the preferred anticoagulant. It is intravenous (IV) bolus administered in the venous line, 2000 to 5000 units, allowing a few minutes to mix. Maintenance is 500 to1000 units/h infused by roller pump into the arterial line. Partial thromboplastin time (PTT) is measured via arterial and venous lines every 6 hours to maintain PTT 40 to 45 or greater than 65, respectively.

In patients with heparin-induced thrombocytopenia direct thrombin inhibitors are used.[45] Argatroban is preferred in renal patients at 0.5 to 1 µg/kg/min,

due to its liver metabolism.[46] Lepirudin is renal eliminated and may be administered as bolus or infusion (0.005-0.025 mg/kg/h). A target activated partial thromboplastin time (aPTT) greater than 1.5 to 2 times normal avoids excessive bleeding and ensures anticoagulation. Fresh frozen plasma is employed for reversal of bleeding attributed to these direct thrombin inhibitors.

Anticoagulation should be reviewed daily between intensivist and nephrologist, and if contraindicated, heparin-free treatments are possible. In SLEDD periodic, every 15 to 30 minutes, saline flushes are instituted. In CVVH, RF is infused prefilter to avoid hemoconcentration.[47] Heparin-free extracorporeal circuits on average clot over 8 hours. Decrease in dialysate/serum BUN levels to less than 0.6 may indicate imminent clotting.

Regional citrate avoids systemic anticoagulation, and is superior in circuit survival and bleeding complications.[9] Citrate can be administered either before or after blood has been exposed to the filter. Commercially available solutions include ACD-A which has 3% trisodium citrate, citric acid, and dextrose. Using calcium-free RF decreases the amount of citrate required for anticoagulation. Periodic assessment of bicarbonate levels and ionized Calcium (iCA), both from the extracorporeal circuit and patient, is mandatory to avoid serious hypocalcemia. The citrate administration or calcium supplementation is titrated to keep the postfilter iCA between 1.21 and 1.45 mmol/L. Infusion of calcium into circuit avoids delivery of hypocalcemic blood to patient. Citrate toxicity can be a concern in patients with liver disease or lactic acidosis.[48]

Staffing CRRT requires intense attention to patient care, necessitating one-to-one nurse-to-patient ratios. Elevating the head of the bed or turning the patient can compromise flow and risk clotting, making positioning an issue. In the case of femoral access, better flow is obtained in the supine position.[47] Also, some institutions require hemodialysis staff to assist at CRRT commencement, interruption, or termination.

Equipment CVVH equipment is smaller in size since water purification filters in RRT requiring dialysate (IHD, CVVHDF, or SLEDD) are not necessary. The basic operating principle is similar to IHD as a blood pump is utilized to circulate blood through the dialyzer/filter to generate UF (see Figure 31–3). CVVH machines are now equipped with temperature regulation mechanisms resulting in added hemodynamic effects of vasoconstriction at lower temperatures. The febrile response to infection can therefore be missed. Despite impressive advancements in practicality and compactness of machines, it is still necessary to interrupt CRRT for transportation.

Access Any preexisting ESRD access can be utilized for CRRT. In AKI requires placement of a double-lumen catheter in either the femoral or internal jugular (IJ) vein regardless of RRT. These catheters have staggered openings allowing blood flow out from the patient via the proximal (insertion site) opening and return via the distal opening. This arrangement diminishes the degree of mixing or recirculation, and hence, inefficiency.

In general, site selection for catheter placement follows similar risks such as bleeding and infection. Subclavian and left IJ veins are avoided when possible due to the angulation necessary for proper placement and flow. The stiffer catheter risks vessel injury, compromising blood flow and clotting. Furthermore, the subclavian catheter can cause stenosis resulting in high venous pressures, making the creation of a permanent AV access difficult. Up to 14% of AKI patients may need permanent chronic dialysis.[5,8]

Sustained Low-Efficiency Daily Dialysis

Also called extended dialysis (ED), it is a hybrid of CRRT and IHD. It is increasingly utilized throughout the world,[49] as well as in the United States, where about 25% of ICU providers reported using SLEDD in 2007.[40]

SLEDD generally runs daily for 8 to 10 hours with low DFR (200-400 cc/min) and BFR (150-200 cc/min). It can utilize the IHD machinery with added software to support a lower BFR allowing for a more gradual solute and/or fluid removal. Time on SLEDD can be extended up to 24 hours, to provide for greater clearance according to perceived needs by providers.[50] The filters have smaller surface areas (1 m² compared with 1.5 m² for IHD), lower UF coefficients (10 mL/h/mm of Hg compared with 45), and lower K0As (maximal theoretical clearance of dialyzer of 600 mL/min compared with 1000 mL/min), but are similarly composed of polysulfone.

SLEDD's hybrid properties support hemodynamics, enhance clearance, and increase convenience while lowering costs. This, as well as its versatility, accounts for a rising popularity.[49] For instance, it often is utilized overnight (nocturnal dialysis) when the probability for interruption from procedures or radiologic examinations is less likely. Such maneuvers better guarantee the prescribed dialysis without interruption. Still another important benefit is the decreased need for heparin, not being continuous.

Most importantly, these benefits come without compromising outcomes in AKI as compared to CRRT.[49] In a recent study,[50] the net 24-hour UF and fluid balances were similar between CVVH and SLEDD, as were hypotensive episodes. Furthermore, SLEDD was associated with a fewer days on mechanical ventilation and in the ICU.

Sustained Continuous UF and Fluid Removal in Severe CHF

Though technically not RRT, extracorporeal modalities for UF are considered in severe CHF with diuretic resistance. In such patients renal impairment is not the overwhelming reason to initiate sustained continuous UF (SCUF) but rather as an alternative to diuretics. To date various studies, the UNLOAD and others, have not demonstrated any renal or length-of-stay advantages.[51] SCUF should probably be relegated to patients who failed medical therapy and are awaiting cardiac transplant (see Table 31–1).[52]

Dosing

Unfortunately, significant questions involving RRT, namely the exact clearance provided, how much is necessary and when to provide it are poorly understood. Dosing should indicate a measured effectiveness of the ridding of waste products from a given volume of blood.[14] Urea kinetic modeling, which is ESRD based, is questionable in assessing efficacy in the critically ill, given their increased catabolism and urea Vd.[14,26]

Treatment dosing (volume of fluid processed) utilizes urea generation (g) over 24 hours (the difference in BUN levels 24 hours apart + loss in urine in nonoliguric AKI) as a marker, divided by the target

BUN (g/L). For a 60-kg individual, water compartment is 33 L (0.55% of body weight). Total body urea = BUN level in g/L X's body water (add edema volume to this). The difference between 2 values 24 hours apart + urine loss of urea is total urea generation (g) in 24 hours. If urea production is 16 g/d and target BUN is 40 mg/dL (0.4 g/L), 16/0.4, 40 L of fluid needs to be processed to achieve the clearance and maintain BUN at 40 mg/dL. This however is not generally done when utilizing these modalities. In fact most providers are uncertain of prescribed dosing.[53]

Past RRT trials have not used urea clearance as a study goal. Guidelines suggest a CRRT KT/V of 3.9/wk or an effluent volume of 20 to 25 mL/Kg/h.[54] To achieve this a higher prescription of 25 to 30 mL/kg/h may be necessary. What's more, CVVHDF studies suggest using doses at 35 mL/kg/h.

Antibiotic Management The most common cause of AKI in the ICU remains sepsis[8] and despite advances, the mortality has not appreciably improved.[3,6,13,29] Though the reasons are likely multifactorial, recent attention on antibiotic (AB) dosing during RRT has identified an important shortcoming (Table 31–3).[55] High-flux membranes with larger surface areas and increased time on RRT (CRRT or SLEDD) remove ABs more efficiently compared to IHD. In these forms of RRT, eGFR provided may be up to 30 mL/min and as many as 25% of patients are not making pharmacokinetic targets.[55] Furthermore, difficulties in dosing are further compounded when considering modality variability and intermittent usage.[56] Given data supporting improved mortality with adequate AB dosing, this is a legitimate concern for septic patients on RRT.

SELECTION OF RRT: SPECIAL CONSIDERATIONS
Avoiding Rapid Changes in Osmolarity and Electrolyte Levels

In patients with hemodynamic uncertainty it may be prudent to select a modality other than IHD. However, there are at least 3 scenarios where a gradual clearance rate may be wise even with hemodynamic stability: in the setting of acute coronary syndromes, elevated ICPs or hypo/hypernatremia. In such cases the issue is avoiding an abrupt solute or osmole change rather than hemodynamics.

Rapid decline of potassium levels in ESRD patients with acute myocardial infarction (MI) may increase the risk for arrhythmias.[57] Longer RRT time with lower BFR achieves a gradual safer decrease in potassium levels. Continuous RRT is ideal for such a presentation.

In patients with raised ICP or its potential, standard IHD should be avoided. Abrupt decreases in urea with resultant fluid shifts in the central nervous system (CNS) can result in worsening cerebral edema. Similarly, gradual decreases in urea concentration using continuous, sustained, or peritoneal dialysis are better tolerated.[38] These modalities also provide some insurance against hypotensive episodes, which by lowering cerebral perfusion pressure adds to the injury. Here too, if other modalities are not available, IHD slowed down to BFR of 150 to 200 cc/h as discussed earlier should be sufficient.

Finally, rapid normalization of sodium levels in patients with hyper- or hyponatremia can induce central pontine myelinolysis and/or edema.

TABLE 31–3 Suggestions to consider when antibiotics (ABs) are to be used.[a]

1. ABs are either time dependent (TD) or concentration dependent (CD) and should be approached and adjusted accordingly.
2. For TD ABs (beta-lactams, linezolid, vancomycin, erythromycin) increase the frequency of the dose to maintain levels. In TD ABs, it is the time spent above the MIC that is crucial.
3. For CD ABs (fluoroquinolones, aminoglycosides, metronidazole, daptomycin, colistin) increasing the dose maintains levels. In CD ABs it is desirable to have high peaks and low troughs to enhance bactericidal activity while diminishing toxicity.
4. The Vd in AKI is altered, often higher than normal. It may be preferable to give the first 1 or 2 doses as if the patient's renal function is normal, then adjust to function. In CRRT assume creatinine clearances of 30 cc/min.
5. Use therapeutic monitoring where possible.
6. Other systems such as ECMO and nonoliguric patients may increase AB clearances.

[a]Data from Eyler RF, Mueller BA: Antibiotic dosing in critically ill patients with acute kidney injury, *Nat Rev Nephrol* 2011:7:226–235; Connor, Jr. M, Salem C, Bauer, S, et al: Therapeutic Drug Monitoring of Piperacillin-Tazobactam using Spent Dialysate Effluent in Patients Receiving Continuous Venovenous Hemodialysis, *Antimicrob Agents Chemother* 2011:55:557-560.

Likewise, dialysis disequilibrium syndrome is due to rapid reduction of high urea levels. Use of gradual RRT, close monitoring, and intravascular fluids can help guarantee safe normalization.

Endotoxin Removal

There are multiple systems studying endotoxin removal in sepsis such as high-volume hemofiltration and hemoperfusion with polymyxin B embedded polystyrene absorbing surfaces. One issue of controversy is that anti-inflammatory cytokines and factors are removed as well.[58] Small studies have shown decreases in cytokines with inconsistent outcome effects.[59]

RRT OUTCOMES: MORTALITY, RENAL RECOVERY, AND COST

Renal Recovery

In general, AKI patients requiring RRT recover significant renal function, not requiring chronic dialysis. However, up to 14%, primarily those with baseline CKD, will continue RRT.[5,8] Recently, Wald et al[60] demonstrated that dialysis-requiring AKI was associated with an increased risk for later ESRD (adjusted heart rate [HR] 3.2; 95% confidence interval [CI] 2.7-3.9) compared with controls matched for age, gender, CKD status, need for mechanical ventilation, and a propensity score for dialysis-requiring AKI.

As to the benefits of one RRT modality versus another in supporting renal recovery, CRRT may be preferred. The suggestion is that better hemodynamic control, solute clearance, and maintenance of acid-base, may be more natural with CRRT. Though not seen in all studies, a recent review of 16 observational and 7 randomized controlled trials (RCTs) suggests CRRT benefits renal recovery (relative risk IHD vs CRRT of 1.73, $P = 0.02$).[61] Significance was not seen when limiting the study to RCTs, and does not distinguish SLEDD from IHD. If this leads to less ESRD, then the use of CRRT may benefit quality of life as well as long-term costs.[62]

Cost

RRT is one of the most expensive interventions used in an already cost burdensome ICU setting.[62]

Cost is primarily personnel, whose need is largely related to the selected modality's degree of complexity. Furthermore, RRT patients inevitably have longer lengths of stay.[5] CRRT modalities being the most complicated and requiring the most supplies (replacement fluid, tubing, etc) are the most expensive, by as much as thousands of dollars per week.[9] Of the RRTs, a number of studies have indicated SLEDD to be the least expensive, largely due to decreased nursing needs.[50]

Mortality and Outcomes

ICU patients with AKI requiring RRT have a higher mortality than other ICU patients including those with ESRD or AKI without need for RRT.[6,8] Despite over 35 years of experience and improvements,[2,30,39] there still remains an unfortunate mortality of between 25% and 50%.[3,6,10,13,29]

The long-standing controversy is whether CRRT is superior to IHD in regards to mortality. At present the predominant evidence, randomized trials, and meta-analyses, do not support a mortality benefit for CRRT.[9] Still the recent KDIGO AKI guidelines prefer CRRT (level 2 recommendation), over IHD, for hemodynamically unstable patients.[54] What's more, there does not seem to be a mortality advantage with larger delivered clearance doses.[9,13,29] Palevsky reviewed 2 cohorts of AKI patients receiving RRT, one attaining a higher intensity and therefore higher RRT dose compared to a second lower dose; no mortality advantage was demonstrated.[13] Similarly, higher CVVH doses have not demonstrated any mortality benefits (Table 31-4).[29]

Shortcomings: What Explains These Shortcomings is Likely Multifactorial

First the modalities themselves: Closer monitoring is vital. In the Palevsky study, which demonstrated a lack of benefit with intense RRT, it is notable that there was a greater need for vasopressor support in this group despite the use of continuous RRT.[13] Moreover, there was significantly more hypokalemia and hypophosphatemia. The latter also seen in the higher UF group of the RENAAL study.[29] In the critically ill, electrolyte abnormalities and/or their rapidity[57] may result in morbidity and even mortality (Table 31-5).

TABLE 31–4 General summary of various aspects of RRT management and potential risks.

1. Early, nonemergent, RRT should be considered in azotemic, oliguric patients with AKI and a high acuity level not likely to timely improve.
   a. Increased consideration made for evidence of CKD and volume overload.
   b. Consider continuous or slowed modalities in severe electrolyte disturbances, azotemia, and in patients with possible elevated ICP.
2. Inadvertent removal and underdosing of antibiotics or other therapeutic agents.
   a. Adjust antibiotics.
   b. Other catheter systems such as ECMO may also increase clearances.
3. Depletion of trace nutrients, adjustment in protein dosing.
   a. Protein restriction should not be used to prevent the need for RRT.
   b. Once RRT begins daily protein intake should return to the suggested needs in critically ill patients without AKI. (1.5 g/kg/d; up to 1.7 g/kg in CRRT).
   c. Protein increases reflect: improved clearances; hypercatabolism; and losses that accrue during RRT.
4. Depletion of electrolytes.
   a. Frequent monitoring in CRRT is important for proper supplementation. In the SLEDD modalities electrolytes should be checked every 4 hours.
   b. Adjustments in the concentrations of electrolytes can be made in the dialysate and/or total parenteral nutrition (TPN) where applicable, to avoid repeated supplemental infusions.
5. Bleeding and need for continuous anticoagulation (see text).
6. Avoid errors in volume management.
   a. This is an important issue and daily changes need discussion between intensivist and nephrologist when calculating the new "dose" of RRT and net UF necessary.
7. Errors can occur in the compounding of replacement fluid or dialysate by local hospital pharmacies or in the addition of additives by bedside nursing staff.
8. Errors can occur in the compounding of fluids for CRRT.

Secondly, the process itself: the water in the dialysate, catheter and tubing plastic, and dialyzers are all capable of initiating inflammatory responses. Modifying dialysate water to ultrapure status, for instance can decrease inflammation and morbidity.[63] Finally as discussed earlier, better attention to antibiotic dosing is needed.

Thirdly, it may be that even with all these RRTs, present clearances are simply inadequate in the severely critically ill patient. Recent data demonstrate eGFR rising up by 40%, and over 130 cc/min in some critically ill patients.[64] Critically ill patients may need elevated clearances to help them survive their catabolic state, where the uremic toxin burden may be high.[16] RRT modalities at best approach 30 cc/min or stage 4 CKD. Data that more intense RRT does not improve outcomes further support this.[13] Even with higher-intensity RRT, our attempts may not even begin to provide what is needed.

RRT: FUTURE

Reviewing the shortcomings of present RRT systems prompts possible future research endeavors to optimize present systems. These include pharmacokinetic studies, improved biocompatible materials, and possibly water purification. Improving monitoring accuracy is also needed to minimize electrolyte and hemodynamic deficits.

Care in the design of proper future studies[65] is also paramount to understand outcomes. Biomarkers of AKI such as cystatin need to be studied to not only assess earlier response but if RRT is necessary. Recognition of the important consequences of AKI appears to be at hand and has prompted research in these areas.

TABLE 31–5 Outcome benefits.

Cost	[a]SLEDD
Elevated ICP	[b]CRRT, SLEDD, [c]PD
Hyperkalemia; hyper/hyponatremia	CRRT, SLEDD, PD
Volume control/hemodynamics	CRRT, SLEDD
Mortality	Comparable

[a]SLEDD, sustained low-efficiency daily dialysis.
[b]CRRT, continuous renal replacement therapy.
[c]PD, peritoneal dialysis.

REFERENCES

1. Smith LH, Post RS, Teschan PE, et al. Post-traumatic renal insufficiency in military casualties. II. Management, use of artificial kidney, prognosis. *Am J Med.* 1955:18:187-198.

2. Kramer P, Wigger W, Reiger J, Matthaei D, Scheler F. Arteriovenous haemofiltration: a new and simple method for treatment of over hydrated patients resistant to diuretics. *Klin Wochenschr.* 1977;55:1121-1122.

3. Hsu RK, McCulloch CE, Dudley RA, Lo LJ, Hsu CY. Temporal changes in incidence of dialysis-requiring AKI. *J Am Soc Nephrol.* 2013;24(1):37-42.

4. Collins AJ, Foley RN, Chavers B, et al. United States Renal Data System 2011 Annual Data Report: atlas of chronic kidney disease and end-stage renal disease in the United States. *Am J Kidney Dis.* 2012;59(suppl 1):A7, e1-e420.

5. Liangos O, Wald R, O'Bell JW, et al. Epidemiology and outcomes of acute renal failure in hospitalized patients: a national survey. *Clin J Am Soc Nephrol.* 2006;1:43-51.

6. Strijack B, Mojica J, Sood M, et al. Outcomes of chronic dialysis patients admitted to the intensive care unit. *J Am Soc Nephrol.* 2009;20:2441-2447.

7. Coritsidis G, Guru K, Ward L, Bashir R, Feinfeld DA, Carvounis CP. Differences in prediction of acute renal failure in medical and surgical intensive care patients. *Ren Fail.* 2000;22:235-244.

8. Uchino S, Kellum JA, Bellomo R, et al. Acute renal failure in critically patients: a multinational, multicenter study. *JAMA.* 2005;294:813-818.

9. Pannu N, Klarenbach S, Wiebe N, et al. For the Alberta kidney disease network. Renal replacement therapy in patients with acute renal failure: a systematic review. *JAMA.* 2008;299(7):793-805.

10. Ympa YP, Sakr Y, Reinhart K, et al. Has mortality from acute renal failure decreased? A systemic review of the literature. *Am J Med.* 2005;118:827-832.

11. Van Berendoncks AM, Elseviers MM, Lins RL; SHARF Study Group. Long-term follow-up. *Clin J Am Soc Nephrol.* 2010;5:1755-1762.

12. Mehta RL, McDonald B, Gabbai F, et al. Nephrology consultation in acute renal failure: does timing matter? *Am J Med.* 2002;113:456-461.

13. Palevsky PM, Zhang JH, O'Connor TZ, et al. Intensity of renal support in critically ill patients with acute kidney injury. *N Engl J Med.* 2008;359:7-20.

14. Ricci Z, Ronco C. Dose and efficiency of renal replacement therapy: continuous renal replacement therapy versus intermittent hemodialysis versus slow extended daily dialysis. *Crit Care Med.* 2008;36(suppl 4):S229-S237.

15. Daugirdas JT, Van Stone JC. Physiologic principles and urea kinetic modeling. In: Daugirdas JT, Blake PG, Ing TS, eds. *Handbook of Dialysis.* 3rd ed. Philadelphia, PA: Lippincott, Williams & Wilkins; 2001:15-45.

16. Meyer TW, Hostetter TH. Uremia. *N Engl J Med.* 2007;357:1316-1325.

17. Hutchison CA, Crowe AV, Stevens PE, Harrison DA, Lipkin GW. Case mix, outcome and activity for patients admitted to intensive care units requiring chronic renal dialysis: a secondary analysis of the ICNARC Case Mix Programme Database. *Crit Care.* 2007;11:R50.

18. Bellomo R, Wan L, Langenberg C, Ishikawa K, May CN. Septic acute kidney injury: the glomerular arterioles. *Contrib Nephrol.* 2011;174:98-107.

19. Coca SG, Peixoto AJ, Garg AX, Krumholz HM, Parikh CR. The prognostic importance of a small acute decrement in kidney function in hospitalized patients: a systematic review and meta-analysis. *Am J Kidney Dis.* 2007;50:712-720.

20. Thakar CV, Rousseau J, Leonard AC. Timing of dialysis initiation in AKI in ICU: international survey. *Crit Care.* 2012;16:R237.

21. Faubel S. Have we reached the limit of mortality benefit with our approach to renal replacement therapy in acute kidney injury? *Am J Kidney Dis.* 2013;62:1030-1033.

22. Karvellas CJ, Farhat MR, Sajjad I, et al. A comparison of early versus late initiation of renal replacement therapy in critically ill patients with acute kidney injury: a systematic review and meta-analysis. *Crit Care.* 2011;15:R72.

23. Gaudry S, Hajage D, Schortgen F, Martin-Lefevre L, Pons B, Boulet E, Boyer A, Chevrel G, Lerolle N, Carpentier D, et al. Initiation strategies for renal-replacement therapy in the intensive care unit. *N Engl J Med.* 2016;375(2):122-33

24. Zarbock A, Kellum JA, Schmidt C, Van Aken H, Wempe C, Pavenstadt H, Boanta A, Gerss J, Meersch M. Effect of early vs delayed initiation of renal replacement therapy on mortality in critically ill patients with acute kidney injury: the ELAIN randomized clinical trial. *JAMA.* 2016;315(20):2190–9

25. Bagshaw SM, Uchino S, Kellum JA, et al. Association between renal replacement therapy in critically ill patients with severe acute kidney injury and mortality. *J Crit Care.* 2013;28:1011-1018.

26. Waikar SS, Bonventre J. Can we rely on blood urea nitrogen as a biomarker to determine when to initiate dialysis? *Clin J Am Soc Nephrol.* 2006;1:903-904.

27. Liu KD, Himmelfarb J, Paganini E, et al. Timing of initiation of dialysis in critically ill patients with acute kidney injury. *Clin J Am Soc Nephrol.* 2006;1:915-919.

28. Bagshaw SM, Uchino S, Bellomo R, et al. Timing of renal replacement therapy and clinical outcomes in critically ill patients with severe acute kidney injury. *J Crit Care.* 2009;24:129-140.

29. RENAL Replacement Therapy Study Investigators, Bellomo R, Cass A. Intensity of continuous renal-replacement therapy in critically ill patients. *N Engl J Med.* 2009;361:1627-1638.

30. Hakim RM, Wingard RL, Parker RA. Effect of the dialysis membrane in the treatment of patients with acute renal failure. *N Engl J Med.* 1994;17:1338-1342.

31. Bouchard J, Soroko SB, Chertow GM, et al. Fluid accumulation, survival and recovery of kidney function in critically ill patients with acute kidney injury. *Kidney Int.* 2009;76:422-427.

32. Payen D, de Pont AC, Sakr Y, et al. A positive fluid balance is associated with a worse outcome in patients with acute renal failure. *Crit Care.* 2008;12:R74.

33. Sutherland SM, Zappitelli M, Alexander SR, et al. Fluid overload and mortality in children receiving continuous renal replacement therapy: the prospective pediatric continuous renal replacement therapy registry. *Am J Kidney Dis.* 2010;55:316-325.

34. Vaara ST, Korhonen AM, Kaukonen KM, et al. Fluid overload is associated with an increased risk for 90-day mortality in critically ill patients with renal replacement therapy: data from the prospective FINNAKI study. *Crit Care.* 2012;16:R197.

35. Vanholder R, Baurmeister U, Brunet P, Cohen G, Glorieux G, Jankowski J; European Uremic Toxin Work Group. A bench to bedside view of uremic toxins. *J Am Soc Nephrol.* 2008;19:863-870.

36. Siddiqui NF, Coca SG, Devereaux PJ, et al. Secular trends in acute dialysis after elective major surgery—1995 to 2009. *CMAJ.* 2012;184(11):1237-1245.

37. Ponce D, Berbel MN, Regina de Goes C, et al. High volume peritoneal dialysis in acute kidney injury: indications and limitations. *Clin J Am Soc Nephrol.* 2012;7:887-894.

38. Davenport A. Practical guidance for dialyzing a hemodialysis patient following acute brain injury. *Hemodial Int.* 2008;12:307-312.

39. Schortgen F, Soubrier N, Delclaux C, et al. Hemodynamic tolerance of intermittent hemodialysis in critically ill patients: usefulness of practice guidelines. *Am J Respir Crit Care Med.* 2000;162:197-202.

40. Overberger P, Pesacreta M, Palevsky PM; VA/NIH Acute Renal Failure Trial Network. Management of renal replacement therapy in acute kidney injury: a survey of practitioner prescribing practices. *Clin J Am Soc Nephrol.* 2007;2:623-630.

41. Yagi N, Leblanc M, Sakai K, et al. Cooling effect of continuous renal replacement therapy in critically ill patients. *Am J Kidney Dis.* 1998;32:1023-1030.

42. Barenbrock M, Hausberg M, Matzkies F, de la Motte S, Schaefer RM. Effects of bicarbonate- and lactate-buffered replacement fluids on cardiovascular outcome in CVVH patients. *Kidney Int.* 2000;58(4):1751-1757.

43. Uchino S, Fealy N, Baldwin I, Morimatsu H, Bellomo R. Pre-dilution vs. post-dilution during continuous veno-venous hemofiltration: impact on filter life and azotemic control. *Nephron Clin Pract.* 2003;94(4):c94-c98.

44. Friedrich JO, Wald R, Bagshaw SM, Burns KE, Adhikari NK. Hemofiltration compared to hemodialysis for acute kidney injury: systematic review and meta-analysis. *Crit Care.* 2012;16:R146.

45. Steinfeldt T, Rolfes C. Heparin induced thrombocytopenia and anticoagulation in renal replacement therapy. *Anasthesiol Intensivmed Notfallmed Schmerzther.* 2008;43(4):304-310; quiz 312.

46. Reddy BV, Grossman EJ, Trevino SA, Hursting MJ, Murray PT. Argatroban anticoagulation in patients with heparin-induced thrombocytopenia requiring renal replacement therapy. *Ann Pharmacother.* 2005;39(10):1601-1605.

47. Joannidis M, Oudemans-van Straaten HM. Clinical review: patency of the circuit in continuous renal replacement therapy. *Crit Care.* 2007;11(4):218.

48. Zhang Z, Hongying N. Efficacy and safety of regional citrate anticoagulation in critically ill patients undergoing continuous renal replacement therapy. *Intensive Care Med.* 2012;38(1):20-28.

49. Fliser D, Kielstein JT. Technology insight: treatment of renal failure in the intensive care unit with extended dialysis. *Nat Clin Pract Nephrol.* 2006;2:32-39.

50. Schwenger V, Weigand MA, Hoffman O, et al. Sustained low efficiency dialysis using single batch system in acute kidney injury—a randomized interventional trial: the REnal Replacement Therapy in Intensive Care Unit PatiEnts. *Crit Care.* 2012;16:R140.

51. Costanzo MR, Guglin ME, Saltzberg MT, et al; UNLOAD Trial Investigators. Ultrafiltration versus intravenous diuretics for patients hospitalized for acute decompensated heart failure. *J Am Coll Cardiol.* 2007;49:675-683.

52. Adams KF, Lindenfield J, Arnold JMO, et al. Executive summary: HFSA 2006 comprehensive heart failure practice guideline. *J Card Fail.* 2006;12:29-32.

53. Ricci Z, Ronco C, D'amico G, et al. Practice patterns in the management of acute renal failure in the critically ill patient: an international survey. *Nephrol Dial Transplant.* 2006;21:690-696.

54. KDIGO Clinical Practice Guideline for Acute Kidney Injury. Kidney International Supplements (2012) 2, 1; doi:10.1038/kisup.2012.1

55. Seyler L, Cotton F, Taccone FS, et al. Recommended beta-lactam regimens are inadequate in septic patients treated with continuous renal replacement therapy. *Crit Care.* 2011;15:R137.

56. Bogard KN, Peterson NT, Plumb TJ, et al. Antibiotic dosing during sustained low-efficiency dialysis: special considerations in adult critically ill patients. *Crit Care Med.* 2011;39:560-570.

57. Coritsidis GN, Dharmeshkumar S, Gupta G, et al. Does timing of dialysis in ESRD patients with acute myocardial infarcts affect morbidity or mortality? *Clin J Am Soc Nephrol.* 2009;4:1302-1311.

58. Pertosa G, Grandaliano G, Loreto G, et al. Clinical relevance of cytokine production in hemodialysis. *Kidney Int.* 2000;58(suppl 76):S104-S111.

59. Payen D, Mateo J, Cavaillon JM, et al. Impact of continuous venovenous hemofiltration on organ failure during the early phase of severe sepsis: a randomized controlled trial. *Crit Care Med.* 2009;37:803-810.

60. Wald R, Quinn RR, Luo J, et al. Chronic dialysis and death among survivors of acute kidney injury requiring dialysis. *JAMA.* 2009;302:1179-1185.

61. Schneider AG, Bellomo R, Bagshaw SM, Glassford NJ, Lo S, Jun M, Cass A, Gallagher M. Choice of renal replacement therapy modality and dialysis dependence after acute kidney injury: a systematic review and meta-analysis. *Intensive Care Med.* 2013 Jun;39(6):987-97

62. Parikh A, Shaw A. The economics of renal failure and kidney disease in critically ill patients. *Crit Care Clin.* 2012;28:99-111.

63. Rahamati MA, Homel P, Hoenich NA, et al. The role of improved water quality on inflammatory markers in patients undergoing regular dialysis. *Int J Artif Organs.* 2004;27:723-727.

64. Udy AA, Roberts JA, Shorr A, et al. Augmented renal clearance in septic and traumatized patients with normal plasma creatinine concentrations: identifying at-risk patients. *Nat Rev Nephrol.* 2011;7:539-543.

65. Palevsky PM, Molitoris BA, Okusa MD, et al. Design of clinical trials in acute kidney injury: report from an NIDDK workshop on trial methodology. *Clin J Am Soc Nephrol.* 2012;7:844-850.

Hematologic Dysfunction in the ICU

32

John C. Chapin, MD and Maria T. Desancho, MD, MSc

KEY POINTS

1. The most common reasons for hematologic consultation in critically ill patients include thrombocytopenia, anemia, and less commonly, evaluation of leukocytosis and thrombocytosis.

2. Coagulopathies including severe bleeding and thrombotic disorders are very prevalent in intensive care unit (ICU) patients due to their underlying conditions including liver dysfunction and acquired vitamin K deficiency. Bleeding can occur due to renal insufficiency and the use of antiplatelet agents and anticoagulant therapy.

3. Inflammation occurs in sepsis, systemic inflammatory response syndrome, and other critical illnesses, and causes alterations in both hemostasis and fibrinolysis.

4. Disseminated intravascular coagulation (DIC) is observed in approximately 50% of patients with sepsis, and is an independent predictor of morbidity and mortality.

5. Thrombocytopenia (platelet count < 150,000/L) occurs in 15% to 58% of ICU patients and may be due to medications, infections, DIC, thrombotic microangiopathies (thrombotic thrombocytopenic purpura [TTP] and atypical hemolytic uremic syndrome), heparin-induced thrombocytopenia (HIT), catastrophic antiphospholipid syndrome, and immune thrombocytopenic purpura.

6. HIT is a clinicopathologic diagnosis that occurs in 1% to 4% of patients on unfractionated heparin (UFH), and less than 1% of patients on low-molecular-weight heparin (LMWH). It is more common in postsurgical patients than medical inpatients and in females.

7. Prompt interaction between the intensivist and the hematologist is key to optimize the care of critically ill patients with hematologic dysfunction.

INTRODUCTION

Patients admitted to the ICU have frequent hematologic dysfunction as a result of critical illness leading to multiorgan dysfunction and failure. A hematology consultation is often requested for evaluation of hematologic complications in these critically ill patients. The most common reasons for hematologic consultation include evaluation of cytopenias mainly thrombocytopenia, anemia, and less commonly, evaluation of leukocytosis and thrombocytosis. Coagulopathies including severe bleeding and thrombotic disorders are very prevalent in the ICU patients due to their underlying conditions. These patients frequently develop DIC or severe coagulopathy secondary to liver dysfunction or acquired vitamin K deficiency. Bleeding can also be seen as a consequence of renal insufficiency, and the use of antiplatelet agents causing an acquired thrombocytopathy. The administration of anticoagulants in these patients is challenging as the bleeding risk is increased. Hemostasis is frequently disrupted, as these patients often require invasive and/or surgical procedures. Thrombotic complications either venous, arterial, or microvascular are commonly seen as a result of indwelling catheter placement or other invasive procedures, prolonged immobilization, underlying malignancy, autoimmune disorder, or medication related. Frequent exposure to blood products, increases the risk of transfusion reactions including transfusion-related acute lung injury (TRALI) and hemolytic, febrile, and allergic transfusion reactions. In addition dilution coagulopathies are seen in patients who are massively transfused. Prompt interaction between the intensivist and the hematologist is key to optimize the care of these challenging patients.

Overview of Hemostasis

Hemostasis maintains a closed system of vascular integrity and prevents blood loss from injury.[1] The hemostatic response is initiated by injury to endothelial cell surfaces that leads to exposure of tissue factor (TF), collagen, von Willebrand factor (vWF), and fibronectin on the subendothelial matrix. Primary hemostasis consists of platelet adhesion by binding to collagen and vWF on the exposed endothelial surface. Platelets then aggregate via glycoprotein IIb-IIIa receptors, which bind fibrinogen and form platelet thrombi. When activated, platelets release vasoactive, inflammatory, and thrombogenic mediators. For example, ADP binds to the purinergic receptors P2Y2 and P2Y12 to promote aggregation. Thromboxane A2 is also synthesized in the platelets by cyclooxygenase (COX) enzymes and stimulates vasoconstriction and platelet aggregation.

Secondary hemostasis is the process of thrombin generation by coagulation proteins, which are classified into extrinsic, intrinsic, and common pathways (Figure 32–1). The initial step in secondary hemostasis occurs when TF binds to activated factor VII (extrinsic pathway). The intrinsic pathway is composed of factors XII, XI, IX, and VIII, also known as the contact activation pathway.

Both pathways activate thrombin (factor IIa) from prothrombin (factor II) through the prothrombinase complex, which is composed of factors Xa, Va, calcium, and phospholipids. Thrombin generation leads to the conversion of fibrinogen to fibrin, which polymerizes and is cross-linked by factor XIIIa, creating a thrombus.

Thrombin activates fibrinogen, platelets, and acts as its own regulator by activating the natural anticoagulants protein C (PC), protein S (PS), and antithrombin (AT) that in turn inactivate coagulation at multiple steps and limit fibrin deposition (see Figure 32–1).

Vitamin K, an essential cofactor for the conversion of glutamic acid residues to gama-carboxyl glutamate (Gla) residues, allows factors II, VII, IX, X, PC, and PS to bind to the surface of plasma membranes and perform their functions. Vitamin K antagonists like warfarin cause multisite blockade of the coagulation cascade by impairing the creation of Gla domains. Fibrinolysis is the process of thrombi dissolution, a necessary step to prevent undesired excess fibrin deposition and pathologic thrombus formation.[2,3] Plasminogen is activated by tissue plasminogen activator (tPA) and urokinase plasminogen activator (uPA) in conjunction with annexin II, which cleave fibrin into fibrin degradation products including D-dimers.

Evaluation of Primary and Secondary Hemostasis

Platelet functional assays and aggregometry measure qualitative defects in platelet hemostasis. These tests include platelet functional assay 100 (PFA-100) and platelet aggregometry (Table 32–1). PFA-100 testing uses special collagen-epinephrine and collagen-ADP cartridges where in whole blood pass through a chamber and aggregate. If one or both of the cartridge closure times are prolonged, it suggests a qualitative platelet defect. Aspirin and nonsteroidal anti-inflammatory drugs (NSAIDs) cause prolongation of the collagen-epinephrine time. Both tests will be prolonged in von Willebrand disease (vWD), congenital or acquired thrombocytopathies seen in renal and hepatic disease. Platelet aggregation and secretion studies either using whole blood or platelet-rich plasma evaluates specific platelet defects. It should be

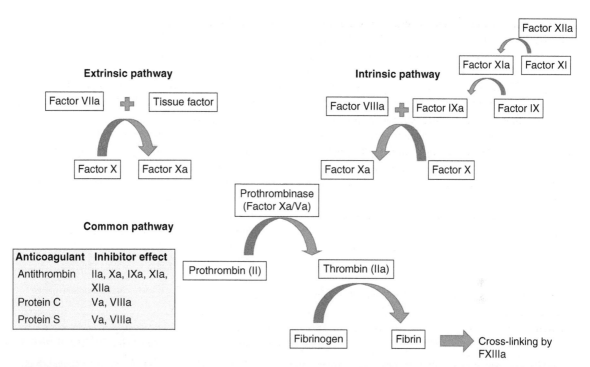

FIGURE 32-1 The coagulation cascade model of hemostasis. The extrinsic pathway is activated by exposure of tissue factor. The intrinsic pathway begins when factor XIIa is activated by contact pathway activators. Both pathways result in the generation of factor Xa and the formation of the prothrombinase complex. Thrombin activates fibrinogen to fibrin, which is cross-linked and polymerizes.

noted that platelet function tests might be abnormal when the platelet count is less than 100,000/L unless the concentrations are adjusted in plasma.

The screening tests of blood coagulation are the prothrombin time (PT) and the activated partial thromboplastin time (aPTT). These tests become prolonged when coagulation factor activities are 20% or less. The PT is used to determine risks of bleeding from defects in the extrinsic and common pathways. The international normalized ratio (INR) is the PT normalized to a pool of known PTs in a population of patients on vitamin K antagonists and adjusted for thromboplastin reagent types. It should be noted that the INR is standardized for bleeding and thrombotic risks for patients on warfarin and does not accurately reflect coagulation dysfunction in liver disease or other coagulopathies.[4,5]

The aPTT is a test of the intrinsic and common pathways of coagulation. The aPTT is also used to measure therapeutic levels of intravenous anticoagulants like heparin and direct thrombin inhibitors like argatroban and bivalirudin. When a prolonged PT or aPTT is detected, a variety of diagnoses are implicated and should be related to the patient's clinical presentation and history (Table 32–2). Further evaluation consist on a mixing PT and/or aPTT test that is performed by adding the patient's plasma to a pool of normal plasma in a 1:1 ratio and measuring the PT and /or aPTT immediately and after incubation of 60 to 120 minutes at 37°C. If the clotting time corrects into the normal range upon mixing, this is referred to as an immediate correction. Incubation is performed to detect slow-acting coagulation inhibitors, characteristic of an acquired factor VIII deficiency, which will cause prolongation of the aPTT after initial correction. A failure of the mixing study to correct immediately and after incubation is consistent with the presence of a lupus or lupus-like anticoagulant (LA). A sustained correction is consistent with a

TABLE 32-1   Coagulation tests methodology and diagnostic use.

Thrombin time	Add thrombin to citrated plasma, cleaves fibrinogen to fibrinopeptides A and B	Detects defect in thrombin or fibrinogen, affected by anticoagulation
Reptilase time	Add reptilase to citrated plasma, cleaves fibrinogen to fibrinopeptide A	Detects fibrinogen deficiency, not affected by heparin or other anticoagulants
Dilute Russell viper venom time (DRVVT)	Add RVV to plasma to activate factor X in the presence of phospholipid	Detects presence of a lupus anticoagulant, requires confirmation by addition of excess phospholipids
Euglobulin lysis time	Measure time to clot lysis	Detects increased fibrinolysis, factor XIII deficiency
Ecarin clot time	Add ecarin to citrated plasma + thrombin inhibitor, activates prothrombin	Detects direct thrombin inhibitors, not widely available
Thrombin generation assay	Add thrombin to citrated plasma, measure substrate cleavage	Detects quantitative thrombin activity, interlaboratory variability, research tool
Thromboelastography	Can be performed on whole blood	Detects multiple parameters of hemostasis and fibrinolysis, interlaboratory variability, research tool
Bleeding time[a]	Cutaneous lancet injury, measure time to stop bleeding	Detects in vivo qualitative platelet defect, poor reproducibility
PFA-100[a]	Platelet function assay for collagen and ADP	Detects mild platelet binding disorders and aspirin exposure, does not detect platelet secretion defects
Platelet aggregometry[a]	Measures platelet aggregation and secretion to multiple agonists	Detects platelet secretion defects and aggregation defects which are agonist-specific, high variability
Verify now[a]	Measures platelet aggregation and response to P2Y12 inhibitors	Detects clopidogrel, prasugrel, ticagrelor, ticlopidine-induced platelet inhibition, interference with inherited platelet disorders and VWD

[a]Any test of platelet in whole blood must be performed with platelet counts more than 100,000/L to avoid false-positives from thrombocytopenia.

coagulation factor deficiency. Falsely positive LA is seen in the presence of heparin, direct thrombin, and Xa inhibitors and may be falsely positive when the patient is on warfarin and the INR is supratherapeutic. Therefore an LA test should not be

TABLE 32-2   Prolonged coagulation tests and diagnosis.

Prolonged PT	Factor VII deficiency, vitamin K antagonist use, vitamin K deficiency, lupus anticoagulant
Prolonged aPTT	Factor deficiency (factors VIII, IX, XI), heparin anticoagulation, argatroban, bivalirudin anticoagulation, lupus anticoagulant
Prolonged PT and aPTT	Factor deficiency (factors II, V, X, fibrinogen), vitamin K deficiency

requested when the patient is receiving these anticoagulants. Bethesda units (BU) are used to measure inhibitor titers to clotting factors and reflect the strength of inhibitors that are detected on mixing studies. One BU is equivalent to the reciprocal dilution of the patient's plasma at which 50% of the specific factor activity is inhibited. For example, in the case of acquired hemophilia A, a BU titer of 5 indicates a dilution of 1:5 where 50% of the factor VIIIa activity was inhibited.

Occasionally, a shortened PT or aPTT is observed in critical illness. A shortened PT is the result of an increase in circulating TF after central nervous system (CNS) injury, stroke, or sickle cell crisis. Similarly, inflammation-induced elevations of factor VIII may result in a shortened aPTT. More specific coagulation testing and their indications are described in Table 32-1.

Inflammation in the ICU

Inflammation occurs in sepsis, systemic inflammatory response syndrome, and other critical illnesses, and causes alterations in both hemostasis and fibrinolysis. Platelets are activated and may become prothrombotic in inflammatory states, white cells are more adhesive to vessel walls by expressing vessel adhesion molecules, and toxic degranulation occurs. Oxidative damage as the result of free radical generation causes decreased red cell membrane flexibility and expression of adhesion molecules on the surface of endothelial cells. Hypoxia is also a prothrombotic trigger. Inflammation may worsen anemia as red blood cells are subjected to cytokines and turbulent blood flow, ultimately leading to hemolysis. Inflammatory cytokines also increase expression of TF on the surface of monocytes and in circulating microparticles. Coagulation factors like fibrinogen, factor VIII, and vWF are acute-phase reactants and their levels may increase secondary to inflammation.

Targeting Inflammation

Initial clinical trials to treat sepsis with drotrecogin-alfa (Xigris), a recombinant activated protein C suggested improvement in outcomes in some critically ill patients. However, reevaluation of this agent in the PROWESS-SHOCK trial showed no benefit of drotrecogin-alfa in patients with septic shock and the drug was withdrawn from the market.[6,7]

Disseminated Intravascular Coagulation

DIC is a consumptive coagulopathy that is frequently encountered in critically ill patients. DIC is observed in approximately 50% of patients with sepsis, and is an independent predictor of morbidity and mortality. Other common etiologies of DIC are shown in Table 32–3. DIC occurs as the result of increased circulating procoagulant factors that lead to high levels of thrombin generation and cytokine activation. Systemic activation of thrombin and platelets causes thrombosis in both small and large vessels. Platelets become activated and then aggregate in response to increased thrombin generation causing progressive thrombocytopenia. As the regulatory proteins of thrombin generation and coagulation are progressively overwhelmed,

TABLE 32–3 Etiologies of disseminated intravascular coagulation.

Tissue injury	Neoplasms	Obstetrical
• Trauma • Crush and CNS injuries • Heat stroke • Burns • Hemolytic transfusion reaction • Acute transplant rejection	• Solid tumors • Leukemias (mainly acute promyelocytic leukemia) • Cancer chemotherapy • Tumor lysis syndrome **Infections** • Gram-positive bacteria • Gram-negative bacteria • Spirochetes • Rickettsia • Protozoa • Fungi • Viruses	• Abruptio placenta • Placenta previa • Retained death fetus • Amniotic fluid embolism • Uterine atomy • Therapeutic abortion • Severe preeclampsia and eclampsia **Other** • Shock • Cardiac arrest • Fat embolism • Aortic aneurysm • Giant hemangiomas • Snake bites • Near drowning

the systemic circulation becomes more thrombogenic. Coagulation factors are consumed in diffuse thromboses, leading to organ failure, ischemia, and tissue damage. Deep venous, arterial, and cerebrovascular thromboses also occur. Fibrinogen levels decrease as DIC continues, resulting in a fibrinogen deficiency and increased bleeding tendency.[8] In severe cases, gangrene and limb ischemia (purpura fulminans) develops. No single test or clinical finding is able to accurately diagnose DIC. The diagnosis must be based on underlying clinical predisposition. A combination of prolonged PT, prolonged aPTT, and thrombocytopenia are suggestive of DIC, as is a decreased level of fibrinogen.[9] Approximately 50% of patients with DIC will have prolongation of the PT or aPTT at some point during the course of DIC. The aPTT may initially be shortened as a result of inflammatory increases in FVIII and fibrinogen. Elevated fibrin degradation product (FDP) and D-dimer levels indicate increased thrombin and plasmin generation. However, D-dimer is also elevated in the postsurgical state, after trauma, in the setting of deep vein thrombosis and with liver and renal dysfunction. The platelet count is of particular utility in DIC as thrombocytopenia correlates with thrombin generation.[9,10] Thrombocytopenia may develop rapidly (within 1-4 hours) of the onset of DIC and is an independent predictor of mortality and length of ICU stay.[10] Once the platelet count reaches a nadir, it suggests stabilization of thrombin generation. A platelet count less than 100,000/L is seen in 50% to 60% of patients with DIC, and counts less than 50,000/L are seen in approximately 10% of patients. Several scoring systems for DIC have been developed, and are dependent on clinical presentation and laboratory values. The International Society for Thrombosis and Haemostasis (ISTH) score for overt DIC is shown in Table 32–4, and has a specificity of 91% and a sensitivity of 97%.[11] This score is meant to be calculated daily based on serial laboratory measurements and guide clinicians to the improvement or worsening of their patients. The scoring system should be used only when the patient's clinical history is compatible with DIC.

The cornerstone of treating DIC is correction of the underlying cause. Platelets and plasma transfusions should be used for bleeding patients and not solely to correct laboratory values. In the setting of bleeding, plasma should be administered at 15 to 20 mL/kg, and platelets should be transfused to over 50,000/L. Hypofibrinogenemia (fibrinogen concentration 100 mg/L) should be corrected by 10 donor pools (2 units) of cryoprecipitate or 3 g of a fibrinogen concentrate. Antifibrinolytics (tranexamic acid, ε-aminocaproic acid), activated prothrombin complex concentrates (FEIBA) and recombinant factor VIIa (rFVIIa) should be avoided, as they can worsen thrombosis. Anticoagulation should not be withheld in patients with DIC unless the bleeding risk is significant. DIC patients without bleeding should have routine pharmacologic thromboprophylaxis.

Bleeding

Bleeding disorders occur in critically ill patients and their etiology is usually multifactorial. Bleeding is seen as a consequence of thrombocytopenia and/or thrombocytopathies or is related to acquired coagulation factor deficiencies. Thrombocytopenia is commonly drug related, or caused by severe liver disease, or DIC. Thrombocytopathies are secondary to the use of antiplatelet agents such as aspirin, NSAID, and PY212 inhibitors, also seen with liver and renal dysfunction and in patients with congenital thrombocytopathies or vWD. The bleeding pattern may point to a specific etiology. For example, patients with severe thrombocytopenia, thrombocytopathies, and vWF defects present with mucocutaneous bleeding. Conversely patients with severe inherited coagulation factor defects (eg, factors VIII and IX) present with hemarthrosis, muscle, and soft tissue bleeding. Interestingly, the bleeding pattern in patients with acquired factor VIII inhibitors is also mucocutaneous. Some patients may have no known personal or family history of bleeding disorders, but hemostatic challenges that occur in the hospital setting (biopsies, surgeries, placement of intravascular devices) may unmask mild congenital bleeding disorders such as thrombocytopathies, factor XI deficiency, and fibrinolytic defects.

A diagnostic approach to the bleeding patient should include thorough examination of patient's skin, flank, hips, and mucosal surfaces for petechiae, ecchymoses, or hematomas. Inspection of the digits

TABLE 32–4 ISTH DIC scoring system for overt DIC.

1. Risk assessment: Does the patient have an underlying disorder known to be associated with overt DIC?[a] If yes, proceed. If no, do not use this algorithm

2. Order global coagulation tests (platelet count, PT, fibrinogen, soluble fibrin monomers/fibrin degradation products/D-dimer)

3. Score global coagulation test results
   Platelet count (> 100 = 0, < 100 = 1, < 50 = 2)
   Elevated fibrin-related marker (eg, soluble fibrin monomers/fibrin degradation **products**/D-dimer; no increase = 0, moderate increase = 2, strong increase = 3)
   Prolonged PT (< 3 s = 0, > 3 but < 6 s = 1, > 6 s = 2)
   Fibrinogen level (> 1 g/L = 0, < 1 g/L = 1)

4. Calculate score
   > 5 = compatible with overt DIC, repeat score daily
   < 5 = suggestive of nonovert DIC, repeat in next 1-2 d

*e.g. bacterial sepsis, trauma (esp CNS), fat embolism, burn injury , pancreatitis, malignancies (esp acute *e.g.
[a]For example, bacterial sepsis, trauma (esp CNS), fat embolism, burn injury, pancreatitis, malignancies (esp acute promyelocytic leukemia), obstetric complications (preeclampsia, placental abruption, amniotic fluid embolism, intrauterine fetal demise), vascular aneurysms, hemangiomata (eg, Kasabach-Merritt syndrome), advanced liver failure, illicit drug use, snake bites, severe transfusion reactions, transplant organ rejection.

may reveal evidence of ischemia or embolism that reflects a systemic disorder.

In addition careful inspection of chest and endotracheal tubes, urinary catheters, surgical drains, and suction devices should be carefully performed. A high suspicion for local wound complications should be maintained, especially if the patient is within 48 hours of an invasive or surgical procedure. Hemoccult testing is useful in assessment of gastrointestinal bleeding.

The Initial laboratory evaluation should include a complete blood count, PT, aPTT, and fibrinogen. A manual platelet count should be performed by manual examination of the peripheral blood smear if thrombocytopenia is reported in a patient with no signs of bleeding. Pseudothrombocytopenia is a laboratory artifact characterized by platelet aggregation in response to ethylenediaminetetraacetic acid (EDTA), heparin, or citrate, and should be excluded early in the diagnostic evaluation. If large clumps of platelets are observed on the peripheral smear, the platelet count should be repeated using a different anticoagulant tube or by peripheral finger stick to obtain a more accurate platelet count.

Acute management of a bleeding includes discontinuation of all medications that contribute to bleeding, evaluation of a bleeding site, and reversal of hemostatic abnormalities. In addition to local cauterization or compression when a bleeding site is identified, platelets are used for patients with severe thrombocytopenia or thrombocytopathy. Vitamin K is administered for correction of acquired vitamin K deficiency either due to vitamin K antagonists or other acquired etiologies of vitamin K deficiency. Vitamin K is administered at 10 mg intravenously over 15 to 30 minutes and takes effect within 6 to 12 hours. Plasma is used to correct coagulopathy secondary to liver disease and for rapid reversal or vitamin K antagonists. Plasma is infused at doses of 10 to 15 mL/kg given every 6 hours until hemostasis is achieved. Plasma contains approximately 0.7 to 1 unit/mL of clotting factor activity and 1 to 2 mg/unit of fibrinogen. Cryoprecipitate is a protein fraction of plasma, enriched in factor VIII, vWF, fibrinogen, fibronectin, and factor XIII. One unit of cryoprecipitate is obtained from 1 unit of plasma. Cryoprecipitate is indicated to correct hypofibrinogenemia in patients with DIC presenting with bleeding and it is also used in managing dysfibrinogenemia or hypofibrinogenemia in patients with severe liver disease. Cryoprecipitate is administered at 1 unit per 5 kg of body weight, with the goal of increasing fibrinogen to greater than 100 mg/dL.

If excessive fibrinolysis is suspected, antifibrinolytic lysine analogues should be administered. These drugs act as competitive analogues of fibrin and bind plasminogen. Tranexamic acid is given orally at 25 mg/kg or 10 mg/kg IV every 8 hours, ε-aminocaproic acid is given at 50 mg/kg every 6 hours orally or IV 5 g bolus followed by 1 g/h continuous infusion. Tranexamic acid must be dose reduced in patients with renal failure. Both of these agents should be avoided in DIC and in genitourinary bleeding, where the risk for thrombosis is significant. Tranexamic acid has been shown to reduce bleeding and death related to bleeding if administered within 3 hours.

Transfusions of red blood cells should be restricted to actively bleeding patients and the decision to transfuse blood products must be carefully weighed against the risk of transfusion-related fever, circulatory overload, lung injury, and alloimmunization.[12]

Specific Bleeding Diagnoses

Acquired Hemophilia A

Acquired hemophilia A is a rare disorder with an incidence of 1 in 1 million, where patients develop autoantibodies to endogenous factor VIII. This disease is characterized by ecchymoses, soft tissue hematomas, and petechiae, but CNS bleeding can develop. Predisposing factors are poorly understood. In some cases, the identified trigger is pregnancy, new-onset malignancy, and autoimmune disorders and is more commonly seen in the elderly. In nearly 50% of cases, it appears to be idiopathic. Acquired hemophilia A is diagnosed by a prolonged aPTT with initial partial correction by a mixing study, which prolongs after incubation. Treatment should be aimed at controlling bleeding and eradicating the inhibitor. Bleeding is managed with activated prothrombinase complex concentrates (FEIBA at 60-100 IU/kg every 12-24 hours) or rFVIIa (90-100 µg/kg given every 2-3 hours). Simultaneously, treatment to eradicate the inhibitor is initiated with either high-dose prednisone (1 mg/kg) and cyclophosphamide (2 mg/kg daily) or rituximab

(375 mg/m^2) administered as 4 weekly doses. The inhibitor is eradicated in approximately half of all patients but may take several months, and careful observation for bleeding and complications of immunosuppression is warranted during this time.[13]

Congenital Bleeding Disorders

Congenital bleeding disorders include hemophilia A and B, vWD, and other factor deficiencies. In the presence of a known coagulopathy, factor-specific assays should be sent to determine the baseline activity. Severe hemophilia patients should be maintained on a factor replacement prophylaxis strategy, consisting of factor VIII products administered at doses of 25 to 35 IU/kg every other day (hemophilia A), or factor IX doses of 40 to 60 IU/kg twice a week (hemophilia B). One specific concern with hemophilia B replacement products is the development of anaphylaxis in 5% of patients. Prior to invasive procedures or surgeries, factor VIII or IX activity should be elevated to approximately 100% by the administration of factor-specific products. In mild hemophilia A and vWD, desmopressin acetate (DDAVP) may be administered by IV (0.3 μg/kg) or intranasally 150 μg (1 puff in each nostril) to increase vWF and FVIII activity by 2 to 5 times the baseline within 15 to 30 minutes. Severe vWD patients may require vWF-containing factor replacement (Humate P, Wilate, Alphanate). Hemophilia patients with inhibitors are treated with FEIBA or rFVIIa. New longer acting hemophilia concentrates are now available that can prolong the detectable activity of factors VIII and FIX. (ref 36)

Liver Disease and Coagulation

The liver is the source of synthesis of most coagulation factors. Clues to hepatic dysfunction as the cause of a coagulopathy are a decreased albumin, prolonged PT, or known cirrhosis. Liver coagulopathy may present as both bleeding and clotting disorders. In addition to having reduced procoagulant factors, liver dysfunction results in decreased synthesis of natural anticoagulants namely protein C, S, and antithrombin and impaired fibrinolysis, which can lead to a prothrombotic state. A patient with bleeding should receive plasma and cryoprecipitate, and a patient with thrombosis should be anticoagulated, even in the setting of a prolonged PT.[5]

Aside from liver transplantation, there is no cure for hepatic coagulopathies.

Vitamin K Deficiency

Vitamin K is a fat-soluble vitamin that exists in 2 important forms: vitamin K_1, found in green leafy vegetables, and vitamin K_2, is synthesized by normal gut flora. Antibiotic exposure alters the natural gut flora, decreasing the reserve of bacteria-producing vitamin K. Deficiencies of vitamin K occur in the hospital when the diet is not well balanced or the patient is on broad-spectrum antibiotics for over a week.[14] Other causes are poor oral intake, impaired absorption of fat-soluble vitamins (occurring in pancreatitis and cholestyramine treatment), and the use of nasogastric suction. Vitamin K deficiency leads to gastrointestinal, and postsurgical hemorrhage. Excessive bleeding from needle punctures, and intramuscular hematomas can also be noted. Both the PT and aPTT are prolonged as in DIC, but in vitamin K deficiency plasma activity levels of factors II, VII, IX, and X are less than 50%, while fibrinogen, factor V, and VIII are normal. D-Dimer is also normal in vitamin K deficiency. A 1:1 mixing study should completely correct in this setting. If a vitamin K deficiency is suspected, repletion with 5 to 10 mg of vitamin K should begin by intravenous administration. Correction of the PT should occur 6 to 12 hours after vitamin K administration. Critically ill patients at risk for coagulopathies from vitamin K deficiency should be supplemented by administering 5 mg of vitamin K 2 or 3 times weekly, either orally or intravenously.[14]

Anticoagulant Overdose

Overdosing of anticoagulants can result in serious bleeding complications in critically ill patients. Intravenous and subcutaneous UFHs are preferable to oral anticoagulation in the ICU because of their short half-life and reversibility (Table 32–5). If a bleed occurs, heparin must be stopped immediately. Heparin is reversed by administering protamine sulfate 1 mg per 100 units of heparin every 2 to 8 hours, to a maximum dose of 50 mg in 24 hours. If there is an ongoing need for anticoagulation, the heparin should be restarted without bolus at a reduced dose once the bleeding has been controlled. Protamine is less effective at reversing LMWHs and is not effective in reversing fondaparinux.

TABLE 32–5 Anticoagulation reversal.

Anticoagulant	Half-Life (hours)	Reversal Agents
Vitamin K antagonists	20-60	Vitamin K 10 mg IV or po, plasma, 4-factor PCCs (eg, Kcentra)
Unfractionated heparin (IV or sq)	1-3	Protamine 1 mg per 100 units of UFH, do not exceed 50 mg
Low-molecular-weight heparin	4 5	Last dose 0-8 h: protamine 1 mg per 100 units of heparin, do not exceed 50 mg, last dose 8-12 h: protamine 0.5 mg per 100 units of heparin, last dose > 12 h, no protamine indicated
Dabigatran[1]	12-14	Local compression, dialysis, activated charcoal if within 2 h, transfusion support, FEIBA, rFVIIa, idaruciumab (Praxbind)
Edoxaban	10-14	Local compression, activated charcoal if within 2-3 h, transfusion support, PCCs, rFVIIa, FEIBA
Rivaroxaban[a2]	5-9	Local compression, activated charcoal if within 2-3 h, transfusion support, PCCs, rFVIIa, FEIBA
Fondaparinux[a]	17-21	Local compression, transfusion support, PCCs, rVIIa, FEIBA
Apixaban[a]	9-14	Local compression, activated charcoal if within 1 h, transfusion support, PCCs, rFVIIa, FEIBA
Argatroban[a]	1-3	Local compression, transfusion support, PCCs, rFVIIa, FEIBA
Bivalirudin[a]	25 min	Local compression, transfusion support, PCCs, rFVIIa, FEIBA

[a]To date there are no effective reversal agents for these drugs.
1. Dialysis eliminates 60% of dabigatran from circulation.
2. Doses rFVIIa 45-90 µg/kg, FEIBA 25-50 IU/kg, PCCs 50 IU/kg.

Warfarin-induced bleeding can be mild or severe. However, supratherapeutic INRs may not need aggressive reversal in the absence of bleeding. Patients with a supratherapeutic INR without bleeding should have their warfarin held and their INR monitored daily until it reaches the therapeutic range. Vitamin K reversal should be given when the INR is 10 or greater in the absence of bleeding. Any bleeding that occurs while on warfarin should be reversed with vitamin K, regardless of the INR. An intracranial bleed should be treated immediately with vitamin K (10 mg IV), plasma (25-35 mL/kg), and 4 factors prothrombin complex concentrate (PCCs) like Kcentra. Kcentra contains factors II, VII, IX, X, PC, and PS, which is, concentrated 25-fold, equivalent to 2 L of plasma. As Kcentra contains heparin, it is contraindicated in patients with HIT. Kcentra is administered over 10 to 15 minutes at doses of 25 to 50 IU/kg, and normalizes the INR within 30 to 60 minutes of administration.[15]

The Food and Drug Administration (FDA) approved idarucizumab (Praxbind) , a monoclonal Fab fragment for reversal of dabigatran, in 2015 based on the results of the RE-VERSE AD trial (Pollack N Engl J Med 2015, PMID: 26095746). This drug is administered by IV injection at a single dose of 5g. Repeat doses can be considered in consultation with a hematologist and pharmacist. Development of reversal agents for anti-Xa inhibitors are currently in development, including the recombinant protein factor Xa mimic andexanet (Segal DM N Engl J Med 2015; PMID 26559317). In the event of bleeding, besides discontinuation of the offending agent, evaluation for the source of bleeding and supportive therapy including transfusion of red blood cells, activated charcoal (25 g) can be administered orally if ingestion of dabigatran was within 3 hours and within 2 to 3 hours after ingestion of rivaroxaban and apixaban, particularly if intentional overdose. In addition, approximately 60% of dabigatran can be removed by hemodialysis over 2 to 3 hours. Activated prothrombin complex concentrates (FEIBA) 25 units/kg can be considered for dabigatran-related life-threatening bleeds, and rFVIIa has been used as well to control bleeding.[16] Kcentra at a dose of 50 units/kg can be considered for life-threatening bleeds related to rivaroxaban and apixaban. Plasma does not reverse dabigatran, rivaroxaban, or apixaban bleeds, thus is not recommended for reversal. Platelet transfusions are used if the patient was using concomitant antiplatelet agents.

Acquired von Willebrand Disease

Acquired vWD generally manifests as mucocutaneous bleeding. Different mechanisms are responsible for the loss of vWF multimers in acquired vWD, and this disease should be suspected in patients with myeloproliferative neoplasias, plasma cell dyscrasias, hypothyroidism, lymphoproliferative disorders, and solid tumors. Acquired vWD also result from flow obstructions and increased shear that occurs in hypertrophic cardiomyopathy, aortic valve stenosis, and ventricular assist devices. Valve-induced acquired vWD can present with gastrointestinal bleeding, also known as Heyde syndrome. Decreased vWF antigen and loss of high-molecular-weight vWF multimers are suggestive of acquired vWD. Management of bleeding involves using DDAVP or vWF concentrates, but acquired vWD will only resolve after correction of the underlying disorder.[17] Caution must be exercised with DDAVP administration, as patients may develop hypotension, flushing, and fluid retention. Fluid should be restricted to maintenance rate for 24 hours, and electrolytes should to be monitored every 6 to 8 hours. DDAVP should not be administered for more than 3 days because of the development of tachyphylaxis.

Hemodilution

Critically ill patients frequently are exposed to very high volumes of crystalloid and colloid for volume resuscitation and administration of blood products. The resultant volume changes may affect blood count measurements and cause a dilution in hemoglobin, platelets, and coagulation factors. Prior to evaluation for coagulopathy, these tests should be repeated and drawn peripherally, or off lines that are not receiving fluids or medications. Prior studies

suggest the amount of crystalloid fluid needed to cause true hemodilution is significant, usually from several liters of normal saline given as bolus dosing.[18-20] Maintenance fluids alone are insufficient to cause dilution. A recent and more clinical relevant definition of massive bleeding patient proposed by Savage et al refers to patients transfused with greater than 3 units of RBCs in any 60-minute period (within 24 hours of admission). This new definition includes a clinically relevant rate of transfusion and includes the majority of patients who rapidly exsanguinate.[21] The Trauma Outcomes Group collected data from 466 massive transfusion patients from 16 level 1 centers from 2005 to 2006 across the United States. This study demonstrated that outcomes were improved with a more balanced ratio of at least 1:1:2 of plasma:platelets:RBC. Subsequently, the Prospective Observational Multicenter Major Trauma Transfusion (PROMMTT) study was performed at 10 level 1 trauma centers where in-house 24/7 research assistants recorded the sequence and timing of all infused fluids in bleeding trauma patients in 2009 to 2010. A balanced use of plasma early in resuscitation was associated with improved early survival. The median time to hemorrhagic death was 2.6 hours, whereas platelets were infused at a median time of 2.7 hours and 30% of patients who died from hemorrhage never received any platelets. An ongoing prospective randomized clinical trial at 12 centers in North America Pragmatic Randomized Optimal Platelet and Plasma Ratios (PROPPR) trial (www.clinicaltrials.gov identifier: NCT01545232) compares a 1:1:1 ratio of plasma:platelets:RBCs with a 1:1:2 ratio in patients predicted to receive a massive transfusion.[22] The colloid solution hydroxyethyl starch has also been associated with both a dilutional coagulopathy and an acquired vWD.[23]

Using Recombinant Factor VIIa in Critical Illness

The use of rFVIIa has been used in ICU patients to control bleeding. This short-acting activated coagulation factor binds directly to activated platelets and improves systemic hemostasis. It is currently approved for use in hemophilia patients with inhibitors and in patients with congenital factor VII deficiency. The advantages of rFVIIa are rapid onset of hemostasis and minimal volume. However, this drug must be used with caution in patients who do not have congenital coagulopathies, especially in patients over the age of 65, where the risk of arterial thrombotic events was 5.5%.[24]

Acquired Platelet Dysfunction

Acquired platelet dysfunction may occur as a result of medication use (nonsteroidal anti-inflammatory agents, aspirin, clopidogrel, prasugrel, ticagrelor) or uremia. Uremic platelet dysfunction is multifactorial, resulting from decreased aggregation, displacement from the endothelium, and impaired secretion of granules. Dialysis is used to correct platelet dysfunction. Although desmopressin can shorten the skin-bleeding time in patients with uremia, the use of recombinant erythropoietin stimulating agents has made this abnormality of hemostasis much less frequent than it was previously. The beneficial effect of erythropoietin on hemostasis is based on the increase in red-cell mass, which affects the blood-fluid dynamics, leading to a more intense interaction between circulating platelets and the vessel wall.[25] Conjugated estrogens may also be used to correct uremic dysfunction, given at 0.6 mg/kg IV over 30 to 40 minutes for 5 days.

Multiple antiplatelet agents are used in cardiac patients, including aspirin, ibuprofen, ticlopidine, clopidogrel, prasugrel, ticagrelor, dipyridamole, abciximab, tirofiban, eptifibatide, and vorapaxar (Table 32–6). All of these medications create a qualitative platelet dysfunction and can cause bleeding. If bleeding develops, they should be held while the patient receives platelet transfusions to restore the pool of functional platelets.

Thrombocytopenias

Platelets are synthesized from megakaryocytes in the bone marrow by stimulation of the thrombopoietin receptor by thrombopoietin and other cytokines. The megakaryocytes then release platelets into circulation, which are ultimately cleared in the spleen and liver. Splenomegaly or platelet-specific antibody binding may result in increased clearance of platelets and result in thrombocytopenia, defined as a platelet count less than 150,000/L. Thrombocytopenia occurs in 15% to 58% of ICU patients. In medical ICU patients and in septic patients, platelet counts may decrease within 3 to 5 days of admission, dropping to levels 40% to 90% below baseline. Persistent

TABLE 32–6 Antiplatelet agents.

	Half-life	Mechanism
Aspirin	3 h	Irreversible inhibition of COX-2, decreased thromboxane synthesis
NSAIDs (eg, ibuprofen)	1.8-2 h	Reversible COX-2 inhibition
Clopidogrel	7-8 h	ADP P2Y12 receptor inhibitor
Prasugrel	7-8 h	ADP P2Y12 receptor inhibitor
Ticlopidine	12 h	ADP P2Y12 receptor inhibitor
Ticagrelor	7-8 h	ADP P2Y12 receptor inhibitor
Abciximab	10-30 min	GP IIb-IIIa inhibitor
Tirofiban	2 h	GP IIb-IIIa inhibitor
Eptifibatide	2.5 h	GP IIb-IIIa inhibitor
Aggrenox (aspirin and dipyridamole)	3 h	Irreversible COX-2 inhibitor & thromboxane receptor inhibitor, Vasodilator
Voraxapar	5-13 days	PAR-1 inhibitor

thrombocytopenia at day 14 predicts increased mortality, irrespective of an identified etiology.[26] In the absence of thrombotic disease, platelet transfusions may be used to prevent or correct bleeding.[27]

When the platelet count falls below 50,000/L, patients are at an increased risk of bleeding from procedures. Furthermore, patients may bleed spontaneously when the platelet count drops below 10,000/L. The differential is broad for thrombocytopenia in critical illness, as numerous medications, infections, and concomitant illnesses can be implicated. However, decreases in the platelet count can also be manifestations of severe thrombotic diseases. A diagnostic strategy must take the clinical scenario into consideration. Platelet counts under 100,000/L are associated with increased 30-day mortality and disturbed immune responses to sepsis in critically ill patients.

Initially, the most important diseases to consider and diagnose are the thrombotic microangiopathies

(TTP and atypical hemolytic uremic syndrome), HIT, catastrophic antiphospholipid syndrome, and immune thrombocytopenic purpura (ITP). These disorders can be fatal if not immediately diagnosed and treated. After these disorders have been evaluated and ruled out, a more detailed review of causes of thrombocytopenia can be accomplished. Disseminated intravascular coagulation should always be considered as the cause of thrombocytopenia in a patient with sepsis, prolonged PT, elevated D-dimer, and low fibrinogen.

Thrombotic Microangiopathies

Thrombotic microangiopathies (TMA) are characterized by microvascular injury to endothelial cells, which can be provoked by infection, inflammation, drugs, and other factors. These injuries promote endothelial cell injury, platelet aggregation, and hemolysis. Inhibition of the vWF-cleaving protease ADAMTS13 is implicated in the pathology of some types of TMAs. The accumulation of ultra-large vWF multimers causes microvascular thrombi that result in multiple organ failure and dialysis dependence. Rapid recognition and treatment of TMAs is essential, as the mortality can approach 90%. Two important TMAs that must be distinguished acutely are atypical hemolytic uremic syndrome (aHUS) and TTP. Differentiating TTP from aHUS is difficult since the 2 diseases have overlapping manifestations. Higher platelet counts and worse degrees of renal failure are associated with aHUS, whereas platelet counts will almost invariably be low (< 40,000) in TTP and only mild renal failure is seen.[24]

The initial evaluation of TMAs should include review of a peripheral smear to confirm decreased platelet count and to identify schistocytes. Markers of hemolysis should be requested including lactate dehydrogenase (LDH), haptoglobin, and a direct antiglobulin test. Stool antigens to evaluate for shiga toxins, like O157:H7 and ADAMTS13 activity should be sent prior to treatments. Undetectable ADAMTS13 activity may indicate either a congenital absence of ADAMTS13 caused by mutation of the *ADAMTS13* gene (Upshaw-Schulman syndrome), or the presence of an acquired anti-ADAMTS13 IgG inhibitor. Liver disease, vasculopathies, and peripheral artery disease may also have an ADAMTS13 deficiency, and caution should be used in interpreting these results of such patients.[28]

Plasma exchange restores ADAMTS13 activity in the majority of TTP patients.[29] If plasma exchange is not available, simple plasma transfusions should be initiated at doses of 30 mL/kg. If a response to plasma exchange is not seen within approximately 20 exchange sessions or 45 L of plasma, an alternate diagnosis should be considered, including aHUS. Treatment of refractory TTP is less effective and no current standard exists. Second-line therapies include immunosuppression with rituximab, vincristine, mycophenolate, cyclosporine, bortezomib, and splenectomy. Rituximab (375 mg/m²) for 4 weekly doses has been used successfully to induce remission in patients with persistently low ADAMTS13 activity despite plasma exchange.[30]

aHUS is a TMA that presents like TTP, but ADAMTS13 activity may be normal. This syndrome is caused by complement protein mutations resulting in hyperactivation of the complement system. The anticomplement C5a antibody eculizumab is approved to treat aHUS with an initial dose of 900 mg IV weekly for 4 weeks, followed by maintenance dosing of 1200 mg every 2 weeks. Prior to eculizumab treatment, it is important to ensure the patient is vaccinated against *Neisseria meningitidis* or covered with antibacterial prophylaxis for the duration of treatment. Clinical and hematologic improvement is usually seen within 1 to 2 weeks.[28]

Heparin-induced Thrombocytopenia

HIT is a diagnosis not to be missed in a hospitalized patient with new-onset thrombocytopenia. The formation of HIT antibodies occurs when heparin binds to platelet factor 4 and causes a rapid prothrombotic antibody reaction by activating platelet FcγIIaR receptors and increasing thrombin generation. The severity of thrombotic disease in HIT cannot be underestimated. HIT occurs in 1% to 4% of patients on UFH, and fewer than 1% of patients on LMWH, and is more common in postsurgical patients than medical inpatients and in females compared to males.[31] HIT is a clinicopathologic diagnosis. The first step in evaluation is calculating the 4T score by using the clinical prediction rule (Table 32–7). A low score effectively excludes HIT, and no further workup is needed. If the score is intermediate or high, heparin products, including heparin flushes, and catheters coated with heparin

TABLE 32–7 HIT 4T score.

Parameter	2 points	1 point	0 point
Thrombocytopenia	Platelet count > 50% of baseline and nadir > 20,000/L	Platelet count 30%-50% of baseline or nadir 10-19,000/L	Platelet count < 30% of baseline or < 10,000/L
Timing of platelet count fall	5-14 d after heparin exposure or < 1 d if heparin exposure within 30 d	5-14 d with missing data points, or onset after day 14, or < 1 d with prior exposure to heparin 30-100 d prior	Platelet count fall < 4 d without heparin exposure
Thrombosis	New thrombosis, skin necrosis at heparin site, anaphylaxis to heparin after IV bolus	Progressive or recurrent thrombosis, erythematous skin lesions, suspected thrombosis	None
Other causes of thrombocytopenia	None	Possible	Definite

High probability 6-8 points, intermediate probability 4-5 points, low probability 0-3 points.
Reproduced with permission from Lo GK, Juhl D, Warkentin TE, et al: Evaluation of pretest clinical score (4 T's) for the diagnosis of heparin-induced thrombocytopenia in two clinical settings, *J Thromb Haemost.* 2006 Apr;4(4):759-765.

should be discontinued immediately and the patient should be initiated on an alternate nonheparin anticoagulant. Both the heparin antibody ELISA assays and the serotonin release assay (SRA) test should be sent at presentation. If the antibody test is negative but the clinical prediction score remains high, the patient should remain on heparin-free anticoagulant until the SRA is reported. If the SRA is negative, this effectively rules out HIT and heparin can be resumed. If both tests are positive, the patient should remain on an alternate anticoagulant until the platelet count recovers. The patient may be transitioned to warfarin when the platelet count is over 150,000/L. Argatroban, dosed intravenously at 2 ug/kg/min to an aPTT goal of 1.5 to 3 times baseline, is the only anticoagulant currently approved for treatment of HIT in the USA. Dosing needs to be reduced to 25% (0.5 ug/kg/min) of the indicated dose in case of hepatic insufficiency. In a retrospective analysis of 12 ICU patients with multiple organ dysfunction syndrome (MODS) treated with argatroban for suspected or diagnosed HIT, the mean argatroban dose was significantly lower in patients with hepatic insufficiency compared with patients without hepatic impairment (0.10 ± 0.06 μg/kg/min versus 0.31 ± 0.14 μg/kg/min).[32]

Immune Thrombocytopenic Purpura

ITP is characterized by isolated thrombocytopenia often occurring in the absence of identifiable and specific triggers. ITP is caused by autoantibody-mediated clearance of platelets. The thrombocytopenia is usually severe, with platelet counts often less than 10,000/L. Physical examination may reveal petechiae on the soft palate and the extremities. The peripheral smear may reveal large platelets, which result from the egress of immature platelets from the bone marrow to compensate for platelet destruction. The most feared clinical complication of ITP is intracranial hemorrhage. Secondary causes of ITP, including HIV, hepatitis C, and autoimmune diseases like systemic lupus erythematosus (SLE) should be identified and treated. The first line of treatment in severe ITP is glucocorticoids (prednisone1 mg/kg daily), intravenous immunoglobulins (IVIg) 1 g/kg given over 1 to 2 days or anti-D for Rh-positive, nonsplenectomized individuals. Treatment options of patients who are unresponsive to or relapse after initial corticosteroid therapies include, rituximab, and the thrombopoietin receptor mimetics romiplostim and eltrombopag. Splenectomy remains a mainstay of therapy in providing sustained remission rates in patients with ITP, although long-term remissions have been attained with Rituximab and other immunosuppressive agents. However, infection and thrombosis remain long-term risks.[33]

Medication-related Thrombocytopenia

Drug-induced thrombocytopenia occurs by a variety of mechanisms including direct bone marrow damage and immune-mediated destruction.[34] The bleeding rate is approximately 9% secondary to drug-induced thrombocytopenia and is related to the degree of thrombocytopenia. Nonimmune causes are the result of drug toxins on the bone marrow in patients receiving antineoplastic drugs, antivirals, ethanol, and thiazide diuretics that develop slowly over several weeks of exposure. Immune-mediated thrombocytopenia develops within 14 days, and within 1 to 3 days if the patient had been previously exposed to this drug. The causes of drug-induced immune-mediated thrombocytopenia are multiple and are related to the interaction of the drug, the antibody, and the platelet. Penicillin and cephalosporin drugs act as haptens to initiate an immune response. Quinine and related drugs act as binding agents for platelets and antibodies. Tirofiban, eptifibatide, and abciximab bind directly to GP IIb-IIIa. Gold and procainamide induce the production of platelet-specific autoantibodies. The diagnosis of drug-induced thrombocytopenia should start with the timing of thrombocytopenia and duration of exposure to the medication, with careful notation of the platelet trends. This trend will indicate the trajectory of thrombocytopenia. An excellent resource for reports of drug-induced thrombocytopenia and a grading system is available at www.ouhsc.edu/platelets.

It is prudent to suspect a drug-induced thrombocytopenia after exposures of approximately 9 to 10 days (exceptions noted below). Platelet counts may be severe in some cases, resembling ITP. Improvement is seen after 10 to 14 days of discontinuing the offending medication, but can take up to several months. In severe thrombocytopenia with bleeding, stress doses of prednisone (1 mg/kg) and platelet transfusions should be used in conjunction with stopping the offending drug. Bleeding will resolve in 1 to 2 days after discontinuation of the drug, even though improvements in platelet counts may take longer. In the case that a mild thrombocytopenia develops without bleeding, careful risk-benefit assessment should be made as to the indication for the drug compared to the risk for bleeding.

Posttransfusion Purpura

Posttransfusion purpura occurs as a thrombocytopenia that develops 7 to 14 days after blood transfusions, often in postpartum women. These women had been preimmunized during pregnancy against a platelet antigen (HPA-1a). When they receive blood products this increases the production of alloantibodies that binds to and clears their platelets, promoting a platelet transfusion-refractory state. This disorder presents with patients having purpura or petechiae, platelet counts are often less than 10,000/L. Platelet clearance should be measured to determine appropriate response to platelet transfusions as follows:

Corrected Count Increment (CCI): (platelet count posttransfusion – platelet count pretransfusion) × (body surface area)/(number of platelet units transfused × 10^{11}). If the **CCI** is normal after 1 hour but decreased at 24 hours this suggests a nonimmune mechanism.

If CCIs at 1 hour and 24 hours are less than 7500, the patient is considered platelet refractory and human leukocyte antigen (HLA)-matched platelet transfusions should be considered. Acute bleeding from posttransfusion purpura is treated similarly to ITP, and first-line therapy should be IVIg 1 g/kg for 2 days.

Postsurgery Thrombocytopenia

Platelet counts decline to a nadir within 1 to 4 days after cardiac, vascular, abdominal, or orthopedic surgery as a result of tissue trauma and blood loss, which lead to platelet consumption. Platelet counts should begin to increase after day 4 and reach presurgery levels usually between 5 and 7 days postoperation and may continue to increase for 10 days as a result of reactive thrombocytosis before return to baseline by day 14.

Thrombocytosis

Elevated platelet counts (> 450,000/L) may be seen in the ICU patient. Thrombocytosis should be divided into primary and secondary causes. Elevated platelet counts may occur as a result of myeloproliferative neoplasms including essential thrombocythemia (ET) and polycythemia vera (PV). JAK2 mutations in V617F, exon 12 and exon 13 occur in greater than 95% of PV and 50% of ET patients. Myeloproliferative neoplasms are thrombotic risk factors, especially in patients older than 60 years with prior thrombosis and underlying cardiovascular risk factors. Significant elevation of platelet counts more than 1.5 million may also present with a bleeding diathesis secondary to acquired thrombocytopathy or acquired vWD. Symptomatic patients with elevated platelet counts may benefit from treatment with plateletpheresis and cytoreduction with hydroxyurea, interferon, or anagrelide. Low-dose aspirin 81 mg may be used as primary prevention of thrombosis in some patients without another indication for anticoagulation.[35] Secondary thrombocytosis may result from prior splenectomy, postsurgery, and as a result of inflammation. Secondary thrombocytosis does not constitute a significant thrombotic risk.

REFERENCES

1. Furie B, Furie BC. Mechanisms of thrombus formation. *N Engl J Med.* 2008;359(9):938-949.
2. Cesarman-Maus G, Hajjar K. Molecular mechanisms of fibrinolysis. *Br J Haematol.* 2005;129(3):307-321.
3. Hajjar K, Acharya S. Annexin II and regulation of cell surface fibrinolysis. *Ann NY Acad Sci.* 2006;902:265-271.
4. Tripodi A, Chantarangkul V, Mannucci PM. The international normalized ratio to prioritize patients for liver transplantation: problems and possible solutions. *J Thromb Haemost.* 2008;6(2):243-248.
5. Tripodi A, Mannucci PM. The coagulopathy of chronic liver disease. *N Engl J Med.* 2011;365:147-156.
6. Marco Ranieri V, Taylor Thompson B, Barie PS, et al. Drotrecogin alfa (activated) in adults with septic shock. *N Engl J Med.* 2012;366(22):2055-2064.
7. Thachil J, Toh CH, Levi M, Watson H. The withdrawal of activated protein C from the use in patients with severe sepsis and DIC [amendment to the BCSH guideline on disseminated intravascular coagulation]. *Br J Haematol.* 2012;157:493-516.
8. Thachil J, Toh CH. Current concepts in the management of disseminated intravascular coagulation. *Thromb Res.* 2012;129(S1):554-559.
9. Levi M, Meijers JC. DIC: which laboratory tests are most useful. *Blood Rev.* 2011;25:33-37.
10. Favaloro E. Laboratory testing in disseminated intravascular coagulation. *Semin Thromb Haemost.* 2010;36:458-468.
11. Bakhtiari K, Meijers JC, de Jonge E, et al. Prospective validation of the International Society of Thrombosis and Haemostasis scoring system for disseminated intravascular coagulation. *Crit Care Med.* 2004;32(12):2416-2421.
12. Carson J, Grossman B, Kleinman S, et al. Red blood cell transfusion: a clinical practice guideline from the AABB. *Ann Intern Med.* 2012;157:49-58.
13. Collins P, Baudo F, Knoebl P, et al. Immunosuppression for acquired hemophilia A: results from the European Acquired Haemophilia Registry (EACH2). *Blood.* 2012;120(1):47-55.
14. Alperin J. Coagulopathy caused by vitamin K deficiency in critically ill, hospitalized patients. *JAMA.* 1987;258:1916-1919.
15. Pabinger J, Brenner B, Kalina U, et al. Prothrombin complex concentrate (Beriplex P/N) for emergency anticoagulation reversal: a prospective multinational clinical trial. *J Thromb Haemost.* 2008;6:622-631.
16. Marlu R, Hodaj E, Paris A, Albaladejo P, Cracowski JL, Pernod G. Effect of non-specific reversal agents on anticoagulant activity of dabigatran and rivaroxaban: a randomized cross over ex vivo study in healthy volunteers. *Thromb Haemost.* 2012;108:217-224.
17. Tiede A, Rand JH, Budde U, Ganser A, Federici AB. How I treat acquired von Willebrand syndrome. *Blood.* 2011;117(25):6777-6785.
18. Grathwohl KW, Bruns BJ, LeBrun J, et al. Does hemodilution exist? Effects of saline infusion on hematologic parameters in euvolemic subjects. *South Med J.* 1996;89(1):51-55.
19. Stamler KD. Effect of crystalloid infusion on hematocrit in nonbleeding patients, with applications to clinical traumatology. *Ann Emerg Med.* 1989;18(7):747-749.
20. Bolliger D, Goerlinger K, Tanaka KA. Pathophysiology and treatment of coagulopathy in massive hemorrhage and hemodilution. *Anesthesiology.* 2010;113:1016-1018.
21. Savage SA, Zarzaur BL, Croce MA, Fabian TC. Redefining massive transfusion when every second counts. *J Trauma Acute Care Surg.* 2013;74(2):396-400; discussion 400-392.
22. Holcomb JB, Pati S. Optimal trauma resuscitation with plasma as the primary resuscitative fluid: the surgeon's perspective. *Hematology Am Soc Hematol Educ Program.* 2013;2013:656-659.
23. Fenger-Eriksen C, Tonnesen E, Ingerslev J, Sorensen B. Mechanisms of hydroxyethyl starch-induced dilutional coagulopathy. *J Thromb Haemost.* 2009;7:1099-1105.
24. Levi M, Levy JH, Andersen HF, Truloff D. Safety of recombinant activated factor VII

in randomized clinical trials. *N Engl J Med.*
2010;363(19):1791-1800.

25. Mannucci PM, Levi M. Prevention and treatment of major blood loss. *N Engl J Med.* 2007;356:2301-2311.

26. Thiele T, Selleng K, Selleng S, Greinacher A, Bakchouf T. Thrombocytopenia in the intensive care unit-diagnostic approach and management. *Semin Hematol.* 2013;50:239-250.

27. Slichter S. Evidence-based platelet transfusion guidelines. *Hematology Am Soc Hematol Educ Program.* 2007:172-178.

28. Laurence J. Atypical hemolytic uremic syndrome (aHUS): making the diagnosis. *Clin Advan Hematol Oncol.* 2012;10(S17):1-12.

29. Rangarajan S, Kessler C, Aledort L. The clinical implications of ADAMTS13 function: the perspectives of haemostaseologists. *Thromb Res.* 2013;132:403-407.

30. Scully M, Cohen H, Cavenagh J, et al. Remission in acute refractory and relapsing thrombotic thrombocytopenic purpura following rituximab is associated with a reduction in IgG antibodies to ADAMTS13. *Br J Haematol.* 2007;136(3):451-461.

31. Warkentin TE. HITlights: a career perspective on heparin-induced thrombocytopenia. *Am J Hematol.* 2012;87(suppl 1):S92-S99.

32. Saugel B, Phillip V, Moessmer G, Schmid RM, Huber W. Argatroban therapy for heparin-induced thrombocytopenia in ICU patients with multiple organ dysfunction syndrome: a retrospective study. *Crit Care.* 2010;14(3):R90.

33. Neunert C, Lim W, Crowther M, Cohen A, Solberg L Jr, Crowther MA. The American Society of Hematology 2011 evidence-based practice guideline for immune thrombocytopenia. *Blood.* 2011;117:4190-4207.

34. Priziola J, Smythe M, Dager W. Drug-induced thrombocytopenia in critically ill patients. *Crit Care Med.* 2010;38:S145-S154.

35. Cervantes F. Current issues in myeloproliferative neoplasms management of essential thrombocythemia. *Hematology.* 2011;2011:215-221.

36. Powell JS et al N Engle J Med 2013-PMID 24304002; Mahlangu et al Blood 2014, PMID: 24227821; Konkle B et al Blood 2015, PMID 26157075

Transfusion Medicine in Critical Care

33

Aryeh Shander, MD; Carmine Gianatiempo, MD and Lawrence T. Goodnough, MD

KEY POINTS

1 Patient blood management (PBM) is the timely application of evidence-based medical and surgical concepts designed to maintain hemoglobin (Hb) concentration, optimize hemostasis, and minimize blood loss in an effort to improve patient outcome.

2 Anemia in the critically ill patients is often multifactorial and can be traced to one or a combination of iron deficiency, inflammatory responses, blunt response to endogenous erythropoietin, bleeding and aggressive diagnostic blood draws that are common in many intensive care units (ICUs).

3 The use of hemoglobin as the only "trigger" for red blood cell (RBC) transfusion should

be avoided, and transfusion decisions should be made based on other parameters such as patient's volume status, evidence of shock, duration, and severity of anemia, and cardiopulmonary status of the patient.

4 The benefit of fresh frozen plasma (FFP) administration remains controversial and with the advent of more specific factor concentrates, its indications are on the decline.

5 Higher plasma (and platelet) to RBC ratios as part of "balanced" transfusion protocols during early resuscitation of trauma patients may be associated with better survival, but is still under investigation.

INTRODUCTION TO PATIENT BLOOD MANAGEMENT

Blood transfusion occurs in 1 of every 10 hospital admissions that includes an invasive procedure, and has been identified as one of the top 5 most frequently overused therapeutic procedures in the United States.[1,2] Allogeneic blood transfusions have been associated with unfavorable patient outcomes, including morbidity and mortality[3]; and a significant percentage of transfusions to hospitalized patients have been identified to be inappropriate.[4] These observations have led to proposals that exposure to blood transfusion should be regarded as quality indicators for clinical services.

Awareness of the risks, costs, and trends of blood inventory has stimulated interest in examining clinical implications of transfusions. Established in 2000, the Society for the Advancement of Blood Management (SABM, www.sabm.org) recognized the unmet need and developed the concept of PBM that changed the focus from transfusion of products (blood) to the patients' needs with the emphasis on improving patients' outcome. PBM is defined by SABM as "the timely application of evidence-based medical and surgical concepts designed to maintain hemoglobin concentration, optimize hemostasis, and minimize blood loss in an effort to improve patient outcome."[i] The concept has been adopted by organizations globally, ranging from the National Blood Transfusion Committee in the United Kingdom, AABB in the United States, and National Blood Authority in Australia, to the World Health Organization (WHO) as put forward in Declaration 63.12 by the 63rd World Health Assembly.[5,6]

The PBM strategies in general have included management of anemia, minimization of blood loss, and increased focus on evidence-based transfusion practices, 3 strategies which form the pillars of PBM.[7] It should be noted that despite many similarities, the "product-centered" concept of blood management—the predecessor to PBM—primarily addresses improving blood utilization which results in improved patient safety and reduced costs with reduced exposure to RBC transfusions and their inherent risks.[6] PBM took this concept to a higher level by giving priority to improving the patient outcomes.

Blood management has been cited as 1 of the 10 key advances in transfusion medicine over the last 50 years,[8] and it is being increasingly adopted as a standard of care across the globe.[5] We have reported successful implementation of a system of clinical decision support (CDS) using a best practice alert (BPA) at computerized provider order entry (CPOE)[9] in order to improve blood utilization at our institution. As already indicated, this is just one aspect of numerous strategies that are utilized as part of a PBM program, and below we address some other PBM strategies.

Anemia Prevention, Screening, and Management

Anemia is a major risk factor for transfusion and an independent predictor of increased morbidity and mortality and diminished quality of life in many patient populations including the critically ill.[10] Anemia is particularly prevalent in critically ill patients, with a tendency to exacerbate during ICU stay.[11] The reported prevalence of anemia in the ICU is

understandably variable, and it usually ranges from 50% to almost 100%.[11-13] Anemia in the critically ill patients is often multifactorial and can be traced to one or a combination of iron deficiency, inflammatory responses, blunt response to endogenous erythropoietin, bleeding, and aggressive diagnostic blood draws that are common in many ICUs.[14,15]

Anemia should not be left unmanaged and proper screening for and management of anemia is a key strategy in patient blood management. This is particularly important during the perioperative period. Guidelines developed under the auspices of the Network for Advancement of Transfusion Alternatives (NATA) recommend routine screening for anemia in patients scheduled for elective surgery as early as 4 weeks prior to the scheduled surgery.[16] This approach will allow time for proper diagnostic workup of the anemia and its treatment, and the treating clinicians can consider rescheduling of the elective surgery if needed.[6] While these guidelines primarily target patients undergoing elective surgeries, they can also be useful in the critical care setting, particularly for proper diagnosis and management of anemia in the critically ill patients.

Understanding the etiology of anemia is necessary to guide the treatment, although more than one etiology often coexist. The NATA guidelines propose an algorithm for detection and management of preoperative anemia with primary emphasis on assessment of iron status (serum ferritin and transferrin saturation).[6] Iron deficiency syndromes (a spectrum including absolute iron deficiency, functional iron deficiency, and iron sequestration) are commonly present in patients. Iron deficiency can be effectively treated with iron, with several intravenous iron preparations available.[17] Erythropoiesis-stimulating agents (ESAs) are another group of medications that can be used to rapidly increase red blood cell mass and hemoglobin level. These are highly useful and potent agents that should be used appropriately to balance their benefits against their documented side effects, such as increased risk of thromboembolic events.[18]

Reduction and Avoidance of Blood Loss

Blood loss is another important predictor and risk factor for blood transfusion is the amount of surgical

---

[i] What is patient blood management? PROFESSIONAL DEFINITION. Society for the Advancement of Blood Management. http://www.sabm.org. Accessed August 2, 2014.

blood loss.[19] This issue is most commonly encountered in surgical patients (including critically ill surgical patients), but it can also affect all other critically ill patients. Efforts should be made to avoid any unnecessary blood loss, and to retrieve and salvage the shed blood if blood loss occurs (red cell salvage). Several studies have supported the safety and efficacy of red cell salvage in intra- and postoperative periods.[20] Hemostatic agents, tools such as electrocautery, and approaches such as minimally invasive procedures are other important strategies for reducing surgical blood loss.[21] Of particular interest is the use of lysine analogues including tranexamic acid in reducing blood loss and improving patient outcomes in various settings including surgical and critically ill trauma patients.[22,23]

Close surveillance and monitoring of patients in the postoperative period for signs of bleeding and immediate attention to control it is very important. Last but not least, special consideration should be given to diagnostic blood draws which can be a significant source of blood loss, with reports indicating an average of 40 mL per day of blood draws in the ICUs.[24] Measures to control and reduce this source of blood loss in the critically ill patients include elimination of unnecessary and standing orders and limiting the volume of the blood draws to the minimum needed to achieve the results.[24]

Evidence-Based Transfusion Practices

Another important aspect of PBM is the justified utilization of allogeneic blood components to achieve clear clinical end points. Several physiologic mechanisms are in place to maintain the oxygen delivery to the tissues despite reduced blood oxygen-carrying capacity in anemia. These include improved ventilation-perfusion matching in the lungs, increased heart function and cardiac output, redistribution of vascular flow toward more critical tissues, and increased extraction of oxygen from blood at tissue site. Thanks to these and other physiologic adaptations, oxygen consumption at the tissues remains relatively unchanged despite substantial changes in oxygen-carrying capacity of blood due to anemia. With progress of anemia, however, a point is reached that these compensatory mechanisms are no further sufficient, and tissue oxygen consumption drops as

hypoxia develops.[10] In such situations, transfusion of red blood cells alongside other management strategies to increase oxygen delivery (eg, supplemental oxygen therapy) or decreased oxygen need (eg, neuromuscular block or control of heart rate) is critical in avoiding ischemia.[7,10]

The issue is further complicated in the critically ill patients, as many of these compensatory mechanisms can already be disrupted (eg, respiratory or cardiac failure). Critical illness is often associated with increased oxygen demand and consumption at tissues, further compromising the tolerance of anemia and increasing the likelihood of the patients becoming hypoxic.[24] Judicious use of allogeneic blood products when the potential benefits outweigh the risks remains an important aspect of PBM, and evidence-based guidelines for use of these treatments in the critically ill patients are discussed in subsequent sections.

UTILIZATION OF BLOOD COMPONENTS IN ICU

Anemia—preexisting or new onset—is common in the critical care units (ICUs), and blood transfusions are routinely employed to "correct" anemia in this setting. In a surgical ICU, about 19% of the patients had Hb less than 7 g/dL and 30% had Hb levels between 7 and 9 g/dL,[12] indicating that a significant number of ICU patients were anemic (many, moderately or severely anemic) according to the WHO definition of anemia.[10] The reported incidence and prevalence were 46.6% and 68%, respectively among cancer patients admitted to another ICU.[13] Another prospective study reported that almost all consecutive patients admitted to a general ICU were anemic, and patients' Hb level continued to drop during their ICU stay.[11] The etiology of anemia in the ICU is varied and often multifactorial, and can include iron deficiency, inflammatory responses, blunt response to endogenous erythropoietin, bleeding and aggressive diagnostic blood draws.[14,15] A large and evergrowing body of evidence supports the independent link between anemia and unfavorable clinical outcomes in various patient populations including the critically ill.[10]

Although transfusion of blood components in ICU is common, the clinical evidence to guide the use of these products is limited. It has been estimated that greater than 40% of patients receive one or more RBC transfusions while in the ICU, and about 90% of transfusions are provided in the context of stable anemia without evidence of need or benefit of the transfused blood.[25] In a matched-cohort study of nonbleeding critically ill patients with moderate anemia (Hb between 7 and 9.5 g/dL), RBC transfusions were associated with increased mortality and nosocomial infections.[26] Several other studies have indicated that transfusions are associated with worsening of clinical outcomes, and they are often ineffective in improving oxygen consumption, questioning the main reason they are given to the patients in the first place.[10,27]

In a single-center study it was reported that about 50% of patients received blood products during their ICU stay: 48.3% received packed red blood cells; 18.3% received FFP, and 8.4% of patients received platelet transfusion. Interestingly, approximately one-fourth to one-half of these transfusions were not medically indicated.[28] According to a study performed in 29 ICUs in the United Kingdom, 9% of the patients received platelet transfusion in ICU, one-third of which occurred in patients with platelet counts above 50×10^9/L and in absence of clinically significant bleeding.[29] In a prospective cohort study of septic shock patients, 57% of the patients received FFP transfusion during ICU stay; one-third of the plasma transfusions were given without any evidence of bleeding or any planned invasive procedures.[30] A survey has also shown substantial variations in transfusion practices and uncertainties toward indications of plasma transfusions in ICU among clinicians.[31]

On the other hand, one study in 47 ICUs in Australia and New Zealand indicated (although somewhat broadly interpreted) that 98% of RBC transfusions were performed according to the national transfusion guidelines, while only 47% of platelet, 71% of FFP, and 12% of cryoprecipitate transfusions were done according to the guidelines.[32] Of note, in this study 40.2% of the RBC transfusions were given to improve oxygen delivery (DO_2) and 43.6% of the RBC transfusions were given for bleeding (nearly half of which were considered to be "minor").[32] As will be discussed later, these numbers may not be necessarily consistent with current evidence or guidelines for use of RBC transfusions in critically ill patients.

Somewhat similar results were observed in a single-center study in Spain where RBC transfusion seem to be more restrictive than any of the other blood components.[33] These findings are also consistent with the high frequency of blood product transfusion and high variability in transfusion practices reported in many other studies and reviews.[34]

Evidence-based general recommendations for transfusion of RBCs, plasma, and platelets were discussed in previous sections. Here we take a closer look at these blood components and their usage in ICU.

Red Blood Cells

RBC is a heterogeneous group of products that includes packed red blood cells (PRBCs), gamma-irradiated blood, washed RBCs, and whole blood. PRBC is the preparation used in most clinical situations. One unit PRBC has an average volume of 300 mL, of which two-thirds is consisted of RBCs, and the remaining is mostly the preservative solution. Each unit has a hematocrit of approximately 55% to 60% and approximately 200 mg of iron.[35] PRBCs undergo leukoreduction (removal of leukocytes) and hence are known as *leukoreduced* PRBCs. Universal leukoreduction of allogeneic blood as part of blood banking process has been implemented in an increasing number of nations. Leukoreduction has been suggested to improve the safety profile of allogeneic blood by reducing the risk of febrile transfusion reactions, alloimmunization and transmission of some pathogens (cytomegalovirus [CMV] and possibly prions), but the overall impact on patient outcomes and its cost-benefits are still a matter of debate.[36] Although leukoreduced PRBC units are gaining universal acceptance, these units are more costly, and in some instances may be preferred for chronically transfused patients, potential transplant recipients, patients with previous transfusion reactions, patients undergoing cardiopulmonary bypass, and CMV seronegative patients at risk for CMV infection.

Gamma-irradiated RBC units are produced by subjecting the units of blood to external-beam radiation. This process results in destruction of donor T-lymphocytes in the blood and is effective for prevention of graft-versus-host disease (GVHD) in the transfused patients, particularly the transplant patients and severely immunocompromised patients. However, irradiation is associated with several changes in the RBCs which could result in reduced life span of these units.[37]

As the name suggests, washed RBCs are produced by "washing" the donor cells with normal saline solution to remove as much of the proteins and macromolecules of the donor plasma as possible. These units are preferred for patients with immunoglobulin A deficiency and those at high risk for anaphylactic reaction.[38] Lastly, whole blood is rarely indicated and seldom available and it is most often considered in the context of massive blood transfusion. The rationale is to avoid dilutional deficiencies that can be caused with transfusion of other components.[39]

For many decades, transfusion of RBCs was used to maintain a blood hemoglobin level above 10 g/dL or a hematocrit above 30% (the 10/30 rule), even though these thresholds were arbitrary numbers with no proven physiologic or clinical significance. Emergence of a large body of work and clinical evidence, especially within the last 25 years, has changed transfusion practice to balance the benefit of treating anemia with the desire to avoid unnecessary transfusion and its associated risks and complications in various medical settings including in the ICU.[40] However, there is evidence to suggest that considerable variation in RBC transfusion practices in critical care still exists. A Canadian scenario-based national survey sent to critical care practitioners demonstrated that transfusion thresholds differed significantly ($P < 0.0001$) when faced with different medical scenarios.[41] A study by Herbert and colleagues examined blood use in 5298 consecutive patients admitted to 6 tertiary level ICUs.[42] The overall number of transfusions per patient day ranged from 0.82 ± 1.69 to 1.08 ± 1.27 between institutions ($P < 0.001$).

The multicenter Transfusion Requirements in Critical Care (TRICC) trial showed that a restrictive strategy, that is, a threshold for transfusion for hemoglobin less than 7 g/dL in critically ill patients is safe.[43] Furthermore, there is a trend toward decreased hospital morbidity and mortality when compared to patients with a more liberal (transfusion for a hemoglobin < 10 g/dL) transfusion strategy. An exception to this strategy is patients with

acute myocardial ischemia. The optimal transfusion threshold for these patients has not been determined because such patients were excluded from most clinical trials. Similarly, the Transfusion Requirements in Pediatric ICU (TRIPICU) study showed that in stable, critically ill children, using a Hb threshold of 7 g/dL for transfusion can reduce the transfusions compared with a Hb threshold of 9.5 g/dL without negatively affecting the outcomes.[44] Subsequent subgroup analyses of this trial further supported the restrictive transfusion strategy in patients with higher severity of illness, postsurgical patients and those with respiratory dysfunction, sepsis, neurologic disorders, and severe trauma.[45]

The joint taskforce of Eastern Association for Surgery of Trauma (EAST) and the American College of Critical Care Medicine (ACCM) of the Society of Critical Care Medicine (SCCM) have developed clinical practice guidelines for RBC transfusion in the critically ill patients.[36] Based on these guidelines, RBC transfusion is indicated for patients with evidence of hemorrhagic shock, and it may also be indicated for those with evidence of acute hemorrhage and hemodynamic instability or inadequate DO_2. According to these guidelines, in hemodynamically stable critically ill patients, transfusion of RBC at hemoglobin level of less than 7 g/dL is as effective as using a more liberal trigger of Hb less than 10 g/dL, with the possible exception of patients with acute myocardial infarction or unstable myocardial ischemia, given the paucity of data on these patients. However, the guidelines emphasize that use of hemoglobin as the only "trigger" for RBC transfusion should be avoided, and transfusion decisions should be made based on other parameters such as patient's volume status, evidence of shock, duration and severity of anemia, and cardiopulmonary status of the patient.[36] Based on these guidelines, RBC transfusion should be **considered** in critically ill patients with Hb less than 7 g/dL in following conditions: patients who require mechanical ventilation (despite lack of conclusive evidence), resuscitated trauma patients, and patients with stable cardiac disease. Despite lack of supportive evidence, the guidelines recommend that RBC transfusion may be considered in critically ill patients with acute coronary syndrome with Hb less than or equal to 8 g/dL. The guidelines recommend against RBC transfusion as an absolute method to improve tissue oxygen consumption (VO_2). When indicated and with exception of acute hemorrhage, RBC transfusion should be given 1 unit at a time, with reevaluation of the patient prior to giving the next unit.[36] The guidelines call for individual assessment of transfusion needs in each septic patient given that optimal transfusion threshold and the impact of transfusion on oxygen consumption in these patients are not well established.[36]

In critically ill patients with or at risk of acute respiratory distress or lung injury, the guidelines call for making all efforts to avoid RBC transfusions after completion of resuscitation, and to appropriately diagnose transfusion-related acute lung injury (TRALI) given its prominence as a leading cause of morbidity and mortality in transfused patients. The guidelines proscribe against use of RBC transfusion with the goal of facilitating weaning patients from mechanical ventilation.[36]

The guidelines indicate no benefit for liberal transfusion (at Hb > 10 g/dL) in patients with moderate-to-severe traumatic brain injury (TBI). In patients with subarachnoid hemorrhage (SAH), transfusion decisions must be made on case-by-case basis since the optimal transfusion threshold and the impact of transfusion on outcomes in these patients are undetermined.[36] The guidelines provide an overview of various blood management strategies that can be used in critically ill patients to reduce the avoidable allogeneic transfusions and improve the outcomes of the patients.[36] Of note, the guidelines emphasize the insufficiency of the available evidence in many of the discussed topics,[36] underscoring the importance of further research in the field.

Similar to general critically ill patient populations, evidence regarding transfusion in critically ill children is very limited. Anemia and transfusion are both common in these patients, and in addition to proper management of anemia, transfusion decisions should be made based on the individual patient's factors and characteristics, rather than using general transfusion triggers, and appropriate blood management strategies should be utilized.[46]

Another set of transfusion guidelines for the critically ill adult patients has recently been developed by the British Committee for Standards in Haematology (BCSH).[24] These guidelines share many similarities with the ACCM/SCCM transfusion guidelines discussed above.[36] They recommend a Hb level of less than or equal to 7 g/dL (with a target Hb range of 7-9 g/dL) as the default transfusion threshold in critically ill patients in general. Again, despite lack of evidence, a target Hb level of 7 to 9 g/dL has been recommended in patients with TBI as well as during later stages of severe sepsis (vs a Hb target of 9-10 g/dL during early resuscitation of severe sepsis with evidence of inadequate DO_2). Similarly, despite lack of supporting data, the guidelines recommend that Hb level of patients with stable angina should be maintained above 7 g/dL. In addition, a target Hb level of 8 to 10 g/dL is recommended in patients with SAH and the Hb should be kept greater than 8 to 9 g/dL in patients with acute coronary syndrome. Finally, a target Hb level of greater than 9 g/dL is recommended in TBI patients with evidence of cerebral ischemia and patients with acute ischemic stroke.[24] Similar to the ACCM/SCCM guidelines, the BCSH guidelines recommend against use of RBC transfusion to facilitate weaning patients from mechanical ventilation if Hb greater than 7 g/dL.[24]

Most recently and as part of its evidence-based "Choosing Wisely" recommendations, the Critical Care Societies Collaborative (CCSC)—a multidisciplinary group composed of the American Association of Critical-Care Nurses (AACN), American College of Chest Physicians (ACCP), American Thoracic Society (ATS), and SCCM—have identified transfusion of RBCs as one of routine practices in the ICUs that should be questioned, given its doubtful benefits and certain harms. The group has made the recommendation to not transfuse RBCs in hemodynamically stable, nonbleeding critically ill patients with Hb greater than 7 mg/dL.[ii] The AACN—as part of the CCSC—has identified 5 routine critical care practices that should be questioned because they may not always be necessary and could, in fact, be harmful.

Plasma Products

Plasma is the portion of whole blood that remains after white cells, red cells, and platelets are removed

---

[ii] Critical Care Societies Collaborative (CCSC)—Critical Care. Five things physicians and patients should question. http://www.choosingwisely.org/doctor-patient-lists/critical-care-societies-collaborative-critical-care/. Accessed February 20, 2014.

by centrifugation. Plasma contains various macromolecules namely procoagulation and anticoagulation factors, albumin, and immunoglobulins. It is indicated when inadequate hemostasis is present and the benefits of correction outweighs risks of transfusion. However, the benefit of plasma administration remains controversial, and with the advent of more specific factor concentrates, its indications are on the decline.

Plasma products come in a number of forms. FFP is separated from freshly drawn blood by removing the cellular components. It is frozen for storage and thawed when needed for transfusion. Once thawed, FFP needs to be transfused within 24 hours as factors V and VIII decline with time. Also, FFP must be cross-matched to confirm ABO compatibility. Thawed plasma is a plasma not transfused within 24 hours of thawing. It can be transfused for up to 5 days if it is kept refrigerated at 1°C to 6°C. Other plasma products include jumbo apheresis plasma, single-donor, liquid plasma, and solvent/detergent-treated (SD) plasma (Octaplas). Cryoprecipitate is a by-product of FFP and it is obtained by thawing FFP at 4°C and collecting the white precipitate. It is rich in von Willebrand factor (vWF), factors VIII and XIII, and fibrinogen. It allows replacement of these factors using much smaller volumes compared with plasma volumes needed to achieve the same level of factors.

A prospective, observational study of an adult ICU determined that the incidence of laboratory evidence of coagulopathy was 67% of patients and 14% of patients received transfusion of FFP.[47] Approximately one-third of FFP usage is for correction of elevated international normalized ratio (INR) prior to invasive and surgical procedures[48]; however, there is a paucity of evidence to support this practice. Furthermore, plasma should not be used to reverse supratherapeutic warfarin effects, unless in the presence of active bleeding or need for invasive or surgical procedures because plasma products are only partially effective,[49] its action is of short duration and it could increase the risk of hypervolemia (transfusion-associated circulatory overload [TACO]) and other complications such as TRALI).[50]

The response to plasma transfusion is directly proportional to the difference between the patient level of coagulation factors and that of the infused plasma. Thus, patients with severe deficiencies are more likely to see a more significant change in their INR than patients with mild deficiencies. It is worth noting that the INR of a unit of plasma is usually elevated itself and tends to be around 1.3.[51] The dose of FFP transfused to patients is also commonly erroneous and often inadequate to achieve the desire impact on coagulation. The response to cryoprecipitate transfusion is even more difficult to predict; 10 bags of cryoprecipitate is expected to increase fibrinogen level by approximately 70 mg/dL. With availability of prothrombin complex concentrates (PCC)—particularly the 4-factor products—there is less need to plasma for reversing the effects of warfarin.[52] Use of plasma in conjunction with other blood components to create a "balanced" transfusion strategy in trauma resuscitation has been gaining more interest. The Prospective, Observational, Multicenter, Major Trauma Transfusion (PROMMTT) study has indicated that higher plasma (and platelet) to RBC ratios during early resuscitation of trauma patients were associated with better survival in patients who received at least 3 units of RBC during the first 24 hours.[53] Another phase III trial in massively transfused trauma patients, Pragmatic, Randomized Optimal Platelets and Plasma Ratios (PROPPR) study compared the effectiveness of transfusing patients with severe trauma and major bleeding using plasma, platelets and red blood cells in a 1:1:1 ratio compared with a 1:1:2 ratio. No significant differences in mortality were detected at 24 hours or at 30 days. However, exsanguination, which was the prominent cause of death within the first 24 hours, was significantly decreased in the 1:1:1 group (9.2% vs 14.6% in the 1:1:2 group, P = 0.03) and more patients achieved hemostasis in the 1:1:1 group (86% vs 78%, P = 0.006).[54] Of note, rapid anatomic control of bleeding (e.g., primary surgical hemostasis) was not reported and might have influenced the hemostasis results. Furthermore, ratio-based transfusion is not intended to replace transfusion based on coagulation testing but rather to supplement it with the goal of more effective control of acute trauma coagulopathy and hemorrhagic shock.[55]

Platelets

Platelet concentrates are prepared from whole blood by centrifugation at low speeds to separate the erythrocytes. The supernatant, "platelet-rich plasma" is then centrifuged at high speeds to separate the platelets. This results in "pooled concentrates." It is less expensive to produce, but more donors are required because the yield is lower; 6 to 10 donors are required per platelet transfusion. Single-donor apheresis platelet concentrates are obtained by apheresis; that is, whole blood from a donor passes through a device that separates the platelets while returning the remainder to the donor. This process is more expensive, but it has a higher yield, fewer donors are necessary (one donor per platelets transfusion), and hence the risk of transmission of infection is lower compared with pooled platelets. Platelet concentrates can be stored for up to 7 days, but platelets start losing their efficacy (viability) after 3 days.[56]

The generally expected response to transfusion of 1 unit of platelets is a rise in platelet count by 5 to 10,000; presence of platelet destruction or consumption at the bleeding site can blunt this response. Efficacy is reduced by the presence of antibodies to ABO antigens on platelets or to leukocyte antigens. This can be ameliorated with transfusions of ABO-compatible platelets or using single-donor concentrates.

Current indications for platelet transfusions in thrombocytopenic patients can be therapeutic or prophylactic.[56] These include the following:

- Platelet count less than 10,000, to reduce the risk of spontaneous bleeding
- Platelet count less than 50,000, in patients who are actively bleeding, or are scheduled for invasive procedures, or have a qualitative platelet defect
- Platelet count between 70,000 and 100,000, with a central nervous system (CNS) injury, or undergoing neurosurgery or intrathecal catheter insertion
- Normal platelet count, with active bleeding due to platelet dysfunction (although platelet transfusion is not consistently effective in these patients)

As discussed earlier, the most efficient use of platelets (alongside plasma) as part of "balanced" transfusion protocols to supplement RBCs during trauma resuscitation is still under investigation.

Complications

A number of complications can result from transfusions of blood products. Often, the greater the volume of transfusion, the greater is the risk or severity of the complication. These complications can be infectious (human immunodeficiency virus [HIV], hepatitis B virus [HBV], hepatitis C virus [HCV], hepatitis A virus [HAV], human T-cell leukemia/lymphoma virus [HTLV], parvovirus B19, bacterial) or noninfectious which include acute hemolytic reactions, delayed hemolytic reactions, febrile reactions, allergic reactions, posttransfusion purpura (rare), acute lung injury (TRALI), immunomodulation, that is, the immunosuppressive activity of allogeneic blood transfusion, and transfusion-related GVHD.[57] Other complications include volume overload (TACO) with consequent pulmonary edema due to expansion of the intravascular volume especially in patients with compromised cardiac or renal function or due to fluids shift due to increased oncotic pressure particularly with FFP; hypothermia if large volumes are transfused rapidly (blood products are stored at cold temperatures); coagulopathy presumably as a result of hemodilution from resuscitative fluids and acidosis secondary to tissue hypoxia; and life-threatening hyperkalemia (especially in pediatric population with relatively large transfusion volume). Citrate is present in stored blood products and can lead to metabolic alkalosis and hypocalcemia.[57]

With significant advances in the screening and testing of donors for transmittable diseases, the infectious risks are very rare with an incidence ranging from 1 for every 7,800,000 units of RBC units transfused for HIV to 1 in 50,000 units transfused for bacterial contamination. However, the incidence of bacterial contamination is much more common with platelet transfusion with a reported incidence of 1 infection per 1000 units of platelets transfused,[57] and septic transfusion reactions remain a concern with platelet transfusions, making the case for additional testing. The American Association of Blood Banks (now referred to as AABB) standards call for the use of enhanced bacteria detection methods and require blood banks or transfusion services to employ methods to detect bacteria in all platelet components.[iii] The nature of allogeneic blood and reliance on donors and screening tests means that the risk of transmitting infections through blood can never be fully eliminated and some residual risk of undetected and/or emerging pathogens remains.[57]

Acute hemolytic reactions occur due to antibodies, usually IgM in the recipient's serum against major antigens present on the donor's RBCs. These are almost always due to ABO incompatibility. The frequency has been described to range from 1 in 40,000 to 1 in a 1,000,000. These occur within the first several minutes of transfusion and manifest acutely with fever, tachycardia, hypotension, dyspnea, and back and chest pain.[57]

Delayed hemolytic reactions usually occur more than 24 to 48 hours, and up to 7 to 10 days after the transfusion. They result from antibodies in the recipient's serum directed toward minor antigens on the donor's RBCs. These reactions occur with a frequency of 1 in 7000 with a sudden decrease in hemoglobin. They are often mild and frequently undetected and require no specific therapy.[57]

Febrile nonhemolytic reactions result from the presence of antileukocyte antibodies induced by previous transfusions acting against leukocytes in the donor's product or secondary to accumulated cytokines in stored blood components. It is relatively frequent, ranging from 1 in 20 (with platelets transfusion) to 1 in 300. These reactions are manifested acutely by an increase in body temperature. These are usually self-limited, but can be treated with antipyretics and the transfusion allowed to be completed. Leukoreduction of stored blood can reduce the incidence of febrile nonhemolytic reactions.[57]

Allergic reactions occur because of presence of allergens in the donor's blood component to which the patient has preexisting antibodies; they do not require previous blood exposure. These reactions can vary from urticaria and/or bronchospasm with a frequency of 1 in 100 to anaphylaxis, with a frequency of 1 in 40,000. Patients with IgA deficiency are especially at risk for severe anaphylactic reactions. These reactions are best prevented with washed RBCs, but

can be treated with high-dose corticosteroids, antihistamines, and airway protection.[57]

TRALI is related to presence of alloreactive plasma antibodies within red blood cell products or FFP which can lead to agglutination and diffuse activation of leukocytes with subsequent diffuse capillary damage of the pulmonary vasculature and rapid onset of acute pulmonary injury and development of inflammatory pulmonary edema. The pulmonary dysfunction may not manifest for hours to, less frequently, days after the transfusion was administered. The incidence of TRALI varies from 1 in 700, especially with FFP to 1 in 5000; however, this incidence may be underestimated as the reaction may go unrecognized.[57]

The adverse events discussed here are often recognized as known immediate complications of allogeneic blood transfusion, and most of the time, a causal link can be established and recognized. In critically ill patients, it is difficult at time to recognize these events because of the underlying acuity of the illness. Hypotension, sepsis, and shock can accompany some of the complications stated earlier or can occur independent of transfusion and due to the underlying disease. What complicates this picture is the delayed adverse outcomes that are associated with allogeneic transfusions. Several studies have shown that blood transfusions are independently associated with increased risk of wound infection, pneumonia, sepsis, and other nosocomial infections, multiorgan failure, systemic inflammatory response syndrome (SIRS), and other morbidities and mortality.[10,36]

CONCLUSIONS

Anemia and transfusion are common in critically ill patients and both are independently associated with worsening of patient outcome. Substantial variations in transfusion practices have been documented. Evidence-based guidelines for transfusion of blood components have been developed and available, even though the underlying "evidence" is often limited. Additionally, several PBM strategies are available to reduce and avoid unnecessary transfusions and improve the outcomes of critically ill patients. Use of these strategies alongside adherence to evidence-based transfusion guidelines are effective measures that can reduce inappropriate transfusions,[32,33] and improve the patients' outcomes.

[iii] AABB Standards. Interim standard 5.1.5.1.1. http://www.aabb.org/resources/governmentregulatory/bloodcomponents/platelets/Pages/default.aspx. Accessed February 20, 2014.

REFERENCES

1. Proceedings from the National Summit on Overuse. September 24, 2012. The Joint Commission. February 4, 2014 (http://www.jointcommission.org/assets/1/6/National_Summit_Overuse.pdf). Accessed: 7/14/2016.
2. Bulger J, Nickel W, Messler J, et al. Choosing wisely in adult hospital medicine: five opportunities for improved healthcare value. *J Hosp Med.* 2013;8:486-492.
3. Vamvakas EC. Establishing causation in transfusion medicine and related tribulations. *Transfus Med Rev.* 2011;25:81-88.
4. Spahn DR, Goodnough LT. Alternatives to blood transfusion. *Lancet.* 2013;381:1855-1865.
5. Farmer SL, Towler SC, Leahy MF, Hofmann A. Drivers for change: Western Australia Patient Blood Management Program (WA PBMP), World Health Assembly (WHA) and Advisory Committee on Blood Safety and Availability (ACBSA). *Best Pract Res Clin Anaesthesiol.* 2013;27:43-58.
6. Goodnough LT, Shander A. Patient blood management. *Anesthesiology.* 2012;116:1367-1376.
7. Shander A, Javidroozi M, Perelman S, Puzio T, Lobel G. From bloodless surgery to patient blood management. *Mt Sinai J Med.* 2012;79:56-65.
8. McCullough J. Innovation in transfusion medicine and blood banking: documenting the record in 50 years of TRANSFUSION. *Transfusion.* 2010;50:2542-2546.
9. Goodnough LT, Shieh L, Hadhazy E, Cheng N, Khari P, Maggio P. Improved blood utilization using real-time clinical decision support. *Transfusion.* 2014;54;1358-1365.
10. Shander A, Javidroozi M, Ozawa S, Hare GM. What is really dangerous: anaemia or transfusion? *Br J Anaesth.* 2011;107(suppl 1):i41-i59.
11. Thomas J, Jensen L, Nahirniak S, Gibney RT. Anemia and blood transfusion practices in the critically ill: a prospective cohort review. *Heart Lung.* 2010;39:217-225.
12. Sakr Y, Lobo S, Knuepfer S, et al. Anemia and blood transfusion in a surgical intensive care unit. *Crit Care.* 2010;14:R92.
13. Cardenas-Turanzas M, Cesta MA, Wakefield C, et al. Factors associated with anemia in patients with cancer admitted to an intensive care unit. *J Crit Care.* 2010;25:112-119.
14. Prakash D. Anemia in the ICU: anemia of chronic disease versus anemia of acute illness. *Crit Care Clin.* 2012;28:333-343.
15. Branco BC, Inaba K, Doughty R, et al. The increasing burden of phlebotomy in the development of

anaemia and need for blood transfusion amongst trauma patients. *Injury.* 2012;43:78-83.
16. Goodnough LT, Maniatis A, Earnshaw P, et al. Detection, evaluation, and management of preoperative anaemia in the elective orthopaedic surgical patient: NATA guidelines. *Br J Anaesth.* 2011;106:13-22.
17. Auerbach M, Goodnough LT, Shander A. Iron: the new advances in therapy. *Best Pract Res Clin Anaesthesiol.* 2013;27:131-140.
18. Goodnough LT, Shander A. Update on erythropoiesis-stimulating agents. *Best Pract Res Clin Anaesthesiol.* 2013;27:121-129.
19. Gombotz H, Rehak PH, Shander A, Hofmann A. Blood use in elective surgery: the Austrian benchmark study. *Transfusion.* 2007;47:1468-1480.
20. Carless PA, Henry DA, Moxey AJ, O'Connell D, Brown T, Fergusson DA. Cell salvage for minimising perioperative allogeneic blood transfusion. *Cochrane Database Syst Rev.* 2010;(4):CD001888.
21. Goodnough LT, Shander A. Current status of pharmacologic therapies in patient blood management. *Anesth Analg.* 2013;116:15-34.
22. Ker K, Prieto-Merino D, Roberts I. Systematic review, meta-analysis and meta-regression of the effect of tranexamic acid on surgical blood loss. *Br J Surg.* 2013;100:1271-1279.
23. Faraoni D, Van Der LP. A systematic review of antifibrinolytics and massive injury. *Minerva Anestesiol.* 2014;80:1115-1122.
24. Retter A, Wyncoll D, Pearse R, et al. Guidelines on the management of anaemia and red cell transfusion in adult critically ill patients. *Br J Haematol.* 2013;160:445-464.
25. Walsh TS, Garrioch M, Maciver C, et al. Red cell requirements for intensive care units adhering to evidence-based transfusion guidelines. *Transfusion.* 2004;44:1405-1411.
26. Leal-Noval SR, Munoz-Gomez M, Jimenez-Sanchez M, et al. Red blood cell transfusion in non-bleeding critically ill patients with moderate anemia: is there a benefit? *Intensive Care Med.* 2013;39:445-453.
27. Lelubre C, Vincent JL. Red blood cell transfusion in the critically ill patient. *Ann Intensive Care.* 2011;1:43.
28. Makroo RN, Mani RK, Vimarsh R, Kansal S, Pushkar K, Tyagi S. Use of blood components in critically ill patients in the medical intensive care unit of a tertiary care hospital. *Asian J Transfus Sci.* 2009;3:82-85.
29. Stanworth SJ, Walsh TS, Prescott RJ, Lee RJ, Watson DM, Wyncoll DL. Thrombocytopenia and platelet transfusion in UK critical care: a multicenter observational study. *Transfusion.* 2013;53:1050-1058.

30. Reiter N, Wesche N, Perner A. The majority of patients in septic shock are transfused with fresh-frozen plasma. *Dan Med J*. 2013;60:A4606.

31. Watson DM, Stanworth SJ, Wyncoll D, et al. A national clinical scenario-based survey of clinicians' attitudes towards fresh frozen plasma transfusion for critically ill patients. *Transfus Med*. 2011;21:124-129.

32. Westbrook A, Pettila V, Nichol A, et al. Transfusion practice and guidelines in Australian and New Zealand intensive care units. *Intensive Care Med*. 2010;36:1138-1146.

33. Leal-Noval SR, rellano-Orden V, Maestre-Romero A, et al. Impact of national transfusion indicators on appropriate blood usage in critically ill patients. *Transfusion*. 2011;51:1957-1965.

34. Shander A, Puzio T, Javidroozi M. Variability in transfusion practice and effectiveness of strategies to improve it. *J Cardiothorac Vasc Anesth*. 2012;26:541-544.

35. Shander A, Berth U, Betta J, Javidroozi M. Iron overload and toxicity: implications for anesthesiologists. *J Clin Anesth*. 2012;24:419-425.

36. Napolitano LM, Kurek S, Luchette FA, et al. Clinical practice guideline: red blood cell transfusion in adult trauma and critical care. *Crit Care Med*. 2009;37:3124-3157.

37. Mintz PD, Anderson G. Effect of gamma irradiation on the in vivo recovery of stored red blood cells. *Ann Clin Lab Sci*. 1993;23:216-220.

38. Popovsky MA. Frozen and washed red blood cells: new approaches and applications. *Transfus Apher Sci*. 2001;25:193-194.

39. Pham HP, Shaz BH. Update on massive transfusion. *Br J Anaesth*. 2013;111(suppl 1):i71-i82.

40. Marik PE, Corwin HL. Efficacy of red blood cell transfusion in the critically ill: a systematic review of the literature. *Crit Care Med*. 2008;36:2667-2674.

41. Hebert PC, Wells G, Martin C, et al. A Canadian survey of transfusion practices in critically ill patients. Transfusion Requirements in Critical Care Investigators and the Canadian Critical Care Trials Group. *Crit Care Med*. 1998;26:482-487.

42. Hebert PC, Wells G, Martin C, et al. Variation in red cell transfusion practice in the intensive care unit: a multicentre cohort study. *Crit Care*. 1999;3:57-63.

43. Hebert PC, Wells G, Blajchman MA, et al. A multicenter, randomized, controlled clinical trial of transfusion requirements in critical care. Transfusion Requirements in Critical Care Investigators, Canadian Critical Care Trials Group. *N Engl J Med*. 1999;340:409-417.

44. Lacroix J, Hebert PC, Hutchison JS, et al. Transfusion strategies for patients in pediatric intensive care units. *N Engl J Med*. 2007;356:1609-1619.

45. Lacroix J, Demaret P, Tucci M. Red blood cell transfusion: decision making in pediatric intensive care units. *Semin Perinatol*. 2012;36:225-231.

46. Istaphanous GK, Wheeler DS, Lisco SJ, Shander A. Red blood cell transfusion in critically ill children: a narrative review. *Pediatr Crit Care Med*. 2011;12:174-183.

47. Chakraverty R, Davidson S, Peggs K, Stross P, Garrard C, Littlewood TJ. The incidence and cause of coagulopathies in an intensive care population. *Br J Haematol*. 1996;93:460-463.

48. Vlaar AP, In der Maur AL, Binnekade JM, Schultz MJ, Juffermans NP. Determinants of transfusion decisions in a mixed medical-surgical intensive care unit: a prospective cohort study. *Blood Transfus*. 2009;7:106-110.

49. Yang L, Stanworth S, Hopewell S, Doree C, Murphy M. Is fresh-frozen plasma clinically effective? An update of a systematic review of randomized controlled trials. *Transfusion*. 2012;52:1673-1686.

50. Roback JD, Caldwell S, Carson J, et al. Evidence-based practice guidelines for plasma transfusion. *Transfusion*. 2010;50:1227-1239.

51. Abdel-Wahab OI, Healy B, Dzik WH. Effect of fresh-frozen plasma transfusion on prothrombin time and bleeding in patients with mild coagulation abnormalities. *Transfusion*. 2006;46:1279-1285.

52. Tran HA, Chunilal SD, Harper PL, Tran H, Wood EM, Gallus AS. An update of consensus guidelines for warfarin reversal. *Med J Aust*. 2013;198:198-199.

53. Holcomb JB, del Junco DJ, Fox EE, et al. The prospective, observational, multicenter, major trauma transfusion (PROMMTT) study: comparative effectiveness of a time-varying treatment with competing risks. *JAMA Surg*. 2013;148:127-136.

54. Holcomb JB, Tilley BC, et. al. Transfusion of Plasma, Platelets, and Red Blood Cells in a 1:1:1 vs a 1:1:2 Ratio and Mortality in Patients With Severe Trauma. the PROPPR Randomized Clinical Study. *JAMA*. 2015; 313 (5): 471-482.

55. Janelle GM, Shore-Lesserson L, et. al. What is the PROPPR Transfusion Strategy in Trauma resuscitation?. *Aneshtesia & Analgesia*. 2016; 12: 1216-1219.

56. Delinas JP, Stoddard LV, Snyder EL. Thrombocytopenia and critical care medicine. *J Intensive Care Med*. 2001;16:1-21.

57. Shander A, Goodnough LT. Why an alternative to blood transfusion? *Crit Care Clin*. 2009;25:261-277.

Anticoagulation

Victor F. Tapson, MD and Shant Shirvanian, MD

KEY POINTS

1 Anticoagulation is the key in the management of venous thromboembolism (VTE), atrial fibrillation (AF), mechanical heart valves, and idiopathic pulmonary arterial hypertension (IPAH).

2 Critically ill patients are at increased risk for complications with anticoagulant therapy due to their underlying disease states, presence of thrombocytopenia, coagulopathy, renal and hepatic failure, need for invasive procedures, and the potential for major surgery.

3 Intravenous unfractionated heparin (UFH) remains the most commonly utilized parenteral therapy when therapeutic doses are needed in the critically ill. Monitoring with the activated partial thromboplastin time (aPTT) or heparin level (anti–factor Xa assay) is required.

4 Heparin resistance may occur due to nonspecific binding of the drug to various plasma proteins, altered intravascular volume, and/or increased heparin clearance. In cases of heparin resistance, anti-Xa level should be utilized for monitoring.

5 Low-molecular-weight heparins (LMWHs) have several advantages over UFH including greater bioavailability and more

predictable effects, lesser incidence of thrombocytopenia, and in general do not require monitoring except in patients who are morbidly obese, pregnant, or with severe renal insufficiency.

6 Argatroban is a synthetic direct thrombin inhibitor that is approved for prevention and treatment of VTE in patients with heparin-induced thrombocytopenia (HIT).

7 Novel oral anticoagulants inhibit either thrombin (factor IIa) or factor Xa. They include rivaroxaban, apixaban, edoxaban and dabigatran etexilate. These agents do not require routine monitoring.

8 The risk/benefit of anticoagulant discontinuation for emergent procedures including surgery depends on the reason the patient is anticoagulated, the bleeding risk imparted by the procedure, and concomitant comorbidities.

9 Warfarin and other vitamin K antagonists (VKAs) may be reversed with vitamin K and/or fresh frozen plasma (FFP).

10 Four-factor prothrombin complex concentrate (PCC) is approved for use in the United States for warfarin reversal in the setting of severe bleeding.

INTRODUCTION

Anticoagulation is the mainstay of therapy for VTE and is a key therapeutic component for a number of other clinical settings including atrial fibrillation (AF), mechanical heart valves, and idiopathic pulmonary arterial hypertension (IPAH). In the critical care setting, the use of anticoagulation is frequently warranted, but is often associated with an increased risk for complications based on underlying disease states, necessary invasive procedures, trauma, thrombocytopenia, coagulopathy, renal failure and hepatic failure, and the potential for major surgery. Reversing anticoagulation must be considered in certain clinical scenarios. The focus of this chapter will be anticoagulation in the intensive care unit (ICU), with a particular focus on therapeutic anticoagulation.

Anticoagulation in the critically ill patient requires therapeutic levels when treating an acute condition such as acute VTE. Given the high risk of morbidity and mortality caused by VTE, patients in the ICU, almost without exception, require VTE prophylaxis. Mechanical prophylaxis is used when pharmacologic prophylaxis is contraindicated or in certain lower-risk settings.

The ideal anticoagulant would be effective, easily administered with a predictable anticoagulant effect (oral, if the patient is capable) and rapid in onset, require no monitoring, and be easily reversible. Ideally, it would cause no significant adverse effects, including thrombocytopenia, and would not cause bleeding. The latter is a virtual impossibility, based on the clinical effect required. The direct oral anticoagulants (DOACs) are a significant advance, reminiscent of how LMWH dramatically changed the anticoagulation world nearly 2 decades ago.

PARENTERAL ANTICOAGULATION

Standard, Unfractionated Heparin

In spite of its limitations, intravenous (IV) standard UFH remains the most commonly utilized parenteral therapy when therapeutic doses of anticoagulants are required in the ICU. Monitoring with the aPTT is required. Heparin is a "promiscuous" molecule. It binds almost indiscriminately to various plasma proteins, monocytes, and endothelial cells.

Because it binds to a number of circulating proteins and cell types, different clinical conditions can significantly affect the heparin levels. The response can be thus, difficult to predict. Weight-basing heparin is crucial to hasten the achievement of therapeutic levels but monitoring is still essential (Figure 34–1). The aPTT is a clot-based, in vitro assay using citrated, platelet-depleted plasma. While the aPTT is sensitive to the inactivation of thrombin and factor Xa by UFH, it is a nonspecific assay. The therapeutic range should be a heparin concentration of 0.3 to 0.7 anti-Xa units/mL, using plasma samples from patients being treated with UFH for VTE. This aPTT range is specific for the reagent used by a given manufacturer lot. Alternatively, heparin levels (anti–factor Xa assay) can be monitored.

Decades ago, IV UFH dosing was routinely a 5000 unit bolus followed by an infusion of 1000 units/h followed by aPTT monitoring. In 1993, Raschke and colleagues[1] demonstrated that dosing heparin based on actual body weight (bolus of 80 units/kg followed by 18 units/kg/h) achieved a therapeutic aPTT at 24 hours more often than the standard dosing regimen. Furthermore, there was no difference between the 2 regimens with regard to bleeding events, although the weight-based subjects had a higher percentage of supratherapeutic aPTTs. The rate of recurrent VTE was statistically significantly higher in the non-weight-based regimen.

In this study, only 9 patients in the weight-based arm weighed more than 100 kg, and the largest patient was 131 kg making it difficult to extrapolate these findings to obese patients in general.[1] The volume of distribution of heparin is about the same as blood volume. Blood volume is increased in obesity, but adipose tissue has less blood volume compared with lean body tissue. This suggests that using actual body weight for the morbidly obese could increase the incidence of supratherapeutic aPTTs as well as the bleeding risk.

Several studies and reviews have attempted to address the dilemma of heparinization in the obese. One concluded that actual body weight in both non-obese and obese patients should be used to calculate heparin infusion rates, as long as a dosing cap of 10,000 units and infusion rate limit of 15,000 units/h was utilized.[2] A smaller study also found that actual body weight in both nonobese and obese patients was appropriate.[3] Still another study concluded that

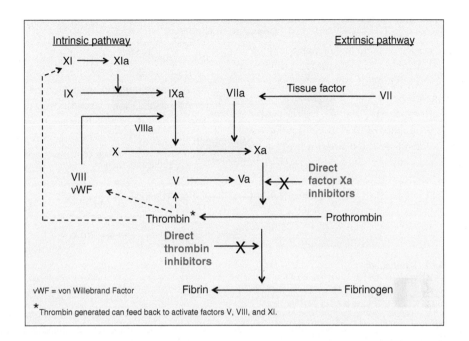

Novel oral anticoagulants and the coagulation cascade

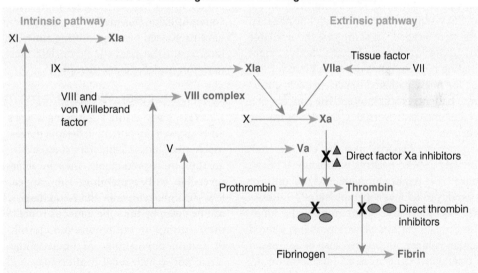

FIGURE 34–1 Thrombin (factor IIa), a serine protease, activates factors V, VIII, and XI (in turn, generating more thrombin), catalyzes the conversion of fibrinogen to fibrin, and stimulates platelet aggregation. This key role in the final steps of the coagulation cascade makes it an attractive target for new direct thrombin inhibitors such as dabigatran.

Factor Xa is also a serine protease that plays a pivotal role in the coagulation process. It represents the convergence point for the extrinsic and the intrinsic coagulation pathways. It converts prothrombin to thrombin. Thus, it is a very desirable target for the direct factor Xa inhibitors rivaroxaban and apixaban.

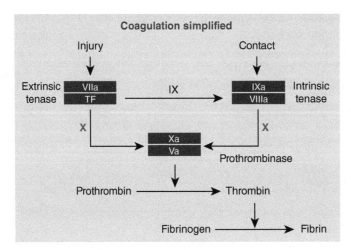

FIGURE 34–1 (*Continued*)

morbidly obese patients dosed according to actual body weight on a weight-based heparin nomogram were more likely to experience supratherapeutic aPTT values compared to nonmorbidly obese patients.[4] They suggested a dosing cap but believed more data were needed. In summary, the available evidence supports the use of actual body weight for calculating heparin bolus doses and initial infusion rates for obese patients. Experience with morbidly obese patients is still limited. The concept of a dose cap remains controversial. Careful monitoring remains crucial.

Resistance to heparin may be encountered. Approximately 25% of patients with acute VTE on IV standard UFH require more than 35,000 units of heparin per day to achieve a therapeutic aPTT. Resistance may occur because of the nonspecific binding of the drug to various plasma proteins, altered intravascular volume, and/or because of increased heparin clearance.[5] Other reasons for alterations in the aPTT dose-response include increased concentrations of clotting factors, including thrombin or factor VIII, or a reduction in anticoagulation factors such as antithrombin which may occur in the critically ill setting. In the case of apparent heparin resistance, the anti-Xa level should be utilized.[6] This may help differentiate pharmacokinetic from biochemical heparin resistance in patients requiring high infusion rates.

Another option is to simply monitor anti-Xa levels in *any* ICU patient on heparin since such patients appear more susceptible to variable aPTTs.[7] No data thus far, however, have proven better outcomes utilizing this method. In any patient found to have prolonged baseline clotting times, the heparin level by anti-Xa assay should be determined prior to initiating anticoagulant therapy.

Low-Molecular-Weight Heparins

LMWHs have distinct advantages over standard UFH as well as potential disadvantages. They are much more bioavailable than standard heparin, and are thus, more predictable. They are at least partially reversible with protamine. They appear to cause less thrombocytopenia than standard UFH. They can be given by the subcutaneous route (SC) and in most settings do not require monitoring. However, in certain populations, particularly the morbidly obese, those with renal insufficiency, and pregnant patients, these drugs may be less predictable. A creatinine clearance less than 30 mL/min requires a dose reduction or discontinuation.

While in most prophylactic and therapeutic anticoagulation settings, no monitoring of LMWH is necessary, critically ill patients who have marked metabolic derangements may be less predictable. A number of factors including hypotension, particularly requiring vasopressor therapy, renal insufficiency, and variable absorption may affect drug efficacy. Furthermore, such conditions may rapidly change in severity, making prediction of appropriate levels more difficult.[8] In such scenarios, when therapeutic anticoagulation is required, the goal should be a chromogenic anti-Xa assay level of 0.5 to 1.0 units/mL 4 hours after SC dosing, if the patient is on an every 12-hour dosing regimen. A higher level of 2 units/mL is recommended for a once-daily regimen.[9] Trough or even random anti-Xa levels may also be useful when there are concerns, for example, that a LMWH may be accumulating in renal failure. The anti-Xa assay should be calibrated to the specific LMWH being utilized. Finally, while levels are generally not checked in patients on deep venous thrombosis (DVT) prophylaxis, a level of approximately 0.1 to 0.3 units/mL measured 3 to 4 hours after a SC injection would appear reasonable.[10] Despite some limitations of antifactor Xa monitoring for LMWH therapy, the unreliability of SC drug administration in critically ill patients warrants the routine use of monitoring to assure adequate drug exposure.

Fondaparinux

Fondaparinux, a selective factor Xa inhibitor, has a longer half-life than the LMWHs and thus, is less useful in the ICU. For prophylaxis in total joint arthroplasty, it is prescribed as 2.5 mg SC once-daily and is as effective as LMWH. It does not appear to be associated with HIT.

Argatroban

Argatroban, a small molecule synthetic direct thrombin inhibitor (DTI) administered IV, is Food and Drug Administration (FDA) approved for prevention and treatment of thrombosis in patients with HIT. Plasma concentrations reach steady state in 1 to 3 hours. This drug is hepatically metabolized which must be considered. However, this also allows its use in renal insufficiency. Its half-life is about 50 minutes. The recommended range for the aPTT to monitor argatroban is 1.5 to 3 times control, not to exceed 100 seconds. The ecarin clotting time may have certain advantages in monitoring DTI therapy, but it is not routinely available. It has not yet been adequately evaluated to be used in place of the aPTT. Lepirudin, a recombinant hirudin, is no longer available.

Warfarin

Warfarin is impractical in the critical care setting. It is very long acting and associated with innumerable drug interactions. Although reversible with vitamin K, it is not immediately reversible. It is still used by some orthopedic surgeons as prophylaxis for total knee or hip arthroplasty is used less commonly since the advent of LMWH and DOACs (see "Anticoagulant Reversal").

Aspirin

Aspirin has been studied for long-term secondary prevention of DVT/pulmonary embolism (PE). In this setting, it appears more effective than placebo but less effective than all other available anticoagulants drugs. While it is used in the setting of acute coronary syndromes and AF, it has no real role in the ICU patient with acute VTE.

Direct Oral Anticoagulants

DOACs inhibit either thrombin (factor IIa) or factor Xa. Thrombin is a serine protease and activates factors V, VIII, and XI and catalyzes the conversion of fibrinogen to fibrin, as well as stimulating platelet aggregation. Factor Xa is also a serine protease that represents the intersection of the extrinsic and the intrinsic coagulation pathways. It catalyzes the conversion of prothrombin to thrombin (see Figure 34–1).

Four DOACs are approved for use in the United States, including the Xa inhibitors rivaroxaban (Xarelto) and apixaban (Eliquis), and the direct thrombin inhibitor, dabigatran etexilate (Pradaxa). All 4 are approved for stroke prevention in nonvalvular AF, as well as for treatment of established DVT and/or PE. Rivaroxaban and apixaban are also approved for prophylaxis for total hip and knee arthroplasty (Table 34–1). Others, including betrixaban could follow. The safety and efficacy of these drugs have not been studied for mechanical prosthetic heart valves and thus are not recommended in this setting.

A major advantage of these DOACs includes the lack of need for monitoring although this could be useful in emergencies. There is a marked reduction in drug interactions compared with warfarin, although cytochrome P450 (CYP) metabolism

TABLE 34–1 New oral anticoagulants: indications and comparative pharmacology.

	Dabigatran	Rivaroxaban	Apixaban	Edoxaban
FDA approved for acute VTE therapy	Yes	Yes	Yes	Yes
FDA approved for AF	Yes	Yes	Yes	Yes
FDA approved for VTE prophylaxis for total hip/knee arthroplasty	Yes	Yes	Yes	No
Target	IIa (thrombin)	Xa	Xa	Xa
Time to C_{max}	1.25-3 h	2-4 h	3-4 h	
CYP metabolism	None	32%	Minimal	Minimal
Transporters	P-gp	P-gp/BCRP	P-gp/BCRP	P-gp
Bioavailability	6%	80%	60%	60%
Plasma protein binding	35%	93%	87%	55%
Half-life	14-17 h	5-13 h	8-15 h	10-14h

AF, atrial fibrillation; C_{max}, maximum concentration; CYP, cytochrome; P-gp, P-glycoprotein; BRCP, breast cancer–related protein; VTE, venous thromboembolism.
[a]5-9 h in healthy subjects and 11-13 h in the elderly.

is important for factor Xa inhibitor metabolism and P-glycoprotein (P-gp) metabolism affects the metabolism of all 4 of these agents. Renal metabolism also must be considered. Dosing for dabigatran, rivaroxaban, and apixaban, for treatment of established VTE and AF is outlined in Table 34–2 and the potential for drug interactions is further outlined in Table 34–3.

Large, randomized clinical trials in thousands of patients with AF and acute DVT and/or PE have been completed with these agents, indicating that they are at least as effective as warfarin. They appear to be at least as safe, and in some instances safer, with regard to bleeding.

Concomitant use of other drugs affecting hemostasis increases the risk of bleeding, including other anticoagulants, aspirin, other antiplatelet agents, thrombolytic agents, and nonsteroidal anti-inflammatory drugs.

Edoxaban

Edoxaban is the most recently approved direct factor Xa inhibitor in the United States. It is indicated to reduce risk of stroke and systemic embolism in patients with nonvalvular AF and for the treatment of DVT and PE following 5 to 10 days of initial

therapy with a parenteral anticoagulant (references 1 and 2 below). For AF, the recommended dose is 60 mg PO once daily. It should not be prescribed in patients when the CrCL is > 95 mL/min because of an increased risk of stroke compared with warfarin. The dose must be reduced to 30 mg once daily in patients with CrCl of 15 to 50 mL/min. In the nonvalvular AF trial, major bleeding occurred with a significantly lower incidence with edoxaban compared with warfarin. The endpoint of death or ICH also occurred in significantly fewer patients receiving edoxaban. Importantly, fatal bleeding and life-threatening bleeding occurred significantly less often with edoxaban, as did gastrointestinal bleeding with the lower dose. In contrast, the higher edoxaban dose led to more gastrointestinal bleeding than warfarin. For DVT and PE, the recommended dose is 60 mg once daily. The dose should be similarly reduced to 30 mg once daily for patients with CrCL 15 to 50 mL/min, body weight ≤ 60 kg, or in patients on certain P-gp inhibitors.

Dabigatran

Thrombin is a logical target for an anticoagulant. When it is activated from prothrombin, it converts soluble fibrinogen to insoluble fibrin, activates

TABLE 34-2 Dosing of new oral anticoagulants for therapy of acute VTE and AF.

Drug	Oral Dose	Renal Dosing	Heparin Bridge
Rivaroxaban (Xarelto)	VTE: 15 mg q12h x 21 d, then 20 mg once daily AF: 20 mg once daily Take with food	**Acute VTE:** Do not use with marked renal impairment (CrCl < 30 mL/min) **AF:** For CrCl 15-50 mL/min, 15 mg orally, once daily	No
Apixaban (Eliquis)	10 mg q12h x 1 wk, then 5 mg q12h After at least 6 mo of therapy, decrease to 2.5 mg once daily	**Acute VTE:** No dose reduction **AF:** Decrease dose to 2.5 mg q12h if any 2 of the following are present: -Creatinine ≥ 1.5 mg/dL -Age ≥ 80 -Weight ≤ 60 kg ESRD on HD: 5 mg q12h; decrease dose to 2.5 mg q12h if age ≥ 80 or weight ≤ 60 kg	No
Dabigatran (Pradaxa)	150 mg twice daily	**All patients:** CrCl < 30 mL/min with concomitant use of P-gp inhibitors: Do not use P-gp inducers (eg, rifampin): Do not use **HD patients:** No dosing recommendations can be offered **Acute VTE:** CrCl < 30 mL/min: Do not use CrCl < 50 mL/min with concomitant use of P-gp inhibitors: **AF:** CrCl 15-30 mL/min: 75 mg q12h CrCl 30-50 mL/min with concomitant use of P-gp inhibitors: • P-gp inhibitors dronedarone or ketoconazole: Consider reducing dose to 75 mg q12h • Dose adjustment not necessary when coadministered with other P-gp inhibitors	Yes
Edoxaban (Savaysa)	60 mg once daily	**Acute VTE:** Reduce to 30 mg once daily for patients with CrCL 15 to 50 mL/min, body weight ≤ 60 kg, or in patients on certain P-gp inhibitors (see below). **AF:** Should not be prescribed when CrCL is > 95 mL/min. Reduce dose to 30 mg once daily in patients with CrCl of 15 to 50 mL/min.	

AF, atrial fibrillation; CrCl, creatinine clearance; ESRD, end-stage renal disease; HD, hemodialysis; P-gp, P-glycoprotein; VTE, venous thromboembolism.

TABLE 34-3 New oral anticoagulants: drug interactions.[a]

Drug	
Rivaroxaban (Xarelto)	Concomitant use of rivaroxaban with combined P-gp and strong CYP3A4 inhibitors (eg, ketoconazole, itraconazole, lopinavir/ritonavir, ritonavir, indinavir, and conivaptan) should be avoided. Concomitant use of rivaroxaban with drugs that are combined P-gp and strong CYP3A4 inducers (eg, carbamazepine, phenytoin, rifampin, St. John's wort) should also be avoided.
Apixaban (Eliquis)	If on strong dual CYP3A4/P-gp inhibitors (eg, ketoconazole, itraconazole, ritonavir, or clarithromycin): -If apixaban dose > 2.5 mg q12h, decrease dose by 50% -If apixaban dose 2.5 mg q12h, avoid coadministration If on strong dual CYP3A4/P-gp inducers (eg, rifampin, carbamazepine, phenytoin, St. John's wort) avoid use.
Dabigatran (Pradaxa)	Concomitant P-gp inducers (eg, rifampin) should not be used. AF: With moderate renal impairment (CrCl 30-50 mL/min), reduce dose to 75 mg twice daily when administered concomitantly with the P-gp inhibitors dronedarone or systemic ketoconazole. Concomitant use of P-gp inhibitors in severe renal impairment (CrCl 15-30 mL/min) should be avoided. VTE: Avoid use with P-gp inhibitors in patients with CrCl in patients with CrCl < 50 mL/min
Edoxaban (Savaysa)	No dose reduction when P-gp inhibitors are coadministered. Avoid concomitant use of rifampin, a P-gp inducer.

CYP, cytochrome; P-gp, P-glycoprotein.
[a]See also Table 34–2 (regarding adjustments for renal dosing).

coagulation factors V, VIII, and XI, thus, generating more thrombin, and activates platelets. Dabigatran etexilate is a synthetic, orally available prodrug that is rapidly absorbed and converted by esterases to its active form, dabigatran, a potent direct inhibitor of both free thrombin and clot-bound thrombin. This drug has a rapid onset of action, very few drug interactions, no reported food interactions, and does not require routine coagulation monitoring.

Dabigatran is 35% bound to plasma proteins and is renally excreted, with 80% of the drug entering the urine unchanged. The anticoagulant effect accumulates in the setting of renal insufficiency, and such bioaccumulation correlates well with the degree of renal dysfunction.[11] In cases of moderate hepatic impairment, dabigatran can be administered safely and no dose adjustment is necessary.[12]

P-gp inhibition and renal insufficiency are major independent factors in increased exposure to dabigatran. There is no significant cytochrome P450 metabolism. Concomitant use of P-gp inhibitors in patients with renal impairment is expected to produce increased exposure of dabigatran compared to that seen with either factor alone (see Table 34–2). Absorption of dabigatran etexilate is mediated by P-gp; dabigatran etexilate is a substrate for P-gp, but active dabigatran is not. Thus, P-gp inhibitors can increase dabigatran absorption, increasing both area under curve (AUC) and C_{max} and P-gp inducers can reduce its absorption, resulting in inadequate levels. Concomitant P-gp inducers (eg, rifampin) should not be used in patients on dabigatran (see Table 34–3).

This drug is FDA approved for stroke prevention in patients with nonvalvular AF and for acute VTE at a dose of 150 mg twice daily. It is not approved, at present, for prophylaxis following total hip or knee replacement in the United States.

For AF, dabigatran was shown to be superior to dose-adjusted warfarin with a similar rate of major bleeding.[13] A dose of 75 mg twice daily, is approved in the United States for patients with nonvalvular AF and severe renal insufficiency; that is, creatinine clearance (CrCl) of 15 to 30 mL/min.

Over 9000 patients were evaluated in studies involving dabigatran leading to the approval of this drug for the treatment of acute VTE, including RE-COVER, RE-COVER II, RE-MEDY, and RE-SONATE.[14-16] The first 2 studies were initial VTE therapy studies utilizing a parenteral anticoagulant bridge. Dabigatran proved effective standard therapy, and while major bleeding rates were similar, there were fewer episodes of nonmajor bleeding with dabigatran than with warfarin. There was, however, a higher rate of gastrointestinal (GI) bleeding.[14,15] The extension studies in patients who had completed a course of anticoagulation demonstrated not surprisingly, that extended duration of anticoagulation with dabigatran was noninferior to warfarin but superior to placebo in reducing recurrent VTE. Based on the way these clinical trials were conducted, for acute VTE, the parenteral anticoagulant bridge is required for 5 to 10 days prior to oral dabigatran alone. Dabigatran is rated pregnancy category C.

Rivaroxaban

Factor Xa represents the rate-limiting factor in thrombin generation and amplification, generating the Xa complex that converts prothrombin to thrombin. The direct factor Xa inhibitors inhibit free factor Xa, factor Xa in the prothrombinase complex, and factor Xa found in clots, and this is independent of antithrombin. In contrast, LMWHs, UFH, and fondaparinux, are dependent on antithrombin to inhibit factor Xa.

Clearance of this drug is decreased to some extent in patients with renal impairment, but two-thirds of its primary mode of clearance is nonrenal. While approximately 67% of rivaroxaban is *eliminated* by the kidney, half of this is clearance of active drug and half of it is clearance of inactive rivaroxaban, which is not clinically important. CYP450, P-gp and breast cancer–related protein (BCRP) are all involved with metabolism. It is 93% protein bound and thus, not dialyzable. Rivaroxaban is a substrate of CYP3A4/5, CYP2J2, and the P-gp and ATP-binding cassette G2 (ABCG2) transporters. Inhibitors and inducers of these CYP450 enzymes or transporters, such as P-gp, may result in changes in rivaroxaban exposure.

Concomitant use of rivaroxaban with combined P-gp and strong CYP3A4 inhibitors (eg, ketoconazole, itraconazole, lopinavir/ritonavir, ritonavir, indinavir, and conivaptan) should be avoided. In addition, concomitant use of rivaroxaban with drugs that are combined P-gp and strong CYP3A4 inducers (eg, carbamazepine, phenytoin, rifampin, St. John's wort) should also be avoided (see Tables 34–2 and 34–3).

For stroke prevention, the randomized, double-blinded ROCKET AF trial found that rivaroxaban 20 mg daily (15 mg daily if CrCl is 15-50 mL/min) was noninferior to warfarin in efficacy, with no significant difference in major bleeding events.[17] Due to high plasma protein binding (> 90%), rivaroxaban is not eliminated during hemodialysis.

The Einstein DVT and PE studies (> 8000 patients) led to FDA approval for rivaroxaban for the treatment of established DVT and/or PE.[18,19] These large prospective, randomized trials demonstrated noninferiority to warfarin with regard to recurrent VTE, and in the PE study, the risk of major bleeding was significantly lower. For acute VTE, the drug is dosed as 15 mg q12h for 3 weeks and then 20 mg once daily. Unlike in AF, where the dose can be reduced with a CrCl of 15 to 50 mL/min, this has not been recommended in VTE. However, in acute VTE with CrCl less than 30 mL/min, the drug should not be used (see Table 34-2).

Rivaroxaban is also approved in the United States for VTE prophylaxis after hip or knee replacement surgery based on superiority over enoxaparin, and at least comparable safety. At present, however, no NOAC is approved specifically for VTE prophylaxis in the ICU.

When changing from warfarin, rivaroxaban should be initiated when the INR is less than or equal to 3. Finally, tablets may be crushed and either mixed in applesauce or suspended in water and administered via an nasogastric (NG) tube to appropriate patients who have difficulty swallowing a whole tablet. This drug is pregnancy category B and should be used during pregnancy only if the potential benefit outweighs the potential risk to the mother and the fetus.

Apixaban

Like rivaroxaban, apixaban is FDA approved for stroke prevention in AF, acute VTE, and for prophylaxis in total knee and hip replacement. Apixaban is an oral, direct factor Xa inhibitor that is highly bioavailable (80%), is highly protein bound, and reaches peak plasma concentration within 2 to 3 hours after intake. It is 75% hepatically metabolized with the rest renally excreted. Dosing including renal dosing is outlined in Table 34-2. No dose adjustment is required in patients with mild hepatic impairment.

It has the least renal dependence of the three FDA-approved NOACs and has limited drug interactions. While there is minimal CYP3A4 metabolism, the drug does have potential interactions with potent CYP3A4 inhibitors. For patients on doses of apixaban greater than 2.5 mg twice daily, the dose should be decreased by 50% when it is administered with drugs that are strong dual inhibitors of CYP3A4 and P-gp (eg, ketoconazole, itraconazole, clarithromycin, or ritonavir). For patients receiving a dose of 2.5 mg twice daily, strong dual inhibitors of CYP3A4 and P-gp should be avoided (see Table 34-3).

In the setting of nonvalvular AF, the ARISTOTLE trial demonstrated that apixaban was superior to dose-adjusted warfarin in preventing stroke and systemic embolism. There was a lower rate of bleeding complications, and a lower mortality.[20] In the AVERROES trial, apixaban 5 mg twice daily was compared with aspirin (81-325 mg) for stroke prevention.[21] There was a lower risk of stroke with apixaban but, interestingly, no difference in the bleeding rate compared with aspirin.

FDA approval of apixaban for acute DVT/PE was based on 2 large, prospective, phase 3 trials, AMPLIFY[22] and AMPLIFY-EXTENSION.[23] There was no 5 to 10 day heparin bridge required. Apixaban proved noninferior to standard therapy with LMWH followed by warfarin with regard to recurrent VTE events, and was associated with significantly less major bleeding, and less clinically relevant nonmajor bleeding than standard therapy. The FDA-approved dose of apixaban for the treatment of acute DVT and/or PE is 10 mg twice daily for 1 week followed by 5 mg twice daily. Based on the extension study, a dose of 2.5 mg twice daily is indicated to reduce the risk of recurrent DVT and PE following initial 6 months treatment for DVT and/or PE.

In the setting of total joint replacement, apixaban is administered as 2.5 mg orally 12 to 24 hours after surgery. For hip replacement, the dose is 2.5 mg twice daily for 35 days and for total knee replacement (TKR), the dose is 2.5 mg po twice daily for 12 days. As noted, none of the NOACs are approved for use as prophylaxis other than TKR and total hip replacement (THR). Importantly for ICU patients, when patients cannot swallow whole tablets, 5 mg and 2.5 mg apixaban tablets may be crushed and suspended in 60 mL D_5W and immediately administered through a nasogastric tube. There are no data regarding crushed and suspended apixaban tablets swallowed by mouth. Like rivaroxaban, apixaban is pregnancy category B.

Anticoagulant Monitoring for Novel Oral Anticoagulants

The NOACs do not require routine monitoring in the setting of AF, acute VTE, or in the setting of VTE prophylaxis. However, it is important to check coagulation tests when a patient is admitted to the ICU on a NOAC, particularly if it is unclear whether or not the patient has been taking one. This may also be useful if there is bleeding or a high risk of bleeding. Thus, coagulation assays are not helpful in adjusting doses of NOACs but may help determine whether there is significant ongoing anticoagulant effect. With acute bleeding, or with emergency invasive surgical procedure, this is particularly important.

Dabigatran catalyzes the conversion of fibrinogen to fibrin, and thus, results in prolongation of most routine coagulation assays except the prothrombin time (PT). The ecarin clotting time is useful but less widely available. Because the thrombin time increases linearly with increasing dabigatran concentration, it seems intuitive that this measurement would provide the best direct assessment of thrombin activity. However, the thrombin time is overly sensitive to dabigatran levels and may be prolonged in the setting of a clinically insignificant dabigatran effect. The dilute thrombin time (Hemoclot assay) has very good linear correlation to plasma levels of dabigatran and is probably the most reliable method to measure the anticoagulant effect of dabigatran.[24] The aPTT can also be used; however, the relationship between dabigatran concentration and the aPTT is nonlinear and so is less reliable. A normal aPTT will likely indicate the absence of a clinically important anticoagulant effect. It is crucial to develop additional laboratory studies to correlate coagulation assay results with plasma levels of dabigatran.

Rivaroxaban and apixaban directly inhibit factor Xa, complexing with factor Va, independent of antithrombin. An increased PT tells us it is likely there is rivaroxaban in the bloodstream. There is less effect on the aPTT. A specific assay has been developed for direct Xa inhibitors that differs from the anti-Xa assay used to monitor LMWH, and this could potentially provide an effective method to determine the effect of rivaroxaban.[25] More data are needed, however. At present, there is no precise means by which to accurately assess the degree of anticoagulation in a patient on an Xa inhibitor.

Surgery and Procedures in the Critically Ill Patient

When urgent or emergent procedures arise, there are a number of potential anticoagulant considerations. The risk/benefit of anticoagulant discontinuation depends on the reason the patient is anticoagulated, the bleeding risk imparted by the procedure, and concomitant comorbidities. A patient with submassive or massive acute PE with another life-threatening condition requiring immediate surgery should simply have an inferior vena cava filter (IVCF) placed and have anticoagulation discontinued. Patients should be individualized.

As described earlier, neither the aPTT nor PT can determine the anticoagulant effects of dabigatran, rivaroxaban, or apixaban at any given time. A normal aPTT suggests that hemostatic function is not impaired by dabigatran, and a normal PT or lack of antifactor Xa activity would indicate that hemostatic function is not impaired on rivaroxaban or apixaban. Thus, these tests are useful when upcoming surgical procedures impart a significant bleeding risk. A normal thrombin time excludes a significant dabigatran effect; this measurement may be useful when a high-risk procedure is emergent.

Dabigatran is primarily renally eliminated so the timing of discontinuation should be based on the CrCl and the bleeding risk associated with the procedure. The pharmacodynamic effect of dabigatran declines in parallel with its plasma concentration, so surgery may only need to be delayed for about 12 hours after the last dabigatran dose.

If the CrCl is 31 to 50 mL/min, the last dose of dabigatran should be at least 48 hours before the procedure for low-risk surgery, and even longer (consider 4 days) before a procedure that poses a high risk of bleeding.[11] Mild or moderate renal impairment would appear to be of less concern in patients on rivaroxaban, in whom a decreased CrCl appears to have a more limited effect on the half-life of the drug, but it should still be considered when stopping the drug preoperatively.

A large nonrandomized study examined perioperative bleeding rates from 7 days prior until 30 days after invasive procedures for patients on warfarin or dabigatran.[26] The procedures included pacemaker/defibrillator insertion, dental procedures, diagnostic procedures, cataract removal, colonoscopy, and joint replacement. The last dose of dabigatran was given a mean of 49 hours (range 35-85) before the procedure, compared to 114 hours (range 87-144) for the last preprocedure dose of warfarin ($P < 0.001$). There was no significant difference in the rates of periprocedural major bleeding between the drugs. Among patients having urgent surgery, major bleeding occurred in 21.6% with warfarin, 17.7% with dabigatran at 150 mg, and 17.8% with dabigatran at 110 mg.[26]

While there are no large studies examining perioperative bleeding rates in patients receiving rivaroxaban or apixaban, the same general principles should apply with regard to procedure bleeding risk and drug elimination based on the characteristics of these drugs. It should be recognized that these guidelines are approximate and that patients should be carefully scrutinized based on the specific procedure, perceived bleeding risk, and comorbidities including renal function.

For rivaroxaban and apixaban, it appears acceptable to delay low-risk surgery for approximately 24 hours after the previous dose. When the bleeding risk is higher, 48 hours would appear to be safer. With a more significant decrease in CrCl (ie, < 30 mL/min), an approximately 4 day delay would be appropriate. Resumption of a NOAC in a low bleeding risk scenario should be at least 24 hours after the procedure. The European Society of Anaesthesiology and the French Study Group on Thrombosis and Hemostasis have published recommendations about perioperative management of NOACs.[27,28]

The general principles described above also apply to neuraxial anesthesia but it should be realized that bleeding in this setting has tremendous implications. Catheter placement should be considered when the anticoagulant level is at its trough and while removal may be less critical; it should also be timed as carefully as possible. At least 2 half-lives should be allowed to pass before catheter removal, at which point only 25% of the drug remains active. Patients should be monitored carefully for bleeding after catheter removal. Recommendations for the use of the NOACs in the setting of neuraxial anesthesia have been proposed by Llau and colleagues based on existing guidelines and the pharmacokinetics of each drug.[29]

Anticoagulant Reversal

With the much shorter half-lives of the NOACs, discontinuing a NOAC and providing supportive care may be all that is required depending on the type and severity of the bleed, or whether an invasive procedure can be delayed. The half-life of dabigatran after multiple doses is approximately 14 to 17 hours and is not dose dependent; if there is no active bleeding after an overdose, stopping the drug may be sufficient. The shorter half-life proven in younger healthy patients on rivaroxaban or apixaban compared with elderly patients may also be favorable with regard to simply stopping the drug.

When a bleeding event occurs, initial measures include control of the bleeding site, volume resuscitation with fluids and/or packed red blood cells, as well as determination of the source of bleeding. Minor bleeding such as epistaxis, or other mucosal or superficial bleeding can often be managed symptomatically with compression/nasal packing and drug discontinuation. Gastrointestinal bleeding is managed by anticoagulant discontinuation, blood transfusion as needed, and aggressive endoscopic and other specific therapy. Life-threatening bleeding including intracerebral hemorrhage (ICH) requires not only withdrawal of the anticoagulant and supportive measures but also ICU transfer and potentially interventional procedures as well as consideration for reversal. Nonspecific reversal agents can be considered in patients with major or life-threatening bleeding.[30,31]

Warfarin and other VKAs may be reversed with vitamin K and/or FFP. Reversal is not instantaneous. Four-component PCCs are recommended in recent guidelines.[28] Four-factor PCC is FDA approved for use in the United States for warfarin reversal in the setting of severe bleeding.

In the case of overdose with an anticoagulant, activated charcoal may prevent additional oral drug absorption when administered within 1 to 2 hours of ingestion. The minimal data available suggest that activated charcoal may be useful in dabigatran and apixaban overdose or accidental ingestion, and probably this applies to rivaroxaban as well.[32,33] Hemodialysis may reverse the anticoagulant effects of dabigatran overdose in severe bleeding because only about 35% of dabigatran is bound to plasma proteins.[11] Rivaroxaban and apixaban are highly protein bound (95% and 87%, respectively) precluding removal with dialysis.

While FFP is frequently administered for initial control of bleeding in anticoagulated patients, its use as a NOAC reversal agent has not undergone detailed evaluation in humans. The 2011 American College of Cardiology Foundation/American Heart Association guidelines recommended that severe bleeding from dabigatran merits transfusion of FFP, packed red cells, and surgical intervention as appropriate.[34] Studies in mice suggest that FFP may help limit ICH hematoma expansion.[35] In humans, data are inadequate to support the use of FFP in ICH caused by dabigatran.

While FFP may be useful in cases of coagulation factor *depletion*, it is not generally effective in reversing bleeding resulting from *inhibition* of coagulation factors.[30] However, it may be that delivery of clotting factors may overwhelm an ongoing inhibitory effect (see "Nonspecific Reversal Agents"). Still, overall, FFP remains controversial based on a lack of clear supportive data.

Specific NOAC Reversal Agents

Idarucizumab is a monoclonal antibody fragment that binds dabigatran with an affinity that is 350 times higher than that observed with thrombin. (REF 1 BELOW) Thus, this drug binds free and thrombin-bound dabigatran and neutralizes its activity (SAME REF 1 AS BELOW). In a clinical trial leading to FDA approval, idarucizumab completely reversed the anticoagulant effect of dabigatran within minutes.

Andexanet alfa is a novel recombinant, modified factor Xa molecule that acts as a factor Xa decoy that binds and sequesters direct Xa inhibitors in the blood (REF 2 BELOW). The native factor Xa is then be available to participate in the coagulation process and restore hemostasis. In a preliminary report of an ongoing cohort study in patients with acute major bleeding associated with the use of factor Xa inhibitors, andexanet rapidly reversed anti–factor Xa activity and was not associated with serious side effects (SAME REF 2 AS BELOW). Effective hemostasis was achieved 12 hours after an infusion of andexanet in 79% of the patients. Thrombotic events occurred in 18% of the patients in the safety population. Additional data are pending as is consideration for FDA approval.

Finally, another agent, ciraparantag (PER977), is being evaluated as a more universal anticoagulant reversal agent (REF 3 BELOW). This small, synthetic, water-soluble, cationic molecule is designed to bind specifically to unfractionated heparin an LMWH through noncovalent hydrogen bonding and charge–charge interactions. This drug binds in a similar way to the new oral factor Xa inhibitors and to dabigatran.

Nonspecific Reversal Agents

Nonspecific agents have been used for reversal of major bleeding in this setting[37,38]; however, more data are needed. Recombinant factor VIIa (NovoSeven) initiates thrombin generation by activating factor X. Prothrombin complex concentrates were originally utilized for treating patients with hemophilia B. More recently, data have been published related to the treatment of VKA-related bleeding for their ability to rapidly and effectively correct the INR. These preparations are concentrated solutions derived from human plasma containing coagulation factors II, IX, X, and/or VII. They exist as either 3-factor or 4-factor PCCs depending on their factor VII content. Three-factor PCCs contain the inactivated vitamin K–dependent coagulation factors II, IX, and X, with minimal to no factor VII. Four-factor PCCs contain the same 3 coagulation factors with inactivated factor VII concentrations similar to their factor IX content. Thus, thrombin formation is stimulated. Both 3-factor and 4-factor PCCs have been studied in major bleeding with VKAs, although none have been compared head-to-head.

There is only one 4-factor PCC available in the United States, marketed under the name Kcentra (marketed as Beriplex P/N in 25 other counties) and the only PCC in the United States that is FDA-approved indication for the urgent reversal of acquired coagulation factor deficiency in the setting of *vitamin K–related* acute major bleeding. In addition to clotting factors, it also contains proteins C and S, antithrombin III, human albumin, and heparin. In view of the latter, it is contraindicated in HIT.[39]

There are two 3-factor PCCs available in the United States—Profilnine SD and Bebulin. Another PCC, an activated PCC (aPCC, also referred to as anti-inhibitor coagulant complex) is available in the United States under the name FEIBA NF. It differs from other PCCs in that it contains inactivated factors II, IX, and X and small amounts of activated factor VII; this combines the effect of both recombinant factor VIIa and 4-factor PCC.

van Ryn and colleagues found that recombinant factor VIIa and activated prothrombin complex concentrate may be potential antidotes for dabigatran-induced severe bleeding in humans.[38] Marlu and associates determined that activated prothrombin complex concentrate as well as 4-factor PCC could be reasonable antidotes to dabigatran and rivaroxaban.[37]

Thus far, it appears that 3-factor PCC products may be less effective than 4-factor PCCs in reversing elevated INRs in patients with warfarin overdose, but more data are needed for the NOACs. Finally, more data are needed with regard to the thrombotic risk associated with the use of these nonspecific prohemostatic agents.

SUMMARY AND THE FUTURE

Critically ill patients continue to require careful consideration with regard to anticoagulation and bleeding risk. Parenteral anticoagulants are favored in the ICU and we have substantial experience with these agents with regard to monitoring, perioperative dosing, and reversal. The NOAC era is upon us. The learning curve remains steep. Renal dosing and drug interactions must be considered. As with LMWHs, antifactor Xa activity monitoring may become a more available validated means of testing for exposure to rivaroxaban and apixaban. Newer assays derived from INR testing may become more useful methods to monitor NOACs. More studies are needed to examine reversal.

REFERENCES

1. Raschke RA, Reilly BM, Guidry JR, et al. The weight-based heparin dosing nomogram compared with a "standard care" nomogram. *Ann Intern Med.* 1993;119(9):874-881.
2. Yee WP, Norton LL. Optimal weight base for a weight-based heparin dosing protocol. *Am J Health Syst Pharm.* 1998;55(2):159-162.
3. Spruill WJ, Wade WE, Huckaby WG, Leslie RB. Achievement of anticoagulation by using a weight-based heparin dosing protocol for obese and nonobese patients. *Am J Health Syst Pharm.* 2001;58(22):2143-2146.
4. Barletta JF, DeYoung JL, McAllen K, et al. Limitations of a standardized weight-based nomogram for heparin dosing in patients with morbid obesity. *Surg Obes Relat Dis.* 2008;4(6):748-753.
5. Young E, Prins M, Levine MN, Hirsh J. Heparin binding to plasma proteins, and important mechanism for heparin resistance. *Thromb Haemost.* 1992;67:639.
6. Levine MN, Hirsh J, Gent M, et al. A randomized trial comparing activated thromboplastin time with heparin assay in patients with acute venous thromboembolism requiring large daily doses of heparin. *Arch Int Med.* 1994;154:49.
7. Baker BA, Adelman MD, Smith PA, Osborn JC. Inability of the activated partial thromboplastin time to predict heparin levels. Time to reassess guidelines for heparin assays. *Arch Intern Med.* 1997;157:2475.
8. Priglinger U, Karth D, Geppert A, et al. Prophylactic anticoagulation with enoxaparin: is the subcutaneous route appropriate in the critically ill? *Crit Care Med.* 2003;31:1405.
9. Bates SM, Weitz JI. Coagulation assays. *Circulation.* 2005;112:e53.
10. Mayr A, Dunser M, Jochberger S, et al. Antifactor Xa activity in intensive care patients receiving thromboembolic prophylaxis with standard doses of enoxaparin. *Thromb Res.* 2002;105:201.
11. Stangier J, Rathgen K, Stähle H, Mazur D. Influence of renal impairment on the pharmacokinetics and pharmacodynamics of oral dabigatran etexilate: an open-label, parallel-group, single-centre study. *Clin Pharmacokinet.* 2010;49:259-268.
12. Stangier J, Stähle H, Rathgen K, Roth W, Shakeri-Nejad K. Pharmacokinetics and pharmacodynamics of dabigatran etexilate, an oral direct thrombin inhibitor, are not affected by moderate hepatic impairment. *J Clin Pharmacol.* 2008;48:1411-1419.
13. Connolly SJ, Ezekowitz MD, Yusuf S, et al; the RE-LY Steering Committee and Investigators. Dabigatran versus warfarin in patients with atrial fibrillation. *N Engl J Med.* 2009;361:1139-1151.
14. Schulman S, Kearon C, Kakkar AK, et al. Dabigatran versus warfarin in the treatment of acute venous thromboembolism. *N Engl J Med.* 2009;361:2342-2352.
15. Schulman S, Kakkar AK, Goldhaber SZ, et al; RE-COVER II Investigators. Treatment of acute venous thromboembolism with dabigatran or warfarin, and pooled analysis. *Circulation.* 2014;129:764-782.
16. Schulman S, Kearon C, Kakkar AK, et al; RE-MEDY and RE-SONATE trials investigators. Extended

use of dabigatran, warfarin, or placebo in venous thromboembolism. *N Engl J Med*. 2013;368:709-718.

17. Patel MR, Mahaffey KW, Garg J, et al; ROCKET AF Steering Committee, for the ROCKET AF Investigators. Rivaroxaban versus warfarin in nonvalvular atrial fibrillation. *N Engl J Med*. 2011;365(10):883-891.

18. Bauersachs R, Berkowitz SD, Brenner B, et al; The Einstein Investigators. Oral rivaroxaban for symptomatic venous thromboembolism. *N Engl J Med*. 2010;363:2499-2510.

19. Büller HR, Prins MH, Lensin AW, et al; The Einstein-PE Investigators. Oral rivaroxaban for the treatment of symptomatic pulmonary embolism. *N Engl J Med*. 2012;366:1287-1297.

20. Granger CB, Alexander JH, McMurray JJ, et al. Apixaban versus warfarin in patients with atrial fibrillation. *N Engl J Med*. 2011;365:981-992.

21. Connolly SJ, Eikelboom J, Joyner C, et al; AVERROES Steering Committee and Investigators. Apixaban in patients with atrial fibrillation. *N Engl J Med*. 2011;364:806-817.

22. Agnelli G, Buller HR, Cohen A, et al. Oral apixaban for the treatment of acute venous thromboembolism. *N Engl J Med*. 2013;369:799-808.

23. Agnelli G, Buller HR, Cohen A, et al. Apixaban for extended treatment of venous thromboembolism. *N Engl J Med*. 2013;368(8):699-708.

24. Stangier J, Feuring M. Using the HEMOCLOT direct thrombin inhibitor assay to determine plasma concentrations of dabigatran. *Blood Coagul Fibrinolysis*. 2012;23:138-143.

25. Samama MM, Amiral J, Guinet C, Perzborn E, Depasse F. An optimised, rapid chromogenic assay, specific for measuring direct factor Xa inhibitors (rivaroxaban) in plasma. *Thromb Haemost*. 2010;104:1078-1079.

26. Healey JS, Eikelboom J, Douketis J, et al. Periprocedural bleeding and thromboembolic events with dabigatran compared with warfarin: results from the Randomized Evaluation of Long-Term Anticoagulation Therapy (RE-LY) randomized trial. *Circulation*. 2012;126:343-348.

27. Gogarten W, Vandermeulen E, Van Aken H, et al. European Society of Anaesthesiology. Regional anaesthesia and antithrombotic agents: recommendations of the European Society of Anaesthesiology. *Eur J Anaesthesiol*. 2010;27:999-1015.

28. Sié P, Samama CM, Godier A, et al. Working Group on Perioperative Haemostasis; French Study Group on Thrombosis and Haemostasis. Surgery and invasive procedures in patients on long-term treatment with direct oral anticoagulants: thrombin or factor-Xa inhibitors. Recommendations of the Working Group on Perioperative Haemostasis and the French Study Group on Thrombosis and Haemostasis. *Arch Cardiovasc Dis*. 2011;104:669-676.

29. Llau JV, Ferrandis R. New anticoagulants and regional anesthesia. *Curr Opin Anaesthesiol*. 2009;22:661-666.

30. Crowther MA, Warkentin TE. Managing bleeding in anticoagulated patients with a focus on novel therapeutic agents. *J Thromb Haemost*. 2009; 7(suppl 1):107-110.

31. Levy JH, Tanaka KA, Dietrich W. Perioperative hemostatic management of patients treated with vitamin K antagonists. *Anesthesiology*. 2008;109:918-926.

32. van Ryn J, Neubauer M, Flieg R, et al. Successful removal of dabigatran in flowing blood with an activated charcoal hemoperfusion column in an in vitro test system. *Haematologica*. 2010;95(suppl 2):293.

33. Wang X, Mondal S, Wang J, et al. Effect of activated charcoal on apixaban pharmacokinetics in healthy subjects. *Am J Cardiovasc Drugs*. 2014;14(2):147-154.

34. Wann LS, Curtis AB, Ellenbogen KA, et al. 2011 ACCF/AHA/HRS focused update on the management of patients with atrial fibrillation (update on dabigatran): a report of the American College of Cardiology Foundation/American Heart Association Task Force on practice guidelines. *J Am Coll Cardiol*. 2011;57:1330-1337.

35. Zhou W, Schwarting S, Illanes S, et al. Hemostatic therapy in experimental intracranial hemorrhage associated with the direct thrombin inhibitor dabigatran. *Stroke*. 2011;42:3594-3599.

36. Lu G, DeGuzman FR, Hollenbach SJ, et al. A specific antidote for reversal of anticoagulation by direct and indirect inhibitors of coagulation factor Xa. *Nat Med*. 2013;19:446-451.

37. Marlu R, Hodaj E, Paris A, et al. Effect of non-specific reversal agents on anticoagulant activity of dabigatran and rivaroxaban: a randomised crossover ex vivo study in healthy volunteers. *Thromb Haemost*. 2012;108:217-224.

38. van Ryn J, Ruehl D, Priepke H, Hauel N, Wienen W. Reversibility of the anticoagulant effect of high doses of the direct thrombin inhibitor dabigatran, by recombinant factor VIIa or activated prothrombin complex concentrate. *Hematologica*. 2008;93(suppl 1):148.

39. Eerenberg ES, Kamphuisen PW, Sijpkens MK, et al. Reversal of rivaroxaban and dabigatran by prothrombin complex concentrate: a randomized, placebo-controlled, crossover study in healthy subjects. *Circulation*. 2011;124:1573-1579.

Acute Abdominal Dysfunction

Vanessa P. Ho, MD, MPH and
Philip S. Barie, MD, MBA, FIDSA, FCCM, FACS

KEY POINTS

1 Causes of acute abdominal pathology in the intensive care unit (ICU) patient include acute acalculous cholecystitis (AAC), severe acute pancreatitis, feeding intolerance, paralytic ileus and diarrhea, and abdominal compartment syndrome (ACS).

2 An emergent bedside laparotomy may be indicated for patients with a high suspicion for intra-abdominal pathology; however, this is a high-risk procedure, requires substantial resources to be mobilized, and has a risk of mortality.

3 Modern management of pancreatic necrosis and infected necrosis, known as the "step-up" approach, consists of initial medical management with fluid resuscitation and antibiotic administration, followed by percutaneous catheters for drainage of infected fluid.

4 Feeding intolerance in the critically ill patient can be attributable to the patient's critical illness, medications, intra-abdominal pathology, or underlying disease.

5 Treatment and management of ACS consists of serial monitoring of intra-abdominal pressures (IAP); optimization of systemic perfusion and organ function in the presence of intra-abdominal hypertension (IAH); institution of medical procedures to decrease IAP and reduce end-organ dysfunction; and prompt surgical decompression for refractory IAH or ACS.

INTRODUCTION

Critically ill patients are susceptible to a variety of causes and manifestations of abdominal dysfunction. However, the diagnosis and treatment of these conditions can be challenging secondary to nonspecific clinical findings, concurrent complex disease processes, and altered mental status. The purpose of this chapter is to discuss select causes of abdominal dysfunction in the critically ill patient, including evaluation for acute abdominal pathology in the critically ill patient, AAC, severe acute pancreatitis, feeding intolerance, paralytic ileus and diarrhea, ACS, and care of the long-term open abdomen.

Evaluation for Acute Abdominal Pathology in the Intensive Care Unit

Critically ill patients are susceptible to acute abdominal pathology, including bowel perforation, biliary tract disease, pancreatitis, ischemia, and hemorrhage. Acute abdominal pathology may be the patient's initial insult, or the patient may develop abdominal dysfunction as a complication of critical illness. Patients with recent surgery may manifest intra-abdominal complications such as anastomotic leak or abscess, or may develop iatrogenic abdominal complications such as bowel perforation from paracentesis, or pancreatitis after endoscopic retrograde cholangiopancreatography (ERCP). Critically ill patients may pose a diagnostic dilemma, as some patients may be challenging to evaluate due to concomitant critical illness; even patients with evaluable mental status may have unreliable clinical examinations. Steroid use and immunosuppression may blunt a patient's clinical examination even in the presence of an intra-abdominal catastrophe. Evaluation of the patient with suspicion for acute abdominal pathology should occur expeditiously; failure to consider the abdomen as a potential source of sepsis or hemorrhage can lead to missed diagnoses and poor outcomes.

Although physical examination findings in this population can be nonspecific, patients with unexplained sepsis or abdominal pain (if they can communicate same) should undergo a thorough physical examination to evaluate for abdominal distension, tenderness, and inspection of all wounds and incisions. Laboratory findings will be nonspecific as well, but may provide important clues to the diagnosis and should be obtained and trended; white blood cell count, liver enzymes, amylase, lipase, lactate, and arterial blood gases may be of value.

Evaluation of the abdomen in the critically ill patient should include diagnostic radiologic imaging if clinically tolerable (in terms of positioning, or the need to transport the patient to the radiology suite) and appropriate for the suspected underlying process.[1] In general, computed tomography (CT) is the test of choice for patients with a suspected intra-abdominal source of sepsis. Pancreatitis, diverticulitis, and other inflammatory bowel processes; intra-abdominal abscesses; and bowel obstructions are visualized easily with contrast-enhanced CT. Patients with recent abdominal surgery and postoperative intra-abdominal infection typically manifest signs and symptoms of dehiscence, leak, or abscess after 5 to 10 days and CT scan can be instrumental for the diagnosis; CT scans performed earlier than 5 to 7 days in postoperative patients are of limited value due to identification of nonspecific abdominal fluid, inflammation, and even residual pneumoperitoneum introduced during celiotomy. CT scans are sensitive for detecting the presence of air, which can be pathologically located outside the bowel in the peritoneal cavity, within the bowel wall (pneumatosis intestinalis), or in the portal venous system.

In order to obtain the most useful images, both oral and intravenous contrast should be utilized. Oral contrast allows differentiation of the intraluminal bowel fluid from extraluminal fluid collections and will help to identify the transition point in cases of bowel obstruction. Intravenous contrast optimizes visualization of infectious processes by highlighting areas of inflammation; additionally, intravenous contrast aids in the assessment of solid organs and areas of potential ischemia or hemorrhage. Intravenous contrast is especially useful in cases of acute pancreatitis to delineate areas of devitalized or necrotic pancreatic tissue or retroperitoneal fat. Allergy or the patient's renal function may limit the ability to utilize intravenous contrast.

Specific conditions may require targeted diagnostic evaluation. Patients with a suspected biliary infection may benefit more from ultrasound (US) evaluation of the abdomen, rather than CT scan. Calculous or acalculous cholecystitis or dilation of bile ducts can be evaluated easily with US. Patients with gastrointestinal bleeding or suspicion of ischemic colitis or *Clostridium difficile* infection would benefit from endoscopy. Endoscopy for bleeding can be both diagnostic and therapeutic and can be performed at the bedside if necessary. Angiography with interventional radiology techniques can also be diagnostic and therapeutic for arterial bleeding.

Patients who are too unstable hemodynamically or clinically for imaging pose a greater diagnostic predicament. Patients requiring multiple or increasing doses of vasopressors, patients with ongoing hemorrhage, or patients with severely compromised respiratory status may have excess or unacceptable risk of morbidity from transport to radiology for testing.[2] These patients should be given goal-directed resuscitation and stabilized with fluids and antibiotics if possible and imaged when feasible. For patients with a high suspicion for intra-abdominal pathology, an emergent bedside laparotomy may be indicated; however, this is a high-risk procedure, requires substantial resources to be mobilized, and has a risk of mortality. Other described diagnostic options for these patients include diagnostic peritoneal lavage (DPL), which places a catheter through the abdominal wall into the peritoneal cavity to allow evaluation of peritoneal fluid; some centers also advocate bedside diagnostic laparoscopy. These techniques have been used in the ICU to evaluate the abdomen for otherwise unevaluable patients with some success, but are not yet standard of care.[1,3,4]

Acute Acalculous Cholecystitis

AAC is the development of acute inflammation of the gallbladder in the absence of gallstones. AAC is generally considered to be a complication of serious medical and surgical illnesses, especially in the setting of trauma, burns, sepsis, prolonged fasting, or total parenteral nutrition. Among medical patients, a variety of systemic diseases have been associated with the development of AAC such as diabetes mellitus, abdominal vasculitis, congestive heart failure, and cholesterol embolization of the cystic artery. Resuscitation from hemorrhagic shock or cardiac arrest has been associated with AAC.[5,6] Acalculous cholecystitis may also develop as a secondary infection of the gallbladder during systemic sepsis for a wide range of infections.

AAC poses major diagnostic challenges. Most afflicted patients are critically ill and unable to communicate their symptoms. Cholecystitis is but one of many potential causes in the differential diagnosis of systemic inflammatory response syndrome (SIRS) or sepsis in such patients. Rapid and accurate diagnosis is essential, as gallbladder ischemia can progress rapidly to gangrene and perforation. Acalculous cholecystitis is sufficiently common that the diagnosis should be considered in every critically ill or injured patient with a clinical picture of sepsis or jaundice and no other obvious source.

US and CT are generally useful for the diagnosis of AAC. Ultrasound of the gallbladder is generally the first-line modality for the diagnosis of AAC in the critically ill patient as it is rapid, low risk, and portable. In calculous cholecystitis, US is useful for detecting gallstones and measuring bile duct diameter; in AAC, these measurements are not valuable. Thickening of the gallbladder wall is the single most reliable criterion, with reported specificity of 90% at 3 mm and 98.5% at 3.5-mm wall thickness, and sensitivity of 100% at 3 mm and 80% at 3.5 mm.[7] Accordingly, gallbladder wall thickness greater than or equal to 3.5 mm is generally accepted to be diagnostic of AAC. Other helpful US findings for AAC include pericholecystic fluid or the presence of intramural gas or a sonolucent intramural

layer, or "halo," that represents intramural edema. Distension of the gallbladder of more than 5 cm in transverse diameter has also been described.[6,7] False-positive US examinations may occur in particular when conditions including sludge, nonshadowing stones, cholesterolosis, hypoalbuminemia, or ascites mimic a thickened gallbladder wall. CT appears to be as accurate as US in the diagnosis of AAC. Diagnostic criteria for AAC by CT are similar to those described for US. Low cost and the ability to perform US rapidly at the bedside make it the preferred diagnostic modality in possible AAC in the ICU setting. Preference may be given to CT if other thoracic or abdominal diagnoses are under consideration.

Historically, the treatment for AAC was cholecystectomy, owing to the ostensible need to inspect the gallbladder and perform a resection if gangrene or perforation was discovered. In the modern era, percutaneous cholecystostomy can be a lifesaving, minimally invasive approach, as it controls the AAC in 70% to 90% of patients.[8,9] For this procedure, the gallbladder is intubated under US (occasionally laparoscopic) guidance via an anterior or transhepatic approach (through the right hepatic lobe) in order to minimize leakage of bile. Rapid improvement should be expected when percutaneous cholecystostomy is successful. Percutaneous treatment is an especially useful modality in the elderly patient with sepsis or patients who are unstable for a surgical procedure. Cholecystostomy will not decompress the common bile duct if cystic duct obstruction is present, therefore the common duct must be decompressed in addition by some manner (eg, ERCP) with sphincterotomy, or laparoscopic or open common bile duct exploration if cholangitis is suspected.

If percutaneous cholecystostomy does not lead to rapid improvement, the tube may be malpositioned, not draining properly, or the patient may have gangrenous cholecystitis. Other reported causes of failure include catheter dislodgement, bile leakage with peritonitis, or an erroneous diagnosis. Perforated ulcer, pancreatic abscess, pneumonia, and pericarditis have been discovered in the aftermath of percutaneous cholecystostomy when patients failed to improve. Reported major complications occur after 8% to 10% of procedures, including dislodgment of the catheter, acute respiratory distress syndrome (ARDS), bile peritonitis, hemorrhage, cardiac arrhythmia, and hypotension due to procedure-related bacteremia.[8,9] A cholecystostomy or cholecystectomy may be required if other sources of sepsis are ruled out and the patient continues to deteriorate. If an operation is warranted, open cholecystostomy may be accomplished under local anesthesia through a short right subcostal incision, but the ability to visualize elsewhere in the abdomen is limited. A laparotomy or laparoscopy would be required to drain distant fluid collections or identify other pathology that may mimic acute cholecystitis in the case of a misdiagnosis (eg, perforated ulcer, cholangitis, pancreatitis). In stable patients with AAC who require surgery, laparoscopic cholecystectomy has been described.

Antibiotic therapy does not substitute for drainage of AAC, but is an important adjunct. The most common bacteria isolated from bile in acute cholecystitis are *Escherichia coli*, *Klebsiella* spp., and *Enterococcus faecalis*, although prior antibiotic administration may allow for other opportunistic pathogens to be present.[5] However, critical illness and prior antibiotic therapy alter host flora, and resistant or opportunistic pathogens may be encountered. Anaerobes are particularly likely to be isolated from bile of patients with diabetes mellitus, in those older than 70 years, and from patients whose biliary tracts have been instrumented previously.

Patency of the cystic duct can be determined immediately after the cholecystostomy is performed by tube cholangiography. This should be performed again after the patient has recovered to determine the presence of gallstones that may not have been detected initially. If gallstones are present, an elective cholecystectomy is usually recommended, with the drainage tube remaining in place during the interprocedure interval. For patients without gallstones, interval cholecystectomy is usually not indicated, and the cholecystostomy tube can be removed 4 to 6 weeks postcholecystostomy after tube cholangiography confirms that gallstones are absent. Recurrent episodes warrant cholecystectomy.

Acute Pancreatitis

Acute pancreatitis can vary in presentation from mild to severe. Patients with severe acute pancreatitis often require a prolonged ICU stay to provide supportive therapy as patients may develop sepsis and progressive organ failure. The pancreas can develop focal or diffuse areas of nonviability, known as necrotizing pancreatitis; when bacteria from the gut infiltrate the nonviable tissue, it becomes infected necrosis. Whereas mild acute pancreatitis has a low mortality rate and usually resolves after a short period of bowel rest, mortality from severe acute pancreatitis with sterile necrosis is estimated to be 10% and can be as high as 70% in the presence of infected pancreatic necrosis.[10,11]

Acute pancreatitis typically presents with epigastric pain that radiates to the back or shoulder, concomitant with nausea, vomiting, fever, and leukocytosis. Laboratory evaluation should include a complete blood count, a complete metabolic panel with liver enzymes, amylase, lipase, and lactate dehydrogenase. For diagnosis of pancreatitis, amylase has a higher sensitivity and lipase has higher specificity; levels greater than 3 times the upper limit of normal support the diagnosis. However, the magnitude of elevation of these laboratory values does not correlate with severity of illness; similarly, normalization of values does not signify resolution of disease. Concurrently elevated liver enzymes, especially alanine aminotransferase, can suggest a biliary etiology.

The most important first step in evaluation of patients with pancreatitis is to identify risk of progression to severe pancreatitis so that aggressive treatment can be instituted expeditiously. Multiple scoring systems exit that are designed to assess the disease severity, although no one system is universally accepted as superior. Common scoring systems include the Ranson criteria, Acute Physiology and Chronic Health Evaluation (APACHE)-II, and the CT severity index (also known as the Balthazar score) (Table 35–1). Although the Ranson criteria were first described in 1974, the score remains clinically useful. Early CT scans for prognostic reasons are not indicated in patients with pancreatitis, as early imaging lacks sensitivity to detect necrosis and infected necrosis is not typically present early in the course of the disease. Patients who develop persistent SIRS or clinical deterioration after 72 hours may benefit from further characterization of disease by CT.

The initial treatment of severe acute pancreatitis is supportive and includes aggressive fluid resuscitation, pain control, and supplemental oxygen administration. A substantial inflammatory response leads to

TABLE 35-1 Severe acute pancreatitis scoring systems.

System	Criteria	Scoring and Interpretation

Ranson criteria	On admission
	  1. Age > 55
	  2. WBC > 16 × 10⁹/L
	  3. LDH > 350/L
	  4. AST > 250/L
	  5. Glucose > 200 mg/dL
	During initial 48 h
	  1. Hgb falls below 10 mg/dL
	  2. BUN rises by > 5 mg/dL
	  3. Calcium < 8 mg/dL
	  4. PaO_2 < 60 mm Hg
	  5. Base deficit > 4
	  6. Fluid sequestration > 6 L
		1 point for each factor listed
		Score > 3 indicates severe acute pancreatitis
		Requires 48 h to calculate entire score

Acute physiology and chronic health evaluation II score (APACHE II)	Calculated from 12 measurements
	  1. Age
	  2. Temperature (rectal)
	  3. Mean arterial pressure
	  4. pH arterial
	  5. Heart rate
	  6. Respiratory rate
	  7. Sodium (serum)
	  8. Potassium (serum)
	  9. Creatinine (serum)
	  10. Hematocrit
	  11. White blood cell count
	  12. Glasgow Coma Scale
		Score > 8 predicts increased risk for complications and mortality
		Score calculated at 24 h

Computer tomography scoring index (CTSI, or Balthazar index)	Based on CT scan
	  1. Pancreas appearance
	    a. Normal pancreas (0 point)
	    b. Enlarged pancreas (1 point)
	    c. Pancreatic/peripancreatic inflammation (2 points)
	    d. One peripancreatic collection (3 points)
	    e. 2 or more peripancreatic collections or retroperitoneal air (4 points)
	  2. Percentage of necrosis
	    a. None (0 point)
	    b. < 30% necrosis (2 points)
	    c. 30%-50% necrosis (4 points)
	    d. > 50% necrosis (6 points)
		Grade points are added to necrosis points to determine the total score
		Cannot be performed prior to 72-96 h after the onset of symptoms because initially pancreatic necrosis is indistinguishable from edema

increased vascular permeability and fluid sequestration within the intra-abdominal space. Resuscitation should target adequate end-organ perfusion to maintain acceptable physiologic targets such as blood pressure, heart rate, and urine output. Patients with severe acute pancreatitis are at risk for development of multiple organ dysfunction syndrome (MODS); acute respiratory failure, circulatory shock, and acute kidney injury are observed in severe cases. In extremely ill patients, central venous pressure and mixed venous oxygen saturation may be of additional value. Sequential bladder pressure measurements are advisable to monitor for ACS.

Historically, a mainstay of treatment for severe acute pancreatitis was bowel and pancreatic rest, as pancreatic stimulation from enteral nutrition was believed to exacerbate pancreatic inflammation. Accordingly, patients with severe acute pancreatitis were given parenteral nutrition until the pancreas recovered. However, over the last decade, several randomized controlled trials comparing enteral to parenteral nutrition have demonstrated that enteral nutrition is associated with decreased infectious morbidity, shorter length of stay, fewer overall complications, and faster resolution of the disease process.[12] Accordingly, enteral nutrition is preferred over parenteral nutrition. Enteral nutrition should be administered early; while the exact timing for initiating enteral nutrition is unknown, it is currently believed that feeding should be commenced soon after admission. Delays in initiation of enteral nutrition can lead to prolonged ileus and decrease tolerance to feeding; additionally, small studies suggest that the benefits of enteral nutrition may be reduced if the enteral nutrition is delayed. The preferred route of enteral administration is also unknown; several trials have failed to detect a difference between nasogastric and nasojejunal feeding.[11] It has been suggested that probiotics could protect patients from overwhelming sepsis from opportunistic pathogens. Ultimately, probiotics have not proved to be effective and may actually increase mortality; routine administration of probiotics is not recommended.[13]

The most common cause of death from severe acute pancreatitis is MODS that develops as a result of infected pancreatic necrosis. This led to the hypothesis that antibiotic prophylaxis for patients with pancreatic necrosis might prevent the later sequelae and morbidity of infection. Early studies in the 1990s showed lower rates of infected pancreatic necrosis with lower mortality; subsequently, administration of antibiotics for prophylaxis became common.[14,15] More recently, 3 double-blind randomized trials were published that could not confirm any beneficial effects of antibiotic prophylaxis; these well-done studies showed that prophylaxis is not associated with a statistically significant reduction in mortality, in the incidence of infected pancreatic necrosis, in the incidence of nonpancreatic infections, or in need for surgical interventions.[16-18] Therefore, antibiotic prophylaxis for severe acute pancreatitis is not recommended.

It can be challenging clinically to differentiate if a severe SIRS response from active infection of pancreatic necrosis as patients will appear ill in both circumstances. Patients suspected of having infected necrosis should have the tissue sampled for culture via percutaneous fine-needle aspiration. Patients with infected necrosis should have antibiotic treatment and management of the infected tissue.

Traditionally, open debridement with pancreatic necrosectomy was performed to remove infected tissue but this procedure was associated with high morbidity and mortality, as well as high rates of long-term pancreatic insufficiency for survivors.[10,11] Overall, there has been a trend toward less invasive approaches to management of necrosis and infected necrosis with or without delayed surgical intervention, known as the "step-up" approach. Patients receive initial medical management with fluid resuscitation and antibiotic administration, followed by percutaneous catheters for drainage of infected fluid. The percutaneous catheters can be irrigated using large volumes of sterile saline and patients are monitored for improvement. Patients who fail to improve may be candidates for operative debridement. In general, postponement of operative debridement for as long as possible is encouraged, as it is associated with decreased morbidity and mortality; however, prolonged antibiotic treatment leads to increased infections with resistant organisms and fungi.[19] Skilled endoscopists have also started to explore transgastric and transduodenal necrosectomy, although these methods are not yet standard of care.

Feeding Intolerance

It is well established that enteral nutrition, provided as early as possible, is beneficial to patients in the ICU. Malnutrition is associated with increased infections, reduced wound healing, increased mortality, prolonged hospital stay, and increased cost. Many critically ill patients present to the hospital with preexisting protein-calorie malnutrition, which is exacerbated by their acute illness. ICU admission leads to periods of starvation (*nil per os* for a variety of reasons), with simultaneous increased metabolic demand from the acute illness. Early enteral nutrition is encouraged and most studies support the dictum "if the gut works, use it." The indications and methods for enteral feeding are discussed elsewhere in this text.

Studies have demonstrated that a substantial percentage of patients in the ICU develop intolerance to enteral feeding, which can be manifested by high gastric residuals, emesis, abdominal distension, or abdominal pain.[20] Most studies of critically ill patients report the ability to deliver only 40% to 60% of goal nutrients secondary to gastrointestinal dysmotility or other barriers to early nutrition.[21] Once mechanical reasons for obstruction are ruled out, feeding intolerance in the critically ill patient stems from the presence of gastric dysmotility or ileus. Rapid resolution of dysmotility is crucial to allow progression of enteral feeding.

Gastric residual volumes are used as a surrogate marker for feeding intolerance, and thus "high gastric residuals" are frequently the rationale for interruption of feeding. Unfortunately, the relationship between gastric residual volumes and delayed gastric emptying is unclear, and the residual volumes that should trigger the cessation of enteral feeding are controversial.[22,23] Some consensus groups agree that a gastric residual volume greater than 200 mL is abnormally high, but still recommend that this threshold should not trigger automatic cessation of enteral nutrition. Because there is no accepted definition for high gastric residuals, thresholds for holding enteral nutrition can vary among institutions, and caregivers at the same institution. Creation of an enteral tube feeding protocol that is not physician-dependent may also improve delivery of nutrients by minimizing feeding interruptions and standardizing the thresholds of residual volumes within an ICU.[24]

Feeding intolerance in the critically ill patient can be attributable to the patient's critical illness, medications, intra-abdominal pathology, or underlying disease. Feeding intolerance may also be due to ileus or bowel obstruction; mechanical obstruction must be ruled out prior to administering enteral nutrition aggressively. Gastric emptying is believed to be delayed in patients with traumatic brain injuries (TBIs) and elevated intracranial pressure (ICP); hyperglycemia may also contribute to delayed gastric emptying.[25] Endogenous or exogenous catecholamines are likely to decrease gastric emptying, whereas dopamine reduces antral contractions. Anticholinergics, calcium channel blockers, sedatives, and opiates, all of which are used commonly in the ICU, also slow gastric motility.

Therapeutic options for the treatment of delayed gastric emptying are imperfect. Prokinetic options are most widely used, but no regimen is perfect. Common prokinetic agents include metoclopramide or erythromycin as monotherapy, or in combination. Metoclopramide antagonizes the effect of dopamine on the gastric antrum and improves gastric motility when given as a 10 mg q6h, although the effect is blunted in TBI patients. With repeated administration, tachyphylaxis develops quickly and reliably such that after 7 days of routine metoclopramide administration, only 20% to 25% of patients continue to have successful nasogastric feeding.[25,26] Another commonly utilized promotility agent, erythromycin, acts as a motilin agonist and can be given intravenously in doses of 1 to 3 mg/kg/d and likely has better prokinetic activity than metoclopramide. Unfortunately, patients also become resistant to the effects of erythromycin over time, such that after 7 days, only 30% to 45% of patients can be successfully fed via a nasogastric tube. Additionally, there are concerns that erythromycin can exacerbate antibiotic resistance or lead to cardiotoxicity. Cardiac toxicity can be minimized by using smaller doses; reportedly, an intravenous dose of 70 mg of erythromycin is as effective as a 200-mg dose in accelerating gastric emptying. Once feedings are tolerated, the prokinetic agent can be discontinued.

Combination therapy of metoclopramide plus erythromycin may be superior to the use of either drug alone and decreases the incidence of tachyphylaxis as first-line treatment of feeding intolerance or after the failure of monotherapy.[25-27] Newer therapies with potential to improve gastric emptying include opioid antagonists such as methylnaltrexone or alvimopan. Methylnaltrexone and alvimopan theoretically do not cross the blood-brain barrier so that analgesia is maintained while the effects of opioids on the gastrointestinal tract are blunted. Both drugs have been tested in in postoperative elective bowel resection patients and help accelerate recovery of bowel function or decrease postoperative ileus without increased pain. Unfortunately, these opioid antagonist agents have not been proved in the critically ill patient.[28] When drug treatment fails, alternatives can include parenteral nutrition or postpyloric feeding access. In fact, some clinicians advocate enteral feeding into the small bowel as first-line enteral access. Controversy exists on the optimal anatomic location for feeding access, and this is discussed elsewhere in this text.

Other Enteral Feeding Issues: Hemodynamic Instability, Ileus, and Diarrhea

Patients in the ICU may undergo prolonged periods of starvation for reasons other than feeding intolerance, including imminent or recent surgical procedures, hemodynamic instability, diarrhea, and lack of functional enteral access. Some clinicians are reluctant to initiate early enteral feeding until the "acute" phase of the injury response has subsided, owing to the fear that immediate feeding will result in higher complications from delayed gastric emptying, such as aspiration of gastric contents. Despite this, large studies suggest that the benefits of early feeding outweigh the risks and the practice of early nutrition is becoming more common.

Giving enteral feeds on vasopressors continues to be contentious. Hemodynamic instability requiring vasopressors is often considered to be a relative contraindication to enteral feeding; however, the data supporting this are inconclusive. In healthy adults, enteral nutrition is associated with an increase in blood flow to the intestines. The concerns for feeding patients who are on vasopressors are 2-fold: Patients can develop intestinal ischemia from the increased demand when the circulatory system is not able to increase blood flow, or patients may experience a "steal" phenomenon, where blood is diverted to the splanchnic circulation leading to ischemia of other end organs. There have been a few case reports of very early enteral feeding being associated with intestinal ischemia in underresuscitated trauma patients but it is unclear whether the feeding or the inadequate resuscitation was the culprit leading to intestinal ischemia.[29] Whereas it is probably prudent to not feed patients in hemorrhagic shock or with rapidly escalating vasopressor requirements, some data suggest that enteral feeding is safe in patients receiving vasopressors.[30]

Another common reason for delay of enteral nutrition is adynamic or paralytic ileus of the small bowel. Ileus can be caused by a number of intra-abdominal and retroperitoneal processes, including intestinal ischemia, ruptured viscus, hemorrhage, pancreatitis, peritonitis, medications (opioids, anticholinergics), and electrolyte abnormalities. It may also occur after abdominal surgery. Ileus is heralded by abdominal pain, vomiting, and abdominal distension with obstipation and must be differentiated from a mechanical small bowel obstruction. Radiographic studies may help differentiate obstruction from ileus. Laboratory studies should be obtained, including a complete blood count, chemistries, and perhaps an arterial blood gas and lactate if there is concern for intestinal ischemia, although no laboratory test is definitive. Patients with worsening signs on serial abdominal examinations, or who develop a fluid requirement and acidosis, should have a surgical evaluation for obstruction or ischemia. Plain abdominal films performed at the bedside have limited value. On plain radiographs, ileus will show diffuse small bowel dilation (> 3 cm) with air-fluid levels and no distinct cutoff point. Air and stool present in the colon on a plain radiograph can be a reassuring sign that there is no mechanical obstruction present but is not particularly specific, as a patient with acute obstruction or a closed loop obstruction may not have had time to decompress the distal bowel. Patients who are suspected of having a mechanical obstruction should undergo a CT scan with oral and intravenous contrast. Nasogastric tube decompression can be used to ease symptoms of nausea and may help resolve the ileus.

Colonic pseudo-obstruction (Ogilvie syndrome) occurs typically in bedridden or elderly patients, but may also happen as a sequela of spinal cord injury, prolonged opioid use, or postoperatively from abdominal or nonabdominal surgery. This manifests characteristically with abdominal distension, abdominal pain, obstipation, and possibly tenderness; vomiting may or not be present. Plain radiographs demonstrate a dilated colon, usually most pronounced at the cecum, and should be performed as an initial diagnostic test to rule out a mechanical cause of obstruction such as volvulus. Perforation risk is approximately 3% but risk increases if the diameter of the cecum exceeds 12 cm or if the distension has been present for more than 6 days. Therapy should include correction of electrolyte abnormalities, cessation of narcotics, and nasogastric decompression. Neostigmine, 2 mg IV over a period of 5 minutes, can be utilized to resolve the ileus. Administration of neostigmine should take place in the ICU, as some patients develop symptomatic bradycardia and require administration of atropine. A repeat dose of neostigmine may be administered after 3 hours.[31] If neostigmine does not resolve the pseudo-obstruction (~ 15% of cases), colonoscopic decompression may be considered as success rates are high (~ 70%); complications include perforation, inability to decompress the colon, and recurrence. Surgical intervention may be necessary for patients who have perforated, patients who have had unsuccessful attempts at decompression, or patients with recurrent pseudo-obstruction after decompression.

Critically ill patients often develop diarrhea, defined as an increase in the fluidity, frequency, or quantity of bowel movements. The actual volume of stool that constitutes diarrhea is debated but typically is described as greater than 300 mL/d or greater than 4 loose stools per day. Diarrhea can lead to electrolyte imbalance, wound contamination, and dehydration, and may prompt providers to hold enteral nutrition, which can exacerbate malnutrition. Diarrhea may be attributable to one or multiple simultaneous causes, including enteral feeding formulas or regimens, malabsorption, underlying disease, medications, or infections.[32] Medications that may cause diarrhea should be discontinued, such as metoclopramide, erythromycin, oral magnesium or phosphorus, or antibiotics. Diarrhea is the most commonly reported complication of enteral tube feeding; research on various feeding formula issues have been studied, including temperature, osmolality, fiber content and type, density, delivery rate, and formula content, but no factor in the feeding formula is consistently associated with development of diarrhea.[32] Infectious diarrhea in the ICU can be secondary to *C difficile*, *Klebsiella oxytoca*, *Clostridium perfringens*, *Salmonella* spp., *Staphylococcus aureus*, or gastrointestinal viruses.

For patients with profuse diarrhea, all possible offending medications should be discontinued and infectious sources should be treated. Several nutritional interventions have been studied, with limited success. Fiber-enriched formulas are supported by the Society of Critical Care Medicine and the American Society for Parenteral and Enteral Nutrition in patients who have developed diarrhea,[33] but not all clinical trials demonstrate an effect of fiber on diarrhea. Probiotics have been suggested as a way to recolonize the intestine and normalize the intestinal flora. However, the administration of probiotics is controversial in critically ill patients with abnormal immune responses; one study of patients with severe acute pancreatitis even showed increased mortality with probiotic prophylaxis.[13] For patients with diarrhea that is deemed noninfectious, antidiarrheal agents may be considered but should be used with great caution. Opioid analogs may be considered; the most common form is dephenoxylate with atropine (1 tablet 3-4 times/d) or loperamide (up to 4 mg, 4 times/d).

Abdominal Compartment Syndrome

In the critically ill patient, pressure within the abdominal cavity can be increased pathologically above the patient's baseline. Prolonged elevations of intra-abdominal pressure can result in organ dysfunction and failure, known as ACS. In the healthy patient, physiologic intra-abdominal pressure is close to 0 mm Hg, although this can be increased chronically to 10 to 15 mm Hg in obesity or pregnancy. In the critically ill patient, pressures are generally increased to levels of 5 to 7 mm Hg.[34] Acidosis, multiple blood transfusions, sepsis, major trauma or burns, pancreatitis, ileus, liver dysfunction, and aggressive ventilator settings with high positive end expiratory pressures are factors that can further increase intra-abdominal pressure. IAH is defined as intra-abdominal pressure greater than 12 mm Hg. ACS is defined as intra-abdominal pressure greater than 20 mm Hg with evidence of end-organ dysfunction or failure.[34] Clinically, this may manifest with a tense, distended abdomen, progressive hypotension, oliguria, and increased airway pressures. Primary abdominal compartment syndrome is characterized by acute or subacute development of intra-abdominal hypertension in a relatively brief period of time secondary to pathology within the abdominopelvic cavity, usually due to abdominal trauma, ruptured abdominal aneurysm, hemoperitoneum, acute pancreatitis, acute peritonitis, or retroperitoneal hemorrhage. Secondary ACS is characterized by IAH that develops over a subacute or chronic time period as a result of an extra-abdominal cause such as sepsis, capillary leak syndrome, or aggressive fluid resuscitation following a major burn. Patients may develop recurrent ACS after abdominal decompression, even with an open abdomen, if resuscitation is ongoing or dressings are too tight, or if abdominal closure was performed and intra-abdominal pressure becomes elevated again.

Intra-abdominal pressure monitoring is essential to the diagnosis of ACS. A variety of methods exist to measure pressure within the abdominal cavity, which include direct (via needle puncture into the abdominal cavity) or indirect (transduction of intra-abdominal pressure through a surrogate, such as the bladder or colon). Bladder pressure measurement has the most widespread adoption owing to the simplicity and minimal cost; additionally most critically ill patients already have a bladder catheter in place, so the measurement of pressure is relatively noninvasive. However, there is increased risk of urinary tract infection. Regardless of the technique utilized, several key principles need to be followed as outlined by the International Conference of Experts on Intra-abdominal Hypertension and Abdominal Compartment Syndrome in 2004.[34] Intra-abdominal pressure should be expressed in mm Hg and measured at the end of end expiration, with the transducer zeroed at the midaxillary line and ensuring that there are no abdominal muscle contractions. There reference standard is instillation of 25 mL sterile saline into the bladder; higher volumes of instilled fluid can overfill the bladder such that the transduced pressure becomes the pressure of the bladder wall instead of the intra-abdominal pressure. Changes in body position, and the presence of abdominal or bladder wall contractions have been demonstrated to impact the accuracy of intra-abdominal pressure measurements.[35]

Treatment and management of ACS consists of 4 general principles: (1) serial monitoring of intra-abdominal pressures, (2) optimization of systemic perfusion and organ function in the presence of intra-abdominal hypertension, (3) institution of medical procedures to decrease intra-abdominal pressure and reduce end-organ dysfunction, and (4) prompt surgical decompression for refractory intra-abdominal hypertension or ACS. Generally, the "critical" intra-abdominal pressure at which end-organ dysfunction occurs differs among patients, but some trials have evaluated abdominal perfusion pressure (similar in concept to ICP monitoring and cerebral perfusion pressure), where the abdominal

perfusion pressure is equal to the mean arterial pressure minus the intra-abdominal pressure. Several retrospective trials have suggested that abdominal perfusion pressure above 50 to 60 mm Hg is associated with improved survival, but this has yet to be validated prospectively.[35]

Several medical therapies have been hypothesized to temporize and treat mild IAH; however, if a patient is showing signs of end-organ damage, medical therapies are unlikely to have beneficial or expeditious enough effects to prevent the need for decompressive laparotomy. Pain, agitation, ventilator dyssynchrony, and use of accessory muscles during work of breathing all may contribute to increased intra-abdominal pressure. Patients at risk for ACS must be afforded adequate sedation and pain control. It has been suggested that neuromuscular blockade may allow for muscle relaxation to decrease the compliance of the abdominal wall, thus decreasing intra-abdominal pressure. However, the risks of pharmacologic paralysis must be weighed carefully against the uncertain benefits. Body positioning may also contribute to intra-abdominal pressure; elevation of the head of the bed and supine positioning may increase intra-abdominal pressure, but again the benefits of these positions in specific patient populations may outweigh the risk of supine and flat positioning. Other interventions that may theoretically decrease intra-abdominal pressure such as nasogastric and colonic decompression, diuretics, and renal replacement therapy have not been adequately studied in this patient population.

Surgical decompressive laparotomy is the standard treatment for patients who develop ACS. Once a patient's IAH has become refractory to medical therapies, laparotomy is a lifesaving intervention. Surgical decompression results in an "open abdomen," which is discussed further in the next section. Decompressive laparotomy is also a reasonable therapeutic option in a patient with intra-abdominal hypertension for whom the risk of ACS is high but the patient has not yet manifested end-organ damage.[35]

The Long-Term Open Abdomen

Use of damage control surgery with temporary abdominal closure has gained popularity since the late 1980s as a way to salvage critically ill trauma patients with physiologic compromise due to massive hemorrhage in the abdomen. This approach has been adapted for use in other nontrauma surgical patients with abdominal catastrophes, such as ACS or pancreatic necrosectomy with expected serial debridement procedures. There are generally 3 stages to damage control surgery: abbreviated surgery, resuscitation, and delayed definitive closure. The initial surgery is abbreviated to allow for rapid control of hemorrhage or abdominal contamination, and may require packing for hemostasis. At this point, the abdominal contents are covered with a temporary dressing. This is followed by resuscitation, warming, and correction of any existing coagulopathy in order to allow the patient to have normalization of physiology. Implicit in this approach is the planned surgical reexploration, which typically occurs 12 to 72 hours after the index operation. Aggressive resuscitation between the first and second operation may render the abdomen unable to be closed and serial dressing changes and staged operations may be necessary to obtain closure or coverage of the abdominal contents. Ideally, patients should undergo definitive fascial closure whenever possible, even if closure must be performed in stages; in some cases, closure is impossible. Surgical options for these patients are limited and unappealing but include temporary mesh closure, skin-only closure, or split-thickness skin grafts with planned ventral hernia. Many of these patients develop severe loss of domain and loss of function of the abdominal wall, eventually necessitating extensive reconstructive surgery to regain some abdominal wall functionality.

All patients who undergo damage control surgery with an open abdomen are at high risk for infectious complications. Surgical site infections have been reported to occur in as many as 83% of cases, and postoperative fascial dehiscence is reported in up to 25% of patients who have had an open abdomen.[36] However, no data support antibiotic prophylaxis of the open abdomen. Particularly concerning in patients who are unable to undergo fascial closure is the development of bowel fistulae. The incidence of fistulae in patients with an open abdomen is approximately 5% to 19%, and varies according to the initial indication for damage control surgery.[37] Of unique concern in this patient population is the "enteroatmospheric" fistula, which occurs because there is no tissue that overlies the exposed bowel and spontaneous healing becomes impossible. Patients with enteroatmospheric fistulae should have radiologic evaluation with enteral contrast to clarify the location of the fistula (proximal or distal bowel) to create strategies for enteral nutrition, if possible, and minimize fluid and electrolyte losses. Continuous leakage of enteric contents into the wound contributes to elevated catabolism, protein loss, infection/sepsis, and increased mortality. These patients likely require serial abdominal operations to control enteric leakage and reestablish bowel continuity.

CONCLUSIONS

Critically ill patients are susceptible to a variety of sources of abdominal dysfunction. These issues must be diagnosed quickly and addressed in a way that considers each patient's current clinical status and concurrent critical issues.

REFERENCES

1. Crandall M, West MA. Evaluation of the abdomen in the critically ill patient: opening the black box. *Curr Opin Crit Care.* 2006;12(4):333-339.
2. Warren J, Fromm RE Jr, Orr RA, Rotello LC, Horst HM; American College of Critical Care Medicine. Guidelines for the inter- and intrahospital transport of critically ill patients. *Crit Care Med.* 2004;32(1):256-262.
3. Karasakalides A, Triantafillidou S, Anthimidis G, et al. The use of bedside diagnostic laparoscopy in the intensive care unit. *J Laparoendoscop Adv Surg Tech Part A.* 2009;19(3):333-338.
4. Walsh RM, Popovich MJ, Hoadley J. Bedside diagnostic laparoscopy and peritoneal lavage in the intensive care unit. *Surg Endosc.* 1998;12(12):1405-1409.
5. Barie PS, Eachempati SR. Acute acalculous cholecystitis. *Gastroenterol Clin North Am.* 2010;39(2):343-357.
6. Huffman JL, Schenker S. Acute acalculous cholecystitis: a review. *Clin Gastroenterol Hepatol.* 2010;8(1):15-22.
7. Deitch EA, Engel JM. Acute acalculous cholecystitis. Ultrasonic diagnosis. *Am J Surg.* 1981;142(2):290-292.
8. Joseph T, Unver K, Hwang GL, et al. Percutaneous cholecystostomy for acute cholecystitis: ten-year

experience. *J Vasc Intervent Radiol*. 2012; 23(1):83-88.e1.

9. McLoughlin RF, Patterson EJ, Mathieson JR, Cooperberg PL, MacFarlane JK. Radiologically guided percutaneous cholecystostomy for acute cholecystitis: long-term outcome in 50 patients. *Can Assoc Radiologists J*. 1994;45(6):455-459.

10. Babu RY, Gupta R, Kang M, Bhasin DK, Rana SS, Singh R. Predictors of surgery in patients with severe acute pancreatitis managed by the step-up approach. *Ann Surg*. 2013;257(4):737-750.

11. Anand N, Park JH, Wu BU. Modern management of acute pancreatitis. *Gastroenterol Clin North Am*. 2012;41(1):1-8.

12. Ong JP, Fock KM. Nutritional support in acute pancreatitis. *J Dig Dis*. 2012;13(9):445-452.

13. Besselink MG, van Santvoort HC, Buskens E, et al. Probiotic prophylaxis in predicted severe acute pancreatitis: a randomised, double-blind, placebo-controlled trial. *Lancet*. 2008;371(9613):651-659.

14. Pederzoli P, Bassi C, Vesentini S, Campedelli A. A randomized multicenter clinical trial of antibiotic prophylaxis of septic complications in acute necrotizing pancreatitis with imipenem. *Surg Gynecol Obstet*. 1993;176(5):480-483.

15. Sainio V, Kemppainen E, Puolakkainen P, et al. Early antibiotic treatment in acute necrotising pancreatitis. *Lancet*. 1995;346(8976):663-667.

16. Isenmann R, Runzi M, Kron M, et al. Prophylactic antibiotic treatment in patients with predicted severe acute pancreatitis: a placebo-controlled, double-blind trial. *Gastroenterology*. 2004;126(4):997-1004.

17. Dellinger EP, Tellado JM, Soto NE, et al. Early antibiotic treatment for severe acute necrotizing pancreatitis: a randomized, double-blind, placebo-controlled study. *Ann Surg*. 2007;245(5):674-683.

18. Garcia-Barrasa A, Borobia FG, Pallares R, et al. A double-blind, placebo-controlled trial of ciprofloxacin prophylaxis in patients with acute necrotizing pancreatitis. *J Gastrointest Surg*. 2009;13(4):768-774.

19. Besselink MG, Verwer TJ, Schoenmaeckers EJ, et al. Timing of surgical intervention in necrotizing pancreatitis. *Arch Surg*. 2007;142(12):1194-1201.

20. Kim H, Stotts NA, Froelicher ES, Engler MM, Porter C. Why patients in critical care do not receive adequate enteral nutrition? A review of the literature. *J Crit Care*. 2012;27(6):702-713.

21. Ukleja A. Altered GI motility in critically Ill patients: current understanding of pathophysiology, clinical impact, and diagnostic approach. *Nutr Clin Pract*. 2010;25(1):16-25.

22. Dive A, Moulart M, Jonard P, Jamart J, Mahieu P. Gastroduodenal motility in mechanically ventilated critically ill patients: a manometric study. *Crit Care Med*. 1994;22(3):441-447.

23. Nguyen NQ, Fraser RJ, Chapman M, et al. Proximal gastric response to small intestinal nutrients is abnormal in mechanically ventilated critically ill patients. *World J Gastroenterol*. 2006;12(27):4383-4388.

24. Arabi Y, Haddad S, Sakkijha M, Al Shimemeri A. The impact of implementing an enteral tube feeding protocol on caloric and protein delivery in intensive care unit patients. *Nutr Clin Pract*. 2004;19(5):523-530.

25. Chapman MJ, Nguyen NQ, Fraser RJ. Gastrointestinal motility and prokinetics in the critically ill. *Curr Opin Crit Care*. 2007;13(2):187-194.

26. Nguyen NQ, Chapman MJ, Fraser RJ, Bryant LK, Holloway RH. Erythromycin is more effective than metoclopramide in the treatment of feed intolerance in critical illness. *Crit Care Med*. 2007;35(2):483-489.

27. Nguyen NQ, Chapman M, Fraser RJ, Bryant LK, Burgstad C, Holloway RH. Prokinetic therapy for feed intolerance in critical illness: one drug or two? *Crit Care Med*. 2007;35(11):2561-2567.

28. Roberts DJ, Banh HL, Hall RI. Use of novel prokinetic agents to facilitate return of gastrointestinal motility in adult critically ill patients. *Curr Opin Crit Care*. 2006;12(4):295-302.

29. Zaloga GP, Roberts PR, Marik P. Feeding the hemodynamically unstable patient: a critical evaluation of the evidence. *Nutr Clin Pract*. 2003;18(4):285-293.

30. Khalid I, Doshi P, DiGiovine B. Early enteral nutrition and outcomes of critically ill patients treated with vasopressors and mechanical ventilation. *Am J Crit Care*. 2010;19(3):261-268.

31. Ponec RJ, Saunders MD, Kimmey MB. Neostigmine for the treatment of acute colonic pseudo-obstruction. *N Engl J Med*. 1999;341(3):137-141.

32. Chang SJ, Huang HH. Diarrhea in enterally fed patients: blame the diet? *Curr Opin Clin Nutr Metab Care*. 2013;16(5):588-594.

33. Martindale RG, McClave SA, Vanek VW, et al. Guidelines for the provision and assessment of nutrition support therapy in the adult critically ill patient: Society of Critical Care Medicine and American Society for Parenteral and Enteral Nutrition: executive summary. *Crit Care Med*. 2009;37(5):1757-1761.

34. Malbrain ML, Cheatham ML, Kirkpatrick A, et al. Results from the International Conference of Experts on Intra-abdominal Hypertension and Abdominal Compartment Syndrome. I. Definitions. *Intensive Care Med.* 2006;32(11):1722-1732.

35. Cheatham ML, Malbrain ML, Kirkpatrick A, et al. Results from the International Conference of Experts on Intra-abdominal Hypertension and Abdominal Compartment Syndrome. II. Recommendations. *Intensive Care Med.* 2007;33(6):951-962.

36. Smith BP, Adams RC, Doraiswamy VA, et al. Review of abdominal damage control and open abdomens: focus on gastrointestinal complications. *J Gastrointest Liver Dis.* 2010;19(4):425-435.

37. Stawicki SP, Brooks A, Bilski T, et al. The concept of damage control: extending the paradigm to emergency general surgery. *Injury.* 2008;39(1):93-101.

Gastrointestinal Hemorrhage (Upper and Lower)

36

Pari Shah, MD, MSCE

Gastrointestinal (GI) bleeding accounts for a significant number of hospitalizations every year with a median length of stay of 4 days and with greater than 30% of patients requiring intensive care unit (ICU) care.[1] Early diagnosis of the cause and appropriate intervention can significantly reduce ICU and hospital stays and improve morbidity and mortality. This chapter focuses on a discussion of the differential diagnosis of upper and lower GI bleeding and management principles.

UPPER GI BLEEDING

KEY POINTS

1. The first step in the management of upper GI bleeding (UGIB) is to assess hemodynamic status and resuscitate if there is any instability. Restricted transfusion strategies (transfusion for hemoglobin [Hb] < 7) yield better outcomes than aggressive transfusion strategies.

2. Patients should be stratified for risk of rebleeding and mortality based on clinical predictors and endoscopic findings.

3. Early endoscopy (within 24 hours) for UGIB improves outcomes and length of hospital stay; endoscopic treatment is warranted for high-risk lesions (active bleeding vessel, oozing vessel, visible vessel). Angiography with embolization or surgery can be used as rescue therapy for patients who fail endoscopic therapy.

4. Patients with acute hemorrhage suspected from varices should undergo early endoscopy and endoscopic band ligation for treatment of varices that have stigmata of bleeding; transjugular intrahepatic portosystemic shunting (TIPS) can be used as rescue therapy for patients who fail endoscopic therapy.

5. Pharmacologic therapy in conjunction with endoscopic therapy can improve rebleeding rates and survival.

INTRODUCTION

UGIB has an incidence of 48 to 160 cases/100,000 adults per year.[2] Bleeding from an upper GI source is defined by overt presentation of bleeding represented as melena, hematemesis, or occasionally hematochezia, with localization of the bleeding lesion to the esophagus, stomach, or duodenum. UGIB is 5 to 6 times more common than lower GI bleeding (LGIB). The clinical presentation of UGIB can vary widely from clinically insignificant bleeding to life-threatening bleeding. Mortality from UGIB is generally between 10% and 14%.[3] The management principles of UGIB focus on the risk stratification of patients and the early diagnosis and treatment of underlying causes.

HISTORY

UGIB is generally described as the presentation of melena, black tarry stools, or the description of hematemesis, vomiting of blood. The presentation may be insidious in onset or abrupt. Details obtained on history will suggest the duration of the bleeding and whether it is acute or chronic. Patients will often describe the presence of diarrhea associated with UGIB because blood passing through the GI tract often results in multiple loose bowel movements. Rapid UGIB may present as hematochezia (bright red blood or maroon stools from below) in addition to melena. Approximately 10% of patients with hematochezia may have upper GI sources of their bleeding.

Symptoms that accompany UGIB may reflect significant hemodynamic compromise; these include dizziness, light-headedness, chest pain, shortness of breath or dyspnea on exertion, weakness, or fatigue. Symptoms such as chest pain or shortness of breath suggest a more acute hemodynamic compromise and clinically significant blood loss. Patients without accompanying hemodynamic symptoms suggest a slow bleeding rate or a more chronic process. Symptoms such as abdominal pain, abdominal cramping, or postprandial pain may be helpful in narrowing the differential diagnosis of the source of the bleeding.

Essential to the history taking is obtaining information of comorbid conditions the patient may have and any medications the patient may be taking. Comorbid conditions can help in diagnosis, for example, liver disease may suggest a possible diagnosis of varices. Comorbid conditions are also important in treatment; for example underlying cardiac or pulmonary disease may be significant to the management of the patient. Medications that may play a role in UGIB include nonsteroidal anti-inflammatory drugs (NSAIDs), or antithrombotic agents, such as antiplatelet medication or anticoagulants. NSAIDs may cause UGIB through the formation of peptic ulcers, while therapy with

antithrombotic agents may exacerbate UGIB from underlying lesions. A recent meta-analysis evaluated 35 randomized controlled trials (RCTs) and demonstrated that antiplatelet therapy with aspirin (ASA) (defined as 75-325 mg/d) increased the risk of UGIB 1.5 times compared to nonusers. The odds ratio (OR) of UGIB in patients taking ASA and clopidogrel was 1.86 when compared to ASA alone and the OR of GI bleeding with anticoagulants was 1.93 when compared to ASA alone.[4] New anticoagulants, such as thrombin and factor Xa inhibitors, have also been shown to increase risk of GI bleeding; a meta-analysis analyzing 43 RCTs revealed an overall OR of GI bleeding of 1.45 when compared to traditional anticoagulants and an OR as high as 5 when used in the setting of acute coronary syndrome.[5] Information about the dose, duration, and effects of these medications can help direct further care.

PHYSICAL EXAMINATION AND INITIAL ASSESSMENT

The physical examination focuses initially on hemodynamic evaluation. Assessing a patient's volume status with blood pressure monitoring and heart rate (HR) evaluation is crucial to determining the critical nature of the GI bleed. Patients with hemodynamic instability, suggested by HR greater than 100 beats/min, systolic blood pressure (SBP) less than 100 mm Hb, or the presence of orthostatic hypotension (defined by drop in SBP of > 20 mm Hb or rise in HR of > 20 beats/min from lying to sitting or sitting to standing) or the presence of syncope suggest a loss of blood volume of greater than 10% and indicates an urgency for volume resuscitation.

Other aspects of initial examination include assessment of the abdomen and rectum. Abdominal auscultation and palpation may help to narrow down the differential diagnosis. Patients with physical examination findings of peritonitis or clinical concern for perforation should be triaged for computed tomographic (CT) scan prior to further workup. Rectal examination is essential to confirm the presence of melena and support the etiology of UGIB and to help distinguish UGIB from lower gastrointestinal bleeding (LGIB). Patients in whom UGIB needs to be further confirmed and in whom endoscopy is being considered may benefit from nasogastric (NG) tube placement and gastric lavage. NG lavage provides supporting information of UGIB by witnessing the return of bright red blood or coffee ground material. It allows for the determination of ongoing UGIB: bright red blood that does not clear with lavage suggests active UGIB while clearance of red blood and return of coffee ground material suggest recent UGIB that may have stopped. Finally, NG lavage may allow for clearance of gastric contents facilitating views of the stomach on upper endoscopy. Some physicians advocate for NG lavage in all patients suspected of UGIB; in our practice, we determine its role in diagnosis and management on a case-by-case basis.

Laboratory studies supplement the assessment made on initial physical examination. The patient's Hb should be assessed immediately with a complete blood count (CBC) and compared to previous Hb levels to assess change; however the Hb level can be misleading in acute UGIB if there has not been sufficient time for the cardiovascular system to equilibrate and reflect the blood loss. Other laboratory values that may assist in the assessment are the blood urea nitrogen (BUN) and creatinine, the ratio of which can often be greater than 20:1 in patients with UGIB. All patients with evidence of GI bleeding should have a type-and-cross match sent to establish blood type given the possible need for blood transfusion.

Initial Management

The goals of initial management focus on resuscitation. Additionally, management decisions must be made to minimize ongoing bleeding and to minimize the impact of the UGIB on other organ systems (Figure 36–1).

Resuscitation is initiated and driven by amount of blood loss as assessed on CBC and by hemodynamic compromise. All patients should have 2 large-bore peripheral venous access catheters or a central venous access placed. Patients with altered mental status or respiratory compromise should be intubated for airway protection. Patients with significant hemodynamic compromise should be admitted to

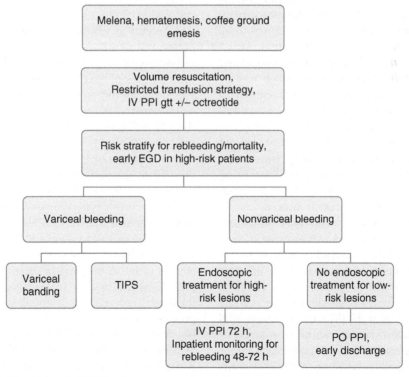

FIGURE 36–1 Management of UGIB.

the ICU for close monitoring and management. Volume replacement should be initiated immediately with normal saline or lactated Ringer solution. Colloid solutions can be given.

The goal of blood transfusion is to increase the delivery of oxygen to the tissues. The need for blood transfusion is based on initial Hb and assessment of whether UGIB is ongoing and significant. Patients with massive UGIB may benefit from an aggressive transfusion strategy; patients with clinically stable UGIB and low-risk or intermediate-risk UGIB are more likely to benefit from a restrictive transfusion strategy. A recent RCT of patients with acute UGIB comparing a restrictive transfusion strategy (transfusion for Hb < 7) versus a liberal transfusion strategy (transfusion for Hb < 9) found that patients with a restrictive transfusion strategy had higher probability of survival at 6 weeks, decreased rates of rebleeding, and lower number of adverse events. This benefit is most clearly understood in patients with cirrhosis and portal hypertension-related variceal bleeding.[6] Aggressive reconstitution of blood volume has previously been shown to induce rebound increases in portal pressure, which may precipitate rebleeding of varices; a restrictive transfusion strategy was shown to be beneficial in these patients. Additionally, a restrictive transfusion strategy was shown to be beneficial in patients with nonvariceal UGIB, which may be due to decreased transfusion-related complications, decreased transfusion-related abnormalities in coagulation, or decreased cardiac complications such as pulmonary edema.[6] Patients should be evaluated on a case-by-case basis for transfusion needs, taking into consideration age, coexisting comorbidities, and hemodynamic status; however, a restrictive transfusion strategy is favored.

Patients should concurrently have prothrombin time (PT) and activated partial thromboplastin time (aPTT) levels checked and corrected as necessary. In patients with ongoing GI bleeding, the goal international normalized ratio (INR) is less than 1.5 and fresh frozen plasma (FFP) can be given to achieve this in the short term. Patients who are hemodynamically stable can proceed to upper endoscopy while transfusion is being given. A recent study demonstrated no difference in risk of rebleeding following endoscopic therapy in patients with mild-to-moderate elevated INR compared to normal INR.[7] Patients with history of thrombocytopenia should have platelet levels checked and corrected to values greater than 50,000/mm³.

After the initial management, the focus is on minimizing ongoing UGIB. UGIB is often divided between nonvariceal bleeding and variceal bleeding and initial assessment for chronic liver disease helps to differentiate these possibilities. The most common cause of nonvariceal UGIB is peptic ulcer disease (PUD). Thus, to reduce ongoing bleeding from this potential cause, all patients are recommended to receive intravenous (IV) proton pump inhibitor (PPI) therapy until further risk stratification is completed. This is generally given in the form of intravenous pantoprazole starting with a bolus of 80 mg followed by a continuous infusion of 8 mg/h. A RCT of patients receiving PPI infusion versus placebo prior to endoscopy revealed lower need for endoscopic intervention and decreased length of hospital stay in patients treated with pre-endoscopic PPI.[8] PPI therapy is thought to stabilize blood clot and reduce risk of bleeding by decreasing levels of gastric acid, which can inhibit platelet aggregation and lead to clot lysis.[9]

Patients in whom chronic liver disease is suspected and who have a risk of variceal bleeding are recommended to receive pharmacologic therapy in conjunction with endoscopic therapy as well. Somatostatin and somatostatin analogues such as octreotide and vapreotide have been evaluated in the pre-endoscopic period for patients in whom variceal bleeding is suspected. Octreotide is the only medication of this class currently available in the United States; intravenous octreotide infusion starting with 50 μg bolus followed by 50 μg/h continuous infusion is recommended to be given in all patients in whom variceal bleeding is suspected followed by early endoscopy. A meta-analysis of 8 randomized trials revealed improved endoscopic control of initial bleeding in patients who received pharmacologic therapy in addition to endoscopic therapy.[10] Terlipressin, a synthetic analogue of vasopressin, has also been evaluated and been shown to be effective in acute variceal bleeding; however, this medication is not yet available in the United States. A recent study comparing somatostatin, octreotide, and terlipressin in a randomized fashion showed no difference in the hemostatic effects or safety between these medications.[11]

Additionally, patients with cirrhosis and suspected UGIB are recommended to receive short-term prophylactic antibiotics. Prophylactic antibiotics are intended to decrease the risk of bacterial infection such as spontaneous bacterial peritonitis and other infections; studies evaluating the role of prophylactic antibiotics have shown decreased rates of infection and improved survival.[12] Norfloxacin 400 mg twice daily given orally for 7 days is the recommended antibiotic, though other fluoroquinolones have also been shown to be effective. Additionally, IV ceftriaxone 1 g/d has been studied and shown to be effective.

RISK STRATIFICATION

An estimated 80% of patients with UGIB will spontaneously stop without intervention other than those described earlier. Patients who have completed initial resuscitation should be evaluated for evidence of ongoing bleeding, risk of rebleeding, and risk of mortality. This assessment should be made first based on clinical and laboratory findings, and then may be modified after endoscopic findings. Several scoring systems have been developed to stratify patients into high risk or low risk for rebleeding and mortality (Table 36–1). In previous studies, clinical predictors of rebleeding and mortality include age greater than 65, shock, comorbid

TABLE 36–1 Rockall score.

Variable	Age	Shock	Comorbidity	Diagnosis	Evidence of Bleeding
0 point	< 60	No shock	None		None
1 point	60-79	Pulse > 100 SBP > 100		MWT	
2 points	> 80	SBP < 100	CHF CAD Other	All other diseases	Blood Adherent clot Spurting vessel
3 points			ARF Liver disease Metastatic cancer		

Score < 3 points—good prognosis; score > 8—poor prognosis.
ARF, acure renal failure; CAD, coronary artery disease; CHF, congestive heart failure; MWT, Mallory-Weiss tear; SBP, systolic blood pressure.

Glasgow-blatchford score

Variable	Blood Urea	Hb—Men (g/L)	Hb—Women (g/L)	SBP (mm Hb)	Pulse (Beats/min)	Presentation	Comorbidity
0 point							
1 point		≥ 12, < 13	≥ 10, < 12	100-109	≥ 100	Melena	
2 points	≥ 6.5, < 8			90-99		Syncope	Liver disease CHF
3 points	≥ 8, < 10	≥ 10, < 12		< 90			
4 points	≥ 10, < 25						
5 points							
6 points	≥ 25	< 10	< 10				

illnesses, and clinically significant UGIB as evidenced by hematemesis, hematochezia, or melena; low initial Hb or high transfusion requirements; and hemodynamic instability or syncope. Additionally, sepsis, elevated urea, creatinine, or serum aminotransferase levels have been predictors of poor clinical outcome.[2,3] Two scoring systems commonly used to risk-stratify patients are the Blatchford score and the Rockall score, which can be initially calculated on clinical and laboratory data and updated based on endoscopic findings. Patients considered high risk should undergo upper endoscopy immediately after resuscitation is complete and the patient is clinically stable to undergo a procedure. These patients often require ICU stay, either for monitoring or to facilitate bedside endoscopy. If patients demonstrate evidence of active UGIB, we will often recommend intubation in the ICU for airway protection. Prior to endoscopy, it is often helpful to consider use of a promotility agent such as metoclopramide or erythromycin to facilitate clearance of the stomach and improve endoscopic visualization. Patients should be monitored closely in the interval between presentation and endoscopy with every 6- to 8-hour CBC depending on the clinical presentation.

For nonvariceal UGIB, endoscopic features can also be used to predict risk of rebleeding and mortality. The presence of high-risk stigmata as defined by the Forest classification has been associated with higher rates of rebleeding and mortality. High-risk stigmata include actively bleeding vessel (Forest class IA), oozing blood (IB), and nonbleeding visible vessel (IIA). Adherent clot (IIB) is felt to be moderate risk. Flat pigmented spots (IIC) and clean-based ulcers (III) are low-risk lesions for rebleeding. The complete Rockwell score (see Table 36–1) can be used when clinical criteria and endoscopic criteria are available to determine risk of rebleeding and mortality.

Varices are present in approximately 50% of patients with cirrhosis and their presence correlates with severity of liver disease. Variceal hemorrhage occurs at a rate of 5% to 15% per year; predictors of variceal hemorrhage include size of varices, decompensated cirrhosis (Child-Pugh class B/C), and the endoscopic presence of red wale signs at the time of screening endoscopy (citation). Patients who have variceal bleeding have a median rebleeding rate of

63% within 1 to 2 years and mortality of at least 20% at 6 weeks.[13] Predictors of rebleeding and mortality include Child-Pugh class, Model for End-Stage Liver Disease (MELD) score, renal failure, bacterial infection, hypovolemic shock, active bleeding at endoscopy, hepatocellular carcinoma, and hepatic venous pressure gradients (HPVGs) of greater than 20 mm Hb when measured within 24 hours of variceal bleed. A recent study described a MELD-based model to predict risk of mortality among patients with acute variceal bleeding and was demonstrated to be more accurate than other proposed prediction models.[14]

DIFFERENTIAL DIAGNOSIS

The most common causes of UGIB remain similar over time; a recent study reviewing the most common causes of UGIB at a large urban hospital cited PUD as the diagnosis in 34% of cases followed by variceal bleeding in 33% of cases.[1] Ninety percent of all PUD is caused by either infection with the gram-negative bacterium *Helicobacter pylori* or by the use of NSAIDs. *H pylori* is found in as many as 90% of patients with duodenal ulcers and 70% of patients with gastric ulcers. The bacteria are transmitted via the fecal-oral route and are most commonly acquired in childhood. Most infected individuals are asymptomatic with no clinical consequence; a subset of patients can develop decreased mucosal barriers and increased mucosal susceptibility to gastric acid damage. Patients with persistent infection and chronic inflammatory changes can develop ulcers.

NSAIDs are a widespread and commonly used class of medications. Chronic use with even low-dose aspirin for cardioprotective measures can lead to mucosal changes throughout the GI system with ulcerations in the stomach, duodenum, and even the distal small bowel and colon. NSAIDs result in prostaglandin inhibition with subsequent decreased mucosal barriers and increased mucosal susceptibility to gastric acid injury. In addition, NSAIDs can cause direct mucosal injury resulting in erosions and ulcerations. PUD can also be seen in patients with severe stress, trauma, burns, sepsis, and prolonged ICU stays.

Variceal formation is caused by collateral vessels in the GI tract as a consequence of portal hypertension in patients with chronic liver disease. The most common site of varices is the esophagus though varices can also form in the gastric fundus and cardia. Portal hypertension can cause other gastric changes in the form of portal hypertensive gastropathy, a diffuse mucosal change in the stomach. Variceal bleeding can present as acute-onset severe UGIB with associated hemodynamic compromise. The decrease in portal pressures by bleeding can lead to self-resolution; however, the risk of rebleeding remains high and can be exacerbated by aggressive volume resuscitation, as described earlier.

Other causes of UGIB include vascular malformations such as arteriovenous malformations (AVMs) or Dieulafoy lesions, traumatic lesions such as Mallory-Weiss tears of the esophagus, or malignant lesions such as gastric cancer or esophageal cancer.

FURTHER MANAGEMENT

Endoscopic therapy, in combination with pharmacologic therapy, is the main tool used for diagnosis and treatment of UGIB. Early endoscopy, defined by esophagogastroduodenoscopy (EGD) within the first 24 hours after presentation, to localize the site of bleeding and treat bleeding lesions has been shown to improve outcomes and reduce lengths of hospitalization. Most endoscopic findings can be treated within the same setting to stop active bleeding and reduce risks of rebleeding.

Nonvariceal UGIB

In patients with nonvariceal UGIB, high-risk stigmata, such as actively bleeding vessel, oozing vessel, or nonbleeding visible vessel, should be treated endoscopically. It is unclear whether treatment of adherent clot is beneficial; generally accepted practice is to attempt to gently dislodge the clot and treat the lesion based on appearance underneath. Low-risk lesions, such as pigmented spots or clean-based ulcers, do not require endoscopic treatment.

Endoscopic treatment consists of one or more techniques to attempt to stop active bleeding and prevent rebleeding. Tools available to the endoscopist include injection of epinephrine at a concentration of 1:10,000, thermocoagulation of the lesion with bipolar electrocautery probe, or placement of clips. A recent meta-analysis suggested that injection

therapy is better than no therapy but that combined therapy (injection plus thermocoagulation or injection plus clips) is better than monotherapy with injection alone. Monotherapy with thermocoagulation or clips is equivalent in efficacy to combined modality therapy.[15] Routine second look endoscopy is not recommended and should be considered on a case-by-case basis. Evidence of rebleeding or inability to identify the bleeding lesion on initial endoscopy is generally considered indication for second endoscopy.

Patients with bleeding that cannot be localized on endoscopic evaluation or patients who have ongoing bleeding despite endoscopic therapy should be considered for surgery or for interventional radiology directed angiography and percutaneous embolization.

Patients with low-risk clinical features and low-risk endoscopic features may be discharged home after endoscopy; RCTs of this highly select group of patients suggest no difference in outcomes with a policy of early discharge versus inpatient observation. These patients need to have close outpatient monitoring and follow-up.

All patients should be discharged with oral PPI therapy to decrease risk of rebleeding with dosage and duration determined by etiology of bleeding; most patients are given once-daily PPI therapy for 8 weeks with close outpatient follow-up. Patients with PUD should be evaluated for *H pylori* with treatment of any positive results to minimize risk of recurrent ulcers and facilitate ulcer healing. These patients should have eradication confirmed 2 weeks after completion of their PPI therapy. Patients with NSAID use should discontinue use if possible. Patients who require low-dose ASA for cardiovascular protection should resume therapy when the risk of cardiovascular complications outweighs the risk of rebleeding; this appears to occur as early as 5 days after the onset of bleeding and decisions about timing of ASA resumption should be made with a multidisciplinary approach. Patients who require ASA and clopidogrel who have UGIB should continue on PPI therapy. The role of PPI therapy in combination with ASA and clopidogrel was evaluated in a RCT (COGENT trial), which examined the risk of adverse GI events and adverse cardiovascular events in patients taking ASA and clopidogrel randomized to PPI use or placebo. This study found a statistically significant reduction in adverse GI events in patients taking once-daily omeprazole with no difference in cardiovascular events between the 2 groups.[16] This study supports the benefit of PPI use in prevention of primary GI events. The benefit of PPI in preventing rebleeding is also likely to outweigh the hypothesized increase in risk of cardiovascular events attributable to the interaction between PPI therapy and clopidogrel. Recent guidelines on antiplatelet therapy management have been changed to reflect this consensus.

Variceal UGIB

Early endoscopy and endoscopic intervention has also been shown to improve outcomes in patients with variceal bleed. Variceal bleeding is identified when active bleeding is seen from a varix, when a "white nipple" is seen overlying the varix, when clots are seen overlying a varix, or when varices are seen with no other source of UGIB identified. Varices are described as number of columns and are graded into categories of small or large based on their appearance. Endoscopic interventions available for the treatment of variceal bleeding includes endoscopic variceal ligation (EVL) with the use of rubber bands placed at the base of the varix or use of sclerotherapy with injection of agents such as N-butyl-cyanoacrylate or isobutyl-2-cyanoacrylate. Endoscopic therapy in conjunction with pharmacologic therapy is the treatment of choice for bleeding varices; in general, endoscopic treatment with EVL is the preferred form of treatment by consensus. Sclerotherapy is recommended if EVL is not technically feasible.

Patients who fail endoscopic therapy or patients in whom early rebleeding occurs should be evaluated for shunt therapy, either through transjugular intrahepatic portosystemic shunt (TIPS) placement or through surgical shunt placement. One recent study demonstrated survival benefit with early TIPS placement (within 24 hours of bleeding) in patients with acute variceal bleeding and HVPG greater than 20 mm Hb.[17] Patients who undergo shunt placement experience higher rates of hepatic encephalopathy; thus, while TIPS is felt to be equally effective in treatment of variceal bleeding with no difference in overall survival, it is recommended as a rescue therapy

in patients who have failed EVL and pharmacologic therapy because of this significant side effect. Balloon tamponade via placement of a Blakemore or Minnesota tube may be used to temporarily control bleeding prior to definitive therapy in patients with acute variceal bleeding; this is generally only recommended in patients with massive variceal bleeding as part of temporizing measures until definitive therapy with endoscopy or TIPS is available.

Patients who survive an episode of acute variceal hemorrhage are at high risk of rebleeding and death. Thus it is important that patients be treated to minimize risk of recurrence. Patients who undergo EVL should be started on a nonselective betablocker as soon as they have remained 24 hours without evidence of rebleeding to reduce portal pressures. Patients who have EVL are recommended to undergo repeat EGD at 7- to 14-day intervals until complete obliteration of varices is seen, usually requiring between 2 and 4 sessions. Combination of endoscopic therapy plus pharmacologic therapy with nonselective beta-blocker has been shown to be more effective than EVL alone with decreased rebleeding rates in 2 RCTs. Patients who undergo TIPS for treatment of variceal bleeding do not require any further therapy. All patients with clinically significant variceal bleeding should be referred for liver transplant evaluation if they are appropriate candidates.[18]

CONCLUSIONS

UGIB should be confirmed quickly by clinical examination with identification of melena or evidence of hematemesis or evidence of positive NG lavage. The patient's hemodynamic status should be assessed and resuscitation initiated rapidly to correct abnormalities. Empiric therapy with intravenous PPI and/or intravenous octreotide can help to reduce active bleeding and/or stabilize clot. Early endoscopic evaluation and therapy of high-risk lesions improve outcomes and reduces length of hospital stay. Patients should be managed endoscopically if high-risk lesions are identified. Patients should be monitored after intervention for rebleeding with continued adjuvant pharmacologic therapy (PPI, octreotide, nonselective beta-blockers, antibiotics) as indicated to decrease rates of rebleeding and mortality.

Lower GI Bleeding

INTRODUCTION

LGIB is defined as bleeding from a lesion distal to the ligament of Treitz. The most common site of LGIB is the colon; bleeding from the small intestine is much less common. LGIB generally presents clinically as hematochezia or bright red blood from the rectum. LGIB can present in an acute manner or a subacute manner and is managed with many of the same principles used to manage UGIB.

HISTORY

As described, most patients with LGIB will describe the presentation of hematochezia that occurs acutely or subacutely. Hematochezia can present as large quantity or small quantity, can be described in isolation or to be mixed in with brown stool. Patients may have associated symptoms that can help narrow the differential diagnosis such as symptoms of diarrhea, abdominal pain, or tenesmus. Eliciting past medical history and medication use is as important in LGIB as it is in UGIB and may help to narrow the differential diagnosis. Understanding and managing comorbid conditions are similar to that in patients with UGIB and patients should be evaluated for the presence of underlying cardiac or pulmonary diseases.

PHYSICAL EXAMINATION AND INITIAL MANAGEMENT

Similar to UGIB, patients' initial evaluation includes evaluation of vital signs and clinical status. This involves evaluation of heart rate, blood pressure, and orthostatic measurements. Assessing the volume status and proceeding with resuscitation are similar as in patients with UGIB. Patients should have 2 large-bore IVs placed, followed by infusion of crystalloid, colloids, and blood to correct the volume status. Patients with severe volume loss and clinical consequences should be admitted to the ICU for closer monitoring and management. Patients with clinically significant hematochezia should be evaluated for the possibility of UGIB; approximately 10% of patients with UGIB will present with hematochezia. These patients should be evaluated with NG lavage for risk stratification and may require EGD prior to any additional workup to rule out UGIB causes.

Patients who are clinically stable can be further evaluated based on clinical presentation. As with UGIB, checking serum Hb further differentiates the clinical impact of bleeding. Restrictive transfusion strategies are recommended in patients with low or intermediate risk. Additional laboratory studies such as lactic acid may assist in narrowing the differential diagnosis.

DIFFERENTIAL DIAGNOSIS

The differential diagnosis of overt LGIB is broad. Diverticular bleeding is the most common cause of LGIB and accounts for 40% of all LGIB.[19] Diverticulosis increases with age and the overall prevalence is estimated to be 30% to 50% with as many as 60% of people over 80 years being affected. The incidence of bleeding is estimated to be 5% to 50% in patients with diverticulosis. The clinical presentation of diverticular bleeding is generally consistent with arterial bleeding. Patients may have acute onset of painless hematochezia that ceases spontaneously in most cases with recurrent bleeding in 14% to 38% of cases. Diverticular bleeding can come from either the left colon or the right colon and localization of the site of bleeding can often be challenging. Because most cases resolve spontaneously without rebleeding, diagnosis is often made after exclusion of other potential cases of bleeding.

Ischemic colitis accounts for 1% to 19% of LGIB. This results from sudden loss of blood flow to the mesenteric vessels and most commonly affects the areas of the colon described as "watershed" areas: the splenic flexure and the rectosigmoid junction. Ischemic colitis may occur as a result of an embolic or a thrombotic event or because of transient hypoperfusion or vasospasm of the mesenteric vessels. Patients generally describe sudden onset of abdominal pain accompanied by hematochezia and may have advanced age, or significant cardiovascular disease. Ischemic colitis is diagnosed by a classic appearance of segmental inflamed mucosa on colonoscopy and is generally treated with supportive measures and reversal of the underlying etiology.

Other lesions that can less commonly lead to LGIB include AVMs or Dieulafoy lesions. AVMs are ectatic blood vessels that can be located anywhere in the GI tract but are predominantly found in the cecum and ascending colon. They account for approximately 11% of LGIBs. They may appear as isolated lesions or in clusters of multiple small, flat, red telangiectasias. Dieulafoy lesions are arterial blood vessels that appear close to the mucosal surface that intermittently bleed. Identifying these vascular lesions can be challenging.

Finally, hemorrhoidal bleeding represents 5% to 10% of acute LGIB. Hematochezia tends to be low volume with little to no clinical significance. Episodes can be isolated or sporadic and often is described by the appearance of blood on the toilet paper or on the outside of stool.

Other causes of LGIB represent a wide variety of possible diagnoses including hemorrhagic infectious diarrhea, colitis from infection, inflammatory bowel disease or radiation change, and malignancy, among others.

DIAGNOSTIC STUDIES AND MANAGEMENT

Similar to UGIB, the gold standard for evaluation of LGIB is endoscopic assessment via colonoscopy, though several other diagnostic tools are available. Patients who present with hematochezia hemodynamic compromise should be evaluated for the possibility of UGIB source. These patients should have NG tube placement with NG lavage to assist in localizing the source of bleeding. Patients with clinical evidence of rapid/ongoing GI blood loss should undergo emergent EGD to rule out UGI etiologies (Figure 36–2).

Patients with hemodynamic stability and hematochezia should be evaluated first by colonoscopy. The patient should be prepared by using a polyethylene glycol-based solution to cleanse the colon prior to procedure. This can be consumed by having the patient drink the preparation or by administering it through the NG tube. Preparation prior to colonoscopy is essential to facilitate visualization, increase the diagnostic yield of the procedure, and minimize the risk of complication such as perforation. The diagnostic yield of colonoscopy varies widely; patients with diverticular bleeding often have low yield at localization of the bleeding site. Alternate etiologies such as ischemic colitis, vascular lesions, infectious/inflammatory colitis, or malignancy can be diagnosed by colonoscopy. Identification of bleeding diverticula or vascular lesions can be treated endoscopically using the same modalities as

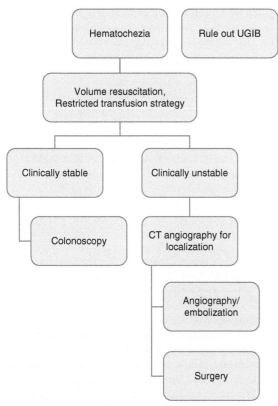

FIGURE 36–2 Management of LGIB.

previously described such as a combination of injection therapy, thermocoagulation, or clip placement.

Patients with nonlocalization of bleeding site and high clinical suspicion for diverticular bleeding can be managed conservatively with close follow-up to assess for ongoing bleeding. If massive bleeding is present, clinical compromise is noted, or ongoing bleeding is suspected, patients may benefit from evaluation by one of several radiologic tests such as CT angiogram, standard angiography, or tagged red blood cell scanning.

The widespread availability of CT angiography has made this a common first test to localize bleeding site. Several studies have demonstrated the high accuracy of CT angiography in identifying and localizing active bleeding either through identification of active extravasation of blood or to localization of intraluminal contents consistent with recent bleeding. The advantage of CT angiography is largely in the ability to perform this evaluation

quickly. If localization is successful, patients are able to undergo subsequent management either through IR-directed percutaneous embolization or through surgical resection. IR-directed embolization is highly effective at treating LGIB and often is used with priority over colonoscopy or surgery in patients who have clinically significant GI bleeding. Tagged red blood cell scans are also able to aid in localization of LGIB but are less in favor than CT angiogram because of the time required to perform the evaluation and its inability to localize the precise source of bleeding/lack of structural imaging.

The determination of which localization modality is optimal in LGIB remains an ongoing discussion and should be handled with a multidisciplinary approach between gastroenterologists, radiologists, and surgeons taking into account the clinical stability of the patient and the time required to prepare for colonoscopy.

CONCLUSIONS

LGIB follows similar principles for management as UGIB; evaluation begins with confirmation of hematochezia and evaluation for a possible UGIB. Evaluating blood loss and resuscitation is the first step in management. Patients who are clinically stable are recommended to undergo preparation followed by colonoscopy for localization and possible treatment of bleeding lesions; patients with hemodynamic instability or ongoing GI blood loss are recommended to undergo CT angiogram for localization of bleeding site followed by conventional angiography and embolization of bleeding vessel or surgery for definitive treatment.

REFERENCES

1. Kim JJ, Sheibani S, Park S, Buxbaum J, Laine L. Causes of bleeding and outcomes in patients hospitalized with upper gastrointestinal bleeding. *J Clin Gastroenterol.* 2014;48(2):113-118.
2. Greenspoon J, Barkun A, Bardou M, et al. Management of patients with nonvariceal upper gastrointestinal bleeding. *Clin Gastroenterol Hepatol.* 2012;10(3):234-239.
3. Barkun AN, Bardou M, Kuipers EJ, et al. International consensus recommendations on

the management of patients with nonvariceal upper gastrointestinal bleeding. *Ann Intern Med.* 2010;152(2):101-113.

4. Lanas A, Wu P, Medin J, Mills EJ. Low doses of acetylsalicylic acid increase risk of gastrointestinal bleeding in a meta-analysis. *Clin Gastroenterol Hepatol.* 2011;9(9):762-768.e6.

5. Holster IL, Valkhoff VE, Kuipers EJ, Tjwa ET. New oral anticoagulants increase risk for gastrointestinal bleeding: a systematic review and meta-analysis. *Gastroenterology.* 2013;145(1):105-112.e15.

6. Villanueva C, Colomo A, Bosch A, et al. Transfusion strategies for acute upper gastrointestinal bleeding. *N Engl J Med.* 2013;368(1):11-21.

7. Wolf AT, Wasan SK, Saltzman JR. Impact of anticoagulation on rebleeding following endoscopic therapy for nonvariceal upper gastrointestinal hemorrhage. *Am J Gastroenterol.* 2007;102(2):290-296.

8. Lau JY, Leung WK, Wu JC, et al. Omeprazole before endoscopy in patients with gastrointestinal bleeding. *N Engl J Med.* 2007;356(16):1631-1640.

9. Green FW Jr, Kaplan MM, Curtis LE, Levine PH. Effect of acid and pepsin on blood coagulation and platelet aggregation. A possible contributor prolonged gastroduodenal mucosal hemorrhage. *Gastroenterology.* 1978;74(1):38-43.

10. Banares R, et al. Endoscopic treatment versus endoscopic plus pharmacologic treatment for acute variceal bleeding: a meta-analysis. *Hepatology.* 2002;35(3):609-615.

11. Seo YS, Park SY, Kim MY, et al. Lack of difference among terlipressin, somatostatin, and octreotide in the control of acute gastroesophageal variceal hemorrhage. *Hepatology.* 2014;60(3):954-963.

12. Garcia-Tsao G, Sanyal AJ, Grace ND, et al. Prevention and management of gastroesophageal varices and variceal hemorrhage in cirrhosis. *Hepatology.* 2007;46(3):922-938.

13. Puente A, Hernandez-Gea V, Graupera I, et al. Drugs plus ligation to prevent rebleeding in cirrhosis: an updated systemic review. *Liver Int.* 2014 Jul;34(6):823-833.

14. Reverter E, Tandon P, Augustin S, et al. A MELD-based model to determine risk of mortality among patients with acute variceal bleeding. *Gastroenterology.* 2014;146(2):412-419.e3.

15. Laine L, McQuaid KR. Endoscopic therapy for bleeding ulcers: an evidence-based approach based on meta-analyses of randomized controlled trials. *Clin Gastroenterol Hepatol.* 2009;7(1):33-47; quiz 1-2.

16. Bhatt DL, Cryer BL, Contant CF, et al. Clopidogrel with or without omeprazole in coronary artery disease. *N Engl J Med.* 2010;363(20):1909-1917.

17. Monescillo A, Martínez-Lagares F, Ruiz-del-Arbol L, et al. Influence of portal hypertension and its early decompression by TIPS placement on the outcome of variceal bleeding. *Hepatology.* 2004;40(4):793-801.

18. Garcia-Tsao G, Sanyal AJ, Grace ND, et al. Prevention and management of gastroesophageal varices and variceal hemorrhage in cirrhosis. *Hepatology.* 2007;46(3):922-938.

19. Davila RE, Rajan E, Adler DG, et al. ASGE guideline: the role of endoscopy in the patient with lower-GI bleeding. *Gastrointest Endosc.* 2005;62(5):656-660.

Liver Failure:
Acute and Chronic

Brian Kim, MD and Leona Kim-Schluger, MD

KEY POINTS

1 Acute liver failure (ALF) is defined as the rapid and severe development of liver dysfunction, marked by encephalopathy and coagulopathy in an individual without a prior history of cirrhosis or liver disease.

2 Acetaminophen is the most common cause of ALF in the United States, and prompt administration of N-acetylcysteine helps to decrease mortality in acetaminophen hepatotoxicity. N-acetylcysteine may also have some benefit in nonacetaminophen hepatotoxicity.

3 Supportive care remains the mainstay of ALF management. Spontaneous survival rate from ALF is 40% and liver transplantation (LT) remains the only definitive therapy for patients who are unable to achieve timely regeneration of liver mass to maintain life despite adequate supportive care.

4 Cirrhosis is characterized by progressive hepatic fibrosis that can lead to consequences of portal hypertension including variceal hemorrhage, ascites, renal failure, and encephalopathy.

5 The combination of pharmacologic therapy and endoscopic variceal ligation is effective in controlling bleeding in up to 90% of patients presenting with acute variceal hemorrhage.

6 Hepatic encephalopathy is a frequent reason for hospital admissions. Common precipitants, such as infection, dehydration, and bleeding, should be ruled out in any patient presenting with hepatic encephalopathy.

INTRODUCTION

Liver disease results in approximately 35,000 deaths each year, making it the 12th leading cause of death in the United States.[1] Patients suffering from ALF or consequences of chronic liver disease are among the sickest in the hospital. These patients often develop problems that require critical care, and physicians should be knowledgeable about the various complications of liver disease that can be encountered in the intensive care unit (ICU).

Acute Liver Failure

General Considerations

There are an estimated 2000 cases of acute liver failure (ALF) annually, which accounts for 0.1% of all deaths in the United States. Approximately 6% to 7% of all LTs performed in the United States are secondary to ALF.[2,3]

ALF is defined as the rapid and severe development of liver dysfunction, marked by encephalopathy and coagulopathy with an elevated prothrombin time (PT) or international normalized ratio (INR), in an individual without a prior history of cirrhosis or liver disease. The exceptions to this definition are in patients who have had previously undiagnosed hepatitis B virus (HBV) infection, hepatitis D virus (HDV) infection with underlying chronic HBV infection, autoimmune hepatitis, or Wilson disease. In these patients, underlying cirrhosis may be present, provided the disease has been recognized for less than 26 weeks.

ALF can be subcategorized by the interval between the development of jaundice and onset of encephalopathy. Common classification cutoffs are: hyperacute (< 7 days), acute (8-28 days), and subacute (28 days-26 weeks). This classification can be clinically useful as cerebral edema is common in hyperacute and acute liver failure whereas complications of portal hypertension are more commonly seen in subacute liver failure.

In the United States, drug-induced hepatitis, especially acetaminophen overdose is the most common cause of ALF in adults. Other causes of ALF are listed in Table 37–1.

Clinical Features

Signs and Symptoms—The symptoms of ALF may vary depending on the severity and etiology. In the case of acetaminophen toxicity, patients may present with rapid onset of abdominal pain, nausea, vomiting, and confusion, several hours after ingestion of acetaminophen. The presentation of ALF due to other etiologies can be more insidious. Patients may present with nonspecific symptoms such as malaise, fatigue, or subtle changes in personality and behavior. New-onset ascites, pruritus, or asymptomatic jaundice can also be seen.

Encephalopathy is a prerequisite to the diagnosis of ALF, and the degree of encephalopathy may be variable from mild to severe (Table 37–2).

Patients with encephalopathy grade I may have mild asterixis whereas patients with grades II, III, or IV may have overt asterixis or clonus on physical examination. The development of encephalopathy grade III and IV usually heralds the development of cerebral edema and increased intracranial pressure (ICP).

Laboratory Findings—Laboratory testing will reveal a prolonged PT and increased INR greater than 1.5, not correctable by the administration of intravenous (IV) or subcutaneous (SC) vitamin

TABLE 37–1 Causes of acute liver failure.

Drug toxicity
- Acetaminophen
- *Amanita* poisoning
- Carbon tetrachloride
- Antimicrobials (eg, ampicillin-clavulanate, isoniazid, ciprofloxacin, erythromycin, tetracycline)
- Valproate
- Halothane
- Troglitazone
- Reye syndrome (salicylic acid)
- Herbal medications (eg, ginseng, pennyroyal oil)

Other toxins
- *Amanita* poisoning
- Ecstasy (methylenedioxymethamphetamine)
- Organic solvents

Acute viral hepatitis
- Hepatitis A virus
- Hepatitis B virus +/– hepatitis D virus
- Hepatitis C virus
- Hepatitis E virus
- Cytomegalovirus in immunocompromised patients
- Herpes simplex virus in immunocompromised patients

Miscellaneous causes
- Wilson disease
- Budd-Chiari syndrome
- Sinusoidal obstruction syndrome
- Ischemic (shock) liver
- Autoimmune hepatitis
- Acute fatty liver of pregnancy
- HELLP syndrome (hemolysis, elevated liver function tests, low platelets)
- Malignant infiltration of the liver
- Indeterminate

K. Bilirubin and aminotransferase levels are often elevated. Elevated serum creatinine (Cr) and blood urea nitrogen (BUN) levels can be seen with

TABLE 37–2 Grades of hepatic encephalopathy.[4]

I	Changes in behavior minimal change in level of consciousness
II	Gross disorientation, drowsiness, possibly asterixis, inappropriate behavior
III	Marked confusion, incoherent speech, sleeping most of the time but arousable to vocal stimuli
IV	Comatose, unresponsive to pain, decorticate or decerebrate posturing

Reproduced with permission from Conn HO, Leevy CM, Vlahcevic ZR, et al: Comparison of lactulose and neomycin in the treatment of chronic portal-systemic encephalopathy. A double blind controlled trial, Gastroenterology. 1977 Apr;72(4 Pt 1):573-583.

TABLE 37–3 Predictors of poor outcome in patients with acute liver failure (King's College Criteria).[7]

Acetaminophen-induced acute liver failure
- Arterial pH < 7.30 (irrespective of grade of encephalopathy) *or*
- A combination of encephalopathy grade III or IV, PT > 100 s (INR > 6.5), and serum Cr > 3.4 mg/dL

Nonacetaminophen-induced acute liver failure
- PT > 100 s (INR > 6.5) (irrespective of grade of encephalopathy) *or*
- Any 3 of the following (irrespective of grade of encephalopathy):
  - Age < 10 or > 40
  - Unfavorable etiology such as non-HAV, non-HBV, idiosyncratic drug reaction, or Wilson disease
  - Duration of jaundice before onset of encephalopathy > 7 d
  - PT > 50 s (INR > 3.5)
  - Serum bilirubin level > 17.5 mg/dL

Cr, creatinine; HAV, hepatitis A virus; HBV, hepatitis B virus; INR, international normalized ratio; PT, prothrombin time.
Adapted with permission from O'Grady JG, Alexander GJ, Hayllar KM, et al: Early indicators of prognosis in fulminant hepatic failure, Gastroenterology. 1989 Aug;97(2):439-445.

concurrent acute kidney injury (AKI). AKI occurs in up to 80% of patients with ALF and can occur secondary to hypovolemia, sepsis, or acute tubular necrosis (ATN).[5] ATN can occur as a result of severe hypotension or, in the case of acetaminophen ingestion, as a result of direct tubular toxicity.[6] Acidosis is common in ALF as a result of the body's inability to clear lactic acid in the setting of severe hepatic necrosis and concurrent AKI. The severity of laboratory abnormalities and encephalopathy can be used to help predict patient outcomes (Table 37–3).

Treatment

ALF is a medical emergency with high rates of multisystem organ failure and high mortality without appropriate management. Only 40% of patients diagnosed with ALF have spontaneous recovery.[8] Thus, all patients presenting with ALF should be managed in a center with an active liver transplant program.

Patients with grade I encephalopathy can be managed with care in a general medical ward, provided that they undergo frequent neurologic checks (every 2 hours) to identify signs of progression to higher grades of encephalopathy. Grade II encephalopathy and higher should be managed in the ICU.

Specific etiologies of ALF may have specific management options that can help avoid LT and decrease mortality (Table 37–4). Of special note, N-acetylcysteine, which is the antidote of choice for acetaminophen toxicity, may also be of benefit in other forms of ALF. The administration of NAC has been shown to increase transplant-free survival in patients with grade I and II encephalopathy, presenting with nonacetaminophen ALF.[9]

Regardless of the etiology, supportive measures remain essential in the management of ALF patients.
Supportive Measures
Cerebral Edema and Intracranial Hypertension— Cerebral edema leading to intracranial hypertension remains the major cause of mortality in patients presenting with ALF. The pathogenesis of cerebral edema is not clearly understood in ALF and likely is secondary to multiple factors including the breakdown of the blood-brain barrier, neurotoxin release, and resultant osmotic disturbances. The predictors

TABLE 37–4 Specific etiologies of acute liver failure and potential treatments.

Acetaminophen toxicity	N-acetylcysteine
Mushroom toxicity (*Amanita phalloides*)	Penicillin G or silymarin
Valproate	Carnitine
Hepatitis B virus +/– hepatitis D virus	Antiviral nucleo(s)tide (eg, entecavir, tenofovir, lamivudine, adefovir, telbivudine)
Herpes simplex virus	Acyclovir
Budd-Chiari syndrome	Transjugular intrahepatic portosystemic shunt placement, surgical shunt placement, or thrombolysis
Autoimmune hepatitis	Prednisone
Wilson disease	Usually will require liver transplantation but plasma exchange can be a temporizing measure
Acute fatty liver of pregnancy	Expedited delivery of the fetus

of cerebral edema include high-grade encephalopathy (grade III/IV) and increased arterial ammonia concentration (> 200 µmol/L).[10,11]

Simple interventions may be beneficial to reduce intracranial hypertension in patients with grade III/IV encephalopathy. Tracheal intubation with sedation, elevation of the head to 30°, minimization of painful stimuli, and control of arterial hypertension should be initiated universally. A quiet environment should be maintained to reduce external stimuli, and premedication should be given prior to tracheal suctioning or patient positioning to minimize changes in ICP.

The use of ICP monitoring devices in ALF is controversial, and its use is largely dependent on local practices. The decision to place an ICP monitoring device should be made after discussion with the ICU, transplant hepatology, and neurosurgery teams.

If the patient does develop increased ICP as evident by direct ICP monitoring or neurologic examination (pupillary abnormality or decerebrate posturing), further measures to reduce ICP should be initiated. The goal of therapy is to reduce the ICP to below 20 to 25 mm Hg while maintaining cerebral perfusion pressure (CPP) above 50 to 60 mm Hg.

Mannitol causes osmotic diuresis and has been shown to decrease ICP. Its use has been associated with improved survival in ALF.[12,13] Patients can be given bolus doses of mannitol to decrease ICP, provided that serum osmolality does not exceed 320 mOsm/L. The use of mannitol is limited in the setting of volume overload and renal failure. Hypertonic sodium chloride (30% normal salaine [NS]) can also be considered to maintain serum (Na) levels of 145 to 155, to prevent a rise in ICP.[14]

Hyperventilation to reduce $Paco_2$ quickly lowers ICP via vasoconstriction and decrease in cerebral blood flow. However, this effect is short lived and does not adequately lower ICP long term.[15]

Seizure—Seizure activity in patients with ALF is common but difficult to detect in intubated and sedated patients. Seizures should be treated promptly as seizure activity can acutely increase ICP and cause cerebral edema.[16]

Infection—Infection is a major contributor to mortality in patients presenting with ALF. All patients with ALF are at increased risk for bacterial and fungal infections. Common sites of infection include the respiratory tract, urinary tract, and blood. Routine surveillance cultures should be obtained from the sputum, urine, and blood along with chest radiograph to detect infections early, as severe sepsis increases mortality as well as precludes potential LT. Prophylactic antibiotic use is controversial but can be considered in patients with severe encephalopathy. Empiric antibacterial and antifungal antibiotics should be started if patients present with worsening hypotension or renal failure, as early signs of infection.

Coagulopathy—Coagulopathy, marked by prolonged PT and INR, is universal in patients presenting with ALF. PT/INR is one of the predictors of outcomes in ALF (see Table 37–3), and thus, empiric correction of PT/INR with fresh frozen plasma (FFP) should be held unless patients have signs of overt bleeding or are in need of an invasive procedure. If a patient has signs of overt bleeding or is in need of an invasive procedure, such as ICP monitoring device placement, FFP and/or recombinant human factor VIIa can be used to help reverse the coagulopathy. However an increasing body of data suggests that routine correction of PT/INR is not necessary prior to percutaneous vascular access procedures, paracentesis, and other nonneurosurgical procedures in patients with liver disease.

Renal Failure—AKI can be seen in 55% to 80% of patients presenting with ALF.[5,17] Maintenance of euvolemia is critical and determination of preload responsiveness via echocardiography should be considered to manage volume status. Nephrotoxic drugs such as aminoglycosides should be avoided and renal replacement therapy (RRT) may need to be initiated in setting of worsening renal function. If patient requires RRT, continuous rather than intermittent RRT is recommended to avoid large fluid shifts that may impact ICP.

Cardiovascular Support—ALF is characterized by high cardiac output with low systemic vascular resistance secondary to decreased clearance of vasoactive metabolites. Vasopressor drugs may be required to maintain adequate systemic mean arterial pressure (MAP) and CPP.

Respiratory Failure—Acute respiratory distress syndrome (ARDS) occurs in one-third of patients presenting with ALF and can cause significant hypoxemia that requires low tidal volume and high positive end-expiratory pressure (PEEP) to achieve adequate tissue oxygenation.[10] The lowest possible PEEP should be used as high PEEP ventilation can exacerbate cerebral edema and hepatic congestion. *Nutrition*—Hypoglycemia is common in ALF due to severe hepatic necrosis that impairs glycogenolysis and gluconeogenesis. Frequent serum glucose monitoring should be instituted, and profound hypoglycemia should be managed with continuous glucose infusion. Hyperglycemia should be avoided as it may contribute to poor ICP control.

Owing to the catabolic state of ALF, enteral nutrition should be initiated as early as possible. **Liver Transplantation**—Liver transplantation remains the only definitive therapy for patients who are unable to achieve timely regeneration of liver mass to maintain life. Spontaneous survival rate from ALF is 40%, as compared to posttransplantation survival rate of greater than 80%.[8] Although imperfect, the King's College Criteria is most often used to help triage those that may benefit from LT (see Table 37–3).

Early involvement of a multidisciplinary LT team is essential to determine if a patient is a suitable organ recipient, medically, psychologically, and socially. Timely evaluation for LT is essential; as high as 37% of patients die despite being listed for LT due to the shortage of available organs.[18]

Chronic Liver Failure

General Considerations

Cirrhosis is characterized by progressive hepatic fibrosis and represents the final, common pathway of a variety of chronic liver diseases (Table 37–5). With progressive injury to the liver, patients with cirrhosis can have consequences of liver dysfunction, such as jaundice, coagulopathy, and hypoalbuminemia. Scarring and architectural distortion of the liver lead to portal hypertension with resultant ascites, variceal formation, hepatic encephalopathy (HE), thrombocytopenia, and renal failure. These consequences of cirrhosis lead to increased morbidity and mortality, especially in patients with high Model for End-Stage Liver Disease (MELD) scores. Liver transplantation remains the only definitive treatment for complications from cirrhosis.

TABLE 37–5 Causes of liver fibrosis and cirrhosis.

Drug and toxins
• Alcohol
• Methotrexate
• Amiodarone
• Vitamin A
Viral hepatitis
• Hepatitis B virus +/– hepatitis D virus
• Hepatitis C virus
Metabolic/genetic disease
• Hemochromatosis
• Wilson disease
• α_1-Antitrypsin deficiency
• Nonalcoholic steatohepatitis
• Congenital biliary cysts
• Biliary atresia
• Cystic fibrosis
Autoimmune disease
• Autoimmune hepatitis
• Primary biliary cirrhosis
• Primary sclerosing cholangitis
Vascular abnormalities
• Budd-Chiari
• Right-sided heart failure
• Sinusoidal obstruction syndrome
• Hereditary hemorrhagic telangiectasia
Miscellaneous causes
• Granulomatous liver disease
• Idiopathic portal fibrosis

Acute Gastrointestinal Bleeding From Esophageal Varices

General Considerations

Gastroesophageal varices form as a result of increased portal pressures and occur in about 50% of patients with cirrhosis. Usually, the hepatic venous pressure gradient (HVPG) must be at least 12 mm Hg for varices to form.[19] Hemorrhage from varices occurs at a yearly rate of 6% to 76%, depending on the size of the varices and the severity of the underlying liver disease.[20] The mortality of patients presenting with variceal hemorrhage approaches 20%.[21] Early identification of gastroesophageal varices is important as prophylaxis with beta-blockade or endoscopic variceal ligation (EVL) decreases the risk of variceal hemorrhage.

Clinical Features

Signs and Symptoms—Patients with hemorrhage from gastroesophageal varices present with hematemesis or melena. Patients often present with hemodynamic instability marked by tachycardia and hypotension.

Laboratory Findings—Anemia occurs frequently, but a decrease in hemoglobin level may not be detected early in the course of hemorrhage.

Differential Diagnosis

Similar clinical presentation can be seen in other etiologies of upper gastrointestinal hemorrhage such as from peptic ulcer diseases, Mallory-Weiss tears, and Dieulafoy lesions.

Treatment

Patients with suspected acute variceal hemorrhage should be managed in an ICU. The need for airway protection with tracheal intubation should be assessed early. Adequate peripheral venous access should be obtained and volume resuscitation started to maintain hemodynamic stability. Transfusions with FFP and platelets should be considered in patients with severe coagulopathy and thrombocytopenia.

However, red blood cell transfusion should be used cautiously in patients with suspected variceal hemorrhage. Overtransfusion may propagate bleeding due to increased portal pressures. Prospective, randomized data suggest that restricting red blood cell transfusions improves outcomes in acute variceal hemorrhage. A restrictive transfusion strategy (transfusion when hemoglobin falls below 7 g/dL) compared to a liberal transfusion strategy (transfusion when hemoglobin falls below 9 g/dL) resulted in lower rates of death, rebleeding, and adverse events.[22] Of note, the study excluded patients presenting with massive exsanguination. In these patients, it may be prudent to initiate volume resuscitation and transfuse blood products to help maintain hemodynamic stability prior to obtaining hemoglobin levels.

Pharmacologic Therapy

Vasoactive Drugs—Vasoactive drugs should be started as soon as a variceal hemorrhage is suspected. These drugs can temporize bleeding prior to more definitive treatment modalities.

The somatostatin analog, octreotide, causes splanchnic vasoconstriction and is a safe pharmacologic therapy to decrease portal pressures. It is given as a bolus infusion of 50 µg IV followed by a continuous infusion at 25 to 50 µg/h. Meta-analysis suggests improved outcomes with the use of octreotide as compared to placebo when paired with EVL.[23]

Despite routine outpatient use to reduce portal pressures, beta-blockers should not be used during acute hemorrhage as it decreases systemic blood pressure and blunts physiologic increase in heart rate associated with acute hemorrhage.

Antibiotic Prophylaxis—Cirrhotic patients with upper gastrointestinal bleeding have high rates of developing severe bacterial infections including spontaneous bacterial peritonitis (SBP), urinary tract infection, and bacteremia. Trials have shown that short-term antibiotic prophylaxis given at presentation and continued for 7 days improves infection rates as well as survival after variceal hemorrhage.[24] Oral norfloxacin 400 mg twice daily or IV ceftriaxone 1 g once daily can be used.

Endoscopic Treatment—For suspected variceal hemorrhage, early endoscopy (< 12 hours after presentation) is recommended. For esophageal variceal hemorrhage, EVL should be used to control bleeding. When combined with pharmacologic therapy, EVL is effective in controlling bleeding in up to 90% of patients.[25]

Gastric type varices are seen in about 20% of patients with portal hypertension.[26] Active gastric variceal hemorrhage has a poor response to EVL and sclerotherapy. Endoscopic variceal obturation with tissue adhesive such as N-butyl-cyanoacrylate, isobutyl-2-cyanoacrylate, or thrombin is more effective, controlling bleeding in 90% of patients.[27] However, variceal obturation is not routinely practiced, and its use may be limited by local expertise.

In those with early rebleeding, repeat attempt at endoscopic intervention can be considered. If hemorrhage cannot be controlled, balloon tamponade can be used as a temporizing measure to control bleeding in 80% of patients.[28]

Shunt Procedures—The placement of a transjugular intrahepatic portosystemic shunt (TIPS) is an effective way to decrease portal pressures and is now widely used as an option to control refractory bleeding from esophageal and gastric type varices. A reduction in HVPG to below 12 mm Hg or a reduction in HVPG greater than 20% from baseline appears to effectively eliminate the risk of rebleeding.[29,30] Caution should be taken in patients with heart failure, pulmonary hypertension, and intrinsic renal failure as the extra shunting of blood volume into the systemic circulation may not be handled appropriately in these patients. By increasing shunting from the portal vasculature to the systemic vasculature, TIPS placement may also worsen symptoms of HE. Elective TIPS procedure in a patient with a high MELD score (> 18) is relatively contraindicated as it may precipitate worsening liver dysfunction.[31] The presence of hepatocellular carcinoma (HCC) is also a relative contraindication to TIPS placement as it may promote vascular seeding.

Surgical shunt procedures such as portacaval, mesocaval, and splenorenal shunt procedures have been used successfully to control refractory bleeding but have now fallen out of favor given the effectiveness of the TIPS procedure.

Balloon-Occluded Retrograde Transvenous Obliteration—Balloon-occluded retrograde transvenous obliteration (BRTO) is a technique that is widely used in Asia to treat gastric varices. BRTO is a fluoroscopically guided transcatheter procedure used to introduce sclerosants into gastric varices. It relies on the presence of a gastrorenal or gastrocaval shunt to access the varices. If the appropriate shunt is identified on cross-sectional imaging, BRTO can be considered to treat gastric varices in select centers with local expertise.[32] BRTO has been shown to control bleeding in up to 88% of patients with active gastric variceal bleeding.[33]

Ascites

General Considerations

Ascites is the pathologic accumulation of fluid in the peritoneal space, and cirrhosis accounts for 85% of cases.[34] Ascites is one of the most common complications of cirrhosis, developing in 58% of patients within 10 years of the diagnosis of cirrhosis.[35] Patients who develop ascites have a 1-year mortality of 15% and 5-year mortality of 44%.[36]

Clinical Features

Symptoms and Signs—Patients presenting with large-volume ascites complain of increased abdominal girth and discomfort. Nausea, early satiety, and anorexia are common symptoms. Clinical examination can reveal a distended abdomen with shifting dullness and the presence of fluid waves.

Laboratory Findings—A diagnostic paracentesis should be performed in all patients presenting with new-onset ascites. Inspection of the ascitic fluid can help determine the etiology of ascites. A serum albumin-ascites gradient (SAAG) should be calculated in all new-onset ascites. A SAAG greater than or equal to 1.1 g/dL has a 97% sensitive for the detection of portal-hypertensive ascites.[34] A protein level greater than 2.5 g/dL in the ascitic fluid can further help classify portal-hypertensive ascites into the category of cardiac ascites.[37]

Treatment

Medical Treatment

Diuretics—Minimal ascites can be managed effectively with a Na-restricted diet (2 g/d). In patients with moderate ascites, the addition of diuretic regimen consisting of a loop diuretic (eg, furosemide) and aldosterone inhibitor (eg, spironolactone) is effective in controlling ascites in 90% of patients.[38] The combination works better than either diuretic alone and helps to maintain normokalemia. Initial dose of 40 mg daily of furosemide and 100 mg daily of spironolactone is usually well tolerated by patients. If serum Cr and electrolytes remain stable, the diuretic dose can be increased in a step-wise fashion up to 160 mg daily for furosemide and 400 mg daily for spironolactone. Daily weight loss of 1 kg until euvolemia is appropriate.

Paracentesis—In less than 10% of patients, ascites can be refractory to Na-restricted diet and diuretics. These patients may benefit from serial large-volume paracentesis (LVP). LVP is safe and effective in removing large amounts of ascites at one time. Even in the absence of urine output, ascites can be well controlled when performed every other week.[39] LVP can significantly increase plasma renin and serum Cr; however, this effect can be tempered by the use of albumin replacement.[40] Typically 25% IV albumin at a dose of 8 g per 1 L of ascites removed is given to attenuate the electrolyte and fluid shift changes seen after LVP.

Shunt Procedures—An alternative to serial LVP is the TIPS procedure. Several trials have shown improved control of ascites in the TIPS group as compared to serial LVP.[41,42] However, TIPS should be placed with extreme caution in patients with severe HE, heart failure, pulmonary hypertension, intrinsic renal disease, HCC, and high MELD scores (> 18).

Spontaneous Bacterial Peritonitis

General Considerations

SBP is an infection of the ascitic fluid without a surgically treatable intra-abdominal source and most commonly occurs as a complication of ascites from advanced cirrhosis.[43] SBP is diagnosed in 12% of hospitalized patients with cirrhosis and ascites.[44] In-hospital mortality of SBP can be up to 33%.[45]

Clinical Features

Symptoms and Signs—Patients may present with fever and abdominal tenderness, but often the presenting symptoms may be subtle, such as confusion and fatigue. Approximately 13% of patients with the diagnosis of SBP have no signs or symptoms of infection.[46] SBP should be suspected in any patients presenting with signs of hepatic decompensation in the setting of cirrhosis and ascites.

Laboratory Findings—Diagnosis of SBP is by the presence of an ascitic fluid absolute polymorphonuclear leukocyte (PMN) count greater than 250 cells/mm³.[47] Gram stain and cultures should be sent from the ascitic fluid, but the yield can be low in identifying the offending organism. Concurrent blood culture can increase the diagnostic yield of identifying an organism.

Treatment

As PMN count results are available more quickly than culture results, patients with ascitic PMN counts greater than 250 cells/mm³ should be treated with broad-spectrum antibiotics. The 3 most common organism isolates are *Escherichia coli*, *Klebsiella pneumoniae*, and *Streptococcal pneumoniae*. Empiric treatment with third-generation cephalosporin such as ceftriaxone or cefotaxime appears to be effective in covering 95% of cases.[48] After antibiotic sensitivities of the organism are obtained, the antibiotic

coverage can be adjusted accordingly. If no clinical improvement is seen in 48 hours, a repeat diagnostic paracentesis should be considered to assess the PMN response and to document sterility of the ascites.

Hepatorenal Syndrome

General Considerations

Hepatorenal syndrome (HRS) is the development of renal dysfunction in the setting of cirrhosis and ascites. Progressive portal hypertension and splanchnic vasodilatation are followed by fall in systemic vascular resistance. Relative renal hypoperfusion occurs with resultant vasoconstriction of the renal circulation and drop in glomerular filtration rate (GFR).

HRS is divided into 2 types. Type I is characterized by the rapid and progressive impairment in renal function with associated oliguria. Without treatment, type I HRS is uniformly fatal. Type II HRS develops more slowly and is marked by relatively mild reduction in renal function. Typically, patients with type II HRS present with diuretic-resistant ascites. The diagnostic criteria for HRS are listed in Table 37–6.

Clinical Features

Signs and Symptoms—Patients present with signs of progressive renal failure. Volume overload can be seen with oliguria. Signs of uremia may be present, including progressive confusion.

Laboratory Findings—Serum Cr is greater than 1.5 mg/dL with concurrent BUN elevation. Urinary Na concentration less than 10 mEq/L and serum Na

TABLE 37–6 Diagnostic criteria for the hepatorenal syndrome.[49]

1. Presence of cirrhosis with ascites
2. Serum creatinine greater than 1.5 mg/dL
3. No improvement of serum creatinine (decrease to level < 1.5 mg/dL) after at least 2 ds with diuretic withdrawal and volume expansion with albumin (1 g/kg of body weight per day up to a maximum of 100 g/d).
4. Absence of shock
5. No current or recent treatment with nephrotoxic drugs
6. Absence of parenchymal kidney disease as indicated by proteinuria greater than 500 g/d, microhematuria (> 50 red blood cells per high-power field), and/or abnormal renal ultrasonography

Reproduced with permission from Salerno F, Gerbes A, Ginès P, et al: Diagnosis, prevention and treatment of hepatorenal syndrome in cirrhosis, *Postgrad Med J.* 2008 Dec;84(998):662-670.

concentration less than 130 mEq/L are often seen in patients with HRS.

Differential Diagnosis

Other causes of AKI should be excluded, as patients with cirrhosis may be especially susceptible to prerenal azotemia and ATN. Patients should be questioned about recent use of nephrotoxic drugs such as nonsteroidal anti-inflammatory drugs or aminoglycosides.

Treatment

Pharmacologic Therapy—Initial management of patients presenting with renal failure should be volume resuscitation to exclude prerenal azotemia. Albumin (1 g/kg of body weight per day, up to a maximum of 100 g/d) should be given. If no improvement in renal function is seen and HRS is suspected, an attempt at pharmacologic therapy should be attempted.

Terlipressin is the drug studied most extensively to treat HRS. In combination with albumin, it has been shown to have 50% efficacy in reversing HRS.[50] Terlipressin is currently not available in the United States.

The combination of oral midodrine (7.5-12.5 mg 3 times daily), SC octreotide (100-200 μg 3 times daily), and IV albumin may be utilized as an alternative to terlipressin. The combination appears to be effective in lowering serum creatinine and 30-day mortality.[51]

For patients in the ICU, albumin and continuous IV norepinephrine can be attempted to reverse type I HRS.[52]

Renal Replacement Therapy—More often, patients with type I HRS are unresponsive to pharmacologic therapy, and RRT is required to manage electrolyte imbalance and volume overload. Expedited LT evaluation should be performed in these patients, as the development of type I HRS is a predictor of poor outcome.

Hepatic Encephalopathy

General Considerations

Hepatic encephalopathy is a reversible impairment in neuropsychiatric function associated with hepatic dysfunction. The exact pathophysiology of HE in chronic liver disease remains unclear, but a

TABLE 37-7 Precipitating factors of hepatic encephalopathy.

Infection
Dehydration
Renal failure
Hypokalemia
Hypoglycemia
Hypoxia
Sedative use
Gastrointestinal bleeding
Constipation
Portal decompression procedure
Portal vein or hepatic vein thrombosis
Malignancy
Medication noncompliance

combination of elevated ammonia level along with alteration in blood-brain barrier leads to changes that activate inhibitory neurotransmitters (gamma-aminobutyric acid, [GABA], serotonin) and impair excitatory neurotransmitters (glutamate, catecholamine). Overt HE is present in 30% of patients with cirrhosis and is a frequent reason for hospital admissions.[53] Common precipitants of HE are listed in Table 37–7.

Clinical Features

Symptoms and Signs—Patients can present with varying degrees of neuropsychiatric dysfunction, ranging from subtle cognitive deficits to overt coma (see Table 37–2).

Laboratory Findings—Patients will have abnormal liver function tests, reflective of their underlying liver disease. Electrolyte disturbances may be seen that can precipitate HE. Patients may have elevated arterial and venous ammonia levels. However, an elevated ammonia level is not required to make the diagnosis of HE, and the level often does not correlate with the degree of encephalopathy.

Treatment

General supportive care should be provided to patients presenting with HE. Appropriate triage of patients should be made depending on the severity of encephalopathy. Patients with agitation or confusion may need close supervision to avoid injury. In patients presenting with grade IV encephalopathy, observation in an ICU may be appropriate with consideration for tracheal intubation for airway protection.

The treatment of HE begins with the correction of any underlying, precipitating factors, including infection, bleeding, dehydration, electrolyte abnormality, and renal dysfunction.

Treatment with lactulose, a synthetic disaccharide, is the mainstay of therapy for overt HE despite limited evidence from randomized trials.[54] Lactulose is metabolized by the colonic flora and lowers colonic pH. The resultant pH favors the formation of nonabsorbable NH4+ from NH_3, thus reducing plasma ammonia concentration. Lactulose also works to clear ammonia via its osmotic laxative effect. Oral or rectal lactulose can be given for acute overt HE until mental status improves. Once HE resolves, the drug dose can be titrated to achieve 2 to 3 soft bowel movements per day.

In combination with lactulose, rifaximin, a nonabsorbable antibiotic, has been shown to maintain remission of HE.[55] Rifaximin 550 mg twice daily or 400 mg 3 times daily is effective in controlling HE with minimal reported adverse effects. Other antibiotics such as metronidazole and neomycin have been used for HE. However, concern for long-term side effects including neuropathy for metronidazole and ototoxicity for neomycin has limited their chronic use in HE.

L-Ornithine L-aspartate, zinc, branched-chain amino acids, flumazenil, and sodium benzoate have all been used with variable success in HE and may be options in the setting of brittle encephalopathy.

REFERENCES

1. Hoyert DL, Xu J. Deaths: preliminary data for 2011. *Nat Vital Stat Rep.* 2011;61(6):1-52.
2. Hoofnagle JH, Carithers RLJ, Shapiro C, Ascher N. Fulminant hepatic failure: summary of a workshop. *Hepatology.* 1995;21(1):240-252.
3. Khashab M, Tector AJ, Kwo PY. Epidemiology of acute liver failure. *Curr Gastroenterol Rep.* 2007;9(1):66-73.
4. Conn HO, Leevy CM, Vlahcevic ZR, et al. Comparison of lactulose and neomycin in the treatment of chronic portal-systemic encephalopathy. A double blind controlled trial. *Gastroenterology.* 1977;72(4):573-583.
5. Wilkinson SP, Blendis LM, Williams R. Frequency and type of renal and electrolyte disorders in fulminant hepatic failure. *Br Med J.* 1974;1(5900):186-189.
6. Cobden I, Record CO, Ward MK, Kerr DN. Paracetamol-induced acute renal failure in the absence of fulminant liver damage. *Br Med J.* 1982;284(6308):21-22.
7. O'Grady JG, Alexander GJ, Hayllar KM, William R. Early indicators of prognosis in fulminant hepatic failure. *Gastroenterology.* 1989;97(2):439-445.
8. Ostapowicz G, Fontana RJ, Schiodt FV, et al. Results of a prospective study of acute liver failure at 17 tertiary care centers in the United States. *Ann Intern Med.* 2002;137(12):947-954.
9. Lee WM, Hynan LS, Rossaro L, et al. Intravenous N-acetylcysteine improves transplant-free survival in early stage non-acetaminophen acute liver failure. *Gastroenterology.* 2009;137(3):856-864.
10. Munoz SJ. Difficult management problems in fulminant hepatic failure. *Semin Liver Dis.* 1993;13(4):395-413.
11. Bernal W, Hall C, Karvellas CJ, et al. Arterial ammonia and clinical risk factors for encephalopathy and intracranial hypertension in acute liver failure. *Hepatology.* 2007;46(6):1844-1852.
12. Nath F, Galbraith S. The effect of mannitol on cerebral white matter water content. *J Neurosurg.* 1986;65(1):41-43.
13. Canalese J, Gimson AE, Davis C, et al. Controlled trial of dexamethasone and mannitol for the cerebral oedema of fulminant hepatic failure. *Gut.* 1982;23(7):625-629.
14. Murphy N, Auzinger G, Bernel W, Wendon J. *Hepatology.* 2004;39(2):464-470.
15. Laffey JG, Kavanagh BP. Hypocapnia. *N Engl J Med.* 2002;347(1):43-53.
16. Gabor AJ, Brooks AG, Scobey RP, Parsons GH. Intracranial pressure during epileptic seizures. *Electroencephalogr Clin Neurophysiol.* 1984;57(6):497-506.
17. Ring-Larsen H, Palazzo U. Renal failure in fulminant hepatic failure and terminal cirrhosis: a comparison between incidence, types, and prognosis. *Gut.* 1981;22:585-591.
18. Bismuth H, Samuel D, Castaing D, et al. Orthotopic liver transplantation in fulminant and subfulminant hepatitis. The Paul Brousse experience. *Ann Surg.* 1995;222(2):109-119.
19. Garcia-Tsao G, Groszmann RJ, Fisher RL, et al. Portal pressure, presence of gastroesophageal varices and variceal bleeding. *Hepatology.* 1985;5(3):419-424.
20. The North Italian Endoscopic Club for the Study and Treatment of Esophageal Varices. Prediction of the

first variceal hemorrhage in patients with cirrhosis of the liver and esophageal varices. *N Eng J Med.* 1988;319(15):983-989.

21. El-Serag HB, Everhart JE. Improved survival after variceal hemorrhage over an 11-year period in the Department of Veterans Affairs. *Am J Gastroenterol.* 2000;95:3566-3573.

22. Villanueva C, Colomo A, Bosch A, et al. Transfusion strategies for acute upper gastrointestinal bleeding. *N Eng J Med.* 2013;368(1):11-21.

23. D'Amico G, Pagliaro L, Bosch J. Pharmacological treatment of portal hypertension: an evidence-based approach. *Semin Liver Dis.* 1999;19:475-505.

24. Chavez-Tapia NC, Barrientos-Gutierrez T, Tellez-Avila F, et al. Meta-analysis: antibiotic prophylaxis for cirrhotic patients with upper gastrointestinal bleeding—an updated Cochrane review. *Aliment Pharmacol Ther.* 2011;34(5):509-518.

25. Banares R, Albillos A, Rincon D, et al. Endoscopic treatment versus endoscopic plus pharmacologic treatment for acute variceal bleeding: a meta-analysis. *Hepatology.* 2002;35(3):609-615.

26. Sarin SK, Lahoti D, Saxena SP, Murthy NS, Makwana UK. Prevalence, classification and natural history of gastric varices: a long-term follow-up study in 568 portal hypertension patients. *Hepatology.* 1992;16(6):1343-1349.

27. Sarin SK, Jain AK, Jain M, Gupta R. A randomized controlled trial of cyanoacrylate versus alcohol injection in patients with isolated fundic varices. *Am J Gastroenterol.* 2002;97(4):1010-1015.

28. Avgerinos A, Armonis A. Balloon tamponade techniques and efficacy in variceal hemorrhage. *Scand J Gastroenterol Suppl.* 1994;207:11-16.

29. Feu F, Garcia-Pagan JC, Bosch J, et al. Relationship between portal pressure response to pharmacotherapy and risk of recurrent variceal haemorrhage in patients with cirrhosis. *Lancet.* 1995;346(8982):1056-1059.

30. Casado M, Bosch J, Garcia-Pagan JC, et al. Clinical events after transjugular intrahepatic portosystemic shunt: correlation with hemodynamic findings. *Gastroenterology.* 1998;114(6):1296-1303.

31. Malinchoc M, Kamath PS, Gordon FD, et al. A model to predict poor survival in patients undergoing transjugular intrahepatic portosystemic shunts. *Hepatology.* 2000;31(4):864-871.

32. Saad WE. Balloon-occluded retrograde transvenous obliteration of gastric varices: concept, basic techniques, and outcomes. *Semin Intervent Radiol.* 2012;29(2):118-128.

33. Kitamoto M, Imamura M, Kamada K, et al. Balloon-occluded retrograde transvenous obliteration of

gastric fundal varices with hemorrhage. *AJR AM J Roentgenol.* 2002;178(5):1167-1174.

34. Runyon BA, Montano AA, Akriviadis EA, et al. The serum-ascites albumin gradient is superior to the exudate-transudate concept in the differential diagnosis of ascites. *Ann Intern Med.* 1992;117(3):215-220.

35. Gines P, Quintero E, Arroyo V, et al. Compensated cirrhosis: natural history and prognostic factors. *Hepatology.* 1987;7(1):122-128.

36. Planas R, Montoliu S, Balleste B, et al. Natural history of patients hospitalized for management of cirrhotic ascites. *Clin Gastroenterol Hepatol.* 2006;4(11):1385-1394.

37. Runyon BA. Cardiac ascites: a characterization. *J Clin Gastoenterol.* 1988;10(4):10-12.

38. Perez-Ayuso RM, Arroyo V, Planas R, et al. Randomized comparative study of efficacy of furosemide versus spironolactone in nonazotemic cirrhosis with ascites. Relationship between the diuretic response and the activity of the renin-aldosterone system. *Gastroenterology.* 1983;84(5):961-968.

39. Runyon BA. Care of patients with ascites. *N Engl J Med.* 1994;330(5):337-342.

40. Gines P, Tito L, Arroyo V, et al. Randomized comparative study of therapeutic paracentesis with and without intravenous albumin in cirrhosis. *Gastroenterology.* 1988;94(6):1493-1502.

41. Rossle M, Ochs A, Gulberg V, et al. A comparison of paracentesis and transjugular intrahepatic portosystemic shunting in patients with ascites. *N Engl J Med.* 2000;342(23):1701-1707.

42. Salerno F, Merli M, Riggio O, et al. Randomized controlled study of TIPS versus paracentesis plus albumin in cirrhosis with severe ascites. *Hepatology.* 2004;40(3):629-635.

43. Such J, Runyon BA. Spontaneous bacterial peritonitis. *Clin Infect Dis.* 1998;27(4):669-674.

44. Chinnock B, Hendey GW, Minnigan H, Butler J, Afarian H. Clinical impression and ascites appearance do not rule out bacterial peritonitis. *J Emerg Med.* 2013;44(5):903-909.

45. Thuluvath PJ, Morss S, Thompson R. Spontaneous bacterial peritonitis-in-hospital mortality, predictors of survival, and health care costs from 1988 to 1998. *Am J Gastroenterol.* 2001;96(4):1232-1236.

46. Runyon BA. Monomicrobial nonneutrocytic bacterascites: a variant of spontaneous bacterial peritonitis. *Hepatology.* 1990;12(4):710-715.

47. Runyon BA, Antillon MR. Ascitic fluid pH and lactate: insensitive and nonspecific tests

in detecting ascitic fluid infection. *Hepatology.* 1991;13(5):929-935.

48. Felisart J, Rimola A, Arroyo V, et al. Cefotaxime is more effective than is ampicillin-tobramycin in cirrhotics with severe infections. *Hepatology.* 1985;5(3):457-462.

49. Salerno F, Gerbes, A, Gines P, Wong F, Arroyo V. Diagnosis, prevention and treatment of hepatorenal syndrome in cirrhosis. *Postgrad Med J.* 2008;84(998):662-670.

50. Dobre M, Demirjian S, Sehgal AR, Navaneethan SD. Terlipressin in hepatorenal syndrome: a systematic review and meta-analysis. *Int Urol Nephrol.* 2011;43(1):175-184.

51. Esrailian E, Pantangco ER, Kyulo NL, Hu KQ, Runyon BA. Octerotide/midodrine therapy significantly improves renal function and 30-day survival in patients with type 1 hepatorenal syndrome. *Dig Dis Sci.* 2007;52(3):742-748.

52. Sharma P, Kumar A, Shrama BC, Sarin SK. An open label, pilot, randomized controlled trial of noradrenaline versus terlipressin in the treatment of type 1 hepatorenal syndrome and predictors of response. *Am J Gastroenterol.* 2008;103(7):1689-1697.

53. Romero-Gomez M, Boza F, Garcia-Valdecasas MS, Garcia E, Aguilar-Reina J. Subclinical hepatic encephalopathy predicts the development of overt hepatic encephalopathy. *Am J Gastroenterol.* 2001;96(9):2718-2723.

54. Als-Nielsen B, Gluud LL, Gludd C. Non-absorbable disaccharides for hepatic encephalopathy: systemic review of randomised trials. *Br Med J.* 2004;328(7447):1046-1051.

55. Bass NM, Mullen KD, Sanyal A, et al. Rifaximin treatment in hepatic encephalopathy. *N Engl J Med.* 2010;362(12):1071-1081.

Fever in the ICU

Anuja Pradhan, MD and Daniel Caplivski, MD

38

KEY POINTS

1. Fever should prompt investigation into potential infectious as well as noninfectious etiologies.

2. Treatment with empiric antibiotics may be indicated in particular in patients with other signs of sepsis such as tachycardia and hypotension.

3. Fever may also be caused by potentially life-threatening noninfectious syndromes such as thromboembolic disease and it is important to investigate these possibilities as well.

INTRODUCTION

Fever is a state of elevated core temperature that is often a sign of infection in patients admitted to the intensive care unit (ICU). It should prompt investigation into potential infectious as well as noninfectious etiologies. Treatment with empiric antibiotics may be indicated in particular in patients with other signs of sepsis such as tachycardia and hypotension. Fever may also be caused by potentially life-threatening noninfectious syndromes such as thromboembolic disease and it is important to investigate these possibilities as well.

PATHOPHYSIOLOGY

The febrile response, of which temperature rise is a component, is a complex physiologic reaction to disease, involving cytokine-mediated rise in core temperature, generation of acute phase reactants, and activation of numerous physiologic, endocrinologic, and immunologic systems. In contrast, simple heat illness or malignant hyperthermia is an unregulated rise in body temperature caused by inability to eliminate heat adequately. Fever begins with the production of one or more proinflammatory cytokines in response to exogenous pyrogens (microorganisms, toxic agents) or immunologic mediators. Interleukin 1 (IL-1), tumor necrosis factor (TNF), lymphotoxin, interferons (IFNs), and interleukin 6 (IL-6) are known and documented to induce fever independently. Cytokines interact with receptors located at the organum vasculosum of the lamina terminalis causing synthesis and release of prostaglandins, chiefly prostaglandin E_2, which raises body temperature by initiating local cAMP production, which resets the thermoregulatory set point of the hypothalamus and by coordinating other adaptive responses such as shivering and peripheral vasoconstriction. Fever induces the production of heat shock proteins (HSPs), a class of proteins critical for cellular survival during stress. HSPs may have an anti-inflammatory role and indirectly decrease the level of proinflammatory cytokines. Core body temperature may be influenced by numerous external factors including cooling blankets or continuous venovenous hemofiltration. Patients who have suffered neurologic injury or central nervous system (CNS) hemorrhage may also have hypothalamic dysfunction that could lead to elevated body temperature.

EPIDEMIOLOGY

The incidence of fever in the ICU ranges from 28% to 70%. Infectious as well as noninfectious etiologies contribute almost equally to the causation of febrile episodes. The finding of a new fever in an ICU patient has a significant impact on health care costs due to the blood cultures, radiologic imaging, and antibiotics that are often empirically initiated. It is therefore important to have a good understanding of the mechanisms and etiology of fever in ICU patients, how and when to initiate a diagnostic workup, and when initiation of antibiotics is indicated.

DIAGNOSTIC APPROACH TO THE FEBRILE PATIENT IN THE ICU

A new fever in a patient in the ICU should trigger a careful clinical assessment rather than automatic orders for laboratory and radiologic tests. A cost-conscious approach to obtaining cultures and imaging studies should be undertaken if indicated after a clinical evaluation.

History and Physical Examination

Many patients admitted to the ICU are not able to provide direct information about localizing complaints. In patients who are intubated or obtunded information should be obtained from medical records regarding relevant antecedent problems (eg, previous infections, cancer, allergic reactions to drugs, immunosuppression etc). Relatives and friends of the patient may also provide pertinent epidemiologic information related to the patient's exposures and risk factors for infections. Physical examination of the febrile ICU patient should include examination of devices including intravenous catheters, endotracheal and nasogastric tubes, and bladder catheters. Skin examination may demonstrate findings suggestive of drug reaction,

vasculitis, infective endocarditis, or soft tissue infection. All intravenous and intra-arterial line sites should be inspected for signs of erythema, warmth, tenderness, and purulence. All surgical wounds should be examined 24 hours postoperatively. Head and neck examination may reveal important signs of localized and systemic infection. Funduscopic examination may provide clues to systemic viral or fungal infection, particularly in immunocompromised patients. Oral lesions of recrudescent herpetic stomatitis are common in the ICU setting and may be obscured by the presence of oral endotracheal tubes or orogastric feeding tubes. These lesions may be extensive, more ulcerated and necrotic, and less vesicular in appearance in a seriously ill patient. Examination of the lungs can be difficult in the intubated ICU patient and often is unrewardingly nonlocalizing and nonspecific. Abdominal findings can be misleadingly unremarkable in the elderly, in the patient with obtunded sensorium, and in the patient receiving sedatives and can be confounding in the patient with recent abdominal or thoracic surgery. Abdominal pain and tenderness may be localized (cholecystitis, intra-abdominal abscess, diverticulitis) or generalized (diffuse peritonitis, ischemic bowel, antibiotic-associated colitis). Examination of the genitalia and rectum may demonstrate unsuspected epididymitis, prostatitis, prostatic abscess, or perirectal abscess.

INFECTIOUS CAUSES OF FEVER IN THE ICU

Catheter-Associated Bloodstream Infections

Catheter-associated bloodstream infections are one of the most common reasons for patients to have fever in the ICU. Central venous and arterial catheters are important tools for monitoring patients and delivering fluids, antibiotics, nutrition, and other therapies. Bacteria and yeast that colonize the skin of the patient or the hands of health care providers can easily gain access to the circulation via these devices. The risk of infection from these catheters is variable and depends on several factors such as length of the catheter, type of catheter such as arterial versus venous, tunneled versus nontunneled, technique of insertion, site of insertion, duration they have been in place, frequency of manipulation, patient population etc (Table 38–1). The highest risk is with short-term, noncuffed central venous catheters, in the range of 2 to 5 per 1000 catheter-days. There are several mechanisms, which may lead to the infection of an indwelling catheter. Skin pathogens can infect the catheter exit site or contaminate the catheter hub, leading to intraluminal catheter colonization and infection. Parenteral fluid, blood products, or intravenous medications can also be a source of infection. The catheter exit site should be inspected daily for evidence of erythema or pus; however these signs are absent in most cases with catheter-related bloodstream infection. Any expressible purulence or exudate should be sent for Gram stain and culture. Gram-positive organisms such as *Staphylococcus aureus*, coagulase-negative *Staphylococcus*, and *Enterococcus* species are commonly responsible for catheter-associated bloodstream infections. Increasingly these organisms have acquired resistance to beta-lactam antibiotics and even vancomycin. Many gram-positive organisms are also capable of forming biofilms which make them difficult to eradicate and removal of the central venous catheter is

generally necessary for successful treatment of these infections.

Gram-negative organisms are also important cause of catheter-associated bloodstream infections. Enterobacteriaceae such *Escherichia coli*, *Klebsiella pneumoniae*, and *Enterobacter* species are considered normal flora of the gastrointestinal (GI) tract; however they may colonize the hubs and tubing of central catheters and they may eventually be a cause of bacteremia. *Pseudomonas aeruginosa* is another important gram-negative organism that is often associated with nosocomial infection, including catheter-associated bacteremia. Because of the production of endotoxin gram-negative organisms are likely to trigger the release of cytokines that clinically manifest with signs of sepsis. In the hospital environment many gram-negative organisms have acquired multiple antibiotic resistance mechanisms. In addition to production of extended-spectrum beta-lactamase, several gram-negative species have also acquired carbapenemases that have made them resistant to the carbapenem class of antibiotics. The spread of these organisms within ICUs and throughout health care institutions more generally has been a particular challenge for infection control programs.

Candida bloodstream infections are also a common source of fever in the ICU. The use of central venous catheters to deliver total parenteral nutrition and empiric broad-spectrum antibacterial agents are important risk factors for *Candida* bloodstream infections. Catheter removal is of particular importance in the setting of fungemia as these infections are typically very difficult to eradicate when the infected catheter has not been removed. *Candida albicans* is frequently recovered from blood cultures in these patients; however increasingly nonalbicans species are responsible for these types of infection. Empiric therapy for *Candida* bloodstream infections should be guided initially by the severity of the infection as well as the epidemiology of *Candida* species as several nonalbicans species are resistant to fluconazole.

Pulmonary Infection Including Ventilator-Associated Pneumonia

Pneumonia is the second most common cause of infection acquired in the ICU and ventilator-associated pneumonia (VAP) is a common source of

TABLE 38–1 Infectious causes of fever in the ICU.

Most common
Catheter-related bloodstream infection
Ventilator-associated pneumonia
Primary septicemia/bacteremia
Surgical site/wound infection
Other causes
Sinusitis
Intra-abdominal abscess
Empyema
Diverticulitis
Cholangitis
Cellulitis
Soft tissue infections including necrotizing fasciitis and myonecrosis
Infected decubitus ulcer
Endocarditis
Suppurative thrombophlebitis
Septic arthritis
Urinary tract infections
Septic arthritis
Clostridium difficile colitis

fever in the intubated patient. Between 10% and 25% of patients on mechanical ventilation will develop VAP during their ICU stay. Several factors increase the risk of patients in the ICU for developing pneumonia including endotracheal intubation and altered levels of consciousness associated with primary processes or with sedation for mechanical ventilation. Cough responses normally important as a host defense may be impaired by these and other factors, including age over 60, male gender, chronic lung disease, aspiration, acute respiratory distress syndrome (ARDS), sinusitis, nasogastric tube use, delayed extubation, continuous sedation, use of paralytic agents, and endotracheal cuff pressures less than 20 cm of H_2O.

Nosocomial pathogens such as *Pseudomonas* and methicillin-resistant *S aureus* are more commonly associated with patients in the ICU. Precise microbiologic diagnosis is often challenging since obtaining an appropriate sputum sample or endotracheal aspirate is difficult in patients who are intubated. Organisms that colonize the airways may not reflect the true etiology of a lower respiratory tract infection in a patient with nosocomial pneumonia and sputum cultures should be interpreted with caution. High-quality sputum or bronchoalveolar lavage specimens with few squamous epithelial cells and many polymorphonuclear cells may be useful to guide antibiotic therapy. A higher-resolution study such as computerized tomography (CT) may be pursued if clinical suspicion is high enough and it may be helpful for detecting infiltrates in the posterior-inferior lung bases. Fiberoptic bronchoscopy with transbronchial biopsy may be especially useful for the detection of pathogens such as *Pneumocystis jiroveci*, *Aspergillus* species and other filamentous fungi, *Nocardia*, *Legionella*, cytomegalovirus (CMV), and *Mycobacterium* species. Thoracentesis can also be performed on patients with significant pleural effusions. Fluid should be sent for cell count, chemical analysis, and culture, especially if there is adjacent pulmonary infiltrate, suspicion of tuberculosis, or possible contamination of the pleural space due to surgery, trauma, or a fistula.

Urinary Tract Infection

Catheterization of the bladder is a common practice in ICUs for several reasons including close monitoring of fluid balance. Urinary tract infection can be a cause of fever for patients in the ICU, particularly if there is some obstruction to urinary flow such as nephrolithiasis or ureteral blockage by tumor. Colonization of urinary catheters by resistant organisms such as vancomycin-resistant *Enterococcus* (VRE) is also very common in patients in the ICU and interpretation of urine cultures must be made with caution with this caveat in mind. It is important to distinguish between asymptomatic bacteriuria from a genuine urinary tract infection.

Clostridium Difficile

The frequent use of empiric systemic antibiotics puts many patients in the ICU at risk for *C difficile* infection. In patients with *C difficile* infection watery diarrhea is generally accompanied by marked leukocytosis; however some patients with toxic megacolon may also present with abdominal distension and reduced bowel sounds. The diagnosis can be confirmed with stool polymerase chain reaction (PCR) testing for *C difficile* toxin. If sigmoidoscopy is performed, pseudomembranes may also be noted, but stool assays are generally adequate for diagnosis. In addition to therapy with oral vancomycin or metronidazole, systemic antibiotics should be discontinued if possible. Stool transplant has emerged as a potentially useful therapy in particular for patients with refractory *C difficile* infection.

Central Nervous System Infections

Nosocomial meningitis is most commonly seen in hospitalized patients who have undergone neurosurgical procedures. When an infection is suspected in a febrile patient with an intracranial device, cerebrospinal fluid (CSF) should be obtained for analysis from the CSF reservoir. In patients with ventriculostomies who develop stupor or signs of meningitis, the catheter tip should be removed and cultured. CSF should be analyzed with Gram stain, cell count, protein, and glucose measurements. The most common organisms are *S aureus* and coagulase-negative staphylococci; however, Gram-negative organisms such as *Pseudomonas* and *Klebsiella* may also be responsible for CNS infections in this setting. Additional testing for tuberculosis, viral and fungal disease should be performed if there is a clinical suspicion of these less common organisms.

Postoperative Infections

Surgical site infections can be important causes of fever in patients recovering from recent surgery. These infections will often present with erythema and purulence at a surgical site and eventually may lead to dehiscence of the wound. Prompt surgical debridement is generally required for patients with this etiology of fever. Deeper infections may also occur in particular in patients with recent bowel surgery where intraluminal organisms can leak into the peritoneum and cause abscesses. Evaluation with CT or direct examination in the operating room may be necessary for patients with abdominal or pelvic collections. Drainage of collections and correction of anastomotic leaks are generally required in addition to appropriate antibiotic therapy.

Sinusitis

Sinusitis is a less frequent infectious cause of fever in the ICU. Most ICU patients have nasogastric tubes and endotracheal tubes which predispose them to nosocomial sinusitis. Other risk factors include facial fractures or nasal packing. The most common organisms causing nosocomial sinusitis are those that colonize the naso-oropharynx. Gram-negative bacilli (especially *P aeruginosa*) constitute 60% of the bacteria isolated from nosocomial sinusitis. Gram-positive cocci such as *S aureus* are also common, and many infections are polymicrobial. Diagnosis may be made supported by imaging such as CT scan or confirmed with puncture and aspiration of the involved sinuses for culture and susceptibility if invasive testing is warranted.

NONINFECTIOUS CAUSES OF FEVER

A large number of noninfectious causes can cause tissue injury with inflammation and a febrile reaction (Table 38–2).

Postoperative Fever

Fever is common in the postoperative period during the first 48 hours and is due to release of endogenous pyrogens into the bloodstream. Usually fever this early in the postoperative period is noninfectious

TABLE 38–2 Noninfectious causes of fever in the ICU.

Drug fever
Neuroleptic malignant syndrome
Malignant hyperthermia
Acalculous cholecystitis
Intracranial hemorrhage
Early postoperative fever
Gout
Serotonin syndrome
Thromboembolic disease
Vasculitis
Malignancy
Ischemic colitis
Pancreatitis
Thyroid storm
Heat stroke
Seizures
Pheochromocytoma
Transfusion reaction
Mesenteric ischemia
Adrenal insufficiency
Hematoma
Seizures
Myocardial infarction
Acute respiratory distress syndrome
Aspiration pneumonitis
Thyroid storm
Immune reconstitution inflammatory response
Stroke
Alcohol and drug withdrawal

in origin; however fever more than 96 hours after surgery is more likely to represent an infection and needs full evaluation. Although atelectasis is considered to be the most common cause of postoperative fever, clinical evidence regarding this association is scarce.

Medication Allergy

Numerous medications may be associated with an allergic response that includes fever. Any medication can cause fever due to hypersensitivity, which may manifest as fever alone to life-threatening hypersensitivity. Most common drugs known to cause fever are beta-lactam antibiotics, phenytoin, quinidine, procainamide, and methyldopa. Reactions to antiepileptic medications such as phenytoin may also include elevated liver enzymes and skin eruptions but often fever is the only clinical manifestation of this problem. A high clinical suspicion is needed for diagnosing drug fever since there is nothing characteristic about these fever patterns and they do not invariably occur immediately after drug administration. They may occur days after commencing a new medication, but a temporal relationship of the fever to starting and stopping the medication is supportive of this diagnosis.

Acalculous Cholecystitis

Acute acalculous cholecystitis is a condition of inflammation of the gall bladder in the absence of calculi. It is a disease with significant morbidity and mortality as it can lead to complications such as empyema of the gallbladder, gangrene, or perforation. A high index of suspicion is necessary, as it may be a difficult diagnosis to make in the sedated and intubated patient. The pathophysiology of this disorder is complex and involves hypoperfusion and biliary stasis. Risk factors include trauma, surgery, positive-pressure ventilation, total parenteral nutrition, sedation, immunosuppression, transfusion of blood products, and hypotension. Ultrasound or CT scan can be supportive of the diagnosis. As soon as the diagnosis is suspected, blood cultures should be drawn and broad-spectrum antibiotics commenced. Surgical intervention may be necessary, but may not be feasible in unstable patients.

Thromboembolic Disease and Hematoma

Deep venous thrombosis may be another noninfectious cause of fever. Patients with immobility, vascular injury, and underlying malignancies are at particular risk for thromboembolism. Large hematomas may also produce fevers and may be difficult to detect when they occur in the retroperitoneal space. Thrombotic thrombocytopenic purpura (TTP) is another syndrome associated with fever that also includes microvascular injury, platelet destruction, altered mental status, and renal injury.

Malignancies and Central fever

Certain malignancies such as lymphoma are associated with "B symptoms" such as weight loss, fevers, and sweats that may mimic infection. Brain injury or hemorrhage in the CNS may lead to hypothalamic dysfunction. Central fever and tumor fever are generally established as an etiology when infectious etiologies and other noninfectious etiologies have been excluded.

EVALUATION OF THE FEBRILE ICU PATIENT

Initial Empiric Therapy

Once an infectious cause is suspected source control and early initiation of appropriate antimicrobial therapy are often the most important interventions for management. Infected catheters should be removed and abscesses should be drained. Empiric therapy should be based on the site of infection as well as local hospital epidemiology. Antimicrobials should be evaluated daily to reassess their need and potential de-escalation to avoid toxicity and emergence of resistant organisms. Positive cultures may help to narrow antibiotic coverage (Table 38–3).

Gram-Positive Organisms

S aureus, *Enterococcus*, and coagulase-negative staphylococci are among the common gram-positive pathogens involved in nosocomial ICU infections. Vancomycin can be included in the initial empiric regimen if these organisms are suspected. Linezolid or daptomycin may be used if there is a history of vancomycin-resistant *Enterococcus*, or vancomycin allergy. If methicillin-susceptible *S aureus* is isolated therapy should be switched to nafcillin or cefazolin.

Streptococcus pneumoniae and alpha-hemolytic streptococci (*Streptococcus viridans* group) are more common in community-acquired infections such as pneumonia or infective endocarditis. Empiric therapy for nosocomial pneumonia often includes broad-spectrum antibiotics with good levels of penetration in the lung tissue. Gram-positive coverage with vancomycin or linezolid is favored over

TABLE 38–3 Preliminary evaluation of the febrile ICU patient.

Blood cultures
Imaging studies
Urine cultures
Stool testing for *Clostridium difficile* (if diarrhea is present)
Sputum cultures/endotracheal aspirate
Peripheral blood smear evaluation

daptomycin due to surfactant binding of daptomycin. Broad-spectrum antibiotics with gram-negative activity may include cefepime or imipenem. In cases in which *Legionella* is suspected, fluoroquinolones or macrolides are appropriate.

Necrotizing fasciitis with group A *Streptococcus* may be seen in surgical site infections postoperatively and have a devastating outcome without surgical debridement and early appropriate antibiotic therapy. Penicillin G is usual drug of choice, as most streptococci are sensitive to penicillin. Clindamycin should be added for decreased toxin production effect for necrotizing fasciitis secondary to group A *Streptococcus*. Combination therapy may be necessary in certain infections such as enterococcal endocarditis which usually requires synergy with aminoglycoside in addition to vancomycin or penicillin.

Gram-Negative Organisms

Gram-negative organisms commonly encountered in an ICU-acquired infection include *P aeruginosa*, *E coli*, *K pneumoniae*, *Acinetobacter* species, and *Stenotrophomonas*. Abdominal infections usually have mixed bacteriology including anaerobes. The emergence of multidrug-resistant gram-negative organisms has been a challenging problem in the ICUs in recent times. These organisms may produce carbapenemase enzymes that confer resistance to broad-spectrum agents such as imipenem and meropenem. When gram-negative infections are suspected, empiric antimicrobial agents should be chosen with knowledge of the local ICU resistance pattern.

Extended-spectrum beta-lactam penicillins such as piperacillin combined with a beta-lactamase inhibitor such as tazobactam have good activity against *Pseudomonas*, *E coli*, *Proteus*, *Serratia*, *Klebsiella*, and most commonly encountered gram negatives. It also has excellent anaerobic activity comparable to metronidazole. Pharyngeal colonization with gram-negative bacilli rapidly develops in patients in the ICU, and initial therapy of nosocomial aspiration pneumonia requires the addition of an antipseudomonal penicillin, carbapenem, or cephalosporin. Higher doses of piperacillin/tazobactam should be considered for serious infections due to *Pseudomonas*. Although traditionally aminoglycosides have been added for synergy or double coverage for *Pseudomonas*, there is little data to support this approach routinely.

Fungal Infections

Invasive and disseminated fungal infections are becoming increasingly common in the ICU. Risk factors for invasive fungal infections include broad-spectrum antibiotic use, immunosuppression, and use of total parenteral nutrition. Patients with lymphoproliferative disease, transplant patients, and advanced HIV disease are also at risk. Bloodstream infections with *C albicans* remain the most commonly seen fungal infections and are usually susceptible to triazoles. *Candida krusei* and *Candida glabrata* may be resistant to fluconazole and voriconazole or caspofungin should be used when these organisms are suspected. Lipid preparations of amphotericin B are the initial drug of choice for empiric therapy of life-threatening, invasive, or systemic fungal infections including mucormycosis, cryptococcosis, histoplasmosis, and coccidioidomycosis.

REFERENCES

1. O'Grady NP, Barie PS, Bartlett JG, et al. Guidelines for evaluation of new fever in critically ill adult patients: 2008 update from the American College of Critical Care Medicine and the Infectious Diseases Society of America. *Crit Care Med.* 2008;36(4):1330-1349.
2. Principles and practice of Infectious Diseases: Temperature regulation and the Pathogenesis of Fever, 7th edition chapter 50; 765-778.
3. Irwin & Rippe's Intensive Care Medicine: Approach to fever in the ICU patient, 7th edition, chapter 76; 932-938.
4. Niven DJ, Léger C, Stelfox HT, Laupland KB. Fever in the critically ill: a review of epidemiology, immunology, and management. *J Intensive Care Med.* 2012;27:290-297.

Community-Acquired Infections in the ICU

Meenakshi M. Rana, MD

Community-acquired infections and concomitant sepsis are commonly a reason for admission to the ICU. In these infections, patients typically present with symptoms and signs prior to admission. The most common infections managed in the ICU are described below—CAP, UTIs, IAIs, necrotizing skin and soft tissue infections (NSTIs), and IE.

COMMUNITY-ACQUIRED PNEUMONIA

Introduction and Epidemiology

CAP is one of the most frequent causes of infection-related death in the United States. It occurs in approximately 4 million adults per year, accounting for 1.1 million hospitalizations and 50,000 deaths per year. Of the 20% to 60% of patients who require hospital admission for CAP, anywhere between 10% and 22% may require critical care.[1] Mortality rates remain high despite advances in antibiotics and critical care.

Pathogenesis

The lower respiratory tract remains sterile because of a combination of pulmonary defense mechanisms that involve anatomic and mechanical barriers, and humoral and cell-mediated immunity. The development of CAP is therefore a result of either a defect in the host pulmonary defense system, an exposure to a virulent or large inoculum of microorganisms, or a combination of these factors.[2] Certain risk factors for CAP have previously been described. These include increased age, male sex, malnutrition or poor dental hygiene, high alcohol consumption, smoking, immunosuppression including HIV, asplenia, and other underlying comorbidities.[3]

Microbiology

The most common etiology of CAP remains bacterial or viral; other fungal or parasitic organisms are isolated infrequently and are usually related to various geographic and host factors. Causes of bacterial CAP can be divided into typical or atypical organisms. The most common cause of CAP is *Streptococcus pneumoniae*; other typical bacterial pathogens include *Haemophilus influenzae*, *Moraxella catarrhalis*, *Staphylococcus aureus*, and gram-negative organisms such as *Klebsiella pneumoniae* and *Pseudomonas aeruginosa*, seen in patients with previous exposure to antimicrobials or structural lung disease. Community-associated methicillin-resistant *S aureus* (CA-MRSA) as an etiology of CAP should be considered in the appropriate clinical situation, usually in patients presenting with cavitary pneumonia, lung necrosis, or concurrent influenza.[4] Atypical organisms, such as *Mycoplasma pneumoniae*, *Chlamydophila* spp. (*Chlamydophila pneumoniae* and *Chlamydophila psittaci*), and *Legionella*, can often result in admission to the ICU. Viral etiologies should not be overlooked and include influenza and respiratory syncytial virus; other viruses such as parainfluenza, human metapneumovirus, and adenovirus should also be considered. Influenza specifically should be included in the differential of anyone presenting with CAP in the typical season, especially given that a significant number of patients can have concomitant bacterial infection. Other pathogens in the appropriate host include *Mycobacterium tuberculosis*, specifically in patients who are homeless, recently incarcerated, have HIV, or are from a country where tuberculosis is considered prevalent. Endemic fungi such as *Histoplasma capsulatum*, *Coccidioides immitis*, and *Blastocystis hominis* should be considered in patients from the appropriate geographic region. Immunocompromised hosts, such as solid organ transplant recipients, hematopoietic stem cell transplant recipients, patients with HIV/AIDS, and patients on chemotherapy may be at risk for other opportunistic pathogens such as *Aspergillus*, *Cryptococcus*, and *Pneumocystis jiroveci* pneumonia.

Diagnosis

CAP is defined as acute infection of the lungs in patients who are not hospitalized or residents of long-term care facilities. Patients can present with symptoms of cough, fever, dyspnea, sputum production, and pleuritic chest pain. Other nonrespiratory symptoms may also be present. On physical examination, vital signs are notable for fever and associated tachycardia; hypotension is also present in severe CAP and concomitant septic shock. Tachypnea, the use of accessory muscles, or cyanosis and hypoxia are seen in respiratory compromise. Rales, bronchial breath sounds, and egophony are present on auscultation. On laboratory examination, leukocytosis with neutrophilic predominance is typically seen, although leukopenia can also occur in septic shock. Other signs of organ dysfunction such as acute kidney injury, hepatic dysfunction, lactic acidosis, and disseminated intravascular coagulation can also be seen with severe CAP and concomitant sepsis.

A chest radiograph should be performed and is critical to differentiating between upper respiratory and lower respiratory tract infection. Typically, a lobar infiltrate is present in bacterial pneumonia such as those seen in pneumococcal pneumonia; an interstitial pattern is typically seen with Mycoplasma and a bilateral mixed interstitial-alveolar pattern can be seen in viral pneumonia.[2] For patients hospitalized with suspected CAP but a negative chest x-ray, occasionally an infiltrate can be seen when the chest x-ray is repeated in 24 to 48 hours.[5] Computed tomography (CT) of the chest is not routinely recommended given radiation exposure and expense; however, it may be useful in certain situations, such as nonresponse to initial therapy or in the immunocompromised host where certain infections such as *Aspergillus* and *M tuberculosis* have a classic appearance.[2]

In patients admitted to the ICU, certain diagnostic tests are recommended by Infectious Diseases Society of America (IDSA)/American Thoracic Society (ATS) guidelines. All patients with severe CAP should have blood cultures done to guide antibiotic therapy. In addition, urinary antigens for *Legionella pneumophila* and *S pneumoniae* should be performed. These may be especially useful in pneumococcal pneumonia when initial antibiotics have been given and the utility of a positive blood culture may be reduced. In *Legionella*, culture is less sensitive and urinary antigen testing is a useful tool for diagnosis, although only positive in serogroup 1. In addition, rapid antigen or PCR testing for viruses such as influenza should be performed in the appropriate clinical setting. If expectorated sputum of good quality with minimal oropharyngeal contamination can be obtained, it should be sent for Gram stain and culture. In intubated patients with severe CAP, endotracheal aspirates or bronchoscopy can be done to obtain respiratory samples for culture, with significantly more yield.[5]

Management

Severity Scoring Systems

For each patient being evaluated for pneumonia, the following 2 questions need to be asked—"Should the patient be hospitalized?" and if so, "Should the patient be admitted to the ICU?" Several scoring systems have been developed to assess severity of illness in order to identify patients with severe CAP. The first 2 tools, the Pneumonia Severity Index (PSI) and CURB-65, can aid in the diagnostic decision of whether or not to admit someone to the hospital. The PSI, which has been validated in several large studies, uses age, comorbidity, and vital signs to determine if the patient can be discharged and treated as an outpatient. The second tool, the British Thoracic Society CURB-65 system, uses fewer variables—confusion, urea, respiratory rate, blood pressure (BP), and age, to determine if patients can be treated as an outpatient or should be admitted.[6]

In addition, the IDSA/ATS has developed criteria to aid in identifying patients that would require admission to the ICU (Table 39–1). Any patient with one of the major criteria, either vasopressor use or respiratory failure requiring intubation and mechanical ventilation, require admission to the ICU. Patients with 3 of the minor criteria should also be considered for direct admission to an ICU.

TABLE 39–1 Criteria for severe community-acquired pneumonia.

Major Criteria	Minor Criteria
Septic shock requiring vasopressors	Respiratory rate ≥ 30 breaths/min
Acute respiratory failure requiring intubation and mechanical ventilation	PaO_2/FIO_2 ratio ≤ 250
	Multilobar infiltrates
	Confusion/disorientation
	Uremia (BUN level ≥ 20 mg/dL)
	Leukopenia (WBC count < 4000 cells/mm³)
	Thrombocytopenia (platelet count < 100,000 cells/mm³)
	Hypothermia (core temperature < 36°C)
	Hypotension requiring aggressive fluid resuscitation

BUN, blood urea nitrogen; WBC, white blood cell.
Adapted with permission from Mandell LA, Wundering RG, Anzueto A, Bartlett JF, et al. Infectious Diseases Society of America/American Thoracic Society Consensus Guidelines on the Management of Community-Acquired Pneumonia in Adults, *Clin Infect Dis* 2007 Mar 1;44 Suppl 2:S27-S72.

Validation studies support the use of the criteria in Table 39–1. Other scoring systems have been developed and include the SMART-COP, which aims to predict the need for respiratory or vasopressor support and the PIRO score, which aims to predict 28-day mortality.[1]

Antimicrobial Therapy

The initial treatment for CAP is empiric therapy directed at the most common pathogens; specific risk factors based on the host as well as local hospital epidemiology should be taken into account when considering initial therapy. For patients admitted to the ICU with severe CAP, a beta-lactam for initial pneumococcal coverage and plus either azithromycin or a respiratory fluoroquinolone for atypical coverage is recommended. In patients with a severe penicillin allergy, a respiratory fluoroquinolone or aztreonam is recommended. If *Pseudomonas* is suspected based on risk factors such as structural lung disease in bronchiectasis or severe chronic obstructive pulmonary disease (COPD) with frequent steroid or antibiotic use, then an antipseudomonal beta-lactam is recommended (ie, cefepime, piperacillin-tazobactam or a carbapenem).

Drug-resistant pneumococcus has been reported, with about 85% of isolates susceptible to penicillin and up to 30% of isolates demonstrating resistance to macrolides.[1] Respiratory fluoroquinolone resistance remains low in North America. In cases where CA-MRSA is suspected, such as necrotizing pneumonia or lung abscess, linezolid or vancomycin should be added.[5] In one randomized control trial for nosocomial pneumonia, linezolid has been shown to have clinical superiority to vancomycin although there was no difference in 60-day mortality.[7] It is unclear if this data can be generalized to patients with CAP. Ceftaroline, which has activity against MRSA in addition to other gram-positive and gram-negative pathogens, was approved for the treatment of CAP based on phase III trials which demonstrated noninferiority to ceftriaxone for the treatment of non-ICU hospitalized CAP.[8] Telavancin, a new gram-positive agent, which has activity against MRSA, has also been approved for hospital-acquired pneumonia.[9] Daptomcyin is not effective in the treatment of MRSA pneumonia because it is inactivated by surfactant.

Antimicrobial therapy should be administered in the emergency department as quickly as possible in order to avoid delayed treatment, which has been associated with adverse outcomes. If a microbiological etiology is identified, treatment should be narrowed appropriately. In general, patients with CAP should be treated for at least 5 days,[5] with the majority receiving around 7 to 10 days for severe CAP. Treatment can be continued with oral therapy once there has been clinical improvement. While studies on duration of therapy are generally limited, a randomized controlled trial looking at duration of therapy for ventilator-associated pneumonia (VAP) showed that 8 days of therapy were as effective as 15 days of therapy.[10]

URINARY TRACT INFECTIONS

Introduction and Epidemiology

UTI can be a challenging diagnosis and can present as various clinical syndromes ranging from acute

TABLE 39–2 Various urinary clinical syndromes.

Urinary Clinical Syndrome	
Asymptomatic bacteriuria	Significant bacteria in the urine in the absence of symptoms which is not treated
Uncomplicated urinary tract infection	Infection in a structurally and neurologically normal urinary tract
Complicated urinary tract infection	Infection in a urinary tract with functional or structural abnormalities, such as indwelling catheters and calculi
Acute pyelonephritis	Infection of the kidney and renal pelvis
Emphysematous pyelonephritis	Uncommon, severe, necrotizing infection of the kidney in which gas is seen in the renal parenchyma
Prostatitis	Infection or inflammation of the prostate

uncomplicated UTI to acute pyelonephritis, complicated UTI, and prostatitis (Table 39–2). Severe infection and sepsis usually occur in patients with complicated UTI who have functional or structural abnormalities of the urinary tract.[11]

The urinary tract is a common source of sepsis in critically ill patients, ranging from 9% to 30% in different cohorts.[12] Risk factors typically include obstruction or hydronephrosis, and mucosal trauma including presence of indwelling catheters or manipulation of the urogenital tract with surgery. Other studies have shown that older age, female gender, and other comorbidities such as liver cirrhosis and diabetes are risk factors for severe infection.[11]

Pathogenesis

UTIs occur through 3 different mechanisms by which bacteria invade the urinary tract—ascending, hematogenous, lymphatic. The ascending route accounts for the majority of UTIs in women and involves bacterial pathogens that colonize the vagina and periurethral area that ascend to the bladder, for example after vaginal intercourse. The hematogenous route of infection involves seeding of the kidney in the setting of a bloodstream infection. The lymphatic route is uncommon and involves increased pressure in the bladder that directs lymphatic flow toward the kidney.[13]

Microbiology

The majority of UTIs are caused by *Escherichia coli*, isolated in 80% to 85% of episodes of community-acquired infections. In patients with complicated UTI who may have obstructive uropathy or neurogenic bladder, other Enterobacteriaceae such as *Klebsiella* or *Enterobacter* spp., *Pseudomonas* or *Proteus* are more likely to be isolated. Occasionally, gram-positive organisms such as *Enterococcus* or *Staphylococcus* as well as *Candida* spp. may be isolated, especially in patients with indwelling devices.[11] Renal abscesses have been described in patients with *S aureus* bacteremia and candidemia, presumably as a result of hematogenous infection. Antimicrobial resistance has been increasingly reported in community-acquired UTIs, specifically trimethoprim-sulfamethoxazole and fluoroquinolone resistance. The emergence of extended-spectrum beta-lactamase producing gram-negative organisms in community-acquired UTIs has also been described and renders limited treatment options.[14]

Diagnosis

The diagnosis of UTI can be challenging, especially in patients presenting with signs of sepsis. Patients should have symptoms of a UTI or history suggestive of a urinary source along with a positive urine culture. Symptoms of uncomplicated UTI include dysuria, urinary frequency, urgency, suprapubic pain, hematuria, or fever. Patients who present with symptoms of pyelonephritis may also have nausea, vomiting, flank pain, and concomitant bacteremia along with a positive urine culture. In addition, symptoms consistent with renal colic suggesting ureteral calculus or obstruction are also relevant in addition to history regarding recent urologic intervention, indwelling ureteral catheter, or presence of ureteral devices such as stents and nephrostomy tubes.[11]

Physical examination should assess for costovertebral angle tenderness, hematuria, or presence of an indwelling device.[11] A clean catch urine sample should be sent for urinalysis and urine culture, and a positive urine culture is required for diagnosis of a urinary tract infection. Urine and blood cultures should be sent prior to administration of antimicrobial therapy, otherwise culture data may be falsely negative. If a patient has an indwelling urinary catheter in place, the urine sample should be sampled through the catheter port using aseptic technique or obtained from a freshly placed catheter, to avoid contamination of the urine sample. Typically, patients with a urinary source of infection have a single uropathogen isolated with greater than 10^5 colony-forming units/mL. A blood culture isolate with similar susceptibilities as the urine culture typically confirms a urinary source of infection. Urinalysis with pyuria alone is not helpful in making the diagnosis of symptomatic UTI as often times pyuria, accompanies asymptomatic bacteriuria, is present after an urologic procedure or in the presence of a urinary catheter. Imaging of the kidneys and bladder is helpful to identify structural abnormalities that may require source control, such as a perinephric abscess or emphysematous pyelonephritis that may require drainage or obstruction that may require decompression.[1]

Management

Antimicrobial therapy and source control should guide the management of critically ill patients with sepsis due to UTI. For pyelonephritis requiring hospitalization, the IDSA guidelines recommend an intravenous fluoroquinolone with renal excretion such as levofloxacin or ciprofloxacin, an extended-spectrum cephalosporin (ceftriaxone, cefepime, ceftazidime), piperacillin-tazobactam, or a carbapenem.[15] Local resistance data should be used to guide choice about initial therapy; for example, if fluoroquinolone resistance is known to be high, an extended-spectrum cephalosporin may be preferred. If there is a history of health care exposure or extended-spectrum beta-lactamase–producing organisms, then a carbapenem would be considered the drug of choice. Antibiotics should be administered rapidly, as this has previously been shown to improve outcomes in both severe UTI and sepsis.[12]

If a complicating factor in the urinary tract is identified, source control is warranted. In the management of an obstruction for example, decompression with percutaneous nephrostomy may be necessary; a large abscess may require drainage. In emphysematous pyelonephritis, initial percutaneous drainage is recommended with antimicrobial therapy, followed by nephrectomy if needed after the patient is stabilized.[11]

Antibiotics should be narrowed based on urine culture and susceptibilities and can be transitioned to oral therapy once the patient has clinically improved. Traditionally, antibiotics for a 10- to 14-day course have been recommended for pyelonephritis and complicated UTI. However, recent data show that shorter courses of 7 days of treatment for acute pyelonephritis is equivalent to longer courses[16] and the European Urology guidelines have recommended 3 to 5 days following defervescence and control of the complicating factor.[11] Treatment for acute bacterial prostatitis or abscess may require longer courses.

INTRA-ABDOMINAL INFECTIONS

Introduction and Epidemiology

IAIs represent a diverse group of infections and are a common source of sepsis in patients hospitalized in the ICU. Mortality rates range from 30% to greater than 50% in patients with increased severity of illness at presentation and organ dysfunction.[17]

Pathogenesis

IAIs refer to the invasion of enteric bacteria into the wall of a hollow viscus. There are 2 types of IAI—uncomplicated or complicated. An uncomplicated IAI refers to an inflammatory process confined to the wall of an abdominal organ. It can often times be managed with surgical resection and perioperative antibiotic prophylaxis alone, that is, cholecystitis and appendicitis.[18] A complicated IAI extends beyond the organ through a perforated viscus, into the peritoneal cavity. It is associated with peritonitis and/or the formation of an abscess.[19]

Microbiology

The microbiology of the gastrointestinal (GI) tract is complex and contains a wide variety of gram-positive, gram-negative, and anaerobic organisms. In the oral cavity, gram-positive cocci harbor the mouth and oropharynx, but in the distal small intestine gram-negative organisms begin to predominate. Bacterial colony counts increase further down in the GI tract, with the largest colony counts being in the colon, with a predominance of anaerobic organisms. Most IAI are therefore usually polymicrobial in nature. Often times, all organisms may not be identified in the laboratory, especially anaerobes. The most common organism isolated in patients with community-acquired intraabdominal infections is *E coli*, followed by other Enterobacteriaceae, such as *Klebsiella* and *Enterobacter*. Typically gram-positive organisms, such as *Enterococcus*, are seen in patients with nosocomial infection or in patients who are immunocompromised or have previously received broad-spectrum antibiotics or cephalosporins.[20] Anaerobic organisms most frequently isolated include members of the *Bacteroides* family. Those patients who have a prolonged exposure to antimicrobial therapy often develop colonization and subsequent infection with other organisms such as *Pseudomonas* or *Candida* spp., and may develop infection with multidrug-resistant organisms such as multidrug-resistant *Acinetobacter* or vancomycin-resistant *Enterococcus faecium*.[19]

Clinical Presentation

The clinical presentation of IAI varies widely depending on location of the infection within the GI tract. In critically ill patients, the diagnosis can be especially difficult to make, given that history and physical examination may be limited in a sedated patient. Nonetheless, key history, physical examination, and laboratory and imaging findings together are essential to localizing intra-abdominal infection (Table 39–3).

Management

Management of IAIs is critical, especially in complicated IAI where morbidity and mortality are high in the ICU. Appropriate management involves both a

TABLE 39–3 Clinical manifestations of various intra-abdominal infections.[21,22]

	Pathogenesis	History	Physical Examination	Diagnosis	Management Options
Appendicitis	Obstruction of the appendiceal lumen, resulting in ischemia and inflammation	Vague periumbilical pain that migrates to right lower quadrant	Tenderness with localized peritonitis Pain with flexion and internal rotation of R hip (obturator sign) Pain with passive extension of R hip (Psoas sign) Pain in RLQ with palpation of LLQ (Rovsing sign)	Leukocytosis with left shift CT scan with contrast	Appendectomy (laparoscopic vs open) Antibiotics (in cases with phlegmon) Percutaneous drainage and antibiotics in patients with appendiceal abscess
Cholecystitis	Calculous obstruction of the cystic duct or acalculous inflammation of the biliary tree in critically ill patients	RUQ pain, nausea, vomiting, fever; more subtle in acalculous presentation	RUQ tenderness with tenderness on inspiration (Murphy sign)	Leukocytosis, mild elevation of LFTs Ultrasound of RUQ shows thickened GB wall, pericholecystic fluid, sonographic Murphy sign	Cholecystectomy (laparoscopic or open) Percutaneous cholecystostomy as temporizing measure in poor surgical candidates
Cholangitis	Obstruction and stasis leading to bacteria ascending to the biliary tract	Charcot triad of fever, RUQ pain, jaundice	Fevers with rigors, RUQ tenderness, hypotension/sepsis	Increased total and direct bilirubin	Antibiotics and decompression of biliary system
Pancreatitis	Inflammation of the pancreas either mechanical (ie, gallstones, ERCP) or systemic (EtOH, medication-related, increased calcium, increased triglycerides)	Central upper abdominal pain, associated with nausea/vomiting, radiating to the back	Epigastric tenderness	Elevated serum amylase/lipase CT with contrast to assess for local complications or severity/necrosis	Fluid resuscitation/nutritional supplementation Systemic antibiotics and drainage/debridement in infected necrosis only
Diverticulitis	Acute inflammation of a diverticulum; can lead to perforation causing complicated disease	Pain in the lower abdomen; history of prior episodes	Pain in the LLQ or suprapubic tenderness	CT with contrast	Antibiotics and bowel rest for uncomplicated disease Drainage for abscess Sigmoid colectomy rare but may be needed in complicated disease

(Continued)

TABLE 39–3 Clinical manifestations of various intra-abdominal infections.[21,22] (*Continued*)

	Pathogenesis	History	Physical Examination	Diagnosis	Management Options
Primary peritonitis	Not directly related to another intra-abdominal infection, ie, bacterial translocation in spontaneous bacterial peritonitis	Pain and fever, eg, in patients with cirrhosis/ ascites	Diffuse abdominal tenderness with rebound; may be more subtle in some patients, ie, patients on steroids	Elevated WBC count of ascitic fluid (> 250 PMNs) along with Gram stain and culture; typically monomicrobial	Antibiotics
Secondary peritonitis	Perforation of viscus in GI tract; may result in formation of abscess or walled-off cavity	Abdominal pain worse with movement, fever, nausea/ vomiting	High fever, signs of sepsis Significant abdominal tenderness on palpation with rigidity of the abdominal wall produced by guarding, direct and referred rebound tenderness	Free air beneath the diaphragm on CXR; CT scan except in cases where RUQ source is suspected in which case ultrasound may be more helpful Typically polymicrobial	Antibiotics along with source control (see Table 39–5)

CT, computed tomography; CXR, chest x-ray; EtOH, ethyl alcohol; GI, gastrointestinal; LFT, liver function test; LLQ, left lower quadrant; PMN, polymorphonuclear; R, right; RLQ, right lower quadrant; RUQ, right upper quadrant; WBC, white blood cell.

combination of source control and appropriate antimicrobial therapy.

Source control refers to the concept of mechanical control of the source of infection, the elimination of ongoing contamination, and ultimately restoration of anatomy and function. In uncomplicated IAI, source control is sufficient to control infection and prevent development of complications, for example, an appendectomy. In complicated IAI, drainage or debridement along with a 5- to 7-day course of antimicrobials may be required. Drainage is used in the setting of an abscess and is commonly performed percutaneously using imaging. Surgical debridement is required in the setting of infected necrotic tissue.

Initial appropriate antimicrobial therapy is critical and has been shown to be associated with clinical outcome.[23] Empiric antimicrobial therapy should be directed against both aerobic and anaerobic gram-negative and gram-positive bacteria. Recommended empiric therapy includes a beta-lactam/beta-lactamase inhibitor such as piperacillin/tazobactam, a third- or fourth-generation cephalosporin with metronidazole, or a carbapenem.[24] Duration of therapy is 5 to 7 days if appropriate source control has been achieved.

NECROTIZING SKIN AND SOFT TISSUE INFECTIONS

Introduction and Epidemiology

NSTIs refer to the process of soft tissue necrosis secondary to toxin-secreting bacteria, and were first described by Hippocrates in 500 BC. During the Civil War, NSTI were further reported as "hospital gangrene" and noted to have high mortality rate. Since then, the pathogenesis of NSTI has been further described but is still associated with a high mortality rate anywhere from 25% to 35%.[25] Approximately 500 to 1500 cases have been described per year in the United States. Fournier gangrene is a variant of NSTI involving the penis, scrotum, or vulva. Risk factors such as diabetes mellitus, peripheral vascular disease, intravenous drug use, and other immunocompromising factors such as HIV and malignancy have been associated with NSTI.[25]

Pathogenesis and Microbiology

NSTI is typically described as 2 types, type I and type II. Type I infections are monomicrobial and are caused by streptococci or clostridia species, and type

II infections are polymicrobial. Other organisms associated with NSTI in specific clinical situations include *Vibrio vulnificus*, *Aeromonas hydrophila*, and MRSA. Necrosis of the fascial and muscle layers is caused by exotoxin production of these pathogens and results in a rapid progression of infection and cytokine production causing septic shock.[26]

Diagnosis

The diagnosis of NSTI can be challenging; initial skin findings can vary from skin discoloration or cellulitis to gangrene or necrosis. Symptoms progress quickly and are usually associated with ecchymosis, blisters or bullae, edema, crepitus, or necrosis. Pain may be out of proportion to what is seen on physical examination, and there may be a hard, wooden feel to the subcutaneous tissues. Systemic findings include fever and signs of sepsis such as tachycardia and hypotension. Laboratory examination is significant for a leukocytosis with left shift, electrolyte disturbances such as acidosis and elevated creatine kinase. Radiologic findings include soft tissue stranding or edema in the deep fascial layers and the presence of gas is highly specific. Frozen section biopsy can also be done to confirm diagnosis of NSTI. If clinical suspicion is high for NSTI, early surgical evaluation is indicated.[25]

Management

NSTI is considered a surgical emergency and requires aggressive resuscitation along with surgical debridement and broad-spectrum antibiotics. Surgical debridement of all necrotic tissue is paramount and should be done as early as possible in order to improve outcome. Antimicrobial therapy serves as an adjunct to source control and should cover gram-positive, gram-negative aerobic and anaerobic organisms. Initially, empiric coverage includes a broad-spectrum beta-lactam such as piperacillin-tazobactam or carbapenem along with empiric vancomycin. In streptococcal toxic shock syndrome or necrotizing fasciitis caused by group A streptococci, therapy should be penicillin along with clindamycin, which is added for suppression of streptococcal toxin and cytokine production. Antimicrobial therapy should be continued until operative treatment is no longer needed and there has been clinical improvement without fever for 42 to 78 hours.[27] Close monitoring in the ICU is important in order to provide supportive care with fluid resuscitation and optimal nutritional support.

INFECTIVE ENDOCARDITIS

Introduction and Epidemiology

IE remains relatively uncommon and affects about 10,000 to 15,000 people annually.[28] Men are affected more commonly and the median age of patients with IE is greater than 60. Common reasons for admission to the ICU include the development of congestive heart failure, septic shock, and neurologic deterioration.[29]

Pathogenesis

The pathogenesis of IE involves initial damage to the endothelial surface of the valve, followed by platelet and fibrin deposition. This allows bacteria to subsequently adhere to the valve surface and produce disease at a lower inoculum.[30] Typical risk factors for IE include rheumatic heart disease, injection drug use, degenerative valve disease, prosthetic devices, and immunosuppression.[29]

Microbiology

IE can be caused by several organisms, but is usually associated with *S aureus* and streptococci infection. *S aureus* is the most common cause of IE in the developed world, and is frequently associated with health care–associated infection. The streptococci make up a wide variety of organisms, but the viridans group streptococci are the most common pathogens associated with endocarditis, followed by *Enterococcus* and *Streptococcus bovis*. Coagulase-negative staphylococci, such as *Staphylococcus lugdunensis* have also increasingly been described. The HACEK organisms, *Haemophilus* spp., *Aggregatibacter* spp., *Cardiobacterium* spp., *Eikenella corrodens*, and *Kingella*, have been associated with culture-negative endocarditis, although sterile blood cultures in the setting of endocarditis can be due to several different factors.[30] Lastly, organisms other than bacteria, such as fungi, can also be a rare cause of endocarditis, the most common of which is *Candida* spp.[29]

Diagnosis

The diagnosis of IE involves pathologic diagnosis on examination of the valve or the presence of major or minor criteria as described by the modified Duke criteria (Table 39–4). Blood cultures are critical to the diagnosis and 3 sets should be obtained in the first 24 hours. If the patient received antibiotics previously, more blood cultures may be required. Echocardiography is central to the diagnosis of IE, and transesophageal echocardiography (TEE) is more sensitive than transthoracic echocardiography (TTE).

TABLE 39–4 Modified Duke criteria.

Definite infective endocarditis
Pathologic criteria
• Microorganisms demonstrated by culture or histologic examination of vegetation or intracardiac abscess or • Pathologic lesions: vegetation or intracardiac abscess confirmed by histologic examination
Clinical criteria
• 2 major criteria or • 1 major criterion and 3 minor criteria or • 5 minor criteria
Possible IE
• 1 major criterion and 1 minor criterion or • 3 minor criteria
Rejected
Firm alternative diagnosis explaining evidence of IE Resolution of IE syndrome with antibiotic therapy for ≤ 4 d No pathologic evidence of IE at surgery or autopsy with antibiotic therapy for ≤ 4 d
Major criteria
Blood culture positive for IE—typical microorganisms from 2 separate blood cultures Echocardiography positive for IE
Minor criteria
Predisposing heart condition or IDU
Fever greater than 38°C
Vascular phenomena, ie, arterial emboli, mycotic aneurysm, conjunctival or intracranial hemorrhage
Immunologic phenomena, ie, glomerulonephritis, Osler nodes, Roth spots
Microbiological evidence not meeting criteria above or serologic evidence of active infection

A good-quality TTE with a low clinical suspicion usually excludes the diagnosis of IE. However in cases where there is high clinical suspicion and TTE is negative or a suboptimal examination, TEE may be required. Occasionally repeat TEE after 7 to 10 days is needed to reassess for a vegetation in the setting of an initial negative examination.

Clinical Manifestations

Patients present with fever and other nonspecific symptoms, such as anorexia, weight loss, and malaise, especially in subacute cases. On examination, an audible heart murmur is heard about 85% of the time.[30] Other findings on physical examination include splinter hemorrhages (linear streaks in the fingernails or toenails), conjuctival petechiae, Osler nodes (small, painful nodular lesions on pads of fingers or toes), Janeway lesions (macular, painless plaques seen on palms or soles), and Roth spots (retinal lesions surrounded by hemorrhage).

The most common complication of IE is severe valvular regurgitation or heart failure. Major embolic phenomena are the second most common complication and may reflect the initial clinical presentation. Splenic emboli with infarction may cause left upper quadrant abdominal pain and renal infarction may present with hematuria. Renal abscess or glomerulonephritis may also be seen in the setting of IE. Mycotic aneurysms, or direct bacterial invasion or immune complex deposition in the arterial wall, can be seen in cerebral vessels or in the abdominal aorta. Neurologic complications are a common cause of initial ICU admission and include ischemic cerebrovascular accident (CVA), cerebral hemorrhage, or brain abscess. Right-sided IE may present as pulmonary embolism or infarction.[30] Anemia is almost always seen and erythrocyte sedimentation rate (ESR) is usually elevated, although laboratory parameters are not diagnostic.[29]

Management

American Heart Association (AHA) and IDSA guidelines include recommended pathogen-guided antimicrobial therapy for IE, as listed in Table 39–5.[31] Surgical indications in IE include heart failure not responsive to medical therapy, severe aortic or mitral regurgitation, endocarditis due to highly resistant

TABLE 39–5 Management of native-valve endocarditis.

Organism	Susceptibility Testing	Treatment Options	Duration	Comments
Staphylococcus aureus	Oxacillin-susceptible	Nafcillin	6 wk	Addition of gentamicin no longer routinely recommended given nephrotoxicity[32]
		Cefazolin	6 wk	
	Oxacillin-resistant	Vancomycin	6 wk	
		Daptomycin	6 wk	Approved for right-sided endocarditis
Streptococcal IE (ie, viridans group *Streptococcus* or *Streptococcus bovis*)	Penicillin highly susceptible (MIC < 0.12)	Penicillin (PCN)	4 wk	
		Ceftriaxone (CTX)	4 wk	
		PCN/CTX plus gentamicin	2 wk	Selected patients without intracardiac or extracardiac complications and no preexisting renal disease may be given shorter course of combination therapy[28]
Streptococcal IE	Penicillin relatively resistant (MIC 0.12-0.5)	PCN/CTX plus gentamicin	4 wk of PCN/CTX 2 wk of gentamicin	
Streptococcal IE	Penicillin resistant (MIC > 0.5)	Same as *Enterococcus*		
Enterococcus	Penicillin susceptible	Ampicillin or penicillin plus gentamicin (if susceptible)	4-6 wk	No randomized control trials comparing treatments in enterococcal IE; recent data suggest shorter duration of gentamicin may be as effective with less nephrotoxicity[33]
	Penicillin susceptible	Ampicillin plus ceftriaxone	4-6 wk	Recent data suggest this may be an alternative to combined beta-lactam/aminoglycoside therapy, especially in the setting of gentamicin resistance[33]
	Penicillin resistance	Vancomycin plus gentamicin	6 wk	
	Penicillin resistance/ vancomycin resistance	Daptomycin or linezolid	6 wk	Should be done in consultation with infectious disease specialist given side effects associated with prolonged therapy and cardiac valve replacement may be necessary[31]
HACEK		Ceftriaxone	4 wk	
		Ampicillin-sulbactam	4 wk	
		Ciprofloxacin	4 wk	

organisms or persistent bacteremia, perivalvular infection with abscess, recurrent emboli or persistent vegetations, and large, mobile vegetations greater than 10 mm.[28]

REFERENCES

1. Sligl WI, Marrie TJ. Severe community-acquired pneumonia. *Crit Care Clin.* 2013;29(3):563-601.
2. Donowitz GR. Acute pneumonia. *Mandell, Douglas and Bennett's Principles and Practice of Infectious Diseases.* 7th ed. 2010, Philadelphia, PA: Churchill Livingstone/Elsevier.
3. Torres A, Peetermans WE, Viegi G, Blasi F. Risk factors for community-acquired pneumonia in adults in Europe: a literature review. *Thorax.* 2013;68:1057-1065.
4. Wunderink RG. How important is methicillin-resistant Staphylococcus aureus as a cause of community-acquired pneumonia and what is best antimicrobial therapy? *Infect Dis Clin North Am.* 2013;2(1):177-188.
5. Mandell LA, Wundering RG, Anzueto A, et al. Infectious Diseases Society of America/American Thoracic Society Consensus guidelines on the management of community-acquired pneumonia in adults. *Clin Infect Dis.* 2007;44:S27-S72.
6. Rellos J. Demographics, guidelines, and clinical experience in severe community-acquired pneumonia. *Crit Care.* 2008;12(suppl 6):S2.
7. Wunderink RG, Niederman MS, Kollef MH, et al. Linezolid in methicillin-resistant Staphylococcus aureus nosocomial pneumonia: a randomized, controlled study. *Clin Infect Dis.* 2012;54(5):621-629.
8. File TM, Jr, Low DE, Eckburg PB, et al. Integrated analysis of FOCUS 1 and FOCUS 2: randomized, doubled-blinded, multicenter phase 3 trials of the efficacy and safety of ceftaroline fosamil versus ceftriaxone in patients with CAP. *Clin Infect Dis.* 2010;51(12):1395-1405.
9. Rubinstein E, Lalani T, Corey GR, et al; the ATTAIN study group. Telavancin versus vancomycin for hospital-acquired pneumonia due to gram-positive pathogens. *Clin Infect Dis.* 2011;52(1):31-40.
10. Chastre J, Wolff M, Fagon JY, et al. Comparison of 8 vs 15 days of antibiotic therapy for ventilator-associated pneumonia in adults: a randomized trial. *JAMA.* 2003;290(19):2588-2598.
11. Nicolle LE. Urinary tract infection. *Crit Care Clin.* 2013;29:699-715.
12. Wagenlehner FM, Lichtenstern C, Rolfes C, et al. Diagnosis and management for urosepsis. *Int J Urol.* 2013;20:963-970.
13. Sobel JD, Kaye D. Urinary tract infections. *Mandell, Douglas and Bennett's Principles and Practice of Infectious Diseases.* 7th ed. 2010, Philadelphia, PA: Churchill Livingstone/Elsevier.
14. Meier S, Weber R, Zbinden R, Ruef C, Hasse B. Extended-spectrum B-lactamase-producing gram-negative pathogens in community-acquired urinary tract infections: an increasing challenge for antimicrobial therapy. *Infection.* 2011;39(4):333-340.
15. Gupta K, Hooton TM, Naber KG, et al. International clinical practice guidelines for the treatment of acute uncomplicated cystitis and pyelonephritis in women: a 2010 update by the Infectious Disease Society of America and the European Society for Microbiology and Infectious Diseases. *Clin Infect Dis.* 2011;52(5):e103-e120.
16. Eliakim-Raz N, Yahav D, Paul M, Leibovici L. Duration of antibiotic treatment for acute pyelonephritis and septic urinary tract infection—7 days or less versus longer treatment: systematic review and meta-analysis of randomized controlled trials. *J Antimicrob Chemother.* 2013;68:2183-2191.
17. Marshall J, Innes M. Intensive care unit management of intra-abdominal infection. *Crit Care Med.* 2003;31(8):2228-2237.
18. Blot S, De Waele JJ. Critical issues in the clinical management of complicated intra-abdominal infections. *Drugs.* 2005;65(12):1611-1620.
19. Mazuski JE, Solomkin JS. Intra-abdominal infections. *Surg Clin North Am.* 2009;89:421-437.
20. Solomkin JS, Mazuski J. Intra-abdominal sepsis: newer interventional and antimicrobial therapies. *Infect Dis Clin N Am.* 2009;23:593-608.
21. Fagenholz PJ, de Moya MA. Acute inflammatory surgical disease. *Surg Clin North Am.* 2014;94:1-30.
22. Intra-abdominal infection. *Mandell, Douglas and Bennett's Principles and Practice of Infectious Diseases.* 7th ed. 2010, Philadelphia, PA: Churchill Livingstone/Elsevier.
23. Krobot K, Yin D, Zhang Q, et al. Effect of inappropriate initial empiric antibiotic therapy on outcome of patients with community-acquired intra-abdominal infections requiring surgery. *Eur J Clin Microbiol Infect Dis.* 2004;23:682-687.
24. Pieracci FM, Barie PS. Intra-abdominal infections. *Curr Opin Crit Care.* 2007;13:440-449.

25. Hussein QA, Anaya DA. Necrotizing soft tissue infections. *Crit Care Clin*. 2013;29:795-806.

26. Kaafarani HM, King DR. Necrotizing skin and soft tissue infections. *Surg Clin North Am*. 2014;94:155-163.

27. Stevens DL, Bisno AL, Chambers HF, et al. Practice guidelines for the diagnosis and management of skin and soft tissue infections: 2014 update by the Infectious Diseases Society of America. *Clin Infect Dis*. 2014;59(2):e10-e52.

28. Chopra T, Kaatz GW. Treatment strategies for infective endocarditis. *Expert Opin Pharmacother*. 2010;11(3):345-360.

29. Keynan Y, Singal R, Kumar K, Arora R, Rubinstein E. Infective endocarditis in the intensive care unit. *Crit Care Clin*. 2013;29:923-951.

30. Endocarditis and intravascular infections. *Mandell, Douglas and Bennett's Principles and Practice of Infectious Diseases*. 7th ed. 2010, Philadelphia, PA: Churchill Livingstone/Elsevier.

31. Baddour L, Wilson WR, Bayer AS, et al. Infective endocarditis: diagnosis, antimicrobial therapy, and management of complications. *Circulation*. 2005;111:e394-e434.

32. Cosgrove SE, Vigliani GA, Campion M, et al. Initial low-dose gentamicin for Staphylococcus aureus bacteremia and endocarditis is nephrotoxic. *Clin Infect Dis*. 2009;48(6):713-721.

33. Dahl A, Bruun NE. *Enterococcal faecalis* infective endocarditis: focus on clinical aspects. *Expert Rev Cardiovasc Ther*. 2013;11(9):1247-1257.

Health Care–Associated Infections

40

Subani Chandra, MD and David Chong, MD

KEY POINTS

1 Health care–associated infections (HCAIs) contribute significantly to morbidity and mortality, and health care costs.

2 The most frequent HAIs are catheter-related bloodstream infections (CRBSIs), ventilator-associated pneumonias (VAPs), infections with *Clostridium difficile*, surgical site infections (SSIs), and catheter-associated urinary tract infections (CAUTIs).

3 Major preventive strategies to reduce CRBSIs include optimal catheter site selection; proper hand hygiene; maximal barrier precautions at the time of insertion; chlorhexidine skin antisepsis, use of chlorhexidine-impregnated dressings, or use of antiseptic or antimicrobial-coated catheters; tunneled insertion; catheter site care and limited manipulation of the catheter; and daily review of line necessity and prompt removal of unnecessary lines.

4 The most common causes for VAPs are aerobic gram-negative bacilli such as *Pseudomonas aeruginosa, Klebsiella pneumoniae,* and *Acinetobacter* species and less commonly gram-positive organisms such as *Staphylococcus aureus.*

5 *C difficile* can cause a wide range of disease from asymptomatic infection in a silent carrier state to fulminant disease associated with severe sepsis and death.

6 Essential elements of the SSI bundle include appropriate use of prophylactic antibiotics; appropriate hair removal, controlled postoperative serum glucose in patients after cardiac surgery, and immediate postoperative normothermia in patients with colorectal surgery.

7 The single most significant risk factor for a CAUTI is the prolonged use of the urinary catheter.

INTRODUCTION

HCAIs, particularly those acquired in a critical care setting contribute significantly to morbidity and mortality, and health care costs. Critically ill patients have more comorbid diagnoses and higher severity of acute illness making them particularly susceptible to new infections while hospitalized. Indwelling catheters and increasing prevalence of multidrug-resistant (MDR) pathogens add to the risk and negative consequences of HCAIs. One in 20 patients acquires a HCAI while receiving medical care.[1] The most frequent HCAIs include bloodstream infections (BSIs), VAPs, infections with *C difficile*, SSIs, and CAUTIs.

Bloodstream Infections

BSIs or bacteremias remain common in hospitalized patients both within the intensive care units (ICUs) and in hospital wards. About 90% of these BSIs are associated with a catheter in the bloodstream, usually a central line.[2] CRBSIs are considered a preventable cause of morbidity and mortality and are a target of interventions aimed at improving quality of health care and cost-effectiveness.

Risk Factors and Microbiology

Central lines are at risk for infection both during the process of insertion and subsequent access and maintenance. Factors associated with a lower incidence of CRBSIs include the following:

- Optimal catheter site selection (subclavian vs internal jugular, or femoral veins)
- Use of proper hand hygiene
- Maximal barrier precautions at the time of insertion
- Chlorhexidine skin antisepsis, use of chlorhexidine-impregnated dressings, or use of catheters coated with antiseptic or antimicrobials
- Tunneled insertion
- Catheter site care and limited manipulation of the catheter
- Daily review of line necessity and prompt removal of unnecessary lines

Gram-positive aerobes are the most frequently isolated pathogens from the bloodstream of hospitalized patients. Coagulase-negative staphylococci and S aureus account for just over half of all nosocomial bacteremias (51%). Candida species and enterococci were each responsible for 9% of BSIs. Gram-negative bacteria, including many MDR species, accounted for most of the remainder.[3]

Certain patient populations are at increased risk of CRBSIs and may have greater susceptibility to microbial pathogens not commonly responsible for infections otherwise. Patients receiving intravenous hyperalimentation or high concentrations of glucose via a central line are particularly susceptible to fungal infections especially Candida species. Gram-positive aerobes are the most commonly isolated pathogens from the bloodstream of patients who receive hemodialysis. Immunocompromised hosts, especially those who are neutropenic or receiving chemotherapy may translocate microbes from their gut into the bloodstream and therefore have a disproportionately high rate of infection with gram-negative bacilli. Burn victims are particularly susceptible to infections due to Pseudomonas species.

Diagnosis

The diagnosis of CRBSI is based on clinical criteria and microbiological confirmation. The clinical symptoms and signs of CRBSI can be protean and need not include typical indicators of infection such as fever, especially in critically ill patients. A high degree of suspicion should be maintained in a patient with a central line and clinical changes. Positive blood cultures in the absence of other identifiable source of infection suggest a CRBSI. Proper specimen collection prior to initiation of antimicrobial therapy and repeat sampling can help increase the yield of microbial cultures. Positive cultures taken from a peripheral site have the highest specificity; cultures drawn from the catheter have a high false-positive rate but excellent negative predictive value.

Treatment

Once CRBSI is confirmed, the treatment is focused on catheter management and antimicrobial treatment. In critically ill patients with a CRBSI and signs of sepsis or hemodynamic instability, the catheter should be removed promptly. Additionally, clinical practice guidelines recommend catheter removal if there is endocarditis or persistent bacteremia after 72 hours of appropriate antibiotic treatment, or fungemia.[4] Catheter removal is also recommended in cases of infection with most organisms encountered in critical care settings: S aureus, gram-negative bacilli (including Pseudomonas), mycobacteria, and low-virulence organisms such as Bacillus species or Propionibacterium.

Infrequently, salvage of long-term catheters with systemic antimicrobial therapy with or without an antibiotic lock may be attempted if none of the criteria for removal are met. Similarly, in a patient without sepsis or hemodynamic instability, a catheter may be exchanged over a guidewire if the risks of catheter reinsertion are considered to be unacceptably high. However, it is important to note that the success rate of these strategies is low and unpredictable and the data supporting catheter exchange are sparse and present only in small, uncontrolled studies.

Empiric antimicrobial therapy for CRBSIs usually includes antibiotics to cover resistant gram-positive organisms including *S aureus*, such as vancomycin. Additionally, empiric therapy should be tailored to the patient, based on host risk factors and susceptibility to certain infections as discussed earlier. Antimicrobial therapy should be reassessed and narrowed based on microbiological profile as soon as culture results are available.

Typical duration of antimicrobial therapy in uncomplicated CRBSI is 10 to 14 days from the first day blood cultures turned negative. In suspected or confirmed endocarditis, treatment is usually continued for 4 to 6 weeks.

Follow-Up and Outcomes

After initiation of antimicrobial therapy, patients with BSIs should be followed closely and monitored with surveillance cultures until the bacteremia or fungemia resolves. Persistently positive cultures or lack of clinical improvement should prompt investigation of the causes of treatment failure: inappropriate antimicrobial therapy, failure to remove the catheter, or development of an associated complication such as a persistent secondary source of infection or a septic focus, endocarditis, or suppurative thrombophlebitis.

CRBSIs are associated with increased hospital length of stay and costs and have an associated mortality of 25%.[5] Every effort should be made to prevent CRBSIs.

Pneumonia

Definitions

Hospital-acquired pneumonia (HAP) is defined as a pneumonia that occurs 48 hours or more after hospital admission that did not exist at the time of admission. VAP is defined as a pneumonia that occurs 48 hours after intubation and institution of mechanical ventilation. Health care–associated pneumonia (HCAP) includes pneumonia that occurs within 48 hours of hospital admission in patients who were hospitalized for 2 or more days within 90 days of the infection, or resided in a nursing home or long-term care facility, or received recent intravenous antibiotic therapy, chemotherapy or wound care within the past 30 days, or attended a hospital or hemodialysis clinic.

Ventilator-associated event (VAE) is a recent surveillance definition developed by the Centers for Disease Control and Prevention (CDC) to create a more objective and systematic way of measuring VAPs. VAEs may not represent true clinical VAPs. In the VAE algorithm there are sequential tiers. The first tier is ventilator-associated condition (VAC) defined as an increase in the fraction of inspired oxygen (FIO_2) of 0.20 for 2 or more days or an increase in positive end-expiratory pressure (PEEP) of greater than or equal to 3 cm H_2O for 2 days after 2 or more days of stable or decreasing daily minimal values. Tier two is infection-related ventilator-associated condition (IVAC) which includes VAC plus a temperature greater than 38°C or less than 36°C or white blood cell count greater than or equal to 12,000 or less than or equal to 4000 cells/mm^3, and initiation of a new antimicrobial agent that is continued for 4 or more days. The third tier is for patients that meet the IVAC definition and have purulent secretions (defined as $\geq$ 25 neutrophils and $\leq$ 10 squamous epithelial cells per low power field) or have a positive sputum or other specimen culture, for a designation of possible VAP. Qualification as a probable VAP does not allow use of sputum, instead the patient must have purulent secretions and a positive quantitative or semiquantitative aspirate or lavage or biopsy, or in the absence of purulent secretions, a positive pleural culture, lung pathology, or diagnostic serology for virus or *Legionella*.[6] Note that the CDC VAE definitions exclude chest radiographs due to their subjectivity and variability in their technique, interpretation, and reporting.

Epidemiology

HAP is the second most common nosocomial infection in the United States and accounts for up to 16% of all hospital-acquired infections (HAIs) and up to 27% of HAIs in the ICU.[7] HAPs can increase hospital stays up to 9 days and cost as much as $40,000 per patient. VAP can occur in 9% to 26% of all intubated patients. Attributable mortality ranges from 0% to 50%. In 2002, an estimated 250,000 HAPs developed in US hospitals and 36,000 of these were associated with deaths.[6] Major risk factors for HAP include age more than 70, underlying chronic lung disease, immunosuppression, prolonged intubation, enteral feeding, and prior thoracoabdominal surgery.

Pathogenesis

The common causes of VAPs are microaspiration of oropharyngeal organisms, inhalation of aerosols containing bacteria, infected biofilm in the endotracheal tube with subsequent embolization to the distal airways, and less commonly hematogenous spread via infected intravenous catheters and gut translocation. Aspiration is the most common cause of HAP and VAP in hospitalized patients with risks that are often increased due to intubation, sedation, and bacterial colonization of the oropharynx with gram-negative organisms. Intubated patients are at the highest risk for VAP due to the common use of sedation, reduced cough, and the leakage of oropharyngeal contents and organisms around the high volume, low-pressure cuffs of the endotracheal tube, as well as the formation of a biofilm and subsequent colonization with bacteria. The risk of pneumonia increases each day the patient is intubated and can be as high as 3% for the first 5 days, 2% from days 5 to 10, and 1% per day afterward. The most common causes for HAP/HCAP/VAP are aerobic gram-negative bacilli such as *P aeruginosa, K pneumoniae,* and *Acinetobacter* species and less commonly gram-positive organisms such as *S aureus.* Anaerobes are an uncommon cause of VAP. Early-onset VAP occurs within 96 hours of admission, is usually caused by antibiotic-sensitive bacteria, and has a more favorable prognosis. Late-onset VAP occurs after 96 of ICU admission and is commonly caused by MDR pathogens. Risk factors for MDR pathogens include immunosuppression, prior antibiotic use, HCAP risk factors, and high frequency of resistance in the community or hospital unit.

Diagnosis

The diagnosis of HAP or VAP can be challenging. The clinical approach includes a chest radiograph that shows a new infiltrate plus at least 2 of the following features: temperature greater than 38°C or less than 36°C, leukocytosis greater than 12,000 or leukopenia less than 4000 cells/mm³, and purulent secretions. As opposed to the VAE surveillance criteria, chest radiographs are clinically recommended to assess for the severity of pneumonia (such as multilobar involvement), and to detect complications like pleural effusion, cavitation, and pneumothorax. Given the high sensitivity but very low specificity of

this approach as well as the emergence of more MDR pathogens and the polymicrobial nature of HAPs and VAPs, the search for the causative organism(s) should be attempted with blood cultures and semi-quantitative sputum cultures prior to the start of empiric antibiotics. Furthermore, if available and logistically possible the ideal approach is a quantitative sampling of the lower respiratory tract with an endotracheal aspirate, bronchoalveolar lavage (BAL), or protected brush sampling. The diagnostic thresholds for BAL are 10^4 to 10^5 CFU/mL, and for protected brush sample 10^3 CFU/mL. A diagnostic thoracentesis should be performed if the pleural effusion is large or if the patient appears toxic. The Clinical Pulmonary Infection Score (CPIS) includes temperature, white blood cell count, tracheal secretions, oxygenation (PaO_2/FiO_2), chest radiography, and microbiological data. A score of greater than or equal to 6 suggests pneumonia and a score less than 6 suggests that antibiotics can be safely discontinued. However, due to the overall low sensitivity and specificity of the CPIS it has not been widely used clinically to diagnose VAP. Procalcitonin (PCT) is a biomarker that has been studied in hospitalized as well as outpatients to help diagnose sepsis and pneumonia. It has shown to have a high specificity for bacterial infections rather than for viral infections. Unfortunately, PCT is elevated in many noninfectious inflammatory disorders such as burns, major surgery, trauma, and pancreatitis, as well as sepsis from any etiology. The use of PCT in the critically ill has yet to be fully realized. There is data suggesting that a very low or a significant decrease in PCT levels can allow for safe and earlier discontinuation of antibiotics.

Treatment

The key decision in the initial empiric antimicrobial treatment of patients with VAP or HAP rests on whether the patient has risk factors for MDR pathogens. If patients have the previously mentioned risk factors or if they have been intubated or in the hospital for more than 96 hours, coverage for MDR pathogens is required. Several studies have showed an increase in mortality by 2- to 3-fold if inappropriate or delayed (> 24 hours) antibiotics are given. The American Thoracic Society/Infectious Diseases Society of America guidelines published in 2005 can

TABLE 40–1 2005 ATS/IDSA guidelines.

Empiric Antibiotic Treatment in Patients With no Known Risk Factors for MDR Pathogens	
Potential Pathogens	**Antibiotics**
Streptococcus pneumoniae *Haemophilus influenzae* Methicillin-sensitive *Staphylococcus aureus* **Antibiotic sensitive enteric GNB** *Escherichia coli* *Klebsiella pneumoniae* *Enterobacter spp* *Proteus spp* *Serratia marcescens*	Ceftriaxone 2 g daily OR Ampicillin-sulbactam 3 g every 6 hours OR Levofloxacin 750 mg daily OR Moxifloxacin 400 mg daily OR Ertapenem 1 g daily
Empiric Antibiotic Treatment in Patients Known Risk Factors for MDR Pathogens	
Potential MDR Pathogens Gram Negatives	**Combination Antibiotics Therapy***
Pseudomonas aeruginosa *Acinetobacter baumannii* **Antibiotic resistant enteric GNB** *Escherichia coli* *Klebsiella pneumoniae* *Enterobacter spp* *Proteus spp* *Serratia marcescens*	**Beta-lactam/beta-lactamase inhibitor** Piperacillin/tazobactam 4.5 g every 6 hours OR **Antipseudomonal cephalosporins** Ceftazidime 2 g every 8 hours Cefepime 2 g every 8 hours OR **Antipseudomonal carbapenems** Imipinem 500 mg every 8 hours Meropenem 1 g every 8 hours PLUS **Antipseudomonal fluoroquinolone** Levofloxacin 750 mg daily Moxifloxacin 400 mg daily Ciprofloxacin 400 mg every 8 hours OR **Aminoglycosides†** Gentamicin 7 mg/kg daily Tobramycin 7 mg/kg daily Amikacin 20 mg/kg daily
Gram positives Methicillin-resistant *Staphylococcus aureus*	PLUS Linezolid 600 mg every 12 hours Vancomycin 15-20 mg/kg every 12 hours‡

*Dosages based on normal renal and hepatic function.
† Trough levels for gentamicin and tobramycin should be < 1µg/ml, and for amikacin, they should be < 4-5 µg/ml.
‡ Trough levels for vancomycin should be 15-20 µg/ml.
Data from American Thoracic Society; Infectious Diseases Society of America: Guidelines for the management of adults with hospital-acquired, ventilator-associated, and healthcare-associated pneumonia, *Am J Respir Crit Care Med* 2005 Feb 15;171(4):388-416.

help with the initial choice of antimicrobial agents and are shown in Table 40–1.

Prevention

General strategies that have been found to influence the risk of VAP include active surveillance for VAP. The Institute for Healthcare Improvement (IHI) endorses the ventilator bundle checklist. Although not all the elements are aimed at VAP prevention, it represents the best practices for patients on mechanical ventilation. The elements include keeping the head of the bed elevated 30° to 45°, daily sedation interruption and assessment of readiness to extubate, daily oral care with chlorhexidine, peptic ulcer disease prophylaxis, and deep venous thrombosis prophylaxis. Another essential element is the emphasis on adherence to the hand hygiene guidelines. Other strategies that appear helpful include using standardized weaning protocols, using non-invasive positive pressure ventilation (NIPPV) whenever possible, educating the staff about VAP prevention, using subglottic drainage (shown to decrease early-onset VAP),[8] changing the ventilator circuit only when visibly soiled or malfunctioning, using a closed in-line suctioning system, and avoiding nasotracheal intubation (which may result is sinusitis that will increase the risk of VAP). However, the most important element of all is the implementation strategy. For such a strategy to be effective it is important to have complete buy-in and accountability of the senior clinical and administrative leadership on the importance of VAP prevention, education of the staff, monitoring of practice, and feedback to all staff on the outcomes, risk factors, and local epidemiology. It is essential to measure the occurrence of VAP as well as compliance with performance measures such as adherence to the ventilator bundle elements and hand hygiene.[9] A checklist is not enough; there must be cultural (adaptive) change to effect true change in practice.

Infection With *C Difficile*

C difficile is the most commonly reported nosocomial pathogen and causes about 12% of HCAIs.[10] The spectrum of disease caused by *C difficile* can range from an asymptomatic carrier state to varying severity of colitis with diarrhea. Both the incidence and severity of *C difficile* infections (CDIs) have increased dramatically since the late 1990s. In North America, the overall incidence of CDI went up 5-fold and the attributable mortality rate has increased 4-fold. Those above the age of 65 are particularly susceptible and the incidence of CDI in the elderly increased 8-fold.[11] In the United States alone, an estimated 500,000 cases of CDI occur annually and about 15,000 to 20,000 patients die from CDI each year.[5]

Risk Factors

The single greatest risk factor for CDI is antibiotic use. Antibiotics disrupt the natural flora in the gut, and this along with high resistance of *C difficile* to the most commonly used antibiotic agents allows *C difficile* to proliferate and CDI to occur. The risk of CDI is higher with the use of multiple antibiotics, broader-spectrum agents, and longer duration of therapy. Almost all antibiotics have been associated with CDI but the risk is highest with clindamycin, broad-spectrum cephalosporins, and fluoroquinolones.

Notably, fluoroquinolone resistance of the NAP1/BI/027 strain is believed to be an important factor in the increased virulence of *C difficile*.

Patients above the age of 65 are at increased risk of severe CDI. Use of gastric acid suppressants (proton pump inhibitors and H_2 receptor blockers) is also a possible risk factor for CDI. Immunosuppressive agents such as methotrexate and the presence of chronic inflammatory bowel disease have also been associated with CDI. Hospitalization or residence in a long-term care facility bring together multiple risk factors for CDI and are therefore responsible for almost all the cases.

Spectrum of Disease

C difficile can cause a wide range of disease in patients: at one end is asymptomatic infection in a silent carrier state, and at the other end, fulminant disease associated with severe sepsis and death.

Asymptomatic carriage: About 20% to 30% of hospitalized patients and 50% of residents of long-term care facilities are silent carriers of *C difficile*. They have no symptoms but serve as a reservoir of infection and can play an important role in transmission of *C difficile*.[12]

C difficile diarrhea (CDAD): This presents as antibiotic-associated diarrhea and is one of the most frequent manifestations of CDI. Systemic symptoms such as fever and leukocytosis are less frequent.

C difficile colitis: This is a more severe form of CDAD and presents with high-volume watery, foul-smelling diarrhea with fever and leukocytosis. Pseudomembranes are not seen.

Pseudomembranous colitis: Diarrhea is more severe and may progress to a protein-losing enteropathy. Fever and leukocytosis are common. Pseudomembranes are seen on sigmoidoscopy.

Fulminant colitis: This is the most serious, life-threatening form of CDI occurring in about 3% of patients. Prolonged ileus, toxic megacolon, colonic perforation, severe sepsis, and death may occur. Diarrhea may be much less prominent due to ileus.

Diagnosis

CDI should be suspected in any patient with diarrhea and antibiotic exposure or another risk factor.

Different methods for laboratory confirmation of CDI are available. A cytotoxin assay that detects the cell toxicity of toxin B is considered the gold standard with a sensitivity of 67% to 100% and a specificity of 85% to 100%.[13] It is a tissue culture test and results can take up to 3 days.

An enzyme-linked immunosorbent assay (ELISA) is also available. While the ELISA is rapid and can provide results within a few hours, it has a relatively low sensitivity (75%-85%) but a high specificity (95%-100%); thus false-negative results are not infrequent.[13] C difficile can be isolated in anaerobic stool culture but cannot distinguish between toxigenic and nontoxigenic strains. Molecular methods such as polymerase chain reaction (PCR) are rapid and sensitive tests for detection of C difficile that are being increasingly used.

Treatment

First-line treatment is based on the severity of CDI. Oral metronidazole is the initial treatment recommended for mild and moderate CDI. Oral vancomycin is superior to metronidazole for treatment for severe CDI. For patients with the most severe form of disease, or complications such as ileus or toxic megacolon, current guidelines recommend treatment with a combination of oral vancomycin and intravenous metronidazole. Surgery with colectomy may be needed as a lifesaving measure in extreme cases. Many newer approaches and antimicrobial agents for the treatment of CDI are under development but none are recommended for routine use at this time. Studies of probiotics aimed at restoring normal gut flora are inconclusive for treatment of CDI. Supportive care and management of fluid status and electrolytes are important adjuncts to treatment of CDI. Antibiotics that may have contributed to the development of CDI should be stopped as soon as possible.

Recurrence

Twenty percent of patients with one episode of CDI develop recurrent infection and 60% of those who have had 2 episodes will develop recurrence. About half of the recurrences are due to new infections and not relapses per se. Persistence of risk factors for CDI and depletion of normal gut flora contribute to recurrence. The first recurrence is treated in a manner similar to the initial episode with metronidazole and/or vancomycin based on the severity of illness. Further recurrences may benefit from a prolonged taper of oral vancomycin. Fecal transplant can help restore normal flora and may be effective in the management of recurrent CDI.

Prevention

Prevention of CDI involves measures targeted at the individual patient and other interventions designed to prevent the spread of C difficile spores within the hospital environment. Judicious use of antibiotics and avoidance of high-risk agents can help reduce the incidence of CDI. Acid suppressants should only be used when clearly indicated.

On a broader scale, containment of C difficile infections within hospital and health care facilities is essential to prevent spread between patients. C difficile is transmitted when spores infect patients via the fecal-oral route. The spores can be transferred between patents via equipment or the hands of health care providers. Rapid and reliable detection of CDI is critical to early isolation of infected patients. Contact precautions with the use of gowns and gloves for all visitors and health care providers should be strictly enforced. Hand washing with soap and water is essential after caring for a patient with CDI since commonly used antimicrobial hand gels are ineffective against spores of C difficile. These spores are hardy and resistant to desiccation, chemicals, and extremes of temperatures. They can survive on surfaces for months. Environmental decontamination should be diligently performed to prevent transmission of CDI.

Surgical Site Infections

SSIs are a very common cause of HCAIs. From 2007 to 2010, SSIs accounted for approximately 23% of all HCAIs.[14] More than 5% of all surgical patients acquire an SSI and many (40%-60%) are preventable.[15] SSIs are classified as being either incisional or organ/space infections. Incisional SSIs are further divided into those involving only skin and subcutaneous tissue (superficial incisional SSI) and those involving deeper soft tissues of the incision (deep incisional SSI). Organ/space SSIs involve any part of the anatomy that was opened or manipulated during an operation, other than incised body wall layers.

Microbiology

S aureus, coagulase-negative staphylococci, *Enterococcus* spp., and *Escherichia coli* remain the most frequently isolated pathogens. An increasing proportion of SSIs are caused by MDR pathogens, such as methicillin-resistant *S aureus* (MRSA), or by *Candida albicans*.

Pathogenesis

Microbial contamination of the surgical site is a necessary precursor of SSI. The risk of SSI can be conceptualized according to the following relationship[16]:

$$\frac{\text{Dose of bacterial contamination} \times \text{virulence}}{\text{Resistance of the host patient}}$$
$$= \text{Risk of surgical site infection}$$

Quantitatively, if a surgical site is contaminated with greater than 10^5 microorganisms per gram of tissue, the risk of SSI is markedly increased. However, the dose of contaminating microorganisms required to produce infection may be much lower when foreign material is present at the site (ie, 100 staphylococci per gram of tissue introduced on silk sutures).

Outcomes

SSIs are associated with considerable morbidity with over one-third of postoperative deaths related, at least in part, to SSIs. SSIs can double the length of time a patient stays in the hospital and thereby can increase the cost of health care.

Prevention

Essential processes for prevention of SSIs are core measures in the Surgical Care Improvement Project: Hospital Compare Hospital Quality Initiatives.[17] The essential elements of the SSI bundle[18] are appropriate use of prophylactic antibiotics; appropriate hair removal, controlled postoperative serum glucose in patients after cardiac surgery, and immediate postoperative normothermia in patients with colorectal surgery.

It is important to standardize the administration process of delivering prophylaxis so that antibiotics can consistently be given within 1 hour prior to incision. Overuse, underuse, improper timing, and misuse of antibiotics occurs in 25% to 50% of operations. A large number of hospitalized patients develop infections caused by *C difficile* and inappropriate use of broad-spectrum antibiotics or prolonged courses of prophylactic antibiotics puts all patients at risk of developing antibiotic-resistant pathogens.

Avoid hair removal unless necessary for the procedure. Razors should never be used and generally shaving should be avoided before surgery. When necessary, hair should be removed with clippers right before surgery—but not in the operating room itself.

Tight glucose control is important in patients who undergo cardiac surgery. Note that "glucose control" here is defined as serum glucose levels below 200 mg/dL, collected at or closest to 6:00 AM on each of the first 2 postoperative days.

The literature indicates that patients undergoing colorectal surgery have a decreased risk of SSI and other complications if they are not allowed to become hypothermic during the perioperative period.[19]

The CDC recommends the following practices as those with the best evidence to minimize the risk of SSIs:

- Whenever possible, identify and treat all infections remote to the surgical site before elective operation and postpone elective operations on patients with remote site infections until the infection has resolved.

- Encourage tobacco cessation. At a minimum, instruct patients to abstain for at least 30 days before elective operation from smoking cigarettes, cigars, pipes, or any other form of tobacco consumption.

- Require patients to shower or bathe with an antiseptic agent on at least the night before the operative day.

- Thoroughly wash and clean at and around the incision site to remove gross contamination before performing antiseptic skin preparation.

- Keep nails short and do not wear artificial nails.

- Perform a preoperative surgical scrub for at least 2 to 5 minutes using an appropriate antiseptic and scrub the hands and forearms up to the elbows.

- Protect an incision that has been closed primarily with a sterile dressing for 24 to 48 hours postoperatively.

- Provide positive pressure ventilation in the operating room with at least 15 air changes per hour, of which 3 should be of fresh air.

- Keep the operating rooms' doors closed and minimize traffic.

- Sterilize all surgical instruments according to published guidelines. Perform flash sterilization only for patient care items that will be used immediately (eg, to reprocess an inadvertently dropped instrument). Do not use flash sterilization for reasons of convenience, as an alternative to purchasing additional instrument sets, or to save time.

- Wear a surgical mask that fully covers the mouth and nose when entering the operating room if an operation is about to begin or already under way, or if sterile instruments are exposed. Wear the mask throughout the operation.

- Wear a cap or hood to fully cover hair on the head and face when entering the operating room.

- Handle tissue gently, maintain effective hemostasis, minimize devitalized tissue and foreign bodies (ie, sutures, charred tissues, necrotic debris), and eradicate dead space at the surgical site.

- Use delayed primary skin closure or leave an incision open to heal by second intention if the surgeon considers the surgical site to be heavily contaminated.

- Obtain cultures and exclude from duty, surgical personnel who have draining skin lesions until infection has been ruled, out or personnel have received adequate therapy and infection has resolved.

- If drainage is necessary, use a closed suction drain. Place a drain through a separate incision distant from the operative incision. Remove the drain as soon as possible.

- Report appropriately stratified operation-specific, SSI rates to surgical team members. The optimum frequency and format for such rate computations will be determined by stratified caseload sizes (denominators) and the objectives of local, continuous quality improvement initiatives.

Many of these elements have been incorporated in a systemic fashion using the surgical checklist. There have been studies that use a before-and-after methodology demonstrating the effectiveness of a surgical checklist. In 2009, Haynes and Gawande reported the effective use of a 19-item checklist in 8 countries in reducing mortality by 46%, complications by 36%, and SSIs by 45%.[20] To date there have been few randomized trials that have shown benefits of surgical checklists. The most recent clustered randomized trial was a study of 2 Norwegian hospitals and more than 4000 operations, where complications dropped 42% and length of stay was reduced by 0.8 days with the use of a surgical checklist. Mortality did not change significantly.[21] The value of the checklists and their elements are based on the best evidence we have to date, but their implementation may be the key to minimizing surgical complications including SSIs.

Catheter-Associated Urinary Tract Infections

CAUTIs are extremely common and costly complications in hospitalized patients. CAUTIs are the most common type of HCAI accounting for more than 30% of all hospital infections. An estimated 13,000 deaths are associated with UTIs each year.[5] According to the CDC, 75% of UTIs are catheter associated, and 15% to 25% of patients receive a urinary catheter during their hospital stay.[22] In the ICU, the incidence of CAUTIs can range from 3.1 to 7.4 per 1000 urinary catheter days.[23] Over $340 million is estimated to be spent in health care costs attributable to CAUTIs in the United States each year.[24] As of October 1, 2008, the Centers for Medicare and Medicaid Services (CMS) no longer reimburse hospitals for the additional costs for caring for patients with CAUTI and consider CAUTI a "reasonably preventable" infection. Since the single most significant risk factor for a CAUTI is the prolonged use of the urinary catheter, the overriding principle for the prevention of CAUTIs is to minimize any unnecessary catheters by employing systems that ensure that patients have an acceptable indication for a urinary catheter and that catheters are removed as soon as possible.

Appropriate indications for the use of indwelling urinary catheters include urinary tract obstruction, neurogenic bladder dysfunction and urinary retention, and urologic studies or surgery on contiguous structures. Additionally, urinary catheter use is considered appropriate in patients with urinary incontinence and stage III or IV sacral pressure ulcers, as well as for end-of-life care.[23] Other indications for the placement of a urinary catheter in critically ill patient on mechanical ventilation include sepsis (for the first 24 hours), acute respiratory distress syndrome on continuous sedation or who require paralytic agents, continuous renal replacement therapy, acute renal failure, use of vasopressors with titration, temperature management systems, intra-aortic balloon pump, and subarachnoid hemorrhage with triple-H therapy (hypertension, hypervolemia, and hemodilution). Other strategies that are thought to be effective in reducing catheter use and thereby preventing infection include the routine use of a bladder scan to help caregivers identify patients who have urinary obstruction, daily review of the necessity of the urinary catheter, proper insertion technique and maintenance, and decision support tools (both electronic or with paper stop order sets) that are either nurse initiated or nurse prompted to ensure early removal of unnecessary urinary catheters.

In 2007, The Michigan Health and Hospital Association Keystone Center implemented a statewide initiative to reduce unnecessary urinary catheters. The initiative was based on nurse-led multidisciplinary rounds with the use of the "bladder bundle" to aid in the prompt removal of catheters. The efforts lead to a 45% reduction in inappropriate catheter use. The key elements of the "bladder bundle" include the following[25]:

1. Nurse-initiated urinary catheter discontinuation protocol

2. Urinary catheter reminders and removal prompts

3. Alternatives to indwelling urinary catheterization (such a condom catheters)

4. Portable bladder ultrasound monitoring

5. Insertion care and maintenance

Unfortunately, data from the CDC's National Healthcare Safety Network (NHSN) reveal that CAUTI rates remain high. There are many possible reasons for this; priority is given to other infections such as VAP, CRBSI, and SSI, and the morbidity and mortality of CAUTI is underappreciated. Most hospitals in the United States do not have a program for CAUTI surveillance, education, or adopt any of the previously mentioned prevention strategies.[26]

In 2013, the federal government released *The National and State Healthcare-Associated Infections Progress Report* revealing a 3% increase in CAUTIs between 2009 and 2012.[27] At the 2013 Action Planning Conference, a document proposing new targets for the prevention of HAIs was identified in the *National Action Plan to Prevent Healthcare-Associated Infections (HAI): Road Map to Elimination.* One of the proposal's goals was to reduce CAUTIs in ICU and ward patients. Based on the CDC's NHSN data, the proposed 2020 target is a 25% reduction from the 2015 baseline.[28]

REFERENCES

1. Making Healthcare safer: CDC, 2011.
2. Chandra S, Chong DH. New cost-effective treatment strategies for acute emergency situations. *Annu Rev Med.* 2014;65:459-469.
3. Wisplinghoff H, Bischoff T, Tallent SM, et al. Nosocomial bloodstream infections in US hospitals: analysis of 24,179 cases from a prospective nationwide surveillance study. *Clin Infect Dis.* 2004;39:309-317.
4. Mermel LA, Allon M, Bouza E, et al. Clinical practice guidelines for the diagnosis and management of intravascular catheter-related infection: 2009 update by the Infectious Diseases Society of America. *Clin Infect Dis.* 2009;49:1-45.
5. Klevens RM, Edwards JR, Richards CL, Jr, et al. Estimating health care-associated infections and deaths in U.S. hospitals, 2002. *Public Health Rep.* 2007;122:160-166.
6. Ventilator associated Event: CDC.
7. Richards MJ, Edwards JR, Culver DH, et al. Nosocomial infections in medical intensive care units in the United States. National Nosocomial Infections Surveillance System. *Crit Care Med.* 1999;27:887-892.

8. Dezfulian C, Shojania K, Collard HR, et al. Subglottic secretion drainage for preventing ventilator-associated pneumonia: a meta-analysis. *Am J Med.* 2005;118:11-18.

9. Klompas M, Branson R, Eichenwald EC, et al. Strategies to prevent ventilator-associated pneumonia in acute care hospitals: 2014 update. *Infect Control Hosp Epidemiol.* 2014;35(suppl 2):S133-S154.

10. Magill SS, Edwards JR, Bamberg W, et al. Multistate point-prevalence survey of health care-associated infections. *N Engl J Med.* 2014;370:1198-1208.

11. Pepin J, Valiquette L, Cossette B. Mortality attributable to nosocomial Clostridium difficile-associated disease during an epidemic caused by a hypervirulent strain in Quebec. *CMAJ.* 2005;173:1037-1042.

12. Riggs MM, Sethi AK, Zabarsky TF, et al. Asymptomatic carriers are a potential source for transmission of epidemic and nonepidemic Clostridium difficile strains among long-term care facility residents. *Clin Infect Dis.* 2007;45:992-998.

13. Crobach MJ, Dekkers OM, Wilcox MH, et al. European Society of Clinical Microbiology and Infectious Diseases (ESCMID): data review and recommendations for diagnosing Clostridium difficile-infection (CDI). *Clin Microbiol Infect.* 2009;15:1053-1066.

14. Sievert DM, Ricks P, Edwards JR, et al. Antimicrobial-resistant pathogens associated with healthcare-associated infections: summary of data reported to the National Healthcare Safety Network at the Centers for Disease Control and Prevention, 2009-2010. *Infect Control Hosp Epidemiol.* 2013;34:1-14.

15. Smyth ET, McIlvenny G, Enstone JE, et al. Four country healthcare associated infection prevalence survey 2006: overview of the results. *J Hosp Infect.* 2008;69:230-248.

16. Mangram AJ, Horan TC, Pearson ML, et al. Guideline for prevention of surgical site infection, 1999. Hospital Infection Control Practices Advisory Committee. *Infect Control Hosp Epidemiol.* 1999;20:250-278; quiz 279-280.

17. http://www.cms.gov/HospitalQualityInits/11_HospitalCompare.asp.

18. How-to Guide: prevent surgical site infections: Institute for Healthcare Improvement, 2012.

19. Kurz A, Sessler DI, Lenhardt R. Perioperative normothermia to reduce the incidence of surgical-wound infection and shorten hospitalization. Study of Wound Infection and Temperature Group. *N Engl J Med.* 1996;334:1209-1215.

20. Haynes AB, Weiser TG, Berry WR, et al. A surgical safety checklist to reduce morbidity and mortality in a global population. *N Engl J Med.* 2009;360:491-499.

21. Haugen AS, Softeland E, Almeland SK, et al. Effect of the World Health Organization Checklist on Patient Outcomes: a stepped wedge cluster randomized controlled trial. *Ann Surg.* 2015;261:821-828.

22. Catheter-associated Urinary Tract Infections (CAUTI): CDC.

23. Edwards JR, Peterson KD, Mu Y, et al. National Healthcare Safety Network (NHSN) report: data summary for 2006 through 2008, issued December 2009. *Am J Infect Control.* 2009;37:783-805.

24. Scott R. The direct medical costs of healthcare-associated infections in U.S. hospitals and the benefits of prevention. http://www.cdc.gov/HAI/pdfs/hai/Scott_CostPaper.pdf

25. Saint S, Olmsted RN, Fakih MG, et al. Translating health care-associated urinary tract infection prevention research into practice via the bladder bundle. *Jt Comm J Qual Patient Saf.* 2009;35:449-455.

26. Conway LJ, Pogorzelska M, Larson E, et al. Adoption of policies to prevent catheter-associated urinary tract infections in United States intensive care units. *Am J Infect Control.* 2012;40:705-710.

27. http://www.cdc.gov/HAI/pdfs/progress-report/hai-progress-report.pdf.

28. http://www.health.gov/hai/pdfs/HAI-Targets.pdf.

HIV Infection in Critically Ill Patients

41

Mekeleya Yimen, MD

KEY POINTS

1. The acquired immunodeficiency syndrome (AIDS) is caused by human immunodeficiency virus (HIV), a sexually transmitted retrovirus, and characterized by depletion of T-helper (CD4) cells and severe immunodeficiency. Clinically, AIDS is defined as depletion of CD4 cells less than 200 cells/mm^3 or development of AIDS qualifying opportunistic infection.

2. Effective antiretroviral therapy and chemoprophylaxis has increased the latency phase of HIV infection prolonging asymptomatic disease to several decades.

3. Pulmonary complications remain the leading cause of morbidity and mortality in HIV-infected patients. Bacterial pneumonia caused by streptoccocus pneumoniae, staphylococcus aureus and tuberculosis are common causes of respiratory illness.

4. The prevalence of respiratory failure from *Pneumocystis jiroveci* pneumonia (PCP) has significantly decreased over the past 2 decades with the use of highly active antiretroviral therapy and prophylaxis with trimethoprim-sulfamethoxazole.

5. Adjunctive corticosteroid therapy is recommended to prevent lung injury in severe cases of PCP pneumonia, defined as those with PaO$_2$ of less than 70 mm Hg or alveolar-arterial oxygen gradient more than 35 mm Hg on room air.

6. HIV-infected patients have a higher incidence of pancreatitis due to older nucleoside reverse transcriptase agents, pentamidine, sulfa drugs, isoniazid as well as pathogens, such as cytomegalovirus and cryptosporidium.

7. Co-infection with hepatitis B and C viruses is common in HIV patients and can lead to chronic infection, high level of viremia, and early progression to end stage liver disease.

8. Neurological complications in HIV and AIDS patients can range from neurocognitive disorders (eg, HIV dementia) to life-threatening opportunistic infections associated with changes in mental status or seizures.

9. Metabolic and cardiovascular disorders are common in HIV-infected patients and are frequent causes of morbidity and mortality in the post-highly active antiretroviral treatment era.

10. It is usually safer to withhold HIV medications in the critically ill patient. However, if continuing or initiation of antiretroviral agents is warranted, consultation with an infectious disease specialist is recommended.

—Continued next page

Continued—

 Immune reconstitution inflammatory syndrome is commonly seen 4 to 6 weeks after initiation of highly active antiretroviral treatment in treatment naive patients

who are severely immune suppressed (CD4 < 50-100 cells/mm^3) and have an opportunistic infection at the time of HIV diagnosis.

INTRODUCTION

Human immunodeficiency virus (HIV) is a sexually transmitted retrovirus composed of RNA (ribonucleic acid) genome and enzymes such as protease, reverse transcriptase and integrase; enveloped within an outer shell that has binding sites for two cell receptors, CCR5 and CXCR4. CXCR4 is a coreceptor found on CD4+ T cells and CCR5 is found on CD4+ T helper cells, macrophages, and dendritic cells. In the first 2 to 3 weeks of acute infection, macrophages and CD4+ T cells are depleted rapidly as the virus replicates within these cells. Clinically, this period manifests as a febrile viral syndrome commonly with symptoms of atypical rash and lymphadenopathy. Seroconversion eventually follows 2 to 4 weeks after primary HIV infection as humoral immunity develops. As the immune system recognizes and destroys systemic viral particles and infected cells, the body enters a long phase of clinical latency and asymptomatic disease. Using the enzyme reverse transcriptase the viral RNA genome is used as a template to make DNA replica which is integrated into human DNA genome by the enzyme integrase leading to chronic viral replication. Over time, the body loses the ability to replenish infected cell pools especially helper T cells resulting in immune deficiency known as acquired immunodeficiency syndrome (AIDS). Table 41–1 lists common infections that are seen in HIV-infected persons.

AIDS is defined clinically as depletion of CD4 cells less than 200 cells/mm^3 (normal > 800) or development of AIDS-qualifying opportunistic infection. Without antiretroviral treatment, progression to AIDS occurs within an average of 8 to 10 years. The availability of effective antiretroviral therapy and chemoprophylaxis for opportunistic infections has increased the latency phase of HIV infection prolonging asymptomatic disease to several decades. Nonetheless, it is estimated that 1 in 6 newly HIV-infected persons are unaware of their infection status and will present with AIDS associated complications at the time of initial diagnosis.

Current armamentarium of antiretroviral drugs successfully suppress viral replication hence delaying loss of CD4 cells and progression to AIDS. But some anatomical sites are poorly penetrated by drugs and act as viral reservoirs (such as latent CD4 cells, central nervous system [CNS] tissue, and lymphoid tissues in

TABLE 41–1 Opportunistic infections in HIV/AIDS patients.

Respiratory Infections	CAP TB	PCP Endemic Fungi	KS Primary Effusion Lymphoma (HHV 8)	CMV Pneumonitis
CNS infection	Community-acquired meningitis	Syphilis HSV	Toxoplasmosis	Cryptococcus PML (JC virus) CMV PCNSL
GI disordered	Salmonellosis Cryptosporidiosis	Listeria Oropharyngeal candidiasis	Bartonella (*Peliosis Hepatis*) Diarrheal illnesses (*Cryptosporidiosis, Microspora, Isospora*)	Cryptosporidiosis MAI

the GI and genital tracts). Within these sites, ongoing viral spread and replication can occur via cell-to-cell transmission and syncytium formation, leading to a chronic proinflammatory state, which in turn has been linked to increased risk of malignancy, autoimmune, and early cardiovascular disease in HIV patients.

Antiretroviral therapy has dramatically changed the spectrum of illness seen in HIV-infected patients. Studies have shown that hospital and ICU admission rates remain unchanged in HIV-infected persons, although their admitting diagnoses appears to have shifted from infectious to noninfectious illnesses. Following is a summary of frequently encountered ICU diagnoses in HIV-infected patients in the current highly active antiretroviral treatment (HAART) era.

PULMONARY COMPLICATIONS

Pulmonary complication in the form of infectious and noninfectious disease remains the leading cause of morbidity and mortality in HIV-infected individuals. The spectrum of infectious complications appears to have changed since the introduction of combination antiretroviral drugs in the mid-1990s. In the early AIDS epidemic, respiratory failure due to *Pneumocystis jiroveci* pneumonia (PCP) was the leading cause of death. Although respiratory failure remains the most common indication for ICU admission, the rates of PCP have decline. Bacterial pathogens such as streptococcus pneumoniae, stapylococcus aureus and tuberculosis are common causes of respiratory failure. In fact, TB is responsible for 1 of 10 HIV/AIDS-related deaths worldwide. As HIV infection is becoming a chronic medical condition with a long-life expectancy, its association with noninfectious respiratory complications is also becoming widely recognized. Reactive airway disease, lung cancer (irrespective of smoking history) and pulmonary arterial hypertension (PAH) are increasingly becoming common indications for ICU admission in HIV-infected patients. Table 41–2 lists the pulmonary complications frequently encountered in critically ill HIV-infected patients.

Pneumonia

Alterations in host defense mechanisms, such as B lymphocyte dysfunction, abnormal secretion of

TABLE 41-2 Pulmonary complications associated with HIV infection.

Infectious	Noninfectious
Bacterial • **Streptococcus pneumoniae** • **Haemophilus spp** • **Staphylococcus aureus** • Mycobacterial—**M. tuberculosis** and NTM	Malignancy • Lymphoma • Kaposi sarcoma • Other lung cancers
Viral • Seasonal influenza • CMV	Cardiovascular • CHF exacerbation • Pulmonary arterial hypertension
Fungal • **Pneumocystis jiroveci** • Endemic fungi—**Histoplasma capsulatum**, *Coccidioidomycosis*, **Cryptococcus spp**	Others • IRIS • Pneumonitis • COPD/reactive airway diseases

NTM, nontuberculous mycobacteria

immunoglobulin and mucociliary dysfunction, and other risk behaviors, such as tobacco use appear to increase the risk of pneumonia in HIV-infected patients irrespective of CD4 counts or antiretroviral use. *Streptococcus pneumoniae* and *Mycobacterium tuberculosis* are the leading cause of pneumonia but other bacterial, viral, and fungal (especially endemic fungi) pathogens are also prevalent.

Acute respiratory failure is commonly seen with viral and bacterial pneumonias, whereas tuberculosis, PCP, and other fungal infections have more of a subacute presentation. Chemoprophylaxis, vaccination history (pneumococcal and influenza), travel, and endemic exposures are clues when developing a differential diagnosis. Cough, fever, and dyspnea are the most common presenting symptoms.

Basic laboratory workup including lactate dehydrogenase (LDH) and sputum Gram stain and cultures (bacterial, mycobacterial, and fungal) should be obtained. Chest radiography (CXR) showing lobar pneumonia is suggestive of common community-acquired bacterial pathogens including *Streptococcus pneumoniae, Hemophilus influenzae,* and *Staphylococcus aureus.* Bronchoscopy is of limited value in establishing the diagnosis of bacterial pneumonia in HIV-infected patients with the exception of cases where there is high suspicion for mycobacterial disease or fungal process. Ancillary testing with urine antigen detection for *Pneumococcus* and *Legionella* have high specificity, but low sensitivity. For the endemic fungi, *Histoplasma*, *Coccidioidomycosis*, and *Cryptococcus* urine or serum antigen detection tests are available but have better yield in the setting of disseminated disease.

Community-acquired pneumonia coverage with third- or fourth-generation cephalosporin plus a respiratory fluoroquinolone (eg, levofloxacin or moxifloxacin) or macrolide (eg, azithromycin) should be initiated in patients presenting with suspected bacterial pneumonia. In severe respiratory failure requiring ICU admission, initial empiric coverage for gram-negative organisms (eg, *Pseudomonas spp.*) and resistant pathogens such as methicillin-resistant *Staphylococcus aureus* should be considered until culture data is available to guide therapy.

Pneumocystis Jiroveci Pneumonia

Since the widespread use of HAART and prophylaxis with trimethoprim-sulfamethoxazole (TMP-SMX), the prevalence of PCP-associated respiratory failure has decreased. Commonly presenting symptoms are nonproductive cough, fever, and anorexia evolving over 2 to 4 weeks in an AIDS patient (CD4 < 200). Hypoxia is the most common symptomatic and laboratory finding. Elevated LDH along with an alveolar-arterial (A-a) gradient more than 35 mm Hg is suggestive of PCP pneumonia. CXR commonly shows interstitial infiltrates with classic "butterfly" pattern or an atypical presentation with nodular, cavitary, or cystic lesions. In 20% of the cases, the CXR may be normal. Spontaneous pneumothorax in a patient with HIV should raise the suspicion for PCP.

Special stains of induced sputum for cysts or trophozoites are sensitive in less than 60% of cases; thus negative results warrant further investigation with bronchoscopy and bronchoalveolar lavage. Standard stains and techniques used for PCP diagnosis include Giemsa or modified Wright–Giemsa (also known as Diff–Quik), Gomori-methanamine silver, and immunofluorescent staining (direct fluorescent antibody). Recently, polymerase chain reaction (PCR) detection and measurement of 1-3 β-D-glucan levels are gaining wide acceptance in the diagnosis of PCP associated with AIDS although the utility in non-HIV patients is not yet well defined.

TMP-SMX remains the first-line therapeutic agent for PCP pneumonia. Adjunctive corticosteroid therapy is recommended to prevent lung injury in severe cases, clinically defined as PaO_2 of less than 70 mm Hg or A-a oxygen gradient of more than 35 mm Hg on room air. For those patients who are intolerant to sulfa drugs, IV pentamidine is an alternate choice, but serious side effects including pancreatitis, renal failure, and hypoglycemia limit its use. Other alternative agents include the combination of clindamycin and primaquine, dapsone, and TMX or atovaquone. These regimens may not be ideal in critically ill patients, as primaquine, dapsone, and atovaquone are only available orally. Duration of therapy for PCP pneumonia is 21 days and clinical response is expected within 3 to 5 days. Treatment failure should be suspected if response lags more than 8 days. TMP-SMX is commonly associated with atypical adverse reactions such as fever, hepatitis, and leukopenia, which can be mistaken for treatment failure. The most common side effect reported with TMX-SMX is a rash.

Viral Pneumonitis

HIV-infected individuals are at increased risk of developing serious complications from respiratory viruses especially with the influenza virus. During influenza season, HIV-infected patients are hospitalized at increased rates with influenza-related complications so aggressive preventive care with vaccination should be sought. Unlike the influenza virus, the significance of other viral pathogens such as herpes simplex virus (HSV), cytomegalovirus (CMV), and adenovirus when isolated from respiratory secretions is difficult to interpret and may represent viral shedding. For most patients, this may represent severe immunosuppression and is a sign of poor prognosis. The role of antiviral therapy has been debated and does not seem to show survival improvement.

HIV-Related Pulmonary Arterial Hypertension

The increased prevalence of PAH in HIV-infected patients has been recognized since the 1980s and seems to occur independent of the severity of immune deficiency or antiretroviral use. These patients usually present with clinical symptoms of chronic dyspnea and lower extremity edema. Doppler echocardiography shows elevated right ventricular and pulmonary pressures but confirmation of the diagnosis of PAH requires right heart catheterization showing mean pulmonary artery pressure more than 25 mm Hg at rest and normal pulmonary capillary wedge pressure less than 15 mm Hg. Conventional treatment with calcium channel blockers is not effective in HIV-PAH and antiretroviral therapy also does not seem to alter the disease course. Standard treatment agents available for PAH seem to have similar efficacy in HIV-infected patients but drug–drug interactions with antiretroviral agents (especially protease inhibitors, PIs) must be considered.

GASTROINTESTINAL COMPLICATIONS

Most gastrointestinal (GI) manifestations associated with HIV infection do not warrant ICU level of care. Infections that have predilection for the GI tract, such as *Candida*, *CMV*, *HSV*, and *Mycobacterium avium intracellulare* (MAI) cause mucosal disease and commonly manifest with symptoms of odynophagia, dysphagia, and anorexia. Catastrophic complications rarely can develop, such as bowel perforation, obstruction, and life-threatening hemorrhage. In addition, compromise of the mucosal integrity of the GI tract allows gut translocation of bacteria leading to sepsis and septic shock. Pancreatitis and complications of liver disease are also frequent and common indications for ICU admission.

Pancreatitis

A higher incidence of pancreatitis has been reported in HIV patients related to multiple factors. Medications especially older nucleoside reverse transcriptase agents, such as didanosine/stavudine are common culprits. As a class, PIs are known to cause dyslipidemia including hypertriglyceridemia, which may increase the risk of hyperlipidemic injury to the pancreas. Drugs used to treat opportunistic infections, such as pentamidine, sulfa drugs, and isoniazid also cause pancreatitis. Certain pathogens

associated with HIV/AIDS, such as CMV and *Cryptosporidium* have a predilection for the pancreas.

A common presenting complaint is abdominal pain with laboratory data showing elevated amylase or lipase levels. Imaging with CT shows inflammation of the pancreas. Further workup with fine needle aspiration may be helpful in ruling out infectious causes of pancreatitis but is seldom performed. Treatment in most cases is supportive.

Liver Disease

Due to shared risk factors, coinfection with hepatitis B and C is common in HIV patients. HIV virus is known to accelerate liver disease in coinfected patients leading to chronic infection, high levels of viremia and early progression to end-stage liver disease. Hepatic steatosis in association with and without alcohol and medications is also common in HIV patients. Liver disease accounts for 20% of non-AIDS-related mortality in HIV patients. Complications associated with end-stage liver disease, such as hepatic encephalopathy, variceal bleeding, and other organ failures are common indications for ICU admission. Management does not differ from the general population and focuses on preventing further liver damage, slowing the progression of liver disease, and management of cirrhotic complications.

Hepatitis B and HIV Coinfection

Initiation and discontinuation of antiviral therapy in HIV-HBV coinfected patients should be cautiously performed. The choice of antiretroviral agent must also consider treatment of both infections and must avoid monotherapy of hepatitis B virus due to the increased rates of acquiring drug resistance. Table 41–3 lists the medications that are effective

TABLE 41–3 Medications effective against HIV and HBV.

HIV/HBV	HBV Treatment, But Some Activity Against HIV
Lamivudine	Adefovir
Emtricitabine	Entecavir
Tenofovir	

against both HIV and HBV. Ideally, two of the combination antiretroviral HIV medications should be active against HBV. Treatment discontinuation should be avoided if possible, as severe a flare of HBV has been reported with withdrawal. Immune reconstitution syndrome, which commonly presents within 2 months of antiretroviral initiation can also present with hepatitis flare.

Hepatitis C and HIV Coinfection

Hepatitis C infection does not appear to affect the course of HIV disease, but as in the case of HBV infection, liver disease is accelerated with HIV-HCV coinfection. Drug-induced liver injury is also common in coinfected patients. The mainstay of HCV therapy is PEG interferon and ribavirin, but a newer class of agents has recently been introduced for specific genotypes of HCV. These agents are PIs that are metabolized by the liver cytochrome P450 system and may interact with many drugs including antiretroviral agents. Complications from cirrhosis and end-stage liver disease are also of concern in the ICU setting. Many studies have shown acceleration to liver failure, noncirrhotic portal hypertension, and hepatocellular carcinoma with HIV-HCV coinfection. Early consideration for liver transplantation is warranted in these settings. Management of these complications is identical as in non-HIV-infected patients.

CENTRAL NERVOUS SYSTEM COMPLICATIONS

Neuro-AIDS is a terminology used to describe the neurological complications in HIV and AIDS patients. These complications range from neurocognitive disorders, such as HIV dementia to opportunistic infections that cause life-threatening acute illnesses that most commonly present with change in mental status, seizures, or weakness. Evaluation of these symptoms frequently mandates hospitalization and with severe symptoms, ICU admission is indicated.

Neurological manifestations of HIV have changed since the widespread availability of HAART. Neurocognitive disorders and neuropathies are becoming more prevalent as opportunistic infections and malignancies of the CNS remain fatal, but

less frequently encountered in the Western world. Cerebral toxoplasmosis, primary CNS lymphoma (PCNSL), and Cryptococcal meningitis are frequently encountered in HIV/AIDS patients in the ICU setting as severe symptoms, such as acute encephalopathy, seizures, cerebral edema, or increased intracranial pressure are associated with these diagnosis. Nonetheless, HIV-infected patients are also at risk for community-acquired meningitis/encephalitis and vascular disorders, such as strokes. The primary goal in management is securing the airway and symptomatic treatment, such as seizure control while undergoing the appropriate workup.

Cerebral Toxoplasmosis

Toxoplasma gondii is an obligate intracellular protozoa acquired via consumption of undercooked meats (commonly beef or pork) or via exposure to cat feces (usual carriers of oocytes). Primary infection usually presents with a mononucleosis-like illness and is usually subclinical and self-limiting. Prior exposure to toxoplasmosis is diagnosed by antibody detection (IgG for *T. gondii*). Seroprevalence is variable throughout the world. In the United States, 15% of the population has prior exposure. In France and developing countries, higher seroprevalence rates (> 50%) have been reported. Latent cysts can reactivate in the setting of severe immune suppression and cause devastating illness, such as encephalitis, chorioretinitis, myocarditis, and pneumonitis.

Toxoplasma encephalitis (TE) is the most common manifestation in AIDS patients (CD4 counts < 50). It usually presents with fever, headache, and change in mental status. Imaging with contrast MRI or CT shows single or multiple ring-enhancing lesions. Unfortunately, these radiographic findings are nonspecific and may be seen with other CNS infections and malignancies, such as PCNSL. TE is usually a clinical diagnosis in AIDS patients. The presence of multiple lesions or a single ring-enhancing lesion (especially basal ganglia lesions) in a Toxoplasma IgG seropositive patient warrants presumptive treatment. The preferred treatment regimen is sulfadiazine/pyrimethamine with leucovorin (to prevent bone marrow suppression commonly seen with prolonged pyrimethamine use). Treatment duration is 6 weeks with follow-up imaging after 2 weeks to document radiographic improvement. If clinical improvement is not seen at this point, further diagnostic workup, usually a brain biopsy is warranted to rule out PCNSL. In the pre-HAART era, life-long suppressive therapy was mandatory following diagnosis of TE, but with effective antiretroviral therapy, it is now generally continued until immune reconstitution (CD4 rise > 200). It is also worth noting that rates of TE have decreased with widespread use of chemoprophylaxis with sulfa-based drugs for PCP, which is also effecting in preventing toxoplasmosis.

Primary CNS Lymphoma

Primary CNS lymphoma (PCNSL) is an AIDS-defining illness with a prevalence of approximately 5% pre-HAART, but a significant reduction has been seen in recent years. PCNSL is a non-Hodgkin's B-cell lymphoma that is thought to result from malignant transformation of chronically activated EBV infected B cells. Clinical presentation and radiographic findings are similar between TE and PCNSL. Patients present with headache, change in mental status, and visual disturbances, and CT/MRI usually shows a contrast-enhancing lesion. CSF fluid with EBV PCR presence or cytology showing malignant cells is also supportive of diagnosis, but has low yield. Some studies have supported the use of functional imaging studies such as single photon emission computed tomography or positron emission tomography scan to differentiate between TE and PCNSL (especially when a single CNS mass lesion is present). Increased tracer uptake with these studies is suggestive of PCNSL, but should not be used as a definitive diagnosis. In clinical practice, AIDS patients presenting with a contrast enhancing lesion are treated with a trial of toxoplasma therapy with close clinical and imaging follow up, and brain biopsy is pursued if clinical improvement is not attained after 2 weeks.

Treatment for PCNSL is whole brain radiation and chemotherapy, which includes high dose corticosteroids, which are effective as antitumor agents but also treat tumor-associated edema.

Cryptococcal Meningitis

Cryptococcus neoformans is a saprophytic fungus abundant in the environment. Disease results from inhalation of spores, which usually causes self-limited acute respiratory infection. In immunocompromised hosts, disseminated disease to multiple sites including skin, prostate, bone marrow, and CNS can develop. In HIV/AIDS patients, cryptococcal meningitis is the most common presentation and is thought to arise from hematogenous spread following cryptoccocemia in acute infection or from reactivation of latent disease (especially in those with CD4 counts < 100). Patients commonly present with indolent symptoms, such as headache, malaise, and fevers, but in delayed diagnosis obtundation and seizures may warrant ICU level of care. Imaging with CT or MRI of the brain should be performed first to rule out intracranial lesions, but rarely hydrocephalus or infectious granulomas (cryptococcoma), which present as non-contrast enhancing well-circumscribed lesions may be present. CSF analysis should be performed when *Cryptococcus* is suspected along with measurement of opening pressure. Lumbar puncture may show CSF pleocytosis with low glucose and elevated opening pressure (> 20 cm H_2O). Cryptococcal antigen from both serum and CSF are highly sensitive and specific tests. Cryptococcal CSF antigen is nearly 100% sensitive as compared to India ink stains (75% sensitivity) in the case of meningitis, and serum is approximately 95% sensitive and useful when lumbar puncture cannot be performed. Treatment of cryptococcal meningitis includes antifungal therapy and management of intracranial pressure. Treatment duration is for 10 weeks starting with liposomal preparation of amphotericin plus flucytosine induction for the first 2 weeks followed by consolidation therapy with fluconazole for the next 8 weeks. Maintenance with lower dose fluconazole should be continued until sustained immune reconstitution is attained (CD4 > 200). In those patients with opening pressure more than 25 cm H_2O, daily lumbar puncture needs to be performed to reduce pressure (< 20 cm H_2O or by 50%); lumbar drain or ventriculoperitoneal shunt may be warranted for persistently elevated ICP.

HEMATOLOGIC COMPLICATIONS

Cytopenias are the most common complication of HIV disease and develop as a result dysregulated of cytokine release encountered in HIV infection, bone marrow suppression due to medication and infiltration of bone marrow by opportunistic infections that is, *CMV*, *Cryptococcus*, *Histoplasma*, *Mycobacteria*

(*MTB*, *MAI*), or malignancy (ie, lymphoma and Kaposi sarcoma).

Anemia

Anemia of chronic disease is the most common cytopenia encountered, and is frequently associated with use of drugs such as Zidovudine (AZT). Discontinuation of medication and supportive care is the standard of care. Rarely severe anemia may mandate ICU admission as in the case of parvovirus B19 infection or drug-induced hemolytic anemia (eg, use of dapsone in G6PD-deficient patients, primaquine, and ribavirin). Although parvovirus B19 infection causes a self-limited disease in immunocompetent hosts, AIDS patients (especially with CD4 count < 100) are unable to eradicate the infection and may develop pure red cell aplasia. Management includes transfusions, supportive care, and a 5-day course of IV immune globulin.

Hemolytic anemia is rare in HIV disease, but can be seen in association with medication use as in the case of G6PD deficiency and in the setting of thrombotic thrombocytopenic purpura (TTP). Because G6PD deficiency is the most common enzymatic disorder worldwide (especially in African and Mediterranean descendants), preemptive evaluation of patients for G6PD deficiency prior to initiation of drugs known to cause hemolysis is the best management approach. Once complications develop, treatment is usually supportive.

Neutropenia

Prolonged neutropenia is common especially in end-stage HIV disease. HIV associated neutropenia is highly responsive to colony stimulating factors. Neutropenic sepsis is a rare complication, as HIV patients develop gradual neutrophil depletion and mucosal integrity is usually preserved unlike the neutropenia that occurs in cancer patients.

Thrombocytopenia

Thrombocytopenia can develop as a result of idiopathic (immune) thrombocytopenic purpura (ITP) and TTP. The pathogenesis of ITP is related to autoantibodies generated during HIV infection. For most patients, it may be the initial manifestation of HIV disease. Management is with pulse dose corticosteroids and if unresponsive to corticosteroid therapy, splenectomy may be warranted.

HIV is also known to be one of the triggers for TTP. TTP is a rare but life-threatening hemolytic process characterized by pentad of fever, neurologic changes (altered mental status and seizures), renal failure, microangiopathic hemolytic anemia, and thrombocytopenia. Standard diagnostic tests to evaluate for hemolysis and renal failure should be obtained. Since disease may progress to fatal outcomes, prompt recognition and initiation of treatment with plasmapheresis and possibly corticosteroids is essential.

METABOLIC AND CARDIOVASCULAR DISORDERS

Insulin resistance, dyslipidemia, and abnormal fat distribution are common metabolic changes encountered in HIV-infected individuals that are not only directly related to the pathogenesis of HIV infection, but also medications used to treat HIV disease. Several studies have shown an increased rate of early cardiovascular disease associated with prolonged exposure to certain classes of antiretroviral agents (PIs and nucleoside reverse transcriptase agents), but also with their discontinuation. The pathogenesis of heart disease in HIV patients is multifactorial and likely related to the proinflammatory state caused by HIV infection along with the metabolic changes and accelerated rate of atherosclerotic disease. Cardiac events are the leading cause of morbidity and mortality in HIV patients in the post-HAART era. Traditional risk factors along with the socioeconomic status of the HIV population also heighten this risk. Therapeutic measures do not differ in HIV patients with the exception of the need for increased awareness of drug–drug interactions when initiating medical management.

HAART IN THE ICU

Initiation of antiretroviral therapy usually is reserved for the outpatient setting, as genotypic and resistance testing must be performed even in treatment-naïve patients. A common concern encountered in the ICU setting is the question of continuing HIV therapy in the critically ill patient. Critical care providers should be aware of the numerous drug interactions associated with antiretroviral agents. In addition, the erratic drug absorption from the GI tract in the critically ill, need for dose adjustment in the setting of renal and hepatic dysfunction, risk for Immune Reconstitution Inflammatory Syndrome (IRIS) should be considered. It is usually safer to withhold HIV medications in the critically ill patient, but in the rare instances where continuing or initiation of antiretroviral agents is warranted, it should be done in consultation with an infectious disease specialist.

IRIS is a rare atypical inflammatory disorder usually associated with immune recovery. Patients may present with paradoxical worsening or development of an opportunistic infection, or a new autoimmune process. The pathogenesis is thought to be recovery of cellular and humoral immunity with improvement in CD4 cell counts. It is commonly seen 4 to 6 weeks after initiation of HAART in treatment-naïve patients who are severely immunosuppressed (CD4 < 50-100) and have an opportunistic infection at the time of HIV diagnosis. Common disease processes presenting in the setting of IRIS are mycobacterial diseases (MTB, MAI), Cryptococcus, and CMV. Treatment requires close observation, while continuing HAART and treating the opportunistic infection. The role of corticosteroids and nonsteroidal anti-inflammatory drugs is unclear, but commonly utilized in an attempt to subdue the inflammatory reaction.

REFERENCES

1. Deng H, Liu R, Ellmeier W, et al. Identification of a major co-receptor for primary isolates of HIV-1. *Nature.* 1996;381:661-666.
2. Bartlett J, Gallant J, Pham P. The Medical Management of HIV Infection 2009-2010 ed. *Knowledge Source Solutions*, LLC. 2009.
3. Powell K, Davis J, Morris A, et al. Survival for patients admitted to the intensive care unit continues to improve in the current era of highly active antiretroviral therapy. *Chest.* 2009;135(1):11-17.
4. Morris A, Masur H, Huang L. Current issues in critical care of the human immunodeficiency virus-infected patients. *Crit Care Med.* 2006;34:42-49.
5. Huang L, Quartin A, Jones D, et al. Intensive care of patients with HIV infection. *N Engl J Med.* 2006;355:173-181.
6. Masur H. Management of patients with HIV in the intensive care unit. *Proc Am Thorac Soc.* 2006;3:96-102.
7. Corona A, Raimondi F. Critical care of HIV infection patients in the highly active antiretroviral era. *Minerva Anestesiol.* 2007;73:635-645.
8. Barbier F, Legriel S, Pavie J, et al. Etiologies and outcomes of acute respiratory failure in HIV infected patients. *Intensive Care Med.* 2009;35(10):1678-1686.
9. Gordin I, Roediger M, Girard PM, et al. Pneumonia in HIV-infected patients. Increased risk with cigarette smoking and treatment interruption. *Am J Resp Med.* 2008;178:630-636.
10. Bozette SA, Sattler FR, Chiu J, et al. A controlled trial of early adjunctive treatment with steroids for pneumocystis carinii pneumonia in acquired immune deficiency syndrome. *N Engl J Med.* 1990;323:1451-1457.
11. Sitbon O, Lascoux-Combe C, Delfraissy JF, et al. Prevalence of HIV related pulmonary arterial hypertension in the current antiretroviral therapy era. *Am J Respir Crit Care.* 2008;177:108-113.
12. Dragovic G. Acute pancreatitis in HIV/AIDS patients; an issue of concern. *Asian Pac J Trop Biomed.* 2013;3(6):422-435.
13. Price J, Thio C. Liver disease in HIV-infected individuals. *Clin Gastroenterol Hepatol.* 2010;8(12):1002-1012.
14. Price R, Brew BJ. The AIDS dementia complex. *J Infect Dis.* 1988;158(5):1079-1083.
15. Skiest D. Focal neurological diseases in HIV patients with acquired immunodeficiency syndrome. *Clin Infect Dis.* 2002;34:103-105.
16. Perfect J, Dismukes W, Dromer F. Clinical practice guidelines for management of Cryptococcal diseases; 2010 update by Infectious Disease Society of America. *Clin Infect Dis.* 2010;50(3):291-322.
17. Hsue P, Deeks S, Hunt P. Immunologic bases of cardiovascular disease in HIV infected patients. *J Infect Dis.* 2012;205:S375-S383.
18. The data collection on Adverse Events of Anti-HIV Drugs (DAD) Study Group. Combination antiretroviral therapy and risk of myocardial infarction. *N Engl J Med.* 2003;349:1993-2003.

Sepsis, Septic Shock, and Multiple Organ Failure

Russell J. McCulloh, MD and Steven M. Opal, MD

KEY POINTS

1 Sepsis is increasing in incidence worldwide. This is the result of a number of factors including: the aging of the population with a large increase in patients more than 65 years; progressive increase in antibiotic resistance; increased reliance on implanted devices, organ transplantation and other invasive surgical procedures; and increasing prevalence of patients with long-term immunosuppressive diseases and medications who are at risk for severe infection and sepsis.

2 Sepsis is a syndrome consisting of a constellation of signs, symptoms, hemodynamic, and laboratory findings caused by an excessive and/or dysfunctional host immune response to severe infection. There is currently no single diagnostic test sufficient to make a definitive diagnosis of sepsis.

3 The key to optimal care of the septic patient is early recognition and early initiation of appropriate treatment. This places the responsibility for early recognition on the health care team in managing acutely ill patients. The lack of a rapid diagnostic test and the often subtle initial presentation of sepsis make the early detection of sepsis a real challenge.

4 Septic shock is a medical emergency and should be treated as such. The major therapeutic approach is aggressive fluid resuscitation, early and appropriate antibiotic therapy, early determination of the source of the causative infection site and source control if possible (drain abscess, remove necrotic tissue or infected catheters or other devices, etc).

5 The prevention and expert management of organ dysfunction as a result of sepsis is critical for survival and prevention of long-term disability. Expert supportive care by critical care specialists will improve outcomes.

INTRODUCTION

Sepsis and the multiorgan failure that often accompanies the systemic inflammatory response syndrome (SIRS) is a leading cause of mortality in the intensive care unit. Over 750,000 patients develop sepsis annually in the United States accounting for about 10% of all intensive care unit (ICU) admissions. Of these patients, 5% to 15% will be diagnosed with septic shock. The hospital mortality for septic shock remains approximately 35% to 54%, despite concerted efforts to improve the treatment options and outcome.

Although modest improvements in the prognosis have been made over the past 2 decades and promising new therapies continue to be investigated, innovations in the management of septic shock are still required. This chapter will describe the molecular pathophysiology of sepsis, current diagnostic and therapeutic strategies, and the management of septic shock.

SEPSIS DEFINITIONS

New definitions for sepsis were published by the Third International Sepsis Task Force in 2016. According to these updated definitions, sepsis is defined as a life-threatening condition caused by a dysregulated host response to infection accompanied by acute organ dysfunction. Septic shock is a subset of sepsis in which underlying cellular metabolism abnormalities are sufficiently profound to significantly increase mortality. Septic shock is clinically recognized as arterial hypotension, refractory to simple fluid resuscitation, with evidence of hyperlactatemia. Multiple other clinical entities related to sepsis, including SIRS and multiple organ dysfunction syndrome (MODS) are defined in Table 42–1. These definitions account for the finding that sepsis can result from various infectious agents and microbial mediators and is not necessarily associated with bloodstream infection. The goal of the updated definitions is to increase consistency for epidemiologic studies and clinical trials and to help improve earlier recognition and timely management of patients with sepsis or at risk for developing sepsis.

Current sepsis definitions are based upon the fact that the dysregulated immune response itself, not the infectious agent, underlies the pathophysiology of the septic process. The nature of the causative microorganism also clearly contributes to the ultimate fate of the patient. Pathogens differ in their susceptibility to host defenses, their potential for developing antimicrobial resistance, and their ability to generate toxins—all of which affect pathogenicity.

TABLE 42–1 Common definitions and terms used in sepsis.

Term	Definition	Comments
ARDS* (acute respiratory distress syndrome)	Acute onset (< 7 days) respiratory symptoms; bilateral infiltrates on chest radiograph not explained by other pleural or lung disease; infiltrates not due to cardiac failure or fluid overload (must exclude hydrostatic edema if suspected)	A severity score divides patients into 3 groups depending on PaO_2/FiO_2 ratio and predict outcome: 200 to ≤ 300 mm Hg (mild 27 ± 3% mortality); 100 to ≤ 200 mm Hg (moderate 32 ± 3% mortality) or ≤ 100 mm Hg (severe 45 ± 2% mortality)
Bacteremia	Detection of viable bacteria in the bloodstream	Transient bacteremia without clinical symptoms can occur; bacteremia may or may not be present in sepsis
SIRS (systemic inflammatory response syndrome)	Temperature > 38.5°C (101.3°F) or < 36° C (96.8°F) Tachypnea (> 20 breath/min) Tachycardia (> 90 beat/min) WBC count > 12,000 cells/mm³ or > 10% immature forms or < 4000 cells/mm³	Two or more criteria needed; may be caused by infectious and noninfectious etiologies; clinical features attributable to systemic release of inflammatory mediators into the circulation
Sepsis	Life-threatening acute organ dysfunction caused by a dysregulated host response to infection. Organ dysfunction: acute change in SOFA score ≥ 2 points from infection	May be caused by viral, bacterial, fungal, or parasitic pathogens; bloodstream infection need not be present
Septic shock	Sepsis with hypotension requiring vasopressors to maintain MAP ≥ 65 mm Hg and having a serum lactate level > 2 mmol/dL despite adequate volume resuscitation	Hospital mortality in septic shock exceeds 40%

The 2012 Berlin definition (JAMA 307; 2526, 2012) now supersedes the former 1994 European-American Consensus Committee on ARDS definition.
P_aO_2, arterial oxygen tension; F_IO_2, fraction of inspired oxygen; WBC, white blood count.

Failing to account for these differences in microbial virulence limits the utility of current sepsis definitions.

Many patients who present with sepsis have multiple predisposing factors, a variety of preexisting illnesses, and have major underlying organ dysfunction from comorbid diseases. The degree to which sepsis contributes to further disordered organ function is be difficult to accurately determine. Similarly, the degree to which sepsis contributes to the mortality in patients with other serious underlying diseases (attributable risk of mortality) can be difficult to quantify. Further refinements in sepsis terminology may be possible when rapid diagnostic techniques become available to assess the immune status of septic patients. Functional genomics and proteomics may assist in characterizing septic patients in the future.

EPIDEMIOLOGY

Between 1979 and 2000, the incidence of sepsis in the United States increased by 8.7% annually, from 82.7 to 240.4 per 100,000 population. These trends are observed worldwide and will likely continue because sepsis incidence increases with the aging of the population. Innovations in organ transplantation, implanted prosthetic devices, and long-term vascular access devices continue to expand this vulnerable patient population at risk for sepsis. The gradual aging of the population in many developed and developing countries and the increasing prevalence of antibiotic-resistant microbial pathogens also contribute to the rising incidence of septic shock.

PATHOGENESIS: MICROBIAL FACTORS

Causative Microorganisms

The microbiology of sepsis continues to evolve due to changes in microbial epidemiology, pathogen virulence, and pathogens' susceptibility to antimicrobials. The predominant microbial pathogens responsible for sepsis in the 1960s and 1970s were enteric gram-negative bacilli and *Pseudomonas aeruginosa*, but switched to predominantly gram-positive bacterial pathogens in the mid-1980s through 2010, due mostly to the rapid development of antibiotic resistance in gram-positive pathogens and their strong association with vascular-catheter-associated infections. Gram-negative bacterial pathogens are now returning as the dominant cause of sepsis, due largely to progressive antibiotic resistance and the lack of new antibacterial agents effective against gram-negative bacterial pathogens. Opportunistic fungal pathogens are also increasing in frequency as a cause of sepsis.

Bacterial Endotoxin and Other Pathogen-Associated Molecular Pattern Molecules

Bacterial endotoxin, or lipopolysaccharide (LPS), is an intrinsic component of the outer membrane of gram-negative bacteria and is essential for the viability of enteric bacteria. Endotoxin functions as an alarm molecule alerting the host to invasion by gram-negative bacteria. Endotoxin in the circulation provokes a vigorous systemic inflammatory response. Humans are especially susceptible to the profound immunostimulant properties of endotoxin; even minute doses may be lethal. Other highly conserved pathogen-associated molecular pattern molecules such as bacterial lipoteichoic acid, lipopeptides and even sequences of bacterial and viral DNA can be detected by the immune system and activate innate immune responses.

The Toll-like receptor (TLR) family is the most important cellular, pathogen-associated pattern recognition receptor system in humans. The TLRs are transmembrane receptors for detecting endotoxin and many other microbial mediators, such as peptidoglycan, lipopeptides, bacterial flagellin, lipoteichoic acid, microbial-derived nucleic acids, and viral and fungal cell components. Nucleoside oligomerization domain proteins recognize specific components of bacterial peptidoglycan and other microbial elements with the cytosol and activate the acute phase response with the release of the proinflammatory cytokine interleukin-1 beta.

Other pattern-recognition molecules include alternative complement components, mannose-binding lectin, and CD14. The innate immune system is a nonspecific, rapid response system, making this system a critical survival mechanism in the initial stages of infection. However, widespread activation of the innate immune system and its cellular components (neutrophils, monocytes, macrophages, and natural killer [NK] cells) can cause collateral damage to host tissues and contributes to the induction of multiorgan injury and septic shock.

In human blood and body fluids, LPS signaling is mediated by interactions with the acute-phase plasma protein LPS-binding protein (LBP). LBP binds to polymeric LPS aggregates and transfers LPS monomers to CD14. After docking to membrane-bound CD14, LPS is delivered to the extracellular adaptor protein MD2. The LPS-MD2 complex is then presented to the extracellular domain of TLR4. This subsequently triggers a signal to the intracellular space that activates LPS-responsive genes. CD14 also binds to bacterial peptidoglycan and lipopeptides and delivers these ligands to TLR2.

TLR4 binding to LPS leads to sequential activation of specific tyrosine and threonine/serine kinases and phosphorylation, ubiquitylation, and degradation of inhibitory κB (I-κB) along with other transcriptional activators. IκB degradation releases nuclear factor κB (NF-κB) from the cytoplasm. NF-κB then translocates into the nucleus and increases transcription of genes encoding clotting elements, complement, other acute phase proteins, cytokines, chemokines, and nitric oxide synthase. The outpouring of inflammatory cytokines and other inflammatory mediators after LPS exposure contributes to SIRS and is central to the pathogenesis of septic shock induced by gram-negative bacteria.

Bacterial Superantigens

Bacterial superantigens comprise a diverse group of protein-based exotoxins from streptococci, staphylococci, and other pathogens that all share the capacity to bind to specific sites on major histocompatibility class II molecules on antigen presenting cells and activate large numbers of CD4+ T cells, bypassing the usual mechanism of antigen processing and presentation. Superantigens bind to and cross-link to a limited number of Vβ regions of the T cell receptor on CD4+ T cells, along with the costimulatory molecule CD28. This bridging complex brings CD4+ T cells and macrophages into close proximity, which activates both the monocyte-macrophage and T cell populations.

Superantigens can stimulate up to 10% to 20% of the entire circulating lymphocyte population, compared to only about one in 10^5 circulating lymphocytes stimulated by typical bacterial antigens. This stimulation results in excessive activation of lymphocytes and macrophages, which leads to uncontrolled inflammatory cytokine synthesis and release. Superantigen-induced immune activation may terminate in septic shock (eg, streptococcal toxic shock syndrome) if the process is left unchecked. Infections associated with release of both bacterial superantigens and endotoxin may be particularly injurious to the host; the toxicity of bacterial endotoxin is greatly enhanced by superantigens that prime the immune system to react to endotoxin in an overly sensitized manner.

Other Microbial Mediators

During periods of prolonged systemic hypotension such as septic shock, redistribution of blood flow to the tissues results in splanchnic vasoconstriction. The ischemia and subsequent reperfusion of the gastrointestinal tract disrupts the intestinal mucosal barrier to bacterial products and damaged tissue releases host-derived alarmins that further activate inflammatory signaling. Translocation of microbial components such as bacterial endotoxin occurs from the GI tract to the circulation during periods of severe stress and hypoperfusion of the GI mucosa. Bacterial endotoxin and perhaps other gut-derived microbial mediators might play a pathogenic role in the ongoing inflammatory process after systemic hypotension produced by infectious or noninfectious insults. This finding has initiated interest in attempts to strengthen the GI mucosal barrier function through immunonutrition, epithelial growth factors, and selective decontamination of the GI tract in critical illness, which remain active areas of research.

PATHOGENESIS: HOST-DERIVED MEDIATORS
Cytokine Networks

Inflammatory cytokines play a pivotal role in sepsis pathogenesis. The major proinflammatory cytokines, TNF-α and IL-1β, induce their hemodynamic and metabolic effects in concert with an expanding group of host-derived inflammatory mediators that work in a coordinated fashion to produce the systemic inflammatory response (see Table 42–2). The cytokine system functions as a network of communication signals between neutrophils, monocytes, macrophages, and endothelial cells. Autocrine and paracrine activation results in synergistic potentiation of the inflammatory response once it is activated by a systemic microbial challenge. Much of the inflammatory response is localized and compartmentalized in the primary region of initial inflammation. If left unchecked, the inflammatory response enters the systemic circulation, resulting in a generalized reaction culminating in diffuse endothelial injury, coagulation activation, and septic shock. The endocrine-like effect of systemic cytokine and chemokine release drives the inflammatory process and causes coagulation activation throughout the body.

TABLE 42–2 Host-derived inflammatory mediators in septic shock.

Proinflammatory Mediators	Anti-Inflammatory Mediators
Tumor necrosis factor-α	Interleukin-1 receptor antagonist
Interferon gamma	Soluble tumor necrosis factor receptor
Lymphotoxin-α	
Interleukin-2	Soluble interleukin-1 receptor
Interleukin-8	
Interleukin-12	Type II interleukin-1 receptor
Interleukin-17	
Interleukin-18	Transforming growth factor-β
sCD14, MD2	
Complement components (C5a and C3a)	Interleukin-4
Mannose binding lectin	Interleukin-6
Leukotriene B₄	Interleukin-10
Platelet-activating factor	Interleukin-11
Bradykinin	Interleukin-13
Nitric oxide	Prostaglandin E2α
Reactive oxygen species	Granulocyte colony-stimulating factor
Granulocyte macrophage colony-stimulating factor	Antioxidants
Chemokines	Anticoagulants (antithrombin, activated protein C, tissue factor pathway inhibitor)
Macrophage inhibitory factor	
High mobility group box I	Interferon alfa
Histamine, thrombin, other clotting factors	Interferon beta
	Glucocorticoids
TREM-1 (triggering receptor expressed on myeloid cells)	Epinephrine
	Cholinergic agonists
	Resolvins, protectins
	Lipoxygenase pathway

The inflammatory cytokines and chemokines found in excess quantities in the bloodstream in patients with septic shock are matched by a group of anti-inflammatory mediators (see Table 42–2). The proinflammatory mediators tend to predominate locally and in the first 12 to 24 hours of sepsis, whereas the endogenous anti-inflammatory components often prevail systemically in the later phases. Monocyte-macrophage–generated cytokines and chemokines primarily promote sepsis early on; the lymphocyte-derived cytokines and interferons become important in the regulation of later phases of sepsis and may ultimately determine the outcome in septic shock.

CD4+ T Helper Cells

Activated, yet uncommitted, T cells (TH0 cells) have four major pathways of functional differentiation (TH1, TH2, TH17, or Treg cells). TH0 cells exposed to IL-12 in the presence of IL-2 are driven toward a TH1-type functional development. These cells produce IFN-γ, TNF-α, and IL-2 and promote an inflammatory, cell-mediated immune response. TH0 cells exposed to IL-4 will preferentially develop into a TH2-type phenotype; TH2 cells secrete IL-4, IL-10, and IL-13, which promote humoral immune responses and attenuate T helper cells, and myeloid cell activity. Sepsis is often accompanied by a TH2-type response after an initial septic insult, likely due in part to the expression of adrenocorticotropic hormone, corticosteroids, and catecholamines that promote a TH2 response. CD4 cells are selectively depleted by apoptosis in sepsis further limiting cell-mediated immunity and T helper cell capacity.

A phase of relative immune refractoriness occurs in septic patients that place them at increased risk for secondary bacterial or fungal infection. Part of the pathophysiology of sepsis-induced immunosuppression is mediated by Th17 cells and regulatory T cells. Th17 cells are stimulated by dendritic cell-derived interleukin-23 to produce IL-17, chemokines, and antibacterial and antifungal peptides. Th17 cells are depleted in sepsis and might explain the propensity of septic patients to develop late, opportunistic bacterial and fungal infections. Regulatory T cells expand during sepsis and produce anti-inflammatory cytokines such as IL-10 and transforming growth factor beta contributing to

T cell exhaustion. This pathophysiologic state is associated with endotoxin tolerance, anti-inflammatory cytokine synthesis, and deactivation of monocytes, macrophages, and neutrophils.

The Coagulation System

Activation of the coagulation cascade and generation of a consumptive coagulopathy and diffuse microthrombi are well-recognized events in sepsis. The tissue factor pathway (also known as the extrinsic pathway) is the predominant mechanism by which the coagulation system is activated. The contact factors in the intrinsic pathway are also activated, which helps perpetuate clotting and secondarily initiates vasodilation through bradykinin generation. Activation of intravascular coagulation results in microthrombi and contributes to microcirculatory dysfunction and the multiorgan failure that occur in septic patients. Depletion of coagulation factors and activation of plasmin, antithrombin III, and protein C may subsequently lead to a hemorrhagic diathesis. Depletion of these endogenous anticoagulants may secondarily lead to a procoagulant state and portend a poor prognosis.

Neutrophil–Endothelial Cell Interactions

The recruitment of neutrophils to an area of localized infection is an essential component of the host inflammatory response. Localization and eradication of invading microbial pathogens at the site of initial infection is the principal objective of the immune response to microbial pathogens. This physiologic process becomes deleterious if diffuse neutrophil–endothelial cell interactions occur throughout the circulation in response to systemic inflammation.

Complex mechanisms govern the migration of neutrophils from the intravascular space into the interstitium, where invasive microorganisms may reside. Activated neutrophils degranulate, exposing endothelial surfaces and surrounding structures to reactive oxygen intermediates, nitric oxide, and a variety of proteases. This process contributes not only to microbial clearance but also to diffuse endothelial injury in the setting of systemic inflammation.

Nitric Oxide

Nitric oxide is a highly reactive free radical that plays an essential role in the pathophysiology of septic shock. Its half-life of 1 to 3 seconds limits its activity to local tissues, where it is first generated by nitric oxide synthase. Full expression of inducible nitric oxide synthase requires TNF-α, IL-1, LPS, and probably other regulatory elements.

Nitric oxide is the major endothelial-derived relaxing factor that initiates the vasodilation and systemic hypotension observed in septic shock. Nitric oxide activates guanylate cyclase, which increases cyclic guanosine monophosphate levels inside vascular smooth muscle cells. This results in systemic vasodilation and decreased vascular resistance. Excessive and prolonged release of nitric oxide results in generalized vasodilatation and systemic hypotension.

Nitric oxide also helps increase intracellular killing of microbial pathogens and regulation of platelet and neutrophil adherence in septic patients. It is a highly diffusible gas that does not require specific receptors to cross cell membranes. In the presence of superoxide anion, nitric oxide leads to the formation of peroxynitrite and highly cytotoxic molecules, such as hydroxyl radicals and nitrosyl chloride, which then initiate lipid peroxidation and cause irreversible cellular damage. Nitric oxide inhibits a variety of key enzymes in the tricarboxylic acid pathway, the glycolytic pathway, DNA repair systems, electron transport pathways, and energy-exchange pathways. Because of its potent reactivity, nitric oxide alters the function of many metallo-enzymes, carrier proteins, and structural elements.

Late Host-Derived Mediators

Macrophage migration inhibitory factor is a late mediator that activates immune cells, upregulates TLR4 expression, and contributes to lethal septic shock. This corticosteroid-regulated mediator promotes inflammation and has become a target for therapeutic agents in sepsis. The nuclear protein high-mobility group box–1 protein is released into the extracellular space with cell injury and necrosis and also participates in late-onset inflammatory phase of septic shock.

Pathogenesis: Organ Dysfunction

The diffuse endothelial injury accompanying septic shock results in organ dysfunction distant from the original site of the septic insult. The signal that results in diffuse endovascular injury is thought to be relayed by plasma factors (eg, inflammatory cytokines, complement, kinins, and other host-derived inflammatory mediators) or cellular signals from immune effector cells.

Inadequate tissue blood supply and repeated episodes of ischemia-reperfusion produces MODS. The failure of the microcirculation to support tissue maintenance may result from capillary bed hypoperfusion, blood flow redistribution within vascular beds, functional arteriovenous shunting, blood flow obstruction from microthrombi, platelet or white blood cell aggregates, or abnormal red blood cell deformability. Nitric oxide, reactive oxygen intermediates, inflammatory cytokines, and apoptosis inducers may directly damage endothelial surfaces. Endothelial swelling shifts intravascular fluid into extravascular and intracellular spaces, mechanically obstructing capillary lumens and further limiting microvascular blood flow.

Myocardial performance and pulmonary function also diminish over the course of septic shock and may contribute to the development of MODS. Myocardial contractility decreases in response to various myocardial depressant factors. TNF-α is a prominent cause of myocardial dysfunction; IL-1, IL-6, nitric oxide, and other host-derived inflammatory mediators may be contributing factors. Acute lung injury occurs in septic shock as a result of damage to pulmonary vascular circulation and excess permeability of alveolar capillary membranes. A supply-dependent dysoxia, along with altered capacity for oxidative phosphorylation (cytopathic hypoxia), likely contributes to tissue injury and multiorgan failure in sepsis.

DIAGNOSTIC APPROACH TO SEPSIS

Clinical Features

In his classic treatise on human nature (*The Prince*, circa 1505), Machiavelli states, "Hectic fever [meaning sepsis] at its inception is difficult to recognize but easy to treat; left untended, it becomes easy to recognize but difficult to treat." This statement is as true today as it was 500 years ago. Fully developed septic shock is a readily apparent clinical syndrome that is seldom confused with other pathologic states. However, the early phases of septic shock may be quite subtle even in carefully monitored patients. Although fever is characteristic, hypothermia may occur and connotes a poor prognosis. Unexplained tachycardia and tachypnea are often part of the systemic inflammatory response seen in sepsis. It is important to note that many noninfectious diseases may masquerade as sepsis such as acute pancreatitis, pulmonary emboli, myocardial infarction, blood transfusion reactions, and organ transplant rejection. A summary of the major hemodynamic findings of sepsis is provided in Table 42–3.

Laboratory Indicators of Sepsis and Septic Shock

The updated international guidelines use the Sequential [Sepsis-Related] Organ Failure Assessment Score to define sepsis (SOFA, see Table 42–4). Laboratory criteria included in the SOFA focus on the presence of coagulopathy, hepatic dysfunction, and/or renal dysfunction. Other nonspecific laboratory criteria, such as peripheral white blood cell count can aid in the general diagnosis of infection but are no longer used to define sepsis or septic shock.

White Blood Cell Count and Differential

Either leukocytosis or leukopenia may occur in sepsis. An absolute lymphocyte count less than 1200 cells/mm^3 and a ANC:ALC ratio more than 10 have been found to be better predictors of bacteremia than the total white blood cell count or absolute neutrophil count. Interesting, eosinopenia (< 40%) is as useful as C reactive protein in distinguishing SIRS as an immunologically regulated response to infection and SIRS from sepsis.

Coagulation Parameters

Systemic inflammation induced during sepsis can activate the coagulation cascade. In a clinical trial of recombinant human activated Protein C in patients with severe sepsis more than 95% of patients had

TABLE 42–3 Common hemodynamic findings in sepsis.

Parameter	Typical Findings	Comments
Heart rate	≥ 100 beat/min	Major compensatory mechanism for low systemic vascular resistance
Mean arterial blood pressure	< 65 mm Hg	Hallmark of septic shock if it remains low after adequate fluid resuscitation
Cardiac index (cardiac output/m² [surface area])	> 4 L/min/m²	Cardiac index usually elevated in early septic shock; may be depressed in late septic shock
Pulmonary arterial occlusion pressure (PAOP)	8-16 mm Hg	Assure that hypovolemia is not the cause of hypotension; perform fluid resuscitation until PAOP returns to normal
Central venous pressure (CVP)	6-12 mm Hg	Reliable resuscitation goal indicating adequate blood volume for ventricular filling pressure
Systemic vascular resistance (SVR)	< 800 dyne/s/cm⁻⁵	SVR often low in early septic shock; may become elevated in later phases of septic shock
Oxygen delivery (DO_2) Cardiac index (CI) × arterial O_2 content (A)	< 550 mL/min/m²	Try to provide sufficient DO^2 to maintain adequate mixed venous O_2 saturation
Mixed venous O_2 saturation (SvO_2) or Central venous O_2 saturation ($ScvO_2$)	< 70% < 65%	Low mixed venous O_2 saturation or central venous O_2 saturation (from superior vena cava) indicates poor oxygen delivery to tissues
Oxygen consumption (VO_2) (CI) × (A-VO_2) × 10	> 180 L/min/m²	Typically increased in early septic shock

coagulation abnormalities at the time of study entry. Thrombocytosis may occur early as an acute phase response, while thrombocytopenia may occur as a late ominous sign. Additional coagulation findings in severe sepsis are prolongation of the prothrombin time and an increase in fibrin split products or D-dimer. Greater aberrations in coagulation markers are noted in patients with severe sepsis with bloodstream infections compared with those without bloodstream infections. Two endogenous anticoagulants, Protein C and Antithrombin become depleted early on in the development of sepsis far in advance of the development of organ dysfunction.

Chemistries

Unexplained lactic acidemia as a sign of global tissue hypoperfusion occurs in sepsis; a level of more than 2 mmol/dL (18 mg/dL) is a poor prognostic factor and may indicate septic shock as noted earlier. Failure to clear lactate after early fluid resuscitation (> 30 mL/kg intravenous crystalloid) at a rate of at least 10% per hour is a very poor prognostic sign. Chemistry panels can also be used to detect the presence of sepsis-induced organ dysfunction. Acute kidney injury can be recognized by a rise in the serum creatinine of 0.3 mg/dL or more in 48 hours or a serum creatinine that rise more than 1.5 times baseline levels within the previous 7 days. A total plasma bilirubin more than 4 mg/dL is indicative of sepsis-induced hepatic dysfunction.

Acute Phase Reactants/Biomarkers

Biomarkers that are readily available to most clinicians are the ESR (erythrocyte sedimentation rate) and C-reactive protein (CRP). The use of the ESR has largely been supplanted by the CRP in the evaluation of acute infectious diseases like sepsis. CRP is helpful when normal but is not specific for infection when elevated. CRP can be elevated for days following surgery and will also be elevated in rheumatologic and neoplastic illnesses. Very high CRP levels (> 85 mg/L) is useful in distinguishing

TABLE 42–4 Common laboratory findings in sepsis.

Laboratory Study	Typical Findings	Comments
White blood cell count	Leukocytosis or leukopenia	Stress response, increased margination of neutrophils in sepsis can cause transient neutropenia; toxic granulation
Platelet count	Thrombocytopenia (< 150,000/mm³)	Look for evidence of fragmentation hemolysis; thrombocytopenia may be accompanied by DIC
Total lymphocyte count	Lymphopenia (< 1200/mm³)	All lymphocyte types decreased from trafficking out to extravascular sites and excess apoptosis except Treg cells
Eosinophil count	Eosinopenia (< 40/mm³)	Can suggest infection-related acute inflammatory processes
Coagulation studies	Elevated prothrombin time (INR), aPTT, low fibrinogen levels, elevated D-dimer; evidence of fibrinolysis	Coagulopathy very common, but overt DIC is not common (< 15% of patients)
Liver enzymes	Elevated alkaline phosphatase, bilirubin, and transaminases; low albumin	These are generally a late finding in sepsis
Blood cultures	Bacteremia or fungemia	Positive blood cultures not required for the diagnosis of sepsis
Plasma lactate	> 2.2 mmol/L caused by hypermetabolism, anaerobic metabolism, inhibition of pyruvate dehydrogenase	Poor prognostic feature if not improved rapidly by fluid resuscitation; diagnostic criterion for septic shock
C-reactive protein	Elevated as an acute phase reactant from hepatic synthesis	Acute-phase reactant, sensitive, but not specific for sepsis
Glucose	Hyperglycemia or hypoglycemia	Acute stress response, inhibition of gluconeogenesis can lead to hypoglycemia
Arterial blood gases	Respiratory alkalosis (early); metabolic acidosis (late)	Reduced arterial O_2 content and mixed venous O_2 saturation

DIC, disseminated intravascular coagulation; Treg cells, regulatory T cells; INR, international normalized ratio; aPTT, activated partial thromboplastin time.

infection from non-infectious causes of acute systemic inflammation.

A newer biomarker for the diagnosis of sepsis is serum procalcitonin (PCT). In heath, PCT is precursor peptide in calcitonin synthesis by C cells in the thyroid; in septic patients, PCT is generated in prodigious amounts by numerous extra-thyroidal tissues. Elevated levels of PCT are seen 4 to 6 hours after a systemic challenge with endotoxin or other septic stimuli. PCT levels drop quickly following trauma and surgery and are not elevated by malignancies or rheumatologic diseases. PCT is an FDA approved test to aid in the risk assessment of patients with sepsis. A recent meta-analysis of studies examining confirms the value of PCT to distinguish sepsis

for noninfectious causes of systemic inflammation. Levels of PCT more than 2 ng/mL is the best cutoff value in the early diagnosis of bacterial sepsis.

An additional biomarker approved by the FDA for assessing the risk of sepsis in in the ICU is the endotoxin activity assay (EAA). Endotoxin is a known mediator in the pathogenesis of sepsis and septic shock. The EAA relies upon priming of the endogenous neutrophil population by circulating endotoxin. This chemiluminescent assay compares the respiratory burst by endotoxin in the test sample to the maximum burst when the sample is spiked with excess LPS. In one study, elevated endotoxin levels were found in 58% of patients admitted to a mixed surgical-medical ICU, irrespective of the reason for admission. Elevated EAA in patients admitted to the ICU portends a greater chance of septic shock and excess mortality.

Use of the SOFA to Assess Sepsis Severity

Hallmark strong predictor of sepsis mortality is the development of organ dysfunction. The SOFA score assesses the degree of organ dysfunction across several domains and has been integrated into the 2016 guidelines for diagnosing sepsis (Tables 42–1 and 42–5). A SOFA score of 2 or more reflects an overall mortality risk of roughly 10% in the setting of suspected infection. Additionally, use of the bedside qSOFA (Quick SOFA) criteria has been validated as a reliable bedside tool for identifying adult patients with suspected infection who are likely to have poor outcomes. Presence of any 2 of the following criteria represents a positive qSOFA: (1) respiratory rate of 22/min or more; (2) altered mentation (defined as any Glasgow Coma Scale score < 15); and/or (3) systolic blood pressure of 100 mm Hg or less. The qSOFA is best applied as an early warning sign of infection-induced organ dysfunction for use on the medical or surgical floor, whereas the standard SOFA score has greater predictive power in the critical care setting. It is essential that clinicians recognize these early signs and symptoms because successful management of sepsis depends on early recognition and appropriate intervention. The mortality rate in sepsis increases with an increasing number of organ dysfunctions.

SEPTIC SHOCK

Septic shock occurs in up to 15% of patients with sepsis, and is defined as a hypotension requiring vasopressors to maintain a MAP of 65 or more and a serum lactate level of more than 2 mmol/L (18 mg/dL). The most common hemodynamic findings in early septic shock are a high cardiac output and a low systemic vascular resistance state. Myocardial performance is markedly diminished in septic shock. Without adequate intervention, circulating blood volume is continually lost into the interstitial space and intracellular locations, perpetuating systolic hypotension. Deterioration of myocardial performance, accompanied by diffuse vasoconstriction, marks the late refractory state of septic shock.

TABLE 42–5 The Sequential [Sepsis-Related] Organ Failure Assessment (SOFA) Score.[1]

	Score				
	0	**1**	**2**	**3**	**4**
Respiration PaO$_2$/FiO$_2$ mm Hg (kPa)	≥ 400 (53.3)	< 400 (53.3)	< 300 (40)	< 200 (26.7) with respiratory support	< 100 (13.3) with respiratory support
Coagulation platelets, ×10^3/μL	≥ 150	< 150	< 100	< 50	< 20
Liver bilirubin, mg/dL (μmol/L)	< 1.2 (20)	1.2-1.9 (20-32)	2.0-5.9 (33-101)	6.0-11.9 (102-204)	> 12.0 (204)
Cardiovascular	MAP ≥ 70 mm Hg	MAP < 70 mm Hg	Dopamine < 5 or dobutamine (any dose)[2]	Dopamine 5.1-15 or epinephrine ≤ 0.1 or norepinephrine ≤ 0.1[2]	Dopamine > 15 or epinephrine > 0.1 or norepinephrine > 0.1[2]
Central nervous system Glasgow Coma Scale Score	15	13-14	10-12	6-9	< 6
Renal creatinine, mg/dL (μmol/L) or	<1.2 (110)	1.2-1.9 (110-170)	2.0-3.4 (171-299)	3.5-4.9 (300-440)	> 5.0 (440)
Urine output, mL/d				< 500	< 200

[1]Reproduced with permission from Vincent JL, Moreno R, Takala J, et. al. Working Group on Sepsis-Related Problems of the European Society of Intensive Care Medicine. The SOFA (Sepsis-related Organ Failure Assessment) score to describe organ dysfunction/failure. *Intensive Care Med.* 1996 Jul;22(7):707-710.
[2]Catecholamine doses are given as mcg/kg/min for 1 hour or more.

Acute Respiratory Distress Syndrome

The acute respiratory distress syndrome (ARDS) remains a major cause of morbidity and mortality in septic shock. Increased capillary permeability in these patients results in pulmonary edema, which manifests clinically as dyspnea and cough; standard radiographs will typically show bilateral, symmetrical alveolar opacities in all four quadrants. The initial diagnostic criteria for ARDS include the absence of clinical evidence of left atrial hypertension, the requirement for intubation and positive pressure ventilation, and a PaO_2/FiO_2 ratio of 200 or less. The new Berlin definition of ARDS simplifies the diagnostic criteria for ARDS and classifies the patients into three diagnostic and prognostic categories depending upon the severity of gas exchange based on the PaO_2/FIO_2 ratio (see Table 42–1). A detailed analysis of the Berlin definition of ARDS from a large patient database found that a PaO_2/FiO_2 ratio of between 200 and 300 mm Hg or less (classified as mild ARDS) was associated with a mortality rate 27±3% mortality. Moderately severe ARDS with a PaO_2/FiO_2 ratio of 100 to 200 mm Hg or less was associated with a mortality rate of 32±3%. Severe ARDS manifest by a PaO_2/FiO_2 ratio 100 mm Hg or less is accompanied by a mortality rate of 45±2%.

Management of Septic Shock

The management of a patient with septic shock begins with prompt recognition of the condition and the rapid administration of appropriate antibiotic therapy as well as source control of infection. Attention is simultaneously given to failing organs with institution of measures including fluid resuscitation, vasopressors, blood transfusions, and inotropic agents as needed to maximize oxygen delivery. Patients with ARDS are managed with low tidal volume ventilator strategies to minimize damage induced by overstretching the alveoli. Consideration is also given to the use of low dose corticosteroids in in cases of refractory septic shock. Reasonable glycemic control is utilized in effort to minimize septic complications. Guidelines for the initial management of sepsis are provided in the Surviving Sepsis Campaign guidelines.

Microbiologic Workup

A rapid systematic search for infection should include a thorough physical exam, review of pertinent radiographic studies, and microbiologic studies. The three most common sites of infection are the lung followed by infection in the abdomen and genitourinary tract. In approximately 30% of cases a causative organism and focus of infection is never found. Based upon history and physical exam imaging and culturing of normally sterile body sites should be done to define infection. In community-acquired pneumonia obtaining high-quality sputum samples for making an etiologic diagnosis is quite difficult. A rapid immunoassay that detects the C-polysaccharide from the cell wall of *Streptococcus pneumoniae* from the urine is clinically useful for the diagnosis of pneumococcal pneumonia. A similar urine immunoassay is available for *Legionella* spp. pneumonia. Two sets of blood cultures should be collected as soon as possible and preferably before starting antibiotics. If a central venous catheter is present, one blood culture should be drawn from the catheter and one from a peripheral venipuncture. A blood culture drawn from a central line that becomes positive 2 or more hours before a peripheral venipuncture drawn at the same time supports a diagnosis of a catheter-related bloodstream infection. In patients at high risk for candidemia, a beta-D-glucan assay should be obtained. This assay is often positive for 2 or more days before the blood culture grows *Candida* spp.

Appropriate Antibiotic Therapy

Numerous studies in patients with sepsis have demonstrated a survival advantage in patients who have received appropriate versus inappropriate antibiotic therapy. Furthermore, animal and human studies demonstrate a decrease in survival for each hour delay in the administration of antibiotic therapy from the onset of septic shock. Optimal antimicrobial therapy in sepsis depends on the site of infection, local susceptibility patterns, prior antimicrobial exposure, presence or absence of pregnancy, hepatic and renal function, and history of drug allergy. Suggested empiric antibiotic regimens for the different sites of infection are presented in Table 42–6. A propensity matched

TABLE 42–6 Suggested initial empiric antibiotic choices for sepsis.

Source of Infection	Antimicrobial Choice
Community-acquired pneumonia	Third-generation cephalosporin with a macrolide or respiratory fluoroquinolone. Use cefepime or piperacillin-tazobactam in place of third-generation cephalosporin if risk factors for Pseudomonas infection or MDR pathogens
Hospital-acquired pneumonia	Third- or fourth-generation cephalosporin or an extended-spectrum penicillin ± an aminoglycoside or a fluoroquinolone (or: carbapenems, β-lactam—β-lactamase inhibitor); add vancomycin or linezolid if MRSA suspected
Urinary tract infection	Extended-spectrum β-lactam agent ± aminoglycoside or fluoroquinolone). Use cefepime or a carbapenem if history of, or at risk for MDR organism
Intra-abdominal infection	A carbapenem or piperacillin-tazobactam as monotherapy or a third or fourth-generation cephalosporin or fluoroquinolone in combination with metronidazole
Neutropenic sepsis	Monotherapy with an antipseudomonal beta-lactam agent, such as cefepime, a carbapenem (meropenem), or piperacillin-tazobactam is recommended (add vancomycin when there is evidence of gram-positive infection or linezolid if MRSA or VRE suspected); add a triazole (voriconazole or fluconazole) or β-glucan inhibitor (eg, caspofungin or micafungin) if systemic fungal infection suspected
Necrotizing skin/soft tissue infection	Vancomycin and piperacillin-tazobactam ± clindamycin

MDR, multiple antibiotic drug resistant; MRSA, methicillin-resistant *Staphylococcus aureus*; VRE, vancomycin-resistant enterococcus.

analysis comparing monotherapy to combination therapy for sepsis favored combination therapy for both gram-positive and gram-negative infections in severely ill patients at increased risk of death (estimated mortality rate > 25%). Empiric treatment for methicillin-resistant *Staphylococcus aureus* (MRSA) depends upon the clinical context especially given the increasing incidence of infections due community-acquired, methicillin-resistant *Staphylococcus aureus* (CA-MRSA). Empiric antifungal therapy in patients with sepsis is not routinely recommended, but should be reserved for cases where patients have well-described risk factors for fungemia including a history of receiving multiple antibiotics for multiple days, the presence of a central venous catheter for TPN or hemodialysis, elevated beta-D-glucan levels or *Candida* spp. previously isolated from multiple anatomic sites. Initial antimicrobial therapy should be reconsidered at 72 hours and "deescalated" based upon the final culture and susceptibility data.

Optimizing Tissue Oxygenation

In the early phase of sepsis, an imbalance develops between tissue oxygen delivery and oxygen demand.

This can be diagnosed by laboratory testing of lactic acid levels. Rivers and colleagues performed a randomized, clinical trial to see if a protocolized algorithm of early goal directed therapy (EGDT) to meet a resuscitation goal of a central venous oxygen saturation of 70% decreased mortality in septic shock. In this study, patients with septic shock and lactic acidemia were randomized to either a standard therapy arm or EGDT arm. Patients in the EGDT group received crystalloid fluid boluses every 30 minutes in attempt to achieve a CVP of 8 to 12 mm Hg. If the mean arterial pressure remained less than 65 mm Hg vasopressors were then added. If following these maneuvers, the central venous O_2 saturation remained less than 70%, red cell transfusions were given to achieve a hematocrit of more than 30%. If these targets were still not met, dobutamine was then added. The in-hospital mortality was significantly lower in the EGDT group than the standard treatment group (30.5% vs 46.5%, $P = 0009$). This treatment strategy is now widely utilized and is generally followed in the recent 2013 sepsis guidelines. However, three subsequent, large, randomized trials have failed to confirm a clear survival advantage to EGDT versus usual care in the emergency resuscitation of patients in septic shock.

Fluid Resuscitation

Debate continues regarding the appropriateness of colloid versus crystalloid fluids. The lack of clear evidence of benefit of colloid agents (eg, albumin, dextran, and plasma expanders) and their high cost have generally resulted in the use of saline solutions for volume expansion.

Vasopressor Therapy

Failure to improve patient hemodynamics with fluids alone often necessitates the use of vasopressor agents to reestablish adequate tissue perfusion. Dopamine, epinephrine, norepinephrine, phenylephrine, and vasopressin have been used to reverse hypotension in the setting of septic shock. The use of any of these agents in septic shock carries with it certain risks and should be reserved for patients with significant hemodynamic instability that is unresponsive to fluid therapy. The clinical target of vasopressors to maintain organ perfusion is a mean arterial pressure of more than 65 mm Hg. Results of both individual studies and a meta-analysis have revealed that the use of dopamine is associated with a higher mortality and a higher incidence of arrhythmias than norepinephrine. As such, norepinephrine is now considered the agent of first choice for septic shock. Dobutamine remains the inotropic agent of first choice in septic shock in patients with low cardiac output despite adequate fluid resuscitation.

Low-Dose Corticosteroid Therapy for Septic Shock

The value of corticosteroids in the treatment of sepsis have been the subject of a debate for greater than fifty years. Studies have also suggested that a state of relative adrenal insufficiency and glucocorticoid resistance occurs during sepsis and is associated with a poor outcome. A study by Annane observed relative adrenal insufficiency, defined as an increase in serum cortisol less than 9 mg/dL 60 minutes after receiving 250 mg of synthetic ACTH in patients with septic shock. In a clinical study in patients with

vasopressor-dependent refractory septic shock to receive either 50 mg of hydrocortisone every 6 hours and 50 mg/day of fludrocortisone improved survival over placebo treatment. A large follow-up study failed to confirm the benefit of low-dose corticosteroids, with the possible exception of patients with refractory septic shock. The current recommendation is to consider corticosteroids (≤ 200 mg of hydrocortisone/day) in the subpopulation with refractory septic shock. Treatment should be given for at least 5 days followed by a taper to prevent rebound hypotension.

Blood Transfusions

The threshold for blood transfusions in improving the oxygen-carrying capacity of blood is a matter of ongoing research. A large Canadian study, the TRICC trial (Transfusion requirements in Critical Care) showed that maintaining a hemoglobin (Hgb) level of 7 to 9 gm/dL and setting a transfusion threshold as low as 7 gm/dL in volume-resuscitated patients is not associated with a worse outcome than maintaining an Hgb of more than 10 gm/dL. The hemoglobin level may need to be maintained at a higher level include severe coronary artery disease and severe hypoxemia.

Glycemic Control

Reasonable glycemic control in sepsis is now considered glucose control (targeted around 150 mg/dL) is now recommended in patients with sepsis-induced glucose intolerance. Large swings on blood glucose levels are to be avoided and hypoglycemia can be particularly hazardous.

Infection Control

Patients with severe sepsis are at risk for the development of new infections and superinfections. In patients on mechanical ventilation, elevating the head of the bed by 30 to 45 degrees limits the risk of aspiration and ventilator-associated pneumonia. Carts containing all the materials necessary for sterile insertion of central venous catheters should be used and maintained in all ICUs. Universal MRSA decolonization of ICU patients with nasal mupirocin and chlorhexidine baths has been shown to decrease the incidence of bloodstream infections.

Experimental Therapies for Septic Shock

Despite the failure of many agents in the past, studies of additional experimental treatments continue. Late-stage therapies are targeting sepsis-induced DIC and patients with elevated endotoxin activity. Multiple failures using a variety of anti-inflammatory compounds have led to a renewed appreciation of the immunoparalysis of sepsis. The future therapy of sepsis will likely resemble cancer chemotherapy with personalized combinations of agents being used to target each patient's unique situation and needs.

The authors have no commercial relationships with manufacturers of products or providers of services discussed in this chapter.

REFERENCES

1. Dellinger RP, Levy MM, Rhodes A, et al. Surviving Sepsis Campaign: international guidelines for management of severe sepsis and septic shock, 2012. *Intensive Care Med.* 2013;39:165-228.
2. Martin GS, Mannino DM, Eaton S, Moss M. The epidemiology of sepsis in the United States from 1979 through 2000. *N Engl J Med.* 2003;348:1546-1554.
3. Angus DC, Linde-Zwirble WT, Lidicker J, Clermont G, Carcillo J, Pinsky MR. Epidemiology of severe sepsis in the United States: analysis of incidence, outcome, and associated costs of care. *Crit Care Med.* 2001;29:1303-1310.
4. Suffredini AF, Munford RS. Novel therapies for septic shock over the past 4 decades. *JAMA.* 2011;306:194-199.
5. Singer M, Deutschman CS, Seymour CW, et al. The Third International Concensus Definitions for Sepsis and Septic Shock (Sepsis-3). *JAMA.* 2016;315(8):801-810.
6. Cohen J. The immunopathogenesis of sepsis. *Nature.* 2002;420:885-891.
7. Opal SM, Calandra T. Antibiotic usage and resistance: gaining or losing ground on infections in critically ill patients? *JAMA.* 2009;302:2367-2368.
8. Pridmore AC, Wyllie DH, Abdillahi F, et al. A lipopolysaccharide-deficient mutant of Neisseria meningitidis elicits attenuated cytokine release by human macrophages and signals via toll-like receptor (TLR) 2 but not via TLR4/MD2. *J Infect Dis.* 2001;183:89-96.
9. Akira S, Takeda K. Toll-like receptor signalling. *Nature Rev Immunol.* 2004;4:499-511.
10. Hotchkiss RS, Opal S. Immunotherapy for sepsis—a new approach against an ancient foe. *N Engl J Med.* 2010;363:87-89.
11. Vincent JL, Moreno R, Takala J, et al. Working Group on Sepsis-Related Problems of the European Society of Intensive Care Medicine. The SOFA (Sepsis-related Organ Failure Assessment) score to describe organ dysfunction/failure. *Intensive Care Med.* 1996;22(7):707-710.

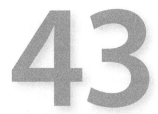

Antimicrobials in the ICU

*Perminder Gulani, MD; Julie Chen, PharmD, BCPS;
and Adam Keene, MD, MS*

KEY POINTS

1 Because therapeutic delay has been clearly shown to increase mortality, prompt empiric broad-spectrum antimicrobial therapy is crucial in patients with shock and new organ dysfunction thought secondary to infection.

2 Overuse of antimicrobials in the ICU is common and is associated with multiple adverse drug reactions, superinfections and the development of antimicrobial resistance; antimicrobial therapy should be tailored as soon as possible and courses of therapy should not be prolonged unnecessarily.

3 Beta-lactams are the most important antibacterial agents used in the ICU; allergic reactions are the most common adverse effects but are frequently misreported so the risks of such reactions must always be weighed against the importance of these agents for severe bacterial infections.

4 The aminoglycosides are potent agents against gram-negative bacteria but their utility is limited by frequent misdosing due to concerns of nephrotoxicity; extended dosing intervals can be helpful in maximizing efficacy and minimizing toxicity.

5 The fluoroquinolones have activity against a variety of bacterial infections in the ICU; they are generally well tolerated but are considered second-line agents for a number of severe sepsis syndromes.

6 Vancomycin, linezolid, and daptomycin are important agents for resistant gram-positive infections in the ICU. Their utility varies by the site of primary infection.

7 Azithromycin and doxycycline are particularly useful for atypical bacterial infections in the ICU and are generally well tolerated. Metronidazole and clindamycin are useful primarily for coverage of anaerobic infections in the ICU.

8 Tigecycline and polymyxin B/colistin are used mainly for resistant gram-negative infections in the ICU; use of the former is limited by lack of potency and the latter is limited by high potential for nephrotoxicity.

9 The three classes of antifungals used in the ICU are the polyenes, the azoles, and the echinocandins. Polyenes are broad spectrum but nephrotoxic; azoles have variable coverage but resistance can be a problem; echinocandins are excellent anticandidal agents and are generally well tolerated.

10 The nucleoside analogues are the primary agents used to treat herpes viruses in the ICU; their efficacy is variable and they may cause hematologic and renal toxicity.

11 The neuraminidase inhibitors are important agents that may improve the outcome of influenza virus infections in the ICU.

INTRODUCTION

The principles used to guide antimicrobial therapy in all patients can be applied to the critically ill patients, with some modification. Patient characteristics including environmental history, immune status, prior antimicrobial exposure, and prior culture results are essential in determining likely organisms and appropriate empiric therapy. In patients who develop infection after hospital admission, knowledge of common local institutional pathogens and their sensitivity patterns is important. Source identification and control are crucial, although imaging tests may be limited by patient instability and organ failure. As discussed further in the Chapter "Pharmacology in Critical Illness," the efficacy and toxicity of antimicrobial agents can be profoundly affected by the alterations in tissue perfusion, volume of distribution, serum protein levels, and renal and hepatic function that occur in the critically ill patients.

In ICU patients with new onset of shock and organ dysfunction thought secondary to infection, prompt empiric broad-spectrum antimicrobial therapy is crucial. Each hour of delay in adequate antimicrobial therapy after the onset of hypotension has been associated with a mean decrease in survival of 7.6%.[1] Although the common infectious syndromes encountered in the ICU are discussed elsewhere, suggested empiric antimicrobial therapy for non-immunocompromised patients based on suspected source is provided in Table 43–1.

Unfortunately, antimicrobials are also the most unnecessarily prescribed medications in the ICU. Antimicrobial overuse has numerous deleterious effects. Allergic reactions, drug fever, and nephrotoxicity are common. In additon, antibiotic overuse has been clearly linked to the development and transmission of multidrug resistant (MDR) organisms.[2] Finally, the development of antibiotic-associated C. difficile colitis is a particular danger to ICU patients that has been worsened by the recent emergence of hypervirulent strains.[3]

A few strategies may help to strike a balance between the seemingly opposing recommendations to provide broad antimicrobial coverage for septic critically ill patients and to avoid antimicrobial overuse in the ICU. While it is important to provide empiric therapy that covers all likely pathogens in the critically ill patient, it is also imperative to step down the antimicrobial regimen as much as possible once culture results are available. Because standard culture techniques have limited sensitivity, it is sometimes necessary to continue broad empiric therapy even in the face of negative cultures. Biomarkers such as procalcitonin tend to become markedly elevated in the face of serious bacterial infections, and normal levels may be useful in rapidly ruling out such a process.[4] Unfortunately, a myriad of non-infectious critical illnesses cause these nonspecific biomarkers to rise as well. Because of this, they are usually unable to safely rule out bacterial infections in the acutely critically ill patients and may actually increase the use of antibiotics when they are used to drive antimicrobial initiation.[5] Molecular tests to detect the presence of invasive pathogens are just beginning to show clinical utility, and in the future may greatly increase our ability to rapidly and safely narrow antimicrobial therapy.

When narrowing antimicrobial coverage it is important to understand that antibiotic spectrum and antibiotic potency are distinct concepts, and that many of the antimicrobials that are reserved to treat MDR infections have both suboptimal efficacy and increased toxicity. For health-care–associated pneumonia (HCAP) caused by pathogens other than methicillin-resistant *Staphylococcus aureus* (MRSA) and nonlactose fermenting gram-negative rods, there is now adequate evidence that antibacterials may be stopped after 8 days, thus decreasing overall antibiotic exposure.[6] Properly organized antibiotic stewardship programs can help clinicians to rationally utilize antimicrobials and have been shown to safely reduce antimicrobial overuse in the ICU.[7]

ANTIMICROBIAL AGENTS COMMONLY USED IN THE ICU

Due to space limitations several agents that are significant but infrequently used will not be discussed here. These include the antibacterial agents quinupristin/dalfopristin and telavancin, the antiviral agents cidofovir and ribavirin, the antifungal agents itraconazole and pentamidine, and the antiparasitic agents albendazole, ivermectin, artesunate, and quinine.

TABLE 43–1 Suggested empiric antimicrobial therapy for adult patients with newly acquired severe sepsis/septic shock.

Suspected Source	Empiric Therapy by Patient Type		Comments
	Community Acquired/ Antibiotic Naive	**Health Care Associated/Prior Antibiotic Exposure**	
Lung	(A) Ceftriaxone plus azithromycin or an antistreptococcal quinolone **plus** (B) Vancomycin or linezolid	(A) Piperacillin/tazobactam or cefepime or imipenem/cilastatin **plus** (B) An aminoglycoside or ciprofloxacin **plus** (C) Vancomycin or linezolid	Consider empiric antiviral therapy (ie, oseltamivir) during seasonal outbreaks.
Heart/intravascular catheter/ bloodstream/ unknown source	(A) Vancomycin **plus** (B) Ceftriaxone	(A) Vancomycin **plus** (B) Piperacillin/tazobactam or cefepime or imipenem/cilastatin **plus/minus** (C) An aminoglycoside	Consider echinocandins if patient with risk factors for candidemia. Consider rifampin if endovascular prosthesis present. Catheter removal whenever possible, particularly for patients in shock.
Intra-abdominal	(A) Cefoxitin, ertapenem, moxifloxacin, or ticarcillin/ clavulanate **or** (B) Ceftriaxone plus metronidazole **or** (C) Ciprofloxacin plus metronidazole	(A) Imipenem/cilastatin or piperacillin/tazobactam **or** (B) Cefepime plus metronidazole **plus/minus** (C) An aminoglycoside	Empiric antipseudomonal therapy may be considered in severely ill patients with community-acquired infections. Always consider C. difficile.
Skin and soft tissue	(A) Vancomycin **plus** (whether diabetic or vasculopath) (B) Piperacillin/tazobactam and (if concern for toxic shock syndrome) clindamycin	(A) Vancomycin **plus** (whether diabetic or vasculopath) (B) Piperacillin/tazobactam and (if concern for toxic shock syndrome) clindamycin	For community-acquired infections, environmental exposures (to water, animals, plants, etc) must be considered.
Genitourinary	(A) Ceftriaxone or (B) Ampicillin/sulbactam	(A) Cefepime or (B) Piperacillin/tazobactam or (C) Imipenem	Consider adding an aminoglycoside to any patient in shock or with a history of recurrent infections.
Central nervous system	(A) Ceftriaxone (2 grams every 12 hours) **plus** (B) Vancomycin **plus** (C) Ampicillin (if age > 60 years)	(A) Cefepime or imipenem/ cilastatin **plus** (B) Vancomycin	High-dose acyclovir should be added if suspicion of encephalitis. Metronidazole should be added if suspicion of brain abscess.

These recommendations do not take into account all clinical scenarios and are not intended for immunocompromised patients, pregnant women, and travelers.
Knowledge of predominant local pathogens and their sensitivity profiles may alter optimal empiric therapeutic regimens.
Appropriate cultures should be drawn before antimicrobials are administered.
Doripenem or meropenem may be substituted for imipenem/cilastatin.

Antibacterials

β-Lactams

The β-lactam group includes the penicillins, cephalosporins, carbapenems, and monobactams. All β-lactams share a common mechanism of action: inhibition of synthesis of the bacterial peptidoglycan cell wall by binding to variety of penicillin-binding proteins (PBPs). All β-lactams are bactericidal and demonstrate time-dependent killing; time for which drug levels exceed the minimum inhibitory concentration (MIC) correlates best with bacterial eradication. β-lactams can be inactivated by bacterial β-lactamases, a process that can be prevented by combining them with β-lactamase inhibitors such as sulbactam, clavulanate, and tazobactam. Bacterial resistance against the β-lactam antibiotics continues to increase at a dramatic rate. Mechanisms of resistance include not only production of β-lactamases but also alterations that cause decreased entry or active efflux of antibiotic and acquisition of novel PBPs.

Penicillins

Natural penicillins (penicillin G)—The use of penicillin G in the ICU is limited to treatment of proven infection due to sensitive organisms. It is active against most streptococci but penicillin-resistant S. viridans and S. pneumonia are becoming more common. It is not active against staphylococci. It continues to be highly active against Neisseria, Clostridia, Corynebacterium, Treponema, Leptospira, and Actinomyces species as well as Treponema pallidum and Borrelia burgdorferi.

Antistaphylococcal penicillins (methicillin, oxacillin, and nafcillin)—The antistaphylococcal penicillins were specifically developed to treat infections due to S. aureus. They are the preferred drugs for infections with methicillin-sensitive strains (MSSA) because their use has been associated with decrease mortality compared to vancomycin.[8] However, in areas where MRSA is broadly prevalent these agents should not be used alone for empiric treatment of suspected S. aureus infections.[9]

Aminopenicillins (ampicillin and ampicillin/sulbactam)—Ampicillin is the drug of choice for infections due to Listeria monocytogenes and those caused by sensitive strains of Enterococcus. Although it has activity against some community-acquired gram-negative organisms, many strains of H. influenza, E. coli, Enterobacter, and Klebsiella species are resistant, as are Serratia, Pseudomonas, and Acinetobacter species. Ampicillin–sulbactam has a wide range of antibacterial activity that includes gram-positive and gram-negative aerobic and anaerobic bacteria. However, the drug is not active against Pseudomonas and pathogens producing ESBLs. In addition, it is no longer recommended as an empiric treatment for community-acquired intra-abdominal infections due to a high prevalence of resistant E. coli.[10] One of the specific advantages of this agent is the inherent activity of sulbactam against Acinetobacter baumannii, making it a valuable option against MDR isolates.[11]

Extended spectrum penicillins (piperacillin–tazobactam and ticarcillin–clavulanate)—Piperacillin–tazobactam and ticarcillin–clavulanate are β-lactam/β-lactamase combinations with a broad spectrum of antibacterial activity. Their gram-positive activity includes MSSA and some strains of Enterococcus. They have good activity against many nosocomial gram-negative organisms including most strains of Pseudomonas, but are not effective against ESBL-producing E. coli and Klebsiella species. Resistance may develop during therapy for Enterobacter and other organisms that produce inducible β-lactamases, so they are not the preferred drugs for serious infections due to these organisms. They are frequently included as part of an empiric regimen for critically ill patients with new-onset sepsis. Piperacillin–tazobactam, in particular, has been shown to be effective in the treatment of patients with intra-abdominal infections, HCAP, complex skin and soft tissue infections (cSSTIs), and febrile neutropenia.[12]

Cephalosporins

The cephalosporins are commonly used in the ICU. They are classified into generations, each having been developed to combat specific groups of resistant organisms.

First-generation cephalosporins (cefazolin)—Cefazolin has good activity against β-hemolytic streptococci, MSSA, and many community-acquired gram-negatives. It is no longer a preferred drug for empiric treatment of skin and soft tissue infections due to the increased prevalence of community- and hospital-acquired MRSA.

Second-generation cephalosporins (cefoxitin, cefotetan, and cefuroxime)—These have broader spectra than the first-generation agents, covering most strains of E. coli, Enterobacter, Proteus, and Klebsiella species. They are less active than the first-generation agents against gram-positives, but both cefoxitin and cefotetan have good anaerobic activity. The use of these agents in the ICU is generally limited to community-acquired intra-abdominal infections. Like nearly all cephalosporins, they are not active against Enterococcus species.

Third-generation cephalosporins (ceftriaxone and ceftazidime)—Ceftriaxone has good activity against Pneumococcus, β-hemolytic streptococci, and MSSA. Its activity is more variable against S. viridans and it has no activity against MRSA. It is highly active against Haemophilus, Moraxella, Neisseria, Salmonella, and Shigella species. However, like other third-generation cephalosporins, it has variable activity against most Enterobacteriaceae. It is not active against Acinetobacter, Pseudomonas, or Stenotrophomonas maltophilia. Extensive data from randomized clinical trials confirm the efficacy of ceftriaxone in treatment of serious and difficult to treat community-acquired infections including pneumonia, pyelonephritis, and (at high dose) meningitis. Ceftriaxone is currently recommended as a first-line empirical treatment option (with the addition of a macrolide) for community-acquired pneumonia (CAP) in both Europe and the United States. Ceftazidime has good coverage against gram-negatives including Pseudomonas. However, its gram-positive activity is poor. In the past it was used extensively for neutropenic fever and for meningitis related to neurosurgical procedures, but its clinical niche has been greatly diminished by the development of cefepime.

Fourth-generation cephalosporins (cefepime)—Cefepime is a broad-spectrum agent with activity against gram-positive organisms such as Streptococcus pyogenes, Streptococcus pneumoniae, and MSSA. It also has good activity against nosocomial gram-negative bacteria including many strains of Pseudomonas, E. coli, and Klebsiella. It has poor activity against agents such as Stenotrophomonas maltophilia, Acinetobacter, and gram-negative anaerobes. Although ESBL-producing organisms are frequently sensitive to this agent in vitro, the clinical efficacy of cefepime in treating serious infections due to these organisms may be inferior to that of the carbapenems. Cefepime is a recommended agent for empiric treatment of HCAP, neutropenic fever, and central nervous system (CNS) infections associated with neurosurgical procedures.

Fifth-generation cephalosporins (ceftaroline)—Ceftaroline, unlike other cephalosporins, possesses bactericidal activity against resistant gram-positive pathogens including MRSA and resistant pneumococci. It also covers many gram-negative pathogens. However, it has poor activity against Pseudomonas, Acinetobacter, and ESBL-producing organisms. Approved indications for ceftaroline include cSSTIs and CAP.

Carbapenems (Imipenem/Cilastatin, Meropenem, Doripenem, and Ertapenem)

Carbapenems are broad-spectrum agents that are frequently reserved for critically ill patients with suspected or proven infection due to resistant nosocomial organisms. They are active against organisms that produce inducible amp-C β-lactamases as well as those that produce ESBLs. With the exception of ertapenem, they are useful in the treatment of Pseudomonas and Acinetobacter infections. However, they are not active against MRSA, Enterococcus faecium, Stenotrophomonas maltophilia, and Burkholderia cepacia. Because of their broad range of activity, imipenem–cilastatin, meropenem, and doripenem are indicated for complicated intra-abdominal infections, HCAP, neutropenic sepsis, and CNS infections related to neurosurgical procedures. Ertapenem is a newer analogue and has a prolonged half-life. It has a narrower spectrum than the other carbapenems and is not active against Pseudomonas or Acinetobacter species. It is indicated for CAP, urinary tract infections (UTIs), and intra-abdominal infections.

Monobactams (Aztreonam)

Aztreonam has broad aerobic gram-negative activity but lacks gram-positive and anaerobic activity. Its spectrum includes Pseudomonas but it is ineffective against ESBL-producing organisms. The majority of Acinetobacter and S. maltophilia strains are resistant. Resistant strains of P. aeruginosa frequently emerge during aztreonam monotherapy.

Aztreonam has minimal cross-allergenicity with the other β-lactams, with the exception of ceftazidime due to structural similarity. Aztreonam is frequently used in treating patients with severe β-lactam allergy, usually in combination with other agents such as vancomycin or an aminoglycoside.

Adverse Effects of β-Lactams

Allergic reactions are the most common serious adverse effects noted with the β-lactams. These may manifest as maculopapular rash, urticarial rash, fever, bronchospasm, vasculitis, serum sickness, exfoliative dermatitis, Stevens–Johnson syndrome, and anaphylaxis. The reported overall incidence of such reactions to the penicillins is 0.7% to 10%. Historical reports of penicillin allergy may be inaccurate; only about 20% of patients with a reported penicillin allergy have such an allergy confirmed on skin testing.[13] There is cross-allergenicity between all the forms of penicillin. Studies have reported 1% to 20% cross-allergenicity between penicillins, cephalosporins, and carbapene-ms. Persons who have had a non-life–threatening reaction to one class of β-lactam may receive a trial agent of a different class for appropriate empiric or definitive therapy. For patients with a history of life-threatening allergy, in whom a β-lactam agent is necessary, desensitization may be required. Other serious adverse effects of the β-lactams include interstitial nephritis, transaminitis, bone marrow suppression, and lowering of the seizure threshold.

Aminoglycosides (Gentamicin, Amikacin, and Tobramycin)

Aminoglycosides are bactericidal agents which bind irreversibly to the 30S subunit of the bacterial ribosome. They have excellent activity against gram-negative aerobic bacteria. They are ineffective against gram-positive and anaerobic bacteria. However, in the presence of a cell-wall active antibiotic, they may have a synergistic effect against aerobic gram-positive organisms. These agents exhibit concentration-dependent killing; bactericidal activity is maximized when the peak serum concentration is 8 to 10 times above the MIC. They also have a significant postantibiotic effect. These two pharmacodynamic properties provide the rationale for high-dose, extended-interval dosing of aminoglycosides.[14]

High dosing (5-7 mg/kg for gentamicin or tobramycin and 15-20 mg/kg for amikacin) assures adequate peak concentrations; this eliminates the need to check peak serum levels. Extended dosing intervals may also limit nephrotoxicity by allowing time for renal recovery. Trough concentrations should be confirmed to be essentially zero when this strategy is used.

The most common indications for the primary use of aminoglycosides in the critically ill patient are complicated UTIs, complicated intra-abdominal infections (in addition to an agent with anaerobic activity), and gram-negative bacteremia. These agents are also recommended in combination with an antipseudomonal β-lactam as empiric therapy for patients with HCAP and as definitive therapy for patients with confirmed pseudomonal bacteremia. Synergistic doses of gentamicin (1-1.5 mg/kg every 8-12 hours for patients with normal renal function) are recommended for combination therapy for enterococcal endocarditis, staphylococcal or streptococcal endocarditis in the presence of a prosthetic valve, and streptococcal endocarditis in the presence of intermediate penicillin resistance.

Aminoglycosides are inactivated in acidic, anaerobic environments such as abscesses and have poor lung tissue penetration. Inhaled aminoglycosides may overcome this latter limitation, although clinical data to support this mode of administration are limited.

The primary toxicities of aminoglycosides are dose-related nephrotoxicity, ototoxicity, and neuromuscular paralysis. With the exception of the ototoxicity, these adverse reactions may be reversible after drug discontinuation. Elevated serum trough levels, hypotension, concurrent nephrotoxic drugs, female sex, and liver disease have been shown to increase the risk of aminoglycoside-induced nephrotoxicity. These agents should be used with caution in patients receiving neuromuscular blocking agents and in patients with neuromuscular disease.

Fluoroquinolones (Ciprofloxacin, Levofloxacin, and Moxifloxacin)

These bactericidal agents act by inhibiting bacterial DNA gyrase and/or topoisomerase-IV, resulting in damage to bacterial DNA and cell death. Quinolones exhibit concentration-dependent killing.

Bactericidal activity becomes more pronounced as the serum drug concentration increases to roughly 30 times the MIC. Ciprofloxacin, a second generation quinolone, has expanded gram-negative activity and atypical pathogen coverage. It is distinguished by its potency against Pseudomonas, for which it is the most useful fluoroquinolone for systemic therapy. It is a valuable agent for treatment of complicated UTIs, prostatitis, and as part of combination therapy for HCAP. However, it is not a preferred agent for CAP because of poor pneumococcal susceptibility. Levofloxacin and moxifloxacin, the third generation quinolones, are characterized by clinically useful antibacterial activity against Chlamydia, Legionella, Mycoplasma, and streptococci including penicillin-resistant pneumococci. They are recommended first-line agents for treatment of CAP, either alone or in combination with extended-spectrum cephalosporin. Moxifloxacin does not concentrate in the urine and thus should not be used for UTIs. Fluoroquinolones are generally well tolerated. Adverse effects include gastrointestinal and CNS symptoms as well as dysglycemia and QT-interval prolongation. Achilles tendon rupture is a rare adverse effect of fluoroquinolones.

Miscellaneous Antibacterials

Vancomycin—The glycopeptide antibiotic vancomycin acts by disrupting the biosynthesis of peptidoglycan, the primary structural polymer of gram-positive cell walls. Vancomycin exhibits time-dependent bactericidal activity. It is active against number of aerobic and anaerobic gram-positive bacteria. Vancomycin is a first-line agent for suspected or proven methicillin-resistant strains of coagulase-negative and coagulase-positive staphylococcal infections, including bacteremia, endocarditis, pneumonia, cSSTI, osteomyelitis, septic arthritis, and CNS infections. It should not be used to treat MSSA infections because it is inferior to β-lactams for these infections. Vancomycin is a drug of choice for infections caused by penicillin-resistant streptococci and enterococci. It is recommended as initial therapy for cases of proved, suspected, or possible pneumococcal meningitis, in combination with a third-generation cephalosporin. Oral vancomycin is the drug of choice for the treatment of severe C. difficile enterocolitis.

Unfortunately, the prevalence of vancomycin resistance is on the rise among Enterococcus species and *S. aureus*. Although plasmid-mediated vancomycin resistance remains rare among *S. aureus*, intermediate sensitivity due to the production of a thickened cell wall is an increasing problem. Intermediate resistance may develop during therapy, so MICs should be rechecked whenever cultures remain persistently positive. *S. aureus* strains with MICs more than 1.5 mcg/mL have been associated with poorer response rates. In addition, strains that display variable sensitivity to vancomycin (hetero-resistance) have been reported and associated with treatment failure.[15]

Rapid infusion of vancomycin can lead to histamine-release-induced "red man" syndrome. Clinical signs and symptoms include pruritus, erythema and flushing of the upper torso, angioedema, and (occasionally) hypotension. Slow infusion (over at least 2 hours) and prophylactic antihistamines may prevent this syndrome. Nephrotoxicity is much less common with modern formulations of the drug but may occur with persistently elevated trough levels (>20 mcg/mL) or with concurrent aminoglycoside therapy. These are also the primary risk factors for ototoxicity, which may be irreversible. Vancomycin-induced neutropenia is rare.

Linezolid—Linezolid is an oxazolidinone antibiotic which acts in a bacteriostatic manner by blocking protein synthesis via the 50S ribosomal subunit. It is active against gram-positive aerobes including *S. aureus* (MSSA, MRSA, VISA, and VRSA), streptococci, and enterococci including vancomycin-resistant strains (VRE). Linezolid is recommended as an initial or alternative therapy for patients with cSSTIs, osteomyelitis, septic arthritis, meningitis, and brain abscesses. In one clinical trial, patients with confirmed MRSA pneumonia treated with linezolid had higher clinical response rates than those who received vancomycin (57% vs 46%).[16] Thus it is a reasonable choice for initial empiric MRSA coverage in patients with HCAP. However, because linezolid is a bacteriostatic agent, it is generally not recommended as first-line therapy for endovascular infections. Some gram-positive organisms have developed resistance to linezolid, but fortunately this is currently at low prevalence (<1%). Irreversible peripheral neuropathy and optic neuritis have been described with prolonged use. Other adverse effects with extended use include thrombocytopenia and lactic acidosis. Linezolid is a weak monoamine oxidase inhibitor. Concurrent serotoninergic medications are contraindicated.

Daptomycin—Daptomycin, a cyclic lipopeptide antibiotic, exerts its bactericidal effects by binding to, damaging, and causing depolarization of the cell membrane of gram-positive bacteria. Its antibacterial spectrum covers staphylococci (MSSA, MRSA, VISA, and VRSA), streptococci, and enterococci including VRE. Daptomycin is indicated for bacteremia and endocarditis caused by these organisms, either as initial therapy or in cases of reduced vancomycin sensitivity or clinical failure. It is also recommended as an initial or alternative therapy for cSSTIs. Its antibacterial activity is inhibited by pulmonary surfactant, and it should not be used for treatment of pneumonia. The prevalence of daptomycin resistance in clinical isolates of *S. aureus* appears to be low (0.3%). Unfortunately, the prevalence of daptomycin resistance appears to be increased in those MRSA isolates with reduced vancomycin sensitivity. Rhabdomyolysis is the primary toxicity of the drug. Concurrent use of statins may increase the risk of this toxicity.

Tigecycline—Tigecycline, a glycylcycline antibiotic closely related to the tetracyclines, has a broad spectrum of activity. It is a bacteriostatic agent that binds to the bacterial 30S ribosomal subunit. Tigecycline covers gram-positive and gram-negative aerobes and anaerobes as well as atypical species. It is active against MRSA, VRE, ESBL-producing organisms, inducible ampC producing organisms, KPC organisms, Stenotrophomonas, and C. difficile. However, it is inherently inactive against Pseudomonas species and is less effective against Proteus and Providencia species. Although it is effective in vitro against Acinetobacter isolates, there is increasing concern with clinical-treatment failures. It is FDA approved for the treatment of CAP.

Tigecycline is a bacteriostatic agent and does not maintain adequate serum concentrations for the treatment of bloodstream infections. In addition, in 2013 the FDA issued a black box warning based on postmarketing analyses suggesting an increased risk of death in patients with pneumonia who receive tigecycline as compared with other antimicrobials.[17] Thus, this agent should only be used when no other antimicrobial options are available. The most frequent side effects associated with the use of tigecycline are gastrointestinal.

Azithromycin—Azithromycin belongs to the macrolide class of antibiotics, which inhibit protein synthesis by binding to the 50S subunits of bacterial ribosomes. It is active against S. pneumonia and Hemophilus as well as atypical pneumonia pathogens including Legionella, Chlamydia, and Mycoplasma. It is recommended in combination with ceftriaxone for the empiric treatment of CAP. Major toxicities of azithromycin include hepatic injury and QT-interval prolongation.

Doxycycline—Doxycycline is the most commonly used tetracyclines which function by binding to the 30S ribosomal subunit. It is a bacteriostatic agent that is active against many aerobic and atypical pathogens including Rickettsia, Borrelia Chlamydia, and Mycoplasma. Due to high rates of pneumococcal resistance in the United States it is not a drug of choice for CAP.

Clindamycin—Clindamycin works primarily by binding to the 50S ribosomal subunit of bacteria and disrupting protein synthesis. It is active against gram-positive organisms including streptococci and *S. aureus* including some strains of community-acquired MRSA. It has excellent anaerobic activity, although some gram-negative anaerobes such as Bacteroides show resistance. It is also frequently used to decrease superantigen production in toxic shock syndromes due to β-hemolytic streptococci and *S. aureus*. Clindamycin use increases the risk of C. difficile colitis.

Metronidazole—Metronidazole is a bactericidal agent that acts by fatal destabilization of the DNA helix. It is active against most anaerobic gram-negative bacilli including Bacteroides, Prevotella, Fusobacterium, and Clostridium species but has minimal activity against many anaerobic gram-positive organisms. It is also active against some protozoa including Entamoeba and Giardia. Oral metronidazole is the drug of choice for treatment of mild to moderate C. difficile colitis. Because of good CNS penetration, it is empirically included to cover anaerobes in the setting of brain abscess. It is a preferred agent for intra-abdominal and genital infections. Taste disturbances and peripheral neuropathy are the major side effects of metronidazole.

Trimethoprim/sulfamethoxazole—Trimethoprim/ sulfamethoxazole (TMP-SMX) is available in a fixed combination of 1:5 and works by sequential blockade of microbial folic acid synthesis. The use of TMP-SMX in the ICU is often limited to patients known to have susceptible organisms or to immuno-compromised patients with suspected Pneumocystis jirovecii infections. TMP-SMX is also a first-line treatment for infections caused by the gram-negative bacilli Stenotrophomonas maltophilia and Burkholderia cepacia. Skin rashes, bone marrow suppression, interstitial nephritis, hyperkalemia, and aseptic meningitis are major side effects.

Polymyxin B and colistin (polymyxin E)— Polymyxins are cationic polypeptides which were originally discovered in 1950s. The use of polymyxins decreased over the next few decades because of their toxicity profile and the development of newer, more tolerable agents. However, recently they have been reintroduced for the treatment of MDR gram-negative bacilli infections. These agents interact with the anionic lipopolysaccharide molecules in the outer membrane of gram-negative bacteria, ultimately resulting in loss of membrane integrity and cell death. Polymyxin B and colistin have identical spectra, and are active against most aerobic gram-negative bacilli including MDR Pseudomonas aeruginosa, Acinetobacter species, Stenotrophomonas maltophilia, ESBL-producing organisms such as Klebsiella species and E. coli, and carbapenemase-producing Enterobacteriaceae. They are not active against Serratia and Proteus species. They are inherently inactive against gram-positive bacteria and anaerobes. Reasonable clinical cure rates (close to 70%) have been reported in critically ill patients treated with the polymyxins for pneumonia and bacteriemia caused by MDR strains of Pseudomonas and Acinetobacter.[18] Although clinical data is limited, these agents may also be administered intrathecally for meningitis and in aerosolized form for pneumonia in cases of resistant or refractory disease. The most common toxicities of the polymyxins are dose-dependent nephrotoxicity and neurotoxicity. In the past, reported incidences of nephrotoxicity were as high as 58%. However, recent data suggest an incidence of 10%. Neurotoxicity occurs in about 5% of patients and includes perioral paresthesias, ataxia, visual disturbances, confusion, vasomotor instability, and neuromuscular blockade.

Antifungals

Polyenes (Amphotericin B Deoxycholate, Liposomal Amphotericin B, Amphotericin B Lipid complex, and Amphotericin B Colloidal Dispersion)

The polyenes act by binding to sterols in the fungal cell membrane, increasing permeability and precipitating cell death. The various formulations of amphotericin B have the broadest antifungal spectra, with resistance among only a few significant species including Aspergillus terreus and Candida lusitaniae. Amphotericin B in combination with flucytosine continues to be the mainstay of initial treatment of CNS or disseminated cryptococcosis. It has been replaced by voriconazole as the first-line agent for treatment of invasive aspergillosis. It is the mainstay of treatment against all forms of invasive mucormycosis as well as against life-threatening forms of histoplasmosis, blastomycosis, and coccidiomycosis. Infusion of amphotericin B is commonly associated with severe febrile reactions, generalized malaise, and gastrointestinal symptoms. These can be minimized by prophylactic antihistamines, antipyretics, and antiemetics. Rapid infusion of amphotericin B has been reported to precipitate life-threatening hyperkalemia and cardiac arrhythmias; therefore, the daily dose of amphotericin B should be infused over 2 to 6 hours. Dose-dependent nephrotoxicity is the major limitation of amphotericin B, and about 80% of the patients receiving the deoxycholate form of the drug show some degree of renal impairment. It manifests as azotemia, decreased urinary concentration ability and a distal renal tubular acidosis with profound potassium and magnesium wasting. The most effective preventative measure is preinfusion and postinfusion crystalloid administration. Although higher doses of the liposomal forms are necessary to achieve equivalent serum levels, they have been shown to be less nephrotoxic than amphotericin B deoxycholate. They are used routinely in critically ill patients despite their higher cost. Anemia is common with long-term amphotericin B therapy. Hepatotoxicity is rare but may be severe.

Azoles (Fluconazole, Voriconazole, and Posaconazole)

Azoles inhibit the enzyme lanosterol 14-alpha-demethylase, which converts lanosterol to ergosterol, a key component of cell membranes. In areas with a low prevalence of azole-resistance, fluconazole is a first-line empiric therapy for candidal infections in non-neutropenic, azole-naïve hemodynamically stable patients. It has no activity against Candida krusei and up to 30% of Candida glabrata; and therefore, should not be used as empiric therapy for invasive candida infections in hemodynamically unstable patients. It has good CNS penetration and may be used in stable patients with endophthalmitis and meningitis due to sensitive Candida species. It is effective in the primary treatment of coccidiomycosis and as maintenance therapy for disseminated cryptococcal infections. It is ineffective against the molds and is not reliable against Histoplasma or Blastomyces. Voriconazole is the first-line agent against invasive Aspergillus fumigatus infections and has been found to be superior to traditional amphotericin B against such infections.[19] It is also active against Fusarium and Scedosporium species as well as some fluconazole resistant Candida species. It has no activity in mucormycosis. The intravenous form should be used with caution in patients with renal insufficiency due to potential accumulation of cyclodextrin, a vehicle used in the formulation. Posaconazole has expanded the spectrum of the triazole agents to include the Zygomycetes while maintaining against yeasts and molds covered by voriconazole. It may show activity against Candida species resistant to fluconazole and Aspergillus species resistant to amphotericin B and voriconazole. Posaconazole has shown promising results as a salvage therapy for the treatment of refractory fungal CNS, lung, oropharyngeal, and esophageal infections. Posaconazole is currently only available in the oral form. Absorption is improved when taken with high fat meals. Azoles are potent cytochrome P-450 enzyme inhibitors, leading to interactions with many drugs including cyclosporine, phenytoin, tacrolimus, and warfarin. The most common adverse effects of the azoles are gastrointestinal upset and reversible transaminitis. Voriconazole has been noted to cause transient visual disturbances.

Echinocandins (Caspofungin, Micafungin, and Anidulafungin)

The echinocandins act by inhibiting β-1,3 glucan synthase, thus disrupting cell wall synthesis.

These agents are rapidly fungicidal against most Candida species and fungistatic against Aspergillus species. They are first-line agents for treatment of invasive Candida infections in critically ill patients, neutropenic patients, and those with prior azole exposure. At present, all 3 echinocandins should be viewed as equally effective for candidemia. In clinical trials, they have shown superior microbiologic and clinical cure rates to fluconazole when treating candidemia, including that caused by fluconazole-sensitive Candida albicans.[20] In addition, they may be used in combination with amphotericin B or voriconazole for treatment of invasive aspergillosis. They have no activity against mucormycosis and cryptococcal species. They are generally well tolerated with the most commonly reported side effects being headaches, chills, elevated liver enzymes, and phlebitis at the infusion site.

Antivirals
Nucleoside Analogues (Acyclovir, Valacyclovir, Ganciclovir, and Valganciclovir)

These drugs require phosphorylation in virally infected cells to become active. They then become competitive substrates for the viral DNA polymerase, causing chain termination. Acyclovir is the drug of choice for all forms of HSV-1 disease including encephalitis, pneumonia, and hepatitis as well as for genital disease due to HSV-2. It is also used for pneumonia or disseminated disease due to VZV. It is not effective for EBV or CMV disease. Valacyclovir is a prodrug which has enhanced oral bioavailability; it is converted to acyclovir after first-pass metabolism. Resistance to acyclovir most commonly develops from mutations in viral thymidine kinase. Ganciclovir is the mainstay of treatment and prophylaxis of CMV retinitis, pneumonitis, and gastrointestinal infections in immune-compromised (HIV, solid organ and bone marrow transplant) patients. Ganciclovir has activity against HSV and VZV, but its toxicity profile precludes its use in these infections. Resistance to ganciclovir results from either reduced phosphorylation because of mutations in viral phosphotransferase gene or secondary to mutations in the gene encoding viral DNA polymerases. Valganciclovir, a prodrug, is converted to ganciclovir providing a potent oral alternative to intravenous ganciclovir. The adverse effects of the nucleoside analogues are primarily seen when the drugs are given in high doses intravenously. Nephrotoxicity can occur with either drug. Acyclovir can precipitate in renal tubules; this can be prevented with adequate volume administration and slow infusion rates. Reversible myelosuppression (neutropenia, thrombocytopenia) is the most notable adverse effect of ganciclovir, occurring in 25% to 30% of recipients. Both drugs can cause CNS toxicity including confusion, seizures, extrapyramidal signs, and autonomic instability.

Pyrophosphate Analogues (Foscarnet)

Foscarnet acts by inhibiting DNA and RNA polymerases. It is active against CMV, HSV, and VZV. Foscarnet is the drug of choice for the treatment of CMV infections in individuals unable to tolerate ganciclovir, for patients with acyclovir-resistant HSV and VZV infection, and for those with ganciclovir-resistant CMV infections. Nephrotoxicity is a common adverse effect of foscarnet. Bone marrow suppression and transaminitis may also occur.

Neuraminidase Inhibitors (Oseltamivir and Zanamivir)

Oseltamivir and zanamivir are active against influenza A and influenza B. They are indicated for suspected or confirmed influenza infection in all critically ill patients. Oseltamivir is only available in oral formulation. Zanamivir can be delivered as an inhalational drug but this form cannot be given to patients on mechanical ventilation. An intravenous formulation of zanamivir exists, but currently can only be obtained from the manufacturer as compassionate release. The prompt receipt of these medications has been associated with improved outcomes in patients with pandemic H1N1 influenza. They are usually well tolerated, with the most common side effects being headache, dizziness, and vertigo. Inhaled zanamivir can cause bronchospasm and is contraindicated in patients with asthma and chronic obstructive pulmonary disease.

REFERENCES

1. Kumar A, Roberts D, Wood KE, et al. Duration of hypotension before initiation of effective antimicrobial therapy is the critical determinant of survival in human septic shock. *Crit Care Med.* 2006;34(6):1589-1596.
2. Barbosa TM, Levy SB. The impact of antibiotic use on resistance development and persistence. *Drug Resist Updat.* 2000;3(5):303-311.
3. McDonald LC, Killgore GE, Thompson A, et al. An epidemic toxin gene-variant strain of Clostridium difficile. *N Engl J Med.* 2005;353(23):2433-2441.
4. Wacker C, Prkno A, Brunkhorst FM, Schlattmann P. Procalcitonin as a diagnostic marker for sepsis: a systematic review and meta-analysis. *Lancet Infect Dis.* 2013;13(5):426-435.
5. Jensen JU, Hein L, Lundgren B, et al. Procalcitonin-guided interventions to increase early appropriate antibiotics and improve survival in the intensive care unit: a randomized trial. *Crit Care Med.* 2011;39(9):2048-2058.
6. Chastre J, Wolff M, Fagon JY, et al. Comparison of 8 vs 15 days of antibiotic therapy for ventilator-associated pneumonia in adults: a randomized trial. *JAMA.* 2003;290(19):2588-2598.
7. Kaki R, Elligsen M, Walker S, et al. Impact of antimicrobial stewardship in critical care: a systematic review. *J Antimicrob Chemother.* 2011;66(6):1223-1230.
8. Schweizer ML, Furuno JP, Harris AD, et al. Comparative effectiveness of nafcillin or cefazolin versus vancomycin in methicillin-susceptible Staphylococcus aureus bacteremia. *BMC Infect Dis.* 2011;11:279-286.
9. Frazee BW, Lynn J, Charlebois ED, et al. High prevalence of methicillin-resistant Staphylococcus aureus in emergency department skin and soft tissue infections. *Ann Emerg Med.* 2005;45(3):311-320.
10. Solomkin J, Mazuski J, Bradley J, et al. Diagnosis and management of complicated intra-abdominal infection in adults and children: guidelines by the Surgical Infection Society and the Infectious Diseases Society of America. *Clin Infect Dis.* 2010;50:133-164.
11. Oliveira MS, Prado GV, Costa SF, Grinbaum RS, Levin AS. Ampicillin/sulbactam compared with polymyxins for the treatment of infections caused by carbapenem-resistant Acinetobacter spp. *J Antimicrob Chemother.* 2008;61(6):1369-1375.
12. Gin A, Dilay L, Karlowsky JA, Walkty A, et al. Piperacillin–tazobactam: a beta-lactam/beta-lactamase inhibitor combination. *Expert Rev Anti Infect Ther.* 2007;5(3):365-383.
13. Stember RH. Prevalence of skin test reactivity in patients with convincing, vague, and unacceptable histories of penicillin allergy. *Allergy Asthma Proc.* 2005;26(1):59-64.

14. Bailey TC, Little JR, Littenberg B, Reichley RM, Dunagan WC. A meta-analysis of extended-interval dosing versus multiple daily dosing of aminoglycosides. *Clin Infect Dis*. 1997;24(5):786-795.

15. Bae IG, Federspiel JJ, Miró JM, et al. Heterogeneous vancomycin-intermediate susceptibility phenotype in bloodstream methicillin-resistant Staphylococcus aureus isolates from an international cohort of patients with infective endocarditis: prevalence, genotype, and clinical significance. *J Infect Dis*. 2009;200(9):1355-1366.

16. Wunderink RG, Niederman MS, Kollef MH, et al. Linezolid in methicillin-resistant Staphylococcus aureus nosocomial pneumonia: a randomized, controlled study. *Clin Infect Dis*. 2012;54(5):621-629.

17. Prasad P, Sun J, Danner RL, Natanson C. Excess deaths associated with tigecycline after approval based on noninferiority trials. *Clin Infect Dis*. 2012;54(12):1699-1709.

18. Markou N, Apostolakos H, Koumoudiou C, et al. Intravenous colistin in the treatment of sepsis from multiresistant gram-negative bacilli in critically ill patients. *Crit Care Med*. 2003;7(5):R78-R83.

19. Herbrecht R, Denning DW, Patterson TF, et al. Voriconazole versus amphotericin B for primary therapy of invasive aspergillosis. *N Engl J Med*. 2002;347(6):408-415.

20. Kett DH, Shorr AF, Reboli AC, et al. Anidulafungin compared with fluconazole in severely ill patients with candidemia and other forms of invasive candidiasis: support for the 2009 IDSA treatment guidelines for candidiasis. *Crit Care Med*. 2011; 15(5):R253.

Endocrine Dysfunction Leading to Critical Illness

Michael A. Via, MD and Jeffrey I. Mechanick, MD

KEY POINTS

1 The immune-neuroendocrine response of critical illness (CI) is marked by hypercatabolism and diminished hypothalamic-pituitary-end-organ function.

2 Despite low circulating growth hormone (GH) levels in CI, the administration of exogenous GH is detrimental.

3 Central adrenal insufficiency typically results from overly rapid tapering of corticosteroid dosing or increased stress in a patient who was recently tapered off of corticosteroids.

4 CI or relative adrenal insufficiency, though real and relevant, is still the subject of great interest among intensivists and changes in definitions and management are likely to change in the near future.

5 Diabetic ketoacidosis typically occurs in patients with type 1 diabetes that are newly diagnosed, acutely ill, or resulting from missed scheduled insulin doses.

INTRODUCTION

The endocrine system of extracellular hormone signaling maintains homeostasis via regulation of metabolic pathways and cellular function in multicellular organisms, including humans. During critical illness (CI), the extreme systemic inflammatory response disrupts normal physiology and alters hormone signaling. The immune-neuroendocrine response of CI is marked by hypercatabolism and diminished hypothalamic-pituitary-end-organ function. In some cases, disorders of the endocrine system directly lead to CI. This chapter reviews the endocrine and metabolic physiology and sequelae of CI as well as specific conditions of the endocrine system that can lead to CI.

PITUITARY FUNCTION AND CRITICAL ILLNESS

The pituitary gland, or hypophysis, is located within the sella turcica, inferior to the optic chiasm and is connected to the hypothalamus via the infundibulum. The pituitary is divided functionally and anatomically into anterior and posterior sections. Although much of its function is controlled by the hypothalamus, the pituitary is considered the "master gland" for its role in regulating many of the other endocrine glands.

The anterior pituitary secretes 6 major peptide hormones: growth hormone (GH), prolactin (PRL), thyroid stimulating hormone (TSH), adrenocorticotrophic hormone (ACTH), luteinizing hormone (LH), and follicle stimulating hormone (FSH). The secretion of each of these hormones is pulsatile and follows a circadian rhythm. PRL synthesis is primarily regulated by inhibitory dopaminergic neurons of the hypothalamus. The other peptide hormones of the pituitary are synthesized primarily in response to stimulatory hypothalamic hormones.

Hypothalamic and anterior pituitary function are greatly reduced in CI as a result of high levels of circulating inflammatory cytokines (Table 44–1).[1] In early CI, circulating GH, LH, and FSH levels diminish to negligible levels. TSH production initially rises sharply, but within 6 to 18 hours of CI, TSH secretion is also impaired as part of the nonthyroidal illness phenomenon. ACTH levels also initially increase as part of a generalized stress response of acute CI, but typically decline to below normal levels on day 3 of CI.[2] Cortisol levels generally remain elevated, even as ACTH levels decline after day 3, suggesting an independent mechanism governing the release of cortisol as patient progress into the prolonged phase of CI.[2-4]

Despite low-circulating GH levels in CI, the administration of exogenous GH is detrimental. Several large randomized controlled trials have studied the use of GH as an attempt to treat hypercatabolism, that is, commonplace among critically ill patients. Results of these trials consistently show

TABLE 44–1 Anterior pituitary response to critical illness.[4]

Thyroid stimulating hormone (TSH)	Elevated briefly then suppressed during CI, elevated during recovery
Adrenocorticotrophic hormone (ACTH)	Elevated for first 3 days of CI, then suppressed
Luteinizing hormone (LH)	Suppressed
Follicle stimulating hormone (FSH)	Suppressed
Prolactin (PRL)	Elevated
Growth hormone (GH)	Suppressed

Data from Mechanick JI, Sacks HS, Cobin RH: Hypothalamic-pituitary axis dysfunction in critically ill patients with a low free thyroxine index, *J Endocrinol Invest* 1997 Sep;20(8):462-470.

an increase in mortality in the group treated with GH, leading to recommendations against the use of GH in patients with CI.[5,6] In another randomized trial in CI, the administration of insulin-like growth factor-1, an important downstream mediator of GH signaling, also failed to show clinical benefit.[7]

The replacement of testosterone or estrogen, which results from low LH and FSH, and replacement of thyroxine, which results from low TSH, remain controversial.[8-10]

The posterior pituitary releases 2 peptide hormones: antidiuretic hormone (ADH) and oxytocin. These hormones are synthesized in neuronal cell bodies located in the hypothalamus and transported within vesicles along the axons to the posterior pituitary for release into the bloodstream. Disorders of ADH secretion are discussed in the sections on diabetes insipidus (DI) and syndrome of inappropriate ADH secretion (SIADH).

PITUITARY FAILURE

Aside from the typical neuroendocrine stress response in CI, the loss of normal pituitary function due to direct insults of the hypothalamus or pituitary itself can lead to loss of end-organ gland dysfunction such as secondary hypothyroidism, adrenal insufficiency, or hypogonadism. Clinical scenarios that commonly interfere with normal pituitary function include head trauma, intracranial hemorrhage, and neurosurgery, especially following procedures that involve manipulation within the sella turcica such as resection of a pituitary adenoma, Rathke's cleft cyst, or craniopharyngioma.[11,12] Patients with any of these conditions may be suspected for pituitary insufficiency.

Pituitary function may be significantly compromised in postpartum women following large amounts of blood loss during delivery (Sheehan's syndrome).[12] Inflammatory conditions, such as lymphocytic hypophysitis, histiocytosis X, or neurosarcoidosis, may involve the pituitary gland and result in hormonal insufficiencies; these conditions are relatively rare but should be considered and then excluded in appropriate at-risk CI patients.[13] Some malignancies (eg, lymphoma and hypernephroma) can metastasize to the pituitary gland and cause significant endocrinopathy; these conditions should also be included in the differential diagnosis when appropriate.

Pituitary apoplexy, which occurs after hemorrhage of an existing pituitary adenoma, is another possible cause for the sudden loss of pituitary function.[12] Patients typically have a sudden severe headache, nausea, near syncope, or changes in vision if there is any mass effect that compresses the optic chiasm.

Acute manifestations of pituitary insufficiency include hypotension secondary to adrenal insufficiency and either hyponatremia or hypernatremia from changes in ADH secretion. Patients with suspected pituitary insufficiency should be given stress dose corticosteroids and evaluated for the SIADH or DI that may develop acutely in pituitary insufficiency. In some patients, the administration of corticosteroids may unmask underlying DI by impairing the release of ADH by the posterior pituitary and by indirectly attenuating ADH function in the renal collecting ducts.[14]

Diagnosing endocrine deficiencies resulting from hypopituitarism includes measurement of the pituitary hormone(s) and end-organ hormone(s), for instance, TSH and thyroxine, or LH, FSH, and either testosterone in men or estradiol in women. In postmenopausal women, pituitary dysfunction may be queried by measuring LH and FSH, which are expected to be elevated 5 to 20 fold.[15]

If deficiencies exist, replacement of end-organ hormones, such as treatment with thyroxine, testosterone, or estrogen, can be considered. In general, these treatments should be withheld until the patient has been stabilized. In the case of hypothyroxinemia with suspected or known pituitary dysfunction, it is also critical to initiate stress dose corticosteroid treatment prior to L-thyroxine (T4) treatment. This strategy minimizes the risk of severe adrenal insufficiency because cortisol catabolism (and, therefore, requirement) is enhanced by augmenting thyroid hormone levels, metabolic rate, and energy expenditure.

ADRENAL INSUFFICIENCY

Insufficient cortisol production by the adrenal cortex is the hallmark of adrenal insufficiency. Primary adrenal insufficiency results when there is adrenal pathology and secondary/tertiary (or "central") adrenal insufficiency results when there is pituitary/hypothalamic pathology affecting ACTH secretion. Decreased aldosterone reserve, as part of primary adrenal insufficiency, may occur in CI in association with cortisol insufficiency, or more rarely, alone as selective aldosterone deficiency.[16] Underproduction of the weak androgen dehydroepiandrosterone, produced mainly in the zona reticularis of the cortex, or underproduction of adrenal catecholamines, produced in the adrenal medulla generally do not contribute to the clinical scenario of adrenal insufficiency.

Cortisol, the main glucocorticoid hormone, exerts its numerous systemic functions by inducing tissue-specific gene expression. During times of physiologic stress, cortisol secretion increases. Patients with insufficient cortisol production may experience signs and symptoms as mild as headache, malaise, abdominal pain, nausea (generally without vomiting), myalgias, and/or lassitude with adrenal withdrawal (associated with steroid tapering and suppression of the hypothalamic-pituitary-adrenal [HPA] axis), to signs as severe as hypotension, incapacitating fatigue, severe hypoglycemia, hyponatremia (with hyperkalemia if primary adrenal insufficiency), and acidosis with adrenal insufficiency or crisis (associated with either primary or central adrenal insufficiency). Primary adrenal insufficiency can result from autoimmune, infectious, or hemorrhagic processes within the adrenal cortex, for example, Waterhouse–Friderichsen syndrome from meningococcal infection or adrenal vein thrombosis resulting from antiphospholipid antibody syndrome. Central adrenal insufficiency typically results from overly rapid tapering of corticosteroid dosing or increased stress in a patient who was recently tapered off of corticosteroids.

During CI, a form of central adrenal insufficiency (also termed "relative adrenal insufficiency" or "adrenal exhaustion" in the medical literature) may develop due to higher systemic cortisol requirements, effects of certain medications that inhibit cortisol synthesis, such as etomidate, and/or an impaired HPA axis during CI. The incidence of this form of central adrenal insufficiency has been reported between 10% and 30% of patients admitted with septic shock.[17] Note that this entity, though real and relevant, is still the subject of great interest among intensivists and changes in definitions and management are likely to change in the near future.

Adrenal insufficiency should be suspected in patients with unexplained or persistent hypotension, hypoglycemia, hyponatremia, or hyperkalemia. An absence of hyperglycemia, that is, expected as a stress response to CI may also be an indication of adrenal insufficiency.[3] The diagnosis is made by cosyntropin (250 mcg) stimulation testing that includes 2 criteria to confirm normal adrenal function: (1) plasma cortisol levels should reach 18 μg/dL/h after administering recombinant ACTH; (2) plasma cortisol levels should increase by at least 9 μg/dL from baseline. If both of these criteria are met, patients should be considered to have normal adrenal function. Patients with severe adrenal insufficiency fail to meet either of these criteria. If only 1 of the 2 criteria is met, adrenal insufficiency may still be suspected based on clinical impression.[17] Unfortunately, there are several legitimate caveats to this approach that account for overdiagnosis and underdiagnosis: (1) measured total cortisol levels may be falsely low due to typically suppressed levels of cortisol-bind globulin (generally paralleling suppressing of albumin), (2) inadequate normative data for different CI patient subsets, and (3) the appearance of cortisol resistance. Consequently, a free cortisol level may be helpful, but this test usually requires several days to obtain a result, rendering the test moot for emergent decision making. Thus, a clinical diagnosis is still paramount to guide management.[18]

Treatment of adrenal insufficiency in CI includes stress-dose corticosteroids, usually hydrocortisone at doses of 50 to 100 mg every 6 to 8 hours. In patients with suspected adrenal insufficiency, corticosteroid treatment should be empirically initiated, and may be discontinued later in the subgroup of patients that do not meet criteria after the results of cosyntropin stimulation or free cortisol testing become available. In the cases of septic shock refractory to fluid resuscitation, and in patients with acute respiratory distress syndrome, several studies demonstrate improvement in clinical outcomes with glucocorticoid therapy regardless of cosyntropin stimulation testing.[18] Treatment with stress dose glucocorticoid therapy is currently recommended in

these groups of patients.[18] Another approach that is more clinically oriented is to provide a lower dose of hydrocortisone (50 mg q 12) to patients suspected of relative adrenal insufficiency (pressor dependence without clear reason), while deferring specific adrenal biochemical testing and then taper empirically.[18]

Patients with adrenal insufficiency should continue to receive steroid treatment until hemodynamically stable. As the patient improves, the corticosteroid dose should be tapered over days to weeks based on clinical judgment, taking into account initial dosing level, dosing chronicity, and setting.

The administration of fludrocortisone, a pure mineralocorticoid, in conjunction with glucocorticoid therapy in patients with septic shock and adrenal insufficiency, was suggested by the results of 1 clinical trial.[19] However, a subsequent study failed to show any benefit with the use of fludrocortisone in this population.[20]

Several conditions that may mimic adrenal insufficiency should be considered if patients do not respond to corticosteroid therapy. Dysautonomia may occur in patients with chronic underlying neurologic disease, such as parkinsonism, which reduces sympathetic control of blood pressure and may lead to hypotension despite fluid resuscitation.[21] Autonomic dysfunction may also be suspected and responsive to midodrine in patients on renal replacement therapy.[22] Cortisol resistance, which may occur in preterminal patients or those with hepatic disease, may also lead to hypotension, but cortisol levels are often extremely high.[23]

DIABETIC KETOACIDOSIS

Insulin signaling modulates a number of metabolic and growth pathways on the cellular level. In addition to the well-known function of insulin to stimulate glucose uptake in endothelial, muscle, and adipose tissues, a low level of basal insulin regulates β-oxidation of fatty acids. In patients with negligible insulin secretion, uncontrolled fatty acid β-oxidation leads to the generation of acidic ketone bodies, including acetone, acetoacetate, and β-hydroxybutyrate. Overproduction and accumulation of ketone bodies, especially β-hydroxybutyrate and acetoacetate that release hydrogen ions in circulation, are the main causes of diabetic ketoacidosis (DKA).

DKA typically occurs in patients with type 1 diabetes that are newly diagnosed, acutely ill, or resulting from missed scheduled insulin doses.[24] Other patients at risk for DKA include those that have undergone surgical pancreatic resection, have pancreatic failure following episodes of pancreatitis, or patients with type 2 diabetes that have severely reduced pancreatic β-cell function during periods of extreme hyperglycemia (atypical or "Flatbush" diabetes).[25]

Patients that develop DKA present with an anion gap acidosis, mental status changes, hyperglycemia, dehydration, and electrolyte abnormalities that commonly include hyponatremia, and initially, hyperkalemia. As DKA is treated with insulin, hypophosphatemia may develop, which can lead to muscle weakness and in extreme cases, respiratory failure. Without appropriate supportive treatments, severe neurologic deficits and death may occur in patients that develop DKA.[24]

Treatment of DKA includes administration of insulin, intravenous fluids, and supportive measures. Additionally, an underlying cause for DKA should be investigated, which may include urinary tract infections or pneumonia, gastroenteritis, myocardial infarction, or simply nonadherence to insulin dosing.

Patients are stabilized with intravenous administration of regular insulin. A loading dose of 0.05 to 0.1 units/kg is recommended, followed by a continuous rate of 0.025 to 0.05 units/kg/h.[26] Normal saline is infused at the rate of 100 to 200 mL/h after a 1.5 to 2 L bolus. Electrolytes should be monitored at regular intervals, every 1 to 2 hours at first, then with declining frequency as the patient stabilizes. Potassium levels are typically elevated initially, but can decline to severely low serum levels as potassium shifts intracellularly with insulin and fluids treatment. Magnesium levels may also decline through a similar mechanism. As insulin drives cellular glucose uptake, glucose-6-phosphate is formed, consuming intracellular phosphate, and leading to passive inward diffusion of free phosphate and hypophosphatemia. Supplementation with potassium, phosphorus, and magnesium may need to be aggressive and should be administered to compensate for these changes.[26]

Capillary blood glucose levels should also be monitored frequently, with adjustment of the insulin infusion as needed. If blood glucose levels normalize but the serum anion gap remains above 16 mEq/L, the insulin infusion should be continued, and a 5% to 10% dextrose infusion should be started. The overall strategy is to render patients as anabolic, thus the provision of dextrose in addition to insulin can help drive a positive nutritional balance in cellular metabolic pathways.

As the anion gap declines to levels consistently less than 16 mEq/L and arterial pH is greater than 7.30, patients should be considered for transition to subcutaneous insulin.[26] In many cases, the home insulin regimen can be restarted. For newly diagnosed type 1 diabetics, a good rule of thumb is to give 0.2 units/kg of long-acting insulin, such as glargine or detemir, and another 0.2 units/kg of rapid-acting insulin, divided into 3 premeal treatments daily. For patients with Flatbush diabetes, a combination of insulin and antihyperglycemic oral medication may be appropriate. Consultation with an endocrinologist can assist in determining the medication regimen for each individual patient.

HYPERGLYCEMIC HYPEROSMOLAR STATE

In contrast to DKA, which primarily occurs in type 1 diabetes, hyperglycemic hyperosmolar state (HHS), previously known as nonketotic coma, is more commonly seen in patients with type 2 diabetes.[24] Patients with type 2 diabetes have both systemic insulin resistance and impaired β-cell function, which, if not adequately treated, may lead to severely elevated blood glucose levels. HHS usually occurs during a period in which medication adherence has lapsed and uncontrolled blood glucose levels that reach extreme heights, often greater than 600 mg/dL, persist. These concentrations overwhelm renal glucose resorption, leading to hyperglycosuria and an osmotic diuresis occurs. Patients present with severe dehydration, with hyponatremia, polyuria, blurred vision, and acute weight loss. There may be a minimal production of ketones owing to a shift to lipid consumption for energy utilization, but this is generally not sufficient to cause acidosis.

If the dehydration and hyponatremia are severe enough, mental status changes may occur, necessitating admission to a closely monitored setting.

Treatment of HHS is generally supportive in nature. Intravenous fluids are given generously. Insulin should be administered, which may be given as an intravenous infusion or as subcutaneous basal/bolus injections. In patients admitted to the intensive care unit with mental status changes, an intravenous infusion of regular insulin is preferred.

As blood glucose normalizes and patients are able to take meals regularly, the insulin regimen should be converted to a combination of long-acting insulin with rapid acting bolus insulin administered with each meal. As a rule of thumb, 80% of the previous 24 hours intravenous insulin given can be used as a total daily subcutaneous insulin dose. This may be divided in half, and given as basal insulin; the remaining half can be divided into thirds and given as premeal rapid-acting insulin. This basal-bolus insulin administration strategy mimics normal pancreatic function and should be considered for optimal glycemic control in patients tolerating an oral diet, or for those on bolused tube feeding.[27] For patients on continuous enteral feeding, long-acting insulin, given 1 to 3 times per day is more suitable to match the infusion and absorption rate of dietary carbohydrates.

In addition, a multidisciplinary approach to the continued care of the patient may involve consultation with nutrition and diabetes educators and close follow up with the patient's diabetes specialist after hospital discharge.

THYROID FUNCTION

The vast majority of thyroid hormone produced by the thyroid gland is released into circulation as T4 and is converted to triiodothyronine (T3) or reverse T3 (rT3) by deiodinase enzymes in the liver and other target tissues. T3, the active form of thyroid hormone, functions as a general regulatory signal of metabolism, whereas rT3 is generally inactive metabolite of T4. Nearly all cells and tissues contain thyroid hormone receptors that modulate gene expression and cellular metabolic function in response to T3.

The controlled release of thyroid hormone occurs in several steps, which includes the secretion of TSH by the anterior pituitary and the secretion of

thyrotropin releasing hormone from the hypothalamus. Thyroid hormone activity is further modulated through control of the deiodination process during the systemic conversion of T4 to either T3 or rT3.

In addition to the metabolic state of the individual, certain medications may influence the regulation of thyroid hormone function. Lithium affects T4 synthesis and release, and deiodination.[28] Corticosteroids and β-adrenergic antagonists alter deiodination.[29] Amiodarone has several effects on thyroid function and is reviewed as follows.

NONTHYROIDAL ILLNESS

Both the hypothalamus activity and pituitary gland function are affected in CI. Patients commonly demonstrate a typical pattern of thyroid function blood tests that are associated with severity of CI rather than alteration in thyroid function. This phenomenon is known as nonthyroidal illness, or previously the "sick-euthyroid" syndrome.[10] In this condition, TSH levels often decrease. T4 levels may remain normal, but are usually decreased. T3 levels decrease as conversion of T4 to rT3 increases. As a patient recovers, the TSH levels begin to rise and can become elevated above the normal range, as high as 15 to 20 mIU/L (milli-international units per liter). Consequently, thyroid function tests can be difficult to interpret in the setting of acute illness or hospitalization. Treatment of nonthyroidal illness with thyroid hormone replacement remains controversial and has not been shown to affect overall outcome.[30,31]

THYROTOXICOSIS

In conditions that lead to excessive thyroid hormone production, hyperthyroidism or thyrotoxicosis develops. Patients may experience excessive warmth, diaphoresis, tachycardia, hyperreflexia, weight loss, hair loss, fine tremor and loose bowel movements. TSH levels are low, with normal to elevated free T4 and T3 levels.

In severe cases, thyrotoxic crisis may be classified under the Burch–Wartofsky scoring system (Table 44–2) as "Thyroid Storm."[32] In addition to the classic symptoms of hyperthyroidism, patients may exhibit altered mental status, psychosis, fevers, nausea, vomiting, high-output heart failure,

TABLE 44–2 Burch–Wartofsky scoring system for thyrotoxic crisis.[32]

Clinical Sign	Score	Clinical Sign	Score
Body Temperature		**Congestive Heart Failure**	
99°F-99.9°F (37.2°C-37.7°C)	5	Absent	0
100.0°F-100.9°F (37.8°C-38.2°C)	10	Peripheral edema	5
101.0°F-101.9°F (38.3°C-38.8°C)	15	Mild respiratory rates	10
102.0°F-102.9°F (38.9°C-39.3°C)	20	Pulmonary edema	15
103.0°F-103.9°F (39.4-39.9°C)	25	**Gastrointestinal Symptoms**	
104.0°F (40.0°C) or greater	30	Absent	0
		Nausea/vomiting/ diarrhea	10
		Jaundice	20
Pulse (beats/min)			
90-109	5	**Central Nervous System**	
110-119	10	Unaltered mental status	0
120-129	15		
130-139	20	Mild agitation	10
140 or greater	25	Lethargy/delirium/ psychosis	20
Atrial Fibrillation		Seizure/coma	30
Absent	0	**History of Precipitating Event**	
Present	10		
		Absent	0
		Present	10

A total score of 45 represents likely thyrotoxic crisis, 25 to 44 represents probable thyrotoxic crisis, and less than 25 is suggestive that thyrotoxic crisis is unlikely.
Adapted with permission from Klubo-Gwiezdzinska J1, Wartofsky L: Thyroid emergencies, *Med Clin North Am*. 2012 Mar;96(2):385-403.

and unstable blood pressure. This may be precipitated by a large physiologic stressor, such as a myocardial infarction, surgery or other CI in a patient with long-standing, inadequately treated thyrotoxicosis.

Patients with severe thyrotoxicosis should be kept in a closely monitored setting and treated with stress-dose corticosteroids, β-adrenergic receptor blocking agents, and propylthiouracil (PTU) or methimazole, which prevent thyroidal synthesis and release of thyroid hormone. In this setting, PTU is given as a loading dose of 500 to 1000 mg orally or via nasogastric tube, followed by 200 to 250 mg every 4 hours. As an alternative to PTU, methimazole is given as 60 to 80 mg daily.[33,34]

The use of other agents such as lithium to prevent thyroid hormone release or cholestyramine to sequester T4 and T3 from portal circulation may be considered. Lithium may be given at doses of 300 mg every 6 hours.[33] Large amounts of potassium iodine may also be administered orally as 3 to 5 drops every 6 hours, which temporarily down regulates thyroid hormone synthesis and release, known as the Wolff–Chaikoff phenomenon.[33] In the case of a patient with a nodular goiter, the administration of iodine should be omitted. This may lead to the undesired Jod–Basedow phenomenon, a condition in which exogenous iodine induces a surge in thyroxine production by an enlarged, nodular thyroid, that is, typically iodine avid.

Surgical resection of the thyroid gland may also be considered in several conditions such as if the patient remains hemodynamically unstable despite medical treatment, if any of the mentioned medical therapies are contraindicated, during pregnancy or other medical conditions that warrant rapid reversal of thyrotoxicosis. In such patients, plasmapheresis has also been suggested as a means of rapidly lowering circulating T4 and T3.[33] In severely thyrotoxic patients, medication half-lives can be affected; higher doses of medications, such as corticosteroids, antihypertensives, or antiseizure medications, may be required.

With supportive care, mortality rates between 10% and 75% have been reported after thyrotoxic crisis. Patients that survive often show marked improvement within 24 hours of hospitalization.[33] After stabilization, treatment of the underlying cause of thyrotoxicosis should be initiated. The most common cause is Graves' disease, in which autoantibodies activate the TSH receptor on thyrocytes.

Amiodarone toxicity may also induce thyrotoxic crisis though 1 of 2 mechanisms. In type 1 amiodarone-induced thyrotoxicosis, the high iodine content of the amiodarone preparation causes a Jod–Basedow phenomenon in patients with a nodular goiter. In type 2 amiodarone-induced thyrotoxicosis, the direct toxicity of amiodarone to thyrocytes induces subacute thyroiditis. Differentiating these 2 responses in the setting of severe thyrotoxicosis can be difficult because diagnostic testing with radioiodine thyroid uptake and scan can take several days to complete and the initiation of treatment may be more urgent. Often both types of amiodarone-induced thyrotoxicosis are addressed with an empiric medical-treatment strategy that includes either methimazole or PTU, and a 2 to 3 months course of corticosteroids.

Other causes of thyrotoxicosis, which include subacute thyroiditis, a hot thyroid nodule, toxic multinodular goiter, and surreptitious use of T4 are less likely to induce thyrotoxic crisis. A thyroid uptake and scan can help to differentiate these conditions if the diagnosis is not clear.

MYXEDEMA COMA

In patients with less than the required thyroxine production, hypothyroidism ensues. Rarely, if left untreated for a prolonged timeframe, severe hypothyroidism may develop, leading to myxedema coma. These patients generally are unresponsive or have severely altered mental status, with cool, clammy skin, decreased body temperature, nonpitting edema, depressed respiratory drive and hypercapnia, bradycardia, and hypotension. A prolonged Q-T interval may increase risk of Torsades de pointes ventricular tachycardia.

The TSH is elevated, with low T3 and T4 levels. Supportive treatment should include the administration of intravenous fluids. Stress dose corticosteroids should also be given to anticipate a temporary adrenal insufficiency that develops as normal thyroid function is restored. After corticosteroids have been started, T4 may be administered. Initial doses should be given intravenously. Some authors favor giving a loading dose of 300 to 600 mcg T4, followed by a maintenance dose of 100 mcg daily.[35] Comparison studies show no difference in outcome, if lower doses are initiated.[36] The administration of T3 has also been suggested on the theoretical basis that conversion of T4 to T3 is impaired in severe illness. T3 may be given at a dose of 10 mcg every 8 to 12 hours, until consciousness is restored.[33] Once able to take medications orally, T4 may be given as an oral preparation during periods of fasting, separated by other medications that may impair absorption by at least 3 to 4 hours. Oral iron supplements, calcium supplements, and soy products can severely impair the absorption of T4.

Despite intensive supportive measures, mortality for myxedema coma remains at 20% to 25%.[33]

DIABETES INSIPIDUS

The loss of ADH function either through impaired central production or by a lack of renal response to ADH signaling results in DI. Without ADH function, the distal collection tubules of the nephron are unable to adequately concentrate the urine that is produced. The dilute urine output often exceeds 300 mL/h and has an osmolality below 200 mOsm (Table 44–3). Consequently, patients lose a substantial amount of free water and experience an increased thirst sensation. Many patients with DI are able to compensate for renal losses by consuming adequate fluids, leading to the classic symptoms of polydipsia and polyuria. However, if a patient either does not have access to water or if their thirst mechanism is impaired, such as during CI, hypernatremia and dehydration may develop.

Common causes of DI include pituitary or other brain surgery, brain tumors, Sheehan's syndrome, neurosarcoid, histiocytosis X, and head trauma. DI can also result if the cells of the renal collecting ducts do not respond to circulating ADH, a condition known as nephrogenic DI.

DI is treated with desmopressin (DDAVP), a synthetic analogue of ADH which preferentially targets the renal vasopressin receptors. DDAVP may be given as oral, inhaled, and intravenous forms. During administration, plasma sodium levels and urine output should be closely monitored. The dose of DDAVP should be slowly titrated to avoid hyponatremia and to maintain a normal urine output.

TABLE 44–3 Clinical features of SIADH versus DI.

SIADH	DI
Hyponatremia	Normal or hypernatremia
Concentrated urine (> 600 mOsm)	Dilute urine (< 200 mOsm)
Urine sodium 40-70 mEq/L	Low urine sodium < 30 mEq/L

SYNDROME OF INAPPROPRIATE ANTIDIURETIC HORMONE

A disproportionate release of ADH by the posterior pituitary can lead to SIADH, causing an inappropriate retention of free water and hyponatremia as the most common presenting finding. Patients with SIADH also exhibit highly concentrated urine and mildly elevated urine sodium levels ranging from 40 to 70 mmol/L (see Table 44–3). Common etiologies of SIADH include: pain, nausea, head trauma, meningitis, encephalitis, brain tumors, intracranial hemorrhage, pituitary, or other brain surgery as well as certain medications (selective serotonin uptake inhibitors, carbamazepine among others). ADH may also be synthesized ectopically in lung tumors, lymphomas, gastrointestinal tumors, and in association with pulmonary infections.

The mainstay of treatment for SIADH includes restriction of free water intake by the patient while the underlying cause is addressed. Daily weights and total volume taken in and put out should be recorded. ADH receptor blockers such as tolvaptan can also be given when fluid restriction fails to raise the plasma sodium adequately. The use of demeclocycline has fallen out of favor with the availability of ADH receptor blockers. In severe cases and in closely monitored settings, hypertonic saline can be administered.

In some patients at risk for SIADH with conditions affecting the central nervous system, cerebral salt wasting may develop. In this condition, high amounts of brain natriuretic peptide and possibly other factors are released from the CNS lead to excessive renal sodium losses and hyponatremia. Cerebral salt wasting may rarely be seen following head trauma, meningitis, encephalitis, and intracranial hemorrhage.[37] To differentiate from SIADH, urine sodium levels are inappropriately elevated. Treatment is with replacement of salt given either orally as sodium chloride tablets or intravenously as hypertonic saline.

CONCLUSION

In addition to the immune-neuroendocrine response, which is generally observed in all forms of CI, the specific disorders of pituitary insufficiency, adrenal insufficiency, DKA, HHS, thyrotoxic crisis, myxedema coma, DI, and syndrome of inappropriate ADH response represent severe conditions of the endocrine system that can lead to CI. Patients with any of these conditions must be monitored closely, treated appropriately, with continued adjustment to the treatment regimen. Understanding the pathophysiology of each of these disorders allows for the anticipation of treatment strategies and improved and patient outcomes.

REFERENCES

1. Ellger B, Debaveye Y, Van den Berghe G. Endocrine interventions in the ICU. *Eur J Intern Med.* 2005;16(2):71-82.
2. Vermes I, Beishuizen A, Hampsink RM, Haanen C. Dissociation of plasma adrenocorticotropin and cortisol levels in critically ill patients: possible role of endothelin and atrial natriuretic hormone. *J Clin Endocrinol Metab.* 1995;80(4):1238-1242.
3. Via MA, Scurlock C, Adams DH, Weiss AJ, Mechanick JI. Impaired postoperative hyperglycemic stress response associated with increased mortality in patients in the cardiothoracic surgery intensive care unit. *Endocr Pract.* 2010;16(5):798-804.
4. Mechanick JI, Sacks HS, Cobin RH. Hypothalamic-pituitary axis dysfunction in critically ill patients with a low free thyroxine index. *J Endocrinol Invest.* 1997;20(8):462-470.
5. Teng Chung T, Hinds CJ. Treatment with GH and IGF-1 in critical illness. *Crit Care Clin.* 2006;22(1):29-40.
6. Takala J, Ruokonen E, Webster NR, et al. Increased mortality associated with growth hormone treatment in critically ill adults. *N Engl J Med.* 1999;341(11):785-792.
7. Goeters C, Mertes N, Tacke J, et al. Repeated administration of recombinant human insulin-like growth factor-I in patients after gastric surgery. Effect on metabolic and hormonal patterns. *Ann Surg.* 1995;222(5):646-653.
8. Nierman DM, Mechanick JI. Hypotestosteronemia in chronically critically ill men. *Crit Care Med.* 1999;27(11):2418-2421.
9. Maggio M, Nicolini F, Cattabiani C, et al. Effects of testosterone supplementation on clinical and rehabilitative outcomes in older men undergoing on-pump CABG. *Contemp Clin Trials.* 2012;33(4):730-738.

10. Economidou F, Douka E, Tzanela M, Nanas S, Kotanidou A. Thyroid function during critical illness. *Hormones (Athens)*. 2011;10(2):117-124.

11. Fleck SK, Wallaschofski H, Rosenstengel C, et al. Prevalence of hypopituitarism after intracranial operations not directly associated with the pituitary gland. *BMC Endocr Disord*. 2013;13(1):51.

12. Tanriverdi F, Dokmetas HS, Kebapci N, et al. Etiology of hypopituitarism in tertiary care institutions in Turkish population: analysis of 773 patients from pituitary study group database. *Endocrine*. 2014;47(1):198-205.

13. Siram AT, Kouvatsos T, Suarez Y, et al. Postoperative cardiac homograft involvement in Erdheim-Chester disease. *J Heart Valve Dis*. 2012;21(3):401-404.

14. Iida M, Takamoto S, Masuo M, Makita K, Saito T. Transient lymphocytic panhypophysitis associated with SIADH leading to diabetes insipidus after glucocorticoid replacement. *Intern Med*. 2003;42(10):991-995.

15. Mechanick JI, Hochberg FH, LaRocque A. Hypothalamic dysfunction following whole-brain irradiation. *J Neurosurg*. 1986;65(4):490-494.

16. Inada M, Iwasaki K, Imai C, Hashimoto S. Hyperpotassemia and bradycardia in a bedridden elderly woman with selective hypoaldosteronism associated with low renin activity. *Intern Med*. 2010;49(4):307-313.

17. Cohen J, Venkatesh B. Relative adrenal insufficiency in the intensive care population; background and critical appraisal of the evidence. *Anaesth Intensive Care*. 2010;38(3):425-436.

18. Marik PE, Pastores SM, Annane D, et al. Recommendations for the diagnosis and management of corticosteroid insufficiency in critically ill adult patients. Consensus statements from an International Task Force by the American College of Critical Care Medicine. *Crit Care Med*. 2008;36(6):1937-1949.

19. Annane D, Sebille V, Charpentier C, et al. Effect of treatment with low doses of hydrocortisone and fludrocortisone on mortality in patients with septic shock. *JAMA*. 2002;288(7):862-871.

20. Annane D, Cariou A, Maxime V, et al. Corticosteroid treatment and intensive insulin therapy for septic shock in adults: a randomized controlled trial. *JAMA*. 2010;303(4):341-348.

21. Koh O, Umapathi T. A retrospective review of autonomic screening tests conducted at a Tertiary General Hospital. *Auton Neurosci*. 2014;181:69-73.

22. Schulman RC, Mechanick JI. Metabolic and nutrition support in the chronic critical illness syndrome. *Respir Care*. 2012;57(6):958-977; discussion 977-958.

23. Charmandari E, Kino T, Chrousos GP. Familial/sporadic glucocorticoid resistance: clinical phenotype and molecular mechanisms. *Ann N Y Acad Sci*. 2004;1024:168-181.

24. Maletkovic J, Drexler A. Diabetic ketoacidosis and hyperglycemic hyperosmolar state. *Endocrinol Metab Clin North Am*. 2013;42(4):677-695.

25. Imran SA, Ur E. Atypical ketosis-prone diabetes. *Can Fam Physician*. 2008;54(11):1553-1554.

26. Kitabchi AE, Umpierrez GE, Murphy MB, Kreisberg RA. Hyperglycemic crises in adult patients with diabetes: a consensus statement from the American Diabetes Association. *Diabetes Care*. 2006;29(12):2739-2748.

27. Via MA, Mechanick JI. Inpatient enteral and parenteral [corrected] nutrition for patients with diabetes. *Curr Diab Rep*. 2011;11(2):99-105.

28. Kibirige D, Luzinda K, Ssekitoleko R. Spectrum of lithium induced thyroid abnormalities: a current perspective. *Thyroid Res*. 2013;6(1):3.

29. Bianco AC, Nunes MT, Hell NS, Maciel RM. The role of glucocorticoids in the stress-induced reduction of extrathyroidal 3,5,3′-triiodothyronine generation in rats. *Endocrinology*. 1987;120(3):1033-1038.

30. DeGroot LJ. "Non-thyroidal illness syndrome" is functional central hypothyroidism, and if severe, hormone replacement is appropriate in light of present knowledge. *J Endocrinol Invest*. 2003;26(12):1163-1170.

31. Portman MA, Slee A, Olson AK, et al. Triiodothyronine supplementation in infants and children undergoing cardiopulmonary bypass (TRICC): a multicenter placebo-controlled randomized trial: age analysis. *Circulation*. 2010;122(11 Suppl):S224-S233.

32. Burch HB, Wartofsky L. Life-threatening thyrotoxicosis. Thyroid storm. *Endocrinol Metab Clin North Am*. 1993;22(2):263-277.

33. Klubo-Gwiezdzinska J, Wartofsky L. Thyroid emergencies. *Med Clin North Am*. 2012;96(2):385-403.

34. Bahn RS, Burch HB, Cooper DS, et al. Hyperthyroidism and other causes of thyrotoxicosis: management guidelines of the American Thyroid Association and American Association of Clinical Endocrinologists. *Endocr Pract*. 2011;17(3):456-520.

35. Holvey DN, Goodner CJ, Nicoloff JT, Dowling JT. Treatment of myxedema coma with intravenous thyroxine. *Arch Intern Med.* 1964;113:89-96.
36. Rodriguez I, Fluiters E, Perez-Mendez LF, Luna R, Paramo C, Garcia-Mayor RV. Factors associated with mortality of patients with myxoedema coma: prospective study in 11 cases treated in a single institution. *J Endocrinol.* 2004;180(2):347-350.
37. Verbalis JG. Hyponatremia with intracranial disease: not often cerebral salt wasting. *J Clin Endocrinol Metab.* 2014;99(1):59-62.

Oncologic Emergencies

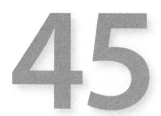

Cristina Gutierrez, MD and
Stephen M. Pastores, MD, FACP, FCCP, FCCM

45

KEY POINTS

1 Oncologic emergencies that may necessitate ICU admission include superior vena cava syndrome (SVCS), cardiac tamponade, malignant spinal cord compression, hypercalcemia, tumor lysis syndrome (TLS), and leukostasis.

2 SVCS is primarily caused by lung cancer and lymphoma. Sudden death is observed only when there is airway compromise or cerebral edema. Management is directed toward restoring the patency of flow in the SVC and stabilizing the airway.

3 Pericardial effusions from malignancies accumulate slowly and may result in large effusions. Lung, breast, melanoma, and lymphoma are the most common malignancies associated with pericardial tamponade. Emergent drainage or pericardial window is the treatment of choice for pericardial tamponade.

4 Early recognition of malignant spinal cord compression with physical exam, magnetic resonance imaging, and angiography is vital to restoring neurologic function.

5 Malignancy-associated hypercalcemia occurs in 20% to 30% of patients and is more common in solid tumors such as breast and lung cancer. Volume repletion with isotonic saline is the initial treatment of choice. Bisphosphonates, calcitonin, and corticosteroids are also useful treatments.

6 TLS is characterized by electrolyte and metabolic derangements from the breakdown of malignant cells. TLS can occur spontaneously or after chemotherapy, radiation, and treatment with corticosteroids. Aggressive hydration and correction of electrolyte abnormalities (hyperkalemia, hyperphosphatemia, hypocalcemia, and hyperuricemia) are keys to management.

7 Hyperleukostasis (WBC > 50,000-100,000/mm^3) is common in patients with acute myelogenous leukemia. Respiratory symptoms include dyspnea, hemoptysis, respiratory distress, and hypoxemia as well as neurologic including dizziness, headache, blurry vision, confusion, and stroke or intracranial hemorrhage. Treatment consists of leukapheresis, hydroxyurea, and chemotherapy.

INTRODUCTION

As the treatments for malignancies continue to improve, so does the long-term survival and prognosis of the oncologic patient. Consequently, an increasing number of patients with cancer face complications that can lead to severe illness and require admission to the intensive care unit (ICU). As in the general population, the majority of ICU admissions for patients with malignancy are due to sepsis and respiratory failure. Intensivists should be familiar with the specific issues relevant to the critically ill oncologic patient so that adequate treatment can be offered (Table 45–1). This chapter will focus on the classic clinical syndromes that represent oncologic emergencies: superior vena cava syndrome (SVCS), cardiac tamponade, spinal cord compression, tumor lysis syndrome, hypercalcemia, and leukostasis.

SUPERIOR VENA CAVA SYNDROME

Superior vena cava syndrome (SVCS) is a group of signs and symptoms that occur when there is obstruction of the SVC. Currently more than 85% to 90% of SVCS cases are associated with malignancy.[1] Ninety percent of malignant causes are due to lung cancer (nonsmall cell lung carcinoma—50%, small cell lung carcinoma—25%) and lymphoma (non-Hodgkin's lymphoma—10%).[2,3] Once SVCS is present in the oncologic patient, life expectancy is not greater than 9 months, although these numbers can vary widely according to the type of malignancy.[3]

Findings on physical exam include facial plethora, neck and superficial chest vein distention, upper extremity edema, dyspnea, orthopnea, and presyncope. In the past, SVCS was considered a medical emergency; however, current data suggests that immediate death is only observed when there is airway compromise (laryngeal or vocal cord edema) or cerebral edema.[2,4]

The diagnosis of SVCS is made clinically with support of imaging studies such as computed tomographic (CT) scan with contrast, magnetic resonance imaging (MRI), or venography. Imaging is used to evaluate the extent of obstruction, possible associated thrombosis, and vascular anatomy in case of any planned interventions.[1,3]

Management of SVCS should be directed toward restoring the patency of flow in the SVC; all other treatments are considered supportive. Management of airway compromise requires oxygenation and rapid stabilization of the airway. Use of corticosteroids has been described but there are no randomized controlled trials suggesting that their use is beneficial.[5] Moreover, the use of corticosteroids prior to any biopsy can alter the yield of pathologic diagnosis, especially if lymphoma is suspected.[1,3] In patients with brain edema, quick restoration of vascular flow should be attempted because morbidity and mortality in these cases is extremely high. Diuretics to decrease edema should not be regularly used; intravascular depletion can adversely affect hemodynamics in these patients; and there is no data to support the effectiveness of diuretics.[2,4]

In recent years, the use of intravascular stents for SVCS treatment has increased significantly. Stenting improves symptoms in the first 24 to 72 hours, making it the treatment of choice for patients with severe SVCS.[5,6] Multiple studies have shown stenting to be efficient, safe, and cost-effective.[5,6] Complications such as stent migration, stenosis, pericardial tamponade, and pulmonary embolism (PE) have been reported in less than 8% of cases.[6] Prolonged use of anticoagulants for this population is controversial. Evidence of PE and risk for stent occlusion have made routine anticoagulation an appealing choice.[7] However, bleeding complications are high and current data do not suggest improved outcomes when using routine anticoagulation.[3]

After stent placement, final treatment for SVCS should be guided toward management of the malignancy. Initiating treatment prior to diagnosis can obscure biopsy results in up to 48% of cases.[3] Therefore, tissue biopsy, pathologic evaluation, and staging should be performed to define adequate treatment. Response to radiation and chemotherapy occurs only after 2 to 3 weeks of initiating treatment and symptoms improve in only 50% to 70% of cases.[1,3] All treatments should be reviewed and their intent, either palliative or curative, should be clear to the clinicians.

CARDIAC TAMPONADE

Accumulation of fluid in the pericardial sac leads to elevated intrapericardial pressures, impaired ventricular filling, decreased preload, low cardiac

TABLE 45–1 Oncologic emergencies.

	Oncologic-Related Causes	
Hemoptysis	*Tumor related* (primary vs metastatic, including germ cell tumors) *DAH*[a] (leukemias, multiple myeloma, HSCT,[b] pretransplant conditioning regimen, and other chemotherapies) *Iatrogenic* (biopsy) *Infectious* (aspergilloma, tuberculosis)	• 30% of all causes of hemoptysis are related to malignancy • Reversal of causes of bleeding diathesis • Response to recombinant factor VIIa administration in cases of DAH has been reported
Status Epilepticus	*Metastasis/primary malignancy* *Leptomeningeal disease* *Paraneoplastic syndromes* *PRES*[c] *Chemotherapy* (cisplatin, cyclophosphamide, bevacizumab, busulfan, intrathecal methotrexate) *Brain radiation* *HSCT* *Electrolyte disorders* (hyponatremia and hypercalcemia)	• Importance of recognizing underlying cause • Management of status should follow guidelines
Intracranial hemorrhage	*Tumor related* *Leptomeningeal disease* *HSCT* *APML*[d] *undergoing chemotherapy* *Radiation* *Coagulopathy* *Leukostasis*	• Reversal of underlying coagulopathy • Role of prophylactic brain radiation in leukostasis is unclear • Higher incidence, and worse outcomes, in hematologic malignancies • No data supporting use of factor VII
Elevated ICP	*Metastasis or primary malignancy* *Leukemic meningitis* *Superior vena cava syndrome*	• Steroids should be initiated in cases of tumor/metastasis • Radiation and surgery as intervention • Avoid lumbar puncture in the case of mass effect • Cautious use of mannitol
ALI/ARDS[g]	*Infectious* (high suspicion for PCP, viral and fungal infections) *Chemotherapy* (eosinophilic pneumonia, acute pneumonitis, pulmonary alveolar proteinosis, BOOP, IPF) *HSCT* (IPS,[e] PERDS,[f] BOOP) *Lymphangitic spread* *DAH*	• Management should follow ARDS recommendations • Poor outcomes on HSCT patients • Refer to pneumotox[i] for further chemotherapy-induced respiratory failure
TTP/HUS[h]	*Chemotherapy induced* (mitomycin-C, bleomycin, cisplatin) *HSCT and lymphomas* *Breast, gastric, lung, prostate carcinoma*	• Overall poor outcomes • Difficult diagnosis due to underlying hematologic disturbances in cancer patients

[a]DAH—Diffuse alveolar damage.
[b]HSCT—Hematopoietic stem cell transplant.
[c]PRES—Posterior reversible encephalopathy syndrome.
[d]APML—Acute promyelocytic leukemia.
[e]IPS—Idiopathic pneumonia syndrome.
[f]PERDS—Periengraftment respiratory distress syndrome.
[g]ALI/ARDS—Acute lung injury/acute respiratory distress syndrome.
[h]TTP/HUS—Thrombotic thrombocytopenic purpura/hemolytic-uremic syndrome.
[i] http://pneumotox.com/

output, and shock, a clinical syndrome known as cardiac tamponade. Pericardial effusions secondary to malignancy usually accumulate slowly giving time for compensatory mechanisms against the elevated intrapericardial pressures. Thus, in the case of malignancy, cardiac tamponade usually occurs in the setting of large pericardial effusions. The most common malignancies associated with pericardial effusions are lung, breast, melanoma, and lymphoma.[8] Primary malignancies of the pericardium, such as mesothelioma, are rare.[8] In addition, treatment for malignancy—including radiation and some chemotherapy agents (eg, cytarabine, daunorubicin)—can cause pericarditis and secondary pericardial effusions.[8] Prognosis of patients with malignant pericardial effusions is poor; at 6 months the survival rate is 45% and at 1 year the survival rate is 10% to 26%.[9] Poor prognostic factors include the presence of primary adenocarcinoma of the lung, positive fluid cytology, and advanced malignancy.[9,10]

The most common symptoms associated with cardiac tamponade are dyspnea, chest discomfort, and chest pain. Beck's triad—pulsus paradoxus, distant heart sounds, and jugular venous distention—is pathognomonic; however, it is present only in a minority of patients.[11] Electrocardiography (EKG) has always been used in the diagnosis of cardiac tamponade. Most specific (86%-99%) EKG signs of cardiac tamponade are low voltage, PR depression, and electric alternans; their sensitivity, however, can be as low as 8% to 42%.[12] Echocardiogram is the gold standard for the diagnosis of cardiac tamponade and should be performed emergently. Signs of tamponade include right ventricular collapse during diastole, exaggerated contraction of the right atrium during atrial systole, swinging motion of the heart, and mitral and tricuspid valve inflow variation with respiration.[8,13]

Emergent drainage by either pericardiocentesis (guided by echocardiogram, fluoroscopy, or CT) or pericardial window is the treatment of choice. Pericardial window is recommended for patients who have a higher risk of recurrence such as those with adenocarcinoma of the lung.[14,15] There is, however, no difference in overall survival or safety when performing any of these 2 procedures.[15] Pericardial radiation and instillation of chemotherapy agents for recurrent effusions have been used safely; however, no survival benefit has been demonstrated with these techniques.[8,14]

After drainage of the effusion, symptoms and hemodynamic instability should improve dramatically. In a small percentage of patients, however, there can be persistent shock due to what is described as a "low cardiac output syndrome."[10] Management should be supportive as resolution is usually gradual; however, it has been associated with a poor prognosis in some studies.[10]

MALIGNANT SPINAL CORD COMPRESSION

Spinal lesions occur in 50% of patients with osseous metastasis.[16] Of these, almost 10% of patients develop malignant spinal cord compression (MSCC).[16,17] Hematologic spread is the most common mechanism of spinal cord involvement. Metastatic solid tumors of the lung, breast, and prostate cancer are the most common malignancies associated with MSCC.[18] Non-Hodgkin's lymphoma, multiple myeloma, renal cancer, sarcomas, and unknown primary tumors are less common causes.[18,19]

Early recognition of MSCC is vital because restoration of neurologic function and prognosis is directly related to the degree of initial neurologic damage.[17,19] Pain is the first symptom in 83% to 90% of cases and studies suggest that 60% of cancer patients complaining of back pain have compression of the epidural space.[18,20,21] Thus, in the setting of metastatic disease and back pain, there should be a high suspicion for MSCC. Motor deficits, ranging from weakness to paralysis, are present in 35% to 68% of cases.[17,20] Sensory deficits are usually not recognized by the patients but are present on physical exam in 70% of cases.[20] Autonomic dysfunction and loss of sphincter tone is a poor prognostic factor for recovery as this presents late in the progression of the disease.[17,18,20]

The gold standard and most cost-effective method for diagnosis of MSCC is MRI.[18] Metastatic lesions to the spine are usually widespread, therefore, a whole spine MRI should be performed in all patients with suspected MSCC.[18] Angiography is useful for hypervascular tumors (sarcoma, melanoma, thyroid, and renal cancer) in which presurgical embolization can be considered.[19,21]

Prognosis after MSCC is poor and survival after diagnosis of MSCC is usually 3 to 6 months.[16,17] The goal of treatment is to decrease pain and preserve neurologic function; therefore, a high suspicion and early recognition is important to improve outcomes.[18,19] Scoring systems that include functional status, type of tumor, number of bone and visceral metastases, degree of neurologic dysfunction, and response to radiotherapy are intended to evaluate prognosis and guide therapy.[17,18] Due to the wide variety of available scores, it is important that treatment is guided by a multidisciplinary team that can assess risks and benefits in an individual manner.

First-line treatment of MSCC are corticosteroids as they have been shown to reduce pain and improve neurologic function.[22] Corticosteroids should be administered promptly to decrease spinal cord edema and in some cases, such as lymphoma, to reduce tumor burden.[18] Administration should be prior to radiotherapy, for a total of 10 days, and low doses seem to be as efficacious as megadoses.[22]

Radiation therapy is also widely used for the treatment of MSCC. It is recommended for patients who are unable to tolerate surgical procedures, have a short life expectancy, have diffuse spinal disease, symptoms present for longer than 48 hours, or those with a known tumor sensitivity to radiotherapy.[17,20] This mode of treatment is known to reduce pain, tumor size, and preserve neurologic function.[17]

Surgical decompression is indicated in patients with progression of tumor and symptoms while undergoing radiation, significant cord compression, medically intractable pain, radioresistant tumors, and evidence of spinal instability.[20] Published meta-analysis and randomized controlled trials (RCTs) have shown that surgical intervention in combination with radiotherapy improves neurologic function, pain control, and survival when compared to radiation alone.[16,18,21] Despite these encouraging results, it is important to take into account the patient's overall status and prognosis before undergoing any surgical procedure.[17,18]

Spinal stereotactic radiosurgery, percutaneous vertebroplasty, and kyphoplasty are being considered as more localized and less invasive methods of treatment of MSCC. Although some studies have shown promising results, they are still not widely used and are still considered experimental.[18,19,21]

Overall, MSCC should be readily recognized in the oncologic population. Management and diagnosis should be immediate, multidisciplinary, and tailored to every patient's diagnosis and overall prognosis.

HYPERCALCEMIA

Malignancy-associated hypercalcemia (MAH) occurs in approximately 20% to 30% of patients and is more common in solid tumors such as breast and lung cancer.[23-25] Patients with hematologic malignancies such as Hodgkins disease, non-Hodgkins lymphoma, adult T-cell leukemia/lymphoma, and multiple myeloma can also rarely present with MAH.[23,24,26] MAH can be divided into humoral, osteolytic, and calcitriol-associated hypercalcemia. Humoral hypercalcemia is the most common presentation of MAH. The main mediator is parathyroid hormone–related protein (PTHrP) which is mostly released by solid tumors but has also been described in cases of non-Hodgkins lymphoma and multiple myeloma.[23,24,26] Osteolytic MAH, observed in 20% of cases, is associated with increased osteoclastic activity secondary to bone metastasis.[24,26] Less than 1% of MAH is mediated by calcitriol production in hematologic malignancies such as lymphomas.[24,27] While these distinctions exist, many cases of MAH are multifactorial. MAH is a marker of poor prognosis and median survival time after its presentation is less than 35 days.[25,28]

Symptoms of hypercalcemia include muscular cramping, constipation, dehydration, polyuria, changes in mental status, and cardiac dysrhythmias. The severity of symptoms is usually associated with the degree of hypercalcemia, and central nervous system symptoms are usually present with calcium levels above 14 mg/dL.[24] Initial workup for hypercalcemia should include measurements of ionized calcium, PTH, PTHrP, and 25-hydroxy vitamin D levels.[25]

Volume repletion should be the initial goal of hypercalcemia as hydration decreases tubular reabsorption of calcium by the renal tubules.[23] Loop diuretics to promote calciuresis are no longer recommended because they do not consistently decrease calcium levels and are associated with further volume depletion and electrolyte disorders.[29]

Glucocorticoids, which inhibit calcitriol production, are effective in the treatment of lymphoma-related hypercalcemia.[25,27]

Bisphosphonates, which block bone resorption by osteoclasts, are recommended for long-term treatment of hypercalcemia.[25] While one study showed zoledronic acid to be more efficient than pamidronate in immediate reduction of calcium levels, the difference seemed to dissipate after 1 week.[24,30] Due to these findings any of the 2 medications can be used according to availability. However, if hypercalcemia is causing severe neurologic and cardiac symptoms, zoledronic acid should be considered as it is more effective in the short term. Renal failure can rarely occur when using bisphosphonates; administration should be avoided, or after discussion or risk benefits, if the glomerular filtration rate is less than 30 mg/dL.[23,25,30]

Because bisphosphonates are effective only after 48 hours and hydration can only aid with calciuresis to a certain degree, other immediate measures such as calcitonin administration should be taken. Calcitonin decreases calcium levels by inhibiting osteoclasts and inducing calciuresis 2 hours after administration.[23,30] Administration should be limited to 2 doses due to resistance and downregulation of its receptors.[28] Cinacalcet, a calcimimetic, rapidly decreases calcium levels in the setting of benign hyperparathyroidism; it's role in MAH, however, is limited only to occasional case reports.[25] Denosumab, a monoclonal antibody that inhibits osteoclast activity, is used in patients with refractory MAH as long-term treatment; its use in the acute setting is also limited and it is not recommended on a regular basis.[25]

As previously mentioned, although hypercalcemia can be reversible and treated with current medications, it is usually associated with poor long-term prognosis. Palliation and goals of care should be discussed with these patients even if their outcome after ICU admission is excellent.

TUMOR LYSIS SYNDROME

Tumor lysis syndrome (TLS) is characterized by electrolyte and metabolic derangements which occur after rapid breakdown of proliferating malignant cells. TLS can be spontaneous in rapidly growing tumors or present after treatment with chemotherapy, corticosteroids, or radiation.[31,32] TLS has an incidence of 5% to 10% and is typically associated with acute leukemias particularly acute lymphoblastic leukemia (ALL) and highly aggressive lymphomas, such as Burkitt's lymphoma.[31,32] TLS can also rarely occurs with solid malignancies and usually occurs weeks after chemotherapy treatment is initiated.[32]

Electrolyte abnormalities associated with TLS include hyperkalemia, hyperphosphatemia, hypocalcemia (due to binding of phosphorus to calcium), and hyperuricemia. Clinical findings include vomiting, diarrhea, cramping, lethargy, seizures, cardiac arrhythmias, and shock. Acute kidney injury (AKI) in TLS is caused by deposition of uric acid and calcium phosphate crystals in the kidney tubules.[31] Early recognition and prevention are extremely important as all of these symptoms and complications progress rapidly and can lead to death.

Recognition of high-risk patients and early detection should be the foundation of TLS management. Common risk factors for TLS include: preexisting hyperuricemia, large tumor burden, rapidly growing malignancies, fluid depletion, and renal dysfunction.[32-34] Patients can be characterized into low, intermediate, and high risk for TLS according to their malignancy, laboratory findings, and presence of pre-existing kidney disease.[31,33] This stratification improves early recognition and serves as a guide for treatment. Moreover, laboratory criteria developed by Cairo and Bishop have helped with the diagnosis and classification according to severity of TLS.[34,35] In their definition, elevations above 25% from baseline of uric acid, potassium, phosphorus, and calcium were included. When 2 or more laboratory abnormalities, 2 days before or 7 days after cytotoxic treatment are present, this is indication of TLS.[35] In addition to these laboratory abnormalities, the presence of AKI, seizures, or arrhythmias classifies the disorder as clinical TLS which carries a higher mortality and should be treated aggressively.[31,34]

Supportive care of patients at risk for TLS should be initiated with aggressive hydration to maintain a urine output of 100 mL/h. Close monitoring of electrolytes, lactate dehydrogenase, and uric acid levels are necessary on days prior and after cytoreduction. Alkalinization of urinary pH has been shown to increase phosphate and xanthine (a uric acid metabolite) precipitation in the renal tubules, therefore, administration of sodium bicarbonate is no longer recommended.[31,34] Diuretics in the setting of oliguria can be administered, however, there is no evidence of improved outcome after its use.[32] Indications for hemodialysis in TLS include signs of uremia, volume overload, persistent hyperkalemia, and acidosis. It is also recommended that patients with severe hyperphosphatemia and symptomatic hypocalcemia be initiated on hemodialysis.[31,34] Prophylactic or early hemodialysis, however, has not been studied for TLS.[34]

Two agents are used in the management of TLS: allopurinol (a xanthine oxidase inhibitor that blocks uric acid production) and rasburicase (a recombinant urate oxidase that degrades formed uric acid into allantoin which is easily excreted in urine).[36] Allopurinol should be started 2 days prior to initiation of cytotoxic treatment in patients at risk for TLS and can be administered both orally and intravenously with the same effectiveness.[31,32] Studies have shown that rasburicase can reduce uric acid levels as fast as 4 hours after the initial dose and treatment required averages 3 days.[36] However, due to its costs and availability, the decision to administer rasburicase should probably be limited to high-risk or severe cases and after further discussion with the oncologist. Secondary effects reported with rasburicase include hypersensitivity, methemoglobinemia, and hemolysis in patients with glucose-6-phosphate dehydrogenase deficiency.[32,36]

Current guidelines on management of TLS are based on the risks and severity of the syndrome.[31,33,34] Although there are no studies comparing outcomes of these different guidelines, they all facilitate early recognition of high-risk patients and initiation of early aggressive treatment.

LEUKOSTASIS

Hyperleukocytosis (WBC > 50,000-100,000/mm^3), common in chronic leukemias, is considered a medical emergency and a sign of poor prognosis when found in acute leukemias.[37,38] Leukostasis occurs when blasts aggregate in the microvasculature leading to endovascular damage, hypoperfusion, cytokine release, and secondary organ dysfunction.[39,40] Incidence of leukostasis is 10% to 30% and is more

common in patients with acute myelogenous leukemia (AML) than ALL.[39] Mortality can be as high as 60% and independent risk factors such as age, creatinine, total bilirubin, and lactic dehydrogenase (LDH) levels have been associated with early death.[37,41]

The diagnosis of leukostasis is challenging as its clinical presentation and radiologic findings cannot be differentiated from common infectious and hemorrhagic complications which affect patients with leukemia. Moreover, some cases have been diagnosed with WBC less than 100,000/mm^3, making this diagnosis even more challenging.[41] Most common symptoms associated to leukostasis are respiratory (hypoxemia, dyspnea, and hemoptysis) and neurologic (dizziness, headache, blurry vision, confusion, and stroke or intracranial hemorrhage). Other clinical findings may include extremity, bowel and cardiac ischemia, renal vein thrombosis, heart failure, and priapism.[40,41] It is important to recognize that in the presence of both respiratory failure and neurologic symptoms, mortality can be as high as 90%.[40]

For the past 2 decades there has been very little progress in the treatment of leukostasis. Current available treatment consists of cytoreduction with leukapheresis, hydroxyurea, and chemotherapy. Leukapheresis is initiated in cases of AML if WBC is more than 50,000/mm^3, and in ALL if WBC is more than 250,000/mm^3.[39,41] Although leukapheresis is still used in many institutions, its timing, number of treatments, and target WBC are not well defined. Reasons for this include the fact that the effectiveness of leukapheresis is not associated with WBC reduction, and its use continues to be based mainly on case reports and retrospective studies.[39,41] Hydroxyurea has comparable efficiency and outcomes to leukapheresis and should be used in all patients with leukostasis.[39]

Early chemotherapy is the only treatment that has shown to improve mortality in the short term.[42] Cranial irradiation was used in the past for neurologic symptoms and as prophylaxis to reduce intracranial hemorrhage; however, this is no longer recommended due to lack of effectiveness.[42] Dexamethasone, which decreases cytokine production and suppresses adhesion markers, has been shown to be effective in acute promyelocytic leukemia; nevertheless, additional studies to look at its role in other hematologic malignancies is necessary.[40]

REFERENCES

1. Wilson LD, Detterbeck FC, Yahalom J. Clinical practice. Superior vena cava syndrome with malignant causes. *N Engl J Med.* 2007;356(18):1862-1869.
2. Lepper PM, Ott SR, Hoppe H, et al. Superior vena cava syndrome in thoracic malignancies. *Respir Care.* 2011;56(5):653-666.
3. Wan JF, Bezjak A. Superior vena cava syndrome. *Hematol Oncol Clin North Am.* 2010;24(3):501-513.
4. Schraufnagel DE, Hill R, Leech JA, Pare JA. Superior vena caval obstruction. Is it a medical emergency? *Am J Med.* 1981;70(6):1169-1174.
5. Rowell NP, Gleeson FV. Steroids, radiotherapy, chemotherapy and stents for superior vena caval obstruction in carcinoma of the bronchus. *Cochrane Database Syst Rev.* 2001;4:CD001316.
6. Nguyen NP, Borok TL, Welsh J, Vinh-Hung V. Safety and effectiveness of vascular endoprosthesis for malignant superior vena cava syndrome. *Thorax.* 2009;64(2):174-178.
7. Otten TR, Stein PD, Patel KC, Mustafa S, Silbergleit A. Thromboembolic disease involving the superior vena cava and brachiocephalic veins. *Chest.* 2003;123(3):809-812.
8. Burazor I, Imazio M, Markel G, Adler Y. Malignant pericardial effusion. *Cardiology.* 2013;124(4):224-232.
9. Dequanter D, Lothaire P, Berghmans T, Sculier JP. Severe pericardial effusion in patients with concurrent malignancy: a retrospective analysis of prognostic factors influencing survival. *Ann Surg Oncol.* 2008;15(11):3268-3271.
10. Wagner PL, McAleer E, Stillwell E, et al. Pericardial effusions in the cancer population: prognostic factors after pericardial window and the impact of paradoxical hemodynamic instability. *J Thorac Cardiovasc Surg.* 2011;141(1):34-38.
11. Jacob S, Sebastian JC, Cherian PK, Abraham A, John SK. Pericardial effusion impending tamponade: a look beyond Beck's triad. *Am J Emerg Med.* 2009;27(2):216-219.
12. Eisenberg MJ, de Romeral LM, Heidenreich PA, Schiller NB, Evans GT, Jr. The diagnosis of pericardial effusion and cardiac tamponade by 12-lead ECG. A technology assessment. *Chest.* 1996;110(2):318-324.
13. Spodick DH. Acute cardiac tamponade. *N Engl J Med.* 2003;349(7):684-690.
14. Kim SH, Kwak MH, Park S, et al. Clinical characteristics of malignant pericardial effusion associated with recurrence and survival. *Cancer Res Treat.* 2010;42(4):210-216.
15. McDonald JM, Meyers BF, Guthrie TJ, Battafarano RJ, Cooper JD, Patterson GA. Comparison of open subxiphoid pericardial drainage with percutaneous catheter drainage for symptomatic pericardial effusion. *Ann Thorac Surg.* 2003;76(3):811-815; discussion 816.
16. Klimo P, Jr, Thompson CJ, Kestle JR, Schmidt MH. A meta-analysis of surgery versus conventional radiotherapy for the treatment of metastatic spinal epidural disease. *Neuro Oncol.* 2005;7(1):64-76.
17. Cole JS, Patchell RA. Metastatic epidural spinal cord compression. *Lancet Neurol.* 2008;7(5):459-466.
18. Sun H, Nemecek AN. Optimal management of malignant epidural spinal cord compression. *Hematol Oncol Clin North Am.* 2010;24(3):537-551.
19. Eleraky M, Papanastassiou I, Vrionis FD. Management of metastatic spine disease. *Curr Opin Support Palliat Care.* 2010;4(3):182-188.
20. Helweg-Larsen S, Sorensen PS. Symptoms and signs in metastatic spinal cord compression: a study of progression from first symptom until diagnosis in 153 patients. *Eur J Cancer.* 1994;30A(3):396-398.
21. Sciubba DM, Gokaslan ZL. Diagnosis and management of metastatic spine disease. *Surg Oncol.* 2006;15(3):141-151.
22. Vecht CJ, Haaxma-Reiche H, van Putten WL, de Visser M, Vries EP, Twijnstra A. Initial bolus of conventional versus high-dose dexamethasone in metastatic spinal cord compression. *Neurology.* 1989;39(9):1255-1257.
23. Body JJ. Hypercalcemia of malignancy. *Semin Nephrol.* 2004;24(1):48-54.
24. Stewart AF. Clinical practice. Hypercalcemia associated with cancer. *N Engl J Med.* 2005;352(4):373-379.
25. Maier JD, Levine SN. Hypercalcemia in the intensive care unit: a review of pathophysiology, diagnosis, and modern therapy. *J Intensive Care Med.* 2013;30(5):235-252.
26. Sargent JT, Smith OP. Haematological emergencies managing hypercalcaemia in adults and children with haematological disorders. *Br J Haematol.* 2010;149(4):465-477.
27. Seymour JF, Gagel RF. Calcitriol: the major humoral mediator of hypercalcemia in Hodgkin's disease and non-Hodgkin's lymphomas. *Blood.* 1993;82(5):1383-1394.
28. Ralston SH, Gallacher SJ, Patel U, Campbell J, Boyle IT. Cancer-associated hypercalcemia: morbidity and mortality. Clinical experience in 126 treated patients. *Ann Intern Med.* 1990;112(7):499-504.

29. LeGrand SB, Leskuski D, Zama I. Narrative review: furosemide for hypercalcemia: an unproven yet common practice. *Ann Intern Med.* 2008;149(4):259-263.

30. Major P, Lortholary A, Hon J, et al. Zoledronic acid is superior to pamidronate in the treatment of hypercalcemia of malignancy: a pooled analysis of two randomized, controlled clinical trials. *J Clin Oncol.* 2001;19(2):558-567.

31. Coiffier B, Altman A, Pui CH, Younes A, Cairo MS. Guidelines for the management of pediatric and adult tumor lysis syndrome: an evidence-based review. *J Clin Oncol.* 2008;26(16):2767-2778.

32. Mughal TI, Ejaz AA, Foringer JR, Coiffier B. An integrated clinical approach for the identification, prevention, and treatment of tumor lysis syndrome. *Cancer Treat Rev.* 2010;36(2):164-176.

33. Cairo MS, Coiffier B, Reiter A, Younes A. Recommendations for the evaluation of risk and prophylaxis of tumour lysis syndrome (TLS) in adults and children with malignant diseases: an expert TLS panel consensus. *Br J Haematol.* 2010;149(4):578-586.

34. Pession A, Masetti R, Gaidano G, et al. Risk evaluation, prophylaxis, and treatment of tumor lysis syndrome: consensus of an Italian expert panel. *Adv Ther.* 2011;28(8):684-697.

35. Cairo MS, Bishop M. Tumour lysis syndrome: new therapeutic strategies and classification. *Br J Haematol.* 2004;127(1):3-11.

36. Jeha S, Kantarjian H, Irwin D, et al. Efficacy and safety of rasburicase, a recombinant urate oxidase (Elitek), in the management of malignancy-associated hyperuricemia in pediatric and adult patients: final results of a multicenter compassionate use trial. *Leukemia.* 2005;19(1):34-38.

37. Novotny JR, Muller-Beissenhirtz H, Herget-Rosenthal S, Kribben A, Duhrsen U. Grading of symptoms in hyperleukocytic leukaemia: a clinical model for the role of different blast types and promyelocytes in the development of leukostasis syndrome. *Eur J Haematol.* 2005;74(6):501-510.

38. Piccirillo N, Laurenti L, Chiusolo P, et al. Reliability of leukostasis grading score to identify patients with high-risk hyperleukocytosis. *Am J Hematol.* 2009;84(6):381-382.

39. Blum W, Porcu P. Therapeutic apheresis in hyperleukocytosis and hyperviscosity syndrome. *Semin Thromb Hemost.* 2007;33(4):350-354.

40. Porcu P, Cripe LD, Ng EW, et al. Hyperleukocytic leukemias and leukostasis: a review of pathophysiology, clinical presentation and management. *Leuk Lymphoma.* 2000;39(1-2):1-18.

41. Ganzel C, Becker J, Mintz PD, Lazarus HM, Rowe JM. Hyperleukocytosis, leukostasis and leukapheresis: practice management. *Blood Rev.* 2012;26(3):117-122.

42. Chang MC, Chen TY, Tang JL, et al. Leukapheresis and cranial irradiation in patients with hyperleukocytic acute myeloid leukemia: no impact on early mortality and intracranial hemorrhage. *Am J Hematol.* 2007;82(11):976-980.

Rheumatologic and Inflammatory Conditions in the ICU

46

Deborah Orsi, MD; Wilma Correa-Lopez, MD and John Cavagnaro, PA

KEY POINTS

1 ICU mortality can be as high as 55% and can reach 79% in the systemic lupus erythematous (SLE) population.

2 Severe sepsis and septic shock represent in fact the primary reason for ICU admission in about half of the rheumatologic patients.

3 The clinical manifestations of autoimmune diseases itself can be very heterogeneous and virtually all organ systems can be affected.

4 Most common adult rheumatologic disease encountered by the intensivist are in order of frequency, according to the most recent literature, SLE, rheumatoid arthritis (RA), systemic vasculitis, and systemic sclerosis (SS).

5 Conditions associated with airway involvement include RA, granulomatosis with polyangiitis (GPA, former Wegener granulomatosis), relapsing polychondritis and SLE.

6 Among all the rheumatologic diseases SS seems to have the highest prevalence (80%) of pulmonary involvement.

7 Rheumatologic patients are at high risk of acute coronary syndromes due to premature atherosclerosis compared to age-match population.

8 Renal involvement occurs in roughly 30% of the overall rheumatologic patients.

9 Chronic steroids therapy used in the treatment of numerous rheumatologic conditions increase the risk of adrenal insufficiency in acutely critically ill patients.

10 No clear prognosticator of in-ICU mortality has been identified as applicable to single patient yet, but intuitively high Apache score, multiorgan failure, comorbidities, advanced age and pancytopenia were all associated with worse outcome.

INTRODUCTION

According to the most recent literature, about a third of rheumatologic patients admitted to the hospital will require admission in an intensive care unit (ICU). Their in-ICU mortality can be as high as 55% and can reach 79% in the systemic lupus erythematous (SLE) population. Such a severe life threatening decompensation may be caused by multiorgan system failure related to disease flare or by the complications of immunosuppressive state or therapy, such as infection.[1-14]

Severe sepsis and septic shock represent in fact the primary reason for ICU admission in about half of the rheumatologic patients. It is the first cause of mortality in SLE patients, therefore, it is crucial to recognize and aggressively treat any infectious process before attempting to achieve diseases control with immunosuppressive therapy.

An increasing number of patients will be recognized ex novo to have a rheumatologic condition during their ICU stay. Such diagnosis can be quite challenging for the intensivist and usually require a multidisciplinary approach.

Few diagnostic tests, that is, autoantibodies, are confirmatory and when negative do not rule out the disease if clinical criteria are met. On the other end of the spectrum, positive autoantibodies can be found in healthy individuals and in extrarheumatologic conditions (Table 46–1). The clinical manifestations of autoimmune diseases itself can be very heterogeneous and virtually all organ systems can be affected.

The most common adult rheumatologic disease encountered by the intensivist are in order of frequency, according to the most recent literature, SLE, rheumatoid arthritis (RA), systemic vasculitis, and systemic sclerosis (SS).

Acute respiratory failure appears to be the most common indication for ICU admission. It remains difficult to estimate from various studies whether related to disease flare involving the respiratory system or to primary pulmonary infectious process or both.

OVERVIEW OF CLINICAL MANIFESTATIONS OF RHEUMATOLOGIC DISEASES BY ORGAN SYSTEMS

Severe Sepsis

Acute respiratory failure due to pneumonia appears to be the most common reason for ICU admission. Chronic inflammatory process and immunosuppressant therapy make rheumatologic patients extremely susceptible to severe infections. Fever and leukocytosis may not be present.

The most common microorganisms involved are the typical bacterial pathogens, therefore treatment for community or hospital acquired

TABLE 46–1 Autoantibodies and associated disorders.

Autoantibody	Associated Disease
RF	RA (80%), LES (10%), MCTD (50%-60%), Sjoegren SD (80%-90%)
	Infections, chronic liver disease, pulmonary disease
	Cryoglobulinemia
Anti-CCP	RA
ANA types:	Also seen in subacute endocarditis, tuberculosis, hematologic Malignancy, chronic infectious disease, other nonconnective tissue Disease (Crohn, autoimmune hepatisis, cholangitis)
Anti-dsDNA	SLE
Anti-Sm	SLE
Anti SS-A	Sjoegren SD (70%), SLE (30%), RA, scleroderma, and MCTD (rare)
Anti SS-B	SJOEGREN SD (60%), SLE (15%), RA, scleroderma, MCTD
Anti RNP	MCTD (95%), SLE (30%)
Anti-Scl-70	Diffuse scleroderma (20%-40%) discord
Anticentromere	Limited scleroderma (60%-90%), diffuse scleroderma (30%)
Anti-histone	Drug-induced SLE
Anti-RNA polymerase	Systemic sclerosis
Anti Jo-1	Polymyositis

RF, rheumatoid factor; anti-CCP, anticyclic citrulline peptide; MCTD, mixed connective tissue disease.

pneumonia should not be delayed. Cases of nonresolving pneumonia must raise suspicion for atypical bacterial infections, reactivation of tuberculosis, disseminated fungal disease (histoplasmosis, cryptococcosis, and aspergillus spp.), listeriosis, and Pneumocystis pneumonia.

Effort should be made to collect all the appropriate body fluids and specimens before initiation of antibiotics treatment. Bronchoalveolar lavage (BAL) should be considered early on in the course of the disease.

Pneumocystis pneumonia prophylaxis should be considered for patient on immunosuppressant agents.

Airway Involvement

Inflammation within the airway, obstruction from inflammation, ankylosis of the cricoarytenoid joints or cervical spine can represent challenging airways for the intensivist.

Conditions associated with airway involvement include RA, granulomatosis with polyangiitis (GPA, former Wegener granulomatosis), relapsing polychondritis and SLE.

Occasionally obstruction caused by angioedema may be seen in its acquired form in lupus patients. Subglottid stenosis can be present in about 10% to 20% of patients with GPA. Relapsing polychondritis of both small and large airways can cause upper or lower airway obstruction due to recurrent cartilage inflammation and destruction. Patients with advanced cutaneous scleroderma may represent difficult airway if mouth opening is narrowed.

Upper airway problems may arise especially in patients with RA and ankylosing spondylitis if airway needs to be secured.

Atlantoaxial subluxation (C1-C2) may be present in RA male patients particularly in those with severe peripheral joint deformities, long disease duration and neck pain. Patients undergoing elective surgery should have cervical radiologic evaluation since subluxation can be asymptomatic and neck manipulation during intubation may be proven to be fatal. In emergent situations, fiberoptic intubation will be the preferred option.

Pulmonary Disease

Respiratory insufficiency is the leading causes of ICU admission. Its manifestation may be expression of autoimmune flare or infection. Interstitial lung disease (ILD), pleuritis, pleural effusion, pulmonary hemorrhage, and embolism can all be encountered in critically ill rheumatologic patients.

RA patients tend to have an increased rate of ILD, cryptogenic organizing pneumonia, obliterative bronchiolitis, and pleural involvement.

Pulmonary hemorrhage seems more prevalent in systemic vasculitis and when associated with SLE.

Among all the rheumatologic diseases SS seems to have the highest prevalence (80%) of pulmonary involvement. ILD (being the nonspecific interstitial pneumonia the most common) and pulmonary arterial hypertension are the most common features and both can coexist. These patients should be screened before symptoms appear since early intervention can slow the disease progression. Doppler echocardiography and right heart catheterization are necessary to estimate pulmonary arterial hypertension. Further lung injury from recurrent aspiration is frequently experienced in scleroderma patients due to an incontinent gastroesophageal sphincter.

Sjogren syndrome (SJ) and polymyositis-dermatomyositis also share a high rate of pulmonary involvement as shown in Table 46–2.

Pleural involvement occurs frequently in RA and SLE patients. The pleural fluid exam is an exudates with low pH, low glucose with a lymphocytic predominance. The level of rheumatoid factor in the pleural fluid parallels that in the serum. Recurrent effusions may require a more definitive treatment (pleurodesis).

Pulmonary embolism and deep vein thrombosis may be the primary manifestation of an underlying prothrombotic state caused by a rheumatologic condition. Lifelong prophylactic anticoagulation is required since new evidence from population-based studies show a 2 to 3 fold increase of thromboembolic phenomena in these patients.

Loss of anticoagulants factor due to concomitant renal impairment can also contribute to a prothrombotic state.

Drug-induced lung toxicity, that is, methotrexate is usually a diagnosis of exclusion.

The general evaluation of pulmonary involvement should include a chest X-ray (CXR), oftentimes not sensitive and a high resolution computed tomography (CT) of the chest. The latter may show pulmonary nodules, ground glass opacity as well as reticular pattern and honeycombing. BAL can help in differentiating between exacerbation of rheumatic disease, infection, drug-induced respiratory failure and alveolar hemorrhage. BAL and lung biopsy can aid the diagnosis but both have no role in prognostication.

TABLE 46–2 Frequency of pulmonary complication in rheumatologic disease.

Clinical Manifestation	RA	SLE	SS	PM-DM	SJ	MCTD
ILD	3+	2+	4+	3	3	2
DAH	1	2	1	1	0	1
COP	2	1	1	3	1	1
OB	2	0	0	0	1	0
PL EFF	3	2	1	0	1	2
ASP PN	0	0	3	3	2	2
VASCUL	2	2	0	1	2	2
PULM HTN	1	2	4	1	0	2
RESP MUSC INVOL	1	2	0	2	0	1

Keys:1+ some, 4+ maximal
DAH, diffuse alveolar hemorrhage; PL EFF, pleural effusion; ASP PN, aspiration pneumonia; VASCUL, vasculitis; PULM HTN, pulmonary hypertension; RESP MUSC INVOLV, respiratory muscle involvement.
Modified with permission from Fischman AP, Elias JA, Fishman JA: Fishman's Manual of Pulmonary Disease and Disorders, 3rd ed. New York: McGraw Hill; 2002.

Aggressive immunosuppressive therapy is warranted to decrease pulmonary inflammation and evolution into acute lung injury as well as multiorgan involvement.

Cardiovascular Disease

Pericardial involvement may affect 12% to 48 % of patients with lupus and as high as 35% in patients with RA. Acute pericarditis may rarely evolve into cardiac tamponade but its progression into chronicity may cause restrictive cardiomyopathy requiring surgical intervention.

Rheumatoid nodules can involve the myocardium and the heart valves causing embolic phenomena and conduction disturbances (RA, SS, and its variant CREST). Myocarditis in lupus and polymyositis-dermatomyositis patients may lead to overt heart failure.

Libman Sacks endocarditis occurs in about 10% of SLE patients. Its fibrinoid vegetations can cause severe valvular regurgitation (mitral and aortic valve most commonly) and thromboembolic phenomena especially if antiphospholipid (APL) syndrome is associated.

Rheumatologic patients are at high risk of acute coronary syndromes due to premature atherosclerosis compared to age-match population. Within the rheumatologic diseases, patients affected by Kawasaki and systemic vasculitis are at the highest risk due to the chronic inflammation of coronary arteries and associated arteritis.

Gatrointestinal Disease

Gastrointestinal hemorrhage is frequently encountered in patients treated with corticosteroids and nonsteroidal anti-inflammatory drugs (NSAIDs). Stress ulcers may provoke brisk bleeding if coagulopathy and thrombocytopenia are associated.

Henoch–Schonlein purpura, SS, necrotizing vasculitis may all cause bleeding from ulceration of small vessels of small bowel or colonic mucosa.

Intestinal ischemia may result as a complication of panarteritis nodosa, RA, SLE, and vasculitides, in general. The clinical manifestation depends on the size and location of the vessel involved. Occasionally profuse bleeding, ulceration with perforation can be seen.

Renal Involvement

Renal involvement occurs in roughly 30% of the overall rheumatologic patients. Lupus nephritis remains the most feared complication of the disease and renal involvement can be detected in as high as 90% of patients before any overt clinical manifestations.

The spectrum of the glomerular involvement varies from minimal to advanced sclerosis. Urine analysis will show proteinuria more than 0.5 g/24 hours and red blood cell cast. Complement levels including C3 and C4 are decreased. Hypertensive crisis can be also present.

Renal biopsy should not be delayed since it can provide diagnosis, staging and therefore treatment. Aggressive immunosuppressive treatment is warranted for advanced stage of glomerulonephritis (GN, staged from I to V, being the III stage usually the initial time for treatment) to prevent further progression of injury and achieve remission. Treatment includes pulse steroids combined with IV or oral cyclophosphamide with possible mycophenolate and cyclosporine in case of refractory response. Occasionally plasma exchange may be instituted for rapid progressive GN. Some patient will recover while some will progress to end stage renal disease requiring dialysis. Renal transplant can be successful if good control of the active disease is achieved.

Scleroderma renal crisis occurs in about 15% of patient with SS. It is a medical emergency presenting with abrupt onset of hypertension and acute renal failure. It can precede the diagnosis of SS. Multisystem involvement with hypertensive encephalopathy, visual disturbances and seizure, pulmonary edema, myocarditis, microangiopathic anemia and thrombocytopenia may be all present. Urine analysis shows granular cast, mild proteinuria and hematuria.

Management includes early treatment with ACE inhibitor such as captopril and lisinopril titrate to decrease blood pressure while avoiding hypoperfusion. Steroids are generally avoided as they are linked to possible risk factor for the development of renal crisis.

Active RA can cause late stage amyloid nephropathy. NSAID, gold and penicillamine can also be responsible for nephritic disease.

Central Nervous System Disease

Primary angiitis of the central nervous system (PACNS), lupus, polyarteritis nodosa (PAN), giant cell arteritis (GCA), and SJ comprise the majority of autoimmune conditions associated with central nervous system (CNS) vasculitis. Patients with primary angiitis will lack the manifestations and the positive inflammatory markers of systemic vasculitis. Symptoms can range from severe headache, seizure, stroke, cognitive impairment, psychosis.

Lupus psychosis is a common manifestation of SLE. Antipsychotic and control of active disease are the treatment of choice. Steroid use may confound as well as precipitate the clinical picture. Lumbar puncture may show mild elevated white blood cell with predominance of lymphocytes, elevated protein and low glucose.

Cerebral venous thrombosis can be seen in patient affected by APS either primary or secondary to lupus.

Headache, diplopia, and stroke in an elderly woman with elevated ESR should raise suspicion for GCA, although a normal ESR does not exclude it. Symmetric stiffness and proximal muscle pain may be expression of the frequently associated polymyalgia rheumatica. Infections and malignancy of the CNS should be ruled out first. Lumbar puncture, brain CT, cerebral magnetic resonance imaging (MRI), and angiographic studies should be performed. Angiogram may reveal arterial stenosis, occlusion, dilatation, or vessel beading.

Hematologic Disorder

A prothrombotic state and anemia of chronic disease are usually present in patient with rheumatologic disease. Microangiopathic anemia, thrombocytopenia and leukopenia may also represent the manifestation of a disease flare that scatters autoantibodies against the hematologic series. Suppressed bone marrow function may also develop from immunosuppressive therapy.

Leukopenia is a clinical defining feature of SLE and is seen in patients with RA complicated by Felty syndrome. Thrombotic thrombocytopenic purpura (TTP) is frequently associated with pediatric SLE. APS is an autoimmune condition characterized by antibodies against phospholipids binding plasma proteins and is clinically manifested by arterial or venous thrombosis. It can occur as a primary condition or associated with other rheumatologic diseases, usually SLE. The affected organ and the clinical manifestation depend on the vessel involved and may manifest as focal neurologic deficit, transverse myelitis, seizure, pulmonary embolism, intra-alveolar hemorrhage, valvular disease, coronary thrombosis, recurrent miscarriages. A catastrophic APS is defined as a wide spread small vessel thrombosis with multiorgan failure. Mortality rate can reach up to 50%. Treatment with anticoagulation, high dose pulse glucocorticoids and plasma exchange with or without IVIG has been associated with 50% to 80% recovery rate.

Coagulation abnormality caused by autoantibodies anticlotting factors may be manifest as disseminated intravascular thrombosis, bleeding or both. Autoantibody antifactor VIII is the most common autoimmune coagulation disorder seen in SLE and RA. Cessation of bleeding will respond to porcine factor VIII which is antigenically different.

A rare but potentially fatal cause of pancytopenia is acute hemophagocytic syndrome, a condition more commonly seen in rheumatologic pediatric patients. It is frequently a diagnosis of exclusion in adults. Pancytopenia, hypertriglyceridemia, elevated transaminase and ferritin characterize the diseases. Overwhelming inflammatory response, coagulopathy, pulmonary involvement and encephalopathy are the most common clinical manifestations. Bone marrow examination is diagnostic. Treatments include high dose steroids, IVIG and cyclosporine.

Musculoskeletal Involvement

Muscular involvement is a characteristic feature of many connective tissue diseases although do not constitute usually an indication for ICU admission except when impairment of the respiratory dynamic is present. Rheumatic inflammatory myopathies can be confused with critical illness myopathy in debilitated patient with prolonged ICU stay.

Immobilization, steroids, and neuromuscular blocking agent are usually associated with the latter. Difficult weaning from mechanical ventilation may contribute further to increase in length of stay in these patients.

Endocrine/Adrenal Insufficiency

Chronic steroids therapy used in the treatment of numerous rheumatologic conditions increase the risk of adrenal insufficiency in acutely critically ill patients. Refractory hypotension and severe electrolytes imbalance may be present.

Stress dose steroids should be initiated (200-300 mg IV daily in divided doses) during an acute illness or high metabolic state.

Vasculitides

The presence of inflammatory leukocytes in a vessel wall and the reactive damage caused to the wall structures define vasculitis. Attack by leukocytes leads to loss of vessel integrity causing bleeding, with subsequent obstruction of the blood vessel lumen ultimately leading to tissue ischemia and necrosis. What triggers this cascade of events is unclear, but it is likely multifactorial. The size and location of the affected vessel and the presence or absence of antineutrophil cytoplasmic antibodies (ANCA) form the basis of the current classification system. The affected organs, and thus the clinical presentation, depend on the presence of the target antigen in the particular organ, on the ability of the endothelial cell to respond to the antigenic presence by activating and recruiting the elements involved in initiating and sustaining the inflammatory cascade.

The American College of Rheumatology (ACR) 1990 criteria was proposed with the intent of facilitating the task of distinguishing the different types of vasculitides. The criteria do not include all the features of each particular form of vasculitis, but mainly focus on those that commonly identify the particular syndrome and to allow for comparable subjects to be included in studies and discussions. The 2012 International Chapel Hill Consensus Conference (CHCC) revised the nomenclature used to categorize the vasculitides. The accompanying tables represent a combination of both the ACR criteria and the CHCC nomenclature, as a general reference point. However, the focus of this discussion is the management of the patient with vasculitis who requires admission to the ICU. Patients with vasculitides are frequently admitted to the ICU because of complications of the immunosuppressive therapy used to control the disease, such as severe infections associated with organ dysfunction, or because of life-threatening manifestations of the disease, such as the pulmonary-renal syndrome. Most patients are admitted to the ICU with a pre-existent diagnosis of vasculitis, but in some cases their ICU admission constitutes the presentation of the disease. Unfortunately, the clinical manifestations of many of the vasculitides are nonspecific and seen in a number of conditions that present with systemic involvement, for example, multiorgan dysfunction seen in conditions such as endocarditis, severe sepsis, meningococcemia, DIC, and TTP. A high index of suspicion is therefore paramount as vasculitides, if severe and untreated, can rapidly deteriorate into life threatening scenarios.

A potentially devastating cause for admission to the ICU for the patient with vasculitis is hemoptysis. Patients with vasculitides are frequently admitted to the ICU with manifestations of the pulmonary-renal syndrome (PRS), the combination of pulmonary hemorrhage and glomerulonephritis. Although anti-GBM disease (Goodpasture's disease) and lupus are responsible for some of the cases of PRS, the small vessel vasculitides account for most. These include the ANCA-positive vasculitides, namely eosinophilic granulomatosis with polyangiitis (EGPA, formerly known as Churg-Strauss syndrome), GPA, and microscopic polyangiitis (MPA). Less common culprits of PRS are the ANCA-negative IgA nephropathy and Henoch–Schonlein purpura. The clinical presentation and diagnostic features of each of the syndrome are summarized in the accompanying tables.

Anti-GBM disease (formerly known as Goodpasture's disease) is an uncommon cause of PRS. It is not a vasculitis, but rather a disorder mediated by antibodies directed against the α3 chain of type IV collagen found in the glomerular basement membrane and the alveolar capillaries. The spectrum of anti-GBM disease includes patients with glomerulonephritis but without pulmonary hemorrhage, or "renal-limited anti-GBM antibody disease," and those with both glomerulonephritis and pulmonary hemorrhage. Patients present with glomerulonephritis, hemoptysis (could be episodic or acute and massive), and constitutional symptoms such as fever, weight loss, malaise, anorexia, and arthralgia. Hemoptysis may be the only presenting complaint, in association with normal renal function. However, rapidly progressive renal failure associated with hematuria is the most common presenting manifestation of anti-GBM disease. Urinalysis shows hematuria with dysmorphic red cells and red

cell casts, and proteinuria, usually non-nephrotic in range. Histologically there is crescent formation within glomeruli. CXR may be normal or may show bilateral alveolar infiltrates, mostly in the perihilar and lower lung areas, which resolve over a few days after cessation of bleeding. Diagnosis depends on the demonstration of anti-GBM antibodies in the appropriate clinical setting. About 20% to 30% of patients are also "ANCA positive," and their disease behaves more like a vasculitis. Renal biopsy is necessary for confirmation of the disease. It shows crescentic glomerulonephritis and linear deposition of IgG along the glomerular basement membrane. Early diagnosis and treatment are crucial in order to prevent progression to ESRD and dialysis dependence. Treatment, as soon as the diagnosis is suspected, involves a combination of steroids, cyclophosphamide, and plasmapheresis. Good outcomes are usually seen in patients with less than 30% crescents on renal biopsy. Prognosis in anti-GBM correlates with the level of renal injury at the time of presentation. Patients with more than 50% crescents on renal biopsy, with serum Cr more than 7 or requiring dialysis with 72 hours of presentation, have poor outcomes. In these patients the benefits of combined therapy are questioned, and many would not recommend it. In these patients, a short course of steroids and plasma exchange is recommended.

The general evaluation of a patient with suspected vasculitis should include routine tests for evaluation of organ dysfunction, such as renal, hematologic, and, liver function tests; ESR and CRP as markers of inflammatory states; ANCA; anti-GBM antibody, for exclusion of Goodpasture's syndrome, Hep B and Hep C serologies; HIV testing; complement levels (C3, C4, CH50; decreased in SLE and cryoglobulinemia), RA (when elevated suggests RA, cryoglobulinemia-associated vasculitis, and SJ); cryoglobulins (seen in mixed essential cryoglobulinemia and in certain forms of vasculitis); CPK to rule out myositis (associated with some vasculitides). Blood cultures should routinely be performed to rule out infection. A CXR, chest CT (if abnormal CXR findings or in cases of pulmonary manifestations not explained by CXR), UA, and EKG may be warranted. If indicated, a lumbar puncture should be performed. Patients with pulmonary hemorrhage usually have pulmonary capillaritis from small vessel vasculitis secondary to GPA and MPA more often than to anti-GBM and cryoglobulinemic vasculitis; it is rare in EGPA and IgAV. Bronchoscopy is performed to rule out other causes of pulmonary hemorrhage, such as infection, malignancy, among others and to establish the presence of alveolar hemorrhage. Tissue biopsy is almost always necessary in order to confirm the presence of a vasculitis.

The management of the patient with PRS involves supportive care and the use of immunosuppressants. Airway management should follow the usual protocols used in the care of patients with respiratory failure, such as lung protective ventilation. The patient with GPA, however, may represent a special challenge due to the occasional occurrence of tracheal stenosis. Infections are a common cause of mortality among these patients, and their occurrence requires diligent surveillance, especially because of the increased risk afforded by the use of immunosuppressants.

Glucocorticoids are the mainstay of therapy in vasculitides. However, the use of cytotoxic agents in addition to steroids has improved the survival of this patient population. The challenge resides in identifying the patient in whom the benefit-risk assessment favors the additional risks of cytotoxic agents. The severity of vasculitis has not been identified as a prognostic marker, in contrast to the presence of respiratory failure, which has been associated with worse outcomes. ANCA titers are not uniformly reflective of disease severity. The revised 2011 Five Factors Score (FFS) has been used to assess the severity of vasculitis and to identify the patient whose survival can be favorably impacted by the addition of cytotoxic agents. In the FFS scoring system a point is given for the presence of each of the following:

- Cardiac involvement
- GI involvement
- Renal injury (peak serum Cr > 1.7 mg/dL)
- Age > 65
- Absence of ENT manifestations (in EGPA)

The 1996 version of the FFS system included proteinuria and CNS involvement. The score ranges from 0 (none of the factors are present) to 2 (2 or more factors are present). The greater the number of factors present, the worse the prognosis, with cardiac and GI involvement being the strongest negative prognostic indicators. The patient with a FFS of 1 has a 26% 5-year mortality risk according to some series. Based on these findings, it follows that patients with FFS of 1 or greater, patients with cardiac and/or gastrointestinal manifestations, as well as the obvious subset of patients with refractory disease, would benefit from the concomitant use of cytotoxic agents.

In general, the treatment of systemic vasculitis entails an induction phase, which typically can last up to 1 to 2 months, and a maintenance phase, which can last 1 to 2 years, or longer. The induction phase uses high dose steroids (IV methylprednisolone 1 g daily for 3 to 5 days, replaced then by prednisone 1 mg/kg/d) and, when indicated, a cytotoxic agent, such as cyclophosphamide, IV or PO. Compared to oral cyclophosphamide, pulse IV cyclophosphamide, every 2 to 4 weeks, is associated with similar rates of induction but a higher risk of relapse. The use of IV cyclophosphamide allows a lower total cumulative dose, and therefore potentially leads to a lower incidence of adverse reactions, especially infectious. Azathioprine and methotrexate have been used in less severe cases of vasculitides and in patients intolerant of cyclophosphamide. These agents are also used after the induction phase with cyclophosphamide in some cases. In patients with life-threatening pulmonary hemorrhage or rapidly progressing glomerulonephritis, plasmapheresis can be used as an adjunct to immunosuppression, although it offers no mortality benefit. The role of plasmapheresis in ANCA-negative glomerulonephritis is not supported by data. Iv IG can be considered in patients with a concurrent, serious infection, in whom cytotoxic agents carry a greater risk of adverse events. In terms of monitoring of the response to therapy, standardized risk scores, decreasing ANCA levels as in the case of GPA and microscopic polyangiitis, can be used to guide therapy aggressiveness and the transition from induction to maintenance phases of treatment. Prophylaxis against opportunistic infections, especially Pneumocystis, is indicated during the period of immunosuppression.

Mortality in patients with vasculitis admitted to the ICU ranges from 11% to 40%, mostly secondary to infections. Early deaths in patients with vasculitis are usually secondary to the disease itself, whereas late mortalities are usually attributed to infectious complications, usually as result of treatment (Table 46–3).

TABLE 46-3 Overview of vasculitides

Small Vessels Vasculitides	Clinical Features/Diagnosis	Treatment
Eosinophilic granulomatosis with polyangiitis, EGPA (previously known as Churg-Strauss vasculitis; allergic granulomatosis with angiitis)	• Most commonly affected: **lungs**, followed by the **skin**. It can be generalized. Atopy/nasal polyps/**allergic rhinitis** and worsening **asthma**, fever, rash, myalgia, arthralgia, weight loss, cough, dyspnea. Rare manifestations: chest pain (secondary to myocarditis, coronary artery involvement; rare), renal dysfunction (less common than in other ANCA-positive vasculitides; most common necrotizing crescentic GN), GI (mesenteric ischemia • CXR: fleeting pulmonary infiltrates • **Peripheral eosinophilia** (> 10%) • **Mono/polyneuropathy** • + ANCA (40%-60%) • **Biopsy**: accumulation of eosinophils in extravascular areas	• Glucocorticoids are the mainstay of therapy (most patients will respond to steroid monotherapy) • Immunosuppressants are recommended for severe and refractory cases • A **Five Factors Score** of 1 or more is associated with increased mortality and benefits from the combination of glucocorticoids and immunosuppressant, usually **cyclophosphamide** • Azathioprine or Methotrexate used commonly for maintenance of induction • Some reports of benefit of IVIG in refractory cases; not the case for plasma exchange
Granulomatosis with polyarteritis (GPA, formerly known as Wegener's)	• Triad of **upper airway disease** (sinusitis, oral ulcers, or bloody or purulent nasal discharge), **lower airway disease** (lung infiltrates/nodules/cavities/hemorrhage, hilar adenopathy tracheal stenosis), **and renal disease** (hematuria, cell casts, non-nephrotic proteinuria, pauci-immune/RPGN). Some cases involve ocular manifestations, heart (pericarditis, myocarditis, conduction abnormalities), GI, CNS involvement • C-ANCA (PR3-ANCA) positivity seen in 65%; a minority are p-ANCA or MPO-ANCA positive 3. About 10% are ANCA negative • **Biopsy**: granulomatous inflammation of artery or perivascular area, necrosis	• Glucocorticoids +/- cyclophosphamide (alternative: rituximab probably as effective as cyclophosphamide according to trials; methotrexate in cases with mild or no extrarenal disease • Response to therapy and mortality correlate to ANCA titers • High rates of relapse • Plasmapheresis may be of benefit in patients with severe disease, especially in patients who also have anti-GBM antibodies • Response to therapy that includes glucocorticoids and cyclophosphamide is seen in more than 90% of patients
Microscopic polyangiitis	• Pulmonary infiltrates/hemorrhage, rapidly progressive glomerulonephritis • p-ANCA positive (antimyeloperoxidase) • Considered to be part of the GPA spectrum	• Same treatment as GPA
IgA vasculitis (Henoch–Schonlein purpura)	• Palpable purpura, arthritis, glomerulonephritis, intestinal ischemia (colic-like abdominal pain)/GI bleeding, hematuria • 10% develop renal insufficiency, 5% progress to renal failure • Pulmonary disease rare • Deposits of IgA in renal or skin biopsy • No new medications	• Usually self-limited • Steroids may be indicated in severe cases with extracutaneous manifestations

(Continued)

TABLE 46–3 Overview of vasculitides (*Continued*)

Small Vessels Vasculitides	Clinical Features/Diagnosis	Treatment
Cryoglobulinemic vasculitis	Purpura, arthralgias, Raynaud's phenomenon, and glomerulonephritis (in severe cases) Low complement levels, cryoglobulins Immune deposits of cryoglobulins in walls of small vessels Seen in association to infections, such as Hep C, autoimmune and lymphoproliferative disorders	• Steroids • Plasmapheresis may be considered in severe cases • Treat associated infection
Hypersensitivity vasculitis	History reveals a possible offending or new drug Palpable purpura, maculopapular rash Skin lesion biopsy shows neutrophils surrounding an arteriole or nodule	• Discontinue offending drug • If more than skin involvement present, steroids may be indicated
Vasculitis secondary to connective tissue disorders	Vasculitis plus diagnosis of a CTD	
Vasculitis associated with viral infection		

Medium Vessel Vasculitides	Clinical Manifestations/Diagnosis	Treatment
Polyarteritis Nodosa	• Peripheral **neuropathy** (mono- or polyneuropathy), testicular pain, **livedo reticularis**, myalgia, **intestinal ischemia**, renal ischemia with elevated BUN and creatinine, new onset diastolic BP > 90 • Most are **ANCA negative** • **Angio:** aneurysmal dilatation of affected arteries • **Biopsy:** polymorphonuclear cells in the arterial wall • **Secondary PAN:** associated with CTD, such as RA, SLE; infections, such as HBV, HCV; and hairy cell leukemia	• Monotherapy with glucocorticoids may be appropriate for patients with mild disease (no renal/neurologic/GI/cardiac involvement) • For severe cases: a combination of glucocorticoids and cyclophosphamide • IFN alpha is used in some cases of PAN associated with HCV and hairy cell leukemia • Plasmapheresis is of no benefit
Kawasaki Disease	• Fever for 5 days or more, bilateral conjunctivitis, desquamating rash with erythema of palms and soles, mucositis, cervical lymphadenopathy, coronary artery aneurysms • Usually seen in children	• High dose aspirin and IVIG

	Clinical Presentation/Diagnosis	Treatment

Primary Central Nervous System Vasculitis	• Noninfectious granulomatous vasculitis limited to the brain, leptomeninges, or spinal cord
	• Insidious onset of persistent headache/cognitive impairment (most common presenting complaints), focal neurologic findings, ICH, seizures, ataxia. SC presentation involves sensory/motor deficits, weakness, pain. Constitutional symptoms uncommon/ESR, CRP normal
	• **Diagnosis requires:**
	  • Acquired neuro deficit of unknown etiology, AND
	  • Angiographic demonstration of CNS vasculitis, AND
	  • No evidence of systemic vasculitis
	• **Imaging:** multiple ischemic lesions over wide spread regions
	• **CSF analysis:** elevated protein, elevated WBCs (LP crucial to exclude alternate diagnoses, esp infectious and malignant)
	• **Angio:** vasospasm, which is helpful, but nondiagnostic (sensitivity: 50%-60%, specificity 30%)
	• **Cerebral/leptomeningeal biopsy:** gold standard for diagnosis
		• Combination therapy with glucocorticoids and cyclophosphamide for induction. Azathioprine or mycophenolate used with steroid taper for maintenance of remission
		• 12-18 months adequate for most patients

Large Vessel Vasculitides	Clinical Presentation/Diagnosis	Treatment
Takayasu arteritis	• Arthralgia, claudication, decreased pulsation of one or both brachial arteries, **difference of at least 10 mm Hg in SBP between the limbs,** bruit over subclavian arteries or abdominal aorta • **Angio:** narrowing or occlusion of aorta, its branches, or large arteries of upper or lower extremities (not secondary to atherosclerosis, fibromuscular dysplasia) • Affects the aorta and its primary branches • Pulmonary arteries affected in 70% of cases, leading to pulm HTN, pulm infarction	• Steroids • Methotrexate or azathioprine added to resistant cases
Giant cell arteritis	• Fever, headache, polymyalgia rheumatica, claudication of jaw, scalp tenderness, vision disturbances • Late sequelae: aortic dilatation and aneurysm	• High dose steroids

CONCLUSION

Overall rheumatologic critically ill patients have very high in-ICU mortality, therefore, early diagnosis and treatment should be sought in order to significantly impact mortality and morbidity. It is necessary to distinguish up front a disease flare versus an infectious process since initiation of immunosuppressive therapy may be fatal in severe septic patients. Aggressive treatment with high dose steroids, disease modifying antirheumatic-cytotoxic drugs and new biological agents must be tailored individually to achieve remission in case of active disease. Adjuvant measures such as plasma exchange and intravenous immunoglobulin are used for nonresponsive patients or for life threatening conditions. No clear prognosticator of in-ICU mortality has been identified as applicable to single patient yet, but intuitively high Apache score, multiorgan failure, comorbidities, advanced age and pancytopenia were all associated with worse outcome.

REFERENCES

1. Quintero OL, Rojas-Villarraga A, Mantilla RD, et al. Autoimmune disease in the intensive care unit. An update. *Autoimmunity Reviews.* 2013;12:380-395.
2. Janssen NM, Karnad DR, Guntupalli KK. Rheumatologic disease in the intensive care unit: epidemiology, clinical approach, management, and outcome. *Crit Care Clin.* 2002;18:729-48.
3. Camargo JF, Tobon GJ, Fonseca N, et al. Autoimmune rheumatic diseases in the intensive care unit: experience from a tertiary referral hospital and review of the literature. *Lupus.* 2005;14:315-20.
4. Cavallasca JA, Del Rosario Mallandi M, Sarquis S, et al. Outcome of patients with systemic rheumatic diseases admitted to a medical intensive unit. *J Clin Rheumatol.* 2010;16:400-402.
5. Olson AL, Swigris JJ, Sprunger DB, et al. Rheumatoid arthritis-Intestitial Lung Disease-associated mortality. *Am J Respir Crit Care Med.* 2011;183;372-378.
6. Neva MH, Hakkinen A, Makinen H, et al. High prevalence of asymptomatic cervical spine subluxation in patients with rheumatoid arthritis waiting for orthopedic surgery. *Ann Rheum Dis.* 2006;65:884.
7. O'Neill S, Cervera R. Systemic lupus erythematous. *Best Practice and Research Clinical Rheumatology.* 2010;24:841-855.
8. Guillevein L, Pagnoux C, Seror R, et al. The Five Factor Score Revisited: assessment of prognoses of systemic necrotizing vasculitides based on the French Vasculitis Study Group (FVSG) cohort. *Medicine.* 2011;90:19.
9. Guillevein L, Cohen P, Gayraud M. Churg-Strauss syndrome: clinical study and long term follow-up of 96 patients. *Medicine.* 1999;78:26.
10. Lahmer T, Heemann U. Anti-glomerular basement membrane antibody disease: a rare autoimmune disorder affecting the kidney and the lung. *Autoimmunity Reviews.* 2012;169:169.
11. McCabe C, Jones Q, Nikolopoulou A, Wathen C, Luqmani R. Pulmonary-renal syndrome: an update for respiratory physicians. *Respir Med.* 2011;105:1413.
12. Rodriguez W, Hanania N, Guy E, Guntupali J. Pulmonary-renal syndromes in the intensive care unit. *Crit Care Clin.* 2002;18:881.
13. Salvarini C, Brown R, Hunder G. Adult primary central nervous system vasculitis. *Lancet.* 2012;380:767.
14. Wilfong E, Seo P. Vasculitis in the intensive care unit. *Best Practice and Research in Clinical Rheumatology.* 2013;27:95.

Skin Complications

Bonnie Koo, MD; John K. Nia, MD and Annette Czernik, MD

47

KEY POINTS

1. Dermatologic diagnoses are associated with longer ICU stays compared to patients with normal skin.

2. Any systemic infection can have cutaneous manifestations that are often nonspecific.

3. There are no mucosal lesions with Staphylococcal scalded skin syndrome distinguishing it from Stevens–Johnson syndrome/toxic epidermal necrolysis.

4. Necrotizing fasciitis is often mistaken for cellulitis. A key feature of necrotizing fasciitis is pain out of proportion to the clinical exam on initial presentation.

5. Meningococcemia should be considered in any patient with fever and petechial rash.

6. When suspecting a drug eruption a drug chart with medications and time courses is extremely helpful in identifying the causative medication.

INTRODUCTION

About 10% of ICU patients have a dermatologic diagnosis, which are associated with longer ICU stays compared to patients with normal skin.[1] This chapter will focus on skin disorders seen in the ICU setting ranging from common relatively benign disorders to life-threatening diseases. One should not hesitate to consult a hospital dermatologist to assist in the diagnosis, workup, and management of these patients.

COMMON DISORDERS

See Table 47–1; Figures 47–1 and 47–2.

Skin Infections

Any systemic infection can have cutaneous manifestations that are often nonspecific. The discussion will be focused on life-threatening infections with distinctive skin findings.

Staphylococcal Scalded Skin Syndrome

Introduction

Staphylococcal scalded skin syndrome (SSSS) is caused by an exfoliative toxin producing staphylococcal species which bind and cleave desmoglein 1, an adhesion molecule that binds keratinocytes. This explains the clinical manifestation of widespread flaccid bullae and exfoliation. Although primarily a disease of infants and young children, adults with renal failure or immunosuppression are at risk for developing SSSS. The initiating event in adults is often a staphylococcal pneumonia or bacteremia.

TABLE 47–1 Common dermatoses in the ICU setting.

Diagnosis	Clinical Features	Workup and Differential Diagnosis	Treatment
Contact dermatitis	Sharply demarcated, erythematous, vesicular, patch or plaque with borders corresponding to the area of contact. Chronic forms are lichenified.	Fungal, scabies, cellulitis, and eczema. No specific workup needed; rule out other conditions.	Discontinue contact with offending agent. Topical steroids (fluocinonide 0.05% ointment) to provide relief and hasten resolution.
Miliara crystallina	Small, fragile, and clear vesicles on the face and trunk appearing as "drops of water."	Consider folliculitis. No specific workup needed; rule out other conditions.	Minimize heat and occlusion to the area.
Miliara rubra	Erythematous macules sometimes with punctate vesicles on the neck and posterior trunk or other dependent areas.	Folliculitis vs infectious such as candida. No specific workup needed; rule out other conditions.	Minimize heat and occlusion to the area. Topical steroids may be used to relieve pruritus as well as oral sedating antihistamines such as hydroxyzine.
Cutaneous candidiasis	Bright erythematous patches that are often accompanied by satellite papules and pustules and maceration often in skin folds.	Seborrheic dermatitis, contact dermatitis, and inverse psoriasis. KOH preparation or fungal culture can be done but rarely performed as lesions are typically classic.	Keep affected areas dry. Topical antifungals such as nystatin powder and/or clotrimazole cream twice a day.

Clinical Features

SSSS begins with widespread erythema beginning on the head and intertriginous areas which then generalize within 48 hours. There is often a preceding prodrome of fever, malaise, and skin tenderness. The skin then takes on a wrinkled appearance due to the superficial flaccid bullae with subsequent exfoliation (Figure 47–3). There are no mucosal lesions distinguishing it from Stevens–Johnson syndrome/toxic epidermal necrolysis (SJS/TEN).

Workup and Differential Diagnosis

SSSS is a clinical diagnosis. Since the condition is due to distant foci of infection, skin cultures are

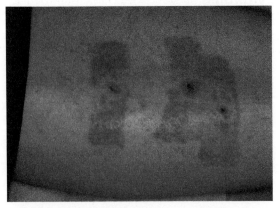

FIGURE 47–1 Contact dermatitis. Typical geometric shape due to adhesive tape.

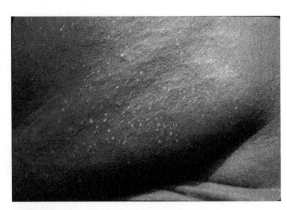

FIGURE 47–2 Miliara crystillina. Clear vesicles on the back.

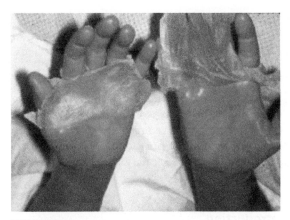

FIGURE 47–3 Staphylococcal scalded skin syndrome. Peeling of the hands.

generally negative. However, blood cultures may be positive. A skin biopsy can be useful and will show disadhesion of keratinocytes due to cleavage of desmoglein 1. Other conditions to consider are extensive sunburns, toxic shock syndrome (TSS, staphylococcal), SJS/TEN, and autoimmune blistering dermatoses.

Treatment

Patients generally require supportive skin care which may best be handled in a burn unit. Parenteral antibiotics with beta-lactamase–resistant penicillins such as dicloxacillin or cephalexin should be given. Clindamycin reduces toxin production and is, therefore, recommended.

Toxic Shock Syndrome

Introduction

Toxic shock syndrome (TSS) is a severe, multisystem disease characterized by fever, hypotension, and multiorgan involvement with skin findings. There are 2 types: (1) classic TSS caused by staphylococcus and (2) streptococcal TSS (sTSS) which is more severe and has a mortality rate of up to 50%. Both tend to affect young healthy adults. Classic TSS was previously associated with tampon use but most recently is associated with surgical (particularly nasal) packing and abscesses, whereas, sTSS is associated with disruption of the skin barrier due to lacerations or bites. Both are due to elaboration of toxins that stimulate massive cytokine release.

Clinical Features

Classic TSS begins with a sudden onset of headache, fever, malaise, myalgias, vomiting, and diarrhea. This can rapidly progress to hypotension and frank shock. Patients generally also have generalized erythema and/or a scarlatiniform exanthema. Conjunctivitis, a red tongue, mucosal involvement and the hands and feet may also be involved.

sTSS often begins with severe pain in an extremity. sTSS is usually due to an invasive soft tissue infection but up to 50% of patients may have only severe extremity pain as the initial symptom. Other nonspecific symptoms such as fever, malaise, myalgias, and diarrhea may also be present. Unlike classic TSS, widespread erythema is often not present. The disease progresses very rapidly with multiorgan failure ensuing in 48 to 72 hours. Disseminated intravascular coagulation (DIC) and acute respiratory distress syndrome may also develop. In both types, desquamation of the hands and feet occur a few weeks after disease onset.

Workup and Differential Diagnosis

Because this condition can progress very rapidly a high index suspicion is needed. Blood cultures and cultures of any visible skin wounds or skin infections should be performed but are often negative in both TSS and sTSS. Laboratory findings may include an elevated creatinine and an elevated white blood count. Other conditions to consider are SSSS and TEN.

Treatment

Supportive care and intensive monitoring are the hallmarks of treatment. Hypotension may require aggressive intravenous fluid resuscitation and vasopressors. In addition parenteral clindamycin should be considered since it reduces toxin load, otherwise a beta-lactamase–resistant penicillin should be given. Surgical packing, if present, should be removed. The use of intravenous immunoglobulin (IVIG) may neutralize toxin.

Necrotizing Fasciitis

Introduction

Necrotizing fasciitis (NF) is a rapidly progressive and life-threatening disease of the subcutaneous fat and fascia. Prompt recognition with surgical intervention and parenteral antibiotics are the mainstay of treatment. Risk factors for NF include diabetes mellitus, immunosuppression, renal failure, peripheral vascular disease, recent surgery and intravenous drug use. NF may also follow penetrating injuries. Mortality is up to 40%. It is generally caused by a polymicrobial infection including streptococci, staphylococci, *E. coli, Bacteroides*, and *Clostridium*.

Clinical Features

NF begins with severe pain, erythema and edema often in an extremity. Initially the skin is taut and shiny. As the condition evolves, the skin then becomes gray-blue with progression to frank necrosis. Hemorrhagic bullae may also form (Figure 47–4). As necrosis of the fascia ensues, a characteristic, malodorous, watery discharge is produced. Anesthesia is a late finding from destroyed nerves. Patients are toxic appearing with fevers, chills, and symptoms of septic shock. A key feature of this condition is pain out of proportion to the clinical exam on initial presentation. Fournier's gangrene refers to NF of the perineum and genitalia that rapidly spreads to the anterior abdominal wall.

Workup and Differential Diagnosis

NF is often mistaken for cellulitis. However, the patient's condition continues to rapidly deteriorate and characteristic skin changes ensue despite antibiotic therapy. Initial evaluation should include a complete white blood cell count, creatinine, electrolytes, and C-reactive protein. Blood cultures and culture of any visible drainage should also be done. NF can be confirmed with MRI but this may not be practical and often a CT scan or echo will show fascial edema.

Treatment

Broad spectrum parenteral antibiotics should be started immediately as workup is in progress and tailored as the causative organism(s) are identified. Surgical debridement is the mainstay of treatment. Amputation may be necessary.

Meningococcemia

Introduction

Meningococcemia is a severe presentation of an infection by *Neisseria meningitidis*. Infections can range from mild upper respiratory infections to meningitis to purpura fulminans. Functional complement is necessary to fight *N. meningitidis*.

Clinical Features

Up to 1/3 of patients with acute meningococcemia will present with a petechial eruption on the trunk and extremities (Figure 47–5). These lesions can progress to large purpuric lesions that are often retiform with a characteristic gunmetal grey color centrally. Bullae may form within these lesions. More extensive and severe skin lesions portend the onset of purpura fulminans.

Patients will have fever and hypotension. Other complications include arthritis, myocarditis, and meningeal symptoms. Of note, meningeal symptoms

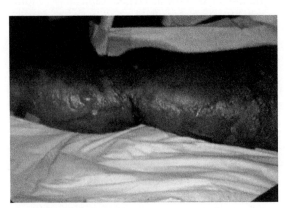

FIGURE 47–4 Necrotizing fasciitis. Confluent bullae. Note the grey-tan color.

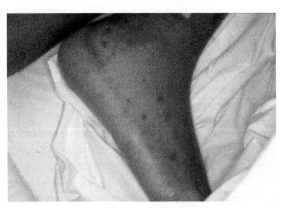

FIGURE 47–5 Meningococcemia. Petechial macules on the lower extremity.

are usually absent in the severe cutaneous presentations of meningococcemia.

Workup and Differential Diagnosis

Diagnosis is made by confirmation of the organism by culture or gram stain. Blood cultures and CSF fluid should be sampled. Other laboratory findings are generally nonspecific except an elevated white blood cell count. Patients with extensive petechial or purpuric lesions should be evaluated for the development of DIC.

Meningococcemia should be considered in any patient with fever and petechial rash. Rocky Mountain spotted fever and West Nile virus and other causes of meningitis also need to be considered.

Treatment

Treatment for acute meningococcemia is high dose intravenous penicillin. Third generation cephalosporins may also be used. Unfortunately, in severe cases, patients may deteriorate rapidly despite aggressive IV antibiotic therapy. All close contacts require prophylaxis with ciprofloxacin or rifampin.

DRUG ERUPTIONS

Drug eruptions are common in the hospitalized patient. The majority of them are relatively benign. When suspecting a drug eruption a drug chart with medications and time courses is extremely helpful in identifying the causative medication. Any medication can cause a drug eruption but the most common offenders are antibiotics (aminopenicillins, cephalosporins, macrolides), sulfonamides, and anticonvulsants.

Morbilliform Drug Eruptions

Introduction

Morbilliform eruptions are the most common type of drug eruptions and follow a benign course. They occur 7 to 12 days after the start of a new medication. The eruption may develop sooner on rechallenge.

Clinical Features

The rash begins as erythematous macules on the trunk that soon generalizes symmetrically (Figure 47–6). The lesions then become more confluent and slightly raised. Morbilliform eruptions

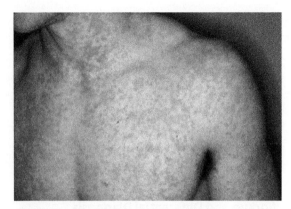

FIGURE 47–6 Morbilliform drug eruption. Symmetric erythematous macules and papules on the trunk.

last 1 to 2 weeks and may be associated with a low grade fever.

Workup and Differential Diagnosis

Morbilliform drug eruption is a clinical diagnosis. A high index of suspicion and recent initiation of culprit medications is often present. There may be a peripheral eosinophilia and mildly elevated white blood cell count. Most importantly, it needs to be watched for possible evolution to a more serious drug eruption such as acute generalized exanthematous pustulosis (AGEP), DRESS, SJS and TEN. Viral exanthems clinically mimic morbilliform eruptions. Skin biopsy is relatively nonspecific but findings such as eosinophils and the presence of interface changes is highly suggestive of a drug eruption.

Treatment

Aside from discontinuing the medication no specific treatment is needed. Topical steroids may be used but will generally not hasten recovery.

Acute Generalized Exanthematous Pustulosis

Introduction

Acute generalized exanthematous pustulosis (AGEP) is characterized by an acute onset of widespread pustules and erythema. The most common causes of AGEP are the beta-lactam antibiotics and macrolides. It can occur as early as 24 hours after exposure to a few days. Other important causes of AGEP include calcium channel blockers and antimalarials.

Clinical Features

The rash begins as erythema, often edematous, usually starting on the face or intertriginous areas. Within days, widespread sterile nonfollicular pustules generalize (Figure 47–7) and are accompanied by high fever. The rash may be asymptomatic, mildly pruritic or burning. Although pustules mainly characterize the rash, blisters, targetoid lesions, and mucous membrane involvement may also occur. AGEP lasts 1 to 2 weeks and resolves with superficial desquamation.

Workup and Differential Diagnosis

The initial presentation may resemble a morbilliform eruption but will be easily distinguished once the pustules appear. High fever is characteristic. There is often an elevated white count. There are generally no other lab abnormalities but mild renal dysfunction, mild hypocalcemia, and mild eosinophilia can occur. Eliciting a personal or family history of psoriasis is helpful since AGEP cannot be clinically distinguished from pustular psoriasis. A skin biopsy will distinguish between the two. A careful review of medications and time course will often reveal the causative drug. AGEP can be distinguished from DRESS by the lack of other organ involvement.

Treatment

Aside from discontinuing the offending medication, treatment is supportive. Topical steroids (such

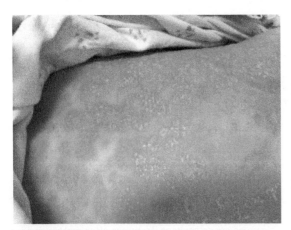

FIGURE 47–7 Acute generalized exanthematous pustulosis. Nonfollicular pustules studding edematous erythematous plaques.

as triamcinolone 0.1% cream) may be helpful if the rash is pruritic and antipyretics for fever.

Drug Reaction with Eosinophilia and Systemic Symptoms

Introduction

Drug reaction with eosinophilia and systemic symptoms (DRESS) is a drug eruption that involves at least one other organ system. The liver is the most commonly affected organ followed by the kidney. The underlying mechanism is most likely due to an impaired ability to detoxify certain drugs. DRESS occurs somewhat later than other drug eruptions at 2 to 6 weeks after starting the medication with a mean of 3 weeks.

DRESS was formally known as phenytoin hypersensitivity syndrome and the anticonvulsants are indeed the most common class of medications to cause DRESS. Other drugs include antibiotics (sulfonamides, minocycline, vancomycin), allopurinol, antiretrovirals, amlodipine, and nonsteroidal antiinflammatory drugs (NSAIDs).

Clinical Features

The rash often begins as a morbilliform eruption but often becomes more edematous and violaceous appearing as it evolves. The face, upper trunk, and upper extremities are most often affected. A hallmark of DRESS is facial edema. Blisters, pustules, purpuric lesions, and an exfoliative dermatitis are other clinical manifestations of DRESS. The mucous membranes can be involved. Fever and lymphadenopathy is almost always present.

Workup and Differential Diagnosis

Laboratory workup for DRESS includes a complete white blood cell count with differential to look for eosinophilia, liver function tests and creatinine. Elevated Aspartate Aminotransferase (AST) and Alanine Aminotransferase (ALT) is often present (70%) and can evolve to a fulminant hepatitis. Kidney involvement is less common (11%). Myocarditis, pneumonitis, and even neurologic symptoms can occur but are fortunately uncommon to rare.[2,3] Skin biopsy is relatively nonspecific.

Treatment

Discontinuing the offending medication is paramount. Depending on the degree of organ involvement, systemic steroids starting at a dose of atleast 1 mg/kg/d may be initiated and tapered slowly over at least a month. Few to several months may be needed. Some advocate the use of IVIG for severe DRESS. Antithyroid antibodies resulting in hypothyroidism can occur a few months after DRESS. A TSH should be checked 1 to 3 months afterward and periodically as indicated.

Stevens–Johnson Syndrome and Toxic Epidermal Necrolysis

Introduction

Stevens–Johnson syndrome (SJS) and TEN are rare, severe, potentially life-threatening drug reactions. The 2 conditions are best thought of as part of a clinical spectrum with SJS associated with milder disease with less than 10% affected body surface area (BSA), SJS-TEN overlap as intermediary disease with 10% to 30% affected BSA and TEN with greater than 30% affected BSA. They are clinically characterized by widespread skin detachment due to keratinocyte apoptosis.

SJS and TEN generally occur about 7 to 21 days after the medication is started. The most common culprits are sulfonamides (particularly trimethoprim-sulfamethoxazole), allopurinol, antibiotics, antiretrovirals, and NSAIDs. Certain risk factors have been identified and include certain Human Leukocyte Antigen types, decreased ability to detoxify drugs, and HIV infection. SJS has a mortality rate of up to 5% vs up to 30% in TEN.

Clinical Features

Initial symptoms include fever, eye pain, and dysphagia. A rash appears a few days later and begins on the trunk and progresses to involve the face and upper extremities. The palms and soles are often involved. The rash initially looks morbilliform then becomes more dusky appearing and/or purpuric. There is mucosal involvement and often appears as hemorrhagic crusting of the lips (Figure 47–8) and painful erosions in the mouth. Patients will often have dysuria. The Nikolsky sign is positive. As the lesions evolve even further they take on a characteristic gray hue with subsequent detachment of the epidermis. This is seen as fragile bullae that break easily revealing raw dermis (Figure 47–9).

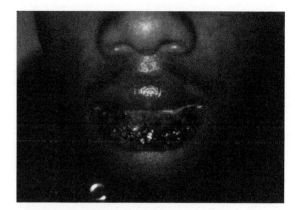

FIGURE 47–8 Stevens–Johnson syndrome. Hemorrhagic crusting of the lips.

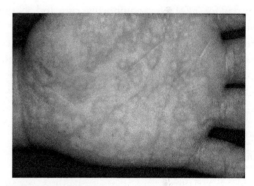

FIGURE 47–9A Stevens–Johnson syndrome. Vesiculobullous lesions with surrounding erythema on the palm.

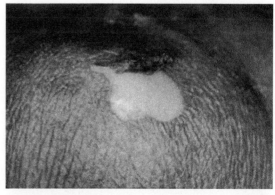

FIGURE 47–9B Toxic epidermal necrolysis. Sloughing of the skin revealing raw dermis.

Workup and Differential Diagnosis

There is no specific laboratory workup for SJS/TEN. There may be electrolyte imbalance due to impaired skin barrier function. Creatinine should be followed regularly to monitor renal function. The clinical presentation is characteristic but a skin biopsy is diagnostic revealing full thickness epidermal necrosis.

Several risk factors that predict worse prognosis have been identified. The SCORTEN represents this prognostic scoring system (Table 47–2).[4-6] Important conditions that need to be distinguished are pemphigus vulgaris, SSSS, and erythema multiforme major.

Treatment

Treatment of SJS/TEN is dependent on early diagnosis and immediate discontinuation of the offending medication. This reduces mortality by up to 30% per day for TEN. Next, supportive care and therapy (outlined below) is instituted. Supportive care is best undertaken in a burn unit familiar with the special needs of patients with SJS/TEN. Nutritional support

TABLE 47–2 SCORTEN. Risk factors to predict mortality risk in TEN.

Risk Factor	Point
Age > 40 years old	1
Malignancy	1
Heart rate > 120 beats/min	1
Serum BUN > 27 mg/dL	1
Detached skin > 20% body surface area	1
Serum bicarbonate > 20 mEq/L	1
Serum glucose > 250 mg/dL	1
Number of Risk Factors	**Mortality Risk**
0-1	3.2%
2	12.1%
3	35.3%
4	58.3%
5 or more	>90%

is paramount. Many patients will require a nasogastric tube due to dysphagia.

Specific treatment is controversial and evolving but for uncom-plicated SJS, prednisone started at 1 mg/kg/d with a slow taper is often used. For SJS/TEN overlap and TEN, cyclosporine or IVIG is advocated. The author uses cyclopsorine starting at 3 mg/kg/day IV or PO in divided BID doses. The data for using cyclosporine is promising. Higher doses of IVIG are used than for autoimmune bullous diseases. We recommend starting IVIG at 1 gm/kg/d for 3 days for a total of 3 g/kg. IVIG is thought to work via inhibition of Fas-Fas ligand mediated keratinocyte death.

For eye involvement, ophthalmology should be consulted. Steroid, antibiotic, and lubricating eye drops are often needed. Long-term sequelae include scarring leading to vision loss. The patient needs to be monitored for infection. Death is mainly due to infection from the impaired skin barrier due to *S. aureus* and *Pseudomonas aeruginosa*.

Purpura

Purpura is hemorrhage into the skin or mucous membranes. The differential diagnosis is extensive and a thorough review of these is outside the scope of this chapter. The two main morphological entities of interest are palpable purpura and retiform purpura. Palpable purpura generally presents as bright red and slightly raised lesions. Discussion will mainly be limited to leukocytoclastic vasculitis (LCV) as the leading clinical entity associated with palpable purpura.

Retiform purpura has a net-like pattern most easily seen at the edges of the lesion. This pattern is due to the pattern of occlusion of the affected vessels. This can be caused by infiltration of the vessel wall by organisms in immunocompromised patients, abnormal coagulation or embolic phenomenon.

Leukocytoclastic Vasculitis

Introduction

Leukocytoclastic vasculitis (LCV) refers to inflammation of predominantly small vessels in the dermis. It is usually idiopathic (~50%) but it can sometimes be attributed to other causes (Table 47–3). It is mediated by the deposition of immune complexes in the vessels. These immune complexes ultimately lead to the release of proteolytic enzymes from neutrophils producing vessel wall inflammation or vasculitis.

TABLE 47–3 Major causes of LCV.

Cause	Incidence	Common Agent/Disease(s)
Idiopathic	50%	
Infectious	15%-20%	**Bacterial:** Group A beta-hemolytic streptococci *Neisseria meningococcus* *Mycobacterium tuberculosis* **Viral:** Upper respiratory infections Hepatitis C > B (including vaccines) Parvovirus B19 HIV **Septic vasculitis:** Infective endocarditis *Neisseria meningitidis* (acute) *Neisseria gonorrhea* *Staphylococcus aureus* Rickettsiae Disseminated fungal infections (immunocompromised patients)
Inflammatory	15%-20%	Autoimmune connective tissue diseases Inflammatory bowel disease
Medication	10%-15%	Allopurinol Bortezimub Cephalosporins (cefaclor) Penicillins NSAIDs* Oral contraceptives Anticonvulsants Sulfonamides Minocycline Cocaine adulterated with levamisole
Malignancy	2%-5%	Plasma cell dyscrasias Lymphoproliferative disorders

*NSAIDs: nonsteroidal anti-inflammatory drugs.

Clinical Features

LCV generally presents as palpable purpura, flat purpuric or petechial lesions, or as urticarial lesions (Figure 47–10). Atypical presentations include pustules and targetoid lesions. They occur 7 to 10 days after the triggering event and tend to favor the extremities and dependent areas. Lower extremity edema may be present. Lesions are usually asymptomatic but may be associated with mild pruritus or burning. Up to 50% of patients will also have mild systemic symptoms such as fevers, myalgias, arthralgias, and weight loss.

Workup and Differential Diagnosis

When LCV is suspected clinically, laboratory workup should be directed at the suspected underlying cause. An initial screening workup could include a complete blood count with differential, ESR, C-reactive protein, blood and urine cultures, cryoglobulins, hepatitis B and C, ANA, C3, C4, ASO titer, and a chest X-ray. Anti-Neutrophil Cytoplasmic Antibodies (ANCAs), further imaging, and a malignancy workup can also be considered. A skin biopsy will confirm the histopathologic diagnosis of vasculitis. Direct immunofluorescence may also be useful.

The main concern will be the presence of a systemic vasculitis or the possibility of cryoglobulinemia. There is no associated vasculitis with Type I cryoglobulinemia since it is due to occlusion of vessels and presents with retiform purpura. It is usually caused by an underlying lymphoproliferative disorder. Types II and III cryoglobulinemia, also known as the mixed cryoglobulinemias, are due to a

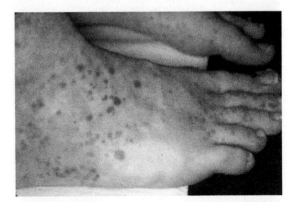

FIGURE 47–10 Leukocytoclastic vasculitis. Palpable purpura on the lower extremity.

vasculitic process and presents as palpable purpura. It is usually due to underlying hepatitis C infection and less likely due to HIV, autoimmune disease, or an underlying lymphoproliferative disorder.

Treatment

Most cases of LCV do not require treatment. Treatment should be directed at the underlying cause, if found. For mild, skin-limited disease, NSAIDs, and antihistamines may be used in addition to other supportive measures such as leg elevation and avoiding tight-fitting clothing. In more severe cases, one can consider a short course of systemic steroids starting at 1 mg/kg/d of oral prednisone. For systemic vasculitis, corticosteroids and other immunosuppressive therapies are the mainstay of treatment.

Calciphylaxis

Introduction

Calciphylaxis is a potentially fatal condition characterized by vessel calcification with necrosis of the skin and soft tissues. It primarily affects obese female patients with diabetes often in the setting of chronic renal failure. Its etiology is poorly understood.

Clinical Features

Calciphylaxis begins with livedoid racemosa, a net-like, mottled discoloration of the skin. The lesions are fixed, unlike the temporary lesions of livedo reticularis. As the lesions progress they become more purpuric (retiform) and necrotic (Figure 47–11). The

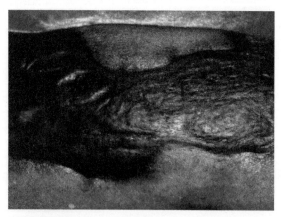

FIGURE 47–11 Calciphylaxis. Necrotic plaques on the lower extremity.

lesions are severely painful and are most common on the lower extremities. Fatty areas such as the abdomen, buttocks, and breasts are also often affected.

Workup and Differential Diagnosis

In the typical patient with diabetes and renal failure, the diagnosis is made easily. Laboratory workup should include serum calcium, phosphate, electrolytes, BUN, creatinine, PTH, and a coagulation factors including PT, aPTT, antithrombin III, proteins C and S, anticardiolipin, antiphospholipid. Other workup to consider is hepatitis C serologies, cryoglobulins, and ANCA to rule out an underlying vasculitis.

Skin biopsy should be taken from the area adjacent to necrosis, preferably an area with early erythema or purpura. An excisional biopsy will provide an adequate sample and should go deep to subcutaneous fat. Other considerations include warfarin necrosis and purpura fulminans.

Treatment

Treatment is mainly directed at correcting calcium dysregulation. This is accomplished with low calcium dialysis, phosphate binders, and possible parathyroidectomy. Intravenous sodium thiosulfate is also commonly used with variable success. Almost all patients will require analgesia for the pain.

Careful wound management with gentle debridement is recommended. Hyperbaric oxygen therapy can be considered for very painful ulcers. Unfortunately, necrotic lesions are very resistant to treatment and often provide a nidus of infection leading to sepsis. This is the leading cause of death in these patients. Even with optimal treatment, the mortality approaches 40% to 80%.

Purpura Fulminans

Introduction

Purpura fulminans is a severe, life-threatening condition due to 3 main etiologies: infection and DIC, postinfectious, and hereditary deficiency of protein C or S (neonatal). Of particular interest is the type caused by infection, usually due to bacterial sepsis but can also be caused by viruses. In the postinfectious kind, it is due to a transient deficiency of protein S due to consumptive processes. Mortality is high at 20% to 40%.

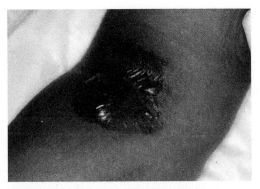

FIGURE 47–12 Purpura fulminans. Necrotic plaque with bullae formation in the antecubital fossa.

Clinical Features

Purpura fulminans presents with an acute onset of large purpuric to ecchymotic areas mainly on the distal extremities and acral surfaces. Its appearance can be gangrenous. The lesions enlarge rapidly and may have overlying hemorrhagic bullae (Figure 47–12). They are quite painful. It is invariably accompanied by fever, chills, shock, and often with DIC.

Workup and Differential Diagnosis

Laboratory workup should include blood and urine cultures, complete white blood cell count with differential, DIC workup.

Few conditions present with a sudden onset of large purpuric lesions. Rocky Mountain spotted fever may present with a purpura fulminans-like picture. In the setting of a patient with known connective tissue disease, the catastrophic antiphospholipid antibody syndrome can be considered.

Treatment

Treatment is mainly supportive but it should also be directed at the underlying cause, if found. Replacement therapy with fresh frozen plasma, platelets, protein, C, and/or antithrombin may be indicated. Heparin may be considered if the patient has a thrombotic process but needs to be used with caution. Surgical debridement of affected extremities may necessary and amputation may sometimes be necessary.

Other Critical Skin Conditions

Erythroderma

Introduction—Erythroderma refers to generalized erythema and scaling. Erythroderma is most commonly due to generalization of a pre-existing skin disease (psoriasis, atopic dermatitis, pemphigus foliaceous), drug reactions, or cutaneous T-cell lymphoma (Sezary syndrome). In approximately 25% of cases, no underlying etiology is found. Erythroderma has serious systemic complications including hypothermia and fluid and electrolyte imbalances.[7]

Clinical Features—Patients present with generalized erythema and scaling of more than 90% of the BSA (Figure 47–13). It is pruritic. Palmoplantar keratoderma may be a clue to underlying pityriasis pilaris rubra. The nails may shed. Eruptive pale seborrheic keratosis may be seen.

Patients are often febrile with chills. Extracellular fluid shifts lead to pedal, pretibial, and facial edema. Increased blood flow through the skin and the loss of a functioning cutaneous barrier lead to extreme

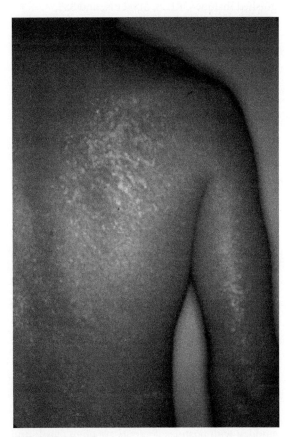

FIGURE 47–13 Erythroderma. Confluent bright erythema.

fluid loss and electrolyte abnormalities. Fluid loss leads to reflex tachycardia as well as disturbances in body temperature regulation (both hyperthermia and hypothermia may be seen). Patients with erythroderma may have secondary cutaneous infections, most commonly with *staphylococcus aureus*.

Workup and Differential Diagnosis—Increased ESR, anemia, and hypoalbuminemia are commonly seen in erythroderma. Electrolytes need to be monitored. Flow cytometry may be useful if Sezary syndrome is suspected.

A history of dermatologic conditions known to cause erythroderma is helpful as well as any recent new medication exposures. A skin biopsy of a primary skin lesion can often differentiate erythrodermic psoriasis, atopic dermatitis, pityriasis rubra pilaris, or bullous disease.[8] However, in many cases a skin biopsy shows a nonspecific hypersensitivity reaction. Important conditions that need be distinguished include DRESS, SJS/TEN, and SSS.

Treatment—Supportive care and treatment of the underlying condition (if found) is the mainstay of treatment. Patients need to be monitored for fluid and electrolyte imbalances, temperature, secondary infections, and nutritional needs. Sedating antihistamines (hydroxyzine) can be used to relieve pruritus. Topical therapy can include wet dressings, low-potency corticosteroid ointments. Systemic corticosteroids at an initial dose of 1 to 2 mg/kg/d may be useful in idiopathic erythroderma and drug reactions. Psoriatic erythroderma is typically treated with cyclosporine, methotrexate, acitretin, or biologic agents. Systemic corticosteroids should not be used in psoriasis as they can cause generalized pustular psoriasis (GPP).

Generalized Pustular Psoriasis

Introduction—Generalized pustular psoriasis (GPP) is a rare, life-threatening form of psoriasis.[9] Usually, patients have a history of stable plaque-type psoriasis that flares into rapidly progressive pustular disease. Know triggers that can lead to a pustular psoriasis include rapid tapering of systemic corticosteroids, hypocalcemia, infections, pregnancy, and irritation such as sunburn.

Clinical Features—GPP presents with erythema studded with pustules. Patients are often febrile and have chills. GPP appears commonly on the trunk,

extremities, face, and can potentially arise on nail beds resulting in onycholysis, lakes of pus with subsequent nail shedding.[10]

Workup and Differential Diagnosis—Initial workup should include a complete white count with differential, electrolytes, ESR and blood cultures. Patients will often have lymphopenia with leukocytosis and an elevated ESR. A skin biopsy can be considered if the patient does not have a pre-existing diagnosis of psoriasis or if the diagnosis is not clear. GPP cannot be clinically distinguished from AGEP. A biopsy will distinguish between the two.

Treatment—Supportive care, including intravenous fluid and temperature regulation is paramount in treating GPP. Intravenous antibiotics may be needed if the patient becomes infected. Specific GPP treatment is with acitretin (considered first line) or cyclosporine and less likely methotrexate due to slower onset of action. It is important to avoid oral corticosteroids unless absolutely necessary, due to withdrawal and worsening of psoriasis.

Pemphigus Vulgaris

Introduction—Pemphigus vulgaris (PV) is a life-threatening autoimmune skin blistering condition. It affects middle-aged adults. Patients frequently develop persistent oral mucosal and/or cutaneous erosions. Lesions may progress to evolve the entire cutaneous surface. The condition runs a relapsing and remitting course over the course over many years.

Clinical Features—PV presents with superficial erosions or flaccid bullae that usually present on the scalp or oral mucosa (Figure 47–14). The blister roof is very

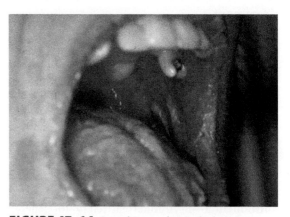

FIGURE 47–14 Pemphigus vulgaris. Oral erosions.

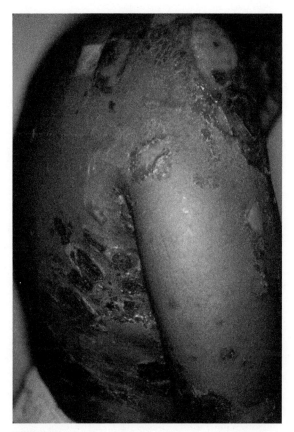

FIGURE 47-15 Pemphigus vulgaris. Eroded plaques.

fragile and often no intact blisters are seen at first presentation. Erosions associated with a collarette of the remains of the prior blister are common. Lesions occur in a seborrheic distribution—involving the central face, chest, and back (Figure 47–15). Involvement of the oral mucosa is associated with significant pain with oral intake. Cutaneous lesions may become superinfected—most commonly with *S. aureus*. However, superficial infections with candida or herpes virus have been reported as well.

Not uncommonly, patients will have a positive Nikolsky sign. This is a test of skin fragility—where firmly stroking the skin induces blister formation. This can be used as a test to determine adequate control of disease activity.

Workup and Differential Diagnosis—All patients must meet clinical, histologic, and immunologic criteria in order to establish the diagnosis. Clinically, the patients must present with a history of chronic mucocutaneous erosions that on exam are consistent with those typically seen in pemphigus. A biopsy for H&E must demonstrate subcorneal or suprabasal acantholysis. Lastly, either direct or indirect immunofluorescence or ELISA autoantibodies to skin antigens must be present. Serum antibodies against intraepidermal adhesion molecules (ie, desmoglein 1 and 3) are present.

Serum may be sent to specialty laboratory (eg, Beutner Laboratories at http://www.beutnerlabs.com) to establish and monitor pemphigus titers. This may distinguish pemphigus from other immunobullous diseases in the differential diagnosis such as paraneoplastic pemphigus and bullous pemphigoid.

Treatment—Prior to the onset of the use of systemic steroids in this condition—pemphigus was uniformly fatal. Treatment involves the use of systemic steroids in combination with a steroid sparing immunosuppressant agent such as mycophenolate mofetil. Steroids are slowly tapered over the course of months to years. In spite of this treatment regimen, a large cohort of patients may be inadequately controlled or develop complications related to treatment.

In recent years, the use of rituximab has shown significant promise.[11,12] Rituximab is an anti-CD 20 antibody that targets pre-B cells for destruction. It removes B-cells destined to become pathogenic antibody producing plasma cells from the circulation. This is often used in combinations with high-dose IVIG. IVIG induces a rapid and selective decrease in pemphigus autoantibodies.[13]

The use of rituximab and IVIG earlier in the course of treatment is becoming increasingly commonplace. Well-designed studies regarding the use of these agents and the weight of their relative toxicities to conventional therapy are lacking.

REFERENCES

1. Badia M, Trujillano J, Gasco E, Casanova JM, Alvarez M, Leon M. Skin lesions in the ICU. *Intensive Care Med.* 1999;25(11):1271-1276.
2. Husain Z, Reddy BY, Schwartz RA. DRESS syndrome: Part II. Management and therapeutics. *J Am Acad Dermatol.* 2013;68(5):709.e1-9; quiz 18-20.
3. Husain Z, Reddy BY, Schwartz RA. DRESS syndrome: Part I. Clinical perspectives. *J Am Acad Dermatol.* 2013;68(5):693.e1-14; quiz 706-708.

4. Schwartz RA, McDonough PH, Lee BW. Toxic epidermal necrolysis: Part II. Prognosis, sequelae, diagnosis, differential diagnosis, prevention, and treatment. *J Am Acad Dermatol.* 2013;69(2):187.e1-16; quiz 203-204.

5. Schwartz RA, McDonough PH, Lee BW. Toxic epidermal necrolysis: Part I. Introduction, history, classification, clinical features, systemic manifestations, etiology, and immunopathogenesis. *J Am Acad Dermatol.* 2013;69(2):173.e1-13; quiz 85-86.

6. Bastuji-Garin S, Fouchard N, Bertocchi M, Roujeau JC, Revuz J, Wolkenstein P. SCORTEN: a severity-of-illness score for toxic epidermal necrolysis. *J Invest Dermatol.* 2000;115(2):149-153.

7. Bolognia JL, Jorizzo J, Rapini R. *Dermatology: 2-Volume Set.* Philadelphia: Mosby; 2007.

8. Sigurdsson V, Toonstra J, Hezemans-Boer M, van Vloten WA. Erythroderma: a clinical and follow-up study of 102 patients, with special emphasis on survival. *J Am Acad Dermatol.* 1996;35(1):53-57.

9. Sugiura K, Takemoto A, Yamaguchi M, et al. The majority of generalized pustular psoriasis without psoriasis vulgaris is caused by deficiency of interleukin-36 receptor antagonist. *J Invest Dermatol.* 2013;133(11):2514-2521.

10. Iizuka H, Takahashi H, Ishida-Yamamoto A. Pathophysiology of generalized pustular psoriasis. *Arch Dermatol Res.* 2003;295:S55-S59.

11. Ahmed AR, Spigelman Z, Cavacini LA, Posner MR. Treatment of pemphigus vulgaris with rituximab and intravenous immune globulin. *N Engl J Med.* 2006;355(17):1772-1779.

12. Joly P, Mouquet H, Roujeau J-C, et al. A single cycle of rituximab for the treatment of severe pemphigus. *N Engl J Med.* 2007;357:545-52.

13. Czernik A, Toosi S, Bystryn J-C, Grando SA. Intravenous immunoglobulin in the treatment of autoimmune bullous dermatoses: an update. *Autoimmunity.* 2012;45(1):111-118.

Principles of Neurosciences Critical Care

Christopher Zammit, MD; Ko Eun Choi, MD and Axel Rosengart, MD, PhD, MPH

More so than any other tissue or organ system, the nervous system is exquisitely sensitive to insults and injuries. The importance of timely recognition, diagnosis, stabilization, and treatment of acute neurologic processes to mitigate or prevent permanent injury, disability, and even death cannot be overemphasized. The most elite resuscitationists will utilize "parallel processing" and ensure that the most time-dependent diagnostics and therapeutics are prioritized.

Neurocritical care (NCC) is a relatively new and rapidly developing subspecialty. Intensive care units (ICUs) dedicated to the care of those with neurologic disorders requiring critical care are rapidly increasing in number. The Neurocritical Care Society (NCS) was established in 1999, and held its first annual meeting in 2003. The United Council for Neurologic Subspecialties, which oversees NCC Fellowship accreditation and NCC certification, hosted its first certification examination in 2007. Most recently, leaders in NCC and Emergency Medicine collaborated to create an educational program establishing guidance on the care for patients during the first critical hours of a neurologic emergency, entitled Emergency Neurologic Life Support (ENLS). Similar to Advance Cardiovascular Life Support offered by the American Heart Association, ENLS Certification is provided to those completing the program.

The expansion in the size and organization of the field has led to advances in the technology available for neuromonitoring and strategies for neurologic resuscitation, making a full introduction to NCC concepts beyond the scope of this chapter, and more appropriately the mission of published textbooks on

NCC. This chapter will provide an initial framework for the recognition, diagnosis, stabilization, and treatment of acute neurologic illness, with focused discussion of specific disease processes, including, encephalopathy and coma, acute ischemic stroke (AIS), intracerebral hemorrhage (ICH), subarachnoid hemorrhage (SAH), neuromuscular disease (NMDz), seizures, and status epilepticus. Other NCC diseases and disorders, such as traumatic brain injury (TBI) and/or spinal cord injury, cardiac arrest (CA), intracranial pressure (ICP) management, fulminant hepatic failure, delirium, encephalitis, and meningitis, are covered elsewhere in this textbook.

COMA AND ENCEPHALOPATHY

Consciousness has two components, arousal or wakefulness and content or awareness. Deficits in *arousal* are the result of either a diffuse, bihemispheric insult to the cerebral cortices or a focal injury to the ascending reticular activating system (ARAS) (see Figure 48A–1). Categories of arousal, in decreasing order, include *awake, drowsy, obtunded* or *lethargic, stuporous,* and *comatose. Drowsy* implies that the patient is prone to long bouts of sleep and hypoactivity during hours when normally expected to be awake and engaged, but they are easily aroused and awake with simple stimulation, such as speaking to them. An *obtunded* or *lethargic* patient requires a greater degree of stimulation to maintain their engagement. They often require a loud voice or gentle tactile stimulation to arouse them to participate in conversation or perform requested tasks. Once engaged, they tend to respond slowly and are prone

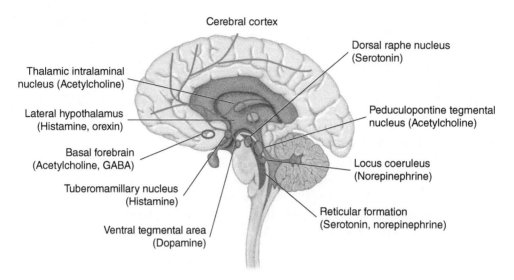

FIGURE 48A–1 Arousal structure and main neurotransmitter.

to disengagement once stimulation is no longer maintained. A *stuporous* patient will require more substantial stimulation to arouse them, such as rigorous tactile or noxious stimulation. At best, they are able to follow simple commands, but more complex tasks are not possible, and may only be capable of localizing to painful stimulation. A *comatose* patient is unable to purposefully engage their environment regardless of the degree of stimulation provided. The best response seen will be a facial grimace and/or stereotyped, posturing, or reflexive movements of the extremities to noxious stimulation. In those with a TBI, a Glasgow Coma Scale (GCS) score of less than 9 (see "Physical Examination," and Table 48A–1A) is often consider to be "coma" despite the possibility that the patient may be able to engage their environment (eg, motor GCS score of 5).

Awareness is a product of the entire neurologic system, both peripheral and central, and whose assessment is a composite of several neurologic functions, including motor, sensory, visual, language, concentration, attention, cognitive, executive,

TABLE 48A–1A   **Glasgow coma scale.**

Eye Opening (E)	Verbal Response (V)	Motor Response (M)
4—Opens spontaneously[a]	5—Alert and oriented	6—Follows commands
3—Opens to voice	4—Disoriented and confused	5—Localizes to pain[b]
2—Opens to pain	3—Incoherent words	4—Withdraws from pain
1—None	2—Incomprehensible sounds, moaning	3—Flexion posturing
	1—None	2—Extension posturing
	"T" or "I"—If patient is intubated or has tracheostomy	1—None

[a]The patient should attend to the examiner in order to score a 4 on (E).
[b]Patient should cross midline to address the noxious stimulus in order to score a 5 on (M).

social, behavioral, and emotional functions. Deficits in awareness are the result of focal neurologic injuries (eg, AIS or NMDz) or diffuse processes that disrupt neural networks (eg, TBI or hypoxic-ischemic encephalopathy after CA). Impairments in arousal, attention, or concentration can adulterate the assessment of awareness, which is most accurately performed in the awake, attentive, and focused patient.

Encephalopathy is a nonspecific term applied to patients with cerebral dysfunction and encompasses scores of possible diagnoses, each with their own requisite diagnostics and therapeutics. Other colloquialisms used to describe encephalopathic patients with overall lesser degrees of precision include "altered mental status," "altered," "delta MS," "changed from baseline," "clouded," or "confused." Clinical features of encephalopathy include abnormalities in arousal ranging from drowsy to hyperactive, with impairments in attention or concentration. A subset of encephalopathic patients will be *delirious*, which is best described as a heterogeneous acute confusional disorder that develops over several hours to days, fluctuates with time, is not attributed to a neurocognitive disorder, and is the result of the exposure to xenobiotics, drug withdrawal, or an acute medical disorder. Disturbances in attention, awareness, and orientation that tend to worsen in the evening and nighttime are hallmark features of delirium. The diagnosis is clinical and outlined in the American Psychiatric Association's Diagnostic and Statistical Manual, 5th edition. Further diagnostic considerations include the delirium etiology, duration of symptoms, and level of psychomotor activity (see Table 48A–1B). Please refer to other chapters in this textbook for a more in-depth discussion of delirium.

When evaluating patients with a change in their neurologic status, it is crucial that a broad differential be maintained that includes both primary medical and neurologic etiologies. As discussed further later, stupor or coma can be the result of many metabolic, toxic, infectious, and inflammatory conditions. Additionally, it is not uncommon for a patient with a primary neurologic insult (eg, AIS) to also be

TABLE 48A–1B Delirium diagnostic criteria, diagnostic and statistical manual, 5th ed.

Diagnostic criteria	A. A disturbance in attention (ie, reduced ability to direct, focus, sustain, and shift attention) and awareness (reduced orientation to the environment).
	B. The disturbance develops over a short period of time (usually hours to a few days), represents a change from baseline attention and awareness, and tends to fluctuate in severity during the course of a day.
	C. An additional disturbance in cognition (eg, memory deficit, disorientation, language, visuospatial ability, or perception).
	D. The disturbances in Criteria A and C are not better explained by another preexisting, established, or evolving neurocognitive disorder and do not occur in the context of a severely reduced level of arousal, such as a coma.
	E. There is evidence from the history, physical examination, or laboratory findings that the disturbance is a direct physiological consequence of another medical condition, substance intoxication or withdrawal (ie, due to a drug of abuse or to a medication), or exposure to a toxin, or is due to multiple etiologies.
Etiology	• Substance intoxication • Substance withdrawal • Medication induced • Due to another medical condition • Due to multiple etiologies
Duration of symptoms	• Acute: hours to days • Persistent: weeks to months
Activity level	• Hyperactive • Hypoactive • Mixed level of activity

Data from the American Psychiatric Association, *Diagnostic and Statistical Manual*, 5th ed. APA Press, Washington, DC 2013.

suffering from an acute medical issue (eg, endocarditis or acute kidney injury). If a diagnosis still exists that can explain the patient's presentation and would require time-dependent treatment, it is important that it be definitively excluded via the expeditious conduction of the appropriate diagnostics.

Historical Considerations

Encephalopathy and coma are not a specific disease or syndrome. They are a physical finding signifying central nervous system (CNS) dysfunction requiring a diagnosis. For acute changes, the last known normal time or last known well time must be established and distinguished from the time that the change was noticed or the patient was found to be abnormal. Dramatic neurologic changes (eg, acute coma) do not preclude preceding subtle changes or stuttering symptoms that should be actively pursued. Historical information should also be sought from a variety of resources including family, friends, neighbors, Emergency Medical Service (EMS) personnel, 911 communication specialists, police, and patient belongings (eg, timed and dated receipts, cell phone text messages, emails, calls, or social media interactions). Clues at the scene of patient discovery should also be sought for consideration of environmental, traumatic, or pharmacologic etiologies.

A catalog of prior medical problems, medications (and compliance), social habits, and hobbies, should be performed. Specific inquiries about use of anticoagulant, antiplatelet, and antiepileptic medications should be made, particularly with the widespread use of target specific oral anticoagulation, such as dabigatran, rivaroxaban, and apixaban. EMS interventions (eg, naloxone) and the patient's response should as be gathered.

Physical Examination

The physical exam commences with observation of the patient prior to interaction to assess for spontaneous movements and general physical condition (eg, healthy, chronically ill, ashen, wasted, cachectic, and disheveled). Violent spontaneous clonic movements may resemble the tonic-clonic activity seen in generalized seizures, but consideration must be given as to whether it is extensor posturing resulting from an acute brainstem injury (eg, basilar

TABLE 48A–1C Odors suggestive of neurotoxin exposure.

Odor	Neurotoxin
Mothballs	Camphor
Garlic	Organophosphates, arsenic, thallium
Peanuts	Vacor
Carrots	Cicutoxin (water hemlock)
Wintergreen	Methyl salicylates
Fruity	Chlorinated hydrocarbons
Glue	Solvents, toluene
Rotten eggs	Dimercaptosuccinic acid, hydrogen sulfide
Shoe polish	Nitrobenzene
Smoke or fire	Carbon monoxide or cyanide

thrombosis). Detection of certain odors can provide clues to neurotoxin exposure (Table 48A–1C). Exposure of the patient will allow for the identification of occult injury, illness, or paraphernalia associated with or causative of the presentation.

Vital signs including heart rate, blood pressure (BP), respiratory rate (RR), and pattern, oxygen saturation (SpO_2), quantitative waveform capnography ($wPetCO_2$), core temperature, and blood glucose should be acquired. Bradycardia may indicate elevated supratentorial pressure in children and infratentorial (posterior fossa) pressure in adults. Tachycardia should be evaluated for possible cardioembolic inducing arrhythmias (eg, atrial fibrillation), which may be the cause or result of a cerebral insult. Hypertension is quite nonspecific, as it may be seen with pain, anxiety, anatomic irritation of the forebrain, insula, limbic system, hypothalamus, descending sympathoexcitatory pathway rostral to the medulla, or intracranial hypertension. Hypotension is suggestive of an injury to the descending sympathoexcitatory pathway (which is anywhere from rostral medulla through the upper thoracic spine). However, if the MAP is less than 60 mm Hg, hypovolemia, neurogenic stunned myocardium, or systemic illness should be considered. $wPetCO_2$ can detect hypercapnia (albeit with limited sensitivity),

TABLE 48A-1D **Respiratory patterns in CNS disease.**

Pattern	Description	Localization	Examples of CNS Disease
Cheyne-Stokes	Several large tidal volume breaths alternating with periods of apnea last 12-30 seconds	Bihemispheric or diencephalon	Bilateral cerebral infarcts, diencephalic shift, early transtentorial herniation, encephalopathy
Hyperventilation	Persistently elevated RR in the absence of metabolic demands, pulmonary disease, or stimulation xenobiotic	Bihemispheric	Bilateral infarcts, encephalopathy
		Brainstem chemoreceptors	SAH or meningitis
		Brainstem (rare)	Glioma or lymphoma
Apneusis	Large tidal volume breaths with breathing holding for 2-3 seconds at end-inspiration and end-expiration	Pons	Basilar artery stroke, transtentorial herniation
Cluster or ataxic	Frequent irregular breaths of varying regularity and tidal volume	Rostral medulla	Transtentorial herniation, cerebellar mass, hemorrhage, swelling
Apnea	No spontaneous breathing	More extensive medullary injury	Late transtentorial herniation, cerebellar mass, hemorrhage, swelling

CNS, central nervous system; RR, respiratory rate; SAH, subarachnoid hemorrhage.

while providing a continuous RR and tracing allowing for the demonstration of respiratory patterns localizable to specific cerebral anatomic locations (Table 48A-1D). Cushing's triad of irregular breathing, bradycardia, and hypertension is an unreliable sign of elevated ICP in adults. If observed, it is much more likely to represent a posterior fossa process or an exceptionally progressed supratentorial process. Hyperthermia may be environmental, suggest infection or signify a toxidrome, such as neuroleptic malignant syndrome, serotonin syndrome, or thyrotoxicosis. Hypothermia may be environmental, or can be seen in sepsis, various intoxications, hypothyroidism, or pituitary apoplexy. A finger stick blood sugar should be obtained immediately to exclude (and potentially emergently treat) symptomatic hypoglycemia.

The following will emphasize the crucial aspects of the neurologic exam in the stuporous or comatose patient. Patients with mild impairments in arousal should undergo a usual neurologic assessment to include visual fields, cranial nerves, motor, language, coordination, reflexes, tone, and attention

(eg, counting backward from 20 to 1 or reciting the months of the year backward).

Level of Arousal (or Wakefulness)

As outlined earlier, a patient's wakefulness can be placed into one of several categories. Clinically, the patient should be described by what they are able to do with a specific type of stimulation, rather than just the category of arousal. This is elicited by progressively escalating the stimulation by first speaking in a normal tone, then a loud voice, then tactile stimulation, then vigorous tactile stimulation (eg, jostling the patient), and finally applying noxious stimulation, and assessing for a response to verbal commands. During this evaluation, one must not assume that the patient is unconscious (eg, they may be locked in). Options for noxious stimulation include a trapezius pinch, nasopharyngeal irritation with a cotton swab, jaw thrust (if not prohibited by a traumatic injury), supraorbital pressure, sternal rub, or nail bed pressure. Grabbing and twisting of the skin or tissue folds is highly discouraged as this may lead to bruising, hematomas, and skin tears.

Prior to providing noxious stimulation, be sure to lift the patient's eyelids and ask him or her to look up/down, left/right to carefully evaluate for a locked-in state.

In acute trauma, the GCS is a validated score of arousal that can be rapidly calculated, with values ranging from 3 to 15. It has three components; eye opening, verbal, and motor function (see Table 48A–1A). A more recently introduced and validated coma scale is the *FOUR (Full Outline of UnResponsiveness) Score*, which ranges from 0 to 16 and include assessments of eye movements, motor function, respiratory pattern, and brainstem function (Table 48A–1H).

Several months to a year after cerebral injury patients may transition from states of depressed arousal to those with near intact arousal, but varying degrees of awareness impairment, such as *vegetative state* and *minimally consciousness state* (Figure 48A–2). These terms can be applied three months after a non-traumatic brain injury (eg, CA) and 1 year after a traumatic brain injury.

Motor Exam

The motor exam in comatose patients assesses appendicular movement, tone, and reflexes to identify asymmetry and/or localize CNS injuries. It occurs simultaneous with the evaluation of arousal. Localization is produced via activation of the cortical inputs to the corticospinal tracts. Therefore, absence of localization is suggestive of cerebral hemispheric dysfunction or an injury along the corticospinal tracts. The careful inspection of nonlocalizing movements provides clues to the presence or absence of a diencephalic or brainstem lesion (Table 48A–1E). To elicit such movements, the stimulus should be sustained until it is clear that the full extent of movement has been observed. Failure to do so may falsely localize the lesion and mischaracterize the problem. If pathologic posturing is observed, the descriptors "flexor" and "extensor" are preferred over "decorticate" and "decerebrate" posturing, respectively.

Repeated identical movements (stereotyped) induced by a variety of stimuli are typical of those with dysfunction of the cerebral hemispheres or diencephalon. More extensive diencephalic lesions or rostral midbrain injury will produce *flexor posturing* in the upper extremities (ie, flexion of the fingers and wrist, forearm supination, elbow flexion, and

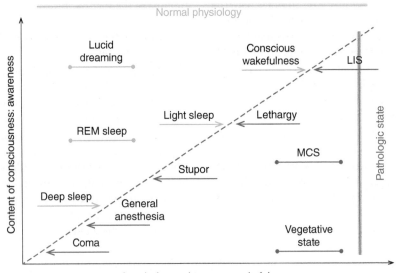

LIS: Locked-in syndrome
MCS: Minimally conscious state

FIGURE 48A–2 State of consciousness by arousal and content.

TABLE 48A-1E Physical exam findings in a comatose patients with brainstem dysfunction.

Anatomic Level	Mental Status	Pupillary Size and Position	Eye Movement	Motor Responses	Respiration
Diencephalon	Drowsy	Small (1-2 mm)	Normal	Abnormalities of flexion	Cheyne-Strokes
Midbrain	Coma	Fixed in mid position (4-5 mm)[a]	Dysconjugate	Abnormalities of extension	Hyperventilation
Pons	Coma	1 mm in primary pontine injury; fixed and 4-5 mm with prior midbrain injury[a]	Complete paralysis	Abnormalities of extension	Hyperventilation or apneusis
Medulla	Variable	Variable	Variable	Flaccid	Cluster, ataxic, or apnea

[a]Fixed and dilated pupil(s) will be seen if brainstem dysfunction is the result of lateral and/or downward compression forces (eg, uncal or transtentorial herniation).

shoulder adduction) and extensor posturing of the lower extremities (ie, extension of the knee, internal rotation and extension of the hip, and plantar flexion of the ankle). More caudal injuries will produce *extensor posturing* of the upper extremities (ie, shoulder adduction, elbow extension, and wrist pronation and flexion) and lower extremities. Extensor posturing can be elicited by trivial internal or external stimulation (eg, distended bladder or ventilator delivering a tidal volume), giving the appearance of spontaneous clonic movements, leading the clinician to falsely suspect they are epileptic in origin. Medullary brainstem lesions will produce flaccidity in all extremities. *Opisthotonic posturing* (ie, clenched teeth, arching of the spine) is an infrequently encountered manifestation of severe brainstem injury.

Tone and reflexes should be examined to discern between upper and lower motor neuron impairment (Table 48A-1F). Upper motor dysfunction leads to

TABLE 48A-1F Neurologic exam findings in lower versus upper motor neuron lesions.

Finding	Upper Motor Neuron	Lower Motor Neuron
Reflexes	Increased	Decreased
Clonus	+	–
Tone	Increased	Decreased
Fasciculations	–	+
Atrophy	–/late	+

increased tone and reflexes, with upgoing toes and clonus, while hypotonicity, hyporeflexia, fasciculations, and mute toes are hallmarks of lower motor neuron dysfunction.

Fundoscopy

The value of fundoscopy in the evaluation of coma is to assess for intracranial hypertension (IC-HTN) and retinal ischemia. IC-HTN slows axoplasmic flow in the optic nerve producing axonal swelling. When sustained over several hours or longer, this is seen on fundoscopy as *papilledema*. Optic nerve demyelination or infarction (ie, *papillitis*), will also be seen as papilledema, as thus should be included in the differential. Dampening or loss of retinal venous pulsations can be seen when ICP exceeds systemic venous pressure. This finding is present in 20% of the population, limiting its specificity for IC-HTN.

Brainstem/Cranial Nerves

The brainstem examination allows for the identification of herniation syndromes, acute treatable lesions of the brainstem (eg, acute basilar thrombosis), and is the crux of brain death examination. The components are pupillary assessment, oculomotor examination, and elicitation of the corneal, gag, and cough reflexes.

Pupillary Evaluation

Components of the pupillary exam include assessment of size and symmetry in ambient light, followed by dim lighting, direct and consensual reactions to

TABLE 48A–1G Physical findings in drug-induced coma.

Drug Class	Pupils	Other changes
Opioids	Miotic	Hypopnea/apneic
Barbiturates and benzodiazepines	Reactive	Hypopnea, mild hypotension
Anticholinergics (scopolamine, etc)	Mydriasis	Tachycardia, seizures
Anticholinesterases (organophosphates)	Miotic	Bradycardia, sweating, salivation, lacrimation, diarrhea, vomiting, urination
Cocaine and amphetamine	Mydriasis	Tachycardia, hypertension, hypotension, arrhythmia
Neuroleptics	Variable	Motor rigidity, hypotension, hyperthermia
Antidepressants	Mydriasis	Rarely seizure

bright light, and the *ciliospinal response*. Pupillary responses in stuporous and comatose patients are often subtle and difficult to detect with the naked eye. The exam can be aided by an ophthalmoscope or otoscope for magnification, or a pupillometer.

An understanding of pupillary innervation is critical to the interpretation of the exam. Parasympathetic innervation, which control pupillary constriction, begins in the medial midbrain at the Edinger-Westphal nucleus (EWN) and runs superficially on the dorsal aspect of the third cranial nerve (CN3). Light detected by the retina sends a signal through the optic nerve to the EWN, producing pupillary constriction. Lesions that stretch or injury CN3, such as a herniating medial temporal lobe or expanding posterior communicating artery aneurysm, impair parasympathetic innervation and produce a unilateral pupillary dilation.

Sympathetic innervation takes a longer and more complicated course. It begins in the hypothalamus, projecting caudally through the brainstem where it receives inputs from several other pathways, proceeds to the upper thoracic spine where it exits and joins the superior cervical ganglion, then branches to the internal carotid artery and finally courses through the cavernous sinus to the pupil. Assessing for the presence of the *ciliospinal reflex* challenges the integrity of the sympathetic pathway. This is done by pinching the face or neck and observing for a 1 to 2 mm dilation of the pupils bilaterally. The painful stimulus is received in the lower brainstem, where it triggers autonomic pathways that

produce a sympathetic discharge. The presence of a ciliospinal reflex implies that if a brainstem lesion is present, it is in the rostral pons or higher, and that the lower brainstem is spared.

Pupils are often observed to be small and reactive in diencephalic dysfunction and metabolic coma/encephalopathy. Notable exceptions to the later are some drug-induced comas (Table 48A–1G). Midbrain dysfunction, whether via a primary lesion or downward or laterally compressive forces, produced 4 mm, mid-position, fixed pupils. If the lesion affects the more dorsal pretectal midbrain (eg, pineal gland mass, enlarged third ventricle, or dorsal midbrain stroke [Parinaud's syndrome]), the pupils tend to be slightly larger (~5 mm) and a downward gaze is observed (sunset eyes). Compressive midbrain lesions that also stretch the CN3 will produce fully dilated (~8 mm) and nonreactive pupils.

Further progressive downward injury or primary pontine injury will produce nonreactive pinpoint (1 mm) pupils. Table 48A–1E summarizes the neurologic exam findings in various brainstem lesions.

Oculomotor Exam

Gaze palsies result from injury to the frontal eye fields (frontal lobes), CN3, sixth cranial nerve (CN6), or the brainstem connections between the CN3 and CN6 nuclei (ie, pontine paramedian reticular formation [PPRF], medial longitudinal fasciculus [MLF]). Symmetric lateral gaze is accomplished by signaling the ipsilateral CN6 via PPRF, and the contralateral

TABLE 48A–1H Full outline of unresponsiveness (FOUR) score.

Score	Eye	Motor	Brainstem	Respiration
4	Open and tracks or blinks to command	Follows command[a]	PR and CR present	Not intubated, normal RP
3	Open, no tracking	Localize	One pupil fixed and dilated	Not intubated, C-S RP
2	Open to loud voice	Flexes to pain	PR or CR present	Not intubated, irregular breathing
1	Open to pain	Extensor posture	PR and CR absent	Breathers over ventilator
0	Do not open	No response or myoclonic status	PR, CR, and cough absent	Breathes at ventilator rate or apnea

PR, pupil reactivity; CR, corneal reflex; RP, respiratory pattern; C-S, Cheyne-Stokes.
Total score ranges from 0 to 16.
[a]Gives thumbs up, makes fist, or shows two fingers.

CN3 through the MLF. Integrity of this system is assessed in conscious patients by having the patient follows the examiner's finger through all extremes of eye movement. The oculocephalic (doll's eyes) reflex is used to assess the oculomotor system in stuporous and comatose patients that are unable to follow commands. It is performed with the patient's neck in 30° of extension and by gently rolling the patient's head from side to side while observing eye movements. The patient's eyes should attempt to move in the opposite direction of head. If this maneuver fails to produce a response or if it cannot be done because of concern for a cervical spine injury, then *caloric oculovestibular testing* (ie, *cold calorics*) can be performed by injecting 30 to 60 mL of cold saline on the tympanic membrane (TM), then observing for 1 to 2 minutes for tonic eye deviation toward stimulus. Before performing this maneuver, be certain that the TM is intact and unobstructed (eg, cerumen impact or hemorrhagic debris in the external auditory canal).

Corneal Reflex, Gag, and Cough

The corneal reflex (CR) is examined by stimulating the cornea with either saline drops or by gently touching the delicate corneal with a cotton swab and observing for a blink and/or elevation of the eye. The CR evaluates CN3, CN5, CN7, the midbrain, and pons. Contact lens wearers will have a suppressed CR. It should not be performed in conscious patients. The gag reflex, which assesses CN9, CN10, and CN12, is assessed by stimulating the posterior pharynx with a tongue blade or a similar object and visually observing for elevation of the ipsilateral soft palate and depression of the tongue. A cough is elicited by carefully advancing the endotracheal suction catheter to the greatest possible depth.

Brain Death Declaration

Patients with loss of all cerebral function due to an irreversible cerebral insult can be evaluated for brain death. The examination components include an assessment of motor function, pupil reactivity, caloric oculovestibular testing, corneal, gag, cough, and oculocephalic reflexes, in the absence of any neuromuscular blockers (NMBs), CNS depressants, metabolic derangements, or physiologic abnormalities. If there is no evident neurologic function, apnea testing is performed to pronounce brain death. Apnea is diagnosed if the $PaCO_2$ rises from a normal level (35-45 mm Hg) to more than 60 mm Hg or by more than 20 mm Hg without evidence of respiratory effort over at least 8 minutes while patient's endotracheal tube is disconnected from the ventilator. A RR greater than the set rate on the ventilator does not imply the patient is not apneic; cardiac pulsations are capable of triggering tidal volumes. Table 48A–1I summarizes the brain death examination conditions and components.

If select components of the neurologic exam cannot be performed (eg, caloric oculovestibular testing due to traumatic TM perforation) or the

TABLE 48A-1I Critical elements of brain death declaration.

Metabolic or Pharmacologic Disturbances Prohibiting Brain Death Assessment	Examination Components
• Severe acid-base abnormalities • Significant electrolyte disturbances • Endocrine abnormalities • Hypo- or hyperthermia • Hypotension • Hypo- or hypercarbia • Hypoxemia • Sedative and paralytics drugs or intoxicants	• Pupillary response • Corneal reflex • Cough reflex • Gag reflex • Oculocephalic reflex • Cold water caloric testing • Grimace or nonreflexive motor movements[a]

Apnea Test Prerequisites	Conditions Mandating Abortion of Apnea Test	Empiric Hypothalamic Hormonal Replacement
• Temperature > 96°F • sBP > 100 mm Hg • Euvolemia • $PaCO_2$ 35-45 mm Hg • PaO_2 > 200 mm Hg	• sBP < 100 mm Hg • Hypoxia (SpO_2 < 90%) • Cardiac dysrhythmias	• Vasopressin 2.4 Unit/h • Levothyoxine 20 mcg IVP, then 10 mcg/h • Methylprednisolone 15 mg/kg IV Q24H

sBP, systolic blood pressure; $PaCO_2$, arterial partial pressure of carbon dioxide; PaO_2, arterial partial pressure of oxygen; IVP, intravenous push.
[a]Apply a central noxious stimulation such as, supraorbital pressure, trapezius pinch, nasopharyngeal irritation with a cotton swab, or jaw thrust (if not prohibited by a traumatic injury).

patient's physiology cannot tolerate at least 8 minutes of apnea, then a confirmatory test can be completed instead. Options include a digital subtraction angiography, CT angiography of the head, cerebral scintigraphy (preferred in most centers), transcranial Dopplers, or electroencephalography (EEG).

The brain death process is prone to institutional idiosyncrasies due to local and state policies. Your institutional policy and state laws should be consulted when pronouncing brain death. Movements in the brain dead have been observed, such as "the undulating toe," lower extremity reflexes, such as "triple flexion" and the "Lazarus sign" (ie, arms raised, then crossed on the chest). These require interpretation. If there is ambivalence, confirmatory testing should be pursued.

Once brain death is pronounced, an organ donation representative may approach the family of the deceased. The clinician should not engage organ donation discussions with patient's surrogate/proxy. If the surrogate/proxy inquires about donation, they should be referred to the organ donation representatives. Leading up to and following brain death declaration, the clinician should continue to optimize the deceased's physiology, as this has been shown to improve the success of transplantation. Physiologic

replacement of hypothalamic hormones can help achieve hemodynamic stability, including vasopressin, levothyroxine, and methylprednisolone. A recent randomized trial found that delayed graft function was decreased in recipients of kidneys from deceased donors that were cooled to 34°C to 35°C.

Pathophysiology and Differential Diagnosis

CNS dysfunction may occur for several reasons. Table 48A-1J breaks them into 7 mechanistic categories that provide a structure for a differential diagnosis. It is not uncommon for multiple etiologies to coexist and synergistically impair CNS function. Asymmetric or lateralizing neurologic findings often suggest a primary CNS disorder, but they can also be seen with systemic illness in patients with a prior CNS insult. Above all, the identification and treatment of etiologies that will lead to irreversible CNS injury with delays in care must be prioritized. This includes failure of systemic substrate delivery, impairment in the local delivery of substrate (eg, AIS or vasospasm), rapidly expanding intracranial masses (eg, ICH), unmitigated deranged physiology (eg, status epilepticus), anatomic neuronal

TABLE 48A-1J Pathophysiologic mechanisms of encephalopathy, stupor, and coma.

Mechanism	Examples
Failure of substrate delivery	Hypoxemia, severe anemia, hypoglycemia, hypotension, cardiogenic shock
Metabolically or pharmacologically induced neuronal dysfunction	Uremia, hyponatremia, liver failure, hypercarbia, drug ingestion, toxidrome, hypothermia
Primary disturbance in neuronal function or physiology	Seizures, convulsive or nonconvulsive status epilepticus
Primary diffuse, bihemispheric cortical pathology	Encephalitis, acute demyelinating Encephalomyelitis, CNS vasculitis
Focal lesion of the ARAS	Acute basilar thrombosis, brainstem intracerebral hemorrhage
Anatomic distortion or compression of the ARAS	Hydrocephalus, SDH with uncal herniation, pineal gland tumor with dorsal midbrain compression
Intracranial hypertension	Acute aSAH, dural sinus thrombosis, meningitis

ARAS, ascending reticular activating system; SDH, subdural hematoma; aSAH, aneurysmal subarachnoid hemorrhage.

distortion (eg, cerebral herniation), and failure of global or focal cerebral perfusion (eg, intracranial hypertension, collapse of perforating vessels causing focal infarction).

Hypotension, hypoxemia, and hypoglycemia warrant immediate exclusion and treatment. Those with evidence of or risk factors for malnutrition should receive thiamine intravenously. wPetCO$_2$ may fail to detect hypercarbia in hypopneic patients; therefore, a blood gas is warranted. Table 48A-1K summarizes theses as well as other metabolic, environmental, and toxicologic processes that require immediate consideration. Table 48A-1G outlines findings in some common toxidromes. Other chapters in this text cover toxicologic and environmental emergencies in greater detail.

Delays of as little as 15 minutes in the diagnosis and treatment of acute primary neurologic emergencies have been associated with worse outcomes. Acute disorders and their corresponding diagnostic tests are found in Table 48A-1L. Neuroimaging, cerebrospinal fluid (CSF) analysis, and EEG will capture nearly all of these conditions. Table 48A-1M lists etiologies of stupor and coma that will require more sophisticated diagnostics, consultative services, and/or unique therapies.

Intracranial Pressure

In adults, the cranial vault is a rigid, noncompliant structure filled with brain tissue, blood, CSF, and meninges. The brain is divided into supratentorial and infratentorial compartments by a dural fold, the *tentorium cerebelli*. The brainstem passes through an opening in the *tentorium*, called the *tentorial incisure or notch*. Another dural fold, the *falx cerebri*, similarly divides the brain into the left and right hemispheres and importantly contains the superior and inferior sagittal sinuses. Cisterns filled with CSF, cranial nerves, and large intracranial arteries surround the brainstem.

Pressure is a function of the amount of mass occupying a fixed amount of space (eg, the human cranium) and is expressed in force per unit area. Alternatively, it is reported in either centimeters of water (cm H$_2$O) or millimeters of mercury (mm Hg). Literally, it is the amount of force applied by a column of either H$_2$O or Hg, with the height of the column being cm with H$_2$O or mm with Hg. When pressures vary at different locations (ie, there is a pressure gradient), objects are liable to be moved from their position by these differences in force. In the brain, pressure gradients cause cerebral tissue to herniate, nerves to stretch, and vascular and ventricular structures to be compressed, displacing CSF and blood and eventually disrupting the circulation of CSF and/or flow of blood. Initial elevations in ICP cause CSF to shift from the ventricles to the spinal subarachnoid space. Next, venous outflow is accelerated when ICP exceeds right atrial pressure. With further increases, cerebral tissue is

TABLE 48A–1K Acute undifferentiated encephalopathy, stupor, and coma: substrate delivery and initial metabolic and environmental considerations.

Condition	Diagnostics and Considerations
Hypoglycemia	FSBG
Hypoxia	Pulse oximetry, arterial blood gas, CO-oximetry
Severe anemia	CBC, inspect conjunctiva, mucus membranes
Hypercarbia	Blood gas (venous or arterial)
Hypotension (absolute or relative)	Palpate pulse, sphygmomanometry, arterial line
Cardiogenic shock	Capillary refill, pulse quality, bedside echocardiography
Severe sepsis or septic shock	Core temperature, physical evidence of infection, WBC, lactate, lipase, U/A
DKA/HONC	BMP, VBG, serum ketones, U/A, serum osm, fruity breath, severe tachypnea without respiratory illness
Myxedema coma/thyrotoxicosis	TSH, free T4, T3; bradycardia, hypothermia or tachycardia, hyperthermia, hypertension
Uremia	BMP
Beriberi/Wernicke's encephalopathy	Evidence or risk factors for malnourishment, empirically treat
Electrolyte derangement	BMP, iCa, PO4, Mg
Hepatic encephalopathy	NH3, LFTs
Carbon monoxide	CO-oximetry, appropriate environmental setting
Methemoglobinemia	CO-oximetry
Cyanide	Lactate, building fire victim, initiate hydroxocobalamin
Hypo- or hyperthermia	Core temperature (bladder, rectal, and esophageal). If hyperthermia considers sepsis, serotonin syndrome, NMS, MH, heat stroke. If hypothermia, consider myxedema, pituitary apoplexy, Addison's disease
Intentional ingestion (suicide attempt)	Serum tylenol, salicylates, toxic alcohols, ethanol, serum Osm, Urine drug screen, evidence of prior or recent self-harm
Electrocution/lightning strike	Total CPK, ferning, entry and exit burns, charred clothing

FSBG, finger stick blood glucose; CBC, complete blood count; WBC, white blood cell count; BMP, basic metabolic panel; VBG, venous blood gas; serum osm, serum osmolality; U/A, urinalysis; DKA, diabetic ketoacidosis; HONC, hyperglycemic hyperosmolar nonketotic coma; TSH, thyroid stimulating hormone; iCa, ionized calcium/free calcium; PO4, serum phosphate; Mg, serum magnesium; NH3, ammonia; LFTs, liver function tests; NMS, neuroleptic malignant syndrome; MH, malignant hyperthermia; CPK, creatine phosphokinase.

displaced (herniated) and arterial perfusion pressures are exceeded, producing ischemia and infarction. The infarcted tissue then swells, leading to further herniation and compromise of arterial blood flow. Once compensatory mechanisms are exhausted (ie, the displacement of CSF and/or venous blood), larger pressure increases occur with small increases in volume (ie, compliance worsens). These are the principles of the *Monro-Kellie doctrine* (Figure 48A–3). When measured via intraparenchymal fiberoptic monitors or intraventricular catheters, ICPs of greater than 20 mm Hg have been associated with worse outcomes. It is important to note that most intracranial disease processes do

TABLE 48A–1L Primary neurologic process and preferred diagnostic tests.

Neurologic Process	First Line Diagnostics
Acute Ischemic stroke	NCHCT (insensitive acutely), CTA head and neck, MRI w/DWI + ADC sequences (difficult to obtain emergently)
Intracerebral hemorrhage	NCHCT
Traumatic brain injury	NCHCT
Extra-axial hemorrhage	NCHCT
Meningitis/encephalitis	LP with CSF analysis
Acute hydrocephalus	NCHCT
Aneurysmal subarachnoid hemorrhage	NCHCT
Dural sinus thrombosis	CTV vs MRV
Status epilepticus	Scalp EEG
Posterior reversible encephalopathy syndrome	NCHCT (limited sensitivity), MRI with FLAIR sequence
Brain abscess/ empyema	Head CT with contrast; MRI ± contrast

NCHCT, noncontract head computed tomography; CTA, computed tomography angiography; MRI, magnetic resonance imaging; DWI, diffusion weighted imaging; ADC, apparent diffusion coefficient; LP, lumbar puncture; CSF, cerebrospinal fluid; CTV, computed tomography venogram; MRV, magnetic resonance venogram; EEG, electroencephalography; FLAIR, fluid attenuated inversion recovery.

TABLE 48A–1M Less common etiologies of stupor and coma.

Brainstem tumor/malignancies
Leptomeningeal carcinomatosis
Pituitary apoplexy
Paraneoplastic encephalopathies
Demyelinating disorders
  Posthypoxic ischemic encephalopathy
  Acute disseminated encephalomyelitis
  Marburg variant of multiple sclerosis
  Central pontine myelinolysis
CNS vasculitis or vasculopathies
Chronic meningitis/CNS infections
Progressive multifocal leukoencephalopathy
Prion disease
Several nutritional deficiencies
Inherited metabolic disorders

not lead to global symmetric increases in pressure. Instead, the aforementioned concepts are frequently localized phenomena that may be under-appreciated by monitors placed in nondiseased tissue (Table 48A–1N). Further details on ICP monitoring, indications, waveforms, and their interpretation can be found in Chapter XY.

Cerebral Herniation Syndromes

Cerebral herniation tends to follow one of several anatomic trajectories, which are accompanied by an expected constellation of neurologic changes, termed *herniation syndromes* (Table 48A–1O and Figure 48A–4). Supratentorial syndromes include subfalcine, diencephalon shift, uncal, and central, while infratentorial syndromes include tonsillar and upward.

Subfalcine herniation and *diencephalon shift* are the result of lateral pressure gradients across the hemispheres. In subfalcine herniation, the cingulate gyrus is forced against and eventually under the inferior margin of the falx cerebri, where the pericallosal branches of the anterior cerebral artery can be compressed, leading to infarction and impaired motor function in the contralateral leg. They are radiographically quantified by the amount of midline shift (MLS) at the septum pellucidum (subfalcine) or pineal gland (diencephalon shift) on axial sequences. Clinically, the level of arousal is depressed in proportion to the degree of MLS.

Uncal herniation occurs when the medial aspect of the temporal lobe is forced over the tentorial edge into the basal cisterns, eventually compressing and pushing the midbrain laterally. The first manifestation is typically impaired consciousness with ipsilateral pupillary dilation due to stretching of the CN3 as it course through the cisterns, followed by contralateral hemiparesis from compression of the midbrain. Approximately 25% of the time, ipsilateral hemiparesis occurs when the midbrain is forced against the contralateral free edge of the tentorium. Arousal is impaired from stretching of the elements of the ARAS. The posterior cerebral artery territory is subject to compression by the uncus with subsequent infarct of its territory.

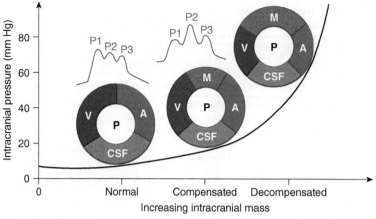

A: Arterial volume
V: Venous volume
P: Parenchyma
M: Mass

FIGURE 48A–3 Monroe-Kellie hypothesis. An increase in cranial volume will lead to an increase in pressure unless an equal amount of volume in cerebrospinal fluid and/or blood is displaced.

Central transtentorial herniation begins with compression of the diencephalon, followed by the midbrain, then the pons, and finally the medulla. It is often the result of obstructive hydrocephalus or other mass located in the midline. Clinically, a *rostrocaudal deterioration* of brainstem function can be appreciated. Initially, compression of the diencephalon causes a depression in arousal with small, minimally reactive pupils. Untreated, midbrain compression ensures, where the pupils enlarge to approximately 4 to 5 mm (mid-position) or dilated and nonreactive, often with flexor posturing. Further progression yields miotic pupils and/or extensor posturing. Finally, once the medulla is compressed, the patient becomes quadriplegic and hypotensive. Neuroendocrine functions can become disturbed at various points along this deterioration as a result of pituitary ischemia or avulsion of the stalk. Additionally, both posterior cerebral arteries are at risk for compression and infarction in this syndrome.

TABLE 48A–1N Regional mass lesion and increasing ICP difference with focal hemispheric lesion.

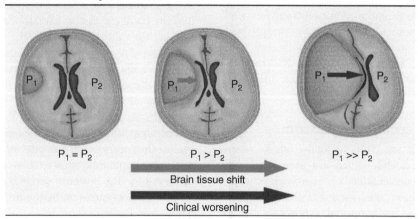

TABLE 48A-10 Herniation syndromes.

Herniation Syndrome	Level of Arousal	Motor Exam	Pupillary Exam	Other Findings
Subfalcine, early	Drowsy to lethargy	Normal to CL LE paresis, paratonia	Normal	
Subfalcine, late	Stupor to coma	CL LE paresis, FP CL > IL	Small, minimally reactive	
Diencephalon shift, early	Drowsy to lethargy	Possible CL HP, paratonic	Small, minimally reactive	
Diencephalon shift, late	Stupor to coma	FP CL > IL to QP	Mid-position, NR, maybe irregular	
Uncal, early	Lethargy to stupor	Localizes IP, paratonic CL	IP Mydriasis, NR[a]	
Uncal, late	Stupor to coma	CL FP/EP to HP (IP ~ 25%)	IP Mydriasis, NR	IP eye is abducted and depressed w/ptosis[a]
Central (transtentorial), diencephalon stage	Lethargy to stupor	Localizes to withdrawal	Small, minimally reactive	
Central (transtentorial), midbrain stage	Coma	FP to EP	Mid-position, NR, maybe irregular	DC gaze w/impaired adduction on VOR
Central (transtentorial), pontine stage	Coma	QP, ± TF of LEs	Miotic	No VOR
Central (transtentorial), medullary stage	Coma	QP, ± TF of LEs	Miotic or Mydriatic and NR	Hypotension and apnea
Tonsillar	Coma	QP, ± TF of LEs	Miotic	Hypotension and apnea
Upward, early	Lethargy	Quadraparesis to QP	Mid-position, NR, maybe irregular	Impaired upward gaze
Upward, late	Coma	EP to QP, ± TF of LEs	Mid-position, NR, maybe irregular	No VOR

CL, contralateral; IL, ipsilateral; UE, upper extremity; LE, lower extremity; QP, quadriplegia; NR, nonreactive; VOR, oculocephalic testing; TF, triple flexion; FP, flexor posturing; EP, extensor posturing; HP, hemiparesis; DC, dysconjugate.
[a]Due to the anatomic location of the third cranial nerve (CN3), the first finding in uncal herniation can be a partial to full CN3 palsy.

Tonsillar herniation can result from posterior fossa masses or advanced transtentorial herniation (uncal or central). The cerebellar tonsils are forced through the foramen magnum, compressing the caudal medulla, causing apnea, hypotension (but often initially hypertension), miotic pupils, and quadriplegia. The fourth ventricle is commonly compressed, leading to obstructive hydrocephalus. In this setting, treating the hydrocephalus first with an *external ventricular drain* can cause the brainstem to *herniate upward*, causing the brainstem to buckle and bend, compressing its perforating arterial supply, leading to infarction. Therefore, it is often prudent to prioritize or simultaneously perform a suboccipital decompression while establishing diversion of CSF.

Neurologic Resuscitation: Treatment of Acute Stupor and Coma

The early treatment goals in undifferentiated acute disturbances in anchor on the empiric optimization of cerebral blood flow (CBF) and delivery of critical substrates, such as oxygen and glucose. To do so, the clinician needs to have a firm understanding of the relationships between MAP, ICP, ventilation, oxygenation, CBF as well as the effects of

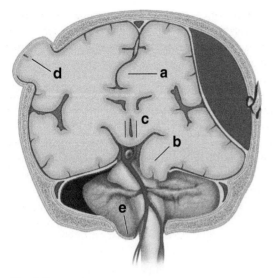

Herniation syndromes
a. Subfalcine
b. Uncal
c. Central transtentorial
d. External
e. Tonsillar

FIGURE 48A–4 Herniation syndromes. (a) Subfalcine, (b) uncal, (c) central transtentorial, (d) external, and (e) tonsillar. (*Adapted with permission from Knoop KJ, Stack LB, Storrow AB, et al: The Atlas of Emergency Medicine, 3rd edition. New York: McGraw-Hill, Inc; 2010.*)

airway management on ICP. Immediate actions are to correct hypoxia, hypoglycemia, hypotension, hypoperfusion, and hypo, or hypercarbia. Prolonged hyperoxia should be avoided, as this is associated with harm. BP reduction and goals are tailored to the etiology of the neurologic change. Prior to definitive diagnostics, it is likely unclear whether the brain is in a hypoperfused state (eg, critical carotid stenosis) or would benefit from aggressive BP reduction (eg, ICH). In those with a diastolic blood pressure (dBP), more than 120 mm Hg or systolic blood pressure (sBP) more than 230 mm Hg, gentle BP reduction to a sBP less than 220 mm Hg and/or dBP less than 120 mm Hg are reasonable, but it represents a low priority therapeutic target, with more risk than reward in the undifferentiated patient. Mildly hypothermic states may not warrant immediately, rapid correct; if ICP proves to be an issue, as rapid normalization can produce herniation. Suggested initial empiric diagnostic and therapeutic targets are summarized in Table 48A–1P.

The $PaCO_2$ heavily influences CBF due to its powerful effects on cerebral vessel diameter. About 1 mm Hg increase in the $PaCO_2$ will increase the CBF by 2% to 4% (and vice versa). Beyond this physiologic relation, hypo- and hypercarbia have been associated with worse outcomes in several

TABLE 48A–1P Empiric diagnostics and therapeutic targets in the patient with undifferentiated disturbance in consciousness.

First-Tier Diagnostics	Second-Tier Diagnostics	Therapeutics
FSBG	CSF Analysis and OP	Airway protection
CBC	Electroencephalography	Correct hypotension[a]
BMP, Mg, Phos, iCa	Brain MRI ± gadolinium	Correct Hypoglycemia
Coagulation panel, fibrinogen	Head CT Venography/MR Venography	Normocarbia
Type and screen		Normoxia
Blood gas, CO, lactate		Thiamine
Beta-hCG		Temperature 32°C-38°C
LFTs, ammonia		
TFTs		
Drug levels (eg, AEDs, digoxin)		
ECG, Troponin		
NCHCT, CTA, head and neck		

FSBG, fingerstick blood glucose; CBC, complete blood count; BMP, basic metabolic panel; Mg, magnesium; Phos, phosphate; iCa, ionized calcium; CO, carbon monoxide; LFTs, liver function panel; TFT, thyroid function tests; AEDs, antiepileptics; ECG, electrocardiogram; NCHCT, noncontrast head computer tomography; CTA, computer tomography angiogram; MRI, magnetic resonance imaging; CSF, cerebrospinal fluid; OP, opening pressure.
[a]Monitor hypertension; correction best determined once the etiology of the neurologic change ascertain/a critical flow limiting stenosis is excluded.

neurologic emergencies. Therefore, vigilant ventilator management is crucial. End-tidal capnography (ETCO$_2$) is a valuable tool to accomplish this, noting that it may prove inaccurate if there is upper airway obstruction, hypopnea, pulmonary disease, hypotension, metabolic acidosis, and/or thoracic trauma. One caveat is the patient with hypocarbia as a compensation for a metabolic acidosis; this patient should have their PaCO$_2$ forcibly normalized, as it will worsen the underlying acidosis and potentially produce cardiovascular collapse.

Via autoregulatory feedback, systemic hypotension will produce cerebral vasodilation, increasing the cerebral blood volume (CBV) (Figure 48A–5). A minimal mean arterial blood pressure (MAP) target of more than 65 mm Hg may be inadequate for those with flow limiting cervical or cerebral vessel stenosis and many not produce the desired cerebral perfusion pressure (CPP) of more than 60 mm Hg in those with IC-HTN (CPP = MAP – ICP); therefore, an initial target MAP of more than 80 mm Hg is often selected. Ensuring euvolemia through clinical intravascular volume assessment and provision of isotonic crystalloids initially pursues MAP targets. Albumin and synthetic colloids have not found a place in the neurologic resuscitation. In fact, a subgroup analysis of the SAFE trial found albumin to be associated with increased mortality in TBI

patients, when compared to crystalloids. Bedside echocardiography is a valuable tool to screen for acute cardiac dysfunction and neurogenic stunned myocardium.

As discussed earlier, ICP is a product of the amount of mass in the intracranial vault. Actions that increase CBV can increase ICP. Hypermetabolic states, such as agitation, seizures, or hyperthermia will increase CBF. Cerebral venous drainage can be impaired when the patient's head is falling to one side or if their cervical collar is tight fitting, causing ICP elevations.

Acute intracranial hemorrhage should remain high on the differential. Inquiries regarding anticoagulant use and serologic assessment of the patient's coagulation status must occur. If intracranial hemorrhage is identified, rapid, immediately correction of any coagulopathy is mandatory and must be conducted with the highest sense of urgency, regardless of any perceived transient stability.

Airway Considerations

Hypoxia, hypercarbia, hypertension, IC-HTN, and hypotension are all known complications of endotracheal intubation (ETI). As described earlier, many acute neurologic conditions are worsened by these physiologic perturbations and must be avoided.

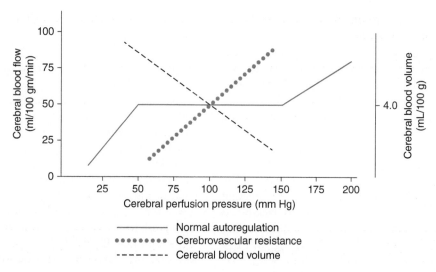

FIGURE 48A–5 Autoregulatory curve.

Hypoxia can be avoided with optimal preoxygenation and utilizing techniques, strategies, and equipment that optimize the probability of first pass success. Similarly, hypercarbia will be minimized with short paralysis to intubation times. The $PaCO_2$ rises by 6 to 7 mm Hg in the first minute of apnea, followed by a 3 to 4 mm Hg rise for every minute thereafter, with greater jumps in those increased metabolism (eg, hyperthermia) and likely with depolarizing NMBs, such as succinylcholine. Hypotension can be avoided via intravascular volume loading with isotonic crystalloids, selection of induction agents with hemodynamic stability (eg, etomidate and ketamine, KET), and using lower doses of induction agents in comatose patients.

Laryngoscopy and endotracheal suctioning are known to increase in ICP via several hypothesized pathways. Weak evidence suggests that administering 1.5 mg/kg of lidocaine IV (up to 150 mg) 3 minutes prior to intubation may mitigate this increase. If provided, note that systemic BP decreases can be seen and the fasciculations normally seen after succinylcholine administration will be blunted or absent. Alternatively, fentanyl (1-3 mcg/kg) IV can be provided to blunt the sympathetic response to laryngoscopy that is blamed for some of the ICP rise.

KET has been reported to dramatically increase ICP and has been contraindicated into those with IC-HTN. More recently, several small, randomized trials have not observed this increased when KET is used in combination with propofol (PRO), benzodiazepines, or barbiturates, although none of these studies used KET for ETI. The overall safety of bolus KET in patients with IC-HTN is still not entirely clear, but its hemodynamic stability makes it an appealing option for those with hypotension or assessed to be high risk for hypotension during intubation.

Extraglottic devices (EGDs) in the acute management of CA have been associated with inferior outcomes, possibly due to compression of the carotid arteries, reducing CBF and exacerbating brain injury. Randomized evidence is lacking to definitely inform the EGD versus ETI decision, but these observations are worth considering with ETI is an option.

Despite some of the speculative physiologic limitations, succinylcholine is the preferred paralytic in these patients, assuming the absence of other contraindications to its use, as its short duration action allows for immediate recovering of the neurologic exam, which is absolutely needed for decisions on further diagnostics and therapeutics. The recent approval of sugammadex (a reversal agent for rocuronium) in the United States does trump this concern, making rocuronium the preferred NMB where sugammadex is available.

SEIZURES AND STATUS EPILEPTICUS

Seizures are a heterogeneous clinical event with scores of etiologies, but a unifying pathophysiologic origin. Seizures that last for more than 5 minutes or sequential seizures without intervening resumption of baseline neurologic function are termed *status epilepticus (SE)*. A comprehensive discussion on seizures in critical illness is beyond the scope of this text and should be sought in other resources. This section will focus on the identification and management of SE.

Definitions and Presentation

Generalized tonic-clonic seizures (GTCs), which consist of generalized convulsions in association with a depressed level of arousal, are the most commonly recognized type of seizures. A patient with GTCs meeting SE criteria is in *generalized convulsive status epilepticus (GCSE).* If GCSE persists despite first and second line antiepileptic drug (AED) therapy (to be discussed further later), it is termed *refractory status epilepticus (RSE).*

Clinical events not uncommonly confused for GTCs are myoclonus, posturing, and psychogenic seizures. It is reasonable to initially treat myoclonus and psychogenic seizures as GTCs, as it is better to err on the side of treatment, since delayed AED administration is associated with an increased likelihood of intubation and being refractory to AEDs. Psychogenic seizures may particularly be difficult to distinguish from a GTC. Confusing the issue further is the high rate of psychogenic seizures in patients with epilepsy. Extensor posturing movements due to acute brain stem injury have been confused with GCSE, as the patient will violently and intermittently extensor posture in response to inconspicuous stimuli, such as a ventilator delivered breath.

Focal seizures (formerly known as "partial" seizures) are a heterogeneous clinical event, with symptoms consistent with area(s) of the brain that are involved. Repetitive, involuntary, and stereotyped movements are the most readily identified clinical demonstration. If a focal seizure persists despite treatment, it is called *epilepsia partialis continua*, which has a very low mortality rate and therefore does not require aggressive treatment. When focal seizures occur in concert with a disturbance in consciousness, they are termed "*complex.*" If this persists, the patient is in *nonconvulsive status epilepticus (NCSE)*. When there is a motor component to the clinical presentation of NCSE, it may also be called "*subtle status epilepticus,*" as it may represent inadequately treated GCSE. A *nonconvulsive seizure (NCSz)* is appreciated electrographically in patients with either vague symptoms or a depressed level of consciousness. Table 48A–1Q lists signs and symptoms seen with NCSz.

TABLE 48A–1Q Symptoms and signs of nonconvulsive seizures.

Negative	Positive
Amnesia	Agitation/aggression
Anorexia	Automatisms
Aphasia/mutism	Blinking
Catatonia	Crying
Coma	Delirium
Confusion	Delusions
Lethargy	Echolalia
Staring	Facial twitching
	Laughter
	Nausea/vomiting
	Nystagmus/eye deviation
	Perseveration
	Psychosis
	Tremulousness

Etiologic Considerations

Distinguishing between *provoked* and *unprovoked* seizures is an important therapeutics step, as the former require resolution of the underlying cause, while treatment of the later is largely dependent on the administration of AEDs, and in very advanced or challenging cases, the consideration of surgical options. The most common cause of SE is AED discontinuation; therefore, AED levels should be obtained immediately. Hypoglycemia, infectious (particularly CNS, but also systemic), metabolic, toxicologic, or environmental etiologies also require immediately consideration. Early neuroimaging (eg, non-contrast head CT (NCHCT)) is warranted to evaluate for a primary neurologic etiologies, such as ICH, SAH, PRES, abscess, tumor, or malignancy. Many medications, particularly when used in combination (ie, polypharmacy) can reduce the seizure threshold. *Serotonin syndrome* and *neuroleptic malignant syndrome* should be considered, as well as ethanol or benzodiazepines withdrawal. Those with a primary neurologic insult, who then suffer from a metabolic or systemic illness, are prone to experiencing provoked seizures (eg, patient with prior ischemic stroke now with sepsis).

SE patients often present with a fever, but this should not delay the attainment of CSF and provision of corticosteroids and meningitic-coverage antimicrobials. Encephalitis, whether it is infectious, inflammatory, autoimmune, or paraneoplastic require early consideration, as the former many benefit from specific antimicrobials, and the later three many require immunomodulatory therapies, such as high-dose corticosteroids, Intravenous Immunoglobulin (IVIG), plasmapheresis, and/or chemotherapeutic agents, such as cyclophosphamide or rituximab. CNS vasculitis, leptomeningeal carcinomatosis, and, rarely, demyelinating disorders, may warrant consideration.

Treatment

The initial approach to the seizing patient includes the principles outlined previously in this Chapter, under "Neurologic Resuscitation," in addition to the cessation of seizure activity, whether it is clinical or electrographic.

Benzodiazepines (BZP) are the first line treatment for SE. When intravenous (IV) access is immediately available, lorazepam (LZP) 4 mg IV is the preferred agent, which may be repeated once, with a success rate of approximately 60%. If an IV is not established, midazolam (MDZ) 10 mg IM has been shown to be noninferior to LZP. Other alternatives include diazepam (DZP) 20 mg per rectum, DZP 10 mg IV, buccal MDZ, or intranasal MDZ.

All patients in SE should be given a second AED. Commonly selected agents include phenytoin (PHT), fosphenytoin (fPHT), valproate (VPA), levetiracetam (LEV), and phenobarbital. If noncompliance with an already prescribed AED is known, it is prudent to reintroduce their home AED. If seizure activity has appeared to clinically resolve and twenty minutes have passed without improvement in their level of consciousness (LOC), continuous video electroencephalogram (ccEEG) should be initiated to exclude NCSE/NCSz.

PHT, while effective, has several drawbacks. If infused too rapidly it can cause heart block, cardiac arrhythmias, hypotension, and cutaneous reactions, including Stevens-Johnson syndrome. fPHT, the prodrug of PHT, is less liable to produce hemodynamic instability during its infusion. PHT is highly protein bound (with free drug providing the clinical activity) displacing other protein bound medications and it induces cytochrome p450 enzymes CYP3A and CYP2C, leading to a variety of drug interactions, particularly in the critically ill patient. Table 48A–1R provides further information on dosing and serum levels.

Limited evidence suggests VPA is likely to be as efficacious as, if not superior to, PHT as a second line agent for SE. Limitations include its potential hepatotoxicity, pancreatitis, CYP2C9 inhibition, and antiplatelet effects, making it unattractive in intracranial hemorrhages. Total and free levels can be monitored. It uncommonly causes hyperammonemic encephalopathy (independent of any hepatic toxicity), which can be treated with L-carnitine, although its efficacy is this regard is questionable. LEV is an attractive option due to its lack of

TABLE 48A–1R Second line antiepileptic drug dosing and serum levels.

AED	Loading Dose (IV)	Postload Level Timing	Maintenance Dose	Trough Level	Level Correction[a]	Toxicities and Interactions
PHT	20 mg/kg	1 hour	5-7 mg/kg/d Q8H, adjust based on trough levels	Total: 15-25 mg/L Free: 1.5-2.5 mg/L	PHT/ ((Adj x Alb) +0.1)[b]	Cardiac arrhythmias, hypotension with infusion; purple glove syndrome, SJS, CYP450 inducer
fPHT	20 PE/kg	2 hours	5-7 PE/kg/day Q8H adjust based on trough levels	Same as PHT	Same as PHT	Same as PHT, but safer infusion
VPA	40 mg/kg up to 3 gm	4-6 hours	30-60 mg/kg/day Q12H	Total: 80-120 ug/mL Free: 7-23 ug/ mL	None clearly agreed on	Hyperammonemia, hepatotoxicity, pancreatitis, anti-platelet, inhibits
LEV	30-60 mg/kg up to 4.5 g	n/a	2-6 g/d Q12H	Not usually obtained[c]	n/a	Minimal
PHB	20 mg/kg	n/a	1-4 mg/kg/d PO/ IV Q12H	30-50 mg/L	n/a	Hypotension, respiratory depression, over sedation, CYP450 inducer

AED, antiepileptic drug; PHT, phenytoin; fPHT, fosphenytoin; VPA, valproic acid; LEV, levetiracetam; PHB, phenobarbital; Adj, adjustment; Alb, albumin; SJS, Steven's Johnson syndrome; Q8H, every 8 hours; Q12H, every 12 hours.
[a]Corrected for protein binding.
[b]Adj = 0.2, unless creatinine clearance < 20 = 0.1.
[c]Typical therapeutic level 25 to 60 mcg/mL in SE/RSE.

TABLE 48A–1S **Continuous infusion anesthetics for RSE and SRSE.**

Anesthetic	Loading Dose	Maintenance Infusion Rate
MDZ	0.2 mg/kg IV, repeat Q5 min until Szs stop (max 2 mg/kg)	Start at 0.2 mg/kg/h and increase by 0.2 with every bolus, up to 2.7 mg/kg/h
PTB	5mg/kg IV, repeat Q5 min until Szs stop or BS achieved (max 15 mg/kg)	Start at 1.0 mg/kg/h and increase by 0.5-1.0 mg/kg, max 10 mg/kg/h
PRO	2 mg/kg IV, repeat Q5 min until Szs stop or BS achieved (max 10 mg/kg)	Start 1 mg/kg/h, max 10 mg/kg/h[a]
KET	0.5-2.0 mg/kg, repeat Q5 min until seizures stop (max 4.5 mg/kg)	Start 1.2 mg/kg/h and increase by 0.6 mg/kg/h, up to 6 mg/kg/h

MDZ, midazolam; PTB, pentobarbital; PRO, propofol; KET, ketamine; Szs, seizures; BS, burst suppression.
[a]If on PRO for more than 48 hours, max rate is 5 mg/kg/h to reduce risk of propofol-related infusion syndrome (PRIS).

life-threatening adverse reactions. Limited available evidence suggests that is has some efficacy in SE, but how that compares with VPA or PHT is unclear.

If seizures persist despite administration of first and second line AEDs, the patient is considered to be in RSE, and a continuous infusion of an anesthetic (cIV) should be initiated and placed on cvEEG. Options include midazolam (cIV-MDZ), PRO, and pentobarbital (PTB). Table 48A–1S outlines dosing of these agents. All of these agents are liable to cause hypotension, so a vasopressor should be prepared and euvolemia ensured. The target for their therapy has not yet been agreed upon, as some centers will increase the dose to achieve burst suppression and others will simply abolish clinical and electrographic seizure activity. The literature is not

strong enough to definitely recommend one agent or strategy over another.

In parallel to the cIV, all current AED dosing should be optimized and a third AED can be considered, with lacosamide (LCS) and topiramate (TOP) being the most common third line agents. LCS is a new AED whose primary reported side effect is PR-prolongation. TOP is only given enterally and causes a metabolic acidosis by inhibiting carbonic anhydrase. See Table 48A–1T for a list of other candidate AEDs and therapies for RSE.

Patients that recrudesce into SE after having been adequately treated with cIV are in *malignant or super RSE*. When this occurs, either the same or an alternative cIV is reinitiated and the goal (burst or seizure suppression) is lengthened by another

TABLE 48A–1T **Fourth line therapies for RSE and SRSE.**

Aeds and Other Medications		Immunomodulatory	Other Interventions
Lacosamide	Pregabalin Gabapentin	High-dose Corticosteroids[a]	Mild hypothermia (33°C)
Topiramate	Inh anesthetics	IVIG[b]	Ketogenic diet
Perampanel	Etomidate	Plasmapheresis (PE)[c]	ECT
Carbamazepine	IV magnesium	Cyclophosphamide[d]	Neurosurgical resection
Oxcarbazepine	IV pyridoxine	Rituximab[d]	VNS
Zonisamide	Lidocaine	ACTH	DBS
Clobazam	Verapamil		TMS
Lamotrigine			

ECT, electroconvulsive therapy; AEDs, antiepileptic drugs; VNS, vagal nerve stimulation; TMS, transcranial magnetic stimulation; DBS, deep brain stimulation; ACTH, adrenocorticotropic hormone; Inh, inhaled.
[a]Common dose is 1 g methylprednisolone IV Q24 for 3 to 5 doses.
[b]Intravenous immunoglobulin, dosing is 0.4 g/kg/d for 5 days.
[c]No agreed upon regimen; often PE on days 1, 2, then every other day for total of 5 to 7.
[d]These agents are selected when an autoimmune or paraneoplastic process have been diagnosed as the etiology of the RSE/SRSE.

24 hours or longer. Small case series have suggested using a continuous infusion of KET in combination with cIV-MDZ or PTB may provide an incremental improvement in efficacy.

As more experience with cvEEG grows, further insight into the significance of different patterns has been to develop. *Periodic epileptiform discharges* of varying arrangements are often seen in the comatose patient, and particularly after SE. Certain characteristics of these patterns may raise concern for persistent epileptic activity, especially if the patient remains comatose. In this instance, some centers advocate for attempting a cIV or a *BZP trial*. The latter involves giving small doses of MDZ in rapid succession and observing the patient for a clinical improvement in association with an improvement in the pattern on the EEG. If the EEG improves, but the patient does not, the result is equivocal.

NEUROMUSCULAR DISORDERS

Neuromuscular disorders are a cohort of diseases (NMDz) that result in skeletal muscle weakness, but differ in their pathophysiology and anatomic localization. The spinal anterior motor neurons, nerve roots, peripheral nerves, neuromuscular junction, and muscles are all potential sites of the different maladies (Table 48A–1U). Intensive care admission is required for those with respiratory failure, significant bulbar dysfunction requiring frequent respiratory care, unstable cardiac arrhythmias, or rapidly progressive symptoms.

More common NMDzs are Guillain-Barré syndrome (GBS), myasthenia gravis (MG), amyotrophic lateral sclerosis, and Duchenne muscular dystrophy (DMD); whereas, Lambert-Eaton myasthenic syndrome (LEMS), botulism, tetanus, porphyria, and diphtheria are less frequent. Neurotoxins can also cause neuromuscular weakness (eg, organophosphates). Chronic NMDz may lead to restrictive pulmonary disease from kyphoscoliosis.

Respiratory failure is due to bulbar muscle weakness resulting in aspiration and compromised upper airway patency and respiratory muscle weakness resulting in atelectasis causing hypoxemia, hypoventilation causing hypercarbia, and a weak cough that impairs alveolar recruitment

TABLE 48A–1U **Neuromuscular disease anatomic location of pathology.**

Disease	Spinal Cord	Anterior Horn Cells	Peripheral Nerve	Neuromuscular Junction	Muscle
Poliomyelitis		+ ± brain			
Amyotrophic lateral sclerosis	+ UMN ± brain	+			
Tick paralysis				+	
Guillain-Barre syndrome			+		
Myasthenia gravis				+	
Botulism				+	
Eaton-Lambert syndrome				+	
Organophosphate intoxication				+	
Aminoglycosides				+	
Muscular dystrophies					+
Inflammatory myopathies					+

UMN, upper motor neuron.

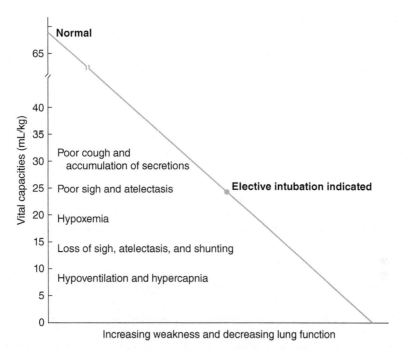

FIGURE 48A-6 Effects of decreasing vital capacities secondary to neuromuscular diseases.

and airway clearance. Respiratory function can be tracked clinically by assessing forced vital capacity (FVC) (ie, the largest volume of air that a patient can exhale), which is a composite measure of inspiratory and expiratory respiratory muscle strength (Figure 48A-6). FVC of less than 20 mL/kg warrant ICU monitoring, while those of less than 10 to 15 mL/kg typically require ETI. Beware of dogmatic statements that mandate intubation for FVC values only; ETI is still a clinically assessment. Noninvasive positive pressure ventilation (NIPPV) and/or high-flow nasal cannula can be considered for the management of mild to moderate respiratory symptoms. FVC values do not provide insight into the quality of secretion clearance or upper airway obstruction, which are more subjective in assessment and must be considered in ETI decisions. Other measures of respiratory function include the negative inspiratory force (also called the maximal inspiratory pressure) and the maximal expiratory pressure or force, which have not been shown to provide any incremental value over FVC. Cough peak flow can be measured by standard peak flow meter and values of less than 270 L/min in an adult suggests inappropriate

clearance of secretions, while results of less than 160 L/min identify profound weakness.

Cardiac complications of NMDz include arrhythmias, autonomic dysfunction (AD), and myopathy. AD is seen in about one quarter of GBS patients and is often provoked by endotracheal suctioning, ETI, or NIPPV. The AD maybe paradoxical and is characterized by severe hypertension, labile BP, postural hypotension, facial flushing, bradycardia, tachycardia, and possible asystole. Patients with SMA may suffer from cardiomyopathy and bradyarrhythmias. AD is much less common in MG patients. Patients with DMD are at increased risk for CA and rhabdomyolysis. Anesthesia-related sudden death and congestive heart failure have well been reported. Patients with myotonic dystrophy may present with cardiac conduction abnormalities such as first degree and paroxysmal complete heart blocks.

The use of NMBs in NMDzs warrants some caution. Nondepolarizing NMBs may lead to prolonged diaphragmatic paralysis with extended need for ventilatory support and smaller doses are suggested. Hyperkalemia is more likely with depolarizing NMBs (eg, succinylcholine), and therefore is best avoided. Additionally, muscular dystrophy patients are at risk for rhabdomyolysis and malignant hyperthermia-like reactions. Frequently encountered gastrointestinal problems included dysphagia, delayed gastric emptying, gastrointestinal dysmotility which are all associated with nutritional impairment.

REFERENCES

1. Plum F, Posner J, Saper C, Schiff N. Pathophysiology of signs and Symptoms of coma. In: Plum F, Posner J, et al., eds. *Plum and Posner's Diagnosis of Stupor and Coma.* 4th Ed. New York: Oxford University Press; 2007.
2. Plum F, Posner J, Saper C, Schiff N. Examination of the comatose patient. In: Plum F, Posner J, et al., eds. *Plum and Posner's Diagnosis of Stupor and Coma.* 4th Ed. New York: Oxford University Press; 2007.
3. Plum F, Posner J, Saper C, Schiff N. Structural causes of stupor and coma. In: Plum F, Posner J, et al., eds. *Plum and Posner's Diagnosis of Stupor and Coma.* 4th Ed. New York: Oxford University Press; 2007.
4. Plum F, Posner J, Saper C, Schiff N. Specific causes of structural coma. In: Plum F, Posner J, et al., eds. *Plum and Posner's Diagnosis of Stupor and Coma.* 4th Ed. New York: Oxford University Press; 2007.
5. Plum F, Posner J, Saper C, Schiff N. Multifocal, diffuse, and metabolic brain diseases causing delirium, stupor, or coma. In: Plum F, Posner J, et al., eds. *Plum and Posner's Diagnosis of Stupor and Coma.* 4th Ed. New York: Oxford University Press; 2007.
6. Plum F, Posner J, Saper C, Schiff N. Approach to the management of the unconscious patient. In: Plum F, Posner J, et al., eds. *Plum and Posner's Diagnosis of Stupor and Coma.* 4th Ed. New York: Oxford University Press; 2007.
7. Plum F, Posner J, Saper C, Schiff N. Brain death. In: Plum F, Posner J, et al., eds. *Plum and Posner's Diagnosis of Stupor and Coma.* 4th Ed. New York: Oxford University Press; 2007.
8. Blazer DG, Petersen RC, Jeste DV et al. Neurocognitive disorders. In: American Psychiatric Association, eds. *Diagnostic and Statistical Manual of Mental Disorders.* 5th ed. DSM-5. Washington, D.C: American Psychiatric Association; 2013:596-602.
9. Wijdicks EF, Varelas PN, Gronseth GS, et al. Evidence-based guideline update: determining brain death in adults: report of the Quality Standards Subcommittee of the American Academy of Neurology. *Neurology.* 2010 Jun 8;74(23):1911-1918.
10. Wijdicks EF. Determining brain death. *Continuum (Minneap Minn).* 2015 Oct;21(5 Neurocritical Care):1411-1424.
11. Wijdicks EF, Bamlet WR, Maramattom BV, et al. Validation of a new coma scale: the FOUR score. *Ann Neurol.* 2005 Oct;58(4):585-593.
12. Teasdale G, Jennett B. Assessment of coma and impaired consciousness. A practical scale. *Lancet.* 1974 Jul 13;2(7872):81-84.
13. Niemann CU, Feiner J, Swain S, et al. Therapeutic hypothermia in deceased organ donors and kidney-graft function. *N Engl J Med.* 2015 Jul 30;373(5):405-414.
14. Bleck TP. Historical aspects of critical care and the nervous system. *Crit Care Clin.* 2009 Jan;25(1):153-164.
15. Jain S, DeGeorgia M. Brain death-associated reflexes and automatisms. *Neurocrit Care.* 2005;3(2):122-126.
16. Nagai M, Hoshide S, Kario K. The insular cortex and cardiovascular system—a new insight into the brain-heart axis. *J Am Soc Hypertens.* 2010 Jul-Aug;4(4):174-182.
17. Stevens RD, Cadena RS, Pineda J. Emergency neurological life support: approach to the patient with coma. *Neurocrit Care.* 2015 Dec;23(Suppl 2):S69-S75.
18. Seder DB, Jagoda A, Riggs B. Emergency neurological life support: airway, ventilation, and sedation. *Neurocrit Care.* 2015 Dec;23(Suppl 2):S5-S22.
19. Benoit JL, Gerecht RB, Steuerwald MT, McMullan JT. Endotracheal intubation versus supraglottic airway placement in out-of-hospital cardiac arrest: a meta-analysis. *Resuscitation.* 2015 Aug;93:20-26.
20. Cohen L, Athaide V, Wickham ME, et al. The effect of ketamine on intracranial and cerebral perfusion pressure and health outcomes: a systematic review. *Ann Emerg Med.* 2015 Jan;65(1):43-51.e2.
21. Yano M, Nishiyama H, Yokota H, et al. Effect of lidocaine on ICP response to endotracheal suctioning. *Anesthesiology.* 1986;64(5):651-653.
22. Rincon F, Kang J, Vibbert M, et al. Significance of arterial hyperoxia and relationship with case fatality in traumatic brain injury: a multicentre cohort study. *J Neurol Neurosurg Psychiatry.* 2013;30;550-555.
23. Lee Sung-Woo, Hong YS, Han C et al. Concordance of end-tidal carbon dioxide and arterial carbon dioxide in severe traumatic brain injury. *J Trauma.* 2009 Sep;67(3):526-530.
24. Ko Sang-Bae. Multimodality monitoring in the neurointensive care unit. *J Stroke.* 2013 May;15(2):99-108.

25. Davis DP, Dunford JV, Poste JC, et al. The impact of hypoxia and hyperventilation on outcome after paramedic rapid sequence intubation of severely head-injured patients. *J Trauma*. 2004;57(1):1-8.

26. Chi JH, Knudson MM, Vassar MJ, et al. Prehospital hypoxia affects outcome in patients with traumatic brain injury: a prospective multicenter study. *J Trauma*. 2006;61(5):1134-1141.

27. White H, Venkatesh B. Cerebral perfusion pressure in neurotrauma: a review. *Anesth Analg*. 2008;107(3):979-988.

28. Myburgh J, Cooper DJ, Finfer S, et al. Saline or albumin for fluid resuscitation in patients with traumatic brain injury. *N Engl J Med*. 2007;357(9):874-884.

29. Kuramatsu JB, Gerner ST, Schellinger PD, et al. Anticoagulant reversal, blood pressure levels, and anticoagulant resumption in patients with anticoagulation-related intracerebral hemorrhage. *JAMA*. 2015 Feb 24;313(8):824-836.

30. Trinka E, Höfler J, Leitinger M, Brigo F. Pharmacotherapy for status epilepticus. *Drugs*. 2015 Sep;75(13):1499-1521.

31. Gaspard N, Foreman BP, Alvarez V, et al. New-onset refractory status epilepticus: etiology, clinical features, and outcome. *Neurology*. 2015 Nov 3;85(18):1604-1613.

32. Hocker SE. Status epilepticus. *Continuum (Minneap Minn)*. 2015 Oct;21(5 Neurocritical Care):1362-1383.

33. Brophy GM, Bell R, Claassen J, et al. Guidelines for the evaluation and management of status epilepticus. *Neurocrit Care*. 2012 Aug;17(1):3-23.

34. Alldredge BK. A comparison of lorazepam, diazepam, and placebo for the treatment of out-of-hospital status epilepticus. *N Engl J Med*. 2001;345(9):631-637.

35. Leppik IE, Derivan AT, Homan RW, Walker J, Ramsay RE, Patrick B. Double-blind study of lorazepam and diazepam in status epilepticus. *JAMA*. 1983;249(11):1452–1454.

36. Silbergleit R, Durkalski V, Lowenstein D, Conwit R, Pancioli A, Palesch Y, Barsan W. Intramuscular versus intravenous therapy for prehospital status epile pticus. *N Engl J Med*. 2012;366(7):591-600.

37. Claassen J, Hirsch LJ, Emerson RJ, Mayer SA. Treatment of refractory status epilepticus with pentobarbital, propofol, or midazolam: a systematic review. *Epilepsia*. 2002;43(2):146-153.

38. Claassen J, Mayer SA, Kowalski RG, Emerson RG, Hirsch LJ. Detection of electrographic seizures with continuous EEG monitoring in critically ill patients. *Neurology*. 2004;62(10):1743-1748.

39. Graus F, Titulaer MJ, Balu R, et al. A clinical approach to diagnosis of autoimmune encephalitis. *Lancet Neurol*. 2016 Apr;15(4):391-404.

40. Claassen J, Taccone FS, Horn P, et al. Recommendations on the use of EEG monitoring in critically ill patients: consensus statement from the neurointensive care section of the ESICM. *Intensive Care Med*. 2013 Aug;39(8):1337-1351.

41. Treiman DM, Meyers PD, Walton NY, et al. A comparison of four treatments for generalized convulsive status epilepticus. Veterans Affairs Status Epilepticus Cooperative Study Group. *N Engl J Med*. 1998 Sep 17;339(12):792-798.

42. Gaspard N, Foreman B, Judd LM, et al. Intravenous ketamine for the treatment of refractory status epilepticus: a retrospective multi-center study. *Epilepsia*. 2013 Aug;54(8):1498-1503.

43. Fernandez A, Lantigua H, Lesch C, et al. High-dose midazolam infusion for refractory status epilepticus. *Neurology*. 2014 Jan 28;82(4):359-365.

44. Claassen J, Riviello JJ Jr, Silbergleit R. Emergency neurological life support: status epilepticus. *Neurocrit Care*. 2015 Dec;23(Suppl 2):S136-S142.

45. Ortega-Gutierrez S, Desai N, Claassen J. Status epilepticus. In: Lee K, ed. *The Neuro ICU Book*. 1st ed. New York, NY: McGraw Hill Medical; 2012.

46. Ortega-Gutierrez S, Gilmore E, Claassen J. Continuous electroencephalogram monitoring in the intensive care unit. In: Lee K, ed. *The Neuro ICU Book*. 1st ed. New York, NY: McGraw Hill Medical; 2012.

47. Frontera J. Neuromuscular disease. In: Lee K, ed. *The Neuro ICU Book*. 1st ed. New York, NY: McGraw Hill Medical; 2012.

48. Flower O, Wainwright MS, Caulfield AF. Emergency neurological life support: acute nontraumatic weakness. *Neurocrit Care*. 2015 Dec;23(Suppl 2):S23-S47.

49. O'Phalen KH, Bunney EB, Kuluz JW. Emergency neurologic life support: spinal cord compression. *Neurocrit Care*. 2015 Dec;23(Suppl 2):S129-S135.

50. Kozak OS, Wijdicks E. Acute neuromuscular respiratory failure in myasthenia gravis and Guillain-Barré syndrome. In: Parrillo JE, Dellinger RP, eds. *Critical Care Medicine*. 3rd ed. Philadelphia, PA: Mosby Elsevier; 2008:1359-1366.

Critical Care of Cerebrovascular Disease

48B

Christopher Zammit, MD; Ko Eun Choi, MD and Axel Rosengart, MD, PhD, MPH

KEY POINTS

1 Stroke is the leading cause of disability and fourth cause of death in the United States. Of the 800,000 annual strokes in the United States, 85% are acute ischemic strokes (AIS).

2 Intensive care issues pertinent to the care of AIS include the recognition and diagnosis of stroke, the provision of fibrinolytics and/or endovascular management, as well the medical management in the 24 hours posttreatment, and management of cerebellar or large hemispheric infarcts (LHIs).

3 Clinical symptoms of stroke are highly heterogeneous and variable and are objectively scored using the National Institutes of Health Stroke Scale (NIHSS).

4 Intravenous recombinant tissue plasminogen activator (IV-rtPA) should be administered as soon as possible to all patients with AIS who meet inclusion/exclusion criteria.

5 Endovascular treatment (EVT) is recommended in AIS patients with an internal carotid artery (ICA) or M1 occlusion who are more than 17 years of age, receiving IV-rtPA and have a prestroke modified Rankin Score (mRS) of 0 to 1, NIHSS greater than 5, and Alberta stroke program early computed tomography score (ASPECTS) greater than 5, and who can have EVT initiated (ie, groin puncture) within 6 hours of their last known well time.

6 During and after the administration of reperfusion therapy (IV-rtPA or endovascular), blood pressure (BP) parameters must be vigilantly maintained (< 180/105 mm Hg). All antiplatelet and anticoagulant medications are held for at least the first 24 hours. Aspirin should be provided 24 hours after IV-rtPA or EVT if the patient is neurologically stable and neuroimaging does not demonstrate hemorrhagic conversion of the infarct.

7 The management of LHI includes therapies aimed to minimize the development of cerebral edema and identifying candidates for decompressive hemicraniectomy (DC).

8 Surgical options in the management of intracerebral hemorrhage (ICH) include craniotomy with or without clot evacuation and, in the setting of obstructive hydrocephalus due to intraventricular hemorrhage, the placement of an intraventricular catheter.

9 Treatment goals for patients with subarachnoid hemorrhage in the first 6 hours include BP control, cardiopulmonary stability, correction of symptomatic hydrocephalus, treatment of intracranial hypertension, reversal of herniation syndromes, and consideration of antifibrinolytics.

ACUTE ISCHEMIC STROKE

Stroke is the leading cause of disability and fourth greatest cause of death in the United States. Of the 800,000 annual strokes in the United States, 85% are acute ischemic strokes (AIS). The remaining 15% are intracerebral hemorrhage (ICH) or subarachnoid hemorrhage (SAH). Intensive care issues pertinent to the care of AIS include the recognition and diagnosis of stroke, the provision of fibrinolytics and/ or endovascular management, as well the medical management in the 24 hours posttreatment, management of cerebellar or large hemispheric infarcts (LHIs), and considerations in the management of a critical stenosis of a cervical arterial vessel.

History and Physical Examination

AIS is the result of a sudden loss of blood flow within a vascular region of the brain, retina, or spinal cord due to arterial vessel occlusion. The flow is most often compromised by the development of an atherosclerotic clot (ie, thrombosis) or sudden occlusion by a clot from a distant source (ie, embolism). The contemporary definition includes imaging findings of an acute infarction, even if clinical symptoms are not observed. Clinical symptoms of stroke are highly heterogeneous and variable (Table 48B–1) and are objectively scored using the National Institutes of Health Stroke Scale (NIHSS) (Table 48B–2). Presentations associated with a delay in stroke diagnosis included mild symptoms (NIHSS < 4), severe symptoms (NIHSS > 25), strokes affecting multiple vascular territories, isolated aphasia,

TABLE 48B–1 Common signs and symptoms of acute ischemic stroke.

- Hemiparesis, monoparesis, or (rarely) quadriparesis (in brainstem stroke)
- Hemisensory deficits
- Monocular or binocular visual loss
- Visual field deficits
- Diplopia
- Dysarthria
- Facial asymmetry
- Ataxia
- Vertigo (rarely in isolation)
- Aphasia
- Sudden decrease in the level of consciousness

posterior circulation symptoms, and young age. Symptoms typically begin suddenly, but a stuttering presentation can be seen in the setting of a partially occluded large vessel. The patient's last known well time (LKWT, ie, when they did not have any stroke symptoms) must be aggressively, thoroughly, and creatively sought (eg, using last social media interaction).

The physical examination is focused on cataloging a very accurate NIHSS, exploring for etiologies of stroke mimics, and findings suggestive of contraindications to intravenous (IV) thrombolysis (eg, scar from recent surgery).

Diagnostics

The ideal diagnostic approach utilizes lean processing, with a prioritization of diagnostics that are critical for the decision to offer thrombolysis with IV recombinant tissue plasminogen activator (IV-rtPA) (see treatment, later). A list of comprehensive diagnostics is found in Table 48B–3. Critical immediate diagnostics are a blood glucose and noncontrast head computed tomography (NCHCT) to rule out hypoglycemia and an intracranial hemorrhage, respectively. The remaining diagnostics should be immediately obtained, but stroke specialists will not uncommonly make decisions to offer IV-rtPA based on patient-related factors, rather than waiting for the results. This is to hasten the provision of thrombolysis, as a 15-minute delay in treatment is associated with worsened outcomes, even if within 3 hours of symptom onset and within an hour of hospital presentation.

The timing of CT angiography (CTA) of the head and neck, CT perfusion, and/or magnetic resonance imaging (MRI) is dependent on local protocols and patient specific conditions. The acquisition of these images should never delay the administration of thrombolysis. A diagnosis of AIS is most commonly confirmed using MRI through interpretation of the diffusion-weighted imaging (DWI) and apparent diffusion coefficient (ADC) sequences. An acute stroke (< 7 days) has occurred when a specific region of the brain is bright (hyperintense) on DWI and dark on ADC. Magnetic resonance angiography (MRA) is also able to characterize the cerebral and cervical vasculatures.

TABLE 48B–2 National institutes of health stroke scale (NIHSS).

Item	Category	Description	Score Range
1a	Level of consciousness (LOC)	Alert, drowsy, stuporous, coma	0-3
1b	LOC questions (month, age)	Answers both, one, or none correctly	0-2
1c	LOC commands (open and close eyes, grip and release hand)	Obeys both, one, or none	0-2
2	Best gaze	Normal, partial palsy, forced deviation	0-2
3	Best visual (visual fields)	Normal, partial hemianopia, complete hemianopia, bilateral hemianopia	0-3
4	Facial palsy	Normal, minor, partial, complete	0-3
5a	Motor arm, left	No drift, drift, some effort against gravity, no effort against gravity, no movement	0-4
5b	Motor arm, right	No drift, drift, some effort against gravity, no effort against gravity, no movement	0-4
6a	Motor leg, left	No drift, drift, some effort against gravity, no effort against gravity, no movement	0-4
6b	Motor leg, right	No drift, drift, some effort against gravity, no effort against gravity, no movement	0-4
7	Limb ataxia	None, present in one limb, present in both	0-2
8	Sensory	Normal, mild to moderate loss, severe to complete loss	0-2
9	Best language	No aphasia, mild to moderate aphasia, severe aphasia, mute with global aphasia	0-3
10	Dysarthria	Normal, mild to moderate dysarthria, severe dysarthria	0-2
11	Extinction and inattention	No neglect, partial, complete	0-2
	Total	n/a	0-42

Data from National Institute of Health (NIH).

Treatment

Acute treatment of AIS consists of restoring blood flow to the compromised neuronal tissue. The first step is to determine eligibility for thrombolysis with IV-rtPA, which should be administered as soon as possible to all patients that meet inclusion/exclusion criteria (Table 48B–4) at a dose of 0.9 mg/kg, maximum dose 90 mg, with 10% bolused over 1 minute, and the remainder dripped over 1 hour. If possible, consent should be obtained, although if the patient is unable to consent and a legal representative is not available, IV-rtPA should be administered, as the benefits outweigh the risks of treatment and

the degree of benefit is time-dependent. If a stroke mimic (ie, neurologic change concerned for AIS) is suspected, but cannot be definitely determined, and no contraindications exist, IV-rtPA administration should not be delayed.

AIS secondary to large vessel occlusions (LVOs), particularly those with large clots (> 8 mm), respond poorly to IV-rtPA alone. Recent randomized controlled trials (RCTs) have concluded that endovascular treatment (EVT) of AIS improves outcomes in those with anterior circulation LVOs (ie, internal carotid artery [ICA] terminus and middle cerebral artery [MCA] M1). Identification and selection of candidates for this therapy can involve clinical

TABLE 48B-3 Acute ischemic stroke diagnostics.

On Presentation	During Admission
• **Finger stick blood glucose**	• Hgb a1c
• Complete blood count	• Lipids
• Basic metabolic panel	• Thyroid studies
• PT/INR/aPTT	• Transthoracic echocardiography (TTE) with bubble study
• Pregnancy test	
• Troponin	• Cervical and intracranial vessel imaging (MRA, CTA, DSA, or Carotid Dopplers[b])
• Electrocardiogram	
• Chest X-ray	
• **Noncontrast head CT**	• Hypercoagulability panel[c]
• CT angiography head and neck[a]	• Cardiac MRI[c]
• CT perfusion head[a]	• Transesophageal echocardiography[c]
	• LE Dopplers/CT pulmonary Angiography[d]
	• Rheumatologic work up[e]
	• CSF studies[e]

MRA, magnetic resonance angiography; CTA, computed tomography angiography; DSA, digital subtraction angiography; CSF, cerebrospinal fluid.
Bold and italics: Most critical diagnostics for IV rtPA decision making. Other studies are required in the appropriate clinical context or when possible contraindication to IV rtPA is suspected based on history, medical record review, and physical examination.
[a]Consult your institutional/regional protocols or stroke team for the role and timing of CT angiography and perfusion studies in AIS. These are critical diagnostics routinely utilized in acute decision making in AIS.
[b]CTA or MRA are preferred over carotid Dopplers, when possible.
[c]Often performed in those less than 50 years with AIS of unknown etiology.
[d]Consider in those with a positive bubble study on TTE and unknown AIS etiology.
[e]Performed in those with AIS presumed or suspected to be due to primary or secondary central nervous system vasculitis.

assessment, CTA, or MRA. The administration of IV-rtPA should never be delayed for the acquisition of angiography. Based on these new data, American Heart Association/American Stroke Association (AHA/ASA) AIS guidelines now make the class 1 recommendation that EVT should be provided to AIS patients with an ICA or M1 occlusion who are more than 17 years of age, receiving IV-rtPA and have a prestoke modified Rankin Score (mRS) of 0 to 1 (see Table 48B-5), NIHSS greater than 5 (Table 48B-2), and Alberta stroke program early CT score (ASPECTS) greater than 5 (see Table 48B-6), and who can have EVT initiated (ie, groin puncture) within 6 hours of their LKWT. Patients should never be observed for a response to IV-rtPA who meet the indications for EVT. As with IV-rtPA, time to

endovascular recanalization has been shown to be a predictor of outcomes.

Of note, the first 3 endovascular trials did not find a benefit, which has been attributed to the poor recanalization rates with the early generation devices. The 5 most recent RCTs, all of which were positive, used newer generation stent retrievers that achieve a much higher rate of vessel recanalization. Although the strongest recommendations were made for those with a mRS of 0 to 1, NIHSS of greater than 5, and ASPECTS of greater than 5, those that fail to meet these criteria should not be interpreted as having an absolute contraindication to EVT. Rather, a class IIb recommendation was issued that it may be reasonable to acutely revascularize some patients with a M1 or ICA occlusion within 6 hours of LKWT, who do not meet all of the ASPECTS, NIHSS, and mRS criteria. More distal MCA (M2, M3), anterior cerebral artery (ACA), basilar artery, and posterior cerebral artery (PCA) occlusions can also be considered for EVT, but the degree of benefit is less certain, as they were either less prevalent or not included in the recent RCTs. Lastly, patients with contraindications to IV-rtPA, but within the 6-hour time window, can be considered for acute EVT (eg, international normalized ratio [INR] > 1.7).

During and after the administration of reperfusion therapy (IV-rtPA or endovascular) the patient requires frequent reassessment, with careful attention to their neurologic status and blood pressure (BP). BP parameters must be vigilantly maintained (< 180/105). All antiplatelet (AP) and anticoagulant (AC) medications are held for at least the first 24 hours. Aspirin, which has been shown to reduce stroke reoccurrence and mortality, should be provided 24 hours after IV-rtPA or EVT if the patient is neurologically stable and neuroimaging does not demonstrate hemorrhagic conversion of the infarct. In some circumstances, BP targets maybe more strict after EVT with full revascularization (thrombolysis in cerebral infarction 3 or 2b flow).

BP targets in patients not receiving IV-rtPA are less clear. Current guidelines support gentle BP reduction if the systolic BP (SBP) greater than 220 mm Hg or the diastolic BP is greater than 120 mm Hg. If performed, a modest goal should be set, so as to avoid expanding the infarct by hypoperfusing penumbral tissue, particularly in those with untreated LVOs.

TABLE 48B–4 Inclusion/exclusion criteria for intravenous recombinant tissue plasminogen activator in acute ischemic stroke.

Inclusion Criteria

- Diagnosis of ischemic stroke causing measurable neurologic deficit
- Neurologic signs not clearing spontaneously to baseline
- Neurologic signs not minor and isolated[a]
- Symptom onset less than 4.5 hours from initiation of IV rtPA (see below additional exclusion criteria for the 3.0-4.5 hour window)

Exclusion Criteria

History and physical
- Symptoms suggest subarachnoid hemorrhage
- Significant head trauma or prior stroke in the previous 3 months
- Arterial puncture at noncompressible site in previous 7 days
- History of previous intracranial hemorrhage
- Intracranial neoplasm, AVM, or aneurysm
- Recent intracranial or intraspinal surgery
- Elevated blood pressure (systolic >185 mm Hg or diastolic >110 mm Hg)
- Active internal bleeding
- Stroke suspected to resulting from a septic embolus (eg, infective endocarditis[a])

Laboratory investigations
- Platelet count less than 100,000/µL
- Heparin received within 48 hours with aPTT above the upper limit of normal
- Current use of Vitamin K Antagonist with INR >1.7 or PT >15 s
- Current use of direct thrombin inhibitors or direct factor Xa inhibitors with elevated sensitive laboratory tests (eg, aPTT, INR, platelet count, ECT, TT, or appropriate factor Xa activity assays)
- Blood glucose concentration less than 50 mg/dL (2.7 mmol/L)

Imaging findings
- Head CT demonstrates multilobar infarction (hypodensity >1/3 cerebral hemisphere)

Relative Exclusion Criteria

- Minor or rapidly improving stroke symptoms
- Pregnancy
- Seizure at onset with postictal residual neurological impairments
- Major surgery or serious trauma within previous 14 days
- Gastrointestinal or urinary tract hemorrhage within previous 21 days
- Acute myocardial infarction within previous 3 months

Exclusion Criteria for the 3 to 4.5 hour Time Window

- More than 80 years of age
- Use of oral anticoagulants, regardless of the INR
- Baseline NIHSS score of more than 25
- History of stroke and diabetes

[a]The threshold for treatment is not based on the score on the NIHSS. Rather it is a subjective determination of the functional impact of the deficit on the patient's outcome.
Data from Demaerschalk BM, Kleindorfer DO, Adeoye OM, et al: Scientific Rationale for the Inclusion and Exclusion Criteria for Intravenous Alteplase in Acute Ischemic Stroke, Stroke 2016 Feb;47(2):581-641.

Large Hemispheric Infarction

AIS secondary to the occlusion of a cervical or large proximal intracranial vessel, such as the carotid terminus (ICA-t) or MCA, is termed LHI. Although LHIs only account for 10% of all AIS, their mortality rate is 15% to 80% and the majority of survivors have significant disability. Clinical manifestations include hemiparesis, homonymous hemianopsia, ipsilateral gaze deviation, aphasia (usually with left LHIs), and agnosia and left-sided neglect (with right LHIs).

TABLE 48B-5 Modified rankin scale.

Score	Clinical Symptoms
0	No symptoms at all
1	No significant disability despite symptoms; able to carry out all usual duties and activities
2	Slight disability; unable to carry out all previous activities, but able to look after own affairs without assistance
3	Moderate disability; requiring some help, but able to walk without assistance
4	Moderately severe disability; unable to walk without assistance and unable to attend to own bodily needs without assistance
5	Severe disability; bedridden, incontinent, and requiring constant nursing care and attention
6	Dead

TABLE 48B-6 Alberta stroke program early CT score (ASPECTS).

Region	Anatomic Location	Head CT Level
C	Caudate head	
LN	Lentiform nuclear or putamen	
IC	Posterior limb of internal capsule	
I	Insular cortex	Third ventricle
M1	Frontal operculum (anterior MCA territory)	
M2	Anterior temporal lobe (lateral to insula)	
M3	Posterior temporal lobe	
M4	Anterior MCA, superior to M1	
M5	Lateral MCA, superior to M2	Lateral ventricles, superior to third ventricle
M6	Posterior MCA, superior to M3	

This score is for anterior circulation ischemic strokes and is used to quantify the amount of territory with ischemic changes on a noncontrast Head CT (NCHCT). Starting from a score of 10 (signifying a NCHCT without ischemic changes) one point is deducted for each of the above areas with ischemic changes (ie, hypodense). Scores of more than 6 are associated with better outcomes. Most recent endovascular treatment trials required a score of more than 5, but there is some evidence that even those with a score of more than 3 may derive benefit from revascularization.

The large area of infarcted brain tissue produces substantial clinical defects at ictus. Over the following 24 to 96 hours (and less commonly up to 10 days) cytotoxic edema (CE) develops, causing the tissue to enlarge, which then compresses, distorts, and herniates neighboring uninfarcted tissues. Unaffected cerebral vessels can be pinched or kinked by the herniating infarcted brain, expanding the territory of infarction.

The first clinical sign of cerebral edema is a decline in the level of arousal. This is followed by ipsilateral or contralateral leg weakness (due to compression of the anterior cerebral artery in the setting of subfalcine herniation). Alternatively or later, findings of uncal herniation (see Chapter 48A—Principles of Neurosciences Critical Care) are seen, during which time the PCA may be compressed expanding the area of infarction. The lateral forces may also compress the third ventricle, producing an obstructive hydrocephalus and its associated symptoms.

The management of LHI includes therapies aimed to minimize the development of CE and identifying candidates for decompressive hemicraniectomy (DC). Strategies that mitigate CE include keeping the head of bed elevated to 30° and the neck in a neutral position, avoiding hypervolemia, and maintaining normothermia, normonatremia, normoglycemia, and normocarbia. The infusion of dextrose containing and hypoosmotic solutions must not occur.

Empiric administration of hyperosmotic solutions is not an uncommon practice, but evidence is lacking to support its efficacy. Aggressively maintaining the serum blood glucose below 125 mg/dL may lead to an increase in infarct size, so a goal of 140 to 180 mg/dL is recommended. Seizure prophylaxis is not indicated, but continuous video electroencephalogram (cvEEG) monitoring can be considered, particularly in patients with fluctuations in mental status. Corticosteroids do not have a proven role in the management of LHI. Dual AP therapy and therapeutic anticoagulation should be held, but subcutaneous heparin or low-molecular-weight heparin should be used for venous thromboembolism (VTE) prophylaxis.

Unfortunately, the available evidence is not able to fully predict which patient is going to have cerebral edema. Intracranial pressure (ICP) monitoring is of limited utility and is not typically performed. Instead the neurologic examination is performed at frequent, regular intervals. Older patients have some degree of cerebral atrophy; therefore they are less likely to deteriorate even if cerebral edema occurs, while the opposite holds true for the younger patient. Risk factors for cerebral edema and subsequent neurologic deterioration include female gender, nausea and vomiting on presentation, congestive heart failure, history of hypertension, leukocytosis, and initial NIHSS greater than 20 in dominant LHI or greater than 15 in nondominant LHI. Neuroimaging findings suggesting increased risk are summarized in Table 48B–7.

In the event that hemispheric swelling occurs causing symptomatic neurologic deterioration, the initial response is to provide therapies that reduce cerebral edema, such as bolus hyperosmolar therapy (eg, 30 mL of 23.4% hypertonic saline or 1-1.5 mg/kg of 20% mannitol). See Chapter _____ for further guidance on the management of cytotoxic cerebral edema/intracranial hypertension. Ultimately, 70% to 80% of patients will die with maximal medical therapy in the absence of early surgical intervention (ie, DC).

Five randomized control trials have explored the efficacy of early DC in LHI. Overall results demonstrate a reduction in mortality (from ~70% to ~20%) and an improvement in functional outcomes in those 18 to 60 years of age. A recent trial demonstrated a similar reduction in mortality in older patients (61-82 years of age), although functional outcomes were not improved. When a DC is performed it should create a bony window of greater than or equal to 12 cm in the anterior-posterior dimension, with a medial border 1 cm lateral to the superior sagittal sinus and inferior border at the floor of the middle cranial fossa. The dura is then opened with cruciate incision (ie, durotomy). Although the timing

TABLE 48B–7 Neuroimaging findings associated with an increased risk of neurologic deterioration in large hemispheric infarction.

Imaging	Timing	Finding
MRI DWI sequence	6 hours after onset	Infarct > 80 mL
MRI DWI sequence	Within 14 hours of onset	Infarct > 145 mL
NCHCT	Within 6 hours of onset	Frank hypodensity > 1/3 of MCA territory
NCHCT	Admission	Dense MCA
NCHCT	Within 48 hours of onset	MLS > or = 5 mm
NCHCT or MRI	Any point	Involvement of multiple vascular territories
NCHCT or MRI	Any point	Infarct of 50% of MCA territory
NCHCT or MRI	Any point	MCA infarct involves the basal ganglia
CTA head, MRA head, catheter angiography	Any point	Occlusion at the carotid terminus
CTA head, MRA head, catheter angiography	Any point	Incomplete circle of Willis
CTA head or catheter angiography	Any point	Marginal leptomeningeal collaterals

MRI DWI, magnetic resonance imaging diffuse weighted imaging; NCHCT, noncontrast head CT; MCA, middle cerebral artery; MLS, mid-line shift; CTA, CT angiography; MRA, magnetic resonance angiography.

of DC was not uniform among the published data, a consistent benefit was seen if it was performed within 48 hours of stroke onset in those experiencing neurologic deterioration. It is uniformly felt that once deterioration occurs, DC should be performed promptly, as unreversed herniation will produce irreversible brainstem injury. Although the evidence for its efficacy is not clear more than 48 hours after stroke onset, it is similarly felt that if deterioration occurs, benefits are likely to be seen.

When considering DC, patients and families must be aware that the procedure is not restorative. That is, it is a lifesaving procedure that may help reduce the degree of loss in functionality in the young patient (< 60 years of age), while strictly striving to save the life of the older patient, who will most likely be left moderately to severely disabled at 12 months (ie, mRS of 4 or 5, see Table 48B–5.) It is best to inform the patient and family of their possible candidacy for the procedure on admission to the ICU. That way if deterioration does occur, they will not be forced to make a hasty decision under duress. Furthermore, neurosurgery should be engaged on admission to avoid unnecessary procedural delays in the event of neurologic deterioration.

Cerebellar Infarctions

Similar to LHI, cerebellar strokes are subject to swelling and mass effect leading to herniation. Although they are smaller infarcts, their infratentorial location and juxtaposition to the fourth ventricle lends less room for their growth. Small increases in volume can compress the fourth ventricle, producing obstructive hydrocephalus. Further swelling will directly compress the brainstem.

As with LHI, similar measures to reduce the likelihood of swelling apply. If neurologic deterioration occurs, ICP lowering therapies can temporarily reverse the mass effect of the swelling, but ultimately surgical intervention is required. Obstructive hydrocephalus from fourth ventricular obstruction is often addressed with the placement of an external ventricular drain (EVD), but this will cause the swollen cerebellum to herniate upward, compressing and kinking the brainstem, producing local ischemia and potentially infarction of the midbrain and pons. Therefore, a suboccipital craniectomy (SOC) should be performed immediately after or simultaneously with EVD placement, which will allow for the swollen cerebellum to temporarily herniate extracranially. In contrast to LHI, nearly 3/4 of patients with large cerebellar infarcts will have very good outcomes.

INTRACEREBRAL HEMORRHAGE

ICH, also referred to as "hemorrhagic stroke," constitutes approximately 15% of all strokes and has an incidence of approximately 25 cases per 100,000 person-years. When compared with AIS of similar presenting severity, the mortality and long-term morbidity of ICH is greater. Management of ICH includes measures to prevent further hematoma expansion, mitigate and treat cerebral edema, prevent further neurologic deterioration, and provide excellent supportive care. Although ICH carries a high morbidity and mortality, decisions on the withdrawal of life sustaining therapy (WLST) and early do-not-resuscitate (DNR) have been found to contribute greatly to outcomes. Prognostication is difficult and ambivalent cases with supportive and willing surrogate decision makers should be allowed time to declare their outcomes, in lieu of the early implementation of WLST.

History and Physical Examination

Those presenting with a headache, unexplained nausea and vomiting, or neurologic change may be harboring an ICH. Clinical features commonly seen in, but not specific to ICH, include nausea, vomiting, impaired level of consciousness, severe hypertension, and headache. As with any neurologic emergency, the LKWT must be expeditious ascertained. Patients presenting within 6 hours of symptom onset are much more likely to experience further enlargement of the hematoma. Hematoma volume is predictive of poor outcomes, therefore those presenting quickly after onset may respond favorable to treatments targeting hemostasis. A history of AC or AP use must be obtained.

Diagnostics

Any patient suspected of having an ICH should immediately receive a NCHCT. MRI can also detect an ICH, particularly when T2*, gradient-recalled echo (GRE), or susceptibility weighted images (SWI) are obtained, but a NCHCT is typically much quicker to obtain. Simultaneous information should be obtained about their hemostatic capacity by obtaining a complete blood count, basic metabolic panel, prothrombin time (PT), INR, and activated partial thromboplastin time (aPTT). Some centers routinely obtain viscoelastic tests, such as thromboelastography, and platelet function assays, but the value of these diagnostics and subsequent therapies targeting their "correction" is as yet unclear.

A critical component of ICH care is determining the etiology of the ICH. Subcortical and pontine ICHs commonly result from hypertension-induced lipohyalinosis of the small perforating arteries in the pons, thalamus, and basal ganglia. Cerebral amyloid angiopathy (CAA) is more common in those more than 70 years of age and involves the cortical regions (lobar ICH). ICHs due to ruptured vascular malformations (arteriovenous malformation [AVM], cavernous, aneurysms, dural arteriovenous fistula [dAVf]) must be promptly identified promptly to allow for prompt surgical interventions that will mitigate rebleeding. Other etiologies are listed in Table 48B–8. CT or MRA is highly sensitive for underlying vascular malformations. Younger patients, those without a history of hypertension or coagulopathy, and females are at greater risk for vascular malformations. The secondary ICH (sICH) score maybe helpful in deciding who should

undergo angiography to rule out an underlying vascular malformation (see Table 48B–9).

CTA may also identify a "spot sign" or evidence of contract extravasation into the hematoma, implying that the hemorrhage is ongoing and the hematoma is enlarging. The clinical utility of this information is as yet unclear. Ongoing trials are exploring the value of administering a prohemostatic agent (either activated factor VIIa [aFVIIa] in STOP-IT and SPOTLIGHT or tranexamic acid [TXA] in the SPOT-AUST) in those with a "spot sign." Other features on the NCHCT suggestive of hematoma expansion include a heterogeneous appearance of the ICH, larger volumes, and those with ventricular extension.

The volume of ICH can be estimated on NCHCT by applying the $(A \times B \times C)/2$ method, where A represents the maximal diameter on an axial image, B is the diameter perpendicular to A, and C is the height of the ICH, as determined by the number of axial slices the ICH is seen on times the width of the slices. Applying this method on serial images provides a quasiobjective was of assessing for hematoma growth. The severity of the ICH is often quantified by determining the ICH score (see Table 48B–10). This score should not be used to assign outcomes, as its correlation with outcomes worsens when excluding those that have undergone WLST.

Treatment

An immediate treatment goal is to stop further hemorrhaging from occurring, as hematoma size is predictive of poor outcome. In parallel, those with acute neurologic deterioration due to cerebral herniation or mass effect may require craniectomy and/or clot evacuation, while those with symptomatic hydrocephalus due to intraventricular hemorrhage (IVH) may undergo ventricular catheterization.

BP control and reduction is a must to mitigate hematoma expansion. Two large randomized trials have been completed in this realm. Second Intensive Blood Pressure Reduction in Acute Cerebral Hemorrhage Trial (INTERACT-2) randomized ICH patients presenting within 6 hours of onset and a SBP of 150 to 220 mm Hg to a target SBP of less than 140 mm Hg or less than 180 mm Hg (without a prescribed approach). No difference in mortality or adverse effects were seen, but an ordinal analysis

TABLE 48B-8 Etiologies of intracerebral hemorrhage.

Chronic hypertension
Cerebral amyloid angiopathy (CAA)
Coagulopathy
Sympathomimetic drug abuse (eg, cocaine and methamphetamines)
Arteriovenous malformation
Cavernous malformation
Arterial aneurysm (saccular or mycotic)
Dural arteriovenous fistula
Moyamoya
Hemorrhagic conversion of acute ischemic stroke
Hemorrhagic conversion of venous infarct from cerebral venous thrombosis or dural sinus thrombosis
Primary or metastatic tumor
Vasculitis

TABLE 48B-9 Secondary ICH score.

Determination				Interpretation	
Age (Years)	**NCHCT***	**Gender**	**Hx of HTN or Admission Coagulopathy[a]**	**Total Score**	**% CTA Positive**
> 70 = 0 46-70 = 1 18-45 = 2	Low probability = 0 Indeterminate probability = 1 High probability = 2	Male = 0 Female = 1	Either = 0 Neither = 1	0	0
				1	~1.5
				2	~5
				3	~20
				4	~40
				5	~85
				6	100

Hx, past medical history; HTN, hypertension; CTA, computed tomography angiography; NCHCT, noncontrast head computed tomography.
[a]NCHCT probability determination:
- High-probability NCHCT either:
  1. Enlarged vessels or calcifications along the margins of the ICH
  2. Hyperattenuation within a dural venous sinus or cortical vein along the presumed venous drainage path of the ICH
- Low-probability NCHCT has both of the following:
  1. No high-probability features
  2. ICH is located in the basal ganglia, thalamus, or brain stem
- Indeterminate NCHCT: does not meet high- or low-probability criteria.
[b]Admission INR more than 3, aPTT more than 80 seconds, platelet less than 50,000, or daily antiplatelet therapy.

found a statistically significant reduction in the mRS (Table 48B-5) in the group targeted to a SBP of less than 140 mm Hg. Based on these data, the subsequent AHA/ASA ICH guidelines published in 2015 were updated to state "for ICH patients presenting with SBP between 150 and 220 mm Hg and without contraindication to acute BP treatment, acute lowering of SBP to 140 mm Hg is safe (class I; level of evidence A) and can be effective for improving functional outcome (class IIa; level of evidence B)." The most recent RCT of SBP control in ICH, Antihypertensive Treatment of Acute Cerebral Hemorrhage

TABLE 48B-10 ICH score.

Determination					Interpretation	
GCS	**ICH Volume**	**IVH Present**	**ICH Location**	**Patient Age**	**Total Score**	**Mortality (%)**
< 5 = 2 5-12 = 1 > 12 = 0	> 30 mL = 1 < 30 mL = 0	Yes = 1 No = 0	Infratentorial = 1 Supratentorial = 0	< 80 = 0 > 80 = 1	0	0
					1	13
					2	26
					3	72
					4	97
					5	100
					6	100[a]

GCS, Glasgow Coma Scale; ICH, intracerebral hemorrhage; IVH, intraventricular hemorrhage.
[a]Estimated, insufficient number of cases when described.

(ATACH-2), failed to find any difference in functional outcomes or hematoma growth, but there were more renal adverse events in the intensive control, compared to the conventional control arm (SBP < 140 mm Hg vs < 180 mm Hg, 9% vs 4%, number needed to harm of 20). These conflicting findings maybe explained by how the patients in the each arm of ATACH-2 and INTERACT-2 were actually treated, as the conventional treatment arm in ATACH-2 had SBPs lower than the intensive arm in INTERACT-2. In the absence of updated guidelines, the best recommendation based on available data is to lower the SBP to 140 to 150 mm Hg in those presenting with a SBP of 180 to 240 mm Hg. If the SBP is greater than 240 mm Hg, a 25% reduction is a reasonable goal, followed by reassessment for tolerance of a lower SBP. Additionally, a post-hoc analysis of the INTERACT-2 trial found that increasing degrees of BP variability were associated with worse outcomes, suggesting that continuous SBP management is preferred to reactionary maneuvers by using a continuous infusion of an antihypertensive, such as nicardipine, labetalol, or clevidipine.

Acute ICH complicated by ACs or coagulopathy must be provided reversal or prohemostatic therapy immediately and without delay. The time to "reversal" is predictive of outcome, with those achieving their target BP and antithrombotic reversal within 4 hours of onset having the best outcomes. Table 48B–11 provides a summary of ACs and suggested reversal strategies. The impact of APs on outcomes and how they should be managed in ICH is less clear. A recently completed RCT of platelet transfusion for reversal of AP activity in nonvascular supratentorial ICH patients presenting within 6 hours of onset, a history of AP use (aspirin, $P2Y_{12}$ inhibitor, or adenosine reuptake inhibitor), and not requiring an intraventricular catheter (IVC) or surgery found that not only was platelet transfusion ineffective in reducing hematoma expansion, but it was also observed to worsen outcomes and increase the risk of neurologic deterioration. Therefore, platelet transfusion should not be performed in this subcategory of ICH. Table 48B–12 provides a recommended approach to ICH complicated by AP agents.

After the initial several hours, secondary intracranial and systemic effects are the next layer of complications that are to be managed. Perihematomal edema develops early, and commonly peaks in the following 4 to 7 days, but atypically courses are seen and can last for upward of a month. Management includes the maintenance of normoglycemia, normothermia, normonatremia, and avoidance of elevated central venous pressures. Fever is associated with worsened outcomes, but temperature control has not been proven to improve outcomes, and maybe associated with longer hospital stays and increased tracheostomy.

Seizures, both convulsive and nonconvulsive, are common are ICH, particularly in those with larger more symptomatic and cortical hemorrhages. Prophylaxis with phenytoin has been associated with, but not causational of, worse outcomes. Guidelines recommend against seizure prophylaxis with antiepileptic drugs, but it is not unreasonable to do so in those at higher risk. A low threshold should be kept for evaluation for nonconvulsive seizures with continuous electroencephalography, particularly in those whose neurologic examination is worse than expected.

Up to one quarter of intubated ICH patients will develop acute respiratory distress syndrome (ARDS), therefore lung protective ventilation should be provided after intubation, as long as normocarbia and ICP can be maintained. Hyperoxia is associated with worsen outcomes in ICH, among other acute brain injuries, therefore normoxia should be targeted at all times, sans the peri-intubation period to prevent hypoxia during airway establishment.

The timing of VTE prophylaxis is not clearly guided by available evidence. Best practice at this time is to initiate pharmacologic VTE prophylaxis with unfractionated or low-molecular-weight heparin 24 hours after demonstrated ICH stability (ie, no further hematoma expansion), assuming there is not underlying coagulopathy. Sequential compression devices should be placed immediately. In the case of a newly diagnosed VTE during the course of care, there is a lack of evidence to advise on when it is safe to initiate therapeutic anticoagulation. A common practice is to wait at least 14, if not 30 days after an ICH. Depending on the etiology of the ICH, the patient may never be a candidate for therapeutic anticoagulation (eg, unsecured vascular etiology or CAA).

TABLE 48B–11 Suggested anticoagulant reversal strategies.

Category	Specific Medications	"Reversal"[a]	Notes
Vitamin K antagonists	Warfarin	Vitamin K 10 mg IV AND 3F- or 4F-PCC[b,c]	IF PCC unavailable or CI to PCC, then 15-20 mL/kg of FFP
Xa inhibitors (Xa-Is)	Rivaroxaban, Apixaban, Edoxaban	aPCC (FEIBA) or 4F-PCC, 50 units/kg If < 2 hours from last drug ingestion, 50 g of activated charcoal oral	A pre- and post-4F-PCC PT should be obtained. Studies of 4F-PCC administration for Xa-Is demonstrate complete normalization of the PT
Direct thrombin inhibitors (DTI)	Oral competitive inhibitor—Dabigatran IV, reversible inhibitors—Argatroban, Bivalirudin SC, irreversible inhibitor[d]*—Desirudin	For dabigatran ONLY—Idarucizumab 5 g IV[e] If < 2 hours from last drug ingestion, 50 gm of activated charcoal oral Other DTIs[f]	Pre- and post-PTT should be obtained for dabigatran, as with Xa-Is
Unfractionated heparin (UFH)	Heparin (IV and SC)	Protamine 1 mg IV for every 100 units of heparin administered in the previous 2-3 hours	Protamine dosing must be precise, as excess protamine becomes an anticoagulant itself
Low molecular weight heparin (LMWH)	Enoxaparin, Dalteparin, Nadroparin, Tinzaparin, Danaparoid	Enoxaparin w/in 8 hours: Protamine 1 mg IV per 1 mg Enoxaparin w/in 8-12 hours: Protamine 0.5 mg IV per 1 mg Dalteparin, Nadroparin, and Tinzaparin: w/in 3-5 half-lives of LMWH—Protamine 1 mg IV per 100 units If protamine contraindicated: rFVIIa 90 mcg/kg IV	Protamine dosing must be precise, as excess protamine becomes an anticoagulant itself
Penta saccharides	Fondaparinux	aPCC (FEIBA) 20 units/kg IV or rFVIIa 90 mcg/kg IV	
Thrombolytics	Alteplase, Reteplase, Tenecteplase	If thrombolytic still active, based on half-life of drug, then 1-2 g TXA or 4-5 g ECA IV Check fibrinogen, if low, administer cryoprecipitate	Alteplase is notable for metabolizing fibrinogen in addition to fibrin. AIS patients who receive IV rtPA and have the greatest drop in fibrinogen are at the greatest risk of hemorrhagic complication

IV, intravenous; SC, subcutaneous; 3F-PCC, 3 factor prothrombin complex concentrates; 4F-PCC, 4 factor prothrombin complex concentrates; aPCC, activated prothrombin complex concentrate; FEIBA, factor eight inhibitor bypassing activity; PT, prothrombin time; PTT, partial thromboplastin time; TXA, tranexamic acid; EACA, epsilon aminocaproic acid; AIS, acute ischemic stroke; rtPA, recombinant tissue plasminogen activator, that is, alteplase.

[a]If emergent neurosurgical intervention is required, consider 20 to 40 mcg/kg of recombinant activated factor VII (rFVIIa) just prior to surgery to compliment the administration of the above suggested agents for reversal of VKA, Xa Inhibitors, LMWH, nondabigatran DTIs, and Penta saccharides. Of note: rFVIIa is not to be administered if the patient has received aPCC/FEIBA, as these products already contain FVIIa.

[b]In all cases of PCC use, 4F-PCCs are preferred to 3F-PCCs.

[c]The dose of 4F-PCCs for VKA is dependent on INR; 25 unit/kg if INR 2 to 4, 35 unit/kg if INR 4 to 6, and 50 unit/kg if INR more than 6. A postreversal INR should be obtained. If INR is more than 1.3, more PCC or FFP should be administered. Of note: the manufacturer of K-Centra does not recommend repeat dosing.

[d]Lepirudin is another irreversible DTI. The manufacturer discontinued its production in 2012 for business reasons.

[e]If idarucizumab unavailable, then emergent hemodialysis to hasten drug elimination AND one of the following: FEIBA 50 unit/kg or 50 unit/kg 4F-PCC and 40-80 mcg/kg rFVIIa. If patient supratherapeutic on dabigatran due to overdose or impaired clearance, then redosing of idarucizumab may be required and should be guided by complete correction of the PTT, assuming no other condition (eg, lupus anticoagulant) or anticoagulant (eg, heparin) is present.

[f]The half-life of argatroban (~45 minutes), bivalirudin (~25 minutes), and desirudin (~2 hours) are quite short. Stopping their infusion/administration while administering a short burst of a prothrombotic regimen (eg, FEIBA 50 unit/kg or 50 unit/kg 4F-PCC and 40 mcg/kg rFVIIa) is a reasonable approach, but there is a severe paucity of evidence to guide this recommendation.

TABLE 48B-12 Suggested antiplatelet reversal strategies.

Category	Specific Medications	"Reversal"	Undergoing Neurosurgical Procedure[a]
Salicylates	Aspirin	DDAVP 0.4 mcg/kg IV	Platelet transfusion[b,c]
COX-1 and 2 inhibitors	Ibuprofen, Naproxen	DDAVP 0.4 mcg/kg IV	Nothing further
ADP/P2Y$_{12}$ inhibitors	Clopidogrel, Prasugrel, Ticlopidine, Ticagrelor[d]	DDAVP 0.4 mcg/kg IV	Platelet transfusion[b,c]
Adenosine reuptake inhibitors	Dipyridamole	DDAVP 0.4 mcg/kg IV	Platelet transfusion[b,c]
PDE III inhibitors	Cilostazol, Anagrelide	DDAVP 0.4 mcg/kg IV	Platelet transfusion[b,c]
GIIb/IIIa antagonists	Abciximab[e], Eptifibatide, Tirofiban	Hold agent[f]	10 units cryoprecipitate[g], platelet transfusion[b,c]

[a]In cases of significant clinical coagulopathy due to antiplatelet agents or congenital disorders of platelet function or the need to perform neurosurgical procedure in the setting of significant antiplatelet activity, activated recombinant factor VII (rFVIIa), 20 to 80 mcg/kg IV has been reported to have been used. However, it should be considered as a desperation measure and is not recommended for widespread use.
[b]Transfuse one single-donor apheresis unit (which is the same as 6 pooled units or one random donor unit per 10 kg of body weight).
[c]When possible, obtain platelet function assays before and after transfusion. Correction of the platelet function assay is seen in a minority of cases of attempted reversal with transfusion.
[d]Ticagrelor is a unique member of this category, as it is not a thienopyridine, but it is a P2Y$_{12}$ Inhibitor. Additionally, ticagrelor is the only reversible inhibitor of P2Y$_{12}$ receptor.
[e]In contrast to eptifibatide and tirofiban, abciximab is an irreversible inhibitor of the G IIb/IIIa receptor. Despite its plasma half-life of ~30 minutes, its receptor-binding half-life is 24 to 48 hours.
[f]The short half-lives of these agents leaves a short window of action for their "reversal." An exception is abciximab, as per the comments under **
[g]GIIb/IIIa platelet receptors allow for platelet-fibrinogen crosslinking. Given the larger quantity of fibrinogen in cryoprecipitate, its transfusion has been reported as a possible measure in hemorrhage complicated by GIIb/IIIa inhibitors.

Surgical options in the management of ICH include craniotomy with or without clot evacuation and, in the setting of obstructive hydrocephalus due to IVH, the placement of an IVC. Two randomized trials (Surgical Trial in Lobar Intracerebral Hemorrhage [STICH] and STICH-2) explored the value of craniotomy for supratentorial ICHs and failed to find a benefit, possibly due to the increased cerebral injury caused by the open craniotomy approach. As such, at present, craniotomy with surgical evacuation is largely considered in those with a deteriorating neurologic examination, symptomatic herniation syndromes, or refractory intracranial hypertension not amendable to medical therapy and diversion of cerebrospinal fluid (CSF) (when IVH complicates the ICH). The failure of open craniotomy led to an interest in minimally invasive stereotactic approaches to aspirate the hematoma. An approach currently under investigation is to stereotactically place a catheter into the hemorrhage, aspirate hematoma, and then leave the catheter in place to instill rtPA every 8 hours for 9 total doses (Minimally Invasive Surgery Plus rt-PA for Intracerebral Hemorrhage Evacuation [MISTIE III]).

ICH complicated by IVH causes obstructive hydrocephalus, which maybe aided by enhanced clearance of the ventricular clot with intraventricular rtPA. Clot Lysis: Evaluating Accelerated Resolution of Intraventricular Hemorrhage Phase III (CLEAR-III), a randomized trial of intraventricular rtPA in IVH, failed meet its primary outcome of increasing the proportion of patients with a good outcome (mRS 0-3), but there was a 10% reduction in mortality and a subgroup benefit in those with a large clots or if the catheter was inserted directly into the clot.

SUBARACHNOID HEMORRHAGE

SAH can occur spontaneously, which is often the result of a vascular malformation, such as an arterial aneurysm (aSAH), or from traumatic injury to bridging veins. The incidence of spontaneous SAH, which this section will focus on, is poorly quantified,

TABLE 48B–13 Etiologies of spontaneous SAH.

Type	Proportion (%)
Aneurysm	85
Perimesencephalic	10
Nonaneurysmal other: tumor, dural sinus thrombosis, cortical vein thrombosis, arterial dissection, RCVS, vascular lesion,[a] vasculitis, sickle cell disease, mycotic aneurysm, coagulopathy, sympathomimetic drugs	5

RCVS, reversible cerebral vasoconstriction syndrome.
[a]Arteriovenous malformation, dural arteriovenous fistula, amyloid angiopathy.

but is estimated to occur in 20 out of every 100,000 adults in the United States. A specific subtype of nonaneurysmal SAH is perimesencephalic SAH (PMSAH), which is thought to be due to a spontaneous venous rupture in the basilar cisterns, producing a radiographic pattern of SAH similar to that seen with aSAH, but it has a much more benign course. Table 48B–13 outlines etiologies of spontaneous SAH.

Risk factors for aSAH include hypertension, smoking, alcohol abuse, use of sympathomimetic drugs, such as cocaine, female sex, family history, collagen vascular diseases, such as type IV Ehlers-Danlos syndrome, and polycystic kidney disease. Cerebral arterial aneurysms are present in 3.6% to 6% of the population and more common in the anterior circulation. Rupture risk increases with aneurysm size and posterior circulation aneurysms.

When an aneurysm ruptures, the pressure in the subarachnoid space rapidly increases and approximates the arterial pressure. This can lead to a temporary decrease or cessation in blood flow to the brain, resulting clinically in syncope. During this period of reduced cerebral blood flow, a clot is able to tenuously form in the aneurysm, stopping further hemorrhaging. This sudden increase in ICP, combined with a brief period of cerebral ischemia can lead to the development of cerebral edema in the first several hours after the aneurysm rupture. Additionally, subarachnoid blood can obstruct the flow and absorption of CSF through the foramen of Luschka and Magendie and arachnoid granulations respectively, producing an obstructive and/ or communicating hydrocephalus. The tenuous clot in the recently ruptured aneurysm is a high risk for dislodgement, making early surgical obliteration of the aneurysm a priority. Beginning at about day 4 after the aneurysm bleed, the risk for cerebral vasospasm (VSP) resulting in delayed cerebral ischemia (DCI) begins. This typically lasts for 14 days, with the peak period being 7 to 10 days postbleed, but can be seen up to 28 days from ictus.

Outcomes after aSAH are highly associated with the severity of presenting symptoms, quantity of SAH, comorbidities, and age. Overall mortality rate ranges from 30% to 40%, with nearly half of survivors experiencing some type of permanent disability. More subtle deficits in memory, executive function, and language ability, as well as psychiatric symptoms, such as anxiety or depression are common. Despite the high morbidity and mortality, even patients with severe presentations can experience outcomes that allow them to return to independent living or a high quality of life.

History and Physical Examination

The most common presenting symptom of aSAH is headache. Less common presentations are syncope or new onset lethargy or confusion. Deciding which headaches are concerning for aSAH can be challenging, both for health care providers and patients themselves. Classically, the patient will describe the worst headache of their life that came on very suddenly (ie, "thunderclap"). A careful neurologic examination should be performed with particular attention to the cranial nerve examination and performance of an assessment of concentration (eg, reciting months of the year backward). Unfortunately, in the presence of a normal neurologic examination there are not any highly specific historical features of aSAH. Given the extremely high morbidity and mortality of a missed aSAH, we must be persuaded to seek out highly sensitive tools at the expense of specificity.

A sentinel headache, or milder headache or headache without neurologic change, can occur a few weeks prior in up to 40% those who experience an aSAH. It represents an initial hemorrhage from the aneurysm of less severity.

TABLE 48B-14 **Clinical grading scales for aneurysmal subarachnoid hemorrhage.**

Grade[a]	Hunt and Hess (H/H)	World Federation of Neurological Surgeons (WFNS)
1	Asymptomatic or minimal headache	GCS 15, no motor deficit
2	Moderate to severe headache; may have one isolated cranial nerve deficit	GCS 13-14, no motor deficit
3	Drowsy, confused, or mild focal deficit	GCS 13-14, with motor deficit
4	Stupor, moderate to severe hemiparesis	GCS 7-12
5	Deep coma, decerebrate rigidity	GCS 3-6

GCS, Glasgow Coma Scale.
[a]Score to be assessed after patient is resuscitated.

There are 2 wildly used systems that score the severity of the aSAH and are based on clinical symptoms. Hunt and Hess (H/H) and World Federation of Neurosurgeons (WFNS) are outlined in Table 48B-14.

Diagnostics

The initial diagnostic test is a NCHCT. If performed without 6 hours of symptom onset, it is a modern day CT scanner, and the patient is not anemic or coagulopathic, the sensitivity approaches 100%. There are reports of reduced sensitivity in this time frame on modern scanners when the head CT is read by nonneuroradiologists in the community setting. After this time frame, a lumber puncture (LP) may need to be performed to full exclude the possibility of SAH, depending on the pretest probability/clinical suspicion, as the SAH will begin to degrade and may no longer be hyperdense on a NCHCT. Of note, the LP should be performed at least 12 hours after symptom onset, as the intracerebral subarachnoid blood may not have adequately circulated into the lumbar cistern, from which the CSF will be collected. An aSAH is excluded by the absence of red blood cells and xanthochromia in the CSF. An MRI of the head can also be performed, with particular attention to the GRE, T2*, or SWI images, but LP remains the gold standard when performed more than 12 hours after symptom onset.

Once SAH is diagnosed, an etiology must be pursued, which begins with vascular imaging. A CTA of the head is most common performed, but if contraindications exist to its performance, an MRA can be performed, although it has a lower sensitivity for aneurysms than CTA. If the CTA is nondiagnostic, a digital subtraction angiogram (DSA) should be performed.

The risk of VSP, DCI, and delayed neurologic deterioration (DND) are proportional to the amount of SAH. Two scoring systems are in use to help stratify this risk, based on the initial head CT. The original system was the Fischer Scale, which was modified in 2001 by Claassen et al and then revalidated by Frontera in 2006. Table 48B-15 summarizes each of these scales and their associated risk of DND.

Treatment

Early (the first 6 hours) treatment goals include BP control, cardiopulmonary stability, correction of symptomatic hydrocephalus, treatment of intracranial hypertension, reversal of herniation syndromes, and consideration of antifibrinolytics. Aneurysmal rebleeding is a catastrophic event. It is associated with a more than 50% mortality rate and none of the survivors recover to a mRS of 0 to 2 (good outcome). It occurs in 8% to 23% of aSAH, with 83% of the rebleeds occurring in the first 6 hours. The risk can be mitigated with rapid, smooth, consistent BP control, minimization of patient agitation, and the rapid correction of any coagulopathy. Commonly selected short acting continuous infusion antihypertensives include nicardipine, clevidipine, labetalol, and esmolol. Robust vasodilators, such as

TABLE 48B-15 Fischer scale and modified fisher scale for risk of delayed neurologic deterioration in aneurysmal subarachnoid hemorrhage.

	Fischer			Modified Fischer	
Grade	Description	DND Rate (%)	Grade	Description	DND Rate (%)
–			0	No SAH or IVH	0
1	No blood or focal thin	0-21	1	Thin SAH, no b/l IVH*	12-24
2	Diffuse, thin SAH < 1 mm thick	20-25	2	Thin SAH, b/l IVH	21-33
3	SAH > 1 mm thick	28-37	3	Thick SAH**, no b/l IVH*	19-33
4	ICH or IVH with SAH	19-31	4	Thick SAH**, b/l IVH*	40

SAH, subarachnoid hemorrhage; ICH, intracerebral hemorrhage; IVH, intraventricular hemorrhage; DND, delayed neurologic deterioration; b/l, bilateral.
aFor the modified Fischer Scale, a score of 2 or 4 requires that there is blood layering in both of the lateral ventricles.
bThick SAH = SAH completely fills at least one cistern of fissure.

nitroglycerin, hydralazine, and sodium nitroprusside are typically avoided, as they may cause significant increases in cerebral blood volume and blood flow dynamics. Antifibrinolytics such as TXA or epsilon-aminocaproic acid (EACA) appear to reduce the risk of rebleeding, but have not been definitively shown to improve functional outcomes. If administered, they should be discontinued 4 hours prior to DSA to minimize the risk of iatrogenic ischemic strokes during the procedure from catheter thrombi. If the patient has a depressed level of consciousness or demonstrated intracranial hypertension, a mean arterial pressure of 80 mm Hg (assuming no intracranial monitoring) or cerebral perfusion pressure of 60 mm Hg should be maintained, while controlling the SBP. An epidemiologic BP target has not been clearly established, but many centers use a target SBP of less than 140 mm Hg. The value of seizure prophylaxis is unclear. Similar observations about phenytoin have been made in aSAH. Many centers will provide 7 days of prophylactic levetiracetam in poor grade aSAH and those undergoing open surgical clipping, but the value of this approach is unclear. Any patient with poor neurologic examination or one that is worse than expected for the severity of the hemorrhage should undergo cvEEG monitoring.

Neurogenic stunned myocardium and/or neurogenic pulmonary edema are not uncommon after aSAH, particularly in those with poor grade (ie, high H/H or WFNS scores) aSAHs. Cardiac complications include dramatic (self-limited) reduction in ejection fraction (Takotsubo cardiomyopathy), electrocardiographic changes (ST/T wave, QT prolongation, U waves) and supraventricular and ventricular arrhythmias. In fact, some aSAH will present in cardiac arrest. Ventilatory support with positive pressure along with optimization of serum potassium (> 4.0) and magnesium (> 2.0) are cornerstones in the management of these cases. If an airway needs to be obtained, be sure to minimize patient agitation, physiologic fluctuations, and BP spikes during the procedure to minimize the risk of causing a rebleed.

Early decisions should be made regarding whether to place an IVC to treat a hydrocephalus, particularly if the patient is going to DSA for diagnostics and possible aneurysmal intervention, where they will be laying flat for a prolonged period of time and difficult to monitor. Cerebral edema may require treatment with hyperosmolar agents, such as mannitol or hypertonic saline.

Early surgical or EVT of the aneurysm is recommended as it improves outcome, most commonly with 24 hours or, as identified in a meta-analysis, within 72 hours. The European International Subarachnoid Aneurysm Trial (ISAT; 2002) randomized good neurologic grades (WFNS I-III) aSAH to surgical clipping ($n = 1070$) or coiling ($n = 1073$) with death and dependency at 1 year as the primary outcome measure. The authors reported better outcome for coiling group (23.5%) compared to surgical clipping group (30.9%); however, the rebleeding rate at 1 year was 2.6% in the coiling versus 1% in the clipping group. However, at 5-year follow-up a reduced death rate for coiling (11%) compared to clipping (14%) was observed while the percentage of independent survivors did not differ making the overall death rate in the coiled group 3% at 5 years. Bias in recruitment strategy, aneurysm location, aneurysm size, selection of good grades, treatment time window, operator experience, age exclusion, presurgical evaluations, choice of techniques and questionnaire follow up are cited in order to understand the limitation of this landmark study. A follow up trial (ISAT II) is underway. Currently, most investigators identify equipoise with respect to longer term outcomes and treatment approach and identify that certain patients are not suitable for either surgical or EVT. For example, coiling is the less preferred option in patients with aneurysms of large size, with large mass effect, wide neck (neck-to-dome ratio > 0.5), fusiform appearance, and at arterial bifurcations. In contrast, posterior circulation aneurysms, especially basilar tip aneurysms, locations within or between the cavernous sinuses, or those that can more readily be accessed by an endovascular approach. Age is a relevant factor in the decision making as younger patients have better long-term protection from recurrent SAH with clipping while coiling is preferred in elderly with multiple comorbidities.

As with all critical brain injuries, normoglycemia, normothermia, normonatremia, and normovolemia must be maintained. Fluid and electrolyte abnormalities are common in aSAH patients. Cerebral salt wasting syndrome and syndrome of inappropriate secretion of antidiuretic hormone (SIADH) are common, and may even coexist in the same patient. Fluid balance must be vigilantly maintained, as negative fluid balances in aSAH are associated with worsened outcomes.

As stated aforementioned, VSP occurs commonly during period following rupture of aSAH, with a peak incidence on postbleed days 7 to 10 (with the day of the bleed being day 0). Those with a normal neurologic examination should have serial assessments vigilantly performed. If the neurologic examination is impaired, serial angiographic assessments with transcranial Dopplers (TCDs), CTAs, CT perfusion studies, and/or DSAs. TCDs noninvasively assess for the velocity of blood flow through the large cerebral arteries (MCA, ACA, Basilar), with increase in velocity indicative of VSP. MCA velocities of greater than 200 cm/s or a ratio between the MCA and the extracranial ICA of greater than 6 (Lindegaard ratio [LR]) are suggestive of severe VSP. TCDs also provide a pulsatility index (PI), which is a marker of distal arteriolar resistance, as would be seen in small vessel VSP.

Examination changes related to VSP should be treated immediately by ensure euvolemia and raising the BP, often pharmacologically. If the neurologic change does not resolved, then more aggressive should be expeditiously performed, such as DSA where intra-arterial verapamil or milrinone can be administered or angioplasty can be performed. Medical measures that have been demonstrated to have some effect with the treatment of VSP include IV milrinone, intrathecal nicardipine, IV magnesium, high-dose statins, and endothelin-receptor antagonists. Unfortunately RCTs exploring the value of the later 3 classes failed to meet their primary functional outcomes, despite evidence suggesting that they are effective at treating angiographic VSP.

Most recently, DCI is being better understood as an arteriolar VSP that results in microvascular thrombosis and perfusion mismatch and neurovascular uncoupling, complicated by spreading depolarizations, which begin at the time of the aneurysm rupture and ultimately lead to cortical infarctions. Nimodipine is a stalwart in the management of aSAH. It should be started on day of arrival and continued for 21 days. It has been shown to improve functional outcomes, but interestingly, it failed to produce a statistically significant reduction in VSP. Reasons for this discrepancy are related to other suspected benefits of calcium channel blockage, including the prevention of small vessel VSP, stabilization of the neurovascular unit, prevention of intracellular calcium influx as part of apoptosis, and mild profibrinolysis that mitigates microvascular thrombosis.

REFERENCES

1. Wiley J. Acute ischemic stroke. In: Lee K, ed. *The Neuro ICU Book*. 1st ed. New York: McGraw Hill Medical; 2012.
2. Gross H, Guilliams KP, Sung G. Emergency neurological life support: acute ischemic stroke. *Neurocrit Care*. 2015 Dec;23(Suppl 2):S94-S102.
3. Demaerschalk BM, Kleindorfer DO, Adeoye OM, et al. Scientific rationale for the inclusion and exclusion criteria for intravenous alteplase in acute ischemic stroke. *Stroke*. 2016 Feb;47(2):581-641.
4. Powers WJ, Derdeyn CP, Biller J, et al. 2015 AHA/ASA focused update of the 2013 Guidelines for the Early Management of Patients with Acute Ischemic Stroke Regarding Endovascular Treatment. *Stroke*. 2015 Oct;46(10):3020-3035.
5. Jauch EC, Saver JL, Adams HP, et al. Guidelines for the early management of patients with acute ischemic stroke. *Stroke*. 2013 Mar;44(3):870-947.
6. Wijdicks EF, Sheth KN, Carter BS, et al. Recommendations for the management of cerebral and cerebellar infarction with swelling. *Stroke*. 2014 Apr;45(4):1222-1238.
7. Prabhakaran S, Ruff I, Bernstein R. Acute stroke intervention: a systematic review. *JAMA*. 2015;313(14):1451-1462.
8. Fernandes PM, Whiteley WN, Hart SR, et al. Stroke: mimics and chameleons. *Pract Neurol*. 2013 Feb;13(1):21-28.
9. Hemphill JC, 3rd, Bonovich DC, Besmertis L, et al. The ICH score: a simple, reliable grading scale for intracerebral hemorrhage. *Stroke*. 2001;32(4):891-897.
10. Yazbeck M, Rincon F, Mayer S. Intracerebral hemorrhage. In: Lee K, ed. *The Neuro ICU Book*. 1st ed. New York: McGraw Hill Medical; 2012.
11. Jauch EC, Pineda JA, Hemphill JC. Emergency neurological life support: intracerebral hemorrhage. *Neurocrit Care*. 2015 Dec;23(Suppl 2):S83-S93.
12. Hemphill JC, 3rd, Greenberg SM, Anderson CS, et al. Guidelines for the management of spontaneous intracerebral hemorrhage: a guideline for healthcare professionals from the American Heart Association/American Stroke Association. *Stroke*. 2015 Jul;46(7):2032-2060.
13. Chan S, Hemphill JC, 3rd. Critical care management of intracerebral hemorrhage. *Crit Care Clin*. 2014 Oct;30(4):699-717.
14. Delgado Almandoz JE, Schaefer PW, Goldstein JN, et al. Practical scoring system for the identification of patients with intracerebral hemorrhage at highest risk of harboring an underlying vascular etiology: the Secondary Intracerebral Hemorrhage Score. *AJNR AM J Neuroradiology*. 2010 Oct;31(9):1653-1660.
15. Qureshi AI, Palesch YY, Barsan WG, et al. Intensive blood-pressure lowering in patients with acute cerebral hemorrhage. *N Engl J Med*. 2016 Jun 8.
16. Anderson CS, Heeley E, Huang Y, et al. Rapid blood-pressure lowering in patients with acute intracerebral hemorrhage. *N Engl J Med*. 2013 Jun 20;368(25):2355-2365.
17. Tsivgoulis G, Katsnos AH, Butcher KS, et al. Intensive blood pressure reduction in acute intracerebral hemorrhage: a meta-analysis. *Neurology*. 2014 Oct 21;83(17):1523-1529.
18. Frontera JA, Lewin JJ, Rabinstein AA, et al. Guidelines for reversal of antithrombotics in intracranial hemorrhage. *Neurocrit Care*. 2016;24:6-46.
19. Steiner T, Poli S, Griebe M, et al. Fresh frozen plasma versus prothrombin complex concentrate in patients with intracranial haemorrhage related to vitamin K antagonists (INCH): a randomized trial. *Lancet Neurol*. 2016;15:566-573.
20. Vandelli L, Marietta M, Gambini M, et al. Fibrinogen decrease after intravenous thrombolysis in ischemic stroke patients is a risk factor for intracerebral hemorrhage. *J Stroke CV Dis*. 2015 Feb 24(2):394-400.
21. Manning L, Hirakawa Y, Arima H, et al. Blood pressure variability and outcome after acute intracerebral hemorrhage: post-hoc analysis of INTERACT-2, a randomized controlled trial. *Lancet Neurol*. 2014;13:364-373.
22. Baharoglu MI, Cordonniet C, Al-Shahi Salman R, et al. Platelet transfusion versus standard care after acute stroke due to spontaneous cerebral haemorrhage associated with antiplatelet therapy (PATCH): a randomized, open-label, phase 3 trial. *Lancet Neurol*. Online May 10, 2016.
23. Kuramatsu JB, Gerner ST, Schellinger PD, et al. Anticoagulant reversal, blood pressure levels, and anticoagulant resumption in patients with anticoagulation-related intracerebral hemorrhage. *JAMA*. 2015;313(8):824-836.
24. Mendelow AD, Gregson BA, Rowan EN, et al. STICH II Investigators. Early surgery versus initial conservative treatment in patients with spontaneous supratentorial lobar intracerebral haematomas (STICH II): a randomised trial. *Lancet*. 2013;382(9890):397-408.
25. Mendelow AD, Gregson BA, Fernandes HM, et al; STICH investigators. Early surgery versus initial

conservative treatment in patients with spontaneous supratentorial intracerebral haematomas in the International Surgical Trial in Intracerebral Haemorrhage (STICH): a randomised trial. *Lancet*. 2005;365(9457):387-397.

26. Prasad K, Mendelow AD, Gregson B. Surgery for primary supratentorial intracerebral haemorrhage. *Cochrane Database Syst Rev*. 2008;(4):CD000200.

27. Wang JW, Li JP, Song YL, et al. Stereotactic aspiration versus craniotomy for primary intracerebral hemorrhage: a meta-analysis of randomized controlled trials. *PLoS ONE*. 2014;9(9):e107614.

28. Ziai W, Nyquist P, Hanley D. Surgical strategies for spontaneous intracerebral hemorrhage. *Semin Neurol*. 2016;36:261-268.

29. Lee K. Subarachnoid Hemorrhage. In: Lee K, ed. *The Neuro ICU Book*. 1st ed. New York: McGraw Hill Medical; 2012.

30. Edlow JA, Figaji A, Samuels O. Emergency neurological life support: subarachnoid hemorrhage. *Neurocrit Care*. 2015 Dec;23(Suppl 2):S103-S109.

31. Connolly ES, Rabinstein AA, Carhuapoma JR, et al. Guidelines for the management of aneurysmal subarachnoid hemorrhage. *Stroke*. 2012 Jun;43(6):1711-1737.

32. Diringer MN, Bleck TP, Claude Hemphill J, 3rd, et al. Critical care management of patients following aneurysmal subarachnoid hemorrhage: recommendations from the Neurocritical Care Society's Multidisciplinary Consensus Conference. *Neurocrit Care*. 2011 Sep;15(2):211-240.

33. Rinkel GJ, Djibuti M, Algra A, et al. Prevalence and risk of rupture of intracranial aneurysms: a systematic review. *Stroke*. 1998;29:251-256.

34. Wiebers DO, Whisnant JP, Huston J III, et al. International Study of Unruptured Intracranial Aneurysms Investigators. Unruptured intracranial aneurysms: natural history, clinical outcome, and risks of surgical and endovascular treatment. *Lancet*. 2003;362:103-110.

35. Rosengart AJ, Schultheiss KE, Tolentino J, Macdonald RL. Prognostic factors for outcome in patients with aneurysmal subarachnoid hemorrhage. *Stroke*. 2007; 38(8):2315-2321.

36. Kreiter KT, Rosengart AJ, Claasen J, Fitzsimmons BF, Peery S, Du YE. Depressed mood and quality of life after subarachnoid hemorrhage. *J Neurol Sci*. 2013 Dec 15;335(1-2):64-71.

37. Ingall T, Asplundh K, Mähönen M, et al. A multinational comparison of subarachnoid hemorrhage in the WHO MONICA stroke study. *Stroke*. 2000;31;1054-1061.

38. Ie Roux AA, Wallace MC. Outcome and cost of aneurysmal subarachnoid hemorrhage. *Neurosurg Clin N Am*. 2010;21:235-246.

39. Hunt WE, Hess RM. Surgical risk as related to time of intervention in the repair of intracranial aneurysms. *J Neurosurg*. 1968;28(1):14-20.

40. Perry JJ, Stiell IG, Sivilotti ML, et al. Clinical decision rules to rule out subarachnoid hemorrhage for acute headache. *JAMA*. 2013;310(12):1248-1255.

41. Frontera JA, Claassen J, Schmidt JM, et al. Prediction of symptomatic vasospasm after subarachnoid hemorrhage: the modified fisher scale. *Neurosurgery*. 2006 Jul;59(1):21-27.

42. Claassen J, Bernardini GL, Kreiter K, et al. Effect of cisternal and ventricular blood on risk of delayed cerebral ischemia after subarachnoid hemorrhage. *Stroke*. 2001;32:2012-2020.

43. Phillips TJ, Dowling RJ, Yan B, et al. Does treatment of ruptured intracranial aneurysms within 24 hours improve clinical outcome? *Stroke*. 2011;42:1936-1945.

44. de Gans K, Nieuwkamp DJ, Rinkel GJ, et al. Timing of aneurysm surgery in subarachnoid hemorrhage: a systematic review of the literature. *Neurosurgery*. 2002;50:336-340.

45. Rosengart AJ, Huo DZ, Tolentino J, Novakovic RL, Frank JI, Goldenberg FD, Macdonald RL. Outcome in patients with subarachnoid hemorrhage treated with antiepileptic drugs. *J Neurosurg*. 2007;107(2):253-260.

46. Dorhout Mees S, Rinkel GJE, Feigin VL, Algra A, van den Bergh WM, Vermeulen M, van Gijn J. Calcium antagonists for aneurysmal subarachnoid haemorrhage. Cochrane Database of Systematic Reviews 2007, Issue 3. Art. No.: CD000277. DOI: 10.1002/14651858.CD000277.pub3.

Delirium in the Intensive Care Unit

S. Jean Hsieh, MD

KEY POINTS

1 ICU delirium is a common form of acute "brain failure" that is associated with significant morbidity and mortality. Delirium has a dose response relationship with poor outcomes: the longer the delirium duration, the poorer the outcome.

2 Delirium can be missed in up to 75% of patients if a screening tool is not used, likely because of the high prevalence of hypoactive delirium.

3 Early diagnosis of delirium is imperative for effective delivery of delirium reduction strategies. Therefore, delirium assessments should be part of the ICU admission physical exam and should be incorporated into the daily work-flow.

4 ICU-acquired risk factors for delirium (eg, oversedation, immobilization, uncontrolled pain) are potentially modifiable and closely interrelated. Implementation of nonpharmacologic multicomponent strategies to prevent and reduce delirium on an ICU-wide scale (eg, targeted light/no sedation, early rehabilitation) can shorten the duration of ICU delirium and improve clinical outcomes.

5 Pharmacologic prevention and treatment of delirium (eg, dexmedetomidine over benzodiazepines for sedation) can be considered for individual patients, although the efficacy of these strategies is still unclear.

INTRODUCTION

Delirium is the most common form of acute brain injury in critically ill patients and is associated with potentially long-lasting serious consequences. This chapter reviews the essentials of diagnosis, risk factors, prevention, and treatment of ICU delirium.

GENERAL CONSIDERATIONS

Delirium is a disturbance of consciousness and cognition that develops acutely (ie, hours to days), fluctuates over time, and is generally reversible.[1] It is characterized by an acute change or fluctuation in baseline mental status, inattention, and either disorganized thinking or an altered level of consciousness. ICU delirium is the most common form of acute brain dysfunction in critically ill patients, with estimates of incidences ranging from 20% to 50% in nonventilated patients and 60% to 80% in ventilated ICU patients, depending on the diagnostic criteria used and the patient characteristics.[2-6] It is important to recognize that delirium is not a normal part of critical illness, but rather represents an acute organ failure that is associated with profound short- and long-term consequences.

Pathophysiology

While the pathophysiology of delirium is still poorly understood, it is thought to be a disease-driven process caused by the complex interaction of various factors including (1) the underlying disease itself, (2) predisposing risk factors unique to each patient, and (3) environmental and treatment-related factors.

Neurotransmitter Imbalance

Delirium is hypothesized to be caused by imbalances in neurotransmitters due to factors such as systemic inflammation, metabolic derangements, acute stress responses, and exposure to psychoactive medications.[7] The 2 main neurotransmitters implicated in these derangements are dopamine and acetylcholine, and they work in opposition by increasing and decreasing neuronal excitability, respectively. Other neurotransmitters that have been implicated in the pathogenesis of delirium include g-aminobutyric acid (GABA), serotonin, glutamate, and endorphins. At this time, data supporting these hypotheses are limited and thus pharmacologic treatment of ICU delirium is largely empirical.

Neuroinflammation

Inflammatory cytokines and endotoxins are postulated to contribute to the development of ICU delirium in several ways.[8] Infiltration of leukocytes and cytokines into the central nervous system may lead to neuronal apoptosis, and may interfere with neurotransmitter synthesis and neurotransmission, increase vascular permeability, and reduce cerebral microvascular blood flow through the formation of microaggregates of fibrin, platelets, erythrocytes, and neutrophils. Microglial activation and oxidative injury can also occur.

Alterations of Brain Structure

Preliminary studies using magnetic resonance imaging have shown an association between the duration of ICU delirium and both cerebral white-matter disruption and cerebral atrophy. Because of the lack of imaging before critical illness, these findings suggest that either the presence of these abnormalities makes patients more vulnerable to developing ICU delirium or that ICU delirium leads to abnormalities in brain structure.[9,10]

Risk Factors

Despite our relatively poor understanding of the overall pathophysiology of delirium, clinical studies have shown delirium to be a disease-driven process caused by a complex interaction of factors including: (1) baseline risk factors unique to each patient; (2) the patient's acute illness and illness-related factors; and (3) ICU-environment and treatment-related factors (Figure 49–1). These risk factors can be further classified as nonmodifiable (ie, predisposing factors that are out of the control of the admitting clinician) and modifiable (ie, factors that the clinician may be able to treat). Although over 100 risk factors have been identified in the literature,[11] few have consistently remained associated with delirium across different studies after adjusting for confounding variables. This is likely due to the different underlying pathophysiology of delirium across study populations.[2,3,6,12-14] This chapter will review risk factors that have been most consistently identified in the literature.

Patient-Level Predisposing Risk Factors

Studies have consistently identified pre-existing cognitive impairment, alcohol use, and history of hypertension as risk factors that significantly increase the risk of delirium in ICU patients (Figure 49–2).[2,5,13,15] Although advanced age has been identified as one of most significant risk factors outside of the ICU, this association has remained inconsistent across ICU studies.[16,17] Physiologic dependence from chronic exposure to alcohol, opiates, and benzodiazepines can lead to withdrawal in the setting of abrupt discontinuation of alcohol use. Of the predisposing patient-level risk factors, withdrawal from these substances is the only modifiable factor, and thus should be carefully considered when encountering a delirious patient.

Illness-Related Risk Factors

High severity of illness at ICU admission and medication-induced coma (as opposed to coma due to a primary neurologic condition) have been consistently identified as independent risk factors for development of delirium in ICU patients.[5,13,16-19] Respiratory failure requiring mechanical ventilation has been identified as a risk factor for delirium, although the results have been inconsistent across studies.[2,5,14,16,20]

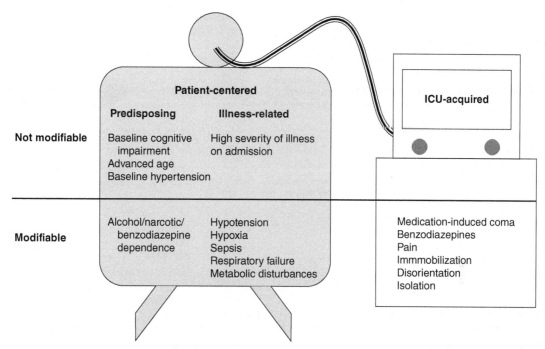

FIGURE 49–1 Risk factors for ICU delirium.
Copyright © 2002, E. Wesley Ely, MD, MPH and Vanderbilt University, all rights reserved (top).
(*Data from Devlin JW, Marquis F, Riker RR, et al: Combined didactic and scenario-based education improves the ability of intensive care unit staff to recognize delirium at the bedside*, Crit Care. 2008;12(1):R19 (bottom).)

Potential reasons for the discrepant findings include exclusion of nonmechanically ventilated patients from observational studies[12,19,21] and lack of measurement of mechanical ventilation as a risk factor in ICU delirium studies.[13,15]

ICU Treatment-Related Risk Factors

An appreciation of the impact of ICU-level risk factors on the development and persistence of delirium is particularly important because (1) these factors are all modifiable, (2) reduction of these risk factors is associated with reduced incidence and duration of ICU delirium and improvements in clinical outcomes, and (3) these factors are closely interrelated.
Sedative Use—Most mechanically ventilated patients receive sedatives in the ICU. Both sedative choice and sedative-induced coma are independently associated with an increased risk of delirium.[13] Benzodiazepines are most consistently associated with delirium across different ICU populations and have demonstrated a dose-dependent relationship, although a few studies have found no significant relationship.[12,16,17,22-24] Most studies on opiates and propofol report an increased risk of delirium, particularly when used in combination with other sedatives or when associated with coma.[2,13,14,16,25] In contrast, recent studies suggest that use of dexmedetomidine and/or avoidance of benzodiazepines may be associated with both a lower risk of developing delirium and a shorter duration of delirium.[26,27] Preliminary data in cardiac surgery patients suggests that dexmedetomidine may also be associated with a lower incidence of delirium compared to propofol and shorter duration of delirium compared to morphine.[28,29]

Immobility—A number of observational studies suggest that neuromuscular function and ICU delirium are closely interconnected.[30] For instance, observational and clinical trial data suggest that immobility is an independent risk factor for delirium in ICU and non-ICU hospitalized patients.[5,22,30-33] Studies show that ICU's that institute early mobilization programs have a lower prevalence and shorter duration of ICU delirium.[33,34]

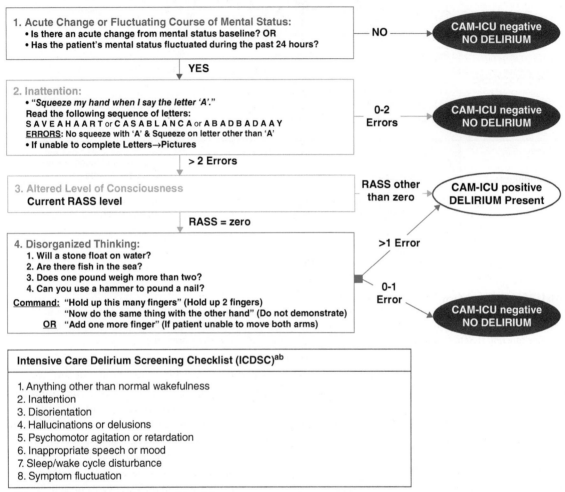

Confusion Assessment Method for the ICU (CAM-ICU) Flowsheet

1. Acute Change or Fluctuating Course of Mental Status:
• Is there an acute change from mental status baseline? OR
• Has the patient's mental status fluctuated during the past 24 hours?

— NO ——► **CAM-ICU negative NO DELIRIUM**

YES

2. Inattention:
• *"Squeeze my hand when I say the letter 'A'."*
Read the following sequence of letters:
S A V E A H A A R T or C A S A B L A N C A or A B A D B A D A A Y
ERRORS: No squeeze with 'A' & Squeeze on letter other than 'A'
• If unable to complete Letters→Pictures

0-2 Errors ——► **CAM-ICU negative NO DELIRIUM**

> 2 Errors

3. Altered Level of Consciousness
Current RASS level

RASS other than zero ——► **CAM-ICU positive DELIRIUM Present**

RASS = zero

4. Disorganized Thinking:
1. Will a stone float on water?
2. Are there fish in the sea?
3. Does one pound weigh more than two?
4. Can you use a hammer to pound a nail?
Command: "Hold up this many fingers" (Hold up 2 fingers)
"Now do the same thing with the other hand" (Do not demonstrate)
OR "Add one more finger" (If patient unable to move both arms)

>1 Error ——► **CAM-ICU positive DELIRIUM Present**

0-1 Error ——► **CAM-ICU negative NO DELIRIUM**

Intensive Care Delirium Screening Checklist (ICDSC)[ab]

1. Anything other than normal wakefulness
2. Inattention
3. Disorientation
4. Hallucinations or delusions
5. Psychomotor agitation or retardation
6. Inappropriate speech or mood
7. Sleep/wake cycle disturbance
8. Symptom fluctuation

[a]Each positive component is scored 1 point
[b]A total score ≥ 4 is positive for delirium; scores 1-3 is termed "subsyndromal" delirium

FIGURE 49–2   Delirium assessment tools. (*Reproduced with permission from Hsieh SJ, Ely EW, Gong MN: Can intensive care unit delirium be prevented and reduced? Lessons learned and future directions, Ann Am Thorac Soc 2013 Dec;10(6):648-656.*)

Clinical Features

ICU delirium is characterized by the following 4 DSM-V criteria: (1) inattention (the most common feature), (2) an acute change or fluctuation in baseline mental status, and either (3) disorganized thinking *or* (4) an altered level of consciousness.[1] Notably, while delusions and hallucinations can be present in delirious patients, these symptoms are not defining features of delirium. Patients with delirium can present in 3 different ways: calm or somnolent (ie, hypoactive), agitated (ie, hyperactive), or alternating between the 2 states (ie, mixed).[24] While hyperactive delirium can be more easily identified without a screening tool, only 2% of patients have purely hyperactive delirium. In contrast, hypoactive and mixed forms are much more common in critically ill patients,[35] and are associated with worse clinical outcomes.[35]

Diagnosis

ICU delirium is a clinical diagnosis; no diagnostic lab, imaging, or electroencephalographic test can accurately diagnose delirium. However, without the use of a delirium assessment tool, over 3/4 of delirium can be missed in routine practice because patients more often present with hypoactive rather than hyperactive delirium.[36] This highlights the importance of integrating a structured tool into clinical practice to rapidly and accurately detect delirium, rather than relying on clinical impressions. Indeed, delirium assessment in the ICU is now considered to be a requisite part of high-quality ICU care.

All patients should be screened for delirium as soon as they are admitted to the ICU and then at least once per nursing shift. Because delirium can only be assessed in patients who are arousable to voice, level of consciousness needs to be determined first. Therefore, delirium screening is a 2-step process.

Step 1: Determine Level of Consciousness—The level of consciousness needs to be determined using a sedation-agitation scale. The 2013 American College of Critical Care Medicine (ACCM) clinical practice guidelines recommended the Richmond agitation-sedation scale (RASS)[37] and Riker sedation-agitation scale (SAS)[38] as the 2 most valid and reliable sedation assessment tools (Table 49–1 and 1B).

Step 2: Screen for Delirium—If the patient is not comatose (ie, RASS –3 or more or SAS 3 or more), delirium can be assessed using a screening tool. Many tools for delirium screening have been published. This chapter will review the 2 most well-studied and commonly used ICU delirium screening tools, that were also recommended by the recently updated ACCM clinical practice guidelines: the Confusion Assessment Method-ICU (CAM-ICU) and Intensive Care Delirium Screening Checklist (ISDSC) (Figure 49–1).[24,40] Both tools have (1) high sensitivity, specificity (ranging from 74% to 96%) and (2) excellent clinical feasibility in both nonventilated and ventilated critically ill patients in mixed ICUs.[41]

Confusion Assessment Method-ICU (CAM-ICU)

The CAM-ICU provides a dichotomous assessment (ie, delirious vs not delirious) at a single time point and can be performed in less than 1 minute. Advantages of the CAM-ICU are its discrete defined measures that

TABLE 49–1A

Richmond Agitation-Sedation Scale (RASS)[88]	
+4: Combative	Overtly combative, violent, immediate danger to self
+3: Very agitated	Pulls or removes tubes or catheters; aggressive
+2: Agitated	Frequent nonpurposeful movement, fights ventilator
+1: Restless	Anxious but movements not aggressive or vigorous
0: Alert and calm	Alert and calm
–1: Drowsy	Not fully alert but has sustained awakening to voice (eye opening or eye contact >10 s)
–2: Light sedation	Briefly awakens with eye contact to voice (< 10 s)
–3: Moderate sedation	Movement or eye opening to voice but no eye contact
–4: Deep sedation	No response to voice but movement or eye opening to physical stimulation
–5: Unarousable	No response to voice or physical stimulation

Adapted with permission from Sessler CN, Gosnell MS, Grap MJ, et al: The Richmond Agitation-Sedation Scale: validity and reliability in adult intensive care unit patients, *Am J Respir Crit Care Med* 2002 Nov 15;166(10):1338-1344.

are obtained from physical assessment of the patient. A disadvantage is that, given delirium's fluctuating course, the periodic nature of the CAM-ICU may miss an episode of delirium. Therefore, it should be performed on a regular basis (eg, every 4 to 12 hours) and with changes in the patient's mental status.

ICDSC

The ICDSC is an 8-item checklist of symptoms observed over an 8-hour to 24-hour period in which a score of 4 or more is positive for delirium and scores of 1 to 3 are defined as "subsyndromal" delirium. Advantages of the ISDSC are its ability to detect "subsyndromal delirium" and a longer assessment period which decreases the chance of missing signs of delirium. A disadvantage is that the ISDSC relies on more subjective observations in the setting of mechanically ventilated patients (eg, hallucinations, inappropriate speech) and thus can be more dependent on the clinical experience of the practitioner.

TABLE 49–1B

Riker Sedation-Agitation Scale (SAS)[89]	
7: Dangerous agitation	Pulling at endotracheal tube, trying to remove catheters, climbing over bed rail, striking at staff, thrashing from side to side
6: Very agitated	Requiring restraint and frequent verbal reminding of limits, biting endotracheal tube
5: Agitated	Anxious or physically agitated, calming at verbal instruction
4: Calm and cooperative	Calm, easily arousable, follows commands
3: Sedated	Difficult to arouse but awakens to verbal stimuli or gentle shaking; follows simple commands but drifts off again
2: Very sedated	Arouses to physical stimuli but does not communicate or follow commands, may move spontaneously
1: Cannot be aroused	Minimal or no response to noxious stimuli, does not communicate or follow commands

Adapted with permission from Riker RR, Picard JT, Fraser GL: Prospective evaluation of the Sedation-Agitation Scale for adult critically ill patients, Crit Care Med 1999 Jul;27(7):1325-1329.

Differential Diagnosis

Pain

Untreated pain can be both a risk factor for ICU delirium and a cause of agitation that is not due to delirium. While the standard for pain assessment is self-report, patients in the ICU often are unable to communicate due to respiratory failure or decreased level of consciousness. Because increased vital signs such as tachycardia or hypertension do not always correlate with pain, it is important to use a structured tool for pain monitoring in patients who are unable to communicate, such as Behavioral Pain Scale (BPS)[42] or the Critical-Care Pain Observation Tool (CPOT).[24,43]

Dementia

While dementia is a risk factor for delirium, it can also be confused with delirium because of changes in cognition. However, its course progresses over a much longer period of time (months to years) in contrast to hours to days in delirium, and the symptoms fluctuate much less. In addition, attention remains relatively intact whereas inattention is the most common feature of delirium.

Underlying Psychosis

Agitation due to underlying psychosis or mania, and inattention due to underlying depression can masquerade as delirium. However, the symptoms associated with psychosis, mania and depression can persist for longer periods of time and fluctuate less, and the sensorium is usually clear.

Prevention

Data on effective pharmacologic prevention strategies are limited. A few preliminary studies in patients undergoing elective surgery suggest that low-dose haloperidol and low-dose risperidone reduced the incidence of postoperative delirium.[23,44] Because these studies involved patients with a low severity of illness, it is unclear if these findings can be extrapolated to the general ICU population. Dexmedetomidine may be associated with less incident postoperative delirium in cardiac surgery patients, compared to propofol or midazolam.[28] However, these findings need to be confirmed before broad treatment recommendations can be made.

Several reasons might explain why studies on successful delirium prevention strategies are limited to date. First, up to 70% patients are admitted to the ICU with delirium already present.[16] Second, prevention studies require a larger sample size to detect a differences in incident delirium (which is a binary outcome) compared to duration of delirium (which is a continuous outcome). Finally, most pharmacologic delirium prevention studies did not include concurrent non-pharmacologic delirium prevention strategies such as sedation titration and early mobilization. Because delirium is multifactorial in origin, addressing only a few of the many factors contributing to its development may limit the efficacy of a prevention strategy.

In contrast, preliminary studies suggest that nonpharmacologic strategies targeting multiple risk factors for delirium may be more effective. These strategies include early rehabilitation, sleep-promotion, and structured reorientation. Because these prevention strategies overlap with treatment strategies, they will be discussed in greater detail in the following ICU-level treatment strategies section.

Treatment

Several high-quality intervention studies to halt and limit the duration of delirium in its earliest stages have successfully reduced the duration of delirium and improved other clinical outcomes. This suggests that despite the occurrence of delirium, strategies to reduce the delirium duration may be the first area of focus for ICU teams. In order to maximize the therapeutic potential, a combination of strategies should be used: (1) multicomponent nonpharmacologic interventions that are useful for all ICU patients should be implemented at an ICU level (ICU-level strategies) and (2) pharmacologic interventions that may be useful for specific patients and should be titrated to each individual (patient-level strategies) (Figure 49–3). Each of these strategies will be discussed in the following sections.

ICU-Level Strategies

Given the multifactorial nature of delirium and the interdependency of ICU-treatment–related risk factors, it is not surprising that multicomponent ICU-level strategies have had better success with reducing the duration of delirium compared to pharmacologic strategies that address only a few ICU-level risk factors (Figure 49–4).

Pain Management

Nearly 50% of critically ill patients experience significant pain during their ICU stay.[42] Studies suggest that pain may be a risk factor for delirium.[12,13] Several possible reasons to explain this relationship are: (1) the deleterious cognitive effects of pain itself, (2) agitation due to untreated pain leading to inappropriate sedative administration, and (3) pain medication doses in excess of what is required for pain control. Indeed a study showed that patients who are regularly assessed for pain received less sedation compared to those who did not receive regular pain

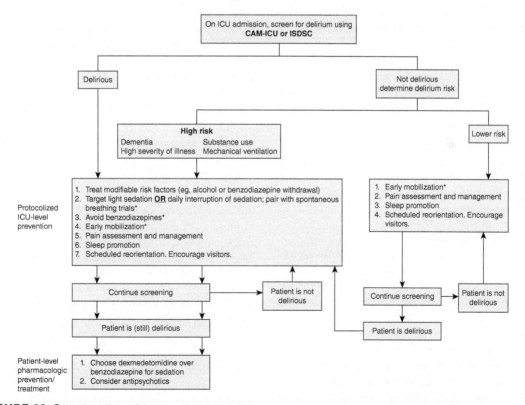

FIGURE 49–3 A clinically useful approach to ICU delirium prevention and treatment. This proposed approach incorporates patient-level delirium prevention and reduction assembled from multiple evidence-based sources, but has not yet been tested in a critically ill population. (*Reproduced with permission from Hsieh SJ, Ely EW, Gong MN: Can intensive care unit delirium be prevented and reduced? Lessons learned and future directions,* Ann Am Thorac Soc *2013 Dec; 10(6):648-656.*)

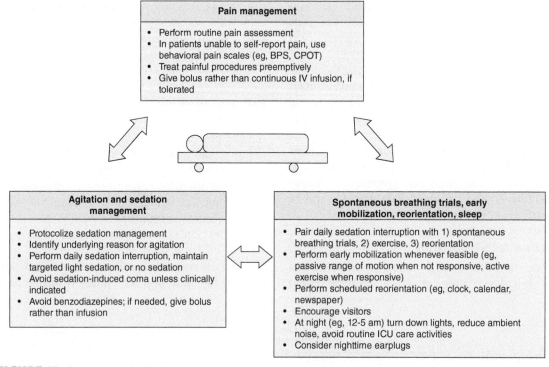

Pain management

- Perform routine pain assessment
- In patients unable to self-report pain, use behavioral pain scales (eg, BPS, CPOT)
- Treat painful procedures preemptively
- Give bolus rather than continuous IV infusion, if tolerated

Agitation and sedation management

- Protocolize sedation management
- Identify underlying reason for agitation
- Perform daily sedation interruption, maintain targeted light sedation, or no sedation
- Avoid sedation-induced coma unless clinically indicated
- Avoid benzodiazepines; if needed, give bolus rather than infusion

Spontaneous breathing trials, early mobilization, reorientation, sleep

- Pair daily sedation interruption with 1) spontaneous breathing trials, 2) exercise, 3) reorientation
- Perform early mobilization whenever feasible (eg, passive range of motion when not responsive, active exercise when responsive)
- Perform scheduled reorientation (eg, clock, calendar, newspaper)
- Encourage visitors
- At night (eg, 12-5 am) turn down lights, reduce ambient noise, avoid routine ICU care activities
- Consider nighttime earplugs

FIGURE 49–4 ICU-level delirium prevention and reduction strategies are interconnected. (*Reproduced with permission from Hsieh SJ, Ely EW, Gong MN: Can intensive care unit delirium be prevented and reduced? Lessons learned and future directions,* Ann Am Thorac Soc *2013 Dec;10(6):648-656.*)

assessments.[45] Therefore, the goal of pain management through routine pain monitoring should be satisfactory pain control without oversedation, and pre-emptive treatment of pain before painful procedures are initiated.

Agitation Management

Agitation is common in critically ill patients. Determining the underlying cause(s) of agitation is essential for determining the appropriate treatment for agitation. Common causes for agitation include untreated pain, anxiety, withdrawal from alcohol or chronic opiates or sedatives, factors associated with the acute illness (eg, hypoxia and hypotension), and delirium. Treatment of agitation that does not address the underlying cause can incite or prolong delirium (eg, a patient with agitation due to uncontrolled pain is given benzodiazepines). Conversely, successful treatment or responsiveness to the underlying cause can potentially reduce sedation use and even improve clinical outcomes.

Sedation Management

Medication-induced coma is a risk factor for ICU delirium. In addition, the prolonged immobility that mechanically ventilated patients experience during deep sedation can lead to complications such as muscle atrophy and weakness, ventilator dependency, pressure sores, and venous thromboembolic disease.[46-48] Rather than routinely providing deep sedation to mechanically ventilated patients without a specific indication, the overall goal of sedation should be to achieve a level of wakefulness so patients can actively participate in rehabilitation and cognitive stimulation during their critical illness. Three different approaches that have demonstrated good outcomes are targeted: (1) daily interruption of sedation, (2) light sedation, and (3) no sedation. Strategies to decrease sedation have led to decreased delirium duration, reduced time on the mechanical ventilator, decreased ICU length of stay, and decreased mortality, and have been demonstrated to be safe, feasible for incorporation into daily care, and acceptable to ICU staff.[49-54] At least one, if not all, of these approaches should be adopted for a "less is more" culture of sedation use.[24,55] Routine monitoring of quality and depth of sedation is needed to guide these strategies. The Richmond agitation-sedation scale (RASS)[37] and sedation-agitation scale (SAS)[38] were identified by the ACCM Clinical Practice Guidelines as the 2 most valid, reliable, and feasible sedation assessment tools for goal-directed sedation delivery.[24]

Early Rehabilitation

Multiple studies have consistently identified immobility as a risk factor for delirium.[5,31] Furthermore, ICU delirium is associated with functional disability after hospital discharge.[56,57] Early delivery of physical and occupational therapy to mechanically ventilated ICU patients (eg, passive range of motion in unresponsive patients, active exercises in interactive patients) has been associated with reduced delirium prevalence and duration, and is safe and well-tolerated.[33,58] In addition, early rehabilitation is associated with less time on mechanical ventilation, improved return to functional status, and may lead to cost savings.[59] Of note, studies demonstrating the benefits of early mobilization also targeted other ICU delirium risk factors such as sedation reduction coordinated with mechanical ventilator weaning.

Sleep Promotion

Critically ill patients frequently experience poor sleep quality in the ICU.[60-62] Sleep deprivation has been postulated to be a risk factor for ICU delirium because both sleep-deprived and delirious patients share common clinical and physiologic derangements.[63] Preliminary studies suggest that a combination of nonpharmacologic sleep promoting interventions (eg, earplugs and reducing nighttime procedures and noise, daytime mobilization), and decreased use of sedatives known to alter sleep or precipitate delirium (ie, benzodiazepines, opiates, diphenhydramine, trazodone), can improve self-reported sleep quality and may even reduce incident delirium and delirium duration.[64-67] Although more work is needed in general ICU populations, given the relative ease of implementation, minimal risk, and potential benefit of

these interventions, it would be reasonable to implement these practices into usual care.

Reorientation

Pre-existing cognitive, visual, and hearing impairment are risk factors for delirium, likely because of the disorientation that patients with these impairments experience.[5,15] Reorientation strategies, such as reading newspapers, listening to music, wearing visual and hearing aids, and performing cognitively stimulating activities, have effectively prevented delirium in older non-ICU patients; preliminary studies in ICU patients also suggest a benefit.[68,69]

Patient-Level Pharmacologic Treatment

Data on pharmacologic treatment of ICU delirium is mixed. Current evidence suggests a potential benefit from dexmedetomidine and antipsychotics, but other agents such as cholinesterase inhibitors and melatonin have not been found to be helpful in preventing delirium and may even be harmful in the case of cholinesterase inhibitors.[70-72] The limited success of these therapies in clinical trials may in part be due to the lack of concurrent nonpharmacologic multicomponent delirium prevention strategies such as early rehabilitation and reduced sedation practices.

Sedation With Dexmedetomidine

Dexmedetomidine is a selective a2-adrenoreceptor agonist that has sedative, analgesic and anxiolytic properties. Studies suggest that it is associated with less delirium and may promote better sleep/wake cycle regulation when compared to medications that work through the GABA receptor pathway such as benzodiazepines.[73] Several large, well-designed randomized controlled trials comparing dexmedetomidine vs benzodiazepines for sedation in mechanically ventilated medical and surgical ICU patients have shown that dexmedetomidine was associated with a 30% lower prevalence of delirium[26] and more days alive without delirium and coma (7 vs 3 days).[27] In addition, patients receiving dexmedetomidine spent less time on mechanical ventilation (3.7 vs 5.6 days),[26] and dexmedetomidine was not associated with increased cost.[27] While evidence comparing dexmedetomidine to other sedatives such as opiates or propofol in the general medical and surgical ICU patient population are more limited,[74] these data are encouraging, particularly since the benefit was observed even in the setting of good sedation practices (eg, daily sedation vacation, targeted light-moderate sedation level, delirium monitoring).

While data are currently insufficient to support the widespread use of dexmedetomidine for sedation in all ICU patients, the 2013 ACCM guidelines recommend that dexmedetomidine could be considered for use as a sedative in patients with delirium and in patients who are at high risk for delirium.[24]

Antipsychotics

Antipsychotics (eg, haloperidol, risperidone, quietiapine) are hypothesized to treat delirium by blocking dopamine-mediated neuronal excitability and thus stabilizing cerebral function.[75] Although they were formerly recommended by major guidelines for treatment of ICU delirium (and are still widely used for that indication),[76,77] no large-scale prospective RCTs have tested the impact of antipsychotics on delirium duration, and the 2013 ACCM guidelines no longer recommend for, or against, their use. A small trial in ICU patients with delirium who were already receiving haloperidol found that delirium resolved faster in patients who received haloperidol plus quetiapine, compared to patients who only received haloperidol.[78] Clinical trials are currently underway to determine if antipsychotics are an effective treatment for ICU delirium.

Prognosis

Delirium is a strong predictor of ICU length of stay, even after adjusting for factors such as severity of illness and age,[79] and is independently associated with poor short-term consequences including increased duration of mechanical ventilation, increased hospital length of stay, and institutional placement.[4,80-83] While even 1 day of delirium is associated with poor clinical outcomes, it is also important to recognize that a "dose-dependent" relationship exists between the duration of delirium and poor clinical outcomes. For each day a patient is delirious, the risk of 6-months and 1-year mortality increases by 10%.[4,82] In addition, a longer duration of delirium is an independent predictor of cognitive impairment in both older and younger mechanically ventilated patients.[83,84] A recent study found that up to 34%

of patients had persistent deficits in global cognition and executive function that were similar to mild Alzheimer's disease and moderate traumatic brain injury 1 year after critical illness.[85] Increased delirium duration is also associated with disability in activities of daily living and worse motor-sensory function in the year following critical illness.[86] These adverse consequences can profoundly impact a patient's ability live independently after hospital discharge and can decrease their health-related quality of life. It can also be highly distressing for family members and caregivers and increase their caregiver burden.[87] With an annual cost of $4 to $16 billion in the United States alone,[81] ICU delirium is now recognized as a major public health problem.

Current Controversies and Unresolved Issues

Over the last 10 years, significant advances have been made in understanding risk factors for ICU delirium and have resulted in effective ICU-level strategies that have reduced the adverse impact of delirium. Nonetheless, many questions remain. First, animal models and trials on pathway modulation are needed to elucidate the pathophysiology of delirium. Second, the optimal pharmacologic therapy to prevent and reduce ICU delirium is still unknown, and the optimal protocols for different patient populations still need to be determined. Third, it is unclear if the improved short-term clinical outcomes that are associated with delirium reduction (eg, decreased time on mechanical ventilation, decreased ICU length of stay) translate into improved long-term cognitive, functional, and psychological outcomes. Fourth, more work is needed to elucidate the clinical implications of delirium severity and its subtypes (eg, subsyndromal delirium; hypoactive vs hyperactive delirium). Finally, more studies on cognitive and physical rehabilitation are needed to determine the optimal prescription, timing, and duration for different ICU patient populations.

REFERENCES

1. American Psychiatric Association. *Diagnostic and Statistical Manual of Mental Disorders.* 5th ed. Arlington, VA: American Psychiatric Publishing; 2013.

2. Dubois MJ, Bergeron N, Dumont M, Dial S, Skrobik Y. Delirium in an intensive care unit: a study of risk factors. *Intensive Care Med.* 2001;27(8):1297-1304.

3. Pisani MA, Araujo KL, Van Ness PH, Zhang Y, Ely EW, Inouye SK. A research algorithm to improve detection of delirium in the intensive care unit. *Crit Care.* 2006;10(4):R121.

4. Ely EW, Shintani A, Truman B, et al. Delirium as a predictor of mortality in mechanically ventilated patients in the intensive care unit. *JAMA.* 2004;291(14):1753-1762.

5. Van Rompaey B, Elseviers MM, Schuurmans MJ, Shortridge-Baggett LM, Truijen S, Bossaert L. Risk factors for delirium in intensive care patients: a prospective cohort study. *Crit Care.* 2009;13(3):R77.

6. Rudolph JL, Jones RN, Levkoff SE, et al. Derivation and validation of a preoperative prediction rule for delirium after cardiac surgery. *Circulation.* 2009;119(2):229-236.

7. Fong TG, Tulebaev SR, Inouye SK. Delirium in elderly adults: diagnosis, prevention and treatment. *Nat Rev Neurol.* 2009;5(4):210-220.

8. Hughes CG, Brummel NE, Vasilevskis EE, Girard TD, Pandharipande PP. Future directions of delirium research and management. *Best Pract Res Clin Anaesthesiol.* 2012;26(3):395-405.

9. Morandi A, Gunther ML, Vasilevskis EE, et al. Neuroimaging in delirious intensive care unit patients: a preliminary case series report. *Psychiatry (Edgmont).* 2010;7(9):28-33.

10. Gunther ML, Morandi A, Krauskopf E, et al. The association between brain volumes, delirium duration, and cognitive outcomes in intensive care unit survivors: the VISIONS cohort magnetic resonance imaging study*. *Crit Care Med.* 2012;40(7):2022-2032.

11. Vasilevskis EE, Han JH, Hughes CG, Ely EW. Epidemiology and risk factors for delirium across hospital settings. *Best Pract Res Clin Anaesthesiol.* 2012;26(3):277-287.

12. Pandharipande P, Cotton BA, Shintani A, et al. Prevalence and risk factors for development of delirium in surgical and trauma intensive care unit patients. *J Trauma.* 2008;65(1):34-41.

13. Ouimet S, Kavanagh BP, Gottfried SB, Skrobik Y. Incidence, risk factors and consequences of ICU delirium. *Intensive Care Med.* 2007;33(1):66-73.

14. Hsieh SJ, Soto GJ, Hope AA, Ponea A, Gong MN. The association between acute respiratory distress syndrome, delirium, and in-hospital mortality in

intensive care unit patients. *Am J Respir Crit Care Med.* 2015;191(1):71-78.

15. Pisani MA, Murphy TE, Van Ness PH, Araujo KL, Inouye SK. Characteristics associated with delirium in older patients in a medical intensive care unit. *Arch Intern Med.* 2007;167(15):1629-1634.

16. Pisani MA, Murphy TE, Araujo KL, Slattum P, Van Ness PH, Inouye SK. Benzodiazepine and opioid use and the duration of intensive care unit delirium in an older population. *Crit Care Med.* 2009;37(1):177-183.

17. Pandharipande P, Shintani A, Peterson J, et al. Lorazepam is an independent risk factor for transitioning to delirium in intensive care unit patients. *Anesthesiology.* 2006;104(1):21-26.

18. van den Boogaard M, Pickkers P, Slooter AJ, et al. Development and validation of PRE-DELIRIC (PREdiction of DELIRium in ICu patients) delirium prediction model for intensive care patients: observational multicentre study. *BMJ.* 2012;344:e420.

19. Ely EW, Girard TD, Shintani AK, et al. Apolipoprotein E4 polymorphism as a genetic predisposition to delirium in critically ill patients. *Crit Care Med.* 2007;35(1):112-117.

20. Kamdar BB, Niessen T, Colantuoni E, et al. Delirium transitions in the medical ICU: exploring the role of sleep quality and other factors*. *Crit Care Med.* 2015;43(1):135-141.

21. Agarwal V, O'Neill PJ, Cotton BA, et al. Prevalence and risk factors for development of delirium in burn intensive care unit patients. *J Burn Care Res.* 2010;31(5):706-715.

22. McPherson JA, Wagner CE, Boehm LM, et al. Delirium in the cardiovascular ICU: exploring modifiable risk factors. *Crit Care Med.* 2013;41(2):405-413.

23. Prakanrattana U, Prapaitrakool S. Efficacy of risperidone for prevention of postoperative delirium in cardiac surgery. *Anaesth Intensive Care.* 2007;35(5):714-719.

24. Barr J, Fraser GL, Puntillo K, et al. Clinical practice guidelines for the management of pain, agitation, and delirium in adult patients in the intensive care unit. *Crit Care Med.* 2013;41(1):278-280.

25. Bryczkowski SB, Lopreiato MC, Yonclas PP, Sacca JJ, Mosenthal AC. Risk factors for delirium in older trauma patients admitted to the surgical intensive care unit. *J Trauma Acute Care Surg.* 2014;77(6):944-951.

26. Riker RR, Shehabi Y, Bokesch PM, et al. Dexmedetomidine vs midazolam for sedation of critically ill patients: a randomized trial. *JAMA.* 2009;301(5):489-499.

27. Pandharipande PP, Pun BT, Herr DL, et al. Effect of sedation with dexmedetomidine vs lorazepam on acute brain dysfunction in mechanically ventilated patients: the MENDS randomized controlled trial. *JAMA*. 2007;298(22):2644-2653.

28. Maldonado JR, Wysong A, van der Starre PJ, Block T, Miller C, Reitz BA. Dexmedetomidine and the reduction of postoperative delirium after cardiac surgery. *Psychosomatics*. 2009;50(3):206-217.

29. Shehabi Y, Grant P, Wolfenden H, et al. Prevalence of delirium with dexmedetomidine compared with morphine based therapy after cardiac surgery: a randomized controlled trial (DEXmedetomidine COmpared to Morphine-DEXCOM Study). *Anesthesiology*. 2009;111(5):1075-1084.

30. Hopkins RO, Suchyta MR, Farrer TJ, Needham D. Improving post-intensive care unit neuropsychiatric outcomes: understanding cognitive effects of physical activity. *Am J Respir Crit Care Med*. 2012;186(12):1220-1228.

31. Inouye SK, Charpentier PA. Precipitating factors for delirium in hospitalized elderly persons. Predictive model and interrelationship with baseline vulnerability. *JAMA*. 1996;275(11):852-857.

32. McCusker J, Cole M, Abrahamowicz M, Han L, Podoba JE, Ramman-Haddad L. Environmental risk factors for delirium in hospitalized older people. *J Am Geriatr Soc*. 2001;49(10):1327-1334.

33. Needham DM, Korupolu R, Zanni JM, et al. Early physical medicine and rehabilitation for patients with acute respiratory failure: a quality improvement project. *Arch Phys Med Rehabil*. 2010;91(4):536-542.

34. Balas MC, Vasilevskis EE, Olsen KM, et al. Effectiveness and safety of the awakening and breathing coordination, delirium monitoring/management, and early exercise/mobility bundle. *Crit Care Med*. 2014;42(5):1024-1036.

35. Peterson JF, Pun BT, Dittus RS, et al. Delirium and its motoric subtypes: a study of 614 critically ill patients. *J Am Geriatr Soc*. 2006;54(3):479-484.

36. Spronk PE, Riekerk B, Hofhuis J, Rommes JH. Occurrence of delirium is severely underestimated in the ICU during daily care. *Intensive Care Med*. 2009;35(7):1276-1280.

37. Ely EW, Truman B, Shintani A, et al. Monitoring sedation status over time in ICU patients: reliability and validity of the Richmond Agitation-Sedation Scale (RASS). *JAMA*. 2003;289(22):2983-2991.

38. Riker RR, Fraser GL, Simmons LE, Wilkins ML. Validating the sedation-agitation scale with the bispectral index and visual analog scale in adult ICU

39. Ely EW, Margolin R, Francis J, et al. Evaluation of delirium in critically ill patients: validation of the Confusion Assessment Method for the Intensive Care Unit (CAM-ICU). *Crit Care Med*. 2001;29(7):1370-1379.

40. Bergeron N, Dubois MJ, Dumont M, Dial S, Skrobik Y. Intensive Care Delirium Screening Checklist: evaluation of a new screening tool. *Intensive Care Med*. 2001;27(5):859-864.

41. Brummel NE, Vasilevskis EE, Han JH, Boehm L, Pun BT, Ely EW. Implementing delirium screening in the ICU: secrets to success. *Crit Care Med*. 2013;41(9):2196-2208.

42. Chanques G, Jaber S, Barbotte E, e al. Impact of systematic evaluation of pain and agitation in an intensive care unit. *Crit Care Med*. 2006;34(6):1691-1699.

43. Gelinas C, Johnston C. Pain assessment in the critically ill ventilated adult: validation of the critical-care pain observation tool and physiologic indicators. *Clin J Pain*. 2007;23(6):497-505.

44. Wang W, Li HL, Wang DX, et al. Haloperidol prophylaxis decreases delirium incidence in elderly patients after noncardiac surgery: a randomized controlled trial*. *Crit Care Med*. 2012;40(3):731-739.

45. Payen JF, Bosson JL, Chanques G, Mantz J, Labarere J. Pain assessment is associated with decreased duration of mechanical ventilation in the intensive care unit: a post Hoc analysis of the DOLOREA study. *Anesthesiology*. 2009;111(6):1308-1316.

46. Schweickert WD, Gehlbach BK, Pohlman AS, Hall JB, Kress JP. Daily interruption of sedative infusions and complications of critical illness in mechanically ventilated patients. *Crit Care Med*. 2004;32(6):1272-1276.

47. Schweickert WD, Hall J. ICU-acquired weakness. *Chest*. 2007;131(5):1541-1549.

48. De Jonghe B, Sharshar T, Lefaucheur JP, et al. Paresis acquired in the intensive care unit: a prospective multicenter study. *JAMA*. 2002;288(22):2859-2867.

49. Mehta S, Burry L, Martinez-Motta JC, et al. A randomized trial of daily awakening in critically ill patients managed with a sedation protocol: a pilot trial. *Crit Care Med*. 2008;36(7):2092-2099.

50. Kress JP, Pohlman AS, O'Connor MF, Hall JB. Daily interruption of sedative infusions in critically ill patients undergoing mechanical ventilation. *N Engl J Med*. 2000;342(20):1471-1477.

51. Girard TD, Kress JP, Fuchs BD, et al. Efficacy and safety of a paired sedation and ventilator weaning

protocol for mechanically ventilated patients in intensive care (Awakening and Breathing Controlled Trial): a randomised controlled trial. *Lancet*. 2008;371(9607):126-134.

52. De Jonghe B, Bastuji-Garin S, Fangio P, et al. Sedation algorithm in critically ill patients without acute brain injury. *Crit Care Med*. 2005;33(1):120-127.

53. Strom T, Martinussen T, Toft P. A protocol of no sedation for critically ill patients receiving mechanical ventilation: a randomised trial. *Lancet*. 2010;375(9713):475-480.

54. Hager DN, Dinglas VD, Subhas S, et al. Reducing deep sedation and delirium in acute lung injury patients: a quality improvement project. *Crit Care Med*. 2013;41(6):1435-1442.

55. Critical Care Societies Collaborative – Critical Care, Five Things Physicians and Patients Should Question. http://www.choosingwisely.org/doctor-patient-lists/critical-care-societies-collaborative-critical-care/

56. Quinlan N, Rudolph JL. Postoperative delirium and functional decline after noncardiac surgery. *J Am Geriatr Soc*. 2011;59 (Suppl 2):S301-S304.

57. Inouye SK, Rushing JT, Foreman MD, Palmer RM, Pompei P. Does delirium contribute to poor hospital outcomes? A three-site epidemiologic study. *J Gen Intern Med*. 1998;13(4):234-242.

58. Schweickert WD, Pohlman MC, Pohlman AS, et al. Early physical and occupational therapy in mechanically ventilated, critically ill patients: a randomised controlled trial. *Lancet*. 2009;373(9678):1874-1882.

59. Lord RK, Mayhew CR, Korupolu R, et al. ICU early physical rehabilitation programs: financial modeling of cost savings. *Crit Care Med*. 2013;41(3):717-724.

60. Cooper AB, Thornley KS, Young GB, Slutsky AS, Stewart TE, Hanly PJ. Sleep in critically ill patients requiring mechanical ventilation. *Chest*. 2000;117(3):809-818.

61. Gabor JY, Cooper AB, Crombach SA, et al. Contribution of the intensive care unit environment to sleep disruption in mechanically ventilated patients and healthy subjects. *Am J Respir Crit Care Med*. 2003;167(5):708-715.

62. Pisani MA, Friese RS, Gehlbach BK, Schwab RJ, Weinhouse GL, Jones SF. Sleep in the intensive care unit. *Am J Respir Crit Care Med*. 2015;191(7):731-738.

63. Weinhouse GL, Schwab RJ, Watson PL, et al. Bench-to-bedside review: delirium in ICU patients—importance of sleep deprivation. *Crit Care*. 2009;13(6):234.

64. Kamdar BB, King LM, Collop NA, et al. The effect of a quality improvement intervention on perceived sleep quality and cognition in a medical ICU. *Crit Care Med*. 2013;41(3):800-809.

65. Van Rompaey B, Elseviers MM, Van Drom W, Fromont V, Jorens PG. The effect of earplugs during the night on the onset of delirium and sleep perception: a randomized controlled trial in intensive care patients. *Crit Care*. 2012;16(3):R73.

66. Li SY, Wang TJ, Vivienne Wu SF, Liang SY, Tung HH. Efficacy of controlling night-time noise and activities to improve patients' sleep quality in a surgical intensive care unit. *J Clin Nurs*. 2011;20(3-4):396-407.

67. Dennis CM, Lee R, Woodard EK, Szalaj JJ, Walker CA. Benefits of quiet time for neuro-intensive care patients. *J Neurosci Nurs*. 2010;42(4):217-224.

68. Inouye SK, Bogardus ST, Jr, Charpentier PA, et al. A multicomponent intervention to prevent delirium in hospitalized older patients. *N Engl J Med*. 1999;340(9):669-676.

69. Colombo R, Corona A, Praga F, et al. A reorientation strategy for reducing delirium in the critically ill. Results of an interventional study. *Minerva Anestesiol*. 2012;78(9):1026-1033.

70. Gamberini M, Bolliger D, Lurati Buse GA, et al. Rivastigmine for the prevention of postoperative delirium in elderly patients undergoing elective cardiac surgery—a randomized controlled trial. *Crit Care Med*. 2009;37(5):1762-1768.

71. van Eijk MM, Roes KC, Honing ML, et al. Effect of rivastigmine as an adjunct to usual care with haloperidol on duration of delirium and mortality in critically ill patients: a multicentre, double-blind, placebo-controlled randomised trial. *Lancet*. 2010;376(9755):1829-1837.

72. Bellapart J, Boots R. Potential use of melatonin in sleep and delirium in the critically ill. *Br J Anaesth*. 2012;108(4):572-580.

73. Nelson LE, Lu J, Guo T, Saper CB, Franks NP, Maze M. The alpha2-adrenoceptor agonist dexmedetomidine converges on an endogenous sleep-promoting pathway to exert its sedative effects. *Anesthesiology*. 2003;98(2):428-436.

74. Jakob SM, Ruokonen E, Grounds RM, et al. Dexmedetomidine for long-term sedation I: dexmedetomidine vs midazolam or propofol for sedation during prolonged mechanical ventilation: two randomized controlled trials. *JAMA*. 2012;307(11):1151-1160.

75. Meltzer HY, Matsubara S, Lee JC. Classification of typical and atypical antipsychotic drugs on the basis

of dopamine D-1, D-2 and serotonin2 pKi values. *J Pharmacol Exp Ther*. 1989;251(1):238-246.

76. Jacobi J, Fraser GL, Coursin DB, et al. Clinical practice guidelines for the sustained use of sedatives and analgesics in the critically ill adult. *Crit Care Med*. 2002;30(1):119-141.

77. Mac Sweeney R, Barber V, Page V, et al. A national survey of the management of delirium in UK intensive care units. *QJM*. 2010;103(4):243-251.

78. Devlin JW, Skrobik Y, Riker RR, et al. Impact of quetiapine on resolution of individual delirium symptoms in critically ill patients with delirium: a post-hoc analysis of a double-blind, randomized, placebo-controlled study. *Crit Care*. 2011;15(5):R215.

79. Ely EW, Gautam S, Margolin R, et al. The impact of delirium in the intensive care unit on hospital length of stay. *Intensive Care Med*. 2001;27(12):1892-1900.

80. Rudolph JL, Inouye SK, Jones RN, et al. Delirium: an independent predictor of functional decline after cardiac surgery. *J Am Geriatr Soc*. 2010;58(4):643-649.

81. Milbrandt EB, Deppen S, Harrison PL, et al. Costs associated with delirium in mechanically ventilated patients. *Crit Care Med*. 2004;32(4):955-962.

82. Pisani MA, Kong SY, Kasl SV, Murphy TE, Araujo KL, Van Ness PH. Days of delirium are associated with 1-year mortality in an older intensive care unit population. *Am J Respir Crit Care Med*. 2009;180(11):1092-1097.

83. Saczynski JS, Marcantonio ER, Quach L, et al. Cognitive trajectories after postoperative delirium. *N Engl J Med*. 2012;367(1):30-39.

84. Girard TD, Jackson JC, Pandharipande PP, et al. Delirium as a predictor of long-term cognitive impairment in survivors of critical illness. *Crit Care Med*. 2010;38(7):1513-1520.

85. Pandharipande PP, Girard TD, Jackson JC, et al. Long-term cognitive impairment after critical illness. *N Engl J Med*. 2013;369(14):1306-1316.

86. Brummel NE, Jackson JC, Pandharipande PP, et al. Delirium in the ICU and subsequent long-term disability among survivors of mechanical ventilation*. *Crit Care Med*. 2014;42(2):369-377.

87. Breitbart W, Gibson C, Tremblay A. The delirium experience: delirium recall and delirium-related distress in hospitalized patients with cancer, their spouses/caregivers, and their nurses. *Psychosomatics*. 2002;43(3):183-194.

88. Sessler CN, Gosnell MS, Grap MJ, et al. The Richmond Agitation-Sedation Scale: validity and reliability in adult intensive care unit patients. *Am J Respir Crit Care Med*. 2002;166(10):1338-1344.

89. Riker RR, Picard JT, Fraser GL. Prospective evaluation of the Sedation-Agitation Scale for adult critically ill patients. *Crit Care Med*. 1999;27(7):1325-1329.

Traumatic Brain and Spinal Cord Injury

50

Vikram Dhawan, MD and Jamie S. Ullman, MD, FACS, FAANS

KEY POINTS

1 Traumatic brain injury is primary and secondary. Primary injury is due to the direct impact of the trauma, while secondary is due to hypoxia leading to a cascade of events set off by ischemia/reperfusion. The focus of management is prevention and treatment of secondary injury.

2 Severity of brain injury is assessed both clinically and radiologically. A Glasgow Coma Scale (normal range 3-15) of 13 to 15 is considered mild brain injury, 9 to 12 moderate, and 3 to 8 severe brain injury. The Marshall score using head computed tomography (CT) is also used to predict severity.

3 The CT scan is the fastest and most widely used initial imaging modality available for skull and brain parenchymal lesions. CT angiography and perfusion studies further help to characterize vascular/perfusion deficits.

4 Preventing and treating hypoxia and hypotension to prevent hypoxia and adequate perfusion is of utmost importance.

5 Patients with risk factors for spinal cord injury should be handled with care in the field and their spine stabilized with rigid cervical collars on a board with straps.

TRAUMATIC BRAIN INJURY

Introduction

Traumatic brain injury (TBI) is the leading cause of death in the early decades of life. The estimated number of deaths is 50,000 with 40% of survivors with disability after the injury.[1] The estimated incidence is 17.5 to 24.6 deaths per 100,000 population.[2,3] Men are more likely to suffer TBI compared to women and the majority of injuries are due to falls.

Injury Types

In TBI injuries are classified as primary and secondary. Primary injury (Table 50–1) happens at the time of impact and secondary injury occurs later due to oxygen deprivation to the brain and the cascade of events set off by ischemia and reperfusion leading to further injury. The target of management focuses more on prevention and treatment of secondary brain injury.

In primary injury, depending upon the mechanism of trauma, fractures of the skull can be open or closed, depressed or nondepressed, and linear or comminuted. Most of these fractures are evident on clinical exam but radiography is required for accurate diagnosis. Both plain skull X-ray and computed tomography (CT) scan can be used for skull fractures, although plain radiologic films are better for linear calvarial fractures tangential to the axial plane. Multislice CT, alternatively, can delineate skull fractures

TABLE 50-1 Primary brain injury.

Primary Injury (Direct Impact)
Contusions
Bone fracture
Depressed skull fracture
Intracranial hemorrhage
Subdural
Epidural
Intracerebral
Diffuse axonal injury

better than plain CT scans. Fractures can result in neurologic deficits related to underlying brain injury, cerebral spinal fluid (CSF) leak (suggesting dural laceration) such as otorrhea or rhinorrhea, pituitary gland shearing injuries, and cranial nerve (CN) injuries. Depending on the fracture location, different CNs can be involved. Temporal bone fractures cause facial or acoustic nerve injuries, anterior fossa basal skull fracture can cause olfactory and optic nerve injuries, and clival fractures can cause abducens nerve injuries. Postauricular ecchymosis (Battle's sign) and periorbital ecchymosis (raccoon's eye) may be seen in basal skull fractures.

Most skull fractures are managed conservatively and prophylactic antibiotic use is controversial. Operative or endovascular treatment is indicated in traumatic aneurysms, carotid-cavernous fistula, CSF fistula, abscess management and for CN decompression.

Depending on the type of injury, different types of hemorrhage can occur in TBI as follows:

1. Epidural: Bleeding between dura and skull, usually from disrupted meningeal artery laceration. The mean age of patients with epidural hemorrhage (EDH) is between 20 and 30 years. About 70% to 90% of EDH is associated with skull fracture and in 36% of cases there was found to be a bleeding artery. Diffuse bone bleeding and venous bleeding (middle meningeal vein, diploic veins and dural venous sinuses) also cause EDH. The most common location is temporal because the bone is relatively thin and more vulnerable to fracture. It appears as a lentiform shape on

CT scan and usually stops at the suture lines where the dura is adherent (Figure 50-1).

2. Subdural: Occurs between the dura and the arachnoid space and is caused by disruption of bridging veins due to acceleration, deceleration, and rotational shearing forces. Frontal and parietal convexities are common places for subdural hemorrhage (SDH). The skull suture lines do not limit the bleeding, so on CT scan it can appear as crescent shape, conforming to the brain surface and traversing suture lines. Acute SDH appears hyperdense on CT scan but can have low-attenuation areas representing hyperacute or active hemorrhage. The incidence of SDH after TBI is approximately 11% with most due to motor vehicle accidents (MVAs) in young people and falls in the elderly. Up to 80% of patients with acute SDH may present with a Glasgow Coma Scale (GCS) less than 8 and pupillary abnormalities are seen in 50% of these patients (Figure 50-2).

3. Subarachnoid: Occurs in the space surrounding the brain and blood vessels.

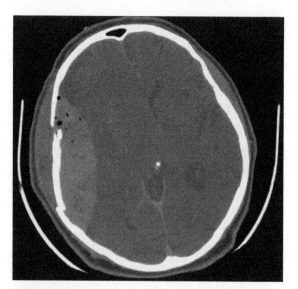

FIGURE 50-1 Epidural hematoma. Patient with significant head injury resulting in a comminuted right temporal bone fracture and underlying large epidural hematoma with pneumocephalus causing midline shift. This hematoma required surgical evacuation.

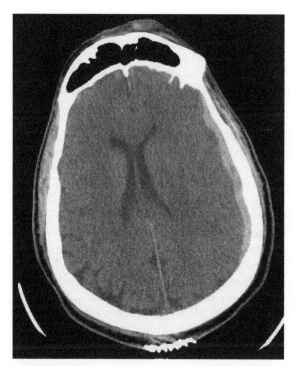

FIGURE 50–2 Subdural hematoma. Patient who fell and sustained an occipital laceration with staples noted in the soft tissues. He has a left frontoparietal subdural hematoma which is less than 1 cm in thickness causing only minimal midline shift. This patient underwent observation in the hospital.

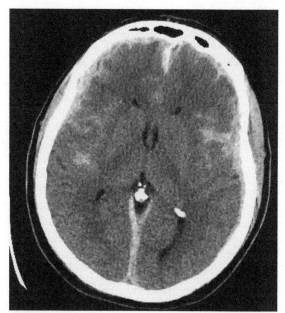

FIGURE 50–3 Subarachnoid hemorrhage. Patient fell after syncope, hit the back of his head, and sustained smaller bilateral subdural hematomas and diffuse subarachnoid blood in both sylvian fissures. There is also subdural hemorrhage along the midline falx cerebri.

Trauma is the most common reason and occurs due to crushed or ruptured small vessels. Bleeding is common on the cortical surface but occasionally in the basal cisterns. Complications of SAH include hydrocephalus, seizures, and cerebral vasospasm, the latter an independent predictor of mortality in severe TBI (Figure 50–3).[4]

4. Intraparenchymal or intracerebral: Bleeding occurs in the parenchyma of the brain. This can vary from contusions to large hematomas in superficial or deep brain areas. Coup injuries are contusions present at the site of impact. For example, an occipital impact may cause frontal contusions. The coup/countercoup phenomenon can also be seen with subdural hematomas, indicating acceleration–deceleration forces. The inferior frontal and temporal areas are most vulnerable to contusion formation due to ridging of the orbital roof and floor of the temporal fossa.[4]

Primary injury causes direct trauma to tissue leading to symptoms. Primary injury to the brain can be due to acceleration, deceleration, or rotational forces. Linear forces cause more superficial grey-matter injuries, while rotational forces cause deeper white-matter injuries leading to diffuse axonal injuries.

Secondary injury occurs due to deprivation of oxygen to the brain, which in turn sets off a cascade of biochemical/molecular events leading to further damage to brain. There are complex cellular and molecular changes including glutamate excitotoxic effects, oxidative stress, metabolic derangements, and inflammatory changes that play a major role in its pathogenesis.[5] Progressive neuronal necrosis and apoptosis may result.

At the beginning of the injury, huge depolarization of neurons and glial cells lead to influx of calcium into the brain cells. This increases oxygen-free radical reactions producing nitric oxide and excitatory amino acids such as glutamate. Glutamate is believed to promote cell death and dysfunction. Mitochondrial influx of calcium causes swelling and loss of ATP generation. As cellular membranes depend on ATP for their integrity, the inability to produce ATP leads to cell wall disruption and cell death.

Apart from the direct compromise of the cranium and outer layers of brain in TBI, disruption of blood brain barrier (BBB) contributes to loss of cerebral autoregulation. Cerebral autoregulation is the maintenance of cerebral blood flow (CBF) over a wide range of blood pressures of which cerebral perfusion pressure (CPP) is an important component. CPP is defined as the difference between mean arterial pressure (MAP) and intracranial pressure (ICP). In TBI, loss of autoregulation results in the inability to maintain adequate cerebral perfusion at CPP below 50. Loss of the BBB causes vasogenic edema from leaking, dilated blood vessels. In the brain, the edema resulting from cellular swelling is called cytotoxic edema.

According to the Monroe–Kellie principle, the cranium has fixed space and is occupied predominantly by brain tissue, CSF, and blood. Any increase in the volume in the cranium will lead to an increase in ICP, unless it is offset by a decrease in the volume of any one of the contents of the cranium. Therefore, intracranial hemorrhage and brain swelling, which increase intracranial mass, cause ICP increase and further brain damage.

In conclusion, production of oxygen-free radicals and calcium ion influx leads to widespread neuronal injury due to oxidation and enhanced enzymatic activity. Shearing of axons causes neurofilament disruption and increases permeability to calcium ions. Calpains are enzymes, which target the cytoskeleton of axons. Apoptosis ensues during TBI and there is proliferation of glial cells and astrocytes.[6]

Diffuse axonal injury is an acceleration–deceleration and rotational injury leading to shearing and disruption of the white-matter axonal transport system pathways. Both functional and anatomic injury can lead to unconsciousness in a patient not explained by other primary injuries (Figures 50–4a and 50–4b).

Injury Severity

The severity of injury determines the outcome of patients with TBI. The GCS (Table 50–2) is the most common tool used to grade severity of TBI at the time of initial injury. It uses 3 parameters—eye opening, motor response, and verbal response—for injury assessment.

A GCS score of 13 to 15 is considered mild TBI, 9 to 12 is moderate TBI, and 3 to 8 is severe TBI (patient in coma). About 70% to 90% of TBI cases are in the mild category. The GCS scoring system is limited when patients are intubated, aphasic, or aphonic as the verbal and eye variables are hard to measure. Other scales have been developed to account for respiratory or pupillary abnormalities.[7] These scales are not as widely used as the GCS.

Neuroimaging can also be used to predict injury severity. Presence of midline shifts, Intracerebral hemorrhage (ICH), SAH, and extra-axial hematomas on CT scan are poor prognostic markers. CT scan grading systems have been used for grading injury on initial presentation. The Marshall (Table 50–3) score is an example.[8,9]

Imaging

Imaging can provide important information regarding severity of injury. The goal of initial imaging is to rapidly diagnose life-threatening injuries in TBI and to treat them in a timely manner.

CT scan is a widely used modality and often the first one to be used in TBI, as it is fast and sensitive. Newer multi-row-detector CT is even faster and can scan a head within seconds. CT scan provides either 2D or 3D reformatted images. CT scans are useful for diagnosing and differentiating different types of brain hemorrhage, hydrocephalus, and mass effect.

In SDH, as mentioned earlier, the bleed can spread beyond skull suture lines and on CT scan blood can appear as crescent-shaped hyperdense in acute stage. Epidural hematomas appear as a lens-shaped hyperdensity not extending beyond suture margins. Subarachnoid hemorrhage usually conforms to the sulcal space of the brain and CT angiography helps in determining aneurysm or vascular malformation as the cause of the bleed.

If hemorrhagic, contusions can be seen on CT scan and if these small hemorrhages coalesce,

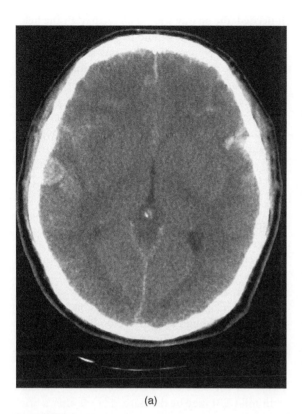
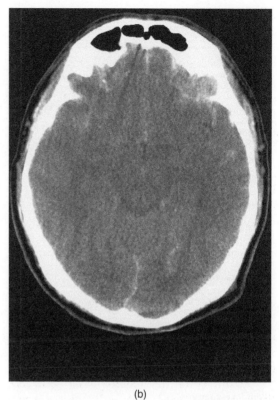

(a) (b)

FIGURE 50–4 Diffuse axonal injury. Patient with a significant diffuse injury after TBI resulting in (A) small right temporal and medial frontal intraparenchymal hemorrhages and (B) compressed/effaced perimesencephalic cisterns resulting in severe diffuse brain swelling. There is also bilateral frontal subarachnoid blood.

they can appear as a hematoma. Small hemorrhages (also called Duret hemorrhages) can be seen in the central pons as a consequence of severe uncal herniation and brainstem compression.

CT angiography is useful for assessing vascular injuries such as aneurysm, pseudoaneurysm, dissection, or thrombus, especially in the face of basilar skull fracture or those crossing a venous sinus. CT perfusion scanning evaluates time to peak (contrast) density, mean transit time, cerebral blood volume, and CBF. Normal CBF is 50 mL/100 g/min (of brain tissue). This modality helps in differentiating between ischemia and infarction, CBF measure 10 to 22 mL/100 g/min and less than 10 mL/100 g/min, respectively.

Magnetic resonance imaging (MRI) evaluates the movement of protons in the tissue when a magnetic field is applied. MR is sensitive in detecting subacute hemorrhage and depending on the appearance of blood on T1 and T2 weighted images, it can detect the timeline of the bleed. Gradient Recalled Echo is a modality of MR that provides information about blood or its degradation products, which appears as a low-intensity signal.

MR angiography is an alternative to CT angiography for characterizing major arterial or venous vascular injuries and can be done with or without contrast. Catheter angiography is the gold standard for diagnosing and treating vascular injuries. Due to long acquisition times, MR imaging may be problematic in critically ill, intubated trauma patients.[10]

Management

Prehospital Management

Management of TBI starts with basic resuscitation efforts. Supplemental oxygen to correct hypoxemia is essential. Hypoxemia should be avoided as it leads to an increase in severe disability and mortality.[11]

TABLE 50-2 Glasgow coma scale (GCS).

	Score
Eye Opening	
Spontaneous	4
Response to verbal command	3
Response to pain	2
No eye opening	1
Best Verbal Response	
Oriented	5
Confused	4
Inappropriate words	3
Incomprehensible	2
No verbal response	1
Best Motor Response	
Obeys commands	6
Localizes to pain	5
Withdraws to pain	4
Flexion response to pain	3
Extensor response to pain	2
No motor response	1

TABLE 50-3 Marshall's CT classification of brain injuries.

Class	Definition	Mortality
Diffuse injury type 1	No visible intracranial abnormality	10%
Diffuse injury type 2	0-5 mm midline shift/ cisterns present/and or lesion density present	14%
Diffuse injury type 3	0-5 mm midline shift/ cisterns compressed or absent/no lesion density > 25 cm³	34%
Diffuse injury type 4	Midline shift > 5 mm/no lesion density > 25 cm³	56%

If needed, the airway should be secured in the field. Volume resuscitation should begin prior to reaching the hospital. Hypertonic solutions such as hypertonic saline (HS) solutions are anti-inflammatory and immunomodulatory.[12] They can be used in case of suspected high ICP.

There is no role for prophylactic hyperventilation that should only be used as a brief temporizing measure when there are visible signs of herniation such as dilated and unreactive pupils, asymmetric pupils, extensor posturing, or no response or decline of 2 or more points from the baseline GCS.

Hospital Management

General Principles—Care should be taken to avoid hypoxemia and hypotension at all costs in TBI patients. Patients with oxygen saturations less than 60% have a 50% incidence of mortality or severe disability. Correction of hypotension improves outcomes. Although a systolic blood pressure value cutoff of 90 is normally targeted, the best systolic blood pressure for optimal outcomes is unknown.

Patients with concussion should be managed based on the severity of the concussion. Patients with mild TBI may be discharged home after a brief observation without any follow-up CT scan or imaging. The only exception is EDH as these patients may have a lucid interval and then rapidly progress to coma and death. Normally, analgesics (avoiding opioids) for headache and meclizine or vestibular exercises for dizziness are sufficient, along with appropriate rest. Some may have a seizure that may be mistaken for a more severe brain injury.

For severe TBI, management is based mainly on treatment of ICP/CPP derangements. Both mannitol and HS can be used to lower ICP. If patients have signs of high ICP such as transtentorial herniation or deteriorating mental status, ICP monitoring is advised for goal directed ICP treatment. Mannitol expands plasma volume and improves blood viscosity and improves oxygen delivery often reducing ICP within a few minutes. The osmotic effect starts within a few minutes and may last for a few hours as a gradient is established between plasma and cells. Mannitol can be given as an intravenous infusion or as a bolus in dosages of 0.25 g/kg to 1 g/kg. HS acts by mobilization of water from the brain across the BBB due to its high osmolality. It also improves plasma volume and hence blood flow. As with mannitol, it can also be given as intravenous infusion or bolus. HS comes in different concentrations ranging from 1.5% to 23.4%. As of this writing, there has been no consensus on the dosing and method of administration. Serum osmolality and serum sodium (Na) levels should be periodically checked, with a goal of not exceeding 320 mOsm/kg and Na of 155, respectively; there is potential for acute kidney injury if these levels are exceeded.

Hyperventilation reduces CO_2 and causes cerebral vasoconstriction, decreasing ICP. Hyperventilation is to be avoided in patients with TBI in the first hours (24-48 hours) as the CBF is decreased. It should only be used as a short-term temporizing measure to delay impending herniation.[13]

Currently, the indications for measuring ICP are GCS less than 8, an abnormal CT scan showing evidence of mass effect in the presence of SDH, EDH, or brain swelling. If the CT scan is normal but injury is severe then monitoring is indicated in patients who have 2 or more of the following:

1. Age above 40 years of age
2. Systolic blood pressure below 90
3. Unilateral or bilateral posturing

Measurement of ICP is useful for prognosis and helpful in guiding therapy. Patients in whom ICP responds to treatment do better than patients who fail to respond, while ICP elevations have been associated with poorer outcomes. The currently proposed threshold to initiate treatment for ICP is 20 to 25 mm Hg.

The devices to monitor ICP range from invasive to less invasive. The gold standard and most accurate ICP monitor is an external ventricular drain (EVD) attached to an external strain gauge pressure transducer. Although being most invasive, EVD confers the benefit of CSF drainage to manage ICP. The risk of hemorrhage is about 0.5% and infection is about 8% with these catheters. Internal transducer devices consisting of a fiber-optic cable or strain-gauge wire can be placed in the brain parenchyma. They are largely accurate but unable to be calibrated once inserted in the parenchyma and are subject to varying degrees of drift after several days of monitoring. Parenchymal devices are also helpful in cases where

intraventricular drain insertion is unsuccessful or when the ventricles are collapsed around the catheter. Subdural, subarachnoid, or epidural space transducers are fluid-coupled systems placed through a hollow bolt in the cranium but are less accurate and are now rarely used.

CPP, the difference between MAP and ICP, is a primary determinant of CBF (along with cerebrovascular resistance). Patients with TBI should be targeted for CPP between 60 and 70 mm Hg. CPP less than 50 mm Hg should be avoided and aggressively treated as patient outcomes are poor. In the same manner, higher CPP should be avoided, as there is an increased risk of acute lung injury, which is thought to be due to increased fluid and inotrope usage.

Besides monitoring and treating ICP/CPP, there are other parameters that can be monitored. These include brain tissue oxygen tension ($PtiO_2$), jugular venous oximetry, near infrared spectroscopy, cerebral microdialysis, CBF assessment, and continuous electroencephalography. Among these parameters, PiO_2 is the most commonly used due to wider commercial availability. TBI patients with optimal ICP/CPP may still have cerebral hypoxia in pericontusional areas according to $PtiO_2$ measurements. Patients who have $PtiO_2$ less than 15 for increased duration have been shown to have poor outcomes and increased mortality. Use of $PtiO_2$ along with use of ICP-based treatment/CPP-based treatment may improve outcomes as compared to only ICP-based management/CPP-based management.[14]

TBI patients may need sedation or analgesia or both for comfort and pain relief. Analgesics such as morphine, fentanyl, or sufentanil provide pain relief, but have minimal effect on ICP. Sedative agents commonly used include propofol and midazolam. The long-term use of propofol or midazolam does not result in significant differences in ICP, CPP, or MAP. In general, sedation decreases ICP in patients with TBI. Propofol infusion may have some side effects such as hypertriglyceridemia (if patients are on TPN, the lipid should be reduced) and the propofol infusion syndrome (rare but usually fatal), especially if used in doses of more than 4 mg/kg/h for more than 48 hours. Barbiturates such as pentobarbital can be used in patients with elevated ICP. For pentobarbital, the following dosing regimen can

TABLE 50-4 Analgesic and sedative dosing.

Morphine sulfate	4 mg/kg infusion with titration
Fentanyl	2-5 mcg/kg/h infusion
Sufentanil	0.05-2 mcg/kg infusion
Midazolam	2-4 mg/h
Propofol	20-75 mcg/kg/min infusion

be used: loading dose 10 mg/kg over 30 min; 5 mg/kg/h for 3 doses; and maintenance of 1 mg/kg/h (see Table 50-4).

Other medications that are used include ketamine and etomidate. The use of any specific analgesics or sedatives, however, has not shown to improve outcome after TBI.[15]

Use of prophylactic hypothermia in patients with TBI has not shown statistically significant mortality benefit,[13] although hypothermia can be used for the management of high ICP.

Patients with TBI and spinal cord injury are at high risk of venous thromboembolism (VTE). The risk ranges from 5% to 6% in patients with spinal cord injury and 3% to 5% in TBI.[16] Currently, the recommendations are to add mechanical thromboprophylaxis to pharmacologic thromboprophylaxis in patients with TBI. When the decision to employ pharmacologic thromboprophylaxis is made after TBI or spinal injury, intravenous unfractionated heparin is the first choice due to the short half-life and rapid reversibility. Low-molecular-weight heparin (LMWH) is an option if the bleeding risks are assessed to be low, but LMWH is avoided in renal failure due to bioaccumulation. There is no data about the timing of VTE prophylaxis, but the sooner it can be safely started, the better. Our protocol is to commence chemoprophylaxis 24 hours after the last stable (no increase in hemorrhage) CT.

Patients with TBI should be started early on nutritional support. Early nutrition support may reduce infectious complications and mortality. If possible enteral nutrition should be started 24 to 48 hours following admission with the aim of reaching goal within 5-7 days.

Post-traumatic seizures (PTS) can occur in patients with TBI with an incidence of 4% to 25% within the first 7 days of injury. Risk factors for PTS after TBI are as follows: GCS less than 10; epidural, subdural, or intracerebral hematoma; cerebral contusion; depressed skull fracture; penetrating head injury; and seizures within the first 24 hours of injury.

Anticonvulsants can be used to decrease the incidence of early PTS during the first week of TBI. They are not recommended for long-term use to prevent late onset PTS. Phenytoin or valproate can be used for seizure prophylaxis. The use of steroids in TBI is not recommended and may be even harmful.

Surgical Management

Surgical options are considered using the following criteria.

Epidural—If EDH volume is more than 30 cm³, it should be evacuated regardless of the GCS score. Patients with anisocoria and coma should undergo hematoma evacuation as soon as possible. Patients can be managed nonoperatively, if they meet all of the following criteria: EDH volume is less than 30 cm³; thickness is less than 15 mm; midline shift is less than 5 mm; GCS is more than 8; and no focal neurologic deficit.[17]

Subdural—Patients with acute traumatic SDH with GCS less than 9 should have ICP monitoring. These patients can be watched nonoperatively if the SDH thickness is less than 10 mm and midline shift is less than 5. If the GCS decreases by 2 points from the time of admission and/or they have asymmetrical or fixed and dilated pupils and/or their ICP rises above 20, they should be taken to operating room (OR). Patients with a hematoma thickness more than 10 mm or midline shift more than 5 mm should be operated upon irrespective of the GCS score. Surgery should be conducted sooner rather than later to improve outcomes.[18]

Parenchymal Lesions—Patients with TBI can have either focal or diffuse parenchymal lesions. Diffuse or nonfocal injuries include cerebral edema or diffuse injury. Focal lesions include contusions, ICH, delayed traumatic ICH (DTICH), and infarctions. DTICH is defined as ICH, which was not initially present on admission CT scan but developed subsequently, mostly in the region of contusions.

Patients with parenchymal lesions should be operated on in the following situations: deteriorating neurologic exam as evidenced by a decrease in GCS by 2 points; refractory ICP; signs of mass effect on CT scan such as basal cistern obliteration; GCS of 6 to 8 and fronto-temporal lesion of more than 20 cm³ with midline shift more than 5 mm and/or cisternal obliteration on CT scan; any patient with a lesion volume more than 50 cm³.

Patients who do not meet the aforementioned criteria and who have their ICP controlled medically can be monitored with serial exams and CT scans. Patients who have diffuse cerebral swelling and difficult to control ICP, can undergo decompressive craniectomy. Others may have focal decompression and lesion resection.[19]

Traumatic Posterior Fossa Mass Lesions—Patients with lesions in the posterior fossa leading to neurologic dysfunction or deterioration require emergent craniotomy as they have a tendency to worsen rapidly. If CT scans show signs of a mass effect such as distortion or compression of the fourth ventricle or hydrocephalus, suboccipital craniotomy should be performed.[20]

Depressed Skull Fractures—Patients with depressed skull fractures may have dural penetration, hematoma formation, and wound contamination. The fracture can involve frontal sinuses and also major cosmetic defects. Surgery may be warranted if any of the aforementioned is present. It is also recommended to operate if the bone is depressed the full thickness of the cranium, or if CSF leak or brain parenchyma is present in the open fractures.[21]

Outcomes

Patients after TBI may follow basic functions of emergence of consciousness, recovery of neuropsychologic functions, and return of functional capacity, or they can progress to coma and further deterioration leading to brain death (Table 50–5).[22]

SPINAL CORD INJURY

Introduction

Traumatic spinal cord injury (TSCI) predominantly affects the young adult (age < 40 years). Annually there are 15 to 40 cases per million. MVA account for the majority (40%-50%) of TSCI. Falls (20%) and violence (14%) account for the rest. The level of injury also determines an individual's functionality. Injuries below T1 are likely to result in independent function, while injury above C6 requires almost complete dependency.[23]

Facial fractures and TBI are not associated with an increased risk of TSCI.[24] Underlying spinal disease such as osteoporosis, rheumatoid arthritis, or ankylosing spondylitis (AS) can predispose to TSCI.

TABLE 50–5 Clinical features of various TBI outcomes.

	Brain Death	Coma	Vegetative State	Minimally Conscious State	Emergence From Minimally Conscious State
Eye Opening	None	None	Occasional	Occasional but inconsistent	Present
Visual Fixation or Pursuit	None	None	None	Occasional but inconsistent	Present
Spontaneous Movement	None	None	Purposeless	Present	Purposeful
Response to Pain	None	None, flexion or extension	Variable	Variable	Variable
Vocalization	None	None	None	Occasional but inconsistent	Present
Functional Communication	None	None	None	Occasional but inconsistent	Consistent

Spinal Cord Anatomy

The spinal cord extends from the medulla in the cervical region to the lumbosacral area. The spinal canal contains the spinal cord, CSF, epidural fat and vessels, and dura mater. On cross-section, the spinal cord fills about 50% of the spinal canal. The corticospinal tracts originating from cerebral cortex (upper motor neuron) cross over to the contralateral side in the medulla and form the lateral corticospinal tract. The corticospinal tract makes synapsis with the lower motor neurons in ventral spinal cord. The sensory input originates in the dorsal grey-matter neurons. Fibers carrying pain and temperature cross over immediately in the spinal cord and ascend up as lateral spinothalamic tracts. Proprioception and vibratory sensation ascend ipsilaterally in the funiculus gracilis and funiculus cuneatus. At the level of L1-L2, there is the conus medullaris, below which the spinal canal is filled by motor and sensory neurons forming the cauda equina.

Pathophysiology

A number of processes occur during spinal cord injury. Primary injury occurs at the time of direct impact to the spinal cord and secondary injury as a cascade of events after the moment of impact. Primary injury can happen due to extension, flexion, or rotation of the spinal cord. It happens when the above movements occur beyond the normal movement capacity of the vertebral column. Most of the information regarding the pathophysiology is derived from animal models and it is still not known how much intact spinal cord is required for neuronal function.

Proposed mechanisms of TSCI include the following:

1. Vascular abnormalities: Most of the impact is due to disruption of the microvasculature. Larger vessels are rarely injured. As the grey matter is highly metabolic, it is more vulnerable to ischemia and gets injured earlier. Further, there may be loss of autoregulation (the ability to maintain blood flow at various pressures) that can lead to further insults to the spinal cord, if the blood pressure varies due to other injuries. Paradoxically, to maintain perfusion to the spinal cord, maintenance of higher pressures may lead to reperfusion injury.

2. Free radicals: Free radicals such as superoxide are produced due to ischemia and these free radicals react with cell membranes causing lipid peroxidation, damaging cell membranes. Superoxides also damage mitochondrial DNA and associated enzymes, inhibiting sodium-potassium ATPase. All this leads to generation of toxic metabolites such as malonyldialdehyde, leading to cell death.

3. Excitotoxic glutamate and electrolyte imbalance: Glutamate accumulates due to ischemia in cells. It acts on N-methyl-D-aspartate receptors and opens calcium channels. The huge influx of calcium causes activation of lethal enzymes. The loss of ATP also leads to an increase in sodium and water within the cell bodies. It is also thought to lead to cell death especially in axonal and glial components of the white matter.

4. Inflammation: At the site of injury in spinal cord, the inflammatory cells secrete lytic enzymes and cytokines such as TNF-α, interleukins, and interferons. These lead to further cell damage.[25]

Histologically, the spinal cord develops microhemorrhages within 30 minutes of trauma beginning anteriorly and moving posteriorly over the next 1 hour. These microhemorrhages coalesce and necrosis of the spinal cord extend beyond the initial impact of the injury. Edema begins within 6 hours of injury, maximizing in 48 to 72 hours.[26]

Neurologic Injury Classification and Clinical Presentation

The American Spinal Injury Association (ASIA) classifies spinal cord injury based on the sensory and motor impairments in the spinal cord after TSCI. It assesses different dermatomes for light touch and pin prick sensation and 10 key muscle movements to establish the grading of TSCI. The maximum score is 100. Any sensory or motor response at the S4-S5 level indicates incomplete spinal cord injury. If both are absent then barring exception of injury at that level, it signifies complete cord

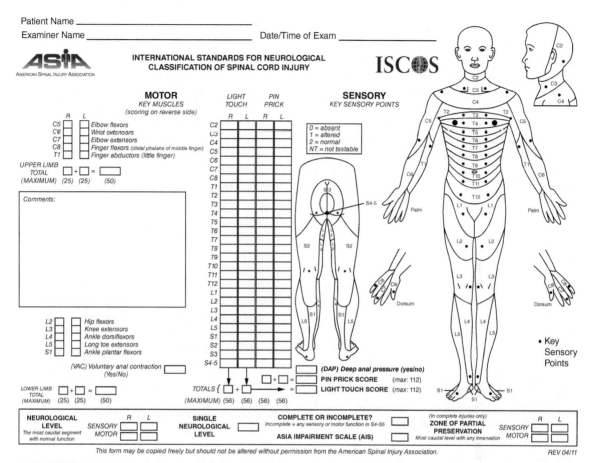

FIGURE 50–5 ASIA (American Spinal Injury Association) classification. (*Reproduced with permission from American Spinal Injury Association (ASIA). International Standards for Neurological Classification of Spinal Cord Injury (ISNCSCI).*)

paralysis. Preservation of perianal sensation, rectal tone, or great toe flexion means intact S2-S5 and is called sacral sparing. "Spinal shock" is the loss of all muscle tone and reflexes. If the S2-S5 reflexes have not returned within 24 hours, the injury is called complete spinal cord injury (ASIA class A), which is associated with a poor prognosis and poor spinal cord function recovery (Figure 50–5).

Incomplete Spinal Cord Syndromes

Central Cord Syndrome

Patients' central grey matter is affected with sparing of the surrounding outer spinal cord. Clinically, patients are often tetraparetic with sacral sparing; upper extremity function is often affected more than that of the lower extremities.

Anterior Cord Syndrome

Occurs due to injury of the anterior spinal artery affecting the anterior two-thirds of the spinal cord. Patients have both motor and sensory loss (pain, temperature). Proprioception is preserved due to sparing of the posterior spinal cord.

Posterior Cord Syndrome

A rare syndrome where there is loss of proprioception in an otherwise normal functioning spinal cord.

Brown-Sequard Syndrome

Injury to one side of the spinal cord leads to ipsilateral motor function and proprioception loss with contralateral pain and temperature loss. This syndrome usually occurs after penetrating spinal cord injury.[26]

Prehospital Management

Emergency medical personnel are often the first responders for suspected spinal cord injury. Three percent to 25% of patients can have TSCI after primary trauma during transport or early management. Patients with suspected cervical TSCI should have their spine secured using a rigid cervical collar and immobilization, which may include a backboard with straps. Patients who are awake and fully oriented (without intoxication) with no complaints of neck pain or tenderness and no neurologic deficit or distracting injuries do not need immobilization as is the case with patients with penetrating spinal injury. After initial resuscitation and, if necessary, spine immobilization, patients should be taken to the nearest medical center equipped to handle such injuries. Delay in transport leads to increased costs and less favorable outcomes.[27]

Hospital Management

Radiography

Once the patient is safely transported to a hospital and undergoes initial resuscitation and clinical examination, the full extent of their spinal injury is assessed by different diagnostic modalities. The following scenarios guide which patient needs radiographic evaluation.

Awake, Asymptomatic Patient—Fully awake, oriented nonintoxicated patients with no neck pain or tenderness, who have no motor or sensory deficit and no major other injuries (which prevent full evaluation), need not have any imaging study.

Awake, Symptomatic Patient—These patients should have good-quality CT scans of the cervical spine. If that is not available, then 3-view cervical spine series (anteroposterior, lateral, and odontoid) should be taken. If there are no radiographic abnormalities and patient is still symptomatic, cervical immobilization can be discontinued in following situations: when the patient is asymptomatic; if dynamic flexion/extension of cervical radiographs are normal; if spine MRI done within 48 hours is normal; at the physician's discretion.

Obtunded Patient—These patients should undergo radiologic imaging. Thin-cut CT with axial, coronal, and sagittal reconstructions, making sure to visualize both bone and soft-tissue imaging, can be used

in the decision to remove cervical spine immobilization, especially if such patients are not expected to regain consciousness within 24 hours. Flexion/extension imaging should not be attempted. High clinical suspicion of TSCI should prompt expert clinical consult. MRI in TSCI has an added benefit of providing information regarding soft-tissue/ligamentous injury in the cervical spine.

Management

General Management

Patients with TSCI frequently have respiratory and cardiovascular dysfunction. Patients have reduced vital and inspiratory capacity. They may have frequent hypoxemia, which may exacerbate cord ischemia. Hypotension is frequent after TSCI and may be due to hypovolemia or neurogenic shock. Neurogenic shock is the sudden loss of sympathetic tone as a result of injury to the cervical and upper thoracic spinal cord. Neurogenic shock is manifested by hypotension and bradycardia. Patients who were aggressively managed with close monitoring of vital signs such as blood pressure and oxygen saturation had improved outcomes. Intensive care unit monitoring is recommended in such cases. Hypoxemia should be treated with supplemental oxygen as necessary. The mean arterial blood pressure should be maintained between 85 and 90 mm Hg for the first 7 days of injury. Vasopressors can be used if required for that purpose.[27]

Pharmacotherapy

Use of steroids such as methylprednisolone is associated with complications such as wound infection, hyperglycemia, and even death and is not recommended according to recent guidelines. GM-1 ganglioside (GM) is a natural compound thought to have antiexcitatory properties and neuronal regeneration. Patients receiving GM initially showed improvement in neurologic recovery, which was subsequently lost. It is, therefore, also not recommended to use in acute TSCI. Other agents studied have not been shown to improve outcomes.[27]

Nutrition

Patients with TSCI have a catabolic state due to the intense reaction of the body to trauma. This leads to breakdown of muscle mass and loss of proteins, immunosuppression, and loss of gastrointestinal barrier breakdown. It makes intuitive sense to start feeding sooner than later. Although early nutrition in these patients have not shown to improve neurologic outcome, nutritional support within the first 72 hours of injury is recommended.[28]

Deep Vein Thrombosis and Thromboprophylaxis

Patients with TSCI have an increased incidence of deep vein thrombosis (DVT) (10%-18%) and the majority occur within the first 3 months of injury. Patients with TSCI should be started on both pharmacologic and mechanical DVT thromboprophylaxis. Low dose heparin, low-molecular-weight heparin or oral anticoagulation can be used but not alone. Mechanical thromboprophylaxis including rotating beds, pneumatic compression stockings, or electrical stimulation should be used additionally. Prophylaxis should be continued for 3 months and then discontinued. Inferior vena cava filters are not recommended unless anticoagulation is contraindicated or the patient has developed DVT or pulmonary embolism while receiving pharmacologic prophylaxis. Ultrasound Doppler studies should be used for diagnosis of DVT.[29]

Management of Specific Injuries

Occipital condyle fractures are rare injuries that should be suspected in patients with high impact trauma, lower CN deficits, and loss of consciousness and neck pain. CT scan is recommended for fracture evaluation. External cervical immobilization is recommended for all types. If bilateral, more rigid immobilization with a halo device is recommended. Surgery (occipitocervical stabilization and fusion) is done in cases with associated atlanto-occipital ligament injury or instability.[30]

Atlanto-occipital dislocation (AOD) is frequently missed and should be suspected in patients with TBI. The condyle-C1 interval should be measured on CT scan for its diagnosis (mostly in pediatric patients). A lateral cervical radiograph showing basion-axial interval-basion dental interval can also demonstrate this injury. Presence of upper cervical prevertebral soft-tissue swelling raises suspicion of AOD. Patients with these injuries often have or may develop neurologic deficits. These injuries should always be treated surgically with internal fixation and fusion.[31]

Isolated atlas fractures can be diagnosed with plain radiography (open mouth radiograph) or CT. They can be of 3 types, anterior or posterior arch fractures (Landell type 1), burst fractures (Landell type 2), and lateral mass fractures (Landell type 3) (Figures 50–6a and 50–6b).

MRI can assess whether the transverse atlantal ligament is intact or not, which will determine if the fracture is stable or not. In general, type 1 and type 3 fractures are considered stable and may be treated with collar or halo. Type 2 fractures may need surgical stabilization and fusion.[32]

C2 dens fracture: Forceful flexion-extension of the head in the sagittal plane may result in fracture of the odontoid process (dens). Three types of fractures are identified; type 1 fracture occurs above the transverse ligament and is stable. Type 2 fracture results in complete disruption of the base of dens and is unstable, requiring surgical management. Type 2 has been further divided into types 2A, 2B, and 2C depending on whether it is nondisplaced, displaced amenable to anterior fixation, and displaced or communicated amenable to posterior fixation/fusion, respectively. Type 3 fractures involve the extension of fracture through the body of C2 and are considered mechanically unstable.[33]

Subaxial cervical spinal injuries can include burst fractures, unilateral or bilateral facet dislocation, and other bony injuries. Patients with these injuries can be managed with external or internal immobilization/fixation. The goal is to restore alignment and decompress the spinal canal. Both anterior and posterior approaches are good surgical options. For patients with incomplete spinal cord injuries and canal compromise, surgical decompression within 24 hours of injury is recommended.[34] Patients who have AS should undergo thorough investigation with CT scan or MRI, even in minor trauma. AS patients requiring surgery should have either posterior fixation or combined anterior and posterior fixation but not stand-alone anterior fixation due to high failure rates.[35]

Acute traumatic central cord syndrome (CCS) is a clinical entity that is suspected when upper extremities are weaker than lower extremities and is most commonly associated with cervical spondylotic disease or ossification of the posterior longitudinal ligament. Patients to be diagnosed with CCS

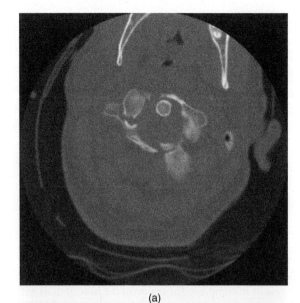

(a)

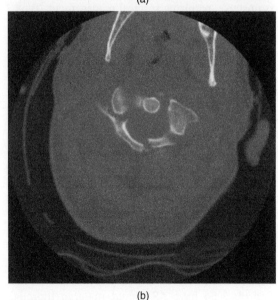

(b)

FIGURE 50–6 C1 comminuted burst fracture involving (A) the right anterior arch and (B) the left posterior arch. This patient was treated in a halo brace.

should have 10 points lower on the ASIA classification motor score in the upper extremities as compared to lower extremities. CCS is thought to be due to disruption of the corticospinal tract. It can be associated with other injuries such as fractures and dislocations. Surgical decompression is considered advisable in many circumstances.[36]

Vertebral artery injuries (VAI) (nonpenetrating cervical trauma) are usually seen in patients with fractures through the foramen transversarium, facet fracture-dislocation, or vertebral subluxation. The modified Denver screening criteria in patients with blunt cervicovertebral injury should prompt VAI evaluation. CT angiography is a good, quick screening tool (Figures 50–7a and 50–7b).

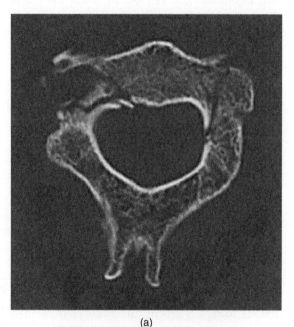

(a)

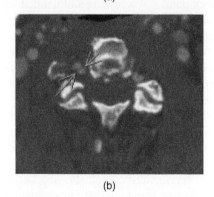

(b)

FIGURE 50–7 (A) C2 vertebral and bipedicular fractures in elderly male after a fall as seen on axial CT. The fracture extends to the right foramen transversarium. (B) CT angiogram reveals luminal hypodensities consistent with a small vertebral artery dissection. The patient was placed on antiplatelet therapy (aspirin).

Angiography or MRI may also be used for diagnosis. Symptomatic patients may be treated with antiplatelet therapy, depending on their risk-benefit ratio. Asymptomatic VAI need not be treated.[37]

REFERENCES

1. Lei J, Gao G, Jiang J. Acute traumatic brain injury: is current management evidence based? An empirical analysis of systematic reviews. *J Neurotrauma*. 2013;30(7):529-537.
2. Adekoya N, et al. Surveillance for traumatic brain injury deaths—United States, 1989-1998. *MMWR Surveill Summ*. 2002;51(10):1-14.
3. Rutland-Brown W, et al. Incidence of traumatic brain injury in the United States, 2003. *J Head Trauma Rehabil*. 2006;21(6):544-548.
4. Stippler M. Trauma of the nervous system. In: Daroff RB, et al., eds. *Bradley's Neurology in Clinical Practice*. Philadelphia: Saunders; 2012:942-956.
5. Rosenfeld JV, et al. Early management of severe traumatic brain injury. *Lancet*. 2012;380(9847):1088-1098.
6. Greve MW, Zink BJ. Pathophysiology of traumatic brain injury. *Mt Sinai J Med*. 2009;76(2):97-104.
7. Stead LG, et al. Validation of a new coma scale, the FOUR score, in the emergency department. *Neurocrit Care*. 2009;10(1):50-54.
8. Marshall LF, et al. The diagnosis of head injury requires a classification based on computed axial tomography. *J Neurotrauma*. 1992;9(Suppl 1):S287-S292.
9. Maas AI, et al. Prediction of outcome in traumatic brain injury with computed tomographic characteristics: a comparison between the computed tomographic classification and combinations of computed tomographic predictors. *Neurosurgery*. 2005;57(6):1173-1182; discussion 1173-1182.
10. Kubal WS. Updated imaging of traumatic brain injury. *Radiol Clin North Am*. 2012;50(1):15-41.
11. Stocchetti N, Furlan A, Volta F. Hypoxemia and arterial hypotension at the accident scene in head injury. *J Trauma*. 1996;40(5):764-767.
12. Scalfani MT, et al. Effect of osmotic agents on regional cerebral blood flow in traumatic brain injury. *J Crit Care*. 2012;27(5):526 e7-e12.
13. Brain Trauma, F., S. American Association of Neurological, and S. Congress of Neurological, Guidelines for the management of severe traumatic brain injury. *J Neurotrauma*. 2007;24(Suppl 1):S1-S106.
14. Stiefel MF, et al. Reduced mortality rate in patients with severe traumatic brain injury treated with brain tissue oxygen monitoring. *J Neurosurg*. 2005;103(5):805-811.
15. Barr J, et al. Clinical practice guidelines for the management of pain, agitation, and delirium in adult patients in the intensive care unit. *Crit Care Med*. 2013;41(1):263-306.
16. Gould MK, et al. Prevention of VTE in nonorthopedic surgical patients: antithrombotic therapy and prevention of thrombosis, 9th ed: American College of Chest Physicians evidence-based clinical practice guidelines. *Chest*. 2012;141(2 Suppl):e227S-e277S.
17. Bullock MR, et al. Surgical management of acute epidural hematomas. *Neurosurgery*. 2006;58(3 Suppl): S7-S15; discussion Si-iv.
18. Bullock MR, et al. Surgical management of acute subdural hematomas. *Neurosurgery*. 2006; 58(3 Suppl):S16-S24; discussion Si-iv.
19. Bullock MR, et al. Surgical management of traumatic parenchymal lesions. *Neurosurgery*. 2006;58(3 Suppl): S25-S46; discussion Si-iv.
20. Bullock MR, et al. Surgical management of posterior fossa mass lesions. *Neurosurgery*. 2006; 58(3 Suppl):S47-S55; discussion Si-iv.
21. Bullock MR, et al. Surgical management of depressed cranial fractures. *Neurosurgery*. 2006;58(3 Suppl): S56-S60; discussion Si-iv.
22. Stevens RD, Sutter R. Prognosis in severe brain injury. *Crit Care Med*. 2013;41(4):1104-1123.
23. Evans LT, Lollis SS, Ball PA. Management of acute spinal cord injury in the neurocritical care unit. *Neurosurg Clin N Am*. 2013;24(3):339-347.
24. Clayton JL, et al. Risk factors for cervical spine injury. *Injury*. 2012;43(4):431-435.
25. Kwon BK, et al. Pathophysiology and pharmacologic treatment of acute spinal cord injury. *Spine J*. 2004;4(4):451-464.
26. Gupta M, Benson D, Keenen T. Initial evaluation and management of spine-injured patients. In: B.D. Browner, et al., eds. *Skeletal Trauma Basic Science, Management, and Reconstruction*. Philadelphia (Pensilvania, Estados Unidos): Saunders/Elsevier; 2008:729-752.
27. Walters BC, et al. Guidelines for the management of acute cervical spine and spinal cord injuries: 2013 update. *Neurosurgery*. 2013;60(Suppl 1):82-91.
28. Dhall SS, et al. Nutritional support after spinal cord injury. *Neurosurgery*. 2013;72(Suppl 2):255-259.
29. Dhall SS, et al. Deep venous thrombosis and thromboembolism in patients with cervical spinal cord injuries. *Neurosurgery*. 2013;72(Suppl 2):244-254.
30. Theodore N, et al. Occipital condyle fractures. *Neurosurgery*. 2013;72(Suppl 2):106-113.

31. Theodore N, et al. The diagnosis and management of traumatic atlanto-occipital dislocation injuries. *Neurosurgery*. 2013;72(Suppl 2):114-126.

32. Ryken TC, et al. Management of isolated fractures of the atlas in adults. *Neurosurgery*. 2013;72(Suppl 2): 127-131.

33. Ryken TC, et al. Management of isolated fractures of the axis in adults. *Neurosurgery*. 2013;72(Suppl 2): 132-150.

34. Fehlings MG, et al. Early versus delayed decompression for traumatic cervical spinal cord injury: results of the Surgical Timing in Acute Spinal Cord Injury Study (STASCIS). *PLoS One*. 2012;7(2):e32037.

35. Aarabi B, et al. Subaxial cervical spine injury classification systems. *Neurosurgery*. 2013;72 (Suppl 2):170-186.

36. Aarabi B, et al. Management of acute traumatic central cord syndrome (ATCCS). *Neurosurgery*. 2013;72(Suppl 2):195-204.

37. Harrigan MR, et al. Management of vertebral artery injuries following nonpenetrating cervical trauma. *Neurosurgery*. 2013;72(Suppl 2):234-243.

General Postoperative Management

Leon Boudourakis, MD, MHS and Adel Bassily-Marcus, MD

KEY POINTS

1. It is of the utmost importance that the staff of the intensive care unit (ICU) understands exactly the type and purpose of each of the foreign bodies and tubes as well as how these tubes should be managed.

2. The aggregate of evidence from the last 15 years generally supports the notion that limited transfusion thresholds are correlated with superior outcomes in most patient populations.

3. Early parenteral nutrition (< 7 days post-ICU admission) has been associated with increased risk of nosocomial infections without benefit.

4. Stress dose steroids should only be considered in refractory septic shock after fluids have been given. There is no benefit to performing adrenocorticotropic hormone (ACTH) stimulation test or random cortisol level.

5. Early mobility decreases length of stay and ventilator duration, and it has been shown to be cost-effective.

INTRODUCTION: INTENSIVE CARE UNIT VERSUS POSTANESTHESIA CARE UNIT

Postoperative patients who require critical care include: those planned for intensive care unit (ICU) admissions because of an anticipated lengthy operative course and recovery and those requiring ICU care because of unforeseen clinical circumstances or emergencies. Patients who require standard immediate postoperative care are generally admitted to a postanesthesia care unit (PACU). Depending on a hospital's unique capabilities, a PACU is capable for caring for the general ongoing mechanical ventilation and hemodynamic needs of a patient, under the supervision of an anesthesiologist.

Though a PACU can and should be capable of functioning at the same level of an ICU, in reality the day-to-day comprehensive multidisciplinary management is efficiently accomplished in the medium and long-term in a formal ICU with trained intensivists. In the circumstance where a PACU cares for patients who are awaiting an ICU bed, formal consultation with an intensivist for ongoing care is highly valuable.

There are some patient populations, such as those undergoing liver transplant, cardiac and trauma surgery, for whom assured direct postoperative admission to an ICU and avoiding the PACU altogether are essential to ensure optimal care by experienced specialized staff.

Hand-Offs

A unique aspect of the critical care management of surgical patients is that the information about the patient needed by the intensivist from the preoperative and intraoperative care is often fragmented. In the United States, surgical patients are always followed primarily by the surgeon(s) who performed the operation. Subspecialists who cared for the patient preoperatively and the anesthesiologist who cared for the patient intraoperatively may have important information relevant to the ICU clinicians. For example, the estimated blood loss value may vary widely depending on who reports these data (surgeons often underestimate blood loss). Data about unforeseen difficult airways, intraoperative hypotension, greater than expected blood loss, and other complications are often not readily available or communicated to the ICU, and the intensivist should be aware of this phenomenon and assured that they have the most accurate and comprehensive picture of the patient admitted to the ICU. When feasible, the intensivist should make every effort to begin their consultation intraoperatively. Although not practical in some situations, this certainly helps the ICU ensure continuity of care for patients who are in the extremes of illness. At our institution, the intensivist has been called as a consultant to the operating room to assist in unusual circumstances such as patients with severe hypoxemia, unusual new echo findings, persistent and increasing vasopressor requirements, etc.

Tubes/Drains/Stoma/Surgical Site

Unlike standard medical ICU patients, the surgical ICU patient can have many foreign bodies in the form of tubes, drains, and surgical-related phenomena such as an open abdomen, stoma, flap, altered anatomy, and complicated surgical incision. It is of the utmost importance that the ICU staff understands exactly the type and purpose of each of these as well as how these tubes should be managed. Some tubes are so-called critical and their inadvertent removal can have potentially devastating consequences. Suction tubes come with a variety of suction methods (self-suction, continuous suction, intermittent suction, suction with concomitant irrigation, etc). The quality of drain output (bilious, bloody, serous, purulent, etc), quantity, and changes to such output overtime can give the intensivist vital information. Though a comprehensive description

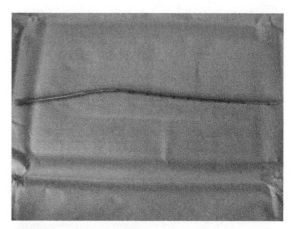

FIGURE 51–1 Chest tube.

and purpose of every possible surgical device is beyond the scope of this text, we describe some of the more common ones.

Chest tube/drain—Flexible plastic tube inserted through chest wall into pleural space usually to remove air or fluid/blood (Figure 51–1).

Pigtail drain—Drain with a coil at the end, which helps keep it in place and allows for more effective drainage through the small holes in the end; typically placed by interventional radiology though sometimes also used as a closed-chest suction drain (Figure 51–2).

Hemovac—Similar to a JP/Blake but much higher suction power; often used in orthopedics

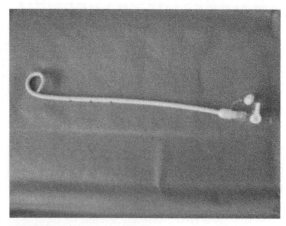

FIGURE 51–2 Pigtail drain.

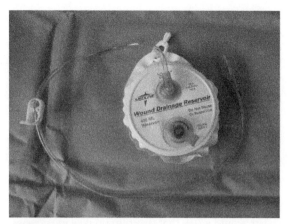

FIGURE 51–3 Hemovac drain.

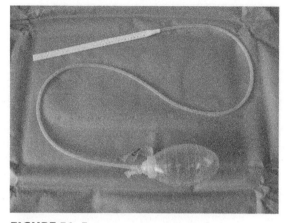

FIGURE 51–5 Jackson Pratt (JP) drain.

and helpful for removing/draining blood (Figure 51–3).

Sump drain—Also known as "Abramson triple lumen drain." This is a large drain with 3 ports, typically used with wall side suction and simultaneous irrigation; often used to continuously irrigate a surgical bed postoperatively (Figure 51–4).

Jackson Pratt—Also called a "JP drain"; closed suction that comes in flat and round forms and in various sizes connected to a grenade-shaped bulb via plastic tubing (Figure 51–5).

Blake—Similar to JP drain, more rigid, designed differently; thought to clot less often. Often

tunneled with a sharp metal applicator that is then removed (Figure 51–6).

Penrose—Yellow-colored soft rubber/floppy tube that is often used to keep a surgical site open for continuous drainage after infection/abscess (Figure 51–7).

Loop ostomy rod—This is a temporary device left under a loop ileostomy or colostomy to prevent retraction into the peritoneum; usually removed by postoperative day 5.

T-tube—A drain shaped like a T placed into the biliary system, usually the common bile duct.

GJ tube/Moss tube—This tube has 2 ports (1 to stomach and 1 to jejunum); often used for feeding in patients not tolerating gastric feeds.

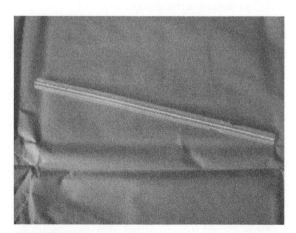

FIGURE 51–4 Sump drain.

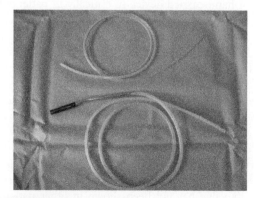

FIGURE 51–6 Blake drain.

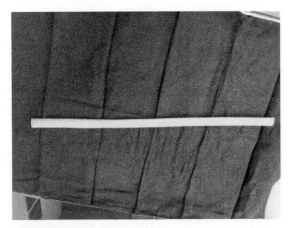

FIGURE 51–7 Penrose drain.

Fluid Management

A detailed discussion of fluid management and fluid responsiveness is a complicated and controversial topic beyond the scope of this chapter. Some key elements are universal to the surgical patient, however. Information about intraoperative fluid and blood loss coupled with fluid/blood-product administration can give the intensivist a clue about the resuscitation status of a newly admitted patient. Physical examination, though always important, is not the most accurate means of assessing volume status in this patient population. Fluid responsiveness can be assessed with a variety of more invasive and noninvasive means such as goal-directed cardiac ultrasound (feasibility and potential clinical utility of goal-directed transthoracic echocardiography performed by noncardiologist intensivists using a small hand-carried device in critically ill patients[1]) and pulse contour analysis. Focused transthoracic cardiac ultrasound is a method that is noninvasive and is gaining popularity in the assessment of fluid status.[2]

Central venous pressure measurement has been proven to not correlate with fluid status when spot-checked or when trended over time.[3] The use of a Swan–Ganz catheter (often called a *pulmonary artery catheter*) is used routinely during cardiac surgery and liver transplantation to measure cardiac index and calculate systemic vascular resistance, but its value has not been shown in other patient populations.

Rapid administration of small boluses of isotonic fluid with real-time monitoring of a patient's clinical response is a time-proven method in the initial resuscitation of postoperative ICU patients. Isotonic fluids should generally be the fluid of choice. pH neutral fluids should be used primarily as massive quantities of sodium chloride will cause an iatrogenic hyperchloremic metabolic acidosis. The intensivist should keep in mind that a patient's output may be substantially higher than urine output given drain output, etc.

Albumin is commonly used as a resuscitative fluid; however, its use is controversial. Most intensivists would agree that its utility makes most sense in patients with hypoalbuminemia secondary to cirrhosis. Synthetic starches are no longer used clinically as they can contribute to renal injury and may contribute to increased mortality.

Blood Transfusion

The aggregate of evidence from the last 15 years generally supports the notion that limited transfusion thresholds are correlated with superior outcomes in most patient populations. These include postoperative patients and patients with resuscitation for septic shock. A recently published study in the *New England Journal of Medicine* randomized 461 patients to a restrictive versus a liberal (hemoglobin threshold of 7 vs 9, respectively) transfusion strategy in patients with acute upper gastrointestinal bleeding. The rate of recurrent bleeding was lower and the survival was higher in the restrictive group.

Patients with active acute coronary syndromes have been shown to do poorly when severely anemic. Likewise, restrictive strategies for transfusion have not been shown to be superior in patients after heart surgery.[4]

Although restrictive transfusion strategies are certainly applicable to most patients in the ICU with anemia or minimal bleeding, it should be noted that aggressive use of packed red blood cells, fresh frozen plasma, and platelets along with minimal to no crystalloid should be the strategy during acute and exsanguinating hemorrhage, particularly in trauma patients. In these circumstances, crystalloid use should be minimized as it contributes to hypothermia, dilution of coagulation factors, and promotes acidosis. Trauma surgeons often say "you don't bleed crystalloid; you bleed blood."

Nutrition

Although historically the surgeon dictated the timing of initiation for feeds based on such things as physical examination, flatus, nasogastric tube output, and bowel movements, such clinical practice is not evidence driven. Although the consequences of this practice may not be substantial in the usual surgical floor, such means of determining when to feed a critically ill patient may lead to deleterious outcomes. The urgency of initiating feeding in large part depends on the preoperative nutritional status of the patient. Patients who have been in the hospital for several days or weeks with inadequate nutritional support who subsequently require ICU care are in more urgent need for expeditious nutritional support. Undernutrition is prevalent in all ICUs and often in surgical ICUs. Having a nutrition protocol helps narrowing the gap between what the patient is getting and what the caloric goal is, though this is less important in the first week of critical illness. Initial low-volume (ie, trophic) enteral nutrition resulted in clinical outcomes similar to those of early full-energy enteral nutrition but with fewer episodes of gastrointestinal intolerance.[5] However, restriction of nonprotein calories (permissive underfeeding) was not associated with lower mortality than that associated with planned delivery of a full amount of nonprotein calories.[6]

A few practices that should be standard are worth mentioning. Intermittent interruption of enteral feeding during an ICU course can contribute to malnutrition in the patient who is in the ICU for over several days. Practices such as NPO before planned procedures, delayed and cancelled operative times, computed tomography (CT) scan, and interruption for various other reasons become cumulative and can substantially contribute to patients receiving suboptimal feeds. It is our practice to minimize this phenomenon by minimizing reasons why patients' feeds are interrupted. For example, patients with endotracheal tubes or a cuffed tracheostomy have protected airways, and several planned procedures or operations can safely be accomplished with enteric feeds continued until the timed event. It is customary to establish an NPO status only if the procedure will entail surgery in the abdomen or airway, or the patient must be positioned in the prone position. Thus patients scheduled for orthopedic, brain, plastic, and extra-abdominal general surgery procedure can be spared unnecessary interruption of feeds. Given the nutritional needs are complex in this population, a dedicated nutrition team trained in critical care nutrition is an essential element to the care of the surgical ICU patient. Early enteral nutrition has been shown to improve infectious complications and mortality when compared to late enteral nutrition including in pancreatitis patients. Early parenteral nutrition (< 7 days post-ICU admission) has been associated with increased risk of nosocomial infections without benefit.[7]

Mechanical Ventilation

Principles of ventilation in a surgical ICU are no different from those in any other ICU. There are, however, different practices based on the expertise and biases of individual ICUs. Cardiac surgery ICUs tend to use pressure control ventilation, whereas trauma ICUs tend to more heavily rely on airway pressure release ventilation. Most standard surgical ICUs use either volume control (guaranteed volume) modes or dynamic hybrid modes such as volume-targeted pressure control mode (eg, pressure-regulated volume control [PRVC]).

Regardless of the mode or ventilator used, the surgical intensivist must be aware of the forces that influence mechanical ventilation in patients who undergo abdominal surgery. This is especially true in trauma and emergency surgery where there is often edema of the internal organs, and the associated increased abdominal pressure pushes upward on the diaphragm, effectively reducing functional residual capacity. This contributes to atelectasis and ventilation/perfusion (V/Q) mismatch.[8,9] When abdominal pressure begins to impair function in the pulmonary, renal, cardiovascular, or gastrointestinal systems, abdominal compartment syndrome should be recognized early and addressed.

Liberation From Ventilator

Successful liberation from mechanical ventilation relies on the application of clinical judgment and medical and nursing intervention. Predictors of successful extubation have significant limitations; some remain complicated and cumbersome to be used at bedside. Paired sedation interruption with daily spontaneous breathing trial[10] (SAT + SBT) has been shown to improve outcome, including more ventilator-free days and less ICU and hospital length of stay (LOS), and 1-year mortality.

Utilizing paired SAT + SBT (spontaneous breathing trial + spontaneous awakening trial) as part of the ABCDEF bundle is an essential part of successful liberation from mechanical ventilation. Tools are available on this website published by the society of critical care medicine: http://www.iculiberation.org/news/Pages/Webcast-Explores-Implementing-New-ABCDEF-Bundle-in-Your-ICU.aspx.

Postextubation Failure

Extubation attempts may fail in up to 23.5% of patients and lead to an increased hospital mortality of 30% to 40%. The use of postextubation noninvasive ventilation (NIV) outside of exacerbation of chronic obstructive pulmonary disease (COPD) should be cautioned as it leads to unnecessary delay in reintubation and worsened outcome particularly in surgical patients.[11,12] High-flow nasal cannula (HFNC) oxygen has been used in hypoxemic respiratory failure and shown to improve 90-day mortality when compared with NIV.[13] The routine application of HFNC to patients in the setting of extubation failure due to hypoxemia is feasible but has not been studied to date.

Sedation

The Society of Critical Care Medicine published updated clinical practice guidelines for adult ICU patients in 2013, which are applicable to the surgical ICU. Although there is variability among ICUs in terms of practice norms, an emphasis on minimizing pain and agitation while also preventing delirium should be the primary goal. The impact of delirium in the ICU on hospital LOS, long-term cognitive impairment, and mortality cannot be overemphasized.[14,15] The Vanderbilt University Medical Center Delirium and Cognitive Impairment Group have created www.icudelirium.org that provides medical professionals with a variety of pearls and tools we use in our practice. For example, ABCDEF is the bundle of measures which includes Assess for and manage pain, Both Spontaneous awake and breathing trials, attention to Choice of sedation and analgesia, Delirium monitoring and management, Early mobility, and Family engagement.

Though any patient who is newly intubated requires analgesia, unique to surgical patients is incisional pain. Analgesia should therefore be the primary and initial focus for patient care. Multimodal therapy including narcotic drip/bolus titration, enteral/IV acetaminophen, and neuroleptics could be utilized. Nonsteroidal agents have a role in the patient without precarious renal function and with low risk of bleeding. Dexmedetomidine, though not a primary analgesia agent, is narcotic sparing and has pain-relieving properties. Low-dose ketamine drips for patients with refractory pain or a significant history of narcotic use previous to admission can attenuate subjective pain scores.

Validated sedation scales such as The Richmond Agitation-Sedation Scale (RASS) or The Riker Sedation-Agitation Scale (SAS) are paramount to goal-directed delivery of sedatives by the nursing staff. We use the RASS that takes less than 20 seconds to perform, and has been shown to be highly reliable and effective. Noncontinuous sedation protocols have been shown to decrease ICU LOS when compared with continuous sedation with daily interruptions.[16]

Abdominal Compartment Syndrome

The surgical intensivist should always keep in mind the phenomenon of abdominal compartment syndrome. The World Abdominal Compartment Society (www.wsacs.org) provides consensus guidelines on this pathology that should be reviewed.

Many postlaparotomy patients have some element of abdominal hypertension. A normal intra-abdominal pressure in most critically ill adults is between 5 and 7 mm Hg. When this pressure is associated with new organ dysfunction and limits perfusion to vital organs (typically when 20 mm Hg with or without an abdominal perfusion pressure < 60 mm Hg), treatment needs to be initiated emergently. Although sedation/analgesia, body positioning, gastric/colonic decompression, and fluid resuscitation/diuresis may be attempted initially, rapid correction with either percutaneous drainage or laparotomy (ie, relaparotomy with abdominal fascia left open) should be performed.

The intensivist should have a low threshold of measuring abdominal pressures with either a standard commercial device, or a Foley catheter with 50 mL injected into bladder connected to standard pressure transducer in the supine and flat patient. It is important to have a baseline pressure and frequent serial abdominal examinations. The intensivist should be aware that abdominal compartment could still develop in a patient with an incompletely open abdomen if the fascia is still under tension or the lapartomy was limited in length. Although these patients often respond seemingly well with initial, intermittent fluid boluses, their underlying pathology worsens over time.

Prophylaxis

Deep Vein Thrombosis

Mechanical and chemical deep vein thrombosis (DVT) prophylaxis is mandatory for the vast majority of patients in the surgical ICU. Although some surgeons are reluctant to begin chemoprophylaxis in the immediate postoperative period, general guidelines should be implemented at each institution to ensure its use. At our hospital, patients with traumatic brain injury are routinely started on chemoprophylaxis 48 to 72 hours after admission if there is no evidence of continued bleeding on CT scan.

Inferior vena cava filters are generally reserved for those patients with a long-term contraindication to chemoprophylaxis, patients with acute DVT and a contraindication to systemic anticoagulation, and patients diagnosed with a new DVT or pulmonary embolism while already on systemic anticoagulation.

Stress Ulcer

The absolute indications for stress ulcer prophylaxis include severe sepsis or septic shock, mechanical ventilation more than 48 hours, major burn injury, and patients with coagulopathy. In practice, stress ulcer prophylaxis is also used for most ICU patients, as well as elderly patients on NSAIDs and those on high-dose steroids (> 250 mg hydrocortisone/d). These recommendations for trauma ICU patients,

which are applicable to most postoperative patients, are readily available at www.east.org.

Effective prophylaxis includes proton pump–inhibiting agents (PPI) and H_2-blocking agents. Although patients who are tolerating feeds are typically at less risk for developing stress ulcers, the indications for its use are not related to the NPO status of the patient. Thus patients who do not meet the aforementioned criteria who are NPO do not need prophylaxis, and patients who do meet criteria who are tolerating enteral feeds still need chemoprophylaxis. PPI use has been linked to increased C diff rates as well as increased ventilator associated pneumonia.[17,18]

Multidrug Resistance

Antibiotic stewardship is of the utmost importance in the surgical ICU. Antibiotic use is divided into its use in surgery for incisional infection prophylaxis and actual treatment. Guidelines mandate less than 24 hours use when used for prophylaxis; whether that dictates one dose intraoperatively only versus continued dosing for less than 24 hours is individual preference. The exception is in cardiac surgery patients following sternotomy and following transplant surgery in whom 48 hours is preferred—though with limited evidence. Notoriously, ENT/OMFS/Ophthalmology/Plastic surgeons often request prophylaxis for extended durations—it should be emphasized this practice is not ideal and institutional guidelines should be established to limit confrontation in these circumstances.

STEROIDS

Steroids are often given to critically ill surgical patients for transplant rejection prevention, vasogenic edema (eg, brain tumors, spinal cord compression, acute pneumococcal meningitis), reduction of edema (eg, airway edema, laryngeal surgery), COPD exacerbation, to improve postoperative nausea, vomiting, headache from vasospasm following subarachnoid hemorrhage.

Administration of steroid to patients with sepsis has been controversial since the 1950s where high-dose (30 mg/kg of methylprednisolone) steroids led to conflicting results.[19] Studies showed improving mortality and others showed worsening mortality rates. In 2002, Annane and colleagues[20] demonstrated that septic-shock patients who have poor response to adrenocorticotropic hormone (ACTH) stimulation test and received low dose stress dose steroids had reduced risk of death without increasing adverse events. This was further tested in a large multicenter randomized controlled trial (CORTICUS)[21] where there was no difference in mortality rates between the treated group and control. Although steroid therapy should not be used in all patients with septic shock, it should be considered in persistent shock despite administration of fluids and vasopressors. The SCCM recommends using a maximum of 200 mg/d of hydrocortisone in refractory septic shock (defined as the need for increasingly higher doses of vasopressors or the need for a second vasopressor after adequate fluid resuscitation). There is no benefit from performing ACTH stimulation tests as critically ill patients with subnormal total cortisol had normal free cortisol.[22] There is insufficient evidence in a meta-analysis to support either gradual or abrupt interruption of steroid treatment following shock reversal.[23]

Recovery after prolonged exposure to oral steroids is highly variable and may take as long as 1 year. Consider stress dose steroids (low dose, 200 mg/d hydrocortisone) for patients who received high-dose steroids (> 200 mg/d hydrocortisone) following a major surgical procedure. Consider 8 mg dexamethasone to prevent adrenal insufficiency from all commonly performed surgeries (hernia repair, cholecystectomy, hysterectomy, bowel resection, joint, and vascular procedures).

A single dose of etomidate blocks cortisol synthesis resulting in primary adrenal insufficiency lasting for up to 48 hours.[24] Hydrocortisone administration following single-dose etomidate did not benefit to overcome etomidate-related adrenal insufficiency.[25] The practical/clinical implications of patient physiology following the administration of etomidate continue to be controversial.

MOBILIZATION

Early mobility includes a spectrum from passive range of motion to active range of motion, to sitting with legs dangling, standing, and walking. For patients in the surgical ICU, early mobilization is particularly an important aspect of recovery. Its use prevents deconditioning and is an integral part of delirium prophylaxis and treatment. Studies clearly show that early mobility decreases days on the ventilator and LOS.[26] It has been shown to be cost-effective and justifies a dedicated mobility team that works in conjunction with primary nursing team particularly in the challenging population.[27]

Short of orthopedic procedures which may limit weight bearing status, the surgical intensivist should not be intimidated by large surgical wounds, number of tubes, etc. At our institution, we routinely get patients out of bed who are intubated on postoperative day 1. Although patients with an open abdomen, brain intraventricular devices, or several drains/tubes, present some logistical nursing challenges, their presence is by no means a contraindication to mobilization. Patients with low dose or deescalating dosing of vasopressors are also safe for mobilization.

"Mobilization teams" have been implemented by some institutions; however, early mobility can be performed by collaboration of the interdisciplinary team members including nurses, physical therapists, occupational therapists, and physicians. Prioritizing the efforts and working as unified team with proper staffing, training and leadership supports are imperative for the success of the mobilization mission.

REFERENCES

1. Manasia AR, Nagaraj HM, Kodali RB, et al. Feasibility and potential clinical utility of goal-directed transthoracic echocardiography performed by noncardiologist intensivists using a small hand-carried device (SonoHeart) in critically ill patients. *J Cardiothor Vasc Anesth*. 2005;19(2):155-159.
2. Kohli-Seth R, Neuman T, Sinha R, Bassily-Marcus A. Use of echocardiography and modalities of patient monitoring of trauma patients. *Curr Opin Anaesthesiol*. 2010;23(2):239-245.
3. Marik PE, Baram M, Vahid B. Does central venous pressure predict fluid responsiveness? A systematic review of the literature and the tale of seven mares. *Chest*. 2008;134(1):172-178.
4. Murphy GJ, Pike K, Rogers CA, et al. Liberal or restrictive transfusion after cardiac surgery. *N Engl J Med*. 2015;372(11):997-1008.
5. Rice TW, Mogan S, Hays MA, Bernard GR, Jensen GL, Wheeler AP. Randomized trial of initial trophic versus full-energy enteral nutrition in mechanically

ventilated patients with acute respiratory failure. *Crit Care Med.* 2011;39(5):967-974.

6. Arabi YM, Aldawood AS, Haddad SH, et al. Permissive underfeeding or standard enteral feeding in critically ill adults. *N Engl J Med.* 2015;372(25):2398-2408.

7. Casaer MP, Mesotten D, Hermans G, et al. Early versus late parenteral nutrition in critically ill adults. *N Engl J Med.* 2011;365(6):506-517.

8. Malbrain ML, Deeren D, De Potter TJ. Intra-abdominal hypertension in the critically ill: it is time to pay attention. *Curr Opin Crit Care.* 2005;11(2):156-171.

9. Habashi NM. Other approaches to open-lung ventilation: airway pressure release ventilation. *Crit Care Med.* 2005;33(3 suppl):S228-S240.

10. Girard TD, Kress JP, Fuchs BD, et al. Efficacy and safety of a paired sedation and ventilator weaning protocol for mechanically ventilated patients in intensive care (Awakening and Breathing Controlled trial): a randomised controlled trial. *Lancet.* 2008;371(9607):126-134.

11. Caples SM, Gay PC. Noninvasive positive pressure ventilation in the intensive care unit: a concise review. *Crit Care Med.* 2005;33(11):2651-2658.

12. Esteban A, Frutos-Vivar F, Ferguson ND, et al. Noninvasive positive-pressure ventilation for respiratory failure after extubation. *New Engl J Med.* 2004;350(24):2452-2460.

13. Frat J-P, Thille AW, Mercat A, et al. High-flow oxygen through nasal cannula in acute hypoxemic respiratory failure. *N Engl J Med.* 2015;372(23):2185-2196.

14. Pandharipande PP, Girard TD, Jackson JC, et al. Long-term cognitive impairment after critical illness. *N Engl J Med.* 2013;369(14):1306-1316.

15. Ely EW, Shintani A, Truman B, et al. Delirium as a predictor of mortality in mechanically ventilated patients in the intensive care unit. *JAMA.* 2004;291(14):1753-1762.

16. Strom T, Martinussen T, Toft P. A protocol of no sedation for critically ill patients receiving mechanical ventilation: a randomised trial. *Lancet.* 2010;375(9713):475-480.

17. Howell MD, Novack V, Grgurich P, et al. Iatrogenic gastric acid suppression and the risk of nosocomial *Clostridium difficile* infection. *Arch Int Med.* 2010;170(9):784-790.

18. Herzig SJ, Howell MD, Ngo LH, Marcantonio ER. Acid-suppressive medication use and the risk for hospital-acquired pneumonia. *JAMA.* 2009;301(20):2120-2128.

19. Spink WW. ACTH and adrenocorticosteroids as therapeutic adjuncts in infectious diseases. *N Engl J Med.* 1957;257(21):1031-1035.

20. Annane D, Sebille V, Charpentier C, et al. Effect of treatment with low doses of hydrocortisone and fludrocortisone on mortality in patients with septic shock. *JAMA.* 2002;288(7):862-871.

21. Sprung CL, Annane D, Keh D, et al. Hydrocortisone therapy for patients with septic shock. *N Engl J Med.* 2008;358(2):111-124.

22. Hamrahian AH, Oseni TS, Arafah BM. Measurements of serum free cortisol in critically ill patients. *N Engl J Med.* 2004;350(16):1629-1638.

23. Annane D, Bellissant E, Bollaert PE, et al. Corticosteroids in the treatment of severe sepsis and septic shock in adults: a systematic review. *JAMA.* 2009;301(22):2362-2375.

24. Vinclair M, Broux C, Faure P, et al. Duration of adrenal inhibition following a single dose of etomidate in critically ill patients. *Int Care Med.* 2008;34(4):714-719.

25. Payen JF, Dupuis C, Trouve-Buisson T, et al. Corticosteroid after etomidate in critically ill patients: a randomized controlled trial. *Crit Care Med.* 2012;40(1):29-35.

26. Brummel NE, Jackson JC, Girard TD, et al. A combined early cognitive and physical rehabilitation program for people who are critically ill: the activity and cognitive therapy in the intensive care unit (ACT-ICU) trial. *Phys Ther.* 2012;92(12):1580-1592.

27. Lord RK, Mayhew CR, Korupolu R, et al. ICU early physical rehabilitation programs: financial modeling of cost savings. *Crit Care Med.* 2013;41(3):717-724.

Posttransplantation Care

Pankaj Kapadia, MD and
John M. Oropello, MD, FACP, FCCP, FCCM

KEY POINTS

1. The main reasons for reoperation after liver transplantation are postoperative bleeding, vascular and biliary complications, and intraabdominal sepsis.

2. Surgical complications after renal transplantation including graft thrombosis, renal artery stenosis, urinary leak, or urinary obstruction have an incidence of 5% to 10% and remain important causes of graft loss.

3. After pancreatic transplant, a sudden increase in amylase and lipase with a change in exogenous insulin requirements is predictor of graft ischemia or rejection.

4. It is important for an intensivist to be familiar with early detection and treatment of infection and immunosuppressive medications and their side effects in the posttransplant patient.

INTRODUCTION

This chapter discusses early postoperative care, early recognition and management of complications, antimicrobial prophylaxis, and immunosuppressant drugs and their side effects in the management of the posttransplant liver, kidney, pancreas, and small intestine recipient.[1-8] Indications for transplantation and preoperative management are not discussed in this chapter.

POSTOPERATIVE CARE AND CRITICAL CARE AFTER LIVER TRANSPLANTATION

There are 3 major types of liver transplantation (LT): cadaveric orthotopic LT (OLT), where a whole organ is transplanted from a deceased donor (most common); cadaveric OLT by split LT, where the recipient receives 1 lobe of the liver from a deceased donor;

and live donor OLT, where the donor undergoes either a right or left hepatic lobectomy. In the case of split or living donor liver transplants, adult recipients usually receive the larger right lobe; children are ordinarily transplanted the smaller left lobe.

OLT requires surgical anastomosis of the hepatic artery, portal vein, bile duct, and inferior vena cava from donor to recipient, and postoperative complications are often related to dysfunction at these anastomotic sites.

Recovery in the Immediate Postoperative Period

Most of the patients after LT, even after an uncomplicated operating room course, are monitored in the ICU. Uncomplicated cases usually transfer to an inpatient liver transplant unit within 24 to 72 hours but complicated cases may require ICU care for weeks. Fifteen percent to 20% of liver transplant patients are taken back to the operating room during the transplant admission. The main reasons for reoperation include postoperative bleeding, vascular and biliary complications, and intraabdominal sepsis.

In the ICU, frequent hemodynamic assessments are commonly performed using vital signs and noninvasive monitoring (eg, ultrasonography). A preexisting pulmonary artery catheter is utilized if placed intraoperatively for more hemodynamically challenging cases or those with pulmonary hypertension. Vital signs, intake, output, physical changes in drain output, bile production (if a biliary drain [eg, T-tube] is present), abdominal drain (eg, Jackson–Pratt) output, and any signs of postoperative bleeding are recorded hourly. The initial postoperative level of liver biochemistries, that is, alanine transaminase (ALT), aspartate aminotransferase (AST), and bilirubin, may not correlate with liver function in the first day or first 2 days after transplant. Therefore, most centers rely on the serial assessment of international normalized ratio (INR) and lactate along with complete blood count, arterial blood gas, electrolytes, glucose, blood urea nitrogen, and creatinine as well as the liver biochemistries (ALT, AST, bilirubin, and alkaline phosphatase) analyzed every 6 hours within the first 2 days. The clinical picture (eg, hemodynamics, renal function, and neurological status) also provides important information about graft function.

Increased INR is usually not treated with fresh frozen plasma (FFP) because it may mask allograft dysfunction and potentially increase the incidence of hepatic artery thrombosis (HAT) or portal vein thrombosis. Thrombocytopenia is also very common after LT, however platelet transfusions are also avoided because they may increase the chances of HAT. If there is significant bleeding, FFP and platelet transfusions may be indicated but the decision to transfuse should be made in concert with the transplant surgeon.

Assessment of Liver Graft Function

Graft edema, any unusual or discolored appearance of the allograft in the operating room, inability of the patient to raise the core body temperature, hemodynamic instability, hypoglycemia, dramatic increases in potassium, prothrombin time or INR, and lactate all signal inadequate allograft function. Inadequate urine output or acute kidney injury is also common

in this setting, but may be caused by factors other than graft dysfunction such as acute tubular necrosis (ATN) or immunosuppressive drugs such as cyclosporine or tacrolimus.

Doppler ultrasonography (DUS) is routinely done on the first postoperative day to assess patency of the hepatic arteries and portal veins to rule out HAT, stenosis, or portal vein thrombosis. DUS also assesses for fluid collections, hematomas, and abscesses. As the hepatic artery supplies blood to the biliary ducts, HAT is associated with bile leaks. Follow up DUS is performed if the initial findings are equivocal or there is a sudden deterioration in graft function or elevation of LFTs.

Split cadaveric and live donor lobe transplants may be associated with initially higher ALT and AST due to raw liver surfaces as well as more prolonged lactate and INR elevation due to smaller liver mass relative to recipient size. Elevated INR may also occur in standard cadaveric OLT when the overall liver mass is small. Recipients of split and living donor transplants often become hypophosphatemic and require rigorous phosphorus supplementation due to the metabolic needs of regenerating liver tissue.

Recognition and Management of Early Complications

Medical Complications

Sepsis—The risk of infections is increased after LT and bacterial infections are more common than fungal infections. Deep surgical space infections and biliary leaks are common sources of infection. All potential sites for infection should be explored and, if possible, eliminated (catheters, hematomas, or fluid collections suspicious for abscess).

Respiratory Complications—Patients that are critically ill prior to LT are at increased risk for prolonged mechanical ventilation due to debilitating conditions and concomitant loss of muscle mass. Those with liver graft dysfunction, extrahepatic organ dysfunction, or sepsis are also more likely to require prolonged ventilator support. Transient severe pulmonary edema may occur due to systemic inflammatory response syndrome (SIRS) or sepsis, or much less commonly transfusion-related lung injury. Although pneumonia is possible early after

LT, pulmonary infiltrates are usually due to noncardiogenic pulmonary edema from systemic inflammation or sepsis originating from the abdomen. Patients intubated postoperatively for more than 7 to 10 days should be evaluated for tracheostomy.

Hepatopulmonary syndrome (HPS) is defined by the triad of liver dysfunction or portal hypertension, abnormal gas exchange, and evidence of pulmonary vascular shunts resulting in hypoxemia. Patients with HPS have an increased length of stay in the ICU (median 4 days) and hospital (median 39 days). LT may be curative, however, the median time to cessation of oxygen is 4.5 months in some series. Right pleural effusions are common after liver transplant due to operation near the right diaphragm, but do not usually cause respiratory failure. Postoperative right pneumothorax may occur less commonly.

Cardiovascular Complications—Liver failure typically results in a hyperdynamic circulation with elevated cardiac index and low blood pressure. A patient receiving a transplant before severe liver failure is manifest, for example, hepatic tumors or living-related donor recipients, may not have a hyperdynamic circulation. If present prior to LT, the hyperdynamic state does not resolve immediately after LT and may persist for weeks or longer. Mild to moderate portopulmonary hypertension in the setting of high cardiac output (CO) usually resolves with successful LT.

The majority of low CO states in the ICU after LT are caused by volume loss usually from bleeding, third spacing, and/or a stunned myocardium due to SIRS or sepsis. Dynamic left ventricular outflow tract obstruction due to decreased LV preload in the setting of inotropes is also a potential cause of low CO post-LT. Rarely, low CO may be caused by an acute myocardial infarction. Other causes of low CO after LT include cirrhotic cardiomyopathy or cardiomyopathies associated with alcohol, hepatitis, or hemochromatosis, although these should have been screened out during the preoperative work up.

Management of hemodynamic instability includes treatment of the causative factors. Central venous pressure measurement is a poor guide for intravascular volume and adequate resuscitation both in the ICU and in the operating room. No relationship between CVP and liver graft outcome has been demonstrated subsequent to an uncontrolled observational study to the contrary. The use of CO trending and mixed venous blood gases via a pulmonary artery catheter (often present in the immediate postoperative period after intraoperative placement), and or serial echocardiography, coupled with lactate trends are helpful to guide hemodynamic management. Although there are no randomized control trials to support the use of colloids over crystalloids after LT, albumin 5% is preferred for volume resuscitation after LT due to hypoalbuminemia and to limit positive fluid balance.

Hypertension may develop posttransplant and is more common in patients with preexisting hypertension. Hypertension can be caused or exacerbated by immunosuppressive drugs such as tacrolimus, cyclosporine, and steroids. The treatment may include diuresis in the setting of fluid overload or the addition of antihypertensive agents.

Renal Dysfunction—The incidence of acute renal failure after LT varies widely in the literature, ranging between 27% and 67%. The most important risk factor for postoperative renal dysfunction is pretransplant renal dysfunction (ie, hepatorenal syndrome or ATN). Most kidneys recover with time and only a small percentage of patients develop chronic kidney failure. Management of renal failure in the posttransplant period includes renal replacement therapy and judicious use of immunosuppressants, particularly, nephrotoxic calcineurin inhibitors (ie, tacrolimus or cyclosporine) or a calcineurin inhibitor-sparing protocol (eg, mycophenolate mofetil, steroids, monoclonal antilymphocyte antibodies) at the discretion of the transplant team. In hemodynamically unstable patients and particularly those with primary nonfunction or poor early graft function, continuous veno-venous hemofiltration is the preferred modality for renal replacement and should be started as early as feasible to maintain metabolic homeostasis during this critical time of multiorgan dysfunction.

Neuropsychiatric Complications—Neuropsychiatric complications occur in up to 30% of liver transplant patients and often require prolonged management in the ICU. Complications include encephalopathy (delirium), tremors, myoclonus and less commonly seizures (including nonconvulsive status epilepticus), meningitis, ischemic stroke, intracerebral hemorrhage, and subarachnoid hemorrhage.

Delirium is common after LT. Treatment with antipsychotic medications may be required (eg, haloperidol or risperidone). It may be due to preexisting hepatic encephalopathy, postoperative liver graft dysfunction, renal failure, sepsis, or side effects of immunosuppressive medications such as steroids and calcineurin inhibitors (see later under Immunosuppressive Drugs). If there are no focal deficits and the patient is hemodynamically and or respiratory unstable, computed tomography (CT) imaging may be postponed or avoided. However, if the patient exhibits focality or seizures, emergent CT should be performed. Ischemic stroke, subarachnoid, and subdural hemorrhages are uncommon but possible. Central nervous system infections such as meningitis and brain abscess are unusual but possible in these immunocompromised patients.

Surgical Complications

HAT occurs in less than 2% to 3% of patients after LT. Thirty percent develop signs of acute hepatic necrosis with high transaminases, sepsis, mental status changes, and coagulopathy, but may the presentation be more subacute with progressive biliary infections and hepatic dysfunction. Suspicion of HAT should be immediately investigated with DUS and potentially confirmed by an arteriogram or exploratory laparotomy depending on the level of surgical concern. HAT within the first week after OLT is an indication for relisting for retransplantation. Portal vein thrombosis is also diagnosed by DUS. If the diagnosis is made during the ICU stay, the patient may undergo thrombectomy depending on the degree of occlusion and collateral circulation.

Biliary complications remain frequent after LT varying between 1.6% and 18% and include bile leaks, bilomas, and strictures. Early bile leaks should be suspected in any patient with constant abdominal pain, or unexplained fever or sepsis after liver transplant. Most leaks occur from the biliary anastomosis and present early. Many require abdominal washout and surgical repair, although endoscopic stenting may be successful. Late bile leaks (after 30 days) are rare, however late strictures are the most frequent cause of biliary complications after LT and are often associated with recurrent cholangitis. Treatment of anastomotic strictures usually requires endoscopic

stenting; intrahepatic strictures are more complex and may lead to retransplantation.

Nutritional Management

In uncomplicated liver transplants an oral diet can be started within the first 1 to 2 days after surgery. A protein-rich diet is recommended, as the liver patient needs 1.5 to 2 g protein per kg body weight per day. If oral intake is not sufficient, postpyloric feeding through a tube should be considered. Parenteral nutrition should be initiated only if tube feeding is not possible due to intestinal complications and prolonged nothing by mouth (NPO) (eg, > 3-7 days) is anticipated. Both steroids and calcineurin inhibitors may cause hyperglycemia and this will be even more pronounced in patients with preexisting diabetes mellitus. Hypoglycemia may be a sign of liver graft dysfunction or excess insulin dosing.

POSTOPERATIVE RENAL TRANSPLANTATION CARE
Early Postoperative Management

Intensive care unit observation is usually not required after renal transplant except under special circumstances involving hemodynamic or respiratory instability.[9] Once the patient is stable hemodynamically and has recovered from anesthesia, transfer to the floor is initiated. Volume status needs to be monitored closely. Additional evaluation includes a full electrolyte panel, complete blood count, chest X-ray, and an electrocardiogram. The intraoperative anesthetic record, blood loss, volume replacement, and the operative report should also be reviewed to identify intraoperative events or complications with potentially adverse sequelae. Voluminous urine output after surgery is a sign of good graft function. A brisk large volume diuresis following graft revascularization may be due to preoperative volume overload, osmotic diuresis in previously uremic patients, intraoperative mannitol or furosemide, or vigorous intraoperative intravenous crystalloid or colloid fluid administration.

In low urine output states, the Foley catheter should be irrigated to rule out obstruction and to flush out blood clots. Evaluation of the kidney by ultrasound to determine blood flow, patency of the renal vessels, and for evidence of urinary tract obstruction is important. The absence of blood flow to the allograft or tract obstruction (eg, ureteral torsion) requires urgent evaluation by the surgical team for possible reexploration. Fluid replacement should equal urine output with 1/2 normal saline because the sodium concentration of the urine from a transplanted kidney is about 60 to 80 mEq/L. Patients who are anuric or oliguric should receive conservative fluid management and diuretics if intravascularly volume repleted or volume overloaded. Renal replacement therapy is necessary if there is inadequate recovery of renal function.

Assessment of Graft Function

Immediate Graft Function—In patients with immediate graft function the serum creatinine commonly decreases by 1.0 to more than 4.0 mg/dL daily. These patients are usually discharged on postoperative day 4 or 5 following successful Foley catheter removal and voiding trial.

Slow Recovery of Graft Function—Patients with slow recovery of graft function are generally non-oliguric and experience a slow decline in serum creatinine. The level typically decreases by 0.2 to 1.0 mg/dL daily. Attention must be given to fluid management. These patients usually do not require dialysis unless complicated by hyperkalemia or fluid overload. Patients who are at high risk for obstruction such as diabetics with neurogenic bladder or male patients with benign prostatic hypertrophy may require a Foley catheter for a longer time period of monitoring.

Delayed Graft Function—The incidence of delayed graft function (DGF) ranges from 10% to 60% and can often be anticipated based on recipient and donor factors. Unless these patients have adequate residual urine output from the native kidneys, most patients are oliguric or anuric and will require temporary dialysis support for volume, hyperkalemia, or uremia. Donor factors for DGF include age (< 10 or > 50), donor macrovascular or microvascular disease, prolonged used of vasopressors, donation after cardiac death, nephrotoxic agents, and prolonged ischemia time. Intraoperative factors include hemodynamic instability and prolonged rewarming time (anastomotic time). Recipient factors include diabetes, age, male gender, African American race, peripheral vascular disease, duration of dialysis before transplant, and early high-dose calcineurin inhibitors.

Surgical Complications

Surgical complications after renal transplantation have an incidence of 5% to 10% and remain an important cause of graft loss.

Graft Thrombosis

Graft thrombosis may be arterial or venous and usually occurs within the first 24 to 72 hours. The incidence ranges from 0.5% to 5%. Renal artery thrombosis may present with sudden cessation of urine output and the diagnosis is made by DUS which shows the absence of arterial inflow and nonperfusion of the transplant kidney. Renal artery thrombosis is a catastrophic complication and almost invariably results in graft loss. With renal vein thrombosis, the clinical presentation includes a sudden decrease in graft function, hematuria, pain, and swelling over the graft. Diagnosis is confirmed by DUS. Urgent exploration and allograft thrombectomy is required.

Renal Artery Stenosis

The incidence of renal artery stenosis ranges from 2% to 10%. The presentation is later, from a few months to 2 years posttransplant with sudden onset of refractory hypertension associated with peripheral edema and graft dysfunction. The anastomotic site is the most common location. Initial screening is performed with DUS and may be followed by magnetic resonance angiogram or CT angiogram. The gold standard for diagnosis remains the arteriogram. The treatment is percutaneous transluminal angioplasty with or without stent placement.

Urological Complications

Urological complications after kidney transplantation have an incidence of 2% to 10%. They may present either as a urinary leak or urinary obstruction. Symptoms and signs include pain and swelling over the graft, fever, decreased urine output, an elevated serum creatinine, and urine draining from the skin incision. Urinary leaks usually occur early after transplantation. Analysis of fluid drainage from the wound will typically demonstrate an elevated creatinine concentration compared to the serum creatinine. Small leaks can be managed by placing a Foley catheter for bladder decompression. Open operative repair and drainage is usually required for larger leaks. Obstruction of the urinary tract often presents with findings similar to acute allograft rejection with a fall in urine output, tenderness over the graft, and fever. Ultrasound confirmation of hydronephrosis is required for diagnosis. Treatment includes percutaneous nephrostomy, balloon dilation of the stricture, and stent placement. If endoscopic techniques fail to resolve the obstruction, open surgical repair is indicated.

POSTOPERATIVE PANCREAS AND SMALL BOWEL TRANSPLANTATION CARE

Only 1 of 10 pancreas transplants are isolated, that is, only pancreas, and these few are performed in complicated diabetics without nephropathy. The majority of pancreas transplants are simultaneous pancreas–kidney transplants in patients with diabetic nephropathy. A pancreas transplant may also be done subsequent to a successful kidney transplant. Occasionally a pancreatic transplant is performed simultaneously with small bowel transplantation.

In terms of exocrine drainage, currently most pancreas transplants are enteric drained rather than bladder drained.

Pancreas Transplant Care

Early Assessment of Allograft Function

The appearance and texture of the pancreas on completion of the procedure is essential because pancreatitis and allograft edema are common at the time of reperfusion. In this setting, osmotic diuretics are frequently administered to decrease edema and improve microvascular perfusion. A similar strategy is used with intestinal allografts to limit edema and bowel distention. The failure of an allograft to respond to intraoperative interventions aimed at reducing edema is a signal to maintain close surveillance of allograft function perioperatively. Donor risk factors associated with intestinal allograft thrombosis include increased donor age,

hemodynamic instability, catecholamine requirements, and acidosis.

Support of the Transplanted Pancreatic Allograft

Optimal support for the pancreatic allograft focuses on the detection and prevention of rejection and thrombosis, the 2 most common causes of pancreatic graft failure.

Although never scientifically validated, prophylactic anticoagulation involving low-dose systemic heparin in the operating room with dose escalation through the first week (due to decreasing bleeding risks) after transplantation, supplemented with aspirin therapy, is routine.

Pancreatitis and pancreatic ischemia typically present as abdominal pain, peritonitis, ileus, and fever. Serum amylase and lipase correlate poorly with the severity of allograft pancreatitis, with post-transplant hyperamylasemia observed in greater than 30% of recipients; however, trend analysis is helpful. In particular, a sudden increase in amylase and lipase with a change in exogenous insulin requirements is predictor of graft ischemia or necrosis. The use of DUS is sensitive in the diagnosis of thrombosis. The "gold standard" for confirming rejection remains a pancreas graft biopsy. Any form of pancreatic rejection is treated aggressively.

Pancreas transplants with exocrine drainage via the bladder have the advantage of closer monitoring for rejection via urine analysis, however more complications occur including urethritis (greater in males), bladder infection, and acid-base abnormalities, specifically metabolic acidosis due to loss of bicarbonate in the urine.

Small Bowel Transplant Care

There are fewer serum markers and radiologic modalities to guide the management of intestinal transplant recipients. In this population, clinicians only have physical examination, ostomy output, laboratory analysis for hyperkalemia, metabolic acidosis and lactate, and endoscopy. Appropriate volume resuscitation is challenging because volume depletion occurs secondary to inflammation and poor fluid absorption from the transplanted intestine in addition to ileostomy losses. These patients are malnourished with low albumin levels. In some cases, the intestinal graft may become very edematous and the transplant surgeon may request fluid restriction and diuresis. Albumin 5% or 25% for fluid resuscitation is preferred in these transplants when volume limitation is the goal. Managing the fluid status requires a clinical assessment of systemic perfusion and a hemodynamic assessment of the intravascular volume. Cardiac and pulmonary ultrasound and lactate trends can help to guide fluid management.

Rejection usually occurs within the first month posttransplant. In many centers, serial endoscopy and biopsy are performed twice a week for the first month. After the first month, endoscopies are performed less frequently. The treatment of rejection involves bolus doses of corticosteroids and intensification of the baseline immunosuppressive regimen. Plasmapheresis may be initiated within 24 hours of transplant to reduce intestinal graft rejection in patients with high levels of donor specific circulating antibodies. The effectiveness of plasmapheresis in this setting is under investigation.

Intestinal transplant recipients typically have malnutrition and protein deficiency that results in low oncotic pressure and further loss of intravascular fluid. If anticipated to be NPO for more than about 3 days, total parenteral nutrition is resumed postoperatively. Once anastomotic integrity is established, enteral feeds are initiated and advanced gradually as tolerated. Most patients continue to need supplemental intravenous fluids and electrolytes due to stoma loss during the first posttransplant year.

Posttransplant Lymphoproliferative Disease

Posttransplant lymphoproliferative disease develops in up to 30% of the recipients of intestinal transplant and is usually associated with Epstein–Barr virus (EBV) infection. Treatment principles include a substantial decrease in the immunosuppression regimen and antiviral therapy.

POSTTRANSPLANTATION INFECTIONS

The risk of infection after transplantation changes over time (Figure 52–1), with modifications in immunosuppression, also depending on the type of organ transplanted. It can be difficult to differentiate rejection or noninfectious inflammation from infection as no assays can accurately distinguish between these entities. Currently, the clinician assesses a recipient's risk of infection while considering the risk of allograft rejection, the intensity of immunosuppression, and other factors that may contribute to infection. Prophylactic strategies are based on the patient's known or likely exposures to infection according to the results of serologic testing and epidemiologic history. The risk of infection in the transplant recipient is a continuous function of the interplay between these factors. Prophylactic antimicrobial regimens vary depending on the transplant center and the type of transplant. All patients receive usual antibacterial surgical prophylaxis and trimethoprim–sulfamethoxazole (Bactrim) prophylaxis against *Pneumocystis jirovecii*. Antifungal prophylaxis is given depending on the organ transplanted, previous infection, and risk factors such as renal failure. Specific antiviral prophylactic regimens are determined by prior history of viral infections in the recipient and the organ donor. The major risks are herpes virus infection or reactivation, particularly cytomegalovirus (CMV) and EBV, hepatitis C virus (HCV) and hepatitis B virus. There is a very high risk of infection in seronegative recipients receiving an organ from a seropositive donor.

Early Posttransplantation Period

The first month after transplant is a vulnerable time for nosocomial bacterial infections including multidrug-resistant organisms related to complicated surgery. Venous and urinary catheterization and intubation add to the risk, as sicker patients tend to have more invasive devices for longer time periods. Opportunistic infections are generally absent during the first month after transplantation because the full effect of immunosuppression is not yet manifest. Unexplained early signs of infection, such as hepatitis, pneumonitis, encephalitis, rash, and leukopenia, may be donor-derived. Therapy may be empiric or determined by antimicrobial susceptibility data.

Intermediate Posttransplantation Period

The full effect of immunosuppressive medications typically manifest in months 1 to 6 posttransplant. This is when opportunistic infections tend to be most common. Viral pathogens and allograft rejection

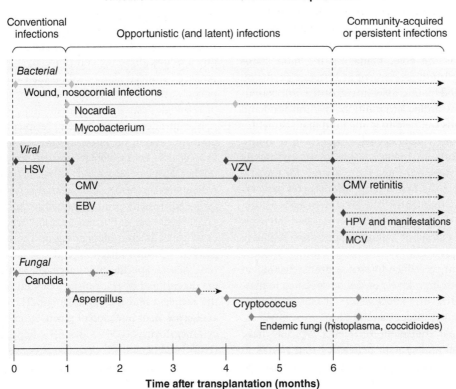

FIGURE 52-1 Timeline of common infections after transplantation.[10] (*Reproduced with permission from Wolff K, Johnson RA, Saavedra AP: Fitzpatrick's Color Atlas and Synopsis of Clinical Dermatology, 7th edition. New York: McGraw-Hill Medical; 2013.*)

are responsible for the majority of febrile episodes that occur during this period. Trimethoprim–sulfamethoxazole prophylaxis generally prevents most urinary tract infections and opportunistic infections such as *P jirovecii* pneumonia, *Listeria monocytogenes* infection, *Toxoplasma gondii* infection, and infection with sulfa susceptible nocardia species. Infection due to endemic fungi, aspergillus, cryptococcus, *Trypanosoma cruzi*, or strongyloides may occur. Herpes virus infections are uncommon with antiviral prophylaxis. However, other viral pathogens, including polyomavirus BK, adenovirus, and recurrent HCV have emerged.

Late Posttransplantation Period

Beyond 6 months posttransplant, most stable patients are on reduced doses of immunosuppression and therefore have decreased risk for

opportunistic infections. CMV, EBV, herpes simplex virus, and hepatitis viruses remain a concern, but more commonly transplant patients are infected with seasonal respiratory and gastrointestinal viruses, community-acquired pneumonias and urinary tract infections during this period. In those who require a higher level of immunosuppression, the risk for opportunistic infections may be as high as during the 1 to 6 months posttransplant period. This includes an increased risk for infections with *P jirovecii*, nocardia, varicella, and aspergillus.

IMMUNOSUPPRESSIVE DRUGS

Immunosuppression protocols vary from center to center and the transplant team determines the immunosuppressive regimens that are used posttransplantation. The intensivist should be familiar with the agents given, what levels to monitor, and the side effects and how they relate to the critical care management. The goal of immunosuppression is to prevent graft rejection while minimizing infection and other side effects. The current initial (ie, for induction) immunosuppression regimens used in solid organ transplants usually consists of a corticosteroid, a calcineurin inhibitor, and an antiproliferative agent. Monoclonal antibodies to lymphocyte receptors may also be used for induction, acute steroid resistant rejection or to reduce calcineurin inhibitors. In patients with corticosteroid intolerance, antiproliferative agents can be increased to reduce corticosteroid use. When renal toxicity is a concern, for example, pretransplant renal failure in a liver transplant patient, corticosteroids and antiproliferative agents may be preferentially used over calcineurin inhibitors.

Corticosteroids

Corticosteroids (eg, methylprednisolone and prednisone) decrease inflammatory proteins and are a cornerstone of immunosuppression. Side effects relevant to postoperative critical care management include mood changes, encephalopathy, hypertension, gastritis, hyperglycemia, hypokalemia, metabolic alkalosis, myopathy, and increased risk of infection.

Calcineurin Inhibitors

Cyclosporine and tacrolimus (Prograf, FK-506) are interleukin-2 (IL-2) inhibitors. They initially require daily monitoring of drug trough levels. The target levels vary with the overall immunosuppressive regimen, the type of transplant, underlying graft function, associated organ function, and the presence of infection. Nephrotoxicity and neurotoxicity remain the most important adverse side effects. Cyclosporine is associated with less neurotoxicity than tacrolimus. Neurotoxic side effects include tremors, headaches, dysarthria, neuropathies, delirium, cognitive impairment, somnolence, seizures, posterior reversible encephalopathy syndrome, and coma. Hypomagnesemia increases neurotoxicity and magnesium replacement with the avoidance of hypomagnesemia is important in patients receiving calcineurin inhibitors.

Antiproliferative Agents

Mycophenolate mofetil (Cellcept) and azathioprine (Imuran) are antimetabolite purine synthesis inhibitors. They are not nephrotoxic or neurotoxic. Side effects include myelosuppression with leukopenia and thrombocytopenia and gastrointestinal symptoms including vomiting, ileus, and oral ulcers. Azathioprine is usually not used as a first-line agent but may be substituted in patients who do not tolerate mycophenolate because of gastrointestinal side effects.

Sirolimus (Rapamune) inhibits IL-2 postreceptor, downstream in the signal cascade, preventing proliferation of T lymphocytes and reducing antibody production. It lacks the neurotoxicity and nephrotoxicity of the calcineurin inhibitors and is a long-term alternative to tacrolimus or cyclosporine in patients with renal dysfunction as a result of calcineurin toxicity. It is avoided in the early posttransplant period due to delayed wound healing and should be avoided in patients with nonhealing wound infections. Other adverse effects include bone-marrow suppression and it has been associated with an increased incidence of HAT after LT.

Monoclonal antibodies (eg, basiliximab) block IL-2 receptors on activated T-lymphocytes thwarting their multiplication and expansion. They have minimal side effects compared to muromonab-CD3 (Orthoclone OKT-3), a monoclonal antibody to T cell CD3 receptors that first activates T cells, causing systemic inflammation, before removing T cells from the circulation thus having significantly more side effects including fever, headache, nausea, and noncardiogenic pulmonary edema.

CONCLUSION

The maturation of solid organ transplantation as a clinical entity has brought new challenges for intensivists managing these patients. The relaxation of recipient criteria combined with expansion of the donor pool has resulted in sicker patients receiving transplants. Donor factors, recipient comorbidities, and intraoperative events play a critical role in determining the postoperative course.

REFERENCES

1. Diaz GC, Wagener G, Renz JF. Postoperative care/ critical care of the transplant patient. *Anesthesiol Clin.* 2013;31(4):723-735.
2. Fishman JA. Infection in solid-organ transplant recipients. *N Engl J Med.* 2007;357(25):2601-2614.
3. Pagalilauan GL, Limaye AP. Infections in transplant patients. *Med Clin North Am.* 2013;97(4):581-600.
4. Feltracco P, Barbieri S, Galligioni H, Michieletto E, Carollo C, Ori C. Intensive care management of liver transplanted patients. *World J Hepatol.* 2011;3(3):61-71.
5. Pham P-TT, Pham P-CT, Danovitch GM. The acute care of the transplant recipient. In: McKay DB, Steinberg SM, eds. *Kidney Transplantation: A Guide to the Care of Kidney Transplant Recipients.* New York: Springer; 2010:207-235.
6. Clavien P-A, Trotter JF. *Medical Care of the Liver Transplant Patient.* 4th ed. Wiley-Blackwell, UK, 2012.
7. Redfield RR, Scalea JR, Odorico JS. Simultaneous pancreas and kidney transplantation: current trends and future directions. *Curr Opin Organ Transplant.* 2015;20(1):94-102.
8. Selvaggi G, Tzakis AG. Small bowel transplantation: technical advances/updates. *Curr Opin Organ Transplant.* 2009;14(3):262-266.
9. Sadaghdar H, Chelluri L, Bowles SA, Shapiro R. Outcome of renal transplant recipients in the ICU. *Chest.* 1995;107(5):1402-1405.
10. Wolff K, Johnson RA, Saavedra AP. *Fitzpatrick's Color Atlas and Synopsis of Clinical Dermatology.* 7th ed. McGraw-Hill Medical, New York; 2013.

Posttrauma Care

J. David Roccaforte, MD

KEY POINTS

1 Survival outcomes in trauma patients over the last 30 years have largely resulted from the adoption of the damage-control strategy than from all other improvements in trauma care combined.

2 Damage-control strategy involves an abbreviated laparotomy, surgical control of arterial bleeding, temporary control of enteric spillage, stabilization of long bone fractures, abdominal packing to control venous bleeding, and temporary wound closures to accommodate swelling and to avoid compartment syndrome.

3 In severely injured trauma patients, the initial hypotension is a consequence of uncontrolled bleeding. Oxygen-carrying capacity must be maintained with red blood cells, the coagulation system must be supported with plasma and platelets, and after meeting those 2 objectives, any remaining hypovolemia can be corrected with balanced crystalloid.

4 Endpoints of resuscitation can monitor regional organ-specific function (eg, urine output, ST-segment abnormalities, and mental status), or global perfusion (lactate, base deficit).

5 An acute traumatic coagulopathy can be observed within 30 minutes postinjury. Thromboelastography-guided resuscitation, using targeted platelets, plasma,

cryoprecipitate, or other directed therapy may be the optimal strategy once the surgical bleeding has been addressed.

6 Abdominal compartment syndrome is important to recognize in the resuscitation of the trauma patient. Definitive treatment is surgical decompression of the abdominal fascia. Intraperitoneal dialysis with a hypertonic glucose solution is a promising intervention to optimize bowel wall perfusion, minimize inflammation, and more rapidly decrease edema.

7 Traumatic brain injury frequently accompanies major blunt trauma. Managing elevated intracranial pressure (ICP) in the setting of severe bleeding, hypovolemia, and shock is particularly challenging. In the presence of elevated ICP, optimizing cerebral perfusion pressure becomes the priority.

8 Corticosteroids for spinal cord injury are no longer recommended.

9 Pulmonary contusion is unique to trauma and can occur directly from blunt injury or indirectly from the blast effect and pressure wave created by a projectile passing through the tissue.

10 Blunt cardiac injury following thoracic trauma is a potentially lethal syndrome. In extreme cases, it can lead to cardiac rupture, valvular dysfunction, or coronary occlusion.

—Continued next page

Continued—

Mortality is typically from malignant arrhythmias.

11 Mechanical limb compression, prolonged ischemia, blast effect, and vascular insufficiency are all factors which can contribute to delayed myonecrosis.

12 Damage-control laparotomy with an open abdomen is not necessarily a contraindication to enteral nutrition.

13 Trauma patients are at elevated risk for posttraumatic stress disorder, and early screening and treatment can begin during their ICU stay.

14 Physical and occupational therapy availability for trauma patients in the ICU enhances their recovery, and eases the transition to their next phase of care.

DAMAGE-CONTROL STRATEGY/INTEGRATION WITH CRITICAL CARE

Despite the publication of over 2000 studies on damage-control strategy for trauma in peer-reviewed journals, not even 1 provides prospective, randomized, and class-1 evidence supporting the practice.[1] Nevertheless, among experienced experts in trauma, the nearly universal opinion is that survival outcomes over the last 30 years have benefitted more from the adoption of the damage-control strategy than from all other improvements in trauma care combined.

Prior to the current era of damage-control strategy, surgeons attempted the definitive operative repair of all injuries in a single, often prolonged procedure. In contrast, the damage-control strategy only temporizes the immediate life-threatening injuries at the first operation, and then addresses lower-acuity injuries later, in multiple, staged procedures. Physiologic stabilization of the severely injured patient in an intensive care unit (ICU) in between, and after the staged surgical procedures is integral to the damage-control strategy. As a consequence, it is imperative that intensivists who manage trauma patients have an overall understanding of the damage-control strategy,[2] as well as in-depth knowledge of critical care objectives and pitfalls specific to trauma patients.

Since the late 1980s, the surgical management of the unstable trauma patient has evolved from a thorough and definitive treatment at the first operation to a damage-control strategy. Specifically, damage-control involves an abbreviated laparotomy, surgical control of arterial bleeding, temporary control of enteric spillage, stabilization of long bone fractures, abdominal packing to control venous bleeding, and temporary wound closures to accommodate swelling and to avoid compartment syndrome. This first operation is completed as expeditiously as possible, ideally within an hour, at which time the patient, likely still in shock, and consequently cold, acidotic, and coagulopathic, is brought to the safe harbor of an ICU where resuscitation is continued, coagulopathy is corrected, and physiologic homeostasis restored.

Early Goals
Resuscitation/Transfusions/Fluid Management
Frequently, with severely injured trauma patients, the initial hypotension is a consequence of uncontrolled bleeding. As described elsewhere, a massive transfusion strategy will have been implemented and continued intraoperatively while surgeons attempt to control the sources of bleeding. The main benefit of massive transfusion protocols is to expedite red cell and blood-product availability to prevent death by exsanguination from uncontrolled surgical bleeding. Although the specific ratios of packed red blood cells (PRBCs) to fresh-frozen plasma (FFP), to platelets are debatable, the objectives of

resuscitation, transfusions, and fluid management are not. Oxygen-carrying capacity must be maintained with PRBCs, the coagulation system must be supported with FFP and platelets, and after meeting those 2 objectives, any remaining hypovolemia can be corrected with balanced crystalloid.[3] During periods of uncontrolled bleeding, oxygen-carrying capacity and coagulation status can change quickly. The inherent delay in obtaining laboratory measurements means that objective data are already old by the time they arrive back to the provider, and thus during periods of rapid, uncontrolled bleeding, presumptions regarding deficits must be inferred (eg, transfusion of PRBC:FFP:platelets in a 1:1:1 ratio) so as to avoid any episodes of undertreatment. Once rapid exsanguination from surgical bleeding has been controlled, the massive transfusion protocols should be terminated. Further blood and blood-product transfusions should be directed at correction of documented deficits in oxygen-carrying capacity or coagulopathy, *not* simply at blindly fulfilling preordained ratios.

The degree of anemia and hypovolemia that any individual patient might be able to tolerate during the early phase of resuscitation is variable, and will depend on the patient's cardiac status, presence or absence of vascular disease, and most importantly, presence or absence of a concomitant head injury with elevated intracranial pressure (ICP). If elevated ICP is suspected, then mean arterial pressure (MAP) should be high enough to maintain a cerebral perfusion pressure (CPP) = (MAP − ICP) of 55 mm Hg or more.

No ideal single marker of resuscitation adequacy exists. Each has its pitfall (see also Chapter 73). For example, serum lactate may be elevated in a perfectly resuscitated patient with baseline liver insufficiency. Base deficit values will be acutely elevated from a benign hyperchloremic acidosis if normal saline (or its equivalents) are used for resuscitation, even though intravascular volume and perfusion may be normal. A safer strategy is to initially collect data for as many endpoints of resuscitation as possible, and over the initial few hours, narrow the focus on those with the best signal-to-noise ratio, individualized to each patient.

Endpoints of resuscitation can monitor regional organ-specific function (eg, urine output, ST-segment

TABLE 53–1 Endpoints of resuscitation— markers of regional perfusion.

Regional Markers	Notes/Pitfalls
Capillary refill	Unknown baseline for comparison
CPK levels	Too slow for acute changes
Echocardiography	Requires special operator skills Absent esophageal or gastric pathology
Electrocardiogram	Unknown baseline for comparison
Jugular bulb saturation	Not routinely available
Mental status	Unavailable during general anesthesia Unreliable with intoxication
NIR spectrometry	Not routinely available
Sublingual tonometry	Not routinely available
Troponin levels	Too slow for acute changes
Urine output	Unreliable with acute or chronic renal failure, SIADH, or neurogenic DI

CPK, creatinine phosphokinase; DI, diabetes insipidus; NIR, near infrared; SIADH, syndrome of inappropriate antidiuretic hormone.

abnormalities, and mental status) (Table 53–1), or global perfusion (lactate, base deficit) (Table 53–2). Ideally, specifically tailored for each patient, 1 global and 1 local marker of resuscitation will be monitored that together optimize sensitivity and specificity for diagnosing shock and recovery.[4]

Coagulopathy/Temperature

The "lethal triad of death" describes the downward spiral of physiologic homeostasis in a patient with uncontrolled hemorrhage and shock. Obviously, if shock is the initial cause of the patient's lactic acidosis, coagulopathy, and hypothermia, even after visible bleeding has been successfully controlled, then inadequate attention to the correction of coagulopathy and hypothermia will lead to continued deterioration. It is during the second phase of damage control, in the ICU, that coagulation system support and aggressive rewarming occur. Classically, the coagulopathy associated with trauma and massive resuscitation was thought to be simply a

TABLE 53-2 Endpoints of resuscitation—markers of global perfusion.

Global Markers	Notes/Pitfalls
Anion gap	May be elevated for reasons other than lactic acidosis
Base deficit	May reflect nonanion gap acidosis
Cardiac output	Requires pulmonary artery catheter Abnormal in shock syndromes in addition to hypovolemia
Core temperature	Hypothermia is a marker of late or advanced shock Fever is the most common transfusion reaction
ET_{CO_2} P_aCO_2-ET_{CO_2} gradient	Elevated with chronic obstructive pulmonary disease
Heart rate	Unknown beta-adrenergic blocker use
Lactate	Impaired clearance with hepatic dysfunction
Mean arterial pressure	Generally well compensated until late Unknown baseline
pH	May reflect respiratory and/or nonanion gap acidosis
P_aO_2 P_aO_2:F_iO_2	Lower from the following: • Shunt (eg, pulmonary contusion, aspiration) • Hypovolemia-related V/Q mismatch Hypoxemia from shunt does not generally respond to supplemental oxygen Hypoxemia from V/Q mismatch easily corrected with supplemental oxygen
Pulse pressure	Difficult to interpret if accompanied by bradycardia
Respiratory systolic pressure variation	Difficult to interpret with obesity or with abdominal compartment syndrome
Sv_{O_2}	Requires pulmonary artery catheter Abnormal in shock syndromes other than hypovolemia

ET_{CO_2}, end-tidal carbon dioxide; F_iO_2, fraction of inspired oxygen concentration; P_aCO_2, partial pressure of arterial carbon dioxide; P_aO_2, partial pressure of arterial oxygen; Sv_{O_2}, mixed venous oxygen saturation; V/Q, ventilation/perfusion.

consequence of clotting factor and platelet dilution, consumption, and dysfunction. More recently, data have emerged which demonstrate that an acute traumatic coagulopathy can be observed within 30 minutes postinjury, more quickly than can be explained by acidosis, consumption, or dilution, indicating that a more complex process is involved. Ongoing research to elucidate the underlying etiology has focused on catecholamine, and inflammatory mediators, protein C activation, and shedding of glycocalyx. Regardless of the underlying complex initial biochemical pathophysiology, by the time a patient survives the first phase of damage control and is transferred to the ICU, the classic concerns of clotting factor and platelet dilution and hypothermia must be addressed.[5]

Thromboelastography (TEG) is a real-time measure of whole blood clotting. Results are available within 10 to 45 minutes—too slow to be useful in the acutely exsanguinating patient, however once surgical bleeding has been addressed, it should be considered. TEG data graphically reveal abnormalities in platelet function, intrinsic, extrinsic pathway integrity as well as fibrinogen deficits and thrombolysis. TEG-guided resuscitation, using targeted platelets, FFP, cryoprecipitate, or other directed therapy may be the optimal strategy during this phase, and likely superior to blindly continuing a massive transfusion protocol following predetermined ratios.[6]

Abdominal Compartment Syndrome

Intra-abdominal hypertension causes symptoms of abdominal compartment syndrome (ACS) when intra-abdominal pressure (IAP) exceeds systemic venous pressure. IAP is traditionally approximated by transducing an indwelling bladder catheter after instillation of saline, which establishes a continuous fluid column from the bladder to the pressure transducer. The transducer is zeroed at the symphysis pubis. Normal IAP is 3 to 10 mm Hg. With mild elevations up to 15 to 20 mm Hg, bowel becomes congested, renal and portal veins may collapse, and urine output may decrease. Provided that the systemic arterial blood pressure and intravascular volume can tolerate it, aggressive diuresis at this stage may be able to break the vicious cycle of increased bowel edema leading to increased venous congestion leading to decreased abdominal organ perfusion, increased edema, and increasing IAP. Because capillary fluid extravasation during the early posttrauma period is largely driven by the inflammatory response to trauma, diuresis usually fails to reverse the progression (Figure 53–1).

Once IAP rises more than 25 mm Hg, urine output is severely impaired, bowel perfusion is compromised, and airway pressures rises as a consequence of cephalad pressure on the diaphragm. At IAP more than 30 mm Hg, bowel ischemia, renal failure, and hypoxia from severe atelectasis are usually observed. The definitive treatment of ACS is to surgically decompress the abdominal fascia. Often at the initial damage-control operation, even if no intra-abdominal injury is found, ACS is anticipated and the abdominal fascia is left open prophylactically until the inflammatory response subsides and sequestered, third-space fluid is mobilized.[7] Intraperitoneal dialysis with a hypertonic glucose solution is a promising intervention to optimize bowel wall perfusion, minimize inflammation, and more rapidly decrease edema.[8]

Other Early Trauma ICU Concerns

During the second phase of damage control, the focus remains on resuscitation. Gradual physiologic improvement should be observed over the subsequent 24 to 48 hours at which time the patient returns to the operating room for definitive repair of remaining injuries. If a patient's condition continues to deteriorate, serious consideration must be given to a missed vascular injury. Interventional radiology may be utilized to diagnose and possibly embolize arterial bleeding that cannot be accessed surgically. Alternatively, a return to the operating room earlier than planned may be required.

The second phase of damage control in the ICU provides the opportunity to repeat and document a thorough baseline head-to-toe physical examination. Commonly, minor extremity fractures may be missed which can be associated with significant long-term disability, if not treated appropriately. Additionally, any extremity swelling should raise the concern of limb compartment syndrome and monitored with serial creatinine kinase (CK) levels or intramuscular pressure transduction as appropriate. Perioperative prophylactic antibiotics should be given[9] and a nutritional plan established.

Any vascular access obtained in the field, or in less-than-sterile conditions, should be removed and replaced if needed. If the patient's cervical spine cannot be cleared, then the extrication collar placed by EMS for cervical immobilization must be replaced with a collar designed for longer-term usage such as a Miami-J or Philadelphia-type collar. Extrication collars are made of thin, hard plastic with minimal padding, designed to be placed in tight quarters and they (as well as backboards) can cause decubitus ulcers within hours.

The patient's family or friends should be updated as to the patient's condition, and also queried regarding the patient's comorbidity, medications, allergies, and social history. Often, details of the patient's history emerge during these conversations which significantly alter the care plan.

Organ-System Supportive Care

Neurologic (See Also Chapters 48 and 50)

Traumatic Brain Injury—Traumatic brain injury (TBI) frequently accompanies major blunt trauma. Managing elevated ICP in the setting of severe bleeding, hypovolemia, and shock is particularly challenging. In the absence of head injury, during resuscitation, the mean arterial blood pressure

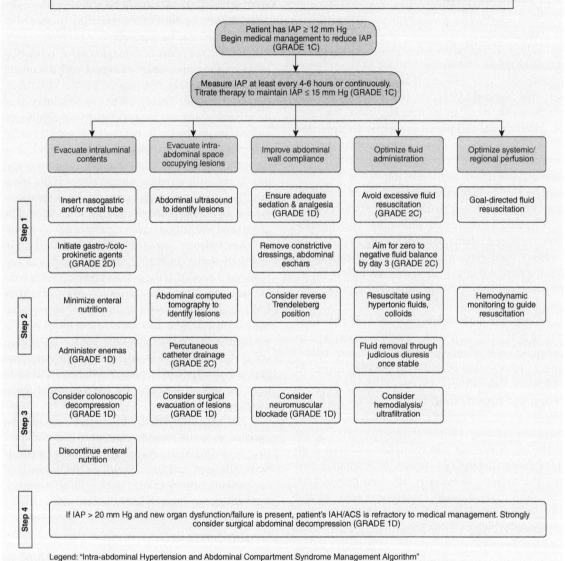

FIGURE 53–1 Intra-abdominal hypertension and abdominal compartment syndrome management algorithm. (*Reproduced with permission from Kirkpatrick AW, Roberts DJ, De Waele J, et al: Intra-abdominal hypertension and the abdominal compartment syndrome: updated consensus definitions and clinical practice guidelines from the World Society of the Abdominal Compartment Syndrome,* Intensive Care Med *2013 Jul;39(7):1190-1206.*)

(MAP) is targeted to be as low as possible so as to minimize additional bleeding while at the same time maintaining organ perfusion. However in the presence of elevated ICP, optimizing CPP becomes the priority.

CPP = MAP – (the higher of ICP or central venous pressure)

In order to accurately calculate CPP, arterial blood pressure, central venous pressure, and ICP must be monitored directly. ICP is monitored either via ventriculostomy and intraventricular catheter or by a parenchymal or subarachnoid transducer (see also Chapter 101). Interventions to consider which optimize CPP are head-of-bed elevation, cerebral spinal fluid drainage (if a ventriculostomy is present), judicious diuresis with osmotic agents such as mannitol (used with discretion in the presence of hypovolemia), intravascular hypertonic saline, deep sedation to achieve burst suppression on EEG, and alpha-agonist vasoconstriction. Interventions which have not shown to be of benefit or which may be harmful include hyperventilation, coticosteroids, and hypothermia.

Current recommendations for the ICU management of TBI can be found in the Guidelines for the Management of Severe Traumatic Brain Injury[10] which is published and updated by the Brain Trauma Foundation and available on-line.

Spinal Cord Injury and C-Spine Clearance— As soon as possible upon admission to the ICU, a thorough neurologic exam should be repeated. Any paraplegias or hemiplegias should raise the suspicion of spinal cord injury (SCI). Cervical and thoracolumbar vertebral immobilization should be maintained until the patient can cooperate with an appropriate examination, or until radiographic studies can be obtained which demonstrate absence of both bony injury (computed tomography [CT] scan) and soft-tissue ligamentous injury (magnetic resonance imaging). If the patient is known to have a spinal cord transection, any accompanying hypotension, bradycardia, or shock should be treated supportively. Anticipate the need for ongoing respiratory support for cervical spinal cord injuries. Corticosteroids for SCI are no longer recommended.

The prerequisite to the clinical clearance of a suspected or potential cervical SCI requires first the evaluation of any radiographic studies and confirmation of the absence of bony fractures or alignment abnormalities. In order for the cervical spine to be clinically cleared, the patient must be able to (1) focus fully on the exam (no distractions), (2) localize and discriminate mildly noxious stimuli, and (3) move and feel all extremities. A practical method of assessing distraction from any cause is to apply a mildly noxious stimulus to the patient's extremities and query if they feel discomfort. This demonstrates the patient's ability to localize sensation, focus on and cooperate with the examination, and communicate adequately with the care provider.

Coma Prognosis—Prognosis for patients with coma following TBI differs from that following anoxic brain injury. Following anoxic brain injury, if no improvement in the patient's neurologic status is observed after 72 hours, it is unlikely that the patient will have a significant recovery. In contrast, following TBI, treatment of concurrent injuries may delay or obscure early recovery from coma. Once the patient has been stabilized from other injuries, most neurologic recovery from TBI can be observed within 6 months with additional incremental improvements up to an year or more following the injury, especially with aggressive rehabilitation.

Sedation/Analgesia/Amnesia (See Also Chapter 16)—Trauma patients often require analgesia for soft-tissue and bony injuries. Intravenous opioids remain the standard means to control pain, either as a continuous or patient-controlled infusion. Appropriate constipation prophylaxis must be initiated. Alternatively, and especially for thoracic trauma and rib fractures, regional anesthesia, nerve blocks, and epidural catheters are effective. Nonsteroidal agents can be used with caution, especially if ongoing bleeding or renal injury is major concern. With few exceptions, a "wake-up" test, or suspension of sedation should be implemented once daily, and the opportunity taken to reassess neurologic function before restarting sedative/hypnotic agents. Utilization of benzodiazepines for amnesia or sedation is controversial. On the one hand, any recall of uncomfortable, upsetting, or delirium-induced memories has a high correlation with development of posttraumatic stress disorder (PTSD). On the other hand, benzodiazepine use is associated with delirium.

Delirium (See also Chapter 49)—Delirium is frequently observed patients following major trauma.

Its etiology is likely multifactorial. Disinhibition can occur from frontal lobe contusions in patients with TBI, systemic inflammatory response or renal failure can cause a metabolic encephalopathy, and given the prevalence of alcohol-related trauma, delirium tremens can occur from ethanol withdrawal. Treatment is largely supportive, with intravenous benzodiazepines for alcohol withdrawal and intravenous haloperidol a typical means of treatment for other causes of delirium in the acute setting. As the inflammatory response subsides, haloperidol can rapidly be tapered off within 2 or 3 days, dystonic reactions and neuroleptic malignant syndrome are rare in this setting. QT-intervals must be monitored closely. Patient recall of delirium episodes is a particularly potent risk factor for PTSD, and an amnestic agent such as a benzodiazepine may be of benefit once delirium has developed. In the absence of head injury, delirium developing in previously healthy trauma patients is temporary, and as they recover from their injuries and inflammation subsides, their mental status also normalizes.

Brain Death Determination—Brain death is the complete and irreversible cessation of all brain and brainstem function. Because cardiopulmonary function may be temporarily suspended and restarted as during cardiopulmonary bypass, even a "cardiac" death is not final until it becomes brain death. The determination of brain death in a patient whose remaining organs can retain function with support enables those organs to be procured for transplantation. The potential for organ transplantation is the only rationale for continuing cardiopulmonary support once brain death has been determined. Occasionally, family members may request continued organ support after death for cultural or religious reasons, and while efforts should be made to accommodate reasonable requests, they should not compromise the care provided to live patients in the ICU.

Specific protocols for the determination of brain death are mandated by individual jurisdictions and adapted at each hospital. In general, the process involves establishing a diagnosis, reviewing radiographs, assessing for potentially reversible causes of coma, conducting a neurologic examination of brain and brainstem function, repeating or confirming the examination, and finally performing an apnea test whereby the arterial carbon dioxide levels

are allowed to rise. The apnea test is performed as the final step because increasing CO_2 will potentially increase ICP and if the patient was not brain dead, the apnea test could theoretically complete a partial herniation, which is not the intention of the test. See Figure 53–2 for a sample protocol for the determination of brain death in adults.

Pulmonary

Pulmonary contusion is a respiratory condition unique to trauma. Contusion can occur directly from blunt injury or indirectly from the blast effect and pressure wave created by a projectile passing through the tissue. The initial chest radiograph may appear normal, however after 4 to 24 hours, the contusions blossom into dense infiltrates. Oxygenation deteriorates as a consequence of shunt, and the degree of hypoxia is proportional to the degree of hypoxic pulmonary vasoconstriction impairment, usually driven by inflammation and thus worse following blunt trauma compared to penetrating. Care is supportive, and an open-lung, protective ventilation strategy should be followed similar to that used to manage acute respiratory distress syndrome (see Chapter 19).

"Flail chest" is a condition whereby 2 or more adjacent ribs are fractured in 2 or more locations following blunt trauma. Historically, mortality was quite high, and thought to be a consequence of compromised respiratory mechanics. Significant effort was directed at stabilizing rib fractures with splints and plates, with minimal outcome benefit. We have come to realize that the true insult in flail chest is the underlying pulmonary contusion, and with adequate epidural analgesia, intubation and supportive ventilator management until the contusions resolve, outcomes have improved.

Cardiovascular

Occasionally a patient's fall or motor vehicle crash is precipitated by loss of consciousness due to another medical condition such as hypoglycemia, seizure, or pulmonary embolism. Commonly, the syncope is cardiac in origin. Myocardial infarction and arrhythmias must be considered, especially in elderly trauma patients. Cardiac monitoring must continue and evaluation undertaken concurrently with the trauma work-up.

The clinical criteria of brain death in adults

Instructions: When Steps 1, 2, and 3 are confirmed, the patient is declared brain dead (legally dead). Step 2 consists of a **First Exam** and a **Second Exam** that are performed at least 6 hours apart (2 hours if a confirmatory test is performed).	Check (✓) Item of Confirmed	
Step 1: Prerequisite to Exam Evaluate and correct potentially reversible causes of the abnormal neurological examination. 1) Hypotension (mean arterial pressure < 60 mm Hg) 2) Hypothermia (core temperature < 32°C or < 90°F) 3) Metabolic disturbances (eg, glucose, electrolyte, acid-base, or endocrine) 4) Significant drugs or medications 5) Confounding diseases (eg, locked-in syndrome, Guillain-Barré)	☐	
The cause of coma is known and sufficient to account for irreversible brain and brainstem death. Clinical history and/or neurological imaging are consistent with brain death.	☐	

	First Exam	Second Exam
Step 2: Absence of Brain and Brainstem Function **Coma:** Absent cerebral motor response in all extremities and face to noxious stimulus (applying firm pressure on the nail-beds and supraorbital ridge)	☐	☐
Absent Brainstem Reflexes: Pupils		
• Size: midposition to dilated (4 to 9 mm)	☐	☐
• Absent response to bright light	☐	☐
Absent corneal reflex (touch edge of cornea)	☐	☐
Absent gag reflex (stimulate pharynx)	☐	☐
Absent cough response (tracheobronchial suction)	☐	☐
Ocular Movement		
• Absent oculocephalic reflex (perform this test only if cervical spine instability is excluded)	☐	☐
• Absent deviation of eyes with cold water stimulation of the tympanic membranes	☐	☐

Step 2a: Consider Confirmatory Test[†] if Steps 1 or 2 cannot be fully performed or adequately interpreted.	
Step 3: Absence of Respiratory Effort[‡] **Positive Apnea Test:** Absent respiratory efforts when the arterial pCO_2 increase by more than 20 mm Hg above the patient's normal baseline.	☐
Step 3a: Consider Confirmatory Test[†] if Step 3 cannot be fully performed or adequately interpreted.	

[†]Confirmatory Testing

These conditions may warrant confirmatory tests: 1) significant levels of drugs, (eg, sedatives, neuromuscular blocking agents, anticholinergics, organophosphates, tricyclic antidepressants, antiepileptic drugs), 2) severe facial trauma, 3) cervical spinal cord injury, 4) preexisting pupillary abnormalities, or 5) severe pulmonary disease and chronic hypercapnia. Confirmatory test options include: cerebral angiography, brain scan with technetium-99m, electroencephalography, transcranial doppler, or somatosensory evoked potentials (See references for details).

[‡]Apnea Test

Prerequisites: 1) Begin test at patient's normal baseline arterial pCO_2 (never less than 40 mm Hg), 2) T ≥ 36.5°C (97°F), systolic BP ≥ 90 mm Hg.
Perform test: 1) Preoxygenate with 100% O_2, 2) monitor BP and pulse oximetry, 3) deliver 100% O_2 via cannula into the trachea to maintain oxygenation, 4) observe for respiratory movements, 5) measure arterial pO_2, pCO_2, and pH after at least 8 minutes and reconnect the ventilator.
Abort test: Draw blood gas and reconnect ventilator for: 1) spontaneous respirations or movement, 2) systolic BP ≤ 90 mm Hg, 3) oxygen desaturation, or 4) cardiac dysrhythmias.

Modified from: Practice parameters for determining brain death in adults. *Neurology*. 1995;45:1012-1014 and Wijdicks EF. The diagnosis of brain death. *N Engl J Med*. 2001;344:1215-1221.

FIGURE 53–2 Algorithm for the determination of brain death. (*Reproduced with permission from Marino PL, Sutin KM: The ICU Book, 3rd ed. Philadelphia: Lippincott Williams & Wilkins; 2007.*)

Blunt cardiac injury (BCI) following thoracic trauma is a potentially lethal syndrome. In extreme cases, it can lead to cardiac rupture, valvular dysfunction, or coronary occlusion; however, most cases manifest as impaired ventricular function. Mortality, when it occurs, is typically from malignant arrhythmias. Consequently, when BCI is suspected, the patient must have a baseline electrocardiogram (ECG) and cardiac troponin level.

The Eastern Association for the Surgery of Trauma publishes updated guidelines[12] for the management of BCI. Among their most recent recommendations (2012):

- If the admission ECG reveals a new abnormality (arrhythmia, ST changes, ischemia, heart block, and unexplained ST changes), the patient should be admitted for continuous ECG monitoring.

- For patients with preexisting abnormalities, comparison should be made to a previous ECG to determine need for monitoring.

- For patients with a normal ECG and normal troponin level, BCI is ruled out.

- Patients with normal ECG results but an elevated troponin level should be admitted to a monitored setting.

- For patients with hemodynamic instability or persistent new arrhythmia, an echocardiogram should be obtained.

If no new arrhythmias develop in a hemodynamically stable patient for 24 to 48 hours, then continuous ECG monitoring may be discontinued. **Tachycardia**—The most common cardiac abnormality in the trauma patient is sinus tachycardia. The finding is nonspecific in trauma patients, and can be a consequence of hypovolemia, anemia, pain, anxiety, inflammation, fever, or elevated catecholamines. Each patient's ability to tolerate tachycardia must be weighed against the stress placed on the heart. Any evidence of strain or ischemia must prompt an investigation to diagnose and treat the underlying cause. If the tachycardia fails to resolve, or is attributable to elevated catecholamines, central fevers, or dysautonomia, then beta blockers should be considered for sustained heart rates more than 130 bpm so as to avoid tachycardia-induced cardiomyopathy.

Anticoagulation Management (See Also Chapters 20 and 34)—Although the early concern during resuscitation is directed at correcting coagulopathy, within hours to days, trauma patients become hypercoagulable and at significantly increased risk for deep vein thrombosis (DVT), especially if other trauma-related risk factors are present (see Table 53–3).

DVT prophylaxis should be initiated as soon as appropriate once bleeding is controlled, and the coagulopathy has been corrected. In patients with TBI, pharmacologic DVT prophylaxis with subcutaneous unfractionated or low-molecular weight heparin is safe to begin once the patient's neurologic exam and head CT scans are stable for 24 hours. Although the combination of mechanical DVT prophylaxis with pharmacologic prophylaxis has not been shown to decrease the incidence of DVT compared to each used alone, because of the high likelihood of missed heparin doses and periods of time where sequential compression devices are removed or turned off, many adopt a "belt and suspenders" approach and implement both modalities concurrently.

General surveillance screening with Doppler evaluation for the presence of DVT in trauma patients has not been shown to be cost-effective provided appropriate DVT prophylaxis is maintained. A notable exception would be a patient at high risk for DVT, who is not a candidate for therapeutic anticoagulation in whom placement of an inferior vena cava (IVC) filter would be considered if a DVT were present.

Unfortunately, definitive data do not exist to guide the appropriate usage of IVC filters in trauma

TABLE 53–3 Trauma-related DVT risk factors.

Trauma-Related DVT Risk Factors
Lower extremity fractures
Pelvic fracture
Spinal cord injury
Traumatic brain injury
Burns
Vascular injury, embolization, or repair

DVT, deep vein thrombosis.

patients.[13] Although retrievable filters are available, for various reasons the actual retrieval rate remains low. The protective benefit of IVC filter placement for pulmonary thromboembolism is temporary, yet the potential IVC complications of erosion and embolization are long-term. On the other hand, for patients with compromised cardiopulmonary function, even a relatively small pulmonary embolus can be fatal.

Musculoskeletal

Fat Embolism Syndrome—Multiple critical care concerns arise as a consequence of bony and soft-tissue injury to the extremities. Fat embolism syndrome (FES) manifests as pulmonary, neurologic, cardiac, and renal dysfunction following pelvic and long-bone fractures.[14] The injurious substances released into systemic circulation are most likely bone marrow constituents rather than purely fat. The diagnosis is one of exclusion and care is supportive. Neither corticosteroids, anticoagulation, nor IVC filter placement are recommended. Because movement of bony fragments is thought to be a contributing factor in the development of FES, the splints, traction, and external fixation devices placed during the first phase of damage control must be assiduously maintained throughout the patient's ICU course.

Crush Injury/Rhabdomyolysis—Mechanical limb compression, prolonged ischemia, blast effect, and vascular insufficiency are all factors which can contribute to delayed myonecrosis. Typically prophylactic fasciotomies are created to prevent limb compartment syndrome. When a limb salvage approach is chosen over early amputation, the intensivist must be aware of the progressive pathophysiology which may follow. Initially the skin and soft tissue of the limb appear normal, however serum CK levels must be monitored closely. If CK levels rise, rhabdomyolysis has begun, and surgical debridement of necrotic tissue (or extension of fasciotomies) must be undertaken before renal failure progresses to multiorgan system failure or worse.[15] If the patient's systemic condition continues to deteriorate, amputation may be necessary. The Mangled Extremity Severity Score (MESS)[16] can aid in anticipating the success or failure of limb salvage (see Table 53–4).

Limb salvage success is significantly diminished when the MESS is greater than 7. Intravenous hydration with close monitoring of electrolytes, directed

TABLE 53-4 Mangled extremity severity score.

Component	Points
Skeletal and Soft-Tissue Injury	
Low energy (stab, simple fracture, "civilian gunshot wound")	1
Medium energy (open or multiplex fractures, dislocation)	2
High energy (close-range shotgun or "military" gunshot wound, crush injury)	3
Very high energy (same as above plus gross contamination, soft-tissue avulsion)	4
Limb Ischemia (score is doubled for ischemia > 6 h)	
Pulse reduced or absent but perfusion normal	1
Pulseless, paresthesias, diminished capillary refill	2
Cool, paralyzed, insensate, numb	3
Shock	
Systolic blood pressure (BP) always > 90 mm Hg	0
Hypotensive transiently	1
Persistent hypotension	2
Age (yr)	
< 30	0
30-50	1
> 50	2
TOTAL	

at maintaining renal function is the mainstay of treatment for rhabdomyolysis. Alkalinization of urine and forced diuresis may be considered.

Renal (See Also Chapters 30 and 31)

Besides the usual factors associated with renal failure in the critically ill (advanced age, hypertension, vascular disease, diabetes), trauma patients have additional risk factors contributing to a high rate of renal insufficiency and need for renal replacement therapy. For instance, direct renal trauma leading to nephrectomy results in an immediate decrease in glomerular filtration rate by half. Multiple exposures to contrast during the radiographic work-up of injuries, or during interventional vascular procedures is common. Rhabdomyolysis, exposure to aminoglycosides, and sepsis are potential additional insults.

Except for hydration therapy for rhabdomyolysis, the evidence supporting renal protective interventions for contrast-induced nephropathy is inconsistent. The potential outcome benefit demonstrated by intravenous hydration, bicarbonate administration, urine alkalinization, and oral N-acetylcysteine administration results in a lower peak creatinine level compared with placebo. Renal prophylactic therapies have neither been shown to improve survival nor to decrease the need for renal replacement therapy. However, because of the low cost, minimal risk, and potential benefit, renal prophylaxis for intravenous contrast exposure is often implemented.

Gastrointestinal Nutrition

In many trauma patients, gastrointestinal ileus develops directly as a consequence of bowel injury or indirectly from an elevated stress response or from narcotic exposure. At the same time, metabolic requirements necessary to heal wounds increase demands significantly following trauma. Interestingly, even relatively minor TBI increases metabolic demands well out of proportion to what might be anticipated from the amount of tissue damaged.

A plan for nutritional support must be established as early as possible. Often, if it can be anticipated that a patient will not be able to eat by mouth for a prolonged period, surgical feeding access may be obtained at the first take-back damage-control operation. Although there appears to be no difference in aspiration risk between nasogastric and postpyloric nasoduodenal tube feeding, a tube placed beyond the ligament of Treitz into the jejunum for feeding, with a proximal gastric port for evacuation may offer some benefit (see also Chapter 70).

Damage-control laparotomy with an open abdomen is not itself a contraindication to enteral nutrition.[17] Intestinal luminal cells derive a portion of their energy from directly absorbed enteral nutrition, so providing even minimal trophic feeding could be expected to increase bowel perfusion and motility, enhance anastomotic integrity and decrease interstitial edema. In fact, in patients without bowel injury, enteral feeding in the open abdomen is associated with increased fascial closure rates, decreased complication rates, and decreased mortality.

Traditionally, enteral feeding is suspended prior to any planned operative procedure. The severely injured trauma patient may return to the operating room almost daily for various staged repairs in a damage-control strategy. As a consequence, nutritional support can become severely compromised. A more prudent approach is to continue enteral nutrition perioperatively, provided that the airway remains protected with a cuffed endotracheal tube, and the planned surgical procedure does not involve the aerodigestive tract.

Long-Term Concerns
Social Support

Unlike the majority of critically ill patients who are admitted to an ICU after a long-term trajectory of deterioration from a chronic disease or condition, most trauma patients are relatively healthy prior to their injury. Indeed, many have never been hospitalized before. Trauma patients require a tremendous amount of social support and assistance ranging from tracking down family members to arranging for pets to be fed. A skilled and experienced trauma social worker is an invaluable member of the team.

Psychologic Issues

As the trauma patient begins to regain consciousness, they often experience retrograde amnesia even if they did not suffer a head injury. The last thing they remember might be events from the day before they were injured. They may not know what happened, where they are, how they got there, nor realize, for instance, that a loved one perished in the same vehicle crash, or that they have lost a limb. As difficult as those conversations are to have, providing truthful information to the patient is the only way to alleviate their extreme anxiety and fear of not knowing. Anticipating how best to compassionately inform a patient of the events surrounding their trauma enables the care team to enroll the expertise of psychologists, social workers, grief counselors, clergy, family members, or even former trauma patient volunteers who can be available to provide support and answer questions for patients and their families.

As gratifying as it can be to care for severely injured trauma patients and enable them to recover from their physical injuries, neglecting their psychologic well-being can undermine an otherwise successful outcome. Trauma patients are at elevated risk for PTSD, and early screening and treatment can begin during their critical care stay.[18] Full-blown PTSD can be incapacitating, but even posttrauma anxiety or depression can lead to substance abuse, alcoholism, and risk-taking that partly explain how trauma can become a chronic, relapsing condition.

Rehabilitation

Early mobility and ambulation, even in the ICU, has been shown to improve outcomes for specific types of injuries, while at the same time prolonged bedrest and immobility have almost universally been associated with increased ICU complications. Physical and occupational therapy availability for trauma patients in the ICU enhances their recovery and eases the transition to their next phase of care.[19]

REFERENCES

1. Cirocchi R, Montedori A, Farinella E, Bonacini I, Tagliabue L, Abraha I. Damage control surgery for abdominal trauma. *Cochrane Database Syst Rev.* 2013;3:CD007438.
2. Sagraves SG, Toschlog EA, Rotondo MF. Damage control surgery—the intensivist's role. *J Intensive Care Med.* 2006;21(1):5-16.
3. Kutcher ME, Kornblith LZ, Narayan R, et al. A paradigm shift in trauma resuscitation: evaluation of evolving massive transfusion practices. *JAMA Surg.* 2013;148(9):834-840.
4. Shere-Wolfe RF, Galvagno SM, Jr, Grissom TE. Critical care considerations in the management of the trauma patient following initial resuscitation. *Scand J Trauma Resusc Emerg Med.* 2012;20:68.
5. Duan K, Yu W, Li N. The pathophysiology and management of acute traumatic coagulopathy. *Clin Appl Thromb Hemost.* 2015;21(7):645-652.
6. Tapia NM, Chang A, Norman M, et al. TEG-guided resuscitation is superior to standardized MTP resuscitation in massively transfused penetrating trauma patients. *J Trauma Acute Care Surg.* 2013;74(2):378-385.
7. Kirkpatrick AW, Roberts DJ, De Waele J, et al. Intra-abdominal hypertension and the abdominal compartment syndrome: updated consensus definitions and clinical practice guidelines from the World Society of the Abdominal Compartment Syndrome. *Intensive Care Med.* 2013;39(7):1190-1206.
8. Smith JW, Garrison RN, Matheson PJ, et al. Direct peritoneal resuscitation accelerates primary abdominal wall closure after damage control surgery. *J Am Coll Surg.* 2010;210(5):658-664.
9. Goldberg SR, Anand RJ, Como JJ, et al. Eastern Association for the Surgery of Trauma. Prophylactic antibiotic use in penetrating abdominal trauma: an Eastern Association for the Surgery of Trauma practice management guideline. *J Trauma Acute Care Surg.* 2012;73(5 suppl 4):S321-S325.
10. Brain Trauma Foundation; American Association of Neurological Surgeons; Congress of Neurological Surgeons. Guidelines for the management of severe traumatic brain injury. *J Neurotrauma.* 2007;24(suppl 1):S1-S106.
11. Marino PL, Sutin KM. *The ICU Book.* 3rd ed. Philadelphia, PA: Lippincott Williams & Wilkins; 2007:920-921.
12. Clancy K, Velopulos C, Bilaniuk JW, et al. Screening for blunt cardiac injury: an Eastern Association for the Surgery of Trauma practice management guideline. *J Trauma Acute Care Surg.* 2012;73(5 suppl 4):S301-S306.
13. Aryafar H, Kinney TB. Optional inferior vena cava filters in the trauma patient. *Semin Intervent Radiol.* 2010;27(1):68-80.
14. Akhtar S. Fat embolism. *Anesthesiol Clin.* 2009;27(3):533-550.
15. Zimmerman JL, Shen MC. Rhabdomyolysis. *Chest.* 2013;144(3):1058-1065.
16. Rozycki GS, Tremblay LN, Feliciano DV, McClelland WB. Blunt vascular trauma in the extremity: diagnosis, management, and outcome. *J Trauma.* 2003;55(5):814-824.
17. Burlew CC, Moore EE, Cuschieri J, et al. Who should we feed? Western Trauma Association multi-institutional study of enteral nutrition in the open abdomen after injury. *J Trauma Acute Care Surg.* 2012;73(6):1380-1387.
18. Zatzick D, Jurkovich G, Rivara FP, et al. A randomized stepped care intervention trial targeting posttraumatic stress disorder for surgically hospitalized injury survivors. *Ann Surg.* 2013;257(3):390-399.
19. Engels PT, Beckett AN, Rubenfeld GD, et al. Physical rehabilitation of the critically ill trauma patient in the ICU. *Crit Care Med.* 2013;41(7):1790-1801.

Postcardiothoracic Surgery Care

Mabel Chung, MD and Anthony Carlese, DO

KEY POINTS

1 Every postcardiac patient should be evaluated for fast tracking, and the decision to proceed with this strategy should be assessed on a case-by-case basis and may be modified by patient comorbidities or situational factors.

2 Subsequent administration of sedatives and analgesics should be done judiciously to keep the patient comfortable while intubated, but to avoid oversedation and respiratory depression that may delay extubation.

3 To conceptualize the hemodynamic changes in the postoperative period is to consider whether the myocardium is pressure overloaded of volume overloaded or particularly with the various valvular surgeries.

4 Viscoelastic whole blood tests such as the thromboelastography (TEG) may pinpoint the hemostatic defect and provide more targeted transfusion therapy.

5 Atrial fibrillation after cardiac surgery is a common phenomenon occurring in 10% to 65% of postoperative patients with a peak incidence occurring 2 to 3 days after surgery.

6 Renal dysfunction is not uncommon after surgery with an incidence of 1.4% for overt renal failure, risk factors being age, New York Heart Association (NYHA) class 3 or 4 heart failure, chronic renal disease, type I diabetes mellitus (DM), prolonged operative time, and poor cardiac performance.

INTRODUCTION

The care of patients after cardiac surgery, particularly in the immediate postoperative period, frequently involves a period of physiologic volatility as the body adapts to the cardiac intervention and recovers from the effects of cardiopulmonary bypass (CPB) and anesthesia. The successful management of this patient population can be facilitated by addressing common issues such as fast-track eligibility and extubation, hypotension and low cardiac output (CO), postoperative bleeding, dysrhythmias, renal function,

and glucose control. This chapter aims to provide an overview of these topics as well as a framework for approaching problems in these areas.

TRANSITION OF CARE

When the postcardiac surgery patient arrives in the intensive care unit (ICU), the optimal transition of care is achieved by direct communication between the ICU team and the surgeons and anesthesiologists involved in the case. If a coronary artery bypass graft (CABG) was performed, the report from the surgeons should include the number of bypasses, the locations of the grafts, and whether the quality of the targets were good, as this has implications for the degree of protection achieved against future myocardial ischemia. Patients very commonly will have had coronary stents placed prior to their CABG. If the grafts did not bypass these stents, then antiplatelet agents such as clopidogrel may need to reinstated as soon as hemostasis is assured. When radial artery or bilateral internal mammary grafts are utilized, some institutions utilize low-dose nitroglycerin or nicardipine to protect against vasospasm, and the need for these agents should be communicated to the ICU team. If a valvular procedure has been performed, the differentiation the surgeon's report should include the valve of interest, whether it was repaired or replaced, and it was replaced, the type of valve that was implanted, that is, bioprosthetic or mechanical. Mechanical valves necessitate anticoagulation once hemostasis is achieved, and a plan for implementation should be made clear. The surgeon should communicate the need for any particular blood pressure goals. A lower blood pressure may be requested in situations where the risk of bleeding is higher than usual, such as when a friable aorta was encountered during the procedure. A higher blood pressure goal may be needed in patients with chronic hypertension or in those with known vascular stenoses of the carotid or renal vasculature. Finally, a plan for devices such as intra-aortic balloon pumps should be communicated.

The transition of care should also include a thorough report from the anesthesiologist. The difficulty of mask ventilation and intubation should be communicated as this has implications for whether a patient might be safely extubated later on. If the intubation was difficult, the details on how intubation was achieved should be obtained. The report should also comment on the difficulty or ease of line placement. Information about CPB should be communicated as well, including prebypass stability, duration of bypass, duration of circulatory arrest, difficulty in arresting the heart and difficulty of weaning off bypass including the number of attempts and the vasoactive medications required for separation. Knowledge of the findings on transthoracic echocardiography are paramount for postoperative

management in the ICU including left and right ventricular functions, thickness of the ventricle, and the presence of any valvular abnormalities. Other details such as rhythm issues and the requirement for pacing as well as baseline hemodynamic measurements such as pulmonary artery pressures and cardiac index (CI) should be obtained. Finally, the number and type of blood products should be communicated to the ICU team.

FAST-TRACK CARE

Once report has been obtained from the surgical and anesthetic teams, the decision of whether to fast track the patient should be made. Fast-track care or fast tracking involves a strategy of early extubation with the aim of promoting an expedient discharge for the purpose of reducing the length of stay in the ICU and hospital and to realize cost savings. It typically starts as an anesthetic strategy of decreased opioid dosage (eg, intraoperative fentanyl usage of less than 20 micrograms/kg vs greater than 20 micrograms/kg) to promote timely awakening and return of respiratory drive, and is executed as an ICU team strategy of achieving extubation within a predetermined timeframe, often with the help of a time-directed extubation protocol, typically within 8 hours of arrival to the unit. One meta-analysis found that fast tracking resulted in a significant mean reduction in time to tracheal extubation of 8.1 hours as well as achievement of a statistically significant decrease in overall ICU length of stay of approximately 5 hours, though not in overall hospital length of stay,[1] a finding echoed by a Cochrane Review on fast-track cardiac care (decreased time to extubation 3.0 to 10.5 hours, decreased length of stay in ICU 0.4-8.7 hours).[2] An earlier trial by Cheng et al found that fast tracking (intraoperative fentanyl 15 g/kg vs 50 g/kg) led to a decrease in time to extubation by approximately 15 hours and a decrease in ICU length of stay of approximately 5 days; in this context, use of fewer higher cost ICU days resulted in a cost savings of per CABG of 25% as well as a decrease in the rate of case cancellations (0.3% vs 2%) due to improved ICU throughput.[3] Fast tracking appears to be safe without evidence of increased mortality or postoperative complications such as myocardial infarction, reintubation, acute renal failure, major bleeding, and stroke.[1,2]

Patient selection for fast tracking must be considered. For example, Cheng et al excluded patients who were older than 75 years of age and who experienced a recent myocardial infarction (within 3 weeks), inotropic therapy within 24 hours before the study, or had an intra-aortic balloon pump as well as patients with severe hepatic disease, significant renal insufficiency, or severe chronic obstructive pulmonary disease (COPD), among other criteria. Every postcardiac patient should be evaluated for eligibility for fast tracking, but the decision to proceed with this strategy should be assessed on a case-by-case basis and may be modified by patient comorbidities or situational factors.

Delays in extubation may be warranted with certain comorbidities. For example, the patient with a low ejection fraction (EF) due to left ventricular dysfunction should be carefully assessed for signs of low CO prior to liberation from the ventilator. CPB induces a temporary deterioration of myocardial contractility[4-6] (see section "Hypotension and Low Cardiac Output"), which may significantly impact a patient with low myocardial reserve. Extubation during this time period, with loss of left ventricular afterload reduction due to withdrawal of positive pressure ventilation, may further compromise a tenuous state of contractility.[7-9] Patients who maintain an adequate CO despite a starting low EF and demonstrate signs of adequate perfusion should be extubated when ready. However, those with myocardial dysfunction resulting in hemodynamic instability with a rising vasopressor requirement, especially with concurrent acidosis, low mixed venous saturation (Svo_2) and oliguria should be kept intubated until stabilized with therapies such as initiation or escalation of inotropic therapy or placement of an intra-aortic balloon pump. Another example is the patient with end-stage renal disease who is dependent on dialysis who may require renal replacement therapy in the immediate postoperative period. In this case, extubation may be better delayed after completion of a therapy that will induce fluid shifts in the early postoperative period.

Situational factors such as bleeding, hemodynamic instability, delayed emergence, difficult intubation, hypothermia, or intraoperative complications may also prevent fast tracking. The bleeding patient with copious output from chest tubes may require a return to the operating room for achievement of surgical hemostasis. The hemodynamically unstable patient with a rising pressor requirement will require assessment for and treatment of hypovolemia or bleeding, tamponade, loss of myocardial contractility, or sepsis. Delayed emergence despite lower doses of narcotic utilization during the operation due to pharmacologic sensitivity may prevent the patient from achieving extubation criteria by 8 hours due to excessive sleepiness and apnea. Although a difficult intubation in and of itself should not be a deterrent to fast tracking as long as extubation criteria are achieved, a difficult airway resulting in trauma due to multiple intubation attempts may warrant a delay in removal of the endotracheal tube in order to institute measures to decrease airway edema (eg, elevation of the head of the bed and steroids), especially if the patient does not demonstrate an air leak with the endotracheal tube balloon deflated. In addition, the patient with the difficult airway with marginal achievement of extubation criteria may benefit from resources that may be more easily available during the daytime rather than the nighttime such as advanced airway equipment and the immediate availability of an anesthesiologist. Hypothermia (core temperature < 36°C) promotes arrhythmias, impairs coagulation, and may cause shivering, which increases oxygen consumption and myocardial oxygen demand and should be rectified prior to extubation. Finally, intraoperative events such as a prolonged (> 2.5 hours) bypass run, bleeding requiring massive transfusion, or difficulty in repairing the aortic cannulation site may merit exemption from fast tracking. In the latter case, avoidance of hypertension both pharmacologically and by preventing rapid awakening with immediate sedation on arrival to the ICU may be requested to decrease the probability of dehiscence of the repair and resultant surgical bleeding.

In general, regardless of whether the patient qualifies for the fast-track strategy, sedatives and analgesics should be held after arrival in the ICU until the patient awakens. Documentation of emergence from the anesthetic with movement of all extremities is an important milestone in the postoperative course, as postoperative stroke may manifest as delayed emergence or hemiplegia. If the patient is to be fast tracked, subsequent administration of sedatives and analgesics should be done judiciously to keep the patient comfortable while intubated but to avoid oversedation and respiratory depression that might delay extubation. In those patients who arrive to the ICU awake or awaken shortly thereafter, a number of agents are available for sedation and analgesia (Table 54–1).[10,11] Dexmedetomidine, an α_2 agonist that decreases sympathetic outflow, produces sedation without respiratory depression and is useful in the patient who expected to be fast tracked. Its cost as well as the potential for inducing bradycardia and resultant hypotension are limiting factors. When dexmedetomidine is not available, propofol provides rapid onset and offset of sedation at low doses; at higher doses propofol will induce respiratory depression. Benzodiazepines such as midazolam are slower in offset and are less favored in the patient expected to be extubated. However, they may provide greater stability in the hemodynamically tenuous patient. The patient in pain may benefit from an array of available analgesics. Intravenous acetaminophen may provide pain relief without concern for inducing apnea. Fentanyl, a μ opioid agonist, provides rapid pain relief with limited duration. Longer acting analgesics such as hydromorphone and morphine should be given judiciously to prevent respiratory depression that may delay extubation. Morphine should not be dosed in patients with significant kidney dysfunction, as the active metabolite morphine-6-glucuronide has additive sedative effects. Certain patients may be candidates for IV ketorolac, a potent nonsteroidal anti-inflammatory drug (NSAID). However, this analgesic should be avoided in patients with renal insufficiency, a history of gastric ulcers, severe or aspirin-sensitive asthma, and in those in whom bleeding is a concern. Lidocaine patches may give relief to the patient who is experiencing great discomfort from chest tubes. The patient who is shivering may benefit from meperidine, although this agent should not be given to the patient on monoamine oxidase inhibitors (MAOIs) or selective serotonin-reuptake inhibitors (SSRIs). Together, these agents should keep the patient comfortable while intubated; ongoing weaning should occur concurrent to completion of an appropriate postoperative evaluation (electrocardiogram, chest X-ray, laboratory values, and continual evaluation of hemodynamics as well as chest tube and urine outputs).

EXTUBATION

In general, extubation of the postcardiac surgery patient can be considered once the patient is warm (temperature > 36.0°C) and has demonstrated hemodynamic stability with regards to heart rate (HR), CI (ideally > 2.2 L/min/m²), and blood pressure. Inotropic and vasopressor requirements should be stable or decreasing and parameters associated with adequate perfusion such as the Svo_2, lactate, and urine output should be acceptable. In addition, chest tube outputs should not be excessive (consider a threshold of > 200 cc/h). As the postoperative evaluation is being completed, the patient should be actively weaned to a fraction of inspired oxygen (Fio_2) 40% and positive end-expiratory pressure (PEEP) 5 cm H_2O while maintaining a peripheral capillary oxygen saturation (Spo_2) greater than 92%. As the spontaneous respiratory drive returns, pressure support ventilation should be instituted and weaned to 5 cm H_2O. The final assessment of extubation should be performed on minimal ventilator settings with evaluation of the following parameters: oxygenation, ventilation and strength, and airway protection (Table 54–2).

Common issues such as atelectasis and pain control may provide barriers to timely extubation. Some patients become atelectatic during the bypass run and develop an alveolar to arterial (A-a) gradient that precludes full weaning of Fio_2. As hemodynamics allow, recruitment maneuvers (ie, PEEP 20 cm H_2O for 20 s) can open up collapsed alveolar units and improve oxygenation. Pain control can pose a challenge, as well. Some patients find inadequate pain relief with opioids and as a result, may splint and breathe shallowly on the ventilator. Other patients demonstrate dose-limiting sleepiness and apnea only to wake up in persistent pain. To those who qualify, adjuncts such as intravenous acetaminophen or ketorolac can be beneficial.

HYPOTENSION AND LOW CARDIAC OUTPUT

The goal mean arterial pressure (MAP) is typically set as greater than 65 mm Hg. A higher goal may be needed with chronic hypertensives in whom the autoregulatory curve of the brain and kidney have shifted to accommodate long-standing elevated

TABLE 54–1 Sedatives and analgesics.

Sedatives and Analgesics	Class	Doses	Considerations
Dexmedetomidine (Precedex)	α_2 agonist	0.5 µg/kg IV over 10 min 0.2-1.5 µg/kg/h	• No respiratory depression • Antishivering, antidelirium properties • Does not accumulate with prolonged infusion • Bradycardia and hypotension; may see transient initial hypertension from crossover α_1 agonism • No active metabolites
Propofol (Diprivan)	GABA$_A$ agonist	5-50 µg/kg/min	• Hypotension, negative inotropy • Respiratory depression • Propofol infusion syndrome (with prolonged infusion rates > 70-85 µg/kg/min) • Accumulates with prolonged infusion • No active metabolites
Midazolam (Versed)	GABA$_A$ agonist (benzodiazepine)	1-5 mg IV 1-5 mg/h	• Possibly greater hemodynamic stability • Respiratory depression • Accumulates with prolonged infusion • Active metabolite 6-hydroxy-midazolam accumulates in renal failure
Fentanyl (Sublimaze)	µ opioid agonist	25-50 µg IV 25-100 µg/h	• Respiratory depression • Accumulates with prolonged infusion • No active metabolite
Hydromorphone (Dilaudid)	µ opioid agonist	0.5 mg IV	• No active metabolite
Morphine	µ opioid agonist	2-4 mg IV	• Histamine release • Active metabolite 6-morphine-glucuronide accumulates in renal failure
Acetaminophen (Tylenol)	Centrally acting analgesic	1 g IV	• No respiratory depression • Antipyretic • Do not exceed 4 g in 24 h • Avoid in hepatic insufficiency
Ketorolac (Toradol)	NSAID	15-30 mg IV	• Avoid in renal insufficiency, gastric ulceration, severe or aspirin-sensitive asthma, and bleeding • Consider lower dose or avoiding in older patients due to decreased GFR
Meperidine (Demerol)	µ opioid agonist	25 mg IV	• Antishivering • Avoid with MAOIs or SSRIs • Neuroexitation w/renal insufficiency or high doses

GFR, glomerular filtration rate; MAOIs, monoamine oxidase inhibitors; NSAID, nonsteroidal anti-inflammatory drug; SSRIs, selective serotonin-reuptake inhibitors.

systemic pressures. In addition, patients with known vascular stenoses of the carotid or renal arteries, as well as those with unrepaired coronary artery disease may require a higher perfusion pressure to overcome these potentially flow-limiting lesions. A lower MAP may be required for a time in patients with a friable aorta to decrease the risk of bleeding.

MAP is defined as MAP = CO × SVR, where SVR denotes systemic vascular resistance. As CO itself is defined as HR times stroke volume (SV), the equation may be further defined as: MAP = HR × SV × SVR.

TABLE 54-2 Extubation criteria.

	Patient Should Achieve
Temperature	36.0°C

Hemodynamics	• Heart rate: absence of excessive bradycardia or tachycardia
	• Cardiac output as follows:
	  • CI > 2.2
	  • Svo_2 > 60%
	  • Normal or downtrending lactate
	  • Urine output > 0.5 cc/kg/h
	• Stable or decreasing inotropic and vasopressor requirements

Chest tube output	< 200 cc/h
Oxygenation	Fio_2 40%, PEEP 5 resulting in Pao_2 > 60-80 mm Hg or SpO_2 > 92%
Ventilation/strength	Pressure support ventilation at 5 cm H_2O • Adequate tidal volume and respiratory rate; rapid shallow breathing index < 105 • Absence of acute respiratory acidosis secondary to rapid and shallow breathing or bradypnea (should achieve pH > 7.35) • Presence of 5 s head lift or strong hand grip
Airway protection	Awake; presence of cough, gag, or swallow
Airway patency	If airway edema a concern, test for presence of air leak while endotracheal tube cuff deflated

CI, cardiac index; Fio_2, fraction of inspired oxygen; Pao_2, partial pressure arterial oxygen; PEEP, positive end-expiratory pressure; Spo_2, peripheral capillary oxygen saturation; Svo_2, mixed venous saturation.

Thus, hypotension may be conceptualized as being affected by 1 of these 3 major variables.

Heart Rate

HR may be a factor in hypotension. The process of cooling and arresting of the myocardium during cardiac surgery renders the muscle less compliant and induces diastolic dysfunction.[12] This resultant increase in the "stiffness" of the ventricles can limit the stroke volume and render the CO more dependent on HR. Thus, a HR that is too slow, even if not strictly bradycardic, may limit CO and decrease MAP. The responsivity of the blood pressure to pacing with epicardial wires to a HR of 90 to 100 beats/minute may be tested. If both atrial and ventricular wires are present, pacing can be accomplished with maintenance of atrial kick. However, if only ventricular wires are available, the hemodynamic benefit of increasing HR with ventricular pacing may be diminished by loss of contribution to stroke volume from loss of atrial kick. In fact, an increased pressor requirement may be observed in patients who lose atrioventricular (AV) synchrony and the atrial contribution to SV due to the development of an arrhythmia such as atrial fibrillation.

Stroke Volume

SV is affected by preload, contractility, and afterload. Hypotension, especially in the patient with a labile blood pressure, may be due to decreased preload and low SV from hypovolemia. Low preload may be due to an obvious process such as chest tube drainage or to a more occult occurrence such as retroperitoneal bleeding in the patient who has undergone femoral arterial cannulation. The volume responsiveness of the patient can be tested empirically by 250 to 500 cc fluid boluses with subsequent assessment of the effect upon blood pressure. Both normal saline and lactated ringers may be used for resuscitation although 5% albumin is frequently utilized with the intention of administering an agent with a greater intravascular half-life. Transfusion with packed red blood cells may be indicated in the setting of significant anemia, especially with a concurrent vasopressor requirement. The data on hydroxyethyl starch (HES) agents discourage its use in the cardiac surgical ICU. One study randomized 45 patients to receive either 15 mL/kg HES solution or 4% albumin after admission to the cardiac ICU and found that the HES group demonstrated thromboelastometry tracings indicative of impaired fibrin formation and clot strength.[13] Although the 2 groups demonstrated similar chest tube outputs, a subsequent meta-analysis of 18 trials comparing HES solutions with albumin for fluid management in CPB surgery found that HES solutions increased blood loss, reoperation for bleeding, and the rate of blood transfusion.[14] Given these results, it seems prudent to avoid the use of HES solutions for resuscitation in the postcardiac surgery patient. Hypotension from decreased preload and low SV may be secondary to mechanical obstructive process rather than hypovolemia. Conditions such as tamponade and tension pneumothorax prevent adequate venous return, depress SV and CO, and can result in hypotension and shock with rising pressor requirement and lactate and oliguria. Tamponade is further discussed under section "Bleeding."

Hypotension may also be secondary to low SV from decreased contractility. A temporary decrease in myocardial function is to be expected in the postcardiac surgery patient.[4-6] One study examining 24 patients undergoing elective coronary artery bypass surgery with serial hemodynamic measurements and radionuclide evaluation of ventricular function found that 96% experienced left- and right-sided myocardial depression postprocedure. The left-sided EF dropped from 58% preoperative to 37% with the nadir occurring 4.4 hours after coronary bypass. Recovery back to 55% occurred approximately 7.1 hours after coronary bypass.[6] An earlier study of 22 patients undergoing coronary artery bypass surgery found that those with an EF of more than 55% recovered ventricular function within 4 hours of bypass but that those with an EF more than 45% demonstrated a more profound decrease in function and a delayed recovery to baseline even after 24 hours.[5] Thus, the immediate postoperative cardiac patient may demonstrate a temporary inotropic or vasopressor requirement until myocardial contractility has fully recovered. However, a high index of suspicion for differentiating between this known and expected decrease in function and concurrent detrimental processes should be maintained.

Other independent causes of decreased myocardial contractility include new onset myocardial infarction from unrepaired disease or from CABG thrombosis or vasospasm. Diagnosis of a new ischemic insult may be accomplished with an electrocardiogram or with echocardiography demonstrating a new wall motion abnormality. In addition to hemodynamic instability, the onset of new arrhythmias such as ventricular tachycardia (VT) may be a manifestation of myocardial supply-demand mismatch. Troponins are of limited utility in detecting ischemia as they are typically elevated postcardiac surgery; however, some advocate trending the values. Management may include the administration of nitroglycerin to vasodilate the coronary arteries and to increase coronary perfusion pressure by decreasing preload and hence left ventricular end-diastolic pressure, cardiac catheterization to remove thrombus, or reexploration in the operating room to visually inspect the grafts.

Systemic Vascular Resistance

Hypotension may also be caused by insufficient systemic vascular resistance. Some patients arrive to the ICU hypothermic despite adequate rewarming on CPB due to a phenomenon called afterdrop—a redistribution hypothermia secondary to a cool periphery. These patients require active rewarming, which results in vasodilation of the peripheral vasculature and can uncover or worsen a vasopressor requirement. CPB causes a systemic inflammatory response that can lead to decreased SVR and a form of postbypass hypotension known as vasodilatory shock,[15,16] generally described as a MAP less than 70 mm Hg in the setting of an adequate CI of more than 2.5 L/min/m². Increased levels of vasodilators such as nitric oxide and bradykinin have been implicated in the pathogenesis of this phenomenon. The increase in bradykinin may be related to lack of deactivation by angiotensin converting enzyme (ACE) due to decreased blood flow to the lungs during CPB.[17,18] Vasodilatory shock may also be caused by a relative vasopressin deficiency.[19,20] One prospective study of 145 patients measured vasopressin levels 5 minutes after weaning from CPB. Those with vasodilatory shock demonstrated lower levels of vasopressin than those with postbypass hypotension due to decreased CI, and infusion with exogenous vasopressin improved MAP.[19] This study found the incidence of vasodilatory shock to be 8%, although the incidence was higher (27%) in those with an EF of less than 35%; in addition, preoperative ACE-inhibitors, commonly part of a heart failure regimen, were found to be a risk factor for the development of vasodilatory shock. A retrospective study of 2823 patients found a 20% rate of vasoplegia; clinical risk factors included observation of a clinically significant decline in MAP at the onset of CPB, length of bypass, and preoperative use of β blockers and ACE-inhibitors among others.[21]

Another way to conceptualize the hemodynamic changes of the postoperative period, especially in patients with valvular lesions, is to consider whether the myocardium is pressure-overloaded or volume-overloaded. Lesions such as aortic stenosis give rise to pressure-overloaded ventricles. In this situation, chronic obstruction to left ventricular ejection results in concentric hypertrophy as a compensatory response to increased wall stress. The increase in ventricular wall thickness results in a ventricle with decreased diastolic compliance or greater "stiffness." As a result, the resultant limitation in SV can result in a decrease in CO with lower HRs. Conversely, excessively high HRs may limit diastolic filling time, SV, and may also compromise CO. The stiffness of the ventricle impedes filling and makes the myocardium more dependent on atrial kick for stroke volume. Hence, the development of a nonsinus rhythm such as atrial fibrillation may result in a decrease in SV that decreases CO and MAP. The pressure-overloaded ventricle is more prone to ischemia than the normal ventricle. The increase in muscle mass increases the basal metabolic rate of the entire ventricle. In addition, the increase in stiffness of the pressure-overloaded myocardium results in an increase in the left ventricular end-diastolic pressure (LVEDP). This results in a decrease in the gradient for coronary perfusion pressure (CPP = aortic diastolic pressure [AoDP] – LVEDP/coronary vascular resistance) rendering the myocardium more vulnerable ischemia with decreases in blood pressure. Tachycardia is particularly detrimental not only because it limits SV by decreasing diastolic filling time but also because it reduces the duration of diastolic coronary perfusion and increases myocardial oxygen demand. The hemodynamic considerations in the pressure-overloaded ventricle are summarized in Table 54–3.

TABLE 54–3 Hemodynamic goals in the pressure-overloaded ventricle.

Rhythm	• Maintain sinus to preserve atrial kick
Heart rate	• Avoid bradycardia to avoid decreased CO (CO = HR × SV) • Avoid tachycardia to avoid ischemia (increased myocardial oxygen demand, decreased duration of diastolic coronary perfusion)
Blood pressure	• Avoid hypotension (CPP = AoDP – LVEDP/coronary vascular resistance)

AoDP, aortic diastolic pressure; CO, cardiac output; CPP, coronary perfusion pressure; HR, heart rate; LVEDP, left ventricular end-diastolic pressure; SV, stroke volume.

Although hypotension is to be carefully avoided in the pressure-overloaded myocardium, patients with preserved LV function often present to the ICU hypertensive, as the left ventricle has not yet had time to adapt to the removal of the stenotic aortic lesion. In this case, institution of a vasodilator such as nicardipine can control blood pressure in the acute setting. The patient with decompensated aortic stenosis may have decreased contractility and may have presented with decompensated heart failure.

Lesions such as aortic and mitral regurgitation result in volume-overloaded ventricles. Chronic volume overload results in eccentric hypertrophy where overall muscle mass is increased but chamber enlargement is greater than the increase in ventricular wall thickness. This gradual increase in LV size and compliance usually causes little change in the LVEDP. Chronic volume overload may result in a dilated cardiomyopathy with decreased LV systolic function and may require the use of inotropes to separate from bypass and their continued use in the ICU until myocardial stunning resolves. Decreased CO after correction of mitral regurgitation may also be secondary to decreased volume loading of the left ventricle from the resolution of regurgitation. Reports of the ejection prior to and after resolution of mitral regurgitation may be somewhat misleading. For example, a preoperative EF of 55% with a postoperative EF of 30% may not reflect any actual change in the contractility. The estimated EF prior to surgery reflects a SV that includes both forward flow and retrograde flow into the left atrium, and the effective EF taking only forward flow into account may have been 30% from the start. Because left ventricular afterload increases acutely after correction of mitral regurgitation, the left ventricle may benefit from pharmacologic afterload reduction. Chronic volume overload differs greatly from the volume overload resulting from acute aortic or mitral insufficiency where LVEDP increases dramatically and can result in sudden pulmonary edema and decreased CO prior to surgical correction.

Mitral regurgitation and stenosis may result in left atrial hypertension and dilation that can predispose to atrial fibrillation. In addition, pulmonary hypertension secondary to chronic venous congestion may be present with concomitant right ventricular dysfunction due to long-standing increases in RV afterload.

The hemodynamic problem of low CO (CO = HR × SV) may be broken down by examining the HR as well as the factors affecting SV (preload, afterload, and contractility). In the situation where low CO is accompanied by bradycardia, the CO may be augmented by increasing the HR. This can be accomplished either by electrical pacing with an external epicardial wire, reprogramming the rate of an internal pacemaker, or increasing the HR chemically with an agent with chronotropic properties. If a low CO is accompanied by a low afterload state and hypotension, the blood pressure should first be supported with vasopressors until more definitive therapies can be instituted. If the patient is volume-responsive, the SV and CO may be augmented with

additional preload. If the patient does not demonstrate improvement with volume, then the depressed CO may be secondary to decreased contractility. Epinephrine, an inoconstrictor, provides inotropic support along with vasoconstriction that should increase MAP. The inodilators dobutamine and milrinone may also be used but because they vasodilate the peripheral vasculature, vasopressor initiation or increase may be necessary to counteract a further drop in blood pressure. SV and CO may also be limited due to excessive afterload. The patient with high MAP and depressed CO may benefit from afterload reduction with a systemic vasodilator.

A high CO in the presence of a low HR does not need any intervention. If accompanied by low MAP, the low SVR state may be counteracted with vasoconstrictors such as norepinephrine and vasopressin. A high CO state with high MAP should be treated, as a high MAP may increase the risk of bleeding and will increase the oxygen demand of the myocardium; a decrease in blood pressure should, however, always be made in the context of baseline blood pressure and with an evaluation of the risk of hypoperfusion to pressure-dependent organs. The various possible therapies for disordered blood pressure and CO are detailed in Table 54–4.[22]

The details of various vasopressors and inotropes are included in Tables 54–5 and 54–6.[23] The vasopressors are utilized for their ability to increase MAP by increasing SVR (MAP = CO × SVR). Norepinephrine, an α_1 agonist that provides β_1 inotropy is typically chosen in favor of phenylephrine, a pure

TABLE 54–4 Therapies for abnormal blood pressure and cardiac output.

Abnormal Blood Pressure	Low Cardiac Output	High Cardiac Output
Low HR	• Electrical pacing • Chemical chronotropy: epinephrine, dopamine, and isoproterenol	—

Low MAP (low afterload state)	• Increase preload: consider volume
	• Increase contractility as follows:
	  • Inoconstrictor: epinephrine
	  • Inodilators: dobutamine, milrinone with norepinephrine, and vasopressin
		• Increase afterload: norepinephrine, vasopressin

High MAP (high afterload state)	• Afterload reduction: nicardipine, and nitroprusside	• Afterload reduction: nicardipine, and nitroprusside

HR, heart rate; MAP, mean arterial pressure.

TABLE 54–5   Vasopressors, inotropes, and afterload reducers (mechanisms and receptors).

	Classification	Receptors					Dose
		DA-1	α_1	β_1	β_2	Other	
Phenylephrine	Vasopressor	0	++	0	0		1-200 μg/min
Vasopressin	Vasopressor	0	0	0	0	V_1 (also V_2)	0.02-0.04 U/min up to 0.1 (1.4-2.4 U/h up to 6)
Norepinephrine	Inoconstrictor	0	+++	++	0		1-20 μg/min
Dopamine	Inoconstrictor	++ ++ ++	0 + ++	+ ++ ++	±		0.5-2 μg/kg/min 2-10 μg/kg/min 10-20 μg/kg/min
Epinephrine	Inoconstrictor	0	+++	+++	++		1-20 μg/min
Dobutamine	Inodilator	0	0	+++	+++		2-20 μg/kg/min
Milrinone	Inodilator	0	0	0	0	PDE3 inhibitor	0.125-0.5 μg/kg/min
Isoproterenol	Inodilator	0	0	+++	+++		1-5 μg/min

Data from Sladen RN: Postoperative Cardiac Care. Philadelphia: Lippincot Williams & Wilkins; 2011.

TABLE 54–6   Vasopressors, inotropes, and afterload reducers (effects).

	Classification	Vasoconstriction	Vasodilation	Contractility	HR	Other
Phenylephrine	Vasopressor	3+	0	0	0	Reflex bradycardia
Vasopressin	Vasopressor	4+	0	0	0	Lacks pulmonary vasoconstrictor activity at doses < 4 U/h
Norepinephrine	Inoconstrictor	4+	0	2+	1+	
Dopamine 0.5-2 μg/kg/min 5-20 μg/kg/min	Inoconstrictor	0 3+	1+ 0	1+ 3+	1+ 2+	
Epinephrine	Inoconstrictor	4+	3+	4+	4+	May induce transient hyperlactatemia
Dobutamine	Inodilator	0	2+	4+	2+	Pulmonary vasodilator
Milrinone	Inodilator	0	3+	3-4+	0	Pulmonary vasodilator; half-life hours, accumulates in renal failure
Isoproterenol	Inodilator	0	4+	4+	4+	

Adapted with permission from St Andre AC, DelRossi A: Hemodynamic management of patients in the first 24 hours after cardiac surgery, Crit Care Med 2005 Sep;33(9):2082-2093.

α_1 agonist that only increases afterload and does not provide inotropic assistance. Vasopressin may be useful in the vasoplegic patient with low SVR post-bypass as a supplement to norepinephrine. In addition, as it has minimal pulmonary vasoconstrictive effects at low doses (< 4 U/h), vasopressin may be useful in patients with significant pulmonary hypertension or right ventricular dysfunction. Dopamine at low doses produces renal and splanchnic vasodilation, an effect that has not been shown to impact outcomes. Dopamine is the precursor to norepinephrine; at higher doses, the effect of dopamine becomes more similar to that of norepinephrine with the addition of inotropic and then vasoconstrictive properties. Epinephrine, dobutamine, and milrinone provide inotropy with varying effects upon the blood pressure. Epinephrine, due to greater α_1 constriction than β_2 vasodilation, has the overall effect of increasing blood pressure. Dobutamine and milrinone, both inodilators, increase inotropy but at the cost of increased vasodilation and the potential need for initiation or escalation of vasopressors. Compared with dobutamine, milrinone produces a greater decrease in SVR. Dobutamine and milrinone both increase levels of cyclic adenosine monophosphate (cAMP) (and subsequently calcium and contractility) in the cardiac myocyte but by different mechanisms: through the β_1 receptor, dobutamine activates the G_s/adenylate cyclase pathway while milrinone inhibits phosphodiesterase III, an enzyme that degrades cAMP. These 2 agents, hence, are synergistic and lower levels of each medication may be coadministered with fewer side effects. Although all β_1 agonists demonstrate some degree of chronotropy, isoproterenol demonstrates a particularly strong ability to increase HR and is colloquially known as the chemical pacemaker.

In addition to chronotropy and inotropy, the different β_1 agonists also demonstrate varying degrees of bathmotropy (arrhythmogenicity) and dromotropy (increased conduction through the AV pathway). High doses of norepinephrine, dopamine, epinephrine, and dobutamine may induce tachycardia or arrhythmias such as atrial fibrillation with rapid ventricular response. Milrinone also has a proarrhythmogenic tendency but is less than that of dobutamine.

The half-lives of these inotropes and vasopressors, with the exception of vasopressin and milrinone, are on the order of minutes, thus enhancing their titratability. Vasopressin has a half-life of approximately 10 to 20 minutes. Milrinone's terminal elimination half-life is approximately 2 hours, which renders it less titratable than other more rapid-offset inotropes such as dobutamine. It accumulates with prolonged infusions as well as in patients with renal insufficiency.

Epinephrine has been associated with the development of hyperglycemia and a type B lactic acidosis, that is, lactate generation in the absence of clinical evidence of tissue hypoperfusion (in contrast to type A which is associated with poor oxygen delivery). One study randomized 36 patients to receive norepinephrine or epinephrine for hypotension after CPB. They found that 6 of 19 patients who received epinephrine developed increased lactate levels peaking between 6 and 10 hours after CPB (lactate to ~3.8 mmol/L, pH 7.34) while 0 of 17 patients who received norepinephrine demonstrated the same phenomenon. The lactate normalized by 22 to 30 hours after bypass. There was no difference in the oxygen-delivery index calculated between the 2 groups. The authors postulated that because epinephrine inhibits the pyruvate dehydrogenase complex, the increased levels of pyruvate get shunted to generate more lactate in order to preserve the normal balance of lactate:pyruvate needed to maintain the oxidized form of nicotinamide adenine dinucleotide (NAD).[24] Another study conducted in a medical ICU studying patients with dopamine-resistant cardiogenic shock randomized patients to receive norepinephrine-dobutamine or epinephrine. This study found that patients in the epinephrine group demonstrated an increase in lactate that peaked at 4.9 mmol/L at 6 hours with a pH of 7.26; this finding was notably absent in the dobutamine-norepinephrine group.[25] Thus, lactic acidosis in the context of epinephrine therapy may not necessarily indicate hypoperfusion as it may reflect generation of endogenous lactate by another unrelated mechanism, especially if oxygen delivery is calculated to be adequate; however, use of epinephrine may obscure the utility of lactate as a marker of hypoperfusion.

The use of a vasodilator may be necessary with excessive hypertension that cannot be resolved with the usual doses of sedative and analgesics (Table 54-7). Nicardipine is a dihydropyridine calcium channel blocker whose main effect is

TABLE 54-7 Vasodilators.

	Classification	Mechanism	Dose	Considerations
Nicardipine	Arterial dilator	Calcium channel blocker	5-15 mg/h	
Nitroglycerin	Venodilator	Nitric oxide	5-400 µg/min	
Nitroprusside	Balance arterial and venodilator	Nitric oxide	0.25-4 µg/kg/min (max 10 µg/kg/min)	Cyanide toxicity, especially with doses > 8 µg/kg/min

vasodilation of the systemic, coronary, and cerebral circulations with essentially no AV nodal blocking activity or negative inotropy. Both nitroglycerin and nitroprusside release nitric oxide, a potent vasodilator that activates guanylyl cyclase, increase cyclic guanosine monophosphate (cGMP), and results in decreased intracellular calcium and vascular smooth muscle relaxation. Nitroglycerin predominantly causes venodilation, which decreases preload and the volume work of the heart. It is particularly useful when myocardial ischemia is suspected as CPP (AoDP – LVEDP/coronary vascular resistance) is improved by 2 mechanisms: by decreasing preload which decreases LVEDP and by decreasing coronary vascular resistance by promoting coronary vasodilation. Nitroprusside causes both venodilation and arterial dilation. High doses may result in cyanide toxicity.

These 3 vasodilators provide rapid onset of action within minutes. Nicardipine has an elimination half-life of approximately 45 minutes while the elimination half life of both nitroglycerin and nitroprusside is approximately 5 minutes. Vasodilators may result in a reflex tachycardia. Tachyphylaxis can be seen, as well as rebound hypertension on sudden discontinuation of the drip. All vasodilators can reverse hypoxic vasoconstriction and worsen hypoxia by increasing shunt in atelectatic areas of the lung. In addition, those with intracranial hypertension may experience an increase in intracranial pressure due to an increase in cerebral blood flow secondary to cerebral vasodilation.

POSTOPERATIVE BLEEDING

Postoperative bleeding is tracked by output from pleural and mediastinal chest tubes. A bleeding rate of 100-400 mL/h may be considered "medical" bleeding that may be successfully treated by correcting postoperative coagulopathy. Cumulative bleeding of more than 200 mL for 2 hours usually mandates intervention for resolution of "medical bleeding." One study of 31 patients found that exposure of blood to the CPB circuit as well as hypothermia-induced activation of platelets resulting in a transient impairment of function and an increase in bleeding time that increased with the duration of bypass. This phenomenon resolved generally within 2 to 4 hours after CPB. However, 10 patients with platelet counts greater than 100,000/µL demonstrated substantial post-CPB bleeding and were found to have persistent platelet dysfunction even to 8 hours postbypass. Platelet transfusion resolved the bleeding in 6 of 10 patients.[26] The patient who has been on aspirin or loaded with clopidogrel due to a recent coronary catheterization (within 5 days) would be expected to have an even more profound platelet plug defect post-CPB due to irreversible inactivation of platelet activation. Significant bleeding in these patients should improve with platelet transfusion. Packed red blood cells should be administered as needed for significant anemia. Fresh frozen plasma may be administered empirically if bleeding is unremitting. Cryoprecipitate for hypofibrinogenemia (< 100 mg/dL) may be warranted. Desmopressin (DDAVP) may aid with bleeding in the context of uremia or in the patient suspected of having a von Willebrand factor deficiency (0.3 µg/kg IV). Recombinant factor VIIa (rFVIIa) may be used as a last resort for life-threatening and intractable bleeding. It activates factor X directly and promotes a thrombin burst that aids in the formation of clot. A phase II dose escalation study was perform in 2009 as an international randomized, double-blind, placebo-controlled study of 172 patients testing placebo against 40 and 80 µg/kg of rFVIIa. The rFVIIa groups experienced a lower rate of reoperation for bleeding (40 µg/kg: 14%, 80 µg/kg: 12% vs placebo: 25%) and a decreased rate of transfusion (40 μg/kg: 640 mL, 80 μg/kg: 500 mL vs placebo: 825 mL). The rate of critical serious adverse events was not statistically significant between the groups, but study was underpowered to assess this outcome; the authors emphasized the trend toward increased serious adverse events in the rFVIIa group and the need for further investigation.[27] Viscoelastic whole blood tests such as thromboelastography (TEG) may pinpoint the hemostatic defect (ie, coagulation factor deficiency, quantitative or qualitative platelet disorders, excessive fibrinolysis) and provide the ability to provide more targeted transfusion therapy.

Bleeding of more than 200 mL for 4 hours or more than 4 to 500 mL in 1 hour that does not respond to blood-product administration is typically designated "surgical bleeding" and may warrant a return to the operating room. Sources of surgical bleeding may include cannulation sites, graft suture lines, vein graft side branches, and small chest wall arterial bleeders.

Copious bleeding increases the risk of tamponade, especially if sudden cessation of chest tube output occurs due to a clot. Tamponade can also occur with removal of pacing wires several days after the procedure or weeks later with the start of anticoagulation for mechanical valves or atrial fibrillation. Cardiac tamponade reduces stroke volume due to restricted diastolic filling and decreased preload ultimately resulting in equalization of filling pressures between the right heart and left heart (including the central venous pressure [CVP], pulmonary artery diastolic pressure, and pulmonary artery wedge pressure). Tamponade should be suspected in the setting of a rising CVP, worsening pressor requirement, oliguria, and acidosis. The likelihood of other similarly presenting clinical entities such as right heart failure, pulmonary embolism, tension pneumothorax, and left heart failure should be assessed. Transthoracic or transesophageal echo may aid greatly in establishing the diagnosis. However, difficulties may be encountered with clotted blood, which is echo-dense and appears similar to myocardium or with effusions localized to a particular area not easily accessible by surface ultrasonography.[28] Ultimately, the patient with suspected tamponade will require a return to the operating room for exploration. Until that occurs, the compensatory tachycardia (increasing the CO due to limited SV)

should not be treated and a high afterload should be maintained. To that end, fluid and inoconstrictors such as epinephrine and norepinephrine may be able to temporize the patient's hemodynamics until the mechanical obstruction can be relieved.

DYSRHYTHMIAS

Atrial fibrillation after cardiac surgery is a common phenomenon, occurring in 10% to 65% of patients.[29] It occurs more frequently in older patients and those undergoing valvular surgery. Those with mitral pathology tend to be at risk for atrial fibrillation due to atrial distension. Agents such as β_1 agonists (dopamine, norepinephrine, epinephrine, dobutamine) as well as milrinone increase the arrhythmogenic potential of the myocardium and may precipitate the onset of atrial fibrillation. The peak incidence of atrial fibrillation is in the second and third postoperative days. Its occurrence increases morbidity, as the rate of stroke is higher, as well as 30-day mortality. In addition, the occurrence of atrial fibrillation increases the length of stay both in the ICU and the hospital.[29] In hemodynamically stable patient who has been weaned-off of inotropes and vasopressors, β-blockade with intravenous or oral (PO) metoprolol is frequently initiated to decrease adrenergic tone that may precipitate atrial fibrillation.

When atrial fibrillation occurs, the stability of the patient should immediately be assessed. If the patient is unstable and is hypotensive or symptomatic (mental status changes, chest pain, or shortness of breath), the patient should be emergently cardioverted. If the patient is stable, the decision with how to proceed often differs based on institution and surgeon. The Atrial Fibrillation Follow-up Investigation of Rhythm Management (AFFIRM) trial[30] showed that there is no mortality benefit to pursuing rhythm control (ie, attempting to convert the patient back to sinus) over HR control. In addition, the natural history of postoperative atrial fibrillation appears to be that of spontaneously converting back to sinus rhythm within 6 weeks. Many take the approach of pursuing rate control and attempting only pharmacologic cardioversion. However, some choose to treat atrial fibrillation aggressively with electrical cardioversion to avoid the need for anticoagulation and to potentially to decrease the risk of stroke, although the risk of stroke does persist for a time after sinus rhythm is achieved (whether via electrical, pharmacologic, or spontaneous cardioversion) due to atrial stunning; more than 80% of thromboembolic events occur during the first 3 days after cardioversion.[31]

Once electrolyte repletion of inadequate potassium and magnesium levels are addressed, first-line medical therapy with hemodynamically stable atrial fibrillation should be β-blockade with an agent such as metoprolol in an attempt to achieve a HR of less than 120. As a class II antiarrhythmic, β-blockade may achieve conversion back to sinus rhythm. Diltiazem, a benzothiazine calcium channel blocker with AV nodal blocking properties, is frequently used in the general hospital setting to control atrial fibrillation with rapid ventricular response; however, its negative inotropic property may induce unwanted hypotension, especially in the immediate postoperative period where postcardiac patients are still recovering from postbypass myocardial stunning, and is not utilized with great frequency in the cardiac ICU. Amiodarone may achieve rate control in the patient with a tenuous blood pressure or who is on vasopressors or inotropes or has a low EF and may achieve chemical cardioversion, as well. It has a long terminal elimination half-life of about 58 days. The patient with a difficult to control HR or with recurrent bouts of atrial fibrillation may benefit from multiple doses of β-blocker or an additional load of amiodarone. Digoxin, an inhibitor of the Na-K ATPase pump, decreases conduction velocity through the AV node and may aid in attaining rate control. In addition, digoxin increases inotropy and may be useful in the patient with a low EF or still on vasopressors. However, its onset of action is slow and requires loading over 1 day. In addition, lower doses must be used in those with renal insufficiency.

The side effects of these aforementioned therapies for atrial fibrillation with rapid ventricular response are hypotension and bradycardia. Thus, those being treated for atrial fibrillation should not have their epicardial pacing wires removed until the therapeutic response is established. Should bradycardia occur, pacing may be required and the therapeutic approach should be reevaluated. Postoperative new onset atrial fibrillation with a slow ventricular response often precludes use of rate-lowering agents. Amiodarone, while ubiquitously used, may with long-term use induce hepatotoxicity, pulmonary disease, and thyroid dysfunction (hyperthyroidism and hypothyroidism). Thus avoidance in patients with liver dysfunction or pulmonary insufficiency may be merited.

Anticoagulation should be considered in those with more than 48 hours of atrial fibrillation to decrease the risk of the development of cardiac thrombus that may embolize to cause stroke. Characteristics that increase the risk of stroke include hypertension, an EF less than 35%, diabetes mellitus (DM), and age 75 years and older. The benefit of anticoagulation must be weighed against the risk of inducing bleeding in the postoperative patient. If the risk is deemed too high, anticoagulation should be held until the risk of bleeding diminishes.

VT is also seen commonly in the postcardiac surgical population. VT may be an expression of myocardial ischemia and its onset should spur an investigation into the presence of a potential myocardial supply-demand imbalance. As with atrial fibrillation, cardiotonic medications such as the β_1 agonists and milrinone may precipitate VT. Prior myocardial infarction and the presence of scar frequently act as anatomic foci of arrhythmogenicity. Finally, VT may manifest in the setting of an unfavorable milieu such as hypoxia, electrolyte imbalances, and acidosis. As with atrial fibrillation, an unstable VT should be electrically cardioverted immediately.

The actual diagnosis of VT may be difficult in the patient with a preexisting bundle branch block. In this situation, a supra-VT (SVT) with aberrancy may be indistinguishable from VT. Provided that the rhythm is regular, adenosine may be utilized to assess whether the tachycardia breaks, in which case the arrhythmia may be diagnosed as SVT.[32] The diagnostic distinction is important as it may have consequences for whether the patient may need invasive therapies such as ablation and an implantable cardioverter defibrillator (ICD). Adenosine should not be given to patients with an irregular wide-complex tachycardia because such arrhythmias may become unstable after administration.

The patient with nonsustained VT (NSVT) or stable VT should be evaluated for the presence of correctable conditions such as hypokalemia and hypomagnesemia, hypoxia, and acidosis. Amiodarone may be administered in an attempt to suppress the arrhythmia. Lidocaine may be used as an antiarrhythmic adjunct. If ischemia is a component of the onset of VT, a trial of a short acting β_1 blocker such as esmolol may be worthwhile to decrease myocardial oxygen demand. Esmolol is degraded by red cell esterases and has a short elimination half-life of 6 minutes. Overdrive pacing may be used in an attempt to suppress reentry circuits at work in the pathogenesis of VT. The patient in VT may ultimately need electrical cardioversion to get back into their native rhythm. Finally, consultation from electrophysiological experts should be obtained as the patient may be a candidate for ablation or may need placement of an ICD. The medications used in the management of dysrhythmias are detailed in Table 54–8.[33]

RENAL FUNCTION

Renal dysfunction is not uncommon after cardiac surgery. Mangano et al conducted a prospective observational study of 2222 patients undergoing CABG and found that the rate of renal dysfunction, defined as a postoperative creatinine of 2.0 mg/dL or more or an increase in creatinine of 0.7 mg/dL or more was about 7.7%. The incidence of oliguric renal failure requiring dialysis was 1.4%. Preoperative risk factor for renal dysfunction included age 70 years or more, New York Heart Association (NYHA) class 3 or 4 heart failure, previous CABG, chronic kidney disease with creatinine 1.4 to 2.0, type I diabetes, and glucose more than 300. Intraoperative and postoperative factors include CPB lasting 3 hours or more, and a low output state with a CI of less than 1.5 or requiring insertion of an intra-aortic balloon pump.[34] Other additional risk factors include preoperative cardiac angiography or angiotensin-converting enzyme inhibitors, angiotensin receptor blockade or diuretic therapy, and perioperative red blood cell transfusion. Additional intraoperative factors include the number of red blood cell units administered, low MAP during CPB, perioperative hemodilution, and postoperative use of norepinephrine.[35]

TABLE 54–8 Agents for rate and rhythm control.

Agents	Mechanism	Dose	Considerations
Diltiazem	Calcium channel blocker	Bolus: 0.25 mg/kg IV over 2 min Continuous: 5-15 mg/h IV PO: 120-360 mg/d in divided doses	• Afib with RVR • Negative inotropic effect may be detrimental in the postcardiac surgical patient and patient with low EF
Metoprolol	β_1-selective blocker	Bolus: 2.5-5 mg IV × 3 Standing: 5 mg IV q4h PO: 12.5-100 mg q12h	• Afib with RVR
Amiodarone	Na^+, K^+, Ca^{2+} and β-blockade	Bolus: 150 mg IV over 10 min × 2 Continuous: 1 mg/min × 6 h then 0.5 mg/min × 18 h PO: 400 mg q12h × 1 wk, then 600 mg daily × 1 wk, then 400 mg daily × 4-6 wk	• Useful in patients on vasopressors, inotropes, or with low EF • Avoid in patients with liver, pulmonary, or thyroid dysfunction
Digoxin	Inhibits Na-K ATPase	Load: 0.25 mg IV then 0.125 × 2 q8h Maintenance: 0.125-0.25 daily or every other day PO: 0.5 mg daily × 2 d, then 0.125-0.375 PO daily or every other day	• Dose cautiously in patients with renal insufficiency • Avoid hypokalemia • Digoxin-specific antibody fragments available for digoxin toxicity
Lidocaine	Na channel blocker	Load: 1 mg/kg Maintenance: 1 mg/h	
Esmolol	β_1-selective blockade	500 µg/kg IV over 1 min 60-200 µg/kg/min	• Short half-life

Afib, atrial fibrillation; EF, ejection fraction; IV, intravenous; PO, oral; RVR, rapid ventricular response.

With regards to outcomes, Mangano et al found that compared with those without renal dysfunction, those with renal dysfunction and failure experienced increased length of stay in the critical care unit (3.1 vs 6.5 and 15.4 days) and the hospital (7.4 vs 11.4 and 14.9 days). In addition, those with renal dysfunction experienced greater mortality (0.9% vs 19% and 63%).

Preventative strategies to decrease the risk of renal dysfunction after cardiac surgery are limited and include minimizing exposure to radiocontrast dyes, delaying the surgery to allow for renal recovery if preoperative renal injury was sustained, and avoidance of intraoperative anemia. Other protective strategies such as urinary alkalinization, glucose control, early continuous renal replacement therapy, statins, and fenoldopam still as of yet need more evidence to elucidate their role in renal protection.[35]

Oliguria, defined as urine output < 0.5 mL/kg/h, as well as increases in creatinine reflective of a decrease glomerular filtration rate occur frequently in the cardiac ICU. Table 54–9 outlines the risk, injury, failure, loss, and end-stage renal disease (RIFLE) criteria and Table 54–10 presents the Acute Kidney Injury Network (AKIN) modifications. The AKIN classification, in particular, highlights how even small increases in creatinine of 0.3 mg/dL indicate some degree of renal injury.

TABLE 54–9 RIFLE classification of acute kidney injury (within 7 days).

Class	GFR	UOP
Risk	↑Cr × 1.5 or ↓GFR by 25%	<0.5 mL/kg/h for >6 h
Injury	↑Cr × 2 or ↓GFR by 50%	<0.5 mL/kg/h for > 12 h
Failure	↑Cr × 3 or ↓GFR by 75% or Cr > 4 mg/dL or acute ↑> 0.5 mg/dL	<0.3 mL/kg/h for > 24 h or anuria > 12 h
Loss	Persistent acute renal failure with complete loss of renal function > 4 wk	
ESRD	Complete loss of renal function without recovery	

Cr, creatinine; ESRD, end-stage renal disease; GFR, glomerular filtration rate; RIFLE, risk, injury, failure, loss, and end-stage renal disease; UOP, urine output.

TABLE 54–10 AKIN classification of acute kidney injury (within 48 hours).

Class	GFR	UOP
Stage 1	↑Cr × 1.5 or ↑Cr by 0.3 mg/dL	< 0.5 mL/kg/h for >6 h
Stage 2	↑Cr × 2	< 0.5 mL/kg/h for > 12 h
Stage 3	↑Cr × 3 or Cr > 4 mg/dL or acute ↑> 0.5 mg/dL	< 0.3 mL/kg/h for > 24 h or anuria > 12 h
Loss	Persistent acute renal failure with complete loss of renal function > 4 wk	
ESRD	Complete loss of renal function without recovery	

AKIN, Acute Kidney Injury Network; Cr, creatinine; ESRD, end-stage renal disease.

The approach to the patient with oliguria and/or rising creatinine may be categorized as postrenal, prerenal, and renal processes.

Postrenal

In the immediate postoperative period, postrenal obstruction may occur if a clogged Foley is preventing the egress of urine. Ultrasonic visualization of a full bladder in the setting of lack of urine output confirms postrenal obstruction. Flushing or changing of the Foley should rectify the problem. Less likely forms of postrenal obstruction such as nephrolithiasis may be formally evaluated by looking for hydronephrosis on a renal ultrasound.

Prerenal

Prerenal causes of oliguria and rising creatinine are secondary to insufficient perfusion pressure or hypovolemia or both. An insufficient MAP may cause oliguria, especially in the patient with chronic uncontrolled hypertension or a renal vascular stenosis and may be caused purely by a vasodilated state with decreased ability of the smooth muscle to constrict or be due to decreased CO due to hypovolemia and insufficient SV. MAP may be supported pharmacologically with vasopressors with concurrent volume loading to address any contribution of hypovolemia. The patient with an adequate MAP may still be hypovolemia. In general, aside from the patient with tenuous pulmonary or right heart function, small boluses of 250 to 500 mL generally incur little harm and can interrogate the volume responsiveness of the patient. Aside from history and calculation of fluid balance, the prerenal state of the patient may be interrogated with the fractional excretion of sodium (FENa) or fractional excretion of urea (FEUrea) if the patient has recently received furosemide.

Renal

Prerenal acute kidney injury, when prolonged, can result in acute tubular necrosis (ATN). Some patients, such as those who underwent cardiac arrest or precipitous operating room courses may have sustained prolonged periods of hypotension and hypovolemia, and will have progressed into ATN. At this point, the patient should be assessed as to whether they are nonoliguric or oliguric. If the patient demonstrates a rising creatinine indicative of ongoing loss of kidney function but are able to generate urine, then not much intervention may be needed except monitoring of volume and electrolyte status and for plateauing of the creatinine level. If the patient has oliguric kidney injury with a poor urine output, they should be assessed for diuretic responsivity. A trial of a loop diuretic such as furosemide (40-100 mg IV) or bumetanide (1-2 mg IV) with or without augmentation with a thiazide diuretic such as metolazone (5-10 mg PO) may be made. If the patient is diuretic responsive, then medical management may be sufficient to manage the volume and electrolyte status of the patient. If the loss of kidney function can be managed pharmacologically, the patient might be able to be maintained only diuretics for management of volume and electrolytes. If the patient is not diuretic-responsive, then renal replacement might be indicated, especially if the patient demonstrates hyperkalemia with peaked T waves on the electrocardiogram, acidosis with pH less than 7.2, blood urea nitrogen (BUN) more than 80 with clinical signs of uremia (bleeding, encephalopathy, pericardial rub or effusion), or volume overload resulting in pulmonary edema and dyspnea/hypoxia.

As mentioned earlier, length of CPB is an intraoperative risk for acute kidney injury. Most patients sustain a small amount of injury from what might be delineated postbypass ATN. The injury incurred is typically small although not infrequently achieves at least stage I by AKIN criteria. However, especially with prolonged bypass runs, the injury to the kidney can be significant. After ruling out prerenal causes of kidney dysfunction, evaluation and treatment of the patient should include an assessment of concurrent oliguria or nonoliguria, diuretic responsiveness, and whether renal replacement therapy is indicated. ATN may be more formally assessed by FENa/FEUrea as well as urine microscopy showing muddy brown casts.

If the patient has not sustained a prerenal injury by history and if MAP and volume status have been deemed to be adequately addressed, oliguria and a rising creatinine be secondary to diuretic dependence. Some patients with preoperative chronic kidney disease with diminished renal function at baseline may be dependent on diuretics for generation of adequate urine. As long as the patient is not suffering from low MAP (absolute or relative) or hypovolemia, reinstating these medications may restore urine production and by providing excretion of creatinine, restore plasma creatinine levels back to baseline.

Other causes of renal injury include toxins (exogenous and endogenous) and sepsis. Exogenous toxins include contrast dye, antibiotics such as the aminoglycosides, and NSAIDs such as ketorolac and ibuprofen. Endogenous toxins include myoglobin from rhabdomyolysis. The septic patient may demonstrate a septic nephropathy that resolves only with source control and antibiotics.

GLUCOSE CONTROL

One landmark single center study of 1548 surgical ICU patients (63% of whom were postcardiac surgical patients) suggested that intense glucose control between 80 and 110 mg/dL versus 180 and 215 mg/dL resulted in a relative reduction in mortality (8% to 4.6%).[36] However, the results of this study could not be replicated in multiple subsequent investigations. In particular, the Normoglycemia in Intensive Care Evaluation and Surviving Using Glucose Algorithm Regulation (NICE-SUGAR) study, a multicenter trial of 6104 medical and surgical patients, randomized the patients to 81 to 108 mg/dL versus 144 to

180 mg/dL and not only found increased mortality with intensive glucose therapy with a 90-day mortality of 27.5% in the treatment group and 24.9% in the control group but also an unacceptably high incidence of severe hypoglycemia (blood glucose $\leq$ 40 mg/dL) with 6.8% in the intensive group and 0.5% in the conventional group.[37] The optimum level of glucose control, thus, is as yet to be defined, and may be better elucidated with the development of technology that may be able to allow for the safer administration of continuous insulin regimens.

SUMMARY

Multiple issues arise in the care of the immediate postoperative cardiac patient. A decision must be made as to the appropriate timing of extubation. In addition, knowledge of normal physiology as well as the pathophysiology resulting from CPB informs the understanding of hypotension and low CO, bleeding, and renal dysfunction in the postcardiac patient. Management of these common postsurgical problems also requires a thorough understanding of the characteristics of the pharmacological tools available to us. This knowledge, as well as good communication with the surgical team, allows for successful management of the postcardiac surgical patient.

REFERENCES

1. Myles PS, et al. A systematic review of the safety and effectiveness of fast-track cardiac anesthesia. *Anesthesiology.* 2003;99(4):982-987.
2. Zhu F, Lee A, Chee YE. Fast-track cardiac care for adult cardiac surgical patients. *Cochrane Database Syst Rev.* 2012;10:CD003587.
3. Cheng DC, et al. Early tracheal extubation after coronary artery bypass graft surgery reduces costs and improves resource use. A prospective, randomized, controlled trial. *Anesthesiology.* 1996;85(6):1300-1310.
4. Roberts AJ, et al. Serial assessment of left ventricular performance following coronary artery bypass grafting. Early postoperative results with myocardial protection afforded by multidose hypothermic potassium crystalloid cardioplegia. *J Thorac Cardiovasc Surg.* 1981;81(1):69-84.
5. Mangano DT. Biventricular function after myocardial revascularization in humans: deterioration and recovery patterns during the first 24 hours. *Anesthesiology.* 1985;62(5):571-577.
6. Breisblatt WM, et al. Acute myocardial dysfunction and recovery: a common occurrence after coronary bypass surgery. *J Am Coll Cardiol.* 1990;15(6):1261-1269.
7. Lemaire F, et al. Acute left ventricular dysfunction during unsuccessful weaning from mechanical ventilation. *Anesthesiology.* 1988;69(2):171-179.
8. Michard F. Changes in arterial pressure during mechanical ventilation. *Anesthesiology.* 2005;103(2):419-428; quiz 449-5.
9. McGregor M. Current concepts: pulsus paradoxus. *N Engl J Med.* 1979;301(9):480-482.
10. Jacobi J, et al. Clinical practice guidelines for the sustained use of sedatives and analgesics in the critically ill adult. *Crit Care Med.* 2002;30(1):119-141.
11. Reade MC and Finfer S. Sedation and delirium in the intensive care unit. *N Engl J Med.* 2014;370(5):444-454.
12. McKenney PA, et al. Increased left ventricular diastolic chamber stiffness immediately after coronary artery bypass surgery. *J Am Coll Cardiol.* 1994;24(5):1189-1194.
13. Schramko AA, et al. Rapidly degradable hydroxyethyl starch solutions impair blood coagulation after cardiac surgery: a prospective randomized trial. *Anesth Analg.* 2009;108(1):30-66.
14. Navickis RJ, Haynes GR, Wilkes MM. Effect of hydroxyethyl starch on bleeding after cardiopulmonary bypass: a meta-analysis of randomized trials. *J Thorac Cardiovasc Surg.* 2012;144(1):223-230.
15. Cremer J, et al. Systemic inflammatory response syndrome after cardiac operations. *Ann Thorac Surg.* 1996;61(6):1714-1720.
16. Kristof AS, Magder S. Low systemic vascular resistance state in patients undergoing cardiopulmonary bypass. *Crit Care Med.* 1999;27(6):1121-1127.
17. Cugno M, et al. Increase of bradykinin in plasma of patients undergoing cardiopulmonary bypass: the importance of lung exclusion. *Chest.* 2001;120(6):1776-1782.
18. Conti VR, McQuitty C. Vasodilation and cardiopulmonary bypass: the role of bradykinin and the pulmonary vascular endothelium. *Chest.* 2001;120(6):1759-1761.
19. Argenziano M, et al. Management of vasodilatory shock after cardiac surgery: identification of

predisposing factors and use of a novel pressor agent. *J Thorac Cardiovasc Surg.* 1998;116(6):973-980.

20. Mekontso-Dessap A, et al. Risk factors for post-cardiopulmonary bypass vasoplegia in patients with preserved left ventricular function. *Ann Thorac Surg.* 2001;71(5):1428-1432.

21. Levin MA, et al. Early on-cardiopulmonary bypass hypotension and other factors associated with vasoplegic syndrome. *Circulation.* 2009;120(17):1664-1671.

22. St Andre AC, DelRossi A. Hemodynamic management of patients in the first 24 hours after cardiac surgery. *Crit Care Med.* 2005;33(9):2082-2093.

23. Sladen RN, ed. *Postoperative Cardiac Care.* Lippincot Williams & Wilkins; 2011:400.

24. Totaro RJ, Raper RF. Epinephrine-induced lactic acidosis following cardiopulmonary bypass. *Crit Care Med.* 1997;25(10):1693-1699.

25. Levy B, et al. Comparison of norepinephrine-dobutamine to epinephrine for hemodynamics, lactate metabolism, and organ function variables in cardiogenic shock. A prospective, randomized pilot study. *Crit Care Med.* 2011;39(3):450-455.

26. Harker LA, et al. Mechanism of abnormal bleeding in patients undergoing cardiopulmonary bypass: acquired transient platelet dysfunction associated with selective alpha-granule release. *Blood.* 1980;56(5):824-834.

27. Gill R, et al. Safety and efficacy of recombinant activated factor VII: a randomized placebo-controlled trial in the setting of bleeding after cardiac surgery. *Circulation.* 2009;120(1):21-27.

28. Ionescu A, Wilde P, Karsch KR. Localized pericardial tamponade: difficult echocardiographic diagnosis of a rare complication after cardiac surgery. *J Am Soc Echocardiogr.* 2001;14(12):1220-1223.

29. Maisel WH, Rawn JD, Stevenson WG. Atrial fibrillation after cardiac surgery. *Ann Intern Med.* 2001;135(12):1061-1073.

30. Wyse DG, et al. A comparison of rate control and rhythm control in patients with atrial fibrillation. *N Engl J Med.* 2002;347(23):1825-1833.

31. Fuster V, et al. ACC/AHA/ESC 2006 guidelines for the management of patients with atrial fibrillation: full text: a report of the American College of Cardiology/American Heart Association Task Force on practice guidelines and the European Society of Cardiology Committee for Practice Guidelines (Writing Committee to Revise the 2001 guidelines for the management of patients with atrial fibrillation) developed in collaboration with the European Heart Rhythm Association and the Heart Rhythm Society. *Europace.* 2006;8(9):651-745.

32. Link MS. Clinical practice. Evaluation and initial treatment of supraventricular tachycardia. *N Engl J Med.* 2012;367(15):1438-1448.

33. Fuster V, et al. ACC/AHA/ESC 2006 guidelines for the management of patients with atrial fibrillation-executive summary: a report of the American College of Cardiology/American Heart Association Task Force on Practice Guidelines and the European Society of Cardiology Committee for Practice Guidelines (Writing Committee to Revise the 2001 Guidelines for the Management of Patients with Atrial Fibrillation). *Eur Heart J.* 2006;27(16):1979-2030.

34. Mangano CM, et al. Renal dysfunction after myocardial revascularization: risk factors, adverse outcomes, and hospital resource utilization. The Multicenter Study of Perioperative Ischemia Research Group. *Ann Intern Med.* 1998;128(3):194-203.

35. Coleman MD, Shaefi S, Sladen RN. Preventing acute kidney injury after cardiac surgery. *Curr Opin Anaesthesiol.* 2011;24(1):70-76.

36. van den Berghe G, et al. Intensive insulin therapy in critically ill patients. *N Engl J Med.* 2001;345(19):1359-1367.

37. NICE-SUGAR Study Investigators, et al. Intensive versus conventional glucose control in critically ill patients. *N Engl J Med.* 2009;360(13):1283-1297.

Postoperative Management After Specialty Surgery

Nagendra Y. Madisi, MD and John M. Oropello, MD, FACP, FCCP, FCCM

KEY POINTS

1. The success of a free-flap transfer is inversely proportional to flap ischemic time and the time to recognition of complications.

2. Dextran infusion syndrome should be suspected in patients on low-molecular-weight dextran that develop noncardiogenic pulmonary edema.

3. The classic triad of fat embolism syndrome is hypoxemia, neurological abnormalities, and petechiae.

4. Bone cement implantation syndrome is a life-threatening complication of orthopedic surgery characterized by hypoxia, hypotension, pulmonary hypertension, arrhythmias, loss of consciousness, and potentially cardiac arrest.

5. Cystectomy is an independent risk factor for venous thromboembolism.

INTRODUCTION

This chapter discusses specific postoperative complications and management in the intensive care unit (ICU) after ENT, orthopedic, and urology surgery. Radical head and neck surgery with free-flap reconstruction, total hip replacement (THR) and total knee replacement (TKR), radical nephrectomy, and radical cystectomy are discussed.

ENT SURGERY

Radical Head and Neck Surgery with Free-Flap Reconstruction

An estimated 55,000 Americans develop head and neck cancer mainly of the pharynx, larynx, and tongue annually and 12,000 die from the disease.[1] Radical head and neck dissection with free-flap reconstruction has evolved over the past 4 decades with free-flap success rates in the 90% to 99% range.

Otolaryngology patients with tumors of the head and neck undergo radical dissection and free-flap microsurgery. These patients are admitted postoperatively to the ICU for neurologic, free flap, and airway monitoring. Complications include flap failure, infections, postoperative bleeding, acute lung injury (noncardiogenic pulmonary edema), and venous thromboembolism (VTE). In addition to comorbid conditions such as chronic obstructive pulmonary disease (COPD) and diabetes, these patients often have a history of alcohol dependence and smoking, hence close monitoring for encephalopathy and alcohol withdrawal syndrome is warranted.

Surgical Factors

Radical head and neck dissection involves en bloc removal of all nodal groups between the mandible and the clavicle with removal of the sternocleidomastoid muscle, internal jugular vein, and spinal accessory nerve.

The free-flap transfer, also called a free tissue transfer, is an autologous transplantation of vascularized tissues that incorporate a direct cutaneous artery and vein in the base. The free flap may contain skin, muscle, bone, or fascia. Free flaps have a higher complication rate than skin grafts. Indications for free flaps include complex defects of the head and neck regions following tumor resection or chemoradiation, reconstruction in patients failing local or regional flaps, or failure of a prior free flap. Common sites of harvest include the anterolateral thigh, fibula, and iliac crest. Fascio-cutaneous flaps are used to repair superficial lesions; and muscle and myocutaneous flaps are used to repair deeper lesions. To reconstruct mandible and floor of the mouth defects, fibular free flaps with overlying skin, or iliac crest bone flaps are usually used.

Patient Risk Factors

Diabetics are at increased risk of flap failure secondary to microangiopathy, increased risk of thrombosis and wound infection. Increasing age is an independent risk factor and smoking is associated with injury to flap vessels causing intimal fibrosis and potentially poorer outcomes.

Postoperative Management

Airway Monitoring

Anatomical changes occur in head and neck cancers that may create a difficult airway. Close monitoring for postoperative airway compromise after head and neck surgery in the ICU is warranted due to complications including soft-tissue edema, bleeding, hematoma, and bilateral laryngeal nerve damage. Securing the airway in head and neck reconstructions may be difficult hence caution should be exercised before extubation. Postoperative soft-tissue edema peaks around the second or third postoperative day.

Once the patient tolerates a spontaneous breathing trial, a cuff-leak test should be considered before extubation. Two cuff-leak methods exist. The qualitative method is listening for air movement with a stethoscope after deflating the endotracheal tube balloon. In the quantitative method the endotracheal balloon is deflated while on volume control ventilation and the difference between the inspired versus expired tidal volume is measured. An at least

110 mL difference or a decrease of 12% to 24% in the expired versus inspired tidal volume supports adequate leakage around the tube and hence less airway edema.[2] However, none of these tests are highly predictive of extubation success or failure and are only adjuncts to the overall clinical assessment.

In the event of respiratory distress or lack of an air-leak, extubation should be deferred for the next 24 hours. Inspection via laryngoscope may be performed to assess airway edema while the patient is still intubated. Steroids may be used in some cases for soft-tissue edema to facilitate extubation.

Intensivists should be prepared for emergent endotracheal intubation or an emergent surgical airway. Anesthesiologists and ENT surgeons should be present at bedside or in close proximity during extubation. Emergent airway equipment should remain at bedside with ENT surgeons on standby to perform emergent bedside tracheostomy if necessary.

In patients with extensive head and neck reconstructions a concomitant tracheostomy is usually done at the time of surgery to overcome airway compromise. Elective tracheostomy is recommended for patients with a high risk of airway obstruction. Multiple scoring systems for elective tracheostomy in head and neck cancer patients have been developed based on various parameters that include tumor size, tumor localization (involving larynx, base of the tongue, pharynx) TNM (tumor, nodes, metastases) staging, mandibulectomy, neck dissection, pathological chest X-ray findings, multiple comorbidities (mostly cardiopulmonary), and chronic alcohol dependence.[3,4] However, there is no gold standard scoring system for determining elective tracheostomy and so clinical judgment is required.

Respiratory Failure

Comorbid conditions such as underlying lung disease, cardiovascular disease, renal disease, alcohol abuse, and malnutrition are significant risk factors for failure to wean from mechanical ventilation.

Fluid Resuscitation

Free-flap tissues can become ischemic and can be sensitive to ischemia/reperfusion injury with different responses to hypotension or vasopressors. Balanced volume resuscitation is very important in microsurgery, because volume overload is associated with flap edema and compromising flap microcirculation. Given the small caliber of blood vessels, hypotension should be avoided because even minimal vasoconstriction in the flap microcirculation leads to decreased blood flow. Low-molecular-weight (LMW) dextran (eg, Dextran 40) is used at some centers because of its rheological properties in reducing viscosity and providing antithrombotic effects thus potentially improving blood flow in the free flap. Increased risk of flap edema and acute lung injury/noncardiogenic pulmonary edema may occur more often in patients receiving higher volume crystalloid administration, for example, more than 130 mL/kg in 24 hours or more than 7 liters intraoperatively as reported in 1 study.[5]

Vasopressors

Vasopressors have been used in clinical practice to increase the mean arterial pressure (MAP) and improve perfusion pressure across the free flap. In a recent study of patients undergoing free flaps receiving mainly phenylephrine or ephedrine, there was no significant relationship between intraoperative vasopressor and major free-flap complications.[6] Prospective studies on the postoperative use of vasopressors have shown that norepinephrine and dobutamine can improve free-flap skin blood flow, with the greatest benefit from norepinephrine. Other pressors such as dopamine and epinephrine decreased flap flow.[6-8] The use of albumin over synthetic colloids to replace intraoperative blood loss has not proven to be beneficial to date. However, the judicious use of pressors in an adequately volume resuscitated patient using norepinephrine is advised; there is no added benefit to use dobutamine which may lead to tachycardia, tachyarrhythmias, and hypotension.

Myocardial Infarction

Coronary ischemia and hemodynamic instability play an important role in flap outcomes. Long-term smoking and tobacco abuse not only increase the risk for cancer but also increase the risk of coronary artery disease (CAD) and myocardial infarction (MI). The risk of MI in the perioperative period is low, but associated with high mortality. High-risk patients with preexisting renal insufficiency, CAD, peripheral vascular disease (PVD), congestive heart failure (CHF), age of above 74, hypertension and prior chemoradiation are at increased risk for troponin elevation in the first 24 hours. Monitoring of troponin levels and the EKG is important in the immediate postoperative period. Elevated troponins post-ENT cancer surgery are associated with an 8 fold increased risk of death.[9]

Harvest Sites

Harvest sites need to be monitored frequently for signs of bleeding, hematoma, ischemia, or infection.

Microvascular Thrombosis

The reexploration rate after free-flap surgery due to circulatory compromise is about 5% to 25%. The success of the flap transfer is inversely proportional to its ischemic time and time to recognition of complications. Venous compromise occurs more often than arterial compromise and is usually seen in the first 2 or 3 postoperative days, while arterial compromise usually occurs later.[10,11] Flaps complicated by postoperative hematomas require early evacuation to avoid vascular pedicle compression and flap engorgement. Good surgical technique, close flap monitoring, and early recognition of flap compromise are the keys to free-flap transfer success.

Data on the success rate of free-flap salvage within the first 1 to 4 hours following vascular compromise are close to 100%, but the success rate drops to 70% to 80% for ischemia times of more than 4 to 8 hours. If circulatory compromise is not addressed within 8 to 12 hours there may be development of no-reflow phenomenon[12] where restoration of blood flow results in initial hyperemia with free-oxygen radicals and complement system activation followed reperfusion injury, a gradual decline in perfusion and cell death.

Flap Monitoring

Flap color, temperature monitoring, color duplex, Doppler ultrasound, and pin-prick testing are a few of the monitoring modalities,[13] but no ideal or gold standard exists. Clinical evaluation and color duplex Doppler has been proven to be more accurate in diagnosing vascular compromise of free-flap transfers.[14] In the first 24 hours, patients are closely monitored in the ICU, kept nil per os (NPO) and are on strict bed rest to prevent potential complications in the event that reexploration is required. Flap checks are initially done half-hourly or hourly to assess flap viability. Avoidance of hypotension, hypoxia, and hypothermia are important. Venous congestion and necrosis in the skin paddle of a free flap might result in loss of the flap. Venous flow can be preserved by using systemic heparin therapy, LMW dextran or medicinal leech therapy.

Clinical observation of flap color, swelling, temperature, and capillary refill remains a vital mode of monitoring. A healthy and a well-perfused flap appears pink, minimally swollen, and warm to touch; a congested flap appears bluish in color, swollen, warm to touch with a short capillary refill time of less than 2 seconds. If the flap is ischemic it appears pale, cold to touch with a delayed capillary refill time of more than 3 seconds. Upon puncturing a viable free flap with a small gauge needle (pin-prick test) bright red blood flows immediately, whereas in a congested flap the blood flow is dark suggesting compromise. This test is usually performed on flaps where clinical monitoring by visualization is difficult. In pharyngo-esophageal reconstruction using small intestine, the sentinel loop that is left outside the neck is used to monitor the viability. A healthy intestinal graft is pink and warm with minimal swelling and visible peristalsis; loss of peristalsis suggests graft compromise.

Compression of the artery will lead to loss of the Doppler signal within the flap, whereas venous compression will lead to augmentation of the venous signal due to increased venous return. Implantable Doppler probes may be used to monitor the flow in buried flaps. A decrease in tissue oxygen partial pressure ($ptiO_2$) monitoring via an implantable oxygen-monitoring probe (eg, Licox) may suggest free-flap compromise. A pitfall of these monitors is that the probes are localized and do not assess viability outside the small sample volume that is monitored.

Microvascular Flap Anticoagulation

Aspirin and LMW heparin alone or in combination are commonly used for postoperative anticoagulation after free tissue transfer. Other strategies to prevent thrombosis include decreasing blood viscosity by LMW dextran infusions and/or hemodilution with IV fluids and avoiding blood-product transfusions unless absolutely necessary. LMW dextran antithrombotic properties are not fully understood but are thought to be secondary to platelet function impairment, destabilizing fibrin, and prolonging bleeding time. Studies report variable efficacy of these anticoagulants in preventing free-flap thrombosis.

Complications of LMW Dextran—Dextran has significant dose-dependent adverse affects. These include anaphylaxis, a rare but potentially life-threatening complication,[15,16] noncardiogenic pulmonary edema, renal insufficiency, and rarely cardiac arrest.

Dextran infusion syndrome should be suspected in patients on LMW dextran that develop noncardiogenic pulmonary edema. They may also develop hypotension, bronchospasm, or coagulopathy. The incidence increases with higher infusion rates and the longer the infusion continues. The treatment is prompt discontinuation of the dextran infusion and initiating symptomatic treatment.

Hirudotherapy—Medicinal leech therapy, called hirudotherapy is commonly used in the setting of free-flap venous congestion or thrombosis to temporarily establish venous outflow until neovascularization of the graft is established. Leeches produce an anticoagulant called hirudin that is a selective thrombin inhibitor; it also secretes vasodilators and hyaluronidase that allow the leech to ingest blood. The regimen is to use about 2 to 4 leeches depending on the size of the flap, attached to the tissue for approximately 20 minutes. Following the leech therapy, blood oozes for the next 24 hours. Complications from this therapy include bleeding, anemia, leech migration to a different body location, and rarely local or systemic infection with the gram-negative bacillus *Aeromonas hydrophila*.[17]

Blood Transfusion

There are no clear transfusion thresholds in free-flap surgery; however, it appears that a restrictive transfusion strategy using a postoperative transfusion trigger of hematocrit of less than 25 is not inferior to a higher transfusion threshold of hematocrit of less than 30 in patients undergoing free-flap surgery, with no increase in flap-related complications in the lower transfusion trigger group.[18]

Wound Infection

Wound infection is not uncommon in tissue transfer surgery involving head and neck tumors. Risk factors for infection include preoperative radiotherapy, blood transfusion, smoking, and the duration of surgery.

Alcohol Withdrawal

The overall flap survival rate with alcohol withdrawal syndrome (AWS) is about 83%. Patients with postoperative AWS have a higher chance of developing non-flap-related complications, especially respiratory problems (prolonged ventilator dependency), encephalopathy, seizures, and hemodynamic instability. The onset of alcohol withdrawal symptoms is usually 1 to 2 days after abstinence (delirium tremens may occur at 2-5 days). Once AWS signs are recognized, prompt treatment should commence with an initial regimen of parenteral thiamine, multivitamins, and folic acid supplements. Effective treatment for AWS involves treatment with benzodiazepines and occasionally antipsychotics.[19] As more data become available, dexmedetomidine appears promising in the treatment of AWS.

ORTHOPEDIC SURGERY

This section reviews critical-care management after THR and TKR.

Admission rates of orthopedic patients to the ICU are rising due to an increasingly elderly population. Approximately 1 of 30 patients undergoing total joint arthroplasty will require critical-care monitoring. Identifying high-risk patients undergoing joint replacement for adverse events and monitoring in ICU can optimize outcome and reduce morbidity and mortality.

Risk factors for requiring critical-care services include advanced age, hip versus knee surgery, general anesthesia, multiple comorbidities, intraoperative or postoperative complications, and surgical indications other than osteoarthritis and rheumatoid arthritis. Smoking is associated with significantly higher perioperative complications and mortality following total hip arthroplasty and total knee arthroplasty.

Surgical Factors

In THR and TKR, the damaged articular cartilage over the bone surfaces is replaced. The bone is cut based on preoperative radiographs and anatomic measurements. These cut bony surfaces are covered by metal, ceramic, or polyethylene components that are sized appropriately to match the alignment, leg length, and range of motion. If all compartments and surfaces of the joint are replaced, the procedure is referred to as a total joint arthroplasty/replacement. If only 1 surface or compartment of the joint is replaced, it is referred to as hemiarthroplasty. In total hip arthroplasty both the femoral head and neck are replaced. In total knee arthroplasty the distal femur, tibia, and patella are resurfaced after any remaining articular cartilage and a layer of subchondral bone are resected.

Blood Transfusion Criteria

Total hip and total knee arthroplasty frequently require blood transfusion with transfusion rates ranging from 18% to 68%. The Function and Overall Cognition in Ultra-High Risk States (FOCUS), largest trial, to address blood transfusion threshold in hip fracture patients suggests that mortality, length of stay, are no different from the general population with a restrictive transfusion threshold of hemoglobin 8 g/dL.[20]

Cardiopulmonary Complications

Risk factors for developing postoperative cardiac complications include age of 80 years or above, hypertension requiring medication and history of cardiac disease. The cardiac complication rate is approximately 0.33% after total knee arthroplasty or total hip arthroplasty. Serious complications such as MI and cardiac arrest constitute 7% to 20% of all major complications. Patients with underlying cardiac disease who receive large volume resuscitation and blood products are at increased risk of noncardiogenic pulmonary edema and supraventricular arrhythmias such as atrial fibrillation and atrial flutter. Risk factors for perioperative development of supraventricular arrhythmias include a history of atrial fibrillation, increasing age, left anterior hemiblock, and atrial premature depolarizations on the preoperative electrocardiogram. In patients aged above 60 years with any one of the above risk factors, the risk of arrhythmia is as high as 18%.[21] Electrolyte abnormalities, hypoxia, and acidosis should be corrected.

Respiratory Failure

Occurrence of postoperative pneumonia is high in elderly patients; atelectasis and secretions, intubation, reintubation, prolonged ventilator support, and use of preoperative proton pump inhibitor use are risk factors for developing pneumonia. The rate of serious pulmonary complications has been reported to be 2.6%, with a 30-day mortality of 17%. Risk factors for developing acute respiratory distress syndrome (ARDS) include aspiration, blood-product administration (including transfusion-related acute lung injury [TRALI]), and lung injury from fat embolism or bone cement, surgical site infection, and sepsis. The mortality rate is approximately 60% in elderly patients above 85 years. Treatment includes supportive care and lung-protective ventilation strategies.

Fat Embolism Syndrome

Fat embolism is defined as occlusion of the microcirculation by presence of fat globules. Common causes of fat embolism syndrome (FES) include orthopedic trauma, particularly involving long-bone fractures in the lower extremity and orthopedic surgeries involving the lower extremity. The incidence of asymptomatic fat embolism in THR and TKR is approximately 46% to 65%.

The development of FES may be secondary to extravasation of fat globules from the bone marrow during the surgical procedure secondary to increased intramedullary pressure. Clinically, the classic triad of FES is hypoxemia, neurological abnormalities (eg, agitated or hypoactive delirium), and petechiae. Occasionally severe cases of FES can be complicated by disseminated intravascular coagulation, right ventricular dysfunction, biventricular failure, ARDS, shock, and death. No gold standard criteria exist to diagnose fat embolism. The incidence of FES thus varies widely. The most frequently used diagnostic criteria are Gurd's criteria (Table 55–1).

Given the systemic complications, high-risk patients need close monitoring. No clear treatment guidelines exist; supportive care with fluid resuscitation and mechanical ventilation are the main stays. Heparin and corticosteroids have not been found to improve morbidity or mortality.[21,22]

Bone Cement Implantation Syndrome

Bone cement implantation syndrome (BCIS) is a life-threatening complication of orthopedic surgery characterized by hypoxia, hypotension, pulmonary

TABLE 55–1 Gurd's criteria for diagnosis of fat embolism syndrome.[21,22]

Major Criteria	Minor Criteria
Axillary or subconjunctival petechiae	Tachycardia < 110 beats/min
Hypoxemia PaO_2 < 60 mm Hg; FIO_2 = 0.4	Pyrexia < 38.5°C
Central nervous system depression disproportionate to hypoxemia	Emboli present in the retina on fundoscopy
Pulmonary edema	Fat present in urine, a sudden inexplicable drop in hematocrit or platelet values Increasing ESR Fat globules present in the sputum

ESR, erythrocyte sedimentation rate; FIO_2, fraction of inspired oxygen; PaO_2, partial pressure arterial oxygen.

hypertension, arrhythmias, loss of consciousness, and potentially cardiac arrest occurring around the time of bone cementation.[23] Complications from acrylic bone cement polymethylmethacrylate (PMMA) have been recognized as early as the 1970s, but recently have been more frequently reported. The majority of complications develop soon after the application of cement or in the immediate postoperative period. Patient risk factors include advanced age, malignancy, osteoporotic bones, renal failure, congestive heart failure, chronic obstructive lung disease, use of diuretics, and angiotensin converting enzyme medications. BCIS increases the 30-day mortality rate by 16 fold.

The pathophysiology is not fully understood but may be secondary to the release of inflammatory markers, anaphylaxis and complement activation leading to increased pulmonary vascular resistance causing ventilation/perfusion disturbances and right ventricular failure. Recently, BCIS has been classified into 3 grades depending on the severity (Table 55–2).[24]

The incidence of BCIS may be reduced by use of noncemented joints, high-volume medullary lavage, intraoperative canal suctioning during cementation, low-viscosity PMMA, and slow controlled insertion of the prosthesis. Use of tobramycin-impregnated

TABLE 55-2 BCIS classification.

BCIS grade I	Moderate hypoxia, (SpO$_2$ < 94%) or hypotension [a decrease in systolic arterial pressure (SAP) > 20%]
BCIS grade II	Severe hypoxia (SpO$_2$ < 88%) or hypotension (a decrease in SAP > 40%) or unexpected loss of consciousness
BCIS grade III	Cardiovascular collapse requiring cardiopulmonary resuscitation

BCIS, bone cement implantation syndrome; SpO$_2$, peripheral capillary oxygen saturation.
Data from Donaldson AJ, Thomson HE, Harper NJ, Kenny NW. Bone cement implantation syndrome, Br J Anaesth 2009 Jan;102(1):12-22.

bone cement decreases the incidence of BCIS but is associated with acute kidney injury (AKI) in patients with underlying renal disease.

ICU admission is warranted in patients with hypotension, hypoxemia, anaphylactic reactions, and right heart failure after undergoing cement joint replacement. Transthoracic echocardiography should be considered in these patients to assess cardiac activity especially, right ventricular function. In patients with hemodynamic instability, fluid resuscitation and vasopressor support should be provided. Patients with symptomatic hypoxia or ARDS should be supported by lung protective mechanical ventilation.

Venous Thromboembolism

The rate of pulmonary embolism (PE) in the nonorthopedic population aged above 65 years is approximately 0.03%, but patients undergoing THR or TKR have a 10 fold or 0.3% increase in PE. Risk factors for VTE are increasing age, immobilization, presence of varicose veins, previous deep vein thrombosis

(DVT), smoking, hormonal therapy, location of surgery (knee > hip) malignancy, type of anesthesia, indwelling venous catheters or pacemaker, surgical time, and joint replacement itself. High-risk patients with evidence of right ventricular dysfunction clinically or echocardiographically are at risk of shock or death and need close ICU monitoring (Table 55-3).

The latest (9th) American College of Chest Physician (ACCP) guidelines from 2012 suggest initiating VTE prophylaxis 12 or more hours preoperatively or postoperatively rather than 4 hours or less preoperatively or postoperatively. LMW heparin is preferred prophylaxis for a minimum of 10 to 14 days along with intermittent pneumatic compression devices. Patients with active signs of bleeding are recommended to receive mechanical VTE prophylaxis. Current evidence does not provide clear guidance about inserting prophylactic inferior vena cava (IVC) filters in patients undergoing elective hip and knee arthroplasty with contraindications to chemoprophylaxis or residual venous thromboembolic disease. Orthopedic surgeons should be consulted prior to initiation of VTE prophylaxis in these patients at all times, especially in patients with acute blood loss anemia requiring ICU admission. Formal discussion with the primary team regarding VTE prophylaxis should be incorporated into team rounds.

UROLOGICAL SURGERY

Most patients undergoing radical nephrectomy and cystectomy do not require intensive care monitoring unless they develop perioperative complications such as hemodynamic instability (from acute blood loss, splenic injury, MI, adrenal insufficiency (AI), hypovolemia, pulmonary embolism) and respiratory failure.

TABLE 55-3 Incidence of VTE in patients with and without VTE prophylaxis after major orthopedic surgery.

	Initial Prophylaxis, Postoperative Days (0-14)	Extended Prophylaxis, Postoperative Days (15-35)	Cumulative, Postoperative Days (0-35)
No prophylaxis	VTE 2.80% (PE 1.00%, DVT 1.80%)	VTE 1.50% (PE 0.50%, DVT 1.00%)	VTE 4.3% (PE 1.50%, DVT 2.80%)
LMWH	VTE 1.15% (PE 0.35%, DVT 0.80%)	VTE 0.65% (PE 0.20%, DVT 0.45%)	VTE 1.8% (PE 0.55%, DVT 1.25%)

DVT, deep vein thrombosis; LMWH, low-molecular-weight heparin; PE, pulmonary embolism; VTE, venous thromboembolism.
Reproduced with permission from Falck-Ytter Y, Francis CW, Johanson NA, et al. Prevention of VTE in orthopedic surgery patients: Antithrombotic Therapy and Prevention of Thrombosis, 9th ed: American College of Chest Physicians Evidence-Based Clinical Practice Guidelines, Chest 2012 Feb;141(2 Suppl):e278S-325S.

Radical Nephrectomy

Renal cell carcinoma (RCC) is the third most common cancer of urinary tract and accounts for 80% to 85% of all primary renal neoplasms, with an annual incidence of over 60,000 in the United States. One third of newly diagnosed patients with RCC present with advanced stage (III/IV) tumors.

Surgical Factors

Radical nephrectomy includes removal of the kidney and Gerota's fascia, ligation of the renal artery and vein, and occasionally removal of the ipsilateral adrenal gland. This procedure is usually done laparoscopically for renal masses smaller than 4 cm, whereas open radical nephrectomy is reserved for large, locally advanced tumors, caval extension, or enlarged lymph nodes.

Complications

In a retrospective analysis from the National Surgical Quality Improvement Program (NSQIP), cystectomy had the highest morbidity (3.2% mortality), followed by nephrectomy, retroperitoneal lymph node dissection, and radical retropubic prostatectomy. Postoperative complications following radical nephrectomy include postoperative bleeding, pneumothorax (PTX), MI, liver injury, pancreatic and splenic injury.

Hypotension is not uncommon in the postoperative period from blood loss, dehydration, and sedation. Prompt recognition of bleeding, achieving hemostasis, fluid resuscitation to maintain intravascular volume and tissue perfusion, MAP greater than 65 and avoidance of fluid overload are the mainstays of treatment.

PTX may occur with surgeries involving the flank; rib resection is not always necessary to cause PTX. In the event of postoperative respiratory or hemodynamic instability, the diagnosis of PTX must be considered. Physical examination, ultrasound, and chest radiography are methods to determine the diagnosis.

The adrenal gland is a highly vascular structure and is occasionally removed during radical nephrectomy. There is no difference in the survival of patients undergoing radical nephrectomy with or without adrenalectomy, whereas in metastatic disease the survival is poor, independent of adrenalectomy.

Monitoring for signs and symptoms of acute Addisonian crisis is important. AI is characterized by hypotension, fever, hyperkalemia, hypoglycemia, weakness, and nausea or vomiting. However, signs of AI may not always be seen in ICU patients who usually present with refractive hypotension with or without hypoglycemia; therefore, a low threshold for the diagnosis of AI is warranted. This is a medical emergency and needs to be treated promptly with corticosteroids without waiting for cortisol levels or an adrenocorticotropic hormone (ACTH) stimulation test.

Left radical nephrectomy is the second most common cause of splenic injury. The incidence is approximately 4.3% to 13.2% and is higher during transperitoneal approach compared to retroperitoneal approach. Common signs and symptoms in an awake patient are abdominal pain, hematocrit drop, hypotension, and Kehr sign (referred pain at left shoulder tip), but these signs may not be recognized in less responsive patients. Splenic injury should be considered in the event of unexplained hypotension or hematocrit drop postnephrectomy. Bedside, ultrasonography can be utilized to quickly diagnose splenic injury in hemodynamically unstable patients (perisplenic fluid or intraperitoneal fluid seen in Morrison's pouch). Splenic injury can be also diagnosed by computed tomography. Nonoperative management of splenic injury includes aggressive volume and blood-product resuscitation and supportive care to keep the hemoglobin greater than 7.0 g/dL. Surgical treatment includes angiography and embolization or emergency splenectomy. Other important differentials for postoperative hemodynamic instability include hypovolemia, acute blood loss, sepsis, acute coronary syndrome, and pulmonary embolism.

Left radical nephrectomy can result in pancreatic injury and bleeding, hence follow up with lipase; amylase and abdominal imaging should be considered in suspected patients. The risk factors for VTE include poor functional status, age of above 60 years, anesthesia time more than 2 hours, steroid usage, metastatic disease, and congestive heart failure.

Patients with underlying chronic kidney disease (CKD) are at increased risk of developing AKI. The overall incidence of AKI in patients undergoing radical or partial nephrectomy is approximately 7%.

Sepsis, urinary obstruction, and bleeding are leading causes of AKI in these patients. The overall mortality increases with severity of AKI (4.8% in stage 1, 9.1% in stage 2, 14.9% in stage 3).

Radical Cystectomy and Urinary Diversion

Open radical cystectomy (ORC) remains the standard treatment for high-grade nonmetastatic invasive bladder cancer. Multiple centers have adopted new operative techniques such as robotic assisted radical cystectomy (RARC) that has increased from 0.6% of all cystectomies in 2004 to 12.8% in 2010.[25]

Surgical Factors

Radical cystectomy involves removal of the bladder, adjacent organs, and regional lymph nodes. In males, radical cystectomy includes removal of the prostate, seminal vesicles, along with the urinary bladder. Advances such as laparoscopic cystectomy and RARC have resulted in technical improvements resulting in less blood loss, fewer blood transfusions, reduced risk of complications and shorter hospital stay, as compared with open surgery.

Using the NSQIP database, the rates of DVT and PE (4.0% and 2.9%) were found to be the highest after cystectomy and urinary diversion[26,27] followed by nephrectomy and prostatectomy. Cystectomy is an independent risk factor for VTE; other risk factors include increased body mass index (BMI), positive surgical margins, older age, and increased length of stay. ACCP guidelines, suggest 4 weeks of low-molecular-weight heparin for VTE prophylaxis in patients at high risk who undergo abdominal and pelvic surgeries.

Gastrointestinal events represent the majority of complications following radical cystectomy with ileal conduit. Intestinal obstruction is most common (23%), followed by ileus (18%) and intestinal anastomotic leakage (3%) in a recent series.[28] Special monitoring is necessary to detect signs and symptoms of urosepsis, urinary leak, and pyelonephritis following urinary diversion surgery.

The use of balanced crystalloid solutions (Plasmalyte, Lactated Ringer's) in patients undergoing radical cystectomy with ileal conduit is preferred over normal saline because 0.9% sodium chloride solution is associated with hyperchloremic metabolic acidosis. Hypervolemia can result in interstitial edema causing deleterious effects on bowel function. One recent report suggested that restrictive fluid administration and preemptive use of norepinephrine to correct hypotension might be beneficial in decreasing postoperative complications.

Infectious events constitute about 25% and are the second most common complications of radical cystectomy according to a recent investigation.[28] Antibiotic prophylaxis (eg, ampicillin) is given for radical cystectomy. Major infections that are encountered following radical cystectomy are urinary tract infection, urosepsis, pyelonephritis, and sepsis. Wound-related complications in the early postoperative period include primary dehiscence and infection.[29]

Urinary diversion is a surgical procedure in which the urinary flow is rerouted from the bladder.[30] Different types of diversion include ileal conduit, continent cutaneous diversion, and orthotopic neobladder (the urine is eliminated by the urethra). Potential complications following urinary diversion include AKI, hydronephrosis, urinary tract infection, nephrolithiasis, and metabolic disturbances. Mucus is often produced by urinary reservoirs and bladder substitutes; hence frequent irrigation of mucus is necessary to avoid mucus accumulation and infection.[31] Orthotopic diversion is a significant predictor of VTE compared to nonorthotropic diversion.

Radical cystectomy often leads to considerable blood loss with an average blood loss of 560 to 3000 mL.

REFERENCES

1. Siegel R, Ma J, Zou Z, Jemal A. Cancer statistics, 2014. *CA Cancer J Clin.* 2014;64(1):9-29.
2. Ochoa ME, Marin Mdel C, Frutos-Vivar F, et al. Cuff-leak test for the diagnosis of upper airway obstruction in adults: a systematic review and meta-analysis. *Intensive Care Med.* 2009;35(7):1171-1179.
3. Cameron M, Corner A, Diba A, Hankins M. Development of a tracheostomy scoring system to guide airway management after major head and neck surgery. *Int J Oral Maxillofac Surg.* 2009;38(8):846-849.
4. Kruse-Losler B, Langer E, Reich A, Joos U, Kleinheinz J. Score system for elective tracheotomy in major head and neck tumour surgery. *Acta Anaesthesiol Scand.* 2005;49(5):654-659.

5. Chappell D, Jacob M, Hofmann-Kiefer K, Conzen P, Rehm M. A rational approach to perioperative fluid management. *Anesthesiology*. 2008;109(4):723-740.

6. Harris L, Goldstein D, Hofer S, Gilbert R. Impact of vasopressors on outcomes in head and neck free tissue transfer. *Microsurgery*. 2012;32(1):15-19.

7. Kelly DA, Reynolds M, Crantford C, Pestana IA. Impact of intraoperative vasopressor use in free tissue transfer for head, neck, and extremity reconstruction. *Ann Plast Surg*. 2014;72(6): S135-S138.

8. Monroe MM, Cannady SB, Ghanem TA, Swide CE, Wax MK. Safety of vasopressor use in head and neck microvascular reconstruction: a prospective observational study. *Otolaryngol Head Neck Surg*. 2011;144(6):877-882.

9. Nagele P, Rao LK, Penta M, et al. Postoperative myocardial injury after major head and neck cancer surgery. *Head Neck*. 2011;33(8):1085-1091.

10. Chen KT, Mardini S, Chuang DC, et al. Timing of presentation of the first signs of vascular compromise dictates the salvage outcome of free flap transfers. *Plast Reconstr Surg*. 2007;120(1):187-195.

11. Kroll SS, Schusterman MA, Reece GP, et al. Timing of pedicle thrombosis and flap loss after free-tissue transfer. *Plast Reconstr Surg*. 1996;98(7):1230-1233.

12. May JW, Jr, Chait LA, O'Brien BM, Hurley JV. The no-reflow phenomenon in experimental free flaps. *Plast Reconstr Surg*. 1978;61(2):256-267.

13. Salgado CJ, Moran SL, Mardini S. Flap monitoring and patient management. *Plast Reconstr Surg*. 2009;124(6 suppl):e295-e302.

14. Holzle F, Loeffelbein DJ, Nolte D, Wolff KD. Free flap monitoring using simultaneous noninvasive laser Doppler flowmetry and tissue spectrophotometry. *J Craniomaxillofac Surg*. 2006;34(1):25-33.

15. Disa JJ, Polvora VP, Pusic AL, Singh B, Cordeiro PG. Dextran-related complications in head and neck microsurgery: do the benefits outweigh the risks? A prospective randomized analysis. *Plast Reconstr Surg*. 2003;112(6):1534-1539.

16. Zinderman CE, Landow L, Wise RP. Anaphylactoid reactions to Dextran 40 and 70: reports to the United States Food and Drug Administration, 1969 to 2004. *J Vasc Surg*. 2006;43(5):1004-1009.

17. Elyassi AR, Terres J, Rowshan HH. Medicinal leech therapy on head and neck patients: a review of literature and proposed protocol. *Oral Surg Oral Med Oral Pathol Oral Radiol*. 2013;116(3):e167-e172.

18. Rossmiller SR, Cannady SB, Ghanem TA, Wax MK. Transfusion criteria in free flap surgery. *Otolaryngol Head Neck Surg*. 2010;142(3):359-364.

19. Chang CC, Kao HK, Huang JJ, Tsao CK, Cheng MH, Wei FC. Postoperative alcohol withdrawal syndrome and neuropsychological disorder in patients after head and neck cancer ablation followed by microsurgical free tissue transfer. *J Reconstr Microsurg*. 2013;29(2):131-136.

20. Brunskill SJ, Millette SL, Shokoohi A, et al. Red blood cell transfusion for people undergoing hip fracture surgery. *Cochrane Database Syst Rev*. 2015;4:CD009699.

21. Memtsoudis SG, Rosenberger P, Walz JM. Critical care issues in the patient after major joint replacement. *J Intensive Care Med*. 2007;22(2):92-104.

22. Kosova E, Bergmark B, Piazza G. Fat embolism syndrome. *Circulation*. 2015;131(3):317-320.

23. Griffiths R, Parker M. Bone cement implantation syndrome and proximal femoral fracture. *Br J Anaesth*. 2015;114(1):6-7.

24. Donaldson AJ, Thomson HE, Harper NJ, Kenny NW. Bone cement implantation syndrome. *Br J Anaesth*. 2009;102(1):12-22.

25. Konety BR, Allareddy V, Herr H. Complications after radical cystectomy: analysis of population-based data. *Urology*. 2006;68(1):58-64.

26. De Martino RR, Goodney PP, Spangler EL, et al. Variation in thromboembolic complications among patients undergoing commonly performed cancer operations. *J Vasc Surg*. 2012;55(4):1035-1040.e4.

27. Tyson MD, Castle EP, Humphreys MR, Andrews PE. Venous thromboembolism after urological surgery. *J Urol*. 2014;192(3):793-797.

28. Shabsigh A, Korets R, Vora KC, et al. Defining early morbidity of radical cystectomy for patients with bladder cancer using a standardized reporting methodology. *Eur Urol*. 2009;55(1):164-174.

29. Wuethrich PY, Burkhard FC. Improved perioperative outcome with norepinephrine and a restrictive fluid administration during open radical cystectomy and urinary diversion. *Urol Oncol*. 2015;33(2):66.e21-4.

30. Roghmann F, Gockel M, Schmidt J, et al. Complications after ileal conduit: urinary diversion-associated complications after radical cystectomy. *Urologe A*. 2015;54(4):533-541.

31. Madersbacher S, Schmidt J, Eberle JM, et al. Long-term outcome of ileal conduit diversion. *J Urol*. 2003;169(3):985-990.

32. Falck-Ytter Y, Francis CW, Johanson NA, et al. Prevention of VTE in orthopedic surgery patients: antithrombotic therapy and prevention of thrombosis, 9th ed: American College of Chest Physicians Evidence-Based Clinical Practice Guidelines. *Chest*. 2012;141(2 suppl):e278S-e325S.

Postoperative Vascular Surgery Care

Charanya Sivaramakrishnan, MD and Rami Tadros, MD

"The tragedies of life are largely arterial"–Sir William Osler

KEY POINTS

1 Permissive hypotension while ensuring adequate organ perfusion is recommended in ruptured abdominal aortic aneurysm (AAA).

2 Acute spinal cord ischemia post-thoraco-AAA repair mandates emergent lumbar CSF catheter placement and monitored drainage in an intensive care unit.

3 High index of suspicion for postoperative ischemic colitis—abdominal pain, rising lactate, fever, and leukocytosis.

4 Management of acute aortic dissections with impulse control by intravenous beta blockers followed by nitroprusside.

5 Early recognition of malperfusion syndromes in type B aortic dissection.

INTRODUCTION

Care of the vascular surgery patient postoperatively presents a challenging clinical scenario to the intensivist. These patients are at a high risk for perioperative complications whether undergoing open or endovascular surgery. Advanced age, comorbidities such as coronary artery disease, congestive heart failure, chronic kidney disease, advanced diabetes, peripheral vascular disease in addition to the insult of major vascular surgery places these patients at a high-risk category and potentially requiring intensive care unit (ICU). Major vascular surgery exposes the patient to extensive tissue damage, elicits a robust inflammatory response and can predispose to profound hemodynamic changes.

This chapter will review the commonly encountered vascular procedures most likely to require subsequent ICU care.

ABDOMINAL AORTIC ANEURYSM

An abdominal aortic aneurysm (AAA) is defined as a pathologic focal dilation of the aorta that is more than 30 mm or 1.5 times the adjacent diameter of the normal aorta. Male aortas tend to be larger than female, and there is a generalized growth of the aortic diameter with each decade of life. Ninety percent of the AAA are infrarenal in location and fusiform in morphology.[1]

Most AAAs are asymptomatic and are found incidentally during workup for chronic back pain or kidney stones. The indications for surgery are any patient who is symptomatic with back pain and/or abdominal pain with a tender pulsatile mass or any asymptomatic aneurysm that is greater than or equal to 5 to 5.5 cm or increases by greater than 0.5 cm/year.

There are 2 approaches to AAA repair—the open surgical approach and endovascular aneurysm repair (EVAR).[2] The majority of AAAs today are managed using EVAR. Therefore, the number of patients requiring ICU care after aneurysm repair has decreased. Currently, those with AAA not treatable with EVAR often have pararenal or juxta-renal morphology increasing the risk of open repair. These aneurysms increase the challenge of repair and often require supraceliac aortic clamping. The physiologic disturbance in this cohort is much greater.

The advantage of open repair (Figure 56–1) is that the AAA is permanently eliminated because it is entirely replaced by a prosthetic graft and risk of recurrence or delayed rupture is less. Consequently, long-term imaging surveillance is not needed in most patients. However, several prospective clinical trials across devices and databases have demonstrated a significantly decreased operative time, blood loss, hospital length of stay, and overall perioperative morbidity and mortality of endovascular repair as compared to open surgical repair.

Endovascular procedures aim to reduce the morbidity and mortality of treating arterial disease in a patient population that is increasingly older and less fit than when major open repairs were developed and popularized. Studies that assign aneurysm patients to treatment with EVAR or traditional open surgery have demonstrated fewer early complications with the minimally invasive approach. Some studies have also observed a lower mortality rate with EVAR. Hence endovascular AAA repair (EVAR) is currently the treatment of choice for repair of uncomplicated infrarenal AAAs. EVAR is also used for ruptured AAA with 1 meta-analysis of 3 recent trials demonstrating a mortality rate of 38.6% with EVAR vs 42.8% in open repair.[3] However, the IMPROVE trial demonstrates no survival benefit, although there is a significant improvement in speed of discharge, quality of life, and cost-effectiveness with EVAR.[4]

There have been advances in the techniques of EVAR allowing treatment of patients with atypical vascular anatomy.

Fenestrated EVAR—When the aneurysm begins close to the renal arteries, standard EVAR may be contraindicated because there will be an inadequate length of suitable aorta for the endograft attachment. In these cases a fenestrated endograft may be useful, where the attachment of the endograft to the aorta may be placed above the renal arteries with each fenestration opposite a renal artery so that blood flow to the kidneys is maintained.[5]

Branched EVAR—A branched endograft has graft limbs that branch off of the main portion of the device to directly provide blood flow to the kidneys or the visceral arteries.[6]

RUPTURED ABDOMINAL AORTIC ANEURYSM

Emergent surgical intervention is indicated for a rupture but despite improvements in perioperative care the mortality rate remains high (approximately 50%) after conventional open repair. Emergency endovascular aneurysm repair (eEVAR) has been used successfully to treat ruptured AAA (RAAA), proving that it is feasible in selected patients.

Management of RAAA discussed as follows:

1. Patients should be resuscitated with fluids (crystalloids, colloids, or blood) to maintain adequate organ perfusion and mentation.

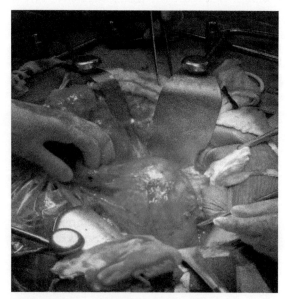

FIGURE 56–1 Large abdominal aortic aneurysm seen in the operating room.

Aggressive resuscitation to a normotensive state is not advised until the aneurysm is repaired. Permissive hypotension is ideal prior to controlling hemorrhage.

2. Hypertension should be avoided to lessen further bleeding.

3. Patients who are relatively stable, with an intact mental status should undergo emergent CT scanning to confirm the diagnosis and to consider EVAR if available.

4. However, those who are persistently unstable should immediately be transferred to the OR for exploration or to a center that can offer the best treatment.

THORACIC AORTIC ANEURYSM

Ascending aortic aneurysms are the most common (~60%) thoracic aortic aneurysm (TAA) followed by aneurysms of the descending aorta (~35%) and of the transverse aortic arch (< 10%). Most descending TAAs begin just distal to the orifice of left subclavian artery.[7]

Most TAA are clinically silent; with nontraumatic TAAs detected as incidental findings on chest imaging obtained for other purposes. A minority of patients may present with chest discomfort or pain that intensifies with aneurysm expansion or rupture, aortic valvular regurgitation, congestive heart failure, compression of adjacent structures (recurrent laryngeal nerve, left main-stem bronchus, esophagus, superior vena cava), erosion into adjacent structures (esophagus, lung, airway), or distal embolization.

Chest X-ray reveals widened mediastinum or an enlarged calcific aortic shadow. Traumatic aneurysms may be associated with skeletal fractures. MR or CT imaging with intravenous (IV) contrast provides precise estimation of the size and extent of aneurysms and facilitates surgical planning (refer to Figure 56–2 for CT evidence of a contained TAAA rupture). Echocardiography may be useful in evaluating aneurysms involving the aortic arch.

Options include open repair and thoracic endovascular aneurysm repair (TEVAR). Surgical management varies based on type and location of TAA. Repair of proximal arch aneurysms requires cardiopulmonary bypass and circulatory arrest. Ascending and transverse arches are repaired through a median

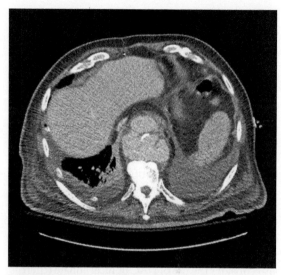

FIGURE 56–2 Contained thoracoabdominal aortic aneurysm rupture.

sternotomy incision. Descending and thoraco-AAAs (TAAAs) are approached through a left posterolateral thoracotomy or thoracoabdominal incision.

Endovascular management of descending TAA: Because of the considerable morbidity and mortality associated with surgical repair of descending thoracic aneurysms, the endovascular approach to aneurysm exclusion is preferred for isolated descending thoracic aneurysms. Newer technologies are being developed for management of TAAA.

Complications

Both open surgical repairs and EVAR are associated with a wide variety of complications ranging from major organ system dysfunction to procedure specific localized complications carrying significant morbidity and mortality.

Cardiac derangements manifest as fatal arrhythmias and myocardial infarction. Myocardial infarction is the most common cause of death following major vascular surgery. Troponin I is a consistent predictor of increased cardiac events and increased mortality following vascular surgery.

Respiratory compromise requiring mechanical ventilation might be needed as a complication secondary to cases with significant intraoperative hemorrhage with ensuing fluid shifts and noncardiogenic pulmonary edema. Respiratory complications are also common due to a history of smoking, COPD, and heart failure.

Acute renal insufficiency negatively impacts hospital length of stay and mortality, with an incidence of 1% to 23% post-EVAR (lower compared to that of open repair).[8] The likely pathophysiology of AKI in EVAR is complex with multiple probable implicated mechanisms—contrast-induced nephropathy, renal microembolization, and acute tubular necrosis. Among the several preventive strategies for AKI, hydration is the mainstay of prevention as it ameliorates the effect of contrast and oxidative stress and increases renal perfusion. Hydration is of crucial importance in ruptured EVAR to correct the associated hypovolemia and decrease the effect of the pronounced oxidative stress onto the kidney. One may also consider the use of NAC or bicarbonate (there is a need for further rigorous clinical trials and studies to validate these 2 measures). Again, these are very relevant in ruptured AAAs where oxidative stress is more significant.

Abdominal compartment syndrome (ACS) is defined by the World Society of Abdominal Compartment Syndrome as intra-abdominal pressure greater than 20 mm Hg with new organ dysfunction. Intra-abdominal hypertension (IAH) is defined as intra-abdominal pressure greater than 12 mm Hg. ACS results in significant cardiac, renal, and respiratory compromise. It is suggested that large retroperitoneal hematoma and diffuse visceral edema postoperatively contribute to the development of IAH/ACS. Intra-abdominal hypertension is noted to be an important risk factor for colonic hypoperfusion and ensuing ischemic colitis after ruptured AAA repair.[9] Monitoring of IAP may be associated with improved mortality postruptured AAA repair treated with open surgery or EVAR.[10]

Intra-abdominal pressures are measured by intermittent or continuous bladder pressure measurement with urethral catheterization. The definitions of the WSACS are used as the diagnostic criteria for both IAH and ACS.

The major pathophysiologic consequences of ACS are listed as follows:

- Decreased preload—compression of IVC
- Increased afterload—aortic impedance, decreased stroke volume

- Decreased extra thoracic compliance—increased shunt fraction, dead space, transalveolar pressures
- Hypoperfusion—hepatic, splanchnic dysfunction
- Increased transmitted intracerebral pressure
- Cessation of renal filtration gradient

Successful outcomes depend on early recognition and management to reduce IAH. Decompressive laparotomy should be used if conservative treatments fail or if the clinical picture warrants decompression (see Table 56–1 for medical management of IAH).

Hypertension—Even brief episodes of hypertension can disrupt suture lines in open surgery and can precipitate bleeding or pseudoaneurysm formation. At the same time, hypotension, after TAA repair, can lead to spinal cord ischemia. Hence it is a delicate, fine balancing act in these cases to maintain mean arterial blood pressure between 80 and 100 mm Hg. Use of IV nitroprusside, IV beta blockers, or IV calcium

TABLE 56–1 Medical management of intra-abdominal hypertension.

Conservative Medical Management of Elevated Intra-abdominal Hypertension Include
Insertion of gastric and rectal decompressive tubes
Administration of promotilic/kinetic GI agents
Percutaneous drainage of fluid collections
Optimize sedation and analgesia
Consider neuromuscular blockade
Consider using reverse Trendelenburg position
Remove abdominal constrictive bandages/dressings
Prevention of positive fluid balance after initial resuscitation
Diuresis or ultrafiltration
Use of hypertonic crystalloids or colloids to expand intravascular compartment
Goal directed resuscitation
Successful outcome depends on early recognition, early conservative treatment to reduce IAH and decompression laparotomy if ACS develops.

channel blockers in cases of hypertension in the first 24 to 48 hours may be needed.

Spinal cord ischemia (SCI)—Surgical and endovascular repair of thoracoabdominal aneurysm is associated with a significant risk of spinal cord ischemia at the rate of 5% to 21%.[11] More common with TAAA and TAA than with AAA, but can occasionally be seen with high AAA or AAA in the setting of prior TAA. The etiology is likely multifactorial involving interference with cord blood supply, prolonged intraoperative hypotension, extended aortic cross-clamping time and aortic embolization. None of these are, however, solely responsible for SCI. The spinal cord depends on more than the artery of Adamkiewicz for perfusion; it relies on a complex network of flow from the vertebral arteries, intercostal arteries, lumbar arteries, and hypogastric arteries. Classical symptoms are lower extremity sensory and motor deficits with bowel/bladder incontinence with conservation of vibration and proprioception sense. SCI can also be seen after TEVAR. The subset of this population that remain at a higher risk are as follows: prior history of aortic surgery, a previous stent graft placement, aortic graft covering more than 20 cm, aortic graft covering the subclavian artery without revascularization, and graft placement in the high-risk zone between T8 and T12.

All patients at a high risk for spinal cord ischemia should be strongly considered for prophylactic CSF drainage with a CSF lumbar catheter placed in the preoperative period to optimize spinal cord perfusion.[12] CSF is drained to achieve target pressures of 10 to 12 mm Hg. The MAP is maintained between 80 and 100 mm Hg to optimize the spinal cord perfusion pressure[13] (MAP – CSF pressure = spinal cord perfusion pressure).

However, patients who develop clinical features suggestive of cord ischemia should have prompt elevation of the blood pressure to maintain mean arterial pressures between 80 and 100 mm Hg using crystalloids, colloids or even vasopressors such as phenylephrine. These patients should then have an emergent CSF drain placed if a preoperative drain is not in place.

Acutely, an initial 20 cc of CSF is drained and opening pressure should be checked. Subsequently 10 cc of CSF is drained every 1 hour to achieve a target spinal fluid pressure of 10 to 12 mm Hg. Careful monitoring of the CSF pressures with intermittent drainage should be done in the ICU to minimize the

TABLE 56–2 Management of spinal cord ischemia.

Management of Spinal Cord Ischemia
Symptoms of acute spinal cord ischemia (lower extremity sensory/motor deficits or bowel/bladder incontinence)
Maintain MAP between 80-100 mm Hg (with crystalloids/colloids/pressures)
Place emergent lumbar CSF catheter
Drain 20 cc CSF and check opening pressure
Subsequently drain 10 cc/h until you achieve opening pressure of 10-12 mm Hg

risk of subdural hematoma. Overaggressive drainage can result in intracranial hemorrhage and/or herniation (see Table 56–2 for management of spinal cord ischemia).

Optimizing spinal cord perfusion has been shown to result in marked clinical improvement if implemented early.

ISCHEMIC COLITIS

Ischemic colitis is a well-described complication following open and endovascular aortic aneurysm repair; however, it is also noted to occur after aortoiliac revascularization and repair of aortic dissection.[14] Ligation of inferior mesenteric artery and subsequent interruption to flow is the commonly implicated etiology of colitis following major aortic surgery.

Following open repair, larger perioperative fluid shifts, longer aortic cross-clamping time, compressive retroperitoneal hematoma and prolonged hypotension; all of which lead to a state of hypoperfusion seems to be the underlying etiology of the ensuing bowel ischemia and subsequent necrosis. However, the implicated pathogenesis following endovascular procedure also includes embolization of the cholesterol plaque. This is suspected to occur after placement of the stent graft or following manipulation of the aortic aneurysmal sac with catheters and guide wires. The inflammatory response is more pronounced following cholesterol embolization and tends to portend a poorer outcome. Peri-EVAR hypogastric occlusion for complex aneurysm morphologies is also a risk factor.

The presentation of ischemic colitis includes fever, abdominal pain, and distension, increased peristalsis with often, but not always, bloody diarrhea in the immediate postoperative phase. Abdominal examination might vary from localized tenderness to diffuse peritonitis. Laboratory values range from leukocytosis with left shift, lactic acidosis (a useful early and consistent marker of bowel ischemia) with metabolic acidosis, significant electrolyte abnormalities, and eventual hemodynamic instability if abdominal sepsis ensues.

Early recognition is vital and the diagnosis requires a high index of suspicion as the initial picture might sometimes only reveal vague abdominal pain and a gradually rising lactate in the setting of fever and leukocytosis. When the diagnosis is suspected, fluid resuscitation and broad spectrum antibiotics aimed at colonic flora should be started.

The diagnostic test of choice is sigmoidoscopy or colonoscopy (done as routine postoperative screening in some centers) with findings ranging from superficial ulcerations, mucosal erythema to mucosal sloughing and full thickness necrosis. CT imaging with contrast is also recommended which might reveal wall thickening, mesenteric fat stranding, mucosal enhancement, intramural air, colonic dilation and in advanced cases portal venous air. CT or endoscopy findings suggestive of mucosal or full thickness transmural involvement, in addition to the patients' hemodynamic status will determine need for surgical intervention versus supportive measures alone, with the unstable patient showing evidence of transmural necrosis necessitating immediate colon resection.

Supportive measures include adequate fluid resuscitation and blood pressure support. Use of vasopressors in the setting of bowel ischemia though controversial is necessary in the background of requiring an adequate blood pressure. If vasopressors are needed then beta adrenergic agonists that improve cardiac output are recommended over alpha agonists. Broad spectrum antibiotics should be initiated empirically covering gram negative and anaerobic organisms, after blood cultures are drawn. There is a high degree of risk of bacterial translocation with a breach in bowel wall mucosa.

In most cases of ischemic colitis, surgical intervention leading to a left colectomy with colostomy is required. Ischemic colitis should be differentiated from acute mesenteric ischemia (AMI). The clinical deterioration in AMI is much more profound and the lactic acidosis is more pronounced. With colitis, the pain may be localized to the LLQ. With AMI, the pain is usually generalized and out of proportion to the physical exam. Eventually frank generalized peritonitis ensues.

AORTIC DISSECTION

Aortic dissection occurs secondary to a tear within the aortic wall that is propagated by the aortic pulse wave.[15] Studies indicate an incidence of 3 cases per 100,000 in a year.

A preceding history of strenuous exercise or drug use (cocaine, amphetamine) is highly suggestive of acute aortic dissection. The presentation is sometimes complicated by malperfusion syndromes, aortic rupture, acute valvular insufficiency, and cardiac tamponade. Malperfusion can manifest in a wide range of organ dysfunctions based on the branch vessel that is obstructed. Malperfusion syndrome is defined as the loss of blood supply to a vital organ caused by a branch arterial obstruction secondary to the dissection. This obstruction can be fixed or dynamic.[16] Fixed obstruction is less common and results in a nonreversible branch vessel occlusion. Commonly, the branch vessel obstruction is dynamic. In this form of obstruction, the branch is compressed with each cardiac pulsation. The result of both forms of obstruction is end-organ ischemia, with possible malfunction and infarction if not corrected in a timely fashion. Reducing the heart rate is first priority. A reduced number of pulsations results in less dynamic compression and reduces the likelihood of propagation. Once the heart rate is controlled then, the blood pressure should be reduced.

Types of Dissections

The classification of aortic dissection is based on anatomic location of entry tear and/or the extent of the dissection flap. This information is crucial to the management of the dissection. It drives the decision to proceed with surgical or medical management. The commonly used classifications are the Stanford[16] and DeBakey[17] systems, as listed in Table 56–3 (see Figure 56–3 for diaphragmatic representation of the above classifications).

TABLE 56–3 DeBakey and Stanford classification.

DeBakey
- Category I: Dissection tear in the ascending aorta propagating distally to include at least the aortic arch and typically the descending aorta
- Category II: Dissection tear only in the ascending aorta
- Category III: Dissection tear in the descending aorta propagating most often distally
- Category IIIa: Dissection tear only in the descending thoracic aorta
- Category IIIb: Tear extending below the diaphragm

Stanford
- Type A: All dissections involving the ascending aorta irrespective of the site of tear
- Type B: All dissections that do not involve the ascending aorta; note that involvement of the aortic arch without involvement of the ascending aorta in the Stanford classificationn is labelled as type B

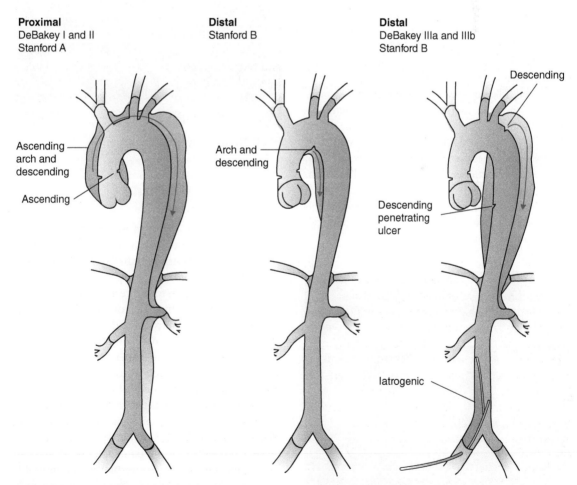

Proximal
DeBakey I and II
Stanford A

Distal
Stanford B

Distal
DeBakey IIIa and IIIb
Stanford B

FIGURE 56–3 Stanford and DeBakey classification. (*Reproduced with permission from Nienaber CA, Clough RE: Management of acute aortic dissection,* Lancet. *2015 Feb 28;385(9970):800-811.*)

The highest mortality is in the first 48 hours, hence early recognition is very important. It becomes especially critical in younger patients, those with connective tissues diseases and in women who can present with atypical symptoms and signs.

Diagnostic Evaluation

Chest X ray: Demonstrates widened mediastinum, double or irregular aortic contour. It may also be normal.

EKG: May show signs of coronary malperfusion.

Labs: Elevated cardiac enzymes, LFT, lactate.

CT angiography (CTA) is the investigation of choice.[18] It is widely available, fast, and noninvasive. It helps to diagnose and classify dissection and also enables early identification of distal complications with detailed views of cardiac, thoracic, and vascular anatomy (see Figure 56–4 for axial and Figure 56–5 for coronal CT scan view of type B dissection).

Transthoracic ECHO (TTE)—In a hemodynamically unstable patient, focused cardiac ultrasound by a trained intensivist can help with time sensitive assessment and evaluation of aortic root size, valvular function and the presence of dissection.

Transesophageal ECHO (TEE)—Offers much better imaging and spatial resolution for evaluation of primary tear, secondary communication and true lumen compression.

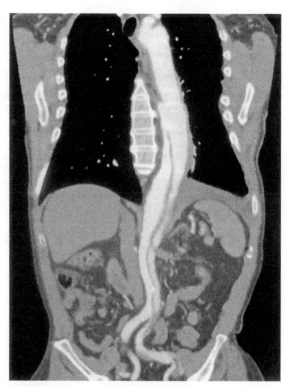

FIGURE 56–5 Type B aortic dissection.

Management of Acute Aortic Dissection

Type A dissection—Patients with acute type A dissection who do not receive treatment die at a rate of 1% to 2% per hour during the first day and almost half die by 1 week. Therefore, emergent surgical repair is an absolute indication for acute ascending aortic dissection as there is a high risk of mortality given the imminent danger of retrograde dissection and all the previously discussed cardiac complications.

Type B dissection—Patients with uncomplicated descending thoracic aortic dissection are traditionally treated with medical therapy. In addition to medical management, complicated dissections (malperfusion, aneurysm, and refractory pain) require early TEVAR ± adjunctive procedures as needed vs open surgical repair. Open surgical repair has a high perioperative morbidity and mortality and is rarely a treatment of choice. More recently, the trend is toward endovascular management of high-risk type B dissections, even if uncomplicated.

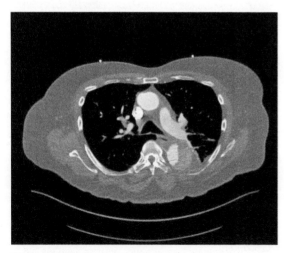

FIGURE 56–4 Type B aortic dissection.

High-risk patients include those with patent and large false lumens (> 22 mm) and those with aortas measuring more than 4 cm at initial presentation. Ideally, this treatment should be offered to those with a life expectancy of approximately 5 years. Endovascular treatment of high-risk uncomplicated type B dissections should be performed during the subacute phase (2-6 weeks) if possible.[19]

ICU Management

Patients with profound hemodynamic instability need to be intubated and ventilated without delay.

Medical therapy is imperative in the management of Stanford type A and type B dissections. Medical management hinges on limiting propagation of the intimal tear and reducing blood pressure over time (dP/dT). Close monitoring in an ICU with an aim to achieve rapid reduction in heart rate and normalization of blood pressure is critical. Importantly, ensuring adequate analgesia to prevent a pain induced catecholamine response, which will cause increased shear stress on the intimal wall, is imperative. Constant vigilance for any evidence of organ or limb malperfusion is also fundamental in the management of these tenuous patients.

Impulse Control

The goal is to reduce left ventricular contractility, prevent and avoid tachycardia to decrease the shear force and hence minimize propagation of the intimal tear. The aim is to achieve a target systolic blood pressure of 100 to 120 mm Hg and a heart rate of 60 to 75. This is best achieved by IV beta blockade such as labetalol and esmolol. Esmolol has the advantage of a shorter half-life and thus potentially less risky to use in patients with intolerance to beta blockade such as those with asthma and heart failure.

If after beta blockade, the blood pressure still remains elevated, then an IV nitroprusside drip or IV calcium channel blockers can be added. Nitroprusside should not be used without prior beta blockade, as the vasodilation alone can cause reflex tachycardia and increased left ventricular contractility and worsening wall shear stress. Hydralazine is generally avoided because it increases aortic wall shear stress. All these patients should be monitored in an ICU setting with an arterial catheter preferably in the arm with the higher blood pressure.

Pain control—In most cases pain is an indication of persistent dissection and resolution of the pain can be a marker of halting dissection. Persistent pain evokes a strong catecholamine response and can aggravate the tachycardia causing an increase in the shear stress. Hence good pain control with narcotics such as morphine or hydromorphone should be given with close monitoring of respiratory status and hemodynamic parameters in an ICU.

Recognition of malperfusion—As previously stated the need for early recognition and high clinical index of suspicion for organ and limb malperfusion is imperative for appropriate management of type B dissection. Always look for evidence of organ malperfusion with laboratory evidence of lactic acidosis, metabolic acidosis, probable rhabdomyolysis (in cases of limb ischemia, abdominal ischemia) such as CPK elevation, urine myoglobin, and organ-specific enzyme elevation. In a system-based approach watching for clinical exam findings as listed in Table 56–4 is necessary.

TABLE 56–4 Malperfusion syndromes.

Anatomic Complications	Symptoms and Signs
Carotid malperfusion	Syncope, focal neurologic deficits
Spinal malperfusion	Paraparesis and paraplegia
Aortic valvular insufficiency	Early diastolic murmur, dyspnea
Coronary malperfusion with myocardial ischemia	Anginal chest pain, dyspnea, ischemic changes in EKG
Pericardial tamponade	Dyspnea, pulsus paradoxus, jugular venous distension, muffled heart sounds
Subclavian or iliofemoral artery malperfusion	Pulse deficit, cold, painful extremity, sensory, motor deficit, syncope
Mesenteric malperfusion	Nausea, vomiting, abdominal pain
Renal malperfusion	Oliguria, anuria, hematuria, AKI

CAROTID ARTERY STENOSIS

The location most frequently affected by carotid atherosclerosis is the carotid bifurcation, often with extension into the proximal internal carotid artery (ie, the origin). Progression of atheromatous plaque at the carotid bifurcation results in luminal narrowing, often accompanied by ulceration. This process can lead to ischemic stroke or transient ischemic attack (TIA) from embolization, thrombosis, or hemodynamic compromise (see Figure 56–6 for CT imaging of severe carotid disease).

Carotid artery stenting is a less invasive alternative to endarterectomy. There is a higher risk of periprocedural stroke with angioplasty and stenting limited to patients who are older than 70 years. There is, however, a greater risk of myocardial infarction (nonfatal), cranial nerve palsy (usually transient), and surgical-site hematoma with endarterectomy.[20]

Postoperatively most of these patients might require closer monitoring and care in an intermediate care unit such as a step down unit.

Carotid surgery is unique in that 1 of the principal components of the physiologic control mechanism of arterial pressure, the baroreceptors in the carotid sinus, are involved in the disease process itself, and may be affected by the surgical procedure, concurrent therapy, and by anesthesia.

Postcarotid endarterectomy—Carotid baroreceptor denervation causes increased arterial pressure variability.[21]

Bradycardia can be seen perioperatively and intraoperatively. Hypotension or hypertension can be seen. It is imperative to aggressively treat postoperative hypertension in these patients, as it can predispose to cerebral edema, cerebral hyperperfusion syndrome and intracerebral hemorrhage. Elevations in blood pressure with SBP more than 160 mm Hg can be controlled by nitroglycerine drip or nicardipine drip. Low blood pressure with SBP less than 90 mm Hg can be treated with phenylephrine drip.

Postcarotid artery stenting—Stretching of the vessel by the balloon or the stent and stimulation of the carotid baroreceptors can lead to a fall in the vascular tone leading to transient hypotension or bradycardia. Most often the hypotension is transient and resolves in time. Acutely, bradycardia can be managed with atropine or glycopyrrolate. If persistent, a phenylephrine drip may be needed until spontaneous hemodynamic stability is achieved. The baroreceptor may take hours to days to regulate. Early ambulation and activity help achieve a new steady state.

Bradycardia can often be observed in a cardiac monitoring unit, however, in rare cases of symptomatic bradycardia with rates below 40, we recommend atropine at doses of 0.5 mg IV push up to a total of 3 mg. Pacing is rarely needed.

ACUTE LIMB ISCHEMIA

Acute arterial insufficiency of the lower extremity presents abruptly with the classical features of ischemia—pain, pallor, pulselessness, paresthesias, and paralysis.

Traditionally, the most common cause was arterial embolization from cardiac sources. With improved anticoagulation and arrhythmia management, arterial thrombosis in the setting of known arterial disease is now the most common cause of arterial ischemia. Other causes include direct arterial trauma, aortic dissection, venous outflow obstruction or low-flow states.

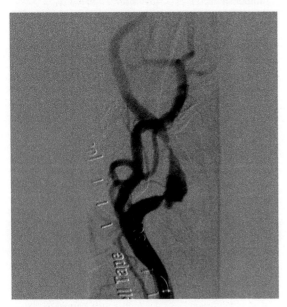

FIGURE 56–6 Severe carotid disease.

TABLE 56–5 Rutherford classification of acute limb ischemia.

Category	Description/Prognosis	Findings		Doppler Signals	
		Sensory loss	Muscle weakness	Arterial	Venous
I. Viable	Not immediately threatened	None	None	Audible	Audible
II. Threatened					
a. Marginally	Salvageable if promptly treated	Minimal (toes) or none	None	Inaudible	Audible
b. Immediately	Salvageable with immediate revascularization	More than toes associated with rest pain	Mild/moderate	Inaudible	Audible
III. Irreversible	Major tissue loss or permanent nerve damage inevitable	Profound anesthetic	Profound paralysis (rigor)	Inaudible	Inaudible

The Rutherford classification of acute limb ischemia is used to correlate the clinical findings and site of arterial occlusion (refer Table 56–5). If history and physical examination are clearly demonstrative of acute limb ischemia there should not be any delay in initiating definitive treatment.

Management is primarily divided into surgical or endovascular revascularization. There are many possible surgical options. Endovascular treatments often include thrombolysis. All patients treated with continuous thrombolytic infusions should be admitted to an ICU or step-down unit bed for closer monitoring.

Continuous thrombolytic therapy is used as an alternative to open surgical procedures or to treat residual clot after percutaneous thrombectomy. Lytic therapy is instilled through an infusion catheter positioned in the thrombus. Despite its association with a higher frequency of hemorrhagic complications, intra-arterial infusion of urokinase reduced the need for open surgical procedures, with no significantly increased risk of amputation or death.[22] Currently used agents are alteplase, reteplase, and urokinase. Doses are as follows:

Alteplase: continuous, 0.5 to 1.0 mg/kg/h (40 mg maximum); bolus, 2 to 5 mg bolus, then continuous infusion; pulse spray, 0.5 mg/mL at 0.2 mL every 30 to 60 seconds.

Reteplase: continuous, 0.25 to 0.5 U/h (20 units maximum); bolus, 2 to 5 U bolus, then continuous infusion.[23]

Based on the TOPAS trial it is now recommended to start the patient on a concurrent subtherapeutic dose of heparin which is given through the arterial sheath to prevent pericatheter arterial thrombosis. Heparin is administered at a subtherapeutic dose to avoid the risk of major intracranial hemorrhage. Heparin is infused at a rate of 200 to 500 units/h when given with intra-arterial TPA with a goal PTT 1.25 to 1.5 times control.

Twenty four hours after initiation of the thrombolytic agents patients are taken back to the angiography suite for reassessment of vessel patency.

In the ICU monitor the following:

1. Blood loss—Assessed by clinical exam and laboratory findings on complete blood count, coagulation parameters (PT, aPTT, fibrinogen, fibrin degradation products). If there is access site bleeding, turn off the thrombolytic agent for 1 hour, and reassess the patient's clinical exam and laboratory parameters. If normal, then restart at the same initial dose or reduced. Any evidence of severe blood loss requires prompt reevaluation by the vascular surgery team, resuscitation, and an early CT scan to assess for retroperitoneal bleeding.

2. Fibrinogen level and coagulation parameters every 6 hours—The risk of major bleeding increases when the fibrinogen level drops to less than 100 mg/dL or the PTT increases to 3 to 5 times the normal. If the fibrinogen

level is less than 100 turn off the thrombolytic infusion and reassess the fibrinogen level in 6 hours. Once normalized then restart the infusion at half the initial dose.

3. Stroke—Neurochecks every hour is needed to assess for hemorrhagic stroke. If a neurologic deficit becomes obvious, all thrombolytics and anticoagulants must be held. Emergency neurology consultation and head CT are needed.

Complications

Rhabdomyolysis secondary to acute reperfusion injury is manifested by markedly elevated CPK levels, lactic acidosis, myoglobinuria, hyperkalemia, and acute kidney injury. All these laboratory parameters should be frequently monitored in an ICU. It is essentially treated with aggressive hydration and if necessary with urinary alkalinization.

Compartment syndrome is a dreaded complication sometimes requiring a 4 compartment fasciotomy. Compartment syndrome can be diagnosed clinically or by finding compartment pressures greater than 30 mm Hg. In the ICU, the diagnosis can be occult and a high index of suspicion is needed. Prophylactic fasciotomy should be done in anyone with more than 6 hours of ischemia or anyone with an unreliable exam.

REFERENCES

1. Kent KC. Clinical practice. Abdominal aortic aneurysms. *N Engl J Med*. 2014;371(22):2101-2108.
2. Badger S, Bedenis R, Blair PH, Ellis P, Kee F, Harkin DW. Endovascular treatment for ruptured abdominal aortic aneurysm. *Cochrane Database Syst Rev*. 2014;7:CD005261.
3. Sweeting MJ, Ulug P, Powell JT, Desgranges P, Balm R; Ruptured Aneurysm Trialists. Ruptured aneurysm trials: the importance of longer-term outcomes and meta-analysis for 1-year mortality. *Eur J Vasc Endovasc Surg*. 2015;50(3):297-302.
4. Grieve R, Gomes M, Sweeting MJ, et al. Endovascular strategy or open repair for ruptured abdominal aortic aneurysm: one-year outcomes from the IMPROVE randomized trial. *Eur Heart J*. 2015;36(31):2061-2069.
5. Health Quality Ontario. Fenestrated endovascular grafts for the repair of juxtarenal aortic aneurysms: an evidence-based analysis. *Ont Health Technol Assess Ser*. 2009;9(4):1-51.
6. Dias NV, Resch TA, Sonesson B, Ivancev K, Malina M. EVAR of aortoiliac aneurysms with branched stent-grafts. *Eur J Vasc Endovasc Surg*. 2008;35(6):677-684.
7. Elefteriades JA, Farkas EA. Thoracic aortic aneurysm: clinically pertinent controversies and uncertainties. *J Am Coll Cardiol*. 2010;55(9):841-857.
8. Saratzis AN, Goodyear S, Sur H, Saedon M, Imray C, Mahmood A. Acute kidney injury after endovascular repair of abdominal aortic aneurysm. *J Endovasc Ther*. 2013;20(3):315-330.
9. Djavani K, Wanhainen A, Valtysson J, Björck M. Colonic ischaemia and intra-abdominal hypertension following open repair of ruptured abdominal aortic aneurysm. *Br J Surg*. 2009;96:621-627.
10. Bajardi G, Pecoraro F, Mirabella D, Bracale UM, Bellisi MG. Abdominal compartment syndrome (ACS) after abdominal aortic aneurysm (AAA) open repair. *Ann Ital Chir*. 2009;80(5):369-374.
11. Gravereaux EC, Faries PL, Burks JA, et al. Risk of spinal cord ischemia after endograft repair of thoracic aortic aneurysms. *J Vasc Surg*. 2001;34(6):997-1003.
12. Kotelis D, Bianchini C, Kovacs B, Müller T, Bischoff M, Böckler D. Early experience with automatic pressure-controlled cerebrospinal fluid drainage during thoracic endovascular aortic repair. *J Endovasc Ther*. 2015;22(3):368-372.
13. Hnath JC, Mehta M, Taggert JB, et al. Strategies to improve spinal cord ischemia in endovascular thoracic aortic repair: outcomes of a prospective cerebrospinal fluid drainage protocol. *J Vasc Surg*. 2008;48(4):836-840.
14. Steele SR. Ischemic colitis complicating major vascular surgery. *Surg Clin North Am*. 2007;87(5):1099-1114.
15. Erbel R, Alfonso F, Boileau C, et al. Diagnosis and management of aortic dissection—recommendations of the Task Force on Aortic Dissection, European Society of Cardiology. *Eur Heart J*. 2001;22:1642-1681.
16. Daily PO, Trueblood HW, Stinson EB, Wuerflein RD, Shumway NE. Management of acute aortic dissections. *Ann Thorac Surg*. 1970;10(3):237-247.
17. Brunner NW, Ignaszewski A. Aortic interlude: Dr Michael DeBakey, aortic dissection, and screening recommendations for abdominal aortic aneurysm. *BCMJ*. 2011;53(2):79-85.

18. Hagan PG, Nienaber CA, Isselbacher EM, et al. The International Registry of Acute Aortic Dissection (IRAD): new insights into an old disease. *JAMA*. 2000;283:897-903.

19. Fattori R, Cao P, De Rango P. Interdisciplinary expert consensus document on management of type B aortic dissection. *J Am Coll Cardiol*. 2013;61(16):1661-1678.

20. Bonati L. Stenting or endarterectomy for patients with symptomatic carotid stenosis. *Neurol Clin*. 2015;33(2):459-474.

21. Stoneham MD, Thompson JP. Arterial pressure management and carotid endarterectomy. *Br J Anaesth*. 2009;102(4):442-452.

22. Ouriel K, Veith FJ, Sasahara AA. A comparison of recombinant urokinase with vascular surgery as initial treatment for acute arterial occlusion of the legs. Thrombolysis or Peripheral Arterial Surgery (TOPAS) Investigators. *N Engl J Med*. 1998;338:1105-1111.

23. Morrison HL. Catheter-directed thrombolysis for acute limb ischemia. *Semin Intervent Radiol*. 2006;23(3):258-269.

24. Nienaber CA, Clough RE. Management of acute aortic dissection. *Lancet*. 2015;385(9970):800-811.

Smoke Exposure Models in COPD

Patrick Geraghty, PhD and Robert Foronjy, MD

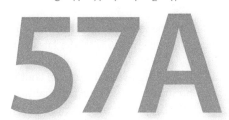

KEY POINTS

1. COPD is a leading cause of death worldwide and the lack of effective therapies and continued smoking prevalence indicate that this will be a major public health challenge confronting physicians for years to come.

2. COPD is a frequent cause of ICU admission and the diagnosis of COPD in ICU patients increases the risk of ICU delirium, ARDS, and in-hospital and postdischarge mortality.

3. Our limited understanding of the pathogenesis of COPD has hindered advancements in treatment of this disease highlighting the need for more basic and clinical research.

4. Animal models of COPD, particularly the cigarette smoke exposure model, reproduce key features of the disease providing the opportunity to gain key disease insights within a relatively short time frame.

5. Findings from animal models have identified the importance of inflammation, proteases, oxidants, and apoptosis in the pathophysiology of this disease. Furthermore, these studies have established key injury repair mechanisms that are activated in the lung in COPD.

6. The findings from these studies could lead to targeted strategies that block damaging injury responses and enhance protective lung repair responses in this disease.

THE SIGNIFICANCE OF CHRONIC OBSTRUCTIVE PULMONARY DISEASE

Chronic obstructive pulmonary disease (COPD) is defined as a disease state characterized by airflow limitation that is not fully reversible.[1] The limitation in airflow is caused by airway inflammation,[2] loss of lung elasticity,[3] lung tissue destruction,[4] and the closure of small airways.[5,6] The airflow obstruction progresses over time and loss of lung function impairs the ability of individuals to carry out routine daily activities and greatly increases their risk of death. Indeed, COPD is now the third leading cause of death in the United States and is projected to become the third leading cause worldwide within the next 20 years.[7,8] While the age-adjusted mortality for cardiovascular diseases had decreased significantly over the past 3 decades, the age-adjusted mortality for COPD has increased over this time period[9] highlighting the need for better therapies[10,11] and increased COPD research. It is well known that exposure to cigarette smoke, both first and second hand, is the primary etiologic factor associated with this disease. Although great strides have been made in reducing smoking prevalence in the United States, 43.8 millions people or 19.0% of the United States population (age 18 or older) continue to smoke.[12]

Moreover, smoking remains a major public health issue for adolescents with the latest surveys showing that 16% of all eighth graders had tried smoking and 17% of high school students continue smoking beyond graduation.[13] Internationally, the picture is even bleaker with a smoking prevalence of 28% in China,[14] 27% in Germany, and 36% in Russia.[15,16] These figures ensure that this disease will be a major public health issue for the foreseeable future.

While cigarette consumption is the main risk factor for COPD, 10% to 15% of COPD cases are not related to cigarette smoke exposure.[17] In the developing world, it is estimated that air pollution from biomass smoke accounts for 2.2 to 2.5 million deaths annually.[18] Epidemiologic studies have implicated biomass use in the development of chronic obstructive pulmonary disease (COPD) in adults and acute lower respiratory infection in children.[19,20] Women are particularly affected given their daily usage of these fuel sources for cooking. Moreover, exposure in women begins early in life and continues for decades.[21] Indeed, several studies have found increased markers of inflammation and oxidative stress in premenopausal women exposed to biomass smoke.[22-24] Worldwide, it is estimated that 3 billion people utilize biomass as their primary source of domestic energy.[25] Though plans are underway to distribute improved cook stoves that emit less harmful particulates, these efforts will take time and a continued commitment on the part of public health authorities to impact on the development of COPD in these impoverished communities. Data obtained from cigarette smoking studies suggest that despite discontinuing smoking the rate of progression of COPD does reduce, but it does not prevent persistent airway inflammation and significant progression of COPD observed by CT scan.[2] Therefore, a large percentage of the current 3 billion people utilizing biomass sources may already have irreversible inflammation and COPD.

THE IMPACT OF COPD ON CRITICAL CARE

Acute episodes of respiratory distress in patients with COPD account for up to 5% to 10% of all emergency medical admissions[26] and almost 10%

of these patients are referred to the ICU for further management.[27] Hospital mortality for those admitted with COPD is 5.6% and approximately 18% of COPD subjects will die within 180 days posthospital discharge. Historically, COPD patients that develop respiratory failure without a precipitating cause (pneumonia, pneumothorax, pulmonary embolism) have been perceived to have very poor outcomes. Indeed, in the United Kingdom, patients with COPD exacerbation were infrequently admitted to the ICU and withdrawal of treatment was the most common cause of death in these individuals after admission.[28] However, the data shows that survival following mechanical ventilation is actually better when no causative factor is identified for an exacerbation.[29] Thus, a COPD patient who presents with isolated respiratory failure cannot be "written off" as a lost cause. Short-term survival following an episode of mechanical ventilation for COPD ranges from 63% to 86%.[30-32] In contrast, long-range survival rates are worse—52%, 42%, and 37% at 1, 2, and 3 years.[28] Determining who will benefit from critical care utilization is difficult. Though medical comorbidities, prolonged (> 72 hours) mechanical ventilation and failure postextubation predict poor outcome,[31] national guidelines do not currently support the use of clinical scoring systems for management of COPD exacerbations.[33] Thus, physicians have little to guide them when judging the appropriateness of critical care intervention in this population.

While many patients make excellent recoveries, others that survive COPD exacerbations suffer with chronic critical illness that impairs their quality of life and causes tremendous financial hardships for their families. Overall, it is estimated that between 5% and 10% of patients requiring mechanical ventilation for acute respiratory failure will develop chronic critical illness.[34-36] The cost of caring for these patients is estimated to be over 20 billion in the United States and will likely rise as the population continues to age.[37] Delirium is a serious adverse event that complicates the management of ICU patients and increases their morbidity and mortality.[38] The diagnosis of COPD has been identified as an independent risk factor for delirium in cardiothoracic ICU patients.[39] In addition, COPD has been reported to increase the risk of developing ARDS in ICU patients.[40,41] The specific mechanisms responsible for this increased susceptibility have yet to be determined. Clearly, an enhanced understanding of the underlying disease pathogenesis is needed for improved prognostication and to develop better means of treating this disease and preventing its associated complications in the ICU.

COPD research funding has been disproportionately low given its impact on public health.[42] This is undoubtedly due to the fact that this is perceived as a "self-inflicted" disease. For the most part, if people did not smoke they would not develop the disease and if they stopped smoking the disease, if present, would not progress as quickly. This naturally raises the question why should scarce public research dollars be used to investigate a disease that has such a clear-cut solution? However, this perspective clearly ignores the history of this product over the past century. Cigarettes are not marketed toward 20, 30, or 40 years olds.[43] Rather, cigarettes, whether in print, sporting events or the movies are aggressively pitched towards adolescents.[44] This is a group that is more susceptible to peer pressure and influence and less able to gauge the true risks of this habit. In fact, billions of dollars are spent annually marketing this product to young people worldwide.[45] Unfortunately, adolescents and the public as a whole have a very poor understanding of the addictive potential of this product. Cigarettes are not ground up tobacco leaves wrapped in paper. They are a carefully engineered product laced with chemicals, such as ammonia that speed the absorption of nicotine in the body.[46] Nicotine reaches the brain within seconds of a puff on a cigarette creating a sensation of euphoria.[47] These rapid effects are powerfully reinforcing psychologically and help to explain why smoking cessation success rates are so poor.[48] There are 17 nicotinic acetylcholine receptor subunits in humans that trigger multiple responses.[49] Cigarettes are a legal product and tobacco companies are permitted to spend billions of dollars to get people to try their product despite the potential of addiction and reliance on this product. Given this current state of affairs, those who suffer from COPD are as deserving of effective treatments as those who suffer from other lifestyle influenced conditions such as diabetes, hypertension, and heart disease. Equally, there are numerous clinical manifestations that occur with second hand smoking, with individuals who involuntarily undergoing smoke exposure. Thus, there is an urgent need to better understand the pathogenic processes that cause this disease so that more effective therapies can be developed.

THE DEVELOPMENT OF ANIMAL MODELS OF COPD

While we know that cigarette smoke exposure will induce pathologic effects in the lungs of smokers, the mechanisms by which cigarette smoke mediates these changes remain incompletely understood. Studies in humans frequently utilize biological materials from patients who are already in the advanced stages of the disease. Although helpful, these studies may not provide insights into the processes by which cigarette smoke promotes the development of the disease state in the lung. Performing prospective studies in humans could address these limitations; however, such studies would be time-consuming and expensive as COPD is an insidious disease that evolves over many years.[50] Over the long term, it would be difficult to perform these analyses in a rigorous scientific manner that would limit the confounding effects of other dietary, genetic and environmental variables. Moreover, obtaining biological specimens over this length of time would be costly and require years to answer scientific questions. For this reason, animal models of COPD are needed to better understand the underlying disease mechanisms. After Laurell and Erickson's observation that A1AT (alpha-1-anti-trypsin) deficiency resulted in the premature development of emphysema,[51,52] the role of elastase in this disease became center focus. A1AT protein is an abundant circulating antiprotease that binds and neutralizes neutrophil elastase within the lung.[53] Thus, it was postulated that the unopposed action of elastase would degrade elastin, which is abundant in the alveolar wall, thereby causing the destruction of lung tissue.[54] This theory was further supported by the finding that intratracheal elastase induced the development of emphysema in rats.[55] This was one of the first animal models of the disease and it had a tremendous influence on the research direction of the pulmonary field for the subsequent 30 years. After this discovery, emphysema was primarily regarded as a disease of elastin degradation that resulted from an elastase/anti-elastase imbalance in the lung. Although this model provided important insights into the disease, it had numerous shortcomings that limited its applicability to the human disease. For one, emphysema in this animal model develops within 3 weeks of exposure.[56] This rapid onset of development does not mimic the human disease, which often takes decades to develop. Thus, it is likely that distinct biological processes are responsible for the pathologic changes that are required for disease initiation and progression to occur. Secondly, by its design, the elastase animal model cannot address the impact of cigarette smoke exposure on the lung. Although cigarette smoke induces expression, release and activation of lung elastases,[57,58] it also triggers a myriad of other effects that will not be replicated by an elastase disease model. Thirdly, the elastase model reproduces the alveolar destruction that occurs in emphysema but it does not replicate other disease features such as mucus plugging, bronchiolitis and altered lung inflammation.[59] Indeed, the hallmark features of human COPD such as chronic lung inflammation, impaired lung function, emphysema, mucus hypersecretion, vascular injury, and small airway remodeling are not well represented in this model. Thus, researchers have sought to utilize smoke exposure models to gain more relevant insights into the disease.

Developing a smoke exposure model that would generate emphysematous changes was a laborious process. The early attempts to develop smoke exposure models were complicated by the long exposure time required to develop the disease and the variable effects of cigarette smoke in the exposed animals. Indeed, some of the first studies reported cellular proliferation and mucus metaplasia but not the classical alveolar destruction seen in the human disease.[60-62] Hautamaki et al were the first group to successfully overcome these challenges in a mouse exposure model.[63] In their model, they used a pump to circulate the cigarette smoke generated by the burning of 2 cigarettes to a Plexiglas chamber containing the mice. Carbon monoxide (CO) measurements showed that the mice had CO levels that were comparable to human smokers. By exposing mice in this manner daily for several months they successfully generated alveolar destruction within the lungs of the exposed mice. Moreover, they demonstrated

that this destruction was dependent on the expression of an elastase, matrix metalloproteinase-12 (MMP-12). Establishing an emphysema model that successfully generated alveolar destruction was one of the most important accomplishments in the pulmonary field in the past 2 decades. Today, investigators are actively using variations of this model to obtain important new insights into the mechanisms of this disease.

The 2 most common smoke exposure models that have been utilized are the nose only and the whole body exposure apparatus.

The nose only system requires restraining the mouse so that their nose is inserted into a cone where they inhale the cigarette smoke.[64] This generates a uniform exposure that produces emphysematous changes. However, the prolonged periods of restraint are stressful for the mice and the machine can usually accommodate only a limited number of mice (eg, the Jaeger system has 18 ports which is depicted in Figure 57A–1A). In contrast, whole body exposure systems expose mice to a mixture of both passive and mainstream smoke released from a burning cigarette and mainstream smoke, which is actually smoke aspirated through the cigarette using a pump.[65] The passive and mainstream smoke streams are mixed and then propelled by a fan to a chamber containing the mice that are housed within their cages. The advantage of this system is that the mice freely move about and have access to food and water (Figure 57A–1B). Thus, mice in this system can be exposed for longer periods of time. In addition, the whole body exposure system allows for the exposure of large groups of mice. Some systems allow the exposure of up to 120 mice at a time enabling researchers to use large numbers of mice and to perform multiple experiments simultaneously. An important note about whole body exposure systems is that the exposure intensity needs to be monitored very carefully. Cigarette smoke is removed from cages via exhaust valves that are typically maintained with a small aperture in order to allow smoke levels to build up within the chambers. Cigarette smoke releases a large amount of tar that can clog these valves and minimize the flow of cigarette smoke, which can allow for smoke levels to build up to toxic levels. If the tar obstruction of the valve becomes too great, all smoke/air flow stops

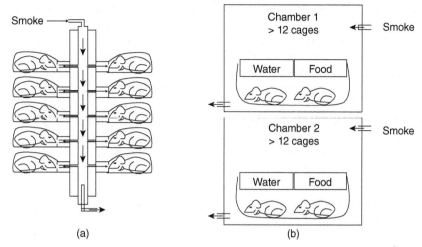

(a)   (b)

FIGURE 57A-1 Typical mouse models for smoke exposure. (A) A nose only cigarette smoke exposure system requires animals to be restrained while they inhale the cigarette smoke. (B) The passive and mainstream smoke streams cigarette smoke exposure system allows animals access to food and water without restraint.

and the mice receive no smoke exposure. Both of these outcomes can ruin a carefully planned experiment. Thus, the mice have to be closely monitored to ensure that airflow is circulating properly and that toxic levels of cigarette smoke are not building up.

This is accomplished by measuring total particulate matter (TPM) concentration within the chamber and carbon monoxide levels in the mice. Typically, the TPM is maintained at 80 to 100 mg/m^3, which will produce CO levels in the mice of 10% to 12%.[65] These levels are well tolerated by the mice and produce the alveolar lung tissue destruction.[63,65] TPM can be monitored using a filter sample unit fitted with a diaphragm pump and a timer. Utilizing sampling air to measure particulate matter in a specific volume sampled over time allows accurate TPM measurements and consistent exposure to animals.

Although many animals have been used in COPD studies, mice offer very clear advantages, which have lead to their becoming the dominant animal model for this disease. For one, mice are small in size and the costs of feeding and housing these animals are far less than dogs, sheep, and large rodents. Also, the mouse genome has been extensively characterized and there is a plethora of antibody, molecular probes and equipment modified for mouse anatomy available for studies in these animals. Likewise, it is far more cost-effective

to generate genetically manipulated mice than it is to do so in other species. The gestational period for a mouse is 21 days compared to a time period of up to 74 days in guinea pigs. This allows investigators to generate large numbers of genetically altered mice in a relatively short period of time. Exposing mice to smoke for 1 year represents approximately 50% of the animal's lifetime, thereby allowing a better representation of lifetime smoke exposure. These cost advantages allow for large numbers of animals to be utilized for smoke exposure studies. This is extremely important when studying this disease, as the effect of cigarette smoke on the lung is highly variable. In humans, some estimates state that only 15% of smokers will develop emphysematous changes in the lung[66] and the susceptibility of mice to cigarette smoke is also quite variable.[65,67] Thus, exposing large numbers of mice increases the power of a study to detect significant differences in emphysema between control and genetically altered mice. The typical enlargement of airways observed after 6 months of smoke exposure is depicted in Figure 57A-2.

Mice provide the best opportunity to investigate the mechanisms of this disease. However, as noted previously, not all strains of mice are equally responsive to cigarette smoke.[65,67] Some strains of mice, such as C57Bl/6J, are relatively resistant to cigarette

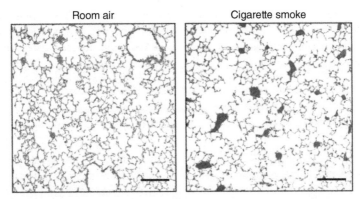

FIGURE 57A-2 Histologic comparison of mouse lung after smoke exposure. H&E-stained lung sections from age-matched room air littermates (C57BL/6J strain) and mice exposed to cigarette smoke for 6 months. Images are at 10× magnification.

smoke and develop increases in their mean linear intercept (MLI), a parameter of airspace enlargement, which range from 15% to 20% after 6 to 12 months of exposure.[67] Because of this, smoke exposure studies using C57Bl/6J mice require large numbers of mice to be exposed for long periods of time. This greatly increases the time and expense needed to carry out these exposure studies. In addition, the C57Bl/6J mice do not develop increased lung compliance following chronic cigarette smoke exposure.[65] Numerous mouse strains have been utilized for smoke exposure studies. However, A/J mice are the most sensitive to cigarette smoke and develop increases in their MLI in the range of 20% to 30%

after only 2 months of exposure,[65] as depicted in Figure 57A–3.

Because of this, the A/J mouse is becoming the preferred strain for smoke exposure studies in mice.[68] Unfortunately, many genetic mouse models are developed in a C57Bl/6J background.

Crossing these mice into a more sensitive A/J background requires several generations of backcrossing. This is a costly and time-consuming endeavor. If the primary endpoint of one's research is emphysema, it may be worthwhile to cross into an A/J background. These mice need less smoke exposure time and develop greater emphysema potentially making it easier to detect changes between

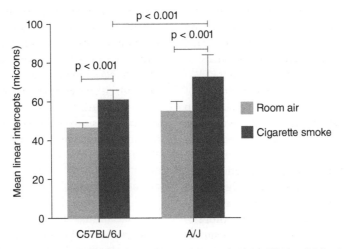

FIGURE 57A-3 Demonstrating the typical MLI, observed in age-matched C57Bl/6J and A/J mice after 6 months of cigarette smoke exposure or their room air controls.

groups. On the other hand, if one's focus is on inflammation, apoptosis, and protease expression then there is no evidence that A/J mice are superior to C57Bl/6J for examining these parameters.

MECHANISTIC INSIGHTS FROM THE SMOKE EXPOSURE MODEL

Inflammation

The smoke exposure model has provided important new insights into the role of inflammation in the development of emphysema. As observed in humans, cigarette smoke induces a pronounced airway and lung parenchymal inflammatory response, particularly in dendritic cells.[65,69] Indeed, smoke studies in mice demonstrated that monocyte chemoattractants, such as granulocyte monocyte chemoattractant factor (GM-CSF), endothelial cell monocyte activating protein (EMAPII) and monocyte chemoattractant protein (MCP-1) play a pivotal role in the development of smoke-induced inflammation and emphysema.[63,70,71] In fact, smoke mediates this inflammatory response by stimulating receptors for advance glycation end-products (RAGE) on the surface of alveolar macrophages.[72] The importance of this cell type was underscored by the fact that deficiencies in macrophage number or function ameliorated the inflammatory and destructive changes to smoke exposure in mice.[63,73]

In addition to macrophages, the murine smoke exposure model has also established that cigarette smoke stimulates the infiltration of CD4+ and CD8+ cells in the lung tissue.[74] This is significant, as T cells have been linked to emphysema development in the human disease.[75-77] In fact, chronic smoke exposure in mice generates an oligoclonal expansion of pathogenic CD4+ and CD8+ cells in a mouse model of COPD.[78] Furthermore, smoke exposure in mice induced IFN-γ expression by NK cells in the lung.[79] By stimulating IFN-γ, these cells promote a Th1 inflammatory response that causes lung remodeling and tissue destruction.[80] More recently, the smoke exposure model identified that IL-17 production by Th17 cells plays an important role in the pathogenesis of this disease.[81,82] These Th17 cells from smoke exposed mice were capable of generating emphysematous changes when transferred into normal recipient mice.[83] While T cells play a central role in the disease pathogenesis, studies in humans show that lymphoid follicles containing B cells are associated with emphysema.[84,85] However, the role of B cells in the development of the disease has been controversial.[86] The smoke exposure model, however, has provided key new insights into the role of these cells in this disease. In mice, the smoke-mediated increase in B-lymphocytes correlated with the development of air space enlargement[87] and neutralizing the B-cell attracting chemokine CXCL13 prevented smoke-induced emphysema.[88] Thus, data from the mouse smoke exposure model suggests that both B and T cells are participating in the evolution of this disease.

While the smoke exposure model has identified new roles for T and B cells in COPD, it has confirmed and expanded our understanding of the effect of neutrophils in this disease. Smoke exposure studies in mice affirmed that proteases released from neutrophils break down matrix elements in the lung[89,90] and inhibiting these proteases exerts a protective effect in this disease.[91] In addition, they demonstrated that cigarette smoke and nicotine sustain inflammatory responses by blocking the spontaneous death of lung neutrophils.[92] Furthermore, the smoke exposure model showed that IL-1α is central to the initiation of smoke-induced neutrophilia.[93] However, though blocking IL-1R1 prior to smoke exposure prevents the influx of neutrophils and the development of emphysema,[94] blocking IL-1 late in the disease course could exacerbate lung injury by preventing the resolution of lung neutrophilia. Stimulation of IL-1R1 induces miR135b, which, in turn, suppresses lung inflammation by down regulating IL-R1 expression in the lung.[95] Thus, the use of IL-1 antagonists as a treatment for COPD will have to be approached with caution as inhibiting IL-1 in the late stages of the disease may accentuate lung tissue injury by heightening and sustaining the influx of neutrophils in the lung.

PROTEASES IN COPD PROGRESSION

Animal models have shown that cigarette smoke triggers the production of damaging proteases in the lung.[96,97] These proteases augment lung inflammation by degrading key structural elements that release chemotactic peptides in lung.[98] Studies in mice show that anti-proteases, such as alpha one antitrypsin, antagonize these effects to prevent the development of smoke-induced emphysema.[99,100] Specifically, A1AT blocks the production of MMP-12 and TNF-α in alveolar macrophages from mice[101] and prevents caspase-3 activity and apoptosis in lung endothelial cells.[102] Animal studies from the mouse smoke exposure model show that both MMP-12 and TNF-α play a central role in the development of smoke-induced emphysema.[63,103] Likewise, endothelial cell death is a key process in the onset and progression of COPD.[104,105] Thus, A1AT, by inhibiting these responses, counteracted key processes responsible for this disease. Alteration on lung signaling can have a profound effect on the protease/antiprotease balance in the lung. Studies in mice show that cigarette smoke inactivates the histone deacetylase SIRT1 leading to the up regulation of MMP-9 and downregulation of TIMP-1.[106] This proteolytic imbalance resulted in the development of smoke-induced emphysema in mice.[107] Furthermore activation of the tyrosine kinase c-Src induced the expression of MMP-9 and MMP-12 both in lung epithelial cells and the lungs from smoke exposed mice.[108] These findings indicate that targeting c-Src may counter the proteolytic process that lead to lung inflammation and tissue destruction in this disease.

Oxidants

The use of animal models has greatly enhanced our understanding of the role of oxidants in the development of emphysema. Chronic smoke exposure studies document the accumulation of oxidative injury in the lungs of exposed mice.[109,110] Importantly, oxidants can inactivate A1AT thereby negating a key protective mechanism in the lung.[111] In fact, oxidized A1AT actually enhances the release of MCP-1 from lung epithelial cells. Although cigarette smoke exposure is associated with oxidative stress and the induction of injury lung responses,[112] direct evidence of the role of smoke-derived oxidants in the pathogenesis of the disease had been lacking. Studies in nuclear factor (erythroid-derived 2)-like 2 (Nrf2) deficient mice demonstrated that lung antioxidant expression was a key determinant of smoke-induced inflammation and tissue destruction. Nrf2

is a transcription factor that is normally bound to its inhibitor Keap1 in the cytosol. In response to oxidative stress, Keap1 dissociates from Nrf2 allowing it to translocate to the nucleus where it turns on the expression of lung antioxidant genes. Thus, Nrf2 knockout mice had deficient antioxidant responses and this resulted in greater oxidative stress, lung inflammation and airspace enlargement.[113] In contrast, Keap1 knockout mice had decreased inflammation and oxidative injury in response to acute smoke exposure.[114] Furthermore, it was demonstrated in mice that enhancing lung antioxidant expression effectively counteracts the inflammation and proteolytic responses to acute and chronic cigarette smoke exposure. Indeed, mice with the transgenic expression of the antioxidant superoxide dismutase-1 (SOD1) were completely protected against smoke-induced inflammation, protease expression, oxidative injury and lung tissue destruction.[56] This was the first direct demonstration that countering smoke-induced oxidants could have a beneficial impact in this disease. Subsequently, it has been shown the extracellular SOD (EC-SOD) similarly protects against smoke-induced emphysema in mice by preventing the oxidative fragmentation of the extracellular matrix.[115] In addition, the antioxidants glutathione peroxidase-1[116,117] and thioredoxin exert similar protective effects in smoke exposed mice.[118,119] These studies offer hope that enhancing the antioxidant defenses of the lung can prevent the damaging effects of chronic smoke exposure in the lung. Current antioxidant approaches in humans are limited by pharmacokinetic factors that restrict the lung bioavailability of exogenously administered antioxidants.[120] Indeed, the n-acetyl cysteine dose used in the BRONCUS study[121] was shown not to significantly enhance lung antioxidant defenses in humans.[122] This may explain the disappointing results from this clinical trial. Lastly, though these studies indicate that oxidants are contributing to the injurious effects of cigarette smoke exposure, the genetic ablation of the NADPH oxidase actually enhances airspace enlargement and inflammation in smoke exposed mice.[123] Free radicals are key mediators of intracellular signaling events. Thus, the complete absence of lung oxidases may alter the ability to the cell to respond to the damaging effects of cigarette smoke exposure in the lung. Rather than an indiscriminate antioxidant approach it may be more effective to identify redox-regulated processes that could be targeted with specific pharmacotherapies.

Apoptosis

Apoptosis is a critical event in the development of lung tissue destruction and remodeling in COPD.[124] However, it is difficult to determine how cigarette smoke induces lung apoptosis using only clinical specimens. Thus, the animal exposure model provides a powerful tool for better understanding the apoptotic mechanisms that are triggered by cigarette smoke. Studies in mice showed that apoptotic responses occur in the lung even after short-term cigarette smoke exposure.[125] Furthermore, these studies show that antioxidant supplementation blocks apoptosis in response to cigarette smoke in these mice. The importance of redox factors on lung apoptosis was further demonstrated in Nrf2 knockout mice. The loss of antioxidant induction in Nrf2 knockouts accentuated the development of apoptosis in both lung epithelial and endothelial cells.[113] Thus, these smoke exposure studies have helped to identify how redox biology influences cell fate in resident lung cells exposed to cigarette smoke.

As observed with oxidants, studies in mice have shown that cytokines, such as IFN-γ, also play a critical role in smoke-induced apoptosis in the lung. Indeed, cigarette smoke up regulates IFN-γ, which then acts through its receptor CCR5 to trigger apoptosis and lung tissue remodeling.[80] Similarly, TNF signaling has been shown to play an important role in the induction of apoptosis in mouse smoke exposure models. Mice that lacked expression of TNF-receptor I or TNF-receptor II (TNFR1 or TNFR2) were protected against the development of smoke-induced apoptosis, particularly within type II pneumocytes.[126] This protection was associated with decreased lung inflammation and the preservation of normal lung architecture. Cigarette smoke also induces IL-6 and this cytokine-triggered alveolar apoptosis and emphysema in smoke exposed mice.[127] In addition to epithelial cells, smoke studies in mice found that IL-18 and the chemokine receptor CXCR3 were important mediators of endothelial cell apoptosis and lung injury.[128,129] Over the past 10 years, there has been an increasing awareness of the role of the lung endothelium

in the pathogenesis of COPD.[59] Vascular endothelial growth factor (VEGF) maintains endothelial integrity and prevents cell death.[130] Impairing VEGF signaling by inhibiting its receptor VEGFR2 augmented inflammation and endothelial dysfunction in smoke exposed mice.[131] This is important as cigarette smoke induces oxidative stress that blocks VEGFR2 activation and impairs VEGF signaling within the endothelium.[132] Studies in both mice and humans show decreased expression of VEGF within the airways in response to cigarette smoke exposure.[133] Moreover, studies in mice show that endothelial VEGF expression is similarly decreased in response to cigarette smoke exposure.[134] Together, these findings establish that altered VEGF signaling within the lung endothelium causes endothelial cell death and tissue destruction in this disease. Future studies are ongoing to determine whether antagonizing these effects can preserve endothelial integrity and ameliorate the inflammatory and destructive changes that occur in this disease.

RECOVERY MECHANISMS IN COPD

As noted in the prior section, the cigarette smoke exposure model has provided key insights into the mechanisms by which cigarette triggers lung inflammation, protease expression, apoptosis, and tissue destruction. These studies have enabled us to better understand why cigarette smoke causes lung disease. Much less attention, however, has been paid to determining how the lung recovers from the damaging effects of cigarette smoke. This is an important question as enhancing recovery mechanisms may be a means of countering or reversing the harmful biological responses that occur in this disease. Several recent reports have begun to address this issue and have laid the groundwork for future study.[135,136]

It is well established that FoxP3+ T regulatory cells mediate the resolution of inflammatory responses in the lung. In an LPS lung injury model, depletion of these cells exacerbated lung inflammation while adoptive transfer of these cells, even 24 hours after LPS challenge, accelerated lung recovery.[137] In smoke exposed mice, there is an accumulation of T regulatory cells in the lung.[138] This suggests that these cells are functioning to limit the inflammatory responses to this stimulus in the lung. Unfortunately, with chronic exposure T cells were skewed to a Th17 phenotype and away from the development of T regulatory cells.[139] While these studies point to a protective role for T regulatory cells in COPD, a recent study in mice found that in utero smoke exposure increased T regulatory activity, which impaired tumor clearance later in life by impeding the function of cytotoxic T cells.[140] Given these conflicting findings, further studies are needed to determine whether augmenting T regulatory cell activity will have a beneficial or adverse effect in this disease.

The clearance of inflammation is not a passive process but rather involves innate resolution mechanisms that are activated at the initiation of injury. In the lung and other organs, a class of natural lipid-derived mediators (lipoxins, resolvins, protectins, maresins) is produced to resolve inflammation in a manner that does not suppress the immune system. Lipoxins are derived from cell membrane arachidonic acid and suppress inflammation in asthma[141] and lung injury models.[142] Serum amyloid A (SAA) protein, which blocks the effects of lipoxins, is increased in COPD and administering SAA enhances neutrophilic responses in mice.[143] Thus, the loss of lipoxin activity may contribute to neutrophilic inflammation in this disease. Resolvins, protectins, and maresins are derivatives of omega-3 polyunsaturated fatty acids (ω-3-PUFA). Eicosapentaenoic acid (EPA) and docosahexaenoic acid (DHA) are 2 essential ω-3-PUFAs that are converted into these bioactive lipid mediators in order to regulate the local resolution of inflammation.[144] Animal models have demonstrated that resolvins promote the resolution of lung inflammation due to bacterial pneumonia,[145] LPS,[146] or asthma.[147] Resolvins exerted these effects by blocking mast cell degranulation,[148] promoting neutrophil clearance[149] and suppressing NF-κB activation.[146] Using the mouse smoke exposure model it was shown that resolvin D1 decreases neutrophilic inflammation and up regulates the anti-inflammatory cytokine IL-10.[135] Given these effects, further studies in this model are needed to determine whether resolvins prevent inflammation and tissue destruction in response to chronic smoke exposure.

The cell contains a tightly coordinated network of kinases and phosphatases that switch proteins from the phosphorylated to the dephosphorylated state in order to cope with various physiologic challenges.[150] Cigarette smoke activates kinases that promote lung disease by stimulating inflammation,[108,151] up regulating proteases[152] and inducing apoptosis.[153] While a significant body of research has elucidated the role that protein kinases exert in these processes,[154] much less is know about the effects of protein phosphatases. Protein phosphatase 2A is the primary serine threonine phosphatase of eukaryotic cells. Cigarette smoke activates PP2A both in human lung epithelial cells and mouse lung.[155] This activation occurs rapidly and limits the intensity and duration of smoke induced inflammation. Indeed, inhibiting PP2A in mice sustained and exacerbated the effects of acute smoke exposure.[155] Though acute smoke exposure activates PP2A, this response is lost with chronic smoke exposure potentially rendering the lung more susceptible to smoke-induced injury.[155] It is important to note that studies from the mouse smoke exposure model showed that PP2A protects against smoke-induced emphysema. In fact, the antioxidant glutathione peroxidase-1 (GPx-1) acted via PP2A to prevent smoke-induced inflammation and lung tissue destruction[117] in mice. PP2A plays a pivotal role in preventing and resolving smoke-induced lung inflammation and injury. Thus, targeting PP2A activity in the lung may be an effective means of preventing the onset and progression of COPD.

FINAL THOUGHTS ON THE SMOKE EXPOSURE MODEL

As noted previously, COPD is a leading cause of death worldwide. Despite its importance, there are few specific therapies for this disease and only oxygen has been shown to impact on disease mortality. The lack of effective treatments is due in large measure to the limited knowledge of the underlying disease mechanisms. Over the past 20 years, the cigarette smoke exposure model in mice has provided valuable insights into the biological processes responsible for the disease pathogenesis. Today, the role of proteases, inflammation and apoptosis in the disease development is much better understood. In addition, researchers have identified key counter inflammatory mechanisms that serve to protect the lung against the damaging effects of cigarette smoke exposure. The knowledge gained from these studies has the potential to translate into effective treatments to prevent or reverse the course of this disease. Additionally, well-established smoke exposure models are now available to test potential new therapies prior to human clinical trials. However, the translational impact of these studies has yet to be realized for a multitude of reasons. For one, COPD is a complex disease that develops over years. Interventions administered during the early or pre stage of disease may not be effective when given to late stage patients. This is a daunting problem for COPD as this is a woefully under diagnosed disease and most cases are not detected till the disease is well established.[156] Unfortunately, most studies that utilize the mouse smoke exposure model administer the intervention before smoke exposure begins or before lung damage is established.[157] This is obviously not what happens with a patient who is newly diagnosed with the disease. Moreover, inhibiting some processes during the early period of exposure may prevent disease but blocking the same pathway in late stage disease may hinder needed compensatory responses. Therefore, the scientific community may be studying the prevention of disease initiation rather than recovery. This may be the case with TNF-α antagonists, which prevented COPD in animal models[158,159] but were ineffective and potentially harmful in clinical studies in humans.[160,161] In the future, animal exposure studies will need to be conducted after the disease is already established. The A/J strain of mice will be well suited for these studies because they develop significant emphysema after only 2 months of smoke exposure. Thus, the intervention could be begun at this time point to assess the potential benefit of an intervention. Though changes in study design will help, the limitations of the murine smoke exposure model have to be recognized. Most obviously, mice are not humans. They have shorter lifespans, less submucosal glands and more airway macrophages than their human counterparts.[162,163] Given these and other biological differences, the mouse model may not fully replicate what occurs in the human lung. Carefully conducted correlative studies in humans are, therefore, needed to confirm promising results obtained with this model. The statistician George E.P. Box once wrote, "All models are wrong, but some models are useful."[164] The smoke exposure

model, by definition, is an approximation of what occurs in the human lung. It can provide useful insights, but if used without discretion it can obfuscate the truth. The challenge for researchers moving forward will be to conduct exposure studies that integrate physiologic, biologic, and architectural endpoints and then to validate these findings with research using complementary in vitro and in vivo models and studies using human samples. Rushing to drug development or testing based on the results from the smoke exposure model alone is shortsighted especially considering the model's limitations. Nevertheless, if used wisely, this model can be an important component of a multifaceted research approach for this disease.

REFERENCES

1. Rabe KF, Hurd S, Anzueto A, et al. Global strategy for the diagnosis, management, and prevention of chronic obstructive pulmonary disease: GOLD executive summary. *Am J Respir Crit Care Med.* 2007;176:532-555.
2. Miller M, Cho JY, Pham A, Friedman PJ, Ramsdell J, Broide DH. Persistent airway inflammation and emphysema progression on CT scan in ex-smokers observed for 4 years. *Chest.* 2011;139:1380-1387.
3. Osman M, Cantor JO, Roffman S, Keller S, Turino GM, Mandl I. Cigarette smoke impairs elastin resynthesis in lungs of hamsters with elastase-induced emphysema. *Am Rev Respir Dis.* 1985;132:640-643.
4. Coxson HO, Rogers RM, Whittall KP, et al. A quantification of the lung surface area in emphysema using computed tomography. *Am J Respir Crit Care Med.* 1999;159:851-856.
5. Stewart JI, Criner GJ. The small airways in chronic obstructive pulmonary disease: pathology and effects on disease progression and survival. *Curr Opin Pulm Med.* 2013;19:109-115.
6. Hogg JC, Chu F, Utokaparch S, et al. The nature of small-airway obstruction in chronic obstructive pulmonary disease. *N Engl J Med.* 2004;350:2645-2653.
7. Murphy BS, Xu J, Kochanek KD. In: Reports NVS, ed. *Deaths: Preliminary Data for 2010*, Vol. 60. Hyattsville, MD: National Center for Health Statistics; 2012.
8. Raherison C, Girodet PO. Epidemiology of COPD. *Eur Respir Rev.* 2009;18:213-221.

9. Miller N, Simoes EJ, Chang JC, Robling AG. Trends in chronic obstructive pulmonary disease mortality. *Mo Med*. 2000;97:87-90.

10. Hogg JC. A brief review of chronic obstructive pulmonary disease. *Can Respir J*. 2012;19:381-384.

11. Kim V, Criner GJ. Chronic bronchitis and chronic obstructive pulmonary disease. *Am J Respir Crit Care Med*. 2013;187:228-237.

12. Schroeder SA, Koh HK. Tobacco control 50 years after the 1964 surgeon general's report. *JAMA*. 2014;311:141-143.

13. Centers for Disease Control and Prevention (CDC). Tobacco product use among middle and high school students—United States, 2011 and 2012. *MMWR Morb Mortal Wkly Rep*. 2013;62:893-897.

14. Li Q, Hsia J, Yang G. Prevalence of smoking in China in 2010. *N Engl J Med*. 2011;364:2469-2470.

15. WHO. Report on the Global Tobacco Epidemic, 2009: Implementing smoke-free environments. In: *Tobacco Free Inititative*. World Health Organization; 2009:1-136.

16. McCartney G, Mahmood L, Leyland AH, Batty GD, Hunt K. Contribution of smoking-related and alcohol-related deaths to the gender gap in mortality: evidence from 30 European countries. *Tob Control*. 2011;20:166-168.

17. Zeng G, Sun B, Zhong N. Non-smoking-related chronic obstructive pulmonary disease: a neglected entity? *Respirology*. 2012;17:908-912.

18. Organization, WWH. Health and environment for sustainable development. (Organization, W. H., ed), Geneva; 1997.

19. Desai M, Mehta S, Smith K. Indoor smoke from solid fuels: assessing the environmental burden of disease at national and local levels; 2004 (Series, W. E. B. o. D., ed).

20. WHO. World Health Report. Geneva; 2002. (Organization, W. H., ed).

21. Behera D, Jindal SK, Malhotra HS. Ventilatory function in nonsmoking rural Indian women using different cooking fuels. *Respiration*. 1994;61:89-92.

22. Banerjee A, Mondal NK, Das D, Ray MR. Neutrophilic inflammatory response and oxidative stress in premenopausal women chronically exposed to indoor air pollution from biomass burning. *Inflammation*. 2012;35:671-683.

23. Dutta A, Roychoudhury S, Chowdhury S, Ray MR. Changes in sputum cytology, airway inflammation and oxidative stress due to chronic inhalation of biomass smoke during cooking in premenopausal rural Indian women. *Int J Hyg Environ Health*. 2013;216(3):301-308.

24. Dutta A, Ray MR, Banerjee A. Systemic inflammatory changes and increased oxidative stress in rural Indian women cooking with biomass fuels. *Toxicol Appl Pharmacol*. 2012;261:255-262.

25. Ezzati M, Kammen D. Indoor air pollution from biomass combustion and acute respiratory infections in Kenya: an exposure-response study. *Lancet*. 2001;358:619-624.

26. Alvarez-Sala J, Cimas E, Masa J, et al. Recommendations for the care of the patient with chronic obstructive pulmonary disease. *Archivos de bronconeumologia*. 2001;37:269-278.

27. Johannesdottir SA, Christiansen CF, Johansen MB, et al. Hospitalization with acute exacerbation of chronic obstructive pulmonary disease and associated health resource utilization: a population-based Danish cohort study. *Journal of Medical Economics*. 2013;16:897-906.

28. Hill AT, Hopkinson RB, Stableforth DE. Ventilation in a Birmingham intensive care unit 1993-1995: outcome for patients with chronic obstructive pulmonary disease. *Respir Med*. 1998;92:156-161.

29. Seneff MG, Wagner DP, Wagner RP, Zimmerman JE, Knaus WA. Hospital and 1-year survival of patients admitted to intensive care units with acute exacerbation of chronic obstructive pulmonary disease. *JAMA*. 1995;274:1852-1857.

30. Hudson LD. Survival data in patients with acute and chronic lung disease requiring mechanical ventilation. *Am Rev Respir Dis*. 1989;140:S19-S24.

31. Nevins ML, Epstein SK. Predictors of outcome for patients with COPD requiring invasive mechanical ventilation. *Chest*. 2001;119:1840-1849.

32. Breen D, Churches T, Hawker F, Torzillo PJ. Acute respiratory failure secondary to chronic obstructive pulmonary disease treated in the intensive care unit: a long term follow up study. *Thorax*. 2002;57:29-33.

33. Society, A. T. S. E. R. Standards for the diagnosis and management of patients with COPD; 2012.

34. Engoren M, Arslanian-Engoren C, Fenn-Buderer N. Hospital and long-term outcome after tracheostomy for respiratory failure. *Chest*. 2004;125:220-227.

35. Seneff MG, Zimmerman JE, Knaus WA, Wagner DP, Draper EA. Predicting the duration of mechanical ventilation. The importance of disease and patient characteristics. *Chest*. 1996;110:469-479.

36. Wagner DP. Economics of prolonged mechanical ventilation. *Am Rev Respir Dis*. 1989;140:S14-S18.

37. Nelson JE, Cox CE, Hope AA, Carson SS. Chronic critical illness. *Am J Respir Crit Care Med*. 2010;182:446-454.

38. Pauley E, Lishmanov A, Schumann S, Gala GJ, van Diepen S, Katz JN. Delirium is a robust predictor of morbidity and mortality among critically ill patients treated in the cardiac intensive care unit. *Am Heart J*. 2015;170:79-86 e71.
39. Mardani D, Bigdelian H. Predictors and clinical outcomes of postoperative delirium after administration of dexamethasone in patients undergoing coronary artery bypass surgery. *Int J Prev Med*. 2012;3:420-427.
40. Veeravagu A, Jiang B, Rincon F, Maltenfort M, Jallo J, Ratliff JK. Acute respiratory distress syndrome and acute lung injury in patients with vertebral column fracture(s) and spinal cord injury: a nationwide inpatient sample study. *Spinal Cord*. 2013;51:461-465.
41. Budweiser S, Jorres RA, Pfeifer M. Treatment of respiratory failure in COPD. *Int J Chron Obstruct Pulmon Dis*. 2008;3:605-618.
42. Peters-Golden M, Klinger JR, Carson SS. The case for increased funding for research in pulmonary and critical care. *Am J Respir Crit Care Med*. 2012;186:213-215.
43. Connolly D. Kids' concept of cigarette code. *JAMA*. 1991;266:3126.
44. Aitken PP, Leathar DS, O'Hagan FJ. Children's perceptions of advertisements for cigarettes. *Soc Sci Med*. 1985;21:785-797.
45. Emmons KM, Kawachi I, Barclay G. Tobacco control: a brief review of its history and prospects for the future. *Hematol Oncol Clin North Am*. 1997;11:177-195.
46. Hall MG, Ribisl KM, Brewer NT. Smokers' and nonsmokers' beliefs about harmful tobacco constituents: implications for FDA communication efforts. *Nicotine Tob Res*. 2014;16(3):343-350.
47. Stolerman IP. Behavioural pharmacology of nicotine: multiple mechanisms. *Br J Addict*. 1991;86:533-536.
48. Tonnesen P. Smoking cessation and COPD. *Eur Respir Rev*. 2013;22:37-43.
49. Graham A, Court JA, Martin-Ruiz CM, et al. Immunohistochemical localisation of nicotinic acetylcholine receptor subunits in human cerebellum. *Neuroscience*. 2002;113:493-507.
50. Maltais F, Dennis N, Chan CK. Rationale for earlier treatment in COPD: a systematic review of published literature in mild-to-moderate COPD. *COPD*. 2013;10:79-103.
51. Laurell CD, Erikson S. The electrophoretic a1-globulin pattern of serum in alpha 1-antitrypsin deficiency. *Scad J Clin Lab Invest*. 1963;15:132-140.
52. Kueppers F, Fallat R, Larson RK. Obstructive lung disease and alpha-1-antitrypsin deficiency gene heterozygosity. *Science*. 1969;165:899-901.
53. Abrams WR, Fein AM, Kucich U, et al. Proteinase inhibitory function in inflammatory lung disease. I. Acute bacterial pneumonia. *Am Rev Respir Dis*. 1984;129:735-741.
54. Abboud RT, Vimalanathan S. Pathogenesis of COPD. Part I. The role of protease-antiprotease imbalance in emphysema. *Int J Tuberc Lung Dis*. 2008;12:361-367.
55. Janoff A. Elastases and emphysema. Current assessment of the protease-antiprotease hypothesis. *Am Rev Respir Dis*. 1985;132:417-433.
56. Foronjy RF, Mirochnitchenko O, Propokenko O, et al. Superoxide dismutase expression attenuates cigarette smoke- or elastase-generated emphysema in mice. *Am J Respir Crit Care Med*. 2006;173:623-631.
57. Shapiro SD, Goldstein NM, Houghton AM, Kobayashi DK, Kelley D, Belaaouaj A. Neutrophil elastase contributes to cigarette smoke-induced emphysema in mice. *Am J Pathol*. 2003;163:2329-2335.
58. Molet S, Belleguic C, Lena H, et al. Increase in macrophage elastase (MMP-12) in lungs from patients with chronic obstructive pulmonary disease. *Inflamm Res*. 2005;54:31-36.
59. Tuder RM, Petrache I. Pathogenesis of chronic obstructive pulmonary disease. *J Clin Invest*. 2012;122:2749-2755.
60. Roe FJ. Certain aspects of the responses of laboratory rats to exposure to (a) nitrogen dioxide and (b) tobacco smoke. *Tokai J Exp Clin Med*. 1985;10:363-369.
61. Rogers DF, Godfrey RW, Majumdar S, Jeffery PK. Oral N-acetylcysteine speeds reversal of cigarette smoke-induced mucous cell hyperplasia in the rat. *Exp Lung Res*. 1988;14:19-35.
62. Wright JL, Ngai T, Churg A. Effect of long-term exposure to cigarette smoke on the small airways of the guinea pig. *Exp Lung Res*. 1992;18:105-114.
63. Hautamaki RD, Kobayashi DK, Senior RM, Shapiro SD. Requirement for macrophage elastase for cigarette smoke-induced emphysema in mice. *Science*. 1997;277:2002-2004.
64. Nemmar A, Raza H, Subramaniyan D, et al. Evaluation of the pulmonary effects of short-term nose-only cigarette smoke exposure in mice. *Exp Biol Med (Maywood)*. 2012;237:1449-1456.
65. Foronjy RF, Mercer BA, Maxfield MW, Powell CA, D'Armiento J, Okada Y. Structural emphysema

does not correlate with lung compliance: lessons from the mouse smoking model. *Exp Lung Res.* 2005;31:547-562.

66. Fletcher C, Peto R. The natural history of chronic airflow obstruction. *Br Med J.* 1977;1:1645-1648.

67. Guerassimov A, Hoshino Y, Takubo Y, et al. The development of emphysema in cigarette smoke-exposed mice is strain dependent. *Am J Respir Crit Care Med.* 2004;170:974-980.

68. Podowski M, Calvi C, Metzger S, et al. Angiotensin receptor blockade attenuates cigarette smoke-induced lung injury and rescues lung architecture in mice. *J Clin Invest.* 2012;122:229-240.

69. D'Hulst AI, Vermaelen KY, Brusselle GG, Joos GF, Pauwels RA. Time course of cigarette smoke-induced pulmonary inflammation in mice. *Eur Respir J.* 2005;26:204-213.

70. Vlahos R, Bozinovski S, Chan SP, et al. Neutralizing granulocyte/macrophage colony-stimulating factor inhibits cigarette smoke-induced lung inflammation. *Am J Respir Crit Care Med.* 2010;182:34-40.

71. Clauss M, Voswinckel R, Rajashekhar G, et al. Lung endothelial monocyte-activating protein 2 is a mediator of cigarette smoke-induced emphysema in mice. *J Clin Invest.* 2011;121:2470-2479.

72. Robinson AB, Johnson KD, Bennion BG, Reynolds PR. RAGE signaling by alveolar macrophages influences tobacco smoke-induced inflammation. *Am J Physiol Lung Cell Mol Physiol.* 2012;302: L1192-L1199.

73. Ofulue A, Ko M. Effects of depletion of neutrophils or macrophages on development of cigarette smoke-induced emphysema. *Am J Physiol.* 1999;277:L97-L105.

74. Moerloose KB, Pauwels RA, Joos GF. Short-term cigarette smoke exposure enhances allergic airway inflammation in mice. *Am J Respir Crit Care Med.* 2005;172:168-172.

75. Finkelstein R, Fraser RS, Ghezzo H, Cosio MG. Alveolar inflammation and its relation to emphysema in smokers. *Am J Respir Crit Care Med.* 1995;152:1666-1672.

76. Majo J, Ghezzo H, Cosio MG. Lymphocyte population and apoptosis in the lungs of smokers and their relation to emphysema. *Eur Respir J.* 2001;17:946-953.

77. Cosio MG, Majo J, Cosio MG. Inflammation of the airways and lung parenchyma in COPD: role of T cells. *Chest.* 2002;121:160S-165S.

78. Motz GT, Eppert BL, Wesselkamper SC, Flury JL, Borchers MT. Chronic cigarette smoke exposure generates pathogenic T cells capable of driving COPD-like disease in Rag2-/- mice. *Am J Respir Crit Care Med.* 2010;181:1223-1233.

79. Motz GT, Eppert BL, Wortham BW, et al. Chronic cigarette smoke exposure primes NK cell activation in a mouse model of chronic obstructive pulmonary disease. *J Immunol.* 2010;184:4460-4469.

80. Ma B, Kang MJ, Lee CG, et al. Role of CCR5 in IFN-gamma-induced and cigarette smoke-induced emphysema. *J Clin Invest.* 2005;115:3460-3472.

81. Shan M, Yuan X, Song LZ, et al. Cigarette smoke induction of osteopontin (SPP1) mediates T(H)17 inflammation in human and experimental emphysema. *Sci Transl Med.* 2012;4:117-119.

82. Chen K, Pociask DA, McAleer JP, et al. IL-17RA is required for CCL2 expression, macrophage recruitment, and emphysema in response to cigarette smoke. *PLoS One.* 2011;6:e20333.

83. Shan M, Cheng HF, Song LZ, et al. Lung myeloid dendritic cells coordinately induce TH1 and TH17 responses in human emphysema. *Sci Transl Med.* 2009;1:4ra10.

84. Gosman MM, Willemse BW, Jansen DF, et al. Increased number of B-cells in bronchial biopsies in COPD. *Eur Respir J.* 2006;27:60-64.

85. Litsiou E, Semitekolou M, Galani IE, et al. CXCL13 production in B cells via Toll-like receptor/lymphotoxin receptor signaling is involved in lymphoid neogenesis in chronic obstructive pulmonary disease. *Am J Respir Crit Care Med.* 2013;187:1194-1202.

86. Brusselle GG, Demoor T, Bracke KR, Brandsma CA, Timens W. Lymphoid follicles in (very) severe COPD: beneficial or harmful? *Eur Respir J.* 2009;34:219-230.

87. van der Strate BW, Postma DS, Brandsma CA, et al. Cigarette smoke-induced emphysema: a role for the B cell? *Am J Respir Crit Care Med.* 2006;173:751-758.

88. Bracke KR, Verhamme FM, Seys LJ, et al. Role of CXCL13 in cigarette smoke-induced lymphoid follicle formation and chronic obstructive pulmonary disease. *Am J Respir Crit Care Med.* 2013;188:343-355.

89. Dhami R, Gilks B, Xie C, Zay K, Wright J, Churg A. Acute cigarette smoke-induced connective tissue breakdown is mediated by neutrophils and prevented by alpha-1-antitrypsin. *Am J Respir Cell Mol Bio.* 2000;22:244-252.

90. Churg A, Zay K, Shay S, et al. Acute cigarette smoke-induced connective tissue breakdown requires both neutrophils and macrophage

metalloelastase in mice. *Am J Respir Cell Mol Biol.* 2002;27:368-374.

91. Stevens T, Ekholm K, Granse M, et al. AZD9668: pharmacological characterization of a novel oral inhibitor of neutrophil elastase. *J Pharmacol Exp Ther.* 2011;339:313-320.

92. Xu Y, Li H, Bajrami B, et al. Cigarette smoke (CS) and nicotine delay neutrophil spontaneous death via suppressing production of diphosphoinositol pentakisphosphate. *Proc Natl Acad Sci U S A.* 2013;110:7726-7731.

93. Botelho FM, Bauer CM, Finch D, et al. IL-1alpha/IL-1R1 expression in chronic obstructive pulmonary disease and mechanistic relevance to smoke-induced neutrophilia in mice. *PLoS One.* 2011;6:e28457.

94. Couillin I, Vasseur V, Charron S, et al. IL-1R1/MyD88 signaling is critical for elastase-induced lung inflammation and emphysema. *J Immunol.* 2009;183:8195-8202.

95. Halappanavar S, Nikota J, Wu D, Williams A, Yauk CL, Stampfli M. IL-1 receptor regulates microRNA-135b expression in a negative feedback mechanism during cigarette smoke-induced inflammation. *J Immunol.* 2013;190:3679-3686.

96. White R, White J, Janoff A. Effects of cigarette smoke on elastase secretion by murine macrophages. *J Lab Clin Med.* 1979;94:489-499.

97. Bracke K, Cataldo D, Maes T, et al. Matrix metalloproteinase-12 and cathepsin D expression in pulmonary macrophages and dendritic cells of cigarette smoke-exposed mice. *Int Arch Allergy Immunol.* 2005;138:169-179.

98. Houghton AM, Quintero PA, Perkins DL, et al. Elastin fragments drive disease progression in a murine model of emphysema. *J Clin Invest.* 2006;116:753-759.

99. Pemberton PA, Kobayashi D, Wilk BJ, Henstrand JM, Shapiro SD, Barr PJ. Inhaled recombinant alpha 1-antitrypsin ameliorates cigarette smoke-induced emphysema in the mouse. *COPD.* 2006;3:101-108.

100. Churg A, Wang RD, Xie C, Wright JL. Alpha-1-antitrypsin ameliorates cigarette smoke-induced emphysema in the mouse. *Am J Respir Crit Care Med.* 2003;168:199-207.

101. Churg A, Wang X, Wang RD, Meixner SC, Pryzdial EL, Wright JL. Alpha1-antitrypsin suppresses TNF-alpha and MMP-12 production by cigarette smoke-stimulated macrophages. *Am J Respir Cell Mol Biol.* 2007;37:144-151.

102. Petrache I, Fijalkowska I, Medler TR, et al. Alpha-1 antitrypsin inhibits caspase-3 activity, preventing lung endothelial cell apoptosis. *Am J Pathol.* 2006;169:1155-1166.

103. Churg A, Dai J, Tai H, Xie C, Wright JL. Tumor necrosis factor-alpha is central to acute cigarette smoke-induced inflammation and connective tissue breakdown. *Am J Respir Crit Care Med.* 2002;166:849-854

104. Petrache I, Natarajan V, Zhen L, et al. Ceramide upregulation causes pulmonary cell apoptosis and emphysema-like disease in mice. *Nat Med.* 2005;11:491-498.

105. Kasahara Y, Tuder RM, Taraseviciene-Stewart L, et al. Inhibition of vascular endothelial growth factor receptors causes lung cell apoptosis and emphysema. *J Clin Invest.* 2000;106:1311-1319.

106. Yao H, Hwang JW, Sundar IK, et al. SIRT1 redresses the imbalance of tissue inhibitor of matrix metalloproteinase-1 and matrix metalloproteinase-9 in the development of mouse emphysema and human COPD. *Am J Physiol Lung Cell Mol Physiol.* 2013;305:L615-624.

107. Yao H, Chung S, Hwang JW, et al. SIRT1 protects against emphysema via FOXO3-mediated reduction of premature senescence in mice. *J Clin Invest.* 2012;122:2032-2045.

108. Geraghty P, Hardigan A, Foronjy RF. Cigarette smoke activates the proto-oncogene c-src to promote airway inflammation and lung tissue destruction. *Am J Respir Cell Mol Biol.* 2014;50(3):559-570.

109. Kuhl P, Grabow-Caspari M, Terpstra P. Comparison of cigarette smoke-induced lipid peroxidation in vitro and in vivo. *Exp Toxicol Pathol.* 1996;48:541-543.

110. Thaiparambil JT, Vadhanam MV, Srinivasan C, Gairola CG, Gupta RC. Time-dependent formation of 8-oxo-deoxyguanosine in the lungs of mice exposed to cigarette smoke. *Chem Res Toxicol.* 2007;20:1737-1740.

111. Li Z, Alam S, Wang J, Sandstrom CS, Janciauskiene S, Mahadeva R. Oxidized {alpha}1-antitrypsin stimulates the release of monocyte chemotactic protein-1 from lung epithelial cells: potential role in emphysema. *Am J Physiol Lung Cell Mol Physiol.* 2009;297:L388-L400.

112. Rangasamy T, Misra V, Zhen L, Tankersley CG, Tuder RM, Biswal S. Cigarette smoke-induced emphysema in A/J mice is associated with pulmonary oxidative stress, apoptosis of lung cells, and global alterations in gene expression. *Am J Physiol Lung Cell Mol Physiol.* 2009;296:L888-L900.

113. Rangasamy T, Cho CY, Thimmulappa RK, et al. Genetic ablation of Nrf2 enhances susceptibility to cigarette smoke-induced emphysema in mice. *J Clin Invest.* 2004;114:1248-1259.

114. Blake DJ, Singh A, Kombairaju P, et al. Deletion of Keap1 in the lung attenuates acute cigarette

smoke-induced oxidative stress and inflammation. *Am J Respir Cell Mol Biol*. 2010;42:524-536.

115. Yao H, Arunachalam G, Hwang JW, et al. Extracellular superoxide dismutase protects against pulmonary emphysema by attenuating oxidative fragmentation of ECM. *Proc Natl Acad Sci U S A*. 2010;107:15571-15576.

116. Duong C, Seow HJ, Bozinovski S, Crack PJ, Anderson GP, Vlahos R. Glutathione peroxidase-1 protects against cigarette smoke-induced lung inflammation in mice. *Am J Physiol Lung Cell Mol Physiol*. 2010;299:L425-L433.

117. Geraghty P, Hardigan AA, Wallace AM, et al. The GPx1-PTP1B-PP2A axis: a key determinant of airway inflammation and alveolar destruction. *Am J Respir Cell Mol Biol*. 2013;49(5):721-730.

118. Tanabe N, Hoshino Y, Marumo S, et al. Thioredoxin-1 protects against neutrophilic inflammation and emphysema progression in a mouse model of chronic obstructive pulmonary disease exacerbation. *PLoS One*. 2013;8:e79016.

119. Sato A, Hoshino Y, Hara T, et al. Thioredoxin-1 ameliorates cigarette smoke-induced lung inflammation and emphysema in mice. *J Pharmacol Exp Ther*. 2008;325:380-388.

120. Foronjy R, Wallace A, D'Armiento J. The pharmokinetic limitations of antioxidant treatment for COPD. *Pulm Pharmacol Ther*. 2007;21:370-379.

121. Decramer M, Rutten-van Molken M, Dekhuijzen PN, et al. Effects of N-acetylcysteine on outcomes in chronic obstructive pulmonary disease (Bronchitis Randomized on NAC Cost-Utility Study, BRONCUS): a randomised placebo-controlled trial. *Lancet*. 2005;365:1552-1560.

122. Bridgeman MM, Marsden M, Selby C, Morrison D, MacNee W. Effect of N-acetyl cysteine on the concentrations of thiols in plasma, bronchoalveolar lavage fluid, and lung tissue. *Thorax*. 1994;49:670-675.

123. Yao H, Edirisinghe I, Yang SR, et al. Genetic ablation of NADPH oxidase enhances susceptibility to cigarette smoke-induced lung inflammation and emphysema in mice. *Am J Pathol*. 2008;172:1222-1237.

124. Segura-Valdez L, Pardo A, Gaxiola M, Uhal BD, Becerril C, Selman M. Upregulation of gelatinases A and B, collagenases 1 and 2, and increased parenchymal cell death in COPD. *Chest*. 2000;117:684-694.

125. Tsuda S, Matsusaka N, Ueno S, Susa N, Sasaki YF. The influence of antioxidants on cigarette smoke-induced DNA single-strand breaks in mouse organs: a preliminary study with the alkaline single cell gel electrophoresis assay. *Toxicol Sci*. 2000;54:104-109.

126. D'Hulst AI, Bracke KR, Maes T, et al. Role of tumour necrosis factor-alpha receptor p75 in cigarette smoke-induced pulmonary inflammation and emphysema. *Eur Respir J*. 2006;28:102-112.

127. Ruwanpura SM, McLeod L, Miller A, et al. Interleukin-6 promotes pulmonary emphysema associated with apoptosis in mice. *Am J Respir Cell Mol Biol*. 2011;45:720-730.

128. Kratzer A, Salys J, Nold-Petry C, et al. Role of IL-18 in second-hand smoke-induced emphysema. *Am J Respir Cell Mol Biol*. 2013;48:725-732.

129. Green LA, Petrusca D, Rajashekhar G, et al. Cigarette smoke-induced CXCR3 receptor up-regulation mediates endothelial apoptosis. *Am J Respir Cell Mol Biol*. 2012;47:807-814.

130. Voelkel NF, Vandivier RW, Tuder RM. Vascular endothelial growth factor in the lung. *Am J Physiol Lung Cell Mol Physiol*. 2006;290:L209-L221.

131. Edirisinghe I, Yang SR, Yao H, et al. VEGFR-2 inhibition augments cigarette smoke-induced oxidative stress and inflammatory responses leading to endothelial dysfunction. *Faseb J*. 2008;22:2297-2310.

132. Edirisinghe I, Arunachalam G, Wong C, et al. Cigarette-smoke-induced oxidative/nitrosative stress impairs VEGF- and fluid-shear-stress-mediated signaling in endothelial cells. *Antioxid Redox Signal*. 2010;12:1355-1369.

133. Suzuki M, Betsuyaku T, Nagai K, et al. Decreased airway expression of vascular endothelial growth factor in cigarette smoke-induced emphysema in mice and COPD patients. *Inhal Toxicol*. 2008;20:349-359.

134. Michaud SE, Menard C, Guy LG, Gennaro G, Rivard A. Inhibition of hypoxia-induced angiogenesis by cigarette smoke exposure: impairment of the HIF-1alpha/VEGF pathway. *Faseb J*. 2003;17:1150-1152.

135. Hsiao HM, Sapinoro RE, Thatcher TH, et al. A novel anti-inflammatory and pro-resolving role for resolvin D1 in acute cigarette smoke-induced lung inflammation. *PLoS One*. 2013;8:e58258.

136. Levy BD, Serhan CN. Resolution of acute inflammation in the lung. *Annu Rev Physiol*. 2014;76:467-492.

137. D'Alessio FR, Tsushima K, Aggarwal NR, et al. CD4+CD25+Foxp3+ Tregs resolve experimental lung injury in mice and are present in humans with acute lung injury. *J Clin Invest*. 2009;119:2898-2913.

138. Botelho FM, Gaschler GJ, Kianpour S, et al. Innate immune processes are sufficient for driving cigarette smoke-induced inflammation in mice. *Am J Respir Cell Mol Biol*. 2010;42:394-403.

139. Wang H, Peng W, Weng Y, et al. Imbalance of Th17/Treg cells in mice with chronic cigarette

smoke exposure. *Int Immunopharmacol.* 2012;14:504-512.

140. Ng SP, Silverstone AE, Lai ZW, Zelikoff JT. Prenatal exposure to cigarette smoke alters later-life antitumor cytotoxic T-lymphocyte (CTL) activity via possible changes in T-regulatory cells. *J Toxicol Environ Health A.* 2013;76:1096-1110.

141. Levy BD, Lukacs NW, Berlin AA, et al. Lipoxin A4 stable analogs reduce allergic airway responses via mechanisms distinct from CysLT1 receptor antagonism. *Faseb J.* 2007;21:3877-3884.

142. Bonnans C, Levy BD. Lipid mediators as agonists for the resolution of acute lung inflammation and injury. *Am J Respir Cell Mol Biol.* 2007;36:201-205.

143. Bozinovski S, Uddin M, Vlahos R, et al. Serum amyloid A opposes lipoxin A(4) to mediate glucocorticoid refractory lung inflammation in chronic obstructive pulmonary disease. *Proc Natl Acad Sci U S A.* 2012;109:935-940.

144. Serhan CN, Chiang N, Van Dyke TE. Resolving inflammation: dual anti-inflammatory and pro-resolution lipid mediators. *Nat Rev Immunol.* 2008;8:349-361.

145. Seki H, Fukunaga K, Arita M, et al. The anti-inflammatory and proresolving mediator resolvin E1 protects mice from bacterial pneumonia and acute lung injury. *J Immunol.* 2010;184:836-843.

146. Liao Z, Dong J, Wu W, et al. Resolvin D1 attenuates inflammation in lipopolysaccharide-induced acute lung injury through a process involving the PPARgamma/NF-kappaB pathway. *Respir Res.* 2012;13:110.

147. Aoki H, Hisada T, Ishizuka T, et al. Resolvin E1 dampens airway inflammation and hyperresponsiveness in a murine model of asthma. *Biochem Biophys Res Commun.* 2008;367:509-515.

148. Martin N, Ruddick A, Arthur GK, et al. Primary human airway epithelial cell-dependent inhibition of human lung mast cell degranulation. *PLoS One.* 2012;7:e43545.

149. El Kebir D, Gjorstrup P, Filep JG. Resolvin E1 promotes phagocytosis-induced neutrophil apoptosis and accelerates resolution of pulmonary inflammation. *Proc Natl Acad Sci U S A.* 2012;109:14983-14988.

150. Hardie DG. Roles of protein kinases and phosphatases in signal transduction. *Symp Soc Exp Biol.* 1990;44:241-255.

151. Mercer BA, D'Armiento JM. Emerging role of MAP kinase pathways as therapeutic targets in COPD. *Int J Chron Obstruct Pulmon Dis.* 2006;1:137-150.

152. Mercer B, Kolesnikova N, Sonett J, D'Armiento J. Extracellular regulated kinase/mitogen activated protein kinase is up-regulated in pulmonary emphysema and mediates matrix metalloproteinase-1 induction by cigarette smoke. *J Biol Chem.* 2004;279:17690-17696.

153. Ryter SW, Kim HP, Hoetzel A, et al. Mechanisms of cell death in oxidative stress. *Antioxid Redox Signal.* 2007;9:49-89.

154. Schemarova IV. The role of tyrosine phosphorylation in regulation of signal transduction pathways in unicellular eukaryotes. *Curr Issues Mol Biol.* 2006;8:27-49.

155. Wallace AM, Hardigan A, Geraghty P, et al. Protein phosphatase 2A regulates innate immune and proteolytic responses to cigarette smoke exposure in the lung. *Toxicol Sci.* 2012;126:589-599.

156. Sandelowsky H, Stallberg B, Nager A, Hasselstrom J. The prevalence of undiagnosed chronic obstructive pulmonary disease in a primary care population with respiratory tract infections—a case finding study. *BMC Fam Pract.* 2011;12:122.

157. Churg A, Sin DD, Wright JL. Everything prevents emphysema: are animal models of cigarette smoke-induced chronic obstructive pulmonary disease any use? *Am J Respir Cell Mol Biol.* 2011;45:1111-1115.

158. Trifilieff A, Walker C, Keller T, Kottirsch G, Neumann U. Pharmacological profile of PKF242-484 and PKF241-466, novel dual inhibitors of TNF-alpha converting enzyme and matrix metalloproteinases, in models of airway inflammation. *Br J Pharmacol.* 2002;135:1655-1664.

159. Zhang C, Chen P, Cai S, Chen JB, Wu J. The effects of recombinant human tumor necrosis factor-Fc on pulmonary function in a rat model of chronic obstructive pulmonary disease. *Zhonghua Jie He He Hu Xi Za Zhi.* 2007;30:432-436.

160. Aaron SD, Vandemheen KL, Maltais F, et al. TNFalpha antagonists for acute exacerbations of COPD: a randomised double-blind controlled trial. *Thorax.* 2013;68:142-148.

161. Rennard SI, Fogarty C, Kelsen S, et al. The safety and efficacy of infliximab in moderate to severe chronic obstructive pulmonary disease. *Am J Respir Crit Care Med.* 2007;175:926-934.

162. Irvin CG, Bates JH. Measuring the lung function in the mouse: the challenge of size. *Respir Res.* 2003;4:4.

163. Shapiro S. The macrophage in chronic obstructive pulmonary disease. *Am J Respir Crit Care Med.* 1999;160:S29-S32.

164. Box GEP, Draper NR. *Empirical Model-Building and Response Surfaces.* New York: Wiley; 1987.

Toxic Pulmonary Inhalation

57B

Jennifer Wang, DO and
John M. Oropello, MD, FACP, FCCP, FCCM

KEY POINTS

1 Accidental and intentional airway inhalation injuries are a major cause of death in the United States.

2 Toxic inhalants include asphyxiants, irritants and systemic toxins that result in airway damage, hypoxia and respiratory failure.

3 Tests and imaging should include arterial blood gas, carboxyhemoglobin level, chest

radiograph, electrocardiogram (EKG), and may include bronchoscopy.

4 Attention should be focused on securing the airway, insuring adequate oxygenation, treating shock, correcting acidemia, cardiac monitoring, and administering available antidotes.

INTRODUCTION

Fires kill more than 3200 and injure approximately 16,000 civilians annually in the United States[1,2] via thermal, chemical and systemic injury to the airway caused by toxic inhalation of carbon monoxide (CO), cyanide (CN), and other toxins. Toxic inhalation is the major cause of death from fires with 80% of cases related to CO poisoning.[3] Complications of toxic inhalation include airway damage, pneumonia, and acute respiratory distress syndrome (ARDS).[4] More than 50,000 patients a year visit the emergency department with CO poisoning in the United States.[5]

PATHOPHYSIOLOGY

Particles greater than 5 μm in diameter are cleared by the nasopharynx,[6] but in smoke inhalation, larger particles may lodge deeper in the airway as patients breathe through the mouth.[4] Thermal injuries from fires primarily affect the upper airways, as air cools as it travels to the carina. Combustion results in decreased oxygen in ambient air and asphyxiation.

Damage to the airway and lung parenchyma result in free radical formation, inflammation, increased capillary permeability, and capillary leakage. Alveoli are filled with fluid and blood. Polymorphonuclear macrophages, IL-1, IL6, IL-8, and tumor necrosis factor-α activation result in atelectasis, bronchospasm, impaired mucociliary function, and in some cases, ARDS. ARDS results from alveolar and lung endothelium capillary injury. Initially inflammation leads to increased capillary endothelial permeability resulting in accumulation of fluid in the alveoli and pulmonary edema. This leads to intrapulmonary shunting as fluid-filled alveoli are perfused but not ventilated, resulting in hypoxemia.

Toxic inhalants can be divided into asphyxiants, irritants and systemic toxins. Asphyxiants induce hypoxia, which can result in headache, dizziness, nausea, dyspnea, altered mental status, cardiac ischemia, respiratory failure, syncope, coma, and seizures. Simple asphyxiants such as helium, argon, carbon dioxide, chlorofluorocarbon refrigerants, methane, and propane displace oxygen and result in oxygen deprivation. Systemic asphyxiants such as CO, CNs, and sulfides impair oxygen transport resulting in tissue hypoxia and reduced oxidative phosphorylation and hence ATP synthesis. Irritants such as ammonia, chlorine, nitrogen oxides, and sulfur dioxide, and systemic toxins such as hydrocarbons, organophosphates, and metal fumes can cause upper and lower airway burns and destruction resulting in respiratory distress and failure.

DIAGNOSIS AND TREATMENT

In all cases of toxic inhalation (Table 57B–1) priorities include securing the airway and insuring adequate oxygenation, treating shock with crystalloids and vasopressors, correcting acidemia, cardiac

monitoring and administering antidotes if available.[7] Tests and imaging should include complete blood count, complete metabolic panel, arterial blood gases (ABG), carboxyhemoglobin to rule out CO poisoning, chest radiograph and an ECG to look for arrhythmias and myocardial ischemia.

Any patient that has the potential to become hemodynamically unstable or have airway compromise should be monitored in the ICU. Patients who appear ill or those with serious comorbidities, other injuries such as hypoxia from smoke inhalation, airway compromise requiring mechanical intubation or burns should be admitted to the ICU. All toxic inhalation victims should receive high (FiO_2 100%) supplemental oxygen, decontamination, airway protection, bronchodilators if necessary and close monitoring.[8,9]

TABLE 57B-1 Potential toxins in inhalational injury.

Category	Substance	Source	Mechanism of Injury	Specific Treatment Considerations
Asphyxiants	Carbon monoxide (CO)	Motor vehicle exhaust fumes, heaters, smoke, gas	Competes for hemoglobin binding sites, impairs oxygen delivery and usage	100% oxygen, hyperbaric oxygen
	Cyanide (CN)	Paint, nylon, silk, wool combustion, smoke	Inhibits cytochrome oxidase	Hydroxycobalamin, thiosulfate; amyl nitrite, sodium nitrite —> methemoglobinemia
	Hydrogen sulfide	Sewer, farm manure, natural hot springs	Inhibits cytochrome oxidase	Amyl nitrite, sodium nitrite —> methemoglobinemia (not as clearly effective as in CN poisoning)
Irritants	Ammonia	Nylon, refrigerant, plastic, fertilizer	Upper airway damage	
	Chlorine	Bleach, germicide	Lower airway damage	
	Nitrogen oxides	Wall paper, lacquered wood, dye, diesel combustion	Lower airway damage	Methylene blue
	Sulfur dioxide	Coal, oil, cooking fuel combustion	Upper airway damage	
Systemic toxins	Hydrocarbons	Glue, paint remover, solvents	CNS depression, bronchospasm, coma	
	Organophosphates	Insecticides, nerve agents	Blocks acetylcholinesterase	Atropine ± pralidoxime
	Metal fumes	Welding	Flu-like symptoms, throat irritation, chest tightness	

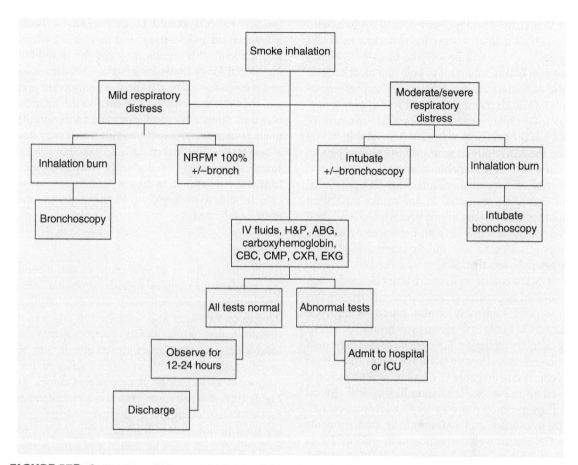

FIGURE 57B-1 Algorithm: Patients with burns in the mouth or difficulty speaking should be evaluated for early intubation. In these patients, laryngoscopy or bronchoscopy can be used to evaluate the extent of airway swelling, ulceration, and structural damage.

Hyperbaric oxygen is useful for CO, CN, and hydrogen sulfide toxicity as it increases the amount of dissolved oxygen in the blood and increases delivery of nonhemoglobin bound oxygen to tissues. Its use is limited by availability. The benefits of hyperbaric oxygen on noncomatose patients are inconclusive.[10] Patients with burns in the mouth or difficulty speaking should be evaluated for early intubation. In these patients, laryngoscopy or bronchoscopy can be used to evaluate the extent of airway swelling, ulceration, and structural damage (Figure 57B-1).

Asphyxiants

CO is the most frequent cause of toxic inhalation in the United States. It is an odorless, colorless gas produced by incomplete combustion of hydrocarbons. Hypoxia results from hemoglobin having a 200-fold greater binding affinity to CO than to oxygen, causing decreased oxygen transport and unloading. Important sources of CO include motor vehicle exhaust, metal and chemical manufacturing, fires, stoves, cigarette smoke, and unvented space heaters. Elevated carboxyhemoglobin levels confirm the diagnosis. However, low carboxyhemoglobin levels do not exclude CO toxic exposure if there is a delay between exposure and testing; oxygen therapy lowers CO levels more rapidly. Severe CO toxicity causes lactic acidosis. The SaO_2 reported from standard ABG (SaO_2 value is calculated from the dissolved oxygen [PaO_2]) will be normal in the presence of CO toxicity; direct measurement of oxyhemoglobin with co-oximetry is needed to accurately detect the SaO_2, which will be lowered by carboxyhemoglobin. It is also important to note that most bedside pulse oximeters cannot differentiate carboxyhemoglobin from oxyhemoglobin and will display a normal SpO_2 (SpO_2 = pulse oximeter measurement of SaO_2) in the presence of low oxyhemoglobin.[11,12] Of note, the ABG findings seen with CO poisoning also occur with methemoglobinemia.

CN toxicity often occurs with CO poisoning and should be suspected in any smoke inhalation patient with elevated carboxyhemoglobin levels and severe lactic acidosis or with persistent neurologic symptoms despite low carboxyhemoglobin levels, for example, less than 30%.

CN is a colorless gas with a bitter almond smell. It is found in plastics, paints, lacquer, polyurethane, nylon, and rubber. It is also found in cigarette smoke. CN binds to ferric on cytochrome a3, arresting cellular respiration. CN toxicity causes persistent hypotension and severe lactic acidemia. There is no specific test to diagnose CN toxicity and suspicion is based on the smoke inhalation history and clinical findings as noted above under CO. Hydroxocobalamin, thiosulfate, and sodium nitrite are treatments for CN toxicity. Hydroxocobalamin directly binds CN, thiosulfate increases the detoxification of CN, and sodium nitrite results in methemoglobin formation increasing the affinity of CN away from the cytochromes and toward hemoglobin. Methemoglobin levels must be checked in these patients. In an event, nitrites should not be administered in patients with significant hypoxemia (eg, as a result of high carboxyhemoglobin levels) that cannot tolerate any further reductions in oxygen delivery (oxyhemoglobin) caused by methemoglobin generation.

Hydrogen sulfide is a colorless, flammable gas that is irritating to eyes and mucous membranes and has a rotten egg odor. It is formed from the decomposition of organic material including crude oil, petroleum, sewers, compost pics, cleaners, sulfur springs, and underground fields of natural gas. Toxicity causes central nervous system (CNS) and respiratory depression. There are no specific tests to diagnose hydrogen sulfide poisoning is suspicion based on the exposure history and clinical findings. There is no specific antidote for hydrogen sulfide

toxicity. Patients should be monitored for ocular inflammation and scarring, and pulmonary edema. Any patient with significant exposure should be monitored for 24 hours for signs of CNS depression and respiratory distress. If these symptoms are present, the patient should be admitted to the intensive care unit. Supportive respiratory and cardiovascular management are primary. Sodium nitrite may have a benefit if administered early in patients without severe hypoxemia by inducing methemoglobin formation to attract hydrogen sulfide away from cytochromes to hemoglobin. Methemoglobin levels must be followed.

Irritants

Irritant inhalation is often a result of manufacturing accidents. Examples include ammonia, chlorine, nitrogen oxide, and sulfur dioxide. Symptoms depend on exposure and solubility. Highly soluble irritants cause upper airway burns whereas low soluble irritants cause lower airway destruction. No specific tests are available to detect irritant toxicity. Ammonia and chlorine have pungent odors, are highly corrosive and cause extensive airway damage, bronchoconstriction and pulmonary edema. Both are used in household cleaners. Ammonia is used in fertilizer and manufacturing. Chlorine is used as a bleach and in manufacturing paper, cloth, and pesticides.[13]

Nitrogen oxides are nonflammable and colorless gases that are found in vehicle exhaust, coal, oil, natural gas combustion, and in manufacturing. Exposure primarily causes lower respiratory tract damage and results in free radical generation, reduced immune function, methemoglobinemia, pulmonary edema, and bronchospasm.

There are no antidotes for ammonia, chlorine, nitrogen oxide, and sulfur dioxide exposure, although methylene blue is used to treat nitrous oxide induced methemoglobinemia.

Methemoglobin and Treatment of Methemoglobinemia

Methemoglobin is an altered form of hemoglobin where iron is oxidized from ferrous to a ferric state, rendering it unable to bind oxygen. It results in decreased oxygen carrying capacity of blood.

Normal methemoglobin levels are 1% to 3%. Methemoglobinemia results in cyanosis which does not improve with oxygenation and ventilation. Levels above 15% cause cardiac, respiratory, and neurologic symptoms, and levels more than 70% are usually fatal. Sources of methemoglobin include nitrates, exhaust, cocaine, dapsone, metoclopramide, primaquine, rasburicase, and sulfonamides.

Pulse oximeters estimate oxygen saturation by comparing the absorbance of light at 2 wavelengths; oxyhemoglobin absorbs infrared light and deoxyhemoglobin absorbs red light. Methemoglobin and oxyhemoglobin absorbance characteristics are similar, thereby, falsely elevating pulse oximeter readings. Specialized pulse oximeters with co-oximetry measure light absorbance at 4 or more wavelengths enabling accurate measurements of oxyhemoglobin, methemoglobin, and carboxyhemoglobin.

The treatment for methemoglobinemia is methylene blue which rapidly reduces methemoglobin to hemoglobin. In high doses, methylene blue can actually induce methemoglobinemia. Methylene blue is contraindicated in patients with glucose-6-phosphate dehydrogenase deficiency because it is ineffective and can cause severe hemolysis.

Systemic Toxins

Hydrocarbons are organic substances that have the potential to be inhaled as recreational drugs or in workplace accidents. Examples include: gasoline, motor oil, paint, glue, and solvents. Inhalation toxicity often results in pneumonitis. Organophosphates are found in insecticides, herbicides, nerve agents, fertilizers, and solvents. Organophosphates inhibit acetylcholinesterase, resulting in cholinergic overstimulation. Toxicity is a clinical diagnosis. Symptoms include sweating, lacrimation, rhinorrhea, salivation, bronchorrhea, miosis, weakness, fasciculations, paralysis, tachycardia, hypertension, and respiratory failure. Metal fumes released by welding cause flu-like illness. Symptoms are often transient and self-limited, and are more likely and severe after a period away from work.

Hydrocarbons and metal fume toxicities are treated with supportive care including supplemental oxygen, decontamination, airway protection and bronchodilators if necessary. Organophosphate antidotes include atropine and pralidoxime.

It is essential to remove any contaminated clothing. Healthcare workers must also take precautions while decontaminating victims.

REFERENCES

1. US Fire Administration NFIRS. Fire loss in the United States (2000-2011). [Excel spreadsheet]. 2015; "Fires & Losses Trends 2002-2011 worksheet." Available at: https://www.usfa.fema.gov/data/statistics/order_download_data.html - download. Accessed 12/10/2015, 2015.
2. Haynes HJG. Fire Loss in the United States During 2014. [PDF]. 2015. Available at: http://www.nfpa.org/~/media/FD0144A044C84FC5BAF90C05C04890B7. Accessed 12/10/2015.
3. Haponik EF, Crapo RO, Herndon DN, Traber DL, Hudson L, Moylan J. Smoke inhalation. *Am Rev Respir Dis*. 1988;138(4):1060-1063.
4. Iberti T, Oropello J. Toxic pulmonary inhalation and thermal burns. In: Callaham ML, ed. *Current Practice of Emergency Medicine*. 2nd ed. Philadelphia B.C.: Decker; 1991:420-426.
5. Hampson NB, Weaver LK. Carbon monoxide poisoning: a new incidence for an old disease. *Undersea Hyperb Med*. 2007;34(3):163-168.
6. Schwab JA, Zenkel M. Filtration of particulates in the human nose. *Laryngoscope*. 1998;108(1 Pt 1): 120-124.
7. Borron SW, Bebarta VS. Asphyxiants. *Emerg Med Clin North Am*. 2015;33(1):89-115.
8. Kales SN, Christiani DC. Acute chemical emergencies. *N Engl J Med*. 2004;350(8):800-808.
9. Rehberg S, Maybauer MO, Enkhbaatar P, Maybauer DM, Yamamoto Y, Traber DL. Pathophysiology, management and treatment of smoke inhalation injury. *Expert Rev Respir Med*. 2009;3(3):283-297.
10. Raphael JC, Elkharrat D, Jars-Guincestre MC, et al. Trial of normobaric and hyperbaric oxygen for acute carbon monoxide intoxication. *Lancet*. 1989;2(8660):414-419.
11. Buckley RG, Aks SE, Eshom JL, Rydman R, Schaider J, Shayne P. The pulse oximetry gap in carbon monoxide intoxication. *Ann Emerg Med*. 1994;24(2):252-255.
12. Vegfors M, Lennmarken C. Carboxyhaemoglobinaemia and pulse oximetry. *Br J Anaesth*. 1991;66(5):625-626.
13. Agency for Toxic Substances and Disease Registry: Cyanide, hydrogen sulfide, ammonia, chlorine, nitrogen oxides, sulfur dioxide. Available at: http://www.atsdr.cdc.gov. Accessed 12/10/2015.

Overdose, Poisoning, and Withdrawal

Edward Mossop, MD and Fred DiBlasio, MD

KEY POINTS

1 Supportive care is most important. "Treat the patient not the poison."

2 Always check for the common and treatable coingestants: alcohol, acetaminophen, and salicylates.

3 Consider decontamination and the use of antidotes.

4 Empiric treatment with glucose, naloxone and thiamine is generally safe in the comatose patient.

5 Always seek help from your regional poison control center.

GENERAL PRINCIPLES OF OVERDOSE AND POISONING

Introduction

Exposures to toxic substances, whether accidental or intentional, remain a significant contributor to morbidity and mortality in the U.S. Approximately 10,830 calls are placed to the Poison Control hotline daily, while The American Association of Poison Control Centers (AAPCC) reported over 2.3 million human exposure calls in 2011, most commonly due to analgesics (12.9%), sedatives and antipsychotics (11%), and antidepressants (6.4%).

The American Academy of Clinical Toxicology (AACT) and the European Association of Poisons Centres and Clinical Toxicologists (EAPCCT) provide detailed guidance regarding overdose, poisoning and withdrawal. In addition assistance should always be obtained from regional poison control centers.

The American Association of Poison Control Centers (AAPCC) can be contacted by the following means: www.aapcc.org or 1-800-222-1222.

History and Physical

Clinicians must follow a systematic and consistent approach throughout evaluation and management. A basic history and physical exam, followed by a more focused poison-specific exam, is vital, from which point management is directed toward the provision of acute stabilization, supportive care, prevention of absorption and, when applicable, the use of antidotes and enhanced elimination techniques.

Due to depressed mentation or reluctance to cooperate useful information may be obtainable from a patient's associates (family, friends, and coworkers), or from first responders and bystanders. Environmental clues such as suicide notes, drug paraphernalia and empty pill bottles can provide valuable information. Once the patient is identified, reviewing prior hospital records may reveal a history of recent prescriptions, previous overdoses and any psychiatric history.

Specificity regarding the type of drug or toxin (including; prescription, illicit, over the counter and herbal medications), the dosage, route of exposure, time of exposure or ingestion and intent requires close attention. Unknown pills or chemicals require

TABLE 58-1   Toxidrome oriented physical exam.

Toxidrome-Oriented Examination
Vital signs
Focused neurologic exam centered on level of consciousness (alert, responsive to voice, responsive to pain, unresponsive)
Pupillary and motor reaction
Skin examination (moisture, cyanosis, rashes)
Respiratory examination
Assessement of bowel sounds

Reproduced with permission from Rumack BH, Matthew H: Acetaminophen poisoning and toxicity, Pediatrics. 1975 Jun;55(6):871-876

identification by consultation with a regional poison control center, computerized drug database, or product manufacturers.

Toxidromes are specific symptoms and physical signs that correlate with the manifestations of a drug class on a particular set of neuroreceptors.

Performed quickly while resuscitative measures are being instituted, a toxidrome-oriented exam should include vital signs, a focused neurological exam centered on level of consciousness, pupillary and motor reaction, broad examination of the skin noting moisture, cyanosis, rashes, and puncture marks, focused evaluation of the respiratory system, and assessment of bowel sounds. See Table 58–1 Toxidromes-oriented physical exam and Table 58–2: Toxidrome clinical findings.

TABLE 58-2   Common toxidromes.

Category	Vital Signs	Mental Status	Physical Signs	Agent/Drug
Sympathomimetic	hypertension, tachycardia hyperthermia, tachypnea	Hyperalert, euphoric agitated, delirium	Mydriasis, tremor, increased peristalsis seizures	Cocaine, MDMA Mephedrone, Methamphetamine
Opioid	Hypotension, bradycardia, apnea, shallow breathing, hypothermia	Stupor, lethargy, coma	Miosis, hyporeflexia	Morphine, oxycodone, fentanyl
Sedative-Hypnotic	Hypotension, bradycardia, apnea	Stupor, coma, slurred speech	Hyporeflexia, ataxia,	Benzodiazepines, zolpidem, barbiturates
Anticholingeric	Hypertension, tachycardia, hyperthermia	Agitated, delirium, hallucinations	Mydriasis, dry flushed skin, urinary retention, decreased bowel sounds, dry mucus membranes, seizures	Atropine, antidepressants, antihistamines
Cholinergic	Bradycardia, apnea, shallow breathing	Confusion, agitation, coma	Miosis, salivation, lacrimation, diaphoresis, nausea, vomiting, urination, defecation, muscle fasciculations, weakness, seizures, arrhythmia	Organophosphates
Hallucinogenic	Hyperthermia, hypertension, tachycardia	Agitated but oriented, psychosis, anxiety	Mydriasis, synesthesia, nystagmus	PCP, LSD, mushrooms, MDMA
Serotonin	Hyperthermia, tachycardia, hypertension, tachypnea	Agitation, confusion	Increased muscle tone, hyperreflexia, clonus	SSRIs, dextromethorphan, TCAs, amphetamines

SSRI: selective serotonin reuptake inhibitor; TCA: tricyclic antidepressants; PCP: phencyclidine; LSD: Lysergic acid diethylamide; MDMA: Methylenedioxymethamphetamine

Investigations

Labs

Bedside serum glucose testing is a requirement for any patient with altered mentation, after which immediate empiric dextrose administration is recommended in cases where measurement result is low, or not available. Thiamine should also be replaced in patients suspected to be deficient, to prevent precipitation of Wernicke encephalopathy (chronic alcoholics). However, it is not recommended to delay glucose administration while thiamine is administered.

Salicylates, acetaminophen, and alcohol are all easily available and commonly used agents, therefore may be co-ingested in addition to other medications in deliberate overdose attempts. Acetaminophen and salicylates are also found in numerous combination preparations of prescription drugs and over-the-counter medications. These agents therefore may worsen outcomes or complicate presenting symptoms and signs in an overdose. Because these agents are so commonly used and potentially treatable, it is recommended to routinely check these blood levels in all overdose patients.

Additional basic investigations should include, complete blood count (CBC), serum electrolytes, blood urea nitrogen, serum creatinine, coagulation profile, liver function tests (LFTs), creatine kinase (CK), arterial blood gas (ABG), serum osmolality, calculated osmolar gap, and a urine analysis (crystals, myo- or hemoglobinuria).

Specific scenarios may necessitate additional testing including specific drug levels, or testing for methemoglobin and carboxyhemoglobin. Serum concentrations may be of utility in the management of salicylate, acetaminophen, barbiturates, digoxin, ethanol, iron, lithium, and theophylline overdose as these serum assays provide rapid result and are widely available.

Urine toxicology screen does not necessarily reflect current intoxication, and may serve in some cases as a distracter rather than a diagnostic aid in patients with change in mental status.

EKG

An electrocardiogram may assist in the evaluation for the presence and severity of specific ingestions, or may demonstrate drug-related cardiotoxicity. Serially, the electrocardiogram (EKG) can facilitate the monitoring of progression of specified toxicities. Performed in all subjects with suspected drug ingestion, the key features to note include heart rate, dysrhythmia, axes, and intervals (QRS and QTc).

Imaging

In some cases, a plain abdominal film may demonstrate radiopaque medications such as iron tablets, and enteric-coated preparations, while indirect visualization of drug packets (body packers and stuffers) may be demonstrated by the alteration of bowel gas patterns. Additionally, visualized radiographic evidence of non-cardiogenic pulmonary edema and/or Adult Respiratory Distress Syndrome on an anterior posterior (AP) chest film, can suggest the exposure to specific toxic agents.

A non-contrast head Computerized Tomography (CT) should be considered in anyone with a change in mental status to exclude non-toxicological causes. In addition significant hypertension and change in mental status, in the setting of overdose with agents with stimulant properties, may be secondary to intracranial complications such as hemorrhage, stroke or encephalopathy.

Initial Hospital Care

"Treat the patient, not the poison" is the adage summating the guiding principle of medical toxicology, and the treatment of this certain population of patients. Still, the methods are generally similar to those utilized frequently in the care of critically ill patients.

In the majority of cases, general supportive care is paramount and frequently sufficient to affect complete recovery, yet initial therapeutic measures will depend on the toxin ingested, severity of illness, and time elapsed between exposure and presentation. Assistance should always be obtained from regional poison control centers.

Airway

Acute respiratory failure and severe acid-base disturbances demand endotracheal intubation and mechanical ventilation. Intubation for the purpose of airway protection should be undertaken early in the poisoned patient with depressed mental status unless a rapidly reversible cause is known given high risk of aspiration, which is increased at times when gastric decontamination must be performed.

Hemodynamic Support

Abnormal hemodynamics such as blood pressure, heart rate, and temperature should be treated in the standard way as per hospital guidelines. An appropriate volume of isotonic intravenous crystalloids should be used to treat hypotension. Refractory hypotension and shock should be treated with direct-acting vasopressors (norepinephrine, epinephrine, or vasopressin) however this may be ineffective in cases of calcium channel overdose (see calcium channel overdose).

Hypertension as sequelae of agitation, or arising directly from ingestion of agents with stimulant properties, can be treated initially with sedatives such as benzodiazepines. Should hypertension require specific therapy due to associated end-organ dysfunction (hypertensive emergency), dihydropyridine subclass calcium-channel blockers are preferable given a profile of potent vasodilatation and few negative effects on cardiac conduction and contractility.

Hyperthermia should be very closely monitored. When the temperature exceeds 39 degrees Celsius urgent cooling is required. Numerous techniques exist and initially should include the use of fans, antipyretic medications (unless contra-indicated), cold IV fluids and ice baths. More specialized methods include the use of intravenous cooling catheters and cooling pads applied to the skin. Those with excessive agitation, recurrent seizures or increased muscular tone may require sedation and paralysis to prevent excessive heat production.

Control of Seizures

Seizures resulting from poisoning or withdrawal are best initially treated with benzodiazepines from which escalation to antiepileptic drugs may be necessitated by persistence of seizures, noting that phenytoin is not recommended in the poisoned patient. In case of refractory seizure, general anesthesia and paralytic agents may be required, and treatment should be monitored with serial or continuous electroencephalography (EEG).

Altered Mental State-Agitation or Coma

Drug associated agitated behavior is best treated with benzodiazepine administration, complimented by high-potency antipsychotics as indicated.

Antipsychotics should however be used with caution as they can lower seizure threshold and worsen hyperthermia and arrhythmias (prolong QT) in certain cases of poisoning. Coma or depressed mental state management should focus on protection of the airway. In those patients with a depressed mental status with no compromise in airway, empiric treatments with naloxone, glucose and thiamine can be administered. The routine use of flumazenil, in the obtunded patient, for potential benzodiazepine overdose is not recommended due to the numerous adverse reactions associated.

Rhabdomyolysis

Rhabdomyolysis is a clinical condition characterized by myocyte injury and leakage of intracellular contents into the extracellular space. The most serious complication is renal failure and it is estimated that 8%-15% of all cases of acute renal failure (ARF) are caused by rhabdomyolysis. There are numerous triggers of rhabdomyolysis, however the final common pathway is depletion of muscle ATP stores causing loss of myocyte integrity causing dysfunction and release of intracellular contents.

Myocyte injury leads to release and increased levels of creatine kinase (CK), myoglobin, potassium, phosphorous, and uric acid. Calcium levels may be low. Myoglobin is excreted in the urine, which becomes a red/brown color. Heme pigment casts cause renal tubular injury and renal failure, which may worsen electrolyte abnormalities and produce an anion gap metabolic acidosis. Other serious complications include cardiac arrhythmias and arrest, compartment syndrome and disseminated intravascular coagulation (DIC). Patients usually report muscle pain, weakness and dark urine. Diagnosis is made by detecting markedly elevated levels of CK (usually greater than 5000 IU/L) with evidence of myoglobinuria on urine dipstick and microscopy.

Drug overdose or poisoning is a common cause of rhabdomyolysis and falls into 3 groups. 1. Trauma: Overdose victims may suffer muscle trauma from accidents or impulsive behavior leading to direct muscle injury. 2. Non-traumatic exertional: Overdose patients may develop extensive muscle activity from agitation or seizures, which can also cause extreme hyperthermia leading to myocyte

TABLE 58-3 Common drugs associated with rhabdomyolysis.

Common drugs associated with rhabdomyolysis	
Lysergic acid diethylamide (LSD)	HIV medications
Alcohol	Statins
Heroin	Macrolides
Cocaine	Colchicine
Amphetamines	Carbon monoxide
Methadone	Cyclosporine
Mushrooms	Antipsychotics
Antihistamines	selective serotonin reuptek inhibitor (SSRIs)

injury. 3. Non-traumatic non-exertional: Certain drugs or toxins can lead to direct myocyte damage. Other drugs may induce coma leading to ischemic compression. Drug induced hyperthermia, without muscle activity, can lead to increased muscle energy demands and subsequent injury. See Table 58–3: Common drugs associated with rhabdomyolysis.

Management of rhabdomyolysis from a poison, drug or toxin initially involves discontinuing the offending agent and using decontamination or enhanced elimination techniques to remove any drug or toxin. Aggressively control any hyperthermia, hyperactivity or agitation. Early and aggressive fluid resuscitation is the mainstay of treatment to prevent renal injury. Fluids should be started if CK levels are > 5000 IU/L. The optimal fluid and rate of repletion are unclear. Fluid repletion should be continued until plasma CK levels decrease to < 5000 IU/L and urine is dipstick negative for hematuria. A forced alkaline diuresis, raising urine pH is raised to above 6.5 with sodium bicarbonate, may diminish the renal toxicity of heme however there is no strong evidence to support this.

Decontamination and Enhanced Elimination

Decontamination involves removal of the toxin/poison from patient surfaces and gastrointestinal (GI) tract. In addition enhanced elimination techniques including ion tapping, chelation therapy, hemodialysis, hemoperfusion, and lipid emulsion can be used to remove poisons/toxins already absorbed.

Decontamination

Surface Decontamination

Surface decontamination involves the removal of dermal and ocular toxins by irrigation. The eye should be irrigated with an isotonic crystalloid until a physiological pH is restored.

Gastrointestinal Decontamination

The practice known as GI decontamination refers to the functional removal of ingested toxins from the GI tract in order to decrease absorption. No controlled clinical studies have demonstrated that the "routine" use of GI decontamination reduces morbidity and mortality in poisoned patients. However, evidence from human volunteer trials and clinical studies suggest that decontamination may reduce the absorption of toxins in the GI tract and may be helpful in select circumstances

Many methods have faded from clinical practice due to evidence based delineation of poor efficacy, and high risks, as well as position papers compiled by AACT and EAPCCT.

1. Ipecac—The only emetic suitable for use in humans is syrup of ipecac, and despite its unique niche, use has significantly declined due to lack of proven efficacy and risk of adverse events and therefore is not recommended.

2. Orogastric lavage—Gastric lavage involves the insertion of a large-bore 36- to 40-French orogastric tube and the subsequent positioning of the patient in the left lateral decubitus position with the head of the bed in Trendelenburg position. The instillation of approximately 250mL of water or saline follows, with the immediate evacuation via suction applied to the distal end of the tube. This cycle is completed until the evacuated solution is free of pill fragments or particulate matter. This method is only considered to be useful in the first hour post ingestion and has been used for agents that do not bind well to activated charcoal as well as for specific life threatening poisons such as tricyclic's, theophylline and cyanide.

Recent papers however, suggest that gastric lavage may be associated with serious complications, namely aspiration, esophageal perforation, hypothermia and death. The American Association of Poison Centers (AAPC) and the European Association of Poisons Centres and Clinical Toxicologists (EAPCCT) have issued a joint statement that gastric lavage should not be employed routinely, if ever, in the management of poisoned patients.

3. Activated charcoal—Activated charcoal (AC) is an organic material, which adsorbs chemicals with a molecular weight range of 100-1000 Daltons, preventing gastrointestinal absorption and subsequent toxicity. The agent can be administered orally or via a nasogastric tube, in single- and multi-dose regimens depending on the toxin ingested, and is administered in a slurry in water containing 25 to 100 g initially (or for single dosing) followed by 25 to 50 g every 2 to 4 hours in adults, unless the toxin dose is known, in which case the dosing of charcoal to toxin is a 10:1 ratio.

Many chemicals adsorb avidly to AC in a dose dependent fashion but certain substances particularly highly ionic compounds with low molecular weight, mineral acids, and strong bases do not bind well. AC has not been shown to adsorb ethanol, even when administered prior to ethanol ingestion. See Table 58–4: Poisons not well bound to activated charcoal.

Those most likely to benefit from single dose activated charcoal (SDAC) must present within one hour of poison ingestion, but despite lack of evidence, potential for benefit later in the course cannot be excluded.

Contraindications include a depressed mental status without airway protection (risk of aspiration), increased risk of severity of aspiration based on ingested toxin (eg, hydrocarbon ingestion), a need for endoscopy, ingestion of a poorly adsorbed toxin (metals including iron, lithium, alkali, mineral acids, alcohols), presence of intestinal obstruction, or concern for decreased peristalsis.

The AACT/EAPCCT recommends multiple-dose activated charcoal (MDAC) be considered only for patients having ingested life threatening amounts of carbamazepine, dapsone, phenobarbital, quinine or theophylline. See Table 58–5: AACT/EAPCCT recommended drugs amenable to repeat dosing of activated charcoal.

TABLE 58–4 Poisons not well bound to activated charcoal.

AC not recommended
Lead
Mercury
Iron
Zinc
Acid/Alkalis
Hydrocarbons
Alcohols
Lithium
Calcium
Magnesium
Potassium

4. Bowel irrigation—Whole bowel irrigation refers to the rapid elimination of unabsorbed toxin from the GI tract through the use of iso-osmotic polyethylene glycol solution at 25 to 40 mL/kg/hr until the rectal effluent is clear. Enteric-coated and extended-release preparations, certain metals, as well as drug packets could be expelled expeditiously in this manner.

Despite an absence of specific evidence to support improved outcomes, sizeable iron overdoses, carrying high morbidity, may benefit from this therapy noting the lack of an alternative.

TABLE 58–5 AACT/EAPCCT recommended drugs amenable to repeat dosing of activated charcoal.

Drugs amenable to repeat dosing of activated charcoal
Carbamazepine
Dapsone
Phenobarbital
Quinine
Theophylline

Enhanced Elimination Techniques

Ion Trapping and Forced Diuresis

The urinary excretion of some drugs can be enhanced by alkalization of the urine with the administration of intravenous sodium bicarbonate to produce urine with a pH $\geq$ 7.5, exploiting the fact that the ionization of a weak acid is increased in an alkaline environment thereby making it lipid in-soluble, reducing reabsorption and enhancing elimination by trapping the toxin in the urine.

Urine alkalization should be considered first line treatment in patients with moderate to severe salicylate poisoning that do not meet criteria for hemodialysis. See Table 58–6: Drugs with enhanced elimination by alkaline diuresis.

Chelation Therapy

Chelation therapy involves intravenous, intramuscular or oral administration of chelation agents to bind heavy metals in the blood stream promoting enhanced renal excretion. See Table 58–7: Different chelation therapies.

Extracorporeal Techniques

Hemodialysis (HD) can be used to remove certain toxins and correct electrolyte and acid-base disturbances induced by toxins. For HD to be effective, the toxin must reside primarily in the extracellular fluid.

Hemoperfusion (HP) refers to the circulation of blood through an extracorporeal circuit containing

TABLE 58–7 Different chelation therapies.

Agent	Route of Administration	Metals Bound
Dimercaprol	IM with urine alkalizing agent	Arsenic, gold, lead, mercury
Penicillamine	Oral	Copper, arsenic, lead
Deferoxamine	IV, IM, or SC	Iron

an adsorbent such as activated charcoal or polystyrene resin. Drugs that are adsorbed by activated charcoal are the same drugs that are amenable to HP.

Hemofiltration, peritoneal dialysis, plasmapheresis, and exchange transfusion can also help eliminate certain toxins. See Table 58–8: Poisons amenable to hemodialysis.

Lipid Emulsion

Intravenous lipid emulsions (ILE) are the fats used in total parenteral nutrition, and ILE has been used to treat toxicity due to lipophilic medication including verapamil, beta blockers, some tricyclic antidepressants, bupivacaine and chlorpromazine.

The proposed mechanism of action is that the ILE acts as a "lipid sink" surrounding a lipophilic drug molecule and rendering it ineffective. A second mechanism proposed is that fatty acids

TABLE 58–6 Drugs with enhanced elimination by alkaline diuresis.

Alkaline diuresis
Salicylates
Methotrexate
Barbiturates
Fluoride
Sulfonamides
Ethylene glycol
Methanol

TABLE 58–8 Poisons amenable to hemodialysis.

Hemodialysis enhanced
Elimination
Alcohols
Lithium
Salicylates
Atenolol
Sot3alol
Theophylline
Procainamide
Barbiturates

within the ILE provide the myocardium with a ready energy source thus improving cardiac function.

Antidotes

While in the majority of poisoning cases supportive care is the key element to improving the survival, a small number of toxins are amenable to a "silver bullet" in the form of an antidote.

By varied means, antidotes reduce or reverse the effects of a poison, but half-life of both the toxin and the antidote must be taken into account during treatment, especially regarding instances of antidotes that antagonize end-organ effects or inhibit conversion to toxic metabolites. See Table 58–9: Common antidotes/treatments.

Disposition

After the initial evaluation, treatment and observation period, patients who suffer from severe toxicity or who are at risk for complications should be admitted to the ICU. Advanced age, abnormal body temperature, and suicidal intent are associated with an increased risk of death.

Sustained-release products, and agents with delayed onset or prolonged action may require up to 24 hrs. of observation to ensure safety.

SEDATIVE-HYPNOTIC OVERDOSE

Sedatives and hypnotics are very commonly abused agents and include; benzodiazepines, barbiturates, and nonbenzodiazepines (zolpidem, zopicline, buspirone, GHB gamma-hydroxybutyric acid). Their use is frequently combined with alcohol and other drugs such as opiates. Typically patients have depressed neurological signs and can develop cardiac, respiratory, renal and gastrointestinal dysfunction. Withdrawal from sedative-hypnotics is often associated with seizures, which can be fatal.

Benzodiazepines

Benzodiazepines (alprazolam, diazepam, lorazepam) are sedative-hypnotic agents used to treat anxiety, seizures, withdrawal states, insomnia and drug associated agitation. Benzodiazepines enhance the inhibitory effect of the neurotransmitter gamma-aminobutyric acid (GABA), which manifests in central nervous system depression.

Clinical Features

Benzodiazepine overdose produces a specific sedative-hypnotic toxidrome. Mild to moderate overdose resembles that of ethanol. The majority of symptoms and signs are neurological and include somnolence, emotional lability, confusion, incoordination, impaired cognition, ataxia, and slurred speech, and may induce horizontal and vertical nystagmus, midriasis and hyporeflexia. Cardiovascular signs include hypotension and bradycardia. Short-term amnesia is a common and often desirable effect especially when used for procedural sedation or general anesthesia. Ingested alone these agents rarely cause significant toxicity, however coma and respiratory and cardiac arrest can be seen in the setting of co-ingestion with other depressants. Rarely patients can exhibit paradoxical excitement, agitation and disinhibition. Predisposition appears to be for younger and older age groups, as well as underlying psychiatric disorders though the mechanism remains unknown.

Differential Diagnosis

Barbiturates, nonbenzodiazepine sedatives (zolpidem, gamma hydroxybutyrate, etc), alcohol and opiates can all cause similar features. Serum and urine toxicological testing is of limited value, as levels do not correlate with clinical findings.

Treatment

Supportive care is the mainstay of treatment including stabilization of the airway, breathing and circulation followed by routine lab tests, control of agitation and seizures and management of any subsequent complications (see general principles of overdose and poisoning). Decontamination with activated charcoal should be considered if ingestion is within 1 hour of presentation. Due to the sedating effects of benzodiazepines and risk of aspiration, the airway should be secured prior to administration. Gastric lavage, forced diuresis and enhanced elimination techniques are not effective.

TABLE 58–9 Common antidotes/treatments.

Common Antidotes/Treatments		
Poison/Condition	**Antidote/Treatment**	**Dose**
Acetaminophen	N-Acetylcysteine	140 mg/kg po load, then 70 mg/kg every 4 hr for 17 doses OR 150 mg/kg IV load over 60 min then 50 mg/kg over 4 hr, then 100 mg/kg over 16 hr
Anticholinergic	Physostigmine	0.5-2 mg IV over 5 min
Benzodiazepines	Flumazenil	0.2 mg/kg IV
Beta blockers	Glucagon	0.05 mg/kg IV bolus may repeat every 10 min
Bupivucaine/local anesthetic	Lipid emulsion 20% IV	100 ml IV over 1 min, then 400 ml IV over 20 min
Calcium channel antagonists	Calcium chloride 10%	0.2-0.25 ml/kg IV
	Insulin	1 unit/kg bolus with 50 ml 50% dextrose followed by 1 unit/kg/hr with D10 W 200 ml/hr
	Glucagon	0.05 mg/kg IV bolus may repeat every 10 min
	Lipid emulsion 20% IV	100 ml IV over 1 min, then 400 ml IV over 20 min
Cholinergic agents	Pralidoxime (2-PAM)	1-2 g IV over 5-10 min, then 500 mg/hr infusion
Chronic alcohol/ Wernicke syndrome	Thiamine	100 mg IV
Cyanide and nitroprusside	Hydroxocobalamin Sodium thiosulfate (25%)	70 mg/kg IV (max 5 g in 30 min) Can repeat up to 3 times 50 ml IV
Digoxin	Digoxin Fab	5-10 vials IV
Ethylene glycol and methanol	Ethanol 10% IV Fomepizole	10 ml/kg IV over 30 min then 1.2 ml/kg/hr 15 mg/kg IV, then 10 mg/kg every 12 hr
Heparin	Protamine	25-50 mg IV
Iron	Deferoxamine	2 g IM, or 15 mg/kg/hr IV (max dose, 6-8 g/day)
Methemoglobin/oxidizing chemicals	Methylene blue	1-2 mg/kg IV
Methotrexate	Folic acid	1-2 mg/kg IV every 4-6 hr
Neuroleptic malignant syndrome	Dantrolene Bromocriptine	1-2.5 mg/kg IV 2.5 mg po every 6 hr
Opioids	Naloxone	0.1-2 mg IV Titrate to response
Serotonin syndrome	Cyproheptadine	4-12 mg po Repeat every 2 hr
Tricyclic antidepressants	Sodium bicarbonate	1-2 mEq/kg IV bolus Repeat as needed

Specific Therapy—Administration of flumazenil, a competitive antagonist of the benzodiazepine receptor, remains controversial due to the low morbidity and mortality associated with overdose, and the potential for inducing withdrawal seizures in patients who chronically take or abuse benzodiazepines, or in cases of pro-convulsant co-ingestion. Therefore flumazenil should not be used empirically for the sedative-hypnotic toxidrome. Its use is reserved for iatrogenic respiratory depression, in a benzodiazepine naïve patient, undergoing procedural sedation with benzodiazepines. The dose is 0.2mg IV over 30 seconds. Onset of action may take 6 to 10 minutes, with repeat dosing sometimes necessary. A maximum of 3 mg should not be exceeded in a one hour period.

Withdrawal

Withdrawal from benzodiazepines may be fatal. Abrupt abstinence is marked by tremor, anxiety, perceptual disturbances, dysphoria, insomnia, sweating, psychosis, and seizures. Onset is usually within 8 to 48 hours dependent on the half-life of the benzodiazepine and the chronicity of use.

Treatment usually involves reintroduction of a benzodiazepine. Tapering of a long-acting benzodiazepine, such as diazepam, over a few months may circumvent withdrawal, and should initially be started at a dose that abates symptoms.

Barbiturates

Barbiturate use is much less common than benzodiazepine use however is associated with greater mortality and morbidity. Barbiturates cause a dose dependent neuronal depression with symptoms and signs similar to benzodiazepines. Blood levels of barbiturates are useful and may help guide therapy. Treatment is supportive. Myocardial depression is more common with barbiturates over other sedatives and may require vasopressor therapy to maintain blood pressure. Decontamination with activated charcoal within 1 hour of ingestion helps reduce absorption. The AACT/EAPCCT recommends multiple-dose activated charcoal should be considered for cases of phenobarbital toxicity. Alkalization of the urine with sodium bicarbonate may enhance renal elimination. Hemodialysis can be used in severe cases of phenobarbital toxicity.

Nonbenzodiazepine Sedative-Hypnotics

This includes medications such as buspirone, carisoprodol, chloral hydrate, melatonin, and zolpidem. In general treatment is supportive. Activated charcoal is recommended within 1 hour of ingestion. Of note flumazenil is ineffective. Gamma hydroxybutyrate (GHB) is a nonbenzodiazepine sedative that is potentially fatal and becoming more popular in Europe and the United States and is discussed in detail below.

Gamma Hydroxybutyrate (GHB)

Gamma hydroxybutyrate or gamma hydroxybutyric acid (GHB) is a naturally occurring 4-carbon central nervous system (CNS) depressant with a structure similar to gamma aminobutyric acid (GABA) capable of crossing the blood brain barrier. GHB is lipid-soluble with no significant protein binding and exerts its effects via a novel GHB receptor as well as GABA B receptors.

Initially it was synthesized in Europe and used as a general anesthetic however, its use was discontinued due to numerous adverse effects. GHB has also been used legitimately as treatment for insomnia, narcolepsy, depression and to help wean people from alcohol. It is currently FDA approved in the USA for treatment of narcolepsy and cataplexy as sodium oxybate. GHB causes numerous different clinical effects and was marketed in the 1980s as a bodybuilding and weight loss supplement due to its effects on increasing growth hormone levels. The drug more recently has become abused in nightclubs for its euphoric, relaxation and sexual stimulation effects. GHB is currently illegal in most countries and is produced illicitly and is easily available on the internet or can be produced at home. The drug is also available as GBL (gamma butyrolactone) and BD (1,4 butanediol) both precursor drugs that are not as tightly controlled, however are rapidly metabolized to GHB in the bloodstream. GBL and BD are found in many industrial organic solvents such as acetone-free nail polish removers, paint strippers, cleaning products, and glue debonders and are often marketed as such to avoid detection. The prevalence of GHB use is not known, partly because the drug is not included in drug surveys or on hospital drug screens. Assays are available but are not easily accessible. However due to the low cost, ease of availability and questionable legal status its use is becoming more popular. Users develop dependence and experience significant withdrawal on discontinuation.

GHB is sold as a sodium salt, in a powder or granular form and dissolves in water to form a clear, colorless, odorless liquid. GBL is sold directly as a colorless, odorless liquid. GHB has a salty taste and is frequently added to various drinks to mask the flavor. GHB is rapidly absorbed and eliminated with a half-life of approximately 30 minutes. It exhibits zero order kinetics at low doses and has a very narrow therapeutic index. Users find it difficult to titrate doses and only need to consume slightly more than their usual dose to develop significant toxicity. GHB manifests a steep dose-effect curve with rapid onset of effect followed by abrupt clearing. Typically the effects last up to 2 hours however, dependent users may dose the drug every 30 minutes to 1 hour.

Clinical Features

Illicit users of GHB and GBL generally fall into two groups. The first group uses the drugs for possible therapeutic health benefits, such as bodybuilders and people attempting self-treatment of insomnia, depression and anxiety. GHB has been shown to increase growth hormone levels and lean body mass. A second group is recreational users, who take the drug at clubs, and bars. At low therapeutic doses GHB has stimulant properties with users experiencing euphoria, disinhibition and enhanced sensuality and empathic states. This can lead to unsafe sexual practices and increased rates of sexually transmitted diseases. Also the drug is often abused concurrently with other illicit drugs such as MDMA, methamphetamine, cocaine, and alcohol.

Due to the narrow therapeutic index acute toxicity is common and users may accidently overdose. Toxicity manifests as a dose dependent CNS depressant. Hypotension, bradycardia, hypothermia, and respiratory depression are common. At lower doses patients can be agitated and show self-destructive behavior. At higher doses rapid sedation and coma is common and patients can be completely unresponsive to painful stimuli. However due to the steep dose-effect curve, abrupt recovery is common, and users can awake suddenly 1-2 hours after

intoxication. Miosis may be evident as well as nystagmus. Respiratory arrest is the most common cause of death. Amnesia after use is common and this combined with its sedating effects makes GHB a choice for drug-facilitated sexual assault.

Differential Diagnosis

GHB toxicity is a clinical diagnosis and assays are not easily available. Agitation followed by obtundation, bradycardia, and hypothermia followed by abrupt recovery points towards GHB. Barbiturates, benzodiazepines, alcohol and opiates can all cause similar features. Urine toxicology screen may not necessarily reflect current intoxication, and may serve as a distracter rather than a diagnostic aid.

Treatment/Work Up

Supportive care is the mainstay of treatment including stabilization of the airway, breathing and circulation followed by routine lab tests, control of agitation and seizures and management of any subsequent complications (see general principles of overdose and poisoning). Decontamination with activated charcoal should be considered if ingestion is within 1 hour of presentation as long as the airway is stable. Other elimination techniques are ineffective.

Specific Therapy—In general the treatment is supportive with no effective antidote. Vasopressors may be required for low blood pressure. Bradycardia should be treated with atropine or temporary pacing if severe. Typically once patients wake up they should be observed for several hours however, patients rarely comply and often leave against medical advice.

Withdrawal and Dependence

Due to the short half-life and dependent nature of the drug users may have to dose every 1 to 6 hours. As a result withdrawal symptoms can develop as early as 1 hour after the last dose and usually last between 4 and 14 days. Patients who use the drug for bodybuilding or to relieve insomnia or other medical conditions are more likely to develop dependence and withdrawal when compared to recreational users that use the drug only when socializing. Users admitted to the ICU for acute intoxication, or other unrelated conditions, may develop withdrawal while an inpatient. Neuropsychiatric symptoms are the most common symptoms experienced during withdrawal.

Initially users may have some autonomic symptoms including tachycardia, hypertension, and diaphoresis however vitals signs can remain normal, unlike in alcohol withdrawal. After 24 hours patients develop extreme agitation, combativeness and anxiety and often will need to be physically restrained. Psychiatric symptoms can develop including paranoia, hallucinations and delirium. On physical exam patients often have a tremor, increased muscle tone, myoclonic jerks and nystagmus. Unlike with alcohol and benzodiazepines seizures are less common. Hyperthermia and rhabdomyolysis can develop from the extreme agitation leading to electrolyte abnormalities and renal failure. Death can occur due to cardiac arrest from electrolyte abnormalities. Supportive care is the mainstay of treatment. Long acting benzodiazepines such as diazepam are titrated to control agitation and anxiety. Extremely large doses may be required which may cause significant respiratory depression and require endotracheal intubation and mechanical ventilation. Baclofen (GABA agonist) can be given in combination with benzodiazepines. Patients resistant to benzodiazepines may require barbiturates or propofol and a secure airway. Creatine kinase (CK) levels should be followed due to the risk of rhabdomyolysis, which should be treated with fluids. The role of urine alkalization with bicarbonate to treat rhabdomylosis in poisoned patients is unclear.

DRUGS OF ABUSE

"Drug of abuse" is a very broad term and is defined as any drug (illicit or prescription), chemical, or plant product that is known to be misused for recreational purposes. The term narcotic generically refers to any psychoactive drug that causes sedation. However, in legal terms it refers to any drug that is prohibited or regulated by the government. Many classes of drugs have potential for abuse, however in this section we will discuss opioids, sympathomimetics and hallucinogens. Sedatives are covered in the sedative-hypnotic section. See Table 58–10: Common drugs of abuse.

Opioids

Opioid refers to any drug, natural or synthetic, that is active upon opioid receptors. Opiate refers to naturally occurring drugs extracted from the opium

TABLE 58–10 Common drugs of abuse.

Class	Drug
Opioids	Morphine, oxycodone, codeine, fentanyl, heroin
Sympathomimetics	Cocaine, methamphetamine, mephedrone, MDMA
Hallucinogens	MDMA, mushrooms, PCP, LSD, cannabis
Sedatives	Benzodiazepines, barbiturates, GHB

poppy plant (morphine and codeine). Opioid receptors are found throughout the central and peripheral nervous system and modulate the release of neurotransmitters with a wide diversity of clinical effects including analgesia, euphoria and anxiolysis. The potency, duration of action and half-life vary widely between different opioids and significant tolerance can develop.

Clinical Features

Opioid overdose produces a specific toxidrome of reduced level of consciousness, respiratory depression, and pinpoint pupils. Other common findings include vomiting, ileus, urinary retention, loss of deep tendon reflexes, bradycardia, and histamine release causing hypotension, urticarial and bronchospasm. Respiratory depression is usually the most serious sequelae. Non-cardiogenic pulmonary edema and ARDS has been associated with heroin (diacetylmorphine) overdose. Opioids may be administered by almost any route, however most are abused intravenously, which can often be associated with cutaneous findings as well as systemic illnesses such as hepatitis, HIV, and endocarditis.

Differential Diagnosis

Opioids are commonly used with other intoxicants such as alcohol or cocaine. The diagnosis of intoxication is largely clinical and is supported by the brisk response to naloxone. Blood and urine toxicology screening can identify coingestants however levels are not helpful. Clonidine can produce a similar clinical picture as opioid intoxication however the response to naloxone is not as pronounced. Sedatives such as benzodiazepines and barbiturates can look very similar to opioids and there coingestion can make diagnosis challenging.

Treatment/Work Up

Supportive care is the mainstay of treatment including stabilization of the airway, breathing, and circulation followed by routine lab tests, control of agitation and seizures and management of any subsequent complications (see general principles of overdose and poisoning). Abdominal imaging may display evidence of body packing or stuffing. Decontamination with activated charcoal is advisable in suspected oral ingestion especially if co-ingestants are suspected and presentation is within 1 hour. It is reasonable to assume that administration of activated charcoal later than 1 hour post ingestion may be beneficial for sustained release oral preparations but there is no clinical trial evidence to support this. Whole bowel irrigation with polyethylene glycol can be used in asymptomatic body packers to help expel packets.

Specific Therapy

1. Transdermal opioids patches should be looked for and removed.

2. An EKG may reveal a prolonged QT interval (in cases of methadone use) with increased risk of developing torsades de pointes, which may require intravenous magnesium sulfate.

3. Naloxone is the primary treatment for respiratory depression. Aim for reversal of respiratory depression, not full reversal of consciousness. For apnea administer 0.4 mg IV, SC or IM, if no response after 60 seconds give additional 0.8 mg every 60 seconds up to 2 mg. If still no response give additional 2 mg. For opioid dependent patients with respiratory depression administer 0.05-0.1 mg doses, to prevent acute withdrawal, until the desired response is achieved. The preferred route of administration of naloxone is intravenous. For large overdoses consider a naloxone infusion at an hourly rate of 2/3 s of the dose required to wake up the patient per hour.

Withdrawal

Withdrawal from opioids produces a surge in catecholamines producing autonomic instability as well as agitation and personality changes. Onset will depend on the individual opiate and can by up to 48 hours when associated with long acting drugs such as methadone or extended release preparations. Symptoms include dysphoria, diaphoresis, rhinorrhea, sneezing, muscle aches and cramps and abdominal pain and diarrhea. Methadone is a long acting opiate and is the mainstay of treatment for withdrawal and dependence. Clonidine has been used to blunt some of the autonomic symptoms. Withdrawal seizures will require high doses of long acting benzodiazepines.

Sympathomimetics

Sympathomimetics drugs are a stimulant class of drug that have similar clinical effects as neurotransmitters of the central nervous system such as catecholamines (norepinephrine, epinephrine, and dopamine). These drugs can act through several mechanisms, such as directly activating alpha and beta adrenergic postsynaptic receptors, blocking breakdown and reuptake of certain neurotransmitters, or stimulating production and release of catecholamines. Sympathomimetic drugs are used routinely in hospitals to help support blood pressure and are available with a prescription to treat common medical conditions such as asthma, narcolepsy or hypotension. Sympathomimetics are also available without a prescription in over the counter cold and flu preparations. Illicit street preparations are commonly abused and include, cocaine and designer drugs such as MDMA (3,4-methylenedioxymethamphetamine), methamphetamine and more recently mephedrone (see Table 58–11).

TABLE 58–11 Common sympathomimetic drugs.

Drug	Use
Norepinephrine, epinephrine, dopamine, midodrine	Blood pressure support
Albuterol, levalbuterol	Bronchodilation
Modafinil	Narcolepsy
Phenylephrine, pseudoephedrine	Over the counter cold and flu preparations
Cocaine, MDMA, methamphetamine, mephedrone	Most commonly used illicitly

Poisoning from sympathomimetic agents can occur secondary to the use of prescription and nonprescription agents. In 2011, approximately 66,540 cases of sympathomimetic and street drug exposures were reported to the American Association of Poison Control Centers.

Cocaine

Other than alcohol, cocaine is the most common cause of acute drug-related emergency department visits in the United States. Extracted from the leaves of the coca plant (Erythroxylum coca) the drug originally found utility as a local anesthetic in eye, nose, and throat surgery in its ability to limit bleeding via blood vessel constriction. Cocaine's effects are primarily medicated by blocking re-uptake of pre-synaptic dopamine, serotonin and norepinephrine. Cocaine has a short half-life and the effects typically last no more than 30 minutes.

Designer Drugs

Designer sympathomimetic drugs are substances commonly used in nightclubs to enhance social intimacy and sensory stimulation. They are synthetic derivatives of federally controlled substances created by slightly altering the molecular structure illegally in clandestine laboratories for illicit use. Many are amphetamine or cathinone analogs, such as mephedrone, methamphetamine and MDMA, with psychoactive properties causing visual disturbances, but are not true hallucinogens.

Mephedrone is a synthetic cathinone derivative of an amphetamine like stimulant, found naturally in the khat plant, which has become extremely popular and is marketed and sold, on the internet and in stores throughout Europe and the USA, as "bath salts." The name derives from instances in which the drugs have been sold disguised as true bath salts. Mephedrone is known to raise both dopamine and norepinephrine, however its exact mechanism of action is unclear.

Methamphetamine is a strong, highly addictive, neurotoxic, amphetamine derived CNS stimulant that has become cheaper and more popular than cocaine in some parts of the USA. Its effects are medicated by both increasing the release and by blocking re-uptake of dopamine, norepinephrine and serotonin. It is more potent and much longer acting than cocaine, with a half-life of approximately 12 hours, and can be produced from over the counter cold and flu medications. Its use, and associated behaviors, has been associated with increased risk of contracting HIV and hepatitis.

MDMA, more commonly known as "ecstasy" or "molly," is a synthetic amphetamine derived drug with both stimulant and hallucinogenic properties that's effects last typically between 4-6 hours. It causes presynaptic release of dopamine, and norepinephrine but also significantly increases the neurotransmitter serotonin which may precipitate serotonin syndrome. One of its more serious complications is alteration of thermoregulation causing significant increases in body temperature. See Table 58-11: Common sympathomimetic drugs.

Clinical Features

Sympathomimetic toxicity, regardless of the specific drug, produces a specific toxidrome of hypertension, tachycardia, hyperthermia with mydriasis and diaphoresis. Hyperthermia is multifactorial and can be caused by extreme agitation in the setting of a hot club environment as well as due to direct toxicity to thermoregulation. CNS toxicity is manifested as psychomotor agitation, teeth grinding, euphoria, anxiety, psychosis, increased sexual stimulation, hallucinations and can progress to seizures. Cardiovascular complications include tachy and bradyarrhythmias and extreme hypertension leading to myocardial ischemia, aortic and coronary artery dissection, intracranial hemorrhage, encephalopathy and ischemic strokes. Other complications include rhabdomyolysis and renal failure. Death is most commonly secondary to seizures, cardiac arrest or hyperthermia. Sympathomimetic drugs are commonly associated with body packers and stuffers, which if associated with rupture of a bag, can lead to extreme systemic symptoms as well as local bowel ischemia and bleeding. Serotonin syndrome (change in mental status, autonomic stimulation and neuromuscular activity) can occur with MDMA, cocaine and amphetamines. In addition to the above symptoms specific drugs can produce unique features:

Cocaine—Cocaine is frequently associated with chest pain and EKG changes. Cocaine use in pregnancy has been associated with spontaneous abortion, placental abruption, and intrauterine growth retardation. Crack cocaine can cause pulmonary complications such as pulmonary edema and bronchospasm. Due to the very short acting nature of cocaine it is typically abused in a binge pattern.

Mephedrone—Patients intoxicated with mephedrone can present with "excited delirium." Although not specific, this may be more common in mephedrone users over other sympathomimetics.

Methamphetamine—Methamphetamine is highly addictive and can be associated with frequent emergency department visits and long-term health problems such as weight loss, dental problems, and skin sores. Its neurotoxic effects can lead to a loss of fine motor skills and impaired verbal learning. Methamphetamine is also associated with increased risk of HIV and hepatitis due to needle sharing and increased sexual stimulation.

MDMA—MDMA use can be associated with more hallucinogenic symptoms and distortions in sensory and time perception. Users can be very emotionally labile and can show extreme empathy towards others. MDMA is often combined with multiple other drugs such as GHB, Viagra and other stimulants. Further more MDMA is commonly associated with serotonin syndrome, extreme hyperthermia and death.

Differential Diagnosis

Diagnosis of sympathomimetic overdose is usually based on clinical signs. Urine drug screens can detect cocaine but are less reliable at detecting amphetamine derivatives. Withdrawal from opiates, sedatives and alcohol can produce a surge in catecholamines that may present like sympathomimetic overdose. Psychopharmacological medication overdose, such as tricyclic's and SSRIs can also raise levels of serotonin and norepinephrine. Any drug causing serotonin syndrome may mimic sympathomimetic overdose. Disease states such as psychosis and thyrotoxicosis can present in a similar way. The use of co-ingestants can complicate the diagnosis.

Treatment/Work Up—Supportive care is the mainstay of treatment including stabilization of the airway, breathing and circulation followed by routine lab tests, control of agitation and seizures and management of any subsequent complications (see general principles of overdose and poisoning). Troponin levels should be trended to assess for cardiac ischemia. CT imaging of the head may be required to exclude intracranial complications. Close attention should be given to suspected body packers or stuffers as a sudden release of large amounts of sympathomimetics can be rapidly fatal. Abdominal imaging may be helpful. Decontamination with activated charcoal is advisable in suspected oral ingestion if presentation is within 1 hour. Whole bowel irrigation with polyethylene glycol can be used in asymptomatic body packers to help expel packets.

Specific Therapy

1. Benzodiazepines are the mainstay of treatment in sympathomimetic overdose for both cardiovascular (hypertension and tachycardia) and neurological effects (agitation and seizures). Lorazepam should be administered IV in 2 mg doses and titrated to response. Alternatively diazepam in 5-10 mg increments can be used. Extremely high doses may be required. Avoid using antipsychotics as they may lower seizure threshold and can worsen arrhythmias and hyperthermia. Status epilepticus may develop and require phenobarbital or phenytoin if unable to be controlled with benzodiazepines. Continuous EEG is recommended in this situation.

2. Hypertension not controlled adequately with benzodiazepines should be treated with intravenous titratable medications such as nitroprusside, phentolamine or calcium channel blockers. Beta-blockers have been used, however they are generally best avoided due to the risk of causing unopposed alpha stimulation and worsening hypertension.

3. Cardiac ischemia should be treated with aspirin, nitrates, morphine, and oxygen with appropriate specialist referral.

4. Arrhythmias are very common and usually respond to benzodiazepines and intravenous fluids. Persistent narrow complex tachyarrhythmia's can be treated with verapamil 5-10 mg IV over 5-10 minutes. Wide complex tachyarrhythmia's should be treated with sodium bicarbonate 1-2 mEq/kg IV titrated to a serum pH of 7.45-7.5.

5. Hyperthermia should be closely monitored. When temperature exceeds 39 degrees Celsius urgent cooling is required.

Numerous techniques exist and initially should include the use of fans, anti-pyretic medications, cold IV fluids, and ice baths. More specialized methods include the use of intravenous cooling catheters and cooling pads applied to the skin. Those with excessive agitation or recurrent seizures may require paralysis to prevent excessive heat production. Renal function and CK levels should be followed closely.

6. Rhabdomyolysis should be treated with intravenous fluids. Urine alkalization has not been shown to be beneficial in rhabdomyolysis secondary to poisoning. See Table 58–12: treatment summary.

Hallucinogens

A hallucinogen is a psychoactive agent that can cause hallucinations, distortions in a person's perception of reality and changes in thought and emotion. Broadly they are divided into 2 categories: classic hallucinogens and dissociative drugs (see Table 58–13). Hallucinogens are found naturally in plants and mushrooms but can also be manmade. Almost all hallucinogens contain nitrogen and are classified as alkaloids. The exact mechanism underlying hallucinogens is unclear but is thought to involve the interaction of numerous neurotransmitters, including serotonin (5-HT), dopamine and glutamate (NMDA). Due to increases in serotonin associated with hallucinogens they increase the risk of developing serotonin syndrome. See Table 58–13: Hallucinogens.

TABLE 58–12 Treatment summary.

Treatment summary of sympathomimetic overdose
Continuous vital signs and serial EKGs
Trend troponin, CK and electrolytes
Consider head CT
Benzodiazepines titrated to response
Nitroprusside or phentolamine for uncontrolled HTN
Sodium bicarbonate for wide complex tachyarrhythmia
Aggressive cooling methods
Consider endotracheal intubation for airway protection

TABLE 58–13 Common hallucinogens.

Classic Hallucinogens	Dissociative Hallucinogens
LSD (d-lysergic acid diethylamide)	PCP (Phencyclidine)
Mushrooms/Psilocybin (4-phosphoryloxy-N, N-dimethyltryptamine)	Ketamine
Peyote (Mescaline)	DXM (Dextromethorphan)
DMT (Dimethyltryptamine)	

The most commonly abused hallucinogens are LSD (d-lysergic acid diethylamide), PCP (phencyclidine) Ketamine and mushrooms (Psilocybin).

LSD

LSD is an alkaloid similar to ergotamine and synthesized from lysergic acid, which is found to occur naturally in several species of plant. LSD is one of the most potent mood-changing chemicals. The most common form is LSD-soaked paper punched into small individual squares, known as "blotters" which are taken orally. The effects can last up to 12 hours.

PCP

PCP is synthetic arylcycloamine developed as a non-narcotic anesthetic to exert a calming effect at low dose and cataplexy at higher dose without suppression of blood pressure or respiration. Use was discontinued due to postoperative dysphoria and hallucination. It is used recreationally, available in powder, crystal, liquid, and tablet forms. PCP is normally snorted, smoked, or orally ingested and the effects typically last for 4-6 hours.

Mushrooms

Psilocybin (4-phosphoryloxy-N,N-dimethyltryptamine) is a naturally occurring tryptamine compound structurally similar to serotonin and is found in dozens of species of mushrooms. These are commonly known as "magic mushrooms" or "shrooms" and may be orally consumed fresh or dried and are usually added to other foods to mask their bitter flavor. Effects typically last up to 6 hours.

Ketamine

Ketamine is a dissociative NMDA receptor antagonist, structurally similar to PCP, which has many uses in medicine. It has anesthetic, analgesic, local anesthetic, amnestic, and bronchodilating properties. It is frequently used by medical professionals for induction and maintenance of anesthesia, procedural sedation and acute and chronic pain relief. Ketamine is usually abused orally and has a short half-life of approximately 2 hours.

Clinical Features

Hallucinogens produce a specific toxidrome dominated by numerous neuropsychiatric symptoms including a heightened perception of sensory input, a distorted sense of time, euphoria, and an enhanced sense of well-being. Users typically report spiritual and out of body experiences and feelings but remain oriented and maintain insight. Negative neuropsychiatric effects include fear, anxiety, dysphoria and an overwhelming sense of dread. Psychosis may occur and may persist for days. Synesthesia is a unique sensation and occurs when a certain sense or part of a sense is activated leading to another unrelated sense or part of a sense to be activated concurrently. For example patients may report "hearing" colors. Vital signs can be normal but usually show tachycardia and hypertension. Hyperthermia can occur with significant overdose. Other physical exam findings include increased muscle tone, dystonic reactions and mydriasis. Serotonin syndrome (change in mental status, autonomic stimulation and neuromuscular activity) can occur directly with LSD. Other hallucinogens raise serotonin, which, in the setting of concurrent use of SSRIs or other serotoninergic agents, can increase the risk of developing serotonin syndrome. Rarely rhabdomyolysis due to hyperthermia and increased muscle activity can occur and lead to renal failure.

Certain clinical signs can point towards specific hallucinogens:

PCP

PCP can be associated with violent destructive behavior and a perception of super human strength, which may lead users to suffer trauma as a result. Physical signs include hypersalivation and horizontal and vertical nystagmus. In high doses patients can be catatonic or in a coma. Users typically experience amnesia, reduced perception of pain, flushing, profuse sweating, and generalized numbness. Elevations in CK are seen more commonly in PCP intoxication.

Mushrooms

Mushroom intoxication is frequently associated with gastrointestinal symptoms such as diarrhea, colicky abdominal pain, nausea, and vomiting. Users also may exhibit muscle weakness and ataxia. Certain mushrooms can also cause hepatotoxicity with elevation of liver enzymes.

LSD—LSD users are more likely to experience synesthesia and extremes of emotion with severe anxiety. As with PCP, users can be very impulsive and suffer serious injuries as a result of poor judgment. Vasospasm leading to strokes and peripheral ischemia has been reported.

Ketamine—Ketamine typically causes tachycardia, hypertension, increased muscle tone, hypersalivation and is associated with amnesia. Rarely users can develop laryngospasm. Once the effects of ketamine begin to dissipate patients may develop an emergence phenomenon characterized by delirium and agitation. Long-term users can develop a chronic cystitis leading to decreased bladder compliance and volume.

Differential Diagnosis

The diagnosis of hallucinogen toxicity is usually based on clinical signs. Drug urine screens can detect PCP but are unreliable. The main differential diagnosis would include sympathomimetic toxicity and acute withdrawal from opiates, benzodiazepines or alcohol. Other causes of altered mental status should be considered such as metabolic derangements, CNS infections and psychiatric conditions.

Treatment/Work Up

Supportive care is the mainstay of treatment including stabilization of the airway, breathing and circulation followed by routine lab tests, control of agitation and seizures and management of any subsequent complications (see general principles of overdose and poisoning). Decontamination with activated charcoal is advisable in suspected oral ingestion, if presentation is within 1 hour.

Specific Therapy

1. Patients should be placed in a quiet darkened room with minimal stimulation.

2. Benzodiazepines should be used to treat agitation, hypertension and tachycardia. Lorazepam 1-2 mg IV or diazepam 5-10 mg IV or PO as needed is recommended.

3. Seizures will require higher doses of lorazepam or diazepam. Avoid using antipsychotics as they may lower seizure threshold and worsen hyperthermia.

4. Hyperthermia should be closely monitored. Persist hyperthermia should be treated with the use of fans, antipyretics, cold IV fluids and ice baths. When temperature exceeds 39 degrees Celsius more urgent cooling is required. More specialized methods including the use of intravenous cooling catheters and cooling pads applied to the skin are rarely needed.

5. Rhabdomyolysis should be treated with intravenous fluids. Urine alkalization has not been shown to be beneficial in rhabdomyolysis secondary to poisoning.

PSYCHIATRIC MEDICATION OVERDOSE

Psychiatric medications are used to treat a wide variety of mental disorders. Mental health medications were first introduced in the mid-20th century. Prior to this psychiatric patients were treated with morphine and sedatives or confined to hospital. Chlorpromazine was developed in Paris in 1951 and was the first drug developed specifically with psychopharmacologic actions. It was the first antipsychotic and worked by indiscriminately blocking central nervous system receptors producing potent anticholinergic, antidopamingeric, antihistaminic and antiadrenergic effects giving rise to the proprietary name of Largactil, that is, large in action.

Antidepressants frequently feature in the top 10 most prescribed medications in the United States. Abilify (antipsychotic) has the highest sales of any drug in the United States generating $6.9 billion in 2013. Due to the widespread use of psychiatric medications accidental and intentional overdose is common. In this section we will focus on tricyclic antidepressants and antipsychotics. Management of stimulants and hypnotics is covered elsewhere.

Tricyclic Antidepressants

Though largely displaced by selective serotonin reuptake inhibitors (SSRIs) and other agents as first line therapy, tricyclic antidepressants (TCAs) are still used to treat depression and poisoning remains a significant clinical issue. Examples include amitriptyline, doxepin, and imipramine.

TCAs work therapeutically by blocking reuptake of norepinephrine and serotonin, however in toxic amounts they have anticholinergic, antiadrenergic, and antihistaminic properties as well as blocking GABA receptors and cardiac sodium channels. In overdose blood levels can become extremely high due to slow GI transit from the anticholingeric effects.

Clinical Features

Ingestion of 15-20 mg/kg would be expected to result in serious, potentially life-threatening symptoms. Patients can present with relatively few symptoms but can deteriorate rapidly and require urgent assessment on presentation. The effects of poisoning are a combination of central and peripheral nervous system toxicity and cardiovascular dysfunction. Central and peripheral nervous system effects are due to anticholingeric and antihistaminic properties. Cardiac toxicity is due to sodium channel blockage and anticholingeric (antimuscarinic, atropine-like) effects. In addition blockage of alpha 1 adrenergic receptors causes peripheral vasodilatation.

Anticholingeric effects produce a combination of peripheral and central nervous system effects including hyperthermia, tachycardia, mydriasis, dry flushed skin, urinary retention, dry mucus membranes, ileus, delirium, agitation, coma and seizures. Other findings include nystagmus, divergent squint, increased muscle tone and respiratory depression. Cardiovascular effects can be fatal and include tachyarrhythmias, heart block, negative inotropy, and vasodilatation causing hypotension. Coma signals a high risk for severe toxic complications (seizures and arrhythmias) more reliably than EKG changes. Common EKG findings include right axis deviation, right bundle branch block (RBBB), sinus tachycardia, QT, PR and QRS prolongation, which can precipitate VF and VT.

Laboratory tests may reveal metabolic acidosis. Death is most commonly due to cardiac arrhythmias.

Differential Diagnosis

Suspect TCA overdose if patients present with the anticholingeric toxidrome but also have cardiovascular abnormalities. Antihistamine and antipsychotic overdose can produce a similar picture. Always consider non-toxicological causes.

Treatment/Work Up

Supportive care is the mainstay of treatment including stabilization of the airway, breathing and circulation followed by routine lab tests, control of agitation and seizures and management of any subsequent complications (see general principles of overdose and poisoning). A urinary catheter is useful to monitor urine pH. Decontamination with activated charcoal should be initiated, if presentation is within 1 hour of ingestion. Gastric lavage should be considered if the patient presents within 1 hour and has ingested a large amount. This will help prevent further absorption from the decreased GI motility. Dialysis is ineffective due to high protein binding.

Specific Therapy

1. TCA overdose is one of the few conditions where bicarbonate has been shown to be beneficial. Alkalization of the blood with sodium bicarbonate IV bolus of 1-2 mEq/kg should be given and repeated until blood pH is 7.5-7.55. This will improve hypotension and cardiac arrhythmias. If intubated transient hyperventilation may be used until bicarbonate is effective. Sodium bicarbonate's effects are mediated by increasing extra-cellular sodium to increase the electrochemical gradient, and by alkalization of the blood, which decreases the amount of ionized drug.

2. Refractory hypotension that does not respond to fluids or bicarbonate may require a vasopressor and inotrope such as norepinephrine. If this fails then hypertonic 3% sodium chloride could be given cautiously, 100 mls over 10 minutes through a central line with close monitoring of sodium levels. This may be repeated no more than 3 times.

3. Arrhythmia's refractory to bicarbonate should be treated with magnesium sulfate 1-2 g IV over 15 minutes. Lidocaine can also be used. If cardiotoxicity is still unresponsive then

intravenous lipid emulsion (ILE) may be given at 1.5 mL/kg of 20% as an IV bolus followed by 0.25-0.5 mL/kg/min for 30-60 minutes to an initial maximum of 500 mL. Any unstable tachyarrhythmia should be treated with synchronized DC cardioversion.

4. Patients with life threatening instability that fail to respond to the above measures should be considered for veno-arterial extracorporeal membrane oxygenation (VA-ECMO) to support cardiac output and oxygen delivery as a bridge to recovery.

Serotonin Agents and Serotonin Syndrome

Newer antidepressants including SSRIs, SNRIs, and SDRIs are much more commonly used than TCAs. SNRIs and SDRIs are more toxic than SSRIs but in general these drugs are much safer than TCAs in overdose.

Serotonin syndrome is a potentially life threatening complication of any medications or illicit substance known to increase serotonin levels (see Table 58-14). Serotonin syndrome can occur from any combination of drugs that increase serotonin levels and does not have to in the setting of a deliberate overdose. The syndrome is classically associated with the simultaneous administration of two serotonergic agents. However, it can occur after initiation of a single serotonergic drug or after increasing

TABLE 58-14 Common drugs known to cause serotonin syndrome.

Drugs of Abuse	Prescription Drugs
MDMA	SSRIs
Amphetamines	SNRIs
Cocaine	SDRIs
LSD	MAOIs
	TCAs
	Linezolid
	Fentanyl

the dose of a previous drug. Serotonin syndrome is usually more pronounced from monoamine oxidase inhibitor use. See Table 58–14: Common drugs known to cause serotonin syndrome.

Clinical Features

Classically serotonin syndrome produces a triad of mental status changes, autonomic hyperactivity, and neuromuscular abnormalities. Mental status changes can be anxiety, delirium, restlessness, and disorientation. Autonomic hyperactivity manifests as diaphoresis, mydriasis, tachycardia, hyperthermia, hypertension, vomiting, and diarrhea. Neuromuscular abnormalities include, tremor, muscle rigidity, myoclonus, hyperreflexia, ocular clonus, and akathesia. Neuromuscular findings are generally more pronounced in the lower extremities.

Differential Diagnosis

Serotonin syndrome is a clinical diagnosis and requires a through history and physical exam. The main differentials include, neuroleptic malignant syndrome (NMS), malignant hyperthermia anticholinergic toxicity, sympathomimetic toxicity, or withdrawal from opioids, sedatives or alcohol. Other non-toxicological causes such as meningitis, hypoglycemia etc should also be considered. To assist with diagnosis you can use the Hunter toxicity criteria. See Table 58–15: Hunter toxicity criteria.

TABLE 58–15 Hunter toxicity criteria for serotonin syndrome.

Hunter Toxicity Criteria
To fulfill the criteria, the patient must have ingested a serotonergic agent and meet one of the stipulated conditions:

• spontaneous clonus	• inducible clonus plus agitation of diaphoresis
• ocular clonus plus agitation or diaphoresis	• tremor plus hyperreflexia
• hypertonia plus temperature abobe 38°C plus ocular clonus or inducible clonus	

The Hunter Toxicity Criteria Decision Rules are 84% sensitive and 97% specific when compared with the gold standard of diagnosis by a medical toxicologist.[7]

Treatment/Work Up

Supportive care is the mainstay of treatment including stabilization of the airway, breathing and circulation followed by routine lab tests, control of agitation and seizures and management of any subsequent complications (see general principles of overdose and poisoning). In cases of deliberate overdose, decontamination with activated charcoal should be initiated, if presentation is within 1 hour of ingestion.

Specific Therapy

1. In mild cases of serotonin syndrome simply discontinuing the medication will result in resolution of symptoms in 24 hours. Of note neuroleptic malignant syndrome may take days to resolve.

2. Prolonged QT and Torsades de pointes should be managed with magnesium sulfate 1-2 g IV over 15 minutes.

3. Hyperthermia should be closely monitored. When temperature exceeds 39 degrees Celsius urgent cooling is required. Numerous techniques exist and initially should include the use of fans, antipyretics, cold IV fluids, and ice baths. More specialized methods include the use of intravenous cooling catheters and cooling pads applied to the skin. Those with excessive agitation, recurrent seizures or increased muscular tone may require paralysis to prevent excessive heat production. Renal function and CK levels should be followed closely.

4. Benzodiazepines not only help with agitation and seizures but also help improve autonomic symptoms such as tachycardia, hypertension, and hyperthermia.

5. If supportive care and benzodiazepines are ineffective then cyproheptadine may be used. This is an antihistamine that has some antiserotonergic properties. The initial dose is 4-12 mg orally, repeated at 12-hour intervals if no response. Propranolol, bromocriptine, chlorpromazine, olanzapine, and dantrolene are not recommended.

6. Rhabdomyolysis should be treated with intravenous fluids. Urine alkalization has not been shown to be beneficial in rhabdomyolysis secondary to poisoning.

Antipsychotics

Antipsychotic, also known as neuroleptics and major tranquilizers, are used to treat a variety of conditions including psychosis, movement disorders, nausea, and agitation. Typical antipsychotics were first developed in 1951 and work by non-specific antagonism of central dopamine receptors. Atypical antipsychotics were developed in 1998 and are much more specific therefore produce much fewer side effects. They selectively antagonize mesolimbic D2 receptors. All classes of antipsychotic medications drugs also have varying degrees of antihistaminic, antiadrenergic, antiserotonergic, and anticholingeric properties leading to numerous side effects, especially in overdose. Aripiprazole is a newer atypical antipsychotic that has a low affinity for serotonin, alpha-1 adrenergic, and histamine-1 receptors and as a result a more favorable side effect profile.

Antipsychotic use is very common in the United States where deliberate and accidental overdose occurs. Mortality from overdose is low. A specific but rare and potentially fatal complication to be aware of is neuroleptic malignant syndrome.

Clinical Features

Symptoms and signs are related to the numerous receptors that are blocked. Histamine receptor antagonism produces lethargy, sedation and coma. Other central effects include ataxia, dysarthria, myoclonus and seizures. Alpha-adrenergic antagonism may produce miosis, tachycardia and orthostatic hypotension. Anticholingeric effects can produce the classic anticholingeric toxidrome of blurry vision, dry mouth, flushed skin, constipation, dilated pupils and urinary retention.

On examination patients may have extrapyramidal signs such as acute dystonic reactions and akathisia. These are common side effects of typical antipsychotics and normal therapeutic doses. These effects can be seen with overdose but are rare. Antipsychotics can also affect cardiac sodium ion channels producing EKG changes including QT, PR and QRS prolongation, ST and T wave abnormalities and right axis deviation. The most common EKG finding is sinus tachycardia.

Neuroleptic Malignant Syndrome (NMS)—NMS is a potentially life threatening neurological emergency due to an idiosyncratic reaction to antipsychotics with a mortality of 10%-20%. It presents with a tetrad of fever (38°C-40°C), muscular rigidity (lead pipe), autonomic dysfunction (tachycardia, diaphoresis, and labile blood pressure), and altered mental status (confusion, delirium and catatonia).

Death usually occurs from complications from autonomic dysfunction including rhabdomyolysis and cardiac and respiratory failure. Onset of symptoms is usually gradual over 3-7 days. CK levels are often significantly elevated > 100,000 IU/L.

Differential Diagnosis

Due to the fact that antipsychotics interact with multiple different receptors producing several clinical toxidromes, diagnosis can be difficult. Anticholingeric toxicity, TCA overdose, sympathomimetic abuse, and sedative-hypnotic overdose can produce similar signs.

Treatment/Work Up

Supportive care is the mainstay of treatment including stabilization of the airway, breathing, and circulation followed by routine lab tests, control of agitation and seizures and management of any subsequent complications (see general principles of overdose and poisoning). In cases of deliberate overdose, decontamination with activated charcoal should be initiated, if presentation is within 1 hour of ingestion.

Specific Therapy

1. Prolonged QT or torsade de pointes should be treated with intravenous magnesium sulfate 1-2 g IV over 15 minutes.

2. Vasopressors such as norepinephrine may be required for hypotension that does not respond to fluid resuscitation.

3. Mild hyperthermia should be treated with conventional cooling methods. When temperature exceeds 39°C urgent cooling is required. Numerous techniques exist and initially should include the use of fans, antipyretics, cold IV fluids, and ice baths. More specialized methods include the use of intravenous cooling catheters and cooling pads applied to the skin.

4. Neuroleptic malignant syndrome is treated as above. In addition high dose

benzodiazepines can help muscle rigidity. Dantrolene 1-2.5 mg/kg IV load may be useful when rigidity is pronounced. Bromocriptine, a dopamine agonist, may be administered orally to counter the dopamine antagonism.

5. Rhabdomyolysis should be treated with intravenous fluids. Urine alkalization has not been shown to be beneficial in rhabdomyolysis secondary to poisoning.

CHOLINERGIC AND ANTI-CHOLINERGIC TOXICITY

Acetylcholine is the most abundant neurotransmitter in the peripheral and central nervous system with actions on both somatic and autonomic nerves via nicotinic and muscarinic receptors.

Anti-cholinergic toxicity is produced by blocking the effects of acetylcholine. Anticholinergic drugs competitively inhibit binding of the neurotransmitter acetylcholine to post synaptic muscarinic acetylcholine receptors found in smooth muscle but not nicotinic acetylcholine receptors found in the neuromuscular junction.

Numerous drugs and classes of drugs have anticholingeric properties at therapeutic levels and in overdose. See Table 58–16: Classes of anticholingeric drugs.

Cholinergic toxicity is produced by an excess of acetylcholine usually by inhibition of the enzyme acetylcholinesterase on the post synaptic membrane. This enzyme is responsible for the breakdown of acetylcholine, which then terminates the nerve signal transmission. This produces nicotinic, muscarinic and CNS effects. Cholinergic toxicity is usually due to exposure to organophosphates in the form of insecticides, herbicides or nerve agents used in chemical warfare or terrorism. Organophosphates cause irreversible inactivation, through phosphorylation, of acetylcholinesterase. Acetylcholinesterase inhibitors are used in medicine for reversal of neuromuscular blockade in general anesthesia and to treat certain neuromuscular disorders such as myasthenia gravis but toxicity from these agents is rare.

Anticholingerics
Clinical Features
Anticholinergic toxicity is usually caused by accidental or deliberate overdose of a prescribed medication and produces a characteristic toxidrome. Patients have tachycardia, mydriasis, urinary retention, dry flushed skin, blurred vision, absent bowel sounds, hyperthermia and can have hypo or hypertension. Mental status changes include confusion, agitation, hallucinations and disorientation. The classic symptoms and signs are described below: See Table 58–17: Classic anti-cholinergic symptoms and signs.

Serious complications of toxicity include status epilepticus, rhabdomyolysis, and cardiovascular collapse.

Differential Diagnosis
Drugs or abuse, psychiatric disorders, encephalitis and withdrawal states can produce similar symptoms and signs. Numerous medications have

TABLE 58–16 Classes of drugs with known anticholinergic properties.

Drug Class/Plant
Antihistamines
Antipsychotics
Antispasmodics
Tricyclic antidepressants
Deadly nightshade

TABLE 58–17 Classic anti-cholingeric symptoms and signs.

Symptom/Sign	Etiology
Dry skin (dry as a bone)	Anhidrosis
Hyperthermia (hot as a hare)	Anhidrosis
AMS (mad as a hatter)	CNS effects
Flushed (red as a beet)	Vasodilatation
Blurred vision (blind as a bat)	Mydriasis
Abdominal pain (full as a flask)	Urinary retention
Tachycardia	Atropine effect

anti-cholinergic properties as part of their toxic profile; therefore clinicians should look for other symptoms and signs associated with other classes of medication.

Treatment/Work Up

Supportive care is the mainstay of treatment including stabilization of the airway, breathing, and circulation followed by routine lab tests, control of agitation and seizures and management of any subsequent complications (see general principles of overdose and poisoning). In cases of deliberate overdose, decontamination with activated charcoal should be initiated, if presentation is within 1 hour of ingestion.

Specific Therapy

1. If toxicity is related to underlying tricyclic overdose then sodium bicarbonate may be required (see TCA overdose).

2. If toxicity is related to anti-psychotics then watch for signs of neuroleptic malignant syndrome (see anti-psychotic overdose).

3. Mild hyperthermia should be treated with conventional cooling methods. When temperature exceeds 39°C urgent cooling is required. Numerous techniques exist and initially should include the use of fans, antipyretics, cold IV fluids, and ice baths. More specialized methods include the use of intravenous cooling catheters and cooling pads applied to the skin.

4. Rhabdomyolysis should be treated with intravenous fluids. Urine alkalization has not been shown to be beneficial in rhabdomyolysis secondary to poisoning.

5. Physostigmine (acetylcholinesterase inhibitor) use is controversial and may be indicated if conventional supportive care is not effective and should only be used in pure anti-cholinergic toxicity. Dose as 0.5-2 mg IV slowly over 5 minutes. Please consult specialist advice before administering.

Organophosphates
Clinical Features

Organophosphate toxicity can be from oral, inhalational (nerve gas) or dermal exposure. This causes an excess of acetylcholine producing a cholinergic crisis and characteristic toxidrome with symptoms due to muscarinic, nicotinic and CNS stimulation.

Peripheral muscarinic effects include bronchorrhea, bronchospasm, salivation, blurred vision, diaphoresis, lacrimation, urinary incontinence, vomiting, and defecation. Nicotinic effects include muscle fasciculations, weakness and paralysis, which can lead to respiratory failure. CNS effects cause headaches, blurred vision, confusion, coma, and seizures. A useful mnemonic for the muscarinic effects is SLUDGE/BBB: salivation, lacrimation, urinary incontinence, defecation and gastric emesis, bradycardia, bronchorrhea and bronchospasm. If muscarinic effects predominate then patients may be bradycardic with miosis versus tachycardic with mydriasis if nicotinic effects predominate. Blood pressure can be either high or low.

Differential Diagnosis

Diagnosis of organophosphate poisoning is a clinical diagnosis. Myasthenia gravis patients who take an excessive amount of their medications can present with a cholinergic crisis.

Treatment/Work Up

Supportive care is the mainstay of treatment including stabilization of the airway, breathing and circulation followed by routine lab tests, control of agitation and seizures and management of any subsequent complications (see general principles of overdose and poisoning). Organophosphate poisoning is often from dermal exposure making surface decontamination important. Personal protective clothing should be worn by medical staff to prevent secondary contamination. The patient should be washed with soap and water and any clothing worn by the patient should be disposed of. Other decontamination and enhanced elimination techniques are ineffective.

Specific Therapy

1. If intubation is required avoid succinylcholine due to the prolonged paralysis effects.

2. Atropine antagonizes the peripheral muscarinic effects of excess acetylcholine and should be given if muscarinic symptoms predominate. Give 1 mg IV every 5 minutes until symptoms improve (most importantly

tracheobronchial secretions should slow down). Large doses of atropine may be required. Of note atropine has no effect on nicotinic receptor function therefore will not effect paralysis or muscle weakness. Tachycardia and mydriasis are not a contraindication to atropine.

3. Pralidoxime is effective at restoring the activity of acetylcholinesterase by reversing the phosphorylation. It predominantly improves the nicotinic effects, such as weakness, and therefore should be used in conjunction with atropine. Give 1-2 g mixed with normal saline over 5 to 10 minutes. Repeat dosing or an infusion may be required.

CARDIAC MEDICATION OVERDOSE

Introduction

Cardiac medications are very commonly prescribed medications with antihypertensives frequently featured in the top 10 most prescribed drugs in the United States. Accidental or deliberate overdose is common and potentially fatal. Cardiac medication toxicity usually presents with hypotension, due to either vasodilatation or decreased myocardial contractility, and arrhythmias, however non-cardiac effects can also present a management challenge. Cardiac medications discussed here include, beta-blockers, calcium channel blockers, and digoxin.

Beta-Blockers

Beta-blockers are competitive antagonists of the B-receptors, with B1-receptors found in the heart, and B2-receptors found in the bronchial tree and blood vessels. They are used to manage acute coronary syndrome, hypertension, thyrotoxicosis, glaucoma, and arrhythmias. Toxicity leads to negative inotropy and chronotropy causing hypotension and bradycardia. Some agents (acebutolol, betaxolol, pindolol, propranolol) demonstrate myocardial membrane stabilizing activity that can cause QRS widening and decrease myocardial contractility as well as potentiate dysrhythmias.

Clinical Features

Patients with significant toxicity present with bradycardia and depressed myocardial contractility causing significant hypotension, which can progress to cardiogenic shock. EKG changes can include atrioventricular blocks, a widened QRS/ventricular arrhythmias and asystole. Global hypoperfusion may cause elevated lactic acid and changes in mental status including seizures. Onset is within 6 hours for immediate release preparations and can be delayed up to 12 hours with extended release. Propranolol may cause more CNS effects independent of hypoperfusion. Other effects include bronchospasm (rare) and hypoglycemia.

Differential Diagnosis

Diagnosis is based on history and physical signs. Beta-blocker overdose may be hard to distinguish from calcium channel blocker (CCB) overdose. Beta-blocker toxicity usually causes hypoglycemia whereas CCB toxicity induces hyperglycemia. Barbiturates can also produce similar signs however patients usually have a significantly depressed mental status.

Treatment/Work Up

Supportive care is the mainstay of treatment including stabilization of the airway, breathing and circulation followed by routine lab tests, control of agitation and seizures and management of any subsequent complications (see general principles of overdose and poisoning). Decontamination with activated charcoal should be initiated, if presentation is within 1 hour of ingestion. Late administration of activated charcoal may be beneficial for sustained release preparations if a potentially toxic amount has been ingested. Gastric lavage performed within 1 hour of ingestion has been used. Whole bowel irrigation, for cases of sustained release preparations, may be affective, however is generally not recommended. Hemodialysis may be beneficial in cases of atenolol, nadolol or sotalol overdose.

Specific Therapy

1. Atropine 0.5-1 mg should be administered for bradycardia.

2. Glucagon has both chronotropic and inotropic effects independent of beta-receptors and should be administered as an IV bolus of 3-5 mg followed by a continuous infusion

of 0.25 ml/kg/min. The main side effect is vomiting which can lead to aspiration.

3. Norepinephrine, epinephrine, or dobutamine can be administered in high doses, for refractory hypotension and bradycardia, to overcome the competitive blockade.

4. Hyperinsulinemia-euglycemia therapy has been shown to improve myocardial contractility and hypotension. Initially administer 50 ml of 50% dextrose. Start high dose regular insulin 1 unit/kg IV bolus followed by a continuous infusion of 0.5-1 unit/kg/hr with dextrose 10% in water at 200 ml/hr. Serum glucose should be monitored every 20 min and the dextrose infusion rate adjusted to maintain serum glucose between 150-300 mg/dL.

5. Calcium supplementation is of limited benefit however should be considered in refractory cases. Calcium chloride is preferred.

6. Intravenous lipid emulsion (ILE) may be considered and administered with a bolus of 1.5 ml/kg followed by a continuous infusion of 0.25 ml/kg/min.

7. For severe cases refractory to the above measures consider transvenous pacing, placement of an intra-aortic balloon pump or veno-arterial extracorporeal membrane oxygenation (VA-ECMO) as a bridge to recovery.

Calcium Channel Blockers

Calcium channel blockers (CCB) are used primarily in the treatment of hypertension, angina pectoris, and supraventricular arrhythmias. CCB all block L-type calcium channels which are known to control myocardial contractility (inotropy), vascular smooth muscle contractility and conduction and pacemaker cells (chronotropy). These agents hold the potential for substantial toxicity and can be fatal in overdose. There are 2 main classes of CCB; dihydropyridines and non-dihydropyridines. At therapeutic dosage, dihydropyridines are potent vasodilators with only a slight negative effect on cardiac contractility and conduction, whereas non-dihydropyridines are weak vasodilators, but exert a depressive effect on

TABLE 58–18 Classes of calcium channel blockers.

Dihydropyridines	Non-Dihydropyridines
Amlodipine	Verapamil
Felodipine	Diltiazem
Nifedipine	
Nicardipine	
Nimodipine	

cardiac conduction and contractility. See Table 58–18: Classes of calcium channel blockers.

Clinical Features

Patients ingesting more than 5 to 10 times the usual dose can develop severe intoxication within 6 hours, or up to 12 hours in extended release formulations. Toxicity causes bradycardia, depressed myocardial contractility and vasodilatation leading to significant hypotension. Dihydropyridines cause more vasodilatation and sometimes induce a reflex tachycardia. Non-dihydropyridines have more myocardial depressing affects however both classes have significant overlap at high doses. Global hypoperfusion may cause drowsiness and elevated lactic acid. Hyperglycemia may develop due to inhibition of calcium-mediated insulin release. EKG findings include PR prolongation and 2nd and 3rd degree atrioventricular block.

Differential Diagnosis

Diagnosis is based on history and physical signs. Beta-blocker overdose may be hard to distinguish from CCB overdose. Beta-blocker toxicity usually causes hypoglycemia whereas CCB toxicity induces hyperglycemia. Barbiturates can also produce similar signs however patients usually have a significantly depressed mental status.

Treatment/Work Up

Supportive care is the mainstay of treatment including stabilization of the airway, breathing and circulation followed by routine lab tests, control of agitation and seizures and management of any subsequent complications (see general principles of overdose and poisoning). Decontamination with activated charcoal should be initiated, if presentation is within 1 hour of ingestion. Late administration of activated charcoal may be beneficial for sustained release preparations if a potentially toxic amount has been ingested. Gastric lavage performed within 1 hour of ingestion has been used. Whole bowel irrigation, for cases of sustained release preparations, may be affective, however is generally not recommended.

Specific Therapy

1. Atropine 0.5-1 mg should be administered for bradycardia, however this is usually ineffective.

2. Calcium should be replaced with calcium gluconate or chloride (10 ml of 10%), however this may also be ineffective. Calcium chloride is preferred because it contains more elemental calcium however may cause irritation and should ideally be given through a central line.

3. Norepinephrine, epinephrine or dobutamine can be administered for refractory hypotension and bradycardia but have varying results.

4. Hyperinsulinemia-euglycemia therapy has been shown to improve myocardial contractility and hypotension. Initially administer 50 ml of 50% dextrose. Start high dose regular insulin 1 unit/kg IV bolus followed by a continuous infusion of 0.5-1 unit/kg/hr with dextrose 10% in water at 200 ml/hr. Serum glucose should be monitored every 20 min and the dextrose infusion rate adjusted to maintain serum glucose between 150-300 mg/dL.

5. Glucagon can be both chronotropic and inotropic and should be administered as an IV bolus of 3-5 mg followed by a continuous infusion of 0.25 ml/kg/min. The main side effect is vomiting which can lead to aspiration.

6. Intravenous lipid emulsion (ILE) may be considered and administered with a bolus of 1.5 ml/kg followed by a continuous infusion of 0.25 ml/kg/min.

7. For severe cases refractory to the above measures consider transvenous pacing, placement of an intra-aortic balloon pump or veno-arterial extracorporeal membrane oxygenation (VA-ECMO) as a bridge to recovery.

Digoxin

Cardiac glycosides are derived from the foxglove plant and are used to treat supraventricular tachyarrhythmia and cardiac heart failure. They increase vagal tone resulting in decreased chronotropy and competitively inhibit the sodium potassium ATPase pump to increase inotropy and extracellular potassium. Toxicity can develop from acute ingestion, drug interactions (amiodarone, diuretics, spironolactone, macrolides, and CCB) leading to elevated digoxin levels or from chronic use in the setting of renal failure and electrolyte abnormalities. Low potassium and magnesium may precipitate toxicity by lack of competition for the sodium potassium ATPase pump.

Clinical Features

Toxicity produces non-specific cardiac, GI, CNS, and electrolyte abnormalities. CNS effects include dizziness, headache, confusion, and visual complaints. The patient may report yellow or green vision or halos. GI effects include nausea and vomiting. Hyperkalemia is a potentially serious complication of digoxin toxicity. EKG changes include tachy and bradyarrhythmias, atrioventricular block, and changes associated with hyperkalemia. Ventricular arrhythmias can occur in severe toxicity. Other non-specific findings include weakness, anorexia, and fatigue.

Differential Diagnosis

Digoxin toxicity may be hard do diagnose clinically due to the numerous non-specific effects. Hyperkalemia is frequently seen in acute toxicity but may be normal in cases of chronic toxicity. EKG changes can help to distinguish toxicity form other more benign conditions. Specific drug levels may be helpful in acute toxicity but may be only minimally elevated in chronic toxicity and therefore the diagnosis may be overlooked by false reassurance. Barbiturate, betablocker and CCB overdose may produce similar features.

Treatment/Work Up

Supportive care is the mainstay of treatment including stabilization of the airway, breathing and circulation followed by routine lab tests, control of agitation and seizures and management of any subsequent complications (see general principles of overdose and poisoning). In cases of acute toxicity activated charcoal should be administered if presentation is within 1 hour of ingestion.

Specific Therapy

1. DC cardioversion should be used for any unstable supraventricular or ventricular tachy-arrhythmias.

2. Brady-arrhythmias should initially be treated with atropine 0.5-1 mg IV or temporary pacing if severe.

3. Stable supraventricular tachy-arrhythmias can be treated with magnesium sulfate IV 1-2 g over 15 minutes. Stable ventricular arrhythmias may be treated with lidocaine IV or phenytoin.

4. Correct any underlying electrolyte abnormalities. Hyperkalemia should be treated with insulin and dextrose, resins or hemodialysis if severe.

5. Digoxin-specific Fab (antigen binding fragment) should be administered to patients who have an unstable arrhythmia that has not responded to conventional therapy, in those who have a potassium of greater than 5 mEq/L after an ingestion of more than 10 mg of digoxin and in patients who have a blood digoxin level of greater than 10 ng/ml.

OVER THE COUNTER ANALGESIC OVERDOSE

Over-the-counter (OTC) drugs as a whole were are the second leading substance type used in suicides representing approximately 10% of suicides due to substance overdose. Prescription drugs are the leading type of drug used in suicides representing 79% of suicides due to substance overdose. Analgesics such as acetaminophen and aspirin (ASA) are easily available cover the counter and at low cost. They can be fatal in overdose but early identification and appropriate treatment can significantly improve outcomes.

Acetaminophen

Background

Acetaminophen is the most widely used antipyretic and analgesic available OTC in the United States and can be found in numerous different preparations. It is rapidly absorbed in the GI tract and metabolized by the liver. At therapeutic doses a very small percentage of acetaminophen is metabolized to a toxic intermediate called N-acetyl-p-benzoquinoneimine (NAPQI), which is rapidly conjugated with hepatic glutathione forming non-toxic compounds. In overdose the metabolic pathways become saturated leading to higher levels of NAPQI, which causes depletion of glutathione stores. NAPQI then begins to react with hepatocytes causing necrosis. The antidote, N-Acetylcysteine (NAC), acts by enhancing glutathione stores and providing a substitute to allow for detoxification. Acetaminophen poisoning has become the most common cause of acute liver failure in the United States.

Clinical Features

Patients can overdose in several different ways: 1. Single acute overdose in < 1 hour, 2. Staggered overdose where doses are taken over more than 1 hour, 3. Therapeutic excess where patients ingest multiple smaller doses over a 24 hour period, 4. Uncertain or unclear knowledge of overdose. For single acute overdose patients may present in less than 4 hours, between 4 and 8 hours or after 24 hours.

Toxic exposure is likely to occur if patients ingest > 150 mg/kg in a single dose or over a 24 hour period. Rarely, toxicity can occur with ingestions between 75 and 150 mg/kg within any 24-hour period in some patients. Clinical features of acetaminophen overdose are detailed in the Table below: See Table 58–19: Four stages of acetaminophen toxicity.

Differential Diagnosis

A full history and physical is important to help establish diagnosis. Acetaminophen levels should be drawn for all patients after a single acute overdose if they present between 4-24 hours post ingestion. The serum level can then be plotted on the Rumack-Matthew normogram to ascertain patient risk of toxicity (see Figure 58–1). If possible levels should be drawn and resulted before 8 hours because NAC is most effective given within the first 8 hours. Levels drawn before 4 hours are unreliable at predicting toxicity. Levels drawn after 24 hours are usually not useful because treatment is likely to be ineffective. This normogram can only be used for acute single

TABLE 58-19 Four stages of acetaminophen toxicity.

Stage	Manifestations
Stage I: 0.5 to 24 hours	Nausea, vomiting diaphoresis, lethargy, and malaise, though some remain asymptomatic. Lab studies are typically normal. CNS depression and elevated anion gap metabolic acidosis can rarely be observed following massive overdose, and if present are likely due to coingestants.
Stage II: 24 to 72 hours	Clinical and laboratory evidence of hepatotoxicity +/− nephrotoxicity become evident. While appearing to improve clinically, elevations of from those who develop hepatic injury, over half will demonstrate aminotransferase elevations within 24 hours and all have elevations by 36 hours.[32] Patients develop right upper quadrant pain with liver enlargement and tenderness. Elevations of prothrombin time (PT) total bilirubin, oliguria and renal function abnormalities become evident.
Stage III: 72 to 96 hours post ingestion	Marked by a peak in liver function abnormalities, systemic symptoms of stage I reappear in conjunction with jaundice, confusion due to hepatic prolongation of PT or INR, hypoglycemia, lactic acidosis, and a total bilirubin concentration above 4.0 mg/dL (primarily indirect). Acute renal failure occurs in 10% to 25% of patients with significant hepatotoxicity and > 50% of those with hepatic failure.[33]
Stage IV: 4 to 14 days	Patients that survive stage III enter a recovery phase by day four that completed by day seven. Symptoms and laboratory abnormalities may not abate for several weeks. When recovery occurs, it is complete; chronic hepatic dysfunction is not a seqyaelae of acetaminophen poising.

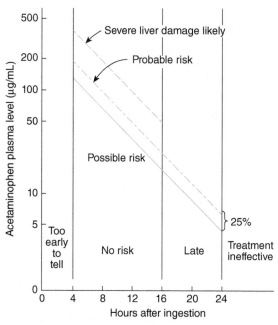

FIGURE 58-1 Acetaminophen treatment protocol normogram. (Adapted with permission from Rumack BH, et al. Acetaminophen overdose: 662 cases with evaluation of oral acetylcystein treatment. *Arch Intern Med.* 1981; 141:382 [PMID: 7469629].)

Treatment/Work Up

Supportive care is the mainstay of treatment including stabilization of the airway, breathing and circulation followed by routine lab tests, control of agitation and seizures and management of any subsequent complications (see general principles of overdose and poisoning). Decontamination with activated charcoal should be initiated if presentation is within 1 hour of ingestion. Activated charcoal may also inadvertently absorb oral NAC in which case the oral dose may need to be adjusted or converted to IV.

Specific Therapy

1. NAC, the antidote, is most effective if given within the first 8 hours after a single acute overdose. Indications for NAC are detailed below (see Table 58-20). NAC can be given intravenously over 21 hours or orally over 72 hours. Intravenous dosing involves an initial load of 150 mg/kg given over 15-60 minutes, followed by 50 mg/kg given over 4 hours, followed by 100 mg/kg in 16 hours. NAC is infused in 5% dextrose in water. Oral dosing

overdose between 4-24 hours. Acetaminophen levels in staggered overdose, therapeutic excess or unknown time of ingestion are misleading and usually not recommended however, some centers recommend treating if acetaminophen levels are over 10 mcg/ml in the setting of an unknown time of ingestion. See Figure 58-1: Acetaminophen treatment protocol normogram.

TABLE 58–20 Indications for NAC therapy.

Indications for NAC Therapy
1	Serum acetaminophen level, drawn after 4 hours after a single ingestion, above the treatment line on the normogram
2	Suspected single ingestion of > 150 mg/kg where serum levels will not be available until after 8 hours of ingestion
3	Staggered overdose
4	Unknown time of ingestion and a serum level of > 10 mcg/ml
5	History of acetaminophen ingestion with ANY evidence of liver injury
6	Delayed presentation of > 24 hours but with evidence of liver injury

involved a loading dose of 140 mg/kg once, followed by 70 mg/kg every 4 hours for 17 doses. NAC can induce histamine release, especially in the intravenous form, resulting in urticaria and bronchoconstriction. See Table 58–20: Indications for NAC.

2. Liver failure and resulting multi-organ failure should be managed in a specialist liver transplant center. Significant complications include coagulopathy, cerebral edema, renal failure, and acidosis.

Salicylates
Background
Salicylic acid derivatives are non-steroidal anti-inflammatories used commonly to treat fever, inflammation, and pain. Aspirin is cheaply and easily available over the counter and is present in many different preparations from cold and flu medications to topical gels. Aspirin is also a widely prescribed antiplatelet therapy as prophylaxis in patients with cardiovascular and cerebrovascular disease. Salicylates are rapidly absorbed, undergoing hepatic metabolism and renal excretion. They exert their effects primarily by inhibition of cyclooxygenase with decreased production of prostaglandins, prostacyclin, and thromboxanes. Aspirin causes a direct stimulation of the respiratory center in the medulla leading to respiratory alkalosis. Aspirin can also interfere with metabolism and oxidative phosphorylation leading to increased oxygen consumption, hyperthermia and an anion gap metabolic acidosis due to increased production of endogenous acids, ketone bodies and lactate.

Clinical Features
Aspirin toxicity can occur from an acute intentional overdose or be more chronic from unintentional gradual misuse. Chronic poisonings tend to occur in the elderly and are associated with a higher mortality. Acute toxicity can be mild < 150 mg/kg ingested, moderate 150-300 mg/kg, or severe > 300 mg/kg. Mild symptoms include nausea, vomiting, tinnitus, and dizziness. Moderate symptoms include hyperventilation, hyperthermia, ataxia, and anxiety. Severe toxicity can result in coma, seizures, agitation, renal failure, cardiac arrhythmia, pulmonary edema, and shock. Chronic toxicity may initially have vague subtle signs that are missed and gradually progress to severe toxicity with behavioral changes, neurological signs, hyperthermia, tachypnea and evidence of pulmonary edema. Acid base disturbances initially show a respiratory alkalosis then a coexisting anion gap metabolic acidosis.

Differential Diagnosis
Aspirin toxicity is a clinical diagnosis supported by acid base changes. Salicylate levels in acute toxicity can be helpful with mild toxicity associated with levels of < 300 mg/L and severe toxicity with > 700 mg/L. However, chronic toxicity develops gradually with lower drug levels, which correlate poorly with toxicity, therefore drug levels may provide false reassurance and should be viewed with caution. Differential diagnosis includes sepsis, encephalitis, stimulant toxicity, and other causes of anion gap metabolic acidosis.

Treatment/Work Up
Supportive care is the mainstay of treatment including stabilization of the airway, breathing and circulation followed by routine lab tests, control of agitation and seizures and management of any subsequent complications (see general principles of overdose and poisoning). Salicylate levels should be checked every 2 hours. Decontamination with activated charcoal should be initiated if presentation is

within 1 hour of ingestion. Consider whole bowel irrigation should be considered with large overdoses or sustained release preparations. Enhanced elimination techniques are discussed below.

Specific Therapy

1. If endotracheal intubation is required care must be taken to prevent worsening acidosis from apnea during intubation or hypoventilation due to a low set respiratory rate. Salicylate is less protein bound in acid environments, with more tissue penetration, and therefore more toxic.

2. Ion trapping with alkaline therapy is effective at removing salicylates. In an alkaline environment weak acids, like salicylates, remain ionized and protein bound, therefore do not penetrate the tissues, and are more easily excreted and trapped in the urine. Administer a bolus of 1-2 mEq/kg of sodium bicarbonate then begin an infusion to maintain urine pH of > 7.5. Potassium levels may need to be supplemented.

3. Hemodialysis should be considered for severe toxicity when levels are > 1000 mg/L in acute poisoning or > 600 mg/L in chronic or in patients who fail to improve despite the above measures.

TOXIC ALCOHOLS

Any alcohol can be toxic if ingested in large enough quantities. The term "*toxic alcohol*" has traditionally referred to isopropanol, methanol, and ethylene glycol. Compared to ethanol use, toxic alcohol use is relatively uncommon, however can be significantly more poisonous.

Alcohols are organic compounds characterized by one or more hydroxyl (–OH) groups attached to a carbon chain. Alcohol as a solute acts as an osmole and increases the serum osmolality. This can be detected by calculating the osmolal gap. This is determined by subtracting the calculated serum osmolality from the measured osmolality. Alcohols are not included in the calculated osmolality; therefore there will be a gap proportionate to the serum concentration of the alcohol and inversely proportionate to the molecular weight.

- Calculated Osmolality (mOsm/kg) = 2x Na+ (mEq/L) + Glucose (mg/dL)/18 + BUN (mg/dL)/2.8

- Osmolal gap = Measured osmolality – calculated osmolality

Ethanol Toxicity

Ethanol use is very common in the United States. Approximately 10% of adults abuse alcohol to become intoxicated with numerous health and social problems associated. The national institute of health reports that in 2013 86.8% of people ages 18 or older reported that they drank alcohol (ethanol) at some point in their lifetime; 70.7% reported that they drank in the past year and 56.4% reported that they drank in the past month. Ethanol use is present in 15% to 40% of unselected emergency department patients. Death can occur from acute overdose but is most likely from trauma associated with being intoxicated. Ethanol is not only found in alcoholic beverages but is present in mouthwash, OTC cold and flu medications, perfume and some cleaning products. Ethanol is rapidly absorbed and metabolized in the liver via alcohol dehydrogenase.

Clinical Features

Over 5 standard alcoholic drinks on one occasion can produce intoxication. Signs and symptoms include slurred speech, nystagmus, disinhibited behavior, incoordination, unsteady gait, memory impairment, stupor, or coma. Hypotension and tachycardia may result from ethanol-induced peripheral vasodilation, or volume loss. Multiple metabolic derangements including hypoglycemia, lactic acidosis, hypokalemia, hypomagnesemia, hypocalcemia and hypophosphatemia may be seen. Intoxicated patients may present with a wide range of traumatic injuries. Alcohol is also a very common coingestant with other drugs of abuse and OTC medications.

Differential Diagnosis

Ethanol intoxication can mimic many causes of altered mental status. Serum ethanol levels will confirm the diagnosis, however due to frequent presence of alcohol in emergency visits, other causes must still be excluded. Acute intoxication will cause an elevated osmolal gap without affecting the anion gap. However chronic alcoholics can develop a starvation ketoacidosis that will lead to an elevated anion gap acidosis. Ethanol levels are diagnostic.

Treatment/Work Up

Supportive care is the mainstay of treatment including stabilization of the airway, breathing and circulation followed by routine lab tests, control of agitation and seizures and management of any subsequent complications (see general principles of overdose and poisoning). Activated charcoal does not bind alcohols.

Specific Therapy

1. If the patient is suspected to be a chronic alcoholic then administer thiamine 100 mg, folic acid 1 mg and a multivitamin to help prevent Wernicke's encephalopathy. These can be given orally or added to IV fluids.

2. Hypoglycemia should be corrected. There is no evidence to suggest delaying glucose administration until thiamine has been repleted.

3. Any other electrolyte abnormalities should be corrected.

Alcohol Withdrawal

The complications related to alcohol withdrawal create a significant demand on healthcare resources and are associated with an increased morbidity and mortality. Alcohol withdrawal syndrome occurs in up to 31% of trauma patients and 16% of postsurgical patients, and there are proximally 500,000 episodes of alcohol withdrawal per year severe enough to require pharmacologic treatment.

Minor symptoms of autonomic hyperactivity can occur within 6 hours of cessation of drinking. This can include tremor, anxiety, palpitations, diaphoresis, and insomnia. Delirium tremens and seizures can develop 12-48 hours after the last alcohol intake and can be accompanied by arrhythmias with a mortality of 5%. Multiple other electrolyte abnormalities can be present. Management should target symptom control and supportive care with correction of metabolic derangements. Escalating doses of long acting benzodiazepines, such as diazepam, are used to control psychomotor agitation and prevent seizures. Patients usually require close observation in an ICU with a symptom triggered approach using the Clinical Institute Withdrawal Assessment for Alcohol Scale (CIWA). This scale provides medication only when required. Thiamine (B1) and other vitamins should always be repleted in chronic alcoholics to help prevent Wernicke-Korsakoff syndrome. Wernicke's classically causes a triad of opthalmoplegia, ataxia, and confusion. Left untreated this can progress to irreversible Korsakoff syndrome of memory loss and confabulation.

Ethylene Glycol and Methanol Toxicity

Ethylene glycol and methanol are toxic alcohols causing CNS depression and multiple other systemic complications. They are toxic in very small amounts (30-60 ml) and can be rapidly fatal. Both these alcohols are present in antifreeze/coolant, paint solvents, and windshield washer fluid or are produced illicitly as an ethanol substitute. Both parent alcohols are relatively non-toxic, however are rapidly absorbed and undergo hepatic metabolism by alcohol dehydrogenase to form severely toxic metabolites. Methanol is converted into formate/formic acid and ethylene glycol is metabolized to glycolate/glycolic acid and oxalate/oxalic acid. Formic acid is toxic to the optic nerve and will eventually cause permanent blindness. Glycolic acid and oxalic acid are toxic to the kidney and can lead to acute tubular necrosis, oxalate crystalluria and calcium oxalate stones. As with all alcohols, the osmolal gap will be elevated early, however as the alcohol is metabolized this may normalize. As the toxic metabolites are produced a severe anion gap metabolic acidosis will develop. Acute ingestions may have a normal anion gap with an elevated osmolal gap because the toxic metabolites have not yet accumulated. Unlike with ethanol, methanol and ethylene glycol do not produce a characteristic odor. Of note the alcohol dehydrogenase enzyme preferentially metabolizes ethanol, so if ethanol has been ingested at the same time this may delay presentation.

Clinical Features

Methanol—Methanol has a half-life of 14-18 hours so toxicity may not develop for 12-24 hours until enough time has passed for toxic metabolites to develop. Presentation may be further delayed if ethanol has also been ingested. Initially patients present with inebriation. Once toxic metabolites have developed patients complain of visual changes including cloudy, blurred vision or the appearance of a snowstorm. Other symptoms include headache, nausea, vomiting and abdominal pain. Fundoscopic exam may reveal retinal edema and a hyperemic optic disc.

Ethylene Glycol

Ethylene glycol has a half-life of 3-8 hours and has 3 distinct clinical phases as toxic metabolites accumulate. Again presentation may be delayed if ethanol has been ingested. The initial stage (CNS) occurs in 12 hours and is characterized by CNS signs including inebriation, slurred speech, ataxia, and coma. The second stage (cardiopulmonary) develops from 12-24 hours and is characterized by tachycardia, tachypnea and hypertension, which can progress to circulatory collapse. The third and final stage (renal) includes flank pain, costovertebral angle tenderness and acute renal failure. Hypocalcemia can develop from calcium oxalate deposition. The urine may show calcium oxalate crystals however this is rarely diagnostic. Of note, ethylene glycol is commonly used in engine coolant where fluorescein may be added to allow the mechanic to use a UV light to detect coolant/radiator leaks. If ethylene glycol is ingested fluorescein may be excreted in the urine causing it to fluoresce under UV light. This is however very rarely helpful. Lactic acid levels may be falsely elevated due to glycolate cross-reacting with lactate in lab assays.

Differential Diagnosis

Diagnosis of toxic alcohol ingestion is clinical with supportive laboratory findings. Initially the osmolal gap will be significantly elevated and will gradually decrease. After several hours patients will begin to develop a progressive anion gap metabolic acidosis. Ethylene glycol toxicity usually shows leukocytosis, elevated lactic acid (not a true lactic acidosis) and hypocalcemia with evidence of renal dysfunction and a normal fundoscopic exam. Urine testing for crystals or florescence is not recommended. Methanol and ethylene glycol levels are diagnostic but may take several hours to result. Other causes of altered mental status and a high anion gap metabolic acidosis should always be considered.

Treatment/Work Up

Supportive care is the mainstay of treatment including stabilization of the airway, breathing, and circulation followed by routine lab tests, control of agitation and seizures and management of any subsequent complications (see general principles of overdose and poisoning). Activated charcoal is ineffective at binding alcohols. Enhanced elimination techniques include hemodialysis to remove both the parent alcohols and toxic metabolites and urine alkalization are discussed below.

Specific Therapy—Treatment is based on: blocking the production of toxic metabolites, removing toxic metabolites and correcting the metabolic acidosis.

1. Sodium bicarbonate 1-2 mEq/kg should be administered and titrated to correct the acidosis and maintain a normal pH. Formic acid and glycolic acid may have enhanced renal clearance by this method.

2. Fomepizole, a competitive inhibitor of alcohol dehydrogenase, can block the formation of toxic metabolites. The AACT recommends starting fomepizole if the ethylene glycol or methanol levels are > 20 mg/dL or if there is a high clinical suspicion. Administer 15 mg/kg IV load followed by 10 mg/kg every 12 hours. If unavailable or contra-indicated then ethanol can be used to preferentially block metabolism. Administer 10 ml/kg IV load of 10% ethanol, followed by 1.2 ml/kg/h. The infusion rate is adjusted to maintain a blood ethanol level of 100-150 mg/dL. Oral dosing can also be used with commercial 80% proof alcohol and dosed to keep the patient mildly inebriated.

3. Hemodialysis is effective at removing the parent compounds and the toxic metabolites and should be initiated in cases of severe poisoning with evidence of renal failure, optic toxicity, refractory acidosis or deteriorating vital signs. Of note if ethanol is being used as a treatment this will also be removed by hemodialysis.

4. Treatment with fomepizole, alcohol and hemodialysis until the levels of toxic alcohol are below 20 mg/dL. Once ethylene glycol levels are < 20 mg/dL administer pyridoxine

TABLE 58-21 Comparison of different alcohols.

	Ethanol	Methanol	Ethylene Glycol	Isopropanol
Metabolites	Acetaldehyde Acetate	Formaldehyde Formate	Glycoaldehyde Glycolate Oxalate	Acetone
Anion gap	Normal (unless develops ketoacidosis)	Early: normal Late: elevated	Early: normal Late: elevated	Normal
Osmolal gap	Elevated (25% more than predicted)	Early: elevated Late: normal	Early: elevated Late: normal	Elevated
Signs	Inebriation	Inebriation, blindness	Inebriation, acute kidney injury, Falsely elevated lactate, Oxalate crystals (urine), Fluorescein presence in urine, Hypocalcemia	Inebriation, Urine ketones, Fruity breath (ketones)

100 mg IV and thiamine 100 mg IV. Once methanol levels are < 20 mg/dL administer folate 40 mg IV. This will shift the metabolism of to less toxic metabolites.

5. Calcium gluconate supplementation may be required in cases of ethylene glycol poisoning.

Isopropyl Alcohol Toxicity

Isopropyl alcohol is commonly used in rubbing alcohol, as a disinfectant, antifreeze, and in solvents. The usual goals of ingestion are intoxication or self-harm but fatality is rare. Isopropyl functions primarily as a central nervous system inebriant and depressant and presents much like ethanol toxicity. It is also a gastric irritant and has been associated with upper GI bleeding. Isopropyl alcohol is metabolized by alcohol dehydrogenase to acetone, a ketone that does not cause acidosis or an elevated anion gap. Urine ketones will be positive and patients may have a fruity odor to their breath. As with all alcohols the osmolal gap will be elevated. Treatment is supportive. Dialysis is rarely required. See Table 58–21: Comparison of different alcohols.

OTHER POISONS

Acquired Methemoglobinemia

Methemoglobin is an abnormal state of hemoglobin and that can be induced by numerous medications. It occurs when the iron in heme is oxidized from Fe2+ (ferrous) to Fe3+ (ferric) which is unable to bind oxygen resulting in a functional anemia due to decreased oxygen carrying capacity and availability to tissues causing the hemoglobin dissociation curve to shift to the left. Topical local anesthetics (benzocaine, lidocaine), dapsone, antimalarials, amyl nitrate, and nitroglycerin are commonly implicated. Patients present with headache, nausea, fatigue and SOB with a slate grey or blue cyanotic discoloration. Symptoms usually occur when methemoglobin levels reach 20%. Levels over 50% can cause loss of consciousness and be life threatening. Levels over 70% can be fatal. Clinically the cyanosis will not respond to increased oxygen administration. Blood will appear a chocolate brown color and cause inaccurate pulse oximetry. Typically the pulse oximeter will always produce a reading of 85%. Arterial blood gas (ABG) analysis will reveal very high PaO_2 (if placed on supplemental oxygen) as this is only a measure of dissolved oxygen, not oxygen bound to hemoglobin. SaO_2 on an ABG may also be 100%, however this only measures saturation of normal ferrous hemoglobin. Newer ABG machines can also measure the percentage of methemoglobin, which is diagnostic. Patients with levels over 25% should be treated with methylene blue, a reducing agent that will convert ferric Fe3+ heme back into ferrous Fe2+. The initial dose is 1-2 mg/kg as a 10% solution given IV over 15 minutes.

Cyanide

Cyanide is a highly toxic substance that causes death via mitochondrial cytochrome dysfunction preventing oxidative phosphorylation. Cyanide exposure is uncommon and usually from the result of fires involving synthetic materials including wool, silk, and plastics. In the hospital setting patients treated with sodium nitroprusside, for hypertension over a prolonged period of time can develop cyanide toxicity. Clinically patients present with headache, anxiety, confusion, vomiting, and abdominal pain. Vital signs may reveal tachycardia, bradycardia, hypotension, hypertension, and hyperventilation. This can progress rapidly to cardiovascular collapse and coma. On exam patients may have flushed skin causing a cherry red appearance. ABG analysis may reveal a severe anion gap metabolic acidosis and elevated lactate due to increased anaerobic metabolism. Diagnosis is based on history and clinical signs. Cyanide levels are not rapidly available. Rapid assessment and treatment is essential to prevent decline. Supportive care with oxygen and fluids should be given. There are different antidotes available that can reduce toxicity by 3 different mechanisms: 1. Binding to cyanide directly, 2. Inducing methemoglobin, and 3. Providing a sulfur donor. Hydroxocobalamin binds directly to intracellular cyanide producing a stable molecule. It is administered as 2 vials, 2.5 grams in 100 ml of saline. Amyl nitrite, an oxidizing agent, can induce formation of methemoglobin. Cyanide can bind to methemoglobin, instead of to mitochondrial cytochromes and forms a less toxic molecule. Amyl nitrate is normally given pre hospital inhaled from a vial over 30 seconds. Sodium thiosulfate provides a source of sulfur that promotes enzymatic formation of less toxic thiocyanate. It is usually administered as 50 ml of a 25% solution IV.

Iron

Iron toxicity usually results from intentional or accident ingestion of iron tablets or multivitamins and is most common in the pediatric population. The amount of elemental iron varies between different preparations. For example ferrous sulfate 325mg tablets only contain 20% of elemental iron. Pre-natal vitamins typically contain the most iron. Ingestions of 60 mg/kg usually will result in blood levels of > 500 mcg/dL causing severe toxicity. Iron toxicity goes through several stages. The first stage (GI) develops within the first 6 hours and causes abdominal pain, nausea, vomiting, and diarrhea and GI bleeding due to the direct toxic effects of iron on the GI mucosa. The second stage (latent) occurs when GI symptoms resolve and there is relative stability or lack of symptoms for up to 24 hours. The third stage (cardiovascular) develops up to 72 hours and is characterized by shock and cardiovascular collapse. The etiology of this stage can be multifactorial from hypovolemia due to diarrhea or blood loss, direct vasodilatation and cardiac dysfunction from direct toxic effects of iron on smooth muscle and the myocardium. Patients can also develop a coagulopathy (direct effect of iron on prothrombin) and metabolic acidosis. This stage is the most common cause of death. The fourth stage (hepatic) involves evidence of hepatotoxicity and develops 2-5 days after ingestion. This can progress to liver failure. The fifth and final stage (delayed) occurs 4-6 weeks after ingestion and involves gastric outlet obstruction caused by scarring of the gastric mucosa. Treatment of iron toxicity initially involves supportive resuscitation. Patients may require aggressive fluid resuscitation and vasopressors to correct hypotension. Decontamination with activated charcoal is not recommended. Gastric lavage may be beneficial if patients present within 60 minutes. Whole bowel irrigation should also be attempted to clear the GI tract. The coagulopathy should be corrected with fresh frozen plasma. Enhanced elimination techniques involve chelation of iron in the plasma with deferoxamine. This can be administered IM or IV however the IV route is preferred. The initial infusion rate is 15 mg/kg/hour as tolerated to provide a total of 1 gram in the first hour. The rate can then be adjusted to provide a total of 6 grams during the first 24 hours. Patients who develop liver failure may require transplant evaluation.

REFERENCES

1. Bailey B. Glucagon in beta-blocker and calcium channel blocker overdose: a systematic review. *Am J Toxicol Clin Toxicol*. 2003;41:595.
2. Boyer EW, Shannon M. Treatment of calcium-channel-blocker intoxication with insulin infusion. *N Engl J Med*. 2001;344:1721.

3. Bradberry SM, Thanacoody HK, Watt BE, et al. Management of the cardiovascular convocations of tricyclic antidepressant poisoning: role of sodium bicarbonate. *Toxicol Rev.* 2005;24:195.

4. Buckley NA, Whyte IM, O'Connell DL, Dawson AH. Oral or intravenous *N*-acetylcysteine: which is the treatment of choice for acetaminophen (paracetamol) poisoning? *J Toxicol Clin Toxicol.* 1999;37:759 67.

5. Christophersen AS. Amphetamine designer drugs – an overview and epidemiology. *Toxicol Lett.* 2000; 112-113:127.

6. Coppola M, Mondola R. Synthetic cathinones: chemistry, pharmacology and toxicology of a new class of designer drugs of abuse marketed as "bath salts" or "plant food." *Toxicol Lett.* 2012;211:144-149.

7. Frederic S Bongard, Darryl Y Sue, Janine RE Vintch. *Current Diagnosis and Treatment Critical Care.* 3rd ed. Lange series.

8. Dyer JE, Roth B, Hyma BA. Gamma hydroxybutyrate withdrawal syndrome. *Ann Emerg Med.* 2001;37:147.

9. Eddleston M, Roberts D, Buckley N. Management of severe organophosphorus pesticide poisoning. *Crit Care.* 2002;6:259.

10. Erikson TB, Thompson TM, Lu JJ. The approach to the patient with an unknown overdose. *Emerg Med Clin North Am.* 2007;25:249.

11. Feldman JA, Fish SS, Beshansky JR, Griffith JL, Woolard RH, Selker HP. Acute cardiac ischemia in patients with cocaine-associated complaints: results of a multicenter trial. *Ann Emerg Med.* 2000 Nov;36(5):469-476.

12. Glauser J, Queen J. An overview of non-cardiac cocaine toxicity. *J Emerg Med.* 2007;32:181-186.

13. Gueret G, Pennec JP, Arvieux CC. Hemodynamic effects of intralipid after verapamil intoxication may be due to a direct effect of fatty acids on myocardial calcium channels. *Acad Emerg Med.* 2007;14:761.

14. http://www.drugabuse.gov

15. http://www.toxbase.org

16. http://www.utdol.com

17. Joranson DE[1], Ryan KM, Gilson AM, Dahl JL. Trends in medical use and abuse of opioid analgesics. *JAMA.* 2000 Apr 5;283(13):1710-1714.

18. Karila L, Megarbane B, Cottencin O, Lejoyeux M. Synthetic cathinones: A New Public Health Problem. *Curr Neuropharmacol.* 2015 Jan;13(1):12-20.

19. Kaufman KR[1], Levitt MJ, Schiltz JF, Sunderram J. Neuroleptic malignant syndrome and serotonin

syndrome in the critical care setting: case analysis. *Ann Clin Psychiatry.* 2006 Jul-Sep;18(3):201-204.

20. Kreshak AA, Cantrell FL, Clark RF, et al. A poison center's ten year experience with flumazenil administration to acutely poisoned adults. *J Emerg Med.* 2012;43:677.

20a. Lynch R. Tricyclic antidepressants overdose. *Emerg Med J.* 2002;19:596.

21. O'Malley GF. Emergency department management of the salicylate poisoned patient. *Emerg Med Clin N Am.* 2007;25:333-346.

22. Olmedo R. Phencyclidine and ketamine. In: Flomenbaume NE, Goldfrank LR, Hoffman RS, et al, eds. *Goldfrank's Toxicologic Emergencies.* 8th ed. New York: McGraw-Hill; 2006:1231.

23. Pali MJ, Tharratt RS, Albertson TE. Phencyclidine and its congeners. In: Brent J, Wallace KL, Burkhart KK, et al, eds. *Critical Care Toxicology.* 1st ed. Philadelphia: Mosby; 2005:777.

24. Position paper On Urine Alkalinization. American Academy of Clinical Toxicology; European Association of Poisons Centres and Clinical Toxicologists. *J Toxicol Clin Toxicol.* 2004;42:1-26.

25. Position paper Update: Gastric Lavage for Gastrointestinal Decontamination. American Academy of Clinical Toxicology; European Association of Poisons Centres and Clinical Toxicologists. *J Toxicol Clin Toxicol.* 2013;51: 140-146.

26. Position paper: Cathartics. American Academy of Clinical Toxicology; European Association of Poisons Centres and Clinical Toxicologists. *J Toxicol Clin Toxicol.* 2004;42:245-253.

27. Position paper: Single-Dose Activated Charcoal. American Academy of Clinical Toxicology; European Association of Poisons Centres and Clinical Toxicologists. *J Toxicol Clin Toxicol.* 2005;43:61-87.

28. Position paper: Whole Bowel Irrigation. American Academy of Clinical Toxicology; European Association of Poisons Centres and Clinical Toxicologists. *J Toxicol Clin Toxicol.* 2004;42: 843-854.

29. Position Statement and Practice Guidelines on the Use of Multi-Dose Activated Charcoal in the Treatment of Acute Poisonings. American Academy of Clinical Toxicology; European Association of Poisons Centres and Clinical Toxicologists. *J Toxicol Clin Toxicol.* 1999;37:731-751.

30. Rietjens SJ[1], de Lange DW, Meulenbelt J. Ethylene glycol or methanol intoxication: which antidote

should be used, fomepizole or ethanol? *Neth J Med.* 2014 Feb;72(2):73-79.

31. Santos-Araujo C, Campos M, Gavina C, et al. Combined use of plasmapheresis and antidigoxin antibodies in a patient with severe digoxin intoxication and acute renal failure. *Nephrol Dial Transplant.* 2007;22:257.

32. Schabelman E, Kuo D. Glucose before thiamine for Wernicke encephalopathy: a literature review. *J Emerg Med.* 2012;42:488.

33. Seger DL. Flumazenil – treatment or toxin? *J Toxicol Clin Toxicol.* 2004;42:209.

33a. Snead OC, Gibson KM. Gamma-hydroxybutyric acid. *N Engl J Med.* 2005;352:2721.

34. *Tintinalli's Emergency Medicine: A Comprehensive Study Guide.* 7th ed.

35. Watson WA, Litovitz TL, Rodgers GC, Jr, Klein-Schwartz W, Reid N, Youniss J, Flanagan A, Wruk KM. Annual report of the American Association of Poison Control Centers Toxic Exposure Surveillance System. *Am J Emerg Med.* 2005;23(5):589.

36. Wolf SJ, Heard K, Sloan EP, Jagoda AS. American College of Emergency Physicians Clinical Policies Subcommittee (Writing Committee) on Acetaminophen Overdose. Clinical policy: critical issues in the management of patients presenting to the emergency department with acetaminophen overdose. *Ann Emerg Med.* September 2007;50:292-313.

Environmental Injuries and Toxic Exposures

Zaffar K. Haque and Tihomir Stefanec

59

KEY POINTS

1 Early recognition and implementation of appropriate therapy is essential in the care of the patient who has suffered environmental injury.

2 The 2 main forms of heat stroke are exertional and nonexertional. Rapid initiation of cooling is essential to management.

3 The mildly hypothermic patient should be rewarmed at a rate of 0.5 to 2°C/h. Indications for a more rapid rate include cardiovascular instability and temperature below 32°C.

4 In the pre-hospital management of frostbite, protect the affected area from thawing; if thawing is inevitable, then prevent refreezing. In the hospital, immerse the affected body part in circulating water 37°C to 39°C.

5 Seek expert toxicology advice if considering administration of antivenom in the management of injury incurred by *Crotalidae* (pit vipers), black widow spiders, or scorpions.

6 A thorough physical examination will dictate the management of lightning injury, with specific attention paid to the integument, tympanic membrane, and eye.

7 The physical examination can be misleading following electrical injury. Deep tissue injury may result in compartment syndrome and rhabdomyolysis.

8 The acute radiation syndrome afflicts 3 systems: hematopoietic, gastrointestinal, and integument.

INTRODUCTION

Man's interactions with the environment may result in an untoward affliction of injury for both. From the patient's standpoint, the common theme in prevention of environmental injury is preparedness and sound awareness of environmental factors. From the practitioner's standpoint, a sound grasp of the diagnosis and management of these relatively rare presentations may aid the patient in these sometimes-critical settings. This chapter will focus on heat stroke, accidental hypothermia, drowning, envenomation, electrical injury and injury due to ionizing radiation. Emphasis will be on basic understanding of the epidemiology, pathophysiology and management of the individual disorders, with some added focus on problems the practitioner might encounter in the critical care setting. For detailed discussions of the individual disorders the reader is advised to consult the references.

One common theme among all disorders included in this chapter is the need for their early recognition and speedy initiation of appropriate therapy in the prehospital environment and emergency department, with critical care continuing such care and management of any associated organ failures in the in-hospital setting. Any deviation from such timely response is likely to result in significant additional injury and increased risk of poor outcome.

HEAT STROKE[1-5]

Essentials of diagnosis are as follows:

- Temperature > 40°C (104°F)
- Central nervous dysfunction

General Considerations

The body's basal rate of metabolism is responsible for heat generation. Almost all energy released in the body will end in heat production. The body's core temperature is maintained in the vicinity of 36°C to 37.5°C to ensure optimal functioning of the enzymatic and molecular machinery. The principal responses to an elevated core temperature are vasodilatation and sweating. Vasodilatation intensifies the rate of heat transfer to the skin, and the evaporation of sweat from the skin surface dissipates this heat. Heat loss via electromagnetic radiation is a negligible form of energy loss, while conduction, that is, heat loss via direct contact with substances of lower temperatures (such as swimming in cool water on a hot day), can play a significant role in maintaining adequate body heat in the right circumstances. Excessive environmental heat and humidity, or increased core heat production (exercise), and interference with sweating (dehydration, hyponatremia, medications), skin perfusion (cardiovascular disorders, medications) or dissipation of heat from the surface of the skin (excessive clothing, such as in firefighters or soldiers) will result in an imbalance of heat production and heat dissipation, exposing the individual to a risk of hyperthermia, and the resulting molecular and subsequent cellular malfunction. This malfunction can manifest itself in a spectrum of presentations, ranging from transient dehydration, hypotension, tachycardia, electrolyte disturbances, heat exhaustion, lower extremity edema and heat cramps, all the way to heat stroke and the associated organ dysfunctions, and death. Pathophysiologically,

temperatures above 42°C are generally thought to result in cessation of adequate function of many enzymes and will be associated with uncoupling of oxidative phosphorylation, with neural tissue, hepatocytes and vascular endothelium being the most sensitive cell types. This will be accompanied by findings that are consistent with systemic inflammatory response syndrome (SIRS) with varying degrees of multiple-organ dysfunction.

Although the critical care practitioner will usually not encounter either heat exhaustion or heat cramps as sole presentations, it is worthwhile expanding on the presentations of these milder disorders.

Heat Exhaustion results from the depletion of water and salt (sweat production and dehydration) in the setting of vasodilated integument and muscles (decreased effective plasma volume). The depletion of salt occurs as the patient consumes fluids without sufficient salt quantities. The patient's presentation will vary, but may include weakness, fatigue, headache, nausea, and vomiting. Laboratory data will demonstrate hyponatremia and hypochloremia. Fluid therapy targeted toward the basic metabolic panel and clinical scenario should correct this syndrome.

Heat Cramps manifest as muscle cramps after strenuous exertion; the patient may endorse a history of copious sweating and consumption of hypotonic fluids. The hyponatremia and hypochloremia will correct with crystalloid infusion, as will the patient's symptoms.

Heat stroke is defined by a body temperature above 40°C (or 104°F) with evidence of central nervous system dysfunction, and is classified as exertional or nonexertional.

The exertional form of heatstroke afflicts the unacclimatized individual performing strenuous activity in hot or excessively humid conditions, such as military recruits, athletes during training or competition and other persons who overexert themselves in conditions of high temperature. In these individuals, the heat loss mechanisms (through the skin and lungs) are overwhelmed by the endogenous heat production (which can rise up to 20 times the baseline of ~100 kcal/h). The reduced effects of vasodilatation and sweating in an excessively hot and humid climate result in a decreased transition of thermal energy to the environment, compounding the situation.

The nonexertional form of heat afflicts typically the elderly, economically disadvantaged and chronically debilitated, and reflects an inability to either liberate oneself from or hydrate oneself in an excessively hot environment. Prescribed therapeutics (diuretics, anticholinergics, psychotropic medications), alcohol and illicit drugs increase one's susceptibility. As opposed to the rapid development of exertional heatstroke, nonexertional heat stroke develops over a longer period.

Clinical Features of Heat Stroke

Symptoms and Signs

Fever above 40°C and central nervous dysfunction must be present to satisfy the definition of heat stroke. The presentation may range from mild confusion in the earliest stages of the illness in an elderly individual to multiorgan failure in the severe extreme. Lethargy, delirium, stupor, obtundation, and seizures, may be seen. Myocardial depression may result in jugular venous distention. The patient may be hypotensive or in a state of high-output cardiac failure, tachycardic and tachypneic, with presence of acute respiratory distress syndrome (ARDS), disseminated intravascular coagulation (DIC), acute kidney injury, hypoglycemia, rhabdomyolysis, and hepatic dysfunction.

Laboratory Findings

Basic metabolic panel, magnesium, and phosphorus, may reveal hyponatremia, hyperkalemia, hypophosphatemia, hypomagnesemia, and acute kidney injury. Complete blood count may initially reveal hemoconcentration. Coagulation panel, fibrin degradation products, and D-dimer may reveal DIC. Elevated creatinine phosphokinase, LDH, urine myoglobin may point toward increased muscle breakdown and rhabdomyolysis. ABG and lactic acid may reveal a metabolic acidosis.

Differential Diagnosis

Hyperthyroidism should be evaluated for on presentation. Drug ingestion and therapeutic prescriptions should be evaluated for by corroborative history and toxicology screen. Malignant hyperthermia,

neuroleptic malignant syndrome, and serotonin syndrome can be included or excluded from the differential after evaluation of drug history. Infection (meningitis, encephalitis, sepsis) should be excluded based on clinical, biochemical, microbiologic, and hematologic evaluation. The exclusion of a cerebral insult (eg, hemorrhage, infarct) may require imaging.

Treatment of Heat Stroke

Following initial assessment and stabilization of vital cardiopulmonary function, it is essential to immediately begin the cooling process. This should take precedence over all additional investigations. The principle of the "golden hour" should guide initial management choices. Cooling should commence as soon as the victim is encountered and should essentially be nearly completed before the patient reaches the critical care environment.

Continual temperature monitoring via rectal or esophageal thermistor is indicated. Although previous recommendations stressed that a target of 38°C should not be exceeded, recent case reports suggest that there may be a role for induction of controlled hypothermia in patients who fail to respond to the initial temperature reduction.[6,7]

Suggested cooling methods include the placement of the naked patient on a net followed by spraying with water in addition to the application of a cooling fan. One can place the naked patient in sheets, which have been submerged in ice-cold water, with the application of a cooling fan. One can also place the patient in ice-cold water, though this may hamper further resuscitative efforts. The recent use of therapeutic hypothermia for patients with cardiac arrest led to the development of protocols for strict temperature control and maintenance in many institutions, and it appears intuitive that the same protocols could be used for rapid temperature reduction from excessively high to normal or near-normal levels in patients who did not suffer from cardiac arrest.[6,7] However, this specific approach will need to be tested before it is adopted as a standard in patients with heat stroke. Additional measures include administration of crystalloid infusions; however, one should avoid overzealous resuscitation, and instead utilize goal-oriented approaches (eg, CVP monitoring, ultrasound evaluation of the inferior vena cava with specific attention to respirophasic variation or urine output). As the vasodilation is addressed with the above stated methods, the intravascular volume status will change accordingly. Other measures may include lavage of various spaces with ice-cold saline (GI tract, pleural space, bladder) and use of cold humidified oxygen. Neither antipyretics (acetaminophen and salicylate) nor dantrolene are indicated, as neither of these drugs' targeted pathways will ameliorate the pathophysiology of heatstroke. Under favorable circumstances failure to respond to simpler measures to cool the patient can be addressed with cardiopulmonary bypass (CPB) or extracorporeal membrane oxygenation (ECMO), although these options are available only in specialized centers. Subsequent standard care for individual organ dysfunctions should not be any different than for other disorders encountered in the critical care setting. Some sources advocate the avoidance of vasopressive agents, with concern that they could diminish skin perfusion and further impede efficient heat removal.[5] However, these recommendations may be difficult to follow in the setting of refractory hypotension that threatens organ perfusion and survival while the patient fails to respond to resuscitative crystalloid infusion.

HYPOTHERMIA[8-10]

Essentials of diagnosis are as follows:

Mild (35°C to 32°C): shivering, impaired judgment, "cold diuresis"

Moderate (less than 32°C to 28°C): CNS depression, loss of shivering, atrial arrhythmias

Severe (less than 28°C to 24°C): coma, ventricular arrhythmias, hypotension, oliguria

Profound (less than 24°C): absence of vital signs

General Considerations

The definition of accidental hypothermia is an unintentional drop of core body temperature to less than 35°C.

Risk factors for accidental hypothermia include extremes of age, alcohol or drug use, homelessness, psychiatric illness, endocrine disorders, and low temperatures during the winter season (in addition to wind-chill). A professional, lifestyle or recreational activity that is based in remote environments (eg, boating, mountain climbing, backcountry skiing, military missions in remote areas) runs the risk of exposure to a frigid environment without easy access to either warm shelter or medical facilities.

Heat loss occurs via 5 mechanisms: convection, conduction, radiation, respiration, and evaporation. The initial response to cold is shivering, a process that serves to generate heat, so long as the energy and glycogen stores permit. Hypothermia results when the environmental cold temperature overwhelms this internal heat generation mechanism.

Clinical Features

Symptoms and Signs

The patient will initially exhibit shivering, tachycardia, and peripheral vasoconstriction. The mental status will be changed to a degree that is roughly correlating with the temperature drop (see above); altered sensorium may be the first subtle feature of hypothermia. Cold-induced diuresis may occur even in the setting of dehydration; it may not be "productive urine" in the sense that the urination does not reflect adequate excretion of nitrogenous waste products. The stiff chest wall will cause increased work of breathing and ultimately contribute to hypoventilation. The hypothermic heart shows a predisposition to develop arrhythmias, and is extremely sensitive to mechanical irritation; any unnecessary movement of the patient may precipitate fatal ventricular fibrillation. The altered level of consciousness favors aspiration. At the most extreme form (< 28°C), "paradoxical undressing" may occur.[11]

Electrocardiography Findings

The bradycardia of hypothermia is caused by decreased pacemaker cell depolarization, and may be refractory to cardiovascular drugs. The characteristic EKG finding in bradycardia is the Osborn (J) wave, which appear at temperatures less than 32°C. As the temperature lowers, the irritable myocardium is predisposed to atrial and ventricular dysrhythmias.

Laboratory Findings

It is essential to monitor serial ABGs (results are typically reported as if the patient has a normal temperature and may be different if corrected for actual body temperature), Basic metabolic panel, Magnesium, Phosphorus, calcium, creatinine phosphokinase, coagulation panel, amylase, and lipase. Endocrine markers such as TSH and Cortisol should be evaluated, as should a toxicology screen. If trauma is suspected, the appropriate imaging should be evaluated.

Temperature Monitoring

The patient should be monitored via a thermistor probe in the esophagus that has been placed 24 cm below the larynx (or in the lower third of the esophagus). The temperature recorded via devices in the bladder or rectum may be markedly different from core temperatures in the proximity of the heart (as measured by a distal esophageal probe). The esophageal probe is the device of choice.

Management

Survival after prolonged CPR, and downtime of up to several hours, in the setting of hypothermia has been described. It is essential that resuscitative efforts be continued until the patient is rewarmed, unless other findings, such as severe injuries incompatible with life, a frozen and nondeformable chest wall, or changes present in prolonged death suggest that such efforts will be futile. Available data suggests that serum potassium can serve as a guide and that levels more than 12 mmol/L are not compatible with survival.[8] While cardiovascular interventions (medications, defibrillation) used in ACLS may show decreased response in the hypothermic patient, current lack of other evidence suggests that it is reasonable to apply the standard ACLS protocol while actively rewarming the patient.[9]

Airway

Orotracheal intubation should be performed unless the patient demonstrates mastery of the airway. As ileus is common in hypothermia, an orogastric tube should be inserted at the time of intubation.

Breathing

Mechanical ventilation with warm humidified air should be delivered.

Circulation

Crystalloids should be warmed and infused with a general assumption that the patient is hypovolemic, while the volume status should be serially assessed. One should ensure that central venous catheters, or guidewires used during their placement, are not inserted into the ventricle, as this may precipitate fatal dysrhythmias.

Rewarming

As wet clothing will strikingly increase heat loss via conduction, these items should be removed. Passive Rewarming consists of simply insulating the patient (eg, with a blanket) with the intent of preventing further heat loss. However, in the typical patient admitted to the ICU with hypothermia, this alone will not be an adequate intervention. In general, the patient should be rewarmed at a rate of 0.5°C to 2°C/h in mild hypothermia cases without significant hemodynamic instability.

Indications for a more expedient rewarming rate (active rewarming) include cardiovascular instability, temperature below 32°C, examination suggestive of peripheral vasodilatation, and endocrine insufficiency. If the patient fails to rewarm in appropriate fashion with "passive rewarming," then "active rewarming" should be performed. Faster rates of rewarming (> 2°C/h) can be achieved with active rewarming.

Active rewarming falls under following 2 categories:

Active external rewarming—involves application of heat to the body surface, and is the method of choice used in Operating rooms (the "Bair Hugger").

Active core rewarming—includes the use of warm humidified oxygen (40°C-45°C), warm intravenous crystalloids (42°C), irrigation of the peritoneal or pleural surfaces with warmed isotonic fluid, hemodialysis, venovenous rewarming circuits, or suitable devices used for therapeutic hypothermia that are capable of active rewarming (eg, endovascular devices commercially available for that purpose). Additional techniques to be considered when core temperature is less than 28°C, or if there is cardiac instability, are extracorporeal membranous oxygenation (ECMO) or cardiopulmonary bypass (CBP).

FROSTBITE[12,13]

Essentials of diagnosis are as follows:

Numbness/paresthesias

Peripheral vasoconstriction

Clumsiness of extremity ("chunk of wood") sensation

Frostbite describes local tissue injury incurred during exposure to cold or freezing temperatures. It occurs when the tissue temperature drops below 0°C. Ice crystal formation will result in disruption of cell structure. Damage to the vascular endothelium promotes stasis and thrombosis. At the macroscopic level, edema, thrombosis, ischemia, and superficial necrosis will result.

Clinical Features

Symptoms and signs always include sensory deficit affecting light touch, pain, and temperature perception, particularly in the acral areas and distal extremities. The hands, feet, nose, ears, and face are especially susceptible. Patients may complain of a clumsy or "chunk of wood" sensation in the extremity. Deep frostbitten tissue may appear waxy, mottled, yellow, or violaceous-white. In advanced cases and delayed presentation there may be bullous formation (the bullae may be filled with clear or hemorrhagic fluid), or changes progressing to eschar formation and tissue necrosis. Superficial frostbite does not entail subsequent tissue loss unless subjected to additional trauma or subsequent infection.

Treatment

Before Thawing

The best field management essentially involves protecting the frozen part, and avoiding attempts at thawing, especially if there is risk of refreezing present, as this will markedly exacerbate any tissue injury.

If thawing is inevitable, then it is essential to prevent refreezing of the injured part. The current literature is quite insistent on forbidding the practitioner from rubbing or massaging the affected part, as this action may exacerbate injury.

During Thawing

Immerse the body part in circulating water 37°C to 39°C (water containing antiseptic flush) for 10 to 45 minutes. Encourage patient to move the body part. If pain is refractory, reduce the temperature to 33°C to 37°C. Parenteral analgesia may be required. Hyperemia is to be expected during the thawing process. In general, these patients may be hypovolemic, and crystalloid infusion should be administered accordingly.

After Thawing

Skin care should be directed by plastic surgery or burn care specialists. The decision about viability of deeper tissue structures, and the need and timing of amputation will also require specialized surgical input. Vascular thrombosis is characteristically present in the affected tissue. Anticoagulation and administration of thrombolytic therapy are options that should be discussed with appropriate surgical consultants.[10,14] Other possible therapies such as pentoxifylline, acetylsalicylic acid (ASA), surgical or chemical sympathectomy to the affected tissue, or use of prostacyclin analogues, are supported by limited data and are not recommended for routine use.

DROWNING[9,15-18]

Essentials of diagnosis are as follows:

- Obtundation
- Asystole
- Hypoxemia
- Hypotension

General Considerations

The WHO defines drowning as: "the process of experiencing respiratory impairment from submersion/immersion in liquid." Immersion syndrome refers to syncope resulting from arrhythmias/vagally mediated asystole induced upon the patient's exposure to cold water.

Risk factors include alcohol, lapses in supervision of children, aquatic sports, boating, seizures, and central nervous system depressants.

In contrast to the general image of the victim waving and shouting for help, the "instinct drowning response" takes over. The individual, in an attempt to increase buoyancy, spreads the arms horizontally under the water surface and breath holds. After this mechanism is overcome by involuntary gasping for air, water is aspirated. The irritation induced by the water induces laryngospasm that results in hypoxemia and hypercapnia. The contents of the water may inactivate the surfactant, promoting alveolar collapse and atelectasis. The actual contents of the water may obstruct the terminal airways. The fluid-filled alveolar sacs are rendered incapable of providing adequate gas exchange. This series of events culminates in cardiac arrest. It is emphasized that it is the hypoxemia that initiates the cascade of events, and is responsible for the cardiac arrest.

Clinical Features

The victim will be cold to touch, and appear mottled and discolored. Water or "foam" may be coming out of the mouth. The respiratory manifestations will be those of distress and will include tachypnea, rhonchi, rales, and cyanosis. The hypoxemia, to an extent, will dictate neurologic sequelae (from altered sensorium to coma). The metabolic state will dictate the arrhythmias.

Management

Taking into account the primary respiratory nature of the event, the current C-A-B approach in resuscitation should be modified to the more traditional A-B-C.[9]

Airway—The act of "mouth-to-mouth" resuscitation should not wait for arrival to the shore, and should instead be initiated immediately upon meeting the victim in the water. The Heimlich maneuver is contraindicated unless there is evidence of a foreign object obstructing the airway. The possibility of cervical injury must be considered in cases of drowning in shallow water after a fall or a dive, and this should prompt appropriate precautions during transport, resuscitation, and airway management. The gastric distention caused by manually ventilating the patient may promote aspiration, and further exacerbate the situation. Chin-lift and rapid orotracheal intubation can prevent gastric inflation. In the same spirit, bag-mask ventilation should be performed by only those experienced in the technique.

Breathing—if Mechanical ventilation is instituted, one generally avoids liberation trials for the first 24 hours. Complications may include the Acute Respiratory Distress Syndrome, hemothorax, and pneumothorax. One should demonstrate findings of pneumonia (infiltrate upon resolution of pulmonary edema, sustained leukocytosis and fever) prior to initiation of antibiotics.

Circulation—CPR must be initiated promptly. Following initial resuscitation or stabilization in the field and the emergency department, the patient will frequently require admission to a critical care area for close monitoring and subsequent management of the expected complications.

Specific manifestations of drowning are as follows:

- Cardiac: arrhythmias may result due to prolonged hypoxia or cardiac arrest may develop

- Pulmonary: mechanical ventilation is frequently necessary for development of pulmonary edema and ARDS. Pulmonary infections may be present and this will be dependent on the characteristics of the aspirated water. Case reports describe the use of ECMO in drowning victims.[19]

- Neurologic: various degrees of anoxic injury with subsequent seizures, and cerebral edema can be expected in prolonged submersion or with associated cardiac arrest

- Hypothermia: can be a complication of prolonged immersion in cold water. This may be associated with additional complications as described above in the separate section of this chapter, but may also contribute to a better outcomes after prolonged immersion due to some degree of associated cerebral protection. However, therapeutic hypothermia has not been associated with improvements in outcome in drowning, and is currently not recommended for routine clinical use.[17]

ENVENOMATION

SNAKEBITES[20-23]

Essentials of diagnosis are as follows:

1. Crotalidae
   - Potential for limb-threatening local reactions
   - Coagulopathy, bleeding
   - Compartment syndrome
   - Rhabdomyolysis
   - Capillary leak with intravascular volume depletion and shock
   - Metallic taste, nerve paralysis and respiratory failure
2. Elapidae
   - Minor local reactions
   - Neurotoxicity
   - Respiratory depression

General Considerations

In North America, venomous snakes include:

- Crotalidae (pit viper): *Crotalus* (rattlesnakes), *Agkistrodon* (copperheads), and cottonmouths. *Crotalidae* are present in most states of the US and are the cause of most snakebites.
- Elapidae (coral snakes). *Elapidae* are present in Gulf Coast states.

Clinical Features: Crotalidae (pit vipers)

Pit viper venom contains numerous proteins with complex and variable effects. Digestive enzymes, myotoxins, metalloproteinases, fibrinolytic and thrombin-like molecules, amongst others, induce extensive local tissue damage, edema, and rhabdomyolysis with a cascade of events that may incorporate acute kidney injury, compartment syndrome, coagulopathy, thrombocytopenia, hemorrhage, diffuse capillary leak, and shock. The rattlesnake may deliver an anticholinergic neurotoxin imparting weakness, cranial nerve palsies, and in some cases respiratory failure. The severity of pit viper envenomation can range from very minimal local reactions with no systemic reactions, to very severe limb-threatening local reactions and vital organ failure-inducing systemic reactions. Generally rattlesnakes cause more systemic

symptoms, sometimes associated with minimal local reactions, while the other Crotalid snakes cause more local reactions.

Treatment in the in-hospital setting and ICU consists of administration of polyvalent Crotalide antivenom for more serious reactions, and additional supportive care and management of the usual complications (hypovolemia, shock, bleeding, compartment syndromes, respiratory failure, acute kidney injury, and others). Initiation and dosing of antivenom is dependent on the severity of reaction observed and should be made with expert toxicologic consultation through the toxicology center network at 1-800-222-1222. Antivenom administration can be associated with immediate life-threatening anaphylaxis and delayed hypersensitivity reactions; preparations should be made for the possibility of severe immediate systemic reactions as the antivenom is prepared for administration. Anaphylaxis and other severe immune reactions associated with antivenom administration are treated in the standard fashion, and may preclude repeat administration of such treatment. Close communications with expert toxicology support is essential for determining the optimal course of action in the individual patient. Some of the above complications of Crotalide envenomation, such as severe local reactions, hemorrhages and compartment syndrome, will require surgical consultation and subsequent management.

Clinical Feature of *Elapidae* (coral snakes)

The venom of these snakes contains phospholipase and a neurotoxin, respectively causing local wound reactions and neurotoxic effects. Systemic reactions can occur in the absence of local reactions and be delayed in onset up to 12 hours. Envenomation from the Eastern coral snake results in predominant systemic reactions consisting of nausea, vomiting, headache, paresthesias or numbness, and may progress to paralysis with respiratory failure. The Texas coral snake causes mostly minor local reactions resulting in local pain, swelling, erythema and paresthesia, requiring mostly management of local pain. Given the delayed systemic reaction that could be associated with respiratory failure and significant paralysis following Elapidae envenomation, close observation in a monitored setting is indicated for the first 12 to

24 hours. Treatment of patients is complicated by limited availability of the antivenom whose production has ceased in 2006. If residual stock of FDA-approved antivenom is available, it should be administered in the presence of any systemic signs of envenomation and this should be done with expert consultative support from the poison control center (1-800-222-1222). The serum used in this antivenom is derived from horse serum and can cause similar hypersensitivity reactions as the Crotalide antivenom; similar degrees of precaution are advised before its use.

SPIDER BITES AND SCORPION STINGS[23-29]

Essentials of Lactrodecism (Black Widow Spider Bite) are as follows:

- Throughout United States
- Intense pain
- Muscle spasms
- Hyperadrenergic response
- Neuromuscular manifestations (fasciculations, ptosis, facial spasm)
- Abdominal pain may mimic surgical abdomen

Essentials of Loxoscelism are as follows:

- Southeastern United States
- Intense local pain and reaction that may result in necrotic eschar formation
- Systemic manifestations (hemolysis, acute kidney injury, rhabdomyolysis)

Essentials of Scorpion Stings are as follows:

- Southern United States
- Intense pain
- Neuromuscular manifestations (muscle jerking, opsoclonus, tongue fasciculations, paralysis, and respiratory failure)

Spider Bite
General Considerations
In North America, the clinically important insults incurred by spider bites are Lacrodectism (bite from Black Widow Spider—Lacrodectus species) and Loxoscelism (bite from the Loxosceles species).

Clinical Features—Lactrodecism (Black Widow Spider Bite)
Present throughout the US, this spider resides mostly in dark places, such as woodpiles or garages. The venom contains a toxin that causes catecholamine and acetylcholine release from presynaptic terminals. The ensuing muscle spasms and severe pain are generally accompanied by a hyperadrenergic response. The resulting presentation may suggest an acute abdomen, a primary cardiovascular condition such as an acute coronary syndrome, as well as rabies or tetanus. Treatment of severe reactions requiring admission to an ICU includes management of symptoms with opiates for pain and benzodiazepines for muscle spasms. Expert toxicology consultation via the regional poison control center (1-800-222-1222) should be sought before administration of the available black widow spider antivenom for severe reactions. As in all animal-derived serums, this antivenom can cause serious immediate and delayed hypersensitivity reactions that have resulted in patient fatalities.

Clinical Features—Loxoscelism (Recluse or Brown Spider Bite)
Loxoscelism is the term used to describe the syndrome caused by the Loxosceles species (the recluse or brown spider) that is present in the Southeastern US. Envenomation is most likely to be incurred by the female upon unintended provocation; sphingomyelinase D and hyaluronidase are the active enzymatic components of the venom. As the initial bites are often painless, the victim will often be unaware of the insult and thus unable to identify the spider. Cutaneous insult is manifested as pain and erythema (within 12-24 hours). Painful edema, irregular areas of ecchymosis and hemorrhagic blisters may form. Within 72 hours, there is a possibility of ulcer and necrosis formation. This may eventually culminate in dry necrotic eschar formation within 5 to 7 days. This progression of events, if it is to occur, will culminate in a fairly well defined ulcer with granulation formation in 2 to 3 weeks. In about 50% of cases, the cutaneous form will be accompanied by nonspecific symptoms such as headache, nausea, and vomiting. The systemic variant of loxoscelism may occur in approximately 10%, and includes renal failure, rhabdomyolysis, and intravascular hemolysis. Systemic loxoscelism

occurs 24 to 72 hours after the bite, and this presentation may require ICU admission.

Management of the rare systemic loxoscelism is supportive, and may include mechanical ventilation and hemodialysis. In other cases, expertise from a wound specialist should be sought. *Loxosceles* antivenom is not available in the United States, but is used in South America.

Scorpion Envenomation

Scorpions, located in the Southern USA, are nocturnal and favor dry environments. Accidental transport of scorpions as stowaways may result in envenomation outside of their endemic area. Only the Centruroides sculpturatus (also known as Centruroides exilcauda or the "bark scorpion") causes clinically relevant presentations in the USA. The intent of the scorpion venom, which acts as a neurotoxin via its action on sodium channels, is to immobilize the victim. Envenomation may result in vomiting, adrenergic effects (tachycardia, hypertension), localized pain, paresthesias, muscle jerking, opsoclonus, tongue fasciculations, rhabdomyolysis, and respiratory failure (loss of airway muscle tone in combination with increased salivation resulting in the inability to handle secretions). In the absence of antivenom administration, 24% may end up requiring mechanical ventilation. Symptom onset will begin 15 minutes after envenomation. Severity of envenomation ranges from self-limited local discomfort and paresthesia, to a more generalized pain with associated skeletal and cranial nerve paralysis, and autonomic nervous dysfunction. Supportive management will include analgesia (opioid analgesia is indicated), benzodiazepines, and intravenous fluid administration. Severe systemic symptoms warrant the administration of the antivenom, immune F(ab')2 (equine) injection, with readministration at 30 minute serial evaluations if symptoms persist. This equine preparation has been successfully demonstrated to resolve Centruroides scorpion envenomation mediated neurotoxicity in children if administered within 4 hours of insult. Expedient administration in the emergency room may altogether obviate the need for ICU admission. For patients admitted to the intensive care unit with persistent symptoms or significant organ dysfunction

expert consultation with toxicology specialists at a regional poison control center (1-800-222-1222) is advised.

Marine Life Envenomations[30,31]

Essentials of diagnosis are as follows:

- Local pain and edema
- Erythema
- Systemic symptoms including cardiovascular collapse are possible

Stingrays (Class *Chondrichthyes*)

Stingrays are found worldwide, and account for around 2000 emergency room visits per year in the United States. The insult inflicted on the human will be the result of an unintended encounter, as opposed to an attack. The stingray is often buried in the sand; the victim may unknowingly step on it, causing the stingray to unleash its tail (decorated with up to 6 barbs) on the extremity. The laceration induced by this may cause hemorrhage if an artery is struck. The embedded spines then release their venom. The venom of the Stingray consists of amino acids, serotonin, 5'-nucleotidase, and phosphodiesterase. The net effect of the venom is potent vasoconstriction and wound necrosis, with the victim experiencing considerable pain and edema. Clinical examination reveals swelling, erythema, and cyanosis. The symptoms peak at 30 to 90 minutes, and last up to 48 hours. The embedded spines, if not removed, remain an active source of venom. The affliction of the heart or secondary trauma accounts for mortality. Systemic symptoms may include excessive salivation, muscle cramps, nausea, and vomiting.

The hallmarks of therapy include hemostasis, hot-water immersion, analgesia, and wound-exploration. Hemostasis should the first priority. The treatment of hot water immersion (43.3°C-45.6°C) takes advantage of the heat-labile nature of the venom. Imaging and exploration should be directed at removing embedded spines.

Spiny Fish

The Scorpaenidae Family (spiny fish) consists of Stonefish and Lionfish. In the United States, the afflicted victims will usually be aquarium owners. The affected extremity will be edematous and painful, with the possibility of wound necrosis development. Systemic effects, though rare, may include myotoxicity, neurotoxicity, and cardiotoxicity. It is suggested that the systemic effects of nausea and syncope may actually be due to the pain inflicted by envenomation from the embedded spines.

As with the envenomation induced by the Stingray, the hallmarks of therapy include hemostasis, hot-water immersion (45°C), analgesia, and wound exploration. In the case of the Stonefish, antivenom may be administered intramuscularly. All spines must be removed (and confirmation should be sought with plain radiographs). The affected extremity must be elevated and washed with water. The wounds may take months to heal, and expert consultation from a Wound specialist should be sought.

Portuguese-man-of-war (*Physalia physalis*)

The Portuguese-man-of-war is found in the Atlantic Ocean, in shallow water and along the shore. Its nematocysts may remain active for months. The victim experiences pain upon exposure; the erythematous skin irritation that accompanies it may eventually progress to wound necrosis. Some may develop a delayed hypersensitivity reaction. Systemic reactions in the form of nausea, vomiting, dyspnea, headache, abdominal pain, and cardiovascular compromise are infrequent but have resulted in death.

The victim should be removed from the water to prevent further envenomation. The tentacles can be removed manually (preferably with forceps or the gloved hand) or by pouring salt water over the affected area. Hot-water immersion will serve to inactivate the heat-labile venom. As of yet, there is no definitive antivenom targeting Physalia physalis.

ELECTRIC SHOCK & LIGHTNING INJURY[32-36]

Essentials of diagnosis are as follows:

- Arrhythmias
- Skin lesions or burns
- Deep tissue injury and rhabdomyolysis

Lightning Injury
General Considerations

Although lightning strikes the earth more than 8 million times per day, its infliction on the human remains relatively rare. Lightning strike occurs when a potential energy gradient (between the clouds and the earth) exceeds the resistance of the air.

Lightning strike can afflict the patient via following 1 of 5 manners:

A. Direct Contact—this is the rarest and deadliest form of injury. Either the person is the direct recipient of the lightning strike. The entire energy of the lightning strike is discharged into the patient (possibly via an open orifice such as the ears).

B. Contact injury—the victim is touching the object (eg, car), which is the strike point of the lightning path.

C. Side Flash or "Side Splash"—Part of the energy from the strike is diverted to the victim, who happens to be within proximity (~6 feet) of the lightning strike's recipient (object or living creature).

D. Ground current or Step Voltage—the lightning strike hits the ground and travels along the ground to the victim, who is within close proximity (usually up one leg and down the other). This is the mechanism that afflicts farm animals.

E. Blunt trauma—the current imposes an opisthotonic contraction on the victim; in addition to the explosive/implosive force that the recipient suffers from the blast effect.

Clinical Features

Cardiac manifestations include Asystole predominantly, Ventricular fibrillation, and myocardial contusion (in those who have suffered blunt injury). Absence of peripheral pulses in the aftermath of a Lightning injury should raise suspicion for significant vasospasm. The Clinician should assess for skin lesions or burns, muscle injury, and compartment syndrome in extreme cases.

Neurologic sequelae include loss of consciousness, headache, amnesia, paresthesias, injuries sustained during blunt trauma (eg, traumatic subdural hematoma), and transient paralysis associated with the hyperadrenergic state (keraunoparalysis). Ophthalmologic evaluation should assess for "lightning cataract" and corneal burns. Tympanic membrane rupture is fairly common and should be evaluated on admission.

Management

A. General Measures—Duration of the lightning strike is measured in milliseconds; the first responder will not be at any risk in approaching the victim. Standard evaluation should address the Airway, Breathing, and Circulatory status, with interventions as indicated. The patient should be evaluated in the same manner as a trauma victim with particular attention paid to the cervical spine.

B. Specific Considerations—Hypotension should prompt an investigation into a possible source of bleeding, resulting from blunt trauma.

If there is concern for rhabdomyolysis or clinical signs of dehydration, adequate tissue perfusion needs to be ensured with intravenous crystalloids. Any resulting kidney injury may require dialysis.

If there is altered sensorium or other neurologic complaints, then evaluate for cerebral edema or traumatic intracranial bleed with CT-brain. Peripheral nerve injury is a common occurrence.

Otolaryngology should be engaged to evaluate for tympanic membrane rupture, as this is fairly common.

In the same spirit, an Ophthalmology opinion should be sought early in the patient's course with the intent of evaluating for cataracts, vitreous hemorrhage, and optic nerve injury.

Standard wound care should be applied to burns. Patients who suffer burns as the result of lightning strike may require referral to a Burn Center.

Electrical Injury

General Considerations

Electrical injury will afflict injury on the patient via 1 of 3 mechanisms:

i. The direct effect of the electrical current on cells and tissues

ii. The conversion of electrical energy to heat injury, with its resultant tissue damage

iii. The electrical current mediated muscle contractions and its subsequent traumatic sequelae.

Clinical Features

Electricity is delivered as direct current (DC) or alternating current (AC). DC induces a single muscle contraction, and its duration of delivery is brief (it will propel the patient away from the source, thus lessening the exposure time). The repetitive delivery of AC, on the other hand, when encountered with the hand will lead to a progressively tighter grip around the source of delivery (the hand flexors are stronger than the extensors). In effect, AC induces sustained contraction or tetany, thus increasing the exposure time and tissue damage.

The physical examination may be misleading, and these patients should be managed as if they are victims of crush injury, as opposed to burn injury.

Well-demarcated partial-thickness and full-thickness burns may be seen, with an evolution toward the latter.

Management

In the field, as opposed to the site of lightning strike, the first responder must be particular about disengaging active hazards such as live wires.

Cardiac arrhythmia and arrest can occur, and respiratory failure is possible, requiring advanced cardiac and mechanical respiratory support.

Deep tissue injury with development of compartment syndrome, bone fracture, osteonecrosis, and spinal injury, and injury to blood vessels may require surgical consultation and management.

Rhabdomyolysis may result in acute kidney injury and should be addressed with adequate volume infusions.

The skin may show significant burn injury at sites of entry and exit of the electrical charge and require expert burn center management.

INJURY DUE TO IONIZING RADIATION[37-39]

Essentials of diagnosis are as follows:

- Nausea, vomiting, diarrhea
- Hypovolemia
- Dermatitis, erythema, blister formation, ulceration
- Pancytopenia, agranulocytosis
- Infections
- SIRS, progression to multiorgan failure

General Considerations

Our clinical knowledge of ionizing radiation injury is largely derived from the occurrences in Hiroshima and Nagasaki (1945), Three Mile Island (1979), Chernobyl (1986), and Fukushima (2011).

Unlike nonionizing radiation, electromagnetic radiation not capable of displacing electrons and thereby generating ions, but with potential for injury via heat production, ionizing radiation (subsequently referred to as "radiation") generates ions via displacement of electrons thereby creating unstable atoms that interact with other molecules. The larger alpha particles are incapable of penetrating clothing or the skin and exert their damaging effects via ingestion or inhalation. The smaller beta particles are capable of limited penetration through skin and can reach the subcutaneous tissue, and will also be harmful when ingested or inhaled. Photons in the form of X-rays or gamma rays are capable of penetration through all tissues. At the biochemical and molecular level, the mechanism of injury is via damage to deoxyribonucleic acid (DNA).

Radiation is measured in units of Gray (Gy) or radiation absorbed dose (rad). (1 Gray = 1 joule of radiation absorbed per kilogram of tissue, with 1 Gray = 100 rads). The exposure of the human body to 1 Gray of radiation may result in acute radiation syndrome (ARS).

Clinical Features

The critical care practitioner may be primarily involved with ARS, a syndrome that involves 3 organ systems: the hematopoietic system, the gastrointestinal tract, and the skin. Exposures of less than 1 Gy are unlikely to result in ARS, doses more than 10 Gy are usually fatal in 5 to 12 days. Massive exposure to more than 20 Gy may result in acute neurovascular compromise, but such exposures may be infrequent in the absence of a nuclear explosion; for comparison, the highest absorbed dose at Chernobyl was 16 Gy.

The hematopoietic system will manifest varying degrees of bone marrow suppression and this will result in the expected complications related to leukopenia, anemia, and thrombocytopenia. Changes in the gastrointestinal tract will result in abdominal pain, nausea, vomiting, diarrhea, ileus, and result in disruptions of the mucosal barrier. The skin will show varying degrees of erythema, edema, blistering, desquamation, ulceration, and necrosis. Changes in all these systems will predispose to infections. The combined effects of injury experienced by these organ systems may be presenting as SIRS or sepsis, and in severe cases as multiorgan failure and lead to death.

The acute radiation syndrome is divided into 3 phases:

- Prodromal phase—nausea, vomiting, diarrhea, erythema, hypotension, hypovolemia, and headache.
- Latent phase—the symptoms will lessen and even disappear. Lymphocyte depletion kinetics may help determine the possible length of this phase.
- Manifestation phase—depending on the intensity and nature of the radiation exposure, this phase will show changes involving the hematopoietic system, the gastrointestinal tract, the skin, and the neurovascular system. This phase may occur after several weeks in case of a mild exposure (1-2 Gy) or may occur immediately following the initial exposure in severe lethal exposures (> 10-20 Gy).

The Combined Injury Syndrome incorporates the generalized trauma, burns, and wounds, inflicted upon the victim, in addition to the radiation exposure.

Management

The culprit radioisotope(s) must be identified, as this will dictate decontamination techniques, helping to maximize the safety of the involved first responders and the victims.

The provider is referred to specific guidance from governmental agencies; latter should direct all aspects of the decontamination process.

Poison Control should be engaged regarding the early administration of blocking agents (eg, Potassium iodide for I^{131} exposure) and chelating agents (eg, Penicillamine for radioactive lead poisoning).

The extreme result of hematopoietic insult is pancytopenia. Transfusion support and colony stimulating factors are used as needed to correct anemia, reduce the risk of or control bleeding, and increase the leukocyte count. Hematopoietic cell transplantation may be considered, with the appropriate triaging and consultations. The immunosuppressed radiation victim is at risk for graft-versus-host disease following transfusions, and all cellular products must be leukoreduced and irradiated.

The cutaneous damage may require specialized care by burn specialists and plastic surgeons in a specialized center.

The management of gastrointestinal symptoms is supportive, and should include prophylaxis against gastric ulceration and avoidance of invasive instrumentation due to the friability of the mucosa that is very prone to bleeding.

The patients are at very high risk of development of infections due to combined effects of damage to the integument and mucosal surfaces, and the immune suppression. Current guidelines advise the use of prophylactic broad-spectrum antimicrobials targeted at bacterial, viral, and fungal organisms. Because control of infections is of critical importance in patients who, otherwise, do not have a lethal exposure to ionizing radiation, specialist input by infectious disease experts may be of critical benefit.

Patients who have been exposed to radiation doses that are more than 10 Gy have a universally fatal outcome and appropriate focus on comfort should be the mainstay of management.

REFERENCES

1. Bouchama A, Knochel JP. Heat Stroke. *N Engl J Med*. 2002;346:1978-1988.
2. Platt M, Vicario S. Heat illness. In: Marx JA, Hockberger RS, Walls RM, et al, eds. *Rosen's Emergency Medicine: Concepts and Clinical Practice*. Philadelphia, PA: Mosby/Elsevier; 2010: 1896-1905.
3. Steiner KM, Curley FJ, Irwin RS. Disorders of temperature control part II: hyperthermia. In: Irwin RS and Rippe JM, eds. *Irwin and Rippe's Intensive Care Medicine*. 7th ed. Lippincott Williams & Wilkins; 2012:745-760.
4. Lipman GS, Eifling KP, Ellis MA, et al. Wilderness Medical Society practice guidelines for the prevention and treatment of heat-related illness. *Wilderness Environ Med*. 2013;24(4):351-361.
5. Atha WF. Heat-related illness. *Emerg Med Clin North Am*. 2013;31(4):1097-1108.
6. Hong JY, Lai YC, Chang CY, Chang SC, Tang GJ. Successful treatment of severe heatstroke with therapeutic hypothermia by noninvasive external cooling system. *Ann Emerg Med*. 2012;59:491-493.
7. Lee EJ, Lee SW, Park JS, Kim SJ, Hong YS. Successful treatment of severe heat stroke with selective therapeutic hypothermia using an automated surface cooling device. *Resuscitation*. 2013;84:e77-e78.
8. Brown DJ, Brugger H, Boyd J, Paal P. Accidental hypothermia. *N Engl J Med*. 2012;367:1930-1938.
9. Vanden Hoek TL, Morrison LJ, Shuster M, et al. Part 12: cardiac arrest in special situations: 2010 American Heart Association guidelines for cardiopulmonary resuscitation and emergency cardiovascular care. *Circulation*. 2010;122:S829-S861.
10. Sheridan RL, Goldstein MA, Stoddard FJ, Walker TG. Case records of the Massachusetts General Hospital. Case 41-2009. A 16-year-old boy with hypothermia and frostbite. *N Engl J Med*. 2009;361(27):2654-2662.
11. Wedin B, Vanggaard L, Hirvonen J. "Paradoxical undressing" in fatal hypothermia. *J Forensic Sci*. 1979;24(3):543-553.
12. Zafren K, Danzl DF. Frostbite. In: Marx JA, Hockberger RS, Walls RM, et al, eds. *Rosen's Emergency Medicine: Concepts and Clinical Practice*. Philadelphia, PA: Mosby/Elsevier; 2010:1877-1882.
13. Zafren K. Frostbite: prevention and initial management. *High Alt Med Biol*. 2013;14(1):9-12.
14. Cauchy E, Cheguillaume B, Chetaille E. A controlled trial of a prostacyclin and rt-PA in the treatment of severe frostbite. *N Engl J Med*. 2011;364(2):189-190.

15. Szpilman D, Bierens JJ, Handley AJ, Orlowski JP. Current concepts: drowning. *N Engl J Med.* 2012;366:2102-2110.

16. Smyrnios NA, Irwin RS. Drowning. In: Irwin RS and Rippe JM, eds. *Irwin and Rippe's Intensive Care Medicine.* 7th ed. Lippincott Williams & Wilkins; 2012:594-600.

17. Topjian AA, Berg RA, Bierens JJ, et al. Brain resuscitation in the drowning victim. *Neurocrit Care.* 2012;17(3):441-467.

18. Bierens J, Scapigliati A. Drowning in swimming pools. *Microchemical J.* 2014;113:53-58.

19. Eich C, Bräuer A, Kettler D. Recovery of a hypothermic drowned child after resuscitation with cardiopulmonary bypass followed by prolonged extracorporeal membrane oxygenation. *Resuscitation.* 2005;67(1):145-148.

20. Ashurst J, Cannon R. Approach and management of venomous snakebites: a guide for the primary care physician. *Osteopathic Family Physician.* 2012;4(5):155-159.

21. Walker P, Morrison R, Stewart R, Gore D. Venomous bites and stings. *Curr Probl Surg.* 2013;50(1):9-44.

22. Toschlog EA, Bauer CR, Hall EL, Dart RC, Khatri V, Lavonas EJ. Surgical considerations in the management of pit viper snake envenomation. *J Am Coll Surg.* 2013;217(4):726-735.

23. Quan D. North American poisonous bites and stings. *Crit Care Clin.* 2012;28(4):633-659.

24. Wasserman GS. Bites of the brown recluse spider. *N Engl J Med.* 2005;352:2029-2030.

25. Swanson DL, Vetter RS. Bites of brown recluse spiders and suspected necrotic arachnidism. *N Engl J Med.* 2005;352:700-707.

26. Boyer LV, Theodorou AA, Berg RA, Mallie J; Arizona Envenomation Investigators, Chávez-Méndez A, García-Ubbelohde W, Hardiman S, Alagón A. Antivenom for critically ill children with neurotoxicity from scorpion stings. *N Engl J Med.* 2009;360(20):2090-2098.

27. Isbister GK, White J. Clinical consequences of spider bites: recent advances in our understanding. *Toxicon.* 2004;43(5):477-492.

28. Isbister GK, Fan HW. Spider bite. *Lancet.* 2011;378(9808):2039-2047.

29. O'Connor A, Ruha AM. Clinical course of bark scorpion envenomation managed without antivenom. *J Med Toxicol.* 2012;8(3):258-262.

30. Fernandez I, Valladolid G, Varon J, Sternbach G. Encounters with venomous sea-life. *J Emerg Med.* 2011;40(1):103-112.

31. Balhara KS, Stolbach A. Marine envenomations. *Emerg Med Clin North Am.* 2014;32:223-243.

32. Price TG, Cooper MA. Electrical and lightning injuries. In: Marx JA, Hockberger RS, Walls RM, et al, eds. *Rosen's Emergency Medicine: Concepts and Clinical Practice.* Philadelphia, PA: Mosby/Elsevier; 2010:1906-1914.

33. Ritenour AE, Morton MJ, McManus JG, Barillo DJ, Cancio LC. Lightning injury: a review. *Burns.* 2008;34(5):585-594.

34. Jain S, Bandi V. Electrical and lightning injuries. *Crit Care Clin.* 1999;15(2):319-331.

35. Cooper MA. Emergent care of lightning and electrical injuries. *Semin Neurol.* 1995;15(3):268-278.

36. Pfortmueller CA, Yikun Y, Haberkern M, Wuest E, Zimmermann H, Exadaktylos AK. Injuries, sequelae, and treatment of lightning-induced injuries: 10 years of experience at a Swiss trauma center. *Emerg Med Int.* 2012;2012:167698.

37. Christodouleas JP, Forrest RD, Ainsley CG, Tochner Z, Hahn SM, Glatstein E. Short-term and long-term health risks of nuclear-power-plant accidents. *N Engl J Med.* 2011;364:2334-2341.

38. Dörr H, Meineke V. Acute radiation syndrome caused by accidental radiation exposure—therapeutic principles. *BMC Med.* 2011;9:126.

39. Waselenko JK, MacVittie TJ, Blakely WF, et al. Medical management of the acute radiation syndrome: recommendations of the Strategic National Stockpile Radiation Working Group. *Ann Intern Med.* 2004;140(12):1037-1051.

Critical Care Issues in Pregnancy

Alina Dulu, MD; Ellie S. Ragsdale, MD and Dena Goffman, MD

60

KEY POINTS

1 Critical illness in obstetrics can be the result of pregnancy-specific conditions or due to commonly seen critical care diagnoses with unique-management considerations in pregnancy as a result of physiologic alterations and fetal concerns.

2 Any pregnant patient requiring ICU level care should be in a facility with obstetric and neonatal teams for collaborative multidisciplinary care.

3 A critically ill pregnant patient is at risk for labor and delivery, regardless of the initial inciting condition.

4 For patients who are still pregnant, in general, the rule is for maternal stabilization prior to delivery of the fetus. In most cases, appropriate treatment of the mother will improve fetal status.

5 The American Heart Association publishes guidelines for cardiac arrest in special situations including pregnancy. Key interventions to prevent arrest in a critically ill pregnant woman include left lateral positioning, 100% oxygen, IV access above diaphragm, and treatment of hypotension.

6 In maternal cardiac arrest not immediately reversed by basic life support and advanced cardiovascular life support (ACLS), prompt consideration for emptying the uterus must be undertaken ("perimortem cesarean"). For this to be feasible, resuscitation teams must activate a protocol for possible cesarean delivery as soon as a maternal cardiac arrest is identified.

7 Important obstetric conditions outlined within the text include preeclampsia, eclampsia, hemolysis, elevated liver enzymes, and low platelets syndrome, acute fatty liver of pregnancy, anaphylactoid syndrome of pregnancy/amniotic fluid embolism, peripartum cardiomyopathy, and obstetric hemorrhage.

8 Nonobstetric conditions with a focus on presentation in pregnancy outlined within the text include thromboembolic disease, severe sepsis, septic shock, and multiorgan failure, pulmonary edema, arrhythmia, diabetic ketoacidosis, and status asthmaticus.

INTRODUCTION

The mortality rate for critically ill obstetric patients ranges from 12% to 20%. A recently published retrospective study described the current leading diagnoses associated with ICU admission in obstetrics.

ICU admissions related to abortions and ectopic pregnancy accounted for 10% of all ICU admissions among pregnant and postpartum women. Leading causes for antepartum admissions included obstetric-related hypertensive disease (23%), trauma

(17%), and cardiac disease (13%). Delivery-related ICU admissions were overwhelmingly related to obstetric-related hypertensive disease (38%), hemorrhage (33%), and cardiac disease (18%). Postpartum admissions were most often attributed to cardiac disease (37%), obstetric-related hypertensive disease (21%), and cerebrovascular disease (20%).

Critical illness in obstetrics can be the result of pregnancy-specific conditions or due to commonly seen critical care diagnoses which may have unique-management considerations in pregnancy as a result of physiologic alterations and fetal concerns. Herein, we will review physiologic adaptations due to pregnancy by systems, general considerations for the critically ill pregnant patient, and management strategies for both pregnancy-specific conditions and critical medical conditions seen most commonly in gravid women.

PHYSIOLOGIC ADAPTATION TO PREGNANCY

Gestation in singleton pregnancies lasts an average of 40 weeks spanning from the first day of the last menstrual period to the estimated date of delivery. Previously, "term pregnancy" was defined as the period between 37 and 42 weeks gestation. However, recent data have shown improved neonatal outcomes with increasing gestation within this window. The American College of Obstetricians and Gynecologists (ACOG) and the Society of Maternal-Fetal Medicine now endorse the use of "early term" (37 0/7 through 38 6/7 weeks of gestation), "full term" (39 0/7 through 40 6/7 weeks of gestation), "late term" (41 0/7 through 41 6/7 weeks of gestation), and "postterm" (greater than 42 0/7 weeks of gestation) for classification.

Major adaptations in maternal physiology are required during gestation to sustain a healthy pregnancy. Many of these adaptations would be considered pathologic in a nonpregnant patient. Understanding of these changes is imperative in clinical decision making when pregnant women become ill.

Cardiovascular System

Pregnancy causes profound physiologic changes in the cardiovascular system. These adaptations begin very early in gestation, often before pregnancy is diagnosed, and are required to maximize oxygen delivery to the uteroplacental unit. In healthy women, these changes are generally well tolerated. However, in certain cardiac diseases, maternal morbidity and even mortality may occur.

Increased uterine volume elevates the diaphragm which displaces the heart up and to the left. The heart rotates along its long axis and the cardiac apex is deviated laterally. This results in an increased cardiac silhouette on routine radiography. Myocardial hypertrophy is observed due to the expanded blood volume and increasing afterload resulting in about a 12% increase in the overall size of the heart. Normal pregnancy can also result in changes in standard echocardiograms and electrocardiograms, including nonspecific T-wave changes and mitral/tricuspid regurgitation.

Cardiac output (CO) is the product of stroke volume and heart rate, both of which increase during pregnancy. The initial rise in heart rate occurs by 5 weeks gestation and continues to rise until it peaks at around 32 weeks gestation at 15 to 20 beats above the pregravid state (16%-20% increase in resting heart rate). The stroke volume begins to rise between 5 and 8 weeks gestation and reaches its maximum at 20 weeks, 20% to 30% above the pregravid state. CO is positional in the second half of pregnancy due the weight of the gravid uterus which compresses the inferior vena cava (IVC) and decreases venous return. The decrease in CO in the supine position compared to the lateral recumbent position is 10% to 30%. The IVC is completely occluded near term in the supine position; venous return from the lower extremities occurs through dilated paravertebral collateral circulation. There is selective distribution of the increased CO with uterine blood flow increasing 10-fold near term. Perfusion to the skin, breasts, and kidneys is also significantly increased.

Blood pressure is the product of CO and systemic vascular resistance (SVR). Despite the significant increase in CO early in gestation, systemic blood pressure is decreased until later in pregnancy as a result of decreased SVR that nadirs midpregnancy and then gradually rises until term. Progesterone-mediated smooth muscle relaxation contributes to the decrease in SVR. Central hemodynamic studies of pregnant women demonstrate a significant decrease in pulmonary vascular resistance. Mean arterial pressure, pulmonary capillary wedge pressure, central venous pressure, and left ventricular stroke work index are unchanged. Colloid osmotic pressure is decreased.

During the intrapartum and immediate postpartum period, the hemodynamic changes of the cardiovascular system reach new heights. CO increases dramatically during labor in part due to increased venous return from 300 to 500 mL autotransfusion that occurs at the onset of each contraction as blood is expressed from the uterus. In addition, mean arterial pressure (MAP) also rises in the first stage of labor and reaches a peak at the beginning of the second stage. The increase in CO and MAP are influenced by maternal pain and anxiety. Regional anesthesia has been shown to reduce the overall increase in CO, but a surge is still present with contractions. Immediately postpartum (10-30 minutes postdelivery) CO reaches its maximum and maternal heart rate declines. Approximately 1 hour postpartum CO returns to pregnancy baseline. Return to prepregnancy levels does not occur until 6 to 8 weeks postpartum.

Respiratory System

Physiologic and structural changes occur throughout the respiratory tract during pregnancy. The nasal mucosa becomes edematous and hyperemic with increased secretions due to a rise in circulating estrogen. These changes cause marked nasal stuffiness and an increased risk of epistaxis. Placement of nasogastric tubes or nasal airways can cause excessive bleeding if adequate lubrication is not used.

The structure of the thoracic cavity is markedly altered in pregnancy and cannot be entirely explained by the mechanical pressure of the gravid uterus. The subcostal angle increases from 68° to 103°, the transverse diameter of the chest expands by 2 cm, and the chest circumference expands by 5 to 7 cm. The resting level of the diaphragm is 4 cm higher at term that in the nongravid state. However, the diaphragmatic excursions are increased by 1 to 2 cm over nonpregnant values.

Intrinsic pulmonary function and static lung volumes are altered throughout the pregnancy. Elevation of the diaphragm decreases the volume of the lungs in the resting state which reduces the total lung capacity by 5% and the functional residual capacity (FRC) by 20%. FRC is the sum of expiratory reserve volume and residual volume; both decrease in pregnancy. Inspiratory capacity, the maximum volume that can be inhaled, increased by 5% to 10% because of the decrease in FRC. The vital capacity does not change (Table 60–1).

Increased progesterone levels during pregnancy leads to a state of chronic hyperventilation, which results in a decrease in $PaCO_2$ to below 30 mm Hg in normal women. Maternal pH does not change because there is a reciprocal decline in the bicarbonate concentration. Total body oxygen uptake at rest increases by 12% to 20%. This increased oxygen is needed to meet the high metabolic demands of pregnancy. The oxygen need is met by increased tidal volume alone because respiratory rate and pulmonary diffusing capacity do not change.

Hematologic System

Blood volume and composition change during pregnancy. Maternal blood volume begins to increase at about 6 weeks gestation and progresses until 30 to 34 weeks and then remains stable until delivery. Average blood volume expansion is 40% to 60% but this varies widely. The increase in blood volume results from a combined expansion of both plasma volume and red blood cell (RBC) mass. Without iron supplementation, RBC mass increases by about 18% by term, supplemental iron causes the increase to rise up to 30%. Plasma volume increases more than the RBC mass leading to a drop in maternal hematocrit, that is, dilutional. This so-called physiologic anemia of pregnancy reaches its nadir at 30 to 34 weeks gestation.

The white blood cell count increases to about 10,000/μL at term and the platelet count decreases slightly. Platelet counts greater than 120,000/μL are generally considered normal in pregnancy. In the third trimester, approximately 8% of gravidas will develop gestational thrombocytopenia with platelet counts between 70,000 and 150,000/μL.

The biochemical characteristics of the blood change in pregnancy. Serum osmolality decreases by 10 mOsm/L early in pregnancy and then remains stable throughout gestation. Minor decreases in sodium, potassium, calcium, magnesium, and zinc occur. Chloride does not change, but bicarbonate markedly decreases. The plasma concentrations of

TABLE 60-1 Pulmonary changes in pregnancy.

Measurement	Definition	Change in Pregnancy
Respiratory Rate (RR)	Breaths per minute	Unchanged
Vital Capacity (VC)	Max amount of air that can be forcibly expired after max inspiration (IC + ERV)	Unchanged
Inspiratory Capacity (IC)	Max amount of air that can be inspired from resting expiratory level (TV + IRV)	Increased 5%-10%
Tidal Volume (TV)	Air inspired and expired in a normal breath	Increased 30%-40%
Inspiratory Reserve Volume (IRV)	Max amount of air that can be inspired at the end of a normal breath	Unchanged
Functional Residual Capacity (FRC)	Air in the lungs at resting expiratory level (ERV + RV)	Decreased 20%
Expiratory Reserve Volume (ERV)	Max amount of air that can be expired from the resting expiratory level	Decreased 15%-20%
Residual Volume (RV)	Air in the lungs after max expiration	Decreased 20%-25%
Total Lung Capacity (TLC)	Total amount of air in the lungs at maximal inspiration (VC + RV)	Decreased 5%

Reproduced with permission from Gabbe SG, Niebyl JR, Simpson JL: Obstetrics: normal and problem pregnancies, 3rd edition. New York: Churchill Livingstone; 1996.

albumin and total protein decrease in proportion to the plasma volume expansion. Alkaline phosphatase increases because of the production of the placental form of the enzyme. Serum lipids increase toward term, with the levels of cholesterol and triglycerides doubling during pregnancy.

Levels of many coagulation factors are altered in pregnancy. Fibrinogen levels increase to as high as 600 mg/dL near term. The prothrombin time, activated partial thromboplastin time, and thrombin time all fall slightly but usually remain within the lower range of normal limits for nonpregnant women. Bleeding time and whole blood clotting times do not change. There is a 5 to 6 fold increased risk for thromboembolic disease in pregnancy. This greater risk is caused by increased venous stasis, vessel wall injury, and changes to the coagulation cascade that lead to hypercoagulability. The overall risk of thromboembolism in pregnancy is estimated to be 1/1500 and accounts for 25% of the maternal deaths in the United States.

Renal System

The kidneys enlarge in size and weight during pregnancy due to increased renal vasculature, interstitial volume, and urinary dead space. The dead space is accounted for in the dilation of the collecting system. Pelvic calyceal dilation is greater on the right than the left. Anatomic changes are also observed in the bladder. The bladder trigone is elevated and increased vascularity is seen throughout the bladder, which increases the incidence of microhematuria.

Renal plasma flow and glomerular filtration rate (GFR) increase significantly early in pregnancy reaching their peak early in the third trimester. The creatinine clearance in pregnancy is increased to values of 150 to 200 mL/min. The increased GFR leads to a reduction in maternal plasma levels of creatinine, blood urea nitrogen, and uric acid. Serum creatinine falls from a nonpregnant level of 0.8 to 0.5 mg/dL by term.

Glucose excretion increases and glycosuria is common. This glycosuria is intermittent and not necessarily related to blood glucose levels or the stage of gestation. No significant increase in proteinuria occurs in a normal pregnancy in women without proteinuria before pregnancy. In women with preexisting proteinuria, the amount of proteinuria increases in both the second and third trimesters.

Other changes in the tubular function include an increase in the excretion of amino acids in the urine and an increase in calcium excretion. This increase in calcium excretion increases the risk of nephrolithiasis in the setting of urinary stasis mediated by progesterone. Finally, the kidney responds to the respiratory alkalosis of pregnancy by increased bicarbonate excretion.

Immune System

The fetus is a semiallograft and a successful pregnancy is dependent on either evasion of immune surveillance or suppression of the maternal-adaptive immune response. A major shift occurs away from cell-mediated cytotoxic immune responses toward increased humoral and innate immune responses.[9] This shift decreases the maternal cytotoxic potential against fetal antigens. The decrease in cellular immunity leads to increased susceptibility to intracellular pathogens such as cytomegalovirus, herpes simplex virus, varicella, and malaria. The changes in the immunologic system of a pregnant woman are complex and not fully understood. Hormones, particularly progesterone, likely play a significant role.

GENERAL CONSIDERATIONS IN THE CARE OF THE CRITICALLY ILL GRAVIDA

Any pregnant patient requiring ICU level care should be in a facility with obstetric and neonatal teams for collaborative multidisciplinary care. The critically ill pregnant patient is at risk for labor and delivery, regardless of the initial inciting condition. In addition, postpartum patients continue to have pregnancy-related physiologic changes and are prone to specific pregnancy-related conditions such as bleeding, hypertensive disorders, venous thromboembolism, and infection from an obstetric source.

For patients who are still pregnant, in general the rule is for maternal stabilization prior to delivery of the fetus. In most cases, appropriate treatment of the mother will improve fetal status. Treatment required to stabilize the mother's critical status should be undertaken, even if such intervention is potentially disadvantageous to the fetus. Short- and long-term morbidity in surviving fetuses is directly related to maternal physiologic status.

There are cases where the obstetric team will be guiding the management of care toward intended delivery (preeclampsia, acute fatty liver, amniotic fluid embolus); however, it is important to know that even in cases where delivery is not recommended, spontaneous labor may ensue. A plan for potential delivery should be made with the obstetric team in case this occurs and should include preferred location, preferred mode (vaginal vs cesarean), need for analgesia or anesthesia and plan for advanced pediatric support for the newborn. Basic supplies should be made available at the ICU bedside. ICU teams must be aware of basic signs of labor including patient pain, leakage of fluid or mucus per vagina, any vaginal bleeding, palpable contractions (tightening at the uterine fundus). Although some of these may be difficult to discern in an intubated and sedated patient, close attention may allow early identification of signs and symptoms of labor in a critically ill patient and can allow for planning and mobilization of appropriate resources to optimize maternal and fetal outcome.

Critical illness can compromise the fetus as a result of maternal hypotension, hypoxemia, and acid-base imbalances. Fetal oxygenation is dependent upon uterine blood flow that is not autoregulated, thus can fall as a result of decrease in maternal systolic blood pressure. Uterine blood flow can also be reduced from vasoconstriction related to vasopressors, maternal hypercarbia or hypocarbia. *Continuous fetal monitoring* of fetuses who have reached viability may be recommended. The fetal heart rate pattern should be monitored by a physician or nurse experienced in fetal heart rate interpretation and information can be used to guide maternal resuscitative strategies.

Oxygen supplementation should be used early with goal maternal oxygen saturation (SaO_2) greater than 95% and PaO_2 greater than 70 mm Hg to maintain a favorable oxygen diffusion gradient from the maternal to the fetal side of the placenta. Early intubation after preoxygenation is recommended if adequate maternal oxygenation cannot be achieved noninvasively. The indications for intubation and ventilation are the same as for nonpregnant patients.

Endotracheal intubation in pregnant women is usually more difficult. Airway edema and hyperemia can contribute to difficult intubation and decreased lower esophageal tone leads to increased aspiration risk during endotracheal intubation. Selecting a size of 6 to 7 ET tube and applying cricoid pressure to prevent aspiration of gastric contents should be considered.

Ventilation of the pregnant patient is similar to that of nonpregnant patients, except that it should be directed to a slightly lower PCO_2 level because the normal pregnant state is a mild respiratory alkalosis with PCO_2 levels of 28 to 32 mm Hg. Excessive hyperventilation will lead to uterine vasoconstriction with decreased placental and fetal perfusion and should be avoided.

If indicated, *chest tube* should be placed 2 intercostal spaces above the usual landmark of the fifth intercostal space due to the elevation of the diaphragm and ideally should be done under ultrasound guidance.

Hypotension management in the parturient requires particular attention to body position and volume status. The uterus reaches the level of the maternal umbilicus by approximately 20 weeks of gestation when it is large enough to compress the IVC when the woman is supine and result in up to a 30% reduction in CO. *Displacing the uterus to the left*, off the vena cava, is critical to restoring CO. This is best accomplished by placing the woman on her left side, putting a wedge or rolled towel under her right side, or adjusting her platform to a 30° left lateral tilt.

Fluid resuscitation must be administered adequately because the addition of vasoconstricting agents will compromise uteroplacental flow if vasoconstriction is imposed on an insufficient circulating volume. All vasoactive agents have the potential to constrict uterine vessels and reduce blood flow to the placenta and fetus despite improving maternal blood pressures. Placental blood flow and uterine perfusion pressure are directly proportional to maternal systemic blood pressure and CO.

Attention should be paid to *glycemic control*, for fetal benefit, particularly if delivery is being considered. Aggressive *venous thromboembolism prophylaxis* should be initiated with sequential compression devices as well as pharmacoprophylaxis if no contraindication exists.

CARDIOPULMONARY ARREST IN THE PREGNANT PATIENT: SPECIAL CONSIDERATIONS

The American Heart Association publishes guidelines for cardiac arrest in special situations including pregnancy. During a maternal resuscitation, providers must consider the mother, the fetus, and anatomic and physiologic changes of pregnancy to optimize resuscitative efforts and outcome. Key interventions to prevent arrest in a critically ill pregnant woman include left lateral positioning, 100% oxygen, IV access above diaphragm and treatment of hypotension. Consideration of reversible causes of critical illness may allow initiation of early aggressive treatment.

Recommended modifications to basic life support (BLS) include patient positioning to optimize venous return and CO. Manual displacement can be accomplished by using a one-handed and two handed technique. A difficult airway should be anticipated due to pregnancy changes and optimal bag-mask ventilation and suctioning should be used while preparing for advanced airway management. Breathing should be supported to ensure adequate oxygenation and ventilation. Chest compressions should be performed the same as most current recommendations. Defibrillation may be utilized as indicated.

Recommended modifications to ACLS include anticipation of difficulty with airway and only attempting intubation with an experienced provider, with bag-mask ventilation with 100% oxygen prior to intubation. Medication and defibrillation should be utilized in the usual doses for the standard indications, however, internal/external fetal monitors should be removed prior to defibrillation. Consider and initiate appropriate therapy for reversible pregnancy-related etiologies for the arrest. Specifically, if the patient is on IV magnesium (a commonly used medication in obstetrics), magnesium should be stopped and IV calcium gluconate should be administered.

In maternal cardiac arrest, not immediately reversed by BLS and ACLS, prompt consideration for emptying the uterus must be undertaken. For this to be feasible, resuscitation teams must activate a protocol for possible cesarean delivery as soon as a maternal cardiac arrest is identified. In general, if the gravid uterus is at the level of the umbilicus (20 weeks size), the uterus may be causing aortocaval compression and impacting maternal hemodynamics. In this case, hysterotomy should be considered for maternal benefit, regardless of exact gestational age and fetal viability. This is an assessment that must be made promptly because the recommendation is to begin the cesarean within 4 minutes of arrest with the goal of delivering a viable fetus within 5 minutes.

PREGNANCY SPECIFIC CONDITIONS

Preeclampsia–Eclampsia

Essentials of diagnosis: hypertension, proteinuria, ± seizures (eclampsia).

Background

Preeclampsia is defined as new onset of hypertension and either proteinuria or end-organ dysfunction at more than 20 weeks gestational age in previously normotensive women or new onset proteinuria, severe hypertension, or symptoms in women with chronic hypertension. Preeclampsia is a common disorder with an incidence of approximately 15% in nulliparous women and 6% in multiparous women. The disease is also more common at extremes of age.

Hypertensive disorders in pregnancy are one of the leading causes of maternal death in the United States and worldwide. Approximately 75% of preeclampsia will be mild and self-limited. Of the remaining 25% that are severe, very few will require ICU care usually due to significant end-organ damage. Preeclampsia affects the cardiovascular, pulmonary, renal, hepatic, hematologic, and neurologic systems.

Early diagnosis of preeclampsia is imperative to optimize maternal and fetal outcomes. The only "cure" for preeclampsia is delivery, the timing of which is determined based on gestational age and severity of disease.

Clinical Features

Symptoms or Signs—Preeclampsia was historically diagnosed based on a triad of hypertension,

proteinuria, and edema. Edema has been removed from the diagnostic criteria because of the frequent occurrence of edema in late pregnancy, but a sudden and dramatic weight gain still conveys a high likelihood of imminent preeclampsia. In 2013, ACOG removed proteinuria as an essential criterion for diagnosis of preeclampsia.

Preeclampsia is defined as with or without severe features. Preeclampsia without severe features, generally, does not cause long-term maternal end-organ damage and thus can be managed expectantly until a later gestational age, that is, 37 weeks. Preeclampsia with severe features can present with a wide variety of signs/symptoms and often requires delivery regardless of gestational age (Table 60–2).

Classically, the minimum criteria for diagnosis of mild preeclampsia are blood pressure greater than 140 mm Hg systolic or 90 mm Hg diastolic on 2 separate occasions greater than 4 hours apart and proteinuria defined as 300 mg of protein in a 24 hours urine collection or at least 30 mg/dL (1+) protein on a spot urine dipstick. There has been a shift to using a urine protein/creatinine ratio of more than or equal to 0.3 to diagnose proteinuria.

Recent guidelines published by the ACOG in December 2013 encourage new diagnostic criteria for preeclampsia excluding the requirement for proteinuria for diagnosis. The authors state that evidence suggests that kidney damage can occur in the setting of preeclampsia without significant proteinuria.

TABLE 60–2 Criteria for severe preeclampsia.

Blood Pressure ≥ 160 or ≥110 (2 values at least 4 hours apart)
Central Nervous System Dysfunction (Cerebral or Visual Disturbances)
Hepatic abnormality (RUQ/epigastric pain, transaminase >= twice normal)
Thrombocytopenia (< 100K platelets/microL)
Renal abnormality (serum creatinine > 1.1 mg/dL or doubling)
Pulmonary Edema
Seizures (Eclampsia)

Laboratory Findings

Preeclampsia is generally a clinical diagnosis. Laboratory data are useful in following the course of the disease, particularly in the case of expectant management due to prematurity of the fetus. Serial monitoring of hemoglobin, platelet count, creatinine, liver function tests, lactate dehydrogenase (LDH), and creatinine are essential.

Management

Delivery—The only definitive management for preeclampsia is delivery of the fetus. In the case of severe preeclampsia, delivery is often expedited except in specific situations including extreme prematurity. Even in these cases, the delay is often brief and used to administer corticosteroids for fetal lung maturity or facilitate transfer to a tertiary care center.

Seizure Prophylaxis—Seizure prophylaxis should be administered to all patients in whom severe preeclampsia is diagnosed or suspected. Seizure prophylaxis is continued through delivery and 24 hours postpartum or until the patient has proven stable enough to attempt expectant management.

In the United States, magnesium sulfate is the most common medication administered for seizure prophylaxis. It is generally administered as an intravenous drip, but can be given intramuscularly if intravenous access is not available. The usual regimen includes a 4 to 6 g loading dose given over 30 minutes, followed by a continuous infusion of 2 g/h. The therapeutic range is wide with goal serum magnesium levels of 4.8 to 8.4 mg/dL.

Magnesium toxicity should be monitored for clinically in alert patients with physical exam (reflexes and cognitive status). Laboratory values can also be monitored. Magnesium is contraindicated in patients with myasthenia gravis and relatively contraindicated with pulmonary edema. It should be used with caution and consideration for dosage modification in the setting of significant renal dysfunction or oliguria. The second-line medication for treatment in these cases is phenytoin.

Control of Hypertension—Severe hypertension (BP > 160/110) should be controlled aggressively. Hydralazine and labetalol are the most common medications used to treat acute hypertension in pregnancy. Hydralazine is administered in 5 to 20 mg doses based on patient response at 30 minute intervals. Labetalol is administered starting at a 20 mg dose and can be doubled every 10 minutes up to an 80 mg dose and a maximum total of 220 mg.

The goal is to lower blood pressure out of the severe range, not to achieve a normal blood pressure. If repetitive IV doses of medication are unable to control the blood pressure, IV drips of nitroglycerin, nicardipine, or nitroprusside can be used in a monitored ICU setting. In the setting of refractory hypertension, delivery is required once the mother is stabilized. Nitroprusside administration can lead to fetal cyanide poisoning and thus should be used with caution prior to delivery of the fetus.

Physicians should exercise caution when using any vasodilators in patients with preeclampsia because patients are often intravascularly depleted making them susceptible to dramatic drops in blood pressure. Significant drops in blood pressure can lead to decreased uteroplacental perfusion and fetal compromise.

Hemodynamic Monitoring—Invasive monitoring is not contraindicated in pregnancy and can be considered in the case of refractory pulmonary edema or oliguria. Historically, it was thought that a pulmonary artery catheter may be favorable because central venous pressures are unreliable. Recently, echocardiography has been the favored method of monitoring for fluid status.

Pulmonary edema in preeclampsia may be due to left ventricular dysfunction secondary to high SVR, iatrogenic volume overload in the face of contracted intravascular space, decreased plasma colloid oncotic pressure, or pulmonary capillary membrane injury. Of note, in the event of respiratory compromise requiring intubation, it is important to note that patients often have laryngeal edema making intubation difficult. Advanced airway devices and a skilled anesthesiologist may be required.

Oliguria in preeclampsia is due to intravascular volume depletion (most common), relative volume overload with decreased left ventricular function secondary to high SVR, or renal arteriolar spasm. Echocardiographic assessment of cardiac function can help determine the cause of oliguria and course of treatment.

HELLP Syndrome—Preeclampsia can be complicated by hemolysis, elevated liver enzymes, and low platelets (HELLP) syndrome. It is unclear if

HELLP syndrome represents a separate clinical entity from preeclampia or is just a part of the spectrum of disease. Women with HELLP syndrome are generally older and multiparous and HELLP syndrome can occur in the absence of proteinuria or hypertension.

Laboratory evidence of HELLP syndrome includes abnormal peripheral smears (burr cells, schistocytes, echinocytes), hemolysis (elevated indirect bilirubin, LDH > 600, low haptoglobin), elevated liver transaminases (2× upper limit of normal), and thrombocytopenia (plt < 100k). Severe thrombocytopenia (plt < 30k) occurs rarely and these patients may require platelet transfusion for delivery.

In the absence of liver rupture, treatment of HELLP syndrome is generally supportive other than delivery. Serial monitoring of laboratory values and magnesium administration for seizure prophylaxis are recommended. Additionally, dexamethasone 10 mg intravenously every 12 hours can be administered to speed the process of laboratory value improvement in the setting of severe thrombocytopenia. Corticosteroids have not been shown to improve maternal morbidity or mortality.

In the event of liver rupture, operative exploration should be expedited as this is a surgical emergency. Exploration should not be delayed for imaging studies. The maternal mortality rate associated with HELLP syndrome has been estimated to be 1% with most mortality occurring in the setting of liver rupture.

Eclampsia—Eclampsia is defined as the presence of grand mal seizures in women with preeclampsia without a seizure disorder or other attributable cause of seizures. Eclampsia carries of maternal mortality rate of 1% to 2% and a fetal mortality rate of 10%. Onset of seizures is often preceded by symptoms including a severe unrelenting headache, nausea, or vomiting. Seizures are usually self-limited and medication is not usually required to break the seizure activity.

Treatment of eclampsia is standard magnesium administration with a 4 to 6 g bolus and then a continuous infusion of 2 g/h. Magnesium should be administered expeditiously in the setting of eclampsia, however, the purpose is to prevent recurrent seizure. Magnesium is superior to phenytoin and diazepam for preventing additional seizures.

Once seizure activity is controlled, delivery should be affected. In many cases, labor can be induced safely and a vaginal delivery can be achieved. Magnesium prophylaxis should be continued throughout delivery and for 24 hours postpartum.

Additional Critical Care Events—Disseminated intravascular coagulation, hypertensive encephalopathy, acute myocardial infarction, acute renal failure, intracranial hemorrhage, and acute aortic dissection can also be associated with hypertensive disorders in pregnancy. In each of these settings, a multidisciplinary approach with critical care, obstetrics, anesthesia and in certain cases other services is required to provide adequate care.

Acute Fatty Liver of Pregnancy

Essentials of diagnosis: hepatic dysfunction and microvesicular fatty infiltration of hepatocytes.

Background

Acute fatty liver of pregnancy (AFLP) is a rare but life-threatening complication of pregnancy with an incidence between 1:7000 and 1:16,000. It occurs late in pregnancy or immediately postpartum, often as fulminant liver failure with sudden onset coagulopathy and encephalopathy in women with no history of liver disease. Microvesicular fatty infiltration of hepatocytes is seen on microscopy.

Historically, AFLP was thought to be universally fatal, but early recognition, aggressive stabilization of the mother, and prompt delivery have improved the prognosis. Maternal and fetal mortality are currently estimated at approximately 15%.

The exact etiology of AFLP remains unknown. In many cases, either the mother or fetus is found to have an autosomal mutation that causes deficiency of the long-chain 3-hydroxyacyl coenzyme-A dehydrogenase (LCHAD), a fatty acid beta-oxidation enzyme. The association of this mutation with AFLP is strong enough that screening for the LCHAD mutation is recommended in the infants of affected mothers. Additional risk factors include nulliparity, multiple pregnancy, male fetus, and coexisting preeclampsia.

Clinical Features

Symptoms or Signs—Patients often present with a history of 1 to 2 weeks of nausea, vomiting, anorexia, and malaise. On physical exam, patients are ill-appearing often with some degree of jaundice. Hypertension with or without proteinuria and transient diabetes insipidus with polydipsia and polyuria are also common.

In severe disease, ascites, progressive hepatic encephalopathy, hypoglycemia, coagulopathy, metabolic acidosis, and renal failure are also often seen. Intrauterine fetal demise occurs frequently, often prior to the diagnosis, likely due to hypoglycemia and uteroplacental insufficiency.

Laboratory Findings—Diagnosis of AFLP is suspected based on clinical presentation and dramatic laboratory changes (Table 60–3), but a definitive diagnosis cannot be made without a liver biopsy, confirming microvesicular fat infiltration of the hepatocytes.

Management

Care of a patient with suspected AFLP has 4 categories: diagnosis, stabilization, delivery, and support. During the diagnosis phase of management, intensive monitoring of the mother and the fetus are required. Because the fetal status can decline rapidly, if AFLP is suspected continuous external fetal monitoring should be applied until the diagnosis is ruled out or delivery is affected. Maternal hemodynamic and metabolic status should be monitored both clinically and with laboratory values.

The stabilization phase includes treatment of the complications of AFLP that are present. This

TABLE 60–3 Laboratory changes in acute fatty liver of pregnancy.

Elevated WBC (> 20 K)	Decreased Fibrinogen
Prolonged PT and aPTT	Decreased Platelets
Elevated Ammonia	Decreased Coagulation Factors
Elevated Uric Acid	Decreased pH (acidosis)
Elevated BUN/Creatinine	Hypoglycemia
Hyperglycemia (if associated with pancreatitis)	Decreased Serum Albumin
Elevated Transaminases (< 2000 IU/L)	

includes establishing stable airway in an obtunded patient, normalizing intravascular volume, correcting electrolyte disturbances, treating hypoglycemia/hyperglycemia and correcting coagulation abnormalities with blood products. In certain cases, dialysis may be required for acute renal failure or desmopressin for diabetes insipidus.

Once the patient is stabilized, an expeditious delivery is recommended within 24 hours. The diagnosis of AFLP does not require a cesarean delivery. In fact, in the setting of significant coagulopathy, operative delivery may increase maternal morbidity and mortality. Regional anesthesia is often prohibited in cases of AFLP due to coagulopathy and thrombocytopenia. Care should be taken with medication choices if general anesthesia is required because certain medications can exacerbate liver failure.

Following delivery, care is supportive until the multisystem organ failure improves. This often requires ICU admission. Fluid balance, electrolyte status, and glycemic management are critical to survival. Blood glucose should be monitored hourly and electrolytes every 2 to 4 hours. Evidence of disseminated intravascular coagulation should be managed aggressively with blood products. Protein intake should be limited with the majority of caloric intake from glucose to decrease the nitrogenous waste. Colonic emptying should be facilitated with promotility agents to increase ammonia loss via stool. Neomycin 6 to 12 g or lactulose 20 to 30 g can also be administered daily to decrease colonic ammonia production. Occasionally, the liver damage from AFLP is so severe that transplantation is required.

Anaphylactoid Syndrome of Pregnancy/Amniotic Fluid Embolism

Essentials of diagnosis: hypotension, hypoxia, coagulopathy and frequently seizures/pulmonary edema/cardiac arrest.

Background

Amniotic fluid embolism (AFE) is a rare but catastrophic complication of pregnancy. The incidence is unknown but is thought to be between 1:8000 and 1:30,000 pregnancies. An AFE is a foreign substance (amniotic fluid with fetal squamous cells) that is introduced into the maternal circulation which causes an acute cardiovascular and pulmonary collapse with associated coagulopathy.

AFE usually occurs during labor, delivery or the first 30 minutes postpartum. The classic presentation is an acute cardiopulmonary arrest in a previously healthy woman laboring or immediately postpartum. Seventy percent of cases occur during labor. Cardiac arrest is common and amniotic fluid emboli account for 5% to 10% of all maternal deaths in the United States. Fetal mortality is approximately 21% and fetal neurologic complications occur in more than half of infants delivered to mothers with an AFE.

Risk factors for amniotic fluid emboli include increased maternal age, uterine overdistension, cesarean delivery, uterine rupture, placental abruption, severe cervical lacerations, and maternal trauma. Links have been suggested between AFE and meconium stained amniotic fluid, augmented labor, and hypertonic contractions but these reports have not been validated.

Clinical Features

Symptoms and Signs—The diagnosis of an AFE is made clinically with the spectrum of disease ranging from mild coagulopathy to sudden and complete cardiopulmonary collapse. Patients most often present with dyspnea, hypotension (100%), and hypoxia (93%). Coagulopathy (83%) and altered mental status (70%) are also common. Seizure activity occurs in approximately 33% of patients and significantly increases maternal morbidity and mortality. Constitutional symptoms (fever, chills, nausea, vomiting, and headache) are also present to varying degrees.

Laboratory Findings—Lab values are nonspecific and do not aid in the diagnosis of AFE. Evidence of coagulopathy without previous blood loss is suggestive and significant hemorrhage is often seen acutely. Fetal squamous cells in the maternal pulmonary circulation at the time of autopsy are diagnostic but cannot always be identified due to prolonged courses following the acute event.

Management

AFE is a rare and unpredictable disorder of pregnancy. Treatment includes prompt initiation of basic and advanced cardiac life support. Continuous cardiac monitoring and pulse oximetry are required with invasive blood pressure monitoring. Coagulopathy must be managed promptly and aggressively with hemorrhage protocol combinations of packed red cells, fresh frozen plasma, cryoprecipitate, and platelets. In catastrophic cases where hemorrhage cannot be controlled, newer procoagulant agents should be used and a hysterectomy may be required. If an AFE is suspected before delivery, delivery should be prompt once the maternal condition is stabilized.

Peripartum Cardiomyopathy

Essentials of diagnosis: heart failure in last month of pregnancy or within 5 months of delivery, no history or other identifiable cause, LV systolic dysfunction.

Background

Peripartum cardiomyopathy (PPCM) occurs in about 1:2200 to 1:3200 pregnancies in the United States but is seen much more commonly globally. It is defined as heart failure in the last month of pregnancy or up to 5 months postpartum in the absence of known heart disease or another identifiable cause. It is characterized by left ventricular systolic dysfunction with an ejection fraction of < 45% or reduced fractional shortening.

Risk factors for peripartum cardiomyopathy include multiparity, black race, maternal age more than 30, hypertensive disorders of pregnancy, multiple gestation, long term tocolytic therapy (terbutaline), and maternal cocaine abuse. The exact etiology is unknown.

About half of patients will have complete resolution of symptoms after delivery with return of normal cardiac size and function. The remainder has continued dilation and often progressive heart failure. Future pregnancies are extremely high risk in women with a history of peripartum cardiomyopathy. In women without complete resolution of symptoms, future pregnancy mortality approaches 50%.

Clinical Features

Symptoms and Signs—Patients present with symptoms of heart failure. Some of the initial nonspecific symptoms may be confusing due to the prevalence of these symptoms in normal pregnancy.

Imaging studies show enlargement of the cardiac silhouette and pulmonary edema. Echocardiography shows decreased universal contractility and left ventricular enlargement without hypertrophy. Diagnostic criteria used include: Left ventricular ejection fraction less than 45% and/or fractional shortening of less than 30% and left ventricular end systolic dimension greater than 2.7 cm/m².

Laboratory Findings—Arterial blood gas shows hypoxemia with respiratory alkalosis. Urinalysis can show concentrated urine. CBC, serum chemistries and liver function tests should be unremarkable. Brain natriuretic peptide (BNP) levels typically increase 2 fold in healthy pregnancy and are usually elevated in heart failure, however limited data are available to support the use of this test in pregnancy. Elevated BNP has been observed in pregnant women with preeclampsia and other clinical conditions associated with volume overload.

Special Considerations—Systemic and pulmonary embolization can be seen more frequently than in other forms of cardiomyopathies.

Management

Treatment of PPCM is similar to that for other types of heart failure. The goal in management is to improve cardiac function by reducing afterload and preload and increasing contractility. It is important to remember to avoid angiotensin inhibition, which is contraindicated in pregnancy.

Initial stabilization may require intravenous diuretics or inotropic support. Loop *diuretics* serve to decrease preload and relieve pulmonary congestion. *Digoxin* may improve myocardial contractility and facilitate rate control when atrial fibrillation is present. *Hydralazine* is the vasodilator of choice and can be used to reduce afterload before delivery and angiotensin-converting enzyme inhibitors can be used postpartum. *Beta blockade* has also been shown to improve cardiac function and survival in chronic heart failure but should not be used in acute decompensated heart failure. Patients with acute decompensated heart failure with hypotension or persistent pulmonary edema despite initial measures may benefit from *intravenous inotropic support* with Dobutamine or Milrinone. An intra-aortic balloon pump, extracorporeal membrane oxygenation, and LV assist devices have been used successfully as

a bridge for recovery or transplantation in patients with PPCM and should be considered in rapidly deteriorating patients who are not responding to medical therapy, including inotropic medications.

Anticoagulation with heparin should be considered if EF is significantly reduced, that is, less than 35% due to the high risk of thrombus formation and thromboembolism in the context of pregnancy-related hypercoaguabllity and stasis due to LV dysfunction.

Early delivery may be necessary if persistent hemodynamic instability is present, but if the mother is stabilized the goal is delivery at term. Cesarean delivery is reserved for obstetric indications. Early pain control is a key in patients with peripartum cardiomyopathy during labor as pain increases cardiac work and causes tachycardia. A carefully dosed epidural that provides adequate pain control and avoids hypotension is vital.

OBSTETRIC HEMORRHAGE
Background

Obstetric hemorrhage is the leading cause of maternal morbidity and mortality worldwide. It is defined as greater than 500 ml blood loss at the time of a vaginal delivery or greater than 1000 ml of blood loss at the time of cesarean birth. Massive hemorrhage is defined as greater than 1500 ml of blood loss. Rates of massive hemorrhage are increasing as the age and comorbidities of the pregnant population increases. Most obstetric ICU admissions will be due to hemorrhage. The most common causes of obstetric hemorrhage are uterine atony, placental abruption, and abnormal placentation (previa/accreta). Less common causes include genital tract lacerations, uterine inversion and coagulopathy.

Clinical Features/Management
1. **Uterine atony**
   a. Signs and symptoms include a boggy, soft uterus after delivery with the lower uterine segment often filled with clot.
   b. Risk factors include precipitous or prolonged labor, labor augmentation, overdistended uterus, grand multiparity, prior history of postpartum hemorrhage from uterine atony.

c. Management include fundal massage and evacuation of the uterus are the first line in treatment of uterine atony. Retained products of conception can prolong the hemorrhage.

Uterotonic drugs are administered during the fundal massage including intravenous oxytocin (10-40 units in 500-1000 ml normal saline), methylergonovine (0.2 mg intramuscularly), carboprost tromethamine (0.25 mg intramuscularly), or misoprostol (1000 mcg/rectum). Methylergonovine may be associated with increases in maternal blood pressure and therefore cannot be used in women with hypertension or preeclampsia. Prostaglandins can cause bronchospasm and therefore should be avoided in asthmatics.

Obstetric balloon devices can also be used temporarily to tamponade uterine bleeding and slow postpartum hemorrhage. Patients may be observed for up to 24 hours with the balloon in situ before deflating and closely observing for recurrent bleeding.

Surgical management options, including uterine compression sutures and uterine artery ligation, can also be pursued prior to hysterectomy.

Additionally, in certain centers angiographic embolization can be performed, however this should not be considered first line therapy to control active obstetric hemorrhage.

2. **Placental abruption**

a. Signs and symptoms include severe persistent abdominal pain differing from the classic crescendo-decrescendo labor pattern; ± vaginal bleeding; retroplacental clot on ultrasound; abnormal fetal heart rate tracing; coagulopathy; bluish "Couvelier's" uterus at the time of cesarean delivery.

b. Risk factors include severe hypertension, preeclampsia, cocaine use, trauma, and rapid decompression of the uterus (ruptured membranes with polyhydramnios, delivery of the first twin).

c. Management include the most important steps in the management of placental abruption are identifying the cause of the abruption, treating the underlying disorder and correction of coagulopathy. In the case of significant abruption, delivery should be affected as soon maternal hemodynamic stability is achieved.

3. **Abnormal placentation (previa/accreta)**

a. Signs and Symptoms include placenta previa (placenta overlying the internal cervical os) often presents with painless third trimester bleeding and is usually diagnosed antepartum if adequate prenatal care is received. Placenta accreta occurs when the placenta invades the myometrium and fails to separate following delivery.

b. Risk factors are similar for previa and accreta and include multiparity and prior uterine procedures (cesarean and curettage). Serial cesarean birth is the single greatest risk factor for abnormal placentation and all women with a prior cesarean delivery should undergo ultrasonographic evaluation for placenta accreta. Often the diagnosis of accreta is suspected on ultrasound based on the lack of integrity in the placenta myometrial border and/or placenta lakes. In cases where the suspicion is high, MRI may help further characterize the extent of invasion.

c. Management include all cases of abnormal placentation should be delivered by cesarean with a skilled pelvic surgeon available. Early notification of the blood bank is imperative as massive transfusion may be required. Some literature has also described preoperative placement of embolization or balloon catheters prophylactically in the highest risk patients.

General Considerations

Obstetric hemorrhage is often underestimated. A stable airway and adequate intravenous access should be established early. Maternal hemodynamic collapse often does not occur until blood loss is greater than 2000 cc and coagulopathy is common. Hemorrhagic shock should be treated early and aggressively with 2:1 replacement with crystalloid and aggressive resuscitation with blood products is imperative. Most academic institutions have created an obstetric hemorrhage protocol to improve communication with the blood bank for release of products. When the hemorrhage protocol is activated packed red cells, fresh frozen plasma and platelets are released together, usually in a 6:4:1 or 4:4:1 ratio. Cryoprecipitate is often added after the first hemorrhage pack is transfused. Identification and correction of bleeding must be accomplished promptly. Newer therapies exist, with limited data regarding safety and effectiveness, which may be advocated for in intractable life-threatening hemorrhage include activated factor VII, prothrombin complex concentrate and tranexamic acid.

When a patient has endured a significant obstetric hemorrhage, she is at risk for significant comorbidities and complications related to the acute blood loss, massive transfusion and indicated therapies. By being aware of these risks, the critical care team can ensure proper posthemorrhage care, with early recognition and appropriate treatment of complications should they arise. Priorities in posthemorrhage management in the ICU include close observation of laboratory parameters (including CBC and coagulation profile) to assure adequate replacement once equilibration has occurred and avoidance of coagulopathy. Close observation is required for evidence of ongoing or recurrent bleeding. Infection is another risk that should be closely monitored for. Recognition of potential hypoperfusion injury to the brain, heart, kidneys and pituitary must be ensured. Additionally, risk for transfusion-related lung injury should be recognized and ventilatory status should be optimized. Aggressive venous thromboembolism prophylaxis must be initiated with sequential compression devices until hemostasis assured, and subsequently pharmacoprophylaxis added.

CRITICAL MEDICAL CONDITIONS IN PREGNANCY

Thromboembolic Disease in Pregnancy

Background

Changes during normal pregnancy promote coagulation, decrease anticoagulation, and inhibit fibrinolysis. Venous thromboembolism (VTE) is the leading cause of maternal death in developed countries. The risk of VTE is increased 4× to 5× in pregnancy and the puerperium with an overall incidence of 1 in 1600 pregnancies. Most (~66%) of deep vein thromboses (DVT) occur during gestation while over half of pulmonary emboli (PE) occur postpartum. The mortality from VTE is higher in black pregnant patient compared with white ones.

Diagnosis

DVT and PE can present with a wide variety of signs and symptoms, many of which can be confused with normal pregnancy-related complaints including shortness of breath and lower extremity edema. Pregnant patients were excluded from the Prospective Investigation of Pulmonary Embolism Diagnosis II (PIOPED II) study that described signs and symptoms of PE in nonpregnant patients. There are no validated clinical prediction guidelines for determining the pretest probability of PE in this population.

Significant clinical debate surrounds the decision between ventilation perfusion scans, computed tomography pulmonary angiography and magnetic resonance angiography for the diagnosis of PE in pregnancy. Every effort should be made to avoid unnecessary radiation exposure to the fetus while providing an accurate and timely diagnosis for the mother. In emergent situations, CT angiography is considered the gold standard for diagnosis of a PE in pregnancy.

American Congress of Obstetricians and Gynecologists (ACOG) committee guidelines state that fetal risks from radiation exposure are negligible when doses are less than 0.05 Gy. CTA delivers slightly lower fetal radiation doses and higher maternal doses of radiation (7.3 vs 0.9 mS) than V/Q scanning (0.003-0.131 mGy vs 0.32-0.74 mGy), in the first through third trimester. Using VQ scans as the initial diagnostic approach may necessitate a second diagnostic scan using CTA, which results in more overall radiation.

1. A normal *arterial blood gas* or alveolar-arterial difference is common with PE. Nonetheless, the presence of hypoxemia with normal chest radiograph should increase the clinical suspicion for PE.

2. *D-dimer* testing in pregnancy has limited value as no pregnancy-related normal values have been established and validated. Kovac and colleagues, proposed new values for D-dimer thresholds in pregnancy that should vary with trimesters: 286, 457, and 644 ng/mL in the first, second, and third trimesters, respectively, but these are not yet validated.

3. *Compression ultrasound (CUS)* is a noninvasive test with a sensitivity of 97% and a specificity of 94% for diagnosing symptomatic, proximal DVT in the general population. CUS appears to have a similar diagnostic accuracy in pregnant patients, with a false-negative rate of approximately 0.7%.[7] The diagnosis of DVT during pregnancy is most often made by demonstrating poor compressibility of the proximal veins with the patient in the left lateral decubitus position. It is important to note that CUS may miss pelvic vein thromboses which are more common in pregnant and postpartum women.

4. *Ventilation/perfusion (V/Q scan)*—For those with a normal chest radiograph, V/Q scanning was can be used for the diagnosis of PE in pregnancy. Very low probability scans are associated with a 0% to 6% chance of having a PE. High probability scans are associated with a 56% to 96% chance of having a PE. Small studies describe *perfusion (Q)* scanning alone with decreases the radiation exposure to mother and fetus, for the diagnosis of PE in pregnancy. In such studies, Q scanning alone had a negative predictive value of 100% and only 7% of scans were nondiagnostic. An abnormal chest radiograph increases the probability of a moderate probability V/Q scan result and should prompt the clinician to avoid V/Q scan and directly proceed to CTPA.[5]

5. *CT pulmonary angiograph (CTA)* is considered the preferred tool for evaluating respiratory complaints and diagnosing PE in pregnancy due to better interobserver agreement for radiologists reading CT than nuclear scans and better imaging of other pulmonary pathology.

6. *Magnetic resonance pulmonary angiography (MRPA)* sensitivity and specificity for the diagnosis of PE during pregnancy has not been evaluated. Although no fetal teratogenicity of gadolinium has been observed in human studies, teratogenicity for high doses or prolonged exposures to gadolinium has been observed in animals, so that gadolinium is classified as a category C agent by the FDA.

Management

Adequate treatment of highly suspected or diagnosed VTE can be achieved using subcutaneous low-molecular-weight heparin (SC LMWH), intravenous unfractionated heparin (IV UFH), or subcutaneous unfractionated heparin (SC UFH). Neither UFH nor LMWH cross the placenta. Warfarin crosses the placenta and is not used for treatment of VTE in pregnancy because of the increased risk of birth defects if used during organogenesis and increased risk of fetal hemorrhage at delivery if used in the third trimester. Direct thrombin inhibitors have been demonstrated to cross the placenta in animal models and are not used in pregnant humans.

Subcutaneous *LMWH*, half-life of 6 hours, is preferred over IV UFH or SC UFH because it is easier to use and more efficacious with a better safety profile, findings extrapolated from clinical trials in nonpregnant patients. Initial doses of SC LMWH include dalteparin 200 units/kg once daily, tinzaparin 175 units/kg once daily, dalteparin 100 units/kg every 12 hours, or enoxaparin 1 mg/kg every 12 hours. While data is limited, many recommend the use of twice daily dosing of LMWH especially after the second trimester due to changes in volume of distribution and increased GFR rate. The dose can be titrated to an anti-Xa level of 0.6 to 1.0 IU/mL for twice daily administration. Controversy exists about monitoring anti-Xa activity in anticipation of the need for dose-escalation as pregnancy progresses. Once a therapeutic dose is achieved, some advocate the performance of periodic anti-Xa levels, particularly in patients at the extremes of body weight or those with altered renal function. The first anti-Xa level is generally measured 6 hours after the third or fourth dose if the dosing is every 12 hours, or 6 hours after the second or third dose if the dosing is once daily. Most adjustments should be an increase or decrease of 10% to 25%.

IV UFH is preferred in critically ill patients and those likely to need delivery due to short half-life (1.5 hours) and easy reversibility with protamine. The impact of protamine on the fetus has not been widely studied, so the use of protamine should be reserved for cases of significant bleeding.

The dose consists of bolus of 80 units/kg, followed by a continuous infusion of 18 units/kg/h. The infusion is titrated every 6 hours to achieve a therapeutic activated partial thromboplastin time (aPTT), that corresponds to an anti-Xa level of 0.3 to 0.7 IU/mL. Once the target aPTT level is achieved, it should be rechecked once or twice daily.

Indications for insertion of an *IVC filter* are the same in pregnant and nonpregnant patients.

Women diagnosed with VTE within 4 weeks of expected delivery, who have high rate of mortality if therapeutic anticoagulation is stopped are transitioned from LMWH to UFH at approximately 36 weeks' gestation The IV UFH can be stopped 4 hours before delivery or when the patient goes into labor, with the PTT and anti-Xa levels used to monitor the coagulation status. In patients with extensive DVT or PE, scheduled induction of labor or cesarean delivery should be considered to minimize the duration of time without anticoagulation and a temporary IVC filter can be inserted. Neuraxial anesthesia is contraindicated in a therapeutically anticoagulated patient; timing delivery can allow patients to receive adequate anesthesia. After uncomplicated delivery heparin may be restarted 12 hours after a cesarean delivery or 6 hours after a vaginal birth.

Thrombolytic therapy. Despite the concern that thrombolytic therapy could lead to placental abruption, this complication has not been reported. Cesarean birth within 10 days is considered a relative contraindication to thrombolytic therapy; however, successful thrombolysis has been reported within an

hour after vaginal and 12 hours after cesarean birth. In a review of 28 cases using thrombolysis in pregnancy, the complication rate was similar to that in nonpregnant patients.

There are case reports of successful use of thrombolytic therapy for massive PE during labor. Cesarean delivery in a patient with massive PE carries a high risk of maternal death and should be performed only in cases where the risks and benefits have been weighed and the mother is stable or perimortem.

In centers with interventional radiology expertise, pulmonary angiography with percutaneous mechanical clot fragmentation and placement of an IV filter may be attempted. Should mechanical and iv thrombolysis not be feasible or fail, ECMO with or without surgical embolectomy followed by cesarean delivery and placement of an IVC filter should be considered.

Severe Sepsis, Septic Shock, and Multiorgan Failure
Background
Severe sepsis and septic shock are not very common conditions, reported to occur in 0.002% to 0.01% of deliveries, but they do carry a high maternal morbidity and mortality with rates between 20% to 30% in pregnant patients with septic shock and multiple organ failure. Pregnancies complicated by severe sepsis are associated with increased rates of preterm labor, fetal infection, and preterm delivery.

Pregnancy predisposes women to specific infectious complications. The most common prenatal infections are chorioamnionitis, septic abortion, pyelonephritis, and pneumonia. The most common postpartum infections are endometritis, wound infection, necrotizing fasciitis, pelvic abscess, septic pelvic thrombophlebitis, and pyogenic sacroiliitis.

The outcome in severe sepsis is improved with early detection, prompt recognition of the infectious source, and early antibiotic therapy. However, there are no pregnancy-specific criteria for sepsis and sepsis criteria are affected by pregnancy physiology.

Diagnosis
Chorioamnionitis—Chorioamnionitis (CA) is an infection of the amniotic fluid, membranes, placenta, and/or decidua. It results from ascending

polymicrobial infection in the setting of rupture of membranes or advanced cervical dilatation, rarely from hematogenous spread or invasive procedures such as amniocentesis, chorionic villus sampling or fetal surgery. Length of labor and ruptured membranes appear to be important risk factors. Signs include typical signs of sepsis associated with uterine tenderness ± foul or purulent amniotic fluid or vaginal discharge. Amniocentesis for amniotic fluid culture, gram stain, glucose concentration, WBC concentration, and leukocyte esterase level can be used to establish a microbiologic diagnosis of intra-amniotic infection

Early treatment with antibiotics covering gram-negative and anaerobic flora and evacuation of the uterus are imperative. The most commonly used antibiotics are ampicillin and gentamicin. Patients who undergo cesarean delivery in the presence of CA, are at increased risk of wound infection, endomyometritis, and venous thrombosis and usually require additional anaerobic antibiotic coverage.

Endometritis—Endometritis occurs postpartum, usually in the first week. It originates from bacterial ascension from the lower genital tract during labor. Symptoms are similar to chorioamnionitis. If there is no improvement within 24 to 48 hours, with broad-spectrum intravenous antibiotic therapy, imaging studies should be undertaken to search for a fluid collection or surgical site infection. The most common antibiotic regimens used to treat endometritis are single agent unasyn or combination ampicillin/gentamicin/clindamycin.

Septic Abortion—Septic abortion is now rare in the United States. Historically, septic abortions commonly occurred prior to national legalization of abortion. After the diagnosis of septic abortion is established, treatment with broad-spectrum antibiotics should be immediately instituted with evaluation for and removal of any retained products of conception. Surgical management should be pursued if the patient becomes hemodynamically unstable or shows no improvement with 24 to 48 hours of broad spectrum antibiotics. Hysterectomy and oophorectomy may be required if a dusky, devitalized uterus or pelvic tissue crepitus is encountered intraoperatively and/or clostridial infection is suspected.

Puerperal Mastitis—Puerperal mastitis is usually unilateral, presents in the first week postpartum,

with septic symptoms, marked breast engorgement, erythema, and severe pain. Cases of toxic shock syndrome secondary to mastitis have been described and recently concern exists over the appearance of community-acquired methicillin-resistant *S aureus* (CA-MRSA). Milk from the affected breast should be aspirated and sent for culture and sensitivity before antibiotic treatment. Breast abscess may require surgical incision and drainage or aspiration. Breast feeding is safe and recommended during episodes of mastitis.

Acute Pyelonephritis—Acute pyelonephritis is common in pregnant patients due to pregnancy physiology; dilation of the ureters secondary to progesterone, lack of protective peristalsis, mechanical compression of the urinary system by the gravid uterus and bacteriuria. It manifests with sepsis symptoms, flank pain, nausea/vomiting, and/or costovertebral angle tenderness in the presence or absence of cystitis symptoms. Microscopic bacteriuria and pyuria on urinalysis are verified by a positive urine culture. Bacteriuria during pregnancy has a greater propensity to progress to pyelonephritis and therefore should be treated. E. coli Klebsiella, Enterobacter, Proteus, and gram-positive organisms, including group B Streptococcus account for approximately 70% of cases. Empiric treatment with a cephalosporin or broad-spectrum penicillin is recommended when pyelonephritis is suspected before a positive culture is confirmed. Failure to improve with first-line antibiotic treatment within 24 to 48 hours should prompt evaluation with ultrasound for obstructive urinary tract lesions, such as urinary calculi or perinephric abscess.

Pneumonia—Pneumonia (PNA) has increased morbidity and mortality in pregnancy. The most common pathogens are the same as those found in nonpregnant patients. Community-acquired MRSA can cause a necrotizing pneumonia or can be a super infection with influenza pneumonia. Standard antibiotics for treatment of PNA can be used in pregnancy with the exception of fluoroquinolones.

Influenza—Influenza in pregnant women is associated with a higher rate of morbidity and mortality. A rapid test can detect Influenza A and B, but the sensitivities differ seasonally. If suspicion is strong, culture should be performed. Oxygen, hydration, and neuraminidase inhibitors zanamivir (Relenza) and oseltamivir (Tamiflu) should be started immediately. Women with suspected or confirmed influenza who are pregnant or who have delivered within the previous 2 weeks should receive aggressive antiviral treatment and undergo close monitoring regardless of the results of rapid antigen tests.

Management

Interventions that improve maternal hemodynamic stability and oxygen delivery to the fetus result in improved maternal and fetal outcomes. Operative intervention on behalf of the fetus in an unstable mother increases maternal morbidity and mortality. To date, no "evidence-based" recommendations are specific to the pregnant patient with septic shock.

1. *Vasopressors* can vasoconstrict uterine blood vessels, reducing fetal blood flow. First line in the management of hypotension is administration of intravenous fluids (normal saline 20 mg/kg) and placing the patient in the left lateral decubitus position to prevent compression of the IVC by the gravid uterus. Hypotension that persists requires vasopressor therapy. Although norepinephrine can reduce uterine blood flow, there is no data to suggest that norepinephrine has an adverse effect on fetal well-being, therefore it is often the first line therapy. Vasopressin may be added in patients with refractory shock at a rate of 0.01 to 0.04 UI/min

2. Bedside *critical care ultrasound* is emerging as a useful tool in the assessment of the hypotensive critically ill patient. Transthoracic echocardiography (TTE) may assist in the differentiation of life-threatening hypotension in the critically ill obstetric patient by allowing the rapid identification of right ventricular versus left ventricular heart failure, pericardial effusion and fluid status.

3. Little evidence exists regarding the management of ARDS specifically in pregnancy, and thus, treatment approaches must be drawn from studies performed in a general patient population. Initial management is the same regardless of the cause of the acute respiratory failure with supplemental oxygen with goal is to maintain the oxyhemoglobin saturation 95% or more and arterial oxygen tension (PaO_2) more than 70 mm Hg, to maintain fetal oxygenation. Mechanical ventilation may be required. Ventilatory goals are different in pregnant patients. The target $PaCO_2$ is 30 to 32 mm Hg, since this is the normal level during pregnancy; more respiratory alkalosis should be avoided because it may decrease uterine blood flow. Maternal permissive hypercapnia may also be deleterious to the fetus because of resultant fetal respiratory acidosis.

4. Sedation is required to tolerate mechanical ventilation. The literature suggests that use of benzodiazepines and narcotics are safe in pregnancy. Transient neurologic deficits and respiratory depression have been reported in neonates born to mothers medicated in the later stages of pregnancy. Propofol classified as a pregnancy category B agent, crosses the placenta and may be associated with neonatal respiratory depression. Data on the clinical use of propofol for pregnant critically ill patients is limited to case reports, so its use should be limited until more prospective data is available.

5. Extracorporeal membrane oxygenation (ECMO) is a technique that provides support to selected patients with severe respiratory failure. Little data exists regarding the long term outcomes for infants born after the use of ECMO during pregnancy. However during the 2009 H1N1 influenza epidemic, ECMO was used with a good impact on survival for pregnant women.

6. *Acute Kidney Injury* is often reversible in pregnancy. Ischemic ATN is usually precipitated by abruptio placentae or postpartum hemorrhage and, less commonly, by AFE and sepsis. The diagnosis of postrenal AKI in the pregnant patient is particularly challenging due to the physiologic dilatation of the collecting system that normally occurs in the second and third trimesters and determining the presence of abnormal findings on renal ultrasonography is more difficult.

Pulmonary Edema

Historically, approximately 50% of the cases of pulmonary edema were attributed to tocolytic therapy or cardiac disease, peripartum cardiomyopathy, mitral stenosis, with the rest due to preeclampsia, eclampsia or iatrogenic volume overload.

The use of tocolytics including calcium channel blockers, to inhibit preterm labor is associated with the pulmonary edema in 0.25% to 5% of treated patients. It is more common among multiple gestations and use of multiple tocolytic agents simultaneously.

The standard therapeutic approach includes discontinuation of potentially contributing tocolytics, supplemental oxygen, fluid restriction, and diuresis. Diuretics should be used with caution in the setting of preeclampsia due to intravascular volume depletion.

Arrhythmia

Arrhythmias are more common in women with heart disease. Arrhythmia with significant hemodynamic effect should be treated urgently and aggressively. If the mother's own perfusion is compromised significantly, uterine vascular constriction will occur. ECG should be done to document the rhythm before treatment and secondary causes for arrhythmia should be ruled out (dehydration, hyperthyroidism, drugs, sepsis, pulmonary emboli).

Paroxysmal supraventricular tachycardia is the most common nonsinus tachycardia in women of childbearing age. Adenosine, verapamil or metoprolol intravenous are highly effective in terminating the rhythm. Paroximal Atrial Fibrillation and Atrial flutter with rapid ventricular response occur more frequently in young women mostly due to successful congenital heart disease treatment. The treatment should be the same as in nonpregnant women, although with a heightened sense of urgency. Intravenous verapamil, metoprolol or diltiazem are usually successful at slowing the ventricular rate. If this is not achieved, cardioversion should be performed.

Ventricular tachycardia does occur in pregnancy especially in patients with history of structural heart disease. Acute treatment should include the usual medications or cardioversion as needed to protect the mother.

All drugs used to treat an arrhythmia cross the placenta resulting in fetal exposure, and most are categorized as Food and Drug Administration (FDA) class C. All beta-blockers have the potential for influencing fetal and newborn size, but only atenolol is singled out as being FDA class D. Digoxin, verapamil, diltiazem, and adenosine have their usual efficacy without adversely affecting the fetus. Experience during pregnancy is greater with quinidine than with all the other antiarrhythmic drugs. Lidocaine has been used without any recognized teratogenic effects, although there has been some concern about fetal bradycardia. A reported series, used Amiodarone in 26 women to treat fetal arrhythmias and also for maternal arrhythmias had no recognized adverse fetal effects. Cardioversion preceeded by moderate sedation has been used in pregnancy without any reported adverse fetal effects.

Symptomatic bradycardia is rare in pregnancy. Temporary and permanent pacing can be performed during pregnancy if required with minimizing irradiation, for maternal and fetal benefit.

Diabetic Ketoacidosis

Diabetic ketoacidosis (DKA) occurs in approximately 1% to 3% of diabetic women who become pregnant and represents a medical emergency with high maternal and fetal mortality. Prompt recognition and resuscitative therapy markedly improves outcome. It can occur in the newly diagnosed diabetic patient, and the hormonal changes of pregnancy, a state of relative insulin resistance may become the background for this phenomenon. The blood glucose levels in pregnant women with DKA are usually lower than those in nonpregnant women with DKA.

The presentation of DKA is similar in pregnant and nonpregnant women, with symptoms of nausea, vomiting, thirst, polyuria, polydipsia, tachypneea, change in mental status.

Maternal hyperglycemia results in fetal hyperglycemia and fetal osmotic diuresis. Maternal acidemia decreases uterine blood flow with a resultant decrease in placental perfusion leading to decreased oxygen delivery to the fetus. Fetal acidosis and fetal volume depletion may occur, which jeopardizes the viability of the fetus. Other than fetal heart rate monitoring, which is used to assess and monitor the fetus, DKA is treated similarly in pregnant and non-pregnant patients.

STATUS ASTHMATICUS

Asthma affects 3% to 8% of pregnant women. Clinical severity of asthma in pregnancy seems to follow the severity before the pregnancy with exacerbations 20% to 36% of pregnancies, most frequently between weeks 14 and 24.

The diagnosis and treatment of acute asthma during pregnancy does not differ from the management in nonpregnant patients. Intensive monitoring of both mother and fetus is essential. Pregnant patients with acute asthma should rest in a seated, rather than supine, position. A severe asthma attack presents more of a risk to the fetus than the use of asthma medications because of the potential for fetal hypoxia, so therapy β2-agonists, anticholinergics, and systemic corticosteroids should be used as indicated to treat exacerbations.

Evidence based data about the management of refractory status asthmaticus in obstetric patients is minimal. Review of 3 case reports with a total of 10 cases, 2 of which were past 32 weeks, revealed 2 patients who underwent cesarean delivery and improved dramatically after the procedure.

SUMMARY

Critical illness in obstetrics may occur due to pregnancy-specific conditions, rarely encountered by the intensivist physician, or due to commonly seen critical care diagnoses with unique-management considerations in pregnancy. A multidisciplinary collaborative approach will help to optimize maternal and fetal outcomes in these high-risk pregnancies.

REFERENCES

1. Wanderer JP, Leffert LR, Mhyre JM, Kuklina EV, Callaghan WM, Bateman BT. Epidemiology of obstetric-related ICU admissions in Maryland: 1999-2008. *Crit Care Med*. 2013;41(8):1844-1852.
2. ACOG Committee Opinion November 2013 "Definition of a Term Pregnancy."
3. Siu S, Sermer M, Colman J, et al. Prospective multicenter study of pregnancy outcomes in women with heart disease. *Circulation*. 2001;104:515.
4. Elkayam U, Gleicher N. *Cardiac Problems in Pregnancy: Diagnosis and Management of Maternal and Fetal Disease*; 1982.
5. Kerr M, Scott D, Samuel E. Studies of the inferior vena cava in late pregnancy. *Br Med J*. 1964;1:532.
6. Thompson K, Cohen M. Studies on the circulation in pregnancy: vital capacity in normal pregnant women. *Surg Gynecol Obstet*. 1938;66:591.
7. Pritchard J. Changes in blood volume during pregnancy and delivery. *Anesthesiology*. 1965;26:393.
8. Burrows R, Kelton J. Incidentally detected thrombocytopenia in healthy mothers and their infants. *N Engl J Med*. 1988;319:142.
9. Foley. *Obstetrical Critical Care: A Practical Manual*; 1997.
10. Sacks G, Sargent J, Redman C. An innate view of human pregnancy. *Immunol Today*. 1999;20:114.
11. ACOG Practice Bulletin 100, 2009. Reaffirmed 2011.
12. Vanden Hoek TL, Morrison LJ, Shuster M, et al. Part 12: cardiac arrest in special situations: 2010 American Heart Association Guidelines for Cardiopulmonary Resuscitation and Emergency Cardiovascular Care. *Circulation*. 2010;122:S829-S861.
13. Gabbe, et al. *Obstetrics: Normal and Problem Pregnancies*. 5th ed.
14. Creasy RK, Resnik R. *Maternal-Fetal Medicine: Principles and Practice*. 5th ed.
15. ACOG Task Force Report: Hypertension in Pregnancy, 2013.
16. Sibai BM. Diagnosis and management of gestational hypertension and preeclampsia. *Obstet Gynecol*. 2003;102:181.
17. Ko HH, Yoshida E. Acute fatty liver of pregnancy. *Can J Gastroen*. 2006;20(1):25-30.
18. Clark SL. Amiotic FLuid Embolism. *Obstet Gynecol*. 2014;123:337-348.
19. Heider A, Kuller J, Straus R, Well S. Peripartum cardiomyopathy: a review of the literature. *Obstet Gynecol Surv*. 1999;54:526.
20. ACOG Practice Bulletin 76, 2006. Reaffirmed 2013.
21. https://www.cmqcc.org/resources/ob_hemorrhage/ ob_hemorrhage_tools_carts_kits_trays_checklists
22. Shields LE, Smalarz K, Reffigee L, Mugg S, Burdumy TJ, Propst M. Comprehensive maternal hemorrhage protocols improve patient safety and reduce utilization of blood products. *Am J Obstet Gynecol*. 2011;205:368.e1-8.
23. Kramer MS, Berg C, Abenhain H, et al. Incidence, risk factors and temporal trends in severe

postpartum hemorrhage. *Am J Obstet Gynecol.* 2013;209:449.e1-7.

24. Bates SM, Greer IA, Middeldorp S, et al. VTE, thrombophilia, antithrombotic therapy, and pregnancy. Antithrombotic Therapy and Prevention of Thrombosis, 9th ed. American College of Chest Physicians Evidence-Based Clinical Practice Guidelines. *Chest.* 2012;141(2 suppl):e691S.

25. Pabinger I, Grafenhofer H, Kyrle PA, et al. Temporary increase in the risk for recurrence during pregnancy in women with a history of venous thromboembolism. *Blood.* 2002;100(3):1060-1062.

26. Kovac M, Mikovic Z, Rakicevic L, et al. The use of D-dimer with new cutoff can be useful in diagnosis of venous thromboembolism in pregnancy. *Eur J Obstet Gynecol Reprod Biol.* 2010;148(1):27-30.

27. Kearon C, Julian JA, Newman TE, Ginsberg JS. Noninvasive diagnosis of deep venous thrombosis. McMaster Diagnostic Imaging Practice Guidelines Initiative. *Ann Intern Med.* 1998;128:663-677.

28. Chan WS, Lee A, Spencer FA, et al. Predicting deep venous thrombosis in pregnancy: out in "LEFt" field? *Ann Intern Med.* 2009;151:85-92.

29. Scarsbrook AF, Bradley KM, Gleeson FV. Perfusion scintigraphy: diagnostic utility in pregnant women with suspected pulmonary embolic disease. *Eur Radiol.* 2007;17(10):2554-2560.

30. Greer IA. Anticoagulants in pregnancy. *J Thromb Thrombolysis.* 2006;21:57-65.

31. Stefanovic BS, Vasiljevic Z, Mitrovic P, Karadzic A, Ostojic M. Thrombolytic therapy for massive pulmonary embolism 12 hours after cesarean delivery despite contraindication? *Am J Emerg Med.* 2006;24:502-504.

32. Leonhardt G, Gaul C, Nietsch HH, Buerke M, Schleussner E. Thrombolytic therapy in pregnancy. *J Thromb Thrombolysis.* 2006;21(3):271-276.

33. Fagher B, Ahlgren M, Astedt B. Acute massive pulmonary embolism treated with streptokinase during labor and the early puerperium. *Acta Obstet Gynecol Scand.* 1990;69:659-661.

34. Hall RJ, Young C, Sutton GC, Cambell S. Treatment of acute massive pulmonary embolism by streptokinase during labor and delivery. *Br Med J.* 1972;4:647-649.

35. Winer-Muram HT, Boone JM, Brown HL, Jennings SG, Mabie WC, Lombardo GT. Pulmonary embolism in pregnant patients: fetal radiation dose with helical CT. *Radiology.* 2002;224(2):487.

36. Bauer ME, Bateman BT, Bauer ST, Shanks AM, Mhyre JM. Maternal sepsis mortality and morbidity during hospitalization for delivery: temporal trends and independent associations for severe sepsis. *Anesth Analg.* 2013;117(4):944-950.

37. Barton JR, Sibai BM. Severe sepsis and septic shock in pregnancy. *Obstet Gynecol.* 2012;120(3):689-706.

38. Dellinger RP, Levy MM, Rhodes A, et al. Surviving sepsis campaign: international guidelines for management of severe sepsis and septic shock: 2012. *Crit Care Med.* 2013;41(2):580-637.

39. Cunningham FG. Urinary tract infections complicating pregnancy. *Clin Obstet Gynecol.* 1987;1:891-908.

40. Laibl VR, Sheffield JS, Roberts SW, McIntire DD, Trevino S, Wendel GD, Jr. Clinical presentation of community-acquired methicillin-resistant Staphylococcus aureus in pregnancy. *Obstet Gynecol.* 2005;106(3):461-465.

41. Cole DE, Taylor TL, McCullough DM, Shoff CT, Derdak S. Acute respiratory distress syndrome in pregnancy. *Crit Care Med.* 2005;33(10 suppl):S269.

42. de La CA, Benoit S, Bouregba M, Durand-Reville M, Raucoules-Aimé M. The treatment of severe pulmonary edema induced by beta adrenergic agonist tocolytic therapy with continuous positive airway pressure delivered by face mask. *Anesth Analg.* 2002;94(6):1593-1594.

43. Strasburger JF, Cuneo BF, Michon MM, et al. Amiodarone therapy for drug-refractory fetal tachycardia. *Circulation.* 2004;109(3):375-379.

44. Carroll MA, Yeomans ER. Diabetic ketoacidosis in pregnancy. *Crit Care Med.* 2005;33(10 suppl):S347.

45. Hardy-Fairbanks AJ, Baker ER. Asthma in pregnancy: pathophysiology, diagnosis and management. *Obstet Gynecol Clin North Am.* 2010;37(2):159-172.

46. Murphy VE. Asthma in pregnancy. *Clin Chest Med.* 2011;32(1):93-110.

Critical Care of Burn Patients

61

Edward Pellerano Guzman, MD and
John M. Oropello, MD, FACP, FCCP, FCCM

KEY POINTS

① Care of the severely burned patient requires prompt resuscitation and definitive surgical management.

② Patients with major burns (≥ 25% total body surface area) require management in an intensive care unit.

③ Burn survival correlates with 3 major factors: patient age, burn size, and presence of inhalation injury.

④ Acute renal failure may result from severe hemodynamic instability, delayed or inadequate resuscitation during the initial burn treatment, or later as a result of sepsis or rhabdomyolysis.

⑤ Compartment syndrome in the extremities, torso, or abdomen have been linked to the presence of deep, full-thickness circumferential burns and to the volume resuscitation.

INTRODUCTION

Caring for critically ill patients is even more challenging when the largest organ, the first barrier against any external insult, is damaged by a burn injury. Care of the severely burned patient requires prompt resuscitation and definitive surgical management to reduce morbidity and mortality. The approach is multidisciplinary and involves intensivists, surgeons, and skilled nursing teams among others. The need for psychologic and social support is considerable.

Mortality rates from severe burn injuries have steadily declined over the last 30 years attributed in part to a multidisciplinary approach and specialized care delivered in burn centers. Most burns are the result of fire or scalding and involve less than 10% of the total body surface area (TBSA) with a mortality of close to 0.5%. Patients with major burns (≥ 25% TBSA) require management in an intensive care unit.

Burn survival correlates with 3 major factors: patient age, burn size, and the presence of inhalational injury.

CLASSIFICATION OF BURNS

Burns are classified as thermal, electrical, chemical, friction, or radiation injuries that result in coagulative necrosis of tissues. The clinical severity is determined by the depth and extent of injury. Depending on the depth of injury, burns are further classified as superficial (first degree), partial thickness (second degree), and full thickness (third degree) when all skin layers are affected (Figure 61–1). A fourth degree burn signifies deeper tissue involvement down to bone or muscle.

Burns affecting the epidermis are usually red with mild pain and no blisters. Burns extending beyond the epidermis tend to be erythematous, painful and with blisters; a dry aspect is seen on deeper dermal burns due to the effect of coagulative

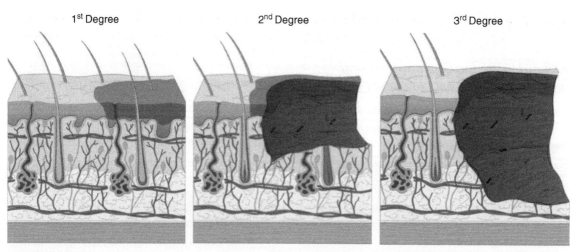

FIGURE 61–1 Classification of burn depth. (*Reproduced with permission from Tintinalli JE, Stapczynski JS, Ma OJ, et al: Tintinalli's Emergency Medicine: A Comprehensive Study Guide, 8th edition. New York: McGraw-Hill Companies, Inc; 2011.*)

necrosis sealing the tissues. Full thickness burns are always dry and in the vast majority insensible, as there is destruction of the entire dermis.

A thermal injury triggers responses in every mayor organ system. Immediately after a burn, intense inflammation and systemic manifestations are generated; inflammatory mediators cause loss of capillary integrity with edema formation mainly in the first hours extending up to 24 hours or more, postburn. The same cascade causes volume depletion, depressed cardiac contractility, and systemic hypoperfusion producing a shock state. Contributing to this process is leukocyte and endothelial activation with cytokine production, complement activation, histamine release, xanthine oxidase, and lysosomal enzyme activation that augment microvascular permeability and wound edema, similar to the cascade that causes acute respiratory distress syndrome (ARDS).

Cortisol, epinephrine, glucagon are also persistently secreted generating glucose intolerance and a hypermetabolic or catabolic state that extends beyond the initial recovery.

INITIAL MANAGEMENT

The initial management is triage and acute resuscitation in the first 24 to 48 hours. Prehospital care and stopping the burning process is the most important component for first responders. Clothes that are burning, smoldering, or soaked with chemicals should be removed. The patient should be removed away from an electrical source. In chemical injuries copious water lavage should be performed. A sequential assessment (primary survey) to avoid missing serious associated injuries as described by the American College of Surgeons in Advanced Trauma Life Support should be followed.

Estimating the total burned body surface area is a key component for resuscitation. Fluid resuscitation by formula is recommended if the TBSA is more than 15%. All current formulas and methods for resuscitation in burned patients are based on body weight and the percentage of TBSA burned. The initial history and physical exam should also include the body weight and an estimate of the second and third degree burn areas used to calculate resuscitation. The "rule of nines" allows a simple, rapid estimate of TBSA: (in an adult [units = % TBSA]): entire head & neck = 9; each arm = 9; upper 1/2 torso front = 9; lower 1/2 torso front = 9; upper 1/2 torso back = 9; lower 1/2 torso back = 9; each leg = 18—anterior leg = 9; and posterior leg = 9.

AIRWAY AND MECHANICAL VENTILATION

In burn patients a reevaluation of the airways and breathing should be done upon hospital arrival. Inhalational injury should be suspected in all patients exposed to smoke, flames, or steam, especially those trapped in a closed environment or rescued in an

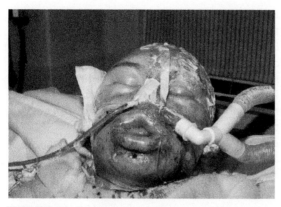

FIGURE 61–2 Edema associated with inhalation injury and resuscitation. Nasotracheal intubation was performed early to prevent accidental loss of airway. (*Reproduced with permission from Kasten KR, Makley AT, Kagan RJ: Update on the critical care management of severe burns,* J Intensive Care Med. *2011 Jul-Aug;26(4):223-236.*)

unconscious state. Early intubation should be performed in the presence of distinct features: deep facial burns, full thickness neck burns, oropharyngeal edema, hypoxemia, stridor, hypercapnia, or a Glasgow Coma Scale less than 8. In the early stages intubation is technically easier if there is minimal or no airway edema. If intubation is performed the internal diameter of the endotracheal tube should be at least 7.5 mm or greater (eg, 8.0-9.0 mm) if possible, in anticipation of the need for later bronchoscopy. Emergency tracheostomy or cricothyroidotomy is rarely needed if intubation is performed early; tissue edema in the head and neck can make these procedures complicated (Figure 61–2).

Pulmonary insufficiency and failure in severely burned patients is multifactorial, due to direct pulmonary and upper airways injury, indirect or secondary injury due to systemic inflammatory response, and delayed injury due to sepsis and pneumonia. Ventilation can also be impaired due to edema within the torso and abdomen; torso escharotomy can avoid laparotomy and improve ventilation.

LUNG INJURY AND ACUTE RESPIRATORY DISTRESS SYNDROME

Severe inflammation and endothelial activation can lead to significant pulmonary capillary leak and ARDS which is common in burn patients with an incidence as high as 30%.[1] It can be exacerbated by sepsis and over resuscitation.

Reduced lung compliance and chest wall rigidity can lead to higher airway pressures. Lung injury may not be a result of higher airway pressures because there is also less stretch on the alveoli as is also seen in other situations where compliance is reduced such as abdominal hypertension. Ventilator strategies may include low tidal volume ventilation with permissive hypercapnia with conventional ventilator modes, airway pressure-release ventilation or high-frequency oscillation in selected patients with inhalational or chest wall injuries. Inhaled nitric oxide may be used for the treatment of hypoxic vasoconstriction improving ventilation/perfusion mismatching and tissue oxygenation. Extracorporeal membrane oxygenation, used more often in pediatrics, may be helpful in selected adults with severe refractory ARDS.[2]

TRACHEOSTOMY

The indications and timing of tracheostomy (either open or percutaneous) after burns are similar to critically ill patients in general, however, caution is needed in the selection of patients with severe facial and neck burns or upper airway edema for tracheostomy because of the increased potential for loss of the airway and local skin complications. Tracheostomy in a burned neck tends to be a difficult procedure due to anatomy disruption, with increased complications such as bleeding, infection, and poor wound site healing.

RESUSCITATION

As in other critical illnesses such as septic shock, prompt and adequate resuscitation is of great importance. However due to external burn injuries, the degree of systemic inflammation and tissue edema, fluid losses are much more prominent. The main focus on resuscitation strategies is to minimize resuscitation complications of under or over resuscitation. Protocols unique to the burned patient take into account fluid losses via the skin.

Two large-bore peripheral intravenous catheters should be inserted through unburned skin if possible and baseline laboratories sent. Frequently unusual peripheral venous sites or central venous access is required. The groins are often spared; so femoral venous cannulation is usually possible. Burns are usually the immediate cause of hypovolemia, however, bleeding from other injuries should also be ruled out.

Fluid resuscitation should be individualized based on age, comorbidities, organ function, burn area and hemodynamics. Fluid resuscitation guidelines are often based on the Parkland burn formula. Typically a lactated Ringer's solution is infused at an initial volume of 4 mL/kg body weight × % burn area in 24 hours with 50% given in the first 8 hours and the remainder over the next 16 hours. However, balanced isotonic crystalloids such as plasmalyte containing acetate, a bicarbonate precursor, may also be used; either Ringer's lactate or plasmalyte will result in less hyperchloremic metabolic acidosis than normal saline. Continuing fluid administration may be based on the formula 0.3 to 0.5 mL/kg × % burn area over 24 hours, but fluid resuscitation must be modified depending on organ function and hemodynamics. In adults, a urine output of at least 30 to 50 mL/h is commonly targeted. Under resuscitation results in reduced cardiac output (CO), inadequate tissue/organ perfusion, oliguria and increasing lactate trends; over resuscitation can result in a constellation of complications including worsening of upper airway edema, pulmonary edema, prolongation of mechanical ventilation, cerebral edema and compartment syndromes (CS) (abdomen, extremities, ocular).[3] Elevated lactate appears to be a biomarker for increased mortality in burn patients but a normal lactate alone does not mean that fluid resuscitation is adequate.

Fluid resuscitation with hypertonic saline (eg, 7.5% NaCl) or colloids (eg, albumin) has not been demonstrated to improve outcomes, although as expected the total resuscitation volume is usually less with colloid administration.

HEMODYNAMICS

Almost immediately after a major thermal injury, CO tends to decrease within an hour. This is, in part, due to myocardial depression from tumor necrosis factor (TNF)-alpha and endotoxin. After adequate resuscitation, the CO tends to normalize and is often followed by a hyperdynamic circulation with vasodilation. Evaluation of hemodynamic parameters typically involves invasive or noninvasive blood pressure measurement and some form of cardiac monitoring. Pulmonary artery catheters are less commonly used, being supplanted by transpulmonary thermodilution devices and noninvasive techniques such as ultrasound of the heart, inferior vena cava (IVC), and lung that can provide accurate information in monitoring resuscitation of the acute burn patient.

BLOOD TRANSFUSION

Restrictive strategies of red blood cell transfusion (hemoglobin 7.0-9.0 g/dL) may be superior or at least equivalent to the liberal strategy (hemoglobin 10.0-12.0 g/dL) in critically ill patients. This appears to also be applicable in burn patients as increased mortality is associated with blood transfusion. The use of erythropoietin is not helpful to prevent or improve anemia in burn patients due blunting of erythropoietic response.

ACUTE RENAL FAILURE AND ELECTROLYTE DERANGEMENTS

Acute renal failure may result from severe hemodynamic instability, delayed or inadequate resuscitation during the initial burn treatment or later as a result of sepsis or rhabdomyolysis. Patients who have sustained high-voltage electrical injuries are at increased risk of acute tubular necrosis, as the large myoglobin molecules released after such an injury can damage the renal tubules. Patients with evidence of myonecrosis or rhabdomyolysis have a reported mortality of more than 70% in severe burns.[4] Intravenous fluid rates should be increased for a target urine output of 1 mL/kg/h, commonly between 75 and 100 mL/h. In difficult cases, diuresis with mannitol or furosemide may be instituted but may result in hypovolemia and invalidates urine output as a reliable measure of resuscitation. Although nothing has been proved to be superior to saline administration, alkalization of the urine with sodium bicarbonate is advocated to prevent precipitation of myoglobin in the renal tubules.

Acute burn patients are at risk for electrolyte derangements, especially hyperkalemia, due to renal failure and rhabdomyolysis. Serum electrolytes—sodium, potassium, calcium, and phosphorus—and creatinine kinase (CK) must be monitored frequently with initial treatment aiming for intravenous (IV) fluid administration and electrolyte management until CK is less than 5000 U/L. In cases that do not respond and develop oliguric or anuric renal failure, fluid resuscitation will no longer be beneficial and if continued will exacerbate volume overload. In this setting with volume overload and/or persistent hyperkalemic acidosis, renal replacement therapy should be initiated.

POSTBURN EDEMA

Edema is almost always present in the burn patient, even in the absence of excessive fluid administration. Edema is seen in tissues affected by the thermal injury and also in unburned areas related to systemic inflammation and resuscitation. Complications due to the edema can be cumbersome; facial and neck swelling create more difficult airway management, requiring prophylactic intubation in some instances.

COMPARTMENT SYNDROME

Compartment syndrome (CS) in the extremities, torso, or abdomen have been linked to the presence of deep, full-thickness circumferential burns and the volume resuscitation.

Limb CS: Clinical suspicion is increased in the presence of delayed capillary refill, cyanosis, paresthesias, and diminished pulses. Compartment pressures can be measured by placement of an 18 grams needle connected to an arterial pressure transducer under the eschar into the subfascial tissue. Pressures above 25 to 30 mm Hg in any compartment are considered diagnostic of CS, but the clinical exam is important in diagnosis regardless of pressure measurements that can be inaccurate or misleading. The diagnosis of CS mandates decompression via escharotomy and/or fasciotomy. Escharotomy includes incision along the full length of eschar with extension into viable unburned tissue, typically using electrocautery. Fasciotomies involve the surgical opening of the full length of fascial compartments.

In both cases, a tissue bulge is often noted indicating adequate release of compartment pressure. Escharotomies are commonly performed at the bedside using mild sedation; fasciotomies may need to be performed in an operating room under general anesthesia. Failure to diagnose and promptly treat CS can lead to ischemia, myonecrosis, and limb loss.

Abdominal CS: Abdominal distention, oliguria, and high airway pressures on mechanical ventilation may signal the development of an abdominal compartment syndrome (ACS). ACS significantly decreases perfusion to vital organs including the small and large bowel, liver, and kidneys, contributing to the development of multisystem organ failure. Early recognition of abdominal hypertension through serial bladder pressure measurement can allow for timely decompressive laparotomy and avoidance of the sequelae caused by prolonged tissue ischemia. In many centers, caring for burned patients there are institutionalized protocols to monitor for abdominal hypertension, especially in patients with greater TBSA percentages, large torso burns, and those who require large volume resuscitation (> 500 mL/h).

Another complication of postburn edema is elevated ocular pressure. Measuring intraocular pressure (IOP) is required in some patients with large facial burns and eyelid edema; when the IOP is persistently high, decompression is indicated to avoid optic nerve damage and visual loss.

INFECTION AND SEPSIS

Sepsis is an independent risk factor for mortality following thermal injury, especially when multiorgan system failure is present. Open wounds, injured lungs, central venous catheters and urinary catheters place the burn patient at increased risk of infection and sepsis, in that order. Signs of systemic inflammatory syndrome (SIRS) are all normal findings induced by burn injury, leading to diagnostic uncertainty. Laboratory markers including peripheral white blood cell (WBC) levels, procalcitonin, C-reactive protein, human leukocyte antigen D-related (DR) expression and others have been proposed as early indicators of sepsis in the burn patient, all with mixed results. Absolute values and trends in WBC, neutrophil percentage and body temperature are unable to predict bloodstream infection in the burn patient. The promise of early markers is to provide earlier diagnosis and treatment of infection. Although controversial, the use of procalcitonin levels has been advocated due to its sensitivity, specificity and mortality correlation in patients with burns having sepsis. However there is insufficient evidence to support the use of procalcitonin as a single diagnostic marker for sepsis in patients with burn injury.

The largest entrance of infection in burns is the breakdown of the skin barrier. The monitoring of wounds and the use of topical and surgical therapies is the first line for prevention of burn wound infection.

Ventilator associated pneumonia (VAP) in severe burn patients is associated with increased mortality but the diagnosis of VAP is nebulous. Due to severe underlying inflammatory pulmonary pathology, accurate clinical diagnosis of VAP can be very difficult in burn patients and infiltrates may be due to noncardiogenic pulmonary edema (ie, ARDS) from SIRS. The emergence of multidrug resistant bacteria is a major problem as is the use of prolonged antibiotherapy.

Bloodstream and urinary tract infections are also of concern. Timing of central access exchange in the patient with burns is determined by the risk of colonization, need for placement through burned versus unburned tissue, and physician preference. The use of peripherally inserted central catheters lines may not decrease the risk of central-line-related bloodstream infections.[3] Prompt removal of all indwelling catheters when no longer warranted provides the best balance between benefit and risk in the patient with burns. Blood and urinary tract infections are treated with removal of the catheter whenever possible and appropriately tailored antibiotic therapy. The use of systemic antibiotic prophylaxis has not been shown to decrease wound infection or any others in the burned patient and may promote infection with multidrug resistant organisms and fungal infections. Protocols vary in when surveillance cultures of burn wounds are performed. Burn wounds often become colonized but may or may not be causing sepsis. Systemic antibiotics are added to standard local wound care if infection is suspected (see Sec. "Wound Care").

Less Common Infections

Acute infective endocarditis has a low prevalence in burn patients, but adds considerable morbidity and mortality. A common pathogen is *Staphylococcus aureus* and persistent bacteremia should prompt investigation for endocarditis. Other less frequent infections in burn patients include parotitis, sinusitis, chondritis of the ear and ocular infections.

Wound Care

Although wound sepsis in burns has steadily decreased, it remains a factor that adds morbidity and mortality. Cleansing and debridement of the wound is accomplished with mild soap and water or with chlorhexadine/normal saline washes. Most burn experts recommend debridement of all blisters larger than 0.5 cm to reduce the risk of bacterial colonization or infection. Burn wounds become colonized in the first few hours with gram-positive bacteria including *S aureus* and epidermidis, and by 5 days are predominantly colonized with gut flora such as *Pseudomonas aeruginosa*, *Enterobacter cloacae*, and *Escherichia coli*.

Health care workers must be vigilant in hand washing and maintenance of a clean environment around the wounds for prevention of cross-contamination in these immunocompromised patients. Culture swabs of all wound beds should be obtained upon admission and repeated serially to monitor for changes in colonization or if there is a clinical suspicion of wound sepsis. Quantitative cultures of the burn to diagnose wound invasion are best obtained by tissue biopsy, either in the operating room or at bedside. Bacterial colonization of burn wounds does not require systemic antibiotics but should be managed with early debridement and/or excision, together with appropriate topical and/or biologic dressings.

Cleansing and debridement is followed by application of a topical antimicrobial agent intended to control colonization, not sterilize the burn wound. Several layers of absorptive gauze and Kerlix cover the wound to decrease evaporative water losses. Minor burns can be managed with biologic dressings, silver-coated dressings, or tribiotic ointment covered with nonadherent gauze. Commonly utilized topical agents include silver sulfadiazine (silvadene), mafenide acetate (sulfamylon), and silver nitrate. Silvadene continues to demonstrate effective control of burn wound colonization, while remaining inexpensive and easy to apply. However, eschar penetration is minimal and complications related to leukopenia and hemolysis have been reported. Mafenide acetate cream (sulfamylon) is painful when applied to superficial partial thickness burns. Eschar penetration is greatest with sulfamylon, making it the topical agent of choice in burns where the eschar will not be excised immediately or when control of *P aeruginosa* is required. Metabolic acidosis may occur, as sulfamylon is a carbonic anhydrase inhibitor. Silver nitrate 0.5% solution has fallen out of favor due to electrolyte abnormalities and poor tissue penetration but may be used as a reasonably effective agent for treatment of gram-negative or fungal colonization. Other alternatives for topical treatment are available especially when patients are allergic to sulfas, such as bacitracin, neosporin, mupirocin (mainly gram-positive coverage), and polymyxin B.

Complications directly related to topical agents, frequent dressing changes often result in traumatized epithelialization and delayed wound healing. Silvadene has been shown to delay wound healing due to a direct toxic effect on keratinocytes. To avoid this silver impregnated dressings have been developed to provide antimicrobial coverage, adequate humidity, and decreased trauma, all with less frequent dressing changes. Biosynthetic products designed as epidermal substitutes are also used, allowing for faster reepithelialization, although their use is limited due to increased infection.

SURGICAL MANAGEMENT

In addition to topical wound care, a great deal of wound care relies on the surgical management. Deep burns are managed with surgical excision and placement of xenograft, allograft, autograft, or cultured skin substitutes.

Most experienced burn centers advocate for an early wound excision within the first 1 to 7 days following thermal injury to attenuate the systemic inflammatory effects of burns and reduce the risk of sepsis. No significant difference in infection or mortality rates was found when burn excision was performed at any point between 2 and 7 days of management. The appropriate timing for burn wound excision and grafting involves a number of important factors including the age of the patient, extent and depth of burn, comorbidities, hospital resources, and physician preference. Mortality and length of stay is decreased in young populations of burn patients (< 30 years and children) with a TBSA more than 30% when early excision is performed.

After the wound is excised, bleeding is controlled and grafting occurs as per institution protocol, after the procedure a proper wound dressing, topical antibiotics are a must to avoid graft failure and infections. Skin substitutes and replacements require adequate wound bed preparation to ensure minimal graft loss.

NUTRITIONAL SUPPORT

Burns are associated with a hypermetabolic state. The increase in metabolic rate is proportional to the extent of the burn and the coexistence of infection; the metabolic rate peaks at 7 to 10 days and can persist for many months postinjury. Overfeeding excess carbohydrate or lipid calories can result in metabolic complications such as hyperglycemia and fatty liver.

Caloric requirements may be estimated using 120% to 150% of the Harris–Benedict formula calculation or 20 to 30 kcal/kg body weight/day, trending toward the higher 30 kcal/kg due to the increased metabolic rate. Supplying 1.5 to 2.0 gram of protein/kg body weight will help in maintaining the nitrogen balance due to excess protein losses via the burn wounds. Enteral nutrition is preferred and early enteral nutrition is beneficial. In patients with gastrointestinal complications (see the following section), unable to tolerate enteral feeding, TPN may be initiated.

MODULATING HORMONAL AND ENDOCRINE RESPONSES

Hyperactive metabolic response in the thermal injury is due to the increased levels of catecholamines and catabolic hormones. The use of betablockers is very common in burn units to attenuate the catabolic state reducing oxygen demand, resting energy expenditure and heart rate. Randomized prospective trials will be needed to assess the impact of beta-blockade after burn injuries.

GASTROINTESTINAL COMPLICATIONS

Multiple complications affecting the gastrointestinal tract arise after the occurrence of severe burns, usually in patients with a Total Body Surface Burn (TBSB) more than 25%. Dysmotility problems vary from diarrhea (very common), mainly while using enteral feeds, high osmotic loads, overfeeding, and infection (*Clostridium difficile*, *Cytomegalovirus*). Ileus may develop due to hypovolemia, use of narcotics, infection, prompting nasogastric decompression and bowel rest.

Within hours of a severe burn injury, the stomach and the duodenal mucosa can develop focal injuries, progressing to larger and multiples lesions and even gastrointestinal bleeding (Curling's ulcers). Rapid resuscitation, the use of proton-pump inhibitors or H-2 blockers and early enteral feeding has decreased this complication to less than 2% in the critically ill population.

The liver seems to be affected immediately following severe burn injury most likely related to severe systemic inflammation, shock, and hemolysis. There is a mild to moderate increase of aminotransferases that should resolve within a few days, the presence of early jaundice is associated with a poor prognosis.

The proposed etiology of hemolysis is the induction of morphologic changes in red cells. Schistocytes and spherocytes are identified due to direct effect of heat on the cells, hemolysis generally takes place during the first 24 to 48 hours and it correlates with the TBSA.

The incidence of pancreatitis has increased in patients with severe burns as more patients survive. Standard diagnostic and therapeutic modalities are used when clinically indicated (amylase, lipase levels) with temporary bowel rest. Acute cholecystitis (mostly acalculous, intestinal necrosis) can occur in any critically ill patient and is increased in patients receiving TPN. Acute cholecystitis is less commonly seen, possibly due to more effective resuscitation and enteral nutrition.

ANALGESIA IN BURNS

Pain as the result of an acute burn is usually a mixed picture (procedural pain and pain directly caused by the injury), multiple procedures from wound dressings changes, debridement, grafting, and physiotherapy will add severe pain to the patient, poor pain management will impede proper patient cooperation and ultimately good rehabilitation. In intubated patients the usual approach is continuous sedation and opiate infusion, in awake patients needing multiple procedures conscious sedation is ideal. Long-acting opiates and patient control analgesia are useful. Evaluation and follow up by an acute pain team can be beneficial by recommending other therapies, anxiolytics, nonopiate medications, and nonpharmaceutical strategies.

DEEP VEIN THROMBOSIS

The incidence of deep vein thrombosis and pulmonary embolism in the burn patient is increased; unless contraindicated all critically ill burn patients should receive both mechanical (intermittent compression devices) and pharmacologic prophylaxis (fractionated or unfractionated heparin) until mobile.

PSYCHOSOCIAL CARE

Psychologic and psychiatric support is often not needed in the acute ICU setting; however, an assessment and treatment should be addressed as soon as needed, taking into account that most of every severe burned patient will live with not only physical sequels from their misfortune but also with a pronounced posttraumatic stress disorder. Caregivers should start a clear and honest conversation with the patient and family when feasible, for a better understanding of the implications of the injuries sustained.

REHABILITATION

A multidisciplinary approach including nurses, physiotherapists, counselors, occupational therapists, and social workers is fundamental to aid rehabilitation and reduce long-term disability. It should start at the time of injury and during the acute care and continue postdischarge. Physical therapy can decrease muscle mass loss and bone mineralization, and improve mobility and function in the burned patient.

REFERENCES

1. Waters JA, Lundy JB, Aden JK, et al. A comparison of acute respiratory distress syndrome outcomes between military and civilian burn patients. *Mil Med.* 2015;180(3 suppl):56-59.

2. Ipaktchi K, Arbabi S. Advances in burn critical care. *Crit Care Med.* 2006;34(9 suppl):S239-S244.

3. Endorf FW, Ahrenholz D. Burn management. *Curr Opin Crit Care.* 2011;17(6):601-605.

4. Coca SG, Bauling P, Schifftner T, Howard CS, Teitelbaum I, Parikh CR. Contribution of acute kidney injury toward morbidity and mortality in burns: a contemporary analysis. *Am J Kidney Dis.* 2007;49(4):517-523.

5. Kasten KR, Makley AT, Kagan RJ. Update on the critical care management of severe burns. *J Intensive Care Med.* 2011;26(4):223-236.

Critical Care of Disaster Victims

Carla Venegas-Borsellino, MD; Sharon Leung, MD, MS and Vladimir Kvetan, MD

KEY POINTS

1. Major natural and manmade disasters have always occurred, but their increasing frequency over the past decade has elevated awareness of the importance of planning and preparing for catastrophic events.

2. The responses of different healthcare systems to major disasters in the past have demonstrated the continued need for a more clearly identified planning process in order to effectively respond to multi-hazard events.

3. The CCM physician should be prepared to provide triage, stabilization, clinical management, teamwork leadership and managing of hospital resources.

4. The goal in mass casualty scenarios is to minimize mortality and morbidity, but an effective response during a disaster situation depends on multiple variables:

nature of the incident, number of victims, resources, and the coordination of efforts, among others.

5. Understanding the characteristics of different disasters and predicting their impact on the healthcare system, integrating the principles of the command center, and participating in the local disaster planning process will improve the appropriate response by the critical care physician to disaster situations.

6. Educational efforts are crucial before and after a disaster. Simulation sessions and mock outbreak/disaster exercises must be instituted on a regular base to understand our current level of preparedness, teach personnel how to respond appropriately to these unique situations, predict and be prepared for unexpected events.

INTRODUCTION

Major natural and manmade disasters have always occurred, but their increasing frequency over the past decade has elevated awareness of the importance of planning and preparing for catastrophic events. Over the past 2 decades, more than 3 million lives have been lost worldwide due to major disasters. In 2008 alone, the total number of deaths caused by disasters with a natural and/or technologic trigger was a staggering 242,662.[1] As populations grow and occupy spaces

that are vulnerable to different hazards, it is expected that disasters will increase in severity and impact. The New York City Panel on Climate Change 2013 states in its executive summary that "Climate change poses significant risks to New York City's communities and infrastructure."[2] Analyses of the response of different healthcare systems to major disasters in the past have demonstrated the continued need for a more clearly identified planning process in order to effectively respond to multihazard events.[3]

In general, the US Critical Care Medicine System receives massive resources in terms of gross national product expenditure when compared with other developed countries, giving it the capacity to provide care to critically ill patients resulting from these disasters. But the question is whether the US critical care system and the intensivists are ready to handle the challenges such events present.[4] The expected percentage of critically injured can vary depending on the nature of the event, but it is estimated to be approximately 16% of the overall number of survivors (range 2.5%-34%).[5,6] However, published experience has shown that in mass casualty situations, the ICU is also commonly utilized as an overflow area for primary triage, as well as initial and overflow postoperative management.[7] Therefore, the CCM physician should be prepared to provide triage, stabilization, clinical management, teamwork leadership and managing of hospital resources.

The responsibility of caring for the most serious salvageable casualties in natural and manmade disasters will ultimately involve the critical care physician.[8] To provide an appropriate response the intensivist should be part of the institutional disaster-planning effort, understand what the resources and capabilities are for the community, hospital, and its ICU on a continual basis, and be able to plan a modular expansion of the critical care services for any successful emergency response.[9]

The goal in mass casualty scenarios is to minimize mortality and morbidity, but an effective response during a disaster situation depends on multiple variables: nature of the incident, number of victims, resources, the coordination of efforts, among others. So one of the most important concepts to guarantee a successful management of disaster victims is understanding the layers of command and control related to which organizations that are responding to any unique event and how to participate within the disaster incident command system.

Through this chapter we want to initially review basic concepts of the nature of the disaster and expected medical complications, and then review the most recent recommendations for critical care providers about disaster medical management and preparedness for local mass casualty situations, based on the 2 most recent publications offering illumination on this topic: the Critical Care Collaborative Initiative's January 2007 Mass Critical Care Summit[10] and the 2007 US Department of Homeland Security National Preparedness Guidelines.[11] The former contains 5 articles which include an executive summary[10] and individual papers on current capabilities,[12] a framework to optimize surge capacity,[3] medical resource guidance,[13] and recommendations for allocating scarce critical care resources in a mass critical care setting.[14] The latter highlights 15 national disaster scenarios, 12 of which have the potential to produce large numbers of critically injured or ill patients.

IMPORTANT DEFINITIONS[15]

Disaster—Currently there is no uniformly accepted definition for the word disaster as it implies individual and local perspective. From a healthcare standpoint, the most important variable that defines a disaster is its functional impact on the healthcare facility.

Hazard—An event with the potential to cause catastrophic damage. It may be a "naturally" or "manmade" occurring phenomena.

Emergency—A natural or manmade event that significantly disrupts the environment of patient care resulting in disrupted care and treatment.

Casualty—Any person suffering physical and/or psychologic damage by outside violence leading to death, injuries, or material losses.

Multicasualty incident—A hazardous event that regardless of its size is containable by local emergency medical services.

Mass casualty incident: A hazardous event that overwhelms local response capability. It is likely to impose a sustained demand for health services rather than a short, intense peak typical of many smaller-scale events.

NATURE OF THE DISASTER

The nature of the disaster is widely variable and can include a terrorist attack, infectious pandemic, mass transit accidents, or natural disaster and all of them can exhaust regional or national critical care systems. As highlighted by the 2007 US Homeland Security Task Force,[11] the scenarios which can generate massive amounts of critically ill victims are broadly divided into 3 general categories: terrorist attacks, epidemic disease, and natural disaster.

Natural disasters arise from forces of nature and include earthquakes, volcanic eruptions, hurricanes, floods, fire, and tornadoes.

Infectious disasters can be classified as epidemic or pandemic.

Manmade disasters are due to identifiable human causes and may be further classified as complex emergencies (eg, wars, terrorist attacks) and technologic disasters (eg, industrial accidents, explosions from hazardous material).

Regardless of the type of classification used to categorize disasters, certain unique features are associated with each type of disaster. It is important to understand the common effects of different natural and manmade disasters to predict their impact and plan effectively.[15]

Natural Disasters

Earthquakes

Earthquakes are common and even predictably frequent especially in many earthquake prone areas of the world and result in significant mortality.[11] Availability of health care providers well trained in basic and advanced trauma and life support and the architectural design and build quality of the stricken area's housing and public facilities are 2 major determinants of outcomes for earthquake victims. Earthquakes also commonly result in damage to health infrastructures and water systems and create disruptions to communication and transportation networks.[11]

Volcanic Eruptions

Different types of eruptive events occur, including pyroclastic explosions, hot ash releases, lava flows, gas emissions, and glowing avalanches (gas and ash releases). Although lava flows tend not to result in high casualties, the "composite" type of volcano is associated with a more violent eruption which is associated with air shock waves, rock projectiles (some with high thermal energy), release of noxious gases, pyroclastic flows, and mud flows (lahars). The morbidity and mortality are related to respiratory-related syndromes and conjunctival and corneal injury, topical irritation of skin and other mucosal surfaces.[15]

Hurricanes, Cyclones, and Typhoons

These are large rotating weather systems that form seasonally over tropical oceans. They are among the most destructive natural phenomena. Many complications are the result of widespread flooding and most hurricane-related deaths occur from storm surge-related drowning. The most common injuries include lacerations, blunt trauma, and puncture wounds. Late morbidity can be due to postdisaster cleanup accidents (eg, electrocution), dehydration, wound infection, and outbreaks of communicable disease.[11]

Floods

There are 3 major types of floods: flash floods (caused by heavy rain and dam failures), coastal floods, and river floods. Together, they are the most common type of disasters and account for at least half of all disaster-related deaths. The primary causes of death are drowning, hypothermia and injury due to floating debris. The impact on the health infrastructures and lifeline systems can be massive and may result in food shortages. Interruption of basic public services (eg, sanitation, drinking water, electricity) may result in outbreaks of communicable disease. Another concern is the increase in both vector-borne diseases and displacement of wildlife.[15]

Landslides

They are defined as downslope transport of soil and rock resulting from natural phenomena or manmade actions and are more widespread than any other geologic event. Landslides cause high mortality but relatively few injuries. Trauma and suffocation by entrapment are common. Pending an assessment needs can be anticipated, such as search and rescue, mass casualty management, and emergency shelter for the homeless.[15]

Other Natural Disasters

Tornadoes occur most commonly in the North American Midwest. They cause widespread destruction of community infrastructure. Injuries most commonly seen are complex contaminated soft-tissue injury, fractures, head injury, and blunt trauma to the chest and abdomen.

Infectious Disasters

Pandemic Respiratory Infections

Pandemic H1N1 2009 was caused by a new strain of influenza A virus that within weeks spread worldwide through human-to-human transmission. During the first month of the emergency, the CDC's Strategic National Stockpile released 25% of the supplies in the stockpile for the treatment and protection from influenza.[6] At the third month the World Health Organization (WHO) declared the 2009 H1N1 influenza a global pandemic, generating the first influenza pandemic of the 21st century. The initial data show that about 8% of H1N1 patients were hospitalized (23 per 100,000 population); 6.5% to 25% of these required being in the ICU (28.7 per million inhabitants) for a median of 7 to 12 days, with a peak bed occupancy of 6.3 to 10.6 per million inhabitants; 65% to 97% of ICU patients required mechanical ventilation, with median ventilator duration in survivors of 7 to 15 days; 5% to 22% required renal replacement therapy; and 28-day ICU mortality was 14% to 40%.[6]

Judicious planning and adoption of protocols for surge capacity and infrastructure considerations are necessary to optimize outcomes during a pandemic.[16,17] Safe practices and respiratory equipment are needed to minimize aerosol generation when caring for patients with influenza. These measures include hand-washing, gloves and gowns, and the use of N95 mask.[16,17]

Manmade Disasters

Transportation Disasters

Transportation accidents can produce injuries and death similar to those seen in major natural disasters. Some of the largest civilian disasters in North America have been related to transportation of hazardous materials, but more commonly they are related to motor vehicle accidents, railway accidents, airplane crashes, and shipwrecks. They cause a wide range of injuries including multiple trauma, fractures, burns, chemical injuries, hypothermia, dehydration, asphyxiation, and CO inhalation.[15]

Weapons of Mass Destruction

Weapons of mass destructions (WMDs) are those nuclear, biological, chemical, incendiary, or conventional explosive agents that pose a potential threat to health, safety, food supply, property, or the environment. Since the terrorist attacks in September 2001 and subsequent intentional release of anthrax spores in the United States, there is growing concern around the world about the possible threat of chemical, biological, or nuclear weapons used against a civilian population. In response to a WMD incident, healthcare personnel should be prepared to manage casualties in an environment of panic, fear, and paranoia.[4] Because most attacks occur without warning, the local healthcare system will be the first and most critical interface for detection, notification, rapid diagnosis, and treatment.[11]

Biological Weapons

Biological weapons can be either pathogens (disease-causing organisms such as viruses or bacteria) or toxins (poisons of biological origin). Compared with other WMDs, biological weapons are characterized by ease of accessibility and dissemination, difficulty in detection because of their slow onset of action, and their ability to cause widespread panic through the fear of contagion.[11,18] Based on these characteristics they require special action for public health preparedness. In the event of a suspected bioterrorist attack, the CDC has issued protocols for early notification of local and state public health department agencies.

Chemical Weapons

Chemical incidents are events that threaten to or do expose responders and members of the public to a chemical hazard. Agents commonly used as chemical weapons are also used in industrial processes. These agents, however, pose serious problems for emergency care providers because of their potential to cause a large number of casualties rapidly and their potential for secondary contamination. Any emergency medical or public health response to a major incident involving a chemical warfare agent will require coordination among local, state, and federal organizations. First responders should be aware of access to specialized local and federal response teams, basic triage and demarcation of the contaminated area, use of handheld devices for agent detection and identification, use of personal protective equipment, and knowledge of appropriate medical treatment and antidotes.[11]

Nuclear Weapons and Radiation Accidents

A variety of terrorist applications of radiation exist that could produce varying degrees of damage to public infrastructure and operations, human casualties and illnesses, and most importantly, fear. Approximately 50% of the energy released from a nuclear bomb is due to the blast and shock waves, giving a majority of the survivors blast-related injuries as well as creating extensive infrastructure damage. About 35% of the energy released is thermal radiation (in orders of tens of millions of degrees), giving rise to high-degree skin lesions. However, the most likely terrorist threat using radiation is the so called "dirty bomb" in which some type of radioactive material is added to a conventional explosive bomb. Among experts in this field it is thought such a bomb would most likely involve the use of more easily accessible but less dangerous forms of radioactive material; thus the likelihood of mass casualties with acute radiation poisoning at this point is not high.[11]

Hazardous Materials Disasters

A hazardous material is a substance potentially toxic to the environment or living organisms. Full-scale disasters from hazardous materials disasters (HazMat) are relatively rare, but isolated incidents are among the most common in the community and are not limited to chemicals but can include various biological and radiologic materials as well. Knowledge of the types of industries present in the community would be helpful in developing a potential plan to deal with likely HazMat situations. Injuries secondary to release of hazardous materials can present as chemical burns, inhalational injury, and a variety of systemic injuries.[11]

Armed Conflict

Armed conflict continues to be the most preventable and destructive of manmade disasters. Specific healthcare issues during these conflicts include trauma from blast injuries and projectiles, crush-related injuries, communicable diseases due to the breakdown of public infrastructure, mass displacement of populations, burns, and radiation-related injury.[15]

PRINCIPLES IN DISASTER PLANNING

Disaster Plan Development

Most of the logistical problems faced in disaster situations are not caused by shortages of medical resources but rather from failure to effectively coordinate their distribution. Planning requires the participation of leaders with clear responsibilities and corresponding skill to coordinate efforts and develop policies to contain the disease; to coordinate resource allocation and manpower; to advise and share information regarding infection control and treatment; to share data and research endeavors; to maintain staff morale; and to provide information to various levels of government, health care institutions, front-line workers and the public.[8]

Existing Preparedness Requirements

In developing disaster plans, hospitals must take into account the national and local requirements imposed by governmental agencies like the Centers for Medicare and Medicaid Services (CMS) and The Joint Commission (TJC). The CMS's conditions for emergency preparedness and services establish minimum requirements for hospitals that participate in Medicare or Medicaid programs. Similarly, TJC standards apply to a full range of hospitals from small rural to large urban academic centers and are focused on 4 main areas: (1) emergency preparedness management plan, (2) security management plan, (3) hazardous materials and waste management plan, and (4) emergency preparedness drills.[19]

Hazard Vulnerability Analysis

Any disaster plan should start with a thorough analysis of potential hazardous events that can occur in or around the healthcare facility. TJC requires a formal documented hazard vulnerability analysis that is integrated with the emergency management plan, setting priorities among potential emergencies and also defining the hospital's role in the local community-wide emergency plan.[19]

Incident Command System

The incident command system (ICS) is designed to provide the basic response in emergency management to avoid the lack of coordination among various public and healthcare agencies and from the lack of operational integration of various medical specialties. The ICS specifies a common terminology and a command structure with 5 functional sections:

Command—Unified command staff responsible for overall management of the incident. This includes a designated person who will have the authority to declare an emergency. All personnel involved in the command system should be aware of the exact predetermined location of the command center.

Operations—Performs the actual response work under the directives of the command center.

Planning—Gathers relevant information and develops response strategies as the situation progresses. The plan should provide protocols that guide notification and the sequence of mobilization of the personnel in a disaster situation.

Logistics—Responsible for facility-wide supplies, equipment, personnel, and services. The command system must have independent telephone lines to ensure uninterrupted communication with the external world in a disaster situation.

Finance—Authorizes expenditures, maintains records, and provides documentation of the incident.

Once initiated, the ICS has a built-in chain of command that would be responsible for triage of patients and allocation of personnel and resources.[19]

TRIAGE

Triage is a dynamic process that includes not only the disaster site or the emergency department but is carried through several levels of the medical response pathway in disaster response. Triaging critically ill patients in the mass casualty situation is challenging, because the medical critical care is provided not necessarily to the sickest patient, but the one who has the best opportunity for long-term survival. Although less applicable in disasters with a gradual onset, patient triaging is extremely important in sudden events like explosions or natural disasters. Frykberg[4] established a direct linear relationship between over-triage (delivery of immediate care to disaster victims who are not critically ill or injured) and higher critical mortality rate.

Problems commonly encountered in the triage process include the following:

Lack of medical direction at the scene—During a mass casualty event, triage is approximately 70% accurate with a tendency to underestimate injury severity.[20] The most important strategy to prevent under or over triage includes the use of an experienced triage officer, usually a senior physician/surgeon, with outstanding leadership and communications skills, who has a clear understanding of the medical resources at hand and the ability to recognize and, if necessary, perform immediate lifesaving measures.

Lack of interorganizational planning—Dynamic management of the triage process requires constant assessment of medical resources and communication between the command center, the scene, and the triage site. This will allow for rational and appropriate triage based on the availability of resources.

Regarding triaging admissions to the ICU, the triage officer will review all patients for inclusion and exclusion criteria (recommended by sequential organ failure assessment [SOFA] scoring system)[21] and facilitate discharge from critical care for patients no longer requiring it. The triage officer will evaluate daily all patients receiving critical care, and evaluate those requested to be considered for critical care as they arise.

Another challenging issue is how to provide critical care management during a prolonged period of time if resources can be limited. In these cases it is important to provide essential rather than limitless critical care to allow many additional community members to have access to key life-sustaining interventions during disasters. The concept of emergency mass critical care (EMCC) involves planning and provision of essential interventions to maximize the number of individuals who receive sufficient critical care.[3] Medical resource planning recommendations for EMCC can be divided into 3 categories: treatment materials, hospital personnel, and facilities; or stuff, staff, and space. Resources include mechanical ventilators, intravenous fluids, vasopressors, antidotes, antimicrobial for specific diseases, sedatives and analgesics, specific therapeutics, and intervention materials (such as those needed in renal replacement therapy and parenteral nutrition). The EMCC recommendations should be used only in overwhelming events, meaning after calls for assistance from local, regional, state, interstate, and federal authorities have been exhausted.[10] The Task Force recommends that hospitals with ICUs should be prepared to provide EMCC for at least 3 times the usual number of critically ill patients and to maintain such care for 10 days without "sufficient external assistance." The panel also offers a progressive list of changes in resource use for coping with shortages. It starts with substitution and runs through adaptation, conservation, reuse, and finally reallocation, the last meaning taking a resource from 1 patient and giving it to another with a better prognosis or greater need.[14]

While the initial triage during a disaster focuses on the patients, the disaster critical care triage focuses on the resources (tertiary triage). Decisions to reallocate critical care resources among patients will require a high degree of transparency and regular reviews to ensure that established processes are being followed.[14] The SOFA score, though not validated, has been proposed to determine qualification for ICU admission during mass critical care.[21] Patients who are excluded from critical care should receive palliative care.[22] It is mandatory that mass disaster preparation anticipates palliation for large numbers of individuals.[10]

The EMCC, to date, is untested, and the real benefits of implementation remain uncertain. Nonetheless, EMCC currently remains the only comprehensive construct for mass critical care preparedness and response.[23]

SURGE CAPACITY

Critical care service and supplies should be assessed and prepared for possible expansion during a major disaster.[7,8] The plan should have a current inventory of all supplies and capabilities of the facility: number of ventilators in use and its absolute capacity, inventory of various ICU supplies; and vendor lists should be readily available if there is sudden demand for supplies. The disaster plan should allow for at least 2 days' worth of supplies. Available computer-base systems can help to predict surge capacity and design the disaster plan response.[24]

Disaster plans should also consider the possibility of internal and external power outages and related disruptions (such as communications), loss of utilities such as power, water, or telephones due to floods, civil disturbances, accidents, or emergencies within the organization or in its community.[10]

Stuff (Medical Equipment and Supplies)

The recommendations focus on the surge-capacity on ventilators because there is little guidance in the medical literature and the anticipation is that most patients who will require mechanical ventilation in a mass critical care event will probably require several days of ventilation.

Ventilators

All predictions are that the need for ventilators in a major pandemic will far exceed the supply.[25] Currently there is an estimated total of 105,000 ventilators in the United States and the US national stockpile has about 4600 ventilators, making them likely insufficient to deal with a pandemic influenza outbreak or lung injury following a widespread terrorist attack.[26,27] Most hospitals cannot afford to stockpile ventilators, and in a catastrophic disaster, transportation and communication disruption may limit the ability to draw from regional and national stockpiles. The guidance includes suggestions on short-term strategies to boost ventilator capacity, such as repurposing other types of ventilators (anesthesia machines, noninvasive devices, and transport devices), and borrowing from other hospitals that are not having critical care shortages. In a surge setting, ventilators should be able to operate without high-pressure medical gas, be able to oxygenate and ventilate pediatric and adult patients with significant airflow obstruction, accurately deliver the prescribed minute ventilation, and have a standard alarms system. Modifying a ventilator to be used for multiple patients is no longer acceptable.[10]

Oxygen Tanks

Oxygen remains the critical consumable resource in disaster management[28] and may run short in a disaster situation due to consumption by large numbers of patients in respiratory failure, or due to damage of oxygen storage and delivery systems. Strategic management of oxygen supplies in disaster scenarios remains a priority because in the case of a shortage, the Strategic National Stockpile will not supply oxygen, and delivery by contracted vendors can be delayed. Medical oxygen sources include bulk and portable liquid systems, compressed gas cylinders, and oxygen concentrators. Most hospitals have sufficient stores of bulk liquid oxygen to support patient needs for the short term. Potential areas of concern include damage to reserve systems that are contiguous with the main system and ventilator models that require a high-pressure gas supply and cannot be supported by small oxygen concentrators.[29]

Medications

The Task Force recommends planning how to optimize availability of medications and safe administration thereof during a disaster response. Planning should include rules for medication substitutions, safe dose or drug frequency reduction, conversion from parenteral administration to oral/enteral when possible, medication restriction, and guidelines for medication shelf-life extension.[13]

Staff

The current shortage of critical care trained personnel is well documented[30] and staffing issues may be further complicated if the crisis is prolonged or affects employees personally (also possible due to staff absenteeism).[8] Staff resources may also be reduced by illness during an influenza epidemic or bioterrorist attack, especially in the critical care setting where the personnel have direct contact with the airway secretions and there can be significant pathogen aerosolization. Strategies for infection control include early identification and triage of at-risk populations, and ensuring adequate supply and strict use of personal protective equipment. Hospitals should also fit-test all staff with negative pressure respirators, such as the n95 mask.[31] Other concerning issues are the exposure to critical care staff at significant risk of sleep deprivation and

exhaustion, the feeling of being isolated working in difficult and demanding conditions, and the worrisome event of them falling ill (like during the Severe Acute Respiratory Syndrome by coronavirus[SARS] SARS epidemic).[31]

A complete disaster management plan should include a regimented shift schedule that balances available staff and skills with current clinical abilities, constant moral support for the team members, a frequent feedback system that allows the personal to get congratulations for their efforts, and the possibility to start a cases group support with help from psychiatric or the emergency response crisis team; treatment for posttraumatic stress disorder that cause long-term disability in the healthcare providers should also be considered.[23]

To extend their ability to provide direct critical care to large numbers of patients, the Task Force guidelines recommend that critical-care-trained physicians and nurses oversee noncritical care staff supported by guidelines of standardize interventions to reduce care variability.[13] The Task Force recommends that any nonintensivist physicians willing to serve in intensivist roles could be encouraged to join critical care teams. These physicians could be assigned to care for up to 6 critically ill patients each with intensivists overseeing 4 to 8 of these nonintensivist clinicians (up to 48 patients), depending on their experience. Noncritical care nurses and pharmacists could become responsible for medication delivery to all of the critical care patients; paramedics could help maintain airways of critical care patients; respiratory therapists (RT) who specialize in critical care could oversee groups of their noncritical care colleagues (1 critical care RT and 1 noncritical care RT to care for perhaps 12-14 patients); and pharmacists could help redistribute scarce pharmaceutical resources.[13]

Space

Hospitals can expand critical care to other areas, but shortages of equipment and staff can limit that option due to the fact that most critical care interventions need specialized machines and equipment which only can be performed in locations with electricity and oxygen.[23] Intensive care units, postanesthesia care units, and emergency rooms are best outfitted to provide mechanical ventilation and close monitoring; step-down units, large procedure suites, telemetry units, and hospital wards may be used for EMCC when capacity in these spaces is exceeded.[13] Facility planning for both backup systems and expansion of services (ie, generator availability) is essential to maximize critical care capacity.

Also because care of noncritical patient requires less infrastructure, strong consideration should be given to the transfer of stable patients to "surge facilities" to maximize dedicated hospital space for critical care delivery in an overflow situation. Finally, another resource is evacuating critical patients to another facility when the hospital exceeds its capacity or is directly affected by the disaster to maximize survival in a mass casualty event[6]; but this is not likely to be a good immediate option while the disaster is in the early stages of its evolution.

Point of Care

There is a constant concern about the delay in identification of complex pathologies which require medical testing and their significant associated mortality and morbidity (eg, myocardial infarctions, acute kidney injury, and sepsis). So, new recommendations are focusing on point-of-care (POC) testing[32] that allows medical testing, early patient stabilization and transfer to a critical care setting for comprehensive critical care management.

Palliative Care

During a catastrophic mass casualty event, there is an important role for palliative care services in the support of individuals not expected to survive and their relatives. These services should be included in the state and local disaster plan to minimize the suffering of the victims, and free up resources to optimize survival of others. In a recent publication,[22] the investigators provide guidance about the role of palliative care in a mass casualty event, stating that even in the context of scarce resources during these events, support and training for healthcare personal deciding treatment for those "likely to die" should be in place.

OTHER CHALLENGES IN DISASTER PLANIING

Planning

It has even been reported that less than 10% of casualties actually require hospital admission[4,5]; in large scale casualty event it is known that field triage stations are often bypassed, causing hospital nearest to the disaster site to receive the bulk of the casualties. This makes it remarkably important to conduct a careful survey of potential sites and types of hazardous events specific to the local area while designing a disaster plan, and include transfer agreements between hospitals and nearby ICUs to meet possible bed shortages.[8]

Communication Devices

The failure of communications systems in major disasters due to excessive demand or possible disruption has been well documented.[10] It is considered the responsibility of local and regional health officers to identify medical disaster communication needs and establish primary and backup systems linking response providers, health care facilities, and emergency operations centers. The Trust for America's Health sponsored by the Robert Woods Johnson Foundation, include streamlined and effective communication channels as 1 of the 8 core goals of a public health emergency response to enhance rapid and accurate transfer of information between health care workers, frontline responders, and the public.[33]

Legal Issues

Resource triage is arguably the most problematic issue in disaster medicine because it inevitably raises the concern of health care rationing that will potentially impact individual survival. The ethical, legal, and social ramifications of resource triage can be quite significant, compelling us to first to make all efforts to obtain scarce resources, transfer patients, or increase surge capacity through EMCC before considering the "rationing" of resources.[14] To ensure appropriate legal and societal support, resource triage should be done in collaboration with regional and federal public health authorities using objective, fair, and transparent criteria for provision of care.[14]

In contemplation of the ethical implications of resource triage, more work is needed to develop a system that is effective, rational, and amenable to society. Several groups, including the Task Force have favored employing the SOFA score to stratify patients with respiratory failure and/or shock with end-organ damage in terms of short-term survival, because it relies on objective data that are relatively easy to obtain and has been validated in a variety of critical illnesses[10,21]; yet, considering finite and potentially dwindling resources consideration must be given to excluding those patients with overall poor prognosis caused by end-organ failure such as end-stage liver disease, end-stage heart failure, or end-stage pulmonary disease.

Education and Simulation Training

Scheduling regular training and exercises in disaster management at different scales is important to enhance preparedness. Regular drills will help identify difficulties and provide knowledge of the absolute capacity of devices, equipment, and services in a disaster situation.[34] Plans to evacuate critically ill patients to nearby hospitals in the event of failure of backup systems should also be addressed in the process. Even though there is no perfect educational tool which exactly replicates a disaster, educational efforts in preparedness are still useful and necessary. Simulation training provides opportunities for teaching, observing and analyzing performance in order to find ways to improve.

Training our staff and our future ICU trainees for such eventualities through the use of simulators and mock disaster codes has become necessary to build on our successes and learn from to avoid the problems we encountered in the past. Educational tools include table exercises, standardize patients, and robotic patient simulators among others. A recent study showed that all critical actions took longer to perform on simulator patients compared to actor patients (standardize patient), and the time required to perform procedures on simulators were similar to published results on real-world patients.[34]

Critical Care in Unconventional Situations

There have been numerous examples in medical literature describing extended critical care through mobile ICU teams, not necessarily restricted to disaster settings. Some of the special factors to consider in the formation of ICU teams are: (1) choosing personnel that are flexible in terms of their availability, (2) having flexible staffing strategies to respond appropriately to each unique situation, (3) providing special training that allows innovative interventions adapted to local needs, and (4) assessing if the mobile ICU team can be implemented quickly enough. The preparation of mobile ICU teams should include review of the overall effort and adequacy of the ICU teams, outcome of victims, operational costs, and analysis of the structure and process of the ICU in the field.[35]

CONCLUSIONS

Critical care is an indispensable part of the medical disaster response not only because intensivists provide care for the sickest of the salvageable patients but also because they can share their clinical expertise in triage, resuscitation, and complex medical care. Understanding the characteristics of different disasters and predicting their impact on the healthcare system, integrating the principles of the command center, and participating in the local disaster-planning process will improve the appropriate response by the critical care physician to disaster situations. Also appropriate interventions for medical syndromes that require specific therapies are critical to minimizing morbidity and mortality during disaster events and their aftermaths.

Educational efforts are crucial before and after a disaster. Simulation sessions and mock outbreak/disaster exercises must be instituted on a regular base to understand our current level of preparedness, teach personnel how to respond appropriately to these unique situations, predict and be prepared for unexpected events. Learning from the successes and failures of past local and global disasters is necessary to prepare our health system for a successful emergency response which can mitigate the inevitable suffer that a mass causally event brings to the community.

General Disaster Resources and Websites

Centers for Disease Control and Prevention, Emergency Preparedness and Response. At http://www.bt.cdc.gov/disasters/

World Health Organization, natural disaster profiles. At http://www.who.int/hac/techguidance/ems/natprofiles/en/index.html

Federal Emergency Management Agency, disaster management. At http://www.fema.gov/hazard/types.shtm

Centers for Disease Control and Prevention, radiation emergencies. At http://www.bt.cdc.gov/radiation/clinicians.asp

Centers for Disease Control and Prevention website for bioterrorism. At http://www.bt.cdc.gov/

REFERENCES

1. Word Disasters Report 2009. Focus on early warning, early action. International Federation of Red Cross and Red Crescent Societies. http://www.ifrc.org/Global/WDR2009-full.pdf.
2. New York City Panel on Climate Change. Climate Risk Information 2013: Observations, Climate Change Projections, and Maps. http://www.nyc.gov/html/planyc2030/downloads/pdf/npcc_climate_risk_information_2013_report.pdf.
3. Rubinson L, Hick JL, Hanfling DG, et al. Definitive care for the critically ill during a disaster: a framework for optimizing critical care surge capacity. *Chest.* 2008;133(5 suppl):18S-31S.
4. Kvetan V. The Word Trade Center Attack: Is critical care prepared for terrorism? *Critical Care.* 2001;5:321-322.
5. Frykberg ER. Medical management of disasters and mass casualties from terrorist bombings: how can we cope? *J Trauma.* 2002;53(2):201-212.
6. Jain S, Kamimoto L, Bramley AM, et al. Hospitalized patients with 2009 H1N1 influenza in the United States, April-June 2009. *N Engl J Med.* 2009;361:1935-1944.
7. Einav S, Limor Aharonson D, Weissman C, Freund HR, Peleg K; Israel Trauma Group. In-Hospital resource utilization during multiple casualty incidents. *Ann Surg.* 2006;243(4):533-540.
8. Corcoran SP, Niven AS, Reese JM. Critical care management of major disasters: a practical guide to disaster preparation in the intensive care unit. *J Intensive Care Med.* 2012;27(1):3-10.
9. Shirley PJ, Mandersloot G. Clinical review: the role of the intensive care physician in mass casualty incidents: planning, organization, and leadership. *Crit Care.* 2008;12(3):214.
10. Christian MD, Devereaux AV, Dichter JR, et al. Definitive care for the critically ill during a disaster. Summary of suggestions from the Task Force for Mass Critical Care summit meeting, January 26-27, 2007. *Chest.* 2008;133(5):1S-7S.
11. US Department of Homeland Security. National preparedness guidelines, 2007. http://www.dhs.gov/xlibrary/assets/National_Preparedness_Guidelines.pdf.
12. Christian MD, Devereaux AV, Dichter JR, Geiling JA, Rubinson L. Definitive care for the critically ill during a disaster: current capabilities and limitations. *Chest.* 2008;133(5 suppl):8S-17S.
13. Rubinson L, Hick JL, Curtis JR, et al. Definitive care for the critically ill during a disaster: medical resources for surge capacity. *Chest.* 2008;133(5 suppl):32S-50S.
14. Devereaux AV, Dichter JR, Christian MD, et al. Definitive care for the critically ill during a disaster: a framework for allocation of scarce resources in mass critical care. *Chest.* 2008;133(5 suppl):51S-66S.
15. Shiloh A, Savel R, Leung S, Carlese A, Kvetan K. Mass critical care. In: Vincent, Abraham, Moore, Kochanek, Finc, eds. *Texbook of Critical Care.* 6th ed. 2011.
16. Hick JL, Christian MD, Sprung CL; European Society of Intensive Care Medicine's Task Force for intensive care unit triage during an influenza epidemic or mass disaster. Chapter 2. Surge capacity and infrastructure considerations for mass critical care. Recommendations and standard operating procedures for intensive care unit and hospital preparations for an influenza epidemic or mass disaster. *Intensive Care Med.* 2010;36(1 suppl):S11-S20.
17. Sprung CL, Zimmerman JL, Christian MD, et al. Recommendations for intensive care unit and hospital preparations for an influenza epidemic or mass disaster: summary report of the European Society of Intensive Care Medicine's Task Force for intensive care unit triage during an influenza epidemic or mass disaster. *Intensive Care Med.* 2010;36(3):428-443.
18. Karwa M, Currie B, Kvetan V. Bioterrorism: preparing for the impossible or the improbable. *Crit Care Med.* 2005;33(1 suppl):S75-S95.
19. 2010 Hospital Accreditation Standards: Joint Commission Resources. http://www.jointcommission.org/

20. Burkle FM, Orebaugh S, Barendse BR. Emergency Medicine in the Persian Gulf War-Part I: preparation for triage and combat casualty care. *Ann Emerg Med.* 1994;23:742-747.

21. Moreno R, Vincent JL, Matos R, et al. The use of maximum SOFA score to quantify organ dysfunction/failure in intensive care-results of a prospective, multicenter study. *Intensive Care Med.* 1999;25:686-696.

22. Matzo M, Wilkinson A, Lynn J, Gatto M, Phillips S. Palliative care considerations in mass casualty events with scarce resources. *Biosecur Bioterror.* 2009;7(2):199-210.

23. Hotchkin DL, Rubinson L. Modified critical care and treatment space considerations for mass casualty critical illness and injury. *Respir Care.* 2008;53(1):67-74.

24. Abir M, Davis MM, Sankar P, Wong AC, Wang SC. Design of a model to predict surge capacity bottlenecks for burn mass casualties at a large academic medical center. *Prehosp Disaster Med.* 2013;28(1):23-32.

25. Halpern NA, Pastores SM, Greenstein RJ. Critical care medicine in the United States 1985-2000: an analysis of bed numbers, use, and costs. *Crit Care Med.* 2004;32:1254-1259.

26. Esbitt D. The Strategic National Stockpile: roles and responsibilities of health care professionals for receiving the stockpile assets. *Disaster Manag Response.* 2003;1:68-70.

27. Strategic National Stockpile. Atlanta, GA: Centers for Disease Control and Prevention. http://www.bt.cdc.gov/stockpile

28. Blakeman TC, Branson RD. Oxygen supplies in disaster management. *Respir Care.* 2013;58(1):173-183.

29. Ritz RH, Previter JE. Oxygen supplies during a mass casualty situation. *Respir Care.* 2008;53(2):215-224.

30. U.S. Health and Human Services, Report to Congress. The Critical Care Workforce: a study of the supply and demand for critical care physicians. http://bhpr.hrsa.gov/healthworkforce/reports/criticalcare/default.htm.

31. Gomersall CD, Tai DY, Loo S, et al. Expanding ICU facilities in an epidemic: recommendations based on experience from the SARS epidemic in Hong Kong and Singapore. *Intensive Care Med.* 2006;32(7):1004-1013.

32. Tran NK, Godwin Z, Bockhold J. Point-of-care testing at the disaster-emergency-critical care interface. *Point Care.* 2012;11(4):180-183.

33. Trust for America's Health. Ready or not: protecting the public's health from diseases, disasters, and bioterrorism. Robert Wood Johnson Foundation; December 2008.

34. Wallace D, Gillett B, Wright B, Stetz J, Arquilla B. Randomized controlled trial of high fidelity patient simulators compared to actor patients in a pandemic influenza drill scenario. *Resuscitation.* 2010;81(7):872-876.

35. Rice DH, Kotti G, Beninati W. Clinical review: critical care transport and austere critical care. *Crit Care.* 2008;12:207.

Controversies: Scoring Systems in Critical Care

Michael Elias, MD and John M. Oropello, MD, FACP, FCCP, FCCM

INTRODUCTION

Management of the critically ill patient is complex. The acuity of illness, multiple organ system derangements, patient heterogeneities such as age, comorbidities, uncharted genomic and epigenetic variability, and the availability of evolving treatments and systems of health care delivery make the prediction of prognosis an elusive, moving target.

Originally created in response to limited ICU resources, an aging population and rising healthcare costs, scoring systems[1-3] (also called scoring models) are intended to provide objective predictions or probabilities of mortality and long-term outcome to aid clinical decision making and planning. Their role has been expanded to benchmark or compare the performance of ICUs and assess the quality of care provided (eg, observed mortality vs predicted mortality), to predict the resources needed or the appropriateness of ICU admission depending on the severity of illness and finally to assess patients for inclusion in research studies or to compare severity of illness and assess case-mix dissimilarities between patients in various study groups.

Although intensivists will increasingly encounter assessments of their ICU patient population, ICU structure and process and physician performance via scoring systems, the application of scoring systems is not without significant controversy. This chapter discusses the main ICU scoring systems in use today,[4-7] how their performance is assessed, how they are utilized, the limitations and the controversial issues surrounding their use.

ICU SCORING SYSTEMS

The type, timing, and quantity of data collected vary significantly among the numerous scoring systems. Some scores, such as the sequential organ failure assessment, measure the organ dysfunction and thus the severity of the disease at any point of time to monitor the clinical evolution. Others, known as general risk prediction scores focus primarily on survival. These systems were developed on the assumption that the severity of illness and mortality are related to acute physiologic derangements that appear early in the course of the disease.[8] The most prevalent are acute physiology score chronic health evaluation (APACHE), mortality probability model (MPM), and simplified acute physiology score (SAPS). They were developed approximately 30 years ago and have since undergone 3 to 4 revisions (Table 63–1). APACHE IV combines a total of 27 variables collected within the first 24 hours of ICU admission, MPM_0III and SAPS III combines, respectively, 16 and 20 variables collected within 1 hour of ICU admission. They all depend on acute physiologic variables collected on admission such as vital signs, electrolytes, cell count, blood gas, etc, in addition to chronic health variables and admission diagnosis.

Scoring systems provide a numerical estimation (score) to quantify the severity of illness, which is correlated to mortality, length of stay (LOS), morbidity, and long-term functional outcome (ie, quality of life). Prognostic models are constructed using prospective cohorts of patients with predefined candidate variables, outcomes and time points. Candidate variables are preselected variables, such as any patient characteristics, lab values or risk factors that are thought to play a role in the prediction of the model. A statistical analysis method, called logistic regression, will then identify and weight the variables that can predict the outcome. Although the original versions of the APACHE and SAPS scoring systems used expert opinions to determine the predictive variables, more recent versions use multiple logistic regression techniques (logistic and Cox regression) to also select and weight the variables.

TABLE 63–1 General risk prediction scoring systems and revisions.

Scoring System (Year Introduced)	Number of Variables	Selection of Variables and Weights	Variables	Comments
Acute Physiology Chronic Health Evaluation (APACHE)				
APACHE I (1981)	34	Panel of expert clinicians	Worst acute physiology variables within the first 32 hours + preadmission chronic health status 3-6 months prior to admission.	The first iteration of the APACHE system. No longer in use.
APACHE II (1985)	12	Panel of expert clinicians	Worst acute physiology variables within the first 24 hours (APS score) + preadmission chronic health status 3-6 months prior to admission	Used for a group of patients, in public domain, limited number of variables, most frequently used system for risk stratification in clinical trials
APACHE III (1991)	17	Multiple logistic regression	See above	Not in public domain, proprietary, available at cost
APACHE IV (2006)	27	Multiple logistic regression (110,518 patients in 104 US ICUs)	Data collected within the first 24 hours Acute physiology variables, age, chronic health variables, ICU admission diagnosis, ICU admission source, length of stay prior to ICU admission, emergency surgery, thrombolytic therapy, FiO_2, mechanical ventilation.	Most accurate for hospital mortality and ICU length of stay, requires considerable data and training. Specific algorithm for mortality prediction after Coronary Artery Bypass Graft (CABG) surgery. Calculator of raw score: in public domain. Real time validation, updated probabilities: proprietary
Mortality Probability Model (MPM)				
MPM I (1985)	11	Multiple logistic regression	First hour and 24 hours of admission	Probability of death
MPM II (1993)	15	Multiple logistic regression	First 24, 48, and 72 hours of admission	Probability of death
MPM_0 III (2007)	16	Multiple logistic regression (124,885 patients in 135 ICUs—mainly US)	Worst values prior to and within 1 hour of ICU admission: Acute physiologic variables, age, chronic health variables, acute diagnoses, admission type (medical, surgical), emergency surgery, CPR within 1 hour of ICU admission, mechanical ventilation, code status	Predicts hospital mortality and ICU length of stay. Least amount of data collection, does not require a diagnosis at ICU admission, collected at lower cost and least time compared to APACHE IV and SAPS III. Predicts ICU LOS
Simplified Acute Physiology Score (SAPS)				
SAPS I (1984)	15	Panel of expert clinicians	Worst values within the first 24 hours	Simple to use, for stratification, not for mortality prediction
SAPS II (1993)	17	Multiple logistic regression	Worst values within the first 24 hours	Simple to use, most widely used in Europe
SAPS III (2005)	20	19,577 patients in 307 ICUs from 35 countries; multiple logistic regression	Worst values prior to and within 1 hour of ICU admission: Acute physiologic variables, age, chronic health variables, ICU admission diagnosis, ICU admission source, length of stay prior to ICU admission, emergency surgery, infection on admission, type of surgery	Simple to use (easy and quick), no cost, wide range of diagnosis represented, worldwide population represented

SCORING SYSTEM PERFORMANCE ASSESSMENT

The performance or ability to predict the outcome, is assessed by comparing the model predictions of mortality risk to the actual mortality in the studied patient populations across different ICUs. The measures used to evaluate outcome prediction include discrimination and calibration. *Discrimination* is the capability to distinguish between patients who will develop the event of interest (eg, death) versus those who will not (eg, survival).[9] Discrimination is represented by the area under the receiver operating characteristic curve (AUROC) (Figure 63–1), where the true positive rate is plotted against the false positive rate. The greater the area under the curve, the more accurate the system is able to discriminate between a given outcome, for example, alive or dead. *Calibration* depicts how the model performs over a wide range of predicted mortality; it estimates the scoring system's accuracy in mortality prediction over a wide spectrum of severity of illness, usually in

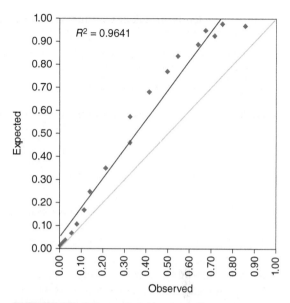

FIGURE 63–2 Legend: Calibration compares the expected and observed death at different deciles of mortality risk. (*Reproduced with permission from Strand K, Flaatten H: Severity scoring in the ICU: a review.* Acta Anaesthesiol Scand. *2008 Apr;52(4):467-478.*)

deciles from low to high (Figure 63–2).[9] For example, scoring systems tend to underestimate mortality in patients with a high severity of illness and underestimate mortality in patients with a low severity of illness.

The predictive performance of models must be validated.[10] *Internal validation* refers to the analysis of the performance of the model in the ICU dataset population from which the model is derived; this is the population in which it will perform the best because the variables were adjusted to optimize the model. This is followed by a process called *external validation* in which the performance of the model is assessed in patients from ICUs that were not part of the original dataset used to develop the model. The ICUs used for external validation should be of the same type (eg, general ICU vs general ICU not general ICU vs specialty ICU [eg, cardiac]) as those used in the internal validation.

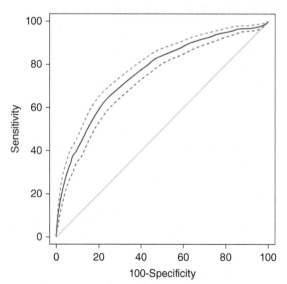

FIGURE 63–1 Discrimination is the ability to distinguish between patients who will and will not develop the event of interest, in this case death. The AUROC represents the accuracy of a scoring system. The true positive rate represents the patients predicted correctly to die. The false positive rate represents the patients predicted to die but survive. AUROC (Area Under the Receiver Operating Characteristic Curve) Sensitivity = true positive rate; 100-Specificity = false positive rate. (*Reproduced with permission from Strand K, Flaatten H: Severity scoring in the ICU: a review.* Acta Anaesthesiol Scand. *2008 Apr;52(4):467-478.*)

UTILIZATION OF SCORING SYSTEMS

Although they were introduced more than 30 years ago, scoring systems have been used in only 10% to 15% of the total yearly ICU admissions in the United

States.[11] This lack of clinical utility at the bedside can be explained by the lack of predictive applicability in the individual patient, the limited practical utility of the models (too complex or cumbersome to implement) and the costs. To be used in clinical practice, the model should be simple, readily available and not expensive. The least expensive and simplest scoring systems to implement have been the most prevalent. For example, the APACHE II system—no cost, in the public domain—is today the most used system to assess patients for inclusion in research studies based on severity of illness or to compare severity of illness between control and treatment groups and assess case mix dissimilarities between patients in various study groups. APACHE II is also used in many ICUs to assess predicted mortality compared to observed mortality, thus as a quality measure of ICU performance to national norms. However, the APACHE II system was created and validated 30 years ago. Ultimately, prognostic scoring systems become obsolete over time if they are not updated to follow the advancement of medical sciences. Due to improvements in medical care and in population health, the mortality predictions of older systems tend to overestimate the current mortality rate. This trend is obvious in inexpensive systems which are almost guaranteed to provide a good result—most ICUs, using APACHE II, will have a lower than predicted mortality and thus favorable benchmarking.

It is important to understand the different components of APACHE IV, which is the paradigm of a more modern system that allows predictions of both hospital mortality and expected ICU LOS. APACHE IV is characterized by an internal validation on a very large database with selected variables determined by multiple logistic regression—a more rigorous statistical method than arbitrary expert opinions. There are 2 versions, 1 in the public domain that is essentially a web-based calculator; 1 enters the patient variables and quickly generates a score that correlates to a predicted mortality. The other version is managed by a company, Cerner (Vienna, VA), which maintains the database and analyzes the APACHE IV data across different hospitals, providing updated and repeated analysis over time with better resolution and potential value. Because the accuracy of the prediction is highly dependent upon the quality

of data collected, this elaborate system is associated with significant costs to avoid any deviation from the precise data-collection methodology that may result in errors in predictions. The cumbersome computer-based data entry requires considerable training, and often, a full time specialist dedicated to collect data on site. Because of the cost, the online "calculator" version of APACHE IV is more commonly used.

Once a scoring system is found to be accurate, one must assess if the prediction obtained has any influence on the management; it becomes beneficial to use in clinical practice if an impact study demonstrates decisional power.[12,13] To date, the impact of APACHE IV (or any other general ICU scoring system for that matter) on patient outcome, on clinical decision-making or cost has not been addressed in any prospective study or a randomized controlled trial.

LIMITATIONS OF SCORING SYSTEMS

Despite the existence of many prognostic models and their attractive potential utility, scoring systems have a limited clinical value at the bedside and are seldom used in clinical practice. There are a number of reasons for this.

Prognostic models should closely follow the advancement of medical sciences and be updated in a timely fashion to avoid becoming obsolete. There may be limitations of the predictive ability after modification of a variable. As diagnosis and treatment evolve scoring systems require repeated recalibration and validation, although this is difficult and time consuming to achieve. Also the lack of collaboration between researchers that might improve upon a single model leads to the multiplication of redundant, often competing and nonvalidated models.[10,13-15]

Most of the available information on scoring systems is based on internal validation, less studies report external validation and almost none report the impact on clinical decision-making and outcome.[16] After the external validation process is completed, the impact of the scoring system on clinical decision-making, patient outcome, or costs should be assessed in a management study or randomized controlled trial[12,13] before being used in clinical practice.

Scoring systems designed for general medical or surgical ICUs would be inappropriate if used in specialized units such as coronary, burn or pediatric where patients differ from the populations of the original and external validation samples from which the system was derived. Clinical judgment remains fundamental because not all relevant variables are included in the models.

The outcome and the time points might be different than those for which the scoring system was designed. For example, changes in hospital practices resulting in earlier discharge of patients to long-term acute care facilities thus reducing the hospital mortality or calculating scores outside of the intended and validated ranges, for example, daily versus within the first hour or first 24 hours.

To be used in clinical practice, the user should understand the existing models, be convinced of their utility and trained in their application. The barriers for the effective use of scoring systems may be related to the limited practical utility of the models. Some models such as APACHE IV are complex and require dedicated personnel and a specific training; they can be expensive to use, therefore, limiting their spread across the healthcare community.

The more data required by the scoring system, both in amount and complexity, the greater the opportunity for errors and missing data. In theory, different users with similar backgrounds in critical care should obtain similar scores for the same patient population, however, low interobserver reliability resulting in dissimilar scoring values by different users can occur.

Scoring systems provide only probabilities, not certainties. It would be inappropriate to deny or withdraw care based solely on a probability derived from any existing scoring system. The course of illness over time is important. Clinical variables may not be included in these models and clinical judgment and ethical principles need to be employed when making decisions regarding prognosis in an individual patient. For example, the physiologic response of sepsis which is linked to unknown genomic factors is not taken into account in any scoring system. Human physiology is complex and clinical assessment prevails over scoring system predictions.

Benchmarking Intensive Care Units Based on Scoring Systems

The ranking of intensive care units and institutions based on severity of illness versus mortality rate is controversial. Different populations of patients in different ICUs are not always comparable even when their severity of illness scores is identical. For example, a hospital with the same mean prognostic score but a higher mortality does not necessarily underperform when compared to another hospital as there may be other elements that are not represented in the dataset captured by these systems. For instance, as the lack of health insurance is associated with increased 30-day mortality and decreased use of common procedures for the critically ill, the insurance status may be an indicator of mortality not picked up by patient and clinical characteristic variables.[17] In elective surgical admissions, there is an association between the socioeconomic status and hospital mortality that is not explained by case mix or the withdrawal of active treatment.[18] Finally, among trauma patients, the uninsured receive less trauma-related care and have a higher mortality rate.[19] These examples illustrate the fact that 2 different populations of patients can have similar severity of illness scores with very different mortality rates.

CONCLUSION

Although scoring systems are numerous and potentially useful, they are not commonly used in clinical practice in part because many flaws exist in their development, validation, and maintenance. The obstacles to the implementation of scoring systems are significant. However, the strategies to overcome many of these barriers are becoming available as clinical information systems become electronic and more sophisticated. In the future, systems may be able to parse notes in the medical record to form alerts in real time and the costs and errors involved with specialized and redundant data entry may be avoided.

REFERENCES

1. Knaus WA, Zimmerman JE, Wagner DP, Draper EA, Lawrence DE. APACHE-acute physiology and chronic health evaluation: a physiologically

based classification system. *Crit Care Med.* 1981;9(8):591-597.

2. Le Gall JR, Loirat P, Alperovitch A. Simplified acute physiological score for intensive care patients. *Lancet.* 1983;2(8352):741.

3. Teres D, Lemeshow S, Avrunin JS, Pastides H. Validation of the mortality prediction model for ICU patients. *Crit Care Med.* 1987;15(3):208-213.

4. Higgins TL, Teres D, Copes WS, Nathanson BH, Stark M, Kramer AA. Assessing contemporary intensive care unit outcome: an updated Mortality Probability Admission Model (MPM0-III). *Crit Care Med.* 2007;35(3):827-835.

5. Metnitz PG, Moreno RP, Almeida E, et al. SAPS 3—From evaluation of the patient to evaluation of the intensive care unit. Part 1: Objectives, methods and cohort description. *Intensive Care Med.* 2005;31(10):1336-1344.

6. Moreno RP, Metnitz PG, Almeida E, et al. SAPS 3—From evaluation of the patient to evaluation of the intensive care unit. Part 2: Development of a prognostic model for hospital mortality at ICU admission. *Intensive Care Med.* 2005;31(10):1345-1355.

7. Zimmerman JE, Kramer AA, McNair DS, Malila FM. Acute Physiology and Chronic Health Evaluation (APACHE) IV: hospital mortality assessment for today's critically ill patients. *Crit Care Med.* 2006;34(5):1297-1310.

8. Strand K, Flaatten H. Severity scoring in the ICU: a review. *Acta Anaesthesiol Scand.* 2008;52(4):467-478.

9. Ohno-Machado L, Resnic FS, Matheny ME. Prognosis in critical care. *Annu Rev Biomed Eng.* 2006;8:567-599.

10. Steyerberg EW. *Clinical Prediction Models: A Practical Approach to Development, Validation, and Updating.* New York, NY: Springer Publishing Company; 2009.

11. Breslow MJ, Badawi O. Severity scoring in the critically ill: part 2: maximizing value from outcome prediction scoring systems. *Chest.* 2012;141(2):518-527.

12. Reilly BM, Evans AT. Translating clinical research into clinical practice: impact of using prediction rules to make decisions. *Ann Intern Med.* 2006;144(3):201-209.

13. Moons KG, Altman DG, Vergouwe Y, Royston P. Prognosis and prognostic research: application and impact of prognostic models in clinical practice. *BMJ.* 2009;338:b606.

14. Janssen KJ, Moons KG, Kalkman CJ, Grobbee DE, Vergouwe Y. Updating methods improved the performance of a clinical prediction model in new patients. *J Clin Epidemiol.* 2008;61(1):76-86.

15. Steyerberg EW, Borsboom GJ, van Houwelingen HC, Eijkemans MJ, Habbema JD. Validation and updating of predictive logistic regression models: a study on sample size and shrinkage. *Stat Med.* 2004;23(16):2567-2586.

16. Steyerberg EW, Moons KG, van der Windt DA, et al. Prognosis Research Strategy (PROGRESS) 3: prognostic model research. *PLoS Med.* 2013;10(2):e1001381.

17. Lyon SM, Benson NM, Cooke CR, Iwashyna TJ, Ratcliffe SJ, Kahn JM. The effect of insurance status on mortality and procedural use in critically ill patients. *Am J Respir Crit Care Med.* 2011;184(7):809-815.

18. Hutchings A, Raine R, Brady A, Wildman M, Rowan K. Socioeconomic status and outcome from intensive care in England and Wales. *Med Care.* 2004;42(10):943-951.

19. Haas JS, Goldman L. Acutely injured patients with trauma in Massachusetts: differences in care and mortality, by insurance status. *Am J Public Health.* 1994;84(10):1605-1608.

Controversies: Patient-Controlled Sedation— Ready for Prime Time?

64

Annie Lynn Penaco, MD and Jay Berger, MD, PhD

KEY POINTS

1 Depth of sedation exists as a continuum from minimal sedation where the patient is able to interact during the sedation to deep sedation which is just short of general anesthesia.

2 Patient-controlled sedation is an extension of patient-controlled analgesia, where the patient is able to control the depth of sedation that is comfortable for them during an invasive procedure.

3 Primary focus on the use of patient-controlled sedation is in the setting of ambulatory procedures that are typically performed under local or regional anesthesia.

4 The highly titratable nature of sedation requires the use of medications that are highly potent with rapid onsets of action.

5 The use of target-controlled infusion allows for more stable plasma concentrations of the sedative medication during the procedure.

6 Patient-maintained sedation utilizing target-controlled infusions is produces more stable plasma concentrations; however, the time to reach adequate sedation is relatively slower as compared to patient-controlled sedation.

7 Most common adverse event encountered during sedation is respiratory depression, manifested as hypoxemia and decreased respiratory rate.

SEDATION

Sedation is an induced altered state of consciousness following the administration of a sedative agent. According to the American Society of Anesthesiologists, depth of sedation exists as a continuum[1] ranging from minimal sedation to deep sedation, just prior to achieving general anesthesia (Table 64–1). With minimal sedation, patients are in a state of anxiolysis and may have impaired cognitive function, but retain protective airway reflexes and the ability to respond normally to verbal commands. Moderate sedation, previously referred to as conscious sedation, refers to a state of depressed consciousness with a purposeful response to verbal commands and light tactile stimulation, such as glabellar tap. In a state of deep sedation, patients are not easily arousable but are able to purposefully respond to repeated or painful stimuli. In cases where the level of sedation becomes deeper

TABLE 64-1 Continuum of depth of sedation.

	Minimal Sedation	Moderate Sedation	Deep Sedation	General Anesthesia
Responsiveness	Normal response to verbal stimulation	Purposeful response to verbal and tactile stimulation	Purposeful response following repeated or painful stimulation	Unarousable to painful stimulation
Spontaneous Ventilation and Airway	Unaffected	Adequate, no intervention required	May be inadequate, may require intervention	Frequently inadequate, intervention required
Cardiovascular Function	Unaffected	Usually maintained	Usually maintained	May be impaired

Reproduced with permission from American Society of Anesthesiologist (ASA): Continuum of depth of sedation: Definition of general anesthesia and levels of sedation/analgesia. ASA House of Delegates, October 30, 1991.

than initially intended, interventions in airway management or hemodynamic support may become necessary. Other similar measures of sedation such as the Observer Assessment of Alertness and Sedation Scale[2] are also commonly used (Table 64–2).

BACKGROUND

Historically, sedation has been widely administered in a clinician-controlled manner as a means of facilitating invasive interventions or making intolerable procedures appropriately acceptable. However, patients often have varying expectations and degrees of anxiety and discomfort as well as different sensitivities to sedative agents. This causes sedation requirements to vary widely, making it clinically challenging to predict and achieve the optimum level of sedation for each individual patient. Clinicians must rely on subjective determinants of adequate sedation with the constant concern for enhancing safety and preventing adverse

TABLE 64-2 Observer assessment of alertness and sedation scale.

Rating	Sedation Level
5	Responds readily to name
4	Lethargic, responds to name
3	Responds if name called loudly
2	Responds after mild shaking
1	Only responds to noxious stimulus
0	Does not respond to noxious stimulus

events. The technique of patient-controlled sedation (PCS) may circumvent these challenges by offering patients the ability to control and titrate their desired levels of sedation.

PATIENT-CONTROLLED ANALGESIA VERSUS PATIENT-CONTROLLED SEDATION

Patient-controlled drug administration is a well-established concept. The more commonly encountered, patient-controlled analgesia (PCA), has been effectively and safely utilized for several decades as a means of providing pain relief especially in the acute postoperative setting. PCA consists of a delivery system with which patients are able to self-administer predetermined doses of analgesic medications as required for pain management. With advances in PCA pump technology, this technique operates safely with the ability to program parameters with respect to bolus dosages and lockout intervals. A similar technique and logical extension of the PCA concept using related technology is PCS.

Initial reports of PCS began independently with investigations by Rudkin et al[3] and Park and Watkins[4] in 1991. Rudkin et al reported a high level of patient satisfaction with PCS using self-administration of propofol during dental extraction surgery under local anesthesia. Meanwhile, Park, and Watkins studied the use of PCS using a combination of midazolam and fentanyl during surgical procedures under epidural anesthesia and compared this to anesthesiologist-administered sedation using the same drugs. The results of the study indicated that PCS is not only a safe and effective technique, but it also leads to higher levels of patient comfort and satisfaction. Subsequent investigations under various clinical conditions have led to similar results using different combinations of medications.[5]

Although seemingly identical in design, PCA and PCS have fundamental differences that limit the similarities in clinical application and associated adverse events. PCA primarily acts on postoperative pain, which tends to be uniform and predictable for each individual. PCA typically utilizes medications with slower onsets of action but with prolonged duration, such as morphine. In this way, PCA is designed to operate safely in the absence of continuous monitoring from an anesthetic-care provider. In contrast, PCS especially in the intraoperative setting requires the flexibility to respond rapidly to constantly changing levels of stimulation. PCS typically utilizes easily titratable medications that have rapid onsets of action that are conducive to the rapidly changing environment in which it is required. Although PCS has been often shown to be generally as safe as conventional anesthetist-administered sedation, experience with PCS in the absence of an anesthetic-care provider has generally not been supported due to the potential for adverse events that are uncommonly seen with PCA.[5] For instance, adverse events such as respiratory depression and excessively deep levels of sedation have been reported to occur in association with PCS, similar to anesthetist-administered sedation.[6] Due to inherent differences, PCA and PCS must differ in the delicate balance between efficacy and safety. Ultimately, with regard to patient safety, as the requirement for effective sedation increases, patient monitoring must also become more intense so that complications can be easily detected and managed expeditiously.

CLINICAL APPLICATIONS

Interest in the use of PCS has generally been focused on a variety of ambulatory procedures which are performed under local or regional anesthesia. Common surgical applications include ambulatory surgery procedures of short duration, dental procedures, ophthalmic surgery, gynecologic or lower abdominal surgery, neurologic surgery, and ortho pedic surgery.[5] PCS is also beneficial for nonoperative procedures associated with discomfort such as endoscopy, colonoscopy, and lithotripsy. Furthermore, PCS may be utilized for perioperative anxiolysis in select patients.

PHARMACOLOGIC AGENTS

PCS typically requires highly potent medications with rapid onsets of action in order to provide effective and reliable sedation in the rapidly changing environment associated with the operating room or procedure room. Several medications such as propofol, benzodiazepines, and opioids have been extensively studied either alone or in various combinations. Each of the agents has been found to be equally safe and effective,[7] but present with varying advantages and disadvantages (Table 64–3).

Propofol (Diprivan)

Propofol has the ideal pharmacokinetic properties for PCS as it has rapid onset, short time to peak effect as well as a short context sensitive half-life that makes it easily titratable. However, its main disadvantage is the high incidence of pain on injection that may make intravenous injection uncomfortable.[5] Propofol in high doses is also associated with apnea and cardiovascular depression. Propofol is often

TABLE 64–3 Commonly used pharmacologic agents for PCS.

	Mechanism of Action	Onset (min)	Duration (min)	Disadvantages
Propofol	Potentiation of GABA receptor activity	< 1	3-10	Causes pain on injection
Benzodiazepines	Enhances GABA receptor function	1-2	30-60	May cause memory impairment
Opioids	Various effects on opioid receptors	1-2	30-60	May cause arterial oxygen desaturation

used successfully as a sole sedative agent but may be supplemented with other agents.

Benzodiazepines

Benzodiazepines, particularly midazolam, are effective sedative agents with the additional effects of amnesia and anxiolysis. However, midazolam has the disadvantage of relatively prolonged recovery.[8] It appears to be associated with the greatest degree of memory impairment, intraoperatively and postoperatively.

Opioids

Opioids, such as fentanyl, alfentanil, and remifentanil, are also commonly used as adjunctive agents in PCS. Opioids are suggested to be useful in treating the discomfort and restlessness from prolonged immobilization[7] during longer procedures, or generally those lasting greater than 2 to 3 hours. The main disadvantages of opioids are transient intraoperative pulse oximetric desaturations and the potential for respiratory depression, especially when given in combination with benzodiazepines. It is also associated with a high incidence of postoperative nausea and vomiting.

PATIENT-CONTROLLED SEDATION

In PCS, patients are clearly instructed preoperatively on the proper use of the infusion device as well as the purpose of sedation. Sedation is carried out via an infusion pump with a reservoir, which is connected to a handheld button that only the patient can control. When the button is pressed, the pump delivers a bolus of a predetermined dosage of medication. A lockout period, or a time interval in which another dose cannot be administered, may or may not be programmed. When present, it appears to offer a safety mechanism by preventing excessive drug administration and subsequent oversedation and loss of consciousness.[7] The patients are instructed to press the button until they reach the desired level of sedation to allow them to be able to tolerate the procedure. In this way, the patients themselves can control and determine the end point of sedation.

In a prospective, randomized, controlled study, Mazanikov et al compared PCS using propofol and remifentanil with anesthesiologist-controlled patient sedation using propofol for ERCP procedures.[9] Between the 2 groups, patient and endoscopist satisfaction were comparable. However, the study found markedly less propofol consumption and faster recovery in the PCS group. Similar results were obtained in a study conducted by Girdler et al on dental patients, with the PCS group requiring a lighter level of sedation compared to a clinician-controlled group.[10] This suggests that anesthesiologist-controlled sedation may result in unnecessary deep sedation while PCS is well-accepted because patients appreciate the ability to maintain control of their sedation.

Target-Controlled Sedation

Due to the short duration of action of sedative agents, particularly propofol, a potential drawback of self-administration in bolus increments is the volatility of plasma concentrations and subsequent varying levels of sedation. Target-controlled infusion (TCI) overcomes this problem of varying blood concentrations. This method of administration utilizes a computer-controlled infusion system that can calculate and maintain target blood concentrations of propofol with great accuracy. TCI uses a pharmacokinetic model to predict the initial bolus dose and infusion rates necessary to achieve and maintain a given target concentration, avoiding peaks and troughs in plasma concentration. The target concentration can then be adjusted accordingly by the patient to achieve the optimal level of sedation.

In a study by Irwin et al, the benefits of TCI were used in combination with patient-controlled feedback[11] in a technique referred to as patient-maintained sedation (PMS). Based on each patient's age and weight, a TCI system calculated the dose necessary to achieve and maintain a selected target concentration of propofol. In this case, an initial target concentration of 1 mcg/mL was chosen. The patient also had control of a handset that when pressed, increased the target concentration by 0.2 mcg/mL increments with a lockout interval of 2 minutes. When no demand boluses were required for several minutes, the system gradually decreased until a baseline target concentration of 0.2 mcg/mL was reached. Although there was wide variability amongst individuals in total consumption of propofol, optimal sedation was found to be achieved at median target concentrations of 0.8 to 0.9 mcg/mL. Following cessation of the infusion at the end of the procedure, recovery was rapid and no delays were reported in meeting discharge criteria from the recovery room. Patients expressed overall satisfaction with the technique and reported interest in using the technique again in the future.

Rodrigo et al performed a randomized study comparing outcomes between PCS and PMS using a TCI of propofol.[12] The study found no significant differences in depth of sedation, operating conditions and patient satisfaction. However, a majority of patients preferred PMS likely because it produces more stable blood concentrations and possibly less oversedation. The main disadvantage of PMS is relatively slower onset in achieving adequate sedation. The time required for adequate sedation was 8.6 minutes in the PMS group, compared to 5.7 minutes in the PCS group.

EFFECT-SITE-CONTROLLED SEDATION

When variable rate infusions of propofol target the plasma concentration, the clinical effect lags behind the plasma concentration, reflecting the fact that the site of action of propofol is the brain rather than the plasma. Because of the inability to measure the concentration of propofol in the brain, or the effect site, it is assumed that the clinical effect of propofol reaches a plateau when the plasma and brain concentrations have equilibrated. This mathematically derived term, the effect-site concentration, therefore, corresponds to the clinical effect of propofol. In an alternative PMS system, where the effect-site compartment is targeted, sedation may be achieved rapidly and safely.

To assess both the efficacy and safety of effect-site-targeted PMS, Anderson et al recruited 20 healthy volunteers and gave them the task of attempting to oversedate themselves using this system.[13] The initial target effect-site concentration was set at 1 mcg/mL. The system was able to overshoot, or increase the target plasma concentration up to 100% over the target effect-site concentration. The predicted plasma concentration was reduced as the target effect-site was approached (Figure 64–1). When the plasma concentration decreased to within 10% of the target effect-site concentration, the patient's demand button was activated. Pressing the button led to an increase in the target effect-site concentration by increments of 0.2 mcg/mL. Although there was no traditional lockout time, further increases

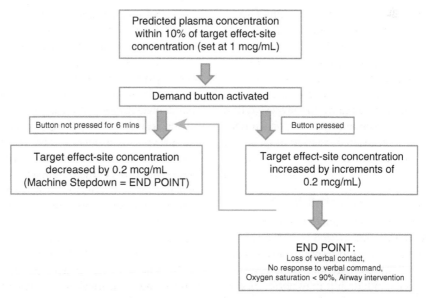

FIGURE 64-1 Effect-site controlled patient-maintained sedation with propofol, study design.[13] To assess PCS safety, study volunteers were instructed to attempt to oversedate themselves using a demand button.

in effect-site concentration could not be requested until plasma concentration fell to within 10% of the target effect-site concentration. The system was programmed with a means of machine stepdown, in which lack of a successful press of the control button after 6 minutes led to a 0.2 mcg/mL reduction in effect-site concentration. Under continuous monitoring, volunteers were instructed to try to make themselves unconscious. End-points of the study included loss of verbal contact, no response to verbal command, machine stepdown, oxygen saturation less than 90% or the requirement for airway intervention. Of the 20 subjects enrolled in the study, 15 terminated the study through machine stepdown, 4 developed oxygen saturation less than 90%, and 1 lost verbal contact. Although the system appeared to function successfully in achieving sedation, when the safety of the system was stressed in the artificial conditions of the study, a significant number reached potentially unsafe end-points. This suggested that anesthetic supervision may be required for safe administration.

Stonell et al studied the use of effect-site PMS with propofol compared to anesthetist-administered sedation with propofol boluses in patients undergoing colonoscopy.[14] Patients in the effect-site PMS group underwent sedation more slowly (13 minutes vs 3 minutes) and less deeply as determined with BIS monitoring. The more rapid induction of sedation in the anesthetist-administered sedation group resulted in a higher incidence of hypotension and oversedation, but overall did not lead to negative outcomes. Between the 2 groups, patient and endoscopist satisfaction was similar. All patients also had similar recall of events. These results suggested that although effect-site-steered PMS may be comparable to anesthetist-controlled sedation in quality, it lacks the efficiency in induction time.

POSSIBLE ADVERSE EVENTS

The most common issue encountered during PCS is respiratory depression, manifested by a decrease in arterial oxygen saturation and respiratory rate. Oxygen supplementation, routinely via nasal cannula, is the standard of care although it may not be necessary especially in young, healthy patients.

Propofol is a known cardiovascular depressant, which may precipitate hypotension especially in elderly patients who are already mildly dehydrated from NPO status.

The potential for respiratory depression and cardiovascular complications highlights the need for close monitoring during PCS. Resuscitation equipment should be made readily available in areas where PCS is practiced and practitioners should be certified in CPR and ACLS.

SPECIAL CONSIDERATIONS

Although PCS has been shown to be safe and effective, most randomized controlled trials have often involved relatively young patients. PCS investigations in elderly patients, while limited, have also resulted in similar outcomes. Herrick et al found that between elderly patients with no intraoperative sedation and those receiving PCS for cataract surgery, satisfaction was higher in the PCS group, whether or not the device was actually used.[15] Many of the patients felt comfortable enough not to need sedation but appreciated the availability of intraoperative sedation, should they desire it. In a prospective, randomized, controlled trial, Lee et al compared conventional clinician-controlled sedation with PCS in elderly patients undergoing outpatient colonoscopy.[16] PCS appeared to be safer with comparable effectiveness and acceptance. PCS must be used cautiously in elderly people, however, as the effect of bolus doses may not be as predictable. Therefore, smaller dosages with longer lockout periods are recommended.

Another application of PCS which may warrant further investigation is the self-administration of sedative medications in critically ill, mechanically ventilated ICU patients. In an investigation by Chlan et al, dexmedetomidine was administered via a basal infusion as well as with patient-triggered boluses.[17] PCS was rated favorably for its ability to safely and adequately relieve anxiety and attain a satisfactory level of comfort.

CLINICAL PRACTICE

PCS has been widely investigated for several years but has yet to achieve widespread clinical application. Reasons for hesitancy in use may involve various factors.[5] Conceptually, the technique of PCS contradicts the traditional tenet of monitored-anesthesia care where an anesthetist proactively administers sedation based on the anticipation for intraoperative events. Also, although many investigators have reported superior outcomes with PCS, others report no difference. With this lack of consistency or definitive benefit, there is a lack of incentive to change current practice and invest in new equipment. Furthermore, not all patients desire control. As patient satisfaction may be associated with degree of control, this may not provide a benefit for all patients.

CONCLUSION

PCS is a technique which allows patients to control and titrate their own level of sedation based on anxiety or perceived discomfort from noxious stimulation during a procedure. Ample evidence has suggested the safety and efficacy of PCS when compared with conventional anesthetist-administered sedation. PCS is also associated with high levels of patient satisfaction which may be related to an increased feeling of control in being able to self-administer sedation as it is required in the rapidly changing environment of the operating room or procedure room. More technologically advanced, alternative techniques of PMS, such as target-controlled sedation or effect-site-controlled sedation, have the added benefit of being able to provide a stable level of sedation uncomplicated by variability of plasma concentration. Despite these perceived advantages, however, PCS has not gained wide acceptance in clinical practice due to a lack of consistent and definitive evidence of superior outcomes compared to the currently utilized sedation techniques. It merits further interest and evaluation because it empowers patients to participate in their own care and challenges anesthetic-care providers to reevaluate sedation practices.

REFERENCES

1. ASA. Continuum of depth of sedation: definition of general anesthesia and levels of sedation/analgesia. ASA House of Delegates. 21 Oct 2009.

2. Chernik DA, Gillings D, Laine H, et al. Validity and reliability of the Observer's Assessment of Alertness/Sedation Scale: a study with intravenous midazolam. *J Clin Psychopharmacol.* 1990;10:244-251.

3. Rudkin GE, Osborne GA, Curtis NJ. Intra-operative patient-controlled sedation. *Anaesthesia.* 1991;46:90-92.

4. Park WY, Watkins PA. Patient-controlled sedation during epidural anesthesia. *Anesth Analg.* 1991;72:304-307.

5. Herrick IA, Ganapathy S, Gelb AW. Patient-controlled sedation. *Best Pract Res Clin Anaesthesiol.* 2001;15:127-135.

6. Mandel JE, Lichtenstein GR, Metz DC, Ginsberg GG, Kochman ML. A prospective, randomized, comparative trial evaluating respiratory depression during patient-controlled versus anesthesiologist-administered propofol-remifentanil sedation for elective colonoscopy. *Gastrointest Endosc.* 2010;72:112-117.

7. Rodrigo C. Patient-controlled sedation. *Anesth Prog.* 1998;45:117-126.

8. Mandel JE, Tanner JW, Lichtenstein GR, et al. A randomized, controlled, double-blind trial of patient-controlled sedation with propofol/remifentanil versus midazolam/fentanyl for colonoscopy. *Anesth Analg.* 2008;106:434-437.

9. Mazanikov M, Udd M, Kylanpaa L, et al. Patient-controlled sedation with propofol and remifentanil for ERCP: a randomized, controlled study. *Gastrointest Endosc.* 2011;73:260-266.

10. Girdler NM, Rynn D, Lyne JP, Wilson KE. A prospective randomized controlled study of patient-controlled propofol sedation in phobic dental patients. *Anaesthesia.* 2000;55:327-333.

11. Irwin MG, Thompson N, Kenny GNC. Patient-maintained propofol sedation. *Anaesthesia.* 1997;52:525-530.

12. Rodrigo MRC, Irwin MG, Tong CKA, Yan SY. A randomized crossover comparison of patient-controlled and patient-maintained sedation using propofol. *Anaesthesia.* 2003;58:333-338.

13. Anderson KJ, Leitch JA, Green JS, Kenny GN. Effect-site controlled patient maintained propofol sedation: a volunteer safety study. *Anaesthesia.* 2005;60:235-238.

14. Stonell CA, Leslie K, Absalom AR. Effect-site targeted patient-controlled sedation with propofol: comparison with anaesthetist administration for colonoscopy. *Anaesthesia.* 2006;61:240-247.

15. Herrick IA, Gelb AW, Nichols B, Kirkby J. Patient-controlled propofol sedation for elderly patients:

safety and patient attitude toward control. *Can J Anaesth*. 1996;43:1014-1018.

16. Lee DWH, Chan ACW, Sze TS, et al. Patient-controlled sedation versus intravenous sedation for colonoscopy in elderly patients: a prospective randomized controlled trial. *Gastrointest Endosc*. 2002;56:629-632.

17. Chlan LL, Weinert CR, Skaar DJ, Tracy MF. Patient-controlled sedation: a novel approach to sedation management in mechanically ventilated patients. *Chest*. 2010:138(5):1045-105.

Controversies: Ventilator Weaning—Which Strategy is Better? RT-RN Versus Physician Driven

65

Ilde Manuel Lee, MD and Louis P. Voigt, MD

INTRODUCTION

The advent of invasive mechanical ventilation (IMV) has been one of the greatest achievements in the field of respiratory and critical care medicine. In the United States alone, there were 790,257 hospitalizations involving IMV in 2005, and that number is expected to steadily increase, outpacing population growth by 2026.[1,2] Although advances in medical technology have facilitated the management of patients who require ventilatory support, mechanical ventilation remains associated with risks and complications.[3] Thus, once clinical improvement occurs, significant emphasis is placed on rapidly weaning the patient from IMV. Over the past 25 years, numerous trials have evaluated the most effective approach to liberate patients from IMV, including the use of protocol-based weaning (PBW). Compared to physician-directed weaning, protocolized strategies driven by nurses and/or respiratory therapists (RTs) have gained general acceptance in many intensive care units (ICUs) because of reduction in morbidity, mortality, and health-care costs (Table 65–1).[4-6]

PAST AND PRESENT WEANING APPROACHES

Prior to the adoption of protocols, conventional weaning was at the sole discretion of the ICU physician(s) overseeing the patient's care.[7] Conventional weaning (ie, no protocol) was highly based on clinical experiences and institutional practices. Thus, the weaning of a particular patient varied considerably among physicians and across institutions. This broad range of traditions and practice patterns underscored an imperfect process of IMV termination. Data from the mid-to-late 1990s highlighted that clinical judgment alone was not always accurate in predicting successful extubation and that physicians were more likely to keep patients on IMV for longer periods than necessary.[6,8,9]

The availability of registered nurses (RNs), RTs, and ancillary staff at the bedside in the ICU coupled with their intimate knowledge of patient's characteristics offered an alternative pathway to liberation from IMV. Subsequent efforts focused on developing conventional, structured, reproducible, and safe methods of liberating patients from IMV, not only to improve patient outcomes but also to decrease existing variations in practice among healthcare providers. Protocol-driven weaning was thus born.[4]

WEANING AND COMPONENTS OF A PROTOCOL

Liberation from IMV is a process composed of several steps including readiness testing (or *screening*), weaning (itself), and extubation.

Readiness testing (or daily screening)—The process uses several criteria to determine if a patient is ready to begin weaning or to undergo a so-called spontaneous breathing trial (SBT). The most frequent criteria include: (1) reversal of the condition(s) that prompted IMV; (2) acceptable PaO_2/FiO_2 ratio; (3) relatively low positive end-expiratory pressure (PEEP);

TABLE 65-1 Benefits of protocolized weaning.

Summary of Benefits of Protocolized Weaning	
Decreased duration of weaning	Reduced costs
Decreased duration of mechanical ventilation	Decreased barotrauma/volutrauma
Decreased ICU LOS	Decreased incidence of VILI
Decreased hospital length of stay	Decreased rates of tracheostomy
Decreased incidence of VAP	Reduced incidence of diaphragmatic dysfunction
Decreased extubation failure rates	Reduced incidence of CIPN/CIPM
Decreased mortality	Reduced incidence of delirium

ICU = intensive care unit; LOS = length of stay; VAP = ventilator-associated pneumonia; VILI = ventilator-induced lung injury; CIPN = critical illness polyneuropathy; CIPM = critical illness polymyopathy.[3,4,6,11,18,27,37]

TABLE 65-2 Commonly used daily screen criteria.[7,10,11]

Criteria for Screening	
(1) Reversal or improvement of clinical conditions that prompted IMV	Yes
(2) Ability to initiate spontaneous breaths	Yes
(3) PaO_2/FiO_2 ratio	> 200
(4) Respiratory rate	≤ 30-35
(5) PEEP	≤ 5-8 cm H_2O
(6) Mental status	Awake, oriented
(7) Hemodynamic stability	HR ≤ 110/min and either off or on low-dose VP agents

PEEP = positive end-expiratory pressure; HR = heart rate; VP = vasopressor.

(4) ability of the patient to initiate spontaneous breaths; and (5) stable hemodynamic parameters (Table 65-2).[7,9-11]

Weaning—It is the practice of either a gradual or total reduction in ventilator support during a SBT, thereby allowing patients to incrementally participate in the work of breathing.[6,8] Weaning a patient from IMV may take up to 40% of the total duration on the ventilator.[6] A SBT is often performed concurrently with daily interruption of sedation.[12] The most popular weaning models are T-piece and continuous positive airway pressure (CPAP) trials, and pressure support ventilation (PSV) either alone or in combination with synchronized intermittent mandatory ventilation (SIMV). These strategies are largely institution-dependent and currently there is no general consensus as to which particular weaning mode leads to faster extubation rates.[6,8]

Extubation—It is the physical act of removing the artificial airway (ie, endotracheal tube) from the patient. Regardless of the weaning model

chosen, extubation is considered once the patient demonstrates the ability to breathe with little or no support from the ventilator and both airway patency and protection have been established. *Liberation* and *discontinuation* of mechanical ventilation are terms used interchangeably to describe the process of *weaning* and *extubation*.[13]

A *weaning protocol* is an algorithm applied to the components of the traditional weaning process highlighted above, with the purpose of consistently identifying and determining the most appropriate time for extubation.[14] A successful protocol usually incorporates the 3 basic components mentioned (ie, daily screening, weaning and criteria for extubation) but 2-step models have also been proposed. A protocol is usually driven by a RN and/or a RT.

Finally, weaning is a fastidious process with sometimes unpredictable outcomes that are dependent on several variables. Patient-specific factors include underlying illness severity, functional status before ICU admission, and comorbid conditions. The application of evidence-based practice by healthcare providers (eg, low tidal volume ventilation strategy for acute respiratory distress syndrome, promotion of sleep hygiene, avoidance of delirium-generating medications and interventions, and early ICU mobilization) has a definite impact on weaning. In reality, some patients are easily and promptly extubated while others linger on the ventilator for long periods of time. To improve standardization, patients who undergo weaning can be classified as simple, difficult and prolonged.[15] The "simple weaning" group incorporates patients that are successfully liberated from IMV after 1 SBT. Patients in the "difficult weaning" group require up to 3 SBTs or up to 7 days on IMV (after failing the first SBT) prior to successful liberation. Those in the "prolonged weaning" group fail at least 3 SBTs and require more than 7 days of weaning before they can be successfully disconnected from the ventilator.[15,16]

EVIDENCE SUPPORTING PROTOCOL-BASED WEANING

The evidence for PBW dates back to the early 1990s. One of the earliest trials was a computer-based protocol that was compared to conventional or physician-controlled weaning. The study reported fewer arterial blood gas samples, shorter weaning times, and less time spent outside acceptable respiratory rate and tidal volume parameters in the group assigned to the computer-based protocol.[17] In 1996, Ely et al demonstrated that, compared to a physician's judgment alone, a protocol executed by nurses and RTs was superior in decreasing the total duration of IMV, associated complications, and costs.[4] Subsequent studies have shown substantial evidence in favor of nursing and/or RT-directed PBW to expedite liberation from IMV.

A 2011 Cochrane systematic review and meta-analysis of 11 randomized and quasi-randomized controlled trials (primarily RN/RT and computerized protocols) concluded that PBW resulted in a decrease in the duration of mechanical ventilation, weaning and ICU length of stay (LOS), without adverse outcomes.[18] A retrospective study of patients mechanically ventilated for more than 24 hours (at an institution with PBW) corroborated a decrease in duration of IMV and a 12.7% reintubation rate, well within the standard of 5% to 15% proposed by the multisociety task force guidelines in 2001.[9,19] Similarly, a multicenter prospective

cohort study by Teixeira et al concluded that incorporating a protocol in difficult-to-wean patients (ie, patients failing their first SBT) led to significantly higher extubation rates and improved mortality.[20] Extubation failure in the protocol group was 13.3% compared to 30.4% in the nonprotocol group.[20] Another prospective randomized controlled trial in a coronary care unit demonstrated significantly faster times to extubation and lower reintubation rates (16.7%), once protocol weaning was initiated.[21]

The majority of the early PBW trials were primarily RT/RN- or RT-driven. Recent evidence from solely RN-driven weaning has emerged (Table 65–3). Danckers et al showed that a protocol for liberation from IMV driven by ICU nurses decreased the duration of IMV and ICU LOS in patients mechanically ventilated for more than 24 hours without adverse effects and was well accepted by ICU physicians.[22]

EVIDENCE AGAINST PROTOCOL-BASED WEANING

In 2001, a study looking at a neurosurgical population found no benefit to an RT-driven protocol (compared to physician judgment alone) in terms of duration of IMV, mortality, reintubation rates, and development of ventilator-associated pneumonia (VAP).[23] Similarly, another study looking at an RT-driven protocol (vs physician judgment) in a trauma ICU also concluded no difference in outcomes (ie, self-extubation rates, ventilator days, ICU LOS, and costs).[24] Krishnan et al studied the outcomes of 2 groups of patients who required mechanical ventilation for more than 24 hours: the experimental group underwent a weaning protocol driven by RTs and/or nursing staff; weaning in the control group was managed by various physicians at different levels of training who staffed a closed ICU.[25] Reported outcomes were successful extubation, duration of mechanical ventilation, hospital mortality, ICU-LOS, and rates of reintubation. The authors reported no difference in outcomes between the 2 groups. Finally, Rose et al found no reduction in duration of IMV in surgical and trauma ICUs that compared Smartcare automated weaning versus usual care.[26]

TABLE 65-3 Summary of various studies on protocol-based weaning.

Author (Date)	Method	Protocol	Conclusions
Strickland (1993)[17]	RCT	Computerized protocol vs physician judgment	Fewer ABGs, ↓ duration MV, less variation in RR and VT parameters
Ely (1996)[4]	RCT	RN-RT driven protocol vs physician judgment	↓ duration MV, ↓ complications* ↓ cost
Kollef (1997)[5]	RCT	RN-RT driven protocol vs physician judgment	Safe; ↓ duration MV
Horst (1998)[37]	Quasi-RCT	RT driven protocol vs physician judgment	↓ duration MV, ↓ cost
Marelich (2000)[38]	RCT	RN-RT driven protocol vs physician judgment and a standardized approach	Safe; ↓ duration MV
Namen (2001)[23]	RCT	RT driven protocol vs physician judgment	No difference in outcomes
Duane (2002)[24]	Retrospective review	RT driven protocol vs physician judgment	No difference in outcomes[a]
Simeone (2002)[39]	RCT	Protocol vs physician judgment	↓ duration MV
Dries (2003)[40]	Quasi-RCT	RN-RT driven protocol vs physician judgment	↓ duration MV, ↓VAP, ↓ unplanned extubations
Krishnan (2004)[25]	RCT	RN-RT driven protocol vs physician judgment	No difference in outcomes
Tonnelier (2005)[41]	Prospective vs retrospective cohort	RN driven protocol vs physician judgment	↓ duration MV
Navalesi (2008)[42]	RCT	RN-RT driven protocol vs physician judgment	↓ reintubation rates; no effect on duration of duration of MV
Piotto (2008)[21]	RCT	RT-driven protocol vs physician judgment	↓ duration MV, ↓ reintubation rates
Rose (2008)[26]	RCT	Computerized protocol vs usual care	No difference in outcomes
Duan (2012)[43]	RCT	RT driven protocol vs physician judgment	↓ duration NIV, ↓ ICU LOS
Roh (2012)[44]	RCT	RN driven protocol vs physician judgment	↓ duration MV
Teixeria (2012)[20]	Prospective	RN-RT driven protocol vs physician judgment	↓ reintubation rates
Danckers (2013)[22]	Prospective vs retrospective cohort	RN driven protocol vs physician judgment	↓ duration MV, no adverse effects

[a]Mortality was not measured.
*Complications included: re-intubation, self-extubations, tracheostomy, mechanical ventilation > 21 days.
Note: RCT = randomized controlled trials; RN = registered nurse; RT = respiratory therapist; ABG = arterial blood gas; MV = mechanical ventilation; RR = respiratory rate; VT = tidal volume; VAP = ventilator-associated pneumonia; ICU = intnsive care unit; LOS = length of stay.

DISCUSSION—WHICH STRATEGY IS BETTER?

The study by Krishnan et al highlighted the importance of the "organizational context," which relates to factors such as staffing, "usual care," type of

ICU (surgical, medical, neurosurgical, etc), bed availability, and even an open versus a closed ICU model. It points to redundancies in hospitals and medical centers where a high staffing level is likely to promote early recognition and transition to weaning and extubation without the need for a choreographed structure.[25,26] *Usual care* refers to the customary practices performed at a particular ICU. At Johns Hopkins Hospital where the Krishnan study was conducted, high-level, evidence-based practice with 24-hour ICU physician coverage (ie, usual care) may explain the lack of difference in outcomes and the apparent ineffectiveness of PBW.[27] Protocolized weaning may be more suitable to hospitals that lack 24-hour coverage by intensivists or other physicians versed in the weaning cultures.

The *type* of ICU can play an important role in the weaning process. For example, a postanesthesia care unit (PACU) or a surgical ICU may not embrace the time-consuming and restrictive PBW. The *daily screen* is often disregarded in favor of an expeditious SBT in the majority of patients in the PACU or surgical ICU, thereby avoiding the burden of fulfilling stringent weaning criteria. No benefits were demonstrated when PBW was tried in neurosurgical and trauma ICUs, reinforcing the limitations associated with certain types of ICU.[23,24] Although safe and effective, PBW may miss many patients that could be extubated sooner than what is predicted by established protocol criteria. As previously reported, half of the patients who self-extubate prematurely, do not require reintubation within a 24-hour period.[28,29]

Another major concern regarding PBW lies in the heterogeneity of the published studies and their conflicting and inconsistent results. Hospital and ICU cultures, resources and settings heavily influence the methodology and protocol designs of these trials, resulting in a vast array of treatment algorithms. In the meta-analysis of 11 randomized controlled trials (RCTs) by Blackwood et al, readiness to wean criteria (*daily screen*) differed in every single study.[18] Likewise, there was variability in the staff members (RTs, RNs, or physicians) involved in the application of the study protocols. Of the 11 studies, only 2 employed the same weaning protocol while the remainder used different combinations of weaning methods for liberation from IMV. The weaning modality (eg, PSV, T-piece trials, SIMV, or CPAP) also differed between the studies but did not impact the process of adequately identifying prospective candidates for liberation from IMV.[10,20] The results of these studies are hardly reproducible and centers should be mindful and perform careful assessment of a protocol before its implementation.

Despite these limitations, a large body of evidence argues in favor of an RN/RT-led approach to weaning when compared to conventional (ie, no protocol) weaning by physicians (Table 65–3). Indeed, RN- and RT-directed protocols appear to be safe, beneficial and cost-effective. Certainly, healthcare providers who spend a lot of time with patients are well equipped to recognize the best time for extubation. PBW is relatively easy to incorporate into the culture of an ICU because RNs and RTs are widely available in many ICUs and they are consistently present at a patient's bedside.

RN/RT-led PBW appears ideal for patients in the "simple weaning" category and for most patients in the "difficult weaning" group. Patients in the "prolonged weaning" group and a few patients in the "difficult weaning" category should undergo further workup to identify barriers to successful liberation from IMV. Imaging studies, electromyography and nerve conduction testing, serologic markers for vasculitides, myopathies and endocrinopathies, esophageal manometry, etc may be necessary to diagnose medical conditions that impede weaning and to develop appropriate plans of treatment.[30,31]

In the past few years, a new paradigm has emerged with the concepts of *limited/no sedation* and *early ICU mobilization (early rehabilitation therapy)* as adjuncts in liberating patients faster from IMV.[32-36] A small number of RCTs and prospective studies have demonstrated that early mobilization of patients requiring mechanical ventilation was not only safe and feasible but also associated with increased ventilator-free days, shorter return time to baseline functional capacity, and reduced ICU and hospital LOS, mortality and costs.[33-35] In the majority of cases, early mobilization was possible at a median of 1.5 days (range of 1-2.1 days) after initiation of IMV.[35]

SUMMARY

Ventilator weaning protocols can aid ICU staff (physicians, RNs, and RTs) in identifying patients ready to be liberated from IMV. However, protocols have limitations. Notwithstanding, protocols are safe and, for the majority of patients, they yield real benefits that reduce morbidity, mortality and costs. RNs and RTs play an instrumental role in successful

PBW strategies but the appropriate weaning strategy is likely dependent on the available resources at a specific institution. We advocate RN/RT PBW for patients in the "simple" and "difficult" to wean groups in hospitals that have limited human and financial resources. At our institution, we use a wide-ranging integrative approach of limited sedation and early mobilization that involves physicians at different levels of experience (ie, residents, fellows, and full-time intensivists), critical care RNs, nurse practitioners, physician assistants, RTs, and physical and occupational therapists to determine readiness to wean and achieve liberation from IMV. We have achieved great success without the need for a specific weaning protocol.

REFERENCES

1. Wunsch H, Linde-Zwirble WT, Angus DC, Hartman ME, Milbrandt EB, Kahn JM. The epidemiology of mechanical ventilation use in the United States. *Crit Care Med.* 2010;38(10):1947-1953.
2. Needham DM, Bronskill SE, Calinawan JR, Sibbald WJ, Pronovost PJ, Laupacis A. Projected incidence of mechanical ventilation in Ontario to 2026: preparing for the aging baby boomers. *Crit Care Med.* 2005;33(3):574-579.
3. Kollef MH. Ventilator-associated complications, including infection-related complications: the way forward. *Crit Care Clin.* 2013;29(1):33-50.
4. Ely EW, Baker AM, Dunagan DP, et al. Effect on the duration of mechanical ventilation of identifying patients capable of breathing spontaneously. *N Engl J Med.* 1996;335(25):1864-1869.
5. Kollef MH, Shapiro SD, Silver P, et al. A randomized, controlled trial of protocol-directed versus physician-directed weaning from mechanical ventilation. *Crit Care Med.* 1997;25(4):567-574.
6. Esteban A, Frutos F, Tobin MJ, et al. A comparison of four methods of weaning patients from mechanical ventilation. Spanish Lung Failure Collaborative Group. *N Engl J Med.* 1995;332(6):345-350.
7. Calhoun CJ, Specht NL. Standardizing the weaning process. *AACN Clin Issues Crit Care Nurs.* 1991;2(3): 398-404.
8. Brochard L, Rauss A, Benito S, et al. Comparison of three methods of gradual withdrawal from ventilatory support during weaning from mechanical ventilation. *Am J Respir Crit Care Med.* 1994;150(4):896-903.
9. MacIntyre NR, Cook DJ, Ely EW, Jr, et al. Evidence-based guidelines for weaning and discontinuing ventilatory support: a collective task force facilitated by the American College of Chest Physicians; the American Association for Respiratory Care; and the American College of Critical Care Medicine. *Chest.* 2001;120(6 Suppl):375s-395s.
10. MacIntyre N. Discontinuing mechanical ventilatory support. *Chest.* 2007;132(3):1049-1056.
11. Haas CF, Loik PS. Ventilator discontinuation protocols. *Respir Care.* 2012;57(10):1649-1662.
12. Girard TD, Kress JP, Fuchs BD, et al. Efficacy and safety of a paired sedation and ventilator weaning protocol for mechanically ventilated patients in intensive care (Awakening and Breathing Controlled trial): a randomised controlled trial. *Lancet.* 2008;371(9607):126-134.
13. Hall JB, Wood LD. Liberation of the patient from mechanical ventilation. *JAMA.* 1987;257(12):1621-1628.
14. Manthous CA, Amoateng-Adjepong Y. Weaning by protocol. *Am J Respir Crit Care Med.* 2004;170(1):98-99.
15. Boles JM, Bion J, Connors A, et al. Weaning from mechanical ventilation. *Eur Respir J.* 2007;29(5):1033-1056.
16. Funk GC, Anders S, Breyer MK, et al. Incidence and outcome of weaning from mechanical ventilation according to new categories. *Eur Respir J.* 2010;35(1):88-94.
17. Strickland JH, Jr, Hasson JH. A computer-controlled ventilator weaning system. A clinical trial. *Chest.* 1993;103(4):1220-1226.
18. Blackwood B, Alderdice F, Burns K, Cardwell C, Lavery G, O'Halloran P. Use of weaning protocols for reducing duration of mechanical ventilation in critically ill adult patients: Cochrane systematic review and meta-analysis. *BMJ.* 2011;342:c7237.
19. Silva CS, Timenetsky KT, Taniguchi C, et al. Low mechanical ventilation times and reintubation rates associated with a specific weaning protocol in an intensive care unit setting: a retrospective study. *Clinics (Sao Paulo).* 2012;67(9):995-1000.
20. Teixeira C, Maccari JG, Vieira SR, et al. Impact of a mechanical ventilation weaning protocol on the extubation failure rate in difficult-to-wean patients. *J Bras Pneumol.* 2012;38(3):364-371.
21. Piotto RF, Maia LN, Machado MN, Orrico SP. Effects of the use of mechanical ventilation weaning protocol in the Coronary Care Unit: randomized study. *Rev Bras Cir Cardiovasc.* 2011;26(2):213-221.
22. Danckers M, Grosu H, Jean R, et al. Nurse-driven, protocol-directed weaning from mechanical

ventilation improves clinical outcomes and is well accepted by intensive care unit physicians. *J Crit Care*. 2013;28(4):433-441.

23. Namen AM, Ely EW, Tatter SB, et al. Predictors of successful extubation in neurosurgical patients. *Am J Respir Crit Care Med*. 2001;163(3 Pt 1): 658-664.

24. Duane TM, Riblet JL, Golay D, Cole FJ, Jr, Weireter LJ, Jr, Britt LD. Protocol-driven ventilator management in a trauma intensive care unit population. *Arch Surg*. 2002;137(11):1223-1227.

25. Krishnan JA, Moore D, Robeson C, Rand CS, Fessler HE. A prospective, controlled trial of a protocol-based strategy to discontinue mechanical ventilation. *Am J Respir Crit Care Med*. 2004;169(6):673-678.

26. Rose L, Presneill JJ, Johnston L, Cade JF. A randomised, controlled trial of conventional versus automated weaning from mechanical ventilation using SmartCare/PS. *Intensive Care Med*. 2008;34(10):1788-1795.

27. Pronovost PJ, Angus DC, Dorman T, Robinson KA, Dremsizov TT, Young TL. Physician staffing patterns and clinical outcomes in critically ill patients: a systematic review. *JAMA*. 2002;288(17):2151-2162.

28. Listello D, Sessler CN. Unplanned extubation. Clinical predictors for reintubation. *Chest*. 1994;105(5):1496-1503.

29. Epstein SK, Nevins ML, Chung J. Effect of unplanned extubation on outcome of mechanical ventilation. *Am J Respir Crit Care Med*. 2000;161(6):1912-1916.

30. Manthous CA, Schmidt GA, Hall JB. Liberation from mechanical ventilation: a decade of progress. *Chest*. 1998;114(3):886-901.

31. Akoumianaki E, Maggiore SM, Valenza F, et al. The application of esophageal pressure measurement in patients with respiratory failure. *Am J Respir Crit Care Med*. 2014;189(5):520-531.

32. Strom T, Martinussen T, Toft P. A protocol of no sedation for critically ill patients receiving mechanical ventilation: a randomised trial. *Lancet*. 2010;375(9713):475-480.

33. Morris PE, Goad A, Thompson C, et al. Early intensive care unit mobility therapy in the treatment of acute respiratory failure. *Crit Care Med*. 2008;36(8):2238-2243.

34. Needham DM, Korupolu R, Zanni JM, et al. Early physical medicine and rehabilitation for patients with acute respiratory failure: a quality improvement project. *Arch Phys Med Rehabil*. 2010; 91(4):536-542.

35. Schweickert WD, Pohlman MC, Pohlman AS, et al. Early physical and occupational therapy in mechanically ventilated, critically ill patients: a randomised controlled trial. *Lancet*. 2009;373(9678):1874-1882.

36. Pandharipande PP, Girard TD, Jackson JC, et al. Long-term cognitive impairment after critical illness. *N Engl J Med*. 2013;369(14):1306-1316.

37. Horst HM, Mouro D, Hall-Jenssens RA, Pamukov N. Decrease in ventilation time with a standardized weaning process. *Arch Surg*. 1998;133(5):483-488.

38. Marelich GP, Murin S, Battistella F, Inciardi J, Vierra T, Roby M. Protocol weaning of mechanical ventilation in medical and surgical patients by respiratory care practitioners and nurses: effect on weaning time and incidence of ventilator-associated pneumonia. *Chest*. 2000;118(2):459-467.

39. Simeone F, Biagioli B, Scolletta S, et al. Optimization of mechanical ventilation support following cardiac surgery. *J Cardiovasc Surg (Torino)*. 2002;43(5):633-641.

40. Dries DJ, McGonigal MD, Malian MS, Bor BJ, Sullivan C. Protocol-driven ventilator weaning reduces use of mechanical ventilation, rate of early reintubation, and ventilator-associated pneumonia. *J Trauma*. 2004;56(5):943-951.

41. Tonnelier JM, Prat G, Le Gal G, et al. Impact of a nurses' protocol-directed weaning procedure on outcomes in patients undergoing mechanical ventilation for longer than 48 hours: a prospective cohort study with a matched historical control group. *Crit Care*. 2005;9(2):R83-R89.

42. Navalesi P, Frigerio P, Moretti MP, et al. Rate of reintubation in mechanically ventilated neurosurgical and neurologic patients: evaluation of a systematic approach to weaning and extubation. *Crit Care Med*. 2008;36(11):2986-2992.

43. Duan J, Tang X, Huang S, Jia J, Guo S. Protocol-directed versus physician-directed weaning from noninvasive ventilation: the impact in chronic obstructive pulmonary disease patients. *J Trauma Acute Care Surg*. 2012;72(5):1271-1275.

44. Roh JH, Synn A, Lim CM, et al. A weaning protocol administered by critical care nurses for the weaning of patients from mechanical ventilation. *J Crit Care*. 2012;27(6):549-555.

Controversies: Invasive Versus Noninvasive Strategy for Diagnosing Respiratory Failure

Anil Singh, MD and Stephen M. Pastores, MD, FACP, FCCP, FCCM

INTRODUCTION

The etiology of acute respiratory failure (ARF) among different patient populations is highly variable.[1] In general, pulmonary infections are the leading cause of ARF followed by heart failure, exacerbation of chronic obstructive pulmonary disease (COPD), and sepsis.[2] Early and appropriate diagnostic strategies are vital for the initial choice of therapy and subsequent treatment decisions. With advances in medicine, aggressive treatments have been introduced to achieve the highest possible cure which in turn, has resulted in the concomitant rise in the incidence of life-threatening toxic and infectious complications, particularly involving the lungs.

There are many practical questions surrounding the diagnostic work-up of critically ill patients with ARF. What is the utility of noninvasive testing? Is empiric treatment enough? What are the risks and benefits of invasive diagnostic procedures? Does invasive testing result in improved outcomes? To answer these questions, a review of the literature has produced mixed results. The apparent dilemma between the need to identify the cause of ARF and complications associated with invasive procedures may have created this uncertainty. To this end, there is some data in hematology and oncology patients which can only be extrapolated to other groups of immunocompromised hosts for whom further testing guided by clinical and epidemiologic data may reveal unsuspected diagnoses. In this chapter, we discuss the utility of noninvasive and invasive testing for diagnosing ARF and provide a diagnostic algorithm based on the best available data (Figure 66–1).

NONINVASIVE STRATEGY

This approach consists of obtaining chest imaging studies, cardiac biomarkers (eg, B-type natriuretic peptide) and echocardiography to exclude cardiogenic pulmonary edema, and serologic and microbiologic studies of sputum, nasopharyngeal (NP) aspirates, blood, and urine to diagnose infection. In addition, newer molecular techniques are being implemented along with conventional methods in order to identify specific pathogens not only faster but more accurately without exposing patients to additional risks.

The most commonly performed noninvasive tests for diagnosing ARF are shown in Table 66–1.

Important causes of ARF such as sepsis, aspiration pneumonia, diffuse alveolar hemorrhage, eosinophilic pneumonia, transfusion-related lung injuries and respiratory failure associated with cancer and other immunocompromised states are diagnosed clinically using a constellation of radiographic and other ancillary investigations.

The clinical presentation of suspected pulmonary infections is usually nonspecific. This is particularly important in immunocompromised patients who are prone to develop pulmonary infections with certain pathogens such as herpes simplex virus, *Cytomegalovirus* (CMV), *Pneumocystis jirovecii* (PCP), *Mycobacterium tuberculosis*, and *Aspergillus* species and hence require specific diagnosis and treatment as opposed to empiric therapy.

Gram stain of respiratory secretions, available within a few hours, may help in narrowing or broadening the antimicrobial spectrum but lacks

Diagnostic Algorithm

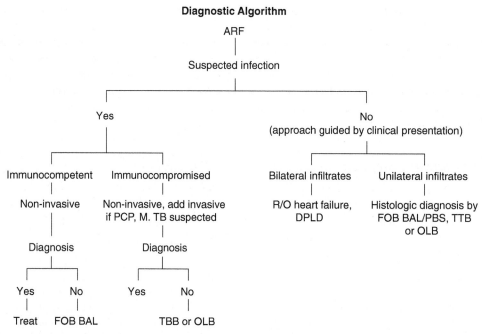

FIGURE 66-1 Diagnostic algorithm for diagnosing acute respiratory failure.
(ARF = acute respiratory failure; FOB = fiberoptic bronchoscopy; BAL = bronchoalveolar lavage; PCP = Pneumocystis jiroveci; MTB = Mycobacterium tuberculosis; TBB = transbronchial biopsy; PBS = protected brush specimen; OLB = open lung biopsy; DPLD = diffuse parenchymal lung disease)

TABLE 66-1   Noninvasive tests for diagnosing acute respiratory failure.

Investigation	Diagnosis/Specific Pathogen
Imaging (chest radiograph, high-resolution CT, chest ultrasound)	Pattern of different radiologic findings may help in narrowing differential diagnosis
Transthoracic echocardiogram	Congestive heart failure, cardiac tamponade, pulmonary embolism
Expectorated sputum	Bacteria (*S pneumoniae, Staphylococcus aureus, Hemophilus influenza, Enterobacteriaceae, Pseudomonas*), *Candida*, other fungi (*Histoplasma, Coccidioides*) and *M tuberculosis*
Induced sputum (smear and cultures)	*P jiroveci, M tuberculosis*
Nasopharyngeal aspirates	*Respiratory viruses, S pneumoniae*
Blood cultures	Various pulmonary infections
Polymerase chain reaction	*Herpes, Cytomegalovirus, P. jiroveci, M. tuberculosis*
Circulating antigens	*Aspergillus, P. jirovecii*
Serum immunoglobulins	*Chlamydia, Mycoplasma, Legionella*
Urine antigens	*Legionella, S pneumoniae*
Pleural fluid analysis (chemistry, microbiology, cytology and other ancillary tests)	Malignancy, pulmonary embolism, collagen vascular disease, pancreatitis, uremia, yellow nail syndrome, sarcoidosis

sensitivity and specificity. Similarly, the yield of conventional stains for the diagnosis of other infections such yeast, other fungi, *Aspergillus*, *M tuberculosis*, and PCP pneumonia have been disappointing and slow which has led to a greater reliance on polymerase chain reaction (PCR)-based techniques. The latter has provided improved insight into the biology and genomic structure of the pathogens.

Azoulay et al[3] performed a multicenter randomized controlled trial (RCT) comparing noninvasive testing (of sputum, induced sputum, NP aspirates, serum and urine as well as chest imaging and echocardiography) with an invasive strategy involving fiberoptic bronchoscopy with bronchoalveolar lavage (FOB-BAL) in 219 hematology and oncology patients with ARF. Bacterial infection was the primary etiology of ARF followed by infections with viruses, yeasts and molds, or *Pneumocystis*. Noninvasive testing provided the diagnosis in 71% of cases and resulted in a change in management in 44% of patients compared to only 34% in those who underwent FOB-BAL. In 20% of cases, no diagnosis was made with either strategy. Additionally, the time to diagnosis of bacterial, non-*Aspergillus*, and viral infection was shorter and available quicker with noninvasive testing as compared to invasive testing. However, the diagnosis of PCP took longer in the noninvasive group (3 [-7] days vs 1 [0-1] day). In both groups, a specific diagnosis was established in 80% of cases. These diagnostic rates were significantly higher than those reported in the earlier observational study conducted by the same authors suggesting the improved utility and advances in noninvasive testing in recent years.[4]

The sensitivity of nasal swab and NP aspirate is comparable for all respiratory viruses except for the detection of respiratory syncytial virus due to the inherent lability and relatively lower viral load present in the nasopharynx.[5] Although serologic testing for CMV IgM and IgG may be used to screen for primary CMV infection or exposure, this is not used for the diagnosis of active CMV infection. Viral load testing in serum, tissue specimens, or BAL fluid using both quantitative nucleic acid amplification testing (QNAT) and antigenemia testing are currently the cornerstone for diagnosis and monitoring for CMV infection and disease.[6] Real-time QNAT testing for CMV is now the standard of care given

its better precision, broader linear range, faster turnaround time, higher throughput, and less risk of contamination compared with conventional PCR tests. In contrast, the antigenemia test is labor intensive, lacks a standardized cutoff value, and the assay performance diminishes when the absolute neutrophil count is less than $1000/mm^3$.[6]

Streptococcus pneumoniae urinary antigen has sensitivity of up to 78% in nonbacteremic patients and 80% in bacteremic cases and a specificity of more than 90% in adults. However, there have been false-positive reports of pneumococcal infection rates ranging from 21% to 54% in children with NP carriage and no evidence of disease.[7] This limitation may be overcome with quantitative real-time PCR testing of NP swab samples to estimate NP colonization density and using cutoff values more than or equal to 8000 copies/mL, which improved the sensitivity to 82% and specificity to 92% for distinguishing pneumococcal pneumonia from asymptomatic colonization.[8] Similarly, detection of *Legionella pneumophila* antigen in urine is rapidly available and requires no specialized laboratory equipment. Sensitivity rates of 73% and 77%, respectively, were reported for the new Meridian TRU Legionella assay and BINAX urinary antigen test. Additionally, the sensitivity of the Meridian TRU Legionella test increased to 81% after 60 minutes of incubation.[9]

PCP cannot be cultured and hence diagnosis relies on visualization of the fungus on microscopic examination of respiratory specimens. The sensitivity of microscopy varies according to the staining technique and type of respiratory sample used. In one study, the sensitivity and specificity of Grocott–Gomori methenamine silver stain for PCP were 79.4% and 99.2%, respectively.[10] A serum assay for beta glucan, a cell wall component of most pathogenic fungi, is currently being used for PCP diagnosis with sensitivity and specificity rates of 100% and 96.4%, respectively, using a cut off value of 100 pg/mL.[11] In a select group of patients the yield of induced sputum-PCR assay for detection of PCP has been shown to be excellent with sensitivity of 100% and specificity of 90% which would make FOB-BAL or lung biopsy practically unnecessary.[12] Of note, respiratory specimens should be collected before or immediately after initiation of therapy because the sputum-PCR assay for detection of PCP may turn negative quickly. A negative PCR may allow for the discontinuation of anti-PCP therapy.[12]

Both direct microscopy and cultures are insensitive methods to diagnose aspergillosis. Galactomannan is an *Aspergillus*-specific polysaccharide which is released during *Aspergillus* growth at the site of infection. This antigen can be detected by quantitative serum galactomannan index and is used as a biomarker of the disease. In addition, galactomannan antigen has a strong correlation with clinical outcome; thus the test is currently repeated frequently during the course of treatment. In contrast, the presence and magnitude of the galactomannan index in BAL fluid does not have any mortality implication.[13] In a study of 500 patients, the diagnostic yield of acid-fast bacilli (AFB) smear, cultures and PCR of induced sputum for *M. tuberculosis* was increased consistently with repeated induction from 64%, 70%, and 89% for AFB smear, and from cultures and PCR, respectively, to 98%, 100%, and 100% on fourth induction.[14] Current amplification techniques can detect *M. tuberculosis* and rifampin resistance directly from clinical specimens in approximately 2 hours with high sensitivity compared to the standard method.[15]

Early molecular detection methods are currently under development. With regards to bacterial pathogens, multiplex amplification assays might include frequently involved microorganisms. Despite the obvious advantages of PCR-based methods (rapidity, sensitivity, convenience), several limitations including the need of cut-off levels to distinguish between colonization and infection, the inability to detect living viruses from prolonged harmless shedding, lack of information about the antibiotic susceptibility and the high cost of these tests still limits their widespread use in clinical decision making. Moreover, studies measuring clinical outcomes and mortality benefits are lacking at this time. These limitations in diagnostic testing with noninvasive strategies have led to the development of antimicrobial guidelines for empiric treatment.[16] At this time, PCR-based testing can supplement rather than replace culture-based methods for pathogens where antibiotic resistance is a concern.

INVASIVE STRATEGY

This approach relies on FOB-BAL and/or protected brush specimens (PBS), transbronchial biopsy (TBB) and lung biopsy (open or video assisted). FOB-BAL and/or PBS permit collection of distal airway secretions with minimal oropharyngeal contamination which is inevitable during specimen collection.

The reported diagnostic yield of FOB in different studies has been variable. This is attributed to the heterogeneity of the patient population, severity of illnesses, regional differences, timing, and techniques of FOB-BAL and/or PBS.[17,18] A summary of these studies is shown in Table 66–2.

In a prospective study of 101 immunocompromised patients with suspected pneumonia, 80% of whom had human immunodeficiency virus infection and/or acquired immunodeficiency syndrome, hematologic and solid organ malignancies, chronic steroid use and neutropenia, FOB-BAL/TBB had a general diagnostic yield of 52% but 76% in infectious diseases.[19] Mycobacterial infections accounted for one third of infections followed by bacterial pathogens and PCP. In contrast, the diagnostic yield of FOB in immunocompetent patients is lower. In one study of nonselected patients, the diagnostic yield of FOB was 53% in immunocompromised patients versus only 19% in immunocompetent patients suggesting that the need of invasive testing in the latter group must be established based on clinical importance and risks of the procedure.[20] The yield was further decreased if patients received antibiotics prior to bronchoscopy. Complications were seen in 5 patients (12%) with a higher proportion of minor self-limited bleeding ($n = 3$), pulmonary edema ($n = 1$), and cardiac arrhythmias ($n = 1$).[20]

In a retrospective study of 501 patients who underwent hematopoietic stem cell transplantation, the mortality rate was lower in the early (< 4 days) FOB-BAL group (6%) versus 14% to the late FOB group (> 5 days). The overall diagnostic yield for clinically significant pathogens was 55% and was highest (75%) if the FOB-BAL was performed with 24 hours.[21] Similarly, a multicenter RCT in patients with suspected hospital-acquired pneumonia (HAP) where an invasive strategy (direct examination of FOB-BAL or PSB samples and quantitative cultures)

TABLE 66–2 Summary of studies comparing noninvasive versus invasive strategy for diagnosing acute respiratory failure.

Authors	Study Design	Patient Population	Results
Jain P, et al[18]	Observational study	Non-HIV infected immunocompromised patients ($n = 104$)	Overall diagnostic yield of FOB: 56.2% (81% yield for an infectious cause vs 56% for a noninfectious cause) FOB+TBB yield: 70% Complication rate: 21%: minor bleeding (13%); pneumothorax (4%)
Azoulay E, et al[3]	RCT	Nonintubated cancer patients ($n = 219$)	Diagnostic yield of FOB-BAL 34% vs 71% with noninvasive tests
Velez L, et al[19]	Prospective study	Immunocompromised predominantly AIDS patients ($n = 101$)	Diagnostic yield of FOB-BAL: 51% (infections accounted for 65%)
Ekdahl K, et al[20]	Prospective study	Nonselected patients ($n = 53$)	Diagnostic yield of FOB 53% in immunocompromised vs 19% in immunocompetent patients
Fagon JY, et al[22]	Randomized uncontrolled trial	Patients suspected of VAP ($n = 413$) FOB BAL/PBS vs nonquantitative endotracheal aspirate cultures	Invasive group had reduced mortality at 14 days (16.2% vs 25.8%) More antibiotic-free days (11.5 ± 9.0 days compared with 7.5 ± 7.6 days)
Papazian L, et al[23]	Prospective study	Medical-surgical patients with negative BAL ($n = 100$) Open lung biopsy performed after 5 days of no improvement of ARDS	Fibrosis 53% (fibrosis with infection 55%) Miscellaneous 14%: systemic lupus erythematosus, rheumatoid arthritis lung, drug toxicity, allograft rejection, lung cancer Complications: 2 pneumothoraces and 8 moderate airleaks
Shannon VR, et al[21]	Retrospective study	HSCT patients < 100 days ($n = 501$) Impact of early vs late FOB (< 4 days vs > 5 days)	Diagnostic yield of FOB-BAL 55%; highest yield (75%) within 24 hour 30-day mortality was 6% in early FOB group vs 14% in late FOB

HIV = human immunodeficiency virus; FOB = fiberoptic bronchoscopy; TBB = transbronchial biopsy; RCT = randomized controlled trial; AIDS = acquired immunodeficiency syndrome; BAL = bronchoalveolar lavage; VAP = ventilator-associated pneumonia; PBS = protected brush specimen; ARDS = acute respiratory distress syndrome; HSCT = hematopoietic stem cell transplant

was utilized compared with patients managed clinically, showed that the invasive approach was associated with reduction in mortality on day 14 (16% vs 25%), decreased organ dysfunction score on day 3 and 7, less use of antibiotics, mean number of antibiotic-free days (7 ± 7 vs 11± 9 days).[22]

Reliance on semiquantitative cultures from endotracheal aspirates which may not distinguish a true pathogen from a colonizer, can lead to more or broader antibiotic use and potential delay in the diagnosis of extrapulmonary infection. Thus, semiquantitative cultures of tracheal aspirates cannot be used reliably as quantitative cultures to define the presence of pneumonia and the need for antibiotic

therapy.[16] However, it is recommended that patients with community-acquired pneumonia should be investigated for specific pathogens only if it would alter the standard (empiric) management decisions when the presence of such pathogen is suspected based on the clinical and epidemiologic clues.[16] For example, such alteration in therapy is likely to benefit patients with psittacosis, tularemia, endemic fungi, *M. tuberculosis* or antibiotic resistance issues.

FOB-BAL is also favored in the presence of noninfectious pulmonary infiltrates causing ARF since as described previously, noninfectious disorders explained most of the missed diagnoses.[3,19] In addition, transbronchial or surgical open lung biopsy

(OLB) may be considered in select patients to obtain a definitive diagnosis and guide therapy when it is believed to make a substantial impact in the management and improvement in the prognosis. These include patients with suspected cryptogenic organizing pneumonia, fungal lung infections, and acute exacerbation of a chronic interstitial lung disease, vasculitis, or disseminated cancer. In a prospective study of 100 nonselected patients with ARF of unknown etiology after a negative BAL, OLB provided a contributive result in 78% of patients. A change in the management was associated with improved survival to 67% compared to 14% when OLB did not help in management. The most common diagnoses obtained by OLB were fibrosis associated with infections (55%), followed by pulmonary infections (42%) (CMV, herpes, *M. tuberculosis*, invasive aspergillosis) and miscellaneous diagnoses such as systemic lupus erythematosus, bronchoalveolar carcinoma, intraalveolar hemorrhage, drug toxicity, and carcinomatous lymphangitis.[23]

FOB is commonly associated with alteration in gas exchange; however, hypoxemia is usually mild and transient.[24] The severity of hypoxemia during bronchoscopy may vary depending on the patient's comorbid conditions, indications of the procedure and the type of bronchoscopic interventions performed. The risk of hypoxemia may be further decreased when using noninvasive ventilation and/or target controlled sedation during bronchoscopy which have both been shown to not only limit discomfort but also reduce the subsequent respiratory worsening.[25] In various studies, the risk of FOB-BAL has been proven to be small with no effect on outcome.[3,26] In few selected patients, the diagnostic yield improves if FOB-BAL is performed in the ICU within 24 hours of admission; thereafter, this benefit seems to fade with less favorable risk/benefit ratio.[3]

A multicenter prospective observational study evaluated the safety of FOB in critically ill non-intubated patients with hypoxemic ARF due to a variety of causes including immunodeficiency (37%), atelectasis (29%), healthcare-associated pneumonia (27%), acute diffuse pneumonia (27%), community-acquired pneumonia (12%), hemoptysis (3%), suspected malignancy (3%), and chronic diffuse infiltrative pneumonia (1%). The patients had a PaO_2/FiO_2 ratio of less than 300 and were on noninvasive ventilation or receiving oxygen supplementation of more than 8 L/min. FOB provided the diagnosis in 59% of cases with subsequent change in the management in 51% of patients. Factors independently associated with the need of invasive ventilatory support were COPD and cancer but not the extent of radiologic opacities, PaO_2/FiO_2 ratio, BAL, or injected BAL volume. The overall incremental risk associated with bronchoscopy is small and has no effect on mortality. It is generally considered safe with arterial oxygen saturation more than 90% on FiO_2 of less than 0.5 and PaO_2 more than 60 mm Hg.

SUMMARY

Recent advances in the sensitivity and specificity of noninvasive diagnostic investigations may change the risk/benefit ratio in favor of conservative noninvasive testing in patients with ARF. However, a subset of patients may still benefit from the addition of FOB-BAL when performed safely in addition to noninvasive testing, particularly when protective procedural strategies such as noninvasive ventilation and/or targeted controlled sedation are used. It is hoped that further refinement of molecular techniques and their enhanced diagnostic yield will decrease the need for invasive procedures in the future. Current evidence suggests that noninvasive and invasive strategies both offer benefits and complement each other. The main consideration in deciding which approach to take is the influence any result would have on management. Noninvasive tests are generally useful in determining the accurate diagnosis in immunocompromised patients. On the other hand, FOB-BAL and other invasive techniques have an advantage especially in the setting of suspected *M. tuberculosis*, PCP, malignancy and interstitial lung diseases. Invasive testing should be reserved for immuncompetent patients only when conservative techniques are likely to miss the diagnosis. We conclude that an individualized approach based on available clinical information and epidemiologic data should facilitate the relevant use of noninvasive and/or invasive testing for diagnosing ARF.

REFERENCES

1. Pastores SM, Voigt LP. Acute respiratory failure in the patient with cancer: diagnostic and management strategies. *Crit Care Clin*. 2010;26(1):21-40.

2. Stefan MS, Shieh MS, Pekow PS, et al. Epidemiology and outcomes of acute respiratory failure in the United States, 2001-2009: a national survey. *J Hosp Med*. 2013;8(2):76-82.

3. Azoulay E, Mokart D, Lambert J, et al. Diagnostic strategy for hematology and oncology patients with acute respiratory failure: randomized controlled trial. *Am J Respir Crit Care Med*. 2010;182(8):1038-1046.

4. Azoulay E, Mokart D, Rabbat A, et al. Diagnostic bronchoscopy in hematology and oncology patients with acute respiratory failure: prospective multicenter data. *Crit Care Med*. 2008;36(1):100-107.

5. Englund JA, Piedra PA, Jewell A, Patel K, Baxter BB, Whimbey E. Rapid diagnosis of respiratory syncytial virus infections in immunocompromised adults. *J Clin Microbiol*. 1996;34(7):1649-1653.

6. Kotton CN, Kumar D, Caliendo AM, et al. Updated international consensus guidelines on the management of cytomegalovirus in solid-organ transplantation. *Transplantation*. 2013;96:333-360.

7. Anh DD, Huong Ple T, Watanabe K, et al. Increased rates of intense nasopharyngeal bacterial colonization of Vietnamese children with radiological pneumonia. *Tohoku J Exp Med*. 2007;213:167-172.

8. Albrich WC, Madhi SA, Adrian PV, et al. Use of a rapid test of pneumococcal colonization density to diagnose pneumococcal pneumonia. *Clin Infect Dis*. 2012;54(5):601-609.

9. Bruin JP, Diederen BM. Evaluation of Meridian TRU Legionella®, a new rapid test for detection of Legionella pneumophila serogroup 1 antigen in urine samples. *Eur J Clin Microbiol Infect Dis*. 2013;32(3):333-334.

10. Procop GW, Haddad S, Quinn J, et al. Detection of Pneumocystis jiroveci in respiratory specimens by four staining methods. *J Clin Microbiol*. 2004;42(7):3333-3335.

11. Desmet S, Van Wijngaerden E, Maertens J, et al. Serum (1-3)-beta-D-glucan as a tool for diagnosis of Pneumocystis jiroveci pneumonia in patients with human immunodeficiency virus infection or hematological malignancy. *J Clin Microbiol*. 2009;47(12):3871-3874.

12. Azoulay E, Bergeron A, Chevret S, Bele N, Schlemmer B, Menotti J. Polymerase chain reaction for diagnosing Pneumocystis pneumonia in non-HIV immunocompromised patients with pulmonary infiltrates. *Chest*. 2009;135(3):655-661.

13. Fisher CE, Stevens AM, Leisenring W, Pergam SA, Boeckh M, Hohl TM. The serum galactomannan index predicts mortality in hematopoietic stem cell transplant recipients with invasive aspergillosis. *Clin Infect Dis*. 2013;57(7):1001-1004.

14. Al zahrani K, Al Jahdali H, Poirier L, René P, Menzies D. Yield of smear, culture and amplification tests from repeated sputum induction for the diagnosis of pulmonary tuberculosis. *Int J Tuberc Lung Dis*. 2001;5(9):855-860.

15. Dorman SE, Chihota VN, Lewis JJ, et al. Performance characteristics of the Cepheid Xpert MTB/RIF test in a tuberculosis prevalence survey. *PLoS One*. 2012;7(8):e43307.

16. American Thoracic Society; Infectious Diseases Society of America. Guidelines for the management of adults with hospital-acquired, ventilator-associated, and healthcare-associated pneumonia. *Am J Respir Crit Care Med*. 2005;171(4):388-416.

17. Pisani RJ, Wright AJ. Clinical utility of bronchoalveolar lavage in immunocompromised hosts. *Mayo Clin Proc*. 1992;67(3):221-227.

18. Jain P, Sandur S, Meli Y, Arroliga AC, Stoller JK, Mehta AC. Role of flexible bronchoscopy in immunocompromised patients with lung infiltrates. *Chest*. 2004;125(2):712-722.

19. Vélez L, Correa LT, Maya MA, et al. Diagnostic accuracy of bronchoalveolar lavage samples in immunosuppressed patients with suspected pneumonia: analysis of a protocol. *Respir Med*. 2007;101(10):2160-2167.

20. Ekdahl K, Eriksson L, Rollof J, Miörner H, Griph H, Löfgren B. Bronchoscopic diagnosis of pulmonary infections in a heterogeneous, nonselected group of patients. *Chest*. 1993;103(6):1743-1748.

21. Shannon VR, Andersson BS, Lei X, Champlin RE, Kontoyiannis DP. Utility of early versus late fiberoptic bronchoscopy in the evaluation of new pulmonary infiltrates following hematopoietic stem cell transplantation. *Bone Marrow Transplant*. 2010;45(4):647-655.

22. Fagon JY, Chastre J, Wolff M, et al. Invasive and noninvasive strategies for management of suspected ventilator-associated pneumonia. a randomized trial. *Ann Intern Med*. 2000;132(8):621-630.

23. Papazian L, Doddoli C, Chetaille B, et al. A contributive result of open-lung biopsy improves survival in acute respiratory distress syndrome patients. *Crit Care Med*. 2007;35(3):755-762.

24. Trouillet JL, Guiguet M, Gibert C, et al. Fiberoptic bronchoscopy in ventilated patients. Evaluation of cardiopulmonary risk under midazolam sedation. *Chest.* 1990;97(4):927-933.

25. Clouzeau B, Bui HN, Guilhon E, et al. Fiberoptic bronchoscopy under noninvasive ventilation and propofol target-controlled infusion in hypoxemic patients. *Intensive Care Med.* 2011;37(12):1969-1975.

26. Cracco C, Fartoukh M, Prodanovic H, et al. Safety of performing fiberoptic bronchoscopy in critically ill hypoxemic patients with acute respiratory failure. *Intensive Care Med.* 2013;39(1):45-52.

"Controversies: Ventilator Management in ARDS: One Size Fits All?"

Muhammad Adrish, MD and Graciela J. Soto, MD, MS

KEY POINTS

1 The pathophysiologic changes in the acute respiratory distress syndrome (ARDS) produce low-compliant lungs containing areas of atelectasis and reduced lung volumes.

2 Positive pressure ventilation in this heterogenous syndrome can lead to overdistension of normally aerated lung regions and stress injury in atelectatic alveoli due to cyclic recruitment and derecruitment.

3 Use of low-tidal-volume ventilation as lung-protection strategy has been studied since 1960s. Despite suggested benefits, concerns regarding additional metabolic abnormalities and hypoxemia in critically ill patients have existed.

4 Results of the landmark ARDS in a large multicentre randomized trial found that the use of low tidal volume (6 mL/kg ideal body weight [IBW]) rather than "standard"

tidal volume (12 mL/kg IBW) significantly reduced mortality. Although the trial was criticized for using excessively large tidal volumes in controls, the trial investigators subsequently published trial data detailing the clinical benefits of tidal volume and plateau pressure reduction across the range of disease severity and plateau pressures.

5 Recent data suggest that many mechanically ventilated patients with ARDS have stress index that indicates alveolar hyperventilation while receiving positive end-expiratory pressure (PEEP) according to the ARDS Network recommendation, advocating even lower tidal volumes.

6 Use of adjunct therapies such as extracorporeal membrane oxygenation may be useful in select patients where lowering tidal volume can lead to serious metabolic abnormalities.

INTRODUCTION

The pathophysiologic changes in the acute respiratory distress syndrome (ARDS) produce low-compliant lungs with atelectasis and reduced lung volumes. Such stiff lungs frequently lead to respiratory failure from severe hypoxemia requiring mechanical ventilation for life support. Computed

tomography shows a heterogeneous involvement of lung injury in ARDS and that approximately only a third of the lung is normally aerated ("baby lung").[1] Positive pressure ventilation can worsen lung injury due to differential distribution of each ventilator-delivered breath. The normally aerated lung regions with the highest compliance receive the largest part of the tidal volume (TV) and are exposed to overdistention from high alveolar wall tension and stress. Conversely, atelectatic nonaerated alveoli are exposed to further damage from shear stress due to cyclic recruitment and derecruitment. Therefore, ventilation strategies in ARDS need to simultaneously reverse life-threatening hypoxemia while protecting the lungs from further injury. Since the first description of ARDS by Ashbaugh in 1967, several decades of experimental and clinical research have shifted the primary goal of mechanical ventilation from a normalization of the arterial-blood gas to a more "lung-protective" ventilation strategy. What follows is a description of the history of mechanical ventilation in ARDS, data on published clinical trials, the debate on low-TV ventilation, barriers for implementation of this approach, and our conclusions and suggestions to the readers.

HISTORY OF VENTILATORY STRATEGIES IN ARDS

In the 1960s, the use of high TVs in all mechanically ventilated patients was considered routine care based on the study by Bendixen et al that showed improved oxygenation, less acidosis and atelectasis in anesthetized patients undergoing laparotomy with high TVs (15 mL/kg) compared to lower TVs (5-7 mL/kg).[2] At that time, experimental data by Greenfield et al were the first to show the adverse consequences of mechanical ventilation of normal lungs with high pressures and volumes (peak airway pressures of approximately 30 cm H_2O).[3] In the following decades, ventilator-induced-lung injury from high TVs were further supported by experimental data from Webb, Tierney, and others showing that ventilation with peak airway pressures more than 30 cm H_2O and high TVs led to pulmonary edema, increased alveolar-capillary permeability, structural abnormalities, translocation of inflammatory mediators, multiple-organ-failure and death. These experimental data were supported by the clinical study by Ranieri et al, showing that ARDS patients who received a lung-protective ventilator strategy that limit airway pressures and TV to 5 to 8 mL/kg of ideal body weight (IBW) had a significant reduction of inflammatory markers in plasma and bronchoalveolar lavage.[4] This preclinical and

clinical data raised concerns in the medical community that what was considered "best practice" at the time could exacerbate lung injury from excessive stress or strain to the lung tissues during mechanical ventilation and aggravate on-going inflammation and diffuse alveolar damage. In the 1990s, the pioneering studies by Hickling et al using low-volume pressure-limited ventilation were the first to demonstrate a reduction in mortality by decreasing TV to 5 to 7 mL/kg in order to lower the end-inspiratory pressure while allowing hypercapnia. In these studies, the mortality was lower than that predicted by the severity of illness (Acute Physiology and Chronic Health Evaluation, APACHE II) and the results suggested that the physiologic derangements from "permissive hypercapnia" could be minimized if the rise in CO_2 is more gradual, allowing the intracellular pH to normalize.[5] The work of Hickling and colleagues led to further clinical trials to address the potential clinical benefits of limiting airway pressures by using a low TV in ARDS. In a prospective randomized controlled trial (RCT) by Amato et al, a "protective strategy" of mechanical ventilation (TV of 6 mL/kg actual body weight and PEEP of +2 cm above the lower inflection poing [LIP]), was associated with 46% decrease in 28-days mortality, higher rate of weaning from mechanical ventilation, and lower rate of barotrauma.[6] However, 3 additional RCTs showed no benefits from a low TV strategy.[7-9] From 1996-1999, the ARDS Network evaluated the effects of a lower TV strategy in patients with ARDS in a large multicentre randomized trial (ARMA) sponsored by the National Institute of Health (NIH).[10] In the ARMA study, a traditional ventilation with a TV of 12 mL/kg of predicted body weight (PBW) and plateau pressure (Ppl) less than or equal to 50 cm H_2O was compared to ventilation with a low TV (6 mL/kg of PBW) and Ppl less than or equal to 30 cm. The trial was stopped after the enrollment of 861 patients because of a significant 22% relative reduction in mortality in the experimental group treated with low TV (31.0% vs 39.8%, $P = 0.007$)—this mortality benefit persisted at 6 months from randomization. Furthermore, the experimental group also had significantly more ventilator-free days (VFDs) at 28 days (12 vs 10, $P = 0.007$), and organ-failure-free days compared to the low TV group.

LOW TIDAL VOLUME STRATEGY CONTROVERSY: DOES ONE SIZE FIT ALL?

Soon after publication of the ARMA trial, the study raised intense debate in the medical community and was criticized by its study design, use of surrogate markers of lung injury, and selection of the control group. Many experts in the field argued that a single ventilator strategy with low TVs may not be beneficial or applicable to all patients with ARDS due to the heterogeneity of the underlying lung injury that characterizes this population of critically ill patients.

One Size Fits All?: CON

The ARMA study was criticized for comparing 2 extremes of TV (6 mL/kg PBW vs 12 mL/kg PBW) rather than a safer range of TV (8-10 mL/kg PBW) which was the routine practice at the time of the trial. In the controversial meta-analysis by Eichacker et al the authors examined the results of 5 RCTs on low TV ventilation in ARDS and questioned the validity of the ARMA trial.[11] The authors argued that in the 2 RCTs that showed a survival benefit from a low TV, the traditional arm received excessively large TVs (≥10 mL/kg) that were not the standard of care (8-9 mL/kg). In contrast, the 3 RCTs that showed no survival benefit from a low TV strategy used TVs in the traditional arm that resulted in lower airway pressures (Ppl 28-32 cm H_2O). Therefore, the mortality benefit from a low TV strategy may reflect an excess mortality in the traditional arm exposed to unconventionally high pulmonary pressures (Ppl 34-37 cm H_2O) rather a benefit from low TVs. This analysis and the authors' conclusions have been vigorously challenged and rebutted by others. However, even though it did not prove the benefit of a low TV approach over traditional practice, this meta-analysis did indicate that using a high TV and high Ppl had deleterious effects.

Two subsequent meta-analyses by 2 independent groups of investigators combined the mortality data from the same 5 RCTs examined by Eichacker et al and performed statistical analysis to account for the overall clinical heterogeneity in these studies.[12,23] The results of the treatment effect on mortality were similar. Petrucci and Lacovelli found that

even though the 28-days mortality was significantly reduced by lung-protective ventilation (RR (relative risk): 0.74, 95%CI: 0.61-0.88), the mortality was not significantly different between low and conventional TV if the control groups kept the Ppl less than or equal to 31 cm H_2O (RR: 1.13, 95%CI: 0.88-1.45).[12] Similarly, the meta-analysis by Moran et al found that the pooled estimate of treatment effect favored protective ventilation but was not statistical significant. However, the treatment effect on 28-days mortality was significant for ARDS patients receiving a TV less than 7.7 mL/kg PBW if the control group had a Ppl more than or equal to 30 cm H_2O but not if the controls had Ppl less than 30 cm H_2O.[23] These results remained unchanged in 2 subsequent meta-analyses by Petrucci et al which included all RCTs available to date.[13,14] The authors suggested that their results may involve variations in transpulmonary pressure in the individual patient. A large TV might induce lung damage when the transpulmonary pressure is high. On the other hand, when transpulmonary pressures are within the safe range, a TV in the middle range (8-10 mL/kg) could be used avoiding deleterious effects. The results of this meta-analysis supports the belief of other leaders in the field that the TV in ARDS patients should be adjusted based on other markers of lung injury such as airway pressures or lung strain. Their rationale is that although some patients, such as those with poor pulmonary compliance and high airway pressures, would benefit from very low TV, others with less severe lung injury may require larger volumes to maintain ventilation and avoid alveolar collapse.

To proof this point, Deans et al provided data to support that the mortality in the ARMA trial depended on the lung compliance prior to randomization into a mechanical ventilation strategy.[15] In patients with less compliant lungs (< 0.6 mL/cm H_2O/kg PBW), there was a direct linear relationship with TV and these patients received lower TVs. There was no association in patients with better lung compliance (≥ 0.6 mL/cm H_2O/kg PBW) and in those patients the TV remained constant. Furthermore, the effect on mortality by changing TV was significantly associated with the prerandomization lung compliance. In patients with more compliant lungs, a lower TV was associated with higher mortality. Conversely, in those patients with less compliant lungs, a low TV was associated with lower mortality compared to a high TV. These associations persisted even after accounting for differences in age, APACHE II, and PaO_2/FiO_2 ratio. Overall, these findings strongly suggest that mechanical ventilation should be managed according to other parameters than TV and Ppl and that a single ventilator strategy with a TV of 6 cc/kg PBW may be not be applicable to all patients with ARDS. To further support their findings, Deans et al also performed a retrospective analysis of 2587 patients screened by the ARDS Network who met enrollment criteria but were ineligible due to technical reasons (eg, difficulties with consent). This group of patients received routine care during the course of the ARMA trial and reflected the standard practice of the time. Remarkably, these ineligible patients for the ARMA trial had a comparable mortality rate to the low TV arm in that study (31.7% and 31%, respectively).

In a recent counterpoint analysis, Gattinoni challenged the use of low TV set at 6 mL/kg PWB because PBW is not an appropriate surrogate for the "resting lung volume" when defining lung strain as the ratio of TV to the resting lung volume.[16] In patients with ARDS, PBW cannot be considered an acceptable surrogate for lung volume because the normal relationship between PBW, lung volume, and height is lost. Even though lung strain always increases with TV, the same applied TV/PBW may lead to completely different strain depending on the available lung volume still open to ventilation ("baby lung" volume) confirming that one size of TV may not fit all patients. In a subgroup of patients with very low "baby lung," a TV 6 cc/kg PBW could be excessively high. In another subgroup of patients with a greater "baby lung," a TV 6 cc/kg PBW could be unnecessarily low increasing the risk of atelectasis, respiratory acidosis, and need for supplementary sedation. This controversy stems from the difficulties of measuring transpulmonary pressure at the bedside—the real distending force of the lung and the cause of alveolar trauma. The ideal ventilation would measure the lung volume and transpulmonary pressure because IBW and Ppl are inadequate surrogates for lung stress and strain. However, it may not be feasible to have these measurements available on a routine basis in most ICUs and a lower TV/PBW might be a better choice than

a higher TV/PBW because the risks associated with an unnecessarily low TV are lower than those associated with an unnecessarily high TV.

One Size Fits All?: PRO

The methodologic and safety concerns raised by Eichacker and colleagues were addressed by the ARDS Network investigators and the Office of Human Research Protections (OHRP). The OHRP conducted a thorough investigation to assess whether the control arm was subjected to a range of TVs that conferred a disadvantage. In their published reports, the OHRP, declared that the risks to the subjects in the ARDS Network trial were minimal and reasonable in relation to the anticipated benefits given the high variability in the care of ARDS patients at the time and the lack of standard of care.[17,18] In their response to Eichacker et al, the ARDS Network investigators challenged the methodology of their critic's meta-analysis and reiterated that at the time of the study there was no standard of ventilator strategy.[19] They indicated that at the time of the ARMA trial the Ppl was not used to adjust TVs in any systematic fashion and that there was disparity in physician-selected TVs and the threshold for a Ppl limit indicating equipoise in the medical community on the most appropriate approach to mechanical ventilation. A "standard control" reflective of prevailing ventilation strategy at that time did not exist and the physician's interpretation of the preclinical data and the resulting clinical practices were highly variable. For instance, in the 5 RCTs evaluated by Eichacker et al, there were 4 different ways to calculate the TV based on PBW, IBW, dry, and measured actual body weight. The ARDS Network investigators indicated that the mean TV of patients in the traditional arm after randomization was 10 mL/kg PBW which was consistent with the prevailing clinical practice in the 1990s. They also challenged the meta-analysis conclusions of lack of efficacy due to the small sample size of the 3 nonbeneficial studies, small differences in TVs between study groups in the 2 beneficial studies, and the lack of a pooled estimate of mortality or clinical heterogeneity. In addition, the ARDS Network investigators subsequently published further data from the ARMA trial that detailed the clinical benefits of TV and Ppl reduction across the range of disease severity and Ppl on day 1 of randomization.[20] They showed greater severity of disease in patients with lower respiratory system compliance and that the Ppl was an independent predictor of mortality—decreasing Ppl decreased mortality in ARDS patients, but the investigators caution that this data should not be interpreted to suggest that TV should be lowered below 6 mL/kg PBW.

A subsequent analysis of the ARMA trial examined the efficacy of a low TV ventilation strategy in patients with different clinical risk factors for ARDS.[21] Even though the risk of death was significantly higher in certain subgroups of patients (sepsis, pneumonia, aspiration), a low TV strategy was equally effective across ARDS patients with different clinical risk factors, pulmonary versus nonpulmonary etiology, or infection-related versus noninfection-related conditions. The results from this study strongly support the beneficial effect of low TV ventilation in patients with diverse clinical risk factors for ARDS.

Further studies have showed a benefit of a low TV approach and a recent meta-analysis of 9 RCTs on lung-protective ventilation by Putensen et al has shed some light on the clinical benefits of this ventilatory strategy.[22] Contrary to prior meta-analysis that did not focus on the comparison between lower and higher TV at similar PEEP,[11,12,23] the authors analyzed data according to the effect of different lung-protective strategies: higher versus lower TV at similar PEEP, higher versus lower PEEP strategies during low TV ventilation, and lower TV and PEEP titrated greater than the LIP of the individual's pressure-volume curve versus higher TV and lower PEEP. The authors showed that compared to higher TV ventilation at similar PEEP, lower TV ventilation-reduced hospital mortality (OR (odds risk): 0.75%, 95%CI: 0.58-0.96), a higher PEEP did not reduce hospital mortality compared with lower PEEP using low TVs but that a higher PEEP reduced the need for rescue therapy to prevent life-threatening hypoxemia. These findings support the hypothesis that the higher heterogeneity found in previous meta-analysis can be partially attributed to the inclusion of RCTs that simultaneously investigated lower TV and higher PEEP strategies. Similar to the data from Moran and Petrucci, the authors also found that a lower TV approach did

not improve outcomes when higher TV ventilation results in Ppl less than 30 cm H_2O. However, none of the analyses demonstrated an advantage of high TV ventilation. The authors concluded that low TV ventilation seems to be beneficial in patients with ARDS for routine clinical practice if potential side effects, such as hypercapnia and respiratory acidosis, are not contraindicated. This recent data indicate that TV is a determinant of lung-injury risk and that a lung-protective ventilator approach in ARDS limits further ventilation-induced damage locally and systemically. In the ARMA trial, low TV ventilation was associated with significant reduction in the plasma level of IL-6 and IL-8 and a more rapid attenuation of the inflammatory response by day.[24] More recently, Determann et al showed a greater decrease in IL-6 levels in patients receiving low TVs as compared to a conventional approach (51 ng/mL to 11 ng/mL vs 50 ng/mL to 21 ng/mL; $P = 0.01$).[25] The CT studies by Terragani et al identified ARDS patients in whom tidal inflation occurred largely in normally aerated compartments (more protected) and those in whom tidal inflation occurred largely in the hyperinflated compartments (less protected). They found that pulmonary cytokines were significantly lower in the more protected patients and concluded that limiting TV to 6 mL/kg PBW and Ppl to 30 cm H_2O may not be sufficient in patients with larger nonaerated compartments.[26] Grasso et al demonstrated that many patients with ARDS have a stress index that indicates alveolar hyperventilation while receiving PEEP according to the ARDS Network recommendations.[27] These data point toward utilization of even lower TVs that may increase the likelihood of hypoxemia and other metabolic abnormalities.

Over the last few years, advances in extracorporeal technology have led to significant rise in the use of extracorporeal membrane oxygenation (ECMO) to minimize these metabolic abnormalities in ARDS.[28] With the adjunctive use of ECMO, even lower TVs can be achieved while removing CO_2 to correct the low-tidal-volume-induced respiratory acidosis. The recent Xtravent RCT in ARDS patients evaluated the effect of low TV (3 mL/kg PBW) using ECMO versus the ARDS Network strategy (TV of 6 mL/kg PBW) without the use of an extracorporeal device.[29] Although there were no significant differences in

VFDs or mortality between the study groups, a post-hoc analysis revealed significantly more VFDs at 60 days in patients with more severe hypoxemia ($PaO_2/FIO_2 \leq 150$) who were in the ECMO group (40.9 ± 12.8 vs 28.2 ± 16.4, $P = 0.033$). Overall, the use of ECMO in ARDS still remains controversial with conflicting survival data and the ongoing EOLIA RCT ("ECMO to rescue lung injury in severe ARDS") will attempt to clarify the role of ECMO in these patients.

CHALLENGES OF A LUNG-PROTECTIVE VENTILATION IN CLINICAL PRACTICE

Although the clinical benefit of lung-protective ventilation has been known for years, many ARDS patients receive large TVs in routine practice. Over a decade ago, the ARMA trial demonstrated a 22% relative reduction in mortality and well-tolerated hypercapnia with a lung-protective approach. Despite the significant benefit and favorable cost-effectiveness profile,[30] implementation of this approach into clinical practice has been slow and only half of eligible patients receive low TV ventilation.[31] Centers participating in mechanical ventilation networks or that use educational tools to improve care have higher compliance; however, this does not reflect real-life practice. Several studies, including a survey in all the ARDS network sites, identified several barriers to implementing lung-protective ventilation such as physician's willingness to relinquish control of ventilator, provider discomfort with low TV, perceptions of patient contraindications to receive low TV, patient discomfort, hypercapnia, acidosis, hypoxemia, and the use of sedatives and paralytics.[32] Implementation of a low TV strategy has been recently challenged by the shifting trend in ICU practice of early mobilization to prevent the long-term neuromuscular and cognitive sequelae of critical illness by limiting the use of sedatives and paralytics. In addition to these factors, many patients with ARDS are either unrecognized or not diagnosed by clinicians in a timely manner, especially if the ARDS is mild, and do not receive lung-protective protective ventilation. Even when ARDS is properly recognized, provider reliance on the actual body weight instead of PBW in the calculation of the set TV is a frequent error, particularly when the calculation yields an apparently too small TV, leading to overtreatment with higher TVs. The patient's actual weight on admission is influenced by obesity, prehospital morbidity, and fluid resuscitation. In many instances, the height of the patient is unknown, particularly outside of the surgical ICUs, and women in particular are mostly affected. Han et al recently showed that patient height is a significant factor in predicting provider adherence with lung-protective ventilation guidelines and women are less likely than men to receive low TV during the first 48 hours of critical illness.[33] Because obesity is more common among adult women than men in the United States, the use of actual body weight would result in larger TVs for women.

Currently, the lung-protective strategy recommends a TV of 6 to 8 mL/kg of PBW in ARDS. Recent data from the United States and Europe indicate that the average TV in ARDS patients receiving lung-protective ventilation is close to 8 cc/kg PBW (the accepted upper limit of a low TV strategy in the ARMA trial).[34-36] Epidemiologic data from the Irish Critical Care Trials group reported a mean TV of 8.4 mL/kg IBW.[37] The ALIEN Network reported a mean TV of 7.2 mL/kg PBW and a mean Ppl of 26 cm H_2O in the Spanish ICUs.[38] In a secondary analysis of 829 patients on mechanical ventilation at 22 centers in the United States, Chang et al found that patients initially intubated with ARDS had a median TV of 7.96 mL/kg PBW which was significantly lower than the median TV in patients without ARDS (8.45 mL/kg PBW) ($P = 0.004$). Although the difference between the 2 groups was statistically significant, the absolute difference in TVs was quite small (< 0.5 mL/kg IBW).[39] This study suggests that in recent years mechanical ventilation practices have moved toward the use of lower TVs even in patients without ARDS and this trend may obscure any differences in ventilator-related outcomes.

CONCLUSIONS

After decades of research, there is still much uncertainty regarding the best ventilator care for patients with ARDS. The ongoing debate on the beneficial effects of the lung-protective strategy using a low TV approach has hindered the implementation of this ventilation strategy in clinical practice. Although recent United States and European data show a shift in mechanical ventilation practices in recent years, there are still multiple barriers to achieve what is considered the best evidence-based medicine.

The evidence to date strongly suggests that ventilation with high TV and high Ppl is associated with increased risk of death and a definite trend has been seen toward using lower TV in ARDS and non-ARDS patients. There is a clear benefit of low TV ventilation on mortality; however, there are no RCTs comparing ventilation with a TV of 6 to 8 mL/kg PBW to a TV of 8 to 10 mL/kg PBW in ARDS patients. ARDS is a heterogeneous disease process and physicians may encounter situations where ventilation with TV even lower than 6 mL/kg PBW might be desired to minimize lung strain, maintain acceptable airway pressures, and hence may risk significant metabolic and hemodynamic instability. Adjunctive techniques aimed at removing excess CO_2 may counteract the metabolic derangements encountered in clinical practice.

Individualization of care is where the true artist of medicine excels and there is no substitute for the clinician's judgment at the bedside monitoring the response to the necessary adjustments in the ventilator. A gentle and safe ventilator strategy requires careful titration of the TV and airway pressures by the clinician in order to minimize lung injury and maintain adequate oxygenation using all available tools and evidence-based medicine at the bedside.

REFERENCES

1. Gattinoni L, Presenti A, Torresin A, et al. Adult respiratory distress syndrome profiles by computed tomography. *J Thorac Imaging*. 1986;1:25-30.
2. Bendixen HH. Atelactasis and shunting. *Anesthesiology*. 1964;25:595-596.
3. Greenfield LJ, Ebert PA, Benson DW. Atelectasis and surface tension properties of lung extracts following positive pressure ventilation and overinflation. *Surg Forum*. 1963;14:239-240.
4. Ranieri VM, Suter PM, Tortorella C, et al. Effect of mechanical ventilation on inflammatory mediators in patients with acute respiratory distress syndrome: a randomized controlled trial. *JAMA*. 1999;282:54-61.
5. Hickling KG. Low volume ventilation with permissive hypercapnia in the adult respiratory distress syndrome. *Clin Intensive Care*. 1992;3(2):67-78.
6. Amato MB, Barbas CS, Medeiros DM, et al. Effect of a protective-ventilation strategy on mortality in the acute respiratory distress syndrome. *N Engl J Med*. 1998;338(6):347-354.
7. Stewart TE, Meade MO, Cook DJ, et al. Pressure- and volume-limited ventilation strategy group. Evaluation of a ventilation strategy to prevent barotrauma in patients at high risk for acute respiratory distress syndrome. *N Engl J Med*. 1998;338(6):355-361.
8. Brochard L, Roudot-Thoraval F, Roupie E, et al. Tidal volume reduction for prevention of ventilator-induced lung injury in acute respiratory distress syndrome. *Am J Respir Crit Care Med*. 1998;158:1831-1838.
9. Brower RG, Shanholtz CB, Fessler HE, et al. Prospective, randomized, controlled clinical trial comparing traditional versus reduced tidal volume ventilation in acute respiratory distress syndrome patients. *Crit Care Med*. 1999;27:1492-1498.
10. Ventilation with lower tidal volumes as compared with traditional tidal volumes for acute lung injury and the acute respiratory distress syndrome. The Acute Respiratory Distress Syndrome Network. *N Engl J Med*. 2000;342(18):1301-1318.
11. Eichacker PQ, Gerstenberger EP, Banks SM, Cui X, Natanson C. Meta-analysis of acute lung injury and acute respiratory distress syndrome trials testing low tidal volumes. *Am J Respir Crit Care Med*. 2002;166(11):1510-1514.
12. Petrucci N, Iacovelli W. Ventilation with smaller tidal volumes: a quantitative systematic review of randomized controlled trials. *Anesth Analg*. 2004;99(1):193-200.
13. Petrucci N, Iacovelli W. Lung protective ventilation strategy for the acute respiratory distress syndrome. *Cochrane Database Syst Rev*. 2007;3:CD003844.
14. Petrucci N, De Feo C. Lung protective ventilation strategy for the acute respiratory distress syndrome. *Cochrane Database Syst Rev*. 2013;2:CD003844.
15. Deans KJ, Minneci PC, Cui X, Banks SM, Natanson C, Eichacker PQ. Mechanical ventilation in ARDS: one size does not fit all. *Crit Care Med*. 2005;33(5):1141-1143.
16. Gattinoni L. Counterpoint: is low tidal volume mechanical ventilation preferred for all patients on ventilation? No. *Chest*. 2011;140:11-13.
17. Steinbrook R. How best to ventilate? Trial design and patient safety in studies of the acute respiratory distress syndrome. *N Engl J Med*. 2003;348(14):1393-1401.

18. Steinbrook R. Trial design and patient safety—the debate continues. *N Engl J Med*. 2003;349(7):629-630.

19. Brower RG, Matthay M, Schoenfeld D. Meta-analysis of acute lung injury and acute respiratory distress syndrome trials. *Am J Respir Crit Care Med*. 2002;166:1515-1517.

20. Hager DN, Krishnan JA, Hayden DL, Brower RG. Tidal volume reduction in patients with acute lung injury when plateau pressures are not high. *Am J Respir Crit Care Med*. 2005;172:1241-1245.

21. Eisner MD, Thompson T, Hudson LD, et al. Efficacy of low tidal volume ventilation in patients with different clinical risk factors for acute lung injury and the acute respiratory distress syndrome. *Am J Respir Crit Care Med*. 2001;164:231-236.

22. Putensen C, Theuerkauf N, Zinserling J, Wrigge H, Pelosi P. Meta-analysis: ventilation strategies and outcomes of the acute respiratory distress syndrome and acute lung injury. *Ann Intern Med*. 2009;151:566-576.

23. Moran JL, Bersten AD, Solomon PJ. Meta-analysis of controlled trials of ventilator therapy in acute lung injury and acute respiratory distress syndrome: an alternative perspective. *Intensive Care Med*. 2005;31:227-235.

24. Parsons P, Eisner M, Thompson B, et al. Lower tidal volume ventilation and plasma cytokine markers of inflammation in patients with acute lung injury. *Crit Care Med*. 2005;33:1-6.

25. Determann RM, Royakkers A, Wolthuis EK, et al. Ventilation with lower tidal volumes as compared with conventional tidal volumes for patients without acute lung injury: a preventive randomized controlled trial. *Crit Care*. 2010;14(1):R1.

26. Terragni PP, Rosboch G, Tealdi A, et al. Tidal hyperinflation during low tidal volume ventilation in acute respiratory distress syndrome. *Am J Respir Crit Care Med*. 2007;175:160-166.

27. Grasso S, Stripoli T, De Michele M, et al. ARDSnet ventilatory protocol and alveolar hyperinflation: role of positive end-expiratory pressure. *Am J Respir Crit Care Med*. 2007;176:761-767.

28. Abrams D, Brodie D, Combes A. What is new in extracorporeal membrane oxygenation for ARDS in adults? *Intensive Care Med*. 2013;39(11):2028-2030.

29. Bein T, Weber-Carstens S, Goldmann A, et al. Lower tidal volume strategy (≈3 mL/kg) combined with extracorporeal CO_2 removal versus "conventional" protective ventilation (6 mL/kg) in severe ARDS: the prospective randomized Xtravent-study. *Intensive Care Med*. 2013;39(5):847-856.

30. Cooke CR, Kahn JM, Watkins TR, Hudson LD, Rubenfeld GD. Cost-effectiveness of implementing low-tidal volume ventilation in patients with acute lung injury. *Chest*. 2009;136:79-88.

31. Umoh NJ, Fan E, Mendez-Tellez PA, et al. Patient and intensive care unit organizational factors associated with low tidal volume ventilation in acute lung injury. *Crit Care Med*. 2008;36:1463-1468.

32. Rubenfeld GD, Cooper C, Carter G, Thompson BT, Hudson LD. Barriers to providing lung-protective ventilation to patients with acute lung injury. *Crit Care Med*. 2004;32(6):1289-1293.

33. Han S, Martin GS, Maloney JP, et al. Short women with severe sepsis-related acute lung injury receive lung protective ventilation less frequently: an observational cohort study. *Crit Care*. 2011;15(6):R262.

34. NIH: NHLBI: ARDS Network. NIH NHLBI ARDS Clinical Network Mechanical Ventilation Protocol Summary. http://www.ardsnet.org/system/files/6mlcardsmall_2008update_final_JULY2008.pdf, Accessed December 29, 2013.

35. Dellinger RP, Levy MM, Carlet JM, et al. Surviving sepsis campaign: international guidelines for management of severe sepsis and septic shock: 2008. *Crit Care Med*. 2008;36:296-327.

36. Girard TD, Bernard GR. Mechanical ventilation in ARDS. A state-of-the-art review. *Chest*. 2007;131:921-929.

37. Irish Critical Care Trials Group. Intensive care for the adult population in Ireland: a multicentre study of intensive care population demographics. *Crit Care*. 2008;12(5):R121.

38. Villar J, Blanco J, Añón JM, et al. The ALIEN study: incidence and outcome of acute respiratory distress syndrome in the era of lung protective ventilation. *Intensive Care Med*. 2011;37(12):1932-1941.

39. Chang SY, Dabbagh O, Gajic O, et al. Contemporary ventilator management in patients with and at risk of ALI/ARDS. *Respir Care*. 2013;58(4):578-588.

Controversies: Corticosteroids for ARDS: Friend or Foe?

68

Paul E. Marik, MD, FCCM, FCCP

INTRODUCTION

The acute respiratory distress syndrome (ARDS) is a common and vexing problem faced by critical care providers worldwide. Despite extensive investigation over the last three decades, the impact of ARDS in terms of morbidity, mortality, and health care costs remains very high. In the United States alone, ARDS affects as many as 200,000 people per year with a mortality rate from 30% to 50% and costs in excess of $60,000 per hospitalization.[1,2] The management of patients with ARDS is essentially supportive using a lung protective ventilatory strategy and treatment of the precipitating cause.[3] The use of corticosteroids in patients with ARDS is controversial with widely dissenting opinions on this topic.[4] At least 6 meta-analyses have been performed with conflicting conclusions.[5-10] However, a summation of this data would suggest that glucocorticoids (GCs) improve oxygenation, increase the number of ventilator-free days, decrease intensive care unit (ICU) and hospital length of stay with a possible mortality benefit with no clear evidence of an increase in complications. Despite the potential benefit of GCs in patients with ARDS, survey data suggest that most clinicians do not prescribe these agents to their patients with ARDS.[11] The purpose of this review is to outline the rationale for GC treatment in ARDS, discuss the factors affecting response to treatment, review the results of clinical trials and the myths concerning GC-related side effects and outline a protocol for GC treatment based on the best available data.

BRIEF REVIEW OF PATHOGENESIS

ARDS develops rapidly, in most patients within 12 to 48 hours of developing an illness associated with severe systemic inflammation. Injury to the alveolar-capillary membrane (ACM) causes exudative neutrophilic inflammatory edema, resulting in severe gas exchange impairment and lung compliance abnormalities. The lung-injury score (LIS) quantifies the impaired respiratory physiology in ARDS by using a 4-point score based on the level of positive end-expiratory pressure (PEEP), ratio of partial arterial oxygen tension (PaO_2) to fraction of inspired oxygen (FiO_2) (PaO_2:FiO_2), the quasistatic lung compliance, and the degree of infiltration on chest radiograph.[12] Using these criteria, the evolution of ARDS can be divided into resolving and unresolving ARDS based on achieving a 1-point reduction in LIS by day 7.[13]

Experimental and clinical evidence has demonstrated a strong cause and effect relationship between persistence in systemic inflammation and progression (unresolving) of ARDS. At the cellular level, patients with unresolving ARDS have inadequate GC-GC receptor (GR)-mediated downregulation of inflammatory transcription factor nuclear factor-κB (NF-κB) despite elevated levels of circulating cortisol, a condition recently defined as *critical-illness-related corticosteroid insufficiency* (CIRCI).[14,15] Patients with unresolving ARDS have persistent elevation in both systemic and bronchoalveolar lavage (BAL) levels of inflammatory mediators, markers of fibrogenesis, and ACM permeability. At the tissue level, uninhibited increased NF-κB activation leads to ongoing tissue injury, intravascular and extravascular coagulation, and proliferation of mesenchymal cells, resulting in maladaptive lung repair and ultimately end-organ dysfunction and failure.[14] The ability of activated GC-GR to downregulate systemic inflammation and restore tissue homeostasis can be significantly enhanced with exogenous GC treatment.[16] In a randomized trial,[17] longitudinal measurements of biomarkers provided compelling evidence that prolonged methylprednisolone treatment modifies CIRCI and positively affects all aspects of ARDS.[18] Treatment with prolonged methylprednisolone was associated with increased GC-GRα activity and reduced NF-κB DNA binding and transcription of inflammatory mediators.[16] In ARDS, methylprednisolone treatment led to rapid and sustained reduction in plasma and BAL levels of proinflammatory mediators,[16,19] chemokines and adhesion molecules, and markers of fibrogenesis[20] and ACM permeability[19] while increasing the anti-inflammatory cytokine interleukin-10 (IL-10) and anti-inflammatory to proinflammatory cytokine ratios.

FACTORS AFFECTING RESPONSE TO PROLONGED GLUCOCORTICOID TREATMENT

Duration of treatment is an important determinant of both efficacy and toxicity. Optimization of GC treatment is affected by 3 factors: (1) actual biological duration of the disease process (systemic inflammation and CIRCI), (2) recovery time of the hypothalamic-pituitary-adrenal (HPA) axis, and (3) cumulative risk associated with prolonged treatment (risk) and the essential role of secondary prevention (risk reduction).

1. Longitudinal measurements of plasma and BAL inflammatory cytokine levels in ARDS showed that inflammation extends well beyond resolution of respiratory failure.[14,21,22] One uncontrolled study found that, despite prolonged methylprednisolone administration, local and systemic inflammation persisted for 14 days (limit of study).[19] Similar findings were reported in an randomized controlled trial (RCT) for inflammatory mediators on day 10 of treatment.[16]

2. Prolonged GC treatment is associated with downregulation of the GR levels and suppression of the HPA axis (reviewed later), affecting systemic inflammation after discontinuing treatment. Experimental and clinical literature underscores the importance of continuing GC treatment beyond clinical resolution of acute respiratory failure (extubation).[9] In the recent ARDS Network

trial, methylprednisolone was removed within 3 to 4 days of extubation and likely contributed, as acknowledged by the authors, to the deterioration in PaO_2:FiO_2 ratio and higher rate of reintubation and associated mortality.[9,23] In 2 other ARDS trials,[17,24] GC treatment was continued for up to 18 days to maintain reduction in inflammation.[17,24] This prolonged GC treatment was not associated with relapse of ARDS.

3. Table 68–1 shows potential complications masked by or associated with prolonged GC treatment and secondary prevention measures.

   Infection surveillance—Failed or delayed recognition of nosocomial infections in the presence of a blunted febrile response represents a serious threat to the recovery

TABLE 68–1 Potential complications associated with prolonged glucocorticoid treatment and secondary prevention measures.

Potential Complications	Secondary Preventive Measures
Glucocorticoids blunt the febrile response leading to failed or delayed recognition of nosocomial infections	Surveillance BAL sampling at 5-7 days intervals in intubated patients. Systematic diagnostic protocol if patient develops signs of infection
Glucocorticoids given in combination with neuromuscular blocking agents increase the risk of prolonged neuromuscular weakness	Avoid concomitant use of neuromuscular blocking agents
Glucocorticoids given as intermittent bolus produce glycemic variability	Following an initial bolus, administer glucocorticoids as a constant infusion
Rapid tapering is associated with rebound inflammation and clinical deterioration	Slow taper over 9-12 days. During and after taper monitor CRP and clinical variables, if patient deteriorates escalate to prior dosage or restart treatment
Suppression of endogenous cortisol synthesis	Avoid concomitant use of etomidate which causes further suppression of cortisol synthesis

of patients receiving prolonged GC treatment. In 2 randomized trials[17,24] that incorporated infection surveillance, nosocomial infections were frequently (56%) identified in the absence of fever. The infection surveillance protocol incorporated bronchoscopy with bilateral BAL at 5 to 7-days intervals in intubated patients (without contraindication) and a systematic diagnostic protocol when patients developed clinical and laboratory signs suggestive of infection in the absence of fever.[25]

Increased risk for neuromuscular weakness with neuromuscular blocking agents—The combination of GCs and neuromuscular blocking agents versus GCs alone increases the risk for prolonged neuromuscular weakness.[26] Consequently the combined use of neuromuscular blocking agents and GCs were considered contraindicated. However, Papazian and colleagues randomized patients with severe ARDS to receive cisatracurium besylate or placebo for 48 hours.[27] In this study, about 40% of patients were concomitantly receiving GCs. The incidence of neuromuscular weakness was similar in both groups. This study suggests that it may be safe to use GCs together with a short course of a neuromuscular blocking agent; however, the prolonged use of a neuromuscular blocking agent should be avoided.

GC treatment can impair glycemic control—It is well established that exogenous GCs administered as a bolus produce hyperglycemic variability, an independent predictor of ICU and hospital mortality.[28] Two studies have shown that GC infusion is superior to intermittent boluses in preventing glycemic variability by decreasing changes in insulin infusion rate.[29,30]

Avoidance of rebound inflammation—There is ample evidence[20,31-37] that early removal of GC treatment may lead to rebound inflammation and an exaggerated cytokine

response to endotoxin.[38] Experimental work has shown that short-term exposure of alveolar macrophages[39] or animals to dexamethasone is followed by enhanced inflammatory cytokine response to endotoxin.[40] Similarly, normal human subjects pretreated with hydrocortisone had significantly higher tumor necrosis factor alpha (TNF-α) and IL-6 response after endotoxin challenge compared to controls.[41] Two potential mechanisms may explain rebound inflammation: homologous downregulation and GC-induced adrenal insufficiency. GC treatment downregulates the GR levels in most cell types, thereby decreasing the efficacy of the treatment. The mechanisms of homologous downregulation have been reviewed elsewhere.[42] Downregulation takes place at both the transcriptional and translational level, and hormone treatment decreases receptor half-life by approximately 50%.[42] In experimental animals, overexpression of GRs improves resistance to endotoxin-mediated septic shock while GR blockade increases mortality.[43] No study (to the best of our knowledge) has investigated recovery of GR levels and function following prolonged GC treatment in patients with sepsis or ARDS.

REVIEW OF CONTROLLED CLINICAL STUDIES

Eight controlled studies (5 RCTs and three cohorts) have evaluated the effectiveness of prolonged GC treatment initiated before day 14 of early ALI/ARDS ($N = 334$)[24,44-46] and late ARDS ($N = 235$).[17,23,47-49] These trials consistently reported that treatment-induced reduction in systemic inflammation[17,23,24,45-47,49] was associated with significant improvement in PaO_2:FiO_2,[17,23,24,45-47,49] and significant reductions in multiple-organ dysfunction score,[17,23,24,45,47,49] duration of mechanical ventilation,[17,23,24,44-46] and ICU length of stay (all with P values < 0.05).[17,23,24,44,45] Four of the 5 randomized trials provided Kaplan Meier curves for continuation of mechanical ventilation; each showed a 2-fold or greater rate of extubation in the first 5 to 7 days of treatment.[17,23,24,45] In the ARDS Network trial, the treated group—before discontinuation of treatment—had a 9.5-days reduction in duration of mechanical ventilation (14.1 ± 1.7 vs 23.6 ± 2.9; $P = 0.006$) and more patients discharged home after initial weaning (62% vs 49%; $P = 0.006$).[23] As shown in Figure 68–1, GC treatment initiated before day 14 of ARDS was associated with a marked reduction in the risk of death (Relative Risk (RR) = 0.68, 95%CI: 0.56-0.81; $P < 0.001$; I^2 56%).[9] There was, however, significant heterogeneity between studies. As a result of the marked differences in study design and patient characteristics, the limited size of the studies (fewer than 200 patients), the cumulative mortality summary of these studies should be interpreted with some caution. For this reason, a recent consensus statement recommended early initiation of prolonged GC treatment for patients with severe ARDS ($PaO_2:FiO_2 < 200$ on PEEP 10 cm H_2O) and before day 14 for patients with unresolving ARDS.[15] The ARDS Network trial reported that treated patients had increased mortality when randomized after day 14 of ARDS (8% vs 35%; $P = 0.01$).[23] This subgroup ($N = 48$), however, had large differences in baseline characteristics, and the mortality difference lost significance ($P = 0.57$) when the analysis was adjusted for these imbalances.[50]

MYTHS ABOUT COMPLICATIONS OF PROLONGED GLUCOCORTICOID TREATMENT

The most commonly cited complications that might temper enthusiasm for GC treatment include increased risks of infection and neuromuscular weakness. Substantial evidence has accumulated showing that systemic inflammation is also implicated in the pathogenesis of these complications,[51-53] suggesting that treatment-induced downregulation of systemic inflammation could theoretically prevent, or partly offset, their development and/or progression.

GC treatment does not increase infection risk—
Contrary to older studies investigating a time-limited (24-48 hours) massive daily dose of GCs (methylprednisolone, up to 120 mg/kg/day),[54,55] recent trials have *not* reported an increased rate of nosocomial infections. In fact, new cumulative evidence indicates that downregulation of life-threatening systemic inflammation with prolonged low-to-moderate dose GC treatment improves innate immunity[37,56] and provides an environment less favorable to the intracellular and extracellular growth of

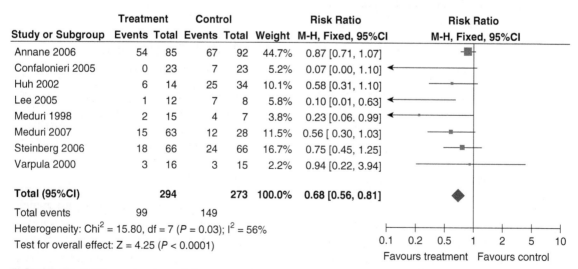

Study or Subgroup	Treatment Events	Total	Control Events	Total	Weight	Risk Ratio M-H, Fixed, 95%CI	Risk Ratio M-H, Fixed, 95%CI
Annane 2006	54	85	67	92	44.7%	0.87 [0.71, 1.07]	
Confalonieri 2005	0	23	7	23	5.2%	0.07 [0.00, 1.10]	
Huh 2002	6	14	25	34	10.1%	0.58 [0.31, 1.10]	
Lee 2005	1	12	7	8	5.8%	0.10 [0.01, 0.63]	
Meduri 1998	2	15	4	7	3.8%	0.23 [0.06. 0.99]	
Meduri 2007	15	63	12	28	11.5%	0.56 [0.30, 1.03]	
Steinberg 2006	18	66	24	66	16.7%	0.75 [0.45, 1.25]	
Varpula 2000	3	16	3	15	2.2%	0.94 [0.22, 3.94]	
Total (95%CI)		**294**		**273**	**100.0%**	**0.68 [0.56, 0.81]**	
Total events	99		149				

Heterogeneity: Chi^2 = 15.80, df = 7 (P = 0.03); I^2 = 56%
Test for overall effect: Z = 4.25 (P < 0.0001)

0.1   0.2   0.5   1   2   5   10
Favours treatment   Favours control

FIGURE 68–1 Effects of prolonged glucocorticoid treatment on acute respiratory distress syndrome survival.

bacteria.[57] GCs, however, do blunt the signs and symptoms of infection as detailed above (Table 68–1).

GC treatment does not increase the risk of neuromuscular weakness—The incidence of neuromuscular weakness is similar between groups treated with or without prolonged GCs (17% vs 18%).[7] Two recent studies found no association between prolonged GC treatment and electrophysiologically or clinically proven neuromuscular dysfunction.[58,59] Given that neuromuscular dysfunction is an independent predictor of prolonged weaning[60] and ARDS randomized trials have consistently reported a significant reduction in duration of mechanical ventilation,[17,23,24,45,46] clinically relevant neuromuscular dysfunction caused by GC or GC-induced hyperglycemia seems highly unlikely. It should be noted that the combination of GCs and neuromuscular blocking agents versus steroids alone significantly increases the risk for prolonged neuromuscular weakness (Table 68–1).[26]

RECOMMENDATIONS FOR TREATMENT

We have reviewed data showing that the benefit-risk of GC treatment in ARDS is largely determined by the drug dosage, timing and duration of administration, weaning protocol, and implementation of secondary preventive measures. The results of one randomized trial in patients with early severe ARDS[24] indicates that 1 mg/kg/day of methylprednisolone given as an infusion and tapered over 4 weeks is associated with a favorable risk-benefit profile when secondary preventive measures are implemented. Treatment response should be monitored with daily measurement of LIS and multiple-organ dysfunction syndrome (MODS) scores and C-reactive protein level.[24,45] Secondary prevention is important to minimize complications. GC treatment should be administered as a continuous infusion (while the patient is in ICU) to minimize glycemic variations.[29,30] GC treatment blunts the febrile response; therefore, infection surveillance is essential to identify early and treat nosocomial

infections (as outlined above). Finally, a slow GC dosage reduction (9-12 days) after a complete course allows recovery of GR numbers and the HPA axis, thereby reducing the risk of rebound inflammation. Laboratory evidence of physiologic deterioration (ie, worsening $PaO_2:FiO_2$) associated with rebound inflammation (increased serum C-reactive protein) after the completion of GC treatment may require reinstitution of treatment.

GLUCOCORTICOIDS TO PREVENT ALI/ARDS

As GCs have demonstrated a benefit in patients with established ARDS is has been postulated that these agents may be useful in preventing ARDS. Four studies have tested this hypothesis; however, this strategy was associated with a trend to an increase in both the odds of developing ARDS and the risk of mortality in those who developed ARDS.[5] The reason for the seemingly differential effect of preventative and therapeutic steroid therapy in ARDS is unclear. In a propensity-based analysis of a large hospital database, the concurrent use of corticosteroids at the time of hospitalization did not reduce the risk of developing ARDS nor did it affect the requirement for mechanical ventilation or influence mortality.[61]

SUMMARY AND CONCLUSIONS

In this review, we presented a rationale for the use of GC treatment in ARDS. Based on molecular mechanisms and physiologic data, a strong association between dysregulated inflammation and progression of ARDS has been established. Further, these data support a strong association between treatment with exogenous GCs leading to regulation of the inflammatory response, improvement in organ physiology (LIS, MODS), and resolution of ARDS. The available clinical trials of prolonged GC treatment show favorable effects on clinical outcomes including ventilator-free days, ICU-free days, and mortality. Although the balance of the available data from controlled trials provides strong evidence for improvement in patient-centered outcomes (sizable reduction in duration of mechanical ventilation and

ICU length of stay) and weak evidence for a survival benefit, the findings recently reported with low-dose methylprednisolone (1 mg/kg/day) in early severe ARDS[24] should be replicated in a larger trial of patients with ALI/ARDS.

REFERENCES

1. Rubenfeld GD, Caldwell E, Peabody E, Weaver J, Martin DP, Neff M, Stern EJ. Incidence and outcomes of acute lung injury. *N Engl J Med.* 2005;353:1685-1693.

2. Angus DC, Clermont G, Linde-Zwirble WT, Musthafa AA, Dremsizov TT, Lidicker J, Lave JR. Healthcare costs and long-term outcomes after acute respiratory distress syndrome: a phase III trial of inhaled nitric oxide. *Crit Care Med.* 2006;34:2883-2890.

3. Ventilation with lower tidal volumes as compared with traditional tidal volumes for acute lung injury and the acute respiratory distress syndrome. *N Engl J Med.* 2000;342:1301-1308.

4. Lamontagne F, Brower R, Meade M. Corticosteroid therapy in acute respiratory distress syndrome. *CMAJ.* 2013;185:216-221.

5. Peter JV, John P, Graham PL, Moran JL, George IA, Bersten A. Corticosteroids in the prevention and treatment of acute respiratory distress syndrome (ARDS) in adults: meta-analysis. *BMJ.* 2008;336:1006-1009.

6. Lamontagne F, Briel M, Guyatt GH, Cook DJ, Bhatnagar N, Meade M. Corticosteroid therapy for acute lung injury, acute respiratory distress syndrome, and severe pneumonia: a meta-analysis of randomized controlled trials. *J Crit Care.* 2010;25:420-435.

7. Tang BM, Craig JC, Eslick GD, Seppelt I, McLean AS. Use of corticosteroids in acute lung injury and acute respiratory distress syndrome: a systematic review and meta-analysis. *Crit Care Med.* 2009;37:1595-1603.

8. Agarwal R, Nath A, Aggarwal AN, Gupta D. Do glucocorticoids decrease mortality in acute respiratory distress syndrome? A meta-analysis. *Respirology.* 2007;12:585-590.

9. Meduri GU, Marik PE, Chrousos GP, Pastores SM, Arlt W, Beishuizen A, Bokhari F. Steroid treatment in ARDS: a critical appraisal of the ARDS network trial and the recent literature. *Intensive Care Med.* 2008;34:61-69.

10. Marik PE, Meduri GU, Rocco PR, Annane D. Glucocorticoid treatment in acute lung injury and acute-respiratory distress syndrome. *Crit Care Clin.* 2011;27:589-607.

11. Lamontagne F, Quiroz MH, Adhikari NK, Cook DJ, Koo KK, Lauzier F, Turgeon AF. Corticosteroid use in the intensive care unit: a survey of intensivists. *Can J Anaesth.* 2013;60:652-659.

12. Murray JF, Mattay MA, Luce J, Flick M. An expanded definition of the adult respiratory distress syndrome. *Am Rev Respir Dis.* 1988;138:720-723.

13. Meduri GU, Annane D, Chrousos G, Marik PE, Sinclair SE. Activation and regulation of systemic inflammation in ARDS. Rationale for prolonged glucocorticoid therapy. *Chest.* 2009;136:1631-1644.

14. Meduri GU, Muthiah MP, Carratu P, Eltorky M, Chrousos GP. Nuclear factor-kappaB- and glucocorticoid receptor alpha-mediated mechanisms in the regulation of systemic and pulmonary inflammation during sepsis and acute respiratory distress syndrome. Evidence for inflammation-induced target tissue resistance to glucocorticoids. *Neuroimmunomodulation.* 2005;12:321-338.

15. Marik PE, Pastores SM, Annane D, Meduri GU, Arlt W, Sprung CL, Keh D. Recommendations for the diagnosis and management of corticosteroid insufficiency in critically ill adult patients: consensus statements from an international task force by the American College of Critical Care Medicine. *Crit Care Med.* 2008;36:1937-1949.

16. Meduri GU, Tolley EA, Chrousos GP, Stentz F. Prolonged methylprednisolone treatment suppresses systemic inflammation in patients with unresolving acute respiratory distress syndrome: evidence for inadequate endogenous glucocorticoid secretion and inflammation-induced immune cell resistance to glucocorticoids. *Am J Respir Crit Care Med.* 2002;165:983-991.

17. Meduri GU, Headley S, Golden E, Carson SJ, Umberger RA, Kelso T, Tolley EA. Effect of prolonged methylprednisolone therapy in unresolving acute respiratory distress syndrome. A randomized controlled trial. *JAMA.* 1998;280:159-165.

18. Meduri GU, Yates CR. Systemic inflammation-associated glucocorticoid resistance and outcome of ARDS. *Ann NY Acad Sci.* 2004;1024:24-53.

19. Meduri GU, Headley S, Tolley E, Shelby M, Stentz F, Postlethwaite A. Plasma and BAL cytokine response to corticosteroid rescue treatment in late ARDS. *Chest.* 1995;108:1315-1325.

20. Meduri GU, Tolley EA, Chinn A, Stentz F, Postlethwaite A. Procollagen types I and III

aminoterminal propeptide levels during acute respiratory distress syndrome and in response to methylprednisolone treatment. *Am J Respir Crit Care Med.* 1998;158:1432-1441.

21. Meduri GU, Headley S, Kohler G, Stentz F, Tolley E, Umberger R, Leeper K. Persistent elevation of inflammatory cytokines predicts a poor outcome in ARDS. Plasma IL-1 beta and IL-6 levels are consistent and efficient predictors of outcome over time. *Chest.* 1995;107:1062-1073.

22. Meduri GU, Kohler G, Headley S, Tolley E, Stentz F, Postlethwaite A. Inflammatory cytokines in the BAL of patients with ARDS. Persistent elevation over time predicts poor outcome. *Chest.* 1995;108:1303-1314.

23. The Acute Respiratory Distress Syndrome Network. Efficacy and safety of corticosteroids for persistent acute respiratory distress syndrome. *N Engl J Med.* 2006;354:1671-1684.

24. Meduri GU, Golden E, Freire AX, Taylor E, Zaman M, Carson SJ, Gibson M. Methyprednisolone infusion in patients with early severe ARDS: results of a randomized trial. *Chest.* 2007;131:954-963.

25. Meduri GU, Mauldin GL, Wunderink RG, Leeper KV, Jones CB, Tolley E, Mayhall G. Causes of fever and pulmonary densities in patients with clinical manifestations of ventilator-associated pneumonia. *Chest.* 1994;106:221-235.

26. Leatherman JW, Fluegle WL, David WS, Davies SF, Iber C. Muscle weakness in mechanically ventilated patients with severe asthma. *Am J Respir Crit Care Med.* 1996;153:1686-1690.

27. Papazian L, Forel JM, Gacouin A, Penot-Ragon C, Perrin G, Loundou A, Jaber S. Neuromuscular blockers in early respiratory distress syndrome. *N Engl J Med.* 2010;363:1107-1116.

28. Egi M, Bellomo R, Stachowski E, French CJ, Hart G. Variability of blood glucose concentration and short-term mortality in critically ill patients. *Anesthesiol.* 2006;105:244-252.

29. Weber-Carstens S, Keh D. Bolus or continuous hydrocortisone—that is the question. *Crit Care.* 2007;11:113.

30. Loisa P, Parviainen I, Tenhunen J, Hovilehto S, Ruokonen E. Effect of mode of hydrocortisone administration on glycemic control in patients with septic shock: a prospective randomized trial. *Crit Care.* 2007;11:R21.

31. Hesterberg TW, Last JA. Ozone-induced acute pulmonary fibrosis in rats. Prevention of increased rates of collagen synthesis by methylprednisolone. *Am Rev Respir Dis.* 1981;123:47-52.

32. Hakkinen PJ, Schmoyer RL, Witschi HP. Potentiation of butylated-hydroxytoluene-induced acute lung damage by oxygen. Effects of prednisolone and indomethacin. *Am Rev Respir Dis.* 1983;128:648-651.

33. Kehrer JP, Klein-Szanto AJ, Sorensen EM, Pearlman R, Rosner MH. Enhanced acute lung damage following corticosteroid treatment. *Am Rev Respir Dis.* 1984;130:256-261.

34. Ashbaugh DG, Maier RV. Idiopathic pulmonary fibrosis in adult respiratory distress syndrome. Diagnosis and treatment. *Arch Surg.* 1985;120: 530-535.

35. Hooper RG, Kearl RA. Established ARDS treated with a sustained course of adrenocortical steroids. *Chest.* 1990;97:138-143.

36. Briegel J, Jochum M, Gippner-Steppert C, Thiel M. Immunomodulation in septic shock: hydrocortisone differentially regulates cytokine responses. *J Am Soc Nephrol.* 2001;12(17 suppl):S70-S74.

37. Keh D, Boehnke T, Weber-Cartens S, Schulz C, Ahlers O, Bercker S, Volk HD. Immunologic and hemodynamic effects of "low-dose" hydrocortisone in septic shock: a double-blind, randomized, placebo-controlled, crossover study. *Am J Respir Crit Care Med.* 2003;167:512-520.

38. Barber AE, Coyle SM, Fischer E, Smith C, van der Poll T, Shires GT, Lowry SF. Influence of hypercortisolemia on soluble tumor necrosis factor receptor II and interleukin-1 receptor antagonist responses to endotoxin in human beings. *Surgery.* 1995;118:406-410.

39. Broug-Holub E, Kraal G. Dose- and time-dependent activation of rat alveolar macrophages by glucocorticoids. *Clin Exp Immunol.* 1996; 104:332-336.

40. Fantuzzi G, Demitri MT, Ghezzi P. Differential effect of glucocorticoids on tumour necrosis factor production in mice: up-regulation by early pretreatment with dexamethasone. *Clin Exp Immunol.* 1994;96:166-169.

41. Barber AE, Coyle SM, Marano MA, Fischer E, Calvano SE, Fong Y, Moldawer LL. Glucocorticoid therapy alters hormonal and cytokine responses to endotoxin in man. *J Immunol.* 1993;150:1999-2006.

42. Schaaf MJ, Cidlowski JA. Molecular mechanisms of glucocorticoid action and resistance. *J Steroid Biochem Mol Biol.* 2002;83:37-48.

43. Cooper MS, Stewart PM. Adrenal insufficiency in critical illness. *J Intensive Care Med.* 2007;22:348-362.

44. Lee HS, Lee JM, Kim MS, Kim HY, Hwangbo B, Zo JI. Low-dose steroid therapy at an early phase of

postoperative acute respiratory distress syndrome. *Ann Thorac Surg.* 2005;79:405-410.

45. Confalonieri M, Urbino R, Potena A, Piattella M, Parigi P, Puccio G, Della PR. Hydrocortisone infusion for severe community-acquired pneumonia: a preliminary randomized study. *Am J Respir Crit Care Med.* 2005;171:242-248.

46. Annane D, Sebille V, Bellissant E. Effect of low doses of corticosteroids in septic shock patients with or without early acute respiratory distress syndrome. *Crit Care Med.* 2006;34:22-30.

47. Huh J, Lim C, Jegal Y. The effect of steroid therapy in patients with late ARDS. *Tuberculosis Respir Dis.* 2002;52:376-384.

48. Keel JB, Hauser M, Stocker R, Baumann PC, Speich R. Established acute respiratory distress syndrome: benefit of corticosteroid rescue therapy. *Respiration.* 1998;65:258-264.

49. Varpula T, Pettila V, Rintala E, Takkunen O, Valtonen V. Late steroid therapy in primary acute lung injury. *Intensive Care Med.* 2000;26:526-531.

50. Thompson BT, Ancukiewics M, Hudson LD, Steinberg KP. Steroid treatment for persistent ARDS: a word of caution [Letter]. *Crit Care.* 2007;11:425.

51. Pustavoitau A, Stevens RD. Mechanisms of neurologic failure in critical illness. *Crit Care Clin.* 2008;24:1-24.

52. Headley AS, Tolley E, Meduri GU. Infections and the inflammatory response in acute respiratory distress syndrome. *Chest.* 1997;111:1306-1321.

53. Meduri GU. Clinical review: a paradigm shift: the bidirectional effect of inflammation on bacterial growth. Clinical implications for patients with acute respiratory distress syndrome. *Crit Care.* 2002;6:24-29.

54. Weigelt JA, Norcross JF, Borman KR, Snyder WH, III. Early steroid therapy for respiratory failure. *Arch Surg.* 1985;120:536-540.

55. Bernard GR, Luce JM, Rinaldo JE, Tate RM, Sibbald WJ, Kariman K, Higgins S. High-dose corticosteroids in patients with the adult respiratory distress syndrome. *N Engl J Med.* 1987;317:1565-1570.

56. Kaufmann I, Briegel J, Schliephake F, Hoelzzl A, Chouker A, Hummel T, Schelling G. Stress doses of hydrocortisone in septic shock: beneficial effects on opsonization-dependent neutrophil functions. *Intensive Care Med.* 2008;34:344-349.

57. Meduri GU, Kanangat S, Bronze M, Patterson DR, Meduri CU, Pak C, Tolley EA. Effects of methylprednisolone on intracellular bacterial growth. *Clin Diagn Lab Immunol.* 2001;8:1156-1163.

58. Stevens RD, Dowdy DW, Michaels RK, Mendez-Tellez PA, Pronovost PJ, Needham DM. Neuromuscular dysfunction acquired in critical illness: a systematic review. *Intensive Care Med.* 2007;33:1876-1891.

59. Hough CL, Steinberg KP, Taylor Thompson B, Rubenfeld GD, Hudson LD. Intensive care unit-acquired neuromyopathy and corticosteroids in survivors of persistent ARDS. *Intensive Care Med.* 2009;35:63-68.

60. De Jonghe B, Bastuji-Garin S, Sharshar T, Outin H, Brochard L. Does ICU-acquired paresis lengthen weaning from mechanical ventilation? *Intensive Care Med.* 2004;30:1117-1121.

61. Karnatovskaia LV, Lee AS, Gajic O, Festic E. The influence of prehospital systemic corticosteroids use on development of acute respiratory distress syndrome and hospital outcomes. *Crit Care Med.* 2013;41:1679-1685.

Thrombolytic Therapy for Submassive Pulmonary Embolism

69

Samarth Beri, MD and Stephen M. Pastores, MD, FACP, FCCP, FCCM

KEY POINTS

1. Acute pulmonary embolism (PE) is the most frequent and potentially fatal venous thromboembolic event.

2. Clinically, acute PE can be classified as either massive or submassive. Thrombolytic therapy is the recommended treatment for patients with acute massive PE who are hemodynamically unstable and do not have a high bleeding risk.

3. In patients with submassive PE, the use of thrombolytic therapy remains controversial.

4. Risk stratification with echocardiography may assist when deciding to use thrombolytic therapy for hemodynamically stable patients with submassive PE and evidence of right ventricular (RV) dysfunction.

5. Echocardiographic findings in patients with acute PE include RV hypokinesis and dilatation, interventricular septal flattening and paradoxical motion toward the left ventricle, tricuspid regurgitation, pulmonary hypertension and loss of inspiratory collapse of the inferior vena cava.

6. The hemodynamic status of the patient with acute PE is the most significant predictor of mortality in the short term.

7. Among patients with submassive PE being treated with unfractionated heparin, the administration of tenecteplase reduced the composite endpoint of all-cause mortality or hemodynamic decompensation at 7 days when compared to placebo but was associated with an increased rate of bleeding.

INTRODUCTION

Acute pulmonary embolism (PE) remains the most frequent and potentially fatal venous thromboembolic event. It is estimated that 100,000 to 180,000 deaths occur annually in the United States from acute PE. The outcome of acute PE depends on both the severity of pulmonary arterial obstruction and the presence and severity of preexisting cardiopulmonary disease in the patient. Acute PE can be classified as massive or submassive. Massive PE accounts

for 5% of patients with acute PE and is associated with hypotension (defined as systolic blood pressure [SBP] less than 90 mm Hg or a decrease in SBP of 40 mm Hg or more from baseline) and frequently results in acute right ventricular (RV) failure. Submassive PE accounts for approximately 20% to 25% of patients with acute PE and is associated with normotension and evidence of RV dysfunction including RV enlargement documented by transthoracic echocardiography or computed tomographic (CT) pulmonary angiography and elevated biomarkers of myocardial injury (troponins I or T- and B-type natriuretic peptide [BNP]).[1-3]

The recent guidelines from the American College of Chest Physicians and American Heart Association recommend treatment with thrombolytic agents for patients with acute massive PE who present with persistent hypotension and do not have a high bleeding risk.[4,5] Several studies have demonstrated that thrombolytic therapy offers angiographic and hemodynamic benefits compared with standard heparin anticoagulation for patients with acute PE.[4,5] The most studied thrombolytic agents for the treatment of PE are recombinant-tissue-type plasminogen activator (TPA, alteplase), streptokinase, and recombinant human urokinase. Other agents include tenecteplase, and reteplase. Absolute contraindications include any prior intracranial hemorrhage, known structural intracranial cerebrovascular disease (eg, arteriovenous malformation), known malignant intracranial neoplasm, ischemic stroke within 3 months, suspected aortic dissection, active bleeding or bleeding diathesis, recent surgery encroaching on the spinal canal or brain, and recent significant closed-head or facial trauma with radiographic evidence of bony fracture or brain injury.[4]

The use of thrombolytic therapy in patients with submassive PE remains controversial. This chapter will discuss the role of thrombolytic therapy in submassive PE focusing on risk stratification and the complex decision to administer systemic thrombolysis in patients with acute submassive PE.

RISK STRATIFICATION IN ACUTE PE

In recent years, there has been an increased appreciation of the need for risk stratification of patients with acute submassive PE who are hemodynamically stable but with evidence of RV dysfunction.[6] In these patients, RV dysfunction is defined as the presence of at least one of the following: RV dilatation (apical 4-chamber RV diameter/left ventricular [LV] diameter more than 0.9 on echocardiography or chest CT, or RV systolic dysfunction on echocardiography); elevation of BNP more than 90 pg/mL or N-terminal pro-BNP more than 500 pg/mL; or

electrocardiographic changes including new complete or incomplete right bundle branch block, anteroseptal ST-segment elevation or depression, or anteroseptal T-wave inversion. Myocardial necrosis is defined as either elevation of troponin I (> 0.4 ng/mL) or troponin T (> 0.1 ng/mL).[4,5] Several studies have shown a 2- to 2.5-fold increased risk of mortality in patients with normal BP and RV dysfunction compared with those without RV dysfunction.[4,5]

Imaging of the RV with echocardiography detects the changes occurring in the morphology and function of the RV as a result of acute pressure overload in PE.[6] Echocardiography also allows for estimation of pulmonary artery pressure. Echocardiographic findings in patients with acute PE include RV hypokinesis and dilatation, interventricular septal flattening and paradoxical motion toward the left ventricle, tricuspid regurgitation, pulmonary hypertension, and loss of inspiratory collapse of the inferior vena cava.[1] Several studies including registries have demonstrated an association between echocardiographic parameters of RV dysfunction and a poor in-hospital outcome.[6-8] Nevertheless, the prognostic value of echocardiography in hemodynamically stable patients appears moderate at best, primarily due to the poor standardization of echocardiographic criteria.[7,8] In a prospective randomized trial, Konstantinides et al reported that normotensive patients with submassive PE defined by echocardiography appeared to have a low early mortality risk, regardless of whether they received thrombolysis plus heparin or heparin alone.[9]

Four-chamber views of the heart on multidetector-row chest CT may, besides visualizing the thrombi in the pulmonary vasculature, also detect RV enlargement and (indirectly) dysfunction.[7] In an international prospective cohort study, Becattini et al confirmed the prognostic value of an enlarged right ventricle on CT in patients with acute PE.[10] However, RV dilatation on CT has been shown to have resulted in only a small ability to classify risk in these patients.[11]

Elevated levels of cardiac biomarkers (troponins I or T and BNP), in combination with the presence of RV dilatation or hypokinesis on echocardiography significantly helps with risk stratification for acute PE.[12-16] Elevated troponins are often found in hemodynamically stable patients with echocardiographic signs of RV overload suggesting myocardial injury.[2] Pruszczyk and colleagues found that an elevated troponin T level more than 0.01 ng/mL was the only parameter to predict adverse events in normotensive patients with acute PE.[13] In a multicenter, multinational study, the high-sensitivity troponin was examined in 526 normotensive patients with PE and demonstrated a high negative predictive value (98%).[14] Similarly, a meta-analysis of 1132 patients showed that 51% of patients with an acute PE had elevated BNP or NT-pro-BNP and were associated with increased early death and complications during hospitalization.[15] However, the positive predictive value of BNP or NT-pro-BNP for higher risk has been rather low.

Heart-type fatty acid-binding protein and growth differentiation factor-15 are 2 promising new cardiac biomarkers that have been shown to provide relevant prognostic information in patients with non-high-risk PE.[6] Both of these biomarkers increase sharply after pressure overload or myocardial ischemia and are undergoing further study.

The most extensively validated clinical score for risk stratification of patients presenting with PE is the Pulmonary Embolism Severity Score (PESI).[17,18] The PESI allows the clinician to rule out an adverse outcome by having a high negative predictive value at the lowest level of PESI classes. The score is however complex to calculate. A more practical approach is the use of the simplified PESI (sPESI) score with 6 parameters: age more than 80 years, history of cancer, history of either heart failure or chronic lung disease, systolic BP less than 100 mm Hg, heart rate more than 110 beats/min, and an arterial oxyhemoglobin saturation less than 90%.[19]

DECISION-MAKING IN ACUTE SUBMASSIVE PE

The hemodynamic status of the patient with PE is the most significant predictor of mortality in the short term. Early mortality rates for PE range from 3% in clinically stable patients to 58% in patients with cardiogenic shock.[20] If the patient survives the initial presentation of PE, the most common cause of death during the first month is PE-associated RV dysfunction.[21] Cardiac failure from PE is due to a combination of the increased wall stress and cardiac ischemia that compromise RV function and impair

LV output.[22] The development of recurrent PE or progression of RV dysfunction in patients with submassive PE may lead to hemodynamic collapse, even though these patients may have initially presented with hemodynamic stability. Thus the practice of evaluating risk in patients with PE based solely upon the presence of hypotension may neglect key prognostic features and may delay further prognostic testing and initiation of more appropriate therapy.[22] Risk stratification is therefore, paramount to differentiate between subsets of patients.

The outcomes of patients with PE who have received thrombolytic therapy have been reviewed from 4 large registries: Management Strategy And Prognosis of Pulmonary Embolism Registry (MAPPET), International Cooperative Pulmonary Embolism Registry, Registro Informatizado de la Enfermedad TromboEmbolica, and Emergency Medicine Pulmonary Embolism in the Real-World Registry (EMPEROR).[4,5,20,23] These registries have reported a trend toward a decrease in all-cause mortality from PE, especially massive PE in those patients who received thrombolytic therapy. The 30-days mortality from PE in normotensive patients in the EMPEROR was 0.9% (95%CI: 0%-1.6%).[23] The recently completed Prognostic Value of Multidetector CT Scan in Hemodynamically Stable Patients With Acute Symptomatic Pulmonary Embolism study of normotensive patients with acute PE showed a 30-days PE-related mortality of 1.3% (95%CI: 0.5%-2.1%).[24] Overall, these studies have showed that short-term mortality directly attributable to submassive PE in patients treated with heparin anticoagulation is less than 3%. The investigators have concluded that even if adjunctive thrombolytic therapy has an extremely high efficacy (eg, 30% relative reduction in mortality), the effect size on mortality due to submassive PE is probably less than 1%. They propose that secondary outcome measures such as persistent RV dysfunction and chronic thromboembolic pulmonary hypertension (CTEPH), and impaired quality of life be used as important surrogate goals of treatment.[4,22] CTEPH is a rare but serious complication, affecting patients who survive acute PE. It can cause severe RV dysfunction and is often lethal. The etiology of CTEPH is unclear but proposed mechanisms include intricate and complex interactions involving thrombotic and thrombolytic processes and cellular remodeling confounded by various predisposing risk factors.[4,25]

A prospective evaluation of RV function and functional status 6 months after acute submassive PE showed that in patients who received heparin only, 27% demonstrated an increase in RV systolic pressures (RVSP) at 6-months follow-up, and 46% had either dyspnea at rest or exercise intolerance.[26] Interestingly, not a single patient treated with TPA showed an increase in RVSP suggesting that thrombolytic therapy may have benefit in reducing the incidence of CTEPH. More recently, the results of the Moderate Pulmonary Embolism Treated with Thrombolysis trial showed that the incidence of pulmonary hypertension was lower in patients who received TPA and concomitant anticoagulation with reduced-dose enoxaparin or unfractionated heparin than in the standard anticoagulation group (16% vs 57%, $P < 0.001$). There were no in-hospital bleeding events reported in either group.[27]

STUDIES OF THROMBOLYTIC THERAPY FOR SUBMASSIVE PE

Three randomized controlled trials (RCTs) were specifically aimed to address the patients with submassive PE benefit from thrombolytic therapy: MAPPET-3, Tenecteplase Italian Pulmonary Embolism Study (TIPES), and the Pulmonary Embolism Thrombolysis (PEITHO) trials.[9,28,29] Of note, tenecteplase is not approved by the Food and Drug Administration in the United States for the treatment of PE.

In the MAPPET-3 trial, 256 hemodynamically stable patients with acute submassive PE were randomized to receive intravenous (IV) recombinant TPA 100 mg over 2 hours followed by unfractionated heparin infusion or placebo TPA plus heparin anticoagulation.[9] The primary endpoint was in-hospital death or clinical deterioration requiring escalation of therapy defined as catecholamine infusion, rescue fibrinolysis, mechanical ventilation, cardiopulmonary resuscitation, or emergency surgical embolectomy. The investigators found that compared with heparin anticoagulation alone, thrombolytic therapy resulted in a significant reduction in the primary endpoint (10.2% vs 24.6%, $P = 0.004$). They ascribed the difference in the primary endpoint to a higher

frequency of escalation of therapy in patients randomized to heparin anticoagulation alone compared to those treated with TPA. Both groups had low rates of major bleeding, although the heparin treatment group, surprisingly, had a trend toward more major bleeding episodes compared to the TPA-treatment group (3.6% vs 0.8%, $P = 0.29$).[9]

The TIPES trial randomized 58 patients to receive weight-adjusted single-bolus IV tenecteplase or placebo.[28] The primary efficacy endpoint was reduction of RV dysfunction on echocardiography at 24 hours. The investigators found that in the tenecteplase group, there was a 0.31 ± 0.08 reduction of the right-to-left ventricle end-diastolic dimension ratio at 24 hours versus a reduction of 0.10 ± 0.07 in the placebo group ($P = 0.04$). At 30 days, 1 patient randomized to tenecteplase suffered a clinical event (recurrent PE), versus 3 patients randomized to placebo (1 recurrent PE, 1 clinical deterioration, and 1 non-PE-related death). Two nonfatal major bleedings occurred with tenecteplase (1 intracranial), and 1 occurred with placebo.

The PEITHO trial was a prospective, multicenter, double-blind, placebo-controlled randomized trial of thrombolysis with a single-bolus injection of tenecteplase plus heparin versus placebo plus heparin in normotensive patients with submassive PE.[29,30] Eligible patients were those with acute symptomatic PE confirmed by CT pulmonary angiography and RV dysfunction on echocardiography or CT *plus* evidence of myocardial injury with a positive troponin I or T value. The primary outcome was the composite of death from any cause or hemodynamic collapse within 7 days of randomization. A total of 1005 patients were included in the intention-to-treat analysis. The investigators found that a single-bolus injection of tenecteplase resulted in a significantly lower risk of early death or hemodynamic decompensation (2.6%) versus 5.6% in the placebo plus heparin group. However, tenecteplase was also associated with a 2% rate of hemorrhagic stroke and a 6.3% rate of major extracranial hemorrhage versus 0.2% and 1.2% in the placebo plus heparin group.

More recently, Kucher et al reported the results of the Ultrasound Accelerated Thrombolysis of Pulmonary Embolism trial.[31] This trial randomized 59 patients with acute main or lower lobe PE and echocardiographic evidence of RV dysfunction to receive unfractionated heparin and an ultrasound-assisted catheter-directed thrombolysis (USAT) regimen of 10 to 20 mg recombinant TPA over 15 hours or unfractionated heparin alone. The primary outcome was the difference in the RV/LV ratio from baseline to 24 hours. The authors found that a standardized USAT regimen was superior to anticoagulation with heparin alone in reversing RV dilatation at 24 hours, without an increase in bleeding complications. However, the study had several limitations including the lack of a thrombolysis control group without ultrasound, possible selection bias, lack of monitoring of quality of anticoagulation therapy with dose adjustments of heparin (based on activated partial thromboplastin time levels) and of vitamin K antagonists (based on international normalized ratio values), poor quality of the echocardiographic images in some patients and the lack of assessment of residual embolic burden by repeated contrast-enhanced CT.[30]

SUMMARY

To date, there has been no adequately powered RCT that has demonstrated that the survival of patients with submassive PE is improved with the administration of thrombolytic therapy. Furthermore, there is currently no validated prediction rule that can identify the subgroup of patients with submassive PE who are at high risk for PE-related complications and who may benefit from thrombolysis. We believe that select patients with acute submassive PE who have severe RV dysfunction on echocardiography and myocardial injury (elevated troponin or BNP levels) and who are at low risk of bleeding complications may be considered for thrombolytic therapy. Ultimately, as other experts have suggested, clinicians should weigh the risks and benefits, consider the patients' preferences, clot burden, acute physiology, comorbidities, and bleeding risk on a case-by-case basis when deciding to use thrombolytic therapy for patients with submassive PE.[31]

REFERENCES

1. Piazza G. Submassive pulmonary embolism. *JAMA.* 2013;309(2):171-180.
2. Stein PD, Matta F, Janjua M, Yaekoub AY, Jaweesh F, Alrifai A. Outcome in stable patients with acute pulmonary embolism who had right ventricular enlargement and/or elevated levels of troponin I. *Am J Cardiol.* 2010;106(4):558-563.
3. Grifoni, S, Olivotto, I, Cecchini, P, et al. Short-term clinical outcome of patients with acute pulmonary embolism, normal blood pressure, and echocardiographic right ventricular dysfunction. *Circulation.* 2000;101:2817-2822.
4. Kearon C, Akl EA, Comerota AJ, et al. Antithrombotic therapy for VTE disease: antithrombotic therapy and prevention of thrombosis, 9th ed: American College of Chest Physicians evidence based clinical practice guidelines. *Chest.* 2012;141(2 suppl):e419S-e494S.
5. Kearon C, Akl EA, Omelas J, et al. Antithrombotic therapy for VTE Disease: CHEST Guideline and Expert Panel Report. *Chest.* 2016;149(2):315-352.
6. Konstantinides S, Goldhaber S. Pulmonary embolism: risk assessment and management. *Eur Heart J.* 2012;33:3014-3022.
7. Sanchez O, Trinquart L, Colombet I, Durieux P, Huisman MV, Chatellier G, Meyer G. Prognostic value of right ventricular dysfunction in patients with hemodynamically stable pulmonary embolism: a systematic review. *Eur Heart J.* 2008;29:1569-1577.
8. ten Wolde M, Sohne M, Quak E, Mac Gillavry MR, Buller HR. Prognostic value of echocardiographically assessed right ventricular dysfunction in patients with pulmonary embolism. *Arch Intern Med.* 2004;164:1685-1689.
9. Konstantinides S, Geibel A, Heusel G, Heinrich F, Kasper W; Management Strategies and Prognosis of Pulmonary Embolism-3 Trial Investigators. Heparin plus alteplase compared with heparin alone in patients with submassive pulmonary embolism. *N Engl J Med.* 2002;347(15);1143-1150.
10. Becattini C, Agnelli G, Vedovati MC, et al. Multidetector computed tomography for acute pulmonary embolism: diagnosis and risk stratification in a single test. *Eur Heart J.* 2011;32:1657-1663.
11. Trujillo-Santos J, den Exter PL, Gomez V, et al. Computed tomography-assessed right ventricular dysfunction and risk stratification of patients with acute non-massive pulmonary embolism: systematic review and meta-analysis. *J Thromb Haemost.* 2013;11:1823-1832.
12. Meyer T, Binder L, Hruska N, Luthe H, Buchwald AB. Cardiac troponin I elevation in acute pulmonary embolism is associated with right ventricular dysfunction. *J Am Cardiol.* 2000;36:1632-1636.

13. Pruszczyk P, Bochowicz A, Torbicki A, Szulc M, Kurzyna M, Fijałkowska A, Kuch-Wocial A. Cardiac troponin T monitoring identifies high risk group of normotensive patients with acute pulmonary embolism. *Chest.* 2003;123:1947-1952.

14. Lnakeit M, Friesen D, Aschoff J, et al. Highly sensitive troponin T assay and the simplified Pulmonary Embolism Severity Index in hemodynamically stable patients with acute pulmonary embolism: a prospective validation study. *Circulation.* 2011;124:2716-2724.

15. Klok FA, Mos IC, Huisman MV. Brain-type natriuretic peptide levels in the prediction of adverse outcome in patients with pulmonary embolism: a systematic review and meta-analysis. *Am J Respir Crit Care Med.* 2008;178:425-430.

16. Kucher N, Goldhaber SZ. Cardiac biomarkers for risk stratification of patients with acute pulmonary embolism. *Circulation.* 2003;108:2191-2194.

17. Donze J, Le Gal G, Gine MJ, et al. Prospective validation of the Pulmonary Severity Index. A clinical prognostic model for pulmonary embolism. *Thromb Haemost.* 2008;100:943-948.

18. Aujesky D, Obrosky DS, Stone RA, et al. A prediction rule to identify low-risk patients with pulmonary embolism. *Arch Intern Med.* 2006;166:169-175.

19. Jimenez D, Aujesky D, Moores L, et al. Simplification of the pulmonary embolism severity index for prognostication in patients with acute symptomatic pulmonary embolism. *Arch Intern Med.* 2010;170:1383-1389.

20. Goldhaber SZ, Visani L, De Rosa M. Acute pulmonary embolism: clinical outcomes in the International Cooperative Pulmonary Embolism Registry (ICOPER). *Lancet.* 1999;353 (9162):1386-1389.

21. Kasper W, Konstantinides S, Geibel A, et al. Management strategies and determinants of outcome in major pulmonary embolism: results of a multicenter registry. *J Am Coll Cardiol.* 1997;30(5):1165-1171.

22. Jimenez, D. Should systemic lytic therapy be used for submassive pulmonary embolism? Yes. *Chest.* 2013;143(2):296-299.

23. Pollack CV, Schreiber D, Goldhaber SZ, et al. Clinical characteristics, management, and outcomes of patients diagnosed with acute pulmonary embolism in the emergency department: initial report of EMPEROR (Multicenter Emergency Medicine Pulmonary Embolism in the Real World Registry). *J Am Coll Cardiol.* 2011;57(6):700-706.

24. Jimenez D, Lobo JL, Monreal M, Otero R, Yusen RD. Prognostic significance of multidetector computed tomography in normotensive patients with pulmonary embolism: rationale, methodology and reproducibility for the PROTECT study. *J Thromb Thrombolysis.* 2012;34(2):187-192.

25. Haythe J. Chronic thromboembolic pulmonary hypertension: a review of current practice. *Prog Cardiovasc Dis.* 2012;5592:134-143.

26. Kline JA, Steuerwald MT, Marchick MR, Hernandez-Nino J, Rose GA. Prospective evaluation of right ventricular function and functional status 6 months after acute submassive pulmonary embolism: frequency of persistent or subsequent elevation in estimated pulmonary artery pressure. *Chest.* 2009;136(5):1202-1210.

27. Sharifi M, Bay C, Skrocki L, Rahimi F, Mehdipour M; "MOPETT" Investigators. Moderate pulmonary embolism treated with thrombolysis (from the "MOPETT" Trial). *Am J Cardiol.* 2013;111(2):273-277.

28. Becattini C, Agnelli G, Salvi A, et al. TIPES Study Group. Bolus tenecteplase for right ventricle dysfunction in hemodynamically stable patients with pulmonary embolism. *Thromb Res.* 2010;125(3):e82-e86.

29. Steering Committee. Single-bolus tenecteplase plus heparin compared with heparin alone for normotensive patients with acute pulmonary embolism who have evidence of right ventricular dysfunction and myocardial injury: rationale and design of the Pulmonary Embolism Thrombolysis (PEITHO) trial. *Am Heart J.* 2012;163(1):33-38.

30. Meyer G, Vicaut E, Danays T, et al; PEITHO Investigators. Fibrinolysis for patients with intermediate-risk pulmonary embolism. *N Engl J Med.* 2014;370(15):1402-11.

31. Kucher N, Boekstegers P, Muller O, et al. Randomized controlled trial of ultrasound-assisted catheter-directed thrombolysis for acute intermediate-risk pulmonary embolism. *Circulation.* 2014;129:479-486.

32. Bilello KL, Murin S. Should systemic lytic therapy be used for submassive pulmonary embolism? No. *Chest.* 2013;143(2);299-302.

Controversies: Enteral Nutrition—Pyloric Versus Postpyloric

70

Amar Anantdeep Singh Sarao and Roopa Kohli-Seth

INTRODUCTION

Critically ill patients are often in hypermetabolic states with increased nutritional needs. At the same time, however, such patients are often unable to take adequate oral intake, necessitating the use of supplementary nutrition. Maintaining adequate nutrition in the critically ill patient has shown to decrease infectious complications.[1] Early enteral nutrition in the critically ill mechanically ventilated patient has shown to decrease ICU and hospital mortality rates with the greatest benefit derived in the sickest of patients.[2] Malnutrition on the other hand is known to adversely impact the length of ICU and hospital stay.[3] It is because of the benefits seen with providing optimal nutrition in the ICU that nutritional support therapy has now become an indispensable component in the management of the critically ill patient. Although nutrition can be provided via the enteral or parenteral route, the enteral route is preferred over the latter due to its lower cost, ease of institution and decreased infectious complications.[4] Not using the gastrointestinal tract predisposes to gut mucosal atrophy, resulting in translocation of the bacteria across the gut wall leading to bacteremia.

Shock, sepsis, traumatic brain injury as well as pharmacologic agents commonly used in the ICU setting (opioid analgesics, vasoactive, and paralytic agents), all predispose critically ill patients to develop impaired gastric emptying and decreased enteral motility that is seen in up to 60% of this patient population.[7] As a consequence of impaired gastrointestinal motility, high gastric residual volumes (GRVs) are frequently encountered. Finding high GRVs is often used clinically, as an indication of intolerance to enteral feeds. Feeds are thus held or stopped altogether upon encountering high GRVs. It is thought that feeding past the pylorus may result in a lower incidence of high GRVs leading to fewer interruptions in enteral feeding and ultimately in increased nutritional delivery to the patient. However, whether routine monitoring of GRVs is warranted in the critically ill is yet another area of controversy.

ENTERAL NUTRITION: SITES OF DELIVERY

Enteral nutrition in the critically ill is usually delivered via an enteric tube which is inserted either through one of the nares or through the oral cavity. The distal tip of this tube may terminate in the stomach (nasogastric or orogastric tube) or in the duodenum (nasoduodenal tube) or alternatively in the jejunum (nasojejunal tube). These feeding tubes can be placed by surgical techniques as well, namely, gastrostomy (percutaneous endoscopic gastrostomy (PEG) if placed via an endoscopic technique) and jejunostomy (percutaneous endoscopic jejunostomy (PEJ) when placed via an endoscopic technique).

Feeding into the stomach is often termed pyloric or prepyloric feeding, where as feeding into the duodenum or the jejunum is appropriately called postpyloric feeding because the distal end of the feeding tube rests past the pylorus. Although there are a relatively few clinical conditions (Table 70–1) in which feeding via the postpyloric route may be indicated, in a vast majority of the critically ill patients, the issue of pyloric versus postpyloric feeding has been an area of debate. Controversies surround issues of delivery of nutritional goals, time, and resources expended in placement of feeding tubes, as well as rates of infectious and noninfectious complications seen with the 2 modes of enteral feeding.

TABLE 70–1 Conditions in which postpyloric feeding may be clinically indicated.

- Proximal gastrointestinal fistulous disease such a trachea-esophageal fistula
- Severe diabetic gastroparesis not responsive to medical therapy[5]
- Jejunal feeding in severe acute pancreatitis
- Hyperemesis gravidarum unresponsive to medical therapy[6]
- Gastric or duodenal outlet obstruction in neoplastic disease
- Certain postoperative states such as after Whipple's procedure

PLACEMENT OF ENTERIC TUBES

Before enteric feeds can be initiated, enteral access must first be obtained. Although the placement of nasogastric or orogastric tubes may be somewhat cumbersome for the patients, they are placed with a relative ease by the clinicians. Often air insufflation, although considered unreliable by many, and pH testing of the gastric contents are undertaken to confirm the placement of the nasogastric tube in the stomach. A chest X-ray (CXR) is also performed in order to confirm that the tip of the feeding tube is in its intended location and not in the lung.

Multiple techniques exist for the placement of postpyloric feeding tubes, and no one technique has been adopted as the standard. Methods employed in the placement of postpyloric feeding tubes range from blind placement at the bedside, placement under fluoroscopy guidance in the radiology suite, to placement by endoscopy under direct visualization. Techniques utilizing prokinetic agents, magnets, weighted-tip tubes, have been well described in literature for small bowel feeding tube placement at the bedside. Recently, CORPAK MedSystems, Inc. have introduced the CORTRAK 2 Enteral Access System to place postpyloric feeding tubes at the bedside. This method uses an electromagnetic sensing device placed on a patient's chest to track the path that the tip of the feeding tube takes and displays it on a visual monitor. Once the tube is placed in its intended location, the electromagnetic transmitting stylet, preinstalled in the feeding tube, is removed.

POINTS OF CONTROVERSY
TIME AND RESOURCES UTILIZED IN PLACING POSTPYLORIC TUBES

Placement of postpyloric enteral tubes may take a considerable amount of time especially when these tubes are placed via endoscopy or fluoroscopic guidance as opposed to bedside techniques. Delays in placing small bowel or duodenal tubes primarily happen when the radiologist or the endoscopist is not available after-hours or during weekends or holidays. Scheduling difficulties with radiology or endoscopy suites also, at times, may contribute to delays in the placement of small bowel tubes. Delays of up to 24 hours to initiate feeds are not uncommon when postpyloric tubes are placed via the endoscopic method.[8] Such delays in the initiation of feeds ultimately affect the amount of nutrition a critically ill patient receives during her or his stay in the ICU. Adequately trained ICU staff skilled in placing postpyloric tubes at the bedside, however, ameliorates the need to take the patient to radiology or endoscopy suites for placement of tubes. Median times as low as 6.6 hours from admission to the ICU or initiation of mechanical ventilation to begin feeding while achieving 80% success rate in placement of postpyloric tubes by bedside nurses has been reported.[8] Placement of postpyloric tubes at the bedside also forgoes the risks associated with transporting a critically ill patient, along with the paraphernalia of tubes and machines, in and out of the ICU. Cost reductions of greater than 60% have been noted when postpyloric tubes are placed at the bedside by dieticians as opposed to placement by the radiologist under fluoroscopic guidance.[9] It is advisable, thus, that an attempt to place a postpyloric feeding tube should ideally be made at the bedside by an adequately trained professional, preferably a nurse or a dietician. If it proves difficult to obtain enteral access at the bedside, only then should alternate means to obtain enteral access be pursued.

ACHIEVING NUTRITIONAL GOALS IN THE CRITICALLY ILL PATIENTS

A number of studies have looked in to whether differences exist in achieving nutritional goals based on whether a patient is fed into the stomach or past the pylorus.

A fair number of studies have found that patients fed past the pylorus received greater amount of nutrition overall[10-13] compared to those fed in to the stomach. Another set of studies, however, found no difference between the 2 groups.[14,15] Evidence also exists which shows that those fed past the pylorus received less overall nutrition than those fed in to the stomach.[8] One study found no difference over all, but upon a subgroup analysis found that in centers which have previous experience with postpyloric feeding, patients fed via the postpyloric route met nutritional goals more frequently than those fed in to the stomach.[14] In a retrospective review of 150 episodes of postpyloric feeding in 146 patients, including 20 patients fed at home for various durations of time, nutritional requirements were met in 90% of the patients.[16] The results of these studies are summarized in Table 70–2.

Meta-analyses that have evaluated this issue have yielded mixed results as well, with some that have reported no difference in achievement of nutritional goals[17,18] while others that have reported a signal toward increased nutritional intake with postpyloric feeding.[19]

PNEUMONIA IN PYLORIC VERSUS POSTPYLORIC FEEDS

Given that critically ill patients have a high incidence of delayed gastric emptying, up to 60% in some studies,[7] high GRVs are frequently

TABLE 70–2 Nutritional outcomes in pyloric versus postpyloric feeding in critically ill patients.

Study	Patient Type	Number of Patients	Results
Montecalvo et al	Mixed, medical, and surgical	38	PP group received higher nutritional intake, P value < 0.05
Kortbeek et al	Trauma (75% had head injury)	80	PP group reached target feed rate faster than P group. 34 vs 43.8 hours, P value < 0.02
Kearns et al	Medical	44	%REE higher in PP group. 69% vs 47%, P value < 0.05
Davies et al	Medical	73	PP group had significantly decreased GRV
Montejo et al	Mixed	101	NSG in caloric intake. Subgroup analysis limited to experienced centers: significantly higher nutritional intake in PP group
Jones et al	Mixed, not all patients critically ill, outpatients included in study also	150 episode of PP feeding in 146 patients	Nutritional goals met in 90% of cases
White et al	Medical	104	Pyloric group reached nutritional goals earlier, average daily energy deficit significantly higher in PP group
Hsu et al	Medical	121	Average daily nutritional intake significantly higher in PP group
Acosta-Escribano et al	Severe traumatic brain injury	104	Mean efficacious volume of diet delivered significantly higher in PP group. P value: 0.01
Davies et al	Mixed, on mechanical ventilation	181	NSG in nutrition delivered

P, pyloric; PP, postpyloric; NSG, no significant difference; %REE, (mean calories delivered/resting energy expenditure) × 100; NJ, naso-jejunal; GRV, gastric residual volume. Note that all studies listed in the table are randomized controlled trials except the study from Jones et al, which is a retrospective analysis.

encountered when these patients are fed in to the stomach. High GRVs are thought to predispose a critically ill patient to a higher chance of developing gastroesophageal reflux, leading to an increased incidence of macroaspiration and microaspiration of gastric contents ultimately resulting in greater incidence of pneumonia. The idea of feeding past the pylorus to decrease reflux, aspiration, and ultimately prevent pneumonia is not an unfounded one. It has been shown in clinical studies that feeding a patient past the pylorus significantly reduces gastroesophageal reflux and results in a trend toward decreased pulmonary aspiration.[20] Whether this decreased incidence of reflux and aspiration of gastric contents leads to clinically important outcomes such as decreased incidence of nosocomial and ventilator associated pneumonias, has been extensively debated in multiple studies.

CURRENT EVIDENCE VALUATING RISK OF PNEUMONIA IN PYLORIC VERSUS POSTPYLORIC FEEDING

A number of studies have found no significant difference in the incidence of pneumonia in patients fed via the pyloric versus the postpyloric route.[8,11,14,15,21] One of the earlier studies did however show a decreased incidence of pneumonia with postpyloric feeding compared to gastric feeding.[10] Two additional studies have also shown a significant decrease in pneumonia with the use of postpyloric feeding as compared to prepyloric feeding.[12,13]

Mostly, studies evaluating controversies surrounding pyloric versus postpyloric feeding have been relatively small. Given the plausibility of how postpyloric feeding can theoretically decrease the incidence of pneumonia and a number of studies showing both benefit and no benefit at all, a number of meta-analyses been carried out to investigate this issue further. Two of the earlier meta-analyses,[17,18] which utilized 9 and 11 studies, respectively; found no difference in rates of pneumonia between the pyloric and postpyloric feeding groups. More recent meta-analyses,[19,22] however, both of which are from 2013, with each including 15 studies, did show significant reduction in incidence of pneumonia with postpyloric feeds. Table 70–3 summarizes the results of the studies exploring pneumonia in pyloric versus postpyloric feeding.

TABLE 70-3 Impact of pyloric versus postpyloric feeding on incidence of pneumonia in critically ill patients.

Study	Year of Publication	Patient Type	Number of Patients	Result
Montecalvo et al	1992	Mixed medical and surgical	38	2 episodes of pneumonia in gastric vs none in jejunal
Kortbeek et al	1999	Trauma (75% had head injury)	80	NSG
Kearns et al	2000	Medical	44	NSG
Montejo et al	2002	Mixed	101	NSG
White et al	2009	Mixed	104	NSG
Hsu et al	2009	Medical	121	8.6 vs 3.1 per 1000 ventilator days for P vs PP, P value: 0.01
Acosta-Escribano et al	2010	Severe traumatic brain injury	104	32% vs 57% for PP vs P, P value: 0.01
Davies et al	2012	Mixed, on ventilator	181	NSG

All studies are randomized controlled trials. P, pyloric; PP, postpyloric; NSG, no significant difference.

COMPLICATIONS OF PYLORIC VERSUS POSTPYLORIC FEEDING TUBES

A few studies have reported *lower* incidence of increased GRVs in the postpyloric group.[13,14,26] Higher incidence of diarrhea, however, has been reported in the postpyloric group.[10] This is at times attributed to the inability of the small bowel to handle high osmotic loads in polymeric feeds. Thus partially hydrolyzed or semielemental feeds may prove to be useful in these instances. Complications related to tube maintenance have been noted to be higher in the postpyloric group.[14,16] Due to their smaller caliber, postpyloric tubes clog more frequently than gastric tubes. Tube blockage with postpyloric feeding tubes can be seen in up to 17% of the cases.[16] Fifty-milliliter water flushes every 4 to 6 hours can help avoid clogging of the tubes. A meta-analysis[18] found that proportion of patients needing an alternate form of feeding because of tube placement or tube blockage was significantly higher in the postpyloric group.

EFFECT ON MORTALITY, ICU AND HOSPITAL LENGTHS OF STAY

Most of the studies done to date have found no statistically significant difference in rates of mortality, ICU, or hospital lengths of stay.[8,11,12,14,21] In addition, none of the meta-analyses conducted to date has a shown a difference in mortality between the 2 groups.

CURRENT GUIDELINES

The 2009 American Society for Parenteral and Enteral Nutrition (ASPEN) guidelines[23] for nutrition support therapy in the critically ill do not make any specific recommendation for gastric or small bowel feeding and note that either of the two is an acceptable strategy. They do, however, recommend small bowel feeding for those at high risk of aspiration or intolerant of gastric feeding (grade C). These guidelines further recommend that withholding enteral feeds for multiple episodes of high gastric residuals is sufficient for one to consider initiating small bowel feeding (grade E).

The 2013 Canadian critical care nutrition guidelines[24] suggest that feeding critically ill patients through the small bowel may be associated with a lower incidence of pneumonia. These guidelines recommend that in ICUs where placement of postpyloric tubes is feasible, critically ill patients should be routinely fed through the postpyloric route. In ICUs where logistical difficulties exist in obtaining postpyloric access, postpyloric feeding should be *considered* only in patients who are at high risk for intolerance to enteric nutrition such as those on continuous infusion of sedatives and opioids, vasoactive agents and paralytics. If small bowel access is not feasible due to lack of fluoroscopy or endoscopy or due to lack of expertise in blind techniques, postpyloric feedings should be considered only in those patients who are intolerant of gastric feeds and those who repeatedly demonstrate high GRVs.

FUTURE WORK NEEDED

With the current evidence that is available, it is clear that the controversy about pyloric versus postpyloric is far from over. Larger studies in the future may show clearer differences in clinical outcomes between pyloric and postpyloric feeding. There is evidence to suggest that differences in clinical outcomes from pyloric versus postpyloric feeding may not be achieved in less critically ill patients and that the benefit of postpyloric feeding may be primarily seen in those with ASPEN II scores greater than 20.[25]

REFERENCES

1. Rubinson L, Diette GB, Song X, Brower RG, Krishnan JA. Low caloric intake is associated with nosocomial bloodstream infections in patients in the medical intensive care unit. *Crit Care Med.* 2004;3(2):350-357.
2. Artinian V, Krayem H, DiGiovine B. Effects of early enteral feeding on the outcome of critically ill mechanically ventilated medical patients. *Chest.* 2006;129(4):960-967.
3. Robinson G, Goldstein M, Levine GM. Impact of nutritional status on DRG length of stay. *JPEN J Parenter Enteral Nutr.* 1987;11:49-51.

4. Moore FA, Moore EE, Jones TN. TEN versus TPN following major abdominal trauma-reduced septic morbidity. *J Trauma*. 1989;29:916-923.

5. Camilleri M. Diabetic gastroparesis. *N Engl J Med*. 2007;356:820-829.

6. Vaisman N, Kaidar R, Levin I, Lessing JB. Nasojejunal feeding in hyperemesis gravidarum—a preliminary study. *Clin Nutr*. 2004;23:53-57.

7. Nguyen NQ, Ng MP, Chapman M, Fraser RJ, Holloway RH. The impact of admission diagnosis on gastric emptying in critically ill patients. *Crit Care*. 2007;11:R16.

8. White H, Sosnowski K, Tran K, Reeves A, Jones M. A randomized controlled comparison of early post-pyloric versus early gastric feeding to meet nutritional targets in ventilated intensive care patients. *Crit Care*. 2009;13(6):R187.

9. Rollins CM. Blind bedside placement of postpyloric feeding tubes by registered dieticians: success rates, outcomes, and cost effectiveness. *Nutr Clin Pract*. 2013;28:506-509.

10. Montecalvo MA, Steger KA, Farber HW, et al. Nutritional outcomes and pneumonia in critical care patients randomized to gastric versus jejunal tube feedings. *Crit Care Med*. 1992;20(10):1377-1387.

11. Kearns PJ, Chin D, Mueller L, et al. The incidence of ventilator associated pneumonia and success in nutrient delivery with gastric versus small intestinal feeding: a randomized clinical trial. *Crit Care Med*. 2000;28(6):1742-1746.

12. Hsu C, Sun S, Lin S, et al. Duodenal versus gastric feeding in medical intensive care unit patients: a prospective, randomized, clinical study. *Crit Care Med*. 2009;37(6):1866-1872.

13. Acosta-Escribano J, Fernandez-Vivas M, Carmona TG, et al. Gastric versus transpyloric feeding in severe traumatic brain injury: a prospective, randomized trial. *Intensive Care Med*. 2010;36:1532-1539.

14. Montejo JC, Grau T, Acosta J, et al. Multicenter, prospective, randomized, single-blind study comparing the efficacy and gastrointestinal complications of early jejunal feeding with early gastric feeding in critically ill patients. *Crit Care Med*. 2002;30(4):796-800.

15. Davies AR, Morrison S, Bailey M, et al. A multicenter, randomized controlled trial comparing early nasojejunal with nasogastric nutrition in critical illness. *Crit Care Med*. 2012;40(8):2342-2348.

16. Boulton-Jones JR, Lewis J, Jobling JC, Teahon K. Experience of post-pyloric feeding in seriously ill patients in clinical practice. *Clin Nutr*. 2004;23:35-41.

17. Marik PE, Zaloga GP. Gastric versus post-pyloric feeding: a systematic review. *Crit Care*. 2003;7(3): R46-R51.

18. Ho KM, Dobb GJ, Webb SAR. A comparison of early gastric and post-pyloric feeding in critically ill patients: a meta-analysis. *Intensive Care Med*. 2006;32:639-649.

19. Deane AM, Dhaliwal R, Day AG, et al. Comparisons between intragastric and small intestinal delivery of enteral nutrition in the critically ill: a systematic review and meta-analysis. *Crit Care*. 2013;17:R125.

20. Heyland DK, Drover JW, MacDonald S, Novak F, Lam M. Effect of postpyloric feeding on gastroesophageal regurgitation and pulmonary microaspiration: results of a randomized control trial. *Crit Care Med*. 2001;29(8):1495-1501.

21. Kortbeek JB, Haigh PI, Doig C. Duodenal versus gastric feeding in ventilated blunt trauma patients: a randomized controlled trial. *J Trauma*. 1999;46(6):992-996.

22. Jiyon J, Tiancha H, Huiqin W, Jingfen J. Effect of gastric versus post-pyloric feeding on the incidence of pneumonia in critically ill patients: observations from traditional and Bayesian random-effects meta-analysis. *Clin Nutr*. 2013;32:8-15.

23. McClave SA, Martindale RG, Vanek VW, et al. Guidelines for the provision and assessment of nutrition support therapy in the adult critically ill patient: Society of Critical Care Medicine (SCCM) and American Society for Parenteral and Enteral Nutrition (A.S.P.E.N.). *JPEN J Parenter Enteral Nutr*. 2009;33(3):277-316.

24. Canadian Clinical Practice guidelines: downloaded from: http://www.criticalcarenutrition.com/docs/ cpgs2012/5.3.pdf. Accessed January 11, 2014.

25. Huang H, Chang S, Hsu C, et al. Severity of illness influences the efficacy of enteral feeding route on clinical outcomes in patients with critical illness. *J Acad Nutr Diet*. 2012;112(8):1138-1146.

26. Davies AR, Froomes PRA, French CJ, et al. Randomized comparison of nasojejunal and nasogastric feeding in critically ill patients. *Crit Care Med*. 2002;30(3):586-590.

Controversies: Continuous Versus Intermittent Renal Replacement in the Critically Ill Patient

71

Min Jung Kim, MD and John M. Oropello, MD, FACP, FCCP, FCCM

INTRODUCTION

Acute kidney injury (AKI) is frequently a part of multiorgan dysfunction syndrome in critically ill patients in the intensive care unit (ICU), and a significant portion, about 2% in some reports,[1] will require renal replacement therapy (RRT). There is controversy about the optimal treatment of AKI regarding modality, dose, and appropriate timing of RRT.

RRT for AKI can be classified as intermittent or continuous, based on the duration of treatment. The duration of intermittent therapy is less than 24 hours, whereas the duration of continuous therapy is at least 24 hours. Intermittent RRT (IRRT) includes intermittent hemodialysis (IHD) and sustained low-efficiency dialysis (SLED). SLED refers to hemodialysis performed with a conventional dialysis machine over a longer time period (usually ≥ 5 hours) than traditional IHD. Continuous therapies include peritoneal dialysis and continuous RRT (CRRT). The 4 main types of CRRT by mechanism of solute removal are slow continuous ultrafiltration (fluid removal only); continuous venovenous hemofiltration (CVVH) (convection); CVV hemodialysis (CVVHD) (diffusion); and CVV hemodiafiltration (CVVHDF) (concurrent diffusion with convection). In developed countries, peritoneal dialysis is rarely used for AKI in the ICU setting because it provides inefficient solute clearance, increases the risk of peritonitis, and compromises respiratory function. In developing countries, peritoneal dialysis is still used for AKI due to low maintenance and cost.

MODALITIES OF RRT: IRRT VERSUS CRRT

Whether IRRT or CRRT influences clinical outcomes remains the subject of debate. Even though the worldwide standard RRT in the ICU is IHD, survey evidence has consistently shown considerable variation in RRT practice patterns. In recent years, the use of SLED has risen and is mainly driven by its convenience and lower cost compared to CRRT.

Several nonrandomized studies have suggested that CRRT may contribute to improved survival and a higher rate of renal recovery; however, other similar studies have failed to show any additional benefit with CRRT. The first randomized controlled trial (RCT) was done in 2001 by Mehta et al.[2] IHD was averaged 5 days/week for 3 to 4 hours per session. Univariate intention-to-treat analysis revealed a higher mortality among patients receiving CRRT. However, multivariate analysis revealed no impact of RRT modality on all-cause mortality or recovery of renal function. Because Mehta et al, there have been 8 RCTs, comparing CRRT and IRRT (Table 71–1) (IHD,[3-8] SLED[9,10]). There is significant variation among these RCTs in terms of study population (exclusion of chronic kidney disease, illness severity, and etiology of AKI), methods of RRT (criteria for RRT, device/technique, doses, and membrane material). Serious concerns have been identified in some trials due to unbalanced baseline characteristics, inappropriate sample size, and significant crossover between dialytic modalities.[11] Most studies[3-5,7,8] used

TABLE 71–1 Characteristics of CRRT and IRRT within randomized controlled trials.

Trial	RRT Decision	IRRT Dose	IRRT Pump Speed	CRRT Dose	Mortality	Renal Recovery	Hypotension	Pressor Requirements	Fluid Balance/Solute Clearance
				RRT Characteristics					
Mehta et al[2]	BUN > 40 mg/dL, serum Cr > 2.0 mg/d	IHD: 4 h/session; 5 days/week	200-300 mL/min	CAVHDF or CVVHDF: urea clearance 22 mL/min	ND[a]	ND	NA	NA	CRRT[b]/CRRT
John et al[5]	serum Cr > 3 mg/dL, UO < 10 mL/h	IHD: 4 h/session	250 mL/min	CVVHF: 2 L/h	ND	NA	IHD > CVVH	ND	NA/CRRT
Gasparovic et al[4]	3X ⇑ Cr, hyperkalemia > 5.5 mmol/L, base deficit > 6	IHD: 3-4 h/session: daily	200-250 mL/min	CVVHF: 18 and 35 mL/kg/h	ND	NA	ND	NA	NA
Augustine et al[3]	Clinical decision	IHD: K+/V 3.6/week; 3 sessions/week	300 mL/min	CVVHD: K+/V 3.6/week	ND	ND	IHD > CVVH	IHD	CRRT/NA
Uehlinger et al[7]	serum Cr > 4 mg/dL, UO < 20 mL/h	IHD: urea clearance 200 mL/min: 3-4 h/session	150-350 mL/min	CVVHDF: 2 L/h or urea clearance 20 mL/min	ND	ND	ND	ND	ND/ND
Vinsonneau et al[8]	urea > 36 mmol/L; serum Cr < 310 μmol/L	IHD: 4 h/session: alternate day	500 mL/min	CVVHDF: 29 mL/kg/h	ND	ND	ND	NA	NA/NA

Lins et al[6]	serum Cr > 2 mg/dL; clinical decision	IHD: 4-6 h/session: daily	100-300 mL/min	CVVH: 1-2 L/h	ND	NA	NA	NA	NA/NA
Kielstein et al[30]	respiratory support in presence of oliguric/anuric ARF (UO < 500 mL)	SLED: urea[c] reduction ratio 53%: 12 h/session; daily	200 mL/min	CVVH: 3.2 L/h (at least 30 mL/kg/h)	NA	ND	ND	ND	NA/ND
Schwenger et al[31]	UO < 500 mL/d; serum potassium > 6.5 mmol/L volume overload nitrogen level above 70 mg/d unresponsiveness to fluid resuscitation acute rise in plasma urea nitrogen level above 70 mg/d	SLED: 12 h/session: daily[c]	100-120 mL/min	CVVH: 35 mL/kg/h	SLED	ND	ND	ND	NA/SLED

[a]After adjustment for the imbalances in group assignment.
[b]P value not reported.
[c]Correction of acidosis was accomplished faster with SLED.
ARF, acute renal failure; BUN, blood urea nitrogen; CAVHDF, continuous arteriovenous hemodiafiltration; CRI, chronic renal insufficiency; CVVHDF, continuous venovenous hemodiafiltration; ESRD, end-stage renal disease; MODS, multiorgan dysfunction syndrome; NA, not applicable; ND, no significant difference; SLED, slow low efficiency dialysis; UO, urine output.

TABLE 71-2 CRRT versus IHD.

	CRRT	IHD
Recovery of renal function	+	
Hemodynamic stability	+	
Control of azotemia and volume overload	+	
Clotting of dialysis filter and bleeding complications		+
Practicality and cost		+

CRRT, continuous renal replacement therapy; IHD, intermittent hemo-dialysis; +, advantage.

IHD 3 times per week; however, recently, Lins et al[6] performed a multicenter prospective RCT comparing IHD (7 days/week, 4-6 hours per session) with CVVH, with a higher sample size, and better control of the severity of illness of the study population. Lins et al reported that after AKI, the modality of RRT had no impact on ICU outcome. However, the dose of IHD (42 hours/week) was far greater than the typical 9 to 12 hours of IHD being delivered in the ICU setting. To date, none of the RCTs and meta-analyses[11-14] has demonstrated any significant difference in mortality between modalities. However, there are other important factors for selecting the RRT modality (Table 71–2).

RECOVERY OF RENAL FUNCTION: CRRT VERSUS IHD

In an animal model of AKI, there was loss of autoregulation of renal blood flow with poor renal perfusion when systolic blood pressure decreased to less than 90 mm Hg.[15] Therefore, improved hemodynamic stability during RRT may be associated with fewer episodes of reduced renal blood flow, less renal ischemia, and more rapid renal recovery. Augustine and colleagues[3] found that renal recovery was influenced by blood pressure changes during RRT; however, the dialysis modality itself did not impact renal recovery. To date, most randomized controlled studies[2,3,6-8] have failed to demonstrate the superiority of CRRT with regard to recovery of renal function. Not surprisingly, results from meta-analyses have been inconsistent.

Three meta-analyses[11,13,14] including RCTs reported no statistical difference in renal recovery with regard to RRT modalities. Most recently, Schneider and colleagues[16] performed a meta-analysis specifically to compare the rate of dialysis dependence among severe AKI survivors according to the choice of initial RRT modality. They found that patients who received IRRT as an initial RRT modality for AKI had 1.7 times increased risk of remaining dialysis dependent as compared with those who initially received CRRT, but this finding did not reach statistical significance. Allocation bias was present in observational trials, with IRRT appearing to be allocated to patients with lesser illness severity, putting them at even less risk for dialysis dependence, potentially favoring CRRT to an even greater degree. In 2014, Wald and colleagues[17] published a large retrospective cohort study, comparing CRRT with IHD in terms of chronic dialysis, defined as the need for dialysis for a consecutive period of 90 days. The risk of chronic dialysis was significantly lower among patients who initially received CRRT versus IHD. This finding was more prominent among those with preexisting chronic kidney disease and heart failure.

In summary, IRRT appears to be associated with a higher rate of chronic dialysis dependence than CRRT. Randomized prospective trials are needed to confirm these findings.

HEMODYNAMIC STABILITY: CRRT VERSUS IHD

Despite the inconsistent results from RCTs and meta-analyses, there might be a hemodynamic benefit for CRRT despite the lack of survival benefit for CRRT. Proponents of CRRT advocate that continuous techniques with a lower ultrafiltration rate provide better hemodynamic stability than with IHD. Augustine and colleagues[3] reported more changes in mean arterial pressure during IHD (3 days/week, treatment times based on a goal of greater than 5 hours on average) as compared to CVVHD. More patients on IHD therapy required an increase in vasopressor dose during the initial therapy. However, Uehlinger and colleagues[7] reported no significant difference between CVVHDF and IHD, in terms of vasopressor requirements, hypotensive episodes, or hemodynamic instability.

However, they used therapeutic maneuvers to enhance hemodynamic stability during IHD (such as lower blood flow rate and lower net ultrafiltration during the initial IHD) with a mean of 5 IHD sessions per week.

In the Cochrane meta-analysis,[14] mean arterial pressure at the end of the study period was significantly higher with CRRT than with IRRT, whereas the number of hypotensive episodes and norepinephrine doses were not different. A meta-analysis by Bagshaw and colleagues[11] reported that CRRT was associated with fewer episodes of hemodynamic instability; however, another systematic review[13] reported nominal differences.

Some argue that improved hemodynamics may be simply related to hypothermic vasoconstriction during CRRT. A similar effect can be obtained in IRRT by cooling the dialysate. Other measures to improve hemodynamics include less aggressive ultrafiltration, more frequent IHD (eg, daily), dialysate sodium and calcium concentrations to 145 and 1.5 mmol/L, respectively, using low blood filter flow (< 150 mL/min), low dialysate flow, and cool dialysate with high sodium concentration.[8,18] Notably, trials reporting no significant difference in hypotensive episodes between CRRT and IHD have used extraordinary measures to reduce hypotensive IHD, which do not reflect standard clinical practice.[7,8] Considering the cost-effectiveness and practicality of IHD as one of its main advantages, applying all these maneuvers to the current IHD technique diminishes the purported advantages in cost and labor intensity.

Patients with cerebral edema or intracranial hypertension have impaired autoregulation of cerebral blood flow. A decrease in systemic blood pressure during RRT can cause decreased cerebral blood flow and cerebral ischemia, possibly exacerbating brain edema. CRRT has been proven superior in maintaining cerebral blood flow in patients with acute liver failure and cerebral edema compared with IHD.[18]

In summary, CRRT is associated with greater hemodynamic stability during RRT, as compared with standard IHD. As expected, increasing the frequency and duration of IHD decreases the differences between IHD and CRRT; however, it does not represent the typical IHD sessions conducted in the ICU. CRRT may be the most beneficial in patients with preexisting hemodynamic instability, brain injury, and fulminant liver failure.

CONTROL OF AZOTEMIA AND VOLUME OVERLOAD: CRRT VERSUS IHD

One of the advantages of CRRT is better control of azotemia and volume overload due to slow, constant blood flow, and ultrafiltration, as compared to IHD. In addition, CRRT may allow administration of medications and nutrition with less concern for volume overload. Mehta et al[2] showed that cumulative solute removal with CRRT is greater than that with IHD. Augustine et al[3] found a marked difference in total fluid balance over 3 days (–4005 mL for the CVVHD group and +1539 mL for the IHD group). However, Uehlinger et al[5] showed that the average daily solute clearance was comparable between the CVVHDF and IHD groups and the amount fluid removed daily by RRT and average fluid balance did not differ between 2 groups. Also, there was no difference in the use of parenteral or enteral nutrition. These inconsistent results may be due to different CRRT techniques used in each study. A retrospective controlled study by Morimatsu et al[19] compared CVVHDF with CVVH in terms of azotemic control. CVVH (ultrafiltration rate: 2 L/h, urea clearance: 28 mL/min) achieved superior control of azotemia when compared to CVVHDF (ultrafiltration rate: 700 mL/h, urea clearance: 27 mL/min). In our institution, CVVH has been used over CVVHDF, due to the past experience that CVVHDF reduced the ultrafiltration rate; CVVH achieved better azotemic control.

In view of all of the uncertainties mentioned earlier and because of the physiologic plausibility, fluid-overloaded patients are among those with the potential to benefit from CRRT.

CONTROL OF ACID-BASE AND ELECTROLYTES: CRRT VERSUS IHD

Constant solute removal with replacement of electrolytes and base (bicarbonate or acetate) in CRRT is more beneficial in stabilizing and maintaining blood pH, which may improve hemodynamic stability and the response to vasopressors. CRRT is also helpful in maintaining electrolyte homeostasis and in providing a more gradual correction of chronic hyponatremia to avoid osmotic demyelination syndrome. CRRT is preferred in patients with cerebral edema and intracranial hypertension[18] to avoid rapid decreases in serum osmolality leading to increased brain edema as well as the hemodynamic benefits on cerebral blood flow.

In contrast to CRRT, IHD can remove small molecules effectively, so it may be more useful in acute life-threatening conditions such as severe hyperkalemia, rhabdomyolysis, tumor lysis syndrome, and certain cases of intoxication.[18]

BLEEDING COMPLICATIONS AND DIALYSIS FILTER CLOTTING: CRRT VERSUS IRRT

Filter clotting is a common problem during RRT, causing poor filter performance. Anticoagulation may be necessary for both IRRT and CRRT to prevent clotting of the dialysis filter. CRRT has a higher risk of filter clotting due to higher rates of ultrafiltration, lower blood flows, and longer duration of RRT. Heparin is the preferred anticoagulant at many institutions but the optimal intensity of heparinization is unknown. Hemodialysis can be performed without anticoagulation, and regular saline flushes can be used in the dialysis circuit instead. Also with CRRT, placement of the replacement fluid before the circuit (predilution hemofiltration) will dilute the blood and decrease filter clotting. Although predilution replacement fluid also dilutes the solute concentration of blood entering the filter, diminishing overall clearance rates, predilution actually increases urea clearance by washing out urea from the red cells. Regional citrate infusion can also be used in CRRT. Citrate chelates calcium in the serum and inhibits activation of the coagulation cascade. Use of citrate anticoagulation, however, increases the complexity of RRT by requiring customized dialysate solutions or replacement fluid and frequent monitoring of laboratory results to minimize metabolic complications. In cases of heparin-induced thrombocytopenia, the direct thrombin-inhibitor argatroban can be used.

In a Cochrane meta-analysis,[14] patients on CRRT had a significantly higher risk of recurrent dialysis filter clotting when compared to those on IRRT, as expected. There was no significant difference in the risk of bleeding between CRRT and IRRT. Another meta-analysis[11] also reported no difference in severe bleeding complications by modality; however, the largest RCT[8] of the meta-analysis excluded patients who had coagulation disorders or uncontrolled hemorrhage. In coagulopathy associated with severe bleeding, continuous replacement of blood products, and FFP coupled with maintenance of fluid balance with CRRT may help to correct coagulopathy and minimize fluid overload and pulmonary edema. In summary, CRRT can often be successfully performed without any anticoagulation; however, in case of frequent filter clotting despite anticoagulation or in the presence of contraindications for systemic anticoagulation, IRRT is preferable.

REMOVAL OF CYTOKINES: CRRT VERSUS IRRT

Experimental and clinical data show that many middle molecules, such as tumor necrosis factor that may be involved in the inflammatory response, can be removed by CRRT modalities.[20] As per the analysis of Ronco et al,[20] septic patients may benefit from a higher dose of treatment (high-volume hemofiltration [HVHF]) allowing blood purification from the inflammatory cytokines during systemic inflammatory and septic states. Oudemans-van Straaten et al[21] conducted a prospective cohort analysis in 306 critically ill patients who received intermittent HVHF at a mean ultrafiltration rate of 4 L/h. Mortality in HVHF patients was lower than that predicted by illness severity scores. In a subgroup analysis, an improvement in cardiac index, blood pressure, and stroke volume was observed after the first HVHF run in patients with low cardiac output. Cole and colleagues[22] measured hemodynamics, serum cytokines, and the complement concentration in 11 patients with septic shock and multiorgan dysfunction syndrome. Patients were randomly assigned to HVHF (8 hours; ultrafiltration rate 6 L/h) or to standard CVVH. HVHF was associated with a greater reduction in norepinephrine requirements than CVVH. HVHF was associated with a greater reduction in the area under the curve for C3a and C5a, but the measured soluble mediators in the ultrafiltrate was negligible, indicating a greater role in filter adsorption of studied mediators. Some drawbacks of HVHF include the large volumes of replacement fluid, the high cost and practicality, should be considered along with the potential benefits.

To date, the significance of inflammatory cytokine removal by standard CRRT is unclear. Some argue that insignificant numbers of these mediators are removed by CRRT in comparison with endogenous clearance, and that CRRT can also remove anti-inflammatory cytokines. In addition, exposure to an extracorporeal circuit can activate proinflammatory cytokines, so a shorter duration of RRT (IHD, SLED) might be more beneficial than CRRT in terms of net clearance of proinflammatory cytokines. Of note, removal of cytokines and other large molecules can be obtained just as well, if not better, with IHD or SLED, under the condition that open membranes with large pore size (so-called high-flux membranes) are applied, even though it removes cytokines intermittently but not continuously.

With regard to cytokine removal, more studies are needed to answer several questions: which technique (IRRT with high-flux dialyzers, standard CRRT, HVHF, and adsorption) gives the best results at the lowest technical cost, and how much cytokine removal has a significant effect (if, any) on mortality and morbidity in critically ill patients.

DOSES OF RRT: INTENSIVE THERAPY VERSUS LESS INTENSIVE THERAPY

The ideal dose of dialytic therapy in critically ill patients has not yet been conclusively determined. Schiffl et al[23] compared daily IHD (6 days/week) with alternate-day IHD (3 days/week) in 160 patients with acute renal failure. The study reported lower mortality (28% vs 46%) and shorter duration of AKI (9 vs 16 days) in the daily IHD group. However, the actual delivered dialysis dose per session was substantially lower than that in usual care practices, and the weekly delivered doses were even lower in the alternate-day IHD group. Ronco et al[24] performed a large single-center prospective RCT to evaluate the impact of different ultrafiltration doses in CRRT on survival and found that doses of 45 and 35 mL/kg/h in CVVH reduced 15-day mortality compared with 20 mL/kg/h in CVVH. A large

multicenter RCT[25] (Acute Renal Failure Trial Network Study) was performed in 2008 to compare intensive RRT (IHD and SLED 6 times per week and CVVHDF at 35 mL/kg/h) with less intensive RRT (IHD and SLED 3 times per week and CVVHDF at 20 mL/kg/h). Sixty-day mortality was 53.6% with intensive therapy and 51.5% with less-intensive therapy (odds ratio, 1.09; $P = 0.47$). There was no significant difference between the 2 groups in the duration of RRT or the rate of recovery of kidney function. A potential reason for this failure could be that the higher intensity of solute removal also has a downside such as greater removal of drugs resulting in inadequate drug concentrations (eg, of antimicrobials) or more electrolyte disturbances.[8,26] Also, in the Acute Renal Failure Trial Network Study,[25] patients in the less-intensive therapy group were better dialyzed than patients receiving usual care in typical clinical practice, the dose delivered during CVVH was 89% of that prescribed for intensive treatment group, 95% for the less intensive treatment group. In usual care practices, CRRT is frequently interrupted owing to clotting of the filter, surgery, diagnostic investigations, or other procedures. In summary, the ideal dose of RRT in critically ill patients remains undetermined to date. It seems that increasing beyond an adequate level of intensity provides no additional benefit in critically ill patients.

PRACTICALITY AND COST: CRRT VERSUS IRRT

The frequency and duration of IRRT can be adjusted according to the patients' condition, allowing more flexibility. IRRT can be performed with the same machines used for chronic IHD, and the same machines can be used for an extended mode (eg, SLED) when needed. This contrasts with CRRT machines, which do not allow an increase of the intensity of the treatment to allow shorter treatments.

Currently, in all of the studies comparing cost, IRRT was less costly than CRRT.[27-29] Even, when the cost of ICU nurses for CRRT was not included into its whole cost, CRRT was more expensive than IHD (at least $3500 per week for CRRT vs $1342 per week for IHD).[24]

Especially, dialysate and replacement fluid costs and extracorporeal circuit costs were in favor of IRRT worldwide.

SUSTAINED LOW-EFFICIENCY DIALYSIS

SLED or extended daily dialysis is a hybrid technique that combines several advantages of both IHD and CRRT. This slower dialytic modality runs for prolonged periods using conventional hemodialysis machines with modification of blood and dialysate flows. Typically, SLED uses lower blood-pump speeds of 200 mL/min and lower dialysate flow rates of 300 mL/min for 6 to 12 hours daily. It allows for improved hemodynamic stability through gradual solute and volume removal as in CRRT, in addition to high solute clearance as in IHD. Still, it is less labor intensive and costly than CRRT. Frequency and duration of therapy can be adjusted based on the needs of the patient as in IHD, and it offers a dialysis-free period, giving opportunities to mobilize patients during their time off dialysis, as in IHD. Kielstein et al[30] compared CVVH with 12-hour daily SLED. Average mean arterial pressure was not significantly different in both therapies. Urea reduction rate was similar with SLED compared with CVVH therapy. Correction of acidosis was accomplished faster with SLED than CVVH, and the amount of heparin used was significantly lower with SLED. A large RCT by Schwenger et al[31] compared CVVH with 12-hour daily SLED. Ninety-day mortality and hemodynamic stability did not differ between groups, whereas duration of mechanical ventilation and time to renal recovery were significantly shorter in the SLED group. Solute clearance was more effective in the SLED group. Patients treated with SLED needed fewer transfusions had substantial reduction in nursing time and costs. However, in usual clinical practice (ie, outside of research protocol), due to time and personnel constraints, SLED can be, and often is, run faster for shorter time periods causing hemodynamic instability similar to IHD.

CONCLUSIONS

To date, neither the modality of RRT the dose, or the timing[32,33] of RRT has been demonstrated to have an impact on patient survival. The benefits of CRRT over IHD in the critically ill patient include hemodynamic stability, potential for decreased need for chronic HD, and improved electrolyte and acid-base homeostasis. IHD is beneficial in the hemodynamically stable patient or and when filter clotting prevents CVVH. CVVHD does not have a clear benefit over CVVH due to reduced filtration. The choice of dialytic modality should be based on the clinical status of the patient, the resources available in the institution, and in the manner that RRT is performed.

REFERENCES

1. Hoste EA, Schurgers M. Epidemiology of acute kidney injury: how big is the problem? *Crit Care Med*. 2008;36(4 suppl):S146-S151.
2. Mehta RL, McDonald B, Gabbai FB, et al. A randomized clinical trial of continuous versus intermittent dialysis for acute renal failure. *Kidney Int*. 2001;60(3):1154-1163.
3. Augustine JJ, Sandy D, Seifert TH, Paganini EP. A randomized controlled trial comparing intermittent with continuous dialysis in patients with ARF. *Am J Kidney Dis*. 2004;44(6):1000-1007.
4. Gasparovic V, Filipovic-Grcic I, Merkler M, Pisl Z. Continuous renal replacement therapy (CRRT) or intermittent hemodialysis (IHD)—what is the procedure of choice in critically ill patients? *Ren Fail*. 2003;25(5):855-862.
5. John S, Griesbach D, Baumgartel M, Weihprecht H, Schmieder RE, Geiger H. Effects of continuous haemofiltration vs intermittent haemodialysis on systemic haemodynamics and splanchnic regional perfusion in septic shock patients: a prospective, randomized clinical trial. *Nephrol Dial Transplant*. 2001;16(2):320-327.
6. Lins RL, Elseviers MM, Van der Niepen P, et al. Intermittent versus continuous renal replacement therapy for acute kidney injury patients admitted to the intensive care unit: results of a randomized clinical trial. *Nephrol Dial Transplant*. 2009;24(2):512-518.
7. Uehlinger DE, Jakob SM, Ferrari P, et al. Comparison of continuous and intermittent renal replacement therapy for acute renal failure. *Nephrol Dial Transplant*. 2005;20(8):1630-1637.
8. Vinsonneau C, Camus C, Combes A, et al. Continuous venovenous haemodiafiltration versus intermittent haemodialysis for acute renal failure in patients with multiple-organ dysfunction syndrome: a multicentre randomised trial. *Lancet*. 2006;368(9533):379-385.
9. Kumar VA, Craig M, Depner TA, Yeun JY. Extended daily dialysis: a new approach to renal replacement

for acute renal failure in the intensive care unit. *Am J Kidney Dis.* 2000;36(2):294-300.

10. Kumar VA, Yeun JY, Depner TA, Don BR. Extended daily dialysis vs. continuous hemodialysis for ICU patients with acute renal failure: a two-year single center report. *Int J Artif Organs.* 2004;27(5):371-379.

11. Bagshaw SM, Berthiaume LR, Delaney A, Bellomo R. Continuous versus intermittent renal replacement therapy for critically ill patients with acute kidney injury: a meta-analysis. *Crit Care Med.* 2008;36(2):610-617.

12. Ghahramani N, Shadrou S, Hollenbeak C. A systematic review of continuous renal replacement therapy and intermittent haemodialysis in management of patients with acute renal failure. *Nephrology (Carlton).* 2008;13(7):570-578.

13. Pannu N, Klarenbach S, Wiebe N, Manns B, Tonelli M. Renal replacement therapy in patients with acute renal failure: a systematic review. *JAMA.* 2008;299(7):793-805.

14. Rabindranath K, Adams J, Macleod AM, Muirhead N. Intermittent versus continuous renal replacement therapy for acute renal failure in adults. *Cochrane Database Syst Rev.* 2007;18(3):CD003773.

15. Kelleher SP, Robinette JB, Miller F, Conger JD. Effect of hemorrhagic reduction in blood pressure on recovery from acute renal failure. *Kidney Int.* 1987;31(3):725-730.

16. Schneider AG, Bellomo R, Bagshaw SM, et al. Choice of renal replacement therapy modality and dialysis dependence after acute kidney injury: a systematic review and meta-analysis. *Intensive Care Med.* 2013;39(6):987-997.

17. Wald R, Shariff SZ, Adhikari NK, et al. The association between renal replacement therapy modality and long-term outcomes among critically ill adults with acute kidney injury: a retrospective cohort study. *Crit Care Med.* 2014;42(4):868-877.

18. Hoste EA, Dhondt A. Clinical review: use of renal replacement therapies in special groups of ICU patients. *Crit Care.* 2012;16(1):201.

19. Morimatsu H, Uchino S, Bellomo R, Ronco C. Continuous renal replacement therapy: does technique influence azotemic control? *Ren Fail.* 2002;24(5):645-653.

20. Bellomo R, Tipping P, Boyce N. Continuous veno-venous hemofiltration with dialysis removes cytokines from the circulation of septic patients. *Crit Care Med.* 1993;21(4):522-526.

21. Oudemans-van Straaten HM, Bosman RJ, van der Spoel JI, Zandstra DF. Outcome of critically ill patients treated with intermittent high-volume

haemofiltration: a prospective cohort analysis. *Intensive Care Med.* 1999;25(8):814-821.

22. Cole L, Bellomo R, Journois D, Davenport P, Baldwin I, Tipping P. High-volume haemofiltration in human septic shock. *Intensive Care Med.* 2001;27(6):978-986.

23. Schiffl H, Lang SM, Fischer R. Daily hemodialysis and the outcome of acute renal failure. *N Engl J Med.* 2002;346(5):305-310.

24. Ronco C, Bellomo R, Homel P, et al. Effects of different doses in continuous veno-venous haemofiltration on outcomes of acute renal failure: a prospective randomised trial. *Lancet.* 2000;356(9223):26-30.

25. Palevsky PM, Zhang JH, O'Connor TZ, et al. Intensity of renal support in critically ill patients with acute kidney injury. *N Engl J Med.* 2008;359(1):7-20.

26. Vanholder R, Van Biesen W, Hoste E, Lameire N. Pro/con debate: continuous versus intermittent dialysis for acute kidney injury: a never-ending story yet approaching the finish? *Crit Care.* 2011;15(1):204.

27. Klarenbach S, Manns B, Pannu N, Clement FM, Wiebe N, Tonelli M. Economic evaluation of continuous renal replacement therapy in acute renal failure. *Int J Technol Assess Health Care.* 2009;25(3):331-338.

28. Manns B, Doig CJ, Lee H, et al. Cost of acute renal failure requiring dialysis in the intensive care unit: clinical and resource implications of renal recovery. *Crit Care Med.* 2003;31(2):449-455.

29. Rauf AA, Long KH, Gajic O, Anderson SS, Swaminathan L, Albright RC. Intermittent hemodialysis versus continuous renal replacement therapy for acute renal failure in the intensive care unit: an observational outcomes analysis. *J Intensive Care Med.* 2008;23(3):195-203.

30. Kielstein JT, Kretschmer U, Ernst T, et al. Efficacy and cardiovascular tolerability of extended dialysis in critically ill patients: a randomized controlled study. *Am J Kidney Dis.* 2004;43(2):342-349.

31. Schwenger V, Weigand MA, Hoffmann O, et al. Sustained low efficiency dialysis using a single-pass batch system in acute kidney injury—a randomized interventional trial: the renal replacement therapy study in intensive care unit patients. *Crit Care.* 2012;16(4):R140.

32. Gaudry S, Hajage D, Schortgen F, et al. Initiation Strategies for Renal-Replacement Therapy in the Intensive Care Unit. *N Engl J Med.* 2016;375(2):122-133.

33. Zarbock A, Kellum JA, Schmidt C, et al. Effect of Early vs Delayed Initiation of Renal Replacement Therapy on Mortality in Critically Ill Patients With Acute Kidney Injury: The ELAIN Randomized Clinical Trial. *JAMA.* 2016;315(20):2190-2199.

Clinical Controversies: Ventilator-Associated Pneumonia: Does It Exist?

72

Kaye Hale, MD

CLINICAL CONTROVERSIES: VAP: DOES VAP EXIST?

In the United States, ventilator-associated pneumonia (VAP) is the most commonly diagnosed hospital-acquired infection in intensive care units (ICUs), affecting upward of 20% of ventilated patients with varyingly estimated attributable mortality ranging from 10% to 55%.[1] Acquisition of VAP is responsible for prolonged ICU and hospital length of stay (LOS), increased hospital costs, and increased utilization of antibiotics. In a post hoc retrospective-matched cohort analysis of microbiologically confirmed cases of VAP in the North American Silver-Coated Endotracheal Tube study, the authors calculate median total charges for patients with VAP were almost $200,000 compared to under $100,000 for patients without VAP. This was accounted for by the patients requiring intubation up to 5 days longer and as a consequence, significantly prolonging their ICU and hospital stays by 11 and 13 days, respectively.[2] A subsequent large, retrospective study comparing 2144 patients who had VAP as determined by International Classification of Diseases, Ninth Revision code to a matched cohort of patients without VAP showed similar findings. The patients with VAP had longer mean durations of mechanical ventilation (21.8 vs 10.3 days), prolonged ICU and hospital LOS (20.5 vs 11.6 and 32.6 vs 19.5, respectively), and an increase in hospital costs of almost $40,000.[3] The high attributable mortality and costs associated with VAP have garnered much attention from national patient safety organizations as well as state and federal health agencies, mandating compliance with preventive measures and reporting metrics.

However, to begin any discussion about VAP, one must first consider by which criteria VAP is defined. Until recently, there was significant discrepancy between medical professional society's definition of VAP and the Centers for Disease Control (CDC)/National Healthcare Safety Network's reportable surveillance definition (Table 72–1). Crucial differences in timing of the onset of pneumonia in a mechanically ventilated patient and whether microbiologic criteria were necessary for diagnosis left these competing criteria at odds. As clinical and reporting definitions of VAP diverged, our ability to reliably estimate rates, costs, and impact of VAP diminished. This is demonstrated in a study by Klompas, where 3 infection control personnel (following the CDC surveillance definition) and 1 physician (used clinical judgment), independently reviewed 50 cases and were only able to agree on a diagnosis of VAP in 3 patients while the range of cases identified varied from 7 to 20 depending on the reviewer.[4] In response to widespread confusion and concern over the discrepancy leading to misleading VAP rates and unclear VAP-associated mortality, the CDC altered its definition to include solely objective data for diagnosis and limited the diagnosis to onset after a minimum of 48 hours of ventilation with stable ventilator settings. This led to an entirely new classification of reportable ventilator-associated events (VAEs): ventilator-associated condition (VAC), infection-related ventilator-associated complication (iVAC), and finally possible VAP and probable VAP.[5] Some would argue, however, that these new diagnoses, VAE, VAC, iVAC, and their criteria have yet to be fully vetted for sensitivity, specificity, preventability, and significant impact on patient outcomes. Therein lies the controversy surrounding VAP, our community of health care providers lacks a unified view of what the real clinical problem is and whether that fairly compares to what

TABLE 72–1 Summary of key differences in diagnostic criteria for VAP according to professional society guidelines (ATD/IDSA) and CDC surveillance definition.

	ATS/IDSA 2005[7]	CDC VAP 2008[8]
Radiographic signs	X-ray presence of a new or progressive infiltrate	*Two or more serial X-rays with at least one* of the following: • New or progressive and persistent infiltrate • Consolidation • Cavitation
Clinical signs	*At least two* of the following: • Fever (> 38°C) • WBC (< 4000 or > 12,000 cells/μL) • Purulent secretions	*At least one* of the following: • Fever or • WBC or • Altered mental status (for adults > 70-year old) *AND at least two* of the following: • New onset purulent or changes in sputum • New onset or worsening tachypnea • Rales/bronchial breath sounds • Worsening gas exchange with increased vent requirements
Microbiologic criteria	Optional qualitative or quantitative culture of respiratory secretions (PSB: 10^3 cfu/mL or BAL: 10^4-10^5 cfu/mL)	*At least one* of the following: • Positive blood culture not related to another infection • Positive pleural fluid culture • Positive quantitative culture (BAL or PSB) • BAL fluid with > 5% cells with intracellular bacteria on microscopy • Positive histopathology

BAL, bronchoalveolar lavage; PSB, protected specimen brush.

regulatory bodies feel should be preventable and thus a marker of ICU quality.

VAP ACCORDING TO WHOM?

As previously stated, the lack of uniformly accepted diagnostic criteria for VAP has led to variability in publically reported rates, difficulty in determining accurate causes, epidemiology, prevention measures, and effective treatment. The Infectious Disease Society of America (IDSA) and American Thoracic Society (ATS) define VAP as pneumonia that develops more than 48 to 72 hours after initiation of ventilation via an endotracheal tube (EET) or tracheostomy tube.[6,7] Pneumonia is suggested by a new or progressive infiltrate on chest X-ray associated with signs or symptoms of infection (fever, leukocytosis, and purulent sputum) and worsening oxygenation. Chest X-ray findings are integral to the clinical diagnosis, wrought as they are with subjectivity, and difficulties in interpretation in the ICU setting due to the presence of overlying lines and tubes, as well as frequently abnormal baseline

radiographs in patients admitted for respiratory failure due to pneumonia and acute respiratory distress syndrome. This constellation of clinical criteria possesses high sensitivity but low specificity. The addition of a lower respiratory tract specimen is recommended as it can improve diagnostic accuracy and guide antimicrobial use. This microbiologic approach, however, is also contentious with regards to how the specimen should be collected (protected specimen brush, bronchoscopically, tracheal aspirate, or mini-bronchoalveolar lavage) and how it should be analyzed (quantitatively or qualitatively). Regardless of the microbiology, the principle of VAP diagnosis according to these professional guidelines focuses on clinical criteria and initiation of empiric antimicrobial therapy pending clinical improvement. The original CDC surveillance definition for VAP also began with chest radiograph interpretation, this time specifying *serial* X-rays, distinguishing findings on whether the patient had an abnormal X-ray at baseline. After meeting radiographic criteria, innumerable combinations from an extensive menu of signs and symptoms of infection (including subjective assessments of character and quantity of sputum, findings on auscultation, and respiratory symptoms such as dyspnea and cough), worsening gas exchange, and laboratory data could arrive one at a diagnosis of VAP on clinical grounds alone or by virtue of positive culture results.[8] The wide array of diagnostic possibilities may have been intended to provide the *infection preventionist* (someone trained in the field of infection control) with a menu of all the possible observed phenomena that could occur as a result of VAP; however, in practice, this was burdensome, impractical, and easily manipulated.

WHAT CAUSES VAP?

Since at least 1987, it has been recognized that the presence of an ETT predisposes patients to the development of pneumonia.[9] In the constant battle between host defense mechanisms and microbial virulence factors, the presence of the ETT and ventilatory circuit present a worthy adversary. Bypassing anatomic barriers such as the glottis with an ETT, impairing cough reflexes with sedatives and hampering mucociliary function by desiccation of secretions from continuous air flow, undermines the body's ability to prevent aspiration of organisms into the normally sterile lower respiratory tract and lung parenchyma. Risk of infection is compounded by eventual biofilm formation on the ETT and colonization of the upper airway with gram-negative organisms and frequently resistant hospital-acquired flora. Additionally, independent risk factors for VAP have been indentified and include nonmodifiable host factors (age > 60 years, underlying pulmonary disease and severity of illness) as well as modifiable risk factors inherent to bedside management of the patient (histamine-2 receptor antagonist use, sedation, duration of mechanical ventilation, maintenance of the ventilatory circuit, head of bed (HOB) position, and presence of a nasogastric tube).[10]

WHAT ARE VAES?

As earlier mentioned, in efforts to simplify VAP surveillance and reporting, the CDC revamped its surveillance definition to include a compilation of

VAC	IVAC	VAP
At least 2 days of sustained rise in PEEP ≥ 3 cm or FiO_2 ≥ 20% following a 2 day period of stable ventilator settings	Meets VAC **plus** temp < 36 or > 38°C or WBC ≤ 4 or ≥ 12 x 10^3 cells /mL **and** at least one new antibiotic initiated and continued for ≥ 4 days	Meets IVAC **plus** sputum/BAL with ≥ 25 PMN and ≤ 10 epithelial cells per hpf **and/or** positive respiratory culture

FIGURE 72-1 Ventilator-associated events: ventilator-associated condition (VAC); infection-related ventilator-associated complication (iVAC); ventilator-associated pneumonia (VAP).

VAEs in January 2013.[5] This shift in surveillance stemmed from the dispute and complexity of defining VAP, nonpneumonic complications associated with the ventilator (eg, ventilator-associated tracheobronchitis) and a desire to develop objective-surveillance criteria for uniformity and ease in reporting. VAEs as listed earlier include VAC (minimum sustained increases in positive end expiratory pressure (PEEP) or FiO_2 after a 2-days period of ventilator stability), iVAC (VAC plus signs of infection and initiation of a new antimicrobial agent that is continued for at least 4 days), possible VAP (iVAC plus symptoms of lower respiratory tract infection or positive cultures from respiratory specimen), and probable VAP (iVAC plus symptoms of lower respiratory tract infection and positive culture results from respiratory specimen).[5] This new surveillance approach depicts VAEs as a spectrum of disease (Figure 72-1). However, Muscedere et al showed that agreement between VAC, iVAC, and VAP was low with positive predictive values of VAC and iVAC for VAP of only 28% and 40%, respectively.[11]

IS VAE A BETTER QUALITY INDICATOR THAN VAP?

A large retrospective multicenter study examining VACs, as evidenced by threshold increases in ventilatory support (> 2 days of sustained increase in PEEP of 2.5 cm H_2O or FiO_2 > 15 points) after a 48-hour period of stability, found a statistically significant association between VAC and duration of mechanical ventilation (median 13 vs 6 days, $P < 0.001$), ICU LOS (median 16.3 vs 8.0 days, $P < 0.001$), and hospital LOS (median 21 vs 16.0 days, $P < 0.001$) as well as hospital mortality (38% + VAC, 23% – VAC, $P = 0.001$) when compared to matched patients without VAC.[12] The authors appropriately cite the concern that it may be difficult to distinguish a VAC from a patent who requires increasing ventilatory support for respiratory failure from a disease that progresses despite intubation. This concern is mirrored by Muscedere's study which showed higher Sequential Organ Failure Assessment (SOFA) scores in patients who subsequently developed VAC and iVAC compared to those who did not.[11] A subsequent small retrospective study by Lewis et al evaluating risk factors for VAEs, identified use of mandatory ventilator modes, positive net daily fluid balance, and benzodiazepine use prior to intubation as independent risk factors for VAC (mode of ventilation and fluid balance) and IVAC (benzodiazepine use).[13] Not surprisingly, there was no impact of the individual ventilator bundle components on VAC or IVAC cases when compared to controls. So, while VAEs are more readily identifiable by objective criteria that can be easily extracted from the medical record, until more, large, prospective studies can be performed the clinical entity of VAEs as preventable, VACs remains debatable.

CAN VAP BE PREVENTED?

There are innumerable reports in the medical literature touting the achievement of "zero VAP" rates with implementation of the "VAP bundle." Except, these publications vary in how they define VAP and no such VAP bundle actually exists. The ventilator bundle was introduced by the Institutes for Healthcare Improvement in 2005 as a means to improve clinical outcomes in mechanically ventilated patients.[14] The elements of the ventilator bundle are well known and now routinely referred to as the VAP bundle despite measures such as deep venous thrombosis and stress ulcer prophylaxes that have no direct benefit to preventing VAP and in the latter case, may even increase risk of pneumonia and other complications such as *Clostridium difficile* infection in critically ill patients.[15] Other bundle elements, including daily sedation "vacation" to limit duration of mechanical ventilation and HOB elevation target well-established independent risk factors for VAP as mentioned earlier but can be difficult to achieve in real practice. Nonetheless, health care quality agencies and state governments require compliance with these ventilator or VAP bundle elements to achieve zero VAP rates. Although all ICUs would aim to provide the best evidence-based care to achieve optimal outcomes for their patients, zero VAP is an unrealistic benchmark. There are nonmodifiable patient and disease-related risk factors that are outside of a care provider's control. By proposing this benchmark, patient safety forums are misleading the public into believing that a patient's course on a ventilator should be brief and uncomplicated, and if not achieved, may speciously reflect poor care and lack of bundle compliance. Furthermore, hospitals may be persuaded to use the subjectivity of some of the surveillance definitions to their advantage in order to report potentially lower VAP rates.

WHAT DOES THE FUTURE HOLD FOR VAP?

As with other hospital-acquired infections, the surveillance definition is not meant to be used clinically and differs out of the necessity to apply the surveillance definition across all hospitals, regardless of resources available, and ideally allows for minimal subjective interpretation to minimize case finding bias and allow for fair comparisons among hospitals. The CDCs replacement of VAP with publically reportable VAEs such as VAC and iVAC will undoubtedly shift focus away from the controversial and subjective VAP and toward establishing VAC and iVAC as the real threat to mechanically ventilated patients. And as with any novel initiative to improve patient safety and outcomes, new and potentially costly ideas for prevention will be brought to light and added to our ventilator bundle. As critical-care practitioners continue to strive to provide the best available evidence-based care for their patients, whether current clinical practice and professional guidelines will reflect this shift remains to be seen.

REFERENCES

1. Dudeck MA, Horan TC, Peterson KD, et al. National Healthcare Safety Network (NHSN) Report, data summary for 2010, device-associated module. *Am J Infect Control.* 2011;39(10):798-816.

2. Restrepo MI, Anzueto A, Arroliga AC, et al. Economic burden of ventilator-associated pneumonia based on total resource utilization. *Infect Control Hosp Epidemiol.* 2010;31(5):509-515.

3. Kollef MH, Hamilton CW, Ernst FR. Economic impact of ventilator-associated pneumonia in a large matched cohort. *Infect Control Hosp Epidemiol.* 2012;33(3):250-256.

4. Klompas M. Interobserver variability in ventilator-associated pneumonia surveillance. *Am J Infect Control.* 2010;38(3):237-239.

5. Magill SS, Klompas M, Balk R, et al. Developing a new, national approach to surveillance for ventilator-associated events. *Crit Care Med.* 2013;41(11):2467-2475.

6. Ventilator-Associated Pneumonia (VAP) Event CDC March 2009.pdf.

7. Guidelines for the management of adults with hospital-acquired, ventilator-associated, and healthcare-associated pneumonia. *Am J Respir Crit Care Med.* 2005;171(4):388-416.

8. Horan TC, Andrus M, Dudeck MA. CDC/NHSN surveillance definition of health care-associated infection and criteria for specific types of infections in the acute care setting. *Am J Infect Control.* 2008;36(5):309-332.

9. Craven DE, Driks MR. Nosocomial pneumonia in the intubated patient. *Semin Respir Infect.* 1987;2(1):20-33.

10. Chastre J, Fagon JY. Ventilator-associated pneumonia. *Am J Respir Crit Care Med.* 2002;165(7):867-903.

11. Muscedere J, Sinuff T, Heyland DK, et al. The c linical impact and preventability of ventilator-associated conditions in critically ill patients who are mechanically ventilated. *Chest.* 2013;144(5): 1453-1460.

12. Klompas M, Khan Y, Kleinman K, et al. Multicenter evaluation of a novel surveillance paradigm for complications of mechanical ventilation. *PloS One.* 2011;6(3):e18062.

13. Lewis SC, Li L, Murphy MV, et al. Risk factors for ventilator-associated events: a case-control multivariable analysis. *Crit Care Med.* 2014;42(8):1839-1848.

14. Berwick DM, Calkins DR, McCannon CJ, et al. The 100,000 lives campaign: setting a goal and a deadline for improving health care quality. *JAMA.* 2006;295(3):324-327.

15. Howell MD, Novack V, Grgurich P, et al. Iatrogenic gastric acid suppression and the risk of nosocomial Clostridium difficile infection. *Arch Intern Med.* 2010;170(9):784-790.

Controversies: ScvO$_2$ Versus Lactate Clearance to Guide Resuscitation in Septic Shock?

73

Jan Bakker, MD, PhD, FCCP

INTRODUCTION

Septic shock has been defined as a state in which hypotension persists despite adequate fluid resuscitation or the presence of a lactate level more than 4 mmol/L (so-called sepsis-induced tissue hypoperfusion) in patients with confirmed or suspected infection.[1] In these conditions, the Surviving Sepsis Campaign Guidelines suggest to restore mean arterial pressure (MAP) more than 65 mm Hg and normalize lactate levels and central or mixed venous hemoglobin saturation (ScvO$_2$/ SvO$_2$).[1] Basically this reflects restoring perfusion pressure, improving tissue perfusion and restoring the balance between oxygen delivery and oxygen demand.

A recent study showed a 46% mortality rate in septic patients with increased lactate levels and hypotension.[2] In addition, a study using ScvO$_2$ as an endpoint of resuscitation[3] and a study using both ScvO$_2$ and lactate clearance as endpoints of resuscitation[4] showed significant improvements in mortality. However, a study (mostly septic-shock patients) comparing the use of either ScvO$_2$ or lactate clearance in early resuscitation with common goals for central venous pressure and MAP did not show differences in mortality.[5] In addition, a recent study in septic-shock patients comparing early goal-directed therapy based on ScvO$_2$ measurements, protocol-based standard therapy based on systolic blood pressure, and heart-rate measurement without mandatory central venous catheter placement and usual-care based on the bedside physician similarly did not show differences in mortality.[6]

Therefore, controversy exists on how to use ScvO$_2$ or lactate levels in the resuscitation of septic-shock patients. In this chapter, both the background physiology of both parameters and their clinical use in the treatment of septic-shock patients is reviewed.

PHYSIOLOGY OF VENOUS OXYGENATION

Many aspects of venous oximetry have recently been reviewed.[7,8] There is an abundance of oxygen available in the circulation. The red blood cells leave the left ventricle with almost 100% saturated hemoglobin to return, after exchanging oxygen in the microcirculation, to the right ventricle with around 75% saturated hemoglobin. When oxygen delivery to the tissues is decreased, stepwise oxygen consumption is maintained by using this surplus of oxygen resulting in a gradual decrease of venous oxygenation.[9] When the decrease in oxygen delivery reaches a critical level, lactate levels generally start to increase.[10,11] In these models, venous oxygenation is proportional to cardiac output (CO) as arterial oxygen saturation and hemoglobin levels are usually stable. Venous oxygenation in these conditions thus reflects the balance between whole body oxygen demand and CO. It is important to realize that SvO$_2$ does not reflects regional venous oxygenation levels.[12] When cardiac function is normal, decreases in oxygen content are met by increases in CO thus minimally affecting venous oxygenation.[13] However, when cardiac function is limited or the decrease in oxygen content is excessive, the surplus of oxygen in the system is mainly used to compensate for changes in oxygen demand so that venous oxygenation decreases.[14] Although in clinical conditions, venous oxygenation is dependent on many factors (Figure 73–1), the response of CO to changes in oxygen content and oxygen demand is probably the main factor.

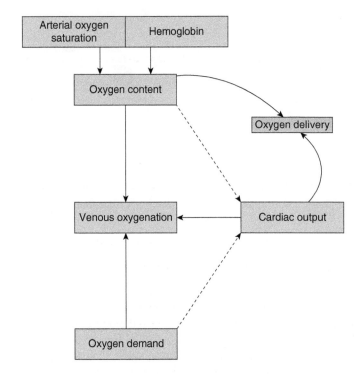

Decrease in venous oxygenation

Loss of oxygen content:
- anemia
- hemorrhage
- hypoxemia

Increase in oxygen content:
- agitation
- shivering
- fever
- pain
- systemic response to injury/infection

Increase in venous oxygenation

Increase in oxygen delivery
- blood transfusion
- supplemental oxygen
- cardiac output

Decrease in oxygen demand
- sedation
- analgesia
- cooling/hypothermia
- mechanical ventilation

Microcirculatory shunting
- change in distribution of flow
- decreased microcirculatory transit time
- cell death

FIGURE 73-1 Factors influencing venous oxygenation. CO plays a central role as this is the only variable that can rapidly adjust for changes in oxygen demand and the different components of oxygen content.

In hyperdynamic septic shock, patients seldom exhibit low levels of venous oxygenation,[15] whereas it is more frequently found in the early unresuscitated patients with severe sepsis.[3]

SCVO$_2$ AS A SURROGATE FOR SVO$_2$

The true venous oxygenation reflecting total body oxygen exchange is the pulmonary artery hemoglobin saturation. However, as pulmonary artery catheters are hardly used anymore and central venous catheters are recommended in the complex septic-shock patients, ScvO$_2$ is frequently used as a surrogate for the SvO$_2$.

In controlled experimental conditions, where usually oxygen demand is stable, ScvO$_2$ and SvO$_2$ highly correlate in various pathologic conditions.[16] However in clinical conditions, significant differences between ScvO$_2$ and SvO$_2$ may exist.[17] This could be related to the interindividual variation in the balance between oxygen demand and oxygen consumption as in low CO states, the ScvO$_2$ adequately reflects SvO$_2$.[18] When conditions are stable and oxygen demand is acutely changed, ScvO$_2$ reflects the decrease in oxygen demand just like SvO$_2$.[19,20]

Other sites for venous sampling (eg, femoral vein) or peripheral tissue oxygen saturation (eg, by near infrared spectroscopy) should not be used to replace ScvO$_2$.[21,22]

Given the relationship of ScvO$_2$ with CO, a normal to high ScvO$_2$ might suggest adequate perfusion. However, normal or high venous oxygenation levels may not reflect adequate tissue oxygenation as microcirculatory shunting may result in increased venous oxygenation levels.[23] In addition, patients with high venous oxygenation levels, independently associated with increased mortality,[24] may have low CO responsive to fluid resuscitation that might contribute to this high mortality.[25] The venous-arterial carbon dioxide difference ($Pv\text{-}aCO_2$) is dependent on CO in septic-shock patients.[26] In the presence of a normal or even increased $ScvO_2$, an increased $Pv\text{-}aCO_2$ may reflect low CO[27] that has been associated with a worse outcome.[28]

PHYSIOLOGY OF LACTATE

Lactate, as a normal end product of glucose metabolism, is produced from pyruvate. When pyruvate concentration exceeds the capacity of the slow metabolic Krebs cycle pathway, the fast metabolic pathway to lactate production is preferred resulting in the net production of 2 mol ATP per mol glucose metabolized. Although this amount of ATP is small compared to the additional 34 mol ATP produced in the Krebs cycle, the lactate pathway is fast and can thus produce large amounts of energy.[29] The increased levels of lactate in these conditions thus do not reflect the pathologic condition where pyruvate accumulates due to hypoxia. Lactate at the level of the organism also acts as an intermediate fuel that can be exchanged between various tissues.[30] In clinical practice, it is frequently difficult to separate these 2 states that clearly have significantly different impact on survival.

Lactate and Tissue Hypoxia

Decreasing oxygen delivery to the cells will ultimately result in decreasing oxygen consumption and increasing lactate levels.[31,32] It is important to realize that lactate levels do not necessarily represent the adequacy of oxygenation in different regional circulations as these have different levels of critical oxygen delivery.[33,34]

When oxygen delivery decreases below a critical level, oxygen consumption starts to decrease and lactate levels increase. This supply-dependent oxygen consumption in relation to increased lactate levels is a key characteristic of shock. Whereas this relationship is easily shown in experimental conditions, clinical circumstances, and ethical considerations limit the possibility to study this in humans. However, a few studies have identified the presence of supply-dependent oxygen consumption in relation to increased lactate levels also in patients with septic shock.[35-37]

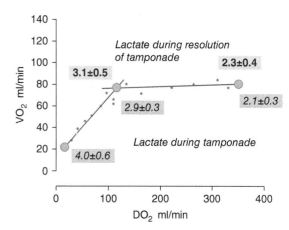

FIGURE 73-2 Effects of progressing tamponade resulting in a decrease in CO and thus oxygen delivery. Beyond a critical point of oxygen delivery, oxygen consumption rapidly falls and lactate levels (measured at 3 time points) start to increase (data in italic). Following the restoration of CO and thus oxygen delivery, oxygen consumption increases and lactate levels return to baseline (data in bold). (*Data from Zhang H, Spapen H, Benlabed M, et al: Systemic oxygen extraction can be improved during repeated episodes of cardiac tamponade, J Crit Care 1993 Jun;8(2):93-99.*)

In a model of tamponade, Zhang et al[32] recently showed that decreasing oxygen delivery beyond the critical value resulted in a rapid increase in lactate levels. Subsequent resolution of the tamponade resulted in supply-independent oxygen consumption and normalization of lactate levels (Figure 73-2). In the same model, van Genderen et al[38] showed that increasing tamponade was associated with decreased microvascular perfusion and increased lactate levels. In this model, resolving tamponade was associated with a normalization of microvascular perfusion and rapidly decreasing lactate levels. In patients with septic shock, Friedman et al showed similar findings.[35] Supply-dependent oxygen consumption was a characteristic of patients early in septic shock with hyperlactatemia, whereas supply-independent oxygen consumption was found following resuscitation and normalization of lactate levels. In addition, improving microvascular perfusion in septic-shock patients with increased lactate levels has been associated with decreasing lactate levels.[39]

Lactate and Aerobic Metabolism

These important observations as mentioned earlier underscore the importance of evaluating increased lactate levels to diagnose and treat supply-dependent oxygen consumption in critically ill patients. However, as lactate is a normal end product of glucose metabolism, increased aerobic glucose metabolism has been shown to increase lactate levels in the presence of adequate tissue oxygenation. Increases in pyruvate either by increasing glycolysis by means of hyperventilation or by infusing pyruvate result in increased lactate levels.[40,41] Similarly, the administration of epinephrine and corticosteroids, known to increase glycolysis, results in dose-dependent increase in lactate.[42,43] Very high lactate levels found in patients suspected of malignant lymphoma may have aerobic lactate production due to what is called the Warburg effect.[44] Treatment of the lymphoma is associated with a decrease in lactate levels, whereas subsequent tumor load leads to rapid increases in lactate levels.[29] In patients with septic shock, the increased activity of the cellular sodium/potassium pump has been associated with increased lactate levels not related to tissue hypoxia.[45] In addition, sepsis is also characterized by increased glycolysis due to cytokine-mediated glucose uptake.[46] Finally, mitochondrial dysfunction, not related to tissue hypoxia, can increase pyruvate levels and thus lactate levels.[47,48] In clinical practice, infusion of Ringer's lactate does not interfere with lactate measurements,[49] whereas high-volume hemofiltration using lactate-buffered solutions do result in transiently increased lactate levels.[50,51] Many other causes of increased lactate levels, not related to the presence of tissue hypoxia, have been identified.[52-56] In the presence of ethylene glycol intoxication, a high lactate level measured with a point-of-care device may be confounded by the adverse reaction to the lactate electrode in the machine.[57] A subsequent normal lactate in the central laboratory can even be used as a diagnostic tool in these circumstances.[58]

Clearance of Lactate

The body is able to clear large lactate loads rapidly as demonstrated by the decrease in lactate levels following exercise, cessation of seizures, or return of circulation in cardiac arrest. However, in specific circumstances, the clearance of lactate maybe limited that could result in prolonged increased lactate levels following resuscitation or in limited increased lactate levels in the case of normal production.

Impaired liver function is known to decrease the clearance of lactate by the liver.[36,59] Also in patients following cardiac surgery, clearance is impaired following a bolus infusion of lactate.[60] The dysfunction of pyruvate dehydrogenase in septic conditions, which can be alleviated by the administration of dichloroacetate, also limits lactate metabolism and results in increased lactate levels, where adequate oxygenation maybe present.[61,62]

HOW AND WHERE TO MEASURE LACTATE LEVELS

Various devices are available to rapidly measure lactate levels. A point-of-care blood gas analyzer has to advantage of delivering both the measurement of $ScvO_2$ and the lactate level. This can be used in clinical practice as the sampling site for lactate measurement (arterial, venous, capillary, etc) does not have a significant impact on the results.[63-65] In addition, hand-held devices to measure lactate have acceptable limits of agreement and clinical value when not used interchangeably with laboratory devices.[66,67]

THE CONTEXT OF LACTATE AND VENOUS OXYGENATION

Physiologically, it is clear that low $ScvO_2$ levels represent a state where the oxygen delivery is not matched to oxygen demand. When this is coincided with an increased lactate level, supply-dependent oxygen consumption might be present. As lactate is not specific for tissue hypoxia and $ScvO_2$ is only specific when very low, the clinical identification of tissue hypoxia represents a challenge. Therefore, clinical context and other signs of abnormal perfusion or limited oxygen transport should be included. Especially in sepsis, no critical values for venous oxygenation exist.[24] This is probably related to the interindividual range of oxygen demand[68] and the microcirculatory shunting that is frequently present.[23] However, other signs also relate to abnormal perfusion and abnormal organ function.[69-73] In the presence of hypotension, patients with normal lactate levels have less organ failure and better preserved microcirculatory perfusion than hypotensive patients with increased lactate levels.[74] Some of these are even strongly related to a worse outcome.[75] Next to other signs of tissue hypoperfusion the context/history of the patient is important. We usually accept low ScvO$_2$ levels in patients with chronic cardiac dysfunction when no signs of impaired organ perfusion exist. In addition, a diabetic patient on metformin presenting with high lactate levels without a clear history that might result in hypovolemia or myocardial dysfunction is likely to have metformin-associated hyperlactatemia even in the presence of acidosis.[76] This is clearly different from a patient admitted with severe trauma and increased lactate levels.[77,78]

As ScvO$_2$ responds immediately to changes in blood flow[79] and lactate clearance takes at least 15 to 20 minutes,[40,80] there is no clear relationship between the change in lactate levels and venous oxygenation levels.[81]

HOW THAN TO USE SCVO$_2$ AND LACTATE LEVELS IN CLINICAL PRACTICE?

Given the increased risk of the presence of tissue hypoperfusion and concomitant hypoxia, the Surviving Sepsis Campaign Guidelines and the Task Force of the European Society of Intensive Care on circulatory shock and hemodynamic monitoring recommend targeting a ScvO$_2$ of 70% and normalization of lactate levels in the resuscitation of septic-shock patients.[82,83]

Given the physiologic coupling of abnormal ScvO$_2$ and increased lactate levels, the Task Force maintained this advice despite the study which showed that either targeting lactate or ScvO$_2$ had no difference in outcome[5] and the study that showed that excluding ScvO$_2$ and lactate measurements from a protocol-based therapy did not affect outcome.[6]

The only study available today showing a significant impact on mortality when combining both ScvO$_2$ and normalization of lactate in the resuscitation of patients with circulatory failure (40% of whom had severe sepsis/septic shock) had a limited time frame of interventions.[84] The aggressive therapy lasted for not more than 8 hours. Given the current possibilities to rapidly improve tissue perfusion and oxygenation by different interventions,[39,85,86] the

changes of persisting tissue hypoxia that responds to optimizing perfusion are small. Recently, Hernandez et al suggested the presence of flow-dependent phase in lactate clearance in survivors of septic shock.[87] This so-called "inflection point" in the lactate versus time graph could identify a point where increased lactate levels are unlikely to be caused by persistent tissue hypoxia. In the study by Jansen et al, where the target was to decrease lactate by 20% every 2 hours (mainly by optimization of the balance between tissue oxygenation and tissue oxygen demand), this goal was met only in the first 2 hours of the study.[84]

CONCLUSIONS

There is a physiologic coupling between decreases in venous oxygenation and increasing lactate levels. However, this relationship is dependent on many factors that are frequently present and can rapidly change in septic-shock patients. Thus, both venous oxygenation and increased lactate levels can have limited specificity and sensitivity to detect tissue hypoperfusion and hypoxia. Other parameters of tissue hypoperfusion are available and should be used to create context to venous oxygenation and increased lactate levels. Although ScvO$_2$ can be used as a surrogate of the true venous compartment, caution should be used in specific circumstances. The venoarterial PCO_2 difference, easily available in these circumstances, can help to disguise a low flow state in the presence of normal to high ScvO$_2$ levels. As the persistence of low ScvO$_2$ values following initial resuscitation is very low[15] and the baseline values for ScvO$_2$ in recent randomized controlled trials were normal,[5,6] lactate monitoring in circumstances where resources and placement of a central venous catheter is limited, represents an easy, cheap, and fast way to assess risk of morbidity and mortality of septic-shock patients.[67,88] The use of both parameters, however, requires adequate understanding of their physiology.

REFERENCES

1. Dellinger RP, Levy MM, Rhodes A, et al. Surviving sepsis campaign: international guidelines for management of severe sepsis and septic shock: 2012. *Crit Care Med.* 2013;41(2):580-637.

2. Levy MM, Dellinger RP, Townsend SR, et al. The Surviving Sepsis Campaign: results of an international guideline-based performance improvement program targeting severe sepsis. *Crit Care Med*. 2010;38(2):367-374.

3. Rivers E, Nguyen B, Havstad S, et al. Early goal-directed therapy in the treatment of severe sepsis and septic shock. *N Engl J Med*. 2001;345(19):1368-1377.

4. Jansen TC, van Bommel J, Schoonderbeek FJ, et al. Early lactate-guided therapy in intensive care unit patients: a multicenter, open-label, randomized controlled trial. *Am J Respir Crit Care Med*. 2010;182(6):752-761.

5. Jones AE, Shapiro NI, Trzeciak S, et al. Lactate clearance vs central venous oxygen saturation as goals of early sepsis therapy: a randomized clinical trial. *JAMA*. 2010;303(8):739-746.

6. The ProCESS Investigators, Yealy DM, Kellum JA, Huang DT, et al. A randomized trial of protocol-based care for early septic shock. *N Engl J Med*. 2014;370(18):1683-1693.

7. Walley KR. Use of central venous oxygen saturation to guide therapy. *Am J Respir Crit Care Med*. 2011;184(5):514-520.

8. van Beest P, Wietasch G, Scheeren T, et al. Clinical review: use of venous oxygen saturations as a goal—a yet unfinished puzzle. *Crit Care*. 2011;15(5):232.

9. Cain SM, Curtis SE. Experimental models of pathologic oxygen supply dependency. *Crit Care Med*. 1991;19(5):603-612.

10. Zhang H, Spapen H, Benlabed M, et al. Systemic oxygen extraction can be improved during repeated episodes of cardiac tamponade. *J Crit Care*. 1993;8(2):93-99.

11. Cain SM, Curtis SE. Systemic and regional oxygen uptake and delivery and lactate flux in endotoxic dogs infused with dopexamine. *Crit Care Med*. 1991;19(12):1552-1560.

12. Meier-Hellmann A, Hannemann L, Specht M, et al. The relationship between mixed venous and hepatic venous O2 saturation in patients with septic shock. *Adv Exp Med Biol*. 1994;345:701-707.

13. Weiskopf RB, Viele MK, Feiner J, et al. Human cardiovascular and metabolic response to acute, severe isovolemic anemia. *JAMA*. 1998;279(3):217-221.

14. Silance PG, Simon C, Vincent JL. The relation between cardiac index and oxygen extraction in acutely ill patients. *Chest*. 1994;105(4):1190-1197.

15. van Beest PA, Hofstra JJ, Schultz MJ, et al. The incidence of low venous oxygen saturation on admission to the intensive care unit: a multi-center observational study in The Netherlands. *Crit Care*. 2008;12(2):R33.

16. Reinhart K, Rudolph T, Bredle DL, et al. Comparison of central-venous to mixed-venous oxygen saturation during changes in oxygen supply/demand. *Chest*. 1989;95(6):1216-1221.

17. Kopterides P, Bonovas S, Mavrou I, et al. Venous oxygen saturation and lactate gradient from superior vena cava to pulmonary artery in patients with septic shock. *Shock*. 2009;31(6):561-567.

18. Berridge JC. Influence of cardiac output on the correlation between mixed venous and central venous oxygen saturation. *Br J Anaesth*. 1992;69(4):409-410.

19. Hernandez G, Pena H, Cornejo R, et al. Impact of emergency intubation on central venous oxygen saturation in critically ill patients: a multicenter observational study. *Crit Care*. 2009;13(3):R63.

20. Weissman C, Kemper M. The oxygen uptake-oxygen delivery relationship during ICU interventions. *Chest*. 1991;99:430-435.

21. Podbregar M, Mozina H. Skeletal muscle oxygen saturation does not estimate mixed venous oxygen saturation in patients with severe left heart failure and additional severe sepsis or septic shock. *Crit Care*. 2007;11(1):R6.

22. van Beest PA, van der Schors A, Liefers H, et al. Femoral venous oxygen saturation is no surrogate for central venous oxygen saturation. *Crit Care Med*. 2012;40(12):3196-3201.

23. Ince C, Sinaasappel M. Microcirculatory oxygenation and shunting in sepsis and shock. *Crit Care Med*. 1999;27(7):1369-1377.

24. Chung KP, Chang HT, Huang YT, et al. Central venous oxygen saturation under non-protocolized resuscitation is not related to survival in severe sepsis or septic shock. *Shock*. 2012;38(6):584-591.

25. Velissaris D, Pierrakos C, Scolletta S, et al. High mixed venous oxygen saturation levels do not exclude fluid responsiveness in critically ill septic patients. *Crit Care*. 2011;15(4):R177.

26. Bakker J, Vincent JL, Gris P, et al. Veno-arterial carbon dioxide gradient in human septic shock. *Chest*. 1992;101(2):509-515.

27. Vallee F, Vallet B, Mathe O, et al. Central venous-to-arterial carbon dioxide difference: an additional target for goal-directed therapy in septic shock? *Intensive Care Med*. 2008;34(12):2218-2225.

28. van Beest PA, Lont MC, Holman ND, et al. Central venous-arterial pCO(2) difference as a tool in resuscitation of septic patients. *Intensive Care Med*. 2013;39(6):1034-1039.

29. Bakker J, Nijsten MW, Jansen TC. Clinical use of lactate monitoring in critically ill patients. *Ann Intensive Care*. 2013;3(1):12.

30. Brooks GA. Lactate shuttles in nature. *Biochem Soc Trans*. 2002;30(2):258-264.

31. Cain SM. Appearance of excess lactate in aneshetized dogs during anemic and hypoxic hypoxia. *Am J Physiol*. 1965;209:604-608.

32. Zhang H, Vincent JL. Oxygen extraction is altered by endotoxin during tamponade-induced stagnant hypoxia in the dog. *Circ Shock*. 1993;40(3):168-176.

33. Cain SM, Curtis SE. Whole body and regional O2 uptake/delivery and lactate flux in endotoxic dogs. *Adv Exp Med Biol*. 1992;316:401-408.

34. Pinsky MR, Schlichtig R. Regional oxygen delivery in oxygen supply-dependent states. *Intensive Care Med*. 1990;16(suppl 2):169-171.

35. Friedman G, De Backer D, Shahla M, et al. Oxygen supply dependency can characterize septic shock. *Intensive Care Med*. 1998;24(2):118-123.

36. Bakker J, Vincent J. The oxygen-supply dependency phenomenon is associated with increased blood lactate levels. *J Crit Care*. 1991;6(3):152-159.

37. Ronco JJ, Fenwick JC, Tweeddale MG, et al. Identification of the critical oxygen delivery for anaerobic metabolism in critically ill septic and nonseptic humans. *JAMA*. 1993;270(14):1724-1730.

38. van Genderen ME, Klijn E, Lima A, et al. Microvascular perfusion as a target for fluid resuscitation in experimental circulatory shock. *Crit Care Med*. 2014;42(2):E96-E105.

39. De Backer D, Creteur J, Dubois MJ, et al. The effects of dobutamine on microcirculatory alterations in patients with septic shock are independent of its systemic effects. *Crit Care Med*. 2006;34(2):403-408.

40. Huckabee WE. Relationships of pyruvate and lactate during anaerobic metabolism. I. Effects of infusion of pyruvate or glucose and of hyperventilation. *J Clin Invest*. 1958;37(2):244-254.

41. Zborowska-Sluis DT, Dossetor JB. Hyperlactatemia of hyperventilation. *J Appl Physiol*. 1967;22(4):746-755.

42. Griffith FR, Jr, Lockwood JE, Emery FE. Adrenalin lactacidemia: proportionality with dose. *Am J Physiol*. 1939;127(3):415-421.

43. Boysen SR, Bozzetti M, Rose L, et al. Effects of prednisone on blood lactate concentrations in healthy dogs. *J Vet Intern Med*. 2009;23(5):1123-1125.

44. Warburg O. On respiratory impairment in cancer cells. *Science*. 1956;124(3215):269-270.

45. Levy B, Gibot S, Franck P, et al. Relation between muscle Na+K+ ATPase activity and raised lactate concentrations in septic shock: a prospective study. *Lancet*. 2005;365(9462):871-875.

46. Taylor DJ, Faragher EB, Evanson JM. Inflammatory cytokines stimulate glucose uptake and glycolysis but reduce glucose oxidation in human dermal fibroblasts in vitro. *Circ Shock*. 1992;37(2):105-110.

47. Brealey D, Brand M, Hargreaves I, et al. Association between mitochondrial dysfunction and severity and outcome of septic shock. *Lancet*. 2002;360(9328):219-223.

48. Crouser ED, Julian MW, Blaho DV, et al. Endotoxin-induced mitochondrial damage correlates with impaired respiratory activity. *Crit Care Med*. 2002;30(2):276-284.

49. Didwania A, Miller J, Kassel D, et al. Effect of intravenous lactated Ringer's solution infusion on the circulating lactate concentration: Part 3. Results of a prospective, randomized, double-blind, placebo-controlled trial. *Crit Care Med*. 1997;25(11):1851-1854.

50. Cole L, Bellomo R, Baldwin I, et al. The impact of lactate-buffered high-volume hemofiltration on acid-base balance. *Intensive Care Med*. 2003;29(7):1113-1120.

51. Bollmann MD, Revelly JP, Tappy L, et al. Effect of bicarbonate and lactate buffer on glucose and lactate metabolism during hemodiafiltration in patients with multiple organ failure. *Intensive Care Med*. 2004;30(6):1103-1110.

52. Lalau JD, Lacroix C, Compagnon P, et al. Role of metformin accumulation in metformin-associated lactic acidosis. *Diabetes Care*. 1995;18(6):779-784.

53. Marinella MA. Lactic acidosis associated with propofol. *Chest*. 1996;109(1):292.

54. Lonergan JT, Behling C, Pfander H, et al. Hyperlactatemia and hepatic abnormalities in 10 human immunodeficiency virus-infected patients receiving nucleoside analogue combination regimens. *Clin Infect Dis*. 2000;31(1):162-166.

55. Claessens YE, Cariou A, Monchi M, et al. Detecting life-threatening lactic acidosis related to nucleoside-analog treatment of human immunodeficiency virus-infected patients, and treatment with L-carnitine. *Crit Care Med*. 2003;31(4):1042-1047.

56. Naidoo DP, Gathiram V, Sadhabiriss A, et al. Clinical diagnosis of cardiac beriberi. *S Afr Med J*. 1990;77(3):125-127.

57. Morgan TJ, Clark C, Clague A. Artifactual elevation of measured plasma L-lactate concentration

in the presence of glycolate. *Crit Care Med.* 1999;27(10):2177-2179.

58. Brindley PG, Butler MS, Cembrowski G, et al. Falsely elevated point-of-care lactate measurement after ingestion of ethylene glycol. *CMAJ.* 2007;176(8):1097-1099.

59. Almenoff PL, Leavy J, Weil MH, et al. Prolongation of the half-life of lactate after maximal exercise in patients with hepatic dysfunction. *Crit Care Med.* 1989;17(9):870-873.

60. Mustafa I, Roth H, Hanafiah A, et al. Effect of cardiopulmonary bypass on lactate metabolism. *Intensive Care Med.* 2003;29(8):1279-1285.

61. Stacpoole PW, Wright EC, Baumgartner TG, et al. A controlled clinical trial of dichloroacetate for treatment of lactic acidosis in adults. The Dichloroacetate-Lactic Acidosis Study Group. *N Engl J Med.* 1992;327(22):1564-1569.

62. Vary TC. Sepsis-induced alterations in pyruvate dehydrogenase complex activity in rat skeletal muscle: effects on plasma lactate. *Shock.* 1996;6(2):89-94.

63. Weil MH, Michaels S, Rackow EC. Comparison of blood lactate concentrations in central venous, pulmonary artery, and arterial blood. *Crit Care Med.* 1987;15(5):489-490.

64. Younger JG, Falk JL, Rothrock SG. Relationship between arterial and peripheral venous lactate levels. *Acad Emerg Med.* 1996;3(7):730-734.

65. Fauchere JC, Bauschatz AS, Arlettaz R, et al. Agreement between capillary and arterial lactate in the newborn. *Acta Paediatr.* 2002;91(1):78-81.

66. Aduen J, Bernstein WK, Khastgir T, et al. The use and clinical importance of a substrate-specific electrode for rapid determination of blood lactate concentrations. *JAMA.* 1994;272(21):1678-1685.

67. Brinkert W, Rommes JH, Bakker J. Lactate measurements in critically ill patients with a hand-held analyser. *Intensive Care Med.* 1999;25(9):966-969.

68. Astiz ME, Rackow EC, Kaufman B, et al. Relationship of oxygen delivery and mixed venous oxygenation to lactic acidosis in patients with sepsis and acute myocardial infarction. *Crit Care Med.* 1988;16(7):655-658.

69. Lima A, Jansen TC, Van BOommel J, et al. The prognostic value of the subjective assessment of peripheral perfusion in critically ill patients. *Crit Care Med.* 2009;37(3):934-938.

70. Lima A, van Bommel J, Jansen TC, et al. Low tissue oxygen saturation at the end of early goal-directed therapy is associated with worse outcome in critically ill patients. *Crit Care.* 2009;13(suppl 5):S13.

71. De Backer D. Lactic acidosis. *Intensive Care Med.* 2003;29(5):699-702.

72. Smith I, Kumar P, Molloy S, et al. Base excess and lactate as prognostic indicators for patients admitted to intensive care. *Intensive Care Med.* 2001;27(1):74-83.

73. Sladen RN. Oliguria in the ICU. Systematic approach to diagnosis and treatment. *Anesthesiol Clin North America.* 2000;18(4):739-752, viii.

74. Hernandez G, Bruhn A, Castro R, et al. Persistent sepsis-induced hypotension without hyperlactatemia: a distinct clinical and physiological profile within the spectrum of septic shock. *Crit Care Res Pract.* 2012;2012:536852.

75. Ait-Oufella H, Lemoinne S, Boelle PY, et al. Mottling score predicts survival in septic shock. *Intensive Care Med.* 2011;37(5):801-807.

76. Kajbaf F, Lalau JD. The prognostic value of blood pH and lactate and metformin concentrations in severe metformin-associated lactic acidosis. *BMC Pharmacol Toxicol.* 2013;14:22.

77. Guyette F, Suffoletto B, Castillo JL, et al. Prehospital serum lactate as a predictor of outcomes in trauma patients: a retrospective observational study. *J Trauma.* 2011;70(4):782-786.

78. Parsikia A, Bones K, Kaplan M, et al. The predictive value of initial serum lactate in trauma patients. *Shock.* 2014;42(3):199-204.

79. Bakker J, Vincent JL. The effects of norepinephrine and dobutamine on oxygentransport and consumption in a dog model of endotoxic shock. *Crit Care Med.* 1993;21:425-432.

80. Vincent JL, Dufaye P, Berre J, et al. Serial lactate determinations during circulatory shock. *Crit Care Med.* 1983;11(6):449-451.

81. Arnold RC, Shapiro NI, Jones AE, et al. Multicenter study of early lactate clearance as a determinant of survival in patients with presumed sepsis. *Shock.* 2009;32(1):35-39.

82. Dellinger RP, Levy MM, Rhodes A, et al. Surviving Sepsis Campaign: international guidelines for management of severe sepsis and septic shock, 2012. *Intensive Care Med.* 2013;39(2):165-228.

83. Cecconi M, De Backer D, Antonelli M, et al. Consensus on circulatory shock and hemodynamic monitoring. Task force of the European Society of Intensive Care Medicine. *Intensive Care Med.* 2014;40(12):1795-1815.

84. Jansen TC, van Bommel J, Schoonderbeek FJ, et al. Early lactate-guided therapy in intensive care unit patients a multicenter, open-label, randomized controlled trial. *Am J Respir Crit Care Med.* 2010;182(6):752-761.

85. Lima A, van Genderen ME, van Bommel J, et al. Nitroglycerin reverts clinical manifestations of poor peripheral perfusion in patients with circulatory shock. *Critical Care.* 2014;18(3):R126.

86. Atasever B, van der Kuil M, Boer C, et al. Red blood cell transfusion compared with gelatin solution and no infusion after cardiac surgery: effect on microvascular perfusion, vascular density, hemoglobin, and oxygen saturation. *Transfusion.* 2012;52(11):2452-2458.

87. Hernandez G, Luengo C, Bruhn A, et al. When to stop septic shock resuscitation: clues from a dynamic perfusion monitoring. *Ann Intensive Care.* 2014;4:30.

88. Bakker J, Coffernils M, Leon M, et al. Blood lactate levels are superior to oxygen-derived variables in predicting outcome in human septic shock. *Chest.* 1991;99(4):956-962.

Controversies: Is Glucose Control Relevant?

Adel Bassily-Marcus, MD and Inga Khachaturova, MD

HYPERGLYCEMIA IN CRITICAL ILLNESS: STRESS HYPERGLYCEMIA

Virtually all adult medical ICU patients experience at least 1 blood glucose value above the normal fasting level (110 mg/dL).[1] The stress of critical illness promotes a state of insulin resistance which is characterized by increased hepatic gluconeogenesis and glycogenolysis, impaired peripheral glucose uptake, and higher circulating concentrations of insulin. There is upregulation of hepatic glucose production triggered by elevated levels of cytokines and counterregulatory hormones such as glucagon, cortisol, growth hormone, and catecholamines. These metabolic disturbances together with common ICU treatments such as corticosteroids, sympathomimetic agents, and glucose-containing infusions explain the frequently observed phenomenon of hyerglycemia irrespective of the disease, diabetes mellitus.

Many practitioners have viewed moderately severe hyperglycemia among critically ill patients to be either an epiphenomenon or an adaptive response, not warranting significant concern or intervention.

Large observational studies in different types of ICU populations reveal a J-shaped relationship between blood glucose levels and mortality of critical illness, with the mortality nadir somewhere between 80 and 140 mg/dL depending on the type of illness and the presence of a history of diabetes mellitus. Observations such as these raised concerns that acute hyperglycemia itself was contributing to poor outcomes, potentially by leaving affected patients susceptible to some of the complications that have long been observed among chronic diabetics, including high infection rates, poor wound healing, and polyneuropathy.

CONTROLLING HYPERGLYCEMIA

The groundbreaking Leuven I study[2] in 2001, conducted in critically ill surgical patients, found a remarkable overall 3.4% ICU mortality reduction, a 9.6% mortality benefit in patients with ICU LOS more than 5 days, and a 34% hospital mortality reduction in the strict normoglycemia group (target glucose 80-110 mg/dL) compared to standard therapy. These beneficial outcomes resulting from the use of intensive insulin therapy targeting normoglycemic levels sparked a strong interest in glycemic management in the ICU. Intensive insulin therapy quickly became the standard of care in both medical and surgical ICUs. However, a follow-up study, done by the same group in 2006,[3] demonstrated that in contrast to the earlier study, intensive insulin therapy did not reduce overall morality and was associated with an even higher rate of serious hypoglycemia (18.7%). In the first study, it was speculated that the benefits seen were primarily due to a surgical patient population and the primary use of parenteral nutrition.

THE HARMFUL EFFECT OF TIGHT GLUCOSE CONTROL

Following 4 consecutive negative trials, the most comprehensive landmark NICE-SUGAR trial[4] results were reported. They found that the intensive insulin therapy groups achieving normoglycemia had an absolute 2.6% increase in mortality ($P = 0.02$) and an increased incidence of hypoglycemia (6.8% vs 0.5%). Furthermore, subsequent meta-analyses demonstrated that intensive insulin therapy provided no survival benefit and was associated with increased morbidity secondary to severe hypoglycemic episodes. These findings are also consistent with observational data reported from ICUs incorporating intensive insulin protocols as part of their hyperglycemic management. The overall consensus from the available evidence suggests that intensive insulin therapy (target glucose 80-110 mg/dL) as compared to standard insulin therapy (target glucose 140-180) does not provide an overall survival benefit, may increase mortality and is associated with a higher incidence of hypoglycemia.

THE IMPACT OF HYPOGLYCEMIA

Hypoglycemia has been shown in the critically ill pateint to be independently associated with a 3-fold increase in mortality. In a trial of intensive insulin therapy, severe hypoglycemia occurred in up to 28% of patients.[5] It is further speculated that the incidence of hypoglycemia is likely to be higher outside of clinical trials if intensive insulin protocols are used. The main consequences of acute and persistent hypoglycemia are neurologic deficits, which at times can be quite difficult to detect but remain a true concern. Hypoglycemia has been shown to cause acute electroencephalographic alterations. In a 4-year follow-up of patients treated with intensive insulin therapy (target blood glucose 80-110 mg/ dL), this population was found to have impairments in quality of life and social functioning as compared to patients who received conventional insulin therapy.[6]

The relationship between hypoglycemia and outcome may be explained by an association with severity of illness and an increased risk of death, or a true deleterious biologic effect in critically ill patients. Hypoglycemia might exert biologic toxicity by increasing the systemic inflammatory response, inducing neuroglycopenia, inhibiting the corticosteroid response to stress, impairing sympathetic nervous system responsiveness, causing cerebral vasodilatation or by unidentified mechanisms. Furthermore, many experimental studies have demonstrated that both insulin and hypoglycemia can induce hypotension, vasodilatation, nitric oxide release, sympathetic system response exhaustion, and decreased ability to respond to repeated stress.

THE RELEVANCE OF HYPERGLYCEMIA

The repeated observation that hyperglycemia is associated with poorer outcomes among critically ill patients, together with the theoretical harm of acutely elevated blood glucose, represents the basis for focusing on glycemic control in the intensive care setting. However, the possibility remains that elevated blood glucose levels are actually beneficial to the critically ill individual, and that stress hyperglycemia is an appropriate and adaptive response to life-threatening illness, as no randomized trial investigating glycemic control has studied the effect of truly permissive hyperglycemia.[7]

Potential benefits of hyperglycemia include promotion of glucose delivery in the face of ischemic insults (enhanced glucose diffusion gradient), with insulin resistance favoring redistribution of available glucose stores toward cells of the immune and nervous systems, and away from peripheral tissues. Recent observational studies have provided some support for this view, reasserting the possibility that hyperglycemia is simply a marker of illness severity when controlled for hyperlactatemia.[8] Our ability to identify patients most likely to suffer harm from hyperglycemia remains incomplete.

Several studies have concluded that the association between hyperglycemia and in-hospital mortality is attenuated among those with preexisting diabetes mellitus, with some even failing to demonstrate any association at all.

GLUCOSE VARIABILITY

Glucose variability (the difference between daily minimum and maximum glucose levels) may be a reflection of dysglycemia induced by severity of illness, inadequate control of glycemia by the treating clinicians resulting in excessive fluctuations of BG levels, or both. Additionally, patients with increased glucose variability are more likely to have experienced hypoglycemia, complicating the assessment of glucose variability versus hypoglycemia and mortality. Over the last several years a plethora of data, from observational studies evaluating a wide variety of acutely and critically ill populations, has confirmed the correlation between glucose variability and increased odds of death. These findings raise the question that attempting to control hyperglycemia may be a major contributing factor in glucose variability and subsequent detrimental outcomes. There has been hope that continuous glucose monitoring will decrease variability and improve outcome, although the one study conducted thus far has failed to show such a relationship.[9]

CONCLUSION

In summary, it was naïve to conclude after a single center study[2] that a single intervention (tight glucose control) would lead to an impressive mortality benefit in our complex critically ill patients with organ failures. A single study should never be followed by widespread promotion and adoption of a basic intervention. For an intervention to be adopted, it should be reproducible in a realistic environment, with a clear benefit that outweighs the risks.

The current recommendations for critically ill patients overall, and for patients with severe sepsis, are that insulin therapy should be started when blood glucose exceeds 180 mg/dL with the goal of maintaining blood glucose between 144 and 180 mg/dL with insulin when necessary. However, even this less stringent advice needs to be validated in future studies.

REFERENCES

1. Cely CM, Arora P, Quartin AA, Kett DH, Schein RM. Relationship of baseline glucose homeostasis to hyperglycemia during medical critical illness. *Chest*. 2004;126(3):879-887.

2. van den Berghe G, Wouters P, Weekers F, et al. Intensive insulin therapy in critically ill patients. *N Engl J Med*. 2001;345(19):1359-1367.

3. Van den Berghe G, Wilmer A, Hermans G, et al. Intensive insulin therapy in the medical ICU. *N Engl J Med*. 2006;354(5):449-461.

4. Finfer S, Chittock DR, Su SY, et al. Intensive versus conventional glucose control in critically ill patients. *N Engl J Med*. 2009;360(13):1283-1297.

5. Arabi YM, Dabbagh OC, Tamim HM, et al. Intensive versus conventional insulin therapy: a randomized controlled trial in medical and surgical critically ill patients. *Crit Care Med*. 2008;36(12):3190-3197.

6. Ingels C, Debaveye Y, Milants I, et al. Strict blood glucose control with insulin during intensive care after cardiac surgery: impact on 4-year survival, dependency on medical care, and quality-of-life. *Eur Heart J*. 2006;27(22):2716-2724.

7. Marik PE, Bellomo R. Stress hyperglycemia: an essential survival response! *Crit Care Med*. 2013;41(6):e93-e94.

8. Kaukonen KM, Bailey M, Egi M, et al. Stress hyperlactatemia modifies the relationship between stress hyperglycemia and outcome: a retrospective observational study. *Crit Care Med*. 2014;42(6):1379-1385.

9. Brunner R, Adelsmayr G, Herkner H, Madl C, Holzinger U. Glycemic variability and glucose complexity in critically ill patients: a retrospective analysis of continuous glucose monitoring data. *Crit Care*. 2012;16(5):R175.

Simulation and Education in the ICU

CHAPTER

75

Maneesha Bangar, MD; Carla Venegas-Borsellino, MD and Lewis A. Eisen, MD

KEY POINTS

1 Simulation training is proven to be beneficial for teaching technical tasks as well as nontechnical skills necessary for the critical care practitioner.

2 Simulation is a broad method of training, which can include standardized patients, partial task trainers, hybrid simulators, advanced task trainers, high-fidelity simulators, screen-based computer simulators, or virtual reality simulators.

3 Simulation training allows the opportunity to learn from errors without jeopardizing patient safety.

4 Debriefing is a key component in any simulation to allow for deliberate practice and improvement.

5 Crisis resource management is a key component of simulation training and should be stressed in all team training scenarios.

INTRODUCTION

Critical care medicine (CCM) specialists face emergencies every day and are required to make decisions in a short span of time. These decisions have a great impact on patient outcomes and physicians may require years of experience in order to be competent in handling such situations. This process poses a real challenge for CCM physicians undergoing training.

As Confucious said: "I hear and I forget, I see and I remember, I do and I understand." Similarly, Edger's cone of experience emphasizes the importance of learning by doing. But, does that mean that physicians in their initial learning curve will continue to learn by doing procedures and executing

management plans on patients? If we were patients, would we want a physician's first ever procedure to be on us? Would it not be better to practice on a model before we practice on a real patient? That is where simulation comes into play.

Simulation is defined as something that is made to look, feel, or behave like something else. Simulation training gives physicians exposure to different case scenarios in a shorter period of time, and imparts knowledge, experience, and skills to deal with them confidently. Learning could be passive such as listening to lectures or active whereby the learner participates verbally by giving comments or physically by participating in the simulation.

Knowles[1] described the adult learner as a self-directed learner who attaches more meaning to learning through experience than through passive learning, is more interested in learning things applicable to real life, is problem-oriented and performance-centric, and always seeks feedback in order to become more efficient. His principles of the ideal way to teach an adult learner have been included in simulation training.

HISTORY OF SIMULATION

Models simulating the brain, heart, airway, and other body organs have been used to teach human anatomy for many years. Medical science has come a long way from using those models to using today's high-fidelity simulation models that can talk, breathe, and have palpable pulses. Simulation-based training has been used in other high-hazard professions, such as aviation, the nuclear industry, and the military, to maximize training safety and minimize risk. Health care has lagged behind in simulation applications for a number of reasons, including cost and resistance to change.[2]

Review of literature shows that flight simulators have been utilized in training since the 1920s. Around the 1960s, the practice of using standardized patients for the training of medical students was started. ResusciAnnie and Harvey for cardiology examinations were developed at the same time that cardiopulmonary resuscitation (CPR) was introduced. The concept of virtual reality was introduced by the entertainment industry in the 1960s via Morton Heilig's Sensorama. Virtual reality entered the medical field through simulated endoscopies in the 1990s. With advancement in computer technology in the 1990s, software-based simulators were developed, leading to the extensive use of simulators in anesthesia.[3]

Before 1990, anesthesiologists were not provided formal training in crisis management, although they were suddenly called upon to manage life-threatening crises. Due to this gap in training, Dr. Howard and Dr. Gaba in the 1990s developed a course in anesthesia crisis resource management (ACRM) analogous to courses in crew (cockpit) resource management (CRM) conducted in commercial and military aviation. Two model demonstration courses in ACRM were conducted using realistic anesthesia simulation systems to test the feasibility and acceptance of this kind of training.[4] Subsequently, simulation was started to be used by many different subspecialties, including critical care, pediatrics, emergency medicine, and obstetrics/gynecology.[5] Around the year 2000, Laerdal introduced a computer-controlled patient simulator mannequin–SimMan, with very realistic features and feedback responses, and subsequently developed more advanced high-quality human simulators. Haptic devices were also used to simulate laparoscopic procedures.

ADVANTAGES OF SIMULATION TRAINING

The main advantages of simulation training are as follows:

- Provides an opportunity to get hands-on experience of real-life scenarios on mannequins before dealing with patients.
- Enables learning of common procedural skills.
- Enables practicing rarely used procedures.
- Enables learning of leadership skills.
- Helps with crew crisis/resource management.
- Enhances communication skills.
- Provides feedback for enhancing the learning process.

Steadman et al[6] conducted a study for training, based on either SIM (learning by simulation) or PBL (practice-based learning), to 31 fourth-year medical students in acute care management; the SIM group performed better than the PBL group (mean PBL 0.53 vs SIM 0.72, $P < 0.0001$). They concluded that SIM was superior to PBL for the acquisition of critical assessment and management skills.

Studies from aviation literature have shown that simulation reduces the number of training hours required to reach a proficiency level compared with other methods of training. Generalizing their results to health care, we can postulate that SIM will be of great help to produce efficient, skillful health care providers in a shorter period of time.[7]

TRANSFER OF TRAINING FROM SIMULATION TO REAL LIFE

This concept is adapted from the aviation literature and involves implementing the gathered knowledge/skills in real-life scenarios (Figure 75–1). Baldwin and Ford[8] define the transfer of training as the application of knowledge and skills gained from training to real-life situations outside training and the maintenance of that transfer over a certain period of time. Later, Ford also mentioned that the factors affecting the transfer of training include trainee characteristics (ability, personality, motivation), training design (learning, sequencing, job relevance of training content), and the work environment (transfer climate, social support from supervisors and peers). Learning does not necessarily equate ability to perform tasks "on the job." If that learning occurs in a simulated environment and does not result in transferable skills, then the training will be of no use.[9] Assessment of this transfer would be by evaluating the trainees' performance in real-life scenarios.

CLASSIFICATION OF SIMULATORS

1. *Standardized patient simulator*: It simulates a person acting as a patient reproducing the history, symptoms, and mien in response to the learner's questions and physical examination. It has been used for years in different scenarios such as the clinical skills examination for USMLE, and recently in palliative care simulations for end-of-life discussions,[10] among others. It is mainly used to evaluate and improve communication skills. It is also being used in institutes in the early mobilization program wherein the multidisciplinary ICU staff members are being trained to mobilize patients on a ventilator by using a standardized patient hooked up to the ventilator.

2. Part task trainers are life-like models of body parts used to enhance procedural skills such as airway management, line placements (Figure 75–2A), chest tube insertions, cricothyroidotomies, and intubations (Figure 75–2B).[11]

3. Hybrid simulators consist of life-like body parts attached to a standardized patient.

4. *Advanced task trainer*: It consists of a body part model linked to a computer; it is used for procedures such as bronchoscopies (Figure 75–3) wherein the practitioner inserts the instrument into the body part and the computer screen displays the internal anatomy as maneuvers are performed. The system is programmed to respond to stimuli (ie, irritation by coughing if adequate analgesia is not given).

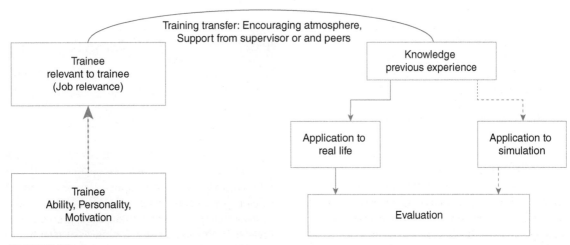

FIGURE 75–1 Transfer of training and its evaluation.

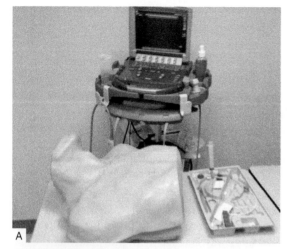

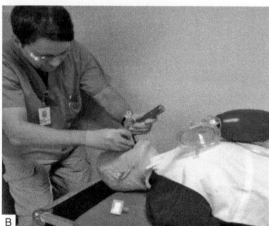

FIGURE 75-2 (A) Part task trainer for ultrasound guided central line placement. (B) Part task trainer for endotracheal intubation.

5. *High-fidelity simulator* (Figure 75–4): A mannequin simulator that very closely mimics real-life responses. It manifests all the physiologic characteristics—breathing, talking, having palpable pulses, and responding to the learner's intervention. Simulation training is carried out on such simulators with real equipment.

6. *Screen-based computer simulator*: A computer screen projecting a patient's history, vitals, details of various medications, for example. It responds realistically to the learner's interventions.

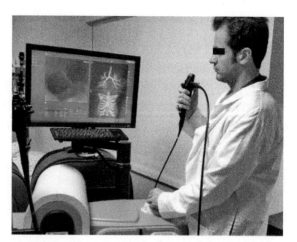

FIGURE 75-3 Advanced task trainer for bronchoscopy.

7. *Virtual reality simulators*: Generally used in surgical fields for a 3-dimensional view of masses/polyps, etc, for laparoscopy, for colonoscopy, etc.

Simulation is not intended to replace the need for learning in a clinical environment, but through improved preparation, it enhances the clinical experience and improves patient care; thus, it is important to integrate it with clinical practice.[12]

The success of a simulator program is not determined primarily by the type of simulator used but more by the enthusiasm, skill, and creativity of instructors, as well as the time and effort devoted to preparing and performing credible simulation scenarios.[13]

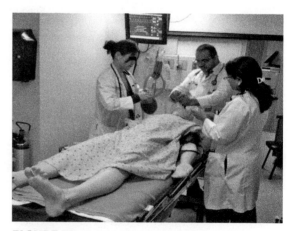

FIGURE 75-4 High-fidelity simulator.

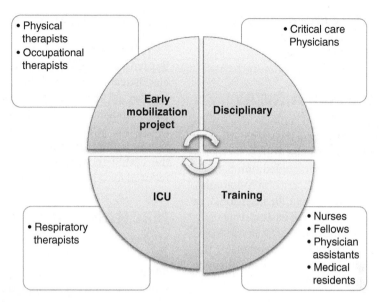

FIGURE 75–5 Interdisciplinary training in ICU.

INTERDISCIPLINARY TRAINING IN ICU

The intensivist has to work as part of a team that includes the nursing staff, respiratory therapist, physical/occupational therapy staff, and other consultants. All medical practitioners can derive benefits from simulation training, not only acquiring knowledge and clinical skills,[14] but also improving team performance and developing leadership skills[15] (Figure 75–5).

SIMULATION TRAINING FOR FELLOWS AND RESIDENTS

Simulation helps physicians improve their performance in highly stressful and life-threatening situations. The diagnosis and management of various shock scenarios, acute coronary syndromes, tachy/bradyarrhythmias, status epileptics, respiratory distress, anaphylaxis, metabolic disturbances, trauma, and post-surgical/cardiothoracic cases can be taught through simulation.

In the study by Sandahl et al,[16] the participants reported that simulation training had increased their awareness of the importance of effective communication for patient safety. However, they caution that the observed improvements will not last, unless organizational features such as staffing rotation and scheduling of rounds and meetings can be changed to enable use of the learned behaviors frequently in the work environment.

Tukey and Wiener[17] in their study surveyed pulmonary and critical care program directors and found that many fellows currently occupied do not get the opportunity to gain proficiency in pulmonary artery catheterization (PAC), and proposed that fellowship training programs should consider alternate means of training fellows in PAC data interpretation, such as simulation.

SIMULATION FOR ULTRASOUND GUIDED LINE PLACEMENTS

With advanced technologies such as ultrasound being used for most ICU procedures, simulation plays an important role in giving trainees skills and confidence to perform procedures. Barsuk et al[18] showed that simulation-based mastery learning increased residents' skills in simulated CVC insertion, decreased the number of needle passes when performing actual procedures, and increased residents' self-confidence.

SIMULATION FOR AIRWAY

The types of airway handling techniques that can be taught in simulation range from the simple (bag and mask ventilation) to the complex (direct laryngoscopy intubations, glidoscope-guided intubations, tube exchangers, bougie use, cricothyrodotomies, and percutaneous tracheostomy tube insertions). In a study with medical residents of basic airway management, Kory et al[19] showed that scenario-based training with a computerized patient simulator was more effective in training medical residents than the traditional experiential method.

SIMULATION FOR BRONCHOSCOPIES

For pulmonary and critical care fellows, simulation allows practicing how to introduce and maneuver the bronchoscope in the simulated airway, thus allowing development of skills before the actual procedure is done on a real patient. The advanced task trainer for bronchoscopy produces natural patient reflexes such as coughing, and responds to sedation and analgesia like a real patient. It helps the new learner to get familiar with the basic techniques of holding and maneuvering the bronchoscope from the upper to the lower airways. If done first on an actual patient, a novice bronchoscopist could expose the patient to untoward events such as hypoxia or hypotension. These simulators may also allow training for bronchoscopic biopsy, brushing, and ultrasound.

Kennedy et al[20] performed a meta-analysis on studies evaluating simulation-based flexible or rigid bronchoscopy training compared to no intervention. In comparison with no intervention, simulation training was associated with large benefits in terms of skills and behaviors (pooled effect size, 1.21 [95%CI, 0.82-1.60]; $n = 8$ studies). They concluded that simulation-based bronchoscopy training is more effective than no intervention and also found that comparative effectiveness studies were few.

SIMULATION AS A TOOL FOR QUALITY IMPROVEMENT

Burden et al[21] collected data for catheter-related bloodstream infection incidence (CRBSI), the number of ICU catheter days, mortality, laboratory pathogen results, and costs pre- and postintervention, which was simulation-based central venous catheter insertion training. They found that the CRBSI incidence and costs were significantly reduced for 2 years postintervention.

MECHANICAL VENTILATION

Mechanical ventilation can be taught by using either screen-based computer simulators or high-fidelity simulators. The screen projects the ventilator screen with waveforms and ventilator settings and pressures. It gives arterial blood gas values and creates scenarios with different airway and ventilation issues. It responds to learner intervention by appropriate changes in arterial blood gases.

SIMULATION IN PALLIATIVE CARE

It is obvious that the patient and their family members in the ICU require emotional support and other comfort measures. An intensivist must conduct family meetings to keep them updated about the patient. They may have to deal with varying responses from the family members. Given the patient's severity of illness, they may also have to discuss end-of-life issues. As mentioned before in this manuscript, simulation is now being used in this field.[11] A standardized patient can act as the patient. Family members' responses can also be simulated. This tool can also be used to evaluate residents'/fellows' baseline communication skills as well as to teach these skills effectively.

A study done by Efstathiou and Walker[22] indicated self-perceived improvements in knowledge, skills, confidence, and competence when dealing with challenging end-of-life care communication situations. A comparison of pre- and post-intervention scores revealed a statistically significant positive change in the students' perceptions about their level of knowledge ($P < 0.02$).

SIMULATION FOR PHYSICAL THERAPY STAFF

Now with early mobilization being implemented in major institutes, physical and occupational therapies are increasingly being followed by the ICU interdisciplinary team. More patients on ventilators are being mobilized out of bed. This could possibly result in more adverse events such as accidental extubations, circuit disconnects, hemodynamic compromise, and falls. So, it is essential that the rehabilitation services staff be trained to anticipate and act on these issues by calling for help early or taking more precautions with tubing and pumps attached to the patients.

Ohtake et al[23] showed that incorporating simulated, interprofessional critical care into a required clinical course improved physical therapist students' confidence in dealing with technical, behavioral, and cognitive performance measures, and was associated with high student satisfaction; using simulation to introduce students to the critical care environment may provide encouragement and increase their interest in this area.

SIMULATION FOR FAMILIARITY WITH EQUIPMENT USE

1. *Pacemaker and defibrillator*: Simulation training will enable health care professionals to better operate the machinery used in this field. Running a scenario on a simulator with different brady/tachyarrhythmias scenarios will give health care providers hands-on training with different equipment so that they are prepared and trained for real-life scenarios. Knowledge of resuscitation algorithms is not sufficient to help patients if operators are not familiar with how to use vital equipment.

2. *Continuous renal replacement therapy* (CRRT): With the technological advancement, there is also a need to train the involved staff in the operation of the new equipment, and the operator should be comfortable with troubleshooting alarms. Mencía et al[24] developed a device and proposed that it may be very useful for training health care

professionals in CRRT management, thus avoiding risk to patients.

3. *Extracorporeal membrane oxygenator circuit* (ECMO): The use of ECMO has increased in recent years. Simulation in ECMO can be used to train surgeons, anesthetists, critical care physicians and nurses, and perfusionists.

SIMULATION TO PREPARE FOR DISASTERS

Simulation with standardized patients during a mass disaster can be used to train health care professionals to be mentally and physically ready. Also with emergency rooms being overcrowded with many sick patients during a disaster, the ICU team should be ready to absorb the very sick patients and provide additional care in unfamiliar settings outside of the ICU. In order for the team to react properly to these kinds of emergencies, simulation training is necessary.

ROLE OF SIMULATION IN PATIENT SAFETY

A medical error is a preventable adverse effect of care, whether it is harmful to the patient or not. Medical errors are one of the main causes of significant morbidity and mortality. They incur a cost burden on the society and health care industry. Medical errors hurt patients physically, economically, and psychologically. They may also cause feelings of inadequacy and guilt in the provider. Decreasing medical errors to improve patient safety is of high importance.

Some of the measures to reduce medical errors and increase patient safety, as suggested by Kohn et al,[25] are to support projects aimed at achieving a better understanding of how the environment affects the ability of the provider to practice safely. Another recommendation is funding researchers and encouraging organizations to develop, demonstrate, and evaluate new approaches to improve provider education in order to reduce errors. Simulation training can be used to fulfill both these purposes. Errors may occur in a team care environment as a result of nontechnical factors (eg, communication), and specific simulation-based training protocols have been developed for enhancing team performance.[16,26]

With the age-old practice of apprenticeship training in the medical field being questioned in light of increased priorities for patient safety, simulation training seems to be a useful tool to help reduce medical errors through training and improve safety. Simulation training allows practitioners to make errors and learn from them in a controlled, simulated environment. This experience can prepare them to face real-life scenarios with confidence and minimize actual errors.

CRISIS RESOURCE MANAGEMENT

Crew resource management, defined as effective utilization of all available equipment and people to carry out safe, efficient flight operations,[27] is a term introduced in the aviation industry during a NASA workshop in 1979. It was designed as a training program to improve air safety and reduce the increasing number of fatal accidents attributable to human error.[28] When errors were analyzed, they were mainly attributed to failure of interpersonal communication, leadership, and decision-making. The same principle can be applied to the medical field where it is called crisis resource management (CRM). Health care industry has now recognized the importance of this training and is slowly and steadily incorporating it into different subspecialties. The traditional medical curriculum does not lay emphasis on nonclinical skills such as communication, leadership, and team building. Now, with human errors being linked to inadequate nonclinical skills, importance has been given for developing and maintaining these skills by simulation training.

How can one evaluate and measure CRM skills? Two validated scales in critical care are the Ottawa Global Rating Scale (GRS) and Mayo High Performance Teamwork Scale (MHPTS).[29] In their study, Kim et al[30] had first- and third-year residents participating in two simulator scenarios, recreating emergencies in acute care settings, and were evaluated using the Ottawa GRS by three different evaluators. With his results, Kim found acceptable inter-rater reliability and validated the Ottawa GRS to evaluate CRM performance during high-fidelity simulations.

Malec et al[30] performed a study to develop and evaluate a scale for assessing teamwork skills in simulated settings. He developed the MHPTS and found that it provides a brief, reliable, and practical measure of CRM skills that can be used by participants in CRM training to reflect on and evaluate their performance as a team.

CRM involves leadership, problem solving, situational awareness, resource utilization, and communication skills. CRM is extremely important for patient safety but is not covered in the traditional learning curriculum. In order to master CRM skills, one has to practice them repeatedly in simulated sessions. Figure 75–6 illustrates how simulation helps improve different skill sets to achieve patient safety.

DEBRIEFING

Debriefing, a term used more often in military scenarios, is a very important component in simulation training. As shown in Figure 75–7, simulation training first involves creating a simulation case scenario (with all pertinent medical details and specific educational goals), then introducing the learner(s) to the simulated scenario, giving them the time to perform a task, and then debriefing them after the scenario is completed. The debriefing should involve the learner's self-evaluation (ideally after viewing a video recording of their performance), and the instructor's feedback (a powerful educational tool). The aim of debriefing is to make learners realize both their strengths and areas that could be improved in an encouraging, healthy manner. Also, during this time the instructor should evaluate and address individual and team performances and gives positive and negative reinforcement as appropriate.

CONCLUSION

Critical care practitioners are increasingly using simulation training. Traditional learning with books and lectures continues to provide a basic fund of knowledge. Simulation helps reinforce and consolidate the knowledge gained from traditional learning. Additionally, simulation helps health care providers develop hands-on clinical and nonclinical skills such as CRM skills. CRM skills cannot be learned from a book or in a lecture hall. Due to the low prevalence yet high complexity of many

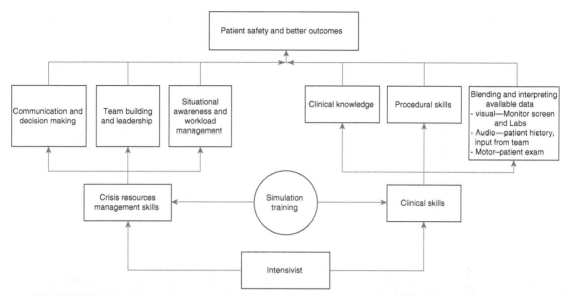

FIGURE 75-6 Combination of clinical and nonclinical skills for patient safety. (Data from Driskel JE, Adams RJ: Crew Resource Management: An Introductory Handbook, August 1992. U.S. Department of Transportation. Federal Aviation Administration.)

disease processes encountered in critical care, critical care performance depends on time-sensitive decision-making, safe procedural skills, and good staff teamwork to ensure positive clinical outcomes. However, the opportunities for young trainees to be present and actively participate during these critical moments are increasingly low. Training in critical care using simulation can make medical education more effective and interesting, providing real benefits to patients. Simulation training enables immediate self-evaluation and provides

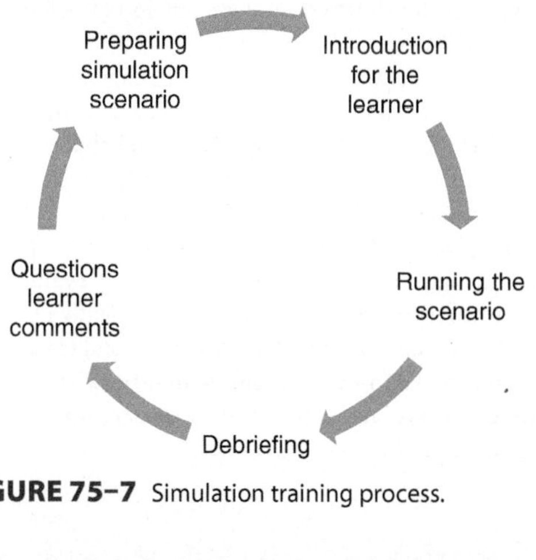

FIGURE 75-7 Simulation training process.

critical feedback, essential for skill development. Simulation training, in all its forms, should be an integral part of the education of all providers who work in the ICU.

REFERENCES

1. Knowles, MS. The Modern Practice of Adult Education; Andragogy versus Pedagogy. (ERIC Document Reproduction Service No.ED043812). 1970.
2. Ziv A, Wolpe PR, Small SD, et al. Simulation-based medical education: an ethical imperative. *Simul Healthcare.* 2006;1:252-256.
3. Kathleen R. History of medical simulation. *J Crit Care.* 2008;23:157-166.
4. Howard SK, Gaba DM, Fish KJ, et al. Anesthesia crisis resource management training: teaching anesthesiologists to handle critical incidents. *Aviat Space Environ Med.* 1992;63:763-770.
5. Fisher N, Eisen LA, Bayya JV, et al. Improved performance of maternal-fetal medicine staff after maternal cardiac arrest simulation-based training. *Am J Obstet Gynecol.* 2011;205:239.e1-e5.
6. Steadman R, Coates W, Huang YM, et al. Simulation-based training is superior to problem-based learning for the acquisition of critical assessment and management skills. *Crit Care Med.* 2006;34:151-157.

7. Eisen LA, Savel RH. What went right: lessons for the intensivist from the crew of US Airways flight 1549. *Chest*. 2009;136:910-917.

8. Baldwin TT, Ford KJ. Transfer of training: a review and directions for future research. *Pers Psychol*. 1988;41:63-105.

9. Hahn SH. The transfer of training from simulations in civilian and military workforces: perspectives from the current body of literatura. The Advanced Distributing Learning (ADL) Research and Evaluation Team. http://www.adlnet.gov/wp-content/uploads/2011/07/Transfer-of-Training-from-Simulations-in-Civilian-and-Military-Workforces-Perspectives-from-the-Current-Body-of-Literature.pdf.

10. Hope A, Howes J, Dow L, et al. Let's talk critical: the development and evaluation of a communication skills training program for critical care trainees. Presented at: American Thoracic Society International Conference. May 2013.

11. Sekiguchi H, Tokita JE, Minami T, Eisen LA, Mayo PH, Narasimhan M. A prerotational, simulation-based workshop improves the safety of central venous catheter insertion: results of a successful internal medicine house staff training program. *Chest*. 2011;140:652-658.

12. Maran NJ, Glavin RJ. Low- to high-fidelity simulation – A continuum of medical education. *Med Educ*. 2003;37:22-28.

13. Gaba D. A brief history of mannequin-based simulation and application. In: Dunn F, ed. *Simulation in Critical Care and Beyond*. Des Plaines, IL: Society of Critical Care Medicine; 2004:7-14.

14. Venegas-Borsellino C, Shiloh A, Dudaie R, et al. Simulation training to improve the performance and confidence of new physician assistants in the critical care environment. *Crit Care Med*. 2012;40:602.

15. Venegas-Borsellino C, Dudaie R, Lizano D, et al. Improving leadership and teamwork in the critical care environment: training physician assistants. *Crit Care Med*. 2012;40:1282.

16. Sandahl C, Gustafsson H, Wallin CJ, et al. Simulation team training for improved teamwork in an intensive care unit. *Int J Health Care Qual Assur*. 2013;26:174-188.

17. Tukey MH, Wiener RS. The current state of fellowship training in pulmonary artery catheter placement and data interpretation: a national survey of pulmonary and critical care fellowship program directors. *J Crit Care*. 2013;28:857-861.

18. Barsuk JH, McGaghie WC, Cohen ER, et al. Use of simulation-based mastery learning to improve the quality of central venous catheter placement in a medical intensive care unit. *J Hosp Med*. 2009;4:397-403.

19. Kory PD, Eisen LA, Adachi M, Ribaudo VA, Rosenthal ME, Mayo PH. Initial airway management skills of senior residents: simulation training compared with traditional training. *Chest*. 2007;132:1927-1931.

20. Kennedy CC, Maldonado F, Cook DA. Simulation-based bronchoscopy training: systematic review and meta-analysis. *Chest*. 2013;144:183-192.

21. Burden AR, Torjman MC, Dy GE, et al. Prevention of central venous catheter-related bloodstream infections: is it time to add simulation training to the prevention bundle? *J Clin Anesth*. 2012;24:555-560.

22. Efstathiou N, Walker WM. Interprofessional, simulation-based training in end of life care communication: a pilot study. *J Interprof Care*. 2014;28:68-70.

23. Ohtake PJ, Lazarus M, Schillo R. Simulation experience enhances physical therapist student confidence in managing a patient in the critical care environment. *Phys Ther*. 2013;93:216-228.

24. Mencía S, López M, López-Herce J, Ferrero L, et al. Simulating continuous renal replacement therapy: usefulness of a new simulator device. *J Artif Organs*. 2014;17:114-117.

25. Kohn LT, Corrigan JM, Donaldson MS. *To Err Is Human: Building a Safer Health System*. Washington, DC: National Academy Press; 1999.

26. Schmidt E, Goldhaber-Fiebert S, Ho LA, et al. *Making Health Care Safer II: An Updated Critical Analysis of the Evidence for Patient Safety Practices*. Rockville, MD: Agency for Healthcare Research and Quality. http://www.ahrq.gov/research/findings/evidence-based-reports/ptsafetyuptp.html.

27. Driskell J, Adams RJ. *Crew Resource Management: An Introductory Handbook*. Washington, DC: Federal Aviation Administration, Research and Development Service; 1992.

28. From the site: www.crewresourcemanagement.net.

29. Malec JF, Torsher LC, Dunn WF, et al. The Mayo High Performance Teamwork Scale: reliability and validity for evaluating key crew resource management skills. *Simul Healthcare*. 2007;2:4-10.

30. Kim J, Neilipovitz D, Cardinal P, et al. A pilot study using high-fidelity simulation to formally evaluate performance in the resuscitation of critically ill patients: The University of Ottawa Critical Care Medicine, High-Fidelity Simulation, and Crisis Resource Management I Study. *Crit Care Med*. 2006;34:2167-2174.

ICU Bed Utilization

Hannah Wunsch, MD, MSc

76

KEY POINTS

1. The lack of an agreed-upon definition of an ICU bed remains a barrier to understanding bed utilization.

2. Small ICUs or systems of ICUs are at a disadvantage due to their size, creating inefficient use of ICU beds.

3. Availability of intermediate-care beds may impact the flow of patients into and out of ICU beds.

4. The casemix of patients admitted to an ICU can vary dramatically. This may be driven by the overall availability of ICU beds, but will also be determined by the casemix of patients in a hospital or system.

5. Use of intensive care beds is often driven by the specific culture of a hospital regarding the "perceived" need of an individual patient, as well as the larger cultural expectations within a given society.

6. Optimization of ICU bed use may include decreasing the number of small ICUs operating separately, standardizing criteria for admission, and increasing alternate care options.

INTRODUCTION

Care of critically ill patients is an integral part of hospital care,[1] but ICU beds are a limited resource in many settings.[2,3] How ICU beds are used has implications for the care of individual patients, as well as resource use and costs at the hospital and regional level. Some aspects of ICU bed utilization may be specific to individual hospitals, but others are more generalizable across hospitals and health care systems. This chapter reviews many of the factors that impact how ICU beds are used, and then discusses potential approaches to optimizing their use.

Definition of an ICU bed: The lack of an agreed on definition of an ICU bed remains a barrier to understanding bed utilization. Some countries, such as the United Kingdom, have a clear definition, describing Level 3 care (ICU-level care) as patients receiving advanced respiratory support alone, or having a minimum of two organs supported.[4] Many countries do not seem to have any definitions. In the United States, there are no standard definitions, but a proposed system of categorization broadly defined the highest level of care as including "sophisticated equipment, specialized nurses, and physicians with critical care training".[5] Across developed countries, the majority of ICU beds have availability of mechanical ventilation and some form of renal support and other organ support. The meaning of an "ICU bed" in developing countries is much more questionable as it does not necessarily include resources to provide specific organ support.[6] This chapter will discuss about the use of ICU beds in systems, with the ability to provide mechanical ventilation and other basic organ support as part of intensive care.

HOW ARE ICU BEDS USED?

The question of the utilization of ICU beds is ultimately one of triage: understanding who is to be admitted to an ICU bed and why, and looking to optimize the use of this expensive resource while providing appropriate care for individual patients. The use of beds is dependent on a number of specific factors: (1) the physical number of ICU beds in a specific ICU, hospital, or system; (2) the ICU bed to hospital bed ratio; (3) other options for care of patients, such as intermediate care units; (3) the casemix of patients cared for in a specific hospital or system, including specific elective surgical patients; (4) hospital culture; and (5) regional culture and norms.

The number of ICU beds: The total number of ICU beds available will clearly have an impact on the use of those beds.[7] This may be due to a number of factors related to the absolute number of beds. First, a hospital with only a few (3-4) ICU beds will not have a high volume of critically ill patients and is likely to have a system for transferring their critically ill patients to larger centers.[8] Some countries or systems may have a formalized regionalization system (such as for trauma),[9] whereas others may be more informal.[8] However, such systems mean that small ICUs may tend to care for patients with only a low severity of illness.[10,11]

Small ICUs or systems of ICUs are also at a disadvantage due to their size, leading to inefficient use of ICU beds. This is due to the concept of queuing theory, which demonstrates that the likelihood of a patient admission being delayed is a function of the occupancy *and* the total number of ICU beds.[12] For example, an ICU that has only 4 beds must operate at 75% occupancy in order to ensure an available bed for the next patient. In contrast, an ICU with 100 beds operating at 75% occupancy has 25 beds available for patients.

The potentially large implications of high occupancy for ICU bed utilization have now been documented in a number of studies. A study by Stelfox et al[13] from Canada demonstrated that when beds are not immediately available, more patients have alterations in their goals of care, with no detectable difference in overall mortality, suggesting that occupancy may drive physicians and patients to choose appropriate alternative care paths. However, the knock-on effect of high occupancy may also depend on the country and the overall availability of beds. For example, data from the United Kingdom suggest that many patients are discharged prematurely due to chronic high occupancy and intense pressure regarding new admissions, with worse hospital mortality for the patients discharged prematurely.[14,15] In contrast, data from the United States suggest that premature discharges associated with "strained" ICUs do not result in increased mortality, and may consequently represent more efficient use of ICU beds.[16]

The ICU bed to hospital bed ratio: Little is understood about the ICU bed-to-overall hospital bed ratio and how this affects ICU bed use. We do know that most systems/countries operate on a relatively fixed ratio of ICU beds to hospital beds of approximately 2 to 5 ICU beds for every 100 hospital beds in total, while the United States operates with a very different ratio of 9 to 10 ICU beds per 100 hospital beds in total.[7] This high ICU bed to hospital bed ratio in the United States may impact ICU bed utilization by decreasing the threshold for use, particularly if other lower acuity beds become the scarce resource. Data from the United States suggest that 40% of patients admitted to an ICU have monitoring needs only (no active treatment), and that only 35% of these patients are considered at high risk of needing active treatment during the ICU stay.[17] Similarly, a study by the Veterans Affairs system in the United States found that many patients (up to 50%) admitted through the emergency room with a predicted risk of death of less than 2% were admitted to ICU beds.[18] This is enabled by an overall high availability of ICU beds and a generous ICU bed to hospital bed ratio, as described above, but also may be driven by inadequate nursing or other resources in other parts of the hospital.

Other options for care of patients: The question of other care options for patients is an important one to understand ICU bed utilization. Intermediate care (also called stepdown care, or high-dependency care) has received little attention in the ICU literature. Yet in a survey of 40 hospitals as far back as 1995, 63% of hospitals reported at least one intermediate care unit.[19] These types of units provide care at a higher level than available in a general ward, but usually without the ability to provide full organ support, such as mechanical ventilation. Evaluation of their use has mostly focused on elective surgical patients,[20-22] but, clearly, the utilization of ICU beds in a system depends on the availability of such beds. The availability of intermediate-care beds may impact both the time patients need to spend in an ICU bed prior to discharge and also the need to admit a patient to an ICU bed at all, particularly when the focus is on better monitoring and/or nursing care, rather than full organ support.

Casemix of patients: The casemix of patients admitted to an ICU can vary dramatically.[23] This may be driven by the overall availability of ICU beds, but may also be determined by the casemix of patients in a hospital or system. This point is related to the one above regarding intermediate care beds, as some individual patients are more amenable to care in alternate settings. One large driver of the routine utilization of ICU beds is specific surgical programs in a hospital. For example, a hospital that routinely performs liver transplants will use ICU beds for the care of those patients (sometimes) before and (always) after the surgical procedure. Similarly, a hospital that has a large population of oncology patients may expect a certain requirement for ICU beds for patients developing complications from chemotherapy or surgery.[24]

Specifics of the hospital culture: Use of ICU beds is often driven by the specific culture of a hospital regarding the "perceived" need of an individual patient. For example, in a study of patients admitted to hospitals in New York State with diabetic keto-acidosis, anywhere from zero to 100% of patients received intensive care during the hospitalization.[25] Although much of this variation may be driven by the factors described above, such as availability of other appropriate care settings and high-level nursing on wards, at least some of this variation is likely attributable to accepted practices. There are similar findings for other diagnoses, such as patients with carotid endarterectomy.[26] One study examined outcomes using their standard practice of admitting almost all (98%) of the patients to the ICU for monitoring after a carotid endarterectomy versus admission based on assessment of risk (22%) and found no difference in outcomes, reinforcing the idea that practices regarding ICU bed utilization may be based on the perceived, rather than actual, need.[26]

Regional culture and norms: Use of ICU beds may be driven not only by the culture or expectations for care within a specific hospital setting, but also by larger cultural expectations. For example, data from the ETHICUS study carried out in Europe found a large variation in the practice of withholding or withdrawing of treatment before death, depending on the region of Europe,[27] and comparison work of cultural expectations in the United States and United Kingdom shows stark differences in expectations and experiences.[28] Some of these cultural norms may be codified into laws that then underpin patterns of ICU bed utilization. In some countries, physicians may make decisions regarding escalation of care and/or end-of-life care choices, such as the placement of a do-not-resuscitate order, without much input from families, while other countries or regions mandate that patients or families must agree to the proposed care plan.[3]

OPTIMIZING ICU BED UTILIZATION

Guidelines: Within the specific culture and laws of a region, a number of approaches may help to optimize ICU bed utilization. The first is to have clear guidelines for admission or refusal. While this approach works well in theory, the reality of such guidelines is that they provide a lot of latitude regarding the appropriateness of admission.[29] For example, the guidelines from the Society of Critical Care Medicine state: "ICU admission criteria should select patients who are likely to benefit from ICU care," going on to try to define groups who may or may not benefit.[30] While such guidelines may help in the most extreme circumstances, the documents themselves acknowledge that they are not particularly useful for individual decision-making.[31]

All guidelines or tools for individual or even diagnosis or procedure-specific decisions are hampered by the lack of data regarding the benefit received from admission to an ICU.[31] Whereas patients who require mechanical ventilation or are in shock requiring systemic circulatory support may be admitted to an ICU and no one doubts the benefit of intensive care for those patients,[32] there are many other circumstances when it is not so straightforward. For example a patient may be too sick to be rescued by the maximal support offered in an ICU or may be too well to benefit from the additional care.[33]

Gatekeepers: Another option that may improve the utilization of ICU beds is designation of appropriate caregivers to act as "gatekeepers." Many ICUs do not have clear designees for this role; particularly for "open" ICUs, this may mean that every physician in the hospital has admitting privileges to the ICU and can decide for themselves whether a patient should be admitted if there is a bed available.[34] Such an approach is clearly problematic, as ICU beds are part of a system, and appropriate use of those beds involves understanding of competing interests and ability to triage based on experience with critical illness and the likely course of an individual's illness. One study has examined the impact of a medical ICU director on resource use, finding that the presence of an active medical ICU director in US ICUs was associated with a lower average occupancy rate and lower probability of patients being "misallocated" to the ICU.[35]

Minimizing small ICUs and specialty ICUs: Along with having appropriate decision-makers, understanding queuing theory (mentioned above)[12,36] and designing a system to minimize the number of small ICUs and maximizing the utilization of available ICU beds are paramount. Cities in England have very few ICU beds, but their utilization is optimized in places such as London by essentially creating a network of all ICU beds across London using the London Ambulance System to track available ICU beds and shift patients to the nearest available bed when needed.[37]

The related problem of many specialty ICU beds may occur particularly in large academic medical centers, with 4 to 5 specialty ICUs (such as a "transplant" ICU). Patients may be left waiting for admission to the "appropriate" specialty ICU, rather than gaining admission to any available ICU bed. Data suggest that for most types of patients, specialty ICUs (compared with general ICUs) may not offer benefit for outcomes.[38] However, with the presence of specialty ICUs, patients who are "boarders" (i.e. admitted to an inappropriate ICU) may also have worse outcomes.[38]

Alternative care options: Another way to optimize the use of ICU beds, particularly in systems such as that in the United States where many patients in ICUs are admitted solely for monitoring purposes, is to create or increase other care options, such as intermediate care areas. This type of approach may also involve such options as increasing the hours a recovery room is open to allow patients to remain in a monitored setting without full admission to an ICU.[39,40] Hand-in-hand with this option is the improvement of nursing on general wards.

High-quality and experienced nursing staff on wards: A large barrier to keeping patients in lower levels of care may often be the perceived lack of quality nursing, rather than the need for any specific interventions provided by an ICU. Many studies suggest that aspects of nursing care, such as the nurse-to-patient ratio, and the level of education of nursing staff, can have a large impact on outcomes for patients.[41-43] Therefore, another approach to optimizing the use of ICU beds may be to ensure quality nursing care in other areas of the hospital so that ICU beds do not become the default destination for any patient who requires good nursing care.

Removing financial misalignment: Finally, in certain systems, such as that in the United States, optimal use of ICU beds may only be achieved once competing financial incentives are removed. For example, a physician who has a salary based on the number of critical care bills generated has a strong incentive to keep patients in the ICU, or admit marginal patients. Similarly, a hospital that is paying nursing staff based on the number of ICU beds in the unit would prefer to have patients in all of those beds to offset the fixed costs of the staff.[44] Or there may be financial penalties for an institution that keeps patients waiting for beds in the Emergency Department, forcing them to use ICU beds for patients who would otherwise go to ward beds. Only once these incentives are removed can other aspects of ICU utilization be optimized.

With the goal of efficient, patient-centered care in hospitals, ICU bed utilization is an important area for further research. Many of the approaches to improve efficiency remain speculative, and warrant further investigation with rigorous study designs to determine optimal approaches.

REFERENCES

1. Coopersmith CM, Wunsch H, Fink MP, et al. A comparison of critical care research funding and the financial burden of critical illness in the United States. *Crit Care Med.* 2012;40:1072-1079.
2. Bion J. Rationing intensive care. *Br Med J.* 1995;310:682-683.
3. Evans T, Nava S, Vazquez M, et al. Critical care rationing: international comparisons. *Chest.* 2011;140:1618-1624.
4. Levels of Care for Adult Patients. In: *Standards And Guidelines, Intensive Care Society. United Kingdom* 2009.
5. Haupt MT, Bekes CE, Brilli RJ, et al. Guidelines on critical care services and personnel: recommendations based on a system of categorization of three levels of care. *Crit Care Med.* 2003;31:2677-2683.
6. Austin S, Murthy S, Wunsch H, et al. Access to urban acute care services in high- vs. middle-income countries: an analysis of seven cities. *Intensive Care Med.* 2014;40:342-352.
7. Wunsch H, Angus DC, Harrison DA, et al. Variation in critical care services across North America and Western Europe. *Crit Care Med.* 2008;36:2787-2789.
8. Iwashyna TJ, Christie JD, Moody J, Kahn JM, Asch DA. The structure of critical care transfer networks. *Med Care.* 2009;47:787-793.
9. MacKenzie EJ, Rivara FP, Jurkovich GJ, et al. A national evaluation of the effect of trauma-center care on mortality. *N Engl J Med.* 2006;354:366-378.
10. Kahn JM, Asch RJ, Iwashyna TJ, et al. Physician attitudes toward regionalization of adult critical care: a national survey. *Crit Care Med.* 2009;37:2149-2154.
11. Kahn JM, Linde-Zwirble WT, Wunsch H, et al. Potential value of regionalized intensive care for mechanically ventilated medical patients. *Am J Respir Crit Care Med.* 2008;177:285-291.
12. Green LV. How many hospital beds? *Inquiry.* 2002;39:400-412.
13. Stelfox HT, Hemmelgarn BR, Bagshaw SM, et al. Intensive care unit bed availability and outcomes for hospitalized patients with sudden clinical deterioration. *Arch Intern Med.* 2012;172:467-474.
14. Goldfrad C, Rowan K. Consequences of discharges from intensive care at night. *Lancet.* 2000;355:1138-1142.
15. Hutchings A, Durand MA, Grieve R, et al. Evaluation of modernisation of adult critical care services in England: time series and cost effectiveness analysis. *Br Med J.* 2009;339:b4353.
16. Wagner J, Gabler NB, Ratcliffe SJ, Brown SE, Strom BL, Halpern SD. Outcomes among patients discharged from busy intensive care units. *Ann Intern Med.* 2013;159:447-455.
17. Zimmerman JE, Kramer AA. A model for identifying patients who may not need intensive care unit admission. *J Crit Care.* 2010;25:205-213.
18. Chen LM, Render M, Sales A, Kennedy EH, Wiitala W, Hofer TP. Intensive care unit admitting patterns in the veterans affairs health care system. *Arch Int Med.* 2012;172:1220-1226.
19. Zimmerman JE, Wagner DP, Knaus WA, Williams JF, Kolakowski D, Draper EA. The use of risk predictions to identify candidates for intermediate care units. Implications for intensive care utilization and cost. *Chest.* 1995;108:490-499.
20. Byrick RJ, Power JD, Ycas JO, Brown KA. Impact of an intermediate care area on ICU utilization after cardiac surgery. *Crit Care Med.* 1986;14:869-872.
21. Bellomo R, Goldsmith D, Uchino S, et al. A before and after trial of the effect of a high-dependency unit on post-operative morbidity and mortality. *Crit Care Resusc.* 2005;7:16-21.
22. Eachempati SR, Hydo LJ, Barie PS. The effect of an intermediate care unit on the demographics and outcomes of a surgical intensive care unit population. *Arch Surg.* 2004;139:315-319.
23. Wunsch H, Angus DC, Harrison DA, Linde-Zwirble WT, Rowan KM. Comparison of medical admissions to intensive care units in the United States and United Kingdom. *Am J Respir Crit Care Med.* 2011;183:1666-1673.
24. Voigt LP, Pastores SM, Raoof ND, Thaler HT, Halpern NA. Review of a large clinical series: Intrahospital transport of critically ill patients: outcomes, timing, and patterns. *J Intensive Care Med.* 2009;24:108-115.
25. Gershengorn HB, Iwashyna TJ, Cooke CR, Scales DC, Kahn JM, Wunsch H. Variation in use of intensive care for adults with diabetic ketoacidosis. *Crit Care Med.* 2012;40:2009-2015.
26. Kraiss LW, Kilberg L, Critch S, Johansen KJ. Short-stay carotid endarterectomy is safe and cost-effective. *Am J Surg.* 1995;169:512-515.
27. Sprung CL, Cohen SL, Sjokvist P, et al. End-of-life practices in European intensive care units: the Ethicus study. *J Am Med Assoc.* 2003;290:790-797.
28. Gusmano M, Allin S. Health care for older persons in England and the United States: a contrast of systems and values. *J Health Polit Policy Law.* 2011;36:89-118.

29. Sprung CL, Baras M, Iapichino G, et al. The Eldicus prospective, observational study of triage decision making in European intensive care units: Part I–European Intensive Care Admission Triage Scores. *Crit Care Med.* 2012;40:125-131.

30. Guidelines for intensive care unit admission, discharge, and triage. *Crit Care Med.* 1999;27:633-638.

31. Wunsch H. A triage score for admission: a holy grail of intensive care. *Crit Care Med.* 2012;40:321-323.

32. Vincent JL, Sakr Y, Sprung CL, et al. Sepsis in European intensive care units: results of the SOAP study. *Crit Care Med.* 2006;34:344-353.

33. Wunsch H. Is there a starling curve for intensive care? *Chest.* 2012;141:1393-1399.

34. Multz AS, Chalfin DB, Samson IM, et al. A "closed" medical intensive care unit (MICU) improves resource utilization when compared with an "open" MICU. *Am J Respir Crit Care Med.* 1998;157:1468-1473.

35. Mallick R, Strosberg M, Lambrinos J, Groeger JS. The intensive care unit medical director as manager. Impact on performance. *Med Care.* 1995;33:611-624.

36. McManus ML, Long MC, Cooper A, Litvak E. Queuing theory accurately models the need for critical care resources. *Anesthesiology.* 2004;100:1271-1276.

37. Aylwin CJ, Konig TC, Brennan NW, et al. Reduction in critical mortality in urban mass casualty incidents: analysis of triage, surge, and resource use after the London bombings on July 7, 2005. *Lancet.* 2006;368:2219-2225.

38. Lott JP, Iwashyna TJ, Christie JD, Asch DA, Kramer AA, Kahn JM. Critical illness outcomes in specialty versus general intensive care units. *Am J Respir Crit Care Med.* 2009;179:676-683.

39. Teres D, Steingrub J. Can intermediate care substitute for intensive care? *Crit Care Med.* 1987;15:280.

40. Franklin CM, Rackow EC, Mamdani B, Nightingale S, Burke G, Weil MH. Decreases in mortality on a large urban medical service by facilitating access to critical care. An alternative to rationing. *Arch Intern Med.* 1988;148:1403-1405.

41. Aiken LH, Clarke SP, Cheung RB, Sloane DM, Silber JH. Educational levels of hospital nurses and surgical patient mortality. *J Am Med Assoc.* 2003;290:1617-1623.

42. Amaravadi RK, Dimick JB, Pronovost PJ, Lipsett PA. ICU nurse-to-patient ratio is associated with complications and resource use after esophagectomy. *Intensive Care Med.* 2000;26:1857-1862.

43. Dimick JB, Swoboda SM, Pronovost PJ, Lipsett PA. Effect of nurse-to-patient ratio in the intensive care unit on pulmonary complications and resource use after hepatectomy. *Am J Crit Care.* 2001;10:376-382.

44. Kahn JM. Understanding economic outcomes in critical care. *Curr Opin Crit Care.* 2006;12:399-404.

The ICU in the Global Hospital Environment

Hayley B. Gershengorn, MD

INTRODUCTION

While the "intensive care unit" (ICU) is a distinct location to which patients with critical illnesses are transferred, in order to optimally manage the ICU and care for the critically ill, it is important to understand the ICU as it functions within the global hospital environment. ICUs in the United States originated during the polio epidemic of the 1950s as a place to cohort patients in need of mechanical ventilation.[1] Over time, however, patients classified as critically ill have become far more heterogeneous and the potential to care for them has increased dramatically.[2] As a result, the role of the ICU in the hospital environment

has necessarily changed. Currently, ICUs cannot be viewed as standalone units that operate in silos. Instead, they must be well integrated into the hospital system to maximize the benefit of what is often a sparse resource—the ICU bed.[3-5]

In this chapter, four aspects of ICU management—(1) the administration of critical care, (2) staffing for critical care, (3) the structure of critical care, and (4) resource utilization for critical care—will be discussed. Some of these topics are addressed in detail in other chapters; herein, I will highlight how they are integral to situating the ICU well within the broader hospital environment.

ADMINISTRATION OF CRITICAL CARE

Critical care medicine has, traditionally, been a specialty without a home. ICU physicians have come from multiple backgrounds (eg, internal medicine, surgery, anesthesiology) and, in larger institutions, the units in which they work have, historically, been separately managed by their individual clinical departments.[6] To make matters more complicated, the administration of nonphysician ICU staff (eg, nurses, respiratory therapists, nonphysician providers) is further fragmented. Instead of having a department unto themselves, critical care practitioners have been scattered throughout the organization. This type of fragmented or "siloed" structure has known drawbacks; silos can detract from teamwork and worsen communication with patients and families.[7,8] An alternate strategy that is gaining favor is that of "service lines" where all aspects of care pertaining to a given clinical entity are grouped under one organizational unit. This organizational methodology has proven beneficial in widely varying clinical settings.[9-12] Administering critical care as a service line is of potential benefit to patients and the hospital as a whole.[13]

Creating a critical care service line can be accomplished through the development of a separate critical care division or department or through the appointment of a director of critical care who helps to oversee a critical care administration that remains housed within distinct clinical departments. While the former is a more drastic change for an institution in which the traditional model is in place, it allows for a more centralized system and, potentially, economies of scale and scope[14] and flexibility in resource use.[15,16] The latter option may not reap the same benefits, yet can make standardization of protocols—known to improve critically ill patient outcomes[17]—more feasible. In either case, all aspects of critical care delivery are managed together. With this model, the mission of the service line may be made clearer and resources may be more easily optimally allocated to achieve consistent goals.

This strategy of collaborative critical care administration has the potential to be beneficial to the hospital. First, if all providers operate under the same administration, collaboration among them is simplified. If a patient in a hospital with more than one ICU is critically ill and in need of an ICU bed at a time when none is available in the ICU most well suited to him/her, coordinated management may facilitate the admission of that patient to another ICU. Additionally, transfer of that patient to the better suited ICU may be more feasible when bed availability permits. In the extreme, ICUs operating under this paradigm can have beds that are flexibly allocated to different care teams (eg, medical or surgical) and/or different care levels, depending on the day-to-day needs of the hospital.[15,16] Second, there is a single person/administration who is responsible for addressing all issues pertaining to critical care delivery. For example, in New York State, a regulation mandating compliance with and documentation of adherence to sepsis bundles of care has been recently passed.[18] With a centralized critical care administration, one single sepsis protocol can be developed and rapidly disseminated. Third, integration across clinical departments within critical care may foster integration outside of it as well. Lines of communication among providers within medicine and surgery, for example, may be bolstered through the existence of an integrated critical care department.

STAFFING FOR CRITICAL CARE

Staffing has become a topic of much focus in intensive care medicine recently. Leapfrog recommendations and Society of Critical Care Medicine (SCCM) guidelines require high-intensity staffing models where intensivists are available and/or onsite 24 hours a day.[19,20] These mandates are difficult to meet for many institutions. Strategies to improve critical care coverage are discussed in detail in the chapter "Alternate Staffing Models in the ICU." As staffing pertains to the ICU as a part of the global hospital environment, two main questions for staffing arise: Is the responsibility of an intensivist only to care for patients in the ICU? Are there advantages and/or disadvantages to having physicians from other service areas be primarily responsible for the care of ICU patients?

An intensivist is a physician with board certification or extensive experience in critical care medicine.[20-22] Traditionally, such a physician may be involved in triage for the critically ill before ICU admission but cares, primarily, for patients within the confines of an ICU. Recently, however, the role of the intensivist has been expanded under the rubric of an "ICU without walls."[23-25] Under this paradigm, the intensivist is expected to consult upon and provide care to critically ill patients prior to, following, and, sometimes, in the absence of, an ICU admission. Rapid response/medical emergency teams are the most commonly used method of delivering critical care expertise to non-ICU patients who become critically ill.[26] While there is no standard structure for these teams, many include an intensivist and/or a critical care nurse.[27-29] In essence, therefore, these teams can be viewed as expanding the ICU. Data on their impact is mixed,[30-33] yet ward staff satisfaction is improved[34,35] and these teams are being used with increasing frequency.[36]

Rather than waiting for a clinical deterioration that merits activation of such emergency response teams, some institutions provide critical care consultation by intensivist-led teams for patients who are either not critical enough to be transferred to an ICU or have been recently transferred out of one.[25,37] These services can create a degree of critical care coverage that, while often lacking in the nursing and monitoring capabilities of an ICU, can benefit less critically ill patients. Staffing these services requires a commitment of an expanded workforce, however. Depending on the specifics of a given institution—available staff, ICU capacity, ICU occupancy, etc—staffing such teams may improve care for the critically ill throughout the hospital.

Bringing the intensivist out of the ICU may be one way to improve care throughout the hospital and another may be having appropriately trained clinicians from other departments work in the ICU. Most ICU patients in the United States do not receive care by an intensivist.[21,38] Instead, many are cared for by physicians with no training in critical care medicine; care often falls to hospitalists[39-41] and emergency medicine physicians.[42] Recently, the SCCM and the Society of Hospitalist Medicine issued a joint position paper on the potential merits of accelerated training of experienced hospitalists in critical care.[40,41] Such training is not currently available, but may be possible in the near future. Over the past several years, emergency medicine physicians have

been granted permission to enter critical care medicine fellowships and sit for the critical care medicine certification examinations administered by the American Boards of Internal Medicine, Surgery, and Anesthesiology.[43] Together, these actions promote an integration of critical care medicine with other disciplines. Hospital administrators can capitalize on the impact of this expanded pool of providers by hiring physicians trained in critical care, whose background makes them well suited to work in non-ICU environments as well. A critical care trained hospitalist will improve care delivery to newly critically ill patients on the general ward; additionally, if he/she also works in the ICU, he/she may enhance communication between the ICU staff and providers in noncritical care areas. Similarly, a critical care trained emergency medicine physician whose responsibilities extend into both environments can bridge care gaps and improve interactions between the ICU and the emergency department. Finally, in times of lower staffing (eg, overnight[21]), having someone available who is willing and able to cover an ICU and another clinical care area may be cost-effective. Critical care staffing can, if done thoughtfully, improve patient care throughout the hospital.

In planning for potentially more diversified ICU staff, hospital administrators must be mindful of competing responsibilities pulling intensivists away from the ICU, however. Most American ICUs have an "open" staffing structure in which there is no unified critical care team of providers looking after all patients in the ICU.[6,39,44] The most common ICU staffing model practiced in other places in the world is a "closed" model in which the primary responsibility for care of all ICU patients is transferred to an intensivist for the time that the patients are in the unit.[45-47] Leapfrog and SCCM advocate for high-intensity staffing, which is more often met by a closed ICU structure, but can be attained using an open model with mandatory critical care consultation. Data on the impact of a high-intensity staffing model on patient outcomes is mixed.[48,49] Most intensivists split time between ICU and other responsibilities.[38] In an open model, almost by definition, the primary physician caring for each patient has *simultaneous* non-critical care responsibilities—to care for either non-critically ill hospitalized patients or outpatients in the office setting. This set-up is often the case even for practitioners in closed model units. A potential disadvantage to having intensivists who have multiple additional skills is that they may be asked to multitask across disciplines; in so doing, needed focus may be inadvertently drawn away from ICU patients. Care must be taken to balance this potential negative consequence with the benefits of diversified staff.

STRUCTURE OF CRITICAL CARE

ICU occupancy is often high[4,5] and patients who are in need of an ICU bed may experience delayed transfers, which are known to result in poor outcomes.[50,51] As touched upon in the section on "Staffing for Critical Care," expansion of critical care services outside of the walls of the ICU itself may be desirable to improve the presence of critical care within the hospital environment. As aforementioned, one method for accomplishing this goal is the creation of rapid response/medical emergency teams or consultation services; others may include telemedicine and/or regionalization of critical care.

Telemedicine involves the use of technology to allow for patient monitoring, review of data, order entry, and, at times, clinical examination using robotic assistants by clinicians not onsite.[52-54] In the ICU, this technology has taken off as a method for expanding coverage of critical care patients nationwide.[55] Numerous studies have been conducted to evaluate the impact of this strategy; a recent meta-analysis demonstrated that while implementation improves ICU mortality and length of stay, hospital mortality and length of stay are unchanged by the introduction of telemedicine.[52] This strategy is often considered as a means of bringing critical care expertise to underserved populations. From a hospital's perspective, however, there are additional potential benefits to offering telemedicine ICU (tele-ICU) services to outlying hospitals. First, ICU patients are often transferred to regional centers from smaller community based institutions when expertise for care is not available at the smaller facility.[56,57] Sometimes the lacked expertise is a subspecialist's opinion or intervention, which can only be provided at the larger center; such transfers likely result in favorable patient outcomes and can be financially attractive to a referral hospital.[58] When patients are transferred

simply for the provision of high-quality critical care, the transfers may overburden the referral center and are less likely to be financially beneficial to it.[59-62] Creation of a tele-ICU service may minimize the need for these latter transfers. Second, despite inconsistent data on its benefits,[63-67] many hospitals have adopted the Leapfrog standard of 24-hour onsite intensivist coverage. For hospitals employing such a model, there may be significant downtime for the in-hospital intensivist in a less busy ICU environment. Consequently, having such providers additionally providing tele-ICU care to outlying hospitals may be a revenue-generating proposition for the hospital. The cost-effectiveness of such a strategy has not been studied, however, and would likely vary greatly across institutions.

Regionalization of critical care is a topic being discussed at the national level.[68-71] Often compared to the regional trauma systems in place in the United States,[72] the purpose would be to identify clear critical care referral centers to which appropriate patients would be triaged by emergency medical personnel prior to hospital arrival. In a survey of physicians who provide acute care, a majority felt such a system would improve patient care (52%) and efficiency (66%); however, 66% also felt that it would place strain on families.[73] Concerns have also been raised about such a system at the national level over (1) the financial implications for referral centers and smaller hospitals as well as (2) the fact that critical illness (unlike trauma) often develops in patients already admitted to the hospital.[62,72] A hospital system may benefit from regionalization of critical care on the more local or even system level, however. In fact, this type of system-based regionalization exists in some instances.[74] Hospital system administrators may be able to use interhospital transfers for critical care expertise as a means to provide better patient care (through optimization of volume-outcome relationships[75-79]) and achieve financial optimization.

RESOURCE UTILIZATION FOR CRITICAL CARE

Resources for critical care include personnel and equipment. Strategies to optimize personnel use are discussed in the section on "Staffing for Critical

Care." Borrowing from economics, equipment can be broken down into "fixed" and "variable" resources where "fixed" resources are those that are permanent/semipermanent and independent of patient volume and "variable" resources are those that are used only when patients are in need of them.[80] Put simply, "fixed" resources can be viewed as ICU beds and large equipment (eg, mechanical ventilators). ICU bed utilization is discussed in detail in the chapter "Utilization of ICU Beds."*** Suffice it to say here that it is important to the hospital's care delivery, operational efficiency, and financial success to consider how many ICU beds and in what configuration (eg, in one mixed specialty unit, spread amongst specialized units, etc) is best to meet the needs of the hospital as a whole. Similarly, the purchase of large mandatory equipment (eg, mechanical ventilators) must be similarly thought through to optimize the return on investment while providing appropriate care to the patients in need.

Allocation of variable resources can often be adjusted more frequently than fixed resources and the potential impact for the hospital environment can be significant. First, decisions must be made about what types of resources to accrue; for instance, there are advanced care devices (eg, continuous veno-venous hemodialysis/filtration, extracorporeal membrane oxygenation) that can be expensive to acquire, but may reap clinical and financial benefits for an institution. Specifically, the possession of such technologies may funnel patients with higher level care needs to the hospital.[81-83] Second, decisions about the availability of "critical care resources" outside of the ICU can impact the hospital as a whole. For example, hospitals with intermediate care/step-down units that allow for higher monitoring than on general wards may improve patient flow out of ICUs.[84-86] In so doing, care for patients in need of ICU beds and costs of patients too ill for the general floor and not sick enough for the ICU may be optimized. Also, there is variability between hospitals in the need for ICU admission for certain illnesses.[87-89] Decisions to determine resource availability throughout the hospital (eg, the ability to administer continuous insulin infusions for patients with diabetic ketoacidosis in settings other than the ICU) can help maximize critical care bed availability for others more in need. The up- and downsides

of these strategies may be different for each hospital and should be evaluated at each institution prior to resource allocation decisions.

CONCLUSIONS

ICUs are often viewed as well-circumscribed units. A simplified model of critical care focuses only on the care delivered by traditional critical care clinicians within the confines of an ICU's walls. Envisioning critical care in this limited fashion, however, benefits neither the critically ill nor the hospital as a whole. Innovative administrative models, staffing strategies, structural plans, and resource allocation can benefit a hospital's patients (both those who are critically ill and those who are not), its ICUs, and the hospital itself.

REFERENCES

1. Grenvik A, Pinsky MR. Evolution of the intensive care unit as a clinical center and critical care medicine as a discipline. *Crit Care Clin.* 2009;25:239-250.
2. Puri N, Puri V, Dellinger RP. History of technology in the intensive care unit. *Crit Care Clin.* 2009;25:185-200.
3. Wunsch H, Angus DC, Harrison DA, et al. Variation in critical care services across North America and Western Europe. *Crit Care Med.* 2008;36:2787-2793.
4. Halpern N, Pastores S. Critical care medicine in the United States 2000-2005: an analysis of bed numbers, occupancy rates, payer mix, and costs. *Crit Care Med.* 2010;38:65-71.
5. Wunsch H, Wagner J, Herlim M, Chong DH, Kramer AA, Halpern SD. ICU occupancy and mechanical ventilator use in the United States. *Crit Care Med.* 2013;41:2712-2719.
6. Groeger JS, Strosberg MA, Halpern NA, et al. Descriptive analysis of critical care units in the United States: patient characteristics and intensive care unit utilization. *Crit Care Med.* 1992;20:846-863.
7. Nelson JE. Identifying and overcoming the barriers to high-quality palliative care in the intensive care unit. *Crit Care Med.* 2006;34:S324-S331.
8. Curtis JR, Shannon SE. Transcending the silos: toward an interdisciplinary approach to end-of-life care in the ICU. *Intensive Care Med.* 2006;32:15-17.
9. Frezza EE, Wachtel M. Metabolic syndrome: a new multidisciplinary service line. *Obes Surg.* 2011;21:379-385.

10. Sussman I, Prystowsky MB. Pathology service line: a model for accountable care organizations at an academic medical center. *Hum Pathol.* 2012;43:629-631.

11. Allen JI. Gastroenterologists and the triple aim: how to become accountable. *Gastrointest Endosc Clin N Am.* 2012;22:85-96.

12. Amir LD, Lukhard KW, Englehart M. UFE program: a service line opportunity for U.S. hospitals. *Health Finance Manage.* 2009;63:104-106, 108, 110 passim.

13. Bekes CE, Dellinger RP, Brooks D, Edmondson R, Olivia CT, Parrillo JE. Critical care medicine as a distinct product line with substantial financial profitability: the role of business planning. *Crit Care Med.* 2004;32:1207-1214.

14. Preyra C, Pink G. Scale and scope efficiencies through hospital consolidations. *J Health Econ.* 2006;25:1049-1068.

15. Iapichino G, Pezzi A, Borotto E, Mistraletti G, Meroni M, Corbella D. Performance determinants and flexible ICU organisation. *Minerva Anestesiol.* 2005;71:273-280.

16. Iapichino G, Radrizzani D, Rossi C, et al. Proposal of a flexible structural-organizing model for the intensive care units. *Minerva Anestesiol.* 2007;73:501-506.

17. Hasibeder WR. Does standardization of critical care work? *Curr Opin Crit Care.* 2010;16:493-498.

18. Amendment of sections 405.2 and 405.4 of Title 10 NYCRR: Sepsis Protocols. New York State Register, 2013.

19. Haupt M, Bekes C, Brilli R, et al. Guidelines on critical care services and personnel: recommendations based on a system of categorization of three levels of care. *Crit Care Med.* 2003;31:2677-2683.

20. Group TL. ICU Physician Staffing Factsheet.

21. Angus DC, Shorr AF, White A, et al. Critical care delivery in the United States: distribution of services and compliance with leapfrog recommendations. *Crit Care Med.* 2006;34:1016-1024.

22. Guidelines for the definition of an intensivist and the practice of critical care medicine. Guidelines Committee, Society of Critical Care Medicine. *Crit Care Med.* 1992;20:540-542.

23. Durand M, Hutchings A, Black N, Green J. 'Not quite Jericho, but more doors than there used to be'. Staff views of the impact of 'modernization' on boundaries around adult critical care services in England. *J Health Serv Res Policy.* 2010;15:229-235.

24. Halpern NA, Pastores SM, Oropello JM, Kvetan V. Critical care medicine in the United States: Addressing the intensivist shortage and image of the specialty. *Crit Care Med.* 2013;41:2754-2761.

25. Abella Álvarez A, Torrejón Psérez I, Enciso Calderón V, et al. ICU without walls project. Effect of the early detection of patients at risk. *Med Intensiva.* 2013;37:12-18.

26. Cretikos MA, Parr MJ. The Medical Emergency Team: 21st century critical care. *Minerva Anestesiol.* 2005;71:259-263.

27. Morris DS, Schweickert W, Holena D, et al. Differences in outcomes between ICU attending and senior resident physician led medical emergency team responses. *Resuscitation.* 2012;83:1434-1437.

28. Rothberg MB, Belforti R, Fitzgerald J, Friderici J, Keyes M.. Four years' experience with a hospitalist-led medical emergency team: An interrupted time series. *J Hosp Med.* 2012;7:98-103.

29. Repasky TM, Pfeil C. Experienced critical care nurse-led rapid response teams rescue patients on in-patient units. *J Emerg Nurs.* 2005;31:376-379.

30. McNeill G, Bryden D. Do either early warning systems or emergency response teams improve hospital patient survival? A systematic review. *Resuscitation.* 2013;84:1652-1667.

31. McGaughey J, Alderdice F, Fowler R, Kapila A, Mayhew A, Moutray M.. Outreach and earlywarning systems (EWS) for the prevention of Intensive Care admission and death of critically ill adult patients on general hospital wards (Review). *Cochrane Database Syst Rev.* 2007;(3):CD005529. http://www.ncbi.nlm.nih.gov/pubmed/17636805.

32. Laurens NH, Dwyer TA. The effect of medical emergency teams on patient outcome: A review of the literature. *Int J Nurs Pract.* 2010;16:533-544.

33. Winters BD, Weaver SJ, Pfoh ER, Yang T, Pham JC, Dy SM. Rapid-response systems as a patient safety strategy: A systematic review. *Ann Intern Med.* 2013;158:417-425.

34. Jones D, Baldwin I, McIntyre T, et al. Nurses' attitudes to a medical emergency team service in a teaching hospital. *Qual Saf Health Care.* 2006;15:427-432.

35. Bagshaw SM, Mondor EE, Scouten C, et al. A survey of nurses' beliefs about the medical emergency team system in a Canadian tertiary hospital. *Am J Crit Care.* 2010;19:74-83.

36. Rapid Response Systems. Washington, DC: Agency for Healthcare Research and Quality: Patient Safety Primers.

37. Niven DJ, Bastos JF, Stelfox HT. Critical care transition programs and the risk of readmission or death after discharge from an ICU: A systematic review and meta-analysis. *Crit Care Med.* 2014;42:179-187.

38. Angus D, Kelley M, Schmitz R, et al. Caring for the critically ill patient. Current and projected workforce requirements for care of the critically ill and patients with pulmonary disease: can we meet the requirements of an aging population? *J Am Med Assoc.* 2000;284:2762-2770.

39. Hyzy RC, Flanders SA, Pronovost PJ, et al. Characteristics of intensive care units in Michigan: not an open and closed case. *J Hosp Med.* 2010;5:4-9.

40. Siegal EM, Dressler DD, Dichter JR, Gorman MJ, Lipsett PA. Training a hospitalist workforce to address the intensivist shortage in American hospitals: a position paper from the Society of Hospital Medicine and the Society of Critical Care Medicine. *Crit Care Med.* 2012;40:1952-1956.

41. Siegal EM, Dressler DD, Dichter JR, Gorman MJ, Lipsett PA. Training a hospitalist workforce to address the intensivist shortage in American hospitals: a position paper from the Society of Hospital Medicine and the Society of Critical Care Medicine. *J Hosp Med.* 2012;7:359-364.

42. Sherwin RL, Garcia AJ, Bilkovski R. Quantifying off-hour emergency physician coverage of in-hospital codes: a survey of community emergency departments. *J Emerg Med.* 2011;41:381-385.

43. Emergency Medicine Residents' Association: Committees and Divisions—Critical Care Division.

44. Treggiari MM, Martin DP, Yanez ND, Caldwell E, Hudson LD, Rubenfeld GD. Effect of intensive care unit organizational model and structure on outcomes in patients with acute lung injury. *Am J Respir Crit Care Med.* 2007;176:685-690.

45. Prin M, Wunsch H. International comparisons of intensive care: informing outcomes and improving standards. *Curr Opin Crit Care.* 2012;18:700-706.

46. Bellomo R, Stow PJ, Hart GK. Why is there such a difference in outcome between Australian intensive care units and others? *Curr Opin Anaesthesiol.* 2007;20:100-105.

47. Graf J, Reinhold A, Brunkhorst FM, et al. Variability of structures in German intensive care units—A representative, nationwide analysis. *Wien Klin Wochenschr.* 2010;122:572-578.

48. Pronovost P, Angus D, Dorman T, Robinson KA, Dremsizov TT, Young TL. Physician staffing patterns and clinical outcomes in critically ill patients: a systematic review. *J Am Med Assoc.* 2002;288:2151-2162.

49. Levy MM, Rapoport J, Lemeshow S, Chalfin DB, Phillips G, Danis M. Association between critical care physician management and patient mortality in the intensive care unit. *Ann Intern Med.* 2008;148:801-809.

50. Sinuff T, Kahnamoui K, Cook DJ, et al. Rationing critical care beds: a systematic review. *Crit Care Med.* 2004;32:1588-1597.

51. Chalfin DB, Trzeciak S, Likourezos A, et al. Impact of delayed transfer of critically ill patients from the emergency department to the intensive care unit. *Crit Care Med.* 2007;35:1477-1483.

52. Young LB, Chan PS, Lu X, Nallamothu BK, Sasson C, Cram PM. Impact of telemedicine intensive care unit coverage on patient outcomes: a systematic review and meta-analysis. *Arch Intern Med.* 2011; 171:498-506.

53. Breslow MJ. Remote ICU care programs: current status. *J Crit Care.* 2007;22:66-76.

54. Sucher JF, Todd SR, Jones SL, Throckmorton T, Turner KL, Moore FA. Robotic telepresence: a helpful adjunct that is viewed favorably by critically ill surgical patients. *Am J Surg.* 2011;202:843-847.

55. Kahn JM, Cicero BD, Wallace DJ, Iwashyna TJ. Adoption of ICU telemedicine in the United States. *Crit Care Med.* 2014;42:362-368.

56. Iwashyna TJ, Christie JD, Moody J, Kahn JM, Asch DA. The structure of critical care transfer networks. *Med Care.* 2009;47:787-793.

57. Horeczko T, Marcin JP, Kahn JM, et al. Urban and rural patterns in emergent pediatric transfer: a call for regionalization. *J Rural Health.* 2014;30:252-258.

58. Veinot TC, Bosk EA, Unnikrishnan KP, Iwashyna TJ. Revenue, relationships and routines: the social organization of acute myocardial infarction patient transfers in the United States. *Soc Sci Med.* 2012;75:1800-1810.

59. Golestanian E, Scruggs JE, Gangnon RE, Mak RP, Wood KE. Effect of interhospital transfer on resource utilization and outcomes at a tertiary care referral center. *Crit Care Med.* 2007;35:1470-1476.

60. Odetola FO, Davis MM, Cohn LM, Clark SJ. Interhospital transfer of critically ill and injured children: an evaluation of transfer patterns, resource utilization, and clinical outcomes. *J Hosp Med.* 2009;4:164-170.

61. Odetola FO, Clark SJ, Gurney JG, Dechert RE, Shanley TP, Freed GL. Effect of interhospital transfer on resource utilization and outcomes at a tertiary pediatric intensive care unit. *J Crit Care.* 2009;24:379-386.

62. Kahn JM, Asch RJ, Iwashyna TJ, Rubenfeld GD, Angus DC, Asch DA. Perceived barriers to the regionalization of adult critical care in the United States: a qualitative preliminary study. *BMC Health Serv Res.* 2008;8:239.

63. Blunt MC, Burchett KR. Out-of-hours consultant cover and case-mix-adjusted mortality in intensive care. *Lancet*. 2000;356:735-736.

64. Gajic O, Afessa B, Hanson A, et al. Effect of 24-hour mandatory versus on-demand critical care specialist presence on quality of care and family and provider satisfaction in the intensive care unit of a teaching hospital. *Crit Care Med*. 2008;36:36-44.

65. Garland A, Roberts D, Graff L. Twenty-four-hour intensivist presence: a pilot study of effects on intensive care unit patients, families, doctors, and nurses. *Am J Respir Crit Care Med*. 2012;185:738-743.

66. Wallace DJ, Angus DC, Barnato AE, et al. Nighttime intensivist staffing and mortality among critically ill patients. *N Engl J Med*. 2012;366:2093-2101.

67. Kerlin MP, Small DS, Cooney E, et al. A randomized trial of nighttime physician staffing in an intensive care unit. *N Engl J Med*. 2013;368:2201-2209.

68. Thompson DR, Clemmer TP, Applefeld JJ, et al. Regionalization of critical care medicine: task force report of the American College of Critical Care Medicine. *Crit Care Med*. 1994;22:1306-1313.

69. Barnato AE, Kahn JM, Rubenfeld GD, et al. Prioritizing the organization and management of intensive care services in the United States: The PrOMIS Conference. *Crit Care Med*. 2007;35:1003-1011.

70. Cairns CB, Glickman SW. Time makes a difference to everyone, everywhere: the need for effective regionalization of emergency and critical care. *Ann Emerg Med*. 2012;60:638-640.

71. Nguyen YL, Kahn JM, Angus DC. Reorganizing adult critical care delivery: the role of regionalization, telemedicine, and community outreach. *Am J Respir Crit Care Med*. 2010;181:1164-1169.

72. Kahn JM, Branas CC, Schwab CW, Asch DA. Regionalization of medical critical care: what can we learn from the trauma experience? *Crit Care Med*. 2008;36:3085-3088.

73. Kahn JM, Asch RJ, Iwashyna TJ, et al. Physician attitudes toward regionalization of adult critical care: a national survey. *Crit Care Med*. 2009;37:2149-2154.

74. Iwashyna TJ, Christie JD, Kahn JM, Asch DA. Uncharted paths: hospital networks in critical care. *Chest*. 2009;135:827-833.

75. Kanhere MH, Kanhere HA, Cameron A, Maddern GJ. Does patient volume affect clinical outcomes in adult intensive care units? *Intensive Care Med*. 2012;38:741-751.

76. Iapichino G, Gattinoni L, Radrizzani D, et al. Volume of activity and occupancy rate in intensive care units.

77. Glance LG, Li Y, Osler TM, Dick A, Mukamel DB. Impact of patient volume on the mortality rate of adult intensive care unit patients. *Crit Care Med*. 2006;34:1925-1934.

78. Kahn JM, Goss CH, Heagerty PJ, Kramer AA, O'Brien CR, Rubenfeld GD. Hospital volume and the outcomes of mechanical ventilation. *N Engl J Med*. 2006;355:41-50.

79. Metnitz B, Metnitz PG, Bauer P, et al. Patient volume affects outcome in critically ill patients. *Wien Klin Wochenschr*. 2009;121:34-40.

80. Kahn JM. Understanding economic outcomes in critical care. *Curr Opin Crit Care*. 2006;12:399-404.

81. Lindén V, Palmér K, Reinhard J, et al. Inter-hospital transportation of patients with severe acute respiratory failure on extracorporeal membrane oxygenation—National and international experience. *Intensive Care Med*. 2001;27:1643-1648.

82. Coppola CP, Tyree M, Larry K, DiGeronimo R. A 22-year experience in global transport extracorporeal membrane oxygenation. *J Pediatr Surg*. 2008;43:46-52.

83. Desebbe O, Rosamel P, Henaine R, et al. Interhospital transport with extracorporeal life support: results and perspectives after 5 years experience. *Ann Fr Anesth Reanim*. 2013;32:225-230.

84. Byrick RJ, Power JD, Ycas JO, Brown KA. Impact of an intermediate care area on ICU utilization after cardiac surgery. *Crit Care Med*. 1986;14:869-872.

85. Byrick RJ, Mazer CD, Caskennette GM. Closure of an intermediate care unit. Impact on critical care utilization. *Chest*. 1993;104:876-881.

86. Mazer CD, Byrick RJ, Sibbald WJ, et al. Postoperative utilization of critical care services by cardiac surgery: a multicenter study in the Canadian healthcare system. *Crit Care Med*. 1993;21:851-859.

87. Chen LM, Render M, Sales A, Kennedy EH, Wiitala W, Hofer TP. Intensive care unit admitting patterns in the veterans affairs health care system. *Arch Intern Med*. 2012;172:1220-1226.

88. Gershengorn HB, Iwashyna TJ, Cooke CR, Scales DC, Kahn JM, Wunsch H. Variation in use of intensive care for adults with diabetic ketoacidosis. *Crit Care Med*. 2012;40:2009-2015.

89. Seymour CW, Iwashyna TJ, Ehlenbach WJ, Wunsch H, Cooke CR. Hospital-level variation in the use of intensive care. *Health Serv Res*. 2012;47:2060-2080.

Association with mortality. *Intensive Care Med*. 2004;30:290-297.

Alternative Staffing Models in the ICU

78

Jibran Majeed, ACNP-BC, CCRN; David Keith, PA-C, MS and Rhonda D'Agostino, ACNP-BC, FCCM

KEY POINTS

1. The nationwide shortage of intensivists has prompted US hospitals to effectively develop and integrate alternative staffing models into their intensive care unit (ICU), including the use of nurse practitioners (NPs), physician assistants (PAs), and hospitalists.

2. Patients managed by NPs, PAs, and hospitalists have been shown to have similar outcomes in hospital mortality and length of stay and greater compliance with evidence-based practice guidelines when compared to those cared for by residents.

3. Hospitalists may serve as the primary providers in ICUs without critical care consultants or assist in the co-management of patients with intensivists.

4. With the myriad of ICU practice models available, additional studies are needed to help sculpt styles based on the particular needs and preferences of an institution.

5. Regardless of the chosen staffing model, the key determinants for the success and growth of the critical care workforce will rely heavily on organization, strategic planning, and communication.

INTRODUCTION

Historically, physician providers in the form of intensivists, critical care fellows, and housestaff trainees delivered care in adult intensive care units (ICUs). In recent years, alternative staffing models, including advance practice providers (APPs) [mainly nurse practitioners (NPs) and physician assistants (PAs)], nonintensivist physicians (hospitalists), and telemedicine, have been increasingly used to manage the critical care physician supply and demand gap.[1] The reasons for this gap are well documented and include an aging and growing population of the chronically ill requiring ICU care,[2] workforce shortage of intensivists,[2-4] and increasing work-hour restrictions on resident duty

hours by the Accreditation Council for Graduate Medical Education (ACGME).[5] A survey of internal medicine housestaff also showed that less than 5% will choose to pursue a career in critical care medicine (CCM) partially as a result of the well-documented intensivist burnout[6] and the sensed mismatch between a heavy work schedule and monetary compensation.[7]

The nationwide shortage of intensivists has been occurring in the midst of ongoing increases in the number of critically ill patients and ICU beds.[8,9] In 2005, there were approximately 94,000 ICU beds in nearly 6500 ICUs in approximately 5000 US acute care hospitals.[8] In order to deal with these realities, institutions need to effectively develop and integrate alternative staffing models into their ICU.

This chapter will focus primarily on the use of advanced practice providers and hospitalists in the adult ICU setting. (*Telemedicine is covered elsewhere in a separate chapter of this textbook.*)

ACUTE CARE NURSE PRACTITIONERS

The acute care nurse practitioner (ACNP) specialty evolved in the late 1980s[1] and is considered the best fit for adult critical care based on the competencies and scope of standards set by the American Association of Critical Care Nurses.[1,10] There are currently more than 192,000 NPs in the United States.[11] In 2012, approximately 14.2% of NPs were prepared in acute care, and 51% of them reported working in an inpatient hospital setting.[11] Their role is not defined necessarily by location but by the patient care needs. The patient population they care for ranges from young adults to the elderly with acute, critical, and complex chronic illnesses.[12] The extent of autonomy and physician oversight for ACNPs in relation to diagnosing and prescription writing privileges vary from state to state.[13]

Perquisites to becoming an NP include obtaining a bachelor's degree in nursing, although some bridge programs from a nonnursing bachelor's degree do exist, and a registered professional nurse license. Completion of an accredited graduate level education program is mandatory.

PHYSICIAN ASSISTANTS

The concept of PAs evolved in the early 1960s in response to a shortage of general practice physicians.[14] PAs are nationally certified, state-licensed, and practice medicine as part of a physician—PA team.[15] The fundamental principle of PA practice is physician-dependent delegated autonomy, defined accountability, and reciprocal responsibility for providing supervision and seeking physician consultation. Supervision is defined by state law and hospital policy, but all states have laws allowing off-site supervision by physicians via telecommunications.[16] In mid-2013, there were 84,064 clinically active PAs (those who held a valid state-issued PA or medical license), and 2% overall were ICU/critical care based.[17,18]

PA programs are based on the medical model, average 27 months in length, and provide broad-based general medicine education with an emphasis in primary care.[19] Most PA programs award a master's degree on completion of the entry-level curriculum.[20] Unlike NP education, PAs do not have different tracks. The expectation is that entry-level PAs will broaden their medical knowledge and clinical skills with practice-based physician teaching and formal continuing medical education programs. A trend in the PA workforce distribution towards specialization is documented.[21] Clinical postgraduate PA programs, in the form of residencies, are available for PAs who want added experience in preparation for practice in a medical or surgical specialty.[22]

HOSPITALISTS

Hospitalist medicine has been the fastest growing specialty in medicine for the past decade. In 2009, 89% of hospitals with over 200 beds had hospitalist presence.[23] Hospital medicine focuses on general medical care for hospitalized patients, allowing primary care physicians to assume responsibilities in the community.[23] The initial intent was to improve patient outcomes and decrease hospital length of stay and costs. Approximately 85% of current hospitalists are board-certified in internal medicine.[23] In 2009, the American Board of Physician Specialists developed the first board certification for the practice of hospital medicine.[23,24]

Hospitalists have mostly replaced primary care physicians as the manager of ICU patients in nontertiary hospitals.[23] In community hospitals, about 87% of the hospitalists are providing care for patients in the ICU, and 30% are providing critical care services in academic medical centers.[25] The primary models of hospitalist care in the ICU include hospitalists serving as primary ICU providers in centers without critical care consultants or assisting in the co-management of patients in collaboration with intensivists.[25]

ROLES AND RESPONSIBILITIES

Delineating the roles and responsibilities of APPs and hospitalists will depend on the institution's needs. The general roles and responsibilities of APPs (Table 78–1) include various levels of autonomy that are dependent on the individual practitioner's experience, capabilities, and granted privileges. In some institutions where ICU staffing is in-house 24/7, their roles may include that of the code team and rapid response team leader.

Hospitalists' roles and responsibilities in the ICU vary depending on the institution policies, whether the ICU is an "open" versus "closed" unit, as well as their own level of experience and competency in providing critical care. Issues such as billing and obtaining credentialing and privileges for critical care are also institution-specific. In some institutions, the hospitalist practices as the sole ICU attending with admitting privileges. In other settings, the hospitalists will follow and provide critical care for their ward patients who are transferred to the ICU. Many hospitalists also seek consultation with intensivists to help manage patients with mechanical ventilatory needs or to manage more complicated critically ill patients.[26] In some institutions, hospitalists are also being utilized as the initial responders of the rapid response team.[27]

BENEFITS

Nonphysician or nonintensivist models in the ICU can offer several institutional benefits. First, these providers can help overcome the current intensivist and resident shortages as well as become a consistent workforce that can positively impact patient care.[1] Regular exposure and practice will help these providers gain knowledge and expertise in CCM and become proficient in performing invasive procedures.[1] A recent national survey of program directors of ACGME-approved critical care fellowship training programs demonstrated that integrating NPs and PAs can positively impact critical care training for the fellows because it allows greater focus and time on fellow educational needs while the NPs/PAs assume daily clinical responsibilities.[28] Additionally, patients managed by NPs, PAs, and hospitalists have been shown to have similar outcomes in hospital mortality[24,29,30] and length of stay[24,29-31] when compared to those cared for by residents. NPs have also been shown to have better communication with nurses[32] and greater compliance with evidence-based practice guidelines[10] that have resulted in decrease in days on mechanical ventilation,[33] rates of urinary tract infections, and skin breakdown.[31] Finally, besides improving the quality of patient care, some studies also suggest that the use of NPs and PAs in acute care may decrease hospital costs[31,34] and improve the financial productivity of the institution.[10]

TABLE 78–1 CCM NP/PA responsibilities.

Clinical daily responsibilities
Obtain history and perform physical examination
Participate in daily rounds
Order and interpret diagnostic test
Prescribe medications
Document in daily progress notes
Manage ventilators
Formulate plan of care with CCM attending
Communicate with patients and families
Communicate with other multidisciplinary team members

Consult and rapid response teams
Act as first responders for the institution's RRT
Participate as team members in medical codes
Provide critical care consultation and follow-up
Coordinate ICU patient admission and discharges

Procedures
Central venous catheters
Arterial line catheters
Intubation
Lumbar puncture
Paracentesis
Thoracentesis
Peripherally inserted central catheter (PICC)

RRT, rapid response team.

INTEGRATING ALTERNATIVE STAFFING PROVIDERS IN THE ICU

Due to the shortages of the traditional ICU workforce, it is evident that APPs and hospitalists are providing care in the ICU. The question then becomes not if but how to successfully integrate them into the ICU. Adding hospitalists, NPs, and PAs into the ICU team as "intensivist extenders" effectively increases

TABLE 78-2 Initial considerations for integrating NP/PAs into the ICU.

Planning
- Define roles and responsibilities
- NP team only versus integration into the existing HS team
- 24/7 coverage versus day shift
- Physical space
- Organizational support
- Budget and billing
- Obtain credential and privileges

Candidate selection
- Experience in critical care
- Motivated learner
- Self-driven
- Humble attitude
- Team player

Benefits
- Financial gain
- Creating a consistent workforce
- Improve communication
- Combating current shortages
- Improve quality of care
- Improve patient outcomes

the availability of adult critical care services.[1-23] However, successfully establishing these alternative providers into an ICU team is not as easy as advertising, hiring a few, and scheduling shifts. Integration of these alternative staffing providers needs effective planning with thoughtful consideration and discussion of many factors, including institutional expectations, financial considerations and rationalization, administrative support, current staff acceptance, governance, recruitment, and retention (Table 78-2).

HOSPITALIST ISSUES

Individual hospitalists' knowledge and skills for managing the critically ill may vary based on differences in training and clinical practice experience prior to becoming a hospitalist.[23] The costs for educating hospitalists in CCM may at times become an employer's expense. A competency-assurance process based on an education and skills training process leading to acquisition of competencies beyond those obtained in internal medicine residency training has been suggested.[25] However, formal opportunities to broaden general critical care knowledge

and obtain skills are reportedly few. Therefore, a traditional critical care fellowship is recommended for those hospitalists who primarily want to work with critically ill patients.[23] In 2012, a position paper endorsed by the Society of Hospital Medicine and the Society of Critical Care Medicine proposed the creation of an expedited ACGME-sanctioned and accredited critical care certification pathway, with the goal of attracting practicing hospitalists to critical care fellowship training.[23] This proposal is still under consideration by the ACGME.

ADVANCE PRACTICE PROVIDER ISSUES

Unlike hospitalists, APPs do not have the preparation and training provided in medical school and residency. They receive less stringent education and therefore have different challenges.[1] However, with a careful selection of motivated individuals and on-the-job training, they can be trained to provide services traditionally performed by ICU physicians. A recent survey showed that NPs and PAs provide care in greater than 50% and approximately 25%, respectively, of adult ICUs in academic medical centers in the United States.[10,35] Thus, teams including APPs or exclusively consisting of APPs, with appropriate physician leadership, can provide critical care that is equivalent to that delivered by traditional teams built around housestaff in a high-intensity ICU setting.[25,28]

INITIAL PLANNING

Integration of APPs into the ICU will require diligent planning and many considerations. These should include the program model one chooses to incorporate APPs into. Will the APPs be integrated into an existing intensivist-led, resident-based team, or as a stand-alone intensivist-APP team? Especially for the novice APPs, the availability of in-hospital physician backup for management decisions and procedural assistance has to be considered.

Staff buy-in is required. This includes the ICU nurses and physicians, hospital staff physicians (particularly if the ICU is transitioning to a "closed" unit), respiratory therapists, dietitians, and pharmacists.

If integrating APPs occurs in a teaching institution, the effect on housestaff and CCM fellow training should be considered. The APP's role and responsibilities need to be clearly defined to avoid any conflict with other team members. The APPs must be presented to all as partners, not competitors.[36]

Organizationally, which department(s) will be responsible for clinical and administrative oversight must also be defined. Generally, NPs fall under the department of nursing and report to nursing leadership, while PAs typically fall under a clinical department and report to the departmental leadership. Dual governance for NPs in the ICU has been described.[37]

ORIENTATION AND MENTORING OF APP

All APPs require orientation and mentoring, regardless of their previous experience and competence. New NPs may have prior experience as ICU nurses, but the transition to a CCM NP can be quite demanding, as described below. New PAs are expected to broaden their knowledge and skills with on-the-job education and training, so experience in a hospital medicine position prior to seeking a CCM PA position is suggested.[38]

Knowledge deficits in basic critical care principles, procedural skills, ultrasonography, and management skills are universal. Thus, a comprehensive, competency-based preparation course, as part of a mentored orientation, is necessary. This will require significant work on the part of the intensivists, consultant attendings, staff APPs, respiratory therapists, nutritionists, physical therapists, and other multidisciplinary team members to ensure success. Several samples of orientation programs are available in the literature.[18,37-39] For programs with less available teaching staff, outsourcing APP training to a regional program has been reported.[40,41]

BUDGETING

Establishing or expanding the multidisciplinary ICU team with APPs requires financial considerations. In 2010, the average salary for an APP working in a hospital-based unit ranged from $93,943 to $94,680 plus 33% benefits totaling ~$125,000. The expense for a postgraduate year-1 resident in 2014 in New York City was $55,900 salary plus 32% benefits, totaling $73,788 dollars, which was reimbursed by Medicare. Using a formula in which 30% of a resident's 80-hour workweek is for educational activities, 56 h/wk is required to replace the resident service hours or ~1.5 full-time equivalents (FTEEs) [42]. At an average cost of $125,000/year (salary + 32% benefits) for an APP, this translates to an additional expense of $187,500 to cover one resident's service time for 1 year. Allowing 5.5 FTEs to cover one 12-bed unit (1:12 provider/patient ratio) each shift (24/7/365), the total expense is $687,500 dollars per unit/year. The cost will vary with geographic location, years of experience for each practitioner, and ratio of providers to patients.

Salary expense may be partially recovered if the APP is on the hospital cost report as an employee, and their services are reimbursed under part A of Medicare. Alternatively, the APP can bill for their services if they are qualified to do so, and not on the hospital cost report, as will be discussed in the Billing section.

Cost rationalization based on potential benefits as discussed below may include cost savings in the long run by improving patient satisfaction, quality, length of stay, and staffing.

BILLING

Billing has to be considered when integrating APPs into the ICU. The Balanced Budget Act of 1997 officially recognized APPs as health care providers. This allowed them to be eligible for their own provider numbers and to submit bills to Medicare Part B for evaluation and management (E/M) services and procedures.[43] As outlined by the Centers for Medicare and Medicaid Services (CMS), qualified APPs can bill for critical care services under their national provider identifier (NPI) at 85% allowable of the physician rate.[44] Billing requires documentation of the encounter and must validate the need for critical care service. For services or procedures that are not regularly part of the critical care services bundle, such as insertion of an arterial line or central line, the provider who performs the procedure bills them separately.[44]

CMS requires a physician supervision agreement for PAs and a collaborative practice agreement for NPs. Individual health insurance companies may have different coding methods and rules for reimbursement when it comes to nonphysician providers. However, most companies follow CMS dictations as a basis for reimbursement.[45]

CREDENTIALING AND PRIVILEGING

APPs have to obtain credentialing and privileges. This process ensures that they have the necessary qualifications to provide safe and quality care in conjunction with federal and state laws, regulations, and standards set by the Joint Commission. Credentialing and privileging are administrative processes driven by the medical staff bylaws and involve obtaining, verifying, and assessing a provider's credentials, based on education, clinical training, certification, licensure, and other professional qualifications for appointment to the medical staff and providing patient care in or for the hospital. Most states require NPs to have a collaborative practice agreement with a supervising physician, and all states require PAs to have a supervising physician agreement. For billing purposes, the APP's scope of practice must include critical care and procedural privileges, and the supervising physician agreement should stipulate that the NP or PA is authorized to provide critical care services.[45]

The evaluation of a practitioner's performance is now an ongoing process that involves an evidence-based approach. The Joint Commission mandates that the hospital attain an initial Focused Professional Practice Evaluation (FPPE) for a non-physician provider who is new to the hospital or an existing one who seeks new privileges. FPPE can also be done when existing credentials and privileges are questioned. The Joint Commission also mandates that providers maintain competence and require periodic review by abiding to the requirement of Ongoing Professional Practice Evaluation (OPPE). The OPPE process consists of periodic evaluations, peer review, quarterly chart review by the collaborating physician, demonstrating ongoing competence for procedures, participating in morbidity and mortality rounds, and reviewing any issues that may be substandard.[43,46]

OVERCOMING COMMON OBSTACLES

Moving from a standard to an alternative ICU staffing model may bring on various issues due to the obstacles naturally associated with a dynamic process and an overall general resistance to change. Although extremely limited, there is literature that describes some of the common obstacles that may occur after a new ICU provider staffing model has been introduced.[37]

RECRUITMENT AND SELECTION

Searching for the right ICU provider can be overwhelming. For example, finding experienced candidates is complicated by the fact that only 2% of PAs and 14.6% of NPs work in acute care settings.[35] Conversely, while 75% of hospitalists are already covering ICUs, many are tied into contracts for their services.[23] As a result, recruitment of these alternative ICU providers must rely on setting up relationships or programs to develop internal candidates. An APP residency/fellowship program, clinical/mentorship rotation, or more recently the emergency medicine and internal medicine pathway into critical care fellowships can help to bridge gaps in employment during the transition year(s) of the staffing model. Regardless of the recruitment method, successful candidates are usually those who demonstrate modesty, flexibility, and eagerness. Typical ideal candidates in the APP track include those with critical care experience (either as a nurse or an NP), PAs who have at least 2 years of in-patient hospital experience (although critical care experience is preferred), and hospitalists who have at least 1 year of practice.[37,47]

Ironically, experience in critical care, although routinely preferred, may have several drawbacks. An "experienced" APP may find assimilation into a new ICU environment, with various degrees of autonomy, different from what he/she may be used to, challenging their comfort level. Experience has shown that objectives for new hires should be predetermined, with weekly goals being outlined and highly structured. If a new candidate fails to meet the objectives or does so with unacceptable delay, the program must have sufficient structure to recognize and support the transition of the new hire out of the ICU setting.[37,48]

RETENTION

ICU "burnout" is well documented; thus, it is not surprising that alternative staffing providers suffer from this similar affliction. It is estimated that 50% of CCM physicians and 33% of critical care nurses suffer ICU burnout.[49] While the implementation of additional alternative staffing, in conjunction with intensivist staff, has helped to reduce burnout, it should be done with caution (Figure 78–1). The majority of burnout is multifactorial, including working long hours (especially on the night shift), prolonged time without vacation, excessive workloads, sleep deprivation, and ICU conflicts. Consequently, it is important for institutions to consider methods to reduce "burnout" in an attempt to provide a stable ICU workforce. These methods may include providing 12 to 16 hour shifts with adequate staffing (ratios of 3-5 patients per APP have

been successful), rotation across various shifts, not reserving day positions for only senior staff, and 4-5 weeks paid and supported vacation. Ultimately, institutional support is mandatory for program success.[50]

ADDRESSING CONFLICTS

Conflicts will arise at some point while implementing a new provider model. These common encounters exist within any discipline, but it has been described (although extremely limited) to occur mostly between the RN and NP, NP and PA, NP/PA and CCM fellow, or between the hospitalist and primary care physician. Regardless of the nature of conflict, structure and processes should be in place to mitigate and provide adequate resolution. Some centers have described preemptive meetings between nursing and medicine, advocating for an advance practice manager and or routine ICU unit meetings. Above all, communication is always of utmost importance in the prevention and resolution of conflicts.

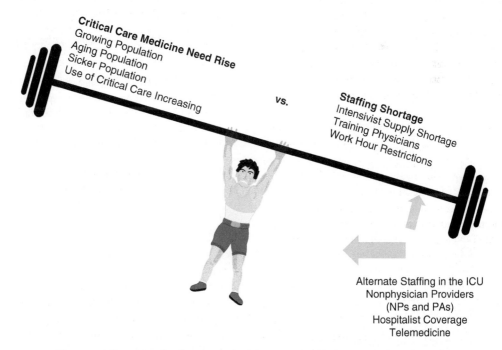

The use of Alternative Staffing can potentially balance critical care supply and demand

FIGURE 78–1 The imbalance between critical care demand and staffing shortage.

SUMMARY

Integrating alternative staffing models into the ICU is a logical, safe, and necessary endeavor to curtail gaps in the workforce as critical care physician shortages increase and available replacements decrease. A recent prospective study showed that outcomes are comparable for critically ill patients cared for by ACNP and resident teams in a medical ICU.[51] The evidence-based studies describe multiple uses of various models to augment staffing, yet there does not seem to be a "best practice" model. With a myriad of coverage and ICU practice models available, additional studies are needed to help sculpt styles based on the particular needs and preferences of an institution; no one model will fit all organizations. However, regardless of the chosen staffing model, the key determinants for the success and growth of the CCM workforce will rely heavily on organization, strategic planning, and communication.

REFERENCES

1. Gershengorn HB, Johnson MP, Factor P. The use of nonphysician providers in adult intensive care units. *Am J Respir Crit Care Med*. 2012;185:600-605.
2. Angus DC, Kelley MA, Schmitz RJ, et al. Caring for the critically ill patient. Current and projected workforce requirements for care of the critically ill and patients with pulmonary disease: can we meet the requirements of an aging population? *J Am Med Assoc*. 2000;284(21): 2762-2770.
3. Kelley MA, Angus DC, Chalfin DB, et al. The critical care crisis in the United States: a report from the profession. *Chest*. 2004;125:1514-1517.
4. Krell K. Critical care workforce. *Crit Care Med*. 2008;36:1350-1353.
5. Pastores SM, O'Connor MF, Kleinpell RM, et al. The Accreditation Council for Graduate Medical Education resident duty hour new standards: history, changes, and impact on staffing of intensive care units. *Crit Care Med*. 2011;39:2540-2549.
6. Lorin S, Heffner J, Carson S. Attitudes and perceptions of internal medicine residents regarding pulmonary and critical care subspecialty training. *Chest*. 2005;127:630-636.
7. Halpern NA, Pastores SM, Oropello JM, Kvetan V. Critical care medicine in the United States: addressing the intensivist shortage and image of the specialty. *Crit Care Med*. 2013;41:2754-2761.
8. Halpern NA, Pastores SM. Critical care medicine in the United States 2000-2005: an analysis of bed numbers, occupancy rates, payer mix, and costs. *Crit Care Med*. 2010;38:65-71.
9. Halpern NA, Pastores SM, Greenstein RJ. Critical care medicine in the United States 1985-2000: an analysis of bed numbers, use, and costs. *Crit Care Med*. 2004;32:1254-1259.
10. Kleinpell RM, Ely EW, Grabenkort R. Nurse practitioners and physician assistants in the intensive care unit: an evidence-based review. *Crit Care Med*. 2008;36:2888-2897.
11. American Association of Nurse Practitioners. National NP sample survey. http://www.aanp.org/research/reports. Accessed November 1, 2014.
12. Bell L. *AACN Scope and Standards for Acute Care Nurse Practitioner Practice AACN Critical Care Publication*. Aliso Viejo, CA: American Association of Critical-Care Nurses; 2012.
13. Yee T, Boukus E, Cross D, et al. Primary Care Workforce Shortages: Nurse Practitioner Scope-of-Practice Laws and Payment Policies. NIHCR Research Brief No. 13, 2013.
14. Physician Assistant History Society. Honoring our History: Ensuring Our Future Timeline, 1957-1970, 1971-1980. http://www.pahx.org/timeline.html. Accessed October 13, 2013.
15. American Academy of Physician Assistants (AAPA). What is a PA? http://www.aapa.org/the_pa_profession/what_is_a_pa.aspx. Accessed October 15, 2013.
16. American Academy of Physician Assistants (AAPA) Physician Assistants in Hospital Practice: Credentialing and Privileging/Medical Staff Membership. Hospital Practice. Issue brief, January 1-4, 2010. http://www.aapa.org/WorkArea/DownloadAsset.aspx?id=513.
17. Hooker RS, Muchow AN. 2013 census of licensed physician assistants. *JAAPA* 2014;27:35-39.
18. Lizano D, Mehta G, Keith D, Shiloh AL, Savel RH. Physician assistants in the ICU: how best to integrate them into the multidisciplinary team. *ICU Dir*. 2011;2:20-24.
19. American Academy of Physician Assistants (AAPA). Physician Assistant Education - Preparation for Excellence. Professional Issues. Issues brief March 1-3, 2011. http://www.aapa.org/WorkArea/DownloadAsset.aspx?id=580.
20. Inside PA Training. Physician Assistant Programs by State. http://www.mypatraining.com/physician-assistant-programs-by-state. Accessed October 2015.

21. Jones PE, et al. Physician assistant education in the United States. *Acad Med*. 2007;82:882-887.

22. Association of Postgraduate PA Programs (APPAP). http://www.appap.org/. Accessed November 12, 2013.

23. Siegal EM, Dressler DD, Dichter JR, et al. Training a hospitalist workforce to address the intensivist shortage in American hospitals: a position paper from the Society of Hospital Medicine and the Society of Critical Care Medicine. *Crit Care Med*. 2012;40:1952-1956.

24. Wise KR, Akopov VA, Williams BR, Jr, et al. Hospitalists and intensivists in the medical ICU: a prospective observational study comparing mortality and length of stay between two staffing models. *J Hosp Med*. 2012;7:183-189.

25. Heisler M. Hospitalists and intensivists: partners in caring for the critically ill–the time has come. *J Hosp Med*. 2010;5(1):1-3.

26. Gesensway D. The tug-of-war over ICU care: hospitalists and intensivists stake out their turf. *Today's Hospitalist*. 2009 April. http://www.todayshospitalist.com/index.php?b=articles_read&cnt=777.

27. Darves B. Can't find an attending? Why hospitalists are taking a hard look at their roles on rapid response teams. *Today's Hospitalist*. 2014. http://www.todayshospitalist.com/index.php?b=articles_read&cnt=623.

28. Joffe AM, Pastores SM, Maerz LL, et al. Utilization and impact on fellowship training of non-physician advanced practice providers in intensive care units of academic medical centers: a survey of critical care program directors. *J Crit Care*. 2014;29:112-115.

29. Gershengorn HB, Wunsch H, Wahab R, et al. Impact of nonphysician staffing on outcomes in a medical ICU. *Chest*. 2011;139(6):1347-1353.

30. Kawar E, DiGiovine B. MICU care delivered by PAs versus residents: do PAs measure up? *JAAPA*. 2011;24:36-41.

31. Russell D, VorderBruegge M, Burns SM. Effect of an outcomes-managed approach to care of neuroscience patients by acute care nurse practitioners. *Am J Crit Care*. 2002;11:353-362.

32. Vazirani S, Hays RD, Shapiro MF, et al. Effect of a multidisciplinary intervention on communication and collaboration among physicians and nurses. *Am J Crit Care*. 2005;14:71-77.

33. Burns SM, Earven S, Fisher C, et al. Implementation of an institutional program to improve clinical and financial outcomes of mechanically ventilated patients: one-year outcomes and lessons learned. *Crit Care Med*. 2003;31:2752-2763.

34. Collins N, Miller R, Kapu A, et al. Outcomes of adding acute care nurse practitioners to a Level I trauma service with the goal of decreased length of stay and improved physician and nursing satisfaction. *J Trauma Acute Care Surg*. 2014;76:353-357.

35. Moote M, Krsek C, Kleinpell R, et al. Physician assistant and nurse practitioner utilization in academic medical centers. *Am J Med Qual*. 2011;26:452-460.

36. Russell JC, Kaplowe J, Heinrich J. One hospital's successful 20-year experience with physician assistants in graduate medical education. *Acad Med*. 1999;74:641-645.

37. Paton A, Stein DE, D'Agostino R, et al. Critical care medicine advanced practice provider model at a comprehensive cancer center: successes and challenges. *Am J Crit Care*. 2013;22:439-443.

38. Grabenkort WR, K.K., Mollenkopf FP, Keith DE. Developing orientation programs for nurse practitioners and physician assistants in the ICU. In: B.W. Kleinpell RM, Buchman TG, eds. *Integrating Nurse Practitioners and Physician Assistants into the ICU*. Mount Prospect, IL: Society of Critical Care Medicine; 2012:47-64.

39. D'Agostino R, P.S., Halpern NA. The NP staffing model in the ICU at Memorial Sloan-Kettering Cancer Center. In: B.W. Kleinpell RM, Buchman TG, eds. *Integrating Nurse Practitioners and Physician Assistants*. Mount Prospect, IL: Society of Critical Care Medicine; 2012:17-26.

40. Venegas-Borsellino C, Dudaie R, Lizano D, et al. 1282: Simulation training improves teamwork and leadership skills among physician assistants new to the critical care environment. *Crit Care Med*. 2012;40:1-328.

41. Venegas-Borsellino C, Shiloh A, Dudaie R, et al. 602: Simulation training to improve the performance and confidence of new physician assistants in the critical care environment. *Crit Care Med*. 2012;40:1-328.

42. Reines HD, Robinson L, Duggan M, et al. Integrating midlevel practitioners into a teaching service. *Am J Surg*. 2006;192:119-124.

43. Boyle III WA, G.A.S., Munro N. Billing, reimbursement, and productivity for nonphysician practitioners in the ICU. In: Kleinpell RM, Buchman TG, Boyle W, eds. *Integrating Nurse Practitioners and Physician Assistants*. Mount Prospect, IL: Society of Critical Care Medicine; 2012:27-46.

44. The Center for Medicare and Medicaid Services (CMS). Physician Quality Reporting: Initiative Medicare Learning Network Matters. http://www.cms.gov/Outreach-and-Education/

Medicare-Learning-Network-MLN/
MLNMattersArticles/downloads/MM5993.pdf.

45. McCarthy C, O'Rourke NC, Madison JM. Integrating advanced practice providers into medical critical care teams. *Chest.* 2013;143:847-850.

46. Kapu AN, Kleinpell R. Developing nurse practitioner associated metrics for outcomes assessment. *J Am Assoc Nurse Pract.* 2013;25:289-296.

47. D'Agostino R, Pastores SM, Halpern NA. The NP Staffing Model in the ICU at Memorial Sloan Kettering Cancer Center. In: Integrating Nurse Practitioners & Physician Assistants Into The ICU. Kleinpell RM, Boyle WA, Buchman TG (eds). 1st ed. Society of Critical Care Medicine, IL. 2012: 17-25.

48. Lizano DM, Keith G, Shiloh D, A,L. Savel R. H., Physician assistants in the ICU. *ICU Dir.* 2011;2:20-24.

49. Hinami K, Whelan CT, Wolosin RJ, et al. Worklife and satisfaction of hospitalists: toward flourishing careers. *J Gen Intern Med.* 2012;27(1):28-36.

50. Embriaco N, Papazian L, Kentish-Barnes N, et al. Burnout syndrome among critical care healthcare workers. *Curr Opin Crit Care.* 2007;13:482-488.

51. Landsperger JS, Semler MW, Wang L, Byrne DW, Wheeler AP. Outcomes of Nurse Practitioner-Delivered Critical Care: A Prospective Cohort Study. *Chest.* 2016;149(5):1146-54.

Governance

Stephen M. Pastores, MD, FACP, FCCP, FCCM and
Vladimir Kvetan, MD, FCCM

79

KEY POINTS

1 The organization and management of critical care services are key to ICU performance and may impact patient outcomes and healthcare costs.

2 Critical care organizations with advanced governance offer several benefits including unifying all ICUs under one leadership with defined accountability; improved opportunities to reduce costs;

standardization of technologies across ICUs; enhanced crtical care research; and improved retention of faculty through a more stale environment.

3 Movement toward unification of governance commences with the education of intensivists during their fellowship training.

INTRODUCTION

Critical care medicine (CCM) has made significant strides since its inception as a unique specialty almost 50 years ago. In the United States, the use and costs of CCM continues to rise. Between 2000 and 2010, critical care beds increased 17.8% (88,235-103,900) in nearly 3000 acute care hospitals with intensive care unit (ICU) beds. In 2010, critical care in the United States accounted for 13.2% of hospital costs, 4.1% of national health expenditures, and 0.74% ($108 billion) of the gross domestic product.[1] As critical care consumes significant portion of hospital beds and resources and plays a major role in throughput of emergency departments and operating rooms, it is of vital interest to hospital leadership to unify, standardize, and control this resource.

In response to the perceived shortage of trained intensivists in the United States,[2] proposals to mitigate this shortfall have been developed including tiered regionalization of critical care services[3] and providing alternative coverage options with

hospitalists,[4] advance practice providers (nurse practitioners and physician assistants),[5] and ICU telemedicine in community hospitals.[6]

In recent years, there has been an increasing tendency for critical care services in academic medical centers to consolidate their staffing and resources, and to form advanced governance organizations, above the level of departmental divisions or sections.[7] The designation varies greatly from service lines, systems, signature programs, centers, institutes, and clinical departments. To date, only one academic university department of critical care exists in North America at the University of Pittsburgh. Introduction of service line models to critical care, mandates to improve quality and safety of healthcare,[8,9] and transparent public disclosure have added momentum to the health care industry recognizing the need for well-governed critical care as an important tool in business management of medical centers. Among the many aspects that need unified critical care governance include patient management, protocol institution, technology acquisition, education, training, and interactions with other hospital areas.

ORGANIZATION AND MANAGEMENT OF CRITICAL CARE SERVICES

The organization and management of critical care services are key components that contribute to ICU performance and may impact patient outcomes and health care costs. The guidelines for critical care delivery, clinical roles, and best practice model in the ICU from the Society of Critical Care Medicine published in 2001 and updated in 2015 are excellent resources for how ICUs should be administered.[10,11] The 2001 recommendations were based on 6 tenets: (1) Medical interventions should be provided by intensivists leading multidisciplinary groups; (2) Patient care should be directed by ICU teams using a "closed" format in which dedicated critical care teams take ownership of all aspects of care in the ICU; (3) ICU physicians should be available for medical and administrative tasks without competing clinical responsibilities; (4) ICU physicians and nurses should have critical care credentials; (5) Care teams should include critical care pharmacists and full-time respiratory care practitioners as well as ICU physicians and nursing staff; and (6) ICU governance should be conducted by multidisciplinary groups.

The most recent guidelines highlighted the importance of process of care and ICU structure to improved outcomes and offered four important recommendations (Table 79–1).[11] The task force

TABLE 79–1 Recommendations from the SCCM task force on models of critical care.[11]

- An intensivist-led, high-performing, multidisciplinary team dedicated to the ICU is an integral part of effective care delivery.
- Process improvement is the backbone of achieving high-quality ICU outcomes.
- Standardized protocols including care bundles and order sets to facilitate measurable processes and outcomes should be used and further developed in the ICU setting.
- Institutional support for comprehensive QI programs as well as tele-ICU programs should be provided.

ICU, intensive care unit; QI, quality improvement; SCCM, Society of Critical Care Medicine.

highlighted, among others, the importance of sustaining process improvements through education of all ICU staff and education of and support from hospital leadership as well as an understanding and use of process improvement methodology to assess the impact of changes in ICU structure.

CRITICAL CARE ORGANIZATIONS WITH ADVANCED GOVERNANCE

Within the past several years, critical care leaders at academic medical centers and large community hospitals have increasingly examined their ICU infrastructure and clinical staff and take on "battles" to pull the ICUs away from departments and place them into a hospital-based environment and political and administrative infrastructure. From the hospital's perspective, a critical care organization (CCO) offers an excellent opportunity to bring together all ICUs under one leadership with defined accountability. Added advantages include improved opportunities to contain costs; implementation of local and national patient safety and quality initiatives through protocols, standardization of technologies across ICUs with resultant savings from volume-based equipment and supply purchases, warranties, and staff training; enhanced critical care research; and improved recruitment or retention of faculty through a more stable environment.[7] We recently reported a descriptive multicenter study on the structure, governance, and experience to date of CCOs in hospitals in North American academic medical centers.[7] We identified very few CCOs (n = 27). Of the 27 CCO physician directors from 23 institutions (19 sites in the United States and 4 in Canada), 24 (89%) completed the survey. Nearly 80% of the CCOs were created in the last 15 years. Majority of these CCOs were located in larger urban hospitals (> 500 beds) and 79% were primary university medical centers. The transition to a CCO was initiated by the hospital administration in 46% and/or existing critical care service or division in 42% and by consensus of department chairmen in 13%. There were various models of CCM governance, reporting structures, hospital support, and general satisfaction. Almost 90% indicated that their CCO governance structure was either moderately or highly effective, and are still evolving. On average, there were 6 ICUs per hospital with an average of 4 ICUs under CCO governance. In-house intensivists were present 24/7 in 49%, nonphysician advanced practice providers (nurse practitioners, physician assistants) in 63%, hospitalists in 21%, and telemedicine coverage in 14%. Nearly 60% indicated that they had a separate hospital budget to support data management and reporting, oversight of all ICUs, and rapid response teams. We attributed the relatively small number of CCOs that currently exist to several factors including, perhaps, the reluctance of department chairpersons to give their ICUs up to a CCO as they perceive potential loss of billing, triage, and patient and staffing control. Furthermore, CCM has been very intertwined with other disciplines in terms of fellowship training and attending staffs (ie, medicine, pulmonary, anesthesiology, surgery, neurosciences, and pediatrics) due to the absence of a unified critical care fellowship track and certification examination. Thus existing departments have come to believe that their ICUs and intensivists especially in specialty ICUs have little in common with each other. Finally, very few CCM graduates have the necessary skill set to champion the creation and lead CCOs despite CCM fellowship program training in management and team leadership.[7]

MANAGEMENT TRAINING FOR CRITICAL CARE FELLOWS AND INTENSIVISTS

Ideally, a properly structured fellowship training program should prepare physicians from any specialty eligible for Accreditation Council for Graduate Medical Education (ACGME)—accredited training to manage a medical, surgical, cardiac surgery, and neuroscience ICU without any problem. The barriers to operating critical care and deriving benefits from economies of scale by full-time intensivists in the United States are frequently derailed by the desire of physicians required to practice their primary specialty/subspecialty (eg, pulmonary medicine, surgery, anesthesiology) creating a system of many part-time intensivists devoting only a small portion of their clinical time to the dedicated care of ICU patients.[2] Other specialists are convinced that only

intensivists with specialized fellowship training are appropriate to work in specialty ICU, such as neurocritical care. Thus, intensivists in US ICUs often have multiple departmental appointments and may be full- or part-time ICU clinicians and hospital-based or voluntary staff members. Whereas large academic institutions have closed model ICUs (ie, intensivists have exclusive or primary authority for patient triage, ICU admission and discharge decisions, and patient care), in nonacademic hospitals, the majority of ICUs are open units with many requiring critical care consultation and intensivists co-managing patients with the primary attending physicians. In contrast, the traditional model of critical care as a division or service of a department is not typical for many European countries where freestanding critical care departments are commonplace. For example, in the United Kingdom, most ICUs are integrated medical-surgical ICUs and the vast majority of intensivists have an anesthesiology background. Similarly, in Canada, most ICUs are combined medical-surgical units; however, the intensivists in many AMCs come from varying training backgrounds (eg, anesthesiology, surgery, internal medicine, emergency medicine) similar to the United States.

Movement toward unification of governance starts with the education of intensivists during their fellowship training. Critical care fellowship programs should focus on administrative and business concepts, including cost containment, finance, and team leadership.[12,13] A few advanced governance organizations have developed professionalism training series to prepare fellowship graduates to deal with the need for a sophisticated approach to budgets and job market needs as they enter the workforce and assume leadership roles.[14]

TOOLS FOR CRITICAL CARE GOVERNANCE

Among the most powerful tools that may be useful to new leaders of critical care in their hospitals are the outreach programs of having intensivists responding rapidly to medical and surgical emergencies outside of the ICU. In addition to expert resuscitation and stabilization, the intensivist controlling the admission to a higher level of care has the ability to select patients who would derive the highest benefit from a trial of

ICU management. In addition, though the opinions vary as to the effectiveness of medical emergency or rapid response teams in modifying outcomes,[15] the clear institutional benefit in rapid decision by the most qualified physicians cannot be denied. The ability to rapidly institute comfort or palliative measures for the patients not likely to benefit from a trial of ICU care is also very important.[16] At the same time, intensivists do have the skills to determine success or failure of a trial of ICU care and provide a time limit to the effort.[17] Unfortunately, despite our best efforts and initiatives, the population of chronically critically ill patients in the United States runs into hundreds of thousands,[18] with most of these patients suffering from prolonged cerebral and neuromuscular dysfunction and risk of early death after failure of a trial of ICU care. Access to, and benefit from, alternative sites, such as long-term acute care (LTAC) facilities, is being questioned[19] and subject to moratoriums, state-level certificate of need, and demonstration of limited benefit to patients and the health care industry.

In conclusion, critical care leaders across the United States are increasingly faced with the rising patient demand for critical care services at a time of intensivist workforce shortage and mandates from external organizations to improve on the efficiency and quality of care. These leaders must also respond to the need to educate new generations of ICU physicians and nonphysician care providers (nurse practitioners and physician assistants); standardize care and technologies in hospitals with many ICUs; optimize ICU integration within the hospital; and participate in cost control, research, and fundraising initiatives. Movement toward unification of governance starts with the education of intensivists during their fellowship training. The creation of more advanced governance CCOs in acute care hospitals led by effective and successful leaders[20] can ensure not only the delivery of high-quality safe patient care but also more effective use of resources and assistance in organizational operations and development.

REFERENCES

1. Halpern NA, Goldman DA, Tan KS, Pastores SM. Trends in critical care beds and use among population groups and Medicare and Medicaid beneficiaries in the United States: 2000-2010. *Crit Care Med.* 2016 Aug;44(8):1490-1499..

2. Halpern NA, Pastores SM, Oropello JM, Kvetan V. Critical care medicine in the United States: addressing the intensivist shortage and image of the specialty. *Crit Care Med.* 2013 Dec;41(12):2754-2761.

3. Nguyen YL, Kahn JM, Angus DC. Reorganizing adult critical care delivery: the role of regionalization, telemedicine, and community outreach. *Am J Respir Crit Care Med.* 2010;181:1164-1169.

4. Siegal EM, Dressler DD, Dichter JR, Gorman MJ, Lipsett PA. Training a hospitalist workforce to address the intensivist shortage in American hospitals: a position paper from the Society of Hospital Medicine and the Society of Critical Care Medicine. *Crit Care Med.* 2012 Jun;40(6):1952-1956.

5. Gershengorn HB, Wunsch H, Wahab R, et al. Impact of nonphysician staffing on outcomes in a medical ICU. *Chest.* 2011;139:1347-1353.

6. Lilly CM, Zubrow MT, Kempner KM, et al. Critical care telemedicine: evolution and state of the art. *Crit Care Med.* 2014 Nov;42(11):2429-2436.

7. Pastores SM, Halpern NA, Oropello JM, Kostelecky N, Kvetan V. Critical care organizations in academic medical centers in North America: a descriptive report. *Crit Care Med.* 2015 Oct;43(10):2239-2244.

8. Kohn LT, Corrigan JM, Donaldson MS; Committee on Quality of Health Care in America, Institute of Medicine. *To Err Is Human: Building a Safer Health System.* Washington, DC: National Academy Press; 2000.

9. Committee on Quality of Health Care in America, Institute of Medicine. *Crossing the Quality Chasm: A New Health System for the 21st Century.* Washington, DC: National Academy Press; 2001.

10. Brilli RJ, Spevetz A, Branson RD, et al. American College of Critical Care Medicine Task Force on Models of Critical Care Delivery; The American College of Critical Care Medicine Guidelines for the Definition of an Intensivist and the Practice of Critical Care Medicine. Critical care delivery in the intensive care unit: defining clinical roles and the best practice model. *Crit Care Med.* 2001;29:2007-2019.

11. Weled BJ, Adzhigirey LA, Hodgman TM, et al. Task Force on Models for Critical Care. Critical care delivery: the importance of process of care and ICU structure to improved outcomes: an update from the American College of Critical Care Medicine Task Force on Models of Critical Care. *Crit Care Med.* 2015 Jul;43(7):1520-1525.

12. Stockwell DC, Pollack MM, Turenne WM, Slonim AD. Leadership and management training of

pediatric intensivists: how do we gain our skills? *Pediatr Crit Care Med*. 2005;6:665-670.

13. Gasperino J, Brilli R, Kvetan V. Teaching intensive care unit administration during critical care medicine training programs. *J Crit Care*. 2008 Jun;23(2):251-252.

14. Moore JE, Pinsky MR. Faculty development for fellows: developing and evaluating a broad-based career development course for critical care medicine trainees. *J Crit Care*. 2015 Oct;30(5):1152.e1-e6.

15. Hillman K, Chen J, Cretikos M, et al; MERIT study investigators. Introduction of the medical emergency team (MET) system: a cluster-randomised controlled trial. *Lancet*. 2005 Jun 18-24;365(9477):2091-2097.

16. Weissman DE, Meier DE. Identifying patients in need of a palliative care assessment in the hospital setting: a consensus report from the Center to Advance Palliative Care. *J Palliat Med*. 2011;14(1):17.

17. Lecuyer L, Chevret S, Thiery G, Darmon M, Schlemmer B, Azoulay E. The ICU trial: a new admission policy for cancer patients requiring mechanical ventilation. *Crit Care Med*. 2007 Mar;35(3):808-814.

18. Kahn JM, Le T, Angus DC, et al; ProVent Study Group Investigators. Chronic critically ill: the epidemiology of chronic critical illness in the United States. *Crit Care Med*. 2015 Feb;43(2):282-287.

19. Kahn JM, Werner RM, David G, Ten Have TR, Benson NM, Asch DA. Effectiveness of long-term acute care hospitalization in elderly patients with chronic critical illness. *Med Care*. 2013 Jan;51(1):4-10.

20. St. Andre A. The formation, elements of success, and challenges in managing a critical care program: Part 1. *Crit Care Med*. 2015 Apr;43:874-879.

Managing the ICU from Afar: Telemedicine

Tzvi Neuman, DO and Baruch Goldstein, MD

KEY POINTS

1. The key to successful telemedicine is communication: telecommunication and interpersonal communication.

2. Telemedicine allows smaller hospitals to provide 24-hour continuity of care by an awake and alert board certified CCM physician, allowing access to an off-site intensivist at any time, day, or night.

3. Telemedicine allows hospitals to be compliant with current medical industry standards.

4. Improvements in delivery of care may lead to improved clinical and financial outcomes.

INTRODUCTION: ADDRESSING A NEED

Telemedicine was developed in the 1960s and 1970s by the US military and aerospace sectors by using information and communication technologies to provide medical care in remote areas.[1] More recently, as telecommunication technologies have significantly advanced, telemedicine can help alleviate the shortage of physicians in certain specialties by allowing instant access to specialists who are not physically available at the location of the patient. Consequently, telemedicine, and in particular, tele-ICU, may help offset several well-known health care delivery challenges within the critical care community. These challenges include the following:

1. A large deficit of board-certified intensivists staffing intensive care units (ICUs) during the day and, especially, at night. It is estimated that currently only one-third of ICU patients are cared for by board-certified critical care

physicians.[2,3] Halpern et al[4] note that many intensivists are also certified in additional specialties and spend a portion of their time in those capacities, thereby reducing the time they spend in the ICU. Furthermore, staffing ICUs in smaller hospitals and those located in rural areas is very challenging. In smaller hospitals, the number of ICU beds is often not sufficient to support a dedicated on-site intensivist, and in rural hospitals, there may be limited access to critical care medicine (CCM) specialists due to issues related to commuting.

2. The aging population is increasing and although the number of trained critical physicians has increased in recent years, it is projected that by 2020 the demand for critical care physicians will exceed the supply.[2]

3. Another concern is the high cost of intensive care. Bartolini and King[5] note that over six million of the sickest patients are treated in ICUs per year. This patient population has the

highest rate of mortality and contributes the most in terms of the cost incurred in health care, consuming $107 billion dollars per year, which is 4.1% of the $2.6 trillion dollars spent on annual health care in the United States.

To the extent that these challenges exist, research has shown that having an intensivist manage the care of ICU patients has significantly reduced mortality and length of stay (LOS) in the ICU.[6,7] Furthermore, the Leapfrog Group, a voluntary employer-based coalition that advocates for improved quality, safety, and affordability in hospitals, notes that due to high mortality rates in ICUs, the quality of care in ICUs is of particular importance. The Leapfrog Group composed a safety standard indicating that intensivists (in particular those specifically trained in critical care medicine) should be present in the ICU during daytime hours and exclusively provide care to these patients and that when physicians are not in-house, the on-call doctor or tele-intensivist needs to return pages at least 95% of the time within 5 minutes and arrange for care to be delivered to a patient by a doctor, physician assistant (PA), nurse practitioner (NP), or registered nurse (RN) within 5 minutes. As of 2010, the Leapfrog Group noted that only 34.5% of the responding hospitals were compliant with this safety standard.

Tele-ICU programs offer one way to improve patient access to critical care specialists and address these issues. In specialized off-site command centers, critical care is delivered by CCM-trained doctors and nurses who provide coverage to patients in academic, community, rural, and critical access facilities. By using telemedicine, specialists can use their expertise to alter patient care plans while constantly monitoring patients with the help of the bedside RN and tele-RN.

Dr. Brian Rosenfeld and Dr. Michael Breslow, critical care physicians for over 20 years at the Johns Hopkins Hospital in Baltimore, developed the initial technology for the electronic ICU (eICU) in 1998. They utilized a physician-focused electronic medical record (EMR), coupled with clinical algorithms of best practices, an early vital sign warning system,[7] and an audio-visual interface to deliver ICU care. The original tele-ICU program was adopted for use by a Virginia hospital system in 2000. As of late 2012, there were 54 tele-ICU monitoring centers utilized by government and civilian health care systems covering over 350 hospitals.[5]

In essence, the tele-intensivist can be thought of as a doctor who is reviewing patients in an office adjacent to the ICU with access to the entire EMR, ICU waveform monitor, and radiologic imaging and who can approach the bedside when alerted by the RN. At night, the tele-intensivist may be better equipped than the day doctor who is on-call from home and is awakened to discuss a patient; the tele-intensivist is awake and alert with all the relevant information in front of him or her in real time. The tele-intensivist, whose only responsibility during a shift is to monitor ICU-level patients using a remotely located eICU workstation, may also be in a better position to provide care when compared to an on-site non-CCM physician who has a number of other responsibilities in the hospital, including those outside the ICU. Tele-intensivists work in different time zones during daytime hours, providing night shift coverage at the location of the patient. For example, the authors of this chapter are located in Israel; they are part of a group of US board certified CCM physicians providing night coverage to ICUs in the United States while working during the day in Israel.

As in all areas of medical care delivery, the key to any successful tele-ICU is proper communication, interpersonal and telecommunication between on-site and off-site staff—whether they are from medical or ancillary services. This includes proper sign-out between the in-house and off-site physicians and nurses, medical consultants, ER and admitting staff, anesthesiologists, and surgeons, and most importantly between the tele-ICU doctor and bedside nurse. Timely and effective communication yields the best results for the patient and their families (Figure 80–1).

TELE-ICU MODELS

There are various types of tele-ICU models (Table 80–1). Some models offer continuous monitoring and management of ICUs during night shift hours or 24 hours a day, where physicians and nurses in a monitoring center work in 8 to 12 hour shifts. During the shift, the tele-ICU team is exclusively dedicated to the care of the patients in the ICUs of that hospital system. In the tele-ICU consultant

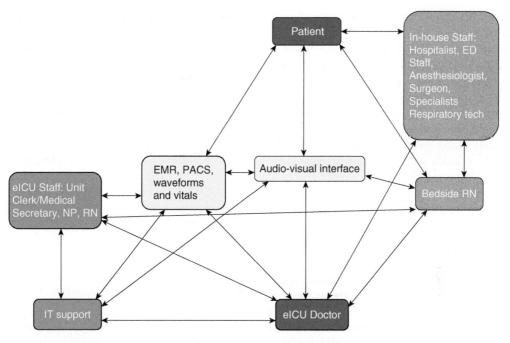

FIGURE 80–1 Schematic presentation of the lines of communication in the tele-ICU.

model, an intensivist provides critical care consultations upon request and is not responsible for continuous monitoring of entire units. Generally, in this model, a mobile cart with audio-video capabilities or a robot is commonly used to gather information followed by treatment recommendations given by the consultant.

TABLE 80–1 Tele-ICU models and brief description of care provided.

Continuous monitoring	• Ongoing 24-hour monitoring by a tele-intensivist and tele-RN in conjunction with in-house staff
Consultation-based monitoring	• Monitoring based on CCM consultation • May be intermittent • Treatment is recommendation based care in conjunction with care plan developed by the primary medical service taking care of the patient
Hospital-defined monitoring	• Uses various EMR programs • May be with or without audio-video capabilities • CCM involvement varies

There are other hospitals that use their own "home-made" tele-ICU monitoring systems by using various EMR programs, with or without audio-video capabilities, for patient assessment. The level of involvement of the tele-intensivist in the care of these patients varies between hospital systems based on the clinical job definition determined by the medical officers of each hospital system.

TECHNOLOGY BASICS

Tele-ICU technology provides access to the hospital's EMR, the radiology image archiving and communication system (PACS), and the ICU hemodynamic monitor, and is coupled with an audio-visual interface allowing the CCM physician to see and communicate with the patient, family, and hospital medical staff.

There are currently several vendors offering different types of ICU EMR systems. The Philips eICU system (Philips Healthcare, Andover, MA) is currently the most commonly used application by health systems that run large tele-ICU programs involving continuous care. This is the system that the authors of this chapter have used in various health systems. When using the Philips eICU system, the ICU rooms are outfitted with high-definition Pan Tilt and Zoom (PTZ) cameras and servers. There is also an option of using a mobile cart with a camera that can be used for patients outside the ICU, such as in an emergency room awaiting ICU admission or during rapid response calls on the wards.

Various EMRs provide the tele-ICU staff with alerts such as sepsis alerts and best practice alerts regarding glycemic control, and DVT and GI prophylaxis, which need to be reviewed. The Philips Tele-ICU software has specialized algorithms that provide alerts when adverse trends in vital signs are noted.

NETWORK REQUIREMENTS

Since the tele-ICU team provides care for critically ill patients, it is crucial that the tele-ICU team is always immediately available for real-time communications and that connectivity with the remote staff is not lost due to technology failure. The tele-ICU center is generally connected to the hospital data center via redundant dedicated T1 lines. Back-up electricity with uninterrupted power supply (UPS) systems and electric generators is used as well to ensure continuous operation even during power failures. Full-time information technology (IT) support is required to address any technical problems that may arise.

STAFF AND SUPPORT

Staff is divided between in-house and off-site personnel, and medical and ancillary services (Table 80-2). The hospital staff available varies from facility to facility and the duties of the tele-intensivist depend on the staff available for that particular ICU.

In-House Staff
Bedside Registered Nurse

The ICU nurse is present at bedside and provides most of the hands-on care to the patient. The bedside RN is the key provider with whom the tele-ICU staff interacts; they discuss any medical events that arise, such as a change in status, or hemodynamic or respiratory issues, and the care plan is delivered per recommendations and orders given by the tele-ICU physician.

TABLE 80-2 In-house and off-site staff.

In-house	Off-Site Tele-ICU Command Center
Bedside RN	Unit Clerk/Medical Secretary
Hospitalist	Tele-RN
Respiratory therapist	NP
Emergency Department physician	Teleintensivist
Information technologies (IT)	IT
Subspecialists, surgeons, and anesthesiologists may be called into hospital as needed	

Hospitalist/Managing Physician

In the majority of hospitals with tele-ICU programs, there is an in-house hospitalist available 24 hours a day. The hospitalist is often responsible for the care of patients admitted to the medical floor, the ICU, as well as any new patients admitted through the ER. In some institutions, there are private internists who are responsible for new admissions and the care of admitted patients; these physicians may not be present on-site all the time. Some hospitals do not employ an on-site hospitalist or internist during the night hours.

Respiratory Therapist

The respiratory therapist helps manage invasive and noninvasive respiratory support. At some facilities, the respiratory therapist is also certified in performing intubations for invasive ventilation. In recent years, some hospitals have expanded the role of the respiratory staff to include critical care procedures such as the placement of central IV access, arterial access, peripherally inserted central catheters (PICC), and conducting focused bedside echocardiography.

ER Physician

In many of the hospitals, there is an emergency medicine physician whose primary responsibility is the emergency room, but the physician can be called to help out on the floors and the ICU for codes, intubations, or other procedures.

Surgeons and Anesthesiologists

Hospitals generally have an anesthesiologist and surgeon on-call. Aside from working in the OR, the anesthesiologist or surgeon can be called to help manage an airway problem or perform other invasive ICU procedures.

Other Specialists

Specialists in other fields may be available for consultation; they generally round in the ICUs during the day and are on-call from home during the night. The types of specialists available vary from hospital to hospital; in some of the more rural facilities, there may not be access to specialists in certain fields of medicine.

Command Center/Tele-ICU Monitoring Site Staff

The off-site center may be located on the premises of one of the hospitals in the system or may be located off-site. The medical staff in these command centers has at their fingertips sophisticated EMR technologies, bedside ICU monitoring, PACS system for imaging, and audio-video access to the patient's room (Figure 80–2). The tele-ICU has medical secretaries, critical care nurses, and critical care physicians. Some tele-ICUs also have acute care NPs. Each member of the medical and nonmedical staff should be oriented, before starting to work in the service, to their own respective roles and duties as well as the roles of the other staff to ensure a cohesive and efficiently run service.

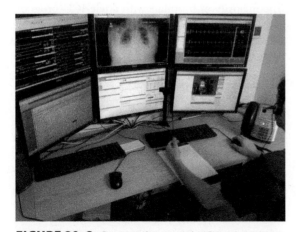

FIGURE 80–2 Command center tele-ICU monitoring.

Unit Clerk/Medical Secretary

The unit clerk or secretary triages phone calls from different hospitals and helps the medical staff communicate with on-site personnel such as the beside nurses, hospitalists, ER physicians, and other on-call specialists. They also ensure that patient data are properly entered into the EMR. When necessary, they also help identify potential or current technical problems in software or hardware that arise with the network and communicate with the IT team.

Tele-ICU RN

The tele-ICU RN has several roles; the most important is to support the bedside RN with any medical concerns that arise. The tele-ICU RN is assigned patients to follow and monitors vital signs, hemodynamics and other tracings, laboratory values and other tests, and can also visually assess the patient using video cameras located in the patient's room. The tele-ICU RN is in close communication with the bedside RN and proactively involves the tele-intensivist with any problems or concerns that arise.

Another tele-ICU RN role is to monitor standards of care and the application of best practices. For instance, the off-site RN can confirm glycemic monitoring and control, GI and DVT prophylaxis, sepsis and delirium alerts, and the VAP bundle. The team is alerted to ensure appropriate protocol-driven care, which can help the hospital meet standards of care developed by national and international medical societies such as the Society of Critical Care Medicine, the American College of Chest Physicians, the American Association of Critical Care Nurses, The Joint Commission (TJC, formerly known as JCAHO), and the World Federation of Societies of Intensive and Critical Care Medicine.

The tele-ICU nursing team also includes a clinical manager, or team leader. The clinical manager, together with the medical director, models the workflow and assigns the specific tasks for the tele-ICU nursing team.

Tele-Intensivist

The tele-intensivist is a board-certified or board-eligible CCM physician who is licensed in the state(s) where the hospital(s) is located. The responsibilities of the tele-intensivist are similar to that of the bedside ICU attending physician. The tele-intensivist is available to triage all matters of medical concern such as electrolyte replacement, pain management, sedation, ventilator management, titration of vasoactive agents, coordination and follow-up with consultants, as well as treat hemodynamic instability and respiratory distress. The tele-intensivist is in close communication with the bedside RN, respiratory therapist, and when applicable, the hospitalist or ER physician. Entering notes into the medical chart is a prudent form of communication and legal recording. Even minor details are recorded in a short note so the bedside staff will know the care provided by the tele-ICU staff.

Nurse Practitioner

Some of the larger or busier tele-ICUs also have acute care NPs, state licensed with specialty certification from the American Association of Critical Care Nurses. The NP, assigned to patients in a fashion similar to the off-site doctor, is responsible for patient care and is in constant communication with the CCM physician. The NP will generally take calls for laboratory orders, medication orders, and radiology requests. The NP may be asked to assist a physician who is attending to other patient care matters. A clear job definition for the NP should be outlined by the medical chief of staff together with the chief of service of each hospital system.

IT Support

IT support is an important component of telemedicine, ensuring that all telecommunications lines, hardware, and software are working reliably and smoothly. IT staff should be available 24/7, in-house and off-site.

PATIENT RATIOS

Monitoring critically ill patients can be labor intensive, especially when there are many high-intensity patients. It is incumbent on the medical chief of staff together with the chief of service and vice-president of nursing for each hospital, in conjunction with the medical director of the tele-ICU service, to find a safe ratio of medical personnel to patient load. The ratio for monitoring that has been recommended for an MD is between 50 and 120 patients, an NP is between 50 and 100 patients, and an RN between 35 and 45 patients.

GENERAL TELE-ICU WORKFLOW

The general workflow in the tele-ICU includes treating all active medical issues that arise and best-practice monitoring. Tele-ICU team involvement occurs when the bedside staff calls them, when they discover medical trends during proactive rounding, or when using the tele-ICU program algorithms.

FACILITIES WITHOUT INTENSIVIST SERVICES

In facilities without intensivist coverage, the tele-intensivist can play a crucial role in the day or night. In these facilities, the hospitalist or internist can review care plans of new admissions with the tele-intensivist by phone or via the audio-video interface from the patient's room. In many hospitals, there are regular daily morning rounds with the tele-intensivist. During the night, the tele-intensivist can be called by the physician or bedside RN to help just as an on-call physician would be called at home. The tele-intensivist can also assist the surgeon in managing patients postoperatively.

FACILITIES WITH AN INTENSIVIST AVAILABLE DURING A PORTION OF THE DAY

The majority of hospitals with a tele-ICU program have an intensivist or a pulmonologist available for consultation to help manage the ICU patients; however, they are not in house all the time. There may be a dedicated intensivist group but without enough staff to allow for in-house night time coverage. Other hospitals have a CCM physician who consults on a daily basis but is not always available to the ICU due to other responsibilities. In those facilities where a dedicated intensivist rounds during the day, the main role of the tele-intensivist is during night-shift hours. Ideally, the managing intensivist will sign out his or her patients at the end of the day to the tele-intensivist just as he would sign out to an in-house night intensivist taking over continuity of care. In the morning, the tele-intensivist signs out major events that occurred over night to the day CCM physician. Should the need arise where the tele-intensivist feels that an intensivist is needed at the bedside, the on-call intensivist can be notified to return to the ICU. Alternatively, the hospitalist, ER physician, or an anesthesiologist, if available, can help at the bedside during the night as well. With more and more facilities having respiratory therapists who are certified in ICU procedures, the tele-intensivist is able, in most cases, to provide appropriate medical management without requiring the help of an on-site intensivist.

FACILITIES WITH 24-HOUR IN-HOUSE INTENSIVIST COVERAGE

Some facilities that have 24-hour in-house intensivist coverage are part of a broader hospital system that utilizes the tele-ICU program. The tele-intensivist is available to assist upon request. This generally happens when the in-house intensivist is covering a large number of patients in a particular ICU or is covering patients in other care areas within the same hospital.

OUTCOMES

Tele-ICU is a relatively new practice in medicine. The greatest theoretical impact that CCM specialists can have is on medical facilities with a deficit of intensivist coverage, facilities with a high severity-adjusted mortality and long LOS, and to facilities located remotely where safe transfer of a critical patient to a higher level care center may not be feasible.[8] Lilly et al[9] reported that early intervention by a tele-intensivist was associated with lower mortality and LOS. Wilmitch et al[10] in their recent 3-year retrospective study found a statistically significant decrease in severity-adjusted hospital LOS by 14.2% and a decreased ICU LOS by 12.6%. The Philips Healthcare company reports,[11] according to company tracking data, that there has been a 37% to 64% decrease in patient mortality, as well as an $8 million consumer savings attributed to reduced ICU days.

BENEFITS AND LIMITATIONS

The main benefit to using a tele-ICU model is real-time access to a CCM specialist who may otherwise not be available to care for ICU patents. The bedside nurses caring for patients who may potentially deteriorate while awaiting a call back from a doctor get an immediate response from the tele-intensivist. The tele-intensivist provides immediate care as orders can be entered efficiently into the medical chart and unnecessary delay is avoided. Implicit in this model is that the nurse is at the bedside while communicating concerns with the tele-intensivist. The patients and their families who are at the bedside, some of whom may have arrived in the middle of the night, can also access a physician upon request. Other benefits include adherence to best practice measures and improved nursing productivity.

Prior to implementing a successful tele-ICU program, there are various issues with cost and culture that need to be addressed. These barriers can be divided into system-based challenges or those related to the CCM specialist. System-based barriers include initial cost to implement a telemedicine program and a smaller hospital's difficulty in putting a program in place. The construction, installation, and training of staff can approach $5 million, while the annual operation of a command center can approach $1 to $2 million for staff, hardware, software, and technology licensing.[8] Although the implementation and maintenance of such a program can be costly, the overall benefit to patients and the hospitals entrusted with their care is tangible.

Another important barrier to implementation is the lack of third-party payer reimbursement for tele-intensivist care. Regarding this, the Leapfrog Group[3] recommends that health care purchasers should encourage hospitals to implement changes and meet their standard by providing marketplace incentives. They call for education of the consumer and purchaser to create a greater demand for care by bedside and tele-intensivists to care for the sickest patients. Such innovations can create financial savings in the health care sector when community hospitals, with the help of telemedicine, can care for critically ill patients in their facilities, as opposed to transferring the patient to a tertiary hospital (unless the community hospital does not have adequate resources, in which case it is appropriate and recommended to transfer care).

Other barriers include acceptance by the in-house CCM community who may be reluctant to have a tele-intensivist intervene in the care of their patients. The tele-ICU staff must be considered by the bedside staff as an integral part of the health care team in order for the system to work and to achieve its benefits.

Another limitation is the inability of the tele-intensivist to perform invasive bedside procedures (such as central access, arterial access, hemodialysis access, or tube thoracostomy) and the potential delay while waiting for another member of the in-house staff to complete these procedures in a timely fashion. Availability of certified staff to perform ICU procedures is an important factor that complements the benefit of having a tele-ICU program.

Maintenance of medical licensing throughout the different states where the tele-ICU service is used is necessary for each physician. This can be facilitated by a dedicated licensing and credentialing coordinator who can ensure continuity of certificates and hospital privileges.

FUTURE CONSIDERATIONS

As the use of focused bedside ultrasound and echocardiography grows in the world of critical care medicine, the tele-intensivist can also utilize this diagnostic modality. Specially trained respiratory therapists have conducted focused bedside transthoracic echocardiography while the tele-intensivist watches the real-time imaging on the high-definition/high-fidelity audio-visual interface, allowing early diagnosis of issues relating to the fluid status and other cardiac abnormalities. As the therapists become more comfortable with ultrasound, they can learn other ultrasound modalities such as lung, renal, and abdominal imaging, and can help diagnose dysfunction in these organ systems. In the future, intensivists may also be able to help stabilize patients being evacuated by mediflight, in dangerous battlefield situations, or conduct international consultations. They may also be able to work with other physicians, such as cardiothoracic surgeons or neurosurgeons, who have accepted patients onto their service from outside hospitals, and help optimize these critical patients in concert with the surgeons prior to or during transfer to the accepting hospital.

REFERENCES

1. Telemedicine: Opportunities and developments in Member States: Report on the second global survey on health; 2009. http://www.who.int/goe/publications/goe_telemedicine_2010.pdf. Accessed February 10, 2014.
2. Duke, EM. Health Resources and Services Administration Report to Congress: The Critical Care Workforce: A Study of the Supply and Demand for Critical Care Physicians. Requested by: Senate Report 108-81. http://bhpr.hrsa.gov/healthworkforce/reports/studycriticalcarephys.pdf. Accessed December 30, 2013.
3. The Leapfrog Group for Patient Safety: Factsheet: ICU Physician Staffing. http://www.leapfroggroup.org. Accessed December 29, 2013.
4. Halpern, NA, Pastores, SM, Oropello, JM, Kvetan V. Critical care medicine in the United States: addressing the intensivist shortage and image of the specialty. *Crit Care Med*. 2013;41:2754-2761.
5. Bartolini, E, King, N. Emerging Best Practices for Tele-ICU Care Nationally. NEHI Issue Brief. http://www.nehi.net/publications/82/emerging_best_practices_for_teleicu_care_nationally. Accessed December 30, 2013.
6. Young MP, Birkmeyer JD. Potential reduction in mortality rates using an intensivist model to manage intensive care units. *Eff Clin Pract*. 2000;3:284-289.
7. Breslow MJ. The eICU® Solution: a technology-enabled care paradigm for ICU performance. In: Reid PP, Compton WD, Grossman JH, Fanjiang G, eds. *Building a Better Delivery System: A New Engineering/Health Care Partnership*. Washington, DC: National Academies Press; 2005:209-213.
8. Ahn Y, Jasmer RM, Shaughnessy T. Perspectives on the Electronic ICU. *ICU Dir*. 2012;3:64-74.
9. Lilly CM, McLaughlin JM, Zhao H, et al. A multicenter study of ICU telemedicine reengineering of adult critical care. *Chest*. 2014;145:500-507.
10. Willmitch, B, Golembeski, S, Kim, SS, Nelson LD, Gidel L. Clinical outcomes after telemedicine intensive care unit implementation. *Crit Care Med*. 2012;40:450-454.
11. eICU-Philips. http://www.healthcare.philips.com. Accessed December 29, 2013.

Ethics and Palliative Care in the Intensive Care Unit

Aluko A. Hope, MD, MSCE

KEY POINTS

1. The four principles of biomedical ethics—beneficence, nonmaleficence, autonomy, and justice can provide a rubric through which clinicians can identify ethical dilemmas in clinical practice.

2. Informed consent is a process of mutual respect between a clinician and a patient that involves (a) ensuring that the patient has the capacity to make the specific medical decision; (b) the skillful disclosure of relevant information to the patient; and (c) ensuring that the patient's expressed choices are voluntary.

3. Advance care planning is a process by which patients, with facilitation by a trained professional, clarifies their current health state, goals, and objectives.

4. A living will is any document where the patient anticipates a specific set of medical circumstances and requests or refuses specific types of treatment under each of these medical circumstances.

5. A health care proxy form allows a patient to name a surrogate decision-maker in the event they become unable to make medical decisions for themselves.

6. In shared decision-making, clinicians are considered the experts on prognosis/treatment options, whereas the patient/family is considered the expert on the patient's values.

7. Palliative care is a multidisciplinary, patient-centered approach to care that focuses on (a) assessing and treating symptoms; (b) providing psychological and spiritual support to patients and families; (c) facilitating treatments that are better aligned with patients' values by ensuring skillful, proactive, and compassionate communication between the clinical team and the patients/families.

8. Most patients die in the ICU after the withdrawal or withholding of some life-sustaining treatments.

9. The withdrawal of life-sustaining treatments should be considered a clinical procedure that requires expertise, careful preparation, appropriate documentation, and ongoing evaluation.

INTRODUCTION

With the inevitable advancement in technological innovation and the aging of the population, more patients with chronic medical problems will face complex medical decisions in intensive care units (ICUs). Although most ICU patients survive, many deaths occur in or directly following an ICU stay.[1] Dying in the ICU has become a negotiated process, most often requiring some limitation of life-sustaining treatments.[2] ICU survivors struggle with physical and psychological symptoms, and functional and cognitive impairments, and their families struggle with caregiver strain in the face of an increasingly fragmented health care system.[3] Patients come to the ICU with diverse expectations and values but are often too incapacitated to fully express them. Families, in the face of their own grief and bereavement, are asked to represent the patient, often weighing the possibility of impaired survival or death with the hope of recovery. All of these factors combine together to make the ICU a clinical arena rife with potential for conflict, making it increasingly important for the ICU clinician to be able to integrate the principles of bioethics and palliative care into the clinical care they provide their patients in the ICU.

This chapter will first discuss the key ethical principles and theories that provide a framework for medical decision-making in the ICU. Second, it will review the key legal cases in the United States that have informed the way in which care is negotiated in the ICU. Third, it will review medical decision-making, focusing on surrogate decision-making and the shared decision-making model in which the patient or the family play an active role in decision-making along with the clinical team. Fourth, it will define palliative care and discuss the integration of its principles into the care of the critically ill patient. Fifth, it will discuss futility conflicts in the ICU. Finally, it will review the principles and practice of withdrawing life-sustaining treatments in the ICU.

ETHICAL FRAMEWORK FOR MEDICAL DECISION-MAKING

Many different approaches to ethical analyses exist. This chapter will review the main approach—principlism—in depth and then briefly summarize other approaches that clinicians can consider.

Principlism

Beauchamp and Childress delineated four principles—beneficence, nonmaleficence, autonomy, and justice—that provide an ethical framework for moral deliberation in medicine.[4]

The principle of beneficence refers to the clinician's duty to act for the benefit of the patient. An extension of beneficence is the principle of nonmaleficence, which imposes an obligation on the clinician to not inflict harm on the patient (associated with the maxim: Primum non nocere, "above all, do no harm"). These principles of beneficence and nonmaleficence underlie the fiduciary relationship between the physician and the patient and are the two oldest ethical principles in medicine.[5] Within the Hippocratic tradition, under the beneficence model, the physician relied exclusively on their own judgment to decide what was best for the patient and would exercise that authority over an obedient patient. In this model, the disclosure of information by the physician to the patient was strictly for the patient's benefit and physicians often practiced "benevolent deception," whereby medical information was withheld or misrepresented to the patient for fear that it might adversely impact the patient's health.

The principle of autonomy in bioethics refers to the fact that the patient should be free of controlling influences and limitations that prevent a meaningful choice (ie, the right of self-determination). The word autonomy is derived from the Greek words *autos* ("self") and *nomos* ("rule"). With the rise of autonomy as an important ethical principle of medical practice, medical decision-making changed significantly: The modern physician must now integrate the patient's choices with his or her own clinical judgment and the patient always has the right to refuse any treatment.[5]

Justice—the fourth ethical principle—is usually defined as the fair distribution of medical resources. This principle, by acknowledging the importance of treating similar patients in a similar fashion, is usually situated in a larger society or organization, rather than in an individual clinician—patient encounter. This principle provides a strong mandate to remove barriers of access to medical care and to eliminate health disparities within health care. In the era of rapidly rising health care costs, questions about how to fairly allocate the expensive, resource-intensive treatments provided in the ICU are often asked under this ethical principle.

Ethical principles alone cannot guide clinical practice; rather, they provide a rubric through which clinicians can identify ethical dilemmas in clinical practice. Respect for autonomy may clash with beneficence when patients refuse treatments that the physician thinks are in their best interest. The ethical responsibility of the individual physician to use medical resources responsibly can put justice in conflict with autonomy when patients request scarce medical resources needed by others who are more likely to benefit from their use.

Other Approaches to Ethical Analysis

There are other approaches to ethical analysis—besides principlism—that may be relevant to ICU care.[6] *Casuistry* approaches ethical reasoning incrementally through the analysis of the features of a specific case and looks to paradigmatic cases for the best resolution of current ethical dilemmas. *Narrative ethics* focuses on the specific story of the actors involved in the ethical dilemma and uses narrative methods to enhance the moral imagination of the clinician to help determine an ethically appropriate course of action. *Virtue ethics* focuses on the moral character of the clinician, his or her attempts to meet a particular standard of action. This theory provides impetus for the development of ethical wisdom in novice clinicians by improving their affective and intellectual reasoning skills. *Relational ethics* emphasizes the care of the whole person in clinical ethical deliberation. Specifically, the patient's personalities, values, pasts, hopes for the future, relationships, roles, and responsibilities are all considered in the ethical analyses.[6] This theory's emphasis on the relational and emotional aspects of medical decision-making is particularly relevant to palliative care and the integration of its principles into the ICU.

INFORMED CONSENT, MEDICAL ETHICS, AND THE LAW

Informed Consent: Legal History

The legal doctrine of informed consent extends from the primacy of autonomy in medical practice. In one of the foundational opinions that would plant the seed for the informed consent doctrine, Judge Cordozo, in *Schloendorff v. Society of New York Hospital* (1914), wrote that "every human being of adult years in sound mind has a right to determine what shall be done with his own body; a surgeon who performs an operation without the patient's consent commits an assault for which he is liable for damages...."[7]

After the travesty of the widespread experimentation on human subjects during World War II, the Nuremberg Code established the voluntary consent of the human subject as an essential step in the ethical conduct of research. With the unveiling of questionable research practices that continued in the United States through the 1950s and 1960s, there was an erosion of the public's trust of the physicians' capacity to ensure the well-being of their patients. Through the then emerging field of medical ethics, an array of voices—lawyers, policy makers, legislators, theologians, philosophers—entered the arena of medical decision-making with the hope of protecting the patient from the imbalance of knowledge inherent in the physician–patient relationship. These voices suggested that medical decisions should include technical as well as value-laden choices that reflect the moral views of the patient, their family, and society.[8]

In *Salgo v. Leland Stanford University Board of Trustees* (1957), the Court of Appeals of California found that the physician in obtaining consent must disclose "all facts which mutually affect his rights and interest." In *Canterbury v. Spence* (1972), another U.S. court ruled that "true consent to what happens to one's self is the informed exercise of a choice, and that entails an opportunity to evaluate knowledgeably the options available," which can only be accomplished when a patient is able to look to the physician "for enlightenment with which to reach an intelligent decision." In the same year, the American Hospital Association published its Patients' Bill of Rights, which enshrined the informed consent doctrine into the lexicon of medical care by establishing that the patient had the right to make decisions about their treatment and the right to refuse any medical treatment.

Informed Consent: The Process

Informed consent is a process of decision-making that requires the participation of the patient and strives for mutual respect between the clinician and the patient. Key elements of informed consent include (1) disclosure of relevant information to the patient; (2) the patient's ability to understand the information; (3) the patient's capacity to make a decision; and (4) the patient's ability to express their choice voluntarily (ie, free of coercion, manipulation, or deception). Patients are deemed to have decisional capacity if they have (1) the ability to communicate a choice freely; (2) the ability to understand the relevant information; (3) the ability to appreciate the situation and its consequences; and (4) the ability to reason and deliberate about the treatment options provided.[9] In the critical care setting, the assessment of the decision-making capacity can be complicated by the need for rapid assessments because of the time pressure in emergency settings and the fact that critically ill patients often have an altered mental status that may make quick assessments difficult. In an emergency situation when the patient lacks any of the requisite abilities for decisional capacity, clinicians turn to surrogate decision-makers or legal documents detailing the patient's desires. If no surrogate decision-maker is found and there is an emergency, the clinician may intervene under the presumption of implied consent.

LEGAL ASPECTS OF END-OF-LIFE CARE AND PALLIATIVE CARE

Some broad understanding of the key legal cases involving the limitation of life-sustaining treatment and the provision of palliative care will help clinicians improve their practice in this important aspect of ICU care.[7,10,11] The first and most important case was the *Quinlan* case decided by the Supreme Court of New Jersey in 1976. Karen Quinlan was a 22-year-old woman in a persistent vegetative state, who was receiving mechanical ventilation in a New Jersey hospital's ICU after presenting with a drug overdose and suffering a cardiac arrest. Her father felt that his daughter would not want to remain alive in such a state and he wanted to be named her guardian so that he could order the removal of the mechanical ventilator. The hospital and the physicians involved in her care refused, arguing that removing the ventilator

would be euthanasia. The Supreme Court of New Jersey reasoned that Quinlan would have refused further treatment and that she had the right to refuse any life-sustaining treatment. Since the patient was incompetent to exercise that right, the court further ruled that the only practical way for that right to be maintained would be for the family to render their best judgment as to whether she would exercise it in these circumstances.

By ruling in this way, the *Quinlan* court rejected any distinction between withholding and withdrawing life-sustaining treatment and acknowledged the importance of surrogate decision-making in end-of-life care. The Quinlan opinion also went further by acknowledging the limitations of the law in resolving future conflicts in this arena and encouraged the use of hospital ethics consultation as a more appropriate mechanism for resolving these conflicts in the future. By 1991, this recommendation for an ethics consultation was operationalized through the Joint Commission on Accreditation of Healthcare Organization's (JCAHO's) requirement that (1) hospitals follow ethical behavior in its care, treatment, services, and business practices, and (2) they establish and maintain structures to support patient rights; these include patients' right to refuse care and patients' wishes relating to end-of-life decisions.[8]

In the years following Quinlan, multiple court cases in the United States firmly established the right of the competent patient to refuse any medical treatment. However, there was considerable variation in how different state courts felt it best to exercise this right of refusal for life-sustaining treatments in patients *without* decisional capacity. The issue of how different U.S. states dealt with the patient's right to refuse life-sustaining treatment first came to the U.S. Supreme Court through the *Cruzan* case.

Nancy Cruzan was a young woman hospitalized in Missouri in a persistent vegetative state after an automobile accident, who required artificial nutrition and hydration to stay alive. The family requested that the feedings be stopped because they felt that Nancy would not have wanted to continue treatment in her health state. The Missouri State Supreme Court ruled in 1988 that since the state had a legitimate interest in preserving life, life-sustaining treatments could only be removed by surrogate decision-makers if there was "clear and convincing evidence" confirming that the particular patient would have rejected such treatment.

The U.S. Supreme Court, in *Cruzan v. Missouri Department of Public Health* (1990), recognized the constitutional right of the competent person to refuse life-sustaining treatments of all types, including life-saving hydration and nutrition. At the same time, the Supreme Court affirmed the Missouri State Supreme Court by ruling that the United States Constitution did not prohibit a state from having a high evidentiary standard (clear and convincing standard lies somewhere between the civil standard of a preponderance of the evidence and the criminal standard of beyond a reasonable doubt) for surrogate decision-making regarding life-sustaining treatments.

In a concurring opinion, Sandra Day O'Connor suggested a larger role for advanced directives as a potential mechanism to safeguard the patient's interest in directing his or her medical care in the event that they become incompetent. Influenced by Sandra Day O'Connor's opinion, Senators Danforth (of Missouri) and Moynihan (of New York) enacted a law entitled the Patient Self Determination Act (PSDA), which became law in 1991 and required health care institutions to provide adult patients with information about advance directives upon admission.

In *Washington v Glucksberg and Quill v. Vacco* (1997), the question presented to the U.S. Supreme Court was whether prohibitions against physician-assisted suicide offended the United States Constitution. The Supreme Court concluded that terminally ill patients do not have the right to physician-assistance in suicide under the United States Constitution.

However, the Supreme Court did rule in favor of a patient's constitutional right to obtain relief from suffering, including terminal sedation. Justice O'Connor in *Glucksberg* inferred a constitutional right to "obtain relief from suffering" and Chief Justice Rehnquist in the majority opinion in *Vacco v. Quill* invoked the doctrine of double effect in his affirmation of the practice by clinicians of relieving pain with medicines, even if those medicines come with the possibility of hastening death.[11] The doctrine of double effect is a Catholic moral argument that tries to make distinctions between intended effects and merely foreseen effects by permitting an act to be done that may have two foreseen effects,

one good (such as relieving pain) and another harmful (such as death), when the intent is to produce the good effect and the harmful effect is foreseen but not intended. This doctrine, although philosophically imperfect, provides justification for the use of opioids and sedatives to maintain the comfort of the patient, even if the clinician sees the potential that the drugs may shorten the time to death.

In general, when asked to resolve disputes between families who request potentially inappropriate treatment and physicians who oppose it, courts in the United States have been reluctant to withdraw treatment that would lead to death over the objection of the family.[11] In the case of *Helga Wanglie*, an 86-year-old woman was in a persistent vegetative state after a series of medical complications over the course of several months, and was chronically dependent on the mechanical ventilator. The hospital wanted to remove the mechanical ventilator citing that the respirator was nonbeneficial. The patient's family objected on moral and religious grounds. The hospital then went to the Court asking for an independent conservator to make medical decisions for the patient instead of the family, but the court rejected the hospital's request. On the other hand, courts have also been reluctant to punish clinicians who act carefully and within professional standard to limit life-sustaining treatments. In *Gilgunn*, a Massachusetts jury imposed no liability on the hospital or the clinicians after they removed the ventilator from a terminally ill patient over the objection of her family.

ADVANCED CARE PLANNING

In response to *Quinlan* and *Cruzan*, U.S. states began to pass laws providing for the use of advance directives in which people could state what they wanted to be done in the event they became seriously ill and could not participate in their own medical decisions. In the *living will*, the patient anticipates a specific set of medical circumstances and can request or refuse specific types of treatment under each of these medical circumstances. With the *durable power of attorney for health care* (or health care proxy) form, the patient can choose in advance a surrogate decision-maker in the event they become unable to make medical decisions for themselves.

Advance care planning is the process by which patients, with facilitation by a trained professional, clarifies their current health state, goals, and objectives. Since living wills cannot be expected to anticipate all of the specific circumstances the patient could face in the ICU, families and/or surrogate decision-makers still need to understand the patient's wishes and values. Studies show that when families are included more upstream in the advance care planning process, advance directives may be helpful in aligning care with patient's preferences and in supporting surrogates during their decision-making for the patient.[12,13]

In the United States, a growing number of states have established templates that allow written directives to be translated into medical orders and can be accessible across multiple venues in the health care system.[14] POLST (Physician Orders for Life Sustaining Treatment) and MOLST (Medical Orders for Life-Sustaining Treatment) are examples of these templates that allow patients with advanced illness or frailty and/or the surrogate decision-maker to have an advanced care planning conversation about whether they want specific life-sustaining treatments in the event of an illness exacerbation.[15] Such forms usually enable a discussion of three categories of life-sustaining treatments: cardiopulmonary resuscitation in the event that the patient becomes pulseless; approaches to medical interventions in the event of an acute illness; and artificially administered nutrition and hydration in the event the patient cannot take fluids by mouth. Within "medical interventions," the POLST cues the clinician to three levels of possible intervention: "comfort measures only"; "limited additional interventions," which add to comfort measure treatments such as antibiotics, intravenous fluids, and cardiac monitoring but avoids mechanical ventilation or ICU level care; and "full treatment," which further adds a trial of life-sustaining treatments with no limitations in treatment (eg, intubation, advanced airway intervention, mechanical ventilation, cardioversion, transfer to the hospital, and ICU). When such forms are completed, they become medical orders immediately but can be changed or updated at any time.

SURROGATE DECISION-MAKING

Many critically ill patients are too sick or impaired neurologically to participate in their own health care decisions, particularly in the complex decisions about life-sustaining therapies. When a patient loses capacity to make medical decisions, their right to informed consent for a treatment is extended to the surrogate decision–maker, who was either previously designated by the patient or is identified by applicable local laws. Wherever they practice, clinicians should be familiar with the applicable local regulations on how surrogate decision-makers are determined when patients have not previously designated someone as their surrogate decision-maker.

Surrogates experience significant distress, anxiety, and guilt in having to be involved in medical decision-making in the ICU and clinicians need to be prepared to give surrogates guidance on the ethical standards for surrogate decision-making.[16,17] When a patient has completed a living will requesting or refusing specific types of care in specific medical situations, even if local laws do not make these requests legally binding, surrogates are expected to make decisions for the patient concordant with the patient's previously expressed wishes. When there is no evidence of the patient's prior wishes, surrogates are expected to make decisions for the patient based on what the patient would have wanted under the circumstances of the illness (ie, substituted judgment standard) by using what they know of the patient's philosophical, religious, and moral beliefs and values. When the surrogate does not have any way of knowing what the patient would have wanted or the patient has never had the capacity to make medical decisions, surrogates are then encouraged to make medical decisions in the patient's best interest, where they weight the risks and benefits of the treatment to the patient (ie, best interest standard).[4]

Some critically ill patients who lack decision-making capacity do not have a surrogate decision-maker or an advanced directive.[18] In such cases, clinicians have an ethical responsibility to act in the patient's best interest, given their understanding of the patient's medical conditions and prognosis. Since there is a great variation in hospital policies and local laws regarding the decision-making process for these patients, clinicians need to be aware of their hospital policies regarding such cases and consider involving ethics consultation to help with complex cases.

SHARED DECISION-MAKING

Critical care guidelines endorse a shared decision-making model in which the patient, if able, and/or the family play an active role in the decision-making in the ICU.[19] Shared decision-making is based on a relationship of mutual respect between the clinical team, who are considered the experts on prognosis and treatment options, and the patient/family, who are experts on the patient's values. The goal in medical decision-making is to reach a consensus regarding the value-laden treatments by discussing the nature of the decision, exchanging the relevant information, and discussing how each party prefers to make decisions. The clinical team shares the burden of the decision-making by being available to help clarify the patient's values and the impact of each option on the patient's goals and interests.[20] Patients and families vary widely in how they prefer to make the value-laden decisions in the ICU, ranging from a preference for complete control of the decision to deference to the clinicians' judgment. The shared decision-making model empowers clinicians to become skillful and flexible communicators who can disclose information, explore expectations, use narrative skills to make sense of complex medical situations, build relationships by explicitly providing emotional support, explore role preferences, and discuss concerns and conflicts openly.[21]

PALLIATIVE CARE IN THE ICU

With the rise of patients' rights movement, researchers conducted the Study to Understand Prognoses and Preferences for Outcomes and Risks of Treatment (SUPPORT), a large multicenter clinical trial that sought to better understand how seriously ill patients were treated in U.S. hospitals. The study found that physicians were not asking seriously ill hospitalized patients about their preferences regarding life-sustaining treatments near the end of life, that a significant percentage of the patients who died spent 10 or more days in the ICU before death, and that the family members remembered significant symptoms, including severe pain in the dying patients.[22] The results of the SUPPORT study generated a robust national discussion in the United States about the inadequacies of end-of-life care in hospitals and, together with the increased polarization around the issue of physician-assisted suicide, helped to catalyze the palliative care movement in the United States.[8]

Palliative care is an approach to care that grew out of a long tradition of hospice care, which provided intensive treatments aimed at relieving suffering in dying patients. Initially, palliative care was seen as a sequel to failed intensive care, and its role was restricted to patients who were actively dying. Over time, ICU clinicians have come to understand that it is difficult to predict survival in the ICU, and that survivors of critical illness often develop profound physical and psychological symptoms and functional and cognitive impairments.[3] Thus, clinicians have come to appreciate that both critically ill patients and survivors of critical illness may benefit from a multidisciplinary, patient-centered approach to care that aims at assessing and treating multiple sources of suffering.[3]

ICUs are increasingly integrating the principles of palliative care into the comprehensive care for all of their patients in an effort to increase the overall quality of care.[23] ICU palliative care focuses on the following principles: assessing and treating the patient's symptoms in the ICU; providing psychological and spiritual support to the patient and their families; facilitating proactive and compassionate communication between the clinical providers and the patient and their families so that treatments are better aligned with the patient's values and interests; planning transition; and support for both patient and family throughout the illness trajectory.[24] The hope is that by integrating palliative care principles into the care of all critically ill patients, the ICU environment will be better suited to support all patients with a high probability of death or impaired recovery.

Over the past decade, there has been a steady increase in the availability of palliative medicine specialists in acute care hospitals in the United States and the trend is seen in other countries as well.[25] Depending on the culture of the institution, some core elements of ICU palliative care can be provided as part of the routine care by members of the ICU team. In addition, a clinician champion in palliative care or use of protocols or order sets can also improve clinical practice in this area. For example, when ICU clinicians conduct routine, proactive meetings within 72 hours of the ICU admission with families of patients at high risk of death, patients spend less time in the ICU without any change in hospital mortality. The reduced length of stay has been attributed to the families and the clinicians reaching a consensus more quickly regarding the plan of care for the patient.[26] Other elements of the ICU palliative care may require consultation from a palliative care specialist (eg, refractory symptom management, conflict resolution regarding goals of treatment, providing support to a family with difficult family dynamics). Specialty palliative care consultation in the ICU has been associated with reduced length of stay, earlier identification of patients who are on a dying trajectory, and more transfer of dying patients to lower intensity care sites when appropriate.[27,28]

MEDICAL FUTILITY

Patients or their surrogates may request treatments in the ICU that the clinicians feel are futile. The root of the word futility (from the Latin *futilis* for leaky, vain, or worthless) suggests a very narrow definition in which a futile intervention literally cannot achieve its goals.[29] The concept of futility can be considered in two different ways. The notion of *quantitative futility* refers to an intervention with a small probability of achieving its physiologic purpose (eg, an intervention might be called futile if it has not worked in the past 100 cases). Clinicians also use futility in a more *qualitative* sense when the treatment in question is being used to achieve goals that the clinician thinks are inappropriate (eg, prolonging an inevitable death or prolonging a minimally conscious state).[29]

The principle of autonomy should not be interpreted to mean that the patient has the right to every requested medical intervention. However, when families or patients request a potentially futile treatment, clinicians should ask themselves what (or whose) goal is the intervention futile to achieve and be careful not to conflate their medical judgments with their value judgments. Clinicians are not ethically obligated to offer or provide treatments that they do not believe will achieve the patient's goals; however, sometimes a clinician's initial sense of what constitutes a benefit to the patient may be broadened by a culturally sensitive, empathic exploration of the patient's values. In the ICU, since the care is interdisciplinary, it is especially important for clinicians to seek consensus among the clinical team members about the appropriateness of a particular treatment approach.

Futility conflicts are often about fundamental differences in values about what makes a life worth living and/or what are the appropriate goals of modern medicine. Other contributory causes of these conflicts may include a misunderstanding of medical facts, including prognosis and the goals of treatment; surrogates' emotional stress; conflicts of interest on the part of the patient/family or clinical team; and intrateam or intrafamily conflict.[30] In most cases, a process-oriented approach to these conflicts that focuses on the best communication practices opens up the possibility for consensus.[31]

When conflicts arise in the ICU over medical decisions, an ethics consultant may be helpful in facilitating an ethically justifiable plan that best integrates the values, perspectives, and interests of the relevant stakeholders. In several studies, proactive ethics consultation in the ICU was associated with fewer days in the ICU and more decisions to forgo life-sustaining treatments without any increase in mortality.[32] Ethics consultants may also be helpful in developing and implementing hospital policies that allow for a "due process" approach to resolving futility conflicts.

PRINCIPLES AND PRACTICE OF LIMITING LIFE-SUSTAINING THERAPIES

Many patients who died in the ICU would have done so in the face of some limitation (withdrawal or withholding) of life-sustaining treatment, although there is a wide variability in this practice across the United State and in other countries.[2,33] ICU clinicians need to be highly skilled and knowledgeable in this aspect of ICU care. Secular ethical principles do not distinguish between withholding (ie, refraining from starting) and withdrawal (ie, stopping a treatment that is already underway) of life-sustaining treatments. In practice, for clinicians and surrogates, stopping a treatment already in place often feels emotionally different from not starting a treatment.

However, when there is a significant uncertainty about prognosis, not starting a treatment may be more difficult and may leave the family with unresolved questions about whether the treatment could have benefitted the patient. The time-limited trial of a particular treatment may be especially useful when the prognosis is uncertain, allowing the clinicians and families to directly assess the benefits of a particular treatment with the recognition that the treatment may be stopped if it does not achieve the patient's goals.[23]

The goal of withdrawing life-sustaining treatment is usually to remove treatments that are no longer wanted or are only serving to prolong the suffering or dying process of the patient.[23,34] In general, guidelines suggest that once a decision has been made to withdraw one life-sustaining treatment (eg, renal replacement therapy or vasopressors), clinicians should carefully consider the utility of other forms of life-sustaining treatment. Clinicians should document the meetings leading up to the decision in the medical record. Interdisciplinary teams should aim for consensus among the team members with direct patient care about how the life-sustaining treatments will be withdrawn. Because the withdrawal of mechanical ventilation has the greatest potential for patient discomfort, some clinicians prefer to remove other life-sustaining treatments (eg, vasopressors, pacemakers, intra-aortic balloon pumps) prior to removing the mechanical ventilator in dying patients, with the hope that death will occur while the patient is on the ventilator.[35]

The withdrawal of life-sustaining treatments is a clinical procedure like any other that is performed in the ICU and it requires expertise, careful preparation, appropriate documentation, and ongoing evaluation.[23,36] The ICU room should be transformed from one equipped to rescue to one more conducive to comfort, dignity, and quiet. Most families will not know what to expect during the process of withdrawal so key information should be provided to alleviate fears, worries, and concerns. Clinicians should be prepared to discuss prognosis and time to death after the withdrawal of a particular treatment. Estimates based on the clinical situation of the patient can sometimes be helpful to families who need more guidance so that they can make arrangements. The possibility of transfer out of the ICU is best discussed openly with families before it is initiated. Spiritual or emotional support should be offered and provided to the patient or family when appropriate.

The mechanical ventilator is the most common treatment that is withdrawn in the anticipation of death in the ICU.[37] There is no optimal strategy for removing the mechanical ventilator from the patient and there is considerable variation in practice. Some clinicians prefer to withdraw the mechanical ventilator and the endotracheal tube in one step, whereas others prefer to maintain the artificial airway to facilitate suctioning and prevent airway obstruction. Effective sedation and analgesia are crucial both before the ventilator is removed and afterwards. Some key steps to this process include ensuring that the patient is comfortable *before* initiating the withdrawal of the mechanical ventilator, assessing the likelihood of imminent death after the withdrawal of the ventilator, and being prepared with bedside medication for analgesia and sedation as appropriate for the clinical scenario.[38] Monitors should probably be turned off and, after the ventilator or endotracheal tube is removed, oral suctioning and intensive symptom management should be initiated. Neuromuscular blocking agents have no role in withdrawal of the mechanical ventilator or any other life-sustaining treatments.[23] Although patients may "look" comfortable during the process of withdrawal with the use of these medications, these drugs preclude any assessment of symptoms and do not have any analgesic or sedative properties. Therefore, their use cannot be justified as part of a comfort-oriented approach. ICU clinicians should become comfortable with the assessment and treatment of end-of-life symptoms (eg, pain, dyspnea, delirium, dry mouth) in patients who cannot self-report, so that the withdrawal of the mechanical ventilator is as comfortable for the patient and the families as possible.[39]

REFERENCES

1. Angus DC, Barnato AE, Linde-Zwirble WT, et al. Use of intensive care at the end of life in the United States: an epidemiologic study. *Crit Care Med*. 2004;32:638-643.
2. Prendergast TJ, Luce JM. Increasing incidence of withholding and withdrawal of life support

from the critically ill. *Am J Respir Crit Care Med.* 1997;155:15-20.

3. Desai SV, Law TJ, Needham DM. Long-term complications of critical care. *Crit Care Med.* 2011;39:371-379.

4. Beauchamp TL, Childress JF. *Principles of Biomedical Ethics.* 6th ed. New York, NY: Oxford University Press; 1999.

5. Will JF. A brief historical and theoretical perspective on patient autonomy and medical decision making: Part I: The beneficence model. *Chest.* 2011;139:669-673.

6. Copp D. *The Oxford Handbook of Ethical Theory.* New York, NY: Oxford University Press; 2006.

7. Menikoff J. *Law and Bioethics: An Introduction.* Washington, DC: Georgetown University Press; 2001.

8. Fins JJ. *A Palliative Ethic of Care: Clinical Wisdom at Life's End.* Sudbhury, MA: Jones and Barlett Publishers; 2006.

9. Appelbaum PS. Clinical practice. Assessment of patients' competence to consent to treatment. *N Engl J Med.* 2007;357:1834-1840.

10. Luce JM, White DB. A history of ethics and law in the intensive care unit. *Crit Care Clin.* 2009;25:221-237, x.

11. Luce JM, Alpers A. Legal aspects of withholding and withdrawing life support from critically ill patients in the United States and providing palliative care to them. *Am J Respir Crit Care Med.* 2000;162:2029-2032.

12. Silveira MJ, Kim SY, Langa KM. Advance directives and outcomes of surrogate decision making before death. *N Engl J Med.* 2010;362:1211-1218.

13. Detering KM, Hancock AD, Reade MC, Silvester W. The impact of advance care planning on end of life care in elderly patients: randomised controlled trial. *Br Med J.* 2010;340:c1345.

14. Sabatino CP. The evolution of health care advance planning law and policy. *Milbank Q.* 2010;88:211-239.

15. Physician Orders for Life-Sustaining Treatment Paradigm. http://www.ohsu.edu/polst/ Accessed February 20, 2014.

16. Wendler D, Rid A. Systematic review: the effect on surrogates of making treatment decisions for others. *Ann Intern Med.* 2011;154:336-346.

17. Curtis JR, Engelberg RA, Wenrich MD, Shannon SE, Treece PD, Rubenfeld GD. Missed opportunities during family conferences about end-of-life care in the intensive care unit. *Am J Respir Crit Care Med.* 2005;171:844-849.

18. White DB, Curtis JR, Wolf LE, et al. Life support for patients without a surrogate decision maker: who decides? *Ann Intern Med.* 2007;147:34-40.

19. Davidson JE, Powers K, Hedayat KM, et al. Clinical practice guidelines for support of the family in the patient-centered intensive care unit: American College of Critical Care Medicine Task Force 2004-2005. *Crit Care Med.* 2007;35:605-622.

20. Scheunemann LP, Arnold RM, White DB. The facilitated values history: helping surrogates make authentic decisions for incapacitated patients with advanced illness. *Am J Respir Crit Care Med.* 2012;186:480-486.

21. Torke AM, Petronio S, Sachs GA, Helft PR, Purnell C. A conceptual model of the role of communication in surrogate decision making for hospitalized adults. *Patient Educ Couns.* 2012;87:54-61.

22. A controlled trial to improve care for seriously ill hospitalized patients. The study to understand prognoses and preferences for outcomes and risks of treatments (SUPPORT). The SUPPORT Principal Investigators. *J Am Med Assoc.* 1995;274:1591-1598.

23. Truog RD, Campbell ML, Curtis JR, et al. Recommendations for end-of-life care in the intensive care unit: a consensus statement by the American College of Critical Care Medicine. *Crit Care Med.* 2008;36:953-963.

24. Clarke EB, Curtis JR, Luce JM, et al. Quality indicators for end-of-life care in the intensive care unit. *Crit Care Med.* 2003;31:2255-2262.

25. Goldsmith B, Dietrich J, Du Q, Morrison RS. Variability in access to hospital palliative care in the United States. *J Palliat Med.* 2008;11:1094-1102.

26. Lilly CM, Sonna LA, Haley KJ, Massaro AF. Intensive communication: four-year follow-up from a clinical practice study. *Crit Care Med.* 2003;31:S394-S399.

27. Norton SA, Hogan LA, Holloway RG, Temkin-Greener H, Buckley MJ, Quill TE. Proactive palliative care in the medical intensive care unit: effects on length of stay for selected high-risk patients. *Crit Care Med.* 2007;35:1530-1535.

28. Campbell ML, Guzman JA. A proactive approach to improve end-of-life care in a medical intensive care unit for patients with terminal dementia. *Crit Care Med.* 2004;32:1839-1843.

29. Schneiderman LJ. Defining medical futility and improving medical care. *J Bioeth Inq.* 2011;8:123-131.

30. Goold SD, Williams B, Arnold RM. Conflicts regarding decisions to limit treatment: a differential diagnosis. *J Am Med Assoc.* 2000;283:909-914.

31. Rubin SB. If we think it's futile, can't we just say no? *HEC Forum*. 2007;19:45-65.

32. Schneiderman LJ, Gilmer T, Teetzel HD, et al. Effect of ethics consultations on nonbeneficial life-sustaining treatments in the intensive care setting: a randomized controlled trial. *J Am Med Assoc*. 2003;290:1166-1172.

33. Sprung CL, Cohen SL, Sjokvist P, et al. End-of-life practices in European intensive care units: the Ethicus Study. *J Am Med Assoc*. 2003;290:790-797.

34. Rubenfeld GD. Implementing effective ventilator practice at the bedside. *Curr Opin Crit Care*. 2004;10:33-39.

35. Faber-Langendoen K. The clinical management of dying patients receiving mechanical ventilation. A survey of physician practice. *Chest*. 1994;106:880-888.

36. Rubenfeld GD. Principles and practice of withdrawing life-sustaining treatments. *Crit Care Clin*. 2004;20:435-451.

37. Cook D, Rocker G, Marshall J, et al. Withdrawal of mechanical ventilation in anticipation of death in the intensive care unit. *N Engl J Med*. 2003;349:1123-1132.

38. Wilson WC, Smedira NG, Fink C, McDowell JA, Luce JM. Ordering and administration of sedatives and analgesics during the withholding and withdrawal of life support from critically ill patients. *J Am Med Assoc*. 1992;267:949-953.

39. Brody H, Campbell ML, Faber-Langendoen K, Ogle KS. Withdrawing intensive life-sustaining treatment – recommendations for compassionate clinical management. *N Engl J Med*. 1997;336:652-657.

Intensive Talk: Delivering Bad News and Setting Goals of Care

Dana Lustbader, MD and Negin Hajizadeh, MD

KEY POINTS

1. Offering palliative care is an integral part of good ICU care.

2. A script for running an effective family meeting in the ICU may include a format like ASK–TELL–ASK.

3. Provide important pieces of information one section at a time, then wait and listen for a response.

4. In addition to disease-targeted interventions, always provide palliative options when appropriate.

5. During a family meeting after you have elicited input from all participants, make treatment recommendations based on the values and preferences expressed.

INTRODUCTION

One of the most important responsibilities of health care providers in the intensive care unit (ICU) is effective communication with seriously ill patients and their family members. Generally, ICU patients are unable to participate in medical decision-making. Therefore, discussions about prognosis and treatments are often held with family members. In this chapter, the term family member will be used to describe related family members, loved ones, or legal surrogates responsible for medical decision-making on behalf of the patient. The ICU family meeting should generally occur within 72 hours of ICU admission. Family meetings are associated with increased patient, family and provider satisfaction with the type of care received, and more preference congruent care. We outline key strategies for conducting meaningful and effective ICU family meetings.

IMPACT OF EFFECTIVE COMMUNICATION

Patients with an advance directive, or patients who participate in discussions with their doctor about their preferences for care as their disease progresses, receive less intensive care in the final weeks of life, are less likely to die in the hospital or ICU, and have improved quality of life.[1] Unfortunately, most patients in the ICU have not had prior discussions regarding their treatment preferences in the outpatient setting or on the medical and surgical floors with health care providers. These difficult conversations are therefore often left to members of the ICU team. Although earlier conversations about treatment preferences is preferred, studies show that patients and family members respond well to anyone with good communication skills, even if the provider does not have an established relationship with the patient or family. In fact, an ICU provider trained in effective communication may conduct a more successful family meeting than the primary physician.

Family satisfaction is directly impacted by effective communication strategies. Factors associated with increased satisfaction include high-quality communication, consistent information from all caregivers, use of empathetic statements, decision-making support, and family-centered care. Patient survival alone is not always correlated with increased family satisfaction.[2] The mnemonic VALUE has been developed to help providers better understand and manage family emotion during interactions and family meetings. The use of VALUE in a large ICU study during family meetings for patients who eventually died in the ICU showed that the surviving family members experienced less post-traumatic stress disorder, anxiety, and depression several months after the death of their loved one when these communication strategies were used. VALUE reminds us to value and appreciate what surrogates communicate (V), acknowledge emotion with reflective statements (A), listen (L), understand who the patient is as a person by asking open-ended questions (eg, "Can you tell me what kind of a person your mom was before she got sick?") (U), and to elicit questions (E).[3] This study highlights the importance of effective family meetings, not only for medical decision-making, but also for mitigating the suffering and bereavement of family members.[4]

IMPACT OF PALLIATIVE CARE

Regardless of the intensity of treatments, palliative care should be fully integrated with intensive care and not separate from potentially life supporting therapies. In fact, the marketing of palliative care as "an extra layer of support to the ICU care already being provided" has increased access to palliative care. In one groundbreaking study, patients with stage IV lung cancer, who had concurrent palliative care with cancer-directed treatment, were less likely to die in the hospital or ICU and had a better quality of life with less depression. Although the patients in the concurrent palliative care arm received less intensive care at the end of life, they lived three months longer than the control group receiving conventional cancer care alone.[5]

THE FAMILY MEETING IN 3 EASY STEPS: ASK–TELL–ASK

The skill of effective communication is as important as the ability to place a central line or treat sepsis and similarly requires practice. There are several key principles for effective family meetings. These include being prepared for the meeting, mindful listening, allowing time for periods of silence, verbal expressions of empathy, avoidance of medical jargon, and ensuring that family members understand the information. These are described below.

Prior to the family meeting, the clinician should review all pertinent information. Prognostic information should be clarified using medical data resources such as eprognosis.org.[6] The physician should consult with the bedside nurse, who often has key pieces of information about the patient's care and about any nuances of family politics that may become evident in the family meeting. The nurse also plays a crucial role in reinforcing concepts discussed during the meeting and answering questions later from family members. Other team members may also be useful during the family meeting such as the ICU social worker or chaplain. The location of the meeting should be in a private space without the concern for interruptions, and all participants should be seated. If a room is not available, the meeting could occur at the end of a hall or an empty waiting room. It is imperative that all participants have the chance to be seated. Most successful meetings last about 30 minutes and those that run beyond this time frame may in fact lose their effectiveness as the ability for family members to take in new information is exhausted.

Start the meeting by introducing everyone in the room and explaining the role of each provider. About half of the meeting time should be spent actively listening to family members. During a 30-minute family meeting, the clinician should be listening for 15 minutes and allow time for questions. This can be hard for some clinicians but listening rather than talking is critically important for an effective meeting and may even mitigate the risk of post-traumatic stress disorder, anxiety, and depression for survivors. Participants feel validated and suffer less guilt later. There may also be periods of silence when family members are grappling with difficult news. The clinician should respect the need to absorb this information and allow time for silence before moving on with an empathetic statement such as: "I know this news is very difficult for you to hear." Verbal expressions of empathy include statements such as: "I wish I had better news about your mom." "I wish his condition could improve." These verbal expressions recognize and legitimize the emotions being felt by family members while creating a relationship of trust with the provider.

Communication should also avoid medical jargon. Phrases like "the prognosis is grim" or "her ARDS is preventing weaning" are meaningless to most lay people and can hijack a well-intentioned family meeting. Instead a clinician could say: "I am worried he is beginning to die." "The scarring in his lungs is preventing him from being able to breathe without the life support machine. I'm concerned his lungs may not get better. We will have to make some difficult decisions in the next few days about what to do." Difficult news can be introduced with a sentence in preparation such as: "Unfortunately I have some bad news to share with you about your father."

To ensure that family members have understood the information, a simple framework for the meeting is ASK–TELL–ASK.

1. ASK—Ask the patient and family member about their own understanding of medical condition and prognosis. This can be done with a question such as:

    "Can you tell me what you know about your mom's condition so far?"

    "What have the doctors told you about your brother?"

    "So I can better understand, can you tell me what you know about your cancer and what is likely to happen now?"

    "What do you think is going on with your son?" "Can you tell me how you came up with this information?"

2. TELL—Provide information about the medical condition, treatment options, and prognosis. Deliver the news in language that is simple and easy to understand. Avoid all medical jargon. Generally, it is advised to summarize the medical condition and major problems to be discussed during the family meeting. Keep in mind that family members are stressed and may have limited ability to understand large blocks of information at one time. Give two or three bits of information at a time and pause to allow families to absorb the information and in case clarifying questions arise. Provide information about treatment options, including risks and benefits for each treatment.

When discussing therapeutic options, it is important to include palliative options in addition to disease-directed therapies, if appropriate, and to frame palliative care as a treatment option. This can be done with statements such as:

"Since the dementia is very advanced, and your mom has not been able to come off the breathing machine, we have two options for our next steps. We can remove the breathing machine and keep her comfortable or we can place a more permanent breathing tube in her neck called a tracheostomy which would allow her to go to a nursing home on the breathing machine in about a week."

When discussing prognosis, always include the range of possible outcomes, given the uncertainty with each individual patient. For example, one might provide information for life expectancy in hours to days, days to weeks, weeks to months, or months to a year at the most. This can be done with statements such as:

"Most patients who have cancer in the lung and liver who are in the ICU for serious infection and low blood pressure like your grandmother die within days to a week."

3. ASK—Provide an opportunity for questions and expressions of emotion. Agree on a plan for next steps. Examples are:

    Can you tell me what you're most worried about right now?

    Given what we've just talked about, what is most important to you now?

    What do you think should be done now?

I wish I had better news for you. How can I help you cope right now?

Structure and reliability can be useful tools to better help families cope with grief and despair. To conclude the meeting, summarize the treatment plan and set up a time for follow-up discussions when appropriate. For example:

So we discussed that we will do a 48 hour trial on the breathing machine with antibiotics for the pneumonia and emphysema. We'll meet again here in two days at 4 PM to re-evaluate how things are going. Is that okay with you?

We will wait for the priest to come later this morning. We will remove the breathing tube and stop the kidney dialysis after his visit and when your other children arrive sometime later today. We will continue to do everything possible to keep your daughter comfortable.

We will start the artificial feeding today through the tube in the nose. We will also get another brain scan today to see if the size of the stroke and bleeding has increased. If so, we will call the neurosurgeon back to help us decide if surgery would be helpful. We will meet again tomorrow around 11 AM after morning rounds to discuss the results of the brain scan with you.

Finally, express empathy again at the end of the meeting. For example:

I wish things were different for your mom. We will work hard to make sure she is as comfortable as possible.

I can see how well you have cared for your dad in your home over the past three years as his dementia and heart failure progressed. Unfortunately this stroke was so large and so sudden, there was nothing anyone could have done to prevent it. We will continue to do everything we can for his comfort. I am so sorry.

MANAGING FAMILY EMOTION

A wide range of family emotions should be expected during family meetings. The clinician should be present emotionally (responsive to the emotions of family members), and mindful of the verbal and nonverbal responses from family members. When emotions escalate, often the best course of action is to listen and to recognize the emotion. If anger at a particular situation is being expressed, one might say: "Let me make sure I understand you correctly—you're angry that the evening nurse did… is that right?" Or you might say: "Thank you for making me aware of that problem; I will speak with him about what you've mentioned." When a problem is brought up during the family meeting that can be validated, one should say something like: "You're right, I wish it didn't take two days for the CT scan to be performed. I can see why you're angry." Often validating or hearing what is of concern in the moment can open doors for a more productive meeting regarding the treatment plan and goals of care by establishing a relationship built on trust.

DISCUSSING PROGNOSIS

Providers are often afraid to discuss accurate prognostic information with patients and their families for fear of removing all hope or causing sadness. A study of hospitalized elderly patients showed that patient preferences for end-of-life care were not documented or incorrectly documented in the medical record 70% of the time.[7] Most studies, however, indicate that discussions of prognosis lead to greater patient satisfaction, improved concordance between treatments wanted and those actually received, less aggressive care at the end of life, and improved psychological outcomes for patients and their families. In fact, inadequate preparation for death is associated with poor bereavement outcomes for survivors with complicated grief, post-traumatic stress disorder, and a sense of regret or guilt.

In providers who do discuss prognosis, survival is often overestimated. In one study physicians overestimated survival by 5-fold.[8] In fact, the longer a physician knows a patient, the more likely they are to provide an overly optimistic survival rate. Therefore, providers should prepare for these discussions with tools that use evidence-based calculators to improve prognostication such as eprognosis.org.[9]

Despite prognostic communication, families may not "hear" what clinicians tell them. Surrogate decision-makers generally believe that their loved one has a better chance of survival than the odds being cited.[10] For example, if a clinician says there is a 10% chance of survival, the family member may believe that their loved one has about a 50% chance. These optimistic biases may be due to the belief that the patient is stronger than most or that the provider is misinformed and does not have all the information.

A family member may say: "My mother is a fighter. She had bad pneumonia before and walked out of here just fine last month." A reasonable response to this may be to highlight why this situation is different from before and the outcome will likely be different as well. One might say: "I understand your mom is a fighter and survived the bad pneumonia last month. This time is different though because your mom is on a life support machine now and the emphysema has progressed. I'm worried she won't be able to breathe on her own again."

Optimistic biases are further reinforced by television shows that depict unrealistic survival rates following cardiopulmonary resuscitation (CPR) and create an expectation by family members of overly hopeful results and superior functional outcomes than are actually possible.[11] Here, the Ask–Tell–Ask framework of communication also allows for clarification.

A family member may ask a question: "How long does she have to live?" The provider should answer honestly if she knows. For example, one might give an accurate range and say: "Most people in her condition can live for days to a week." A follow up might be: "Knowing that time is short, are there others we should call to be here now?"

It is equally important to discuss a patient's likely functional outcome if they do survive their ICU or hospital course. This may significantly impact medical decisions. Uncertainty can be acknowledged with phrases such as:

> I wish I could be more certain right now. Your mom is very sick and the stroke was quite large. We'll have a better understanding of her chances of surviving this over the next two days as we follow her blood pressure. Right now it is dangerously low. In terms of knowing her outcome, it may take weeks to know if she survives.

> We are going to do everything we can to help your daughter's body recover from this serious infection. The kinds of things we'll be looking for are improvement in blood pressure, the lung function and whether she wakes up in the next few days. We will communicate with you at each step along the way.

Finally, when decisions are made for patients to receive life-supporting technologies, they should include clearly defined markers of success or failure of the intervention, and an end-point if unsuccessful. This will facilitate discontinuation of unwanted life-sustaining therapies if the condition fails to improve or deteriorates. Time-limited trials may be warranted if there is uncertainty about the reversibility of the illness. For example, a 48-hour trial of mechanical ventilation and ICU care may be employed to assess whether the pneumonia resolves in an elderly patient with end-stage heart failure, and can be withdrawn if there is no clinical improvement or clinical decline.

It should be noted that the overall goal of effective communication strategies in the ICU is to align medically appropriate treatments with patient and family values. For some, every moment of life has value regardless of quality. For these patients, family members may believe that survival alone, despite the fact that the patient may be ventilator-dependent, comatose with a feeding tube, and discharged to a long-term care facility, is an acceptable outcome.

OFFERING PALLIATIVE CARE

Palliative care is an integral part of good ICU care. One strategy for involving palliative care consultants in the ICU is the use of screening tools to identify patients for whom consultation could benefit.[12] Several clinical triggers exist to prompt a palliative care consultation and include ICU patients with a hospital length of stay greater than 10 days prior to ICU admission, stage IV cancer, age greater than 80 years with two comorbidities, stroke and respiratory failure, terminal dementia, multisystem organ failure, and patients post cardiac arrest.[13] Others have used the surprise question: "Would I be surprised if this patient died in one year?" If the answer to this self-addressed question is no, palliative options should be considered and discussed.[14]

THE DIFFICULT FAMILY— MANAGING CONFLICT

The difficult or hostile family presents unique challenges when leading a family meeting. It is generally advised to start by naming the emotion being observed and allowing the family member to express their anger or frustration. One might say: "I see how angry you are about the care your daughter is receiving in the ICU." "I can see how angry you are that the CT scan wasn't done this morning. Let me find out what time it is scheduled for today?" On the other hand, some recommend to understate the emotion and to instead show curiosity, for example: "I'm wondering if you are concerned." The argument being that "emotion naming" may make patients feel as though they were being labeled.[15] With either style, practice and feedback will help the clinician master this particularly difficult skill.

The family that "wants everything done" in the setting of terminal illness is generally expressing intense grief and sadness at their impending loss. Rather than take the phrase to literally mean the family wants intubation, surgery, chemotherapy, or resuscitation during the dying process, it is best to explore what is medically appropriate for the patient, given the clinical condition, and discuss this with the family while acknowledging their intense pain. Clinicians should only offer and provide treatments that are medically appropriate. There is no medical, ethical, or legal obligation to offer treatments that will not work to benefit the patient and that violate accepted medical guidelines or ethical standards of care. One response to the family that "wants everything done" may be something like: "Can you tell me what you mean by everything done?" "What you are hoping the surgery will accomplish for your brother?" It is very important to understand what the family believes will happen if the requested treatments are done.

The expression of "I want everything done" may also indicate a lack of trust in the clinician or institution. With skillful communication by the clinician, trust is earned over time. Nonetheless, clinicians should only offer medically appropriate therapies that can include disease-directed treatments, palliative care, or both. A provider should feel comfortable making a therapeutic recommendation based on the values and goals expressed during an effectively run family meeting.

Examples of statements limiting the treatment options are:

> Based on what you've told me about your sister, I suggest we do everything we can to treat the infection and keep her comfortable. We will not put her on a life support machine if her breathing fails since this will not reverse the effects of the big stroke she had last week. You have shared with us that she would never want to live in a nursing home dependent on others and unaware of her surroundings.

And, "I know how much you want everything done for your dad's bowel problem now. Unfortunately he cannot have surgery because he is too sick and would die during the operation. I wish there was something we could do to treat the perforation but his other organs have all shut down and his blood pressure is dangerously low right now. We will do everything possible for his comfort today. I wish things were different."

THE DO-NOT-RESUSCITATE (DNR) DISCUSSION

"Getting the DNR" from a distressed family member for a terminally ill patient is a dreaded "task" often delegated to the most junior physician (the intern). This "task" can be very stressful, particularly when prior training has been limited. Several key strategies can make this discussion more effective. First, the clinician should recognize that this may be the first time anyone has addressed preferences for resuscitation with the patient or family member, despite the fact that the patient may have had the diagnosis of terminal illness for weeks or months prior to their current ICU admission. Second, the clinician should remember that resuscitation is a medical treatment aimed at restoring cardiopulmonary function when the heart or lungs stop working temporarily. CPR was never meant to be performed on a patient dying an expected death from a terminal disease. Third, the clinician should feel empowered to make a recommendation about the code status to the family member or patient based on what is known about their personally held values and beliefs:

> As we've discussed, the lung cancer has spread throughout your mom's body. Given what you've told me about the importance of independence and recognizing her grandchildren, I suggest we protect her from CPR if she dies. We will do everything possible to keep her comfortable during that time.
>
> The dementia is very advanced. Your dad got the pneumonia from the terminal dementia that caused an inability to swallow and breathe safely. He is not

responding to the antibiotics for his pneumonia and his blood pressure is dropping now. We need to discuss how his death will be handled here in the ICU. We have two options. We can attempt resuscitation which will not likely work because of his underlying illness, or we can do everything possible to keep him comfortable while he begins to die.

The trauma injuries from the car accident have severely damaged your son's lungs and brain. It does not look like he can survive. I'm worried he may die tonight. We need to discuss how we will handle his death. We can attempt resuscitation which very likely will not work since he is already on a life support machine, or we can keep him very comfortable and do everything possible for your son until that point.

I understand from what you and your rabbi shared with me that every moment of life is valued by your grandfather regardless of quality. Knowing this we will attempt resuscitation when his heart or lungs stop and perform whatever may be medically appropriate at that time. I am afraid those efforts will not likely work to bring your grandfather back, but I understand this resuscitative attempt is important to your grandfather and family.

When a patient suffers cardiopulmonary arrest, the clinician is required to perform resuscitative measures in accordance with medical standards, unless there is a DNR order. These efforts should be medically appropriate and the clinician should not perform medically inappropriate interventions on a patient simply because they are asked to do so. Additionally, there is no legal or ethical obligation to run a code for an arbitrarily defined period of time if the return of spontaneous circulation is unlikely. In situations where there is no DNR order for a terminally ill patient dying of their disease, only appropriate resuscitative measures should be attempted. In addition, the moral distress imposed on providers who are asked to perform procedures that are not medically indicated and are highly unlikely to reverse the disease process in a dying patient must be recognized. This moral distress is felt especially by the youngest team members who are not actively engaged or in control of the decision-making, such as interns, trainees, and new nurses.

Every effort should be made to ensure that treatments align with patient and family preferences, rather than just simply left to chance. Thoughtful

advance directives and DNR conversations ideally should occur in the outpatient setting when a diagnosis of a terminal disease is made.[16] In the absence of advance directives, opportunities often exist during the hospitalization prior to the ICU transfer for less rushed DNR discussions. Since the advent of the rapid response teams nationwide, there has been an increase in DNR discussions occurring and possibly protecting patients from being admitted to the ICU to die. This outcome of rapid response teams may in fact result in reduced intensity of treatment during dying, which may be more closely aligned with patient values and preferences.

CONCLUSION

Nearly 1 in 5 Americans die during or immediately after ICU-level care, often with pain, suffering, and isolation. Intensity of care at the end of life has also increased over the past decade with ICU use in the final 30 days of life in 2009 occurring at a rate of 29.5% for Medicare beneficiaries.[17] Family members of loved ones who die are at risk of experiencing post-traumatic stress disorder and depression. Clinicians should practice conducting effective family conferences as they would for any other ICU procedure. Several websites are available to enhance communication in the ICU with seriously ill patients and their family members, such as Improving Palliative Care in the ICU (IPAL-ICU)[18], Oncotalk Videos,[19] and IntensiveTalk.[20]

Skillfully led family meetings that focus on mindful listening and effective communication increase satisfaction and ensure that patients receive the ICU care they want and value.

REFERENCES

1. Nicholas LH, Langa KM, Iwashyna TJ, et al. Regional variation in the association between advance directives and end-of-life Medicare expenditures. *J Am Med Assoc*. 2011;306:1447-1453.
2. Wall RJ, Curtis JR, Cooke CR, et al. Family satisfaction in the ICU: differences between families of survivors and nonsurvivors. *Chest*. 2007;132:1425-1433.
3. Curtis JR, Engelberg RA, Wenrich MD, et al. Studying communication about end-of-life care

during the ICU family conference: development of a framework. *J Crit Care*. 2002;17:147-160.

4. Lautrette A, Darmon M, Megarbane B, et al. A communication strategy and brochure for relatives of patients dying in the ICU. *N Engl J Med*. 2007;356:469.

5. Temel JS, Greer JA, Muzikansky A, et al. Early palliative care for patients with metastatic non small cell lung cancer. *N Engl J Med*. 2010;363:733-742.

6. http://eprognosis.ucsf.edu/walter.php. Accessed December 25, 2013.

7. Heyland DK, Barwich D, Pichora D, et al. Failure to engage hospitalized elderly patients and their families in advance care planning. *JAMA Intern Med*. 2013;173:778-787.

8. Christakis NA, Lamont EB. Extent and determinants of error in doctors' prognoses in terminally ill patients: prospective cohort study. *Br Med J*. 2000;320:469-473.

9. http://eprognosis.ucsf.edu/walter.php. Accessed December 25, 2013.

10. Zier LS, Sotttile PD, Hong SY, et al. Surrogate decision makers' interpretation of prognostic information. *Ann Intern Med*. 2012;156:360-366.

11. Diem SJ, Lantos JD, Tulsky JA. Cardiopulmonary resuscitation on television, miracles and misinformation. *NEJM*. 1996;13;334:1578-1582.

12. Nelson JE, Curtis RJ, Mulkerin C, et al. Choosing and using screening criteria for palliative care consultation in the ICU: a report from the improving palliative care in the ICU (IPAL-ICU) Advisory Board. *Crit Care Med*. 2013;41:2318-2327.

13. Norton S, Hogan LA, Holloway RG, et al. Proactive palliative care in the medical intensive care unit: effects on length of stay for selected high-risk patients. *Crit Care Med*. 2007;35:1530-1535.

14. Moss A, Lunney JR, Stacey C, et al. Prognostic significance of the surprise question in cancer patients. *J Palliative Med*. 2010;13:837-840.

15. Back A, Arnold R, Tulsky J. *Mastering Communication with Seriously Ill Patients*. 1st ed. Cambridge: Cambridge University Press; 2009:27.

16. The Conversation Project. http://www.ihi.org/offerings/initiatives/conversationproject/Pages/default.aspx. Accessed January 20, 2014.

17. Teno JM, Gozalo PL, Bynum JP, et al. Change in end of life care for Medicare beneficiaries: site of death, place of care, and health care transitions in 2000, 2005, and 2009. *J Am Med Assoc*. 2013;309:470-477.

18. Center to Advance Palliative Care IPAL-ICU Program. http://www.capc.org/ipal. Accessed January 3, 2014.

19. Oncotalk Videos. http://depts.washington.edu/oncotalk/videos/. Accessed January 12, 2014.

20. IntensiveTalk. http://depts.washington.edu/icutalk/. Accessed January 12, 2014.

Can Intensivist Performance Be Measured?

Sharon Leung, MD, MS, FCCP

KEY POINTS

1. CMS launched Physician Compare in December of 2010, and it expanded to include information on the quality of physicians' care in 2013. Measuring and reporting on the performance of doctors represents an effort to move to a more transparent healthcare system.

2. The strategy the IOM recommended to improve quality of care was to pay for performance (P4P) or financial incentives to transform behaviors to achieve greater value.

3. Process measures are more highly sensitive to differences in the quality of care and are easier to interpret. However, a process measure is only of value if it is assumed to have a link to a meaningful outcome. By itself, it has little intrinsic value.

4. One advantage of outcome measurement, for example, mortality rate, is that it is a measure that is important on its own, even if the differences have nothing to do with the quality of care.

5. One of the main issues of measuring intensivist performance is physician attribution. Each episode of care would involve multiple intensivists and other physicians.

6. Using ICU LOS as a process measure would discourage intensivists from providing time-consuming, yet important, end-of-life care for ICU patients, leading to more fragmentation of care.

7. Even though risk adjustment applies, using hospital mortality as a quality-outcome measure would not account for the impact of palliative care and the ability to transfer to LTACs.

8. The current system has not yet been made to link the fragmented entities caring for these patients with critical illnesses around accountability for value.

9. To improve service productivity, measuring and monitoring performance and its variance is a fundamental requirement for identifying efficiencies and best practices and for spreading them throughout the system or organization.

10. Advancing performance measurement at the physician level is the vital strategy on the policy agenda when considerable unexplained variation exists in practices that lead to poor quality, inefficient care delivery, and waste of resources.

INTRODUCTION

The US health system is the most expensive system in the world, and yet numerous developing countries outperform us.[1] Patients with critical illnesses account for the majority of healthcare expenditures per capita. According to a 2009 study by the Medicare Payment Advisory Commission (MedPAC), the top 5% of spenders account for 50% of all healthcare spending, totaling $623 billion, or nearly $41,000 per patient.[2] Since the population is aging and medical technology is advancing, this group of patients is growing rapidly. Managing patients with critical illnesses presents considerable challenges: high-cost care, frequent readmissions, and dissatisfaction of care among them.[3]

ICU care is labor- and resource-intensive. The focus on quality performance and maintaining quality processes is vital to critical care. In the United States, the major players monitoring ICU quality performance include the Agency for Healthcare Research and Quality, the National Quality Forum (NQF), the Volunteer Hospital Association, the Institute for Healthcare Improvement, the Leapfrog Group, and the Joint Commission. In 2010, the NQF endorsed hospital mortality and intensive-care-unit (ICU) length of stay (LOS) as quality indicators.[4] Usually when the NQF measure is endorsed, an exploration of policy around these measures is anticipated. Also, the growing emphasis on processes of care and outcomes is pushing providers to broaden the focus of ICU metrics beyond LOS and mortality to include readmission rates, core measures, and patient satisfaction.

However, can performance indicators such as ICULOS, ICU mortality, and readmission rates be used to measure intensivist performance? If so, what about intensivists working in safety-net hospitals with a high percentage of patients who are uninsured? On the other hand, how can accountability be spread among physicians since each ICU patient is likely to be treated by multiple intensivists and other physicians? What would be the financial implications and consequences of using such measures? The aim of this chapter is to appraise whether these performance measures are appropriate and unbiased in measuring intensivist performance.

BACKGROUND
The ACA

Most of the health systems are now facing the same fundamental challenge: how to deliver broad access to health services while improving quality of care and controlling costs. Greater competition has often been proposed as a solution that addresses each element of this challenge. The performance failures of our healthcare system are largely invisible and will continue to be invisible as long as we do not have systems that allow us to track quality performance of the providers that are the central suppliers of our health care.

The landscape is changing. CMS launched Physician Compare in December of 2010, and it expanded to include information on quality of physicians' care in 2013. Measuring and reporting on the performance of doctors represents an effort to move to a more transparent healthcare system. In the near future, Physician Compare will provide information on physicians whether they provide recommended care to patients or not. New recommendations from the Joint Commission and CMS mandate the tracking of individual provider's competency through the following methods: Ongoing Professional Practice Evaluation on appropriateness of privileges, procedural volume, patient satisfaction, and professional interactions.

The Institute of Medicine (IOM) recognized that payment influences provider behavior. The strategy the IOM recommended to improve quality of care was to pay for performance (P4P) or financial incentives to transform behaviors to achieve greater value.[5,6] Physician Quality Reporting System (PQRS) was a first step in this direction.[7] Value-based purchasing (VBP) is a strategy that links payments to value of care over the entire continuum of patient treatment and hinges on recognizing and rewarding shared accountability among providers.[8] CMS is working to transform the Medicare program from a passive payer to an active purchaser of high-quality healthcare services by linking payment to the value of services delivered.[9]

Quality Indices to Measure ICU Care

The aims of using performance indicators are to inform policy making or strategy at a regional and/or national level, to improve the quality of care, to monitor performance of healthcare funders, to identify poor performers, and to protect public safety. The main issue is which performance indicators are able to differentiate a genuine difference in quality. Process and outcome measures are frequently used in assessing quality care in the ICU. Process measures are more highly sensitive to differences in the quality of care and are easier to interpret. One advantage of outcome measurement, for example, mortality rate, is that it is a measure that is important on its own, even if the differences have nothing to do with the quality of care.[10] It has been used frequently in the critically ill population, but it is important to bear in mind that outcome measures are not a direct measure of quality of care. On the other hand, a process measure is only of value if it is assumed to have a link to a meaningful outcome. By itself, it has little intrinsic value.[10] Thus, robust case-mix adjustment systems are needed before a raw number is evaluated. While it is tempting to use mortality to identify poor performers, its appropriateness needs to be considered for each specific disease and operation.

Quality Performance Tied to Reimbursement

Starting October 1, 2012, the Centers for Medicare and Medicaid Services (CMS) began reducing payments to hospitals with excess 30-day, all-cause, risk-adjusted, hospital readmission rates for pneumonia, acute myocardial infarction, and heart failure. According to MedPAC in 2007: "Readmission is generally more likely the more severely ill a patient is—even within the same diagnosis-related group (DRG)." Severely ill patients whose LOS exceeded the applicable DRG by a factor of two were 26.6% more likely to be readmitted.[11] Patients with a number of co-morbidities are at an increased risk for readmission. Also, patients discharged to an SNF or long-term care facility had twice the risk of 30-day hospital readmission.[11]

QUALITY PERFORMANCE *CANNOT* BE MEASURED IN INTENSIVISTS

Physician Attribution

One of the main issues of measuring intensivist performance is physician attribution. Each episode of

care would involve multiple intensivists and other physicians. How should accountability be spread among all specialists? This issue is especially germane to the ICU population because a majority of patients have multiple conditions and may be treated by multiple physicians. Moreover, nearly three-quarters of the care by intensivists in the United States is delivered in what is considered an "open" or "low-intensity" ICU staffing model: An intensivist makes treatment recommendations but has no authority over patient care.[12] Only in a small percentage of ICUs—mostly medical ICUs and ICUs in teaching hospitals—is critical care provided in a "high-intensity" or "closed" staffing pattern, in which treatment decisions are cohesively managed under the guidance of one intensivist.[12,13]

Therefore, intensivists in the open system more often treat episodes with multiple physicians and to the extent that efficiency varies among the physicians. Intensivists could be unfairly penalized or rewarded if the other physicians are more inefficient or more efficient. Also, multiple attributions could increase the number of episodes attributed (at least partially) to physicians, increasing the statistical precision of performance measures for them.

ICU LOS

ICU LOS is a process measure that can be independent of quality and is easily manipulated. Encouraging earlier transfer out of the ICU could increase the risk of patient harm and increase readmission rate. On the other hand, in states that have access to LTACs, patients can be transferred to LTACs early in their course of treatment. Thus, without another measure, looking at ICU readmission, there may be pressure for clinicians to discharge ICU patients prematurely. There is potential, however, for adverse consequences that may harm patients and ultimately increase healthcare costs. Furthermore, ICU LOS should always account for ICU mortality and ICU readmission. The measures together balance concerns regarding transferring patients faster because, while the LOS measure may improve, the mortality measure is unlikely to improve and may even worsen.[14,15]

There is the potential that hospitals will be rewarded unfairly by transferring a large number of patients to LTACs and encouraging the overuse of post-acute care facilities, which would drive up overall costs. At the same time, the safety-net hospitals will be penalized because the uninsured have no other option for care. Thus, in states without LTACs, both safety-net and non-safety-net hospitals would have increased ICU LOS.

Another issue is coordination of care. In the United States, critical care and palliative care are mutually exclusive entities.[16] After failing a prolonged treatment in the ICU, intensivists are often the first to discuss the goals of care with patients who have reached their end-of-life and their caregivers. Using ICU LOS as a process measure would discourage intensivists from providing time-consuming, yet important, end-of-life care for ICU patients, leading to more fragmentation of care. Having the potential penalty in mind, a goals-of-care conversation is often difficult; intensivists may find it easier simply to transfer the dying patient out of the ICU or into the LTACs.

Hospital Mortality

Even though risk adjustment applies, using hospital mortality as a quality-outcome measure would not account for the impact of palliative care and the ability to transfer to LTACs. Mortality, in general, is higher in safety-net hospitals. Deaths from medical errors and deaths resulting from the decision not to pursue aggressive care are very different things. More than 90% of deaths are unrelated to unsafe care. Most other publicly available quality measures refer only to the in-patient mortality, creating an incentive to move patients to LTACs and other facilities when an end-of-life circumstance arises, an option that is not feasible in a safety-net hospital. Indeed, prior research shows that benchmarking-based in-hospital mortality simply delays death or shifts the site of death to an LTAC, without actually reducing overall mortality.[15]

Readmission Rates

Hospitals that serve economically disadvantaged populations, which presumably have less access to care in the community and lower levels of self-efficacy in navigating a complex, fragmented healthcare system, are going to be penalized the same as hospitals serving populations that do not

struggle with these complexities. On the one hand, the safety-net hospitals cannot afford any reduction in resources. Generally speaking, states with LTACs would have lower readmission rates compared to states without LTACs. These measures reflect a process of care that is independent of quality and that can be misleading.

PERFORMANCE *CAN* BE MEASURED IN INTENSIVISTS
Physician Attribution

Most stakeholders recognize that even with perfect information it would be difficult to equitably divide responsibility for complicated mixtures of resource utilization among multiple physicians treating a single patient in an episode. Therefore, the best way is to try to arrive at a reasonable approximation to reality in these situations. Instead of using single attribution, multiple attribution acknowledges that the decision maker, if there is one, has incomplete control over treatment by intensivists and other physicians, even if the decision maker referred the patient to those other physicians.

ICU LOS

One benefit of performance measurement is to encourage changes—particularly systemic changes—that improve patient outcomes. Public reporting of ICU outcomes can provide the stimulus for needed system changes and appropriate use of resources. The ICU mortality measure has been publicly reported in California since 2007. Developers and implementers of the measure have not received feedback from hospitals identifying unintended consequences. According to MedPAC in March 2011, since reporting of the measure began, patient risk profiles are basically unchanged, but ICU mortality has declined by 0.5%—a statistically significant difference.[17] There has also been excellent engagement in benchmarking and quality-improvement strategies across the ICUs in California as a result of the public reporting of the mortality measure.

The noisy, active ICU is probably not the best environment for end-of-life care, and transfer to other units may be appropriate and desirable. The transfer will only affect the LOS measure since an in-hospital death is still included in the mortality measure.

Hospital Mortality

The suggestion that a 30-day mortality measure would be an alternative to avoid discharge bias has been studied.[18] Comparing in-hospital and 30-day mortality, there was little change in performance, particularly at the high- and low-performance levels. The data from the National Death Index required for 30-day morality measures is expensive, and its availability is delayed by at least 2 years. On balance, the in-hospital measure provides good data in a timely manner.

Readmission Rates

CMS has gone on record as stating that there are several safety-net hospitals that do not show evidence of higher-than-expected readmissions rates. This implies that it is not an unaccomplished act that these hospitals are unable to make improvements in care delivery and services to reduce avoidable rehospitalization.

DISCUSSION

For patients with critical illnesses, improving care coordination does not necessarily mean the index hospitalization would have a shorter LOS and a lower mortality. Whichever variables are chosen must satisfy several preconditions. They must be relevant to deciding whether high-quality care is delivered. Mortality and LOS are simple to measure, but they are only one piece of a larger puzzle. Measuring one process without understanding other processes may be misleading. The current system has not yet been made to link the fragmented entities caring for these patients with critical illnesses around accountability for value. Implementing performance measures such as ICU LOS would only widen the gap between safety and non-safety-net hospitals.

ICU LOS and hospital mortality may be good surrogates for an adverse event: medical errors and hospital-acquired infections; however, there are certain conditions that require longer LOS with better patient outcomes that may lead to reduced

cost overall. The more appropriate indicators should include the total cost of care, outcomes of each chronic disease management separately, management of adverse events, as well as patient and caregiver satisfaction.

To improve coordination and decrease fragmentation of care, intensivists should be encouraged to broaden care beyond the acute episode and to weigh in on quality of life post-ICU care.[16] There should be greater responsibility and accountability placed on physicians to discuss the prognosis and goals of care. Using ICU LOS as a process measure would adversely affect the quality of care in patients with critical and terminal illnesses. On the other hand, if a hospital has a lower mortality rate, it could mean a greater proportion of its discharged patients are eligible for readmission. To some extent, a higher readmission rate may indicate successful care.[19]

To improve service productivity, measuring and monitoring performance and its variance is a fundamental requirement for identifying efficiencies and best practices and for spreading them throughout the system or organization. Although some variance is inevitable, much of it can be controlled if each system properly accounts for differences in the type of patients they serve and then defines and collects data uniformly across different patient populations.[20] To do so, the intensivists in each critical-care service need to compare themselves against their own performance rather than against poorly defined external benchmarks, which only compounds the difficulties for accurate assessment.

Advancing performance measurement at the physician level is the vital strategy on the policy agenda when considerable unexplained variation exists in practices that lead to poor quality, inefficient care delivery, and waste of resources. To move the physician measurement and reporting agenda forward, there is a need for continued development of evidence-based quality measures that can be applied to gauge individual physician performance on a deeper array of medical conditions and specialties. There is a need for research to assess the optimal ways to construct reproducible and unwavering performance scores (eg, levels of aggregation) to assess the optimal ways to provide feedback to physicians and patients to facilitate their understanding and use of the information.[21]

REFERENCES

1. World Health Organization. *World Health Report 2000*. Geneva: WHO; 2000.
2. Schoenman JA. The Concentration of Health Care Spending NIH CM Foundation Data Brief July 2012.
3. Kahn JM, et al. Long-term acute care hospital utilization after critical illness. *J Am Med Assoc.* 2010;303:2253-2259.
4. National Voluntary Consensus Standards for Patient Outcomes. First Report for Phases I and II: A Consensus Report; 2010.
5. Institute of Medicine. *Crossing the Quality Chasm: A New Health System for the 21st Century*. Washington, DC: National Academies Press; 2001.
6. Institute of Medicine. *Rewarding Provider Performance: Aligning Incentives in Medicare.* Washington, DC: National Academies Press; 2007.
7. Centers for Medicare and Medicaid Services. Physician quality reporting system. http://www.cms.gov/Medicare/Quality-Initiatives-Patient-Assessment-Instruments/PQRS/index.html?redirect=/pqrs.
8. Tompkins CP, Higgins AR, Ritter GA. Measuring outcomes and efficiency in Medicare value-based purchasing. *Health Aff. (Millwood)* 2009;28:w251-w261.
9. Physician quality reporting initiative: 2007 reporting experience. http://www.cms.gov/Medicare/Quality-Initiatives-Patient-Assessment-Instruments/PQRS/downloads/PQRI2007ReportFinal12032008CSG.pdf.
10. Mant J. Process versus outcome indicators in the assessment of quality of health care. *Int J Qual Health Care.* 2001;13:475-480.
11. Jweinatt JJ. Hospital readmissions under the spotlight. *J Healthcare Manag.* 2010;55:252-264.
12. Popovich MJ, Esfandiari S, Boutros A. A new ICU paradigm: intensivists as primary critical care physicians. *Cleve Clin J Med.* 2011;78:697-700.
13. Gajic O, Afessa B. Physician staffing models and patient safety in the ICU. *Chest.* 2009;135:1038-1044.
14. Kahn JM, Kramer AA, Rubenfeld GD. Transferring critically ill patients out of hospital improves the standardized mortality ratio: a simulation study. *Chest.* 2007;131:68-75.
15. Vasilevskis EE, Kuzniewicz MW, Dean ML, et al. Relationship between discharge practices and intensive care unit in-hospital mortality performance: evidence of a discharge bias. *Med Care.* 2009;47:803-812.
16. Kahn JM. Quality improvement in end-of-life critical care. *Semin Respir Crit Care Med.* 2012;33:375-381.
17. Report to the Congress. Medicare Payment Advisory Commission. March 2011.
18. Baker DW, Einstadter D, Thomas CL, Husak SS, Gordon NH, Cebul RD. Mortality trends during a program that publicly reported hospital performance. *Med Care.* 2002;40:879-890.
19. Gorodeski EZ, Starling RC, Blackstone EH. Are all readmissions bad readmissions? *N Engl J Med.* 2010; 15:297-298.
20. Thomas JW, Grazier KL, and Ward K. Comparing accuracy of risk-adjustment methodologies used in economic profiling of physicians. *Inquiry.* 2004;41:218-231.
21. McGlynn EA. Selecting common measures of quality and system performance. *Med Care.* 2003;41:I39-I47.

Complications: Never Never or Never Ever

84

Effie Singas, MD and Dana Lustbader, MD

KEY POINTS

1. The ICU can be a dangerous place for patients.

2. Many ICU patients experience hospital acquired infections, medication errors, and procedure related complications.

3. Complications increase morbidity and mortality.

4. ICU complications may be preventable with structured patient handoffs, use of

computerized physician order entry, good hand hygiene, ultrasound guidance for procedures, remote ICU monitoring, use of checklists and standardized treatment protocols.

5. When an error occurs, physicians should disclose the error, document the error in the record and promptly treat any complications arising from it.

INTRODUCTION

Hospitals are a dangerous place. Experts estimate that nearly 100,000 people die every year from medical errors that occur in hospitals, more than die from breast cancer, AIDS or car accidents. The ICU is especially challenging. There are multiple medical personnel including the primary ICU team and usually one or more consultants caring for patients. Critically ill patients are treated with multiple medications and often undergo procedures, thereby increasing the risk for adverse events and drug interactions. Recent trends in medical education have reduced the number of hours that house officers can work each week thereby increasing the number of handoffs, creating more opportunities for communication failures.

In this increasingly complex environment, there will be complications. The stakes are high. Complications increase morbidity and mortality in the critically ill. Furthermore, they erode public trust

in physicians and the medical system as a whole. As a result, physicians may experience stress and loss of confidence in an increasingly complex medical system. One study estimated two serious errors per day for a 10-bed critical care unit. Medication errors accounted for 78% of the serious errors in this study.[1] Medical error is generally defined as the failure of a planned action to be completed as intended (eg, error of execution) or the use of a wrong plan to achieve an aim (eg, error of planning) and an adverse event as an injury caused by a medical intervention rather than the underlying condition of the patient.[2] A recent study reported 1,192 medical errors for 1,369 patients; 27% of patients experienced at least one medical error. Patients experiencing two or more adverse events had a threefold increase in overall mortality.[3]

The landmark report "To Err is Human" published by the Institute of Medicine highlighted the magnitude of the problem and the far reaching cost of medical error. The report heralded an era of patient safety and the development of quality initiatives for the care of hospitalized patients, especially patients in the ICU.[2] Critically ill patients are subject to intensive therapies that are most often associated with highest risk and therefore untoward events. This chapter describes common ICU complications and risk mitigation strategies.

HOSPITAL-ACQUIRED INFECTIONS

Hospital acquired infections (HAIs) are a frequent complication of intensive care accounting for prolonged intensive care unit (ICU) length of stay, morbidity, suffering, and death. According to the Centers for Disease Control and Prevention (CDC), about one in every 20 patients will develop an HAI. Such infections were long recognized by clinicians as an inevitable hazard of hospitalization and are most often associated with invasive medical devices or surgical procedures.[3]

Central line associated bloodstream infections (CLABSI) are common in the United States accounting for nearly 100,000 bloodstream infections annually with half occurring in the ICU setting. While one third of these infections are attributable to gram negative organisms, other organisms like coagulase-negative staphylococci, *Staphylococcus aureus*, and enterococcus predominate. Host factors associated with increased risk for CLABSI include neutropenia, immunosuppression, total parenteral nutrition (TPN) use, chronic illness, and burn. Prolonged catheter use, conditions of insertion, and catheter site care also play a role in the development of CLABSI. For patients with suspected or confirmed CLABSI, the indwelling catheter should be removed and cultured with the institution of empiric antibiotic therapy. The initial selection of antibiotic depends on the severity of the infection, but generally vancomycin is used because of its activity against coagulase negative staphylococci and *Staphylococcus aureus*. Ceftazidime or cefepime may be needed for severely ill or immunocompromised critically ill patients.

Urinary tract infections account for more than 15% of infections reported by hospitals. Virtually all health care associated UTIs are caused by instrumentation of the urinary tract. A catheter-associated UTI (CAUTI) is a UTI where an indwelling urinary catheter was in place for more than two days. The majority of cases are caused by *Escherichia coli* followed by *Pseudomonas aeruginosa*, klebsiella species, and enterobacter species. Cefepime, ceftazidime, piperacillin-tazobactam, aztreonam, ciprofloxacin, and meropenem are generally first-line agents. In addition to sterile unobstructed closed drainage systems, prompt removal of urinary catheters is the single best strategy for CAUTI prevention.

Ventilator associated pneumonia (VAP) is a hospital acquired pneumonia that occurs 48 hours or more after the institution of mechanical ventilation. It is the most common nosocomial infection afflicting patients with respiratory failure and accounts for nearly half of all antibiotics used in the ICU setting. Nearly 20% of mechanically ventilated patients will get a VAP during their ICU course. VAP is caused when the normal host defense mechanisms are bypassed with the endotracheal tube and micro-aspiration of contaminated oropharyngeal secretions occurs. Rapid colonization of the oropharynx with gram negative bacteria occurs following antibiotic use and illness secondary to resultant compromise of host defenses such as ciliated epithelium, mucus, and glottis. Patients are unable to cough and the contaminated secretions pool above the endotracheal tube cuff and migrate along the airway. Biofilm, impervious to systemic antibiotics, forms along the endotracheal tube and serves as a breeding ground for bacterial growth which ultimately leads to infection.

The CDC National Healthcare Safety Network (NHSN) implemented a ventilator-associated events (VAE) surveillance program in 2013.[4] This surveillance algorithm uses objective elements to identify complications associated with mechanical ventilation. VAP is included in the algorithm, which starts with the presence of a ventilator-associated condition (VAC), a period of respiratory deterioration following a sustained period of stability or improvement on the ventilator (eg, changes in PEEP or FiO_2). The second tier definition, infection-related ventilator-associated complication (IVAC), requires that patients with VAC also have an abnormal temperature (temperature > 38°C or < 36°C) or white blood cell count (WBC ≥ 12,000 cells/mm^3 or ≤ 4,000 cells/mm^3), and requires the initiation of a new antibiotic for treatment of presumed infection. The third-tier definition is probable VAP and requires that patients with IVAC also have purulent respiratory secretions or laboratory evidence of respiratory infection. For quantitative cultures, a bacterial density of at least 10^6 CFU/ml for endotracheal aspirate, 10^4 CFU/ml for bronchoalveolar lavage, and 10^3 CFU/ml for protected specimen brush and for semiquantitative cultures, at least moderate growth of bacteria.

Risk factors for VAP include a supine position, previous broad spectrum antibiotic exposure, reintubation, acute respiratory distress syndrome (ARDS), prolonged mechanical ventilation, and trauma. The most common pathogens to consider for VAP are *Pseudomonas aeruginosa*, methicillin-resistant *Staphylococcus aureus* (MRSA), *Klebsiella pneumonia*, acinetobacter species, *Streptococcus pneumonia*, and *Haemophilus influenza*. Polymicrobial pneumonia is common and one should note that multi drug resistance is increasingly frequent in the ICU setting, particularly for patients with prolonged intubation, prior hospitalizations or ICU admissions, immunosuppression or those requiring hemodialysis. All ventilated patients without contraindications should be maintained in the semi recumbent position with the head of the bed raised 45° and be weaned from mechanical ventilation as soon as possible.

Hospital hand hygiene protocols have been shown to reduce the risk of certain HAI. The World Health Organization estimates that nearly 2 million patients each year are affected by poor hand hygiene practices in hospitals. A shocking number of health care providers fail to embrace hand hygiene. Healthcare workers should wash their hands for 15 to 30 seconds with soap and water or an approved alcohol based hand rub before and after patient contact.

MEDICATION ERROR

Medication errors consistently make up the largest group of medical errors. Risk factors include the use of continuous intravenous infusions, polypharmacy with the potential for drug interactions and complex dosing regimens. Medication errors in one study were most commonly associated with treatment, but were also related to prevention (eg, heparin prophylaxis for thromboembolic disease), diagnosis (eg,

intravenous contrast) and monitoring (eg, glucose monitoring). Cardiovascular drugs, anticoagulants and anti-infective agents were most commonly associated with medication errors.[1] Ensuring that medications are used appropriately is a complex process involving professionals from many disciplines. Errors can occur at any stage in the process—from prescribing the correct drug, properly ordering, processing and dispensing the drug, administering the right drug to the right patient, informing the patient about the medication, monitoring the patients response, and identifying adverse events.[2] Errors of omission were most common in both ICU and non ICU settings, whereas errors caused by improper dose or incorrect administration technique were more common in the ICU setting in a national study of voluntarily reported medication errors.[5] In an observational study involving a surgical ICU in a tertiary care hospital, 87.5% of doses for weight-based infusions were calculated based on estimated or unreliable admission weights.[6]

The most common medical error reported in an observational prospective multicenter cohort study of 70 ICUs was related to insulin administration, 186 errors per 1,000 days of insulin treatment.[3] During the time of this study, tight glucose control was advocated in ICUs.[7] Subsequent studies examined the risk-benefit of tight glucose control and the practice remains controversial in ICUs today.[8] Other medication errors included administering anticoagulant medication, prescribing anticoagulant medication, and administering vasoactive agents.[3] A recent review of medication errors in the ICU found substantial differences in medication error rates, varying from 18.6 to 146.1 per 1000 patient care days. Studies that reported higher medication error rates included observation methods and did not rely on voluntary reporting alone suggesting an under reporting of error when self reporting is the only tracking method.[9]

While the use of computerized physician order entry (CPOE) has reduced errors in medication dose, route, substitution, and allergy and has intercepted adverse drug events, its use in the ICU can potentially increase the rates of certain medication errors, or result in entirely new error types. These include medication discontinuation failures, antibiotic renewal failures, unreliable reinstitution of medications following surgery and problems with nonformulary medications.[10] Alert fatigue is another common problem created by computerized entry of orders as the number of cautionary alerts increases, so too does the provider ability to tune them out.

PROCEDURAL COMPLICATIONS

Many ICU patients will be mechanically ventilated at some point during the course of their critical illness. Mechanically ventilated patients can experience complications from the initiation of mechanical ventilation all the way through to their extubation. These complications include esophageal intubation, hemodynamic instability in the peri-intubation period from sedation, hypoxemia, or delay in intubation. Once patients are intubated, endotracheal tubes can become dislodged, clogged or inadvertently removed by the patient. The rate of self-extubation has been reported to occur in about 5% to 15% of intubated patients.

Mechanical ventilation and the positive pressure patients are exposed to can lead to barotrauma and further complications. Use of a video laryngoscope can significantly reduce the number of esophageal intubations and increase first pass success during intubation.[11] The adoption of a combined team approach to urgent endotracheal intubation with designated roles for team members, a mandatory checklist and back-up plan, can minimize peri-intubation complications.[12]

Critically ill patients often require central venous lines for access, monitoring and therapy (eg, dialysis, ECMO). Complications can occur from start to finish—wrong site, improper sterile technique, poor procedural technique, including poor knowledge of the anatomy, resulting in bleeding, local trauma including injury of vessels or underlying lung (eg, pneumothorax), and infectious complications. The presence of a central venous catheter and mechanical ventilation were among the factors independently associated with having at least one medical error in a recent study.[3]

The use of ultrasound to guide invasive procedures such as central line placement and thoracentesis has made them much safer as the anatomy can be directly visualized. A multidisciplinary approach

employing a "time out" can make it difficult for errors of site or identification to occur.

Nasogastric tubes for enteral feeding and medication access can be dislodged or incorrectly positioned, entering the airway instead of the esophagus, resulting in trauma to the lung. Furthermore, patients must be positioned in a semi-recumbent position to minimize the chances of aspiration. Careful monitoring of positioning, securing of these tubes and appropriate sedation of the patient can avoid many complications.

Intern fatigue has been linked to serious medical errors in ICUs. One prospective, randomized study compared the rates of serious medical errors made by interns working a traditional schedule with an every third night call schedule versus an intervention schedule that eliminated extended work shifts and reduced the total number of hours worked per week. Interns made 35.9% more serious medical errors during the traditional schedule than during the intervention schedule. The total rate of serious errors was 22% higher during the traditional schedule.[13] As a result of studies like these, the Accreditation Council for Graduate Medical Education (ACGME) restricted trainees to 16 consecutive hours of work. Shorter work shifts have resulted in a significant increase in the frequency of transitions of care (eg, handoffs) in the ICU. Improving the handoff process with the use of a structured note and face-to-face handoff can reduce medical error.

OH NO, WE HAD A COMPLICATION. NOW WHAT?

Truth telling in the setting of medical error or complication is generally the best approach. Interestingly a recent study showed that one fifth of physicians reported not fully disclosing medical error or mistakes to patients for fear of malpractice lawsuits.[14] The first priority is always to promptly diagnose and treat the complication. Careful documentation in the medical record is a critical next step. Informing the patient, family or surrogate is often difficult but part of good medical care. When discussing the situation, it is helpful to describe the situation, how it happened and the course of action to be taken to resolve the problem whenever possible. Never lie about or cover up a mistake.

CONCLUSION

The ICU is a complex and dangerous place for our patients. Patients are critically ill, require many medications, invasive lines and procedures, and 24/7 multidisciplinary care. This chapter outlines the most frequently encountered complications in ICU patients. Many hospital complications are preventable with good communication, oversight and education. Borrowing from other industries including the airlines and restaurant chains, hospitals have adopted methods and safety checklists to improve the reliability of the health care environment.[15] The use of medical response teams for a faster response to a critically ill patient, remote ICU monitoring for greater oversight (eg, tele-ICU), and the adoption of critical care bundles and protocols are some of the methods being used to improve the safety of our patients in ICUs. The critical question is when will effective quality health care measures be available to every patient every time.

REFERENCES

1. Rothschild JM, Landrigan CP, Cronin JW, et al. The Critical Care Safety Study: the incidence and nature of adverse events and serious medical errors in intensive care. *Crit Care Med.* 2005;33:1694-1700.
2. Kohn LT, Corrigan JM, Donaldson MS. *To Err is Human: Building a Safer Health System.* Washington, DC: National Academy Press; 1999.
3. Garouste-Orgeas M, Tisit JF, Vesin A, et al. Selected medical errors in the intensive care unit. Results of the IATROREF Study: Parts I and II. *Am J Resp Crit Care Med.* 2010;181:134-142.
4. Peleg AY, Hooper DC. Hospital acquired infections due to gram-negative bacteria. *N Engl J Med.* 2010;362:1804-1813.
5. Latif A, Rawat N, Pustavoitau A, et al. National study on the distribution, causes and consequences of voluntarily reported medication errors between the ICU and non-ICU settings. *Crit Care Med.* 2013;41:389-398.
6. Herout P, Erstad BL. Medication errors involving continuously infused medications in a surgical intensive care unit. *Crit Care Med.* 2004;32:428-432.
7. Van Den Berghe G, Wouters P, Weekers F, et al. Intensive insulin therapy in critically ill patients. *NEJM.* 2001;345:1359-1367.
8. Wiener RS, Wiener DC, Larson RJ. Benefits and risks of tight glucose control in critically ill adults. *J Am Med Assoc.* 2008;300:933-944.
9. Wilmer A, Louie K, Dodek P, et al. Incidence of medication errors and adverse drug events in the ICU: a systematic review. *Qual Saf Health Care.* 2010;19:e7.
10. Maslove DM, Rizk N, Lowe HJ. Computerized physician order entry in the critical care environment: a review of current literature. *J Intensive Care Med.* 2011;26:165-171.
11. Lakticova V, Koenig SJ, Narasimhan M, et al. Video laryngoscopy is associated with increased first pass success and decreased rate of esophageal intubations during urgent endotracheal intubation in a medical intensive care unit when compared to direct laryngoscopy. *J Intensive Care Med.* 2013;00:1-5.
12. Mayo PH, Hegde A, Eisen LA, et al. A program to improve the quality of emergency endotracheal intubation. *J Intensive Care Med.* 2011;26:50-56.
13. Landrigan CP, Rothschild JM, Cronin JW, et al. Effect of reducing Interns' work hours on serious medical errors in intensive care units. *N Engl J Med.* 2004;351:1838-1848.
14. Iezzzoni L, Rao SR, DesRoches CM, et al. Survey shows that at least some physicians are not always open or honest with patients. *Health Aff.* 2012;31:383-391.
15. Gawande A. *Big Med.* The New Yorker; 2012.

Controversies: Noninvasive Ventilation at the End-of-Life—Useful or Not?

85

Katerina Rusinova, MD; Alexandre Demoule, MD and Elie Azoulay, MD

INTRODUCTION

Noninvasive ventilation (NIV) has been well described as effective in different patient populations, for example, hypercapnic respiratory failure due to exacerbations of chronic obstructive pulmonary disease (COPD),[1] hypoxic respiratory failure in immunocompromised hosts,[2] or cardiogenic pulmonary edema in the absence of acute coronary ischemia,[3] to cite the most common indications.

Conceptually, the use of noninvasive ventilation can be divided into the following three categories[4]:

1. NIV as a part of "full-code" treatment (life support without preset limits)

2. NIV in patients with do-not-intubate orders (life-support with preset limits)

3. NIV as a comfort measure in patients at the end-of-life (NIV ensuring comfort while dying)

Each category has specific goals of care, response to failure, and main points to communicate with the patient and/or family. Categories 2 and 3 can be defined as *palliative NIV*.[5]

The goals of NIV in patients in category 1 are to alleviate symptoms of respiratory distress, improve oxygenation and/or ventilation, avoid intubation, and reduce the risk of mortality. Endotracheal intubation is performed if necessary.

Patients in category 2 are those who decline endotracheal intubation or patients in whom clinicians feel that intubation would not meet the goals of care. In this group, the use of NIV achieves the same goals as it does in category 1, except that endotracheal intubation is not an option in cases where NIV is ineffective.

The only purpose of NIV in category 3 is symptom palliation and patient comfort.

SYMPTOMS OF RESPIRATORY DISTRESS AT THE END OF LIFE

Respiratory distress is one of the most common symptoms seen in patients approaching the end-of-life. It leads to restrictions in quality of life and increases anxiety and fear.[6]

Terminal dyspnea is a manifestation of an irreversible process, such as carcinomatous lymphangitis in malignant diseases or advanced degenerative neuromuscular disease (amyotrophic lateral sclerosis).

The vast majority of patients with terminal cancer experience symptoms of respiratory distress at some point during the last 6 weeks of life, and they commonly report significantly increased dyspnea during the last two weeks.[7] In patients with a noncancer terminal diagnosis, such as COPD or chronic heart failure (CHF), the severity of respiratory distress can be greater; however, the severity remains relatively stable until death.

RESPIRATORY DISTRESS RELIEF BY USING NIV

The mechanism underlying the relief of respiratory distress through noninvasive ventilation remains the same in all clinical situations.[8] NIV reduces the work of breathing by increasing transpulmonary pressure and reducing inspiratory muscle workloads. Gas exchange is improved by increasing alveolar ventilation, functional residual capacity, opening collapsed alveoli, reducing shunts, and improving the ventilation/perfusion (V/Q) ratio. Altogether, these mechanisms result in a lower respiratory rate, reduced CO_2 retention, and an overall improvement of symptoms of respiratory distress.

RESEARCH FINDINGS

Recently, studies focused on the use of palliative noninvasive ventilation have provided descriptive data, new evidence, and qualitative appraisals of palliative NIV.

A prospective cohort study by Azoulay et al.[9] reported outcomes of patients undergoing NIV in the context of "do-not-intubate" (DNI) orders (ie, category 2). A DNI order is present in about 20% of all patients receiving NIV in intensive care units (ICUs). A substantial hospital survival of 56% was observed, which was most obvious in the COPD patient subgroup. Importantly, for those who survived up to 90 days, health-related quality of life did not significantly change compared to baseline. Moreover, anxiety, depression, and posttraumatic stress disorder (PTSD)-related symptoms in patients and their families were similar to those seen when NIV was used in category 1 (full code) patients. These recent data, together with previously published reports,[10,11] thus support the use of NIV in this clinical context.

A study by Nava et al.[12] that focused on patients with end-stage cancer (ie, category 3 patients) assessed the acceptability and effectiveness of NIV versus oxygen therapy in decreasing dyspnea and its effect on the use of opioids. The study showed that NIV is faster and more effective compared to oxygen in reducing dyspnea and offers the potential to reduce the dose of opioids. Hospital mortality was similar in both groups. NIV was well accepted and well tolerated, again, with the best response in cases of hypercapnic respiratory insufficiency.

Finally, NIV has been evaluated in patients suffering from terminal phase motor neuron disease who are at the end-of-life. A qualitative study by Baxter et al.[13] revealed important variations in patient wishes regarding the use of NIV toward the end-of-life and also a

TABLE 85–1 Expected benefits and possible risks of end-of-life NIV: factors to be considered before NIV initiation (on an individual basis).

Expected Benefits	Possible Risks
Prompt relief of respiratory distress	Discomfort from tight-fitting mask (facial necrosis)
Maintained cognition	Noise exposure (up to 65 dB)
Time to finalize personal affairs (strategy to "buy time")	Possible unnecessary prolongation of the terminal phase of life
Dose of opioids diminished (with fewer or reduced opioid side effects)	Nasal/oral dryness, nasal congestion
Improved ability to communicate due to diminished use of opioids and higher level of consciousness	Limited ability to communicate imposed by the face mask
Reassurance, reduced end-of-life anxiety	Stressful fixation on technology at the end-of-life
Say goodbye to loved-ones	Symptoms of PTSD in family members Complicated grief[15]

degree of uncertainty concerning NIV management among healthcare teams. Nevertheless, end-of-life use of NIV was generally perceived as beneficial, allowing a more peaceful end-of-life, free of choking or struggling to breathe during the final moments.

Even if current research findings support the use of noninvasive ventilation in palliative situations (categories 2 and 3 of the conceptual framework), important questions/objections have been raised, concerning possible discomfort and unnecessary prolongation of the terminal phase of life.[14,15] Some aspects of the current controversies are summarized in Table 85–1.

PRACTICAL CONSIDERATIONS
Prior to NIV Initiation

Palliative noninvasive ventilation, incorporated into a strategy of continuous patient care, should be discussed early, along with the patient's other preferences regarding advanced or terminal stages of their disease. Specific goals of using NIV in the clinical setting should be carefully explained and thoroughly understood by the patient and their family with particular emphasis on concrete measures that can and, if approved, will be taken to quickly achieve patient comfort in cases when NIV fails to achieve the desired results.

Monitoring During NIV

It has been reported that NIV targeted at control of respiratory distress (ie, category 3) can also be successfully used outside the ICU, for example, wards, hospices, and even at home. Monitoring should be oriented toward continually reassessing whether NIV is succeeding or failing to meet therapeutic goals (in category 3, eg, the only monitored aspect would be relief of symptoms).

Discontinuing NIV at the End-of-Life

NIV used to aid patients through the end-of-life should be discontinued when patients feel that the NIV is not making them more comfortable or when patients are no longer able to communicate. This is probably the moment when the benefits of NIV have ceased, since patients have lost control over the decision to continue NIV support.

UNANSWERED QUESTIONS

There are important questions regarding the use of noninvasive ventilation during the end-of-life period that have not yet been addressed. There are no data assessing the quality of NIV–assisted end-of-life care. We also do not have a full appreciation or analysis of life support resource utilization or the effectiveness of palliative NIV on survival.

CONCLUSION

Noninvasive ventilation can and should be considered as a feasible palliative therapeutic option as well as a comfort measure during the dying process. However, there are only limited evidence about what type of patients and what diseases would mostly benefit from palliative NIV. To date, few studies have been published that address this important issue.

Presently, decisions about palliative NIV have to be evaluated carefully and on a case-by-case basis, and oriented on the potential benefits for a given patient.

REFERENCES

1. Keenan SP, Sinuff T, Cook DJ, et al. Which patients with acute exacerbation of chronic obstructive pulmonary disease benefit from noninvasive positive-pressure ventilation? A systematic review of the literature. *Ann Intern Med*. 2003;138:861-870.
2. Hilbert G, Gruson D, Vargas F, et al. Noninvasive ventilation in immunosuppressed patients with pulmonary infiltrates, fever, and acute respiratory failure. *N Engl J Med*. 2001;344:481-487.
3. Vital FMR, Ladeira MT, Atallah AN. Non-invasive positive pressure ventilation (CPAP or bilevel NPPV) for cardiogenic pulmonary oedema. *Cochrane Database Syst Rev*. 2013;5:CD005351.
4. Curtis JR, Cook DJ, Sinuff T, et al. Noninvasive positive pressure ventilation in critical and palliative care settings: understanding the goals of therapy. *Crit Care Med*. 2007;35:932–939.
5. Azoulay E, Demoule A, Jaber S, et al. Palliative noninvasive ventilation in patients with acute respiratory failure. *Intensive Care Med*. 2011;37:1250-1257.
6. Kamal AH, Maguire JM, Wheeler JL, et al. Dyspnea review for the palliative care professional: assessment, burdens, and etiologies. *J Palliat Med*. 2011;14:1167-1172.
7. Shreves A, Pour T. Emergency management of dyspnea in dying patients. *Emerg Med Pract*. 2013;15:1-19.
8. Mehta S, Hill NS. Noninvasive ventilation. *Am J Respir Crit Care Med*. 2001;163:540-577.
9. Azoulay E, Kouatchet A, Jaber S, et al. Noninvasive mechanical ventilation in patients having declined tracheal intubation. *Intensive Care Med*. 2013;39:292-301.
10. Sinuff T, Cook DJ, Keenan SP, et al. Noninvasive ventilation for acute respiratory failure near the end of life. *Crit Care Med*. 2008;36:789-794.
11. Freichels TA. Palliative ventilatory support: use of noninvasive positive pressure ventilation in terminal respiratory insufficiency. *Am J Crit Care Off Publ Am Assoc Crit-Care Nurses*. 1994;3:6-10.
12. Nava S, Ferrer M, Esquinas A, et al. Palliative use of non-invasive ventilation in end-of-life patients with solid tumours: a randomised feasibility trial. *Lancet Oncol*. 2013;14:219-227.

13. Baxter SK, Baird WO, Thompson S, et al. The use of non-invasive ventilation at end of life in patients with motor neurone disease: a qualitative exploration of family carer and health professional experiences. *Palliat Med.* 2013;27:516-523.

14. Clarke DE, Vaughan L, Raffin TA. Noninvasive positive pressure ventilation for patients with terminal respiratory failure: the ethical and economic costs of delaying the inevitable are too great. *Am J Crit Care Off Publ Am Assoc Crit-Care Nurses.* 1994;3:4-5.

15. Azoulay E, Kouatchet A, Jaber S, et al. Non-invasive ventilation for end-of-life oncology patients. *Lancet Oncol.* 2013;14:e200-e201.

CHAPTER

Post-Intensive Care Syndrome

Leonard Lim, MD and Graciela Soto, MD, MS

86

KEY POINTS

1. The number of patients who survive acute critical illness has increased over the last few years and PICS is more common than previously thought.

2. PICS is new or worsening impairment in physical, mental, or cognitive status arising after critical illness and persisting beyond the acute care hospitalization.

3. These impairments are frequently under recognized and adversely impact daily functioning and the quality of life.

4. Decline in lung function parameters and ICU-acquired weakness are some of the physical impairments that can affect health care resource utilization and short- and long-term outcomes.

5. Neurocognitive impairment spans a wide range of dysfunction and is associated with metabolic abnormalities, hypoxemia, fever, sepsis, pharmacological agents, organ dysfunction, and disrupted sleep.

6. The neuro-psychological impairment encountered after ICU care (eg, anxiety, depression, and PTSD) is not associated with an increased severity of illness but rather to both the subjective and objective aspects of the ICU experience.

7. Strategies to minimize or prevent PICS should start during the ICU stay and address those modifiable risk factors known to be associated with the different aspects of PICS (eg, glycemic control, minimizing sedation, early exercise and mobilization, liberation from mechanical ventilation).

INTRODUCTION

Over the past decade, survival from critical illness has dramatically increased due to a better understanding of the pathophysiological mechanisms of disease, improved treatment strategies and advancements in medical technology. Several studies have shown improved survival and long-term outcomes in survivors of critically illness. However, surviving the intensive care unit (ICU) stay is just the start of a long road to recovery for a majority of these patients. The discharge from the ICU opens the path to a long journey of challenging physical rehabilitation, mood disorders, cognitive impairment, psychological distress, financial hardship, and caregiver burden and burnout.

In recent years there has been a growing recognition of impairments that affect the physical, psychological, social, and emotional aspects of the individual after ICU discharge that may adversely impact daily functioning and quality of life (QOL). Recently, the term "post-intensive care syndrome" (PICS) is used to describe any new or worsening impairments in physical, cognitive, or mental health status arising after critical illness and persisting beyond the acute care hospitalization.[1] PICS may persist for months to years after hospital discharge. Most impairments will diminish with time but some may linger on until the patient's actual demise. This chapter will explore in detail the different domains affected in PICS, its impact on the individual and society, and offer insights into future developments.

PHYSICAL IMPAIRMENT

Probably the most obvious and readily recognizable changes in patients immediately after discharge from the ICU are the physical impairments that are the result of the actual critical illness or the direct or indirect side-effects of interventions to treat the disease. An individual patient may lie at a particular point in the spectrum of physical disability according to the patient's age, level of functioning prior to the onset of critical illness, and the burden of co-morbid conditions. At one end of this spectrum, clinicians encounter young, previously working and highly functional patients who develop a severe catastrophic illness. The middle range includes patients who are older and have a greater burden of comorbidities than the previous group. Finally, the opposite end of this spectrum includes those patients who have experienced chronic critical illness, or the very elderly, in whom ICU-level of care may not alter their ultimate outcome but may instead contribute to incremental disability and constitute part of a downward functional trajectory driven by progression of chronic illness.

Lung Function

It has been shown that in critical illness leading to respiratory failure, particularly in acute respiratory distress syndrome (ARDS), that lung function is decreased soon after recovery but improves to normal or near-normal over 6 months to 5 years. The diffusing capacity for carbon monoxide (DLCO) is the lung function parameter that seems to be mostly affected as DLCO values still remain mildly reduced or low-normal even after 5 years of follow-up.[2] This persistent impairment in gas transfer is probably due to injury at the capillary level, which promotes thickening in alveolar capillary interfaces, pulmonary fibrosis, and pulmonary vascular remodeling.

Anatomical changes in the lung are also observed in follow-up imaging studies of ARDS survivors. Localized changes in the nondependent lung zones including reticular changes, ground-glass opacities and minor pulmonary fibrosis are seen on high-resolution computer tomography (CT) scans.[3] The association between the severity of lung injury and length of mechanical ventilation may reflect ventilator-associated lung injury. However, the relationship between the development of lung fibrosis after ARDS and any possible risk factor is not straightforward. Some studies have found significant correlation between CT scan impairment and duration of mechanical ventilation, level of positive end-expiratory pressure (PEEP), and oxygen fraction. These data may only reflect greater severity of ARDS, which can be responsible per se for lung fibrosis.

It is interesting to note that the severity of the patient's dyspnea after recovery from ARDS does not seem to correlate with actual lung dysfunction but may reflect extrapulmonary muscle weakness and sometimes psychological impairments.

Chronic Respiratory Failure

The onset of respiratory failure requiring prolonged mechanical ventilation is associated with increased morbidity, mortality, and health care costs. ICU admission for pneumonia, ARDS, neuromuscular disease, head trauma, or postoperative intracerebral hemorrhage is one of the strongest predictors of prolonged mechanical ventilation.[4] ICU-acquired weakness (ICU-AW) has also been shown to be a predictor of failure to be liberated from the ventilator. The mechanism that is responsible for a majority of ventilator dependence can be explained by an increase in respiratory load coupled with decreased respiratory muscle performance. Chronic ventilator dependence may result in complications similar to those receiving short-term mechanical ventilation. These include infections, tracheal bleeding or malformations, renal failure, pneumothorax, volume overload, ileus, and seizures.

The overall mortality in patients with ventilator-dependent chronic respiratory failure is high and up to 52% at one year from the initial hospitalization.[5] Chronic irreversible neurologic diseases and presence of skin breakdown has been associated with increased risk for mortality. These patients may be discharged to home, long-term acute care (LTAC) facilities, skilled nursing facilities or hospice care centers. The QOL tends to be low but may improve over the years. In particular, ARDS survivors who require prolonged mechanical ventilation have poorer QOL than other ARDS survivors.[6] Health care resource utilization in these patients have been shown to be exceeding high and much of this is spent on ongoing and recurrent medical care.

Weakness

Another important aspect of the physical impairment after recovery from critical illness is weakness. Potential contributors to weakness in survivors of critical illness are listed in Table 86–1. Risk factors for the development of weakness after critical illness are enumerated in Table 86–2. Several contrasting

TABLE 86–1 Contributors to weakness in survivors of critical illness.

Chronic disease
Acute neurologic syndrome, eg, Guillian-Barre syndrome, myasthenia gravis
Persistent organ dysfunction, eg, heart failure, chronic respiratory failure, acute kidney injury
Neuro-muscular pathology, eg, CIP, CIM, ischemic or compression mononeuropathies
Muscle atrophy from prolonged immobility
Deconditioning
Pain
Psychological disturbances

TABLE 86–2 Risk factors for weakness.

Female sex
Advanced age
Severity of illness
Hyperglycemia
Corticosteroids
Neuromuscular blockers

studies have shown variable association between the development of weakness and the severity of illness on ICU admission (eg, SAPS-2, APACHE II/III, SOFA). High blood glucose has been identified as a risk factor through an unknown mechanism while intensive insulin therapy has been shown to be a preventive factor against critical illness-associated weakness and to decrease the risk of critical illness polyneuropathy. The data on the association of corticosteroids with the development of weakness has been conflicting; however one study reported decreased neuromuscular dysfunction in patients on intensive insulin therapy while on corticosteroids, suggesting that when euglycemia is maintained, the anti-inflammatory effect of steroids may benefit the neuromuscular system.[7] Low doses of neuromuscular blockers (eg, paralytics) do not seem to be associated with weakness but larger doses may be independently associated.

Formerly described by different entities such as critical-illness polyneuropathy (CIP), critical-illness myopathy (CIM), and critical-illness neuromyopathy, ICU-AW is the prototypical functional impairment that has been the subject of intense research even prior to the recognition of the other domains of PICS. The incidence of ICU-AW varies from 30% to 90%. It may be missed during the acute phase of critical illness when the patient is sedated, restrained and unable to communicate. Difficulty liberating from mechanical ventilation may be the first indication of an impairment.

CIP is an axonal polyneuropathy that affects both sensory and motor nerves. The causes of axonal degeneration include the systemic inflammatory response syndrome (SIRS), ischemia to nerves from hypotension, microthrombosis, changes in microcirculation, endoneural edema, inflammation, mitochondrial dysfunction causing bioenergetic failure, neurotoxic meds, and metabolic abnormalities. Physical examination may reveal distal sensory deficits, distal weakness, and preserved deep-tendon reflexes (DTRs). Electromyography-Nerve Conduction Velocity (EMG-NCV) studies demonstrate decreased amplitudes of sensory and motor nerve action potentials with normal motor unit potentials and excitability. Pathologic evaluation reveals fiber loss and primary axonal degeneration of both motor and sensory nerve fibers, most severe distally.

CIM includes flaccid tetraparesis with depressed or absent DTRs but sensory function is not affected. The causes include increased muscle breakdown, decreased protein production and abnormal muscle repair, derangement of energy delivery, changes in the muscle membrane with primary inexcitability of muscle fibers, inflammation, steroids, and immobility. NCV studies reveal decreased amplitudes of compound muscle action potentials with preserved sensory nerve action potentials. Direct muscle stimulation demonstrates reduced or absent muscle excitability. Pathology most commonly reveals loss of thick filaments with atrophy of the type II fibers.

In terms of assessing weakness, the six-minute walk test (6MWT) is most widely used as it is an integrated outcome parameter that is dependent on the motor, pulmonary, and circulatory function. This test has proven to be a simple but useful test of global physical recovery in former ICU patients.

NEUROCOGNITIVE IMPAIRMENT

Neuro-cognitive impairment spans a wide range of dysfunction in critically ill patients. From those who are comatose to patients with minor, sometimes subtle dysfunction that may only be revealed using specific tests of cognitive dysfunction, although close relatives may have already recognized behavioral changes in these patients. Among survivors from general, medical and surgical ICU, the incidence of cognitive impairment ranges from 4% to 71%, while the incidence of cognitive impairment in ARDS survivors ranges from 4% to 56%.[3] Two studies in

elderly critically ill patients have reported a prevalence of cognitive impairment varying from 17% to 56%.[8,9] Cognitive impairment is associated with a reduced QOL and is a major determinant of societal health care costs and care-giving needs. The elderly are prone to developing cognitive impairment; however, it appears that younger, relatively healthy patients are also at risk of cognitive impairment following critical illness. Risk factors for the development of cognitive dysfunction after critical illness are listed in Table 86–3. It is unclear whether a low performance on neuropsychological tests reflects impairment in cognitive functioning related to critical illness and ICU admission, or whether it is perhaps merely a marker of patients with poor health and an increased risk of ICU admission. However, studies that include premorbid cognitive data show that at least part of the measured cognitive impairment is related to the ICU admission and critical illness.

Memory, attention, verbal fluency and executive functioning are the domains most frequently impaired after critical illness. The pathogenesis is not fully understood but may represent an accelerated neurodegenerative process that develops in vulnerable patients. Cognitive impairments can also be associated with newly acquired brain damage due to insults from critical illness such as hypoxemia, hypotension, anemia, fever, hyper-/hypoglycemia, systemic inflammation, severe sepsis, pharmacologic agents, disrupted sleep, renal failure, and liver failure. Severe sepsis can lead to a neuroinflammatory response, resulting in increased levels of

TABLE 86–3 Factors associated with neurocognitive impairments in critical illness survivors.

Advanced age
Preexisiting cognitive dysfunction
Genetic predisposition
Higher premorbid IQ (negative risk factor)
Severe sepsis
Lower cognitive reserve

cytokines in the brain.[10] Elevated cytokine levels are associated with impaired memory in healthy volunteers, and neuroinflammation is associated with the development of Alzheimer's disease. Long-term cognitive impairment in patients may therefore represent a maladaptive version of cytokine-induced disease. Delirium in the ICU can cause long-term complications such as cognitive impairment and can also significantly decrease short-term and long-term survival and worsen QOL after critical illness. Increased duration of delirium likewise is associated with worse neurocognitive outcomes in a "dose-dependent" manner.[11]

Radiologic and pathologic findings associated with cognitive dysfunction associated with critical illness include ischemic and hypoxemic hippocampal lesions, brain atrophy, ventricular enlargement, decreased superior frontal lobe and hippocampal volumes, and loss of white matter in the corpus callosum and internal capsule. At 1 year, these anatomical findings were associated with worse overall cognitive performance and worse executive functioning. Left hippocampal volumes on MRI were likewise markedly reduced in a cohort of patients with septic shock.

Individuals who are hospitalized for a critical illness have a greater likelihood of cognitive impairment, even after adjusting for premorbid cognitive screening scores and comorbidity. It has been suggested that critical illness may cause an abrupt loss of cognitive function rather than accelerate the decline in cognitive functioning. Cognitive dysfunction is probably very frequent in the immediate short period after intensive care but tends to normalize in most patients with time. Time to improvement varies from different studies. Improvement towards normal cognitive functioning has been reported to occur as early as 9 months after ICU discharge. Other studies have shown no improvement from 1 up to 5 years of follow-up.

Studies have so far been unable to identify patients at higher risk of cognitive impairment using brief cognitive screening tools at time of hospital discharge. One candidate predictor for cognitive impairment might be quantitative electroencephalogram (EEG). A recent study of sepsis survivors found EEG to be a potential predictor of cognitive impairment in these patients. Deficits in verbal learning and memory were associated with a significant reduction in left hippocampal volume and low-frequency activity on routine EEG. EEG may be able to provide prognostic information, possibly in combination with other modalities. Serum biomarkers may also be useful in predicting cognitive impairment. Elevated serum interleukin (IL)-6 and c-reactive protein (CRP) concentrations are associated with reduced cognition and contribute to accelerated functional decline in both the elderly and in post-operative cardiopulmonary bypass patients. Given the prevalence of delirium in disease states with a higher systemic inflammatory burden, inflammatory biomarkers may be useful for monitoring delirium disease activity and predicting risk of long-term cognitive impairment.

Lower percentages of patients with cognitive impairments were reported in studies using screening tests as compared to studies that utilized extensive neuropsychological testing. A major limitation of most studies is that a baseline assessment of cognitive status before the onset of critical illness is lacking and is oftentimes difficult to determine unless prior premorbid cognitive screening results were available. Ideally, pre-ICU admission cognition should be available because the real interest is not the absolute level of cognitive performance but rather the change in cognitive functioning.

Another limitation is that cognitive testing is seldom standardized from center to center and from cohort to cohort making the comparison between studies difficult. Furthermore, a large number of different tests and combinations have been used making the interpretation and application of the results to critically ill patients challenging. The most widely used tests include the mini-mental status examination (MMSE) for screening patients for cognitive dysfunction and the Cambridge Neuropsychological Test—Automated Battery (developed at the University of Cambridge) as a more in-depth test for cognitive dysfunction in research studies.

PSYCHOLOGICAL AND BEHAVIORAL IMPAIRMENT

The increasing awareness of the PICS has led to the realization that new onset behavioral changes and psychiatric symptoms are the result of the ICU experience in survivors of critical illness. Akin to the psychological trauma experienced by survivors of natural or man-made catastrophes, the time spent in the ICU can be as harrowing as a near-death experience to many. The reported prevalence of anxiety and depression after ICU discharge varies between 6% and 28% among different studies depending on the "cut-off" scores and methodology used. Levels of anxiety and depression appear to decrease in the first year after ICU discharge; however, it is unclear whether this improvement remains or continues to full resolution of symptoms. On the contrary, in patients with ARDS, levels of depression increased from 16% at 1 year after discharge to 23% at 2 years. It has also been suggested that 14% to 27% of critically ill patients may develop a posttraumatic stress reaction or post-traumatic stress disorder (PTSD). Importantly, post-traumatic stress does not appear to decrease over time after ICU discharge and may endure for a number of years. Criteria for the diagnosis of PTSD are defined in the DSM-IV-TR. Factors associated with an increased likelihood of both anxiety, depression and PTSD after ICU discharge are listed in Table 86–4.

Patients who had neuropsychological impairment after ICU care had statistically significantly higher depression scores than those who did not require ICU-level of care.[12] Increased severity of illness does not seem to predict an increased risk of

TABLE 86–4   Factors associated with increased likelihood of psychological dysfunction.

Female sex
Younger age
Longer duration of sedation
Pre-existing anxiety or depressive symptoms
Injuries resulting from trauma
Longer ICU stay
Longer mechanical ventilation
Alcohol dependence prior to critical illness

developing psychological dysfunction, but rather it is both the subjective and objective aspects of the ICU experience that seem to be associated with it. In addition, these subjective and objective indicators are associated with the severity of anxiety and depression experienced by patients after ICU discharge.

The subjective indicators include the reported unpleasant memories of being in the ICU. Patients often report disturbing recollections and these experiences are often persecutory in nature and are associated with feelings of being elsewhere reliving a previous life event or fighting for survival. The lack of memory for actual events may mean that this is the way in which patients process these delusions or unreal experiences that result in longer term psychological problems. In fact, it has been proposed that the content of the ICU memories was more important than their number, and that delusional memories were more likely to result in distress than factual memories, even if these were unpleasant.[13] Patients frequently describe these memories as extremely vivid and real. The traumatic memories may also be linked to the recollection of certain persistent physical symptoms. Some patients may make strenuous efforts to block these traumatic memories but, paradoxically, this may only cause them to occur more frequently.

The objective indicators include variables such as length-of-stay (LOS), duration of sedation and/or neuromuscular blockade, mechanical ventilation, and other respiratory supportive therapies. Some studies show that decreased time under sedation or in mechanical ventilation result in decreased post-traumatic stress symptoms and anxiety. It is interesting to note that there has been some inconclusive evidence to support the role of corticosteroid supplementation during acute illness in preventing PTSD during recovery—as PTSD is associated with abnormalities of the hypothalamic–pituitary–adrenal axis and in stress response in general.

Psychological and behavioral outcome after ICU care has been mainly assessed using standardized questionnaires with demonstrated reliability and validity. Tools used to assess anxiety, depression, and PTSD are listed in Table 86–5.

TABLE 86–5 Questionnaires used to assess psychological impairments.

Anxiety and Depression	Post-traumatic stress and PTSD
Hospital Anxiety and Depression Scale (HADS)	Experience after Treatment in Intensive Care 7-item Scale
Beck Anxiety Inventory	PTSD 10-Questions Inventory
State Trait Anxiety	Davidson Trauma Scale
Beck Depression Inventory	Impact of Event Scale—Revised

CONSEQUENCES OF THE POST-INTENSIVE CARE SYNDROME

Impact on the Patient

Health-related quality of life (HRQoL) sums up the effects of the ICU stay in survivors of critical illness and is probably the best documented of all non-mortality outcomes after hospital discharge. HRQoL encompasses both the physical and psychological aspects of the individual's overall well-being. HRQoL after ICU discharge may range from normal to reduced in different patient populations and are usually compared to the "normal" population in different studies. Elderly survivors tend to have decreased HRQoL mostly in the physical domains. Survivors of severe trauma tend to have more permanent reductions in their HRQoL due to the fact that their HRQoL probably is already reduced at baseline from alcohol and substance abuse, even though these patients are typically younger and frequently do not suffer from prior chronic organ dysfunctions. Studies that compare pre-ICU HRQoL with post-ICU data indicate that ICU patients in general express a reduced HRQoL prior to ICU admission compared to the matched general population. The burden of preexisting medical conditions is one of the most significant factors associated with a reduction in HRQoL after ICU care. This strongly suggests that in most acutely ill ICU patients, their HRQoL after ICU discharge probably will never equal a matched general population. Working status or the ability to return to work is also a frequently reported outcome measure and is in general found to be low and reported to range from 23% to 35% in different studies.

Compounding the already burdened survivor, depression has been associated with poorer HRQoL. However, the direction of this relationship is not clear, and it may be that patients with a poorer HRQoL have a more prolonged recovery and thus are more likely to be depressed. This is an important issue because it suggests that if other aspects of HRQoL are better, then perhaps emotional outcome might be improved. Depression may interfere with the speed of recovery, and in some patients may lead to suicidal attempts.

Impact on Caregivers

There is no question that caregivers have a devastating, parallel, but different experience compared with their loved one. For the family and other caregivers, the daily and overwhelming stress experienced while the patient is in the ICU leaves its mark, and they similarly may experience compromised HRQoL and mental health, including PTSD, emotional distress, caregiver burden, depression and anxiety.[14] There is a strong relationship between high levels of PTSD-related symptoms in family members and those in patients. In some cases, family therapy may be needed. As a result returning to the hospital or doctor's office for outpatient appointments can be very stressful but, at the same time, it may be therapeutic and provide needed reassurance of their loved one's recovery. For bereaved families, the incidence of PTSD may be even higher and often goes completely unrecognized. Even when home care is provided by family members, there is still great opportunity cost, as these individuals must sacrifice other endeavors to free up time at home. Caregivers themselves also may face significant cognitive morbidity simply as a consequence of caring for their chronically ill family members.

Impact on the Health Care System

Along with personal costs, there are significant financial costs associated with surviving an episode of critical illness. ICU survivors face long hospital

LOS and post-discharge care that frequently involves expensive skilled nursing and long-term acute care (LTAC) facilities. Compared with the extensive resources devoted to helping the patient survive their ICU stay, far fewer resources are devoted to improving outcomes in the post-ICU period and systems are not in place to facilitate the patient's transition from the acute to the chronic phase of their illness. Transferring patients to LTACs decreases hospitals costs, but increases total costs, with no consistent improvement in long-term outcomes. In the era of intensivist physician staffing and hospitalist medicine, it is becoming less common that a single physician provides both hospital care and post-discharge care. Instead, the responsibility for post-discharge care falls on busy general practitioners, who are frequently unaware of events in the ICU, and often lack the time and expertise to diagnose the myriad of sequelae of critical illness.

STRATEGIES TO MINIMIZE OR PREVENT PICS

Physical and Neurocognitive Domains

Controlling the modifiable risk factors known to be associated with the different aspects of PICS is probably the first step in mitigating its effects on ICU survivors. These would include maintaining euglycemia, minimizing use of sedation and neuromuscular blockers, early liberation from mechanical ventilation, judicious use of corticosteroids, and early exercise and mobilization.[15] Early identification of ICU-AW will be the key in initiating early physical and occupational therapy. Early exercise and mobilization has been shown to increase the number of patients being discharged from the hospital with an independent functional status. Studies have also demonstrated a link between exercise and cognition through improved cerebrovascular function. Identifying exercise as a mechanism that reverses or alters the trajectory of cognitive impairment would have an important impact on the HRQoL in survivors of critical illness.[16] Furthermore, combining both cognitive and physical rehabilitation has been shown to result in significantly better executive functioning and fewer disabilities in instrumental activities

of daily living. An ICU sleep-promotion initiative has likewise been shown to reduce incident delirium and cognitive impairment. Better sleep efficiency may contribute to improving HRQoL and reducing fatigue to allow more effective participation in physical rehabilitation.

Psychological Domain

The psychological stress resulting from the ICU experience has been shown to be partly contributed by inaccurate memories during the ICU stay. Therefore, it has been suggested that providing survivors with an ICU diary may improve their understanding of their ICU experience and act as a "debriefing" tool. ICU diaries may be compiled by any of the ICU staff members, particularly nurses, and also by family members. It can be a written account complemented by photographs or videos. It should be viewed as a form of exposure to accurate and potentially corrective information, thereby reducing the anxiety caused by inaccurate and oftentimes frightening memories of the ICU stay. Also, reading or viewing of the ICU diary is entirely voluntary at a time of the patient's choosing and should be followed by a discussion of the contents with a member of the ICU staff. This should be viewed as a first step in learning to modify and control feelings and reduce physiological arousal as a step to recovery. Those patients who have received ICU diaries had lower levels of PTSD-related symptoms than those who did not.[17]

A stepped care approach with different degrees of therapeutic intervention depending on patient need may represent a more viable and flexible model for recovering critical illness survivors. This may involve designing or using off the shelf self-help programs to help individuals coping with lower levels of symptoms of anxiety, panic or depression. Those patients not responding to this or who exhibit greater symptom levels may then be referred to specialist psychological services for cognitive behavioral therapy or eye movement desensitization and reprocessing. These are therapies designed to reduce the emotional impact of distressing and traumatic memories and facilitate new ways of thinking. A stepped care approach may offer the appropriate and timely help to the maximum of patients, and may be more cost-effective compared with a more conventional approach of referring all patients to a counselor or clinical psychologist.

FUTURE DIRECTIONS

As the public is slowly becoming more aware of the PCIS because of increased reporting in mainstream media, efforts to further expand knowledge on this syndrome and to implement interventions to treat or mitigate its effects are more important than ever. With the percentage of the elderly population rising to much higher numbers in the next few decades, coupled with increasing survivorship from the ICU, we may be facing a public health emergency. Future research should be geared towards standardizing the definition of cognitive impairment, defining the spectrum of disability after critical illness, refining the associations of risk factors, detailing specific patient and family-centered outcomes, and improving study designs to address long-term patient-centered functional outcomes. In addition, much more research is needed to evaluate the effectiveness of educational strategies that raise awareness and promote treatment of post-ICU morbidity among general practitioners.

A potentially useful post-intensive care recovery intervention is the concept of the post-ICU clinic. From recent experience from the United Kingdom, it has been shown to increase understanding of the longer term recovery from critical illness.[18] However, the provision of services in different clinics is varied, unspecialized and oftentimes inconsistent, and tend to have funding problems hence restricting the number of patients who can be seen. Currently, it is still unclear whether these clinics should be staffed by intensivists or general practitioners.

Nonetheless, a well-designed care model similar to disease management programs for diabetes, heart failure, and COPD, will facilitate the transition of patients and their families to the outpatient setting, allow for early recognition of post-ICU complications and sequelae, increase access to a variety of health care providers, and improve HRQoL. Likewise, principles of longitudinal care models developed from acute stroke care, cardiac rehabilitation, and post-traumatic brain injury may be applied to survivors of critical illness.

CONCLUSIONS

Recent data shows that PCIS is common and involves the physical, cognitive, and mental health status in survivors of critical illness. These impairments are frequently under recognized and adversely impact the daily functioning and overall QOL. It is critical that interventions to prevent the sequelae of acute critical illness begin during the ICU stay and involve not only the ICU staff but those involved in the care of the patient after the acute care hospitalization.

REFERENCES

1. Needham DM, Davidson J, Cohen H, et al. Improving long-term outcomes after discharge from intensive care unit: report from a stakeholders' conference. *Crit Care Med.* 2012;40:502-509.
2. Herridge MS, Tansey CM, Matte A, et al. Functional disability 5 years after acute respiratory distress syndrome. *N Engl J Med.* 2011;364:1293-1304.
3. Wilcox ME, Herridge MS. Long-term outcomes in patients surviving acute respiratory distress syndrome. *Semin Respir Crit Care Med.* 2011;31:55-65.
4. Seneff MG, Zimmerman JE, Knaus WA, Wagner DP, Draper EA. Predicting the duration of mechanical ventilation. The importance of disease and patient characteristics. *Chest.* 1996;110:469-479.
5. Scheinhorn DJ, Hassenpflug MS, Votto JJ, et al. Ventilation Outcomes Study Group. Post-ICU mechanical ventilation at 23 long-term care hospitals: a multicenter outcomes study. *Chest.* 2007;131:85-93.
6. Hopkins RO, Weaver LK, Collingridge D, et al. Two-year cognitive, emotional, and quality-of-life outcomes in acute respiratory distress syndrome. *Am J Respir Crit Care Med.* 2005;171:340-347.
7. Hermans G, Wilmer A, Meersserman W, et al. Impact of intensive insulin therapy on neuromuscular complications and ventilator dependency in the medical intensive care unit. *Am J Respir Crit Care Med.* 2007;175:480-489.
8. Ehlenbach WJ, Hough CL, Crane PK, et al. Association between acute care and critical illness hospitalization and cognitive function in older adults. *J Am Med Assoc.* 2010;303:763-770.
9. Barnato AE, Albert SM, Angus DC, et al. Disability among elderly survivors of mechanical ventilation. *Am J Respir Crit Care Med.* 2011;183:1037-1042.
10. Iwashyna TJ, Ely EW, Smith DM, Langa KM. Long-term cognitive impairment and functional disability

among survivors of severe sepsis. *J Am Med Assoc.* 2010;304:1787-1794.

11. Hsieh SJ, Ely EW, Gong MN. Can intensive care unit delirium be prevented and reduced? Lessons learned and future directions. *Ann Am Thorac Soc.* 2013;10:648-656.

12. Davydow DS, Hough CL, Russo JE, et al. The association between intensive care unit admission and subsequent depression in patients with diabetes. *Int J Geriatr Psychiatry.* 2012;27:22-30.

13. Ringdal M, Johansson L, Lundberg D, Bergbom I. Delusional memories from the intensive care unit experienced by patients with physical trauma. *Intensive Crit Care Nurs.* 2006;22:346-354.

14. Van Pelt DC, Milbrandt EB, Qin L, et al. Informal caregiver burden among survivors of prolonged mechanical ventilation. *Am J Respir Crit Care Med.* 2007;175:167-173.

15. Morris PE, Griffin L, Berry M, et al. Receiving early mobility during an intensive care unit admission is a predictor of improved outcomes in acute respiratory failure. *Am J Med Sci.* 2011;341:373-377.

16. Elliot D, McKinley S, Alison J, et al. Health-related quality of life and physical recovery after a critical illness: a multicentre randomized controlled trial of a home-based physical rehabilitation program. *Crit Care.* 2011;15:R142.

17. Jones C, Backman C, Capuzzo M, et al. Intensive care diaries reduce new onset post-traumatic stress disorder following critical illness: a randomized, controlled trial. *Crit Care.* 2010;14:R168.

18. Griffiths JA, Barber VS, Cuthbertson BH, et al. A national survey of intensive care follow-up clinics. *Anaesthesia.* 2006;61:950-955.

Outcomes Research and Reporting

Angela K. M. Lipshutz, MD, MPH and
Michael A. Gropper, MD, PhD

KEY POINTS

1 Outcomes research evaluates the effects of medical care and the health care process on individual and societal health.

2 Outcomes research seeks to understand the effectiveness of an intervention rather than its efficacy. It is this focus, not the methodology employed, that differentiates outcomes research from traditional clinical research.

3 Commonly used outcome measures include mortality, health status, cost, and quality measures.

4 Although outcomes research is not defined by a specific methodology, outcomes researchers often utilize observational

study designs and methods from the social sciences. The use of large administrative datasets is increasingly popular.

5 The major limitations of observational studies are bias and confounding.

6 Matching, stratification, multivariate analysis, propensity scores, and instrumental variables are tools used to adjust for confounding.

7 Outcomes researchers in the intensive care unit face unique challenges due to the breadth of patients, diseases, therapies, providers, and health care delivery models used in critical care.

INTRODUCTION

Since the Institute of Medicine (IOM) published its first report in the quality series, *To Err is Human*, in 1999, there has been increased awareness of the problems that face health care in the United States and an increased emphasis on improving the quality of care our patients receive.[1] Outcomes research, which "studies the end results of medical care—the effect of the health care process on the health and well-being of patients and populations,"[2] is one type of research used to study, understand, and improve health care quality. Outcomes research differs from more traditional medical research in its focus and endpoints; it seeks to understand the *effectiveness* of

an intervention rather than its *efficacy*. Ultimately, the results of outcomes research can be used to benchmark performance, reduce adverse events, formulate clinical practice guidelines, and inform health policy decisions.[3,4]

In the critical care setting, outcomes research can be particularly impactful for several reasons. First, ICU patients are at a high risk of death and preventable harms due to the acuity of their illnesses and the frequency and complexity of interventions.[5] Additionally, the costs of ICU care are substantial. ICU patients inhabit only 10% of inpatient beds, but account for almost a quarter of acute care hospital costs.[6,7] In 2005, critical care costs in the United States totaled $81.7 billion per year—4.1% of national health expenditures and 0.66% of the gross national product.[8] Furthermore, resource utilization varies significantly, but an association between increased expenditure and quality of care has not been clearly elucidated.[9-12] Therefore, outcomes research in critical care has the potential to make ICU care better, safer, and more cost-effective.

This chapter describes the historical and theoretical basis for outcomes research, methods used by outcomes researchers, endpoints of outcomes research, and common challenges and limitations.

HISTORY AND THEORY

Florence Nightingale and Ernst Codman are often cited as the earliest outcomes researchers— Nightingale for her work studying combat deaths during the Crimean War, and Codman, an early 20th century surgeon at the Massachusetts General Hospital, for advocating hospital reporting of patient outcomes after noting that hospitals routinely reported the number of patients treated, but not the effects of the treatment.[13-15] However, no framework for outcomes research existed until 1966, when Avedis Donabedian put forth a model for evaluating health services and the quality of medical care.[16] The Donabedian model suggests three dimensions for assessing health care quality: structure, process, and outcome (Figure 87–1). Structure refers to the characteristics of the setting or environment in which care is delivered, while process focuses on whether appropriate medical practices are utilized. Outcomes range from mortality and length of stay to functional status and quality of life. Although Donabedian recognized the inherent limitations of outcome measures (see the "Limitations" section), he believed that outcomes "remain the ultimate validators of the effectiveness and quality of medical care."[16]

In 1989, the United States Congress acknowledged the importance of outcomes research when it created the Agency for Health Care Policy and Research [later the Agency for Healthcare Research and Quality (AHRQ)] "for the purpose of enhancing the quality, appropriateness, and effectiveness of health care services and access to care."[17] The Patient-Centered Outcomes Research Institute (PCORI) was established in 2010 as a part of the Patient Protection and Affordable Care Act, further solidifying outcomes research in the American lexicon.

THE FOCUS OF OUTCOMES RESEARCH

Outcomes Research Versus Traditional Clinical Research

Outcomes research "focuses on the effects of medical care on individuals and society."[4] It is this research focus, not necessarily the methodology, that distinguishes outcomes research from traditional clinical research.[4,13,18] Table 87–1 describes the differences between outcomes research and traditional clinical research.[4] Traditional clinical research is hypothesis-driven, and evaluates efficacy, asking whether an intervention works in an idealized setting. Outcomes research is concerned with effectiveness: Does the intervention help an individual patient in a real-world setting?[19] Additionally, outcomes research is patient-centered, rather than disease-centered, and focuses on "what one ultimately wants health care to achieve,"[20] for example, improvements in functional status or quality of life. Furthermore, outcomes research tends to be more inclusive in what it considers an intervention. Traditional clinical research often involves the evaluation of new drugs or devices, while the interventions in outcomes research can range from a new drug to

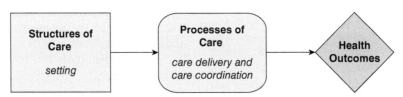

FIGURE 87–1   Donabedian's quality framework. (*Reproduced with permission from McDonald KM, Sundaram V, Bravata DM, et al: Closing the Quality Gap: A Critical Analysis of Quality Improvement Strategies (Vol. 7: Care Coordination). 2007 June.*)

TABLE 87–1 A comparison of features between traditional clinical research and outcomes research.)

Traditional Clinical Research	Outcomes Research
Efficacy	Effectiveness
Mechanisms of disease	Impact of disease on the patient
Experimental	Observational
Feasibility	Cost-effectiveness
The effect of biochemical and physiologic factors on biophysiologic outcomes	The effect of socioeconomic factors on patient-centered outcomes
Disease-centered	Patient- and community-centered
Provider-oriented	Consumer-oriented
Inventing technology	Assessing technology
Drugs and devices	Processes and delivery of care
Methods from the "hard" sciences (physics, biochemistry, physiology)	Methods from the "social" sciences (economics, social and behavioral sciences, epidemiology)

Reproduced with permission from Rubenfeld GD, Angus DC, Pinsky MR, et al: Outcomes research in critical care: Results of the American Thoracic Society critical care assembly workshop on outcomes research, *Am J Respir Crit Care Med* 1999 Jul;160(1):358-367.

a new structure for health care delivery. In order to achieve its goals, outcomes research tends to utilize observational study designs and draw methods from the social sciences more frequently than traditional clinical research (see the "Methods" section).

Commonly Used Outcome Measures

Mortality

Mortality is perhaps the most tangible and meaningful endpoint. It is easy to define and almost uniformly recorded. It sounds relatively simple: Did the patient survive the acute illness or insult? However, using mortality as an endpoint is actually not so straightforward. One must first determine the appropriate time at which to assess mortality: ICU or hospital discharge? 30, 60, or 90 days? Years? Selecting a timeframe that is too short may provide an inaccurate assessment of

the impact of an intervention if the natural history of the condition being studied is longer than the study period. A specific intervention might reduce 30-day mortality, but increase 90-day mortality. Conversely, long-term outcomes may reflect the patient's disease prognosis, age, premorbid conditions,[21] and preexisting functional status[22,23] more than the ICU care they received. Therefore, the appropriate mortality endpoint depends on the specific research question, the study design, and the mechanisms of the disease or treatment being studied.[4]

Even when an appropriate mortality endpoint is chosen, outcomes can be artificially affected by patient choice, as well as ICU and hospital practice patterns. For instance, a patient's decision to transition to comfort care may hasten death; the availability of palliative care suites for transfer of ICU patients receiving comfort measures only alters ICU mortality; and the availability of long-term care facilities for transfer of ventilator-dependent patients could alter hospital mortality. Additionally, comparing mortality rates across different hospitals and ICUs is fraught with problems, largely due to difficulty in adjusting for differences in case-mix.[24] Using mortality as an endpoint may not be feasible if the mortality of the condition being studied is relatively low, as the sample size required to generate adequate power to detect a clinically relevant difference will be quite large. And, of course, the use of mortality as an endpoint does not consider morbidities or the quality of life of the survivor.

Health Status

Health status encompasses several measures of patient-assessed outcomes, including functional status and quality of life. Health status is an important endpoint for critical care outcomes research, as recent data has shown that the long-term consequences of critical illness on physical functional status, cognitive function, and quality of life can be profound.[25-28]

Measurement of health status is not standardized, and relies on patient interviews and questionnaires. Physical functional status can be assessed using the 6-minute-walk test, Medical Outcomes Study Short-Form 36 (SF-36),[25,26] the Karnofsky Performance Status Scale score, the Barthel Index, and the Lawton-Instrumental Activities of Daily Living score.[29,30] Tools to assess mental health status, focusing on symptoms of depression, anxiety, and post-traumatic stress disorder, include the Center for Epidemiologic Studies–Depression Scale,[31] the Hospital Anxiety and Depression Scale,[32] and the Impact of Events Scale-Revised.[33] The Informant Questionnaire on Cognitive Decline in the Elderly, the Trail Making Test, and the Repeatable Battery for the Assessment of Neuropsychological Status have been used to determine cognitive function.[27,28,34] Quality of life can be determined from the results of these various tests, or can be assessed specifically via tools such as the EuroQol-5D[30] or SF-36.[35] Quality of life data can then be used to calculate quality-adjusted life years (QALYs), which take into account both mortality and quality of life.[35]

Of note, completion of these instruments by ICU survivors themselves is not always possible, and the use of surrogates to complete them may not be as useful. Additionally, interpretation of these tests requires knowledge of the patient's baseline prior to ICU admission, which may also require a surrogate for determination, and is subject to recall bias. Nonetheless, data is mounting that ICU patients continue to suffer long after their discharge from the hospital: Depression and anxiety may be present in nearly half of ICU survivors,[36] and post-traumatic stress disorder in one-third.[32,33] Decline in cognitive function is common and can persist for up to eight years.[27] And physical disability is nearly ubiquitous; in one study, 100% of patients reported experiencing subjective weakness and decreased exercise capacity and almost a quarter of patients were unable to return to work at 5 years after discharge from the ICU.[25] Thus, continued work on targeting improvement in health status for ICU survivors is paramount.

Cost

Economic evaluation is "the comparative analysis of alternative health care interventions in their relative costs (resource use) and effectiveness (health effects)."[37] With the aging of the US population, and the availability of new and more expensive treatments, the cost of critical care is increasing.[38,39] As mentioned earlier, ICU care is disproportionately expensive,[6,7] costing over $80 billion per year in the United States alone.[8] Therefore, identifying cost-effective interventions in the ICU is incredibly important. Cost-effectiveness analyses (CEAs)

produce a ratio in which the numerator is the cost of the intervention, and the denominator is the benefit in terms of the clinical outcome.[40] The clinical outcome is often reported in terms of QALYs, such that the ratio produced is cost per QALY.

Given the increasing importance of CEAs, and the increasing frequency with which they are performed, both the US Public Health Service and the American Thoracic Society convened panels to address methodological issues and provide recommendations for the reporting of CEAs.[40,41] Their recommendations include describing the model used; identifying model assumptions; describing how estimates of effectiveness, costs, and health states were obtained; and defining the type of costs, year of costs, inflation adjustment methods, and discount rates used. Even when following these recommendations, critical care outcomes researchers face additional challenges that make CEAs more challenging in the ICU setting. These include the complexity of ICU patients, the lack of data on effectiveness of interventions in the ICU, the unavailability of cost data, and the infrequent collection of ideal outcomes measures for CEAs (eg, long-term quality-adjusted survival rates).[40] The challenge of obtaining accurate cost data can make CEAs difficult to interpret and compare, and limits the generalizability of the results. Charge data (ie, what the patient is billed) are often substituted for cost; however, even when adjusted with cost-per-charge ratios, these data are department and institution specific, and may not reflect actual costs.[37,42] Therefore, interpretation of CEAs must be undertaken with great caution.

Quality Measures

A common focus of outcomes research is quality improvement. Outcome measures for quality improvement research must be "granular enough to be meaningful to clinicians [and to] adequately drive quality improvement interventions."[3] Since preventability is one of the central tenets of quality improvement, outcome measures must also be viewed as preventable.

A recent study by Martinez et al. utilized a consensus process to identify meaningful outcomes measures for quality improvement in the ICU.[3] In the study, 164 ICU providers identified five preventable outcomes: pressure ulcers, central line-associated bloodstream infection, pulmonary embolism, methicillin-resistant *Staphylococcus aureus* infection, and gastrointestinal bleed. Indeed, data support the preventability of these outcomes. For instance, in a landmark study by Pronovost et al., central-line associated bloodstream infections were eradicated in the state of Michigan.[43] However, prior to this study, central-line associated bloodstream infections were not uniformly considered preventable. Therefore, although the development and use of outcomes measures for quality improvement must rely on existing data suggesting preventability, clinicians and researchers must also be creative and innovative, continuing to question our current knowledge base of what is preventable.

Methods

Although the focus of outcomes research differs from that of traditional scientific research, the methods used need not. Outcomes research can take the form of case-control studies, cohort studies, and even randomized controlled trials (RCTs). However, outcomes researchers tend to utilize observational study designs and draw methods from the social sciences more frequently than traditional clinical researchers. The use of large administrative datasets is a growing trend in outcomes research. Additionally, outcomes researchers use qualitative methods to generate hypotheses and describe complex phenomena that do not lend themselves to quantitative methods or traditional hypothesis testing.[4]

Observational Studies

Observational studies can be prospective or retrospective, and include cohort studies, case-control studies, and cross-sectional studies.[44] Such studies seek to identify associations between an exposure (eg, a medication, intervention, or organization of health care delivery) and outcomes, and can utilize primary or secondary data. Primary data are collected to answer a specific research question, while secondary data are data that already exist but are reemployed to answer a novel research question.[45]

Administrative data are a type of secondary data that were originally collected for reasons other than research. Administrative data include health care encounter data, enrollment data, clinical data, data registries, performance data, survey data, and

national data.[4] Examples of data sources utilized in critical care outcomes research include Medicare, the University HealthSystem Consortium, the National Inpatient Sample, and the National Hospital Discharge Database.[46] There are several benefits to using administrative data for outcomes research. First, administrative data may provide answers to research questions that ethically, legally, or practically cannot be answered by RCTs. Second, large registries and administrative data may be broader in scope and thus more generalizable than primary data. Furthermore, large datasets can more efficiently answer questions associated with rare diseases or outcomes. Finally, policymakers may be more interested in outcomes assessed via administrative data. In fact, policy concerns regarding Medicare spending, racial disparities, and unexplained geographic variation in health care are fueled by the results of analysis of administrative data.[46]

However, the use of administrative data is not without its drawbacks. As with all observational studies, studies using administrative data are subject to bias and confounding. Confounding is of particular concern since patients are not randomly assigned to the exposure of interest; thus, any association between the exposure and outcome could be due to a third, unmeasured variable (see the "Limitations" section). However, the primary concern specific to administrative data is data quality. Unlike traditional clinical research, in which the study design is completed before data collection begins, with administrative data, the quality of the data must be assessed before designing the study (but, of course, after the research question is defined).[45] The Directory of Clinical Databases in the United Kingdom recently developed a framework for assessing the quality of administrative data.[47] The framework focuses on data coverage and data accuracy (Table 87–2). Coverage is determined by the representativeness of the data, the completeness of recruitment, the variables included, and the extent of missing variables, while accuracy is determined by the collection of raw data, the definitions and rules utilized, the reliability of coding, the independence of observations, and the method of data validation.[46]

Once the quality of the data has been assessed, the process of research can continue (Figure 87–2). Several aspects of this process are unique to secondary data analyses, and deserve mentioning. First, the

TABLE 87–2 Quality domains important in assessing the quality of administrative data.

Quality Domain	Explanation
Coverage	
Representativeness	How well does the data source represent the population that it intends to?
Completeness of recruitment	This feature measures the extent to which all eligible individuals have been included in the data collection scheme
Variables included	What is the extent of the data collected on each individual? Are demographic, exposure, outcome, and confounding varaibles present?
Completeness of variables	What is the extent of the missing data?
Accuracy	
Collection of raw data	Is the raw data collected are aggregate averages collected?
Explicit definitions	Are the variables explicitly defined?
Explicit rules	Are there explicit rules for deciding how variables are recorded? For example, the timing of physiologic variables
Reliability of coding	Was the reliability of coded conditions and interventions tested?
Independence of observations	Was the data recorder blinded to patient outcome at the time the data were collected?
Data validation	Were data validated using outside sources? Were there consistency checks?

Reproduced with permission from Cooke T, Iwashyna TJ: Using existing data to address important clinical questions in critical care, *Crit Care Med* 2013 Mar;41(3):886-896.

analysis plan must be developed a priori in order to maintain the validity of the study. Since secondary data, by definition, already exists, it can be tempting to perform preliminary analyses before finalizing an analysis plan; this temptation should be avoided as it can bias the results. Similarly, "data-dredging" via post-hoc analyses may result in the identification of erroneous, or at least meaningless, associations, since exploring any 20 associations will, on average, produce one result that is statistically significant to $P < 0.05$.[45] Thus, the number of statistical tests performed should be minimized. In addition, adjustment for bias and confounding must be performed. However, it is important to remember that even the most sophisticated statistics cannot compensate for poor data quality.

Qualitative Research

Qualitative methods are increasingly being used in outcomes research. Qualitative research uses methods such as interviews, focus groups, field observations, and document review (eg, diaries) in order to "understand complex social processes, organizational change, individual health behaviors, and nuanced aspects of environmental context that influence quality of care, health care delivery, and health outcomes for individuals and populations."[48] Qualitative research differs from quantitative research in that it describes the breadth and complexity of a phenomenon rather than measuring occurrences to determine frequency, incidence, prevalence, or magnitude.[49] Given the complexity and nuanced aspects of critical care, qualitative research can be particularly useful in this setting.

Qualitative methods should be considered when: (1) the phenomena of interest are difficult to measure quantitatively, (2) a comprehensive understanding of a problem is desired, (3) the goal is to generate insight as to why an intervention has a specific impact, and (4) special populations are being studied.[49] Once collected, qualitative data can be coded and analyzed. Analysis focuses on identifying taxonomies and themes that can explain and predict outcomes.[50] Although qualitative methods alone can provide interesting and rich data, mixed methods—which combine quantitative and qualitative methods—are even more impactful as they benefit from the strengths of each approach.[49]

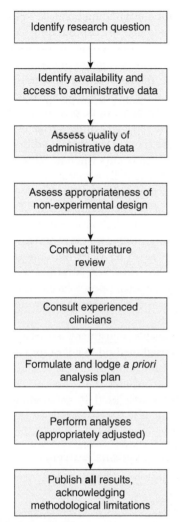

FIGURE 87-2 The process of outcomes research using administrative data. (*Reproduced with permission from Wunsch H, Harrison DA, Rowan K: Health services research in critical care using administrative data, J Crit Care 2005 Sep;20(3):264-269.*)

Randomized Controlled Trials

RCTs are traditionally designed as efficacy studies—assessing the impact of an intervention in an ideal setting—and are thus most commonly used in conventional clinical research. RCTs can also be utilized in outcomes research if the study design focuses on effectiveness—the implications of an intervention or exposure in a "real-world" setting. Unlike observational studies, RCTs do not have the problem of confounding since, by definition, the exposure is

allocated randomly. The lack of confounding makes it easier to conclude causality. However, the use of RCTs in outcomes research is relatively rare for several reasons. First, RCTs are expensive and time-consuming. Second, it may not be legal or ethical to randomize patients to certain exposures or interventions. And, finally, some exposures (eg, socioeconomic status or insurance status) may be impossible to randomize.[4] Nonetheless, RCTs remain the "gold standard," and should be considered by outcomes researchers when feasible. Recently, two RCTs of early mobilization in the ICU, designed as effectiveness studies, showed improved functional status for patients who received physical therapy during their critical illness.[51,52]

LIMITATIONS

As with all scientific research, critical care outcomes research faces its own set of challenges and limitations. Some of these limitations are methodological—for instance, due to issues with bias and confounding—and are common to outcomes research across all fields of medicine, while some limitations are unique to critical care medicine.

Methodological

The methodological challenges inherent to outcomes research are, obviously, specific to the study design being employed. Herein, we will consider the limitations of observational studies, since a large portion of outcomes researchers rely on observational methods.

The primary methodological limitations of observational studies are bias and confounding. Bias is a systematic error in the design or conduct of a study. There are several different types of bias that can obscure the results of observational studies. Selection bias exists when the patients in one group are somehow fundamentally different from the patients in the other group. Observational bias exists when there are systematic differences in the way in which the data was obtained. Recall and recording bias are types of observational bias. Recall bias frequently comes into play in studies evaluating ICU patient and family experiences, since the patient's ultimate outcome may affect how they remember their course of care. Recording bias is especially important when using administrative data, since data collected for coding and billing may be affected by efforts to increase reimbursement.[45]

A confounding variable is an extraneous variable that is correlated with the independent variable being studied; confounding exists when the exposed and unexposed groups being studied differ in some way that is also related to the outcome. Randomized controlled trials obviate the concern for confounding since randomizing attempts to ensure the exposed and unexposed groups are similar. However, observational studies are subject to confounding, and when confounding occurs, the effect of the exposure on the outcome will be distorted.[45] Severity of illness is a common confounder in critical care outcomes research. For instance, consider a comparison of two groups of ICU patients with respiratory failure, where one group received a new mode of mechanical ventilation and the primary outcome measure was ventilator-free days. If the group receiving the intervention was younger and had a significantly higher PaO_2-to-FiO_2 ratio at admission, they may have more ventilator-free days simply because they were less sick.

Unlike bias, which is a systematic error and cannot be fixed, there are five commonly used ways to control for confounding (Table 87–3).[4,53] Matching attempts to identify confounding variables and matches the exposed and unexposed groups based on these variables. Although this technique is relatively simple, the number of confounding variables upon which groups can be matched is limited since an exact match may not be present, and the analysis is limited since matching variables cannot be evaluated as exposure variables. Additionally, overmatching, which occurs when matching for a variable that is not actually a confounder, can decrease the power of the study. Similar to matching, stratification involves the identification of confounding variables and creation of subclasses based on them. Age is a variable that is commonly stratified, for instance 18 to 65 years old and greater than 65 years old. However, stratification becomes unwieldy when attempting to account for multiple confounders as the number of subgroups increases exponentially.

Multivariable adjustment is perhaps the most commonly used method to adjust for confounding. In multivariable adjustment, the researcher creates a model that includes the exposure and outcome of interest, as well as the confounding variables.

TABLE 87–3 Techniques used to adjust for confounding in observational outcomes research.

Technique	Strengths	Weaknesses
Matching	Simple Balances confounding factors	Difficulty finding matches Possibility of overmatching Requires strong understanding of confounders involved Inability to examine effect of confounders used for matching
Stratification	Simple Ability to see effect modification	Difficult to interpret with many subgroups Requires strong understanding of confounders involved
Multivariable adjustment	Can include many confounders Can examine effects of individual confounders Ability to examine multilevel effects	More complicated analysis Potentially poor fit of model Possibility of missing effect modification
Propensity scores	Single number generated for simpler matching Ability to assess for bias between groups	Potentially matching very different patients with similar scores
Instrumental variables	Only single variable needed Ability to look at questions where other types of adjustment can not be easily accomplished	Difficult to ensure variable is not at all associated with the outcome

Reproduced with permission from Wunsch H, Linde-Zwirble WT, Angus DC: Methods to adjust for bias and confounding in critical care health services research involving observational data, *J Crit Care* 2006 Mar;21(1):1-7.

The model used depends on the outcome being studied—logistic regression is used when the outcome is binary, linear regression when the outcome is linear, and proportional hazards when the outcome is time to an event. These techniques hold the confounding variables constant while assessing the relationship between the exposure and the outcome. Severity of illness scores, such as the Acute Physiology and Chronic Health Evaluation Score (APACHE),[54] Simplified Acute Physiology Score (SAPS),[55] or Mortality Prediction Model Score (MPM),[56] is commonly included in multivariate analyses in an attempt to account for how sick patients are on admission to the ICU. These scoring systems take into account a large number of variables and provide a single number. However, one must remember that such scores may not capture all pre-existing comorbidities nor pre-existing frailty, which may have a large impact on the patient's clinical trajectory.[57] Furthermore, multivariate models are not without their pitfalls. Careful attention to which variables are included in the final model, and rigorous testing of model fit are required to avoid erroneous conclusions.

Propensity scores and instrumental variables are two more sophisticated methods of adjusting for confounding. Like severity of illness scores, propensity scores combine multiple variables to create a single value. This value represents a patient's probability of being exposed to the variable of interest.[58] Patients can then be matched or stratified based on their propensity score, or the propensity score can be included in the multivariate model. The use of propensity scores is increasingly common as they are a powerful tool to decrease the effects of confounding. Instrumental variables, like propensity scores, are associated with the exposure, but are selected because they are independent of outcomes. If an outcome is then analyzed by the instrumental variable, a random distribution of patients is created, which simulates randomization to the exposure. Although enticing, the use of instrumental variables is relatively uncommon, largely because it is difficult to identify variables that do not correlate with the outcome being studied.

Unique to Critical Care

In addition to the methodological limitations associated with observational outcomes research

discussed above, ICU outcomes researchers face a unique set of challenges, largely due to the breadth of patients, diseases, therapies, providers, and health care delivery models associated with critical care medicine. Performing research requires identifying a specific question and defining the disease, treatment, patient population, or provider to study. Defining such variables in the ICU can be complex.[4] Disease states, such as sepsis or respiratory failure, may be exceedingly broad and lack exact diagnostic criteria or accepted treatment. The patient population is highly variable, including medical, surgical, cardiac, and neurological patients. And the physicians caring for patients range from pulmonologists and cardiologists to anesthesiologists, surgeons, and surgical subspecialists. Therefore, "critical care" does not have an explicit definition in the literature. Although critical care is often defined geographically as patients cared for in an ICU, this is increasingly problematic as the chronically critically ill may be cared for outside the ICU, and some patients in the ICU may not actually be in critical condition.[4]

Furthermore, as mentioned above, critically ill patients may not be able to consent to or participate fully in research due to the severity of their illness, administration of sedative medications, or use of interventions such as mechanical ventilation that decrease their ability to communicate.

CONCLUSION

Outcomes research studies the end result of medical care on patients and society. Outcomes research in critical care is particularly important due to the severity of illness of ICU patients and complexity of the care they receive, as well as the overwhelming cost of ICU care. Critical care outcomes researchers often utilize observational study designs influenced by the social sciences, and focus on patient-centered outcomes such as mortality, functional status, and quality of life. The limitations of observational study designs can be addressed by several statistical methods. Continued emphasis on critical care outcomes research is of paramount importance as we attempt to understand and improve the long-term outcomes of survivors of critical illness.

REFERENCES

1. Kohn LT, Corrigan J, Donaldson MS. *To Err is Human: Building a Safer Health System*. Washington, DC: National Academies Press.
2. *Health Outcomes Research: A Primer*. Washington, DC: Foundation for Health Services Research; 1994.
3. Martinez EA, Donelan K, Henneman JP, et al. Identifying meaningful outcome measures for the intensive care unit. *Am J Med Qual*. 2014;29:144-152.
4. Rubenfeld GD, Angus DC, Pinsky MR, Curtis JR, Connors Jr AF, Bernard GR. Outcomes research in critical care: results of the American Thoracic Society critical care assembly workshop on outcomes research. *Am J Respir Crit Care Med*. 1999;160:358-367.
5. Bucknall TK. Medical error and decision making: learning from the past and present in intensive care. *Aust Crit Care*. 2010;23:150-156.
6. Halpern NA, Bettes L, Greenstein R. Federal and nationwide intensive care units and healthcare costs: 1986-1992. *Crit Care Med*. 1994;22:2001-2007.
7. Jacobs P, Noseworthy TW. National estimates of intensive care utilization and costs: Canada and the United States. *Crit Care Med*. 1990;18:1282-1286.
8. Halpern NA, Pastores SM. Critical care medicine in the United States 2000–2005: an analysis of bed numbers, occupancy rates, payer mix, and costs*. *Crit Care Med*. 2010;38:65-71.
9. Rothen HU, Stricker K, Einfalt J, et al. Variability in outcome and resource use in intensive care units. *Intensive Care Med*. 2007;33:1329-1336.
10. Dartmouth Atlas of Health Care. http://www.dartmouthatlas.org/. Accessed January 21, 2014.
11. Fisher ES. The implications of regional variations in Medicare spending. Part 1: The content, quality, and accessibility of care. *Ann Intern Med*. 2003;138:273-287.
12. Fisher ES. The implications of regional variations in Medicare spending. Part 2: Health outcomes and satisfaction with care. *Ann Intern Med*. 2003;138:288-298.
13. Chatburn RL. *Handbook for Health Care Research, Second Edition*. Sudbury, MA: Jones & Bartlett Publishers; 2011.
14. Jefford M, Stockler MR, Tattersall MH. Outcomes research: what is it and why does it matter? *Intern Med J*. 2003;33:110-118.
15. Shell CM, Dunlap KD. Florence Nightingale, Dr. Ernest Codman, American College of Surgeons hospital standardization committee, and the Joint Commission: Four pillars in the foundation of patient safety. *Perioper Nurs Clin*. 2008;3:19-26.
16. Donabedian A. Evaluating the quality of medical care. *Milbank Q*. 2005;83:691-729.
17. Reauthorization of the agency for health care policy and research. http://www.hhs.gov/asl/testify/t990429c.html. Accessed January 21, 2014.
18. Kane RL. *Understanding Health Care Outcomes Research*. Sudbury, MA: Jones and Bartlett; 2006.
19. Djulbegovic B, Paul A. From efficacy to effectiveness in the face of uncertainty. *J Am Med Assoc*. 2011;305:2005-2006.
20. Kane RL, Radosevich DM. *Conducting Health Outcomes Research*. Sudbury, MA: Jones and Bartlett Publishers; 2011.
21. Angus DC, Carlet J, 2002 Brussels Roundtable Participants. Surviving intensive care: a report from the 2002 Brussels roundtable. *Intensive Care Med*. 2003;29:368-377.
22. Bagshaw SM, Stelfox HT, McDermid RC, et al. Association between frailty and short- and long-term outcomes among critically ill patients: a multicentre prospective cohort study. *CMAJ*. 2014;186:E95-E102.
23. Bagshaw SM, McDermid RC. The role of frailty in outcomes from critical illness. *Curr Opin Crit Care*. 2013;19:496-503.
24. Glance LG, Osler T, Shinozaki T. Effect of varying the case mix on the standardized mortality ratio and W statistic: a simulation study. *Chest*. 2000;117:1112-1117.
25. Herridge MS, Tansey CM, Matte A, et al. Functional disability 5 years after acute respiratory distress syndrome. *N Engl J Med*. 2011;364:1293-1304.
26. Herridge MS, Cheung AM, Tansey CM, et al. One-year outcomes in survivors of the acute respiratory distress syndrome. *N Engl J Med*. 2003;348:683-693.
27. Iwashyna TJ, Ely EW, Smith DM, Langa KM. Long-term cognitive impairment and functional disability among survivors of severe sepsis. *J Am Med Assoc*. 2010;304:1787-1794.
28. Pandharipande PP, Girard TD, Jackson JC, et al. Long-term cognitive impairment after critical illness. *N Engl J Med*. 2013;369:1306-1316.
29. Haas JS, Teixeira C, Cabral CR, et al. Factors influencing physical functional status in intensive care unit survivors two years after discharge. *BMC Anesthesiol*. 2013;13:11.
30. Sacanella E, Pérez-Castejón JM, Nicolás JM, et al. Functional status and quality of life 12 months after discharge from a medical ICU in healthy elderly patients: a prospective observational study. *Critical Care*. 2011;15:R105.
31. Chelluri L, Im KA, Belle SH, et al. Long-term mortality and quality of life after prolonged mechanical ventilation. *Crit Care Med*. 2004;32:61-69.

32. Myhren H, Ekeberg O, Toien K, Karlsson S, Stokland O. Posttraumatic stress, anxiety and depression symptoms in patients during the first year post intensive care unit discharge. *Crit Care*. 2010;14:R14.

33. Bienvenu OJ, Gellar J, Althouse BM, et al. Post-traumatic stress disorder symptoms after acute lung injury: a 2-year prospective longitudinal study. *Psychol Med*. 2013;43:2657-2671.

34. Girard TD, Jackson JC, Pandharipande PP, et al. Delirium as a predictor of long-term cognitive impairment in survivors of critical illness. *Crit Care Med*. 2010;38:1513-1520.

35. Ferguson ND, Scales DC, Pinto R, et al. Integrating mortality and morbidity outcomes. *Am J Respiratory Crit Care Med*. 2013;187:256-261.

36. Scragg P, Jones A, Fauvel N. Psychological problems following ICU treatment*. *Anaesthesia*. 2001;56:9-14.

37. Cox HL, Laupland KB, Manns BJ. Economic evaluation in critical care medicine. *J Crit Care*. 2006;21:117-124.

38. American Association of Critical-Care Nurses, American College of Chest Physicians, American. Critical care workforce partnership position statement: The aging of the U.S. population and increased need for critical care services. November, 2011.

39. Angus DC, Kelley MA, Schmitz RJ, White A, Popovich Jr J, Committee on Manpower for Pulmonary and Critical Care Societies (COMPACCS). Caring for the critically ill patient. Current and projected workforce requirements for care of the critically ill and patients with pulmonary disease: can we meet the requirements of an aging population? *J Am Med Assoc*. 2000;284:2762-2770.

40. Understanding costs and cost-effectiveness in critical care: report from the second American Thoracic Society workshop on outcomes research. *Am J Respir Crit Care Med*. 2002;165:540-550.

41. Siegel JE. Recommendations for reporting cost-effectiveness analyses. *J Am Med Assoc*. 1996;276:1339.

42. Pines JM, Fager SS, Milzman DP. A review of costing methodologies in critical care studies. *J Crit Care*. 2002;17:181-186.

43. Pronovost P, Needham D, Berenholtz S, et al. An intervention to decrease catheter-related bloodstream infections in the ICU. *N Engl J Med*. 2006;355:2725-2732.

44. Black N. Why we need observational studies to evaluate the effectiveness of health care. *Br Med J*. 1996;312:1215-1218.

45. Wunsch H, Harrison DA, Rowan K. Health services research in critical care using administrative data. *J Crit Care*. 2005;20:264-269.

46. Cooke T, Iwashyna TJ. Using existing data to address important clinical questions in critical care. *Crit Care Med*. 2013;41:886-896.

47. Black N, Payne M. Directory of clinical databases: improving and promoting their use. *Qual Saf Health Care*. 2003;12:348-352.

48. Krumholz HM, Bradley EH, Curry LA. Promoting publication of rigorous qualitative research. *Circ Cardiovasc Qual Outcomes*. 2013;6:133-134.

49. Curry LA, Nembhard IM, Bradley EH. Qualitative and mixed methods provide unique contributions to outcomes research. *Circulation*. 2009;119:1442-1452.

50. Bradley EH, Curry LA, Devers KJ. Qualitative data analysis for health services research: developing taxonomy, themes, and theory. *Health Serv Res*. 2007;42:1758-1772.

51. Schweickert WD, Pohlman MC, Pohlman AS, et al. Early physical and occupational therapy in mechanically ventilated, critically ill patients: a randomised controlled trial. *Lancet*. 2009;373:1874-1882.

52. Burtin C, Clerckx B, Robbeets C, et al. Early exercise in critically ill patients enhances short-term functional recovery. *Crit Care Med*. 2009;37:2499-2505.

53. Wunsch H, Linde-Zwirble WT, Angus DC. Methods to adjust for bias and confounding in critical care health services research involving observational data. *J Crit Care*. 2006;21:1-7.

54. Zimmerman JE, Kramer AA, McNair DS, Malila FM. Acute physiology and chronic health evaluation (APACHE) IV: hospital mortality assessment for today's critically ill patients. *Crit Care Med*. 2006;34:1297-1310.

55. Moreno RP, Metnitz PG, Almeida E, et al. SAPS 3–from evaluation of the patient to evaluation of the intensive care unit. Part 2: Development of a prognostic model for hospital mortality at ICU admission. *Intensive Care Med*. 2005;31:1345-1355.

56. Higgins TL, Teres D, Copes WS, Nathanson BH, Stark M, Kramer AA. Assessing contemporary intensive care unit outcome: an updated mortality probability admission model (MPM0-III). *Crit Care Med*. 2007;35:827-835.

57. Wunsch H. Expanding horizons in critical care outcomes. *Curr Opin Crit Care*. 2013;19:465-466.

58. Austin PC. An introduction to propensity score methods for reducing the effects of confounding in observational studies. *Multivariate Behav Res*. 2011;46:399-424.

C H A P T E R

Critical Care Medicine in the Era of Omics

88

Samantha Strickler, DO and
John M. Oropello, MD, FACP, FCCP, FCCM

KEY POINTS

1 Researchers and physicians are now examining human health and disease in the context of the human genome, epigenome, transcriptome, proteome, and microbiome.

2 In critical illness, disease processes are multifaceted, involving numerous interactions between genes and gene products rather than a single locus.

3 Network medicine focuses on integrating various omic disciplines to create networks that explain healthy and diseased states.

4 Network model analysis of ARDS has revealed redundancy in protein connectivity, with several proteins involved in multiple pathways.

5 More basic research needs to be completed, followed by integration of genomic, epigenomic, transcriptomic, proteomic, microbiomic, and other omic data to create more network models of critical illness.

But nature did not deem it her business to make the discovery of her laws easy for us.
 -Albert Einstein (1911)

Within the human body there exists an incredible complexity, making the practice of medicine extremely challenging. No two individuals manifest illness identically. In critical care medicine, where illness strains human physiology to the brink of collapse, this becomes even more apparent. With critical illness accounting for nearly 39% of total hospital costs, now more than ever there is a demand to understand the multifaceted pathology that contributes to individual critical illness.[1]

For centuries, illness has been studied on a macrolevel with gross anatomy being the epicenter of medicine. However, with the completion of the Human Genome Project (2003), a new paradigm of medicine that focuses on molecular interactions is evolving. Researchers and physicians are now examining human health and disease in the context of the human genome, epigenome, transcriptome, proteome, and microbiome.[2-6] Furthermore, these "omes" are being integrated to create new network models of physiology and pathology (Figure 88–1).

Since the inception of the omic era, multiple disease states have been examined including Alzheimer's disease, cancer, and obesity. However, the

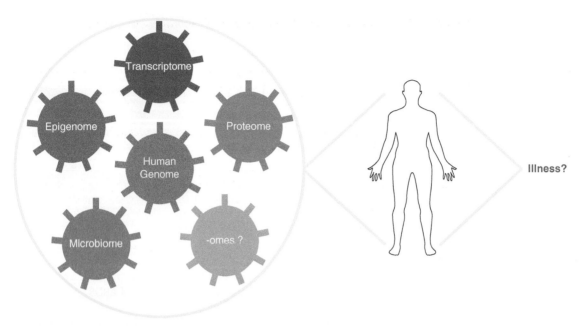

FIGURE 88–1 A new paradigm of medicine is developing, which examines illness through the interactions of the human genome, epigenome, transcriptome, proteome, microbiome, and other developing omes.

application of omics and network medicine to critical illness remains vastly unexplored. The intensive care unit is an uncharted frontier. As omics continues to rapidly expand, the molecular derangements of critical illness will become increasingly apparent. Such insight will evolve the practice of critical care medicine—allowing intensivists to augment their understanding of disease, and to more efficiently diagnose and treat the *individual* with critical illness. (See the "Glossary and Abbreviations" section for key terms.)

FROM MENDEL TO THE HUMAN GENOME PROJECT

For ages mankind has been fascinated by human variability (Table 88–1). Scientists have extensively hypothesized about the origins and variability of man. One of the earliest recognized publications addressing this query came from Dr. William Harvey, an English physician.[7] In 1651 he published, *De Generatione Animaliumi*, which examined the egg and early embryo in different species. In this doctrine, he pronounced, "ex ovo aminum—all things from the egg." His publication was the first to denounce the

concept of spontaneous generation and propose the theory of epigenesis.

Nearly 200 years later, Austrian monk Gregor Mendel expounded further upon the origins of variability.[8] In 1865, Mendel published his well-popularized findings examining flower color and texture of the seed of the garden pea. Through his cross breeding of plants he defined the theory of inheritance, demonstrating that each parent contributes an allele to the offspring for a certain characteristic forming a pair. These pairs further segregate independently of one another.

In the mid-1800s researchers further localized hereditary information to a cellular level. In 1869, Swiss physician and researcher, Friedrich Miescher, isolated nuclein (DNA) from leukocytes collected from soiled bandages from a nearby hospital.[9] In 1882, Walter Flemming, a German physician and professor of anatomy, published the first images of chromosomes in tumor cells (Figure 88–2). Many decades later in 1944, researchers Oswald Avery, Colin MacLeod, and Maclyn McCarty demonstrated that the elemental blocks of inheritance were contained within DNA through experiments with *Streptococcus pneumoniae*.

TABLE 88–1 Timeline of discoveries and establishment of organizations defining the development of omics.

Year	Event
1865	• Gregor Mendel publishes his theory of inheritance and segregation
1869	• Friedrich Miescher isolates DNA (nuclein) from soiled bandages
1944	• Oswald Avery, Colin MacLeod, and Maclyn McCarty demonstrate through experimentation with *Streptococcus pneumoniae* that DNA is the element of inheritance
1953	• Rosalind Franklin and Maurice Wilkins describe the structure of DNA as a double helix • James Watson and Walter Crick describe DNA as a right-handed double helix
1989	• Human Genome Organization (HUGO) created
1990	• Human Genome Project established in the United States, completed in 2000
1996	• The yeast genome, *Saccharomyces cerevisiae*, is sequenced
1998	• The roundworm genome, *Caenorhabditis elegans*, is sequenced
2000	• The fruit fly genome, *Drosophila melanogaster*, is sequenced • The mustard plant genome, *Arabidopsis thaliana*, is sequenced • Mammalian Gene Collection is created, completed in 2009
2002	• International HapMap Project is established, completed in 2005
2003	• ENCyclopedia of DNA Elements (ENCODE) Project created, completed in 2007
2005	• France Human Intestinal Metagenome Initiative established
2007	• Human Microbiome Project initiated
2008	• Roadmap Epigenomics Project started • International Human Microbiome Consortium is formed
2009	• International Human Proteome Organization (HUPO) is established
2010	• Human Proteome Project is created

Following the Avery, MacLeod, and McCarty findings, interest rapidly grew in the scientific community to characterize DNA further. Utilizing x-ray crystallography, English chemist, Rosalind Franklin, and English physicist, Maurice Wilkins, first described the structure of DNA in 1953.[7] Together they revealed a repeating helical structure. In the same year, researchers James Watson and Walter Crick published on the structure of DNA (Figure 88–3).[10] They first described DNA as a right-handed double helix, with base pairing of cytosine with guanine and thymine with adenine.

In the next 30 years, interest in deciphering the DNA sequences of various organisms, including *Homo sapiens*, quickly expanded. In 1989, international efforts collaborated to form the Human Genome Organization (HUGO), which sought to map the entire human genome. At that time, it was estimated that such a project would cost 200 million dollars per year and take 15 years to complete. In 1989, the National Institutes of Health (NIH) also established the National Human Genome Research Institute to participate in the international Human Genome Project (1989). James Watson led the efforts, which were funded by both the NIH and the Department of Energy.

Simultaneously, simpler organisms were being sequenced. In 1996, yeast, *Saccharomyces cerevisiae*,

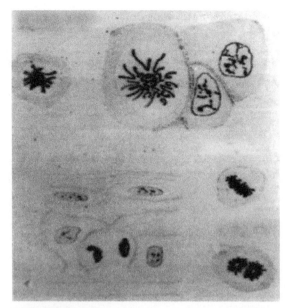

FIGURE 88–2 First illustration of human chromosomes from tumor cells in 1882. (*Reproduced with permission from Rimoin D, Korf RP: Emery and Rimoin's Principles and Practice of Medical Genetics, 6th edition. Oxford: Academic Press; 2013.*)

was the first eukaryote deciphered. The round-worm, *Caenorhabditis elegans,* followed in 1989 and was found to contain 19,000 genes.[11] By 2000, the genome of the fruit fly, *Drosophila melanogaster,* was sequenced and noted to have 14,000 genes.[12] The mustard plant, *Arabidopsis thaliana,* was sequenced in the same year and contained 26,000 genes.[13] Comparing the genomes of these different organisms began to reveal remarkable insight into the functionality and complexity of DNA.

After much anticipation, the first draft of the Human Genome Project (HGP) was announced ahead of schedule in 2000, and made publically available in 2001.[14] Surprisingly, the number of protein coding genes identified was much less than anticipated. Due to the complexity and variation displayed in humans, it was predicted that 100,000 protein-coding genes would be identified. However, only approximately 30,000 protein-coding genes were derived in the first publication of the human genome. A second draft completed in 2003 further delineated the number of protein coding genes. Finally, in 2004 the International Human Genome Sequencing Consortium performed an additional revision of the human genome, further refining

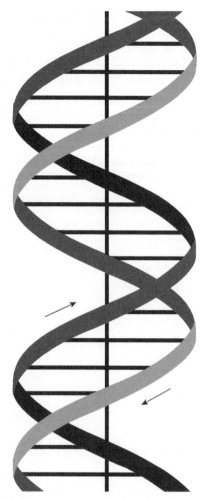

FIGURE 88–3 DNA structure as published by Watson and Crick. (*Reproduced with permission from Watson JD, Crick FH: Molecular structure of nucleic acids; a structure for deoxyribose nucleic acid, Nature 1953 Apr 25;171(4356):737-738.*)

the number of protein coding genes in the range of 20,000 to 25,000. After this revision, the Human Genome Project was deemed complete.[15]

AFTER THE HUMAN GENOME PROJECT: AN ERA OF OMICS

Through the Human Genome Project, a newfound wealth of knowledge was revealed, a blue print for human variability. However, researchers quickly realized that the human genome was a very basic structure, and the protein coding genes could not completely explain the vast differences seen among humans.

Researchers consequently began to search for other parameters that contributed to human variability. In addition to examining the protein-coding regions of DNA, researchers began to analyze the structure, function, and products of the entire human genome. Multiple disciplines quickly developed and flourished, ushering in a new phase of discovery—the era of omics.

Following the completion of the Human Genome Project interest reignited in the already established discipline of epigenetics. Originally termed by British researcher, Conrad Waddington in the early-1940s, epigenetics describes the mechanisms through which undifferentiated cells develop into differentiated cell types such as myocytes, neurons, adipocytes, etc.[16,17] It is now well established that DNA undergoes reversible, non-encoded modifications, which ultimately influence phenotype.[18] Multiple factors, including developmental stage, age, and environment have been linked to epigenetic changes. Research has also revealed that these modifications can be maintained and propagated to daughter cells.

Within the past two decades, efforts have focused on examining the epigenomes (epigenetic changes) of the nearly 200 cell types contained within the human body. Researchers have identified several epigenetic modifications affecting transcription, including DNA methylation, histone modification, nucleosome/chromatin packaging, and RNA transcripts (Figure 88–4).[19] DNA methylation describes the addition of a methyl group to cytosine, creating 5-methylcytosine (5 MeC).[20] Less commonly, cytosine can also undergo hydroxymethylation. Numerous studies have demonstrated that hyper-methylation represses transcription at promoter regions.[21] Histones, which are the scaffolding proteins that support DNA packaging, similarly

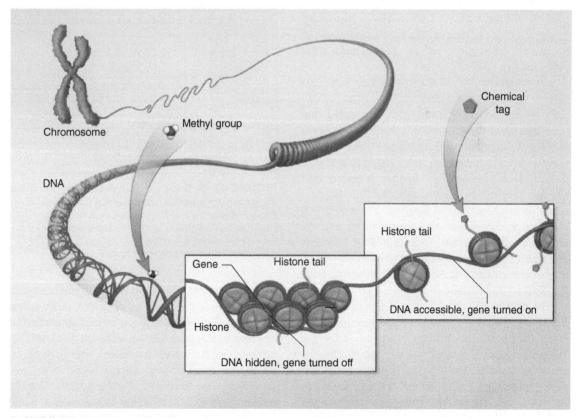

FIGURE 88–4 Epigenetic modifications. Methyl groups bind to both DNA and histones, altering their structure (methylation). Histones also undergo acetylation, phosphorylation, and ubiquitination, which influences coiling of DNA around histones. These modifications consequently influence gene transcription. (*Reproduced with permission from National Human Genome Research Institute.*)

undergo methylation, as well as acetylation, phosphorylation, and ubiquitination. These changes alter the structure of the histone tail, which restricts or facilitates the transcription machinery's access to nucleotides. Nucleosome positioning within the chromatin has also been demonstrated to influence transcription. Akin to histones, the packaging of the nucleosomes exposes certain areas of DNA, which influences binding of transcription factors such as enhancers, silencers, and insulators.

With renewed interest in epigenetics, The National Human Genome Research Institute established two large-scale research projects to examine the human epigenome. In 2003, the ENCyclopedia of DNA Elements (ENCODE) Project was created, with the objective of identifying all functional elements: RNA-transcribed regions, protein-coding regions, transcription-factor-binding sites, chromatin structure, and DNA methylation.[22,23] At its inception, 35 international research groups examined 30 million bases of human DNA, equivalent to about 1% of the genome. In the second phase of the project, researchers analyzed 1640 genome wide data sets, from 147 cell types.

Through the ENCODE project an intricate regulatory system was revealed.[24,25] Among the notable findings was pervasive transcription, meaning that the majority of the genome was transcribed. Areas outside of the protein coding regions that were previously thought to be silent were found to undergo transcription. Researchers further revealed that the majority of the human genome (80.4%) participated in a biochemical function. Much of which was thought to be inert DNA, was found to contain regulators of expression, including RNA elements and transcription factor binding sites. Analysis further demonstrated regulatory elements acting both locally (*cis*) and distally (*trans*).

In 2008, the National Human Genome Research Institute initiated the Roadmap Epigenomics Program (REP) to more thoroughly characterize the human epigenome (Figure 88–5).[26] Specifically, the project sought to examine the temporal changes of the epigenome from stem cells to mature cells in human tissues. The project further aimed to examine the epigenetic changes associated with diseased states. In 2015, the REP published its preliminary integrative analysis of 127 reference human epigenomes.[27]

Sample type	Cell type/ tissue group	EID	Epigenome name
	IMR90	E017	IMR90 fetal lung fibroblast
Primary cultures	**ES cell**	E002	ES-WA7 cells
		E008	H9 cells
		E001	ES-I3 cells
		E015	HUES6 cells
		E014	HUES48 cells
		E016	HUES64 cells
		E003	H1 cells
		E024	ES-UCSF4 cells
	iPSC	E020	iPS-20b cells
		E019	iPS-18 cells
		E018	iPS-15b cells
		E021	iPS DF 6.9 cells
		E022	iPS DF 19.11 cells
ES cell derived	**ES-deriv.**	E007	H1 derived neuronal progenitor cultured cells
		E009	H9 derived neuronal progenitor cultured cells
		E010	H9 derived neuron cultured cells
		E013	HUES64 derived CD56+ mesoderm
		E012	HUES64 derived CD56+ ectoderm
		E011	HUES64 derived CD184+ endoderm
		E004	H1 BMP4 derived mesendoderm
		E005	H1 BMP4 derived trophoblast
		E006	H1 derived mesenchymal stem cells
Primary cells	**Blood & T cell**	E062	Primary mononuclear cells (from PB)
		E034	Primary T cells from primary blood (from PB)
		E045	Primary T cells effector/memory enriched (PB)
		E033	Primary T cells from cord blood
		E044	Primary T regulatory cells (from PB)
		E043	Primary T helper cells (from PB)
		E039	Primary T helper naive cells (from PB)
		E041	Primary T helper cells PMA-I stimulated
		E042	Primary T helper 17 cells PMA-I stimulated
		E040	Primary T helper memory cells (from PB)
		E037	Primary T helper memory cells (from PB)
		E048	Primary T CD8+ memory cells (from PB)
		E038	Primary T helper naive cells (from PB)
		E047	Primary T CD8+ naive cells (from PB)
	HSC & B cell	E029	Primary monocytes (from PB)
		E031	Primary B cells from cord blood
		E035	Primary haematopoietic stem cells (HSCs)
		E051	Primary HSCs G-CSF-mobilized male
		E050	Primary HSCs G-CSF-mobilized female
		E036	Primary HSCs short term culture
		E032	Primary B cells (from PB)
		E046	Primary natural killer cells (from PB)
		E030	Primary neutrophils (from PB)
Primary cultures	**Mesench.**	E026	Bone marrow derived MSCs
		E049	Mesenchymal stem cell deriv. chondrocyte
		E025	Adipose-derived mesenchymal stem cells
		E023	Mesenchymal stem cell derived adipocyte
	Myosat.	E052	Muscle satellite
	Epithelial	E055	Foreskin fibroblast
		E056	Foreskin fibroblast
		E059	Foreskin melanocyte
		E061	Foreskin melanocyte
		E057	Foreskin keratinocyte
		E058	Foreskin keratinocyte

FIGURE 88–5 Tissue and cell types utilized to examine the human epigenome in the Roadmap Epigenome Project. (*Reproduced with permission from Roadmap Epigenomics Consortium, Kundaje A, Meuleman W, et al: Integrative analysis of 111 reference human epigenomes, Nature 2015 Feb 19;518(7539):317-330.*)

REP analysis revealed several epigenetic modifications including histone marks, DNA methylation, DNA accessibility, and RNA expression. As confirmed by previous studies, REP demonstrated that low DNA methylation states were associated with high accessibility for transcription, whereas hypermethylated states were associated with low accessibility. Notably, on average 68% of the reference epigenome was found to be quiescent. Further analysis revealed that embryonic-stem-cell-derived cells and pluripotent cells often exhibited methylation near regulatory elements, whereas differentiated cells exhibited methylation loss. Finally, the REP demonstrated specific epigenetic modifications that are associated with diseased states, including enrichment of enhancers, promoters, and open chromatin.

Following the Human Genome Project, international efforts further collaborated to catalog human genomes of various populations, forming the International HapMap Project (2002–2007). This project sought to identify and catalog human genomes to assist with linking genetic variants to disease states.[28,29] To accomplish this objective the project mapped single nucleotide polymor—phisms (SNPs) of 1184 individuals across 11 populations. Similar to fingerprints, representative SNPs (tag SNPs) were recognized as unique identifiers, allowing for identification of areas linked to individual genes (Figure 88–6).

The database created by the HapMap project has subsequently been utilized to conduct genome wide association studies (GWAS) between healthy and diseased populations. GWAS have allowed researchers to grossly sift through entire genomes and identify allele variants associated with diseases. Thus far, GWAS have facilitated the isolation of genes associated with

cancer, diabetes, obesity, and dyslipidemia.[30-32] Additional GWAS have examined autoimmune diseases such as Crohn disease, ulcerative colitis, and psoriasis. Despite their success, GWAS have demonstrated limitations. Tag SNPs do not precisely localize involved genes; they only serve as general landmarks. Furthermore, disease processes are multifaceted, involving numerous interactions between genes and gene products rather than a single locus.

To better understand human variability and the complexity of disease states, researchers have also examined the human transcriptome. In 2000, the National Human Genome Research Institute initiated the Mammalian Gene Collection (MGC). This project was tasked with creating a database containing at least one complimentary DNA (cDNA) per gene for both human and mouse genomes.[33] The MGC later broadened its initial objective, further constructing rat and cow cDNA databases (completed 2009). The MGC and similar international consortiums anticipated that these databases would facilitate functional and comparative genomics. Specifically, transcript analysis would provide insight into the process of gene transcription, protein

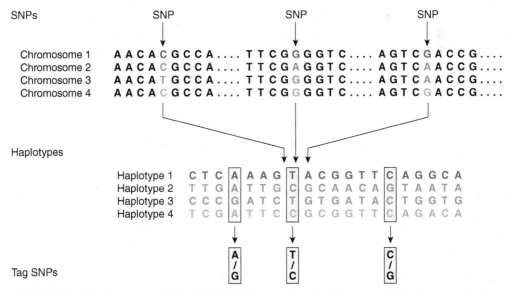

FIGURE 88–6 SNPs, haplotypes, and corresponding tag SNPs. Within short segments of chromosomes, single nucleotide polymorphisms (SNPs) have been identified through sequencing. These variations can be utilized as unique identifiers. Within a series of SNPs, specifically designated polymorphisms known as tag SNPs, can be further utilized to serve as surrogate markers for a specific chromosome. (*Reproduced with permission from International HapMap Consortium: The International HapMap Project, Nature. 2003 Dec 18;426(6968):789-796.*)

expression, and the networks of communication occurring at the molecular level.

Within the human transcriptome, approximately 80,000 transcript products have been identified originating from the 20,000 to 25,000 protein coding genes.[34] This disproportionate relationship of genes to transcription products, spurred considerable research focusing on transcription initiation and termination.[35-37] Researchers have since discovered that an individual gene may contain several transcription start sites (TSS), which can then produce various transcript products. Selection of a specific start site has been found to depend on multiple factors, including a cell's developmental phase, cell-cell signaling, and tissue type. Variation in transcription has also been linked to the terminal processing of transcripts through the addition of adenosine monophosphate moieties. This modification, referred to as polyadenylation, influences processing and nuclear transport of transcripts and has been linked to various developmental phases of the cell. After transcription occurs, transcription products undergo additional processing, where certain areas are spliced out to create various alternative spliced products.

Numerous studies have compared the human transcriptomes during healthy and diseased states.[38] Transcriptomes of neurodegenerative diseases (eg, Alzheimer's disease), malignancies (eg, breast, prostate cancer), and respiratory diseases (eg, asthma, COPD) are a few of the many disease states that have been analyzed.[39] Transcriptome analysis of brain tissue from patients with Alzheimer's disease has revealed alternative promoter regions and transcription start sites.[40] In various malignancies, transcript studies have also identified abnormal fusion transcripts and alternative splicing (Table 88–2). It is theorized that these alternate transcript products result in cellular dysfunction and disease. Although incredibly informative, transcriptomics has limitations. Specifically, transcript products may be extremely fragile and of such small concentrations that current technologies cannot characterize them. Furthermore, transcriptomics primarily identifies genomic metabolites and has limited capabilities to identify the functional properties of transcript products.

After the completion of the Human Genome Project, researchers also focused efforts towards examining the protein products of the human genome. In 2009, the Human Proteome Organization (HUPO) announced an international effort to expand upon previous studies examining the human proteome in healthy and diseased states.[41] In September 2010, HUPO officially initiated the Human Proteomic Project (HPP) to construct a comprehensive library of human proteins. The HPP was also tasked with examining protein expression, splice variants, post-translational modifications, and localization of proteins in cells, tissues, and organs. Furthermore, the project planned to analyze proteins during all developmental stages of adult life and under various physiologic and pathologic conditions. Nearly five years after the induction of the HPP, the first draft of the human proteome was published in 2014.[42] Ongoing efforts continue internationally examining each chromosome to complete a more comprehensive human proteome database.

In the last two decades, research has extended beyond the human chromosome to examine the microorganisms that inhabit the human body, establishing the discipline of microbiomics. One of the first projects examining the human microbiome was the France Human Intestinal Metagenome Initiative (HIMI) established in 2005. The National Institutes of Health (NIH) soon thereafter followed, initiating the Human Microbiome Project (HMP) in 2007.[43] At its inception, the project's initial objective was to examine the microbiomes of the mouth, gastrointestinal tract (stool), skin, and vagina. These databases could then be utilized to identify dysfunction, develop treatments, and possibly prevent illnesses linked to dysbiosis. The HMP project also included an initiative to examine ethical, legal, and social implications associated with genomics. Approximately, one-year after the establishment of the HMP, the International Human Microbiome Consortium formed in 2008 to further foster collaboration worldwide.

Microbiomes of multiple disease processes have since been analyzed.[44,45] Most research to date has focused on the microbiomes of the gut and skin.[46] Numerous studies have repeatedly shown a strong association between diseased states and alterations in the gut microbiome.[47] For example, in obesity and the Crohn disease, there are associated changes

TABLE 88–2 Transcription derangements identified in cancers.

Cancer Type	Analysis Type	Results
Hodgkin lymphoma	PE WT	Identification of gene fusions, among which fusions *CIITA*-involving
Non-Hodgkin lymphoma	PE poly-A$^+$	Detection of 109 genes with multiple somatic mutations, including those involved in histone modifications
MDS	FR small RNA	Discovery of novel miRNA differentially expressed in tumor
Breast cancer	FR poly-A$^+$	Alternative splicing and alterations in gene expression (ie, *LOX*, *ATP5L*, *GALNT3* and *MME*) have been identified in modulated ERBB2 overexpressing mammary cells
	PE poly-A$^+$	Identification of 3 known and 24 novel fusion transcripts (including *VAPB-IKZF3*)
	SE, PE poly-A$^+$	Discovery of gene fusions in breast cancer transcriptomes with BRCAI mutations, including novel in-frame *WWC1-ADRBK2* fusion in HCC3153 cell line and ADNP-C20orf132 in a primary tumor
	FR poly-A$^+$	Investigation of EMT-associated alternative splicing events regulated by different classes of splicing factors (RBFOX, MBNL, CELF, hnRNP, or ESRP)
Prostate cancer	SE poly-A$^+$	Detection of transcription-induced chimeras in prostate adenocarcinoma
	PE WT	Discovery and charcterization of seven novel cancer-specific gene fusions (four involving non-ETS)
	PE poly-A$^+$	Identification of 121 unannotated prostate cancer-associated ncRNA transcripts, including the characterization of *PCAT-1*
	FR poly-A$^+$	25 Previously undescribed alternative splicing events involving known exons, and high-quality singlenucleotide discrepancies, have been detected in prostate cancer cell line LNCaP
Melanoma	PE poly-A$^+$	Identification of 11 novel gene fusions, 12 readthrough transcripts, somatic mutations and unannotated splice variants
	FR poly-A$^+$	Somatic CNVs affecting gene expression and new potential genes and pathways involved in tumorigenesis have been identified in seven human metastatic melanoma cell lines
Ovarian cancer	PE poly-A$^+$	Discovery of the first gene fusions in ovarian cancer through a novel computational method
Sarcoma	PE poly-A$^+$	Detection of novel gene fusions in sarcoma through a novel computational method
	FR ribodepletion	Evidence of a closer relationship between gene expression levels and protein expression in a human osteosarcoma cell line
Oral carcinoma	MP WT	Association of allelic imbalance with copy number mutations and with differential gene expression
Hepatocellular carcinoma	SE WT	Characterization of HBV-related HCC transcriptome, including identification of exon-level expression changes and novel splicing variants

CNVs, copy number variations; EMT, epithelial-mesenchymal transition; FR, fragment library; HCC, hepatocellular carcinoma; MDS, Myelodys plastic syndrome; PE, paired-end; SE, single-end; WT, whole-transcriptome.
Reproduced with permission from Costa V, Aprile M, Esposito R, et al: RNA-Seq and human complex diseases: recent accomplishments and future perspectives, *Eur J Hum Genet* 2013 Feb;21(2):134-142.

in the diversity and composition of gut flora. Environmental stressors have also been shown to induce virulent behavior of bacteria in the gut. Microbiomic research suggests that there are numerous symbiotic and dysbiotic relationships between the human body and microorganisms which appear to directly influence human health and disease.

As omic research develops, it becomes increasingly apparent that the human genome exists within a highly integrated functional complex. Researchers are only beginning to understand the intricacies of the human genome, epigenome, transcriptome, proteome, and microbiome. Omic research is in its formidable years, and growing exponentially. Each discovery raises new questions and hypotheses, giving rise to an ever-expanding discipline.

NETWORK MEDICINE

Throughout the era of omics, the human genome has revealed itself as a multifaceted structure that exists in a constant state of flux. Genomic studies have repeatedly illustrated that the human genome orchestrates thousands of functional elements and metabolites that interact on multiple levels. In order to comprehend what appears chaotic, a new type of medicine has emerged, network medicine. Specifically, this type of medicine focuses on integrating various omic disciplines to create networks that explain healthy and diseased states (Figure 88–7).[19,48,49]

Underlying network medicine are several principles utilized to construct network models.[50] These models assume that biological networks are not random, there is a certain order, and interactions are connected through links or edges. Network medicine designates entities with frequent interactions as nodes. Highly linked nodes are referred to as hubs. Numerous studies have identified hubs as essential functional elements in an organism. Within the nodes there may be subnetworks, or groups of interactions that are referred to as motifs. Networks ultimately create a theoretical model with inherent plasticity amenable to integration of new information.

Various network models have been constructed to explain the functionality of the human genome. Included among them are human diseasome networks (HDN), where various diseases are linked to the same gene. For example, multiple cancers,

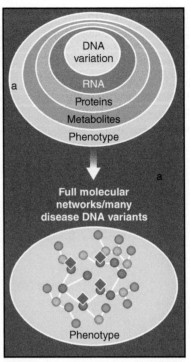

FIGURE 88–7 Network models integrate information from multiple omic technologies to examine relationships between the human genome, its products, and phenotype. (*Modified with permision from Schadt EE, Björkegren JL: NEW: network-enabled wisdom in biology, medicine, and health care, Sci Transl Med. 2012 Jan 4;4(115):115rv1.*)

including breast, head, neck and bladder have been linked to tumor protein 53 gene dysfunction. In another model, referred to as a metabolic disease network (MDN), diseases are linked by a common enzymatic pathway that results in illness. Models have also been constructed based upon phenotype or co-morbidities. Phenotypic disease models (PDM) consider environmental exposures as integral components of variability. These models are relevant to population studies, allowing for analysis in a retrospective manner, from phenotype to genotype.

Newer models have begun to integrate genomic information from multiple platforms to examine common complex diseases utilizing various network algorithms, such as Bayesian models and co-expression gene models.[49,51] Coined network enabled wisdom (NEW) or systems biology, these models utilize supercomputers and distributed processing to systematically integrate vast amounts of data generated by omic technology. Through the integration of omic data, network models illustrate the relationships between the human genome and its metabolites. Once fabricated, these networks are validated by comparison to a new human sample population or by knockout mice models. Several network models for common complex diseases are in development including atherosclerosis, diabetes, Alzheimer disease, allergic rhinitis, asthma, obesity, and coronary artery disease (Figure 88–8).[52,53]

Through the construction and manipulation of network models, the underlying pathology of common complex diseases can be understood. With such information, disease diagnosis and treatment may become infinitely more accurate and personalized. Diseases may also be identified at earlier stages. Network biology can also be utilized to guide development of new pharmaceuticals. By identifying consensual genes or pathways, treatments could be better targeted to address pathologic processes as well as avoid pathways that could result in deleterious side effects. Although in an early phase of

development, network medicine appears to have an incredible potential to expand our understanding of the underlying molecular pathology of illness.

CRITICALOMIC MEDICINE: BRINGING OMICS TO THE INTENSIVE CARE UNIT

The application of omics to critical illness remains vastly unexplored. Most research to date has examined critical illness from a phenotype perspective. Syndromes with multi-organ failure, such as sepsis, trauma, and acute respiratory distress have received the most attention.[54-57] Genome wide association studies and transcription studies have been the most widely applied to critical illness. The majority of studies have been performed in mice models and *in vitro*. Few studies have been conducted in the intensive care unit, and of those completed the population size has predominately been small. In this expanding stage, the application of omics to critical care medicine is just starting to reveal the molecular pathology and complex relationships of critical illnesses.

Sepsis has been the most studied phenotype, and justifiably as it constitutes approximately 37% of ICU admissions and carries the highest mortality in general medical and surgical intensive care units.[58] Efforts have predominately focused on elucidating the molecular pathway of the inflammatory cascade associated with sepsis, with leukocytes being the primary substrate for analysis.[59,60] In transcription studies, several genes involved in pathogen recognition have displayed up-regulation. Included among them are genes encoding toll-like receptors (TLR) and genes involved in cluster of differentiation 14 (CD14) pathways. Upregulation has also been identified in genes involved in signal transduction pathways that induce immune response elements, including nuclear factor kappa-B (NF-KB), mitochondrial activated protein kinase, and Janus kinase (JAK).

Several studies have examined transcription during sepsis in attempt to substantiate the hypothesis of a two-phased model, which describes a proinflammatory state followed by an anti-inflammatory state. Transcription studies have proposed another potential mechanism involved in early sepsis,

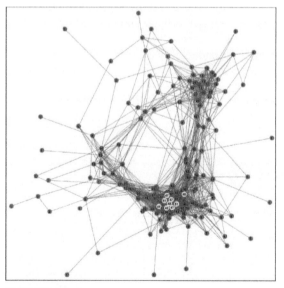

FIGURE 88–8 Arterial wall co-expression gene network constructed from mRNA profiles. In coexpression gene networks, the length of the link between nodes reflects association. Weaker associations have longer links. (*Reproduced with permission from Schadt EE, Björkegren JL: NEW: network-enabled wisdom in biology, medicine, and health care, Sci Transl Med. 2012 Jan 4;4(115):115rv1.*)

adaptive immunity dysfunction. In a small study examining expression profiles of patients with community-acquired pneumonia resulting in severe sepsis or septic shock, genes associated with wounding, inflammatory response, defense response, chemotaxis, and regulation of interleukin-6, exhibited higher expression compared to healthy patients.[61] Notably, this study also found marked variation between gene expression profiles of survivors and non-survivors. In non-survivors, several genes involved in immune response were markedly downregulated after one week compared to initial response (Table 88-3). The deranged gene expression of the immune response system in non-survivors may be reflective of adaptive immunity dysfunction.

In the setting of sepsis, acute kidney injury (AKI) has been analyzed utilizing GWAS.[62] In one large study examining 887 patients with sepsis, GWAS identified several SNPs that appeared to be linked to AKI. Three of the polymorphisms rs8094315 (BCL2 gene), rs12457893 (BCL2 gene), and rs2093266 (SERPINA4 gene) were associated with decreased incidence of AKI. Two additional SNPs, rs625145 (SIK3 gene) and rs1955656 (SERPINA5), were also identified; the former being associated with an increased risk of AKI and the latter noted to be in complete disequilibrium with SERPINA4 gene. In previous research, the BCL2 gene has been shown to express

BCL-2, an anti-apoptosis protein. Previous studies have also demonstrated that the SERPINA4 gene encodes kallistatin, which contains vasodilatory, anti-inflammatory, antioxidant, and antiapoptotic properties. The functional role of the SIK3 gene has yet to be delineated in the context of AKI. These findings correspond with previous research, which has identified apoptosis as a key mechanism contributing to the development of AKI in sepsis.[63]

Omic research has also been utilized to investigate the multi-organ dysfunction that occurs in severe injury. In a multicenter study, examining transcription in severe blunt trauma and burn injuries, lymphocytes displayed remarkably similar patterns of expression as seen in sepsis.[64] After severe blunt trauma, genes involved in innate immunity, pathogen recognition, and inflammatory response had the greatest increase in expression (Figure 88-9). Conversely, genes involved in T-cell receptor function/proliferation, antigen presentation, apoptosis, and natural killer (NK) cell function were downregulated. Examination of the leukocyte transcriptome in burns (> 20% of total surface area), revealed a nearly identical pattern of transcription to severe blunt trauma. These findings suggest similar mediators (ie, damaged cellular component) or receptors (ie, toll-like receptors) that are instrumental in initiating the inflammatory cascade.

TABLE 88-3 Gene ontology terms and their associated genes that were differentially expressed in sepsis.

Term	Genes
Inflammatory response GO:0006954	IL6, TNF, CCL2, OLR1, ADORA2A, KL, CFB, CCR1, CXCL3, CXCL2, IL1RN, NFKB1, CCL7, CXCL10, TNFAIP6, SIGLEC1, IL23A, CCL23, SAA1, PTX3, IL1A
Defense response GO:0006952	TNF, CCL2, ADORA2A, CXCL3, CCR1, CXCL2, NFKB1, CD74, CCL7, CXCL10, IL23A, CCL23, SAA1, PTX3, IL1A, PLD1, IL6, OLR1, KL, CFB, IL1RN, TNFAIP6, SIGLEC1, IFNB1, CLEC5A
Response to wounding GO:0009611	Il6, TNF, CCL2, OLR1, ADOPA2A, KL, CFB, CCR1, CXCL3, CXCL2, IL1RN, NFKB1, CCL7, CXCL10, SIGLEC1, TNFAIP6, IL23A, CCL23, FGA, SAA1, PDGFRA, PTX3, IL1A
Immune response GO:0006955	CSF3, TNF, CCL2, CXCL3, CCR1, CXCL2, OAS3, IFI44L, CCL7, CD74, CXCL10, IL23A, CCL23, PTX3, IL1A, IL6, OLR1, PTGER4, CFB, IL1RN, STXBP2, HLA-DQA2, OASL, TREM1, CLEC5A, GBP1
Chemotaxis GO:0006935	CCRL2, PLD1, IL6, CCL23, CCL2, SAA1, CXCL3, CCR1, CXCL2, ITGA1, CCL7, CXCL10
Cytokine-mediated signaling pathway GO:0019221	CSF3, IL6, TNF, CCL2, CCR1, DUOX1, IL1A

Reproduced with permission from Severino P, Silva E, Baggio-Zappia GL et al: Patterns of gene expression in peripheral blood mononuclear cells and outcomes from patients with sepsis secondary to community acquired pneumonia, PLoS One 2014 Mar 25;9(3):e91886.

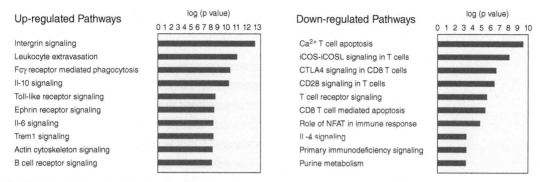

FIGURE 88–9 Transcription of upregulated and downregulated pathways in severe blunt trauma. (*Reproduced with permission from Xiao W, Mindrinos MN, Seok J, et al., A genomic storm in critically injured humans. J Exp Med. 2011 Dec 19; 208(13):2581-2590.*)

Clinical outcomes after severe blunt trauma and burns have been further examined utilizing transcriptomics. Similar to sepsis models, there also appears to be an exaggerated response of gene expression in complicated recoveries. Furthermore, in the above-described multicenter study, uncomplicated recoveries had a return to baseline expression of upregulated and downregulated pathways within 7 to 14 days after insult. In complicated recoveries, gene expression at 28 days continued to be deranged. These results may be interpreted to suggest that resolution of gene expression derangement is associated with recovery. Alternatively, these findings may suggest that adverse outcomes are associated with exaggerated responses of innate immunity and prolonged derangement of adaptive immunity. Further studies are needed to delineate the mechanisms that contribute to outcomes in both sepsis and trauma.

Critical respiratory illnesses, such as acute respiratory distress syndrome (ARDS) and chronic obstructive pulmonary disease (COPD), have also been examined utilizing omic technology. Several proteomic studies have been performed, examining bronchoalveolar lavage fluids (BALF) in humans to elucidate the molecular pathology of ARDS. In one small study examining the expression of proteins in BALFs of ARDS patients ($n = 8$), 22 proteins exhibited increased expression compared to controls ($n = 9$) over seven days. Utilizing gene ontology analysis, these proteins were linked to inflammation, immunity, response to microbials, response to stress/injury, and enzyme inhibitor activity (Table 88–4).[65]

Applying network medicine to these findings has revealed connectivity between multiple proteins, including TNF-α, IL1β, LPS-binding protein, p38 MAPK, β-estradiol, retinoic acid, and the S100 proteins (Figure 88–10). Analysis has also demonstrated temporal changes in protein expression during the progression of ARDS. On day one, complement proteins, antiproteases, annexin A3, S100 proteins, actin, and extracellular matrix proteins increase, whereas surfactant protein-A, annexin A1, fibrinogen, and fatty acid-binding proteins decrease. On day seven annexin A3 and actin decrease, whereas surfactant protein-A increases; these findings may represent regeneration of damaged lung tissue. Network model analysis of ARDs has also revealed redundancy in protein connectivity, with several proteins involved in multiple pathways. These proteins may also assume various functional roles depending upon the time course of ARDS. Specifically, TNF-α has been found to function as both a pro-inflammatory mediator as well as a mediator of lung repair. Thus far, ARDS has been the only critical illness to be examined utilizing network medicine.

Among critical illnesses, chronic obstructive pulmonary disease (COPD) is the first phenotype to be examined for epigenetic modifications that influence disease progression. Until recently, omic research of COPD had predominately focused on identifying risk loci utilizing GWAS.[66] However, more and more omic research has begun to focus on epigenetic changes. Comparison of lung samples from healthy controls to those with COPD has demonstrated increased methylation of multiple genes

TABLE 88–4 Gene ontology analysis of proteins found in bronchoalveolar fluid of patients with acute respiratory distress syndrome that were up-regulated.

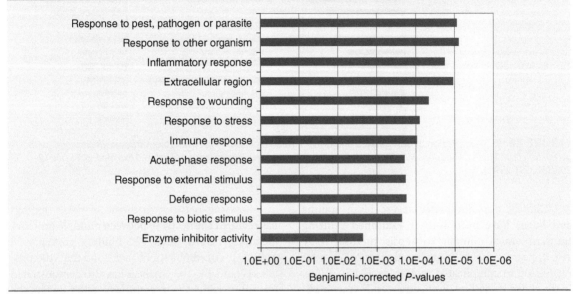

Reproduced with permission from Chang DW, Hayashi S, Gharib SA, et al: Proteomic and computational analysis of bronchoalveolar proteins during the course of the acute respiratory distress syndrome. *Am J Respir Crit Care Med*. 2008 Oct 1;178(7):701-709.

in COPD (EP300, EPAS1, FOXF1, FOXA2, KDR, LAMA5, SHH, NKX2-1, VEGFA, FZD1, NUMB, and PKDCC).[67] Hypermethylation has been shown to be associated with down-regulation of cellular communication, multicellular development, and tissue morphogenesis. It has also been associated with up-regulation of co-translational protein targeting to membranes, protein targeting to endoplasmic reticulum, translational initiation, translation termination, and cellular protein complex disassembly. These changes in transcription induced by methylation appear to be associated with the pathogenesis and progression of COPD.

Microbiomics in critical illness has rapidly gained interest, resulting in numerous studies examining the gut microbiome during this time of extreme physiologic stress. Within the gut microbiome, there are five major phyla of bacteria including actinobacteria, bacterioidetes, firmicutes, fusobacteria, and proteobacteria.[47] During critical illness it has been repeatedly demonstrated that antibiotics, route of nutrition (enteral vs parenteral), vasoactive agents, acid-reducing agents, and opioids induce stress on the gut microbiome altering its phyla composition.

Subsequently, during prolonged critical illness, ultralow diversity communities emerge as well as multidrug-resistant bacteria.[68] It is hypothesized that these multidrug-resistant bacteria are responsible for the development of late sepsis during critical illness.

Additional studies have demonstrated that bacteria and fungi, specifically *Pseudomonas aeroginosa* and *Candida albicans*, can convert from commensal to virulent during physiologic stress. Administration of opioids, hormones, and steroids has been shown to induce virulence through the bacterial quorum-sensing signaling systems. Analysis of critical illness in animal and *in vitro* models has demonstrated that virulence can be mitigated with phosphate supplementation. These findings suggest that the gut microbiome plays an influential role in critical illness and preserving its integrity can improve the outcomes of patients.

During this rapidly developing era of omics, criticalomic medicine is just starting to establish its presence in the intensive care unit as a new conceptualized paradigm of medicine. More and more basic research needs to be done, followed by integration of genomic, epigenomic, transcriptomic, proteomic, microbiomic, and other omic data to create more network

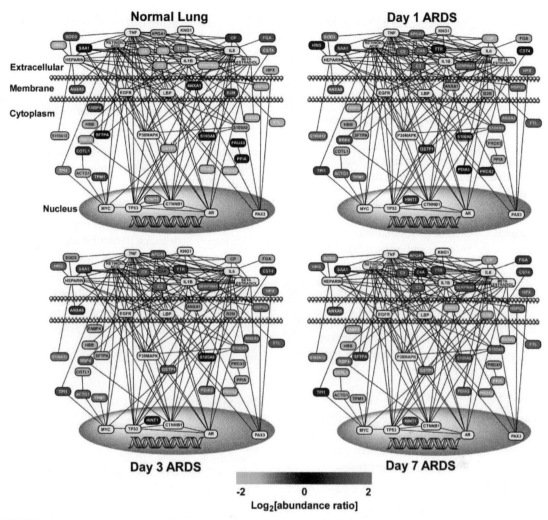

FIGURE 88-10 Network models of proteomes constructed from bronchoalveolar lung fluid from healthy and ARD patients on days 1, 3, and 7. (*Reproduced with permission from Chang DW, Hayashi S, Gharib SA, et al: Proteomic and computational analysis of bronchoalveolar proteins during the course of the acute respiratory distress syndrome,* Am J Respir Crit Care Med *2008 Oct 1;178(7):701-709.*)

models of critical illness. Once established, these models can then be manipulated and applied to the bedside through translational medicine. The ethics of omic research and its applications have also yet to be defined, raising many questions about health privacy and determinism. Omic research holds incredible promise to revolutionize the delivery of health care by individualizing prevention, diagnosis, and treatment of illness. However, it must be done thoughtfully and meticulously to augment the full potential of the secrets contained within our nucleotides.

GLOSSARY AND ABBREVIATIONS

Bayesian network: a network model that is constructed upon an algorithm that reflects probabilities and conditional dependencies.

Epistasis: the effect of one gene being dependent on the presence of one or more modifier genes.

Epigenesis: development of a plant or animal from an egg or spore through a series of processes.

eSNP: expressed single nucleotide polymorphism.

Exons: coding regions of the human genome.

Expression quantitative trait loci (eQTL): genomic loci that regulate expression levels of mRNAs.

Functional elements: include genes that encode proteins and non-coding RNAs, transcripts, protein–nucleic-acid interaction sites, and epigenomic modifications.

Haplotype: contraction for haploid genotypes; specific set of alleles observed on a single chromosome, or part of a chromosome.

Intergenic: between genes.

Introns: any nucleotide sequence within a gene that is removed by RNA splicing while the final mature RNA product is generated.

Microarrays: sometimes called a DNA chip, a small glass slide with short DNA probes attached to it in a specific pattern. When a sample of fragmented DNA is washed over the microarray, pieces of this DNA hybridize to the chip and can then be detected by scanning software.[69]

Nucleosome: a unit containing eight histones wrapped with DNA, which packages into chromatin.

Online Mendelian Inheritance in Man (OMIM): database that contains all of known human diseases linked to genetic component. Funded by NCBI (National Center for Biotechnology Information), established in 1960.

Pseudogenes: genes that have lost their protein-coding ability or are otherwise no longer expressed in the a cell.

Quantitative gene loci: DNA that is linked to or is contained within genes that underlie a quantitative trait.

Single nucleotide polymorphism (SNP or snips): variation in one DNA base, estimated to be about 1 in 10 million bases.

Transcription: first step of gene expression, in which a particular segment of DNA is copied into RNA by the enzyme RNA polymerase.

Translation: process in which mRNA, tRNA and ribosomes coordinate to organize amino acids into proteins.

REFERENCES

1. Coopersmith CM, Wunsch H, Fink MP, et al. A comparison of critical care research funding and the financial burden of critical illness in the United States. *Crit Care Med*. 2012;40:1072-1079.
2. Green ED, Guyer MS. Charting a course for genomic medicine from base pairs to bedside. *Nature*. 2011;270:204-213.
3. Topol EJ. From dissecting cadavers to dissecting genomes. *Sci Transl Med*. 2013;4:1-2.
4. Subramanian G, Adams MD, Venter JC, Broder S. Implications of the human genome for understanding human biology and medicine. *J Am Med Assoc*. 2001;286:2296-3207.
5. Collins FG, Guttmacher AE. Genetics moves into the medical mainstream. *J Am Med Assoc*. 2001;286: 2322-2324.
6. McKusick VA. The anatomy of the human genome: a neo-Vesalian basis for medicine in the 21st century. *J Am Med Assoc*. 2001;286:2289-2295.
7. McKusick VA, Harper PS. History of medical genetics. In: Rimoin D, Korf RP, eds. *Emery and Rimoin's Principles and Practice of Medical Genetics*. 6th ed. Oxford: Academic Press; 2013: 1-39.

8. Correns C. Mendels Regeln qber das Verhalten der Nachkom - menschaft der Rassenbastarde. *Ber Dtsch Bot Ges.* 1900;18:158-168.

9. Dahm R. Friedrich Miescher and the discovery of DNA. *Developmental Biol.* 2005;278:274-288.

10. Watson J, Crick FH. Molecular structure of nucleic acids: a structure for deoxyribose nucleic acid. *Nature.* 1953;4356:737-738.

11. C. elegans Sequencing Consortium. Genome sequence of the nematode C. elegans: a platform for investigating biology. *Science.* 1998;282:2012-2018.

12. Adams MD, Celniker SE, Holt RA, et al. The genome sequence of Drosophila melanogaster. *Nature.* 2000;287:2185-2195.

13. Arabidopsis Genome Initiative. Analysis of the genome sequence of the flowering plant Arabidopsis thaliana. *Nature.* 2000;408:796-815.

14. Lander ES, Linton LM, Birren B, et al. Initial sequencing and analysis of the human genome. *Nature.* 2001;409:861-921.

15. International Human Genome Sequencing Consortium. Finishing the euchromatic sequence of the human genome. *Nature.* 2004;431:931-945.

16. Graves BT, Munro CL. Epigenetics in critical illness: a new frontier. *Nurs Res Pract.* 2013;2013:503-686.

17. Romanoski CE, Glass CK, Stunnenberg HG, Wilson L, Almouzni G. Epigenomics: roadmap for regulation. *Nature.* 2015;518:314-316.

18. Rivera CM, Ren B. Mapping human epigenomes. *Cell.* 2003;155:39-55.

19. Bunyavanich S, Schadt EE. Systems biology of asthma and allergic diseases: a multiscale approach. *J Allergy Clin Immunol.* 2015;135:31-42.

20. Callaway E. Epigenomics starts to make its mark. *Nature.* 2014;508:22.

21. Robinson CM, Neary R, Levendale A, Watson CJ, Baugh JA. Hypoxia-induced DNA hypermethylation in human pulmonary fibroblasts is associated with Thy-1 promoter methylation and the development of a pro-fibrotic phenotype. *Respir Res.* 2012;13:1-9.

22. ENCODE Project Consortium. The ENCODE (ENCyclopedia Of DNA Elements) Project. *Science.* 2004;306:636-640.

23. Birney E. Identification and analysis of functional elements in 1% of the human genome by the ENCODE pilot project. *Nature.* 2007;447:799-816.

24. ENCODE Project Consortium. An integrated encyclopedia of DNA elements in the human genome. *Nature.* 2012;489:57-74.

25. Ecker JR. Genomics: ENCODE explained. *Nature.* 2012;489:52-55.

26. Beyond the genome. *Nature.* 2015;518. doi:10.1038/518273a.

27. Kundaje A. Integrative analysis of 111 reference human epigenomes. *Nature.* 2015;518:317-330.

28. International HapMap Consortium. The International HapMap Project. *Nature.* 2003;426:789-796.

29. International HapMap Project. 2015. http://hapmap.ncbi.nlm.nih.gov/index.html.en. Accessed January 1, 2015.

30. Naidoo N. Human genetics and genomics a decade after the release of the draft sequence of the human genome. *Hum Genomics.* 2011;5:577-622.

31. Locke AE. Genetic studies of body mass index yield new insights for obesity biology. *Nature.* 2015;518:197-209.

32. Zhong H. Liver and adipose expression associated SNPs are enriched for association to type 2 diabetes. *PLoS Genet.* 2010;6:e1000932.

33. MGC Project Team. The completion of the Mammalian Gene Collection (MGC). *Genome Res.* 2009;19:2324-2333.

34. Harrow J. GENCODE: The reference human genome annotation for The ENCODE Project. *Genome Res.* 2012;22:1760-1774.

35. Lindberg J, Lundeberg J. The plasticity of the mammalian transcriptome. *Genomics.* 2010;95:1-6.

36. de Klerk E, Hoen PA. Alternative mRNA transcription, processing, and translation: insights from RNA sequencing. *Trends Genetics.* 2015;31:128-139.

37. Carninci P, Yasuda J Fau-Hayashizaki Y, Hayashizaki Y. Multifaceted mammalian transcriptome. *Curr Opin Cell Biol.* 2008;20:274-280.

38. Costa V. RNA-Seq and human complex diseases: recent accomplishments and future perspectives. *Eur J Hum Genet.* 2013;21:134-142.

39. Pistoni M, Ghigna C Fau-Gabellini D, Gabellini D. Alternative splicing and muscular dystrophy. *RNA Biol.* 2010;7:441-452.

40. Twine NA. Whole transcriptome sequencing reveals gene expression and splicing differences in brain regions affected by Alzheimer's disease. *PLoS One.* 2010;6:e16266.

41. Legrain P, Aebersold R, Archakov A. The human proteome project: current state and future direction. *Mol Cell Proteomics.* 2011;10:M111.009993. doi:10.1074/mcp.M111.009993.

42. Wilhelm M. Mass-spectrometry-based draft of the human proteome. *Nature.* 2014;509:582-587.

43. NIH HMP Working Group. The NIH Human Microbiome Project. *Genome Res.* 2009;19:2317-2323.

44. Muszer M. Human microbiome: when a friend becomes an enemy. *Arch Immunol Ther Exp (Warsz).* 2015;63:287-298.

45. Specter M. Germs Are US, *The New Yorker.* 2012.

46. Mittal R, Coopersmith CM. Redefining the gut as the motor of critical illness. *Trends Mol Biol.* 2014;20:214-223.

47. Dave M. The human gut microbiome: current knowledge, challenges, and future directions. *Trans Res.* 2012;160:246-257.

48. Barabasi AL, Gulbahce N Fau-Loscalzo J, Loscalzo J. Network medicine: a network-based approach to human disease. *Nat Rev Genet.* 2011;12:56-68.

49. Schadt EE, Bjorkegren JL. NEW: Network-enabled wisdom in biology, medicine, and health care. *Sci Transl Med.* 2012;4:1-8.

50. Goh K CM, Valle D, Childs B, Vidal M, Barabasi A. The human disease network. *Proc Nat Acad Sci.* 2007;104:8685-8690.

51. Kidd BA. Unifying immunology with informatics and multiscale biology. *Nat Immunol.* 2014;15:118-127.

52. Zhang B. Integrated systems approach identifies genetic nodes and networks in late-onset Alzheimer's disease. *Cell.* 2013;153:707-720.

53. Bunyavanich S. Integrated genome-wide association, coexpression network, and expression single nucleotide polymorphism analysis identifies novel pathway in allergic rhinitis. *BMC Med Genomics.* 2014;7:1-14.

54. Abraham E. It's all in the genes: moving toward precision medicine in critical illness. *Crit Care Med.* 2013;41:1363-1364.

55. Cuenca AG. Development of a genomic metric that can be rapidly used to predict clinical outcome in severely injured trauma patients. *Crit Care Med.* 2013;41:1175-1185.

56. Wei Y. Platelet count mediates the contribution of a genetic variant in lrrc16a to ards risk. *Chest.* 2015;147:607-617.

57. Villar J, Siminovitch KA. Molecular intensive care medicine. *Intensive Care Med.* 1999;25:652-661.

58. Vincent JL. Sepsis in European intensive care units: results of the SOAP study. *Crit Care Med.* 2006;34:344-353.

59. Tang BM, Huang Sj Fau-McLean AJ, McLean AS. Genome-wide transcription profiling of human sepsis: a systematic review. *Crit Care Med.* 2010;14:3-11.

60. Tang BM. Gene-expression profiling of peripheral blood mononuclear cells in sepsis. *Crit Care Med.* 2009;37:882-888.

61. Severino P. Patterns of gene expression in peripheral blood mononuclear cells and outcomes from patients with sepsis secondary to community acquired pneumonia. *PLoS One.* 2014;9:1-8.

62. Frank AJ. BCL2 genetic variants are associated with acute kidney injury in septic shock*. *Crit Care Med.* 2012;40:2116-2123.

63. Gomez H. A unified theory of sepsis-induced acute kidney injury: inflammation, microcirculatory dysfunction, bioenergetics, and the tubular cell adaptation to injury. *Shock.* 2014;41:3-11.

64. Xiao W. A genomic storm in critically injured humans. *J Exp Med.* 2011;208:2581-2590.

65. Chang DW. Proteomic and computational analysis of bronchoalveolar proteins during the course of the acute respiratory distress syndrome. *Am J Resp Crit Care Med.* 2008;178:701-709.

66. Bosse Y. Updates on the COPD gene list. *Int J COPD.* 2012;7:607-631.

67. Yoo S. Integrative analysis of DNA methylation and gene expression data identifies EPAS1 as a key regulator of COPD. *PLoS Genet.* 2015;11:e1004898.

68. Zaborin A. Membership and behavior of ultra-low-diversity pathogen communities present in the gut of humans during prolonged critical illness. *mBIO.* 2014;5:e01361-e013614.

69. Norrgard K. Genetic variation and disease: GWAS. *Nature Educ.* 2008;1:87.

C H A P T E R

Arterial Line Monitoring and Placement

89

Richard Weiner, MSN, RN, ANP-BC; Erin Ryan, RN, NP and Joanna Yohannes-Tomicich, MSN, RN, NP-C

INTRODUCTION

Arterial catheterization is one of the most frequently performed invasive procedures performed on critically ill patients. It is generally considered to be a safe procedure with few serious complications and a major complication rate ranging between 1% and 5%.[1,2,3,4] Although arterial catheterization was traditionally performed by physicians, contemporary practice in many organizations allows credentialing for this procedure to be performed routinely by non-physician providers including nurse practitioners, certified registered nurse anesthetists, and physician assistants. Arterial line placement remains a readily acceptable intervention for unstable patients requiring continuous monitoring of blood pressure, frequent blood sampling, and blood gas analysis.[1,3,4,5] Newer technologies for hemodynamic monitoring such as measurement of stroke volume variation and cardiac output are also facilitated by the presence of an arterial line. This chapter will review general principles of arterial line placement, monitoring, and care.

INDICATIONS FOR ARTERIAL CANNULATION

In the majority of hospitalized patients, non-invasive indirect monitoring of blood pressure by auscultation of Korotkoff sounds is sufficient. However, in critically ill and hemodynamically unstable patients indirect techniques may underestimate blood pressure[1]; thus the need for more intensive blood pressure monitoring via arterial catheterization may be beneficial. Historically, the indications for placement of arterial lines included: (1) continuous beat-to-beat monitoring of blood pressure; (2) frequent sampling of blood for laboratory analysis and monitoring of ventilatory impairment; (3) arterial administration of drugs such as thrombolytics; and (4) use of an intra-aortic balloon pump.[1,3] These remain compelling indications for placement of arterial catheters, however technological advances in contemporary design of catheter and monitoring systems now allow arterial lines to be used for more advanced hemodynamic monitoring, including real-time calculation of cardiac output, stroke volume, and evaluation of fluid responsiveness in suspected hypovolemic states.[1] The modern practitioner requires adequate knowledge of new technologies and data interpretation in order to effectively use these new modalities to enhance patient care and delivery.

ARTERIAL WAVEFORM ANALYSIS

The waveform seen on bedside monitors is a visual representation of intravascular fluid dynamics as a result of rhythmic pulsation of blood generated by cardiac systole. Changes in intravascular pressure are transmitted through rigid, fluid-filled tubing that propagates the pressure wave to a transducer. This transducer converts the pressure wave from a mechanical process (displacement of fluid) into an electrical signal that is, in turn, amplified, processed,

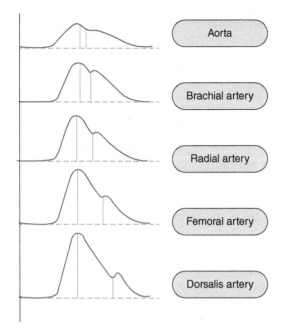

FIGURE 89–1 Normal Arterial Line Waveforms (*Used with permission from Deranged Physiology. http://www. derangedphysiology.com/php/Art-Line/Intensive-Care— Normal-arterial-line-waveforms.php*).

and represented on the monitor as a readily recognizable and characteristic wave. As a result of different pressures through arteries of varying circumference and distance from the heart, the visual representation of the waveform on the monitor will be different based on which artery the catheter has been placed (see Figure 89–1).

EQUIPMENT FOR ARTERIAL LINE PLACEMENT

The basic equipment needed for the placement of an arterial catheter includes (1) a flexible catheter, which selection (long vs short) will depend on site selection (femoral vs radial vs axillary); (2) sterile gown and gloves, hair cap, mask, and drape; (3) sterile connector tubing to attach to the monitoring system; (4) a 2.0 silk suture or tape; (5) a clear biocclusive dressing; and (6) a monitoring system with pressure transduction tubing. A bedside ultrasound device may be used to identify vessels prior and during insertion of the arterial

catheter. Ultrasound guidance may be beneficial in technically challenging procedures, or if there is known or suspected anatomic deviation.

Commercially available arterial catheter kits are present in most organizations. These kits are customizable and contain the equipment routinely used in arterial catheter insertion. The advantages of using customized kits include efficient storing of supplies used for arterial cannulation and avoidance of the need for the operator to gather all the supplies independently. These commercially available kits usually offer supplies needed for placement via in-line guidewire/catheter systems, as well as via the modified Seldinger technique described below.

MONITORING TECHNIQUES AND SOURCES OF ERROR

Proper monitoring of arterial waveforms requires positioning, calibration, and zeroing of the transducer system in order to prevent false elevations in blood pressure measurement or artificial dampening of the waveform. Zeroing of the transducer is accomplished by opening a stopcock located proximal to the transducer to ambient air, followed by pressing the "zero" button on the bedside monitor. This provides the transducer with a pressure reference value (atmospheric pressure) against which intravascular pressure can be measured. Once this is done, the pressure tracing should rest on the zero line of the monitor and a pressure value of zero should be demonstrated. Errors in zeroing the transducer will not result in the desired pressure equilibration; this may occur from technical difficulty related to user error or from electronic difficulty due to the phenomenon of "zero drift." Zero drift is, literally, electronic malfunction of the transducer, transduction cable attached to the monitor, or of the monitor itself, which results in artificial offset of the arterial waveform from the zero line. Sequential manual replacement of each element is indicated to systematically troubleshoot the electronic components.

The arterial transducer system must be calibrated to a point where the monitor accurately reflects the mechanical displacement of blood through the artery. If the system is over- or under-responsive to the amplitude of the pulse wave, it will give a falsely elevated or damped waveform.[1] The test

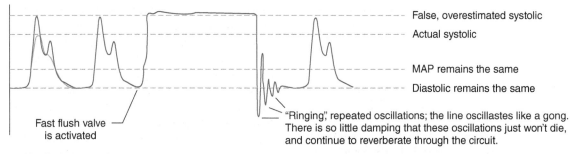

False, overestimated systolic

Actual systolic

MAP remains the same

Diastolic remains the same

Fast flush valve is activated

"Ringing", repeated oscillations; the line oscillastes like a gong. There is so little damping that these oscillations just won't die, and continue to reverberate through the circuit.

FIGURE 89-2 Arterial Line Dynamic Response testing (*Used with permission from Deranged Physiology. http://www. derangedphysiology.com/php/Art-Line/Intensive-Care—Arterial-line-dynamic-response-testing.php*).

most commonly used to determine the accuracy of the damping coefficient and resonant frequency of the tubing-transducer-monitor system is the fast-flush test.[1] This is performed by briefly flushing the system using the manual flush device and observing a square wave while the flush is in progress, followed by a return to the arterial waveform with one or two discrepant waveforms that may vary in amplitude.[1] A larger number of irregular waveforms corresponds to an underdamped or overdamped system that will provide inaccurate arterial pressure monitoring (Figure 89–2).

The transducer system must be leveled to a point parallel with the midaxillary line of the patient. This is easily estimated by visual inspection, limits

technical challenge, and is approximate to the level of the patient's heart.[1] This plane allows for accurate measurement of hydrostatic pressure within the heart. Additionally, this allows for correlation with other measurements of cardiac filling pressures obtained from devices with catheter tips in the great vessels or intracardiac chambers,[1] such as central venous pressure measurement and hemodynamic measurements obtained from a pulmonary artery catheter. Failure to level the catheter to the desired plane being monitored may generate spuriously low or high pressure readings based on whether the transducer is lower or higher than the desired position, with a degree of inaccuracy proportional to the height offset (Figure 89–3).

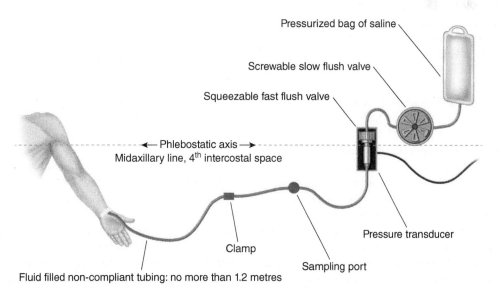

Pressurized bag of saline

Screwable slow flush valve

Squeezable fast flush valve

← Phlebostatic axis →
Midaxillary line, 4th intercostal space

Pressure transducer

Clamp

Sampling port

Fluid filled non-compliant tubing: no more than 1.2 metres

FIGURE 89-3 Arterial Line Mechanics (*Used with permission from Deranged Physiology. http://www.derangedphysiology. com/php/Art-Line/Intensive-Care—Arterial-line-mechanics.php*).

TECHNIQUES OF ARTERIAL CANNULATION

Site selection is the first consideration for arterial cannulation. Common sites for placement include the radial, brachial, axillary, pedal, and femoral arteries; the radial, femoral, and axillary sites are the most frequently cannulated.[3,4] All of these arteries, in the absence of specific patient complications, are of suitable circumference to hold the arterial catheter. However, each of these sites has advantages and disadvantages related to patient comfort during the insertion and once the catheter is in place. For instance, radial catheterization requires little in the way of positioning for insertion, but may leave the affected hand with limited mobility due to the presence of the catheter and tubing. Axillary cannulation is comfortable for the patient, but requires the arm to be immobilized in an unnatural position throughout the procedure. The femoral artery site is arguably the easiest to cannulate and provides an easy access in an emergent situation, but carries the highest risk for infection. Additionally, femoral catheterization severely limits mobility and may prevent ambulation in the alert patient.

MODIFIED SELDINGER TECHNIQUE

The cannulation of deep arteries is frequently achieved using the modified Seldinger technique. This involves the use of a large, hollow introducer needle that is inserted into the artery. The angle, depth, and technique of insertion vary depending on the specific location. A 3-milliliter syringe is attached to the needle prior to insertion. Once the needle penetrates the skin, the syringe is aspirated while the needle is slowly advanced. The operator will recognize that the needle has entered the artery when brisk, pulsatile flow of bright red blood has been obtained. The syringe is then unscrewed while the needle is stabilized with the nondominant hand, and pulsatile flow is seen from the needle. A guidewire is then inserted through the needle, after which the needle is removed. The catheter is then passed over the guidewire, which is then subsequently removed.

Regardless of location, it is vital to maintain visualization of the guidewire while it remains in the patient in order to prevent inadvertent loss within the vessel. Once the catheter is successfully placed in the artery, it should be attached to the tubing–transducer system. Confirmation of an arterial waveform should be noted on the bedside monitor. The catheter should be secured with a suture or tape and an occlusive dressing with antimicrobial properties should be placed over the insertion site.

RADIAL ARTERY CANNULATION

A flexible board or roll of gauze is placed under the wrist in order to obtain dorsiflexion before the arm is abducted and the hand is secured to a flat surface for stability and immobilization with tape. Local anesthesia is achieved with 1% lidocaine infiltrated laterally and medially to the pulsation of the artery. Administration of lidocaine directly into the artery will result in vasospasm, which may preclude placement. Following topical anesthesia, the radial pulse is palpated with either the index or middle finger of the non-dominant hand until the maximal pulsation is felt. The needle is then inserted at a 15° to 30° angle and advanced slowly until return of bright red, pulsatile blood is noted. If using a commercially prepared needle with in-line guidewire and catheter, the guidewire is then advanced into the artery, and the catheter advanced over the wire. The needle–wire device is then removed and the catheter is attached to the tubing and transducer. Alternatively, the modified Seldinger technique can be used in a similar fashion.

FEMORAL ARTERY CANNULATION

The femoral artery is the preferential site for emergent arterial access due to both its large size and central location relative to other potential cannulation sites. These same attributes make the femoral artery the preferred choice for vascular access for surgical and interventional procedures. Thus, the patient's procedural history should be reviewed, and caution must be taken if the femoral vascular system has been previously manipulated. The leg should be placed in a fully extended and abducted position, which can be achieved by laying the patient supine and dangling the lower leg off the edge of the bed. The introducer needle should be inserted at a 45° angle to the skin, bevel up and facing the umbilicus, and distal to the crease of the hip. Subsequent steps for cannulation follow the modified Seldinger technique, as described above.

AXILLARY ARTERY CANNULATION

Similar to the femoral site, the axillary artery is cannulated using the modified Seldinger technique. The arm is properly positioned in a position of abduction, external rotation, flexed at the elbow, and raised; commonly it is suspended above the head by use of a makeshift sling affixed to the head of the bed or IV pole. Successful cannulation is achieved by palpating the artery at the top of a near to the concavity of the axilla. The introducer needle is inserted at a 15° to 30° angle to the skin, aiming for the point where the pulse is most strongly palpable. Once pulsatile blood is obtained, the procedure follows that as described in the Seldinger technique above.

BRACHIAL ARTERY CANNULATION

The brachial artery can be cannulated using either the Seldinger technique as described for the femoral or axillary approach, or by the use of a catheter-over-wire apparatus as described for radial artery catheterization. The artery is access by extending the arm completely and palpating the pulse within the antecubital fossa. Potential disadvantages of this site include distal ischemia and patient discomfort from maintaining the arm in the extended position. Flexing the arm will kink the catheter within the antecubital fossa and preclude proper catheter function.

USE OF ULTRASOUND FOR ARTERIAL CANNULATION

Several studies have shown a reduction in complications and failure rate, as well as an increase in first-pass success with the use of ultrasound guidance during central venous catheter placement compared to traditional landmark technique.[2,4,5,6,7] As a result more ICUs are now equipped with various bedside ultrasound machines and practitioners are becoming more comfortable with its use, especially for insertion of invasive catheters. The use of ultrasound for arterial line placement was initially used as salvage therapy when conventional methods had failed. However, in recent years, the use of ultrasound guidance for radial catheter placement has increased.

Initial ultrasound methodology was based on Doppler techniques, whereas current ultrasound systems use more advanced modes such as B-mode which creates a two-dimensional cross-section of the tissue being imaged.[2,6,7] Other types of images can be displayed to assist the clinician including blood flow. Clinicians use a hand-held probe, typically called a transducer which is placed directly over the area to be imaged. Specific application of ultrasound to arterial cannulation includes differentiating between artery (pulsatile) and vein (nonpulsatile), as well as between blood vessels which appear dark (hypoechoic) in contrast to soft tissue which appears gray (isoechoic). In patients with small arteries or who may be hypotensive, direct visualization of the artery can at times be difficult. In this instance, practitioners can use color flow Doppler to confirm the presence of pulsatile flow within the artery.

Probe selection is also a key component to the proper use of an ultrasound machine. Higher frequency probes (7.5-15 MHz) are used most often for vascular procedures; however, lower frequency probes (5 MHz) may be necessary for deep vessels or obese patients. The ultrasound machine should ideally be positioned on the contralateral side of the patient with the operator on the ipsilateral side. The transducer should be held in the operator nondominant hand and held low on the probe. Various views can also be used during catheter insertion. While direct visualization of the needle at all times can only be accomplished using the longitudinal (long access) view, the transverse (short access) view allows for visualization of smaller and/or more tortous arteries and remains the preferred method for radial artery catheterization.[7]

A meta-analysis of four trials ($n = 311$) by Shiloh et al compared radial artery catheterization using the conventional palpation method (152 patients) versus ultrasound guidance (159 patients). A 71%

improvement (relative risk, 1.71; 95% CI, 1.25-2.32) in the likelihood of first attempt success was noted in the group using ultrasound guidance during radial artery catheterization.[2] In a separate study by Levin et al, 69 patients undergoing elective surgery and requiring arterial catheter placement were randomized into two groups: ultrasound guidance versus palpation alone. There was a significantly higher first pass success rate using ultrasound guidance (62%) versus palpation alone (34%).[8] Several other studies have also shown increased first attempt success rates when comparing conventional palpation methods to ultrasound-guided insertion techniques.[2,4-8]

COMPLICATIONS ASSOCIATED WITH ARTERIAL CANNULATION

Although arterial cannulation is a generally safe procedure, complications can occur. The total complication rate is estimated to range from 15% to 40% of procedures, although clinically significant occurrences are limited to < 5%.[1-4,7,9] Of these, some of the more common incidents include thrombosis and arterial occlusion, embolization and organ ischemia, infection, bleeding, and/or hematoma formation. Less severe but still common complications include vasospasm, diagnostic blood loss, and pain. Heparin-induced thrombocytopenia is also a problem as a result of the heparinized solution sometimes used in continuous flush systems.

Thrombosis

Thrombosis is the most common complication associated with catheter placement.[3,9] It is far more common in the narrow vessels of the distal circulation than in the larger central arteries. In addition to site selection, the incidence of thrombosis increases with duration of indwelling catheter use, length and gauge of arterial catheter selected, and predisposing hypercoagulable state.[9] It is mitigated by use of a continuous flush system, which works to limit stagnation or turbulence of blood flow through the catheter. Although thrombosis may occur, it is usually not a serious complication in that it rarely results in clinically significant ischemia. Furthermore, ischemia usually resolves with catheter

removal, and the thrombus is resorbed within several weeks of catheter removal. Clinically significant ischemia is rare, occurring in < 1% of arterial catheter placements, and usually develops in the setting of preexisting or concurrent circulatory alterations. However, when surgical intervention for ischemia is required, partial to total amputation of the affected extremity is frequently necessary.

Embolization

Cerebral embolization occurs as a result of either air being externally introduced into the systemic circulation, or via dislodgment of a thrombus at the catheter site. It is frequently associated with peripheral cannulation at radial and brachial sites, although has the potential to occur with any catheter. Since gas travels up a fluid-filled system, air will travel up to the cerebral circulation in a sitting or nonrecumbent patient. The rate of instillation of air into the circulation will also predispose to higher rates of embolization. Manual flushing of the arterial catheter with a syringe as opposed to use of the flush valve can cause higher volumes of air to be introduced. Clinical relevance, if any, depends on the site of embolization, the volume of air involved, and the extent of vessel occlusion.

Infection

As with any percutaneous procedure, there is a risk of infection associated with arterial catheterization. The most common routes of arterial infection include contamination with skin flora during catheter insertion, contaminated sterile flush/infusate system, and introduction of bacteria during blood drawing or opening of the tubing–stopcock system to the ambient environment. Common practices to mitigate infection include the use of chlorhexidine solution prior to catheter insertion, use of sterile technique during insertion (including mask, sterile gown and gloves, and hair cap if necessary), and covering stopcocks with diaphragms instead of caps.[1] Routine changing of the tubing/transducer system varies across institutions; 96 hours is a common practice. Routine changing of the arterial catheter itself is infrequently performed as arterial catheterization results in a very low rate of bacteremia (0%-5%),[1] and is rarely the cause of fever. However, repeat cannulation at a new site may be indicated if all other sources of sepsis are ruled out. The most common bacterial isolate from arterial catheters sent for microbial analysis is *Staphylococcus epidermidis*. If bacteremia from the arterial catheter is confirmed, treatment with appropriate antimicrobial agents is indicated.

Hemodynamically Significant Retroperitoneal Bleeding

The femoral artery is a large vessel that is frequently selected in emergent situations due to ease of cannulation. However, improper technique can result in transection of the artery and resultant bleeding into the retroperitoneal space. Large amounts of occult bleeding into the retroperitoneum can occur. Unexplained hemodynamic instability and pallor after femoral arterial catheterization should be promptly evaluated radiographically if hematoma or bleeding is suspected.

Hematoma

Percutaneous puncture of smaller, superficial arteries may result in smaller, visible hematomas; these are more frequently seen at the radial, brachial, and dorsalis pedis sites, but can be seen with axillary puncture. If superficial hematoma develops, direct manual pressure should be held until the hematoma is reduced and the area is soft. The procedure should be aborted, and a new site selected.

Vasospasm

Vasospasm may occur under similar conditions to local hematoma formation. The small, superficial radial, brachial, and dorsalis pedis arteries may become vasospastic after cannulated. If the catheter is unable to be placed due to obstruction or inability to advance the guidewire, the operator may notice diminution of a palpable pulse. In such circumstance, the procedure should be aborted and a new site selected, as further attempts at cannulation of the artery are less likely to be successful and may result in unnecessary patient discomfort.

Diagnostic Blood Loss

Significant blood loss can occur from frequent arterial blood sampling as a result of the need to draw intraarterial blood that is not contaminated by saline diluent or heparinized flush from the transducer system. In order to assure that pure blood is taken, 3 to 5 ml of blood is extracted prior to obtaining the sample for analysis. This can aggregately lead to an increased need for transfusion (with associated morbidity risks). Mitigation of blood loss can be achieved through use of pediatric tubing (smaller volumes), utilization of tubing systems that incorporate a reservoir, and point of care rather than traditional chemical analysis.

Heparin-Induced Thrombocytopenia (HIT)

Some institutions use small amounts of heparin in the arterial flush solution. In critically ill patients with new thrombocytopenia (platelet count decrease of 50% of preheparin levels or absolute platelet count of < 100,000/ml) but no clear etiology, HIT should be considered. If heparin is considered to be a likely cause of thrombocytopenia, all use of heparin in the flush solution should be discontinued. Alternatives include sodium citrate, lactated Ringer's, or 0.9% saline solution.

SUMMARY

Arterial line placement has become a commonly accepted procedure for continuous monitoring of blood pressure and as a reliable access for frequent blood samplings in critical care settings. Although generally considered a safe procedure with few serious complications, consideration of appropriate site selection, contraindications, and potential complications are important prior to insertion of an arterial line.[10] Once the site is selected, use of ultrasound evaluation of the vessel should be considered. Complications associated with arterial catheterization include arterial spasm, thrombosis, embolization and distal ischemia, infection, bleeding and/or hematoma formation. Once accurately placed, continued necessity of the arterial catheter should be evaluated on an ongoing basis, and the catheter should be discontinued as early as possible once the patient is stabilized.

REFERENCES

1. Celinski SA, Seneff MG. Arterial line placement and care. In: Irwin RS, Rippe JM, Lisbon A, Heard SO, eds.

Procedures, Techniques and Minimally Invasive Monitoring in Intensive Care Medicine. 5th ed. Philadelphia, PA: Lippincott Williams and Wilkins; 2010:38-47.

2. Shiloh AL, Savel RH, Paulin LM, Eisen LA. Ultrasound-guided catheterization of the radial artery: a systemic review and meta-analysis of randomized controlled trials. *Chest.* 2011;139:524-529.

3. Scheer B, Perel A, Pfeiffer UJ. Clinical review: complications and risk factors of peripheral arterial catheters used for hemodynamic monitoring in anesthesia and intensive care medicine. *Crit Care.* 2002;6:199-204.

4. Cousins TR, O'Donnell JM. Arterial cannulation: a critical review. *AANA J.* 2004;72:267-271.

5. Shiver S, Blaivas M, Lyon M. A prospective comparison of ultrasound-guided and blindly placed radial arterial catheters. *Acad Emerg Med.* 2006;13:1275-1279.

6. Rahman O, Willis L. Vascular procedures in the critically ill obese patient. *Crit Care Clin.* 2010;26:647-660.

7. Seneff MG. Arterial line placement and care. In: Irwin RS, Rippe JM, eds. *Irwin and Rippe's Intensive Care Medicine.* 5th ed. Philadelphia, PA: Lippincott Williams and Wilkins; 2003:36-45.

8. Esteve F, Pujol M, Perez XL, et al. Bacteremia related with arterial catheter in critically ill patients. *J Infect.* 2011;63:139-143.

9. Milzma D, Janchar T. Arterial puncture and cannulation. In: Roberts JR, Hedges, JR, eds. *Clinical Procedures in Emergency Medicine.* 4th ed. Philadelphia, PA: W.B. Saunders; 2004:384-400.

10. Tegtmeyer K, Brady G, Lai S, et al. Placement of an arterial line. *N Engl J Med.* 2016;354:e13-e14.

Bronchoscopy

Preethi Rajan, MD and
Sanjay Chawla, MD, FACP, FCCP, FCCM

90

KEY POINTS

1. Bronchoscopy is an important and useful tool in the management and care of critically patients.

2. Bronchoscopy can aid in diagnosing pulmonary pathology by direct visualization of the tracheobronchial tree as well as acquisition of deep sampling for culture or in select cases, tissue biopsy.

3. Clinicians need to be aware of the physiologic effects, indications, contraindications and complications of bronchoscopy so that patients can be properly selected and derive benefit from the procedure.

INTRODUCTION

In 1897, Gustav Killian first viewed the trachea and mainstem bronchi via a rigid tube, the prototype for the rigid bronchoscope. Later that year, he removed a bone from the right mainstem of one of his patients, the first known therapeutic use of the bronchoscope. In the early 1900s, Chevalier Jackson added an electrical light source to the distal end of the bronchoscope as well as a suction channel. The flexible bronchoscope was first used in clinical practice in 1967 by Shigeto Ikeda in Japan and by the late 1980s, the videobronchoscope was introduced by Asahi Pentax. For the first time this allowed for visualization of the airways on a screen rather than through the eyepiece of the scope.

Flexible fiberoptic bronchoscopy is an integral and vital skill and has become a common procedure in the intensive care unit (ICU). It allows for real-time imaging of the airways from the vocal cords to the subsegmental bronchi. It can be diagnostic and/or therapeutic such as for airway inspection, foreign body removal, suctioning of secretions, collection of samples and placement of devices or drugs within the airway.

PHYSIOLOGIC EFFECTS OF BRONCHOSCOPY

Bronchoscopy is not a physiologically neutral procedure and continuous monitoring of heart rate, blood pressure and oxygenation must be done during and after the procedure. In ICU patients, ventilator parameters are also monitored to ensure that adequate tidal volumes are delivered and airway pressures are not excessively elevated. The following changes must be taken into account and anticipated during bronchoscopy.

Increased airway resistance. Partial occlusion of the airway by a bronchoscope can increase airway resistance, which can effect peak inspiratory pressure (PIP) and positive end-expiratory pressure (PEEP) as well as delivered tidal volume. These changes can have hemodynamic consequences in patients who may already have cardiovascular instability.

Decreased lung compliance. Bronchoscopy can decrease lung compliance by alveolar collapse from suctioning or surfactant loss after bronchoalveolar lavage (BAL). These effects can be especially significant in patients with decreased compliance, such as acute respiratory distress syndrome (ARDS), pneumonia, atelectasis, and chronic obstructive pulmonary disease (COPD).

Gas exchange. The most common gas exchange abnormality is transient hypoxemia from airway obstruction, alveolar collapse, fluid within the alveoli during BAL or bronchospasm. Oxygenation is likely to worsen in a critically ill patient because of the bronchoscope in the airways or endotracheal tube (ETT) blocking airflow. In patients who are not mechanically ventilated, continuous positive airway pressure (CPAP) applied via full-face mask has been effective in recruiting alveoli and increasing the efficiency of gas exchange in hypoxemic patients.[1] Sedation given to a spontaneously breathing patient can also suppress ventilation and gas exchange. Additionally, small increases in $PaCO_2$ can occur and may need to be monitored in severely hypercapnic patients. Changes in both $PaCO_2$ and PaO_2 may be more dramatic during suctioning.[2] Patients should be preoxygenated with 100% oxygen prior to and during bronchoscopy.

Cardiovascular effects. Changes in intrathoracic pressure especially during coughing may affect venous return and afterload of the left ventricle. Changes in vascular tone from hypoxemia can also result in significant hemodynamic changes. In a small proportion of patients major arrhythmias may develop.[2]

INDICATIONS

The reasons for bronchoscopy in the ICU are generally similar to those in the non-ICU setting but are usually focused to a few specific indications and may be either diagnostic, therapeutic or both. The majority of ICU patients who undergo bronchoscopy are mechanically ventilated.[3] The most common reason for diagnostic bronchoscopy is collection of lower respiratory tract samples for culture while the most common therapeutic indication is removal of mucus plugs or bronchial secretions.[4]

DIAGNOSTIC INDICATIONS

While bronchoscopy can be helpful for many diagnostic purposes, we will focus on the key indications in most ICUs including evaluation for infection, hemoptysis, airway inspection, and inhalation injury.

Evaluation of Parenchymal Infiltrates

Bronchoscopy with collection of samples by BAL or bronchial washings may be helpful to identify infectious pathogens in the lower airways when cultures of tracheobronchial secretions or nasal swab for viral polymerase chain reaction (PCR) are unrevealing. It allows for directed sampling of the lower respiratory tract.[5] Thus, it is more specific than blind methods of obtaining tracheobronchial samples and may help distinguish between infection and colonization. However, this may not be useful in cases of uncomplicated community acquired pneumonia although it may be valuable in cases of poor response to empiric antimicrobial therapy, clinical progression of infection, and in immunocompromised patients in whom the differential diagnosis includes opportunistic pathogens.[6]

In addition to BAL, sterile samples using a protected specimen brush (PSB) can also be obtained by flexible bronchoscopy. Transbronchial lung biopsy remains a controversial procedure when evaluating for infection. It carries a high risk for pneumothorax as well as hemorrhage in mechanically ventilated patients and should be considered only in selected cases.[7] With experienced personnel, transbronchial biopsy while on mechanical ventilation may be preferred over surgical lung biopsy and can provide useful information to impact a change in therapy.[8]

Evaluation of Hemoptysis

Bronchoscopy can rapidly identify the location and extent of bleeding within the airways. If the source of bleeding is not readily discernible, segmental lavages can be performed to locate the area where fresh blood is recovered. In cases of mild to moderate hemoptysis, flexible bronchoscopy has a diagnostic and therapeutic role but rigid bronchoscopy is preferred in massive hemoptysis.

For mild to moderate hemoptysis, cold saline, diluted epinephrine, and fibrin precursors can be instilled into the site of bleeding.[9] In massive hemoptysis, a rigid bronchoscope provides better control of the airway, ventilation during the procedure, visualization and more effective aspiration of blood and clots.[9] Flexible bronchoscopy permits visualization of more distal airways but has limited suctioning capabilities. It does, however, allow for some basic procedures for airway maintenance and immediate control of bleeding, while awaiting more definitive procedures. For example, an endobronchial blocker (a Fogarty balloon-tipped catheter) can be introduced through the flexible bronchoscope in order to tamponade a bleeding bronchial subsegment. In cases where a bleeding endobronchial lesion is identified, electrocautery, cryosurgery and laser photocoagulation can be used.[10]

Airway Inspection

Airway inspection is frequently used in the positioning of an ETT or endobronchial tube, especially when airway management is difficult due to anatomical reasons. It can be performed prior to intubation if a difficult airway is anticipated and can also be used to guide ETT placement when direct laryngoscopy is not possible, such as in cases of head and neck anatomical anomalies due to congenital conditions or as a result of surgery or cancer. It is used in cases where intubation needs to be performed without sedation. Airway inspection can also reveal airway lesions. Finally, flexible bronchoscopy may be used in patients who have undergone lung transplantations to monitor the integrity of anastomotic sites.[11]

Inhalation Injury

Inhalation of large amounts of smoke and particulate matter can result in significant inflammation and irritation of the airways.[12] This in turn can cause pulmonary edema, cast formation, airway obstruction, ventilation/perfusion (V/Q) mismatch and the loss of pulmonary vasoconstriction. Bronchoscopic evaluation helps identify patients with airway obstruction and those with severe airway injury who might require more aggressive airway management.[13] Some patients may benefit from early intubation and mechanical ventilation in anticipation of possible complications as a result of the injury and clinicians should therefore have a low threshold to perform flexible bronchoscopy in these patients.

THERAPEUTIC

Therapeutic uses of flexible bronchoscopy in the ICU sometimes overlap with diagnostic indications and can include treatment of atelectasis, removal of foreign bodies, removal of bronchial secretions and placements of drugs or devices.

Persistent and/or Recurrent Atelectasis

Atelectasis is a common complication in ICU patients and a major cause for delayed recovery due to shunting and worsened hypoxemia. When atelectasis is caused by mucous plugging, flexible bronchoscopy can suction retained secretions, especially those that are thick and tenacious. In this scenario, a bronchial wash or lavage with normal saline can help loosen and access secretions by suctioning. Adjunctive measures such as chest physiotherapy and nebulizers are then instituted to maintain airway patency.[3,11]

Foreign Body Removal

Flexible bronchoscopy can locate foreign bodies within the airways. Removal can be accomplished with small forceps, baskets, and Fogarty balloon catheters that are inserted through the working channel. However, a flexible bronchoscope has limited capacity to grasp and remove objects and a rigid bronchoscope may be necessary if the object is large or if airway protection is necessary during the procedure.

Removal of Bronchial Secretions

Bronchoscopy can also be used to remove secretions that are thick, tenacious, impacted or present distally within the airways, which may not be accessible by in-line suctioning. Clearing of the airways in this manner can improve ventilator parameters and hasten recovery and ventilator weaning.

Placement of Drugs or Devices

Devices including stents, endobronchial blockers, double-lumen ETTs as well as therapeutic coagulants for hemoptysis can be delivered or placed with a flexible bronchoscope. Additionally, while seldom used (< 1%), flexible bronchoscopy may be helpful to better visualize the laryngeal opening and vocal cords during a difficult intubation.[2,4] However, this should be done by an experienced bronchoscopist and preferably in the earlier stages of intubation rather than a rescue maneuver after multiple attempts at direct laryngoscopy.[2]

PROCEDURE IN MECHANICALLY VENTILATED PATIENTS

In mechanically ventilated patients, bronchoscopy is usually performed through the ETT or tracheostomy tube. While the bronchoscope may occupy ~10% of the tracheal lumen it will typically occlude ~50% of the ETT.[14] The bronchoscope is introduced into the airway without disconnection from the mechanical ventilator via an adapted valve, which allows for continued ventilation and maintenance of PEEP during the procedure.

Prior to the procedure, many patients will require increased sedation and analgesia to help minimize coughing, dyspnea and discomfort during the procedure. Clinicians should be skilled and credentialed in delivering conscious sedation. Continuous vital sign monitoring is required to detect physiologic changes as previously described. Additionally, nebulized or instilled 1% lidocaine may help to locally anesthetize the airway as well as reduce the overall dose sedation required during the procedure.[15]

In order to obtain respiratory secretions through BAL, the tip of the flexible bronchoscope is first wedged into the lumen of a target airway, thereby isolating a particular segment from the rest of the tracheobronchial tree. Isotonic saline is then instilled by syringe through the working channel of the bronchoscope and then aspirated back into the same syringe. Several aliquots (3-6) are instilled sequentially and range from 50 to 100 mL each. Each aliquot should have an expected return of 40% to 70% of the initial volume depending on the segment being evaluated.[3] The aliquots from a single lavage can be mixed together and sent for microbiological analysis, including differential cell counts and quantitative cultures and cytopathology.

A PSB is a double lumen catheter brush with an occluding plug to prevent contamination from

TABLE 90-1 Bronchoscopy checklist.

- Obtain consent and perform a time out prior to starting the procedure
- Hold enteral feedings prior to and during the procedure
- Check that the internal diameter of ETT is at least 2 mm larger than the bronchoscope diameter
- Raise FiO_2 to 100%, 10-15 minutes prior to and during the procedure
- Provide continuous monitoring of heart rate, blood pressure, respiratory rate, and oxygenation by noninvasive pulse oximetry
- Assess expired tidal volume and peak airway pressures prior to and during the procedure
- Assess the need for additional sedation, analgesia and possibly muscle relaxation
- Lubricate the bronchoscope prior to use

airway secretions when the catheter is passed through the flexible bronchoscope channel. Samples from a PSB are felt to be more representative of infection since contamination is minimized.

SAFETY

In general, flexible bronchoscopy is a safe and well tolerated procedure. Table 90-1 shows a quick checklist to review prior to the procedure to help minimize complications. Table 90-2 lists general contraindications.

Bronchoscopy should be delayed if a pneumothorax is present and can be reconsidered once it has resolved or addressed by chest tube drainage. Increased intracranial pressure is considered a relative contraindication to bronchoscopy. However, deep sedation with paralysis while monitoring cerebral hemodynamics may minimize complications if the procedure is considered necessary.

TABLE 90-2 Contraindications to bronchoscopy.

- Active/uncontrolled bronchospasm
- Cardiac arrhythmias
- Acute ischemic heart disease/recent myocardial infarction
- Unstable angina
- Hypotension despite vasopressor support
- Increased intracranial pressure
- Severe acidemia with pH < 7.20
- Severe/refractory hypoxemia
- Uncontrolled coagulopathy
- Lack of experienced personnel or staffing

COMPLICATIONS

The complication rate from bronchoscopy is low and reported to range from 0.08% to 1.08%. Most complications are from biopsies especially bleeding and pneumothorax. The risk of pneumothorax related to transbronchial biopsy is somewhat higher in the ICU given the lack of fluoroscopy and positive airway pressure.[16] A chest X-ray is generally recommended for patients undergoing transbronchial biopsy to assess for pneumothorax but is not routinely ordered following flexible bronchoscopy.

Other complications include increased airway resistance related to blockage of airways by the bronchoscope. Bronchospasm/laryngospasm may occur due to airway irritation, especially in patients with known COPD. This, in turn, can result in increased airway resistance with elevated peak airway pressures. Patients may experience hypotension secondary to sedation given for the procedure. Hypoxemia can result from bronchospasm and increased airway resistance. Cardiac arrhythmias are also a known complication and highlight the importance of continuous monitoring of vital signs.

Following the procedure, patients can experience persistent hypoxemia from (V/Q) mismatch due to lavage fluid installation or persistent bronchospasm. Patients may also experience fever, which is usually self-limited and has been reported in 9% to 16% of patients undergoing the procedure.[16]

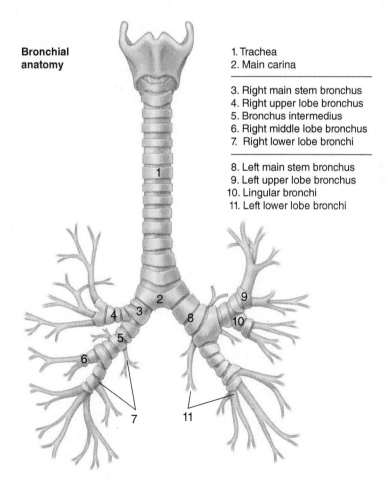

Bronchial anatomy

1. Trachea
2. Main carina

3. Right main stem bronchus
4. Right upper lobe bronchus
5. Bronchus intermedius
6. Right middle lobe bronchus
7. Right lower lobe bronchi

8. Left main stem bronchus
9. Left upper lobe bronchus
10. Lingular bronchi
11. Left lower lobe bronchi

FIGURE 90–1 Airway anatomy. Bronchoscopic pictures: main carina; right mainstem; and left mainstem.

REFERENCES

1. Maitre B, Jaber S, Maggiore SM, et al. Continuous positive airway pressure during fiberoptic bronchoscopy in hypoxemic patients. A randomized double-blind study using a new device. *Am J Respir Crit Care Med*. 2000;162:1063-1067.

2. Jolliet P, Chevrolet JC. Bronchoscopy in the intensive care unit. *Intensive Care Med*. 1992;18:160-169.

3. Guerreiro da Cunha Fragoso E, Goncalves JM. Role of fiberoptic bronchoscopy in intensive care unit: current practice. *J Bronchology Interv Pulmonol*. 2011;18:69-83.

4. Olopade CO, Prakash UB. Bronchoscopy in the critical-care unit. *Mayo Clin Proc*. 1989;64:1255-1263.

5. Luna CM, Vujacich P, Niederman MS, et al. Impact of BAL data on the therapy and outcome of ventilator-associated pneumonia. *Chest*. 1997;111:676-685.

6. Fagon JY. Diagnosis and treatment of ventilator-associated pneumonia: fiberoptic bronchoscopy with bronchoalveolar lavage is essential. *Semin Respir Crit Care Med*. 2006;27:34-44.

7. O'Brien JD, Ettinger NA, Shevlin D, Kollef MH. Safety and yield of transbronchial biopsy in mechanically ventilated patients. *Crit Care Med*. 1997;25:440-446.

8. Bulpa PA, Dive AM, Mertens L, et al. Combined bronchoalveolar lavage and transbronchial lung biopsy: safety and yield in ventilated patients. *Eur Respir J*. 2003;21:489-494.

9. Cahill BC, Ingbar DH. Massive hemoptysis. Assessment and management. *Clin Chest Med*. 1994;15:147-167.

10. Gompelmann D, Eberhardt R, Herth FJ. Interventional pulmonology procedures: an update. *Panminerva Med*. 2013;55:121-129.

11. Raoof S, Mehrishi S, Prakash UB. Role of bronchoscopy in modern medical intensive care unit. *Clin Chest Med*. 2001;22:241-261, vii.

12. Toon MH, Maybauer MO, Greenwood JE, Maybauer DM, Fraser JF. Management of acute smoke inhalation injury. *Crit Care Resusc*. 2010;12:53-61.

13. Dries DJ, Endorf FW. Inhalation injury: epidemiology, pathology, treatment strategies. *Scand J Trauma Resusc Emerg Med*. 2013;21:31.

14. Lindholm CE, Ollman B, Snyder JV, Millen EG, Grenvik A. Cardiorespiratory effects of flexible fiberoptic bronchoscopy in critically ill patients. *Chest*. 1978;74:362-368.

15. Wahidi MM, Jain P, Jantz M, et al. American College of Chest Physicians consensus statement on the use of topical anesthesia, analgesia, and sedation during flexible bronchoscopy in adult patients. *Chest*. 2011;140:1342-1350.

16. Du Rand IA, Blaikley J, Booton R, et al. Summary of the British Thoracic Society guideline for diagnostic flexible bronchoscopy in adults. *Thorax*. 2013;68:786-787.

Cardiac Output Measurement

Paul E. Marik, MD, FCCM, FCCP

KEY POINTS

1 Measurement of stroke volume and cardiac output is fundamental to the hemodynamic management of critically ill patients in the ICU and unstable patients in the operating room.

2 Common methods of measuring cardiac output include the pulmonary artery catheter, transpulmonary thermodilution, pulse contour analysis, esophageal Doppler and bioreactance technology.

3 Perioperative optimization of cardiac output with targeted fluid challenges reduces postoperative complications and mortality.

4 Targeting supranormal hemodynamic targets in patients with traumatic injuries and those with sepsis does not improve outcome and may be harmful.

INTRODUCTION

The management of hemodynamically unstable patients requires an assessment of the cardiac output (CO) and the patients' intravascular volume status (cardiac preload). In most instances the absolute value of the CO is less important than the response of the CO to a therapeutic intervention. In limited circumstances, most notably in the perioperative setting, optimization of CO has been associated with improved patient outcomes. This chapter will review the role of CO monitoring in the ICU and operating room. The most common methods of monitoring CO will be reviewed followed by the utility of CO monitoring.

METHODS OF MEASURING CARDIAC OUTPUT

Pulmonary Artery Catheter

Adolph Fick described the first method of CO estimation in 1870.[1] Fick described how to compute an animal's CO from arterial and venous blood oxygen measurements. Fick's original principle was later adapted in the development of Stewart's indicator-dilution method in 1897,[2] and Fegler's thermodilution method in 1954.[3] The introduction of the PAC in 1970 and its subsequent use in performing thermodilution measurements in humans translated the ability to measure CO from the experimental physiology laboratory to multiple clinical settings.[4] The direct Fick method was the reference standard by which all other methods of determining CO were evaluated until the introduction of the PAC. Currently the PAC is considered the *"gold standard"* against which other devices are compared. Remarkably, the accuracy of the CO measurements as determined by the PAC has never been established. Furthermore, electromagnetometry and ultrasound using aortic flowprobes most closely represent a true "gold standard" for determination of CO but can only be performed in instrumented animals.[5-7] Despite the ubiquitous use of the PAC remarkably few studies have investigated the accuracy of the CO measurements as determined by thermodilution.

A number of studies have compared the thermodilution CO with that measured by the Fick technique. These studies have reported a percentage error of between 56% and 83% (with < 30% being clinically acceptable).[8-10] Philips at al compared thermodilution CO with surgically implanted ultrasonic flow probes in an ovine model.[5] The percentage bias and precision was –17% and 47%, respectively; the PAC under-measured dobutamine-induced CO changes by 20% (relative 66%) compared with the flow probe. This study found that the PAC was an inaccurate measure of CO and was unreliable for detection of CO changes less than 30%. Critchley et al[11] using a similar methodology in pigs reported a precision of 26%. These studies suggest that the true CO has to change by at least 25% to be detected by the PAC. Furthermore, the required change may be as high as 100% depending on the monitor being used.[12] It is likely that multiple factors interact to affect the accuracy of the thermodilution CO calculation.[13] Occult warming of cold indicator before injection can produce indicator loses leading to overestimation of CO. Several physical variables additionally influence the extent of indicator loss through the catheter.[14] In addition, cold indicator losses to surrounding tissue occur during intravascular transit, particularly during low flow states.[15] For thermodilution CO measurements to be "accurate," complete mixing of the thermal indicator must occur in the setting of unidirectional flow within the right ventricle. Incomplete mixing of cold injectate due to tricuspid regurgitation will lead to recirculation of indicator, increased total are under the thermodilution curve and underestimation of CO.[7,16,17] This finding is important as the incidence of tricuspid regurgitation is about 15% in the general population increasing to greater than 70% in elderly patients.[18-20]

Transpulmonary Thermodilution

Transpulmonary thermodilution (TPTD) similar to the PAC calculates the CO by the indicator dilution method using the modified Stewart–Hamilton equation. With this method a known quantity of cold injectate is delivered via a central venous catheter and mixing of the thermal indicator occurs as it passes through the right atrium and ventricle, pulmonary circulation, left atrium, ventricle and aorta. A thermistor-tipped arterial line quantifies the change in temperature over time in a large proximal artery (femoral artery). A monoexponential transformation of the curve with extrapolation of a truncated descending limb back to baseline allows calculation of area under the curve for CO measurement. TPTD suffers from many of the errors and limitations associated with CO determined by the PAC. Compared with PAC thermodilution, the greater transit time and distance between injectate delivery and measurement with TPTD will tend to increase the error associated with conductive loss and recirculation while reducing the potential for the measured CO to be unrepresentative of its true value over the entire respiratory cycle. Nevertheless, several studies have validated the CO measurements obtained by TPTD with the Fick method.[21,22] In addition, the reproducibility of the CO measurements by TPTD appears significantly better than that of the PAC with a precision of about 7% (compared to 25% for the PAC).[23]

Pulse Contour Analysis

The concept of pulse contour analysis is based on the relation between blood pressure, stroke volume (SV), arterial compliance, and systemic vascular resistance (SVR).[24] If arterial compliance remains unchanged the area under the systolic portion of the arterial waveform is proportional to the stroke volume. The SV or CO can be calculated from the arterial pressure waveform if the arterial compliance and SVR is known. Although the pulse contour systems which are commercially available use different pressure–volume conversion algorithms, they are based on this basic principle. These systems can be divided into 3 categories:

1. pulse contour analysis requiring an indicator dilution CO measurement to calibrate the pulse contour, that is, the LiDCO system (LiDCO, Cambridge, UK) and the PiCCO system (Pulsion, Munich, Germany)

2. pulse contour analysis requiring patient demographic and physical characteristics for arterial impedance estimation, that is, the FloTrac system (Edwards Lifesciences, Irvine, California, USA)

3. pulse contour analysis that does not require calibration or preloaded data, that is, the MostCare system (Vyetech Health, Padua, Italy).

Clinical data suggests that only those pulse contour devices that are calibrated to an external method have acceptable clinical accuracy (vascular compliance is measured rather than calculated using predictive algorithms). Furthermore, these devices should be recalibrated when vascular tone changes (eg, use of a vasoconstrictor or vasodilator). The Flotrac™ system has found popular appeal as the system is operator independent, easy to use, needs no external calibration, and only requires a peripheral arterial line (usually radial artery). The accuracy of the first, second, and third generations of this device have been evaluated in over 45 studies; these studies have determined the accuracy of this device to be "clinically unacceptable."[25] This device is particularly inaccurate in patients with a low SVR (eg, sepsis or liver failure). More problematic is the fact that the system does not accurately track changes in SV following a volume challenge or following the use of vasopressors. These limitations significantly restrict the clinical utility of this device.[25]

Esophageal Doppler

The esophageal Doppler technique measures blood flow velocity in the descending aorta by means of a Doppler transducer placed at the tip of a flexible probe. The probe is introduced into the esophagus of sedated, mechanically ventilated patients and then rotated so that the transducer faces the descending aorta and a characteristic aortic velocity signal is obtained. The CO is calculated based on the diameter of the aorta (measured or estimated), the distribution of the CO to the descending aorta and the measured flow velocity of blood in the aorta. As esophageal Doppler probes are inserted blindly, the resulting waveform is highly dependent on correct positioning. The clinician must adjust the depth, rotate the probe and adjust the gain to obtain an optimal signal.[26] Poor positioning of the esophageal probe tends to underestimate the true CO. There is a significant learning curve in obtaining adequate Doppler signals and the correlations are better in studies where the investigator is not blinded to the results of the CO obtained with a PAC.[27]

Bioreactance

Due to the limitations of bioimpedance devices newer methods of processing the impendence signal have been developed. The most promising technology to reach the marketplace is the NICOM device (Cheetah Medical, Portland, OR), which measures the bioreactance or the phase shift in voltage across the thorax. Phase Shifts occur only as a result of pulsatile flow; therefore, the NICOM signal is correlated almost wholly with aortic flow. Furthermore, as the underlying level of thoracic fluid is relatively static, neither the underlying levels of thoracic fluid, nor their change induce any phase shift and do not contribute to the NICOM signal. NICOM is totally noninvasive; the system consists of a high-frequency (75 kHz) sine wave generator and four dual electrode "stickers" that are used to establish electrical contact with the body.[28] Within each sticker, one electrode is used by the high-frequency current generator to inject the high-frequency sine wave into the body, while the other electrode is used by the voltage input amplifier. The system's signal processing unit determines the relative phase shift ($\Delta\Phi$) between the input and output signals. Unlike bioimpedance, bioreactance-based CO measurements do not use the static impedance and do not depend on the distance between the electrodes for the calculations of SV, both factors reducing the reliability of the result.[28] NICOM averages the signal over one minute therefore allowing "accurate" determination of CO in patients with arrhythmias. The CO as measured by bioreactance has been shown to be correlated with flow on cardiac bypass[28] as well as that measured by the Direct Fick method, thermodilution, pulse contour analysis, and carotid Doppler.[10,29-33] Importantly, the device tracks changes in CO closely.[10,29-33]

UTILITY OF CARDIAC OUTPUT MONITORING
Determining Fluid and Inotrope Responsiveness

The measurement of SV and CO is fundamental to the hemodynamic management of critically ill patients in the ICU and unstable patients in the operating room. Fluid resuscitation is generally regarded as the first step in the resuscitation of hemodynamically unstable patients. Fundamentally, the only reason to give a patient a fluid challenge is to increase stroke volume (volume responsiveness).

If the fluid challenge *does not* increase stroke volume, volume loading serves the patient no useful benefit (may be harmful). Clinical studies, however, have demonstrated that only about 50% of hemodynamically unstable patients are volume responsive.[34] According to the Frank–Starling principle as the preload increases left ventricular (LV) stroke volume increases until the optimal preload is achieved at which point the stroke volume remains relatively constant. Once the left ventricle is functioning near the "flat" part of the Frank–Starling curve fluid loading has little effect on the stroke volume. This implies that the measurement of SV and its change with a preload challenge is essential in all patients undergoing fluid resuscitation. Similarly, the use of an ionotropic agent is based on the assumption that these agents will increase CO. CO monitoring is therefore essential when inotropic agents are being used to allow titration of the drug to the desired effect. Previously static pressure measurements, namely the pulmonary capillary wedge pressure (PCWP) and the central venous pressure (CVP), have been used to guide fluid therapy. However, studies performed over the last 2 decades demonstrate that these techniques are unable to accurately assess volume status or fluid responsiveness.[35] Therefore, both fluid challenges and the use of inotropic agent should be based on the response of the SV to either of these challenges.

While a number of definitions exist, an increase in stroke volume (or cardiac output) > 10% to 15% has been used to define volume responsiveness. Interestingly, this rather arbitrary definition was based on the precision of the PAC from studies performed in the 1980s (which we now know are incorrect).[36] Furthermore, although the volume of the fluid bolus has not been well standardized, a volume of between 500 and 1000 mL (or 10 mL/kg) of crystalloid solution has been most studied.[34] As an operational definition we use a > 10% increase in stroke volume following a 500 mL crystalloid bolus (over 10 minutes) as an indicator of fluid responsiveness. Fluid boluses of greater than 500 mL should be avoided as this may lead to volume overload. More importantly, large fluid boluses may acutely increase cardiac filling pressures. Increased cardiac filling pressures trigger the release of natriuretic peptides. Natriuretic peptides cleave membrane-bound

proteoglycans and glycoproteins (most notably syndecan-1 and hyaluronic acid) off the endothelial glycocalyx.[37,38] The endothelial glycocalyx plays a major role in regulating endothelial permeability.[39] Therefore, excessive volume expansion increases the release of natriuretic peptides which in turn damages the endothelial glycocalyx and this is followed by a rapid shift of intravascular fluid into the interstitial space leading to a marked increase in lung water and tissue edema.[37,38] In most circumstances, it would therefore be desirable to determine whether the patient will be fluid responsive without actually administering a fluid bolus. In this regard, the passive leg raising maneuver has received the most attention. Lifting the legs passively from the horizontal position induces a gravitational transfer of blood from the lower limbs toward the intrathoracic compartment. Beyond its ease of use, this method has the advantage of reversing its effects once the legs are tilted down (reversal of the effects on cardiac filling pressures). Therefore, PLR may be considered a reversible "autotransfusion." A recent meta-analysis, which pooled the results of eight studies, confirmed the excellent value of PLR to predict fluid responsiveness in critically ill patients with a global area under the ROC curve of 0.95.[40] It should, however, be noted that intra-abdominal hypertension (an intra-abdominal pressure of > 16 mm Hg) impairs venous return and reduces the ability of PLR to detect fluid responsiveness.[41] Similarly, it is likely (although it has not been studied) that patient's with very thin legs from loss of muscle mass may have a limited "autotransfusion" following a PLR maneuver (and a false negative test). When performing the PLR maneuver, it is important that the method be standardized. The lower limbs should be elevated to 45° (automatic bed elevation or wedge pillow) while at the same time placing the patient in the supine from a 45° semirecumbent position. Starting the PLR maneuver from a total horizontal position may induce an insufficient venous blood shift to significantly elevate cardiac preload.[42] By contrast, starting PLR from a semirecumbent position induces a larger increase in cardiac preload as it induces the shift of venous blood not only from both the legs but also from the abdominal compartment.[43] Since the maximal hemodynamic effects of PLR occur within the first minute of leg elevation,[44] it is important to assess these effects with a method able to track changes in cardiac output or stroke volume on a real-time basis, that is, pulse contour analysis (calibrated), esophageal Doppler, or bioreactance. While the change in SV may be detected within the first minute of the PLR maneuver with pulse contour analysis it may take up to 3 minutes for this change to be detected by bioreactance.

Optimizing Cardiac Output in Elective Surgical Patients

A seminal paper published by Shoemaker et al. in 1982 demonstrated that postoperative patients with an oxygen delivery (DO_2) < 550 mL/min/m² and a cardiac index (CI) < 4.5 L/min/m² were at a significantly greater risk of dying than patients whose DO_2 and CI were above these thresholds.[45] These authors hypothesized that optimizing postoperative DO_2 using the cardiorespiratory pattern of those who survived (DO_2 > 550 mL/min/m² and cardiac index > 4.5 L/min/m²) would improve the outcome of patients undergoing high-risk surgery.[46] This study was followed by a pseudorandomized control trial in which 100 patients were "randomized" to achieve these postoperative DO_2 and VO_2 targets (supranormal) or a control group with standard postoperative hemodynamic goals.[46] The mortality of the control group was 48% compared to 13% in the supranormal group ($P < 0.03$). In 1988 these authors published a now landmark study in which they measured DO_2 and VO_2 in 100 consecutive patients undergoing high-risk surgical operations.[47] They calculated the intraoperative and postoperative oxygen debt (VO_2 debt) by subtracting the measured VO_2 from the estimated VO_2 requirements corrected for temperature and anesthesia. The estimated VO_2 during anesthesia was calculated using the following formula: VO_2 (anesthesia) = 10 x $kg^{0.72}$.[47] This unvalidated equation was published in a textbook by Lowe and Ernst.[48] Shoemaker and colleagues then correlated the calculated VO_2 deficit with the subsequent development of lethal and nonlethal organ failure. In this study the cumulative VO_2 deficit averaged 33.5 ± 36.9 L/m² in nonsurvivors, 26.8 ± 32.1 L/m² in survivors with organ failure, and 8.0 ± 10.9 L/m² in survivors without organ failure ($P < 0.05$). Shoemaker and colleagues noted that the oxygen debt was incurred almost exclusively during the intraoperative period. Based on these findings, the authors proposed that the greater the oxygen debt incurred (during surgery), the greater the risk of organ failure and death.[47] This observation was supported by experimental models of hemorrhagic shock in which the magnitude of VO_2 deficit was related to the risk of death of the study animals.[49] The same year (1988) these authors published the results of two series of patients.[50] The first series was again a pseudo-randomized study in which a DO_2 > 600 mL/min m² and CI > 4.5 L/min m² were targeted in the postoperative period as compared to standard postoperative hemodynamic targets. The reported mortality was 38% in the control group compared to 21% in the protocol group ($P < 0.05$). In the second series, patients were randomized *preoperatively* into one of three treatment groups, namely: (i) a central venous pressure (CVP)-control group, (ii) a pulmonary artery (PAC) control group, and (iii) a PAC protocol group in which "*supranormal*" hemodynamic and oxygen transport values were used as the goals of care (DO_2 > 600 mL/min m² and CI > 4.5 L/min m². The reported mortality was 23% in the CVP control group, 33% in the PA-control group, and 4% in the PA-protocol group ($P < 0.01$). Complications were observed less frequently in patients treated by the protocol in both series. Based on the VO_2 debt incurred intraoperatively and the summation of their outcome data, Shoemaker and colleagues recommended that "in the high-risk patient, PA catheterization should be instituted preoperatively and that the important cardiorespiratory values be prophylactically augmented beginning in the preoperative and continued into the intraoperative and immediate postoperative periods."[51]

The concept of deliberate perioperative supranormal oxygen delivery was subsequently tested in a true randomized controlled clinical trial by Boyd and colleagues published in 1993.[52] In this study 107 high-risk surgical patients were randomized to a control group or a protocol group in which DO_2 was increased to greater than 600 mL/min m² by the use of a dopamine hydrochloride infusion. The mortality was 5.7% in the protocol group compared to 22.2% ($P = 0.01$) in the control group with half the number of complication in the protocol group as compared to the control group ($P = 0.008$). Patients enrolled in this RCT were followed for 15 years following randomization to ascertain their length of survival after surgery.[53] Remarkably 20.7% of the goal directed therapy patients versus 7.5% of the control group were alive at 15 years. The authors concluded that short-term goal directed therapy in the perioperative period may improve long-term outcome, in part due to is ability to reduce the number of perioperative complications. The study of Boyd and colleagues has been followed by at least 30 RCTs which have studied perioperative hemodynamic optimization in a variety of settings using various goals and techniques of hemodynamic optimization.[54-56] The initial preemptive hemodynamic studies used the PAC and targeted the Shoemaker "supranormal" goals while more recent studies have "optimized" CO using esophageal Doppler or dynamic indices of fluid responsiveness. Meta-analyses of these studies have demonstrated that both approaches reduce surgical mortality and morbidity.[54-56] Furthermore, while mortality was reduced only in the high-risk patients' morbidity was reduced across all risk groups. In addition, these meta-analyses have demonstrated that the PAC has been largely replaced by less invasive hemodynamic monitoring techniques.

The original goal directed therapy (GDT) study by Shoemaker et al published in 1982 demonstrated the benefit of achieving postoperative supranormal hemodynamic targets.[46] Following their 1988 study in which they demonstrated that the oxygen debt was incurred intraoperatively,[47] they recommended preemptive perioperative (preoperative or intraoperative) hemodynamic optimization.[50] The studies that followed demonstrated that this approach reduced surgical morbidity and mortality.[54-56] In their 1988 paper Shoemaker and colleagues were unable to determine "which of these influences are operative" to explain the intraoperative oxygen debt.[47] Furthermore, as already mentioned the VO_2 deficit was calculated using a formula that had not been validated.[48] At face value it would appear to be counterintuitive that anesthesia would result in an oxygen debt. General anesthesia and neuromuscular blockade reduce metabolic rate and oxygen consumption while DO_2 remains largely unchanged.[57,58] Hypothermia occurs frequently during anesthesia which further reduces metabolic oxygen requirements.[59,60] Indeed, in Shoemaker's pivotal paper VO_2 fell during

the intra-operative period reaching a nadir and the end of surgery.[47] In this study VO_2 increased sharply after surgery reaching the pre-operative VO_2 at 1 hour with the VO_2 peaking at 4 hours. It is therefore difficult to understand how anesthesia induces an oxygen debt. This apparent contradiction is best resolved by an analysis of the time course of the mixed venous oxygen saturation ($SmvO_2$) or central venous oxygen saturation ($ScvO_2$) during the perioperative period. $SmvO_2$ (or $ScvO_2$) is a reflection of the balance between DO_2 and VO_2; in patients who incur an oxygen debt the $SmvO_2$ should fall. A number of studies have monitored the $SmvO_2$/$ScvO_2$ in the perioperative period.[61-64] These studies have reproducibly demonstrate that the $SmvO_2$/$ScvO_2$ remains stable or increases slightly during anesthesia and surgery but falls sharply in the immediate post-anesthesia period. This data suggests that the oxygen debt is incurred postoperatively with the withdrawal of anesthesia (and NMB) and with the development of postoperative pain, agitation, shivering, and increased sympathetic tone. Furthermore, those patients with limited cardiac reserve and most likely to have the largest postoperative fall in $SmvO_2$/$ScvO_2$ and incur the largest oxygen debt. Indeed, these are the patients that have been demonstrated to be at the greatest risk of death and postoperative morbidity.[62,64] This would suggest that optimization of CO and DO_2 in the immediate postoperative period should be as effective as initiating hemodynamic optimization preoperatively or during the intraoperative period. Meta-analyses have confirmed the benefit of hemodynamic optimization whether initiated pre, intra, or postoperatively.[54,55]

Optimizing Cardiac Output in Trauma Patients

Patients who suffer severe traumatic injuries with blood loss incur an oxygen debt. The early increases in CO and DO_2 following resuscitation of trauma patients is considered compensation in order to replenish the oxygen debt. It has therefore been postulated that hemodynamic optimization following trauma targeting supranormal goals would decreases the incidence of multiple organ failure and death.[65,66] Bishop and coworkers pseudo-randomized 115 patients who had suffered from severe traumatic injuries to normal or supranormal hemodynamic goals (using a PAC) on admission to the SICU.[67] In this study patients in the supranormal group had significantly fewer organ failures and a lower risk of death. Furthermore, the CI and DO_2 of the survivors were significantly higher than those of the patients who died. McKinley and colleagues randomized 36 patients following traumatic shock to a protocol that aimed to achieve a DO_2 > 600 mL/min/m² or a protocol that aimed for a DO_2 of about 500 mL/min/m².[68] The patients in the 500 mL/min/m² group received less fluid and blood; however, there was no difference in outcomes between the groups. Velmahos et al randomized 75 severely injured patients to normal or supranormal hemodynamic goals in the pre-ICU period.[69] Survival rates were identical between the normal and supranormal groups. However, patients from either group who achieved supranormal values had improved survival rates compared with patients who did not. In this study patients in the supranormal group who could not achieve supranormal values had a higher death rate than similar patients in the control group. These findings support the argument that achieving supranormal values is an indicator of physiologic reserve rather than being a useful endpoint of resuscitation. Patients who have the inherent ability to respond to trauma by increasing their CO and oxygen transport capacity beyond normal levels are more likely to eliminate the existing oxygen deficit, avoid organ failure, and survive. Furthermore, attempts to optimize patients who do not have the necessary physiologic reserve may be detrimental. Based on the assimilation of these studies it would appear that targeting supranormal DO_2 does not improve the outcome of patients who have suffered traumatic injuries and that the most appropriate hemodynamic goals would be a MAP > 65 mm Hg with a normal cardiac index (> 2.5 L/min/m²).

Optimizing Cardiac Output in Medical Patients

It is widely believed that patients with sepsis, particularly those with an increased lactate concentration, have an oxygen debt (due to increased oxygen demand) and that increasing oxygen delivery will increase oxygen consumption and improve patient

outcome.[70] This concept was popularized by Edwards et al[71] and Astiz et al[72] in the late 1980s. There is, however, scant evidence that in patients with sepsis tissue hypoxia occurs. Hotchkiss and Karl in a seminal review published by over 20 years ago demonstrated that cellular hypoxia and bioenergetic failure do not occur in sepsis.[73] Using phosphorus 31 NMR spectroscopy to monitor concentrations of high-energy phosphates, Song et al, demonstrated normal concentrations of ATP in the leg muscle of septic rats.[74] Jepson et al confirmed these findings.[75] Similarly, Solomon et al demonstrated that sepsis-induced myocardial depression was not due to bioenergetic failure.[76] Using the hypoxic marker [18F] Fluoromisonidazole, Hotchkiss et al were unable to demonstrate evidence of cellular hypoxia in the muscle, heart, lung, and diaphragm of septic rates.[77] Additional studies support these findings. In a porcine peritonitis model, Regueira et al demonstrated a significant increase in arterial lactate concentration yet there was no significant change in hepatic and muscle mitochondrial oxidative function.[78]

While sepsis is considered to be hypermetabolic condition oxygen consumption and energy expenditure are broadly comparable to that of normal people, with energy expenditure decreasing with increasing sepsis severity.[79-81] Therefore, there is no requirement that oxygen delivery increase with sepsis. Ronco and colleagues determined the critical oxygen delivery threshold for anaerobic metabolism in septic and nonseptic critically ill humans while life support was being discontinued.[82] In this study there was no difference in the critical oxygen delivery threshold between septic and nonseptic patients. The critical oxygen delivery threshold was 3.8 ± 1.5 mL/min/kg (266 mL/min in a 70 kg patient); assuming a hemoglobin concentration of 10 g/L translates into a cardiac output of approximately 2 L/min. It is likely that only preterminal moribund patients with septic shock would have such a low cardiac output.

Several studies performed over four decades ago provide strong evidence that hyperlactacidemia noted during shock states was unlikely to be caused by tissue hypoxia.[83,84] It has now been well established that epinephrine released as part of the stress response in patients with shock stimulates $Na^+ K^+$ ATPase activity. Increased activity of $Na^+ K^+$ ATPase leads to increased lactate production under well-oxygenated conditions in various cells, including erythrocytes, vascular smooth muscle, neurons, glia, and skeletal muscle.[85,86] This concept was confirmed by Levy and colleagues, who in patients with septic shock demonstrated that skeletal muscle was the leading source of lactate formation as a result of exaggerated *aerobic* glycolysis through $Na^+ K^+$ ATPase stimulation.[87] Selective inhibition of $Na^+ K^+$ ATPase with ouabain infusion stopped over-production of muscle lactate and pyruvate. In summary, these data suggest that oxygen requirement are not increased in patients with sepsis, that an oxygen debt does not exist in patients with sepsis, and that lactate is produced aerobically as part of the stress response. This would suggest that increasing oxygen delivery would not be a useful exercise. In a pivotal study published in 1994, Hayes and colleagues randomized 109 fluid resuscitated critically ill patients to receive dobutamine titrated to achieve a $DO_2 > 600$ $mL/min/m^2$ or a control group who received dobutamine only if the CI < 2.8 L/m^2.[88] During treatment there was no difference between groups in the MAP or VO_2, despite a significantly higher CI and DO_2 in the treatment group. The in-hospital mortality was significantly higher in the treatment group (34% vs 54%, $P = 0.04$). In a follow-up publication limited to those patients with sepsis, these authors demonstrated that those patients with normal hemodynamics and those who reached the supranormal DO_2 goal spontaneously (fluid alone) had a significantly lower morality than those in whom the DO_2 goals were achieved with dobutamine.[89] The findings of this study are in keeping with the studies in trauma patients which suggest that attempts at driving up oxygen delivery in patients with limited cardiac reserve is not beneficial and maybe potentially harmful. This concept is supported by the study by Gattinoni and colleagues.[90] These authors randomized 762 critically ill patients to three groups, namely (i) a control group, (ii) a group with a target cardiac index > 4.5 $L/min/m^2$ (supranormal group), and (iii) a group with a target $SmvO_2 > 70\%$. In this study there was no difference in outcome between any of the groups.

In conclusion, fluid challenges and the use of inotropic agents should be guided by the change in cardiac output following these interventions. Perioperative optimization of cardiac output with targeted fluid challenges reduces postoperative complications and mortality. Targeting supranormal hemodynamic targets in patients with traumatic injuries and those with sepsis does not improve outcome and may be harmful. Similarly, in patients with sepsis attempting to increase oxygen delivery in response to an increased lactate concentration is illogical and potentially harmful.

CONFLICT OF INTEREST

The author has no financial interest in any of the products mentioned in this paper.

REFERENCES

1. Fick A. Ueber die Messung des Blutquantums in den Herzventrikeln. *Sitzungsberichte der Physiologisch-Medizinosche Gesellschaft zu Wuerzburg.* 1870;2:16.
2. Stewart GN. Researches on the circulation time and on the influences which affect it. IV. The output of the heart. *J Physiol.* 1897;22:159-183.
3. Fegler G. Measurement of cardiac output in anesthetized animals by a thermodilution method. *Q J Exp Physiol.* 1954;39:153-164.
4. Ganz W, Donosco R, Marcus HS, et al. A new technique for measurment of cardiac output by thermodilution in man. *Am J Cardiol.* 1971;27:392-396.
5. Phillips RA, Hood SG, Jacobson BM, et al. Pulmonary artery catheter (PAC) accuracy and efficacy comparedwith flow probe and transcutaneous Doppler (USCOM): an ovine cardiac output validation. *Crit Care Res Pract.* 2012;62:1494.
6. Heerdt PM, Pond CG, Blessios GA, et al. Comparison of cardiac output measured by intrapulmonary artery Doppler, thermodilution, and electromagnetometry. *Ann Thorac Surg.* 1992;54:959-966.
7. Heerdt PM, Blessios GA, Beach ML, et al. Flow dependency of error in thermodilution measurement of cardiac output during acute tricuspid regurgitation. *J Cardiothorac Vasc Anesth.* 2001;15:183-187.
8. Dhingra VK, Fenwick JC, Walley KR, et al. Lack of agreement between thermodilution and fick cardiac output in critically ill patients. *Chest.* 2002;122:990-997.
9. Espersen K, Jensen EW, Rosenborg D, et al. Comparison of cardiac output measurement techniques: thermodilution, Doppler, CO_2-rebreathing and the direct Fick method. *Acta Anaesthesiol Scand.* 1995;39:245-251.

10. Rich JD, Archer SL, Rich S. Noninvasive cardiac output measurements in patients with pulmonary hypertension. *Eur Resp J*. 2013;42:125-133.

11. Yang XX, Critchley LA, Rowlands DK, et al. Systematic error of cardiac output measured by bolus thermodilution with a pulmonary artery catheter compared with that measured by an aortic flow probe in a pig model. *J Cardiothorac Vasc Anesth*. 2013;27:1133-1139.

12. Yang XX, Critchley LA, Joynt GM. Determination of the precision error of the pulmonary artery thermodilution catheter using an in vitro continuous flow test rig. *Anesth Analg*. 2011;112:70-77.

13. Reuter DA, Huang C, Edrich T, et al. Cardiac output monitoring using indicator-dilution techniques: basics, limits, and perspectives. *Anesth Analg*. 2010;110:799-811.

14. Wong M, Skulsky A, Moon E. Loss of indicator in the thermodilution technique. *Cathet Cardiovasc Diagn*. 1978;4:103-109.

15. Renner LE, Morton MJ, Sakuma GY. Indicator amount, temperature, and intrinsic cardiac output affect thermodilution cardiac output accuracy and reproducibility. *Crit Care Med*. 1993;21:586-597.

16. Cigarroa RG, Lange RA, Williams RH, et al. Underestimation of cardiac output by thermodilution in patients with tricuspid regurgitation. *Am J Med*. 1989;86:417-420.

17. Balik M, Pachl J, Hendl J. Effect of the degree of tricuspid regurgitation on cardiac output measurements by thermodilution. *Intensive Care Med*. 2002;28:1117-1121.

18. Singh JP, Evans JC, Levy D, et al. Prevalence and clinical determinants of mitral, tricuspid, and aortic regurgitation (the Framingham Heart Study). [Erratum appears in *Am J Cardiol*. 1999;84:1143]. *Am J Cardiol*. 1999;83:897-902.

19. Klein AL, Burstow DJ, Tajik AJ, et al. Age-related prevalence of valvular regurgitation in normal subjects: a comprehensive color flow examination of 118 volunteers. *J Am Soc Echocardiogr*. 1990;3:54-63.

20. Fox ER, Wilson RS, Penman AD, et al. Epidemiology of pure valvular regurgitation in the large middle-aged African American cohort of the Atherosclerosis Risk in Communities study. *Am Heart J*. 2007;154:1229-1234.

21. Tibby SM, Hatherill M, Marsh MJ, et al. Clinical validation of cardiac output measurements using femoral artery thermodilution with direct Fick in ventilated children and infants. *Intensive Care Med*. 1997;23:987-991.

22. Pauli C, Fakler U, Genz T, et al. Cardiac output determination in children: equivalence of the transpulmonary thermodilution method to the direct Fick principle. *Intensive Care Med*. 2002;28:947-952.

23. Monnet X, Persichini R, Ktari M, et al. Precision of the transpulmonary thermodilution measurements. *Crit Care*. 2011;15:R204.

24. Montenij LJ, de Waal EE, Buhre WF. Arterial waveform analysis in anesthesia and critical care. *Curr Opin Anaesthesiol*. 2011;24:651-656.

25. Marik PE. Non-invasive cardiac output monitors. A state-of-the-art review. *J Cardiothorac Vasc Anesth*. 2013;27:121-134.

26. Lefrant JY, Bruelle P, Aya AG, et al. Training is required to improve the reliability of esophageal Doppler to measure cardiac output in critically ill patients. *Intensive Care Med*. 1998;24:347-352.

27. Valtier B, Cholley BP, Belot JP, et al. Noninvasive monitoring of cardiac output in critically ill patients using transesophageal doppler. *Am J Respir Crit Care Med*. 1998;158:77-83.

28. Keren H, Burkhoff D, Squara P. Evaluation of a noninvasive continuous cardiac output monitoring system based on thoracic bioreactance. *Am J Physiol*. 2007;293:H583-H589.

29. Raval NY, Squara P, Cleman M, et al. Multicenter evaluation of noninvasive cardiac output measurement by bioreactance technique. *J Clin Monit Comp*. 2008;22:113-119.

30. Squara P, Rotcajg D, Denjean D, et al. Comparison of monitoring performance of Bioreactance vs. pulse contour during lung recruitment maneuvers. *Crit Care*. 2009;13:R125.

31. Squara P, Denjean D, Estagnasie P, et al. Noninvasive cardiac output monitoring (NICOM): a clinical validation. *Intensive Care Med*. 2007;33:1191-1194.

32. Heerdt PM, Wagner CL, DeMais M, et al. Noninvasive cardiac ouput monitoring with bioreactance as an alternative to invasive instrumentation for preclinical drug evaluation in beagles. *J Pharmacol Toxicol Methods*. 2011;64:111-118.

33. Marik PE, Levitov A, Young A, et al. The use of NICOM (Bioreactance) and Carotid Doppler to determine volume responsiveness and blood flow redistribution following passive leg raising in hemodynamically unstable patients. *Chest*. 2013;143:364-370.

34. Marik PE, Cavallazzi R, Vasu T, et al. Dynamic changes in arterial waveform derived variables and fluid responsiveness in mechanically ventilated patients. A systematic review of the literature. *Crit Care Med*. 2009;37:2642-2647.

35. Marik PE, Cavallazzi R. Does the central venous pressure (CVP) predict fluid responsiveness: An update meta-analysis and a plea for some common sense. *Crit Care Med.* 2013;41:1774-1781.

36. Stetz CW, Miller RG, Kelly GE, et al. Reliability of ther thermodilution method in the determination of cardiac output in clinical practice. *Am Rev Respir Dis.* 1982;126:1001-1004.

37. Bruegger D, Jacob M, Rehm M, et al. Atrial natriuretic peptide induces shedding of endothelial glycocalyx in coronary vascular bed of guinea pig hearts. *Am J Physiol Heart Circ Physiol.* 2005;289:H1993-H1999.

38. Bruegger D, Schwartz L, Chappell D, et al. Release of atrial natriuretic peptide precedes shedding of the endothelial glycocalyx equally in patients undergoing on- and off-pump coronary artery bypass surgery. *Basic Res Cardiol.* 2011;106:1111-1121.

39. Jacob M, Chappell D. Reappraising Starling: the physiology of the microcircualtion. *Curr Opin Crit Care.* 2013;19:282-289.

40. Cavallaro F, Sandroni C, Marano C, et al. Diagnostic accuracy of passive leg raising for prediction of fluid responsiveness in adults: systematic review and meta-analysis of clinical studies. *Intensive Care Med.* 2010;36:1475-1483.

41. Mahjoub Y, Touzeau J, Airapetian N, et al. The passive leg-raising maneuver cannot accurately predict fluid responsiveness in patients with intra-abdominal hypertension. *Crit Care Med.* 2010;38:1824-1829.

42. Lakhal K, Ehrmann S, Runge I, et al. Central venous pressure measurements improve the accuracy of leg raising-induced change in pulse pressure to predict fluid responsiveness. *Intensive Care Med.* 2010;36:940-948.

43. Monnet X, Teboul JL. Passive leg raising: keep it easy! *Intensive Care Med.* 2010;36:1445.

44. Monnet X, Rienzo M, Osman D, et al. Passive leg raising predicts fluid responsiveness in the critically ill. *Crit Care Med.* 2006;34:1402-1407.

45. Shoemaker WC, Appel PL, Bland R, et al. Clinical trial of an algorithm for outcome prediction in acute circulatory failure. *Crit Care Med.* 1982;10:390-397.

46. Shoemaker WC, Appel PL, Waxman K, et al. Clinical trial of survivors cardiorespiratory patterns as therapeutic goals in critically ill postoperative patients. *Crit Care Med.* 1982;10:398-403.

47. Shoemaker WC, Appel PL, Kram HB. Tissue oxygen debt as a determinant of lethal and nonlethal postoperative organ failure. *Crit Care Med.* 1988;16:1117-1120.

48. Lowe HJ, Ernst EA. *The Quantitative Practice of Anesthesia: Use of Closed Circuit.* Baltimore, MD: Williams & Wilkins; 1981.

49. Crowell JW, Smith EE. Oxygen deficit and irreversible hemorrhagic shock. *Am J Physiol.* 1964;106:313.

50. Shoemaker WC, Appel PL, Kram HB, et al. Prospective trial of supranormal values of survivors as therapeutic goals in high risk surgical patients. *Chest.* 1988;94:1176-1186.

51. Centers for Disease Control and Prevention. Deaths from motor-vechile-related unintenstional carbon monoxide poisoning-Colorado, 1996, New Mexico, 1980-1995, and United States, 1979-1992. *J Am Med Assoc.* 1996;276:1942-1943.

52. Boyd O, Grounds RM, Bennett ED. A randomized clinical trial of the effects of deliberate perioperative increase of oxygen delivery on mortality in high risk surgical patients. *J Am Med Assoc.* 1993;270:2699-2707.

53. Rhodes A, Cecconi M, Hamilton M, et al. Goal-directed therapy in high-risk surgical patients: a 15-year follow-up study. *Intensive Care Med.* 2010;36:1327-1332.

54. Hamilton MA, Cecconi M, Rhodes A. A systematic review and meta-analysis on the use of preemptive hemodynamic intervention to improve postoperative outcomes in moderate and high-risk surgical patients. *Anesth Analg.* 2011;112:1392-1402.

55. Cecconi M, Corredor C, Arulkumaran N, et al. Clinical review: goal-directed therapy—What is the evidence in surgical patients? The effect on different risk groups. *Crit Care.* 2013;17:209.

56. Corcoran T, Rhodes JE, Clarke S, et al. Perioperative fluid management strategies in major surgery: a stratified meta-analysis. *Anesth Analg.* 2012;114:640-651.

57. Lindahl SG. Energy expenditure and fluid and electrolyte requirements in anesthetized infants and children. *Anesthesiology.* 1988;69:377-382.

58. Marik PE, Kaufman D. The effects of neuromuscular paralysis on systemic and splanchnic oxygen utilization in mechanically ventilated patients. *Chest.* 1996;109:1038-1042.

59. Bacher A, Illievich UM, Fitzgerald R, et al. Changes in oxygenation variables during progressive hypothermia in anesthetized patients. *J Neurosurg Anesthesiol.* 1997;9:205-210.

60. Sessler DI. Temperature monitoring and perioperative thermoregulation. *Anesthesiology.* 2008;109:318-338.

61. Shepherd SJ, Pearse RM. Role of central and mixed venous oxygen saturation measurement in perioperative care. *Anesthesiology*. 2009;111:649-656.

62. Multicenter study on peri- and postoperative central venous oxygen saturation in high-risk surgical patients. *Crit Care*. 2013;10:R158.

63. Futier E, Robib E, Jabaudon M, et al. Central venous O_2 saturation and venous-to-arterial CO_2 difference as complementary tools for goal-directed therapy during high-risk surgery. *Crit Care*. 2010;14:R193.

64. Futier E, Constantin JM, Petit A, et al. Conservative vs restrictive individualized goal-directed fluid replacement strategy in major abdominal surgery: a prospective randomized trial. *Arch Surg*. 2010;145:1193-1200.

65. Moore FA, Haenel JB, Moore EE, et al. Incommensurate oxygen consumption in response to maximal oxygen availability predicts postinjury multiple organ failure. *J Trauma*. 1992;33:58-65.

66. Rady MY, Edwards JD, Nightingale P. Early cardiorespiratory findings after severe blunt thoracic trauma and their relation to outcome. *Br J Surg*. 1992;79:65-68.

67. Bishop MH, Shoemaker WC, Appel PL, et al. Prospective, randomized trial of survivor values of cardiac index, oxygen delivery, and oxygen consumption as resuscitation endpoints in severe trauma. *J Trauma*. 1995;38:780-787.

68. McKinley BA, Kozar RA, Cocanour CS, et al. Normal versus supranormal oxygen delivery goals in shock resuscitation: the response is the same. *J Trauma*. 2002;53:825-832.

69. Velmahos GC, Demetriades D, Shoemaker WC, et al. Endpoints of resuscitation of critically injured patients: normal or supranormal? A prospective randomized trial. *Ann Surg*. 2000;232:409-418.

70. Dellinger RP, Levy MM, Rhodes A, et al. Surviving Sepsis Campaign: International Guielines for Management of Severe Sepsis and Septic Shock: 2012. *Crit Care Med*. 2013;41:580-637.

71. Edwards JD, Brown GCS, Nightingale P, et al. Use of survivors cardiorespiratory values as therapeutic goals in septic shock. *Crit Care Med*. 1989;17:1098-1113.

72. Astiz ME, Rackow EC, Falk JL, et al. Oxygen delivery and consumption in patients with hyperdynamic septic shock. *Crit Care Med*. 1987;15:26-28.

73. Hotchkiss RS, Karl IE. Reevaluation of the role of cellular hypoxia and bioenergetics failure in sepsis. *J Am Med Assoc*. 1992;267:1503-1510.

74. Song SK, Hotchkiss RS, Karl IE, et al. Concurrent quantification of tissue metabolism and blood flow via 2H/31P NMR in vivo. III. Alterations of muscle blood flow and metabolism during sepsis. *Magn Reson Med*. 1992;25:67-77.

75. Jepson MM, Cox M, Bates PC, et al. Regional blood flow and skeletal muscle energy status in endotoxemic rats. *Am J Physiol*. 1987;252:E581-E587.

76. Solomon MA, Correa R, Alexander HR, et al. Myocardial energy metabolism and morphology in a canine model of sepsis. *Am J Physiol*. 1994;266:H757-H768.

77. Hotchkiss RS, Rust RS, Dence CS, et al. Evaluation of the role of cellular hypoxia in sepsis by the hypoxic marker [18F]fluoromisonidazole. *Am J Physiol*. 1991;261:R965-R972.

78. Regueira T, Djafarzadeh S, Brandt S, et al. Oxygen transport and mitochondrial function in porcine septic shock, cardiogenic shock, and hypoxaemia. *Acta Anaesthesiol Scand*. 2012;56:846-859.

79. Uehara M, Plank LD, Hill GL. Components of energy expenditure in patients with severe sepsis and major trauma: a basis for clinical care. *Crit Care Med*. 1999;27:1295-1302.

80. Kreymann G, Grosser S, Buggisch P, et al. Oxygen consumption and resting metabolic rate in sepsis, sepsis syndrome, and septic shock. *Crit Care Med*. 1993;21:1012-1019.

81. Subramaniam A, McPhee M, Nagappan R. Predicting energy expenditure in sepsis: Harris-Benedict and Schofield equations versus the Weir derivation. *Crit Care Resus*. 2012;14:202-210.

82. Ronco JJ, Fenwick JC, Tweeddale MG, et al. Identification of the critical oxygen delivery for anaerobic metabolism in critically ill septic and nonseptic humans. *J Am Med Assoc*. 1993;270:1724-1730.

83. Irving MH. The sympatho-adrenal factor in haemorrhagic shock. *Ann R Coll Surg Engl*. 1968;42:367-386.

84. Daniel AM, Shizgal HM, MacLean LD. The anatomic and metabolic source of lactate in shock. *Surg Gynecol Obstet*. 1978;147:697-700.

85. James JH, Luchette FA, McCarter FD, et al. Lactate is an unreliable indicator of tissue hypoxia in injury or sepsis. *Lancet*. 1999;354:505-508.

86. James JH, Fang CH, Schrantz SJ, et al. Linkage of aerobic glycolysis to sodium-potassium transport in rat skeletal muscle. Implications for increased muscle lactate production in sepsis. *J Clin Invest*. 1996;98:2388-2397.

87. Levy B, Gibot S, Franck P, et al. Relation between muscle Na+K+ ATPase activity and raised lactate

concentrations in septic shock: a prospective study. *Lancet.* 2005;365:871-875.

88. Hayes MA, Timmins AC, Yau E, et al. Elevation of systemic oxygen delivery in the treatment of critically ill patients. *N Engl J Med.* 1994;330:1717-1722.

89. Hayes MA, Timmins AC, Yau EH, et al. Oxygen transport patterns in patients with sepsis syndrome or septic shock: influence of treatment and relationship to outcome. *Crit Care Med.* 1997;25:926-936.

90. Gattinoni L, Brazzi L, Pelosi P, et al. A trial of goal-oriented hemodynamic therapy in critically ill patients. *N Engl J Med.* 1995;333:1025-1032.

Cardioversion and Defibrillation

Rohit R. Gupta, MD and Ylaine Rose T. Aldeguer, MD

KEY POINTS

1. Biphasic waveform cardioversion is safe and equally effective as monophasic cardioversion, using much lower energy with reduced post-shock complications such as cardiac dysfunction, dysrhythmias, and skin burns.

2. Defibrillation or unsynchronized cardioversion is indicated in any patient with pulseless VT/VF or unstable polymorphic VT, where synchronized cardioversion is not possible.

3. Synchronized cardioversion is utilized for the treatment of persistent unstable tachyarrhythmia in patients without

loss of pulse. Amongst this category, AF remains the most frequently encountered.

4. In critically ill patients, unstable supraventricular tachyarrhythmias benefit from individualized therapy such as inotrope and vasopressor support, antiarrhythmic medications or mechanical ventilation and not necessarily electrical cardioversion as the first treatment.

5. It is important to become familiar with the cardioversion device available, the appropriate energy settings and the correct placement of the paddles to ensure effective and timely shock administration.

INTRODUCTION

The incidence of cardiac arrhythmias in critically ill patients has been shown to be considerable, ranging from less than 50% in trauma patients to more than 90% in those admitted with a primary cardiac illness.[1] In the ICU, the most common arrhythmias are atrial fibrillation (AF) and ventricular tachycardia (VT).[2] These arrhythmias vary in their presentation from incidental findings on telemetry to symptomatic episodes with profound compromise in cardiac and pulmonary function. Rapid diagnosis and critical interventions are important as these arrhythmias cause hemodynamic instability, prolong ICU length of stay, and increase morbidity and mortality.[2,3]

Electrical current or shocks delivered to the chest to terminate ventricular fibrillation (VF) was first reported in the 1950s.[4] Today, defibrillation is an established component of the Advanced Cardiovascular Life Support (ACLS) algorithm for pulseless VT/VF. The delivery of an electrical shock results in simultaneous depolarization of the myocardium making the heart refractory to the ongoing disordered electrical activity. This allows for the interruption of the underlying malignant rhythm and reestablishment of the normal electrical rhythm of the heart.[5,6]

In the case of tachyarrhythmias where the rhythm is organized and the patients have a palpable pulse, an electrical shock is given as a synchronized cardioversion. Cardioversion refers to the delivery of an electrical shock that is timed to the peak of the R wave on the EKG. This synchronization ensures that the electrical stimulation occurs only during the refractory period of the cardiac cycle minimizing the risk of iatrogenic arrhythmias. The literature on cardioversion can be confusing as many alternate terms such as external cardioversion, synchronized cardioversion, DC cardioversion, and transthoracic DC cardioversion are used interchangeably.

Traditionally monophasic waveform cardioverters were used until the introduction of biphasic waveform cardioversion in the mid-1990s. Increasingly more cardioverters in the ICU are biphasic. Biphasic waveform cardioversion is safe and as equally effective as monophasic cardioversion, using much lower energy with reduced post-shock complications such as cardiac dysfunction, dysrhythmias, and skin burns.[7-9] It is important for the intensivist to be aware of the type and model of cardioverter/defibrillator available in the units they cover so as to ensure appropriate delivery of electrical shocks.

INDICATIONS

Synchronized cardioversion is utilized for the treatment of persistent unstable tachyarrhythmia in patients without loss of pulse. Amongst this category, AF remains the most frequently encountered. Other unstable tachyarrhythmias with intact pulses where cardioversion has been demonstrated to be effective include atrial flutter, atrial ventricular nodal reentrant tachycardia (AVNRT), atrial ventricular reentrant tachycardia (AVRT) with pre-excitation pathways and monomorphic regular ventricular tachycardia.

Defibrillation or unsynchronized cardioversion is indicated in any patient with pulseless VT/VF or unstable polymorphic VT where synchronized cardioversion is not possible. These are fatal arrhythmias that require prompt recognition and early correction by administration of electrical shock. In these circumstances, defibrillation therapy would take precedence over all other treatments being provided to the ICU patient except when providing the initial cycles of CPR prior to shock delivery per ACLS protocol or establishing an adequate airway when hypoxemia due to an inadequate airway is causing the arrhythmia.

The parameters for defining an unstable arrhythmia as mentioned in the advanced cardiovascular life support guidelines includes any arrhythmia that is causing hypotension, altered mental status, signs of shock, ischemic chest discomfort or acute heart failure. However, ICU patients are frequently admitted with similar symptoms as part of their primary critical illness. In such situations, unstable supraventricular tachyarrhythmias benefit from individualized therapy such as inotrope and vasopressor support, antiarrhythmic medications or mechanical ventilation and not necessarily electrical cardioversion as the first treatment. It is imperative that the intensivist is able to quickly discern if the arrhythmia is the primary cause of a patient's instability, and where it is merely a marker of the patient's illness.

Tachyarrhythmias seen in the ICU setting are often a product of the complex interplay between the patient's severe illness and the interventions being performed. The presence of multi-organ failure, concomitant sympathetic and neurohumoral surges, arrhythmogenic drugs and invasive surgical therapies modulate the pathways for arrhythmia generation as well as their response to conventional therapies. The use of vasopressors and inotropes present a challenge to the control of tachyarrhythmias that requires titrating the dose and duration of these therapies, avoiding more arrhythmogenic agents such as dobutamine or dopamine. Recognizing the need for prompt source control in septic patients, controlling electrolyte disturbances in diabetic ketoacidosis, minimizing autonomic fluctuation following a subarachnoid bleed, and closely monitoring and managing pain, anxiety, agitation, oxygenation, and delirium are some examples of addressing the primary illness which can aid in stabilizing cardiac issues.

Cardioversion is still warranted in situations where the patient's hemodynamic status remains compromised despite the above interventions. While successful, post cardioversion tachyarrhythmias tend to recur in patients with sepsis and multi-organ failure. Furthermore the delivery of successive electrical shocks in these patients may be very poorly tolerated as compared to other patient populations. It is thus for the intensivist to make judicious utilization of cardioversion therapy understanding all the benefits and risks involved.

AF AND ATRIAL FLUTTER

New onset AF occurs in about 46% of patients with septic shock and is associated with prolonged ICU stay and a trend towards increased mortality.[3] It is believed that the increased adrenergic activity during sepsis and septic shock contributes to the frequent occurrence of arrhythmias in the ICU, and in these patients, rate control and maintaining sinus rhythm can be challenging unless the underlying pathology has been addressed. Patients with AF of more than seven days duration, dilated atria on echocardiogram, or heart failure also have an increased risk of recurrence after cardioversion.[10] The use of amiodarone infusion before and after electrical cardioversion increases the chances of maintaining sinus rhythm.

SUPRAVENTRICULAR TACHYCARDIA (SVT)

Narrow complex tachycardias include atrial flutter, atrioventricular nonreentrant tachycardia (AVNRT), atrioventricular reciprocating tachycardia (AVRT) and junctional tachycardia. These rhythms tend to occur in a paroxysmal manner often converting back and forth on their own. Hemodynamic instability or persistent and symptomatic SVT despite medical therapy (IV beta-blocker, calcium channel blocker, or adenosine administration) is an indication for urgent cardioversion.

MONOMORPHIC VT WITH A PULSE

Synchronized cardioversion can be performed in unstable patients with a regular monomorphic VT in the presence of a pulse. Patients with irregular or polymorphic VT should however be managed with defibrillation. It is important to note that synchronization of the electrical discharge with the QRS complex in monomorphic VT may be very challenging to achieve. Thus, patients who present with signs of

clinical instability such as hypotension, chest pain, acute pulmonary edema, heart failure, and change in mental status, should receive urgent unsynchronized defibrillation if attempts at synchronization are unsuccessful.

VF AND PULSELESS VT

VF and pulseless VT are managed by defibrillation and CPR until return of spontaneous circulation (ROSC) with a perfusing rhythm has been established as outlined in the advance cardiac life support (ACLS) protocol. Although improved survival has been linked to early defibrillation in VF, recent guidelines by the American Heart Association (AHA) emphasize the importance of immediate high quality chest compressions during cardiac arrest before attempting defibrillation even in the setting of VF or pulseless VT arrest.[11] Care should be taken to observe for fine VF that can often appear on the cardiac monitor as asystole resulting in an overlooked opportunity for defibrillation.

ENERGY SETTINGS

See Table 92–1 for the initial energy requirements commonly used during cardioversion using monophasic and biphasic waveform cardioverters. In patients with AF causing hemodynamic compromise, start synchronized cardioversion at 120 Joules (J) using a biphasic defibrillator and increase up to 200 J during the subsequent shocks. Unstable atrial flutter or paroxysmal supraventricular tachycardia (PSVT) require much lower energy and cardioversion may be initiated at 50 J biphasic (100 J monophasic) initially, then 100 J if unsuccessful. If it fails to terminate the SVT, a higher follow-up shock of 200 J (360 J monophasic) may be delivered. Monomorphic VT with a pulse is treated with synchronized cardioversion with initial 100 J biphasic (100 J monophasic), and escalation of energy to 200 J biphasic (360 J monophasic) with each successive shock until sinus rhythm is achieved. Delivering an initial 120 J (200 J monophasic) defibrillation shock is usually sufficient to terminate VF or pulseless VT. If unsuccessful, energy can be escalated to 200 J (360 J monophasic) for subsequent shocks. In the case of polymorphic VT with pulse, defibrillation with similar energy

TABLE 92-1 Initial energy requirements commonly used during cardioversion.

Type of Arrhythmia	Type of Cardioversion	Monophasic	Biphasic
Unstable AF	Synchronized	200 J	120–200 J
Unstable atrial flutter	Synchronized	100–200 J	50–100 J
Symptomatic or unstable SVT	Synchronized	100–200 J	50–100 J
Monomorphic VT with pulse	Synchronized	100–360 J	100–200 J
Polymorphic VT with pulse	Unsynchronized	100–360 J	100–200 J
VF or pulseless VT	Unsynchronized	200–360 J	120–200 J

AF: atrial fibrillation; SVT: supraventricular tachycardia; VT: ventricular tachycardia; VF: ventricular fibrillation.

settings (120 to 200J biphasic) are used as with pulseless VT.

PATIENT PREPARATION FOR CARDIOVERSION

Sedation and Analgesia

Delivering shocks can be painful, traumatic and may cause great anxiety in conscious patients receiving synchronized cardioversion or defibrillation. Short acting sedatives such as midazolam (0.02–0.03 mg/kg over 2–3 min) and or ketamine (1–2 mg/kg over 1–2 min), and analgesics such as fentanyl (0.5–1 mcg/kg) can be administered before the procedure. In patients who have a secured airway (eg, endotracheal intubation) and are more hemodynamically stable, propofol (eg, 0.3–1 mg/kg) is an effective short acting sedative that may be used in combination with an analgesic such as fentanyl. Only in the presence of experienced personnel (eg, anesthesiologist, intensivist), propofol can also be administered in smaller doses in nonintubated patients. In the elderly, administering lower doses of sedatives at less frequent intervals and at slower rates may be appropriate.

Application of Electrodes (Paddles or Pads)

The survival rate goes down 2.3% per minute until CPR is started and 1.1% per minute until a defibrillation shock is delivered.[12] The early application of paddles or pads (electrodes) is a critical link in the management of arrhythmias with hemodynamic compromise. It allows for a shorter analysis time and quicker delivery of electric shocks.

The positioning of the electrodes on the thorax determines the transthoracic pathway and the flow of current delivered during cardioversion and defibrillation. Currently, there are two conventional positions accepted for electrode placement: the anterolateral and anteroposterior orientation [Figures 92–1(A) and 1(B)]. In the anterolateral position, a first electrode is placed on the right edge of the sternum along the second or third intercostal space (ICS), while the second electrode is placed laterally on the left at the level of fourth or fifth ICS along the mid-axillary line. In the anteroposterior position, the first paddle is placed as above and the second paddle is placed on the back between the tip of the scapula and the spine. The anteroposterior placement of the electrodes is preferred in patients with implantable cardioverter-defibrillator devices (ICDs) to avoid shunting of energy and damage to the implantable device. The electrodes should be maintained in contact with the skin using either conductive gel (with paddles) or by using self-adhesive pads instead. In the case of pads, care should be taken to ensure that they are well secured. This may be particularly difficult in the patient with excess hair or sweat. The electrode pads are then connected to the cardioverter through a wire with a plastic adaptor (usually colored) as indicated in Figure 92–2. Each cardioverter is provided with disposable electrode pads designed for that model.

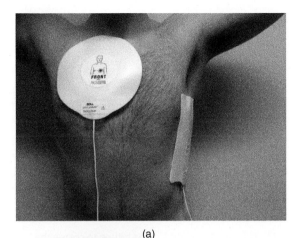

(a)

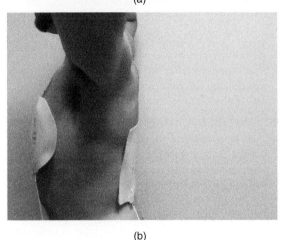

(b)

FIGURE 92-1 Placement of the pads in an (A) anterolateral configuration and (B) anteroposterior configuration.

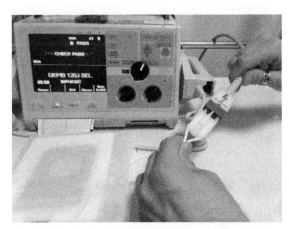

FIGURE 92-2 Attach cables to ensure tight connection between electrode pads and the cardioverter.

CPR Before Cardioversion

In cases such as in VF or pulseless VT, CPR should not be delayed and should be initiated immediately while preparing for defibrillation. The 2010 AHA Guidelines for cardiopulmonary resuscitation (CPR) and emergency cardiovascular care (ECC) recommends high quality CPR to be initiated for at least 90 to 180 seconds while the defibrillator pads and electrodes are being applied and before first defibrillation is attempted. It is believed that during VF, the myocardium is being depleted of oxygen and energy and that delivering CPR during this crucial period will provide the needed oxygen and energy, as well as increase the likelihood of terminating VF during defibrillation and rapid return of spontaneous circulation. Electrolyte imbalances such as hypocalcemia, hypokalemia and hypomagnesemia should also be corrected to improve successful cardioversion.

APPLICATION AND DELIVERY OF CARDIOVERSION

The following are basic steps for using the cardioverter:

1. Press the "ON" button to start operation of the defibrillator.

2. Most defibrillator brands are multifunctional and can be used as an automated external defibrillator (AED), manual defibrillator, external pacer or for ECG monitoring. Make sure that the device is set to defibrillator mode.

3. Apply the self-adhesive electrode pads to the patient's bare chest using anterolateral or anteroposterior orientation [Figure 92-1(A) and 92-1(B)], then connect the electrode pads wire into the cardioverter via a plastic adaptor (usually color-coded, as in Figure 92-2).

4. Place the 3-wire ECG leads on the patient and connect them to the ECG slot of the defibrillator. Once connected, the monitor will display the ECG tracing and the heart rate.

5. Press the "ENERGY SELECT" button to set the initial or preferred energy for defibrillation (Figure 92-3).

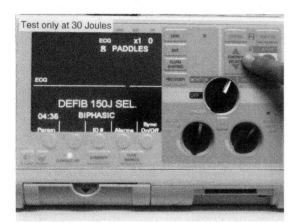

FIGURE 92–3 Use the Energy Select button to choose the energy level delivered during the cardioversion.

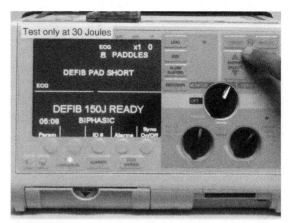

FIGURE 92–4 Use the Charge button to charge the cardioverter.

6. For synchronized cardioversion, press the "SYNC" button and a marker above every QRS is displayed. The monitor also displays "Sync" once this function is turned on. The device automatically returns to asynchronous mode after each synchronized discharge. This means that the "Sync" button needs to be turned on if the first synchronized cardioversion is unsuccessful and a second synchronized shock is indicated. Note again that the defibrillator will not be able to deliver a shock for rhythms requiring unsynchronized cardioversion if the "Sync" button is turned on.

7. Once the preferred energy level is set, pressing the "CHARGE" button charges the defibrillator. A charge tone indicates that the charge is complete to the selected energy level (Figure 92–4).

8. Once the defibrillator is fully charged, a shock can be delivered by pressing the flashing "SHOCK" button. It is utmost important that the person in charge states "all clear" and checks that all personnel are clear of contact with patient, bed, or equipment before delivery of the shock. Occasionally, the defibrillator may not be able to deliver the required shock even after the "Shock" button is pressed. Check to make sure that the defibrillator is connected to a power supply or that battery power is sufficient as displayed by the battery indicator

on the monitor, and that the "Sync" button is not inadvertently on in the setting of rhythms requiring unsynchronized cardioversion (Figure 92–5).

9. After the shock is delivered, the energy for each subsequent shock is automatically selected based on the energy level configured on the set-up. To escalate or change the energy level for the next shock, press the "ENERGY SELECT" button and return to step 5.

10. At anytime, an unwanted charge can be discharged by pressing the "DISARM" button.

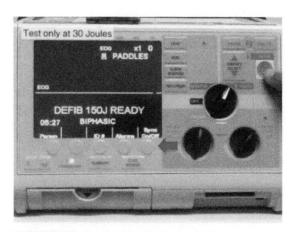

FIGURE 92–5 Arrow- Synchronize Cardioversion On/Off Button.

FACTORS AFFECTING SUCCESS OF CARDIOVERSION AND DEFIBRILLATION

There are a number of variables that influence the outcome of a cardioversion and/or defibrillation attempt. These can be grouped as patient characteristics such as body habitus, device characteristics including paddle size, waveform morphology and iatrogenic factors including administration of medications and ventilator support.

Electric shocks used in cardioversion and defibrillation are quantified by the amount of energy delivered. While this allows for the standardization of shocks delivered, it is important to understand that the determinant of an adequate shock is not the energy itself but the amount of electrical current that travels across the heart depolarizing the myocardium. The transmyocardial current generated is dependent directly on the energy level set and inversely related to the resistance/impedance offered by the circuit.

This resistance, termed as thoracic impedance, is determined by the electrode-to-skin interface, electrode pressure, body habitus and the phase of ventilation. Decreasing the interface between the skin and the paddle by placing more pressure on the paddles, applying adhesive or more conductive gel as well as delivering shocks during expiration decreases thoracic impedance and increases the effectiveness of cardioversion and defibrillation. Hairs should also be shaved off the chest if necessary to facilitate attachment of electrode pads to the skin.

Pad size is also an important determinant of transthoracic flow during delivery of shocks. A paddle or pad size with larger surface area has been associated with less thoracic resistance and less chances of myocardial injury.[10] A standard adult electrode pad size usually measures about 8 to 12 cm and is commercially packaged and available for single use.

Observational studies have shown that persistent AF may be more easily converted using a hand-held paddle and the improved electrode-to-skin contact and reduced thoracic impedance are likely contributing to the higher success rate of cardioversion.[11] However, there is no current data comparing the use of hand-held paddles and self-adhesive pad electrodes for other arrhythmias requiring cardioversion or defibrillation. Therefore, the decision to use which type of electrodes should base on equipment availability and the operator's opinion regarding which electrodes are more likely to be effective in a particular patient.

There has been ongoing debate about the relative impact of the positioning of the electrodes on the outcome of the cardioversion attempt. An initial study from Germany demonstrated a statistically significant difference in the successful cardioversion of AF with anteroposterior positioning of the electrodes (96%) as compared to anterolateral position (78%).[13] However subsequent studies have not demonstrated this benefit in a consistent manner.[14] In the ICU it is often difficult to position patients for placement of posterior pads often resulting in delays in the delivery of shocks. Consequently we do not recommend a particular position for electrode placement over another.

A final point should be made about the use of antiarrhythmic drugs prior to attempted cardioversion. While evidence is limited, in patients who have been pretreated with amiodarone, ibutilide, propafenone or sotalol, the restoration of a sinus rhythm from AF required less electrical energy, fewer attempts and lower number of recurrences.[15-18] Further studies however are required to determine if these findings are representative within the ICU population.

USE OF CARDIOVERSION/ DEFIBRILLATION UNDER SPECIAL CIRCUMSTANCES

Pregnancy

Among the various cardiac pathologies complicating pregnancy, arrhythmias are the most common. Often diagnosed for the first time during pregnancy, tachyarrhythmias are the commonest form of arrhythmias reported during pregnancy. Cardioversion and defibrillation during pregnancy is relatively safe without documented adverse effects to the fetus. However, antepartum fetal monitoring is recommended to monitor fetal heart rate during the procedure. Special consideration of the duration of pregnancy should be made while choosing drugs used for sedation pre-procedure, for example, avoid midazolam. Positioning of patients in the left lateral position if possible also allows the patient to better tolerate the hemodynamic changes associated with cardioversion/defibrillation.

CARDIOVERSION WITH IMPLANTABLE CARDIOVERTER DEFIBRILLATOR

Since the implantation of the first ICD in 1980, there has been a great increase in the use of these instruments and their presence in ICU patients. Occasionally patients continue to have unstable tachyarrhythmias despite having a functioning device. In certain instances, the ICD can be successfully reprogrammed to deliver the shock internally or implement tachycardia-pacing strategies for managing tachyarrhythmia.

The application of electrical current during synchronized and unsynchronized cardioversion in patients with an ICD or permanent pacemaker can potentially cause damage to the ICD circuit and cause malfunction of these devices. However, hemodynamically unstable tachyarrhythmias that are not being controlled by the implanted device need to be treated without hesitation in a manner similar to any other patient in the ICU.

As a strategy for minimizing risk of device damage, it is recommended to place the pads at least 12 cm away from the pulse generator and to use the anteroposterior positioning of electrodes. All ICDs and permanent pacemakers should be interrogated after cardioversion is performed to ensure the proper functioning of these devices.

CARDIOVERSION AND DIGOXIN

A common concern that is raised with the use of cardioversion refers to its use in patients on digoxin and the risk of post-cardioversion ventricular ectopy/arrhythmias. An initial study from 1966 revealed a significant increase in the incidence of serious post-cardioversion ventricular ectopy in patients that had ECG evidence of digitalis toxicity precardioversion.[19]

This however was noted to occur most commonly in patients that received monophasic shocks with energy greater than 200 J. Subsequent studies have confirmed that sustained ventricular ectopy post cardioversion is exceedingly rare and tends to occur with higher energy cardioversion along with other concomitant factors such as hypokalemia. As with all tachyarrhythmias it is important to identify and treat the underlying cause. If cardioversion is deemed necessary it should be carried out starting with a lower energy level and ensuring the correction of any electrolyte abnormalities.

COMPLICATIONS OF CARDIOVERSION

Complications of cardioversion include skin burns, transient hypotension (commonly from sedation), and EKG changes (such as nonspecific ST-T wave changes or transient ST segment elevation). High-energy shocks may also result in myocardial necrosis, which may present as a small rise in cardiac enzymes.[20] In contrast acute myocardial ischemia causes significant elevations of cardiac enzymes and may not be directly related to cardioversion itself. Myocardial dysfunction may also occur due to myocardial stunning and is usually related to ischemia during cardiac arrest. This complication usually improves in 24 to 48 hours post resuscitation. Rarely, pulmonary edema may occur as a result of left atrial standstill or LV dysfunction after cardioversion in patients with longstanding AF.

The two most common potentially life-threatening complications associated with cardioversion and defibrillation are arrhythmia and thromboembolism. Arrhythmias include sinus tachycardia, non-sustained VT, bradycardia and occasionally complete heart block that may require temporary cardiac pacing. Clinically significant VT or VF may also occur infrequently. Previous studies in patients with atrial fibrillation have reported a post cardioversion stroke risk of 1.1% if anticoagulated for 3 weeks and 7% if not anticoagulated.[21]

Much of these studies are retrospective analyses of data from emergency room visits and their results have not been reproduced in the ICU setting. The benefits of cardioversion in unstable AF outweighs the risk of clot embolization and therefore, urgent synchronized cardioversion should not be delayed in these patients. The process of oxygenating at the time of delivery of shock has come under scrutiny as a result of the risk for potential arcing/sparks leading to a fire. Despite defibrillation being used for several decades there have been only 2 reported cases of fire as a result of cardioversion/defibrillation.[22] We do not recommend any special precautions with regards to oxygenation and the delivery of electrical shocks.

REFERENCES

1. Artucio H, Pereira M. Cardiac arrhythmias in critically ill patients: epidemiologic study. *Crit Care Med.* 1990;18:1383-1388.

2. Reinelt P, Delle Karth G, Geppert A, Heinz G. Incidence and type of cardiac arrhythmias in critically ill patients: a single center experience in a medical-cardiological ICU. *Intensive Care Med.* 2001;27:1466-1473.

3. Meierhenrich R, Steinhilber E, Eggermann C, et al. Incidence and prognostic impact of new-onset atrial fibrillation in patients with septic shock: a prospective observational study. *Critical Care.* 2010;14:R108.

4. Zoll PM, Linenthal AJ, Gibson W, Paul MH, Norman LR. Termination of ventricular fibrillation in man by externally applied electric counter shock. *N Engl J Med.* 1956;254:727-732.

5. Zipes DP, Fischer J, King RM, Nicoll A deB, Jolly WW. Termination of ventricular fibrillation in dogs by depolarizing a critical amount of myocardium. *Am J Cardiol.* 1975;36:37-44.

6. Jones JL. Waveforms for implantable cardioverter defibrillators (ICDs) and transchest defibrillation. In: Tacker WA, ed. *Defibrillation of the Heart.* St. Louis: Mosby-Year Book; 1994:46–81.

7. Bardy GH, Ivey TD, Allen MD, Johnson G. A prospective, randomized evaluation of biphasic vs monophasic waveform pulses on defibrillation efficacy in humans. *J Am Coll Cardiol.* 1989;14:728-733.

8. Jones JL, Jones RE. Improved defibrillator safety factor with biphasic waveforms. *Am J Physiol.* 1983;245:H60-H65.

9. Jones JL, Jones RE. Decreased defibrillator-induced dysfunction with biphasic rectangular waveforms. *Am J Physiol.* 1984;247:H792-H796.

10. Abu-El-Haija B1, Giudici MC. Predictors of long-term maintenance of normal sinus rhythm after successful electrical cardioversion. *Clin Cardiol.* 2014;37:381-385.

11. Travers A, Rea T, Bobrow B, et al. 2010 American Heart Association Guidelines for Cardiopulmonary Resuscitation and Emergency Cardiovascular Care. *Circulation.* 2010;122:S676-S684.

12. Kroll MW, Fish RM, Calkins H, Halperin H, Lakkireddy D, Panescu D. Defibrillation success rates for electrically-induced fibrillation: hair of the dog. *Conf Proc IEEE Eng Med Biol Soc.* 2012;2012:689-693.

13. Kirchhof P, Eckardt L, Loh P, et al. Anterior-posterior versus anterior-lateral electrode positions for external cardioversion of atrial fibrillation: a randomised trial. *Lancet.* 2002;360:1275-1279.

14. Stanaitiene G, Babarskiene RM. Impact of electrical shock waveform and paddle positions on efficacy of direct current cardioversion for atrial fibrillation. *Medicina (Kaunas).* 2008;44:665-672.

15. Capucci A, Villani GQ, Aschieri D, Rosi A, Piepoli MF. Oral amiodarone increases the efficacy of direct-current cardioversion in restoration of sinus rhythm in patients with chronic atrial fibrillation. *Eur Heart J.* 2000;21:66-73.

16. Khan IA. Oral loading single dose flecainide for pharmacological cardioversion of recent-onset atrial fibrillation. *Int J Cardiol.* 2003;87:121-128.

17. Lai LP, Lin JL, Lien WP, Tseng YZ, Huang SK. Intravenous sotalol decreases transthoracic cardioversion energy requirement for chronic atrial fibrillation in humans: assessment of the electrophysiological effects by biatrial basket electrodes. *J Am Coll Cardiol.* 2000;5:1434-1441.

18. De Simone A, Stabile G, Vitale DF, et al. Pretreatment with verapamil in patients with persistent or chronic atrial fibrillation who underwent electrical cardioversion. *J Am Coll Cardiol.* 1999;34:810-814.

19. Kleiger R, Lown B. Cardioversion and digitalis. II. Clinical studies. *Circulation.* 1966;33:878-887.

20. Dahl CF, Ewy GA, Warner ED, Thomas ED. Myocardial necrosis from direct current countershock. Effect of paddle size and time interval between discharges. *Circulation.* 1974;50:956.

21. Arnold AZ, Mick MJ, Mazurek RP, Loop FD, Trohman RG. Role of prophylactic anticoagulation for direct current cardioversion in patients with atrial fibrillation or atrial flutter. *J Am Coll Cardiol.* 1992;19:851-885.

22. Hummel RS, Ornato JP, Weinberg SW, et al. Spark-generating properties of electrode gels used during defibrillation. A potential fire hazard. *J Am Med Assoc.* 1988;260:3021-3024.

Central Venous Access

Amit Pandit, MD; Leon Chen, MSc, AGACNP-BC, CCRN, CEN and Daniel Miller, MD

INTRODUCTION

Central venous catheterization is a commonly performed procedure and is an essential skill for critical care physicians. Common indications for placement of a central venous catheter (CVC) include hemodynamic monitoring, lack of peripheral venous access, administration of vasoactive agents, nutritional support, and long-term vascular access. Although traditionally performed by emergency and critical care physicians, anesthesiologists and surgeons, it has been shown that with proper training, this procedure can be safely performed by advanced practice practitioners such as nurse practitioners and physician assistants.[1]

Central venous catheter placement can be attempted via two methods: surface landmark approach or using real-time ultrasound guidance. While the landmark method is the traditional approach taught, real-time ultrasound guided CVC placement has emerged as the preferred and recommended practice, and is endorsed by majority of quality assurance agencies and professional societies. Knowledge of surface and deep anatomy is crucial in minimizing complications related to placement of internal jugular, subclavian, and femoral venous catheters.

ANATOMY

Internal Jugular Vein

The internal jugular (IJ) vein is formed by the inferior petrosal sinus and sigmoid sinus. It forms the brachiocephalic vein after it runs under the clavicle at the level of the sternum. The IJ vein, internal carotid artery and vagus nerve form the carotid sheath which runs under the sternocleidomastoid muscle. The IJ vein runs anterolateral to the common carotid artery, however it may be directly anterior to the common carotid artery on the right side in 26% and in 20% on the left side.[2] The right IJ vein follows a direct course to the superior vena cava (SVC) joining the right subclavian vein and forming a short and steeply angled right brachiocephalic vein. The left IJ vein forms a longer and shallow angled left brachiocephalic vein as it joins the left subclavian vein. The right IJ vein is larger than the left IJ vein given its direct relationship with the right ventricle.

Subclavian Vein

The subclavian vessels are a valveless continuation of the axillary veins. Similar to the IJ veins, the path of the right and left subclavian veins is not symmetrical. The right subclavian vein forms an angled arc as it merges with the right IJ vein forming the right brachiocephalic vein which enters the SVC, whereas the left subclavian vein merges into the left brachiocephalic vein along a shallow trajectory. The subclavian vein lies posterior to the clavicle after crossing the first rib. This isolated region is the only area where the subclavian vein directly communicates with the clavicle. The subclavian artery runs superior and posterior to the subclavian vein. The subclavian artery and vein are separated by the anterior scalene muscle. The phrenic nerve also runs over the lateral aspect of the anterior scalene muscle. The apices of the lungs may reach as far as the first rib.

Femoral Vein

The femoral vein is located in the femoral triangle (of Scarpa). The femoral triangle is a subfascial space secured superiorly by the inguinal ligament, medially by the medial border of the adductor longus muscle, and laterally by the medial border of the sartorius muscle. The femoral vein lies medial to the femoral artery. The femoral nerve travels down the leg lateral to the femoral artery. The pneumonic NAVEL (nerve, artery, vein empty space, and lymphatics) is commonly used to remember the location of the femoral structures from lateral to medial. Cannulation of the femoral vein is performed below the inguinal ligament. Femoral anatomy is the least complex when compared to the neck and the subclavian spaces especially as the course of the femoral veins is symmetric unlike the locations mentioned above. It is important to note that as the femoral vein progresses distally, the artery and vein may rotate on each other and the femoral artery may lie anterior to the vein.

TECHNIQUE

General Considerations

Successful placement of a CVC requires careful pre-procedure setup and patient assessment. A recent complete blood count and coagulation profile should be available to ensure that the platelet count is > 50,000 and the prothrombin time/International Normalized Ratio (INR) is < 2.0 and the activated partial thromboplastin time (aPTT) is < 50 seconds. Consent must be obtained from the patient or a healthcare agent and discussion of the risks, benefits and alternatives to CVC placement must be documented.

Equipment (Figure 93–1)

Typically central venous catheters are available in a prepacked sterile kit. "Bundling" has demonstrated a reduction in central line-associated bloodstream infections (CLABSI).[3] It is important to choose a catheter that has the correct lumen size to deliver medications, blood products, and length to reach the cavoatrial junction. Remember to "know your kit" and the structure of the catheter.

PREPARATION

After pre-procedure laboratory values, consent, and ultrasound (US) imaging have been reviewed, the site of cannulation must be selected. The insertion site must be tailored to the patient's anatomy and clinical scenario. It is advisable to choose insertion sites with easily identifiable anatomical landmarks. If an ultrasound is available, we recommend performing a pre-procedural bedside US survey or

reviewing previously obtained US images to evaluate the selected site's anatomy and vessel patency. Sites with anatomical defects, infections, masses, or areas of recent surgery or trauma should be avoided. Table 93–1 lists the advantages, disadvantages, and complications associated with each anatomical site.

POSITIONING

Position the patient to gain optimal access to the vessel. In all cases, the patient should be placed at a height and position comfortable for the operator.

Internal Jugular Vein

The patient should be placed in a flat supine Trendelenburg position (lower extremities higher than the head) in order to engorge the vein and create a larger target. Additionally, this decreases the risk of an air embolism. The head should be turned to the contralateral side to expose the neck and landmarks. Too generous contralateral rotation of the neck can impede cannulation as the sternocleidomastoid muscle may move into an anterior position over the IJ vein hindering cannulation.[4] Rotation beyond 40° increases the risk of arterial puncture as overlapping of the IJ vein with the carotid artery occurs.[5] Generally rotating the neck by an angle of 15° to 30° to the contralateral side allows for optimal vessel access and does not increase the risk for arterial cannulation. Pillows should be removed from under the head in order to extend the neck.

Subclavian Vein

The patient should be placed in a flat supine Trendelenburg position with the head in a neutral position. Many authors have argued that a roll placed between the scapulae in order to elevate the subclavian vessels anteriorly and widen the sternoclavicular angle. However, magnetic resonance imaging studies have demonstrated that placing a roll between the scapulae leads to compression of the subclavian vein between the first rib and clavicle hindering cannulation. The arm should be placed adducted to the torso.

Femoral Vein

The patient should be placed in a flat supine reverse Trendelenburg position with the targeted side's leg slightly abducted and rotated laterally at the hip.

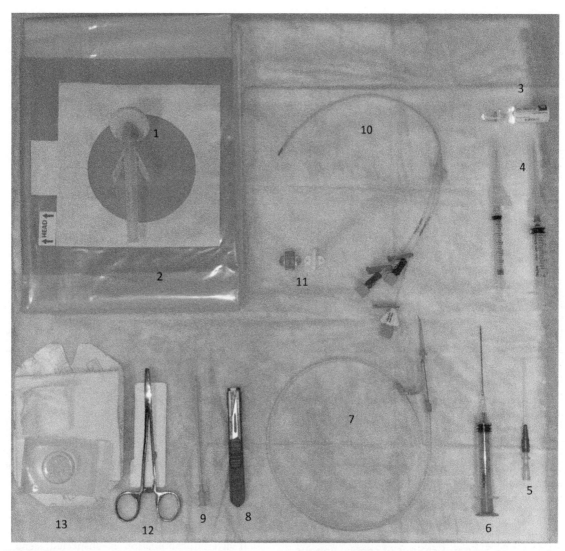

FIGURE 93-1 Central Line Kit (7Fr 20 cm). Legend: 1 = chlorhexidine, 2 = sterile full body drape, 3 = 1% lidocaine without epinephrine, 4 = 22- and 25-gauge needles for local anesthetic, 5 = 18-gauge angiocatheter with an introducer needle, 6 = introducer needle attached to a 5-ml syringe, 7 = guidewire in sheath, 8 = 11-blade scalpel, 9 = tissue dilator, 10 = triple-lumen catheter, 11 = catheter clamps, 12 = needle driver and silk suture, 13 = Tegaderm™ and Biopatch® dressing.

STERILITY

Maximal sterile barriers should be used when central venous cannulation is attempted to decrease the risk of CLABSI. These include using a cap, mask, sterile gown, gloves, and a sterile full-body drape. Chlorhexidine has been shown to be the most efficacious antiseptic.[6] The exposed cutaneous surface should be coated with chlorhexidine thoroughly prior to cannulation.

CANNULATION AND PLACING THE GUIDEWIRE

Prepare the catheter by flushing each lumen it with sterile saline. Anesthetize the cannulation site using 1 to 2 ml of 1% lidocaine or equivalent with a 25-gauge needle. Attach a 10-ml syringe to the finder/introducer needle and puncture the skin applying constant negative pressure approaching

TABLE 93-1 Advantages, disadvantages, and considerations with the CVC insertion site.

	Advantages	Disadvantages	Miscellaneous
Internal jugular vein	Easily visualized with ultrasound External landmarks easily visualized Direct trajectory into the cavoatrial junction Bleeding and hematoma can be recognized and easily controlled Low risk of pneumothorax	Uncomfortable for awake patients Higher risk of infection and thrombosis than subclavian vein Highest risk for arterial cannulation	Left IJ may be slightly challenging to place in the cavoatrial junction A 20-cm catheter should be used when the left IJ is cannulated
Subclavian vein	External landmarks easily visualized Lowest risk for infection and thrombosis Shallow angle of left subclavian is ideal for pacemaker placement	Highest risk for pneumothorax and hemothorax Difficult to achieve hemostasis given non compressibility of the vessel High risk for malpositioning (ascending into IJ or crossing over to the contralateral subclavian vein)	Natural curve of guidewire allows easy threading
Femoral vein	Good external landmarks Easy access during cardiopulmonary arrest Bleeding and hematoma can be identified and controlled	Highest risk for infection Highest risk for thrombosis Should be avoided in the setting of urinary/stool incontinence Close proximity to the peritoneal cavity Cannot measure CVP	

IJ = internal jugular; CVP = central venous pressure.

the target vessel (ultrasound or landmark-guided). As the needle enters the vessel lumen, blood enters the syringe. Ensure that blood is aspirated with good flow. Sluggish blood flow with aspiration suggests that the needle tip is not optimally positioned in the vessel lumen. Stabilize the hub of the needle and remove the syringe. Ensure that the blood flow from the needle is nonpulsatile. Bright red pulsatile blood flow suggests arterial cannulation; however, in states of hemodynamic compromise arterial cannulation may mimic venous cannulation (dark red nonpulsatile blood). Place your thumb over the needle hub to minimize the risk of air embolism before passing the guidewire.

If arterial cannulation is suspected, send a blood gas and compare the results with a confirmed arterial blood gas. Alternatively, introduce the flexible distal end of the guidewire into the cannulated vessel and directly visualize the guidewire in the vein with the ultrasound. Placing a single lumen 18-gauge angiocatheter over the guidewire and then connecting the catheter to a pressure transducer can also confirm venous cannulation in the presence of a transduced venous waveform and pressure. A simpler method of transducing venous pressure can be achieved by using standard IV tubing or the guidewire sheath as a manometer. Connect the IV tubing or remove the connectors of the guidewire sheath and uncurl the plastic guidewire sheath. Attach the

TABLE 93-2 Complications of central venous catheterization by insertion site.

Approach	Complications
Internal jugular and subclavian vein	Neck hematoma Pneumothorax Hemothorax Chylothorax Tracheal perforation Endotracheal cuff perforation Phrenic nerve injury Brachial plexus injury Stroke
Femoral vein	Retroperitoneal hematoma Psoas muscle hematoma Bladder perforation Bowel perforation Femoral nerve injury

IV tubing or uncurled guidewire sheath directly to the hub of the angiocath. The operator should hold the IV tubing or sheath vertically and wait for a blood column to rise in the sheath. If the angiocath is in the vein, the blood column will rise and correspond to the central venous pressure and variate with the respiratory cycle. If the angiocatheter is in the artery, the blood column will fill the entire tubing.[7] Venous cannulation must be confirmed prior to dilation of the soft tissue and vessel. Once venous cannulation is confirmed, introduce the soft end of the guidewire through the needle hub. The guidewire should thread smoothly without resistance. If resistance is met, do not force the wire, but remove it and attach the syringe to the introducer needle and aspirate blood and confirm that the needle tip is in the lumen of the targeted vessel. Retracting the needle slowly and changing the angle of entry may facilitate passing the guidewire. Ultimately, if the guidewire cannot be passed, new cannulation of the same vessel can be attempted or a new site should be chosen. Maintain control of the guidewire throughout the entire process.

Once the wire is placed in the vessel, make an incision at the level of the guidewire entering the skin to ease placement of the tissue dilator. Ensure that the incision completely enters the dermis and is about the width of the catheter. Firmly thread the dilator over the guidewire with a turning motion several centimeters into the vessel, as the dilator does need to be "hubbed." Again, maintain control of the guidewire at all times. Remove the dilator and expect bleeding around the guidewire. Thread the central venous catheter over the guidewire and grasp the guidewire once it emerges from the distal port of the catheter. Advance the catheter into the vessel and remove the guidewire once the catheter has been placed at the correct depth. Remember to cover the open port with the thumb to minimize the risk of air embolization. Next aspirate and flush all ports of the catheter and suture securely into place using non-absorbable silk. Finally clean the skin around the entry site of the catheter, place a Biopatch˚ and a simple transparent dressing. In the nonemergent setting for internal jugular and subclavian approaches, always confirm line placement with a chest X-ray and evaluate for immediate complications.

LANDMARK-GUIDED "BLIND" APPROACH

Internal Jugular Vein

Anterior Approach

Insert needle at an angle of 30° to 45° along the medial border of the sternocleidomastoid muscle 2 to 3 fingerbreadths above the clavicle aiming towards the ipsilateral nipple. Palpate the carotid artery during cannulation and direct the needle away from the carotid pulse.

Central Approach

Insert the needle at angle of 30° at the apex of the triangle formed by the sternocleidomastoid muscle. Direct the needle towards the ipsilateral nipple. Palpate the carotid pulse; the vein lies lateral to the artery.

Posterior Approach

Insert the needle at a 45° angle at the lateral border of the sternocleidomastoid muscle at the midpoint between the mastoid process and the clavicle. The operator should aim towards the suprasternal notch; note that the vein is accessed at a depth of approximately 7 cm.

Subclavian Vein

Infraclavicular Approach

The aim of this approach is to access the subclavian vein as it passes the first rib and travels under the clavicle. The operator places the index finger in the suprasternal notch and places the thumb at the costoclavicular junction. The skin is punctured approximately 2 cm below the junction of the medial two-thirds and the lateral third of the clavicle aiming towards the index finger. The operator "walks the needle" under the clavicle with vessel entry occurring at 3 to 4 cm. Note that entering the skin close to the clavicle makes it difficult to maneuver the needle tip below the clavicle. Prior to puncturing the skin, ensure that the bevel of the needed is pointed inferomedially as this will facilitate directing the guidewire towards the brachiocephalic vein rather than the opposite vessel wall or IJ vein. During cannulation, the risk of pneumothorax is highly dependent on the angle needle. Keeping the trajectory of the needle "parallel to the floor" decreases the risk of hitting the pleural dome and causing a pneumothorax.

Supraclavicular Approach

This less traditional approach to subclavian vein catheterization aims to access the subclavian vein as it meets the internal jugular vein superior to the clavicle. The clavisternomastoid angle is formed by the junction of the lateral head of the sterno-cleidomastoid muscle and the clavicle. The needle is inserted 1 cm posterior to the clavicle and 1 cm lateral to the lateral head of the sternocleidomastoid muscle and aimed towards the contralateral nipple at an angle. The needle tip is angled posteriorly 5° to 15° relative to the coronal plane, following this trajectory the vein is accessed between the clavicle and the anterior scalene muscle. Note the right-sided approach is often preferred given the absence of the thoracic duct and the direct route to the superior vena cava. Additionally the dome of the pleura is lower on the right.[8]

Femoral Vein

The aim of this approach is to access the femoral vessel below the inguinal ligament. The operator palpates the femoral artery pulse 2 fingerbreadths inferior the inguinal ligament and punctures the skin at 45° angle in a cephalad direction 1 cm medial to the femoral pulse. Alternatively, a line can be drawn between the anterior superior iliac spine and midpoint of the pubic symphysis. The femoral artery lies at the midpoint of this line with the corresponding vein 1 cm medial to it. Note that pressure on the femoral artery may distort the anatomy impeding cannulation. The depth of accessing the femoral vein is dependent on body habitus. In a normal sized adult, the vein can be reached at a depth of 2 to 3 cm.

REAL-TIME ULTRASOUND GUIDANCE

In recent years, there has been a significant increase in the use of real-time ultrasonography as a safety-enhancing adjunct during CVC placement. With US guidance, anatomical variations that cannot be readily visualized and pathologies such as vessel stenosis and thrombosis can be detected. The two approaches in US guidance for CVC placement are the short-axis (SA) approach and long-axis (LA) approach. In the SA approach, the operator's US probe is placed perpendicular to the target vessel with the indicator dot pointed to the left, in line with the position of the indicator dot on the US screen. The advantage of the SA approach is that the surrounding structure of the target vessel can be clearly visualized. The disadvantage of the SA approach is that the central line needle shaft can be mistaken for the needle tip on the US screen and as a result, the needle tip can advance beyond US visualization and cause posterior wall puncture. In contrast, in the LA approach, the operator places the US probe parallel and above to the target vessel with the indicator dot cranially. Thus, on the US screen, the left of the screen would represent the cephalic direction and the right would be caudal. The advantage of the LA approach is that the needle tip can be better visualized. However, the surrounding structure cannot be visualized since the US beam is only in line with the vessel. The SA approach is associated with shorter cannulation time while the LA approach is associated with decrease in incidence of posterior wall puncture.[9] With either approach, a standard CVC placement technique such as sterile preparation and Seldinger technique as previously described should be employed.

GENERAL CONSIDERATIONS

Prior to sterilization of the site, the operator should examine the target area with US to determine the size and patency of the target vessel. Alternative target vessel should be selected if pathologies such as thrombosis or stenosis are noted (Figure 93–2). The US machine should be positioned at the ipsilateral side and across from the operator so that direct visualization of the US screen is maintained throughout the procedure (Figure 93–3). The operator should also scan the patient's lung on the ipsilateral side of the procedure for lung sliding prior to procedure to establish the baseline condition (Figure 93–4). In the SA approach, the needle tip should be visualized at all time using the "creep" technique where the US probe is fanned ahead of the needle trajectory to maintain visualization.[10] In the LA approach, the operator must secure the US probe so that the

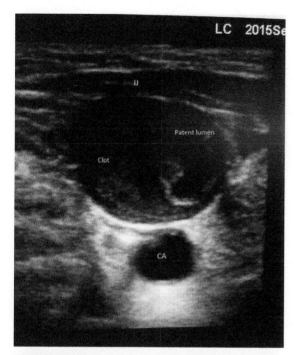

FIGURE 93-2 Clot within internal jugular vein. IJ = internal jugular vein; CA = carotid artery.

entire target vessel in a sagittal plane can be visualized. Visualization of the entire needle shaft and tip should be maintained during cannulation. The target vessel should be centered on the US screen in either approach and proper adjustments should be made to the depth and gain in order to optimize visualization under US.

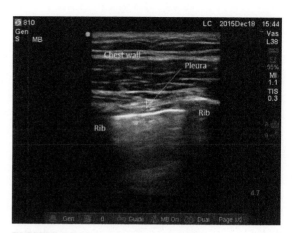

FIGURE 93-4 Ultrasound image of lung.

Internal Jugular Vein

The internal jugular vein is beneath the sternocleidomastoid muscle and is lateral to the trachea and medial to the carotid artery (Figure 93–5). However, anatomical variations exist and the relative position of the vessel may vary. With US guidance, the carotid artery and internal jugular vein can be easily differentiated using direct visualization or with the aid of color flow and Doppler.[11] The needle should be inserted directly beneath the needle guide on the US probe and would appear as a hyperechoic object on the US screen. The US probe should be advanced as the needle is advanced so that the needle tip does not advance beyond the US beam and cause inadvertent posterior wall puncture. Once the

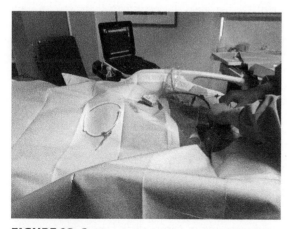

FIGURE 93-3 Ultrasound machine being ipsilateral to the site of procedure.

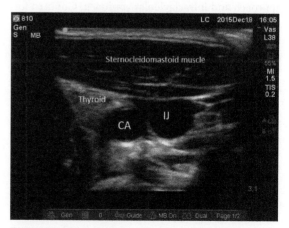

FIGURE 93-5 Ultrasound image of internal jugular vein. IJ = internal jugular vein, CA = carotid artery.

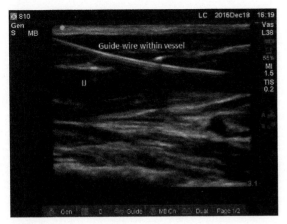

FIGURE 93-6 Ultrasound image of guidewire within the vessel after cannulation. IJ = internal jugular vein.

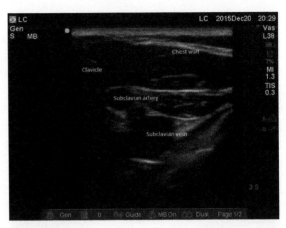

FIGURE 93-7 Subclavian vessels under ultrasound.

needle tip is visualized within the vessel, the operator can release the US probe and proceed with the cannulation. After the guidewire is inserted into the vessel, the operator can use US to visualize the guidewire within the vessel to confirm placement prior to dilation of the vessel (Figure 93–6). After the completion of the procedure, lung sliding on the ipsilateral side can be evaluated using US to look for pneumothorax.

Subclavian Vein

Subclavian vein cannulation using US guidance is difficult technically due to the position of the clavicle in relation to the target vessel.[12] There are two potential approaches to cannulation: supraclavicular approach and infraclavicular approach. Concern for mechanical complications has limited the use of the supraclavicular approach.[13] Although the US-guided infraclavicular approach is technically difficult, it has been shown to be safer than landmark approach in the hands of an experienced operator. Both the short axis (SA) and long axis (LA) approaches can be used. The US probe can be placed over the clavicle perpendicularly with indicator dot directed cranially, and the probe should be moved laterally. As the probe move towards the axilla, the subclavian vein and artery can be visualized to extend beyond the shadow created by the clavicle (Figure 93–7). Color flow and Doppler can be used to differentiate between the artery and vein. After identification of the target vessel, the vessel should be centered on US

screen and the SA or LA approach can be utilized to cannulate the vessel. Due to the proximity of the lungs to the subclavian vein, extra attention should be paid to keep track of the needle tip since losing track can inadvertently result in a pneumothorax.

Femoral Vein

With US guidance, direct visualization of the femoral vein can facilitate CVC placement. The US probe should be placed transverse to the target vessel right below the inguinal crest. The common femoral vein should be in the medial position with the common femoral artery laterally positioned (Figure 93–8). Ideally, the CVC placement should be in the common femoral vein since it is proximal to the branching points and is largest in diameter. Compression of the vessel prior to cannulation attempt should be conducted to evaluate for common femoral vein thrombosis and an alternative site should be selected if there is a positive finding.

IMMEDIATE COMPLICATIONS OF CENTRAL VENOUS CATHETERIZATION

Immediate complications are of mechanical nature and related to operator technique and experience. It is important to know, recognize, and manage the immediate complications as they can become rapidly life-threatening in nature. Risk factors for immediate complications include operator inexperience,

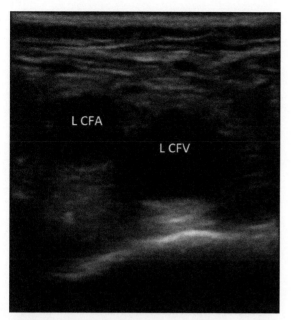

FIGURE 93-8 Ultrasound image of the common femoral vasculature. L CFA = left common femoral artery; L CFV = left common femoral vein.

number of needle passes, and larger catheter size. Mechanical complications include puncture of adjacent artery, hematoma, air embolism, arrhythmia, pneumothorax pericardial tamponade, catheter/wire embolus, arteriovenous fistula, vessel obstruction, vessel perforation, pseudoaneurysm formation, catheter malposition, and catheter knotting.[14-19] Subclavian vein catheterization has been associated with the highest risk of pneumothorax.

DELAYED COMPLICATIONS

Major delayed complications include infection and catheter related thrombosis.[16-19] Some of the rarer late complications include delayed pneumothorax, and vascular and ventricular erosion or perforation, leading to hemothorax or pericardial tamponade. The incidence of delayed pneumothorax occurs around 0.5% to 2%. Time of onset can occur as late as 6 hours after the procedure. The type of damage caused by vascular erosion or perforation depends on the anatomical location of the vascular catheter tip. Erosion leading to pericardial tamponade can occur up to 0.2% of patients and erosion without

pericardial tamponade occurs in 0.4% to 1% of patients.

Infectious complications from CVC placement is a significant cause of increased morbidity and mortality in hospitalized patients. The most common bacterial agents causing catheter-related infections are *Staphylococcus aureus* and *Staphylococcus epidermis,* both of which are natural skin flora. Infection can be caused by catheter contamination from skin flora, contamination from access port or hematogenous spread from other sites. The rate of infection is highest in the femoral site, followed by internal jugular, and finally the subclavian vein.[19] Multiple attempts at CVC are associated with an increased incidence of CLABSI; this can be reduced with US guidance. Thus, professional societies recommend US guided CVC as the preferred method because of the lower incidence of CLABSI.

CVC-related thrombosis after 1 week range from 33% to 67%. There are 2 types of thrombosis: the first type forms as a fibrin sheath around the catheter resulting in the occlusion of the cannulated vessel, whereas the second type forms at the tip of the catheter. Cannulated vessels are at higher risk for thrombosis due to the disrupted endothelium resulting activation of the coagulation cascade. Platelet aggregation subsequently forms at the site of damaged endothelium forming thrombus. Risk factors for thrombus formation include small diameter of the target vessel, site of the cannulation, and difficult cannulation. Less common risk factors include external compression of the target vessel due to mass or tumor. The treatment of choice for catheter-related thrombosis is removal of the catheter and infusion of heparin or injection of low-molecular weight heparin. Instillation of fibrinolytics (eg, tissue plasminogen activator) can also be considered if the thrombus is suspected to be within the catheter lumen.

REFERENCES

1. Sirleaf M, Jefferson B, Christmas AB, et al. Comparison of procedural complications between resident physicians and advanced clinical providers. *J Trauma Acute Care Surg.* 2014;77:143-147.
2. Chandrasekaran S, Chandrasekaran VP. Anatomical variations of the internal jugular vein in relation

to common carotid artery in lesser supraclavicular fossa—A colour Doppler study. *Int J Basic Med Sci.* 2010;1(4). http://www.ijbms.com/anatomy/supra-clavicular-fossa-%e2%80%93-a-colour-doppler-study/****

3. Pronovost P, Needham D, Berenholtz S, et al. An intervention to decrease catheter-related bloodstream infections in the ICU. *N Engl J Med.* 2006;355:2725-2732.

4. Bazaral M, Harlan S. Ultrasonographic anatomy of the internal jugular vein relevant to percutaneous cannulation. *Crit Care Med.* 1981;9:307-310.

5. Sulek CA, Gravenstein N, Blackshear RH, Weiss L. Head rotation during internal jugular vein cannulation and the risk of carotid artery puncture. *Anesth Analg.* 1996;82:125-128.

6. Chaiyakunapruk N, Veenstra DL, Lipsky BA, Saint S. Chlorhexidine compared with povidone-iodine solution for vascular catheter-site care: a meta-analysis. *Ann Intern Med.* 2002;136:792-801.

7. Taira T, Lin M. Tricks of the Trade: Central Venous Line Confirmation Tricks, ACEP News, January 2008. http://www.acep.org/Clinical—Practice-Management/Tricks-of-the-Trade—Central-Venous-Line-Confirmation-Tricks.

8. Patrick SP, Tijunelis MA, Johnson S, Herbert ME. Supraclavicular subclavian vein catheterization: the forgotten central line. *West J Emerg Med.* 2009;10:110-114.

9. Vogel JA. Is long-axis view superior to short-axis view in ultrasound-guided central venous catheterization? *Crit Care Med.* 2015;43:832-839.

10. Stone MB, Moon C, Sutijono D, Blaivas M. Needle tip visualization during ultrasound-guided vascular access: short-axis vs long-axis approach. *Am J Emerg Med.* 2010;28:343-347.

11. Karakitsos D, Labropoulos N, De Groot E, et al. Real-time ultrasound-guided catheterisation of the internal jugular vein: a prospective comparison with the landmark technique in critical care patients. *Crit Care.* 2006;10:R162.

12. Fragou M, Gravvanis A, Dimitriou V, et al. Real-time ultrasound-guided subclavian vein cannulation versus the landmark method in critical care patients: a prospective randomized study. *Crit Care Med.* 2011;39:1607-1612.

13. Bertini P, Frediani M. Ultrasound guided supraclavicular central vein cannulation in adults: a technical report. *J Vasc Access.* 2013;14:89-93.

14. Kornbau C, Lee KC, Hughes GD, Firstenberg MS. Central line complications. *Int J Crit Illness Inj Sci.* 2015;5:170-178.

15. Polderman KH, Girbes AJ. Central venous catheter use. Part 1: Mechanical complications. *Intensive Care Med.* 2002;28:1-17.

16. Deshpande KS, Hatem C, Ulrich HL, et al. The incidence of infectious complications of central venous catheters at the subclavian, internal jugular, and femoral sites in an intensive care unit population. *Crit Care Med.* 2005;33:13-20.

17. Kusminsky RE. Complications of central venous catheterization. *J Am Coll Surg.* 2007;204:681-696.

18. Sznajder JI, Zveibil FR, Bitterman H, Weiner P, Bursztein S. Central vein catheterization: failure and complication rates by three percutaneous approaches. *Arch Intern Med.* 1986;146:259-261.

19. Parienti JJ, Mongardon N, Mégarbane B, et al. 3SITES Study Group. Intravascular complications of central venous catheterization by insertion site. *N Engl J Med.* 2015;373:1220-1229.

Chest Tube Insertion

Lewis Eisen, MD

KEY POINTS

1 Chest tubes vary in size from 6 to 40 French. For patient comfort and to avoid complications, the smallest tube that will drain the pleural space should be chosen.

2 When available bedside ultrasound should be used for pleural diagnosis and to guide chest tube insertion.

3 For a hemothorax, continued drainage of more than 250 mL of blood per hour warrants a surgical consult.

4 The most common complications of chest tube insertion include malposition, blockage, infection, dislodgement, re-expansion pulmonary edema, subcutaneous emphysema, nerve injuries, intrathoracic organ injuries, and residual pneumothorax.

5 Chest tube systems should be examined daily for the amount of drainage, the presence of an air leak and the presence of respiratory variation of the fluid column.

INTRODUCTION

Tube thoracostomy is the procedure of insertion of a sterile tube or catheter into the pleural space. It is used to remove air and/or fluid to restore negative pressure to the pleural space. The various indications, diagnostic techniques, procedural approaches, and complications will be discussed in this chapter.

ANATOMY AND PHYSIOLOGY

The pleural cavity is a closed space that exists between the visceral and the parietal pleura. The visceral and parietal pleura contain a single layer of mesothelial cells with multiple layers of connective tissue.[1] The parietal pleura is innervated by the intercostal nerves while the visceral pleura is not innervated. In a healthy individual, the mesothelial cells on the visceral pleura create a thin film of fluid that allows the pleura to glide smoothy during respiration. See Table 94–1 below for the characteristics of normal pleural fluid versus transudate and exudate.

TYPES OF TUBES

Chest tube sizes are based on the external diameter, ranging from 6 to 40 French (Fr). Adult small bore chest tubes (SBCT) are tubes ≤ 14Fr. Chest tubes also come in a variety of shapes; the majority of chest tubes used in common practice are either straight, right angle, or pigtailed. Each tube has length markers to guide insertion and fenestrations for pleural drainage. Chest tubes can be "tunnelled" to decrease the rate of dislodgement and infection and to allow for long-term, outpatient management of pleural

TABLE 94-1 Characteristics of normal pleural fluid versus transudate and exudate.

	Normal Pleural Fluid	Transudate	Exudate
pH	7.60-7.64	> 7.20	< 7.20
Glucose	Similar to plasma	> 60 mg/L	< 60 mg/L
Protein	1-2 g/dL	Pleural fluid/serum	
		< 0.5	> 0.5
LDH	< 0.5	Pleural fluid/serum	
		< 0.6	> 0.6
Microbiology	< 1000 WBC/mm³, mostly macrophages, no organisms	No organisms present	Organisms possibly found
Appearance	Clear	Clear, free-flowing fluid	Turbid, septations, and loculations may be present

effusions. See Table 94–2 for a summary of choice of tubes based on indication.

INDICATIONS FOR TUBE THORACOSTOMY

When air or fluid enters the pleural space, drainage may be necessary based on the clinical condition of the patient.

Pneumothorax

Pneumothorax occurs when air enters into the pleural cavity. When a pneumothorax occurs unprovoked in a person without any underlying pathology, this is labeled primary spontaneous pneumothorax (PSP). Patients with a PSP can be managed in a number of ways based on their clinical picture and the size of the pneumothorax. To measure the size of a pneumothorax, computed tomography (CT)

TABLE 94-2 Summary of choice of tubes based on indication.

	Intervention	Comments
Primary spontaneous pneumothorax	Small—observation Large or symptomatic— manual aspiration or SBCT	Consult a thoracic surgeon for an air leak > 48 hours Patients on mechanical ventilation may require LBCT if there is a large air leak but SBCT is usually sufficient
Secondary spontaneous pneumothorax	SBCT	
Traumatic pneumothorax	SBCT or LBCT	
Iatrogenic pneumothorax	Manual aspiration or SBCT	
Malignant pleural effusion	SBCT or tunneled catheter	
Parapneumonic pleural effusion or empyema	SBCT or LBCT	Ultrasound guidance important
Hemothorax	LBCT	Evidence is increasing toward use or SBCT
Postoperative	LBCT	Evidence is increasing toward use or SBCT

of the chest gives the most accurate 3-dimensional volume. CT is not always necessary, however, plain upright chest radiographs or bedside ultrasound are generally adequate for clinical decisions. The two most utilized methods of determining the size of a pneumothorax are by the American College of Chest Physicians (ACCP) and the British Thoracic Society (BTS). ACCP guidelines recommend measuring the distance from the outer edge of the pleural space to the most apical portion of the collapsed lung.[3] Using this measurement, ≤ 3cm is considered small. BTS recommends measuring at the level of the hilum from the outer edge of the pleural space to the collapsed lung.[4] According to BTS guidelines, a measurement < 2 cm is considered small.

For clinically stable patents with small pneumothoraces, recommended care includes observation for 3 to 6 hours followed by a repeat chest radiograph. If the repeat radiograph does not show progression of the pneumothorax, the patient can be safely discharged home and should return for a follow-up chest radiograph in 24 hours.[3-6] Uncomplicated pneumothoraces will reabsorb at a rate of 2% of the volume of the hemithorax every 24 hours.[7] For patients with a large PSP or patients experiencing significant symptoms, needle aspiration or SBCT are the recommended treatments. In a study of 60 patients, needle aspiration and small bore catheters had similar failure rates but patients undergoing needle aspiration were hospitalized less.[8] In addition, studies have demonstrated that small catheters are well tolerated and as effective as large bore chest tubes (LBCT).[9] All individuals should have a follow-up within 2 to 4 weeks and avoid all air travel until full resolution of the pneumothorax is confirmed.

Secondary spontaneous pneumothorax (SSP), in contract to PSP, occurs in patients with underlying lung pathology. Patients with a SSP are likely to have worsened clinical symptoms than patients with a PSP. Patients with SSP should be admitted to the hospital and most will require intervention. SBCT have been found to be as effective as LBCT and are thus recommended.[10] It is largely recommended that these patients be admitted but in some circumstances, patients may be discharged home with a Heimlich valve and follow-up within 2 days.[3] If an air leak persists beyond 2 to 4 days, a thoracic surgeon should be consulted for consideration of further intervention.[3,4]

Provoked or traumatic pneumothoraces can occur from blunt or penetrating injuries or from barotrauma. In the case of trauma victims, the number of pneumothoraces being identified has increased with the availability and ease of CT scanning and bedside ultrasonography. Many of these are considered occult pneumothoraces (OP), defined as a pneumothorax identified on CT or ultrasound, which was not suspected on the preceding chest radiographs. Most experts agree that OP in clinically stable patients can be managed conservatively with observation.[11-14] For patients with OP undergoing positive pressure ventilation (PPV), however, there remains controversy regarding whether or not to intervene. The traditional teaching was to perform tube thoracostomy on patients with occult pneumothorax if they were to undergo any period of PPV, including both prolonged mechanical ventilation during an ICU stay or for a limited time under general anesthesia.[15] Recent literature, however, has shown that careful observation and directed intervention when needed of an OP may be safe and there is no difference in mortality or morbidity for these patients.[13-16] For patients chosen for tube thoracostomy, the historical teaching has also been to place a LBCT but recent literature has shown that in many situations, SBCT are considered safe and effective.[17]

The most feared complication of pneumothorax is that it will progress to tension physiology. Tension pneumothorax occurs when there is a disruption in the visceral or parietal pleural or tracheobronchial tree. A one-way valve forms, which allows air to flow into the pleural space with inhalation and prohibits air from flowing out. With each breath, the volume of air in the intrapleural space and pressure within the hemithorax increases. As the pressure increases, the ipsilateral lung collapses and causes hypoxemia. Eventually, the mediastinum will shift toward the contralateral side and impair the venous return to the heart, causing cardiovascular collapse. The treatment is immediate decompression. The historical treatment for a tension pneumothorax is immediate needle decompression in the second intercostal space at the midclavicular line and subsequent tube thoracostomy. However, many studies have shown that the suggested 14-gauge needle for needle decompression is not long enough to penetrate the chest wall in many patients at this location.[18] Alternative approaches for needle decompression are at the fifth intercostal space in the anterior axillary line where the chest wall is generally thinner.[19] Studies have also shown that needle decompression is associated with failure rates as high as 58%.[20] Despite this evidence, needle decompression is still recommended as first line treatment for tension pneumothorax followed by tube thoracostomy.

Hemothorax

Hemothorax is the accumulation of blood in the pleural space. Although the majority of hemothoraces occur as a result of trauma, some do occur in the ICU spontaneously. Also, they may arise as complications from procedures such as thoracentesis and central venous catheterization. These occur due to injuries to the intercostal or internal mammary arteries or pulmonary parenchyma. For traumatic hemothoraces, most surgeons recommend early (within 7 days) drainage of the hemothorax using large bore tubes (36F-42F). If the initial blood drainage is > 1500 mL or > 250 mL/h, surgery may be indicated. Complications such as fibrothorax and empyema can complicate hemothoraces that are not fully drained.

Pleural Effusion

Pleural effusions are abnormal, excessive fluid collections in the pleural space. The differential diagnosis of a pleural effusion is wide and occurs in many conditions, not exclusive to the thoracic cavity. For example, 20% of patients with pancreatitis have accompanying pleural effusion.[21] Pleural effusions are divided into two types: transudative and exudative. Transudative effusions develop when systemic factors affecting the formation and absorption of the pleural fluid are altered, causing the pleural fluid to accumulate.[22] Conditions where transudative effusions form are with increased interstitial fluid (heart failure), increased peritoneal fluid (cirrhosis), and decreased serum oncotic pressure (hypoproteinemia). Exudative effusions, conversely, develop due to the local alteration of the pleural surfaces or capillaries causing fluid to accumulate. The most common causes of exudative effusions are pleural malignancies, infection, and pulmonary embolism.

Traditionally, supine chest radiograph has been used in critically ill patients to identify acute processes such as pleural effusions. This modality, however, has a low sensitivity and specificity and can often miss large effusions. CT scanning is an excellent tool for identifying and characterizing lung, mediastinal, and pleural disease and quantifying the pleural fluid. Often, initial CT scanning has been replaced by bedside ultrasonography. This modality is noninvasive, low risk, and can be repeated as much as necessary. It can be used to evaluate the pleural space for fluid and often can characterize the complexity of the pleural space. In the hands of a trained user, it is highly sensitive and specific and can identify as little as 5 mL of pleural fluid.[23] Figure 94–1 shows ultrasound images of a simple versus complex pleural effusion. If a pleural effusion

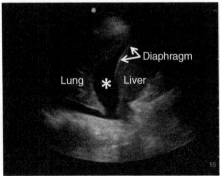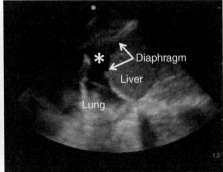

FIGURE 94–1 Ultrasound of the right chest showing a pleural effusion marked with *. The image on the left shows a simple effusion while the image on the right demonstrates a complex effusion.

is identified and if clinically indicated, a thoracentesis and/or tube thoracostomy should be done guided by bedside ultrasonography. For patients with pleural effusion and continued respiratory compromise, drainage of pleural effusions has shown to lead to quick symptomatic improvement in many patients.[24]

Pleural Infections

Parapneumonic effusions are any pleural effusion secondary to pneumonia or lung abscess.[2] Parapneumonic effusions represent a range of disease beginning with a dynamic, often self-resolving exudative effusion to a complex multiloculated fibrotic and often purulent collection to a thick pleural peal. Patients with pneumonia with an associated parapneumonic effusion have a higher morbidity and mortality than patients who have pneumonia without an effusion.[25] Although most simple parapneumonic effusions resolve with antibiotics, about 10% proceed to empyema and fail medical therapy.[2] When the effusion worsens, bacteria will cross the damaged endothelium and propagate pleural inflammation. Neutrophils then migrate into the pleural space and the coagulation cascade will be altered, decreasing fibrinolytic activity, causing septations to form within the fluid. Following this, fibroblasts will proliferate and a solid fibrous pleural peel will form over the lung and re-expansion is prevented, creating a persistent pleural space for continued infection.[26]

For patients with parapneumonic effusions, the current recommendations are to perform a diagnostic thoracentesis to evaluate for empyema.[27] If the diagnostic testing reveals a fluid with a pH < 7.2, LDH > 1000, or a glucose < 60 mg/dL, drainage with tube thoracostomy may be indicated. For drainage of an empyema, LBCT are typically used because smaller pigtail catheters have a higher propensity for becoming clogged or dislodged.[28] For patients with continued symptoms, fibrinolytic enzymes may be attempted followed by consultation with a thoracic surgeon for resection and open drainage or decortication as indicated.

Chylothorax

Chylothorax is a collection of lymphatic fluid in the pleural space. This occurs due to malignancy, congenital abnormalities or injury to the thoracic duct or one of its main branches due to trauma or iatrogenically during a surgical procedure. Diagnosis is made by fluid analysis showing triglyceride level greater than 110 mg/dL or a cholesterol-to-triglyceride ratio of less than 1.[29] Treatment, again, depends on the clinical situation. Most patients require initial drainage due to the large volume (2-4 L/d) of chyle produced. Other strategies range from dietary restrictions to surgery.

CONTRAINDICATIONS

When performing tube thoracostomy, landmark anatomy and bedside ultrasound is generally sufficient for placement. In some instances, however, CT mapping may be indicated. For example, patients with bullous lung disease may be misdiagnosed as a pneumothorax and tube thoracostomy in these patients may cause prolonged air leak from a bronchopleural fisula. For patients who have undergone procedures such as pleurodesis, pleurectomy, and previous thoracotomy, consider CT scanning prior to non-emergent tube thoracostomy to help with directing the tube.[4] Also, patients who have had significant blunt abdominal trauma may be at risk for diaphragmatic injury and again, if the procedure is not emergent, further workup may be indicated.

ULTRASOUND EVALUATION

Ultrasound is a valuable tool when evaluating the thoracic cavity for pathology as well as real-time direction during the procedure. A recent meta-analysis concluded that chest radiography is 39.8% sensitive and 99.3% specific in diagnosing pneumothorax whereas ultrasound is 78.6% sensitive and 98.4% specific.[30] For pleural effusions, ultrasound can help identify the size and characterization of the effusion and localize an area acceptable for tube thoracostomy. Whenever available, bedside ultrasound should be used to identify and map the thoracic anatomy and pathology.

SETUP

Prior to attempting any procedure, it is advisable to review the patient's previous imaging and laboratory results. Appropriate consent should be

TABLE 94-3 Equipment.

Sterile gloves
Sterile gown
Sterile drapes
Skin prep—chlorhexidine or iodine
Gauze
18-, 20-, and 25-gauge needles
Local anesthetic
Scalpel
Suture
Curved clamp
Guidewire with dilators (optional)
Trocar (optional)
Chest tube
Suture
Closed drainage system
Dressing
Silk tape

obtained, when possible. Benefits and risks should be discussed and possible complications should be explained. The patient should be properly pretreated for pain and anxiety associated with the procedure. All of the appropriate equipment should be gathered and a time out should be performed before beginning. See Table 94–3 for a list of common items required at the bedside.

TECHNIQUE

For the mid-axillary approach, place the patient supine, in a position of comfort and place the ipsilateral arm above the head. The BTS guidelines recommend placement of the tube in the "safe triangle" consisting of the anterior border of the latissimus dorsi, the lateral border of the pectoralis major muscle, a line superior to the horizontal level of the nipple, and an apex below the axilla.[31] Identify and mark the fourth and fifth intercostal spaces. For the mid-clavicular approach, place the patient supine, in a position of comfort. Identify and mark the second intercostal space at the midclavicular line.

Using sterile technique, prepare the area with either iodine or chlorhexadine. Infiltrate a 2 to 3 cm wheal one rib space below your mark with 1% lidocaine. Entering below and angling up will create a subcutaneous tunnel that will discourage air

entry into the chest after removal of the tube. Angle the needle cephalad and infiltrate deeper tissues with the lidocaine, aspirating with each advance of the needle to avoid intravascular administration. Once the tip of the needle is over the chosen intercostal space being entered, angle the needle more perpendicular to the chest wall. Continue advancing the needle and anesthetizing until aspiration generates fluid or air, at which point the needle has entered the pleural space. Infuse the remaining lidocaine into the pleural space being careful not to exceed the subcutaneous toxic dose of lidocaine (3-5 mg/kg).

When entering into the thoracic cavity, you must pass first through skin and subcutaneous tissue then through three layers of muscle before entering the parietal pleura. Care must be taken to avoid the intercostal neurovascular bundle that runs inferior to each rib. Traditional teaching has been to place the tube just superior to the rib, however, recent studies show that the anatomy of the intercostal spaces is variable and the tube should be placed in the lower half to two-thirds of the intercostal space.[32]

Blunt Dissection Technique

After the patient has been adequately anesthetized as above, make a 2 to 3 cm incision superior and parallel to the rib. Create a short tunnel using blunt dissection with Kelly clamps, following the previously anesthetized path. Once the parietal pleura is encountered, carefully push the closed clamps through the pleura; this may require some force. Once in the pleural space, do not advance more than 1 cm past the parietal pleura to avoid potential damage to the lung. Widen the pleural defect to accommodate the tube by spreading the clamps to create a defect approximately 1 to 2 cm long. This may cause a gush or air or fluid from the pleural space. Remove the clamps and insert a finger into the pleural space and explore the anatomy, feeling for the lung surface and adhesions. Loose adhesions may be broken, but avoid breaking strong adhesions since this may generate bleeding. Grasp the end of the chest tube with the clamp and gently guide the tube into the pleural space with a finger. Once the tube is in the pleural space, remove the clamp and advance the chest tube. For pneumothorax, advance the tube anteriorly and apically. For pleural effusions, aim the tube basally. Advance the tube until all side ports are within the pleural space. Attach the tube to the closed drainage system and secure into place.

Trocar Technique

This technique involves the use of a sharp tipped rod (trocar) that is inserted into the chest tube prior to placement. A skin incision is made similar to the blunt technique and the trocar/chest tube combination is pushed into the pleural space. Care must be taken not to advance the trocar more than 1 to 2 cm into the pleural space to avoid damage to the intrathoracic organs. The chest tube is then slid off the trocar and left in the pleural space. Since this technique has been associated with increased complication rate, it is generally not recommended for routine situations.

Seldinger Technique

An alternative, often less painful technique, is the Seldinger technique involving a guidewire and serial dilation. Techniques may vary slightly based on kit used. After anesthetizing the subcutaneous tissues as above, make an incision in the skin one rib space below the desired intercostal entry space. Make the incision large enough to accommodate the size of the chosen drain. Following the path of anesthetic, advance the introducer needle and syringe into the pleural space while continuously aspirating until air or fluid is aspirated without resistance. Do not advance the needle more than 1cm past the parietal pleura. Remove the syringe while anchoring the needle in the pleural space. Pass the guidewire through the needle hub and into the pleural space. The guidewire should pass freely without resistance. While holding the guidewire, remove the needle. Dilate the tract with the dilator(s) included in the kit. Only dilate to 1 cm past the parietal pleura. Advance the chest tube into the pleural space over the guidewire, ensuring that all side ports are within the pleural space. Some kits may include an introducer or trocar; pass these cautiously into the pleural space to avoid parenchymal damage. Remove the guidewire and introducer or trocar if included. Attach the tubing to the closed drainage device and secure the tube in place.

Securing the Tube

There are various methods of securing the tube at the site of insertion; none have been compared for failure or complication rate. Mattress sutures with securing ties are often utilized when securing LBCT. Purse string sutures are not recommended because they have been found to be painful and can cause additional scarring.[31] Suture-free holding devices also exist. The tube should be secured to the drainage tubing with silk tape. The insertion site should be covered with sterile or petroleum gauze and taped securely to the patient. Avoid excessive taping or bandage because this may have a restrictive quality on the thoracic wall. Additionally, this may impede the speed that a malfunctioning tube can be evaluated.

Postplacement Management

After placing the tube, a chest radiograph or a lung/pleural ultrasound should be performed. Most chest tubes are designed with a radiopaque strip on the side of the tube to assist in visualization on chest radiographs. The sentinel eye is the most proximal side port; it will appear as a defect in the radiopaque strip. The sentinel eye should be located within the chest cavity.

The chest tube is connected to a closed drainage systems that acts as a one way valve to free air from the pleural space, collect any pleural fluid, and create negative pressure in the pleural space. Most drainage systems use three chambers based on previous three bottle systems. The first chamber is the collection chamber for any fluid drained from the plural space. For hemothorax, initial blood drainage of > 1500 mL or drainage of > 250 mL/h at any time requires emergent thoracic surgery consult and/or open thoracotomy. The second chamber is the water seal that acts as a one way valve. Air in the pleural space will appear as bubbles in the fluid; this is known as an air leak. When performing tube thoracostomy for pneumothorax, an air leak should be expected until the lung fully expands. If an air leak is persistent, surgical consultation may be required. The last chamber regulates the negative pressure being applied to the pleural space.

Frequent monitoring of the tube as well as the drainage system is required. The chamber should always be placed upright and should always be placed below the level of the patient. Monitor the fluid in the tubing for fluctuations during respiration or coughing, this indicates tube patency and placement in the pleural space. Cessation of this "tidaling" may indicate blockage or dislodgement of the tube.

Patients who develop excessive coughing, shortness of breath or chest pain as the pleural space is being drained may have re-expansion pulmonary edema. Temporarily stopping further drainage will be the best management.

Prophylactic antibiotics are recommended for trauma-related thoracic injuries requiring tube thoracostomy.[33] For patients with spontaneous pneumothorax or pleural effusions not related to an infection, antibiotics are not recommended.

Removal of Chest Tubes

Removal of a chest tube is usually a multifactorial decision based on the patient's clinical condition and on the performance of the chest tube. Multiple studies have shown that chest tubes placed after surgery, for hemothorax and for pleural effusions can be safely removed when the drainage is less than 200 mL/d.[34] For pneumothorax, once there is no longer an air leak and the lung is fully expanded, the chest tube can safely be removed.[35] A step-wise practice can also be utilized by first taking the tube off of suction and placing the tube to water seal. If the patient is clinically stable, the tube can then be clamped. If the patient tolerates this and there is no change in chest radiograph, the chest tube can be safely removed. Clamping a chest tube once the air leak has resolved can often detect a small air leak not readily apparent at the bedside. Clamping of a chest tube with an active air leak is never recommended because of the potential for tension physiology to form.

When the clinician decides to remove a chest drain, the patient should be placed supine and in a position of comfort. The bandages should be removed and the sutures should be cut. The tube should be pulled out in one fluid movement. Traditionally, the teaching has been to pull the tube at end expiration or while the patient performs the valsalva maneuver to avoid recurrent pneumothorax. However, in a trial of removal of the tube during inspiration versus at end expiration while performing a valsalva maneuver, there were similar rates of recurrent pneumothorax.[36]

COMPLICATIONS

Tube thoracostomy is a highly effective, and often life-saving technique but it is also associated with a complication rate as high as 30%u.[37] The most common complications include malposition, blockage, infection, dislodgement, re-expansion pulmonary edema, subcutaneous emphysema, nerve injuries, intrathoracic organ injuries, and residual pneumothorax. Less commonly, reports of esophageal perforation, cardiac injury, large vessel injury, chylothorax, fistula formation, and Horner syndrome have all been reported. Many of these complications can be avoided by adequate anxiolytics and analgesia, appropriate training and supervision, adequate technique and use of ultrasound guidance, and proper sterile technique. The most common complication is tube malposition where the tube is placed into somewhere other than the pleural space, including the lung parenchyma, lung fissures, into the chest wall, into the mediastinum, and into the abdomen.[37] The most common site of malposition is in the fissure and the greatest risk factor for this complication is lateral placement.

If fluid within the tube fails to fluctuate with coughing or respiration, the tube should be

TABLE 94–4 Troubleshooting common problems.

Problem	Cause (solution)
No further drainage	Lung fully expanded Tube blocked Tube kinked
No tidaling	Lung fully expanded Chest tube not in pleural space Chest tube blocked
Prolonged air leak	Bronchopleural fistula (consult thoracic surgery to consider surgical or endoscopic therapies)
Increased air leak	Chest tube holes may be outside pleural cavity (remove chest tube and place new tube if indicated) Disconnection

examined for a blockage or kinking tube. It is a common practice to milk or strip the tubes to clear the clot or debris. Although this practice is often effective in clearing the debris, this practice is controversial because it theoretically could cause damage to the lung tissue due to negative pressure.[37] Flushing with sterile saline every 6 to 8 hours can be considered as a method to prevent blockages.

REFERENCES

1. Wang NS. Anatomy of the pleura. *Clin Chest Med.* 1998;19:229-240.
2. Light RW. Parapneumonic effusions and empyema. *Proc Am Thorac Soc.* 2006;3:75-80.
3. Baumann MH, Strange C, Heffner JE, et al. Management of spontaneous pneumothorax: An American College of Chest Physicians Delphi consensus statement. *Chest.* 2001;119:590-602.
4. MacDuff A, Arnold A, Harvey J. Management of spontaneous pneumothorax: British Thoracic Society Pleural Disease Guideline 2010. *Thorax.* 2010;65:ii18-ii31.
5. Stradling P, Poole G. Conservative management of spontaneous pneumothorax. [Thorax. 1966] - PubMed–NCBI. *Thorax.* 1966;145. https://portal.montefiore.org/cvpn/aHR0cDovL3N0YXRpcYy5wd WJtZWQuoZ292LmVsaWJyYXJ5LmVpbnN0ZWlu Lnl1LmVkdQ/pubmed.
6. Clague HW, El-Ansary EH. Conservative management of spontaneous pneumothorax. *Lancet.* 1984;1:687-689.
7. Kelly A-M, Loy J, Tsang AYL, Graham CA. Estimating the rate of re-expansion of spontaneous pneumothorax by a formula derived from computed tomography volumetry studies. *Emerg Med J.* 2006;23:780-782.
8. Wakai A, O'Sullivan RG, McCabe G. Simple aspiration versus intercostal tube drainage for primary spontaneous pneumothorax in adults. *Cochrane Database Syst Rev.* 2007;(1):CD004479.
9. Vedam H, Barnes DJ. Comparison of large- and small-bore intercostal catheters in the management of spontaneous pneumothorax. *Intern Med J.* 2003;33:495-499.
10. Tsai W-K, Chen W, Lee J-C, et al. Pigtail catheters vs large-bore chest tubes for management of secondary spontaneous pneumothoraces in adults. *Am J Emerg Med.* 2006;795-800. https://portal.montefiore.org/cvpn/aHR0cDovL3d3dy5zY2llbmNlZGlyZWN0
LmNvbS5lbGGlicmFyeS5laW5zdGVpbi55dS5lZHU/science/article/pii/S0735675706001422.
11. Wilson H, Ellsmere J, Tallon J, Kirkpatrick A. Occult pneumothorax in the blunt trauma patient: tube thoracostomy or observation? *Injury.* 2009;40:928-931.
12. Moore FO, Goslar PW, Coimbra R, et al. Blunt traumatic occult pneumothorax: Is observation safe?—Results of a prospective, AAST multicenter study. *J Trauma.* 2011;70:1019-1023.
13. Barrios C, Tran T, Malinoski D, et al. Successful management of occult pneumothorax without tube thoracostomy despite positive pressure ventilation. *Am Surg.* 2008;74:958-961.
14. Ball CG, Kirkpatrick AW, Laupland KB, et al. Incidence, risk factors, and outcomes for occult pneumothoraces in victims of major trauma. *J Trauma.* 2005;59:917-924.
15. Enderson BL, Abdalla R, Frame SB, Casey MT, Gould H, Maull KI. Tube thoracostomy for occult pneumothorax: a prospective randomized study of its use. *J Trauma.* 1993;35:726-729.
16. Ouellet JF, Trottier V, Kmet L, et al. The OPTICC trial: a multi-institutional study of occult pneumothoraces in critical care. *Am J Surg.* 2009;197:581-586.
17. Rivera L, O'Reilly EB, Sise MJ, et al. Small catheter tube thoracostomy: effective in managing chest trauma in stable patients. *J Trauma.* 2009;66:393-399.
18. Zengerink I, Brink PR, Laupland KB, Raber EL, Zygun D, Kortbeek JB. Needle thoracostomy in the treatment of a tension pneumothorax in trauma patients: What size needle? *J Trauma.* 2008;64:111-114.
19. Inaba K, Ives C, McClure K, et al. Radiologic evaluation of alternative sites for needle decompression of tension pneumothorax. *Arch Surg.* 2012;147:813-818.
20. Martin M, Satterly S, Inaba K, Blair K. Does needle thoracostomy provide adequate and effective decompression of tension pneumothorax? *J Trauma Acute Care Surg.* 2012;73:1412-1417.
21. Maringhini A, Ciambra M, Patti R, et al. Ascites, pleural, and pericardial effusions in acute pancreatitis. A prospective study of incidence, natural history, and prognostic role. *Dig Dis Sci.* 1996;41:848-852.
22. Light RW. The light criteria: the beginning and why they are useful 40 years later. *Clin Chest Med.* 2013;34:21-26.

23. Gryminski J, Krakówka P, Lypacewicz G. The diagnosis of pleural effusion by ultrasonic and radiologic techniques. *Chest*. 1976;70:33-37.

24. Maslove DM, Chen BT-M, Wang H, Kuschner WG. The diagnosis and management of pleural effusions in the ICU. *J Intensive Care Med*. 28(1):24–36.

25. Hasley PB, Albaum MN, Li YH, et al. Do pulmonary radiographic findings at presentation predict mortality in patients with community-acquired pneumonia? *Arch Intern Med*. 1996;156:2206-2212.

26. Kroegel C, Antony VB. Immunobiology of pleural inflammation: potential implications for pathogenesis, diagnosis and therapy. *Eur Respir J*. 1997;10:2411-2418.

27. Davies C, Gleeson F, Davies R. BTS guidelines for the management of pleural infection. *Thorax*. 2003;58:ii18-ii28.

28. Liang S-J, Tu C-Y, Chen H-J, et al. Application of ultrasound-guided pigtail catheter for drainage of pleural effusions in the ICU. *Intensive Care Med*. 2009;35:350-354.

29. Staats BA, Ellefson RD, Budahn LL, Dines DE, Prakash UB, Offord K. The lipoprotein profile of chylous and nonchylous pleural effusions. *Mayo Clin Proc*. 1980;55:700-704.

30. Alrajab S, Youssef AM, Akkus NI, Caldito G. Pleural ultrasonography versus chest radiography for the diagnosis of pneumothorax: review of the literature and meta-analysis. *Crit Care*. 2013;17:R208.

31. Laws D, Neville E, Duffy J. BTS guidelines for the insertion of a chest drain. *Thorax*. 2003;58:ii53-ii59.

32. Wraight WM, Tweedie DJ, Parkin IG. Neurovascular anatomy and variation in the fourth, fifth, and sixth intercostal spaces in the mid-axillary line: a cadaveric study in respect of chest drain insertion. *Clin Anat*. 2005;18:346-349.

33. Bosman A, de Jong MB, Debeij J, van den Broek PJ, Schipper IB. Systematic review and meta-analysis of antibiotic prophylaxis to prevent infections from chest drains in blunt and penetrating thoracic injuries. *Br J Surg*. 2012;99:506-513.

34. Younes RN, Gross JL, Aguiar S, Haddad FJ, Deheinzelin D. When to remove a chest tube? A randomized study with subsequent prospective consecutive validation. *J Am Coll Surg*. 2002;195:658-662.

35. Davis JW, Mackersie RC, Hoyt DB, Garcia J. Randomized study of algorithms for discontinuing tube thoracostomy drainage. *J Am Coll Surg*. 1994;179:553-557.

36. Bell RL, Ovadia P, Abdullah F, Spector S, Rabinovici R. Chest tube removal: End-inspiration or end-expiration? *J Trauma*. 2001;50:674-677.

37. Kesieme EB, Dongo A, Ezemba N, Irekpita E, Jebbin N, Kesieme C. Tube thoracostomy: complications and its management. *Pulm Med*. 2012;2012:256-878.

Critical Care Echocardiography

95

Yonatan Y. Greenstein, MD and Paul H. Mayo, MD, FCCP

KEY POINTS

1 The frontline intensivist uses echocardiography on a routine basis to aid in the diagnosis and management of patients with hemodynamic failure.

2 Critical care echocardiography (CCE) is divided into basic and advanced levels of competency, with this chapter focusing on the fundamentals of basic CCE.

3 The basic CCE examination comprises five standard transthoracic echocardiography (TTE) views: PSL, PSS, AP4, SCL, and IVC longitudinal axis.

4 The intensivist performing basic CCE is capable of acquiring and interpreting the necessary images, has a strong foundation in the cognitive aspects of CCE, and understands the pitfalls inherent to the various echocardiographic views.

5 Transesophageal echocardiography may be used within the scope of the basic CCE. It is typically used when TTE image quality is suboptimal.

INTRODUCTION

Echocardiography has major applications in the intensive care unit (ICU) for rapid assessment of the patient with hemodynamic failure. Critical care echocardiography (CCE) is an essential skill for the frontline intensivist. This chapter will review key aspects of CCE with emphasis on the basic CCE examination.

LEVELS OF COMPETENCE

The American College of Chest Physicians/Société de Réanimation de Langue Française (ACCP/SRLF) statement on competence in critical care ultrasonography divides CCE competency into basic and advanced levels.[1] Basic CCE requires competence in a limited number of transthoracic echocardiography (TTE) views with an option to use limited transesophageal echocardiography (TEE). Basic CCE is a fundamental skill for all intensivists, and requires a relatively short training period. Competence in advanced CCE requires the intensivist to have a skill level comparable to a cardiology trained echocardiographer in both TTE and TEE, and requires a long training period by comparison to basic TTE.[2-3] Only a small proportion of intensivists need this level of skill, so this chapter will focus on basic CCE. The Accreditation Council of Graduate Medical Education has recently established that knowledge of critical care ultrasonography is a mandatory component of critical care fellowship training in the United States.[4] Within a few years, all graduating fellows will be competent in this essential skill; attending level intensivists will need to develop competence in basic CCE as well.

TABLE 95-1 Required cognitive skills in image interpretation for basic CCE.

Global LV/RV size and systolic function
LV contraction pattern
Echocardiographic patterns
Assessment for pericardial fluid/tamponade
IVC size and respiratory variation
Basic color Doppler assessment for severe valvular regurgitation

TABLE 95-2 Key clinical syndromes.

Recognition of Clinical Syndromes	Key CCE Findings
Hypovolemic shock	End-systolic effacement of the LV; small IVC with significant respiratory variation
Cardiogenic shock	Global LV systolic dysfunction
Obstructive shock from massive pulmonary embolism	RV dilation
Tamponade	Pericardial effusion plus RA/RV diastolic collapse; dilated IVC
Acute massive left-sided valvular regurgitation	Large color Doppler regurgitant jet
Circulatory arrest during resuscitation	Asystole

CCE = critical care echocardiography; LV = left ventricle; RV = right ventricle; RA = right atrium; IVC = inferior vena cava.

TRAINING

Competence in basic CCE requires training. Non-cardiologists can become competent in basic CCE.[5] Exact requirements for training methods have not been standardized, but a recent statement suggests that basic CCE training include at least 10 hours of course work (comprised of lectures, didactic cases, and image interpretation) and a minimum of 30 fully supervised TTE studies (image acquisition and interpretation).[2] While these numbers offer some guidance, they do not guarantee that the trainee is sufficiently trained. Competency based testing at the end of the training period provides assurance that the clinician has achieved the requisite skill. Competence in basic CCE includes the ability to acquire and interpret the necessary images, but also mastery of the cognitive elements of the field (Table 95–1). Key clinical syndromes and their associated CCE findings are summarized in Table 95–2.

THE BASIC CCE EXAMINATION

The ACCP/SRLF Statement on Competence defines the basic CCE examination as including five standard views: parasternal long-axis (PSL) view, parasternal short-axis (PSS) midventricular view, apical four-chamber (AP4) view, subcostal long-axis (SCL) view, and inferior vena cava (IVC) longitudinal axis view. There are several methods described for the performance of a goal directed cardiac examination that have a variety of acronyms. They all have in common a limited number of views designed to rapidly assess cardiac anatomy and function in the patient with hemodynamic failure.

Acquiring adequate CCE views is often challenging due to the nature of ICU patients. Imaging conditions may not be optimal due to the presence of equipment at the bedside and poor lighting conditions. Electrodes and wires may need to be repositioned to allow for optimal placement of the probe. Ribs and aerated lungs do not allow the transmission of ultrasound, and thus can obscure TTE windows. Left-arm abduction may increase the size of the intercostal space, and placing the patient in the left lateral decubitus position may move the heart laterally from behind the sternum making image acquisition easier; however, this may be difficult in the critically ill patient. Image quality may be suboptimal in the obese, edematous, or muscular patient. Frequently, some views may not be obtainable, so every examination must include an attempt at all views. For this reason, the examiner should establish a set scanning routine that includes the same sequence in every patient, as well as a methodical approach to interpreting each image.

With modern-generation portable ultrasonography machines, most medical ICU patients will yield serviceable images. In some situations, image acquisition may not be successful, for example, in the patient who is morbidly obese or following cardiac surgery. In this case, TEE may be required.

TRANSTHORACIC ECHOCARDIOGRAPHY PROBE SELECTION

A convex probe with a small footprint capable of imaging at frequencies between 2.5 and 5 MHz should be used. Harmonic imaging is a preferred feature, which enhances image resolution. The image orientation marker is set in the upper right of the screen.

THE STANDARD VIEWS (TABLE 95–3)

Parasternal Long-Axis View

The transducer is placed in the left 3rd or 4th intercostal space adjacent to the sternum with the orientation marker pointing towards the patient's right shoulder (Figure 95–1). The probe position is adjusted in order to line up the aortic valve (AV), mitral valve (MV), and the largest left ventricular (LV) areas (Figure 95–2).

This view allows for assessment for pericardial effusion, LV/RV size and function, septal kinetics, and valve anatomy. Pitfalls inherent to this view include underestimation of RV size, inaccurate assessment of LV size and function with off-axis

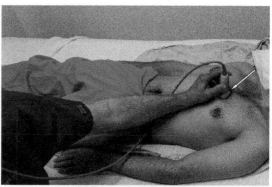

Parasternal Long Axis View
⟹ Probe Orientation Marker

FIGURE 95–1 Parasternal long-axis view—probe positioning.

views (false end-systolic effacement), and underestimation of regurgitant jets with color Doppler.

Parasternal Short-Axis at the Mid-Ventricular Level

From the parasternal long-axis view, the transducer is rotated 90° clockwise without angulation or tilting (Figure 95–3), resulting in a cross-sectional view of the heart at the midventricular/papillary muscle level with the orientation

TABLE 95–3 Utility and pitfalls of basic critical care echocardiography (CCE) views.

Mandatory Views	Utility	Pitfalls
Parasternal long axis	Assessment for pericardial effusion; LV/RV size and function; septal kinetics	Underestimation of RV size; inaccurate assessment of LV size and function with off-axis views; underestimation of regurgitant jets with color Doppler
Parasternal short axis at the mid-ventricular level	Assessment for pericardial effusion; LV/RV size and function; septal kinetics	Inaccurate assessment of LV if off-axis view obtained; difficulty to visualize RV free wall
Apical four chamber	Assessment of LV/RV size and function, particularly identifying RV enlargement by the RV/LV ratio. Assessment of pericardial effusion	Difficult to obtain an on-axis image, which can result in inaccurate assessment of LV/RV size and function and an incorrect ratio
Subcostal four-chamber	Preferred view in a cardiac arrest and often the best view on a mechanically ventilated patient. Assessment of LV/RV size and function, RV/LV ratio	Inaccurate assessment of cardiac structures when view is off-axis
Inferior vena cava longitudinal view	Determination of preload sensitivity in a hypotensive patient	Misidentification of the aorta for the IVC; off-axis view; translational artifact

CCE = critical care echocardiography; LV = left ventricle; RV = right ventricle; RA = right atrium; IVC = inferior vena cava;

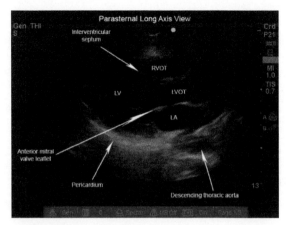

FIGURE 95-2 Parasternal long-axis view.
LV = left ventricle; LA = left atrium; LVOT = left ventricular
outflow tract; RVOT = right ventricular outflow tract;

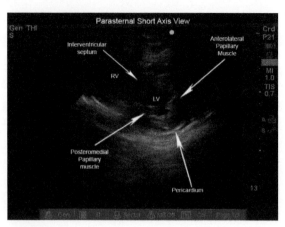

FIGURE 95-4 Parasternal short-axis view.
LV = left ventricle; RV = right ventricle;

marker pointing towards the patient's left shoulder
(Figure 95–4).

This view allows for assessment for pericardial
effusion, LV/RV size and function, and septal kinetics. Pitfalls inherent to this view include inaccurate
assessment of the LV if off-axis views are obtained
(ie, imaging the apex of the LV can create false end-
systolic effacement and overrotation of the transducer may result in septal flattening).

Apical Four-Chamber View

The transducer is placed on the lower lateral chest with
the orientation marker pointed towards the patient's
left shoulder and the tomographic plane adjusted to

bisect the anatomic apex of the LV and the two atria
(Figures 95–5 and 95–6). This view is best achieved
with the patient in the left lateral decubitus position.

This view allows for assessment of LV/RV size
and function, particularly identifying RV enlargement by the RV/LV ratio, and for assessment for
pericardial effusion. Pitfalls inherent to this view
include difficulty obtaining an on-axis image, which
can result in inaccurate assessment of LV/RV size
and function and an incorrect RV/LV ratio.

Subcostal Long-Axis View

The transducer is placed just below the xiphoid process with the orientation marker pointing towards

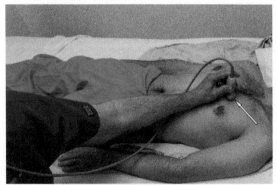

Parasternal Short Axis View
⇒ Probe Orientation Marker

FIGURE 95-3 Parasternal short-axis view—probe
positioning.

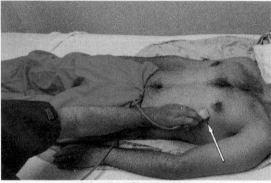

Apical Four Chamber View
⇒ Probe Orientation Marker

FIGURE 95-5 Apical four-chamber view—probe
positioning.

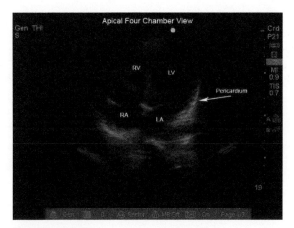

FIGURE 95–6 Apical four-chamber view.
LV = left ventricle; LA = left atrium; RV = right ventricle;
RA = right atrium;

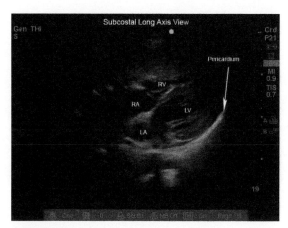

FIGURE 95–8 Subcostal long-axis view.
LV = left ventricle; LA = left atrium; RV = right ventricle;
RA = right atrium;

the 3 to 4 o'clock position and the tomographic plane adjusted to bisect the LV and left atrium (LA). The transducer must be held at the top of its surface in order to allow it to lay as flat as possible on the patient's abdomen (Figures 95–7 and 95–8).

This is often the best view on a mechanically ventilated patient as the liver serves as an acoustic window to the heart and the ultrasound is not blocked by an aerated lung. This view allows for assessment for pericardial effusion, LV/RV size and function, and the RV/LV ratio. This view is the best for a rapid assessment of cardiac function during pulse checks when performing cardiopulmonary resuscitation. Pitfalls include inaccurate assessment of cardiac structures when the view is off-axis.

Inferior Vena Cava Longitudinal View

From the SCL view, the transducer is rotated counterclockwise 90°, tilted inferiorly, and angled laterally to visualize the IVC in the longitudinal axis (Figures 95–9 and 95–10).

This view allows for assessment of preload sensitivity in a hypotensive patient and when assessing a patient for the presence of pericardial tamponade. Pitfalls inherent to this view include the misidentification of the aorta for the IVC, off-axis view of the

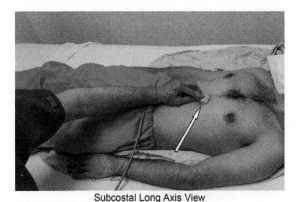

Subcostal Long Axis View
⟹ Probe Orientation Marker

FIGURE 95–7 Subcostal long-axis view—probe positioning.

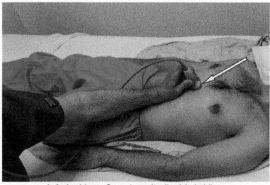

Inferior Vena Cava Longitudinal Axis View
⟹ Probe Orientation Marker

FIGURE 95–9 Inferior vena cava longitudinal view—probe positioning.

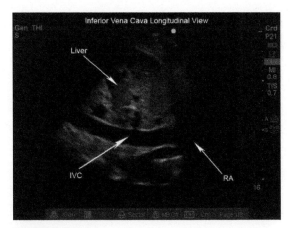

FIGURE 95–10 Inferior vena cava longitudinal view. RA = right atrium; IVC = inferior vena cava.

IVC, and translational artifact mimicking respiratory variation of the IVC.

CLINICAL APPLICATIONS OF BASIC CCE

CCE differs from standard cardiology style echocardiography in that the intensivist personally performs and interprets the examination at point of care and integrates the results into the overall clinical assessment and management plan. The examination is limited in scope and may be repeated as often as needed to track response to therapy and the evolution of illness. This avoids the problems inherent to standard cardiology style echocardiography in the ICU: the delay between ordering and obtaining the study, the time gap before the image is interpreted, the clinical dissociation between the image interpreter from the clinical reality at the bedside, the perception that a full study is required in all circumstances, and the resistance to the performance of repeated study in close succession while the patient is in the ICU.

The basic CCE examination, being performed by the clinician in charge of the case, is always combined with the history, the physical examination, other imaging studies, and laboratory analyses. It is not performed *in vacuo*. When combined with other elements of critical care ultrasonography, Volpicelli et al achieved near perfect concordance with final diagnosis of the cause for shock using an approach that included basic CCE.[6] Laursen et al report similar results with focused ultrasonography diagnosing

previously missed life-threatening conditions.[7] The basic CCE examination may be performed in two to three minutes. When combined with other aspects of critical care ultrasonography, Volpicelli required on average 4.9 minutes to perform an ultrasonography examination, which included basic CCE. Given its ease of use and demonstrated diagnostic utility, the basic CCE examination should be a standard part of the evaluation of every patient with hemodynamic failure. It can be productively combined with other aspects of critical care ultrasonography.

In performing the basic CCE examination, the intensivist needs to consider the following questions:

1. Is there an imminently life-threatening cause for the shock such as cardiac tamponade, marked hypovolemia with an empty ventricle, massive valvular failure, or acute right heart failure?

2. What is the category of shock? Is it hypovolemic, obstructive, cardiogenic (valvular or pump failure), or vasoplegic?

3. What is the best initial management strategy? Does the patient need fluids, inotropes, vasopressors, mechanical assist, thrombolytics, surgery, or another intervention?

4. Is there more than one cause for the shock state or a coexisting condition that will complicate management of the primary cause such as sepsis with aortic stenosis, preexisting LV failure, or pulmonary arterial hypertension with a myocardial infarction?

5. What are the results of repeated CCE studies during the course of treatment? For example, is there improvement in global LV systolic function with treatment of a sepsis induced cardiomyopathy or unloading of the RV with decreasing levels of positive-end expiratory pressure as a patient's acute respiratory distress syndrome improves?

KEY ASPECTS OF THE BASIC CCE EXAMINATION
Global LV Systolic Function

The intensivist who performs basic CCE needs to assess global LV systolic function. Systolic function can be characterized qualitatively as: severely reduced, moderately reduced, normal, or hyperdynamic.[8] Qualitative assessment of LV function is useful for determining a management strategy for the patient with shock, that is, to guide the use of inotropes and/or volume resuscitation. Useful examples of video clips demonstrating degrees of LV dysfunction can be found at www.critcaresono.com. For the purposes of managing an unstable patient in shock, hyperdynamic is defined by end-systolic effacement of the LV cavity. Reduced diastolic excursion of the anterior leaflet of the MV is associated with severely decreased LV function. LV function is best assessed with the PSL view and its orthogonal view, the PSS view at the papillary muscle level. Detailed segmental wall motion analysis is beyond the scope of basic CCE.

Acute Right Heart Failure

There are two findings with basic CCE, which support the diagnosis of right heart failure.[9] Flattening of the interventricular septum during systole is characteristic of RV pressure overload. This is best identified in the PSS view and results in a D-shaped LV (Figure 95–11). Dilatation of the RV is characteristic of RV diastolic overload. This is best identified by comparing the size of the RV and LV at end diastole in the AP4 or SCL views. An RV/LV ratio < 0.6 is normal, between 0.6 and 1 is moderate dilatation, and ≥ 1 is severe RV dilatation (Figure 95–12). Qualitative visual assessment of the ratio is as

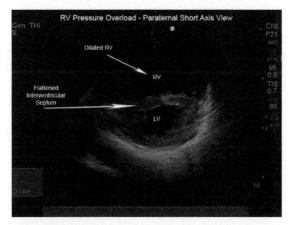

FIGURE 95–11 Right ventricular pressure overload—parasternal short-axis view.
LV = left ventricle; RV = right ventricle;

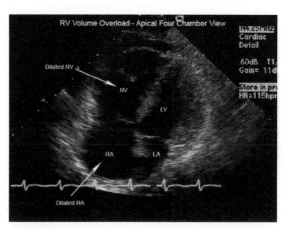

FIGURE 95–12 Right ventricular volume overload—apical four-chamber view.
LV = left ventricle; LA = left atrium; RV = right ventricle; RA = right atrium;

accurate as quantitative planimetry measurement.[10] Normal RV free wall thickness is 3.3 mm ± 0.6 mm. Dilatation of the RV in the setting of normal RV free wall thickness supports an acute process, whereas a thickened RV free wall is likely secondary to a subacute or chronic process.

Pericardial Tamponade

Pericardial tamponade remains a clinical diagnosis and the echocardiographic features associated with it support the diagnosis in the appropriate clinical setting. A pericardial effusion is identified as an echo-free space surrounding the heart. Care must be taken to distinguish a pleural effusion from a pericardial effusion. A pericardial effusion is located anterior to the descending thoracic aorta compared to a pleural effusion which is located posterior to the descending thoracic aorta. Figure 95–13 demonstrates a PSL view of a patient with both a pericardial and pleural effusion.

Pericardial tamponade is associated with a dilated IVC without size variation in the respiratory cycle; swinging of the heart within the large pericardial effusion is characteristic as well. Early diastolic right atrial (RA) collapse has a sensitivity and specificity for tamponade of 92% and 100%, respectively, and occurs earlier than RV diastolic collapse, which carries a sensitivity of 64% and specificity of 100%.[11]

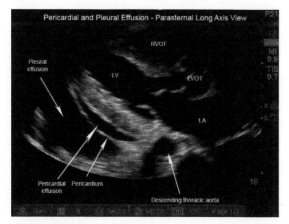

FIGURE 95-13 Pericardial and pleural effusion—PSL view.
LV = left ventricle; LA = left atrium; LVOT = left ventricular outflow tract; RVOT = right ventricular outflow tract;

Assessment of Preload Responsiveness

Inferior vena cava size and its respiratory variation may predict fluid responsiveness in the patient with shock. Acquiring a longitudinal view of the IVC and placing an M-mode scan line through it allows the examiner to measure the size of the IVC during inspiration and expiration (Figure 95–14). Using the IVC size and its respiratory variation to assess fluid responsiveness in passively breathing mechanically ventilated patients is well established.[12-14] Respiratory variation cutoff

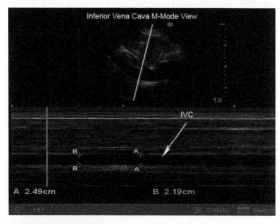

FIGURE 95-14 Inferior vena cava size and respiratory variation—M-mode.
IVC = inferior vena cava.

values of 12% (by using max – min/mean) and 18% (by using max – min/min) separates fluid responders from nonresponders. Data for assessing preload responsiveness in the spontaneously breathing patient are less robust. Expert opinion suggests that if the IVC diameter is < 1 cm, there is a high likelihood of fluid responsiveness; and if the diameter is > 2.5 cm, there is a low probability of fluid responsiveness.[15]

Valve Function and Pathology

Basic CCE allows the intensivist to identify major valve abnormalities that are visible on 2D imaging such as papillary muscle or chordal ruptures, severe aortic stenosis, or large valvular vegetations. Skill at color Doppler analysis of valve function is within the scope of basic CCE; however, more sophisticated Doppler analysis is not. If the clinician suspects significant valve pathology, an advanced CCE examination may be required.

LIMITATIONS OF BASIC CCE

1. Competence in basic CCE requires adequate training. The results of basic CCE may have major implications for the diagnosis and management of the critically ill patient, so it is incumbent upon the intensivist to have a high level of skill. To some trainees, skill at basic CCE appears easy to acquire. This is not the case. The training sequence should include multiple studies initially on normal subjects and then progressing to patients. Recent technological advances now allow trainees to learn on high fidelity TTE and TEE simulators which have the advantage of being able to demonstrate numerous pathologies for the trainee to experience.[16-18] The trainee should have access to a comprehensive image set that features multiple variations of normal and abnormal findings. The trainee must also master the cognitive base of the field, now widely available in articles, textbooks, and internet based resources. In order to assure proficiency, the training sequence should also include formal competency based testing.

2. By definition the basic CCE examination is limited in scope. It does not include a comprehensive image set, nor does it include

Doppler measurements. The intensivist performing basic CCE must understand and accept this limitation and know when to call for a more comprehensive study. Inherent to ICU based echocardiography are the problems related to obtaining high quality images in the critically ill. Often the images of both basic and advanced CCE would be considered inadequate in quality by cardiology standards. Despite this, the critical care clinician needs to be able to interpret and apply the results at the bedside.

3. Documentation for CCE remains a challenge. Ideally, the entire CCE examination image set should be recorded and stored in a durable and accessible format for later review, and a formal report should be entered into the patient's medical record for every study. This requires a well-designed picture archiving and communication system which is fully integrated into the portable ultrasonography machines. To compound the problem, in a busy ICU, the team may perform multiple examinations in rapid sequence in emergency situations, where documentation cannot take precedence over patient care. If the infrastructure to fully integrate CCE studies into the medical record does not yet exist at an institution, at a minimum, a short report should be entered into the medical record documenting the findings of the exam.

TRANSESOPHAGEAL ECHOCARDIOGRAPHY AND ADVANCED CCE

A common indication for TEE in the ICU is when TTE imaging fails due to poor image quality. This may occur due to reasons of body habitus, where TTE images are simply not adequate for interpretation. TEE is also useful in the cardiothoracic ICU, where dressings, wires, and tubes block TTE studies. Depending on the clinical circumstance, the TEE examination may be a comprehensive study; alternatively, a goal directed examination with a limited number of views may suffice.[19]

Advanced CCE requires the intensivist to achieve competence in all aspects of echocardiography that are standard to cardiology-type echocardiography,

in addition to mastering elements of echocardiography that are particular to critical care medicine.[20-22] Competence in advanced CCE requires a long training period similar to the cardiologist who is trained in echocardiography. This includes training in TEE. The majority of intensivists do not have need for advanced level of training; as competence in basic CCE is sufficient for their clinical function. Although it is not known what proportion of intensivists should acquire skill at advanced CCE, one approach for the large ICU operation is for several team members to have advanced CCE training, whereas all other team members have basic CCE skill.

Competence in advanced CCE includes mastery of image acquisition and image interpretation of all standard echocardiography views and Doppler measurements.[23-24] Use of Doppler allows the intensivist to determine hemodynamic function through a wide variety of pressure and flow measurements. This permits the quantitative measurement of stroke volume, cardiac output, intracardiac pressures, preload sensitivity, and valve function.

REFERENCES

1. Mayo PH, Beaulieu Y, Doelken P, et al. American College of Chest Physicians/Société de Réanimation de Langue Française statement on competence in critical care ultrasonography. *Chest.* 2009;135:1050-1060.
2. Cholley BP, Mayo PH, Poelaert J, et al. International expert statement on training standards for critical care ultrasonography. *Intensive Care Med.* 2011;37:1077-1083.
3. Mayo PH. Training in critical care echocardiography. *Mayo Ann Intensive Care.* 2011;1:36.
4. Accreditation Council for Graduate Medical Education. ACGME program requirements for graduate medical education in critical care medicine. www.acgme.org. Accessed July 2013.
5. Labovitz AJ, Noble VE, Bierig M, et al. Focused cardiac ultrasound in the emergent setting: a consensus statement of the American Society of Echocardiography and American College of Emergency Physicians. *J Am Soc Echocardiogr.* 2010;23:1225-1230.
6. Volpicelli G, Lamorte A, Tullio M, et al. Point-of-care multiorgan ultrasonography for the evaluation of undifferentiated hypotension in the emergency department. *Intensive Care Med.* 2013;39:1290-1298.

7. Laursen CB, Sloth E, Lambrechtsen J, et al. Focused sonography of the heart, lungs, and deep veins identifies missed life-threatening conditions in admitted patients with acute respiratory symptoms. *Chest*. 2013;144:1868-1875.

8. Subramanian B, Talmor D. Echocardiographic assessment of left ventricular function and hydration status. In: Levitov A, Mayo PH, Slonim AD, eds. *Critical Care Ultrasonography*. New York: McGraw-Hill; 2009:101-114.

9. Kaplan A. Echocardiographic diagnosis and monitoring of right ventricular function. In: Levitov A, Mayo PH, Slonim AD, eds. *Critical Care Ultrasonography*. New York: McGraw Hill; 2009:125-134.

10. Vieillard-Baron A, Charron C, Chergui K, et al. Bedside echocardiographic evaluation of hemodynamics in sepsis: Is a qualitative evaluation sufficient? *Intensive Care Med*. 2006;32:1547-1552.

11. Sing S, Wann LS, Schuchard GH. Right ventricular and right atrial collapse in patients with cardiac tamponade – A combined echocardiographic and hemodynamic study. *Circulation*. 1984;70:966-971.

12. Barbier C, Loubieres Y, Schmit C, et al. Respiratory changes in inferior vena cava diameter are helpful in predicting fluid responsiveness in ventilated septic patients. *Intensive Care Med*. 2004;30:1740-1746.

13. Feissel M, Michard F, Faller JP, et al. The respiratory variation in the inferior vena cava diameter as a guide to fluid therapy. *Intensive Care Med*. 2004;30:1834-1837.

14. Moretti R, Pizzi B. Inferior vena cava distensibility as a predictor of fluid responsiveness in patients with subarachnoid hemorrhage. *Neurocritical Care*. 2010;13:3-9.

15. Schmidt GS. Ultrasound to guide diagnosis and therapy. *Chest*. 2012;142:1042-1048.

16. Dorfling, J, Hatton KW, Hassan ZU. Integrating echocardiography into human patient simulator training of anesthesiology residents using a severe pulmonary embolism scenario. *Simul Healthcare*. 2006;1:79-83.

17. Platts DG, Humphries J, Burstow DJ, et al. The use of computerised simulators for training of transthoracic and transesophageal echocardiography. The future of echocardiography training? *Heart Lung Circ*. 2012;21:267-274.

18. Neelankavil J, Howard-Quijano K, Hsieh TC, et al. Transthoracic echocardiography simulation is an efficient method to train anesthesiologists in basic transthoracic echocardiography skills. *Anesth Analg*. 2012;115:1042-1051.

19. Benjamin E, Griffin K, Leibowitz AB, et al. Goal-directed transesophageal echocardiography performed by intensivists to assess left ventricular function: comparison with pulmonary artery catheterization. *J Cardiothorac Vasc Anesth*. 1998;12:10-15.

20. De Backer D, Cholley BP, Slama M, et al. *Hemodynamic Monitoring Using Echocardiography in the Critically Ill*. Berlin, Heidelberg: Springer-Verlag; 2011.

21. Narasimhan M, Koenig SJ, Mayo PH. Advanced echocardiography for the critical care physician: part 1. *Chest*. 2014;145:129-134.

22. Narasimhan M, Koenig SJ, Mayo PH. Advanced echocardiography for the critical care physician: part 2. *Chest*. 2014;145:135-142.

23. Koenig S, Mayo PH. Transthoracic echocardiography: image acquisition and transducer manipulation. In: Levitov A, Mayo PH, Slonim AD, eds. *Critical Care Ultrasonography*. New York: McGraw Hill; 2009:79-88.

24. Kory P, Mayo PH. Transesophageal echocardiography: image acquisition and transducer manipulation. In: Levitov A, Mayo PH, Slonim AD, eds. *Critical Care Ultrasonography*. New York: McGraw Hill; 2009:89-100.

Extracorporeal Membrane Oxygenation

Muhammad Adrish, MD; Sharon Leung, MD, MS;
William Jakobleff, MD and Anthony Carlese, DO

KEY POINTS

1. Extracorporeal membrane oxygenation (ECMO) can provide cardiac/cardiopulmonary support via venoarterial (VA) ECMO or pulmonary support via venovenous (VV) ECMO.

2. The indications typically being bridge to recovery, bridge to transplant, or bridge to decision.

3. Early use of ECMO showed poor response leading to a loss of interest in ECMO as a potential therapeutic modality, reappraisal of early results suggests patient selection, and technological limitations precluded successful results.

4. The results of the CESAR trial and H1N1 experience along with technological

improvements and a general improvement in the care of critically ill patients have led to renewed interest in the use of ECMO.

5. Modification of cannulation options either at central or at peripheral locations can affect unloading of the heart as well as impacting the ability to oxygenate the cardiac and cerebral circulations.

6. Improvement in skill of critical care ultrasonography by intensivists has allowed cannulation to move from the operating room and catheterization laboratory to the bedside for VV ECMO and peripherally cannulated VA ECMO.

INTRODUCTION

Extracorporeal membrane oxygenation (ECMO) is a form of partial heart–lung bypass for patients with severe but potentially reversible respiratory and/or cardiac disease who have failed conventional therapies. There are 2 basic types of ECMO: venovenous (VV), which provides the support for the lung only, and venoarterial (VA), which provides support for both heart and lung. In both modalities, blood drained from the venous system is oxygenated outside the body. VA ECMO is similar to standard cardiopulmonary bypass in that both lungs

and heart are bypassed. The purpose of ECMO is to allow time for intrinsic recovery of the lungs and/or the heart, also known as salvage therapy. It can also be used as a bridge to destination therapy such as patients waiting for heart/lung transplant or in certain instances as bridge to decision. During VV ECMO, gas exchange can be supported even in the absence of any pulmonary function but no direct cardiac support is provided. However, the cardiac functions often improve owing to increased oxygen delivery to the heart and concurrently reduced mechanical ventilation. In VA ECMO,

HISTORY OF ECMO

ECMO utilization in adults with respiratory failure dates back to 1970s. A multicenter trial evaluating prolonged venoarterial (VA) ECMO for patients with severe acute respiratory failure failed to show reduction in mortality (> 90% mortality in both groups).[1] The study was later criticized for several reasons such as premature closure, lack of established ECMO experience in some centers, exclusive use of VA ECMO, extensive blood loss during the procedure, and lack of "lung rest" ventilator settings among ECMO patients.[2] ECMO regained cautious attention in the 1990s after several trials showed successful application in neonates and children.[3-5] In an uncontrolled study by Gattinoni and colleagues, venovenous (VV) ECMO improved survival in patients with acute respiratory failure while keeping lungs "at rest" (actual mortality 51.2% vs expected mortality 90%).[6] A subsequent uncontrolled study involving only 10 patients showed similar results but also emphasized that ECMO should be applied early in the course of the disease.[7] In a series of subsequent publications by Bartlett and colleagues showed that ECMO is a successful therapeutic option in patients with severe ARDS who do not respond to conventional mechanical ventilator strategy with survival in such patients in excess of 50%.[8-10] H1N1 influenza emerged as a major cause of respiratory failure during the 2009 epidemic. Favorable outcomes were reported with ECMO use in several studies with survival approaching 80% in patients who were otherwise not responsive to conventional treatment.[11,12] In a multicenter randomized controlled trial published in 2009, ECMO showed a survival benefit at 6 months.[13] Nonetheless, results of this trial need to be interpreted with caution as all patients with ECMO were treated at a different center whereas control patients remained at referring center. More recent meta-analysis published in 2013 concluded that benefit of ECMO on hospital mortality is unclear.[14] Currently, a multicenter randomized trial is underway, evaluating the impact of ECMO instituted early after the diagnosis of ARDS that is not evolving favorably after 3 to 6 hours of maximum medical treatment. (clinicaltrials.gov identifier: NCT014470703).

Clinical Use

ECMO should be considered in patients with life threatening but potentially reversible cardiorespiratory failure who do not have contraindications to extracorporeal support.

Indications

1. **Respiratory indications:**
   A. Inability to ventilate or oxygenate patients in situations where reversal of underlying condition is expected. Some examples include:
      - Pneumonia
      - Pulmonary embolism
      - Adult respiratory distress syndrome
      - Asthma/COPD exacerbation
      - Aspiration pneumonitis
      - Near drowning
      - Wegener granulomatosis
      - Acute chest syndrome, etc
      - Lung transplantation (graft failure)
   B. Bridge to lung transplantation
2. **Cardiac indications:**
   A. Patients with cardiogenic shock as manifested by inadequate tissue perfusion, hypotension and low cardiac output. Typical etiologies include:
      - Acute myocardial infarction
      - Decompensated heart failure
      - Peripartum cardiomyopathy
      - Fulminant myocarditis
      - Heart transplantation (graft failure)
      - Right heart failure
   B. Bridge to heart or heart–lung transplant
   C. During cardiac procedures such as:
      - CABG
      - Aortic valve replacement

Contraindications

ECMO should not be considered for irreversible or non-acute illnesses. Some relative contraindications include:

- Contraindication to anticoagulation
- Preexisting medical conditions affecting quality of life such as advanced malignancies, advanced malignancies

- Multiorgan failure
- End-stage organ failure in a patient not a candidate for destination therapy (ECMO is never used as a destination therapy)
- Medical futility

PHYSIOLOGY OF ECMO

- *VV ECMO*: In VV ECMO, deoxygenated blood is drained from the cannula placed in large central vein, typically inferior vena cava (IVC), and oxygenated blood is returned through a cannula with its tip lying in or at a close proximity to the right atrium (RA). This oxygenated blood mixes with deoxygenated blood from patient's systemic venous return and therefore it is not possible to obtain normal arterial oxygen saturation especially if the lungs are not contributing to the oxygenation. Usual target for oxygen saturation in a patient on ECMO circuit is 86% to 92%. Ideally, the blood from the return cannula passes through the tricuspid valve and then into pulmonary circulation thereby avoiding recirculation through the ECMO circuit. Pulmonary arterial blood is a combination of systemic venous return and oxygenated blood from the return cannula. Preoxygenator oxygen saturation is often used as a surrogate for systemic venous oxygen saturation. As there is always some recirculation present, the preoxygenator oxygen saturation is higher than the venous oxygen saturation. Depending on the positions of cannula, a variable proportion of oxygenated blood from the return cannula enters the drainage cannula, called recirculation. Recirculation reduces the delivery of oxygenated blood into the pulmonary circulation. Recirculation is influenced by several factors such as position of the drainage and return cannula, ECMO circuit flow, intravascular volume status, cardiac output, and position of the patient. High preoxygenator saturation in combination with low systemic arterial saturation suggests clinically significant recirculation. Conversely, low pre-oxygenator saturation along with low arterial saturation suggests that either the cardiac output is abnormally high or ECMO flow is low. High difference between the 2 variables usually suggests minimal recirculation. In the absence of an abnormally high cardiac output or hypermetabolic state, arterial oxygen saturation above 85% can be achieved with VV ECMO even in the absence of pulmonary function.

- *VA ECMO*: In VA ECMO, systemic venous blood drains into the circuit via a cannula placed in vena cava. This blood then passes through the pump and the oxygenator/heat exchanger prior to returning to the patient via a cannula placed in a large artery. This mode works on similar principals to cardiopulmonary bypass in that both heart and lungs are bypassed. Blood is returned to the arterial system and systemic arterial blood pressure is the sum of the ECMO circuit flow plus any ejection from the left ventricle. Likewise, systemic blood pressure is determined by the total blood flow and intrinsic arterial tone. Flow and FiO_2 of the sweep gas which controls the gas exchange by the oxygenator, it is usually the FiO_2 that determines oxygen tension and the flow which determines carbon dioxide tension. In the absence of LV function, the patient's systemic oxygenation depends on the oxygenation in the circuit. However, if there is LV function, the systemic oxygen saturation will depend upon the flow through the ECMO circuit and the amount of blood ejected by the LV. In situations where lung function is severely impaired, placing the return cannula in femoral circulation can lead to upper body hypoxemia as the proximal branches of aorta receive predominantly deoxygenated blood ejected from the LV. Arterial CO_2 tension is determined by balance between carbon dioxide production and its elimination (from the lung or by the oxygenator). It can usually be easily controlled by adjusting flow through the circuit even if the lung is severely damaged.

ECMO CIRCUIT

An ECMO circuit consists of (1) a drainage and return cannula, (2) a oxygenator/heat exchanger, (3) a blood pump, and (4) a tubing. Except for differences in the cannula, identical circuits are used for both VV and VA ECMO.

- *Oxygenator*: Membrane oxygenators can be classified by their structure as either hollow fiber or flat sheet and by their membrane as either microporous or nonmicroporous. Microporous have large number of tiny holes through which gas exchange takes place where in nonmicroporous membrane oxygenators, gas exchanges occurs through diffusion. A decade ago, most of the adult ECMO was performed by using silicone membrane oxygenators that contain nonmicroporous membrane in a rolled flat sheet construction. While having excellent biocompatibility and durability, compared to hollow fiber oxygenators, provided less efficient gas exchange and were more bulky with higher resistance and difficult to prime. Polyprophylene hollow-fiber oxygenators are the standard oxygenators used during CPB. These microporous oxygenators while being highly efficient for gas exchange over short term, but over time the micropores become permeable to fluid causing plasma leaks into the gas phase and out the exhalation port. More recently a new generation of oxygenator containing nonmicroporous hollow fibers constructed of polymethylpentene (PMP) have been introduced. These oxygenators combine the durability of silicone membrane with ease of use and efficient gas exchange of hollow fiber construction. These oxygenators not only have improved durability, but also reduce the requirement of blood transfusion.
- *Blood pump*: There are two basic types of pump: (1) roller and (2) centrifugal. Roller pumps consist of flexible tubing in a curved raceway and are mounted on a rotating arm thus pushing the blood ahead. This pump is usually used with blood-filled bladder that is sited between drainage cannula and the pump to allow continuous pumping despite changes in intravascular volume. As the drainage into the bladder occurs via gravity, these pumps must be kept below the level of the patient. Roller pumps are usually afterload independent; thus, in the presence of obstruction distal to the pump, extremely high pressures can develop leading to circuit rupture. A centrifugal pump consists of a disposable pump head with magnetically driven impeller. The impeller spins rapidly, thus creating a pressure difference across the pump head that causes blood to flow. These are small, easy-to-prime pumps and have a very low volume. The blood flow is preload and afterload dependant such that there is no fixed relation between pump speed and blood flow. For the same reason, a large rise in blood pressure may reduce the blood flow and the pump failure during VA ECMO can even cause flow reversal. Hemolysis occurs with both roller and centrifugal pumps, although it is less with centrifugal pumps.
- *Cannulae and tubing*: Adequate size cannula is essential for adequate blood flow. For most adults, drainage cannula should be 23F to 25F and return cannula should be 17F to 21F. Tubing for the adult ECMO is 3/8 inch in diameter constructed of polyvinylchloride.

INITIATION

In most ECMO centers, perfusionists provide a primed, clamped ECMO circuit into the operative field. The circuit is usually primed with crystalloids, however, for anemic patients a blood prime can be used. It is important to correctly distinguish drainage cannula from return cannula. Both limbs of the circuit are clamped and the tubing is cut 10 cm distal to the clamp. Once connected, all clamps are released except for the clamp between the pump and the oxygenator. The pump is turned on to 1000 to 1500 rpm and the last clamp is slowly released. The sweep gas should initially be set at the same flow as ECMO circuit flow and then adjusted according to $PaCO_2$ and pH. It is common for patients to become hypotensive once ECMO is initiated and appropriate medications for its treatment should be available ahead of time. Patient is heparinized to achieve an activated coagulation time of 1.5 to 2.0 times the normal. Circuit flow is titrated to clinical parameters, which for VA ECMO are mean arterial pressure and arterial oxygen saturation, and, for VV ECMO are arterial oxygen saturation and oxygen saturation in the drainage cannula.

MAINTENANCE

Once ECMO is established, ventilator is set to rest settings. Typical rest ventilator settings are pressure controlled ventilation with peak inflation pressure of 20 to 25 cm H_2O, positive end expiratory pressure of 10 to 15 cm H_2O, and a respiratory rate of 4 to 8 breaths/min. Patients typically develop systemic inflammatory response in the first few days as a consequence on ongoing critical illness and blood contact with ECMO circuit. This may lead to a vasodilator shock, worsening of acute lung injury, and third space fluid losses. If SaO_2 remains low despite adequate circuit flow or if the flow is low despite adequate pump speed, flow pattern in the cannula should be checked using color Doppler with transesophageal echocardiography to rule out any obstruction. The same technique can also be used to check reversibility in the flow. Several other aspects of care need to be managed alongside the ECMO while taking care of these patients. As ECMO support for respiratory failure may extend for weeks, patient may become tolerant to benzodiazepines and opioids. Similarly, weaning off the patients from these medications could be difficult after prolonged use. Thus, administration in low doses is recommended for these medications. Some centers even wake up and extubate some patients although this can be technically challenging. Anticoagulation with unfractionated heparin is required while patient is on ECMO circuit. Patients need to be monitored for the signs of bleeding which can result from anticoagulation, thrombocytopenia (heparin-induced, sepsis), disseminated intravascular coagulation or from gastrointestinal sources. Performing coagulation studies, monitoring the blood counts, and checking a thromboelastogram (TEG) will help in diagnosing the etiology in such circumstances.

In certain instances, ECMO circuit can be run heparin free for around 48 to 72 hours.

Maintaining fluid balance is another important consideration in these patients as they often get flooded with volume during the initial resuscitation period. Thus, it is recommended to limit fluid administration and ideally maintain a negative balance even if it leads to use of vasopressors.

WEANING AND DISCONTINUATION

VV ECMO: Recovery of the pulmonary functions may take days to weeks. Signs such as improvement in oxygen saturation for a given circuit flow, progressive increase in SaO_2 above SvO_2, improving lung compliance and chest radiography. Once a patient is able to maintain a saturation of > 90% at a circuit flow of 1 to 2 L/min, weaning trial can be instituted. Circuit flow is progressively decreased while fully ventilating patient with the ventilator. Once flow is reduced to zero and patient is able to tolerate, ECMO is decannulated.

VA ECMO: Pulsatility is an early sign of recovery of myocardial function. Ionotropic support is started prior to planned weaning and circuit flow are slowly reduced to 1 to 2 L/min. Echocardiography is done during the process to assess cardiac function. Once patient is stable on minimal or no support, ECMO can be discontinued. Majority of the patients who are able to be weaned of VA ECMO do so within 2 to 5 days.[15]

COMPLICATIONS DURING ECMO

Circuit Complications

ECMO is a complex procedure performed on critically ill patients, thus have high potential for complication.

Gas embolism:

Large negative pressure generated with the centrifugal pumps can lead to air entrainment and significant air embolism. A major obstruction in the circuit can also force the gas out solution causing gas embolism. This complication, though life threatening, is rare and occurs in fewer than 2% of adult ECMO runs.[16]

Blood clots: Blood clots can occur at multiple sites in the ECMO circuit. Clot in the pump head usually results in change in sound of the pump and rising plasma hemoglobin. A clot in the oxygenator can result in increasing pressure gradient along with fall in post oxygenator PO_2 and increasing sweep gas needed to maintain $PaCO_2$. Other markers such as increasing d-dimers or fibrin degradation products can also suggest clot formation.

Loss of circuit flow: Loss or reduced flow is most commonly caused by hypovolemia. Other causes such obstructive shock from cardiac tamponade or tension pneumothorax and malpositioned cannula can also decrease the flow. With a roller pump, a decreased flow can lead to slowing or stopping of the pump. In ECMO devices with a centrifugal pump, a decreased flow can lead to increased negative which can progress to suck down at the drainage cannula eventually causing loss of circuit flow.

Circuit failure or breakage: As the name sounds, this complication may lead to a catastrophic complication. Bedside staff trained to check circuit integrity and to react promptly in the case of acute failure can prevent this problem.

Patient Complications

Hemodynamic instability: Circuit flows above 7 L/min are rarely possible even with the optimal cannula. In patients on ECMO support, severe sepsis can lead to significant hypotension as it normally would lead to increase in cardiac output. Left ventricular (LV) distension can occur in patients on VA ECMO especially in patients with mitral or aortic regurgitation, which can lead to pulmonary edema. Increasing pump flow may be helpful in such situations.

Hypoxemia: Upper body hypoxemia can occur in VA ECMO patients with significant LV ejection and impaired lung function. This situation typically occurs when return cannula is placed in lower extremity arteries. Detecting higher saturation in lower extremity compared to upper extremity diagnosis this problem.

Infections: Infective complications related to access sites, indwelling lines or primary pathology can occur. Of note, signs of sepsis may be completely evident; in particular, fever may be absent due to control of temperature via heat exchanger. Thus, any evidence of deteriorating hemodynamics or rising white cell count should be taken seriously. Strict aseptic precautions need to be taken during this process.

Bleeding: Bleeding, in particular from the surgical site, is common during ECMO. In one series, approximately 31.4% patients developed cannulation site bleeding and 26.7% developed surgical site bleeding.[17] Other less common but potentially more serious bleedings could be gastrointestinal and intracranial bleeding which were 7% and just fewer than 3% in same series respectively. Most important mechanism of dealing with this complication is prevention. All unnecessary procedures should be avoided as much as possible while patient is on ECMO.

OTHER USES

VV ECMO may be used as an alternative to cardiopulmonary bypass during procedures involving airway and lungs. Examples include surgical construction of carina,[18] laser resection of tracheal masses,[19] whole lung lavage for alveolar proteinosis,[20] during high risk rigid bronchoscopy,[21] and in adult burn patients with severe inhalational injury.[22] Successful use of VA ECMO has been reported in several different clinical situations such as in patients with toxic shock-induced cardiomyopathy,[23] ARDS with septic cardiomyopathy,[24] to facilitate combined pneumonectomy and transesophageal fistula repair,[25] as a "bridge to bridge" in heart failure patients,[26] in patients with cardiac arrest,[27-29] and as a bridge to organ donation.[30] These examples show that ECMO can be used successfully to support vital organ perfusion in patients with profound but potentially reversible medical conditions.

FUTURE DIRECTIONS

ECMO is highly technical, advanced life support system used for patients with severe cardiac and or pulmonary disease requiring intensive support with a potential for reversibility. With improvements in ECMO device and increasing ECMO experience, there is potential for further improvement in outcomes inpatient on this support. Some experts have started to suggest early implementation of ECMO as a part of lung protection in patients with ARDS.[31,32] ECMO is currently being offered in equipped centers for ARDS patients with severe hypoxemia (PaO_2-to-FiO_2 ratio < 80 mm Hg) who are unresponsive to conventional treatment. The feasibility and efficacy of ECMO for in-hospital cardiac arrest patients have been reported.[33] However such efficacy and cost effectiveness for out-of-hospital cardiac arrest remain unclear and further studies are needed to assess this modality. Extracorporeal removal of CO_2, a function of ECMO circuit, can be potentially used in critically ill patients with acute exacerbation of bronchial asthma and COPD who are unable to tolerate standardized management, although definite guidelines are lacking. Safe application of this device would require multidisciplinary team approach, and experience with its use and improvements to minimize device related complication, before this modality can be applied across the board.

REFERENCES

1. Zapol WM, Snider MT, Hill JD, et al. Extracorporeal membrane oxygenation in severe acute respiratory failure. A randomized prospective study. *J Am Med Assoc.* 1979;242:2193-2196.

2. Peek GJ, Tirouvopaiti R, Firmin RK. ECLS for adult respiratory failure: etiology and indications. In: Van Meurs K, Lally KP, Peek G, Zwischenberger JB, eds. *ECMO Extracorporeal Cardiopulmonary Support in Critical Care.* 3rd ed. Ann Arbor, MI: Extracorporeal Life Support Organization; 2005: 393-402.

3. Bartlett RH, Roloff DW, Cornell RG, Andrews AF, Dillon PW, Zwischenberger JB. Extracorporeal circulation in neonatal respiratory failure: a prospective randomized study. *Pediatrics.* 1985;76:479-487.

4. UK Collaborative ECMO Trial Group. UK collaborative randomised trial of neonatal extracorporeal membrane oxygenation. *Lancet.* 1996;348:75-82.

5. Green TP, Timmons OD, Fackler JC, Moler FW, Thompson AE, Sweeney MF. The impact of extracorporeal membrane oxygenation on survival in pediatric patients with acute respiratory failure. Pediatric Critical Care Study Group. *Crit Care Med.* 1996;24:323-332.

6. Gattinoni L, Pesenti A, Mascheroni D, et al. Low-frequency positive-pressure ventilation with extracorporeal CO_2 removal in severe acute respiratory failure. *J Am Med Assoc.* 1986;256:881-886.

7. Anderson HL III, Delius RE, Sinard JM, et al. Early experience with adult extracorporeal membrane oxygenation in the modern era. *Ann Thorac Surg.* 1992;53:553-563.

8. Kolla S, Awad SS, Rich PB, Schreiner RJ, Hirschl RB, Bartlett RH. Extracorporeal life support for 100 adult patients with severe respiratory failure. *Ann Surg.* 1997;226:544-564.

9. Bartlett RH, Roloff DW, Custer JR, Younger JG, Hirschl RB. Extracorporeal life support. The University of Michigan experience. *J Am Med Assoc.* 2000;283:904-908.

10. Hemmila MR, Rowe SA, Boules TN, et al. Extracorporeal life support for severe acute respiratory distress syndrome in adults. *Ann Surg.* 2004;240:595-607.

11. Beurtheret S, Mastroianni C, Pozzi M, et al. Extracorporeal membrane oxygenation for 2009 influenza A (H1N1) acute respiratory distress syndrome: single-centre experience with 1-year follow-up. *Eur J Cardiothorac Surg.* 2012;41:691-695.

12. Australia and New Zealand Extracorporeal Membrane Oxygenation (ANZ ECMO) Influenza Investigators, et al. Extracorporeal membrane oxygenation for 2009 influenza A (H1N1) acute respiratory distress syndrome. *J Am Med Assoc.* 2009;302:1888-1895.

13. Peek GJ, Mugford M, Tiruvoipati R, et al. Efficacy and economic assessment of conventional ventilatory support versus extracorporeal membrane oxygenation for severe adult respiratory failure (CESAR): a multicentre randomised controlled trial. *Lancet.* 2009;374:1351-1363.

14. Zampieri FG, Mendes PV, Ranzani OT, et al. Extracorporeal membrane oxygenation for severe respiratory failure in adult patients: a systematic review and meta-analysis of current evidence. *J Crit Care.* 2013;28:998-1005.

15. Smedira NG, Moazami N, Golding CM, et al. Clinical experience with 202 adults receiving extracorporeal membrane oxygenation for cardiac failure: survival at five years. *J Thorac Cardiovasc Surg.* 2001;122:92-102.

16. Extracorporeal Life Support Registry Report (International Summary). January 2008 Edition.

Ann Arbor, MI: Extracorporeal Life Support Organization; 2008:30.

17. Hemmila MR, Rowe SA, Boules TN, et al. Extracorporeal life support for severe acute respiratory distress syndrome in adults. *Ann Thorac Surg.* 2004;240:595-605.

18. Horita K, Itoh T, Furukawa K, et al. Carinal reconstruction under veno-venous bypass using a percutaneous cardiopulmonary bypass system. *Thorac Cardiovasc Surg.* 1996;44:46-49.

19. Smith IJ, Sidebotham DA, McGeorge AD, et al. Use of extracorporeal membrane oxygenation during resection of tracheal papillomatosis. *Anesthesiology.* 2009;110:427-429.

20. Kim KH, Kim JH, Kim YW. Use of extracorporeal membrane oxygenation (ECMO) during whole lung lavage in pulmonary alveolar proteinosis associated with lung cancer. *Eur J Cardiothorac Surg.* 2004;26:1050-1051.

21. Gourdin M, Dransart C, Delaunois L, Louagie YA, Gruslin A, Dubois P. Use of venovenous extracorporal membrane oxygenation under regional anesthesia for a high-risk rigid bronchoscopy. *J Cardiothorac Vasc Anesth.* 2012;26:465-467.

22. Chou NK, Chen YS, Ko WJ, et al. Application of extracorporal membrane oxygenation in adult burn patients. *Artif Organs.* 2001;25:622-626.

23. Gabel E, Gudzenko V, Cruz D, Ardehali A, Fink MP. Successful use of extracorporal membrane oxygenation in an adult patient with toxic shock-induced heart failure. *J Intensive Care Med.* 2015;30:115-118.

24. Küstermann J, Gehrmann A, Kredel M, Wurmb T, Roewer N, Muellenbach RM. Acute respiratory distress syndrome and septic cardiomyopathy: successful application of veno-venoarterial extracorporal membrane oxygenation. *Anaesthesist.* 2013;62:639-643.

25. Liston DE, Richards MJ. Venoarterial extracorporal membrane oxygenation (VA ECMO) to facilitate combined pneumonectomy and tracheoesophageal fistula repair. *J Cardiothorac Vasc Anesth.* 2013;pii:S1053-0770(13)00309-1.

26. Fitzgerald D, Ging A, Burton N, Desai S, Elliott T, Edwards L. The use of percutaneous ECMO support as a 'bridge to bridge' in heart failure patients: a case report. *Perfusion.* 2010;25:321-325, 327.

27. Mayette M, Gonda J, Hsu JL, Mihm FG. Propofol infusion syndrome resuscitation with extracorporeal life support: a case report and review of the literature. *Ann Intensive Care.* 2013;3:32.

28. Chiu CW, Yen HH, Chiu CC, Chen YC, Siao FY. Prolonged cardiac arrest: successful resuscitation with extracorporal membrane oxygenation. *Am J Emerg Med.* 2013;31:1627e5-6.

29. Robert Leeper W, Valdis M, Arntfield R, Ray Guo L. Extracorporal membrane oxygenation in the acute treatment of cardiovascular collapse immediately post-partum. *Interact Cardiovasc Thorac Surg.* 2013;17:898-899.

30. Isnardi DI, Olivero F, Lerda R, Guermani A, Cornara G. Extracorporeal membrane oxygenation as a bridge to organ donation: a case report. *Transplant Proc.* 2013;45:2619-2620.

31. Maclaren G, Combes A, Bartlett RH. Contemporary extracorporeal membrane oxygenation for adult respiratory failure: life support in the new era. *Intensive Care Med.* 2012;38:210-220.

32. Checkley W. Extracorporeal membrane oxygenation as a first-line treatment strategy for ARDS: Is the evidence sufficiently strong? *J Am Med Assoc.* 2011;306:1703-1704.

33. Chen YS, Lin JW, Yu HY, et al. Cardiopulmonary resuscitation with assisted extracorporeal life-support versus conventional cardiopulmonary resuscitation in adults with in-hospital cardiac arrest: an observational study and propensity analysis. *Lancet.* 2008;372:554-561.

Airway Management in the Critically Ill Patient

Elvis Umanzor, MD and Andrew Leibowitz, MD

KEY POINTS

1. In the intensive care unit (ICU), endotracheal intubation is usually marked by an urgent need in face of cardiorespiratory instability, poor physiologic reserve, and an unknown airway history.

2. The incidence of difficult intubation and complications during intubation in the ICU are considerably higher than reported in operating room settings.

3. Preoxygenation should take place prior to any airway intervention.

4. Flexing the neck and extending the head at the atlantooccipital joint, called the "sniffing" position is probably the best starting position for direct laryngoscopy.

5. In recent years, the use of bladed indirect laryngoscopes (eg, Glidescope, C-MAC, McGrath) has increased in the operating room, the emergency department, and the ICU.

INTRODUCTION

Endotracheal intubation in the ICU differs significantly from when performed by anesthesiologists in the operating room, with availability of special airway equipment, and trained staff support.[1] In addition, ICU endotracheal intubation is usually marked by an urgent need in face of cardiorespiratory instability, poor physiologic reserve, and an unknown airway history.[2]

The incidence of difficult intubation in the ICU is 12% to 22%, considerably higher than reported in operating room settings.[3-5] The rate of severe complications is very high, including severe hypoxemia (26%), hemodynamic collapse (25%), cardiac arrest (1.6%), and death (0.8%).[2] The Fourth National Audit Project Report (NAP4), a review of major airway-related events occurring in the United Kingdom over a period of a year, revealed that 61% of the airway events that occurred in the ICU resulted in death or brain damage. More concerning is that after qualitative analysis of the events, reviewers assessed airway management as good in only 11%.[3]

AIRWAY ASSESSMENT

Airway assessment must be performed before any procedure. The purpose of this evaluation is to identify possible difficulty with bag-mask ventilation, intubation, supraglottic device placement, or cricothyroidotomy/tracheostomy. Even in the ICU, where most intubations are performed emergently, an abbreviated assessment is warranted.[6-8]

Predicting Difficult Bag-Mask Ventilation

If endotracheal intubation is difficult or impossible, ventilation with a bag-mask will maintain oxygenation until the airway is secured. Difficult ventilation is a serious problem, and every effort should be made to anticipate this complication.[9] Five independent predictors have been identified: age greater than 55, body mass index greater than 26 kg/m², lack of teeth, history of snoring, male gender, and presence of beard.[7,9]

Predicting Difficult Direct Laryngoscopy

Indicators of potentially difficult direct laryngoscopy include inability to prognath (move the lower teeth in front of the upper teeth), high Mallampati-Samsoon classification score (Figure 97–1), interincisor distance of less than 4 cm (~2 fingerbreadths), short thyromental distance (< 6.5 cm or 3 fingerbreadths) measured from the top of the thyroid cartilage to the anterior border of the mandible with the head in full extension, range of neck extension less than 35°, and previous history of a difficult intubation.[7-11]

It is important to note that all these indicators have poor sensitivity and specificity and that no single factor reliably predicts difficulty. The positive predictive value of any of these tests alone is low, but prediction is improved with the presence of multiple concerning factors.[6,10,12]

Predicting a Difficult Surgical Airway

The techniques of needle or surgical cricothyroidotomy depend on the cricothyroid membrane being accessible, which may not always be the case. Some features that may cause difficulty in accessing this membrane include obesity, neck immobility, and local blunt, or penetrating trauma.[6,9]

SECURING AN AIRWAY
Indications for Intubation

Indications for intubation include airway obstruction, airway protection (any cause of depressed level of consciousness, eg, stroke, trauma, or intoxication), facilitation of mechanical support for respiratory failure (hypoxemic or hypercapnic), and circulatory failure (shock).

Equipment

All necessary equipment should be available and checked prior to any intubation attempt regardless of predicted difficulty[7,8] (Table 97–1). The patient should be monitored with at least pulse oximetry, blood pressure cuff, and continuous electrocardiogram. Intravenous access should be secured.

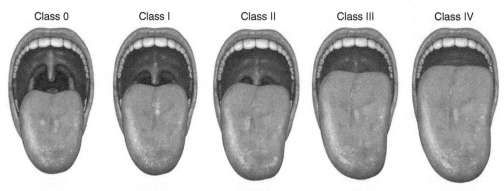

| Class 0 | Class I | Class II | Class III | Class IV |

FIGURE 97–1 The Mallampati-Samsoon classification attempts to correlate the ability to observe intraoral structures and the difficulty to intubate. The patient sits erect with the head in neutral position and is asked to open the mouth as wide as possible and to protrude the tongue maximally. The examiner sits opposite and observes various intraoral structures. Classes I and II predict a low risk of difficulty while with class III or IV there is a greater chance of problems visualizing the glottis during direct laryngoscopy. (*Reproduced with permission from Finucane BT:* Principles of Airway Management. *New York: Springer; 2011.*)

TABLE 97-1 Equipment for endotracheal intubation.

High flow oxygen source
Facemask and bag-mask device
Suction catheters and Yankauer
Oropharyngeal and nasopharyngeal airways
Laryngoscope handles and blades (different types and sizes)
Stylet
Endotracheal tubes (different sizes)
Medications (induction agents, neuromuscular relaxants, vasopressors)
Confirmation placement device

Positioning

The airway contains three visual axes: (1) mouth, (2) oropharynx, and (3) larynx. In the neutral position, these axes form acute and obtuse angles with one another and the glottic opening is not visualized.[11] The traditional teaching is that the "sniffing the morning air" position (Figure 97–2) helps align the oral, pharyngeal, and laryngeal axes.[13] This is achieved by flexing the neck and extending the head at the atlantooccipital joint.[7,8] Cervical flexion approximates the pharyngeal and laryngeal axes, and extension at the atlantooccipital joint brings the oral axis into better alignment with the other two.[11] However, over the past decade, several authors have controversially challenged this issue.[14-16] Adnet et al studied magnetic resonance imaging (MRI) scans of healthy volunteers in 3 anatomic positions (neutral, simple extension, and in the sniffing position) and concluded that the "sniffing position" does not achieve alignment of the 3 important axes.[15] Despite this, we consider that the sniffing position is probably the best starting position for direct laryngoscopy.

In patients at risk of aspiration, compressing the cricoid cartilage posteriorly against the vertebral body (ie, Sellick maneuver) may reduce the diameter of the upper esophageal sphincter and prevent regurgitation of stomach content into the trachea during intubation, but may also interfere with laryngoscopy and endotracheal tube insertion.

Preoxygenation

Preoxygenation should take place prior to any airway intervention. The two primary goals of preoxygenation are (1) maximization of the arterial PaO_2 and (2) denitrogenation of the functional residual capacity. A beneficial secondary goal of the process is hypocarbia.

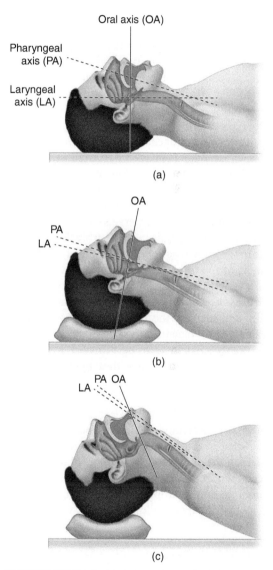

FIGURE 97–2 Three-axis alignment. (**A**) Head in neutral position. (**B**) Elevation of head approximates the laryngeal and pharyngeal axes. (**C**) Extension at the atlantooccipital joint brings the visual axis of the mouth into better alignment with those of larynx and pharynx. (*Reproduced with permission from Hagberg C: Benumof and Hagberg's Airway Management, 3rd edition. Philadelphia: Elsevier Saunders; 2013.*)

Preoxygenation can temporarily raise the SpO_2 and PaO_2, maximizing blood oxygen content. Although dissolved oxygen adds little to the oxygen content of blood as the SpO_2 nears 100%, critically ill patients often suffer from anemia, increased oxygen consumption and regional hypoperfusion, so any increase in dissolved oxygen (eg, 1.5 mL O_2/100 mL of blood) is desirable. More importantly, preoxygenation replaces the nitrogen in the functional residual capacity with oxygen. The functional residual capacity is approximately 30 mL/kg, oxygen consumption is 3 to 4 mL/kg/min, and in healthy patients this "oxygen reserve" may allow up to 8 minutes of apnea before the SpO_2 decreases below 90%. However, efficiency of denitrogenation and the time to critical SpO_2 decrease is markedly reduced in critically ill patients and apnea rarely tolerated for more than 60 to 120 seconds; but, any increase in the time to desaturation will decrease morbidity and mortality.

Encouragement of hyperventilation during preoxygenation may result in hypocarbia that is desirable in the soon to be apneic patient. During the first minute of apnea the Pco_2 will increase by 6 mm Hg and afterward by 3 mm Hg per minute. Hypercarbia will cause hemodynamic instability, cardiac arrhythmias, and increase the intracranial pressure, even while the SpO_2 remains in a safe range.

Preoxygenation may be achieved by administration of 100% oxygen with a tight-fitting face mask, application of continuous positive airway pressure (CPAP) or bilevel positive airway pressure (BiPAP), or manually assisted bag-mask ventilation. The choice of method is highly dependent on personal preference or unit policy and the emergent nature of the procedure. The authors of this chapter recommend that while setting up for intubation at minimum a tight-fitting F_{IO_2} 1.0 face mask should be applied and if time allows BiPAP be initiated.

Face Mask and Bag-Valve Device

Face masks are designed to form a seal around the mouth and nose and connect to a bag-valve device.[6] The operator stands at the patient's head and presses the mask onto the patient's face with the left hand. The thumb should be on the nasal portion of the mask, the index finger near the oral portion, and the rest of the fingers spread on the left side of the patient's mandible so as to pull slightly anterior.[8] The 2 key elements are to establish a tight fit with the mask, covering the patient's mouth and nose to prevent air leaks, and an unobstructed airway.[6,8] The minimum effective insufflation pressure should be used to decrease the risk of insufflating the stomach and increasing the risk of aspiration.[8]

If ventilation is not effective, 2 maneuvers can be performed to improve airflow obstruction. Head extension, by stretching the anterior neck structures and moving the hyoid bone and attached structures anteriorly, is probably the most important single maneuver for maintaining space between the pharyngeal soft tissues (caution is advised in patients with unstable cervical spine). Jaw thrust, achieved by exerting anterior pressure behind the angles of the mandible, can also reduce the airway obstruction.[6]

Airway Adjuncts

If ventilation is not adequate despite proper positioning of the patient and proper use of the bag-valve device, several airway adjuncts may be helpful.[8]

An oropharyngeal airway (Figure 97–3) is semicircular and made of plastic. The 2 types are the Guedel airway, with a hollow tubular design, and the Berman airway, with airway channels along the sides.[7] Both are inserted with the curved portion toward the mouth floor with the help of a tongue depressor to lower the tongue if needed. It should be inserted only when the pharyngeal reflexes are depressed, to minimize the risk of coughing and laryngospasm.[6]

The nasopharyngeal airway is a soft tube approximately 15-cm long that is inserted through

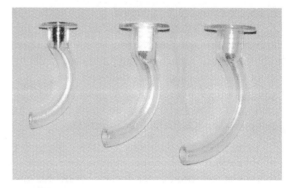

FIGURE 97–3 Oropharyngeal airway (Guedel).

the nostril into the posterior pharynx. This device may be preferable in patients with limited mouth opening and poor dentition. It is also better tolerated in conscious patients. The airway should be lubricated and a vasoconstrictor should be applied before insertion. Its use is contraindicated in patients with skull base trauma, rhinorrhea, and severe coagulopathy.[6,8]

Induction Agents/Muscle Relaxants

Endotracheal intubation is safer and the success rate is higher in the sedated paralyzed state. Given the frequency of difficulty encountered, persons who are not experts and not comfortable with the administration of hypnotics and paralytics should defer to experts.

The choice of sedative hypnotic agent should emphasize hemodynamic stability and short duration of action. Hypotension is best avoided if etomidate (2-3 mg/kg) or ketamine (1-5 mg/kg) are used. Etomidate may cause myoclonus, does not promote muscle relaxation, burns on injection, and is associated with decreased endogenous steroid production, but its hemodynamic stability is unmatched. The administration of propofol to critically ill patients, even in low doses (eg, 1-1.5 mg/kg), almost always causes hypotension.

The choice of paralytic should emphasize short onset of action (ie, "rapid-sequence intubation", ~ 60-75 seconds) and limits the choice to the depolarizing agent succinylcholine, and the nondepolarizing agent rocuronium. Succinylcholine (1-1.5 mg/kg) is the most rapid in onset (30-45 seconds) and shortest in duration (5-10 minutes), but in normal patients may raise the potassium level, and in certain conditions (eg, paralytic stroke, major burns) this rise may be quite profound and result in a hyperkalemic arrest. In these conditions, rocuronium (0.6-1.2 mg/kg) is preferable, although its duration of action is longer than succinylcholine (30-50 minutes).

Given the frequency of hemodynamic instability accompanying intubation in the ICU, preparation and administration of vasoactive medications should occur simultaneously with preparation and probably should precede administration of sedative hypnotics and paralytics. Patients who are already hypotensive prior to endotracheal intubation need reliable venous access through which a vasopressor can be infused. If the mean arterial pressure (MAP) is less than 60 mm Hg the vasopressor infusion should be increased, or alternatively a bolus of vasopressor can be administered. Ephedrine (5-10 mg), phenylephrine (100 μg), and vasopressin (0.5-1 units) have all been frequently used by the authors, usually determined by availability and heart rate. Bradycardic patients should all have at minimum atropine 0.4 mg or glycopyrolate 0.2 mg administered. Hypertensive patients, especially those with intracranial lesions, may benefit from titrated doses of short-acting hypotensive agents such as nitroglycerin (40-100 μg) and esmolol (0.5 mg/kg).

Direct Laryngoscopy and Endotracheal Tubes

Direct laryngoscopy is performed to visualize the laryngeal opening (Figure 97–4). To see through the airway, light must travel from the glottic opening to the laryngoscopist's eye. Since light travels in a straight line, the technique requires an uninterrupted linear path between the larynx and the observer.[11] The tongue and the epiglottis are the anatomic structures that intrude into this line of sight.[6] One of the main objectives of direct laryngoscopy is to move the tongue anteriorly into the mandibular space, allowing direct view of the glottic opening.

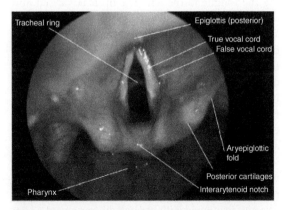

FIGURE 97–4 Glottic opening view. (*Reproduced with permission from Calder I, Pearce A: Core Topics in Airway Management, 2nd edition. New York: Cambridge University Press; 2011.*)

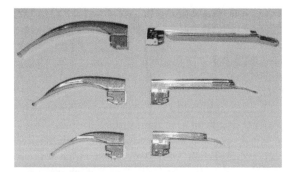

FIGURE 97–5 Macintosh (curved) and Miller (straight) blades.

The laryngoscope has a handle and a blade that snaps securely into the top of the handle. Many blades' shapes and sizes are available, however, 2 types are commonly used (Figure 97–5). The Macintosh blade is curved along its long axis, has a broad, flat surface, and has a right-angled Z-shaped cross-section. The straight blades (Cranwall, Miller, Phillips, Wisconsin) tend to be narrower than the curve blades and have a D-shaped flange.[6-8] Which blade to use is in many cases a matter of personal preference, but the straight blade could be of special use in patients with a larger than normal epiglottis, or with a larynx that is positioned more anterior.

The laryngoscope is held in the left hand and introduced into the right side of the mouth. While advancing the blade to the base of the tongue, the blade is simultaneously moved to the midline sweeping the tongue to the left. The tip is advanced and the epiglottis is lifted away from the glottic opening.[7] With a curved blade the tip rests and applies upward traction to the base of the tongue at the vallecula; the straight blade tip rests in the posterior surface of the epiglottis and lifts it directly.[7,8] Elevating the epiglottis through a lifting motion at 45° from the horizontal using the arm and shoulder exposes the vocal cords. Keeping the wrist stiff to avoid a prying motion that uses the teeth as fulcrum will prevent dental injury.[7,8] Once the vocal cords are visualized, the endotracheal tube is advanced from the right corner of the mouth and into the trachea. The cuff is inflated with enough air to prevent a leak with positive pressure ventilation.

Correct placement is confirmed with visualization of symmetric chest expansion, auscultation over epigastrium and lung fields, and an end-tidal CO_2 detection device (capnography or calorimetric chemical detection of CO_2). After confirmation, the tube is secured in place. A chest radiograph should be ordered in order to confirm correct placement and position of endotracheal tube tip above carina.

Endotracheal tubes are designed to provide a secure channel through the upper airway. The size of the endotracheal tubes is described as the internal diameter in millimeters.[6] Tubes are available in 0.5 mm increments, starting at 2.5 mm. Selection of the proper diameter is important because small-diameter tubes increase airway resistance and work of breathing; moreover, certain procedures like bronchoscopy require large tubes. Common sized tracheal tubes are 8 mm for males and 7.5 mm for females. In general, the larger the patient, the larger the endotracheal tube that should be used.[6,8] For oral intubation, an endotracheal tube insertion depth of 21 cm from the incisors in females and 23 cm from the incisors in males results in proper positioning about 4 cm above the carina in the majority of patients. The endotracheal tubes have a cuff near the distal end that is inflated to provide a seal to protect from aspiration and to allow positive pressure ventilation. Prevention of excessive cuff pressure may reduce the incidence of tracheal damage. Cuff pressure monitoring should be used whenever possible to maintain a pressure in the range of 25 to 30 cm H_2O.[6]

AIRWAY DEVICES

In addition to conventional laryngoscopes, many airway devices and techniques have been developed to manage difficult ventilation or intubation. However, no device or technique is universally successful in all situations.[2,17]

Supraglottic Devices

The laryngeal mask airway (LMA) is a plastic tube attached to a shallow mask with an inflatable ring designed for blind insertion into the pharynx to fit the laryngeal inlet and form a seal around it.[8,17] It was introduced in 1988 and is widely used in the operating room for elective cases. It has also been used as a rescue device and is the key in the adaptive simulated annealing (ASA) algorithm for difficult airway used as a ventilatory device in patients that are difficult to ventilate and intubate, or as a conduit for fiberoptic bronchoscopic intubation in patients that can be ventilated but not intubated.[6,17]

Rigid Indirect Laryngoscopy

Indirect laryngoscopy is a technique in which the glottic view is transmitted through fiberoptic bundles or video technology to the eyepiece of the instrument, or a monitor screen.[18] There are several available devices differing in their design and technical features.

In recent years, the use of bladed indirect laryngoscopes (eg, Glidescope, C-MAC, McGrath) has increased, not only in the operating room, but also in the emergency department and in the ICU (Figure 97–6). Videolaryngoscopes consist of an angled blade with a camera at the tip. The image captured at the distal lens is transmitted to the proximal end of the device into a small screen. It is important to note that the Glidescope and the McGrath have an angulated blade, and provide a view of the glottic opening on the screen while the actual glottis is not directly in the operator's view line. Because of this the endotracheal tube requires the use of a curved stylet to be inserted around and behind the tongue.[18] For this same reason, in some occasions, despite an improved visualization, it is difficult to advance the endotracheal tube into the trachea.

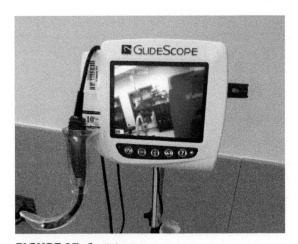

FIGURE 97–6 Glidescope.

Flexible Fiberoptic Bronchoscope Intubation

Fiberoptic bronchoscopes use flexible optical fibers to transmit images from a distal lens as it is steered under vision toward the larynx and into the trachea. The image transmitted is displayed on a monitor by attaching a camera to the eyepiece, or by using a bronchoscope with an integral camera. This device is the most versatile laryngoscope for tracheal intubation and can facilitate intubation that is otherwise impossible.[6]

Unfortunately, many of the relative contraindications for its use are encountered in the ICU, including poor patient cooperation, blood in the airway, and time constraints.

DIFFICULT AIRWAY ALGORITHM

For clinical or anatomic reasons, airway management may be difficult without specialized expertise or tools. One significant advance in the management of patients with difficult airways is the development of algorithms to standardize its approach.[19]

The American Society of Anesthesiologists recently published an update of the *Practice Guidelines for Management of Difficult Airway*. Although these guidelines were designed for its use in the operating room, and in the majority of cases in the ICU the elective pathway is not applicable, they offer a useful stepwise approach to anticipated and unanticipated airway problems (Figure 97–7).[19,20]

AIRWAY MANAGEMENT DURING CARDIOPULMONARY RESUSCITATION

During low-blood-flow states such as patients in cardiac arrest, oxygen delivery is limited by flow rather than by arterial oxygen content. In these circumstances, rescue breaths are less important than chest compressions during the first few minutes of resuscitation. Moreover, rescue breaths could reduce cardiopulmonary resuscitation (CPR) efficacy due to interruption of chest compressions and increases in intrathoracic pressure. Advanced airway placement

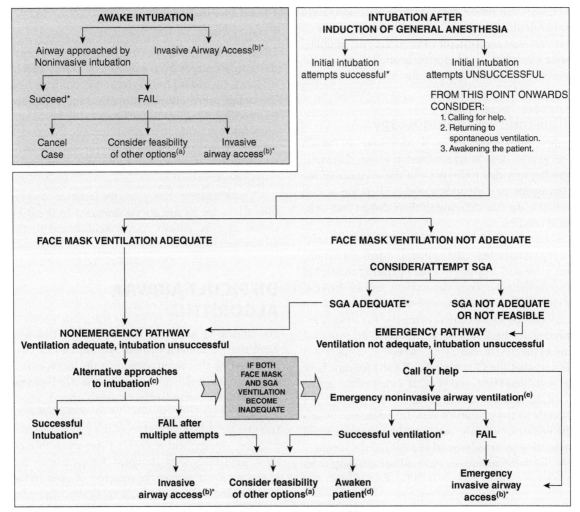

AWAKE INTUBATION

Airway approached by Noninvasive intubation   Invasive Airway Access[(b)]*

Succeed*   FAIL

Cancel Case   Consider feasibility of other options[(a)]   Invasive airway access[(b)]*

INTUBATION AFTER INDUCTION OF GENERAL ANESTHESIA

Initial intubation attempts successful*   Initial intubation attempts UNSUCCESSFUL

FROM THIS POINT ONWARDS CONSIDER:
1. Calling for help.
2. Returning to spontaneous ventilation.
3. Awakening the patient.

FACE MASK VENTILATION ADEQUATE   **FACE MASK VENTILATION NOT ADEQUATE**

CONSIDER/ATTEMPT SGA

SGA ADEQUATE*   SGA NOT ADEQUATE OR NOT FEASIBLE

NONEMERGENCY PATHWAY
Ventilation adequate, intubation unsuccessful   **EMERGENCY PATHWAY**
Ventilation not adequate, intubation unsuccessful

Alternative approaches to intubation[(c)]   IF BOTH FACE MASK AND SGA VENTILATION BECOME INADEQUATE   Call for help

Emergency noninvasive airway ventilation[(e)]

Successful Intubation*   FAIL after multiple attempts   Successful ventilation*   FAIL

Invasive airway access[(b)]*   Consider feasibility of other options[(a)]   Awaken patient[(d)]   Emergency invasive airway access[(b)]*

*Confirm ventilation, tracheal intubation, or SGA placement with exhaled CO_2.

a. Other options include (but are not limited to): surgery utilizing face mask or supraglottic airway (SGA) anesthesia (eg, LMA, ILMA, laryngeal tube), local anesthesia infiltration or regional nerve blockade. Pursuit of these options usually implies that mask ventilation will not be problematic. Therefore, these options may be of limited value if this step in the algorithm has been reached via the Emergency pathway.

b. Invasive airway access includes surgical or percutaneous airway, jet ventilation, and retrograde intubation.

c. Alternative difficult intubation approaches include (but are not limited to): video-assisted laryngoscopy, alternative laryngoscope blades, SGA (eg, LMA or ILMA) as an intubation conduct (with or without fiberoptic guidance), fiberoptic intubation, intubating stylet or tube changer, light wand, and blind oral or nasal intubation.

d. Consider re-preparation of the patient for awake intubation or cancelling surgery.

e. Emergency non-invasive airway ventilation consists of a SGA.

FIGURE 97–7 ASA difficult airway algorithm. (*Reproduced with permission from Apfelbaum JL, Hagberg CA, Caplan RA, et al: Practice guidelines for management of the difficult airway: an updated report by the American Society of Anesthesiologists Task Force on Management of the Difficult Airway, Anesthesiology. 2013 Feb;118(2):251-70.*)

in cardiac arrest should not delay initial CPR and defibrillation.[21]

The current American Heart Association guidelines for CPR included several changes related to airway management.[2,21] The traditional airway, breathing, circulation (ABC) was changed to compressions, airway, breathing (CAB).

Both bag-mask ventilation and ventilation with a bag through an advanced airway are acceptable methods of providing ventilation and oxygenation during CPR. The number and the duration of intubation attempts should be minimized, with a goal of no more than 10 seconds to minimize chest compression interruptions. Supraglottic devices may be reasonable alternatives to tracheal tubes.[21]

EXTUBATION

Extubation can be as challenging as intubation and is also fraught with potential complications. Reintubation can be complicated by the urgency of the situation, changes in airway anatomy (edema), and hemodynamic instability, among other factors already discussed.[2]

Planning for extubation should be performed immediately after intubation. The Difficult Airway Society Extubation guidelines published in 2012 suggest that patients should be approached as "low risk" and "high risk" for extubation. The high-risk patients with history of difficult intubation may be extubated using a supraglottic airway or an airway exchange catheter as a bridge to extubation, but more importantly a highly competent airway person should be at the bedside. Airway exchange catheters can be left in place as needed, are well tolerated by patients, and can be used as a conduit for reintubation.[2,22]

REFERENCES

1. Jaber S, Amraoui J, Lefrant JY, et al. Clinical practice and risk factors for immediate complications of endotracheal intubation in the intensive care unit: a prospective, multiple-center study. *Crit Care Med.* 2006;34(9):2355-2361.
2. Berkow L. What's new in airway management? ASA Refresher Courses. *Anesthesiology.* 2013;41(1):31-37.
3. Cook T, Woodall N, Frerk C. Fourth National Audit Project of the Royal College of Anaesthetists and The Difficult Airway Society. http://www.rcoa.ac.uk/node/4211. Accessed November 23, 2013.
4. Schwartz D, Matthay M, Cohen N. Death and other complications of emergency airway management in critically ill adults. *Anesthesiology.* 1995;82:367-376.
5. Le Tacon S, Wolter P, Rusterholtz T, et al. Complications of difficult tracheal intubation in a critical care unit. *Ann Fr Anesth Reanim.* 2000;19:719-724.
6. Henderson J. Airway management in the adult. In: Miller RD, Eriksson LI, Fleisher LA, eds. *Miller's Anesthesia.* Philadelphia, PA: Churchill Livingstone Elsevier; 2009:1573-1610.
7. Lippmann M. Endotracheal intubation. In: Kollef MH, ed. *The Washington Manual of Critical Care.* Philadelphia, PA: Lippincott Williams and Wilkins; 2012:582-587.
8. Walz JM, Kaur S, Heard SO. Airway management and endotracheal intubation. In: Irwin RS, ed. *Irwin and Rippe's Intensive Care Medicine.* Philadelphia, PA: Lippincott Williams and Wilkins; 2011:3-18.
9. Williamson D, Nolan J. Airway assessment. In: Benger J, ed. *Emergency Airway Management.* New York, NY: Cambridge University Press; 2008:19-23.
10. Finucane BT. Evaluation of the airway. In: Finucane BT, ed. *Principles of Airway Management.* New York, NY: Springer; 2011:27-58.
11. Murphy MF, Walls RM. Identification of the difficult airway. In: Murphy MF, ed. *Manual of Emergency Airway Management.* Philadelphia, PA: Lippincott Williams and Wilkins; 2012:8-21.
12. El-Ganzouri AR, McCarthy RJ, Tuman KJ, et al. Preoperative airway assessment: predictive value of a multivariate risk index. *Anesth Analg.* 1996;82:1197-1204.
13. Bannister FB, Macbeth RG. Direct intubation and tracheal intubation. *Lancet.* 1944;2:651-654.
14. Adnet F, Borron SW, Lapostolle F, Lapandry C. The three axis alignment theory and the "sniffing position": perpetuation of an anatomical myth? *Anesthesiology.* 1999;91:1964-1965.
15. Adnet F, Borron SW, Dumas JL, et al. Study of the "sniffing position" by magnetic resonance imaging. *Anesthesiology.* 2001;94:83-86.
16. Chou HC, Wu TL. Rethinking the three axes alignment theory for direct laryngoscopy. *Acta Anesthesiol Scand.* 2001;45:261-262.
17. Lim MST, Hunt-Smith JJ. Difficult airway management in the intensive care unit: alternative techniques. *Crit Care Resusc.* 2003;5:53-62.
18. Hamaekers AEW, Borg PAJ. Tracheal intubation: rigid indirect laryngoscopy. In: Calder I, Pearce A,

eds. *Core Topics in Airway Management*. New York, NY: Cambridge University Press; 2011:144-150.

19. Zafirova Z, Tung A. The difficult airway: definitions and algorithms. In: Glick DB, Copper RM, eds. *The Difficult Airway: An Atlas of Tools and Techniques for Clinical Management*. New York, NY: Springer; 2013:1-9.

20. Falk JA, Rackow EC, Weil MH. End-tidal carbon dioxide concentration during cardiopulmonary resuscitation. *N Engl J Med*. 1988;318:607-611.

21. Neumar RW, Otto CW, Link MS, et al. Part 8: adult advanced cardiovascular life support 2010 American Heart Association guidelines for cardiopulmonary resuscitation and emergency cardiovascular care. *Circulation*. 2019;122:S729-S767.

22. Popat M, Mitchel V, Dravid R, et al. Difficult Airway Society guidelines for the management of tracheal extubation. *Anaesthesia*. 2012;67:318-340.

Endoscopic Placement of Feeding Tubes

Isaac Soo, MD and Mark Schattner, MD

INTRODUCTION

Nutritional support is an important component of care for the critically ill. There are numerous modalities to provide specialized nutrition support including oral dietary therapy, enteral nutrition, and parenteral nutrition. For patients with a functioning gastrointestinal (GI) tract, enteral nutrition is preferred to parenteral nutrition. It is safer, more physiologic, and economical. In the intensive care unit (ICU) setting, enteral nutrition is associated with a decreased likelihood of developing infections when compared to parenteral nutrition.[1] In patients with acute pancreatitis, use of enteral nutrition is also associated with a reduction in hospital length of stay and a trend toward reduced organ failure when compared to parenteral nutrition.[2] Patients who have a functioning GI tract but are unable to safely ingest oral intake are fed via enteral access. In patients in whom long-term enteral access is required, endoscopically placed enteral access is recommended. Percutaneous endoscopically placed gastrostomy (PEG) and jejunostomy (PEJ) tubes are utilized for long-term enteral nutrition.

ENTERAL FEEDING TUBES

A majority of patients have enteral feeding tubes (EFTs) inserted through the mouth (orogastric) or nares (nasogastric) at the bedside that terminate in the gastric antrum. EFTs allow noninvasive access to the intestinal tract in patients who are unable to eat or drink. Examples of patients requiring EFT include sedated or unconscious patients such as those who are mechanically ventilated or have head injury. Severe oropharyngeal dysfunction that occurs in stroke patients or patients unwilling to have oral intake such as severe depression or anorexia are also candidates for EFT. Use of EFT is short term, typically less than 30 days. If enteral access is required beyond 30 days, a PEG or PEJ tube should be inserted. Contraindications for the placement of EFT include bowel ischemia, intestinal obstruction, and ileus.

Endoscopy is not required for the insertion of most EFTs. Indications for endoscopy include the presence of an esophageal obstruction or to facilitate postpyloric EFT placement. For esophageal obstruction the gastroscope is passed to the stricture, the feeding tube guided through the stricture under direct vision and advanced to the desired depth. Alternatives include placement of a guidewire through the stricture using the gastroscope biopsy channel, exchanging the gastroscope and guidewire to leave the wire in place and then placing an EFT over the guidewire. Also, the stricture can be dilated endoscopically prior to bedside placement.

Postpyloric feeding should be considered in patients with delayed gastric emptying, those with a history of regurgitation[3,4] as well as patients with acute severe pancreatitis. Jejunal feeds minimize pancreatic exocrine secretions by bypassing the upper GI tract and is a core aspect in treating acute severe pancreatitis. Comparisons between gastric and jejunal feedings have shown mixed results and a large prospective study is currently underway.[5–7] Patients with acute severe pancreatitis should receive jejunal feeds until more evidence is available. There are 4 endoscopic methods of postpyloric feeding tube placement:

1. *Drag and pull.* A suture is placed at the distal tip of the feeding tube and then passed via nares to the stomach followed by the gastroscope. Biopsy forceps through the gastroscope grasp the suture and advance together into the small bowel. The feeding tube is then left in position by grasp, advancement,

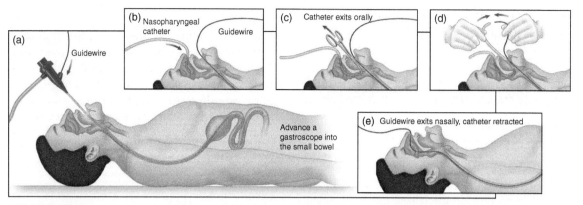

FIGURE 98–1 A-E Endoscopic insertion of feeding tubes. (*Memorial Sloan Kettering Cancer Center © 2014*).

release, and regrasp of the feeding tube while the gastroscope is retracted. Friction of the feeding tube against the gastroscope may lead to retraction of the EFT. Helpful maneuvers include decompression of the stomach to reduce looping within the stomach, liberal lubrication applied to the EFT and gastroscope, and using a feeding tube with an internal guidewire to provide stiffening (one 0.052-in or two 0.035-in guidewires placed through the EFT tube without exiting the tip of the tube). Alternatively, rather than using biopsy forceps an endoscopic clip may be used to grasp the attached suture and advance the EFT as desired. At the desired depth of insertion the hemoclip can then be used to affix the EFT suture to the small bowel mucosa. This approach has been demonstrated to increase the initial success rate of EFT placement and decrease retrograde tube migration with subsequent need for repeat endoscopy.[8]

2. *Over the guidewire.* Advance a gastroscope into the small bowel and exchange with a guidewire down the biopsy channel leaving the guidewire in situ. The guidewire exits orally and is changed to achieve nasal exit. A nasopharyngeal transfer tube is placed via the nares into the pharynx. The distal tip of the tube is grabbed using forceps to allow the distal end to exit orally. The guidewire is fed through this catheter to exit at the nose. Next the catheter is retracted nasally to leave guidewire

in situ (Figure 98–1). The EFT is fed over the guidewire to the small bowel.

3. *Through scope.* A small-diameter feeding tube can be fed through the biopsy channel of a therapeutic scope. A 240-cm 8- or 10-Fr gauge feeding tube is placed through the endoscope biopsy channel. The scope is exchanged with the EFT once the distal end of the feeding tube is in a suitable position. The extended length of the feeding tube allows it to remain in position as the scope is exchanged and removed over the feeding tube. The feeding tube is then cut to the desired length and oronasal transfer performed as presented earlier.

4. *Ultraslim gastroscope.* An ultrathin gastroscope is passed through the nares down the upper GI tract into the small bowel. A soft-tipped guidewire can be inserted in the channel and then exchanged with the gastroscope, leaving the guidewire in place. The EFT is then advanced over the guidewire and guidewire is removed once a suitable depth on EFT insertion is achieved.

PERCUTANEOUS ENDOSCOPIC GASTROSTOMY

Endoscopically placed gastrostomy tubes were first described in 1980 as an alternative to open surgical gastrostomy placement.[9] Since then numerous techniques have been developed and described. The

Ponsky-Pull method is the most commonly practiced method illustrated here.

Indications for PEG

Suitable candidates for insertion of PEG tubes for nutritional supplementation include the following:

- Inability to perform motor mechanisms of oral intake
- Functioning GI tract
- Anticipated requirement of nutritional support for over 30 days

Common indications for the placement of PEG tubes for nutritional supplementation include patients with stroke, head and neck cancer, as well as brain injury or neurologic disorders such as amyotrophic lateral sclerosis. Conversely, feeding tubes in patients with dementia have not shown improved clinical outcomes and are generally ineffective in prolonging life, improving function, or reducing risk of pressure sores or infections.[10]

Contraindications to PEG Placement

Absolute contraindications include a nonfunctional GI tract, active GI bleeding, uncorrected coagulopathy, hemodynamic instability, peritonitis, and abdominal wall infection over insertion site. The presence of ascites is a relative contraindication to PEG placement and depends on the amount, location, and type of ascites.

Complications

PEG tube insertion is a well-tolerated procedure with low incidence of complications; rates up to 4% have been reported. Complications may relate to either the insertion of the PEG tube or complications thereafter. These include stomal site infection, abdominal wall ulceration, necrotizing fasciitis, peristomal leakage, bleeding, transient gastroparesis, bowel perforation, gastric outlet obstruction from the internal bumper, buried bumper syndrome, colocutaneous fistula, peritonitis, and liver puncture. Pneumoperitoneum may be identified on radiologic imaging post-PEG insertion. This is an expected finding and is not worrisome in the absence of clinical signs of peritonitis.

Anesthesia

Insertion of endoscopically placed PEG or PEJ tubes is done with a combination of local anesthesia and sedation. A short-acting benzodiazepine (ie, midazolam) in combination with an opioid such as fentanyl is a common practice. In some instances patients may receive deeper sedation via propofol, or in some cases general anesthesia, under the guidance of a nurse anesthetist or anesthesiologist.

Equipment Required

See Figure 98–2 for typical PEG kit components.

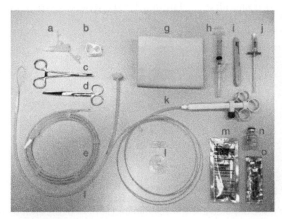

a. Y-Port
b. C-Clamp
c. Curved hemostat
d. Scissors
e. Guidewire
f. PEG tube
g. Drape
h. Syringe
i. Scalpel
j. Trocar cannula
k. Retrieval snare
l. External bolsters
m. Iodine swabs
n. Local anesthetic
o. Lubricating jelly

FIGURE 98–2 A-O Typical PEG kit components.

Personnel

PEG tube insertion generally requires 2 individuals to perform the procedure. One individual functions as the endoscopist and the other as the surgical assistant.

Preparation and Antibiotic Prophylaxis

The patient is kept NPO the night before the procedure. There is creation of a surgical wound during the creation of the gastrostomy and antibiotic prophylaxis is given to prevent abdominal wall infection. A single dose of a first-generation cephalosporin is given prior to PEG tube insertion to reduce the risk of infection. Patients in the ICU often receive significant antimicrobial coverage and as long as there is preexisting gram-positive organism coverage, additional antibiotics are not required. The patient is supine with the head turned to the side and suction available for significant oral secretions. A routine upper GI examination is performed prior to PEG insertion.

Landmarking

The epigastrium is the typical location for PEG placement but can vary. The final site is dependent on appropriate landmarking. The final location for the gastrostomy tube should be at least an inch away from the costal margins and clear of the xiphoid process.

The stomach is inflated to maximally appose the gastric wall with the abdominal wall. This facilitates the 2 maneuvers to identify a suitable PEG insertion site, the absence of any underlying vessel or interposing tissue such as bowel or liver edge. First

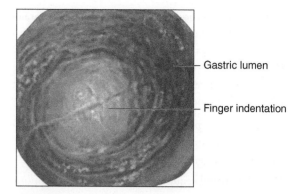

FIGURE 98–4 When point pressure is applied to the abdominal wall, the endoscopic image shows 1:1 transmission of movement. (*Memorial Sloan Kettering Cancer Center ©2014*).

is diaphanoscopy, adequate transillumination of the endoscopy light through the abdominal wall. The endoscopy suite lights are dimmed and transilluminated light from the endoscope should be clearly visible on the anterior abdominal wall (Figure 98–3). The second is 1:1 transmission of abdominal wall pressure. The endoscopic view is directed at the gastric wall corresponding to the point of external point pressure. When point pressure is applied to the abdominal wall, the endoscopic image shows 1:1 transmission of movement (Figure 98–4). Mark the site PEG placement with surgical pen marking.

Site Preparation

PEG placement requires sterile technique with skin disinfection, sterile gloves, and draping. The landmark is washed with povidone/iodine or

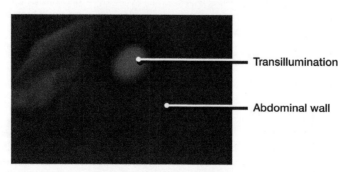

FIGURE 98–3 The endoscopy suite lights are dimmed and transilluminated light from the endoscope should be clearly visible on the anterior abdominal wall.

chlorhexidine wash, 3 times in concentric swirls starting from the landmark site outwards. After the surgical drape is applied local anesthesia with a total of 3 to 5 mL of 1% lidocaine should be injected subcutaneously, followed by injection toward the gastric lumen. Direct the syringe perpendicular to the abdominal wall and apply local anesthesia with periodic suction to inspect for blood return and possible puncture of a blood vessel. Significant heme return should prompt a different site for PEG insertion. The syringe will puncture into the gastric lumen, seen endoscopically to confirm an acceptable PEG location. The depth and direction of the syringe serves as a guide for insertion of the trocar/catheter apparatus.

GASTROSTOMY TUBE INSERTION

Inflate the stomach to facilitate the trocar penetration through the muscular gastric wall. The trocar/catheter apparatus is applied to the abdominal wall in a firm and steady fashion. At all times the endoscope visualizes the point of trocar insertion to monitor the site for location confirmation and applied force of the trocar toward the gastric lumen. This avoids trauma of the posterior gastric wall and underlying structures by overzealous force. Remove the trocar from the trocar/catheter apparatus after it has entered the gastric lumen. A guidewire is inserted through the catheter. Advance a snare through the channel of the gastroscope and grasp the guidewire. One end of the guidewire and gastroscope are pulled out through the mouth. The surgical assistant must ensures that at all times a portion of the guidewire remains external to the catheter on the abdominal wall. Once out of the mouth, the guidewire is released from the snare and affixed to the gastrostomy tube. The loop of the guidewire is inserted through the loop of the gastrostomy tube and then opened and passed over top of the gastrostomy bumper. The 2 pieces of equipment are then pulled, interlocking the loops of the guidewire and gastrostomy tube. The abdominal wall is prepared to allow penetration of the large caliber PEG tube through the abdominal wall. Cut an approximately 1-cm epidermal incision along the trocar puncture site. A deeper incision is not required and will only

worsen postprocedural pain and possible bleeding. Apply a small amount of lubricant onto the gastrostomy tube. Significant amounts may result in pooling of lubricant in the hypopharynx increasing possible aspiration risk and airway compromise. The surgical assistant then pulls the guidewire with the attached gastrostomy tube away from the catheter/abdominal wall. The PEG tube slides down through the mouth and through the abdominal wall. The catheter remains in place during this motion to avoid damage to the surrounding tissue. While pulling on the guidewire resistance is met once the transition from the guidewire to the gastrostomy tube is encountered by the gastric wall. Brace the abdominal wall with taut pressure on the guidewire until the tip of the PEG tube passes through the abdominal wall. Gently continue pulling the PEG tube until resistance is again met, when the internal bumper rests up against the gastric wall (Figure 98–5). An alternative to tactile feedback to indicate appropriate PEG positioning is to insert the gastroscope into the esophagus with direct visualization of the gastrostomy tube while it is pulled into position. In either case the endoscope should visualize the internal gastrostomy site to ensure adequate hemostasis. Cut the guidewire from the PEG tube and slide the external bumper over the tube and down toward the abdominal wall to affix the tube in place. At an appropriate tautness, the external bumper should rest comfortably just above abdominal wall without evidence of significant tension on the skin surrounding the gastrostomy site. There should be no more than 1 cm of PEG tube between the external bumper and abdominal wall when the PEG tube is lifted taut. Decide an appropriate length for the gastrostomy tube, cut and discard the remainder, before placing the clamp and gastrostomy cap onto the PEG tube. The gastrostomy tube can be used for feeding and medication following insertion.

PEG WITH JEJUNAL EXTENSION

Patients with a PEG tube can have an extension placed through the PEG tube into the small bowel. For these cases a large-bore PEG (usually 24 or 28 Fr) is used and the jejunal extensions are 9 to

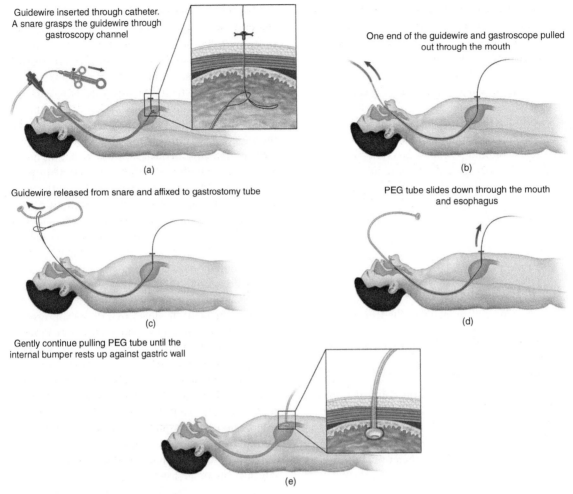

Guidewire inserted through catheter. A snare grasps the guidewire through gastroscopy channel

(a)

One end of the guidewire and gastroscope pulled out through the mouth

(b)

Guidewire released from snare and affixed to gastrostomy tube

(c)

PEG tube slides down through the mouth and esophagus

(d)

Gently continue pulling PEG tube until the internal bumper rests up against gastric wall

(e)

FIGURE 98–5 Gently continue pulling the PEG tube until resistance is again met, when the internal bumper rests up against the gastric wall. (*Memorial Sloan Kettering Cancer Center © 2014*).

12 Fr. For PEG-J extensions there are 3 methods described.

1. *Pull method.* A jejunostomy tube (JT) is advanced through the preexisting PEG tube and grasped by biopsy forceps through the gastroscope channel. The gastroscope is advanced into the small bowel and the biopsy forceps advance the JT distally. After a suitable placement is achieved, as the gastroscope is retracted the biopsy forceps continue to advance the JT until the gastroscope reaches the gastric body and is removed.

2. *Guidewire.* A gastroscope is advanced from the mouth into the stomach and a guidewire is passed through the PEG tube into the stomach. The wire is then grasped by biopsy forceps and pulled as far as possible into the small bowel using the gastroscope. The gastroscope and forceps are removed and a JT is fed over the guidewire into position with subsequent guidewire removal.

3. *Ultrathin gastroscope*: An ultrathin gastroscope is advanced directly through the PEG. Via the biopsy channel a guidewire is placed. The gastroscope is removed via exchange with the

guidewire to leave the guidewire in place. The jejunal extension is passed over the guidewire into the small bowel and the guidewire is subsequently removed.

DIRECT PERCUTANEOUS JEJUNOSTOMY TUBE INSERTION

The placement of direct percutaneous endoscopic jejunostomy (DPEJ) tubes has become more common in recent years. Indications for DPEJ insertion rather than PEG include (1) high risk for aspiration, (2) status postgastric resection, (3) status postesophagectomy, (4) gastric outlet obstruction, (5) obstructed or nonfunctioning gastrojejunostomy, and (6) gastric dysmotility. In comparison to PEG-J and nasojejunal (NJ) tubes, DPEJ has been found to decrease the risk of aspiration in patients.[11] The lack of effectiveness in preventing aspiration in NJ and PEG-J tubes may relate to their smaller caliber with a greater propensity for blockage and tube migration (DPEJ tubes are 18-20 Fr, larger than PEG-J tubes 9-12 Fr). Contraindications to DPEJ insertion are the same as for PEG tubes. Potential complications include bowel perforation, jejunal volvuli, bleeding, aspiration, chronic enterocutaneous fistulae, site infections, and persistent site pain.[12]

Procedure

Many of the maneuvers to insert a DPEJ are similar to PEG tube insertion. However, there are several notable aspects that differ between DPEJ and PEG placement. Employment of a pediatric colonoscope may be required to reach the jejunum; a gastroscope may be used if there has been a prior gastrectomy. For the choice of jejunostomy tube, balloon-type inflatable mechanisms should be avoided as they are prone to obstruct the bowel lumen. Bumper-style jejunostomy tubes are preferred.

Landmarking

In terms of location for DPEJ placement, the site may vary throughout the abdomen. It is not unusual for the DPEJ to be placed in the suprapubic or flank regions. In patients with prior surgery the DPEJ operators should be aware of the altered anatomy and be cognizant for potential limitations or preferences for the site of DPEJ placement (ie, afferent vs efferent jejunal limb). Successful site landmarking requires a greater degree of precision in DPEJ in comparison to PEG. The diaphanoscopy may be falsely reassuring due to the existence of a "periscope effect" from the tortuous course of the small intestine. Transillumination on the abdomen may be the result of the endoscope light source reflecting throughout different points of the bowel wall rather than representing the true position of the endoscope tip. For this reason finger indentation must be particularly precise, in combination with diaphanoscopy, to locate an appropriate DPEJ site. Due to the mobile nature of the small bowel it may take several passes through the jejunum until a suitable location is identified. Once diaphanoscopy and finger indentation prospect a site the negative needle aspiration test can be performed. Following sterile preparation and during local anesthesia, aspiration of the needle is intermittently applied. The operator should look to the syringe now not only for blood that would indicate an underlying blood vessel, but stool as well that would indicate needle insertion into the colon. If this occurs, the needle should be withdrawn and a different location for DPEJ insertion sought. All landmarking maneuvers must be done swiftly due to the mobile nature of the small bowel.

JEJUNOSTOMY TUBE INSERTION

Following successful landmarking and injection of local anesthesia, once the needle has been identified endoscopically it remains held in place in the jejunum. This differs from PEG insertion where the needle is removed. The trocar is then applied beside the needle as close as possible to imitate its course through the abdomen. This reduces the likelihood of inadvertently penetrating abdominal vessels or structures. Once the trocar/catheter apparatus is successfully inserted into the small bowel the needle can be removed and the remainder of DPEJ insertion is similar to PEG insertion via the "pull" technique as presented earlier.

SUMMARY

Nutrition support is a vital component of care for critically ill patients. There are multiple modalities at the disposal of the medical team to ensure adequate nutrient delivery to the patient. The choice of intervention is dictated by the clinical scenario and technical expertise available.

REFERENCES

1. Heyland DK, Dhaliwal R, Drover JW, et al. Canadian clinical practice guidelines for nutrition support in mechanically ventilated, critically ill adult patients. *JPEN J Parenter Enteral Nutr.* 2003;27(5):355-373.
2. McClave SA, Chang WK, Dhaliwal R, et al. Nutrition support in acute pancreatitis: a systematic review of the literature. *JPEN J Parenter Enteral Nutr.* 2006;30(2):143-156.
3. Ho KM, Dobb GJ, Webb SA. A comparison of early gastric and post-pyloric feeding in critically ill patients: a meta-analysis. *Intensive Care Med.* 2006;32(5):639-649.
4. McClave SA, Martindale RG, Vanek VW, et al. Guidelines for the provision and assessment of nutrition support therapy in the adult critically ill patient: Society of Critical Care Medicine (SCCM) and American Society for Parenteral and Enteral Nutrition (A.S.P.E.N.). *JPEN J Parenter Enteral Nutr.* 2009;33(3):277-316.
5. Kumar A, Singh N, Prakash S, et al. Early enteral nutrition in severe acute pancreatitis: a prospective randomized controlled trial comparing nasojejunal and nasogastric routes. *J Clin Gastroenterol.* 2006;40(5):431-434.
6. Eatock FC, Chong P, Menezes N, et al. A randomized study of early nasogastric versus nasojejunal feeding in severe acute pancreatitis. *Am J Gastroenterol.* 2005;100(2):432-439.
7. Eckerwall GE, Axelsson JB, Andersson RG. Early nasogastric feeding in predicted severe acute pancreatitis: a clinical, randomized study. *Ann Surg.* 2006;244(6):959-967.
8. Hirdes MM, Monkelbaan JF, Haringman JJ, et al. Endoscopic clip-assisted feeding tube placement reduces repeat endoscopy rate: results from a randomized controlled trial. *Am J Gastroenterol.* 2012;107(8):1220-1227.
9. Gauderer MW, Ponsky JL, Izant RJ, Jr. Gastrostomy without laparotomy: a percutaneous endoscopic technique. *J Pediatr Surg.* 1980;15(6):872-875.
10. Finucane TE, Christmas C, Travis K. Tube feeding in patients with advanced dementia: a review of the evidence. *JAMA.* 1999;282(14):1365-1370.
11. Panagiotakis PH, DiSario JA, Hilden K, et al. DPEJ tube placement prevents aspiration pneumonia in high-risk patients. *Nutr Clin Pract.* 2008;23(2):172-175.
12. Maple JT, Petersen BT, Baron TH, et al. Direct percutaneous endoscopic jejunostomy: outcomes in 307 consecutive attempts. *Am J Gastroenterol.* 2005;100(12):2681-2688.

Continuous Venovenous Hemofiltration

Anthony Manasia, MD, FCCP and Renzo H. Hidalgo, MD

KEY POINTS

1. Understanding the fundamental principles of continuous venovenous hemofiltration (CVVH), how it differs from hemodialysis, and its use in the critically ill patient is essential for all intensivists.

2. CVVH should be the intensivist's first choice as renal replacement therapy for any intensive care unit (ICU) patient with hemodynamic instability.

3. Continuous renal replacement therapy (CRRT) is most often prescribed based on body weight to an effluent flow rate target

of 20 to 25 mL/kg/h. Effluent flow rates higher than 25 mL/kg/h do not improve outcomes in ICU patients.

4. Anticoagulation is generally recommended, as the clotting cascades are activated when the blood interfaces with the nonendothelial surfaces of the tubing and filter.

5. Administration of replacement fluid (RF) maintains fluid balance and lowers the plasma concentration of solute by dilution. Typical RF rates are 1000 to 2000 mL/h.

INTRODUCTION

CVVH is a form of CRRT that has a slower rate of solute or fluid removal per unit of time. It is generally better tolerated than conventional intermittent hemodialysis as many of the complications of hemodialysis are related to the rapid rate of solute and fluid loss as well as complement-induced hypotension. Acute kidney injury (AKI) occurs in up to 70% of patients admitted to the ICU and is associated with an increased mortality rate.[1] CRRT is the treatment of choice in critically ill septic patients in the ICU.[2,3] Sepsis leads to renal hypoperfusion and subsequent volume resuscitation that cannot be autoregulated by the already insufficient kidney. This is further compounded by the numerous nephrotoxic medications and contrast agents used in diagnosis and treatment. Mortality from AKI is commonly the result of

multiorgan system failure (MOSF). Growing evidence suggests that AKI may also damage the lungs, brain, heart, or liver. Some forms of renal replacement therapy (RRT) may prevent MOSF.[4] There is also evidence that fluid overload increases mortality and that volume control can improve outcomes.[5-7] This has shifted the trend toward more aggressive and earlier RRT.

THE RIFLE AND ACUTE KIDNEY INJURY NETWORK CLASSIFICATIONS OF ACUTE KIDNEY INJURY

The acute dialysis quality initiative (ADQI) developed the following classification of AKI to foster uniformity in both research and clinical practice (Tables 99–1 and 99–2).

TABLE 99–1 RIFLE classification.

	GFR Criteria	Urine Output Criteria
Risk	Increased serum creatinine × 1.5 or GFR decrease > 25%	UO < 0.5 mL/kg/h × 6 h
Injury	Increased serum creatinine × 2 or GFR decrease > 50%	UO < 0.5 mL/kg/h × 12 h
Failure	Increased serum creatinine × 3, GFR decrease > 75% or serum creatinine > 4 mg/dL (acute rise > 0.5 mg/dL)	UO < 0.3 mL/kg/h × 24 h or anuria × 12 h
Loss	Persistent AKI: complete loss of kidney function > 4 wk	
ESKD	End-stage kidney disease: complete loss of kidney function > 3 mo	
AKIN 1	Increased serum creatinine by 1.5-2× above baseline or by 0.3 mg/dL	UO < 0.5 mL/kg/h × 6 h
AKIN 2	Increased serum creatinine by 2-3× above baseline	UO < 0.5 mL/kg/h × 12 h
AKIN 3	Increased serum creatinine by > 3× above baseline or by ≥ 0.3 mg/dL in patients with baseline serum creatinine > 4 mg/dL	UO < 0.3 mL/kg/h × 24 h or anuria for 12 h

AKI, acute kidney injury; AKIN, acute kidney injury network; GFR, glomerular filtration rate; RIFLE, risk, injury, failure, loss, end-stage renal disease; UO, urine output.

The acute kidney injury network (AKIN) classification is based on the risk, injury, failure, loss, end-stage renal disease (RIFLE) system with a few relevant modifications.[8] First, it uses smaller increments in serum creatinine for the diagnosis of AKI. Second, it introduces a 48-hour time for diagnosis. Last, it eliminates the "loss" and "failure" categories as these represent outcomes, and should not be listed as part of the diagnosis. Recent evidence indicates that even minor declines in glomerular filtration rate

TABLE 99–2 The presence of one the following indications suggests, 2 indications strongly suggest, and 3 indications mandate initiation of RRT.

- Anuria/oliguria (diuresis ≤ 200 mL in 12 h)
- Severe metabolic acidosis (pH < 7.10)
- Hyperazotemia (BUN ≥ 80 mg/dL) or creatinine > 4 mg/dL
- Hyperkalemia (K⁺ ≥ 6.5 mEq/L)

- Clinical signs of uremic toxicity
- Severe dysnatremia (Na⁺ ≤ 115 or ≥ 160 mEq/L)
- Hyperthermia (temperature > 40°C without response to medical therapy)
- Anasarca or severe fluid overload
- Multiple organ failure with renal dysfunction and/or systemic inflammatory reaction syndrome (SIRS), sepsis, or septic shock with renal dysfunction

BUN, blood urea nitrogen.
Reproduced with permission from Gabrielli A, Layon AJ, Yu M: Civetta, Taylor, & Kirby's *Manual of Critical Care*. Philadelphia: Lippincott Williams & Wilkins; 2012.

are associated with increased mortality in different populations of hospitalized patients. A meta-analysis of 8 studies observed a graded relationship between the amount of elevation of serum creatinine and mortality in AKI.[9] Regardless of ICU type or clinical scenario, creatinine elevations of 10% to 24% above baseline resulted in a relative risk of 1.8 (1.3-2.5) for short-term mortality (30 days or less); patients with a rise of 25% to 49% had a relative risk of 3 (1.6-5.8), and those with greater than 50% increase had a risk of 6.9 (2-24.5). These data justify the "tighter" criteria proposed in the AKIN classification. Neutrophil gelatinase–associated lipocalin (NGAL) is a protein expressed in multiple tissues that is upregulated in proximal tubular cells immediately following ischemic injury has been studied as a biomarker of early kidney injury.[10] Likewise, interleukin 18 (IL-18), cystatin C, and kidney injury molecule 1 (KIM-1) have all been studied and demonstrated the usefulness in early detection of acute renal injury.

RRT IN ACUTE KIDNEY INJURY

Intermittent hemodialysis has long been the preferred method of RRT in the United States. However, CRRT is gaining in popularity and is now reported to account for 36% of prescribed RRT treatments.[11] Internationally, continuous therapies had become the norm for AKI support.[12] "Beginning and Ending Supportive Therapy for the Kidney" (BEST Kidney), a multinational, prospective study reported that CRRT with RRT support was used in 80% of treatments in the ICU, distantly followed by intermittent hemodialysis (17%).[13] No evidence currently supports the superiority of one continuous modality over another or continuous over intermittent treatment. Choice of RRT modality should be based on clinical judgment and experience of the prescribing physician as well as the technologic, fiscal, and nursing resources available to deliver RRT.

PRINCIPLES OF SOLUTE CLEARANCE AND FLUID REMOVAL BY DIALYSIS AND CONVECTION

Dialysis therapies involve the movement of solute and plasma water across a semipermeable membrane separating a blood compartment and a dialysate compartment. This process occurs within a cartridge called a hemofilter or hemodialyzer. Characteristics such as membrane thickness and pore dimensions determine the size and transfer rate of molecules that move between the blood and dialysate. Removal of solute and water in RRT may occur by diffusion or convection (Figure 99–1). Diffusion involves movement of solute down a concentration gradient, from areas of high concentration to low concentration. Conversely, water will move from an area of low osmolality to an area of high osmolality. Solvent drag is a phenomenon by which large shifts of water pull some solute through the membrane. In a static system, net transfer (dialysis) ceases when solute concentrations equilibrate in the compartments. For RRT, blood and dialysate are continuously replenished to maintain the high concentration gradients favoring maximum transfer of solute and water. Convection involves the transfer of solute across a semipermeable membrane driven by a hydrostatic pressure gradient. Those solutes small enough to pass through pores are swept along with water by solvent drag; substitution fluid is required to prevent excessive fluid removal. The membrane acts as a sieve, retaining molecules that exceed the pore size. All filtered solutes below the membrane pore size are removed at rates proportionate to their concentration. The convective removal of fluid in this manner is termed hemofiltration or ultrafiltration. This technique does not change the plasma concentration of small solutes (blood urea nitrogen [BUN], creatinine, electrolytes, glucose), as water is removed in proportion to solute. In contrast, the concentration of larger molecules, such as albumin, increase as they are sieved off by the smaller membrane pores. Thus, the chemical composition of the filtrate (ultrafiltrate) is almost identical to that of the plasma except for the absence of large molecules such as albumin. The administration of substitution fluid will dilute the plasma concentrations of those solutes (such as urea, creatinine, or potassium) not present in the substitution fluid.

In summary, whether or not a solute is diffused is inversely proportional to its molecular weight. The higher the molecular weight the more inefficient the diffusion.

INDICATIONS FOR INITIATION OF CVVH

The modern paradigm recognizes that AKI is an independent risk factor for death[14-16] and that the aggressive management of RRT may affect outcomes

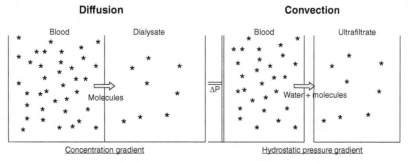

FIGURE 99–1 Renal replacement therapy in the ICU. (*Data from Rimmelé T, Kellum JA: Renal Replacement Therapy in the ICU. PCCSU 24, 2010.*)

and reduce mortality.[17-19] However, there is no consensus on the optimal time to initiate RRT. This has led to a wide variation in clinical practice. Traditionally the indication for RRT[20] has been based on or a combination of the following: volume overload, such as pulmonary edema that is not controlled with diuretic use, hyperkalemia-induced arrhythmias, uncontrolled metabolic acidosis, intoxication with a dialyzable drug or toxin, and overt uremic signs such as encephalopathy, pericarditis, or even uremic bleeding diathesis.

Access for RRT

The optimal access for hemodialysis are arteriovenous fistulas (AVFs) that provide high blood flow (> 500 mL/min), durable long-term vascular access, relatively low thrombosis rates, and low infection rates. AVFs require months to mature and be functional, making them unsuitable for patients with AKI. AVFs cannot withstand prolonged cannulation associated with CCRT. Therefore with CVVH a temporary central venous catheter is needed. These catheters are generally noncuffed, nontunneled, double lumen with a large diameter of 12 to 15 Fr, providing a flow between 200 and 500 mL/min. They contain a venous and an "arterial" lumen although both lumens are in the same vein. The arterial lumen (typically red) withdraws blood from the patient and carries it to the CVVH machine, while the venous lumen (typically blue) returns blood to the patient from the machine. These catheters are typically constructed of materials such as polyurethane and are relatively stiff at room temperature, but become pliable at body temperature. They are inserted at the bedside. The internal jugular or femoral veins are preferred, over the subclavian vein due to the risk of developing venous stenosis after placement precluding future placement of an AVF in the ipsilateral arm.

Dosing

Despite the widespread use of CRRT, there is little consensus regarding the optimum delivery of RRT, resulting in wide variations in clinical practice.[21] Some studies have suggested survival benefit from delivery of higher-intensity CRRT to patients with AKI, whereas other studies have been inconsistent in their results. CRRT is most often prescribed based on the body weight to effluent flow rate target of 20 to 25 mL/kg/h. Recent studies have shown that effluent flow rate higher than 25 mL/kg/h does not improve outcomes in ICU patients.[22] In our institution, the typical rates used for CVVH are a blood flow rate of 200 mL/min and RF rate of 2 L/h with ultrafiltration rate based on the individual need for fluid balance. This rate is variable and changes every hour depending on the total input and output of the previous hour. For example, if the desired fluid balance is –50 mL/h with a total input of 200 mL and output of 100 mL from the previous hour, the balance is +100 mL, therefore the ultrafiltration rate will be set at 150 mL/h.

Anticoagulation

Although CRRT can be run without anticoagulation, filters last much longer if some form of anticoagulation is used. Their fibers are prone to thrombosis, as removal of fluid through ultrafiltration leads to hemoconcentration at the distal end. Anticoagulation is generally recommended, as the clotting cascades are activated when the blood touches the nonendothelial surfaces of the tubing and filter. Multiple options exist for anticoagulation including heparin, prostacyclin, citrate, and even direct thrombin inhibitors. Unfractionated heparin is most commonly used, but can result in systemic anticoagulation and may be contraindicated in patients with active hemorrhage or heparin-induced thrombocytopenia (HIT). Any dose less than 5 units/kg/h is considered low-dose prefilter unfractionated heparin. This dose is reported to have minimal effect on the activated partial thromboplastin time (aPTT). A dose between 8 and 10 units/kg/h is considered medium-dose prefilter unfractionated heparin. This dose mildly elevates the aPTT and is recommended for patients with minimal risk of bleeding. Heparin may be administered using a pump integrated into the CRRT machine, or via a separate volumetric pump. Systemic unfractionated heparin is reserved for patients with other indications for systemic anticoagulation and is administered intravenously and titrated to achieve a target aPTT of about 1.5 to 2.5 times above the patient's baseline. For patients with high risk of bleeding regional unfractionated heparin to the CVVH blood circuit may be used. In this technique, a prefilter dose of 1500 units/h of heparin combined with administration of protamine postfilter at a dose of 10 to 12 mg/h is used. This approach is monitored with the aPTT to keep it as close to normal as possible. Another option for these patients is the use of citrate. Citrate regional anticoagulation is widely used and has become the primary mode of anticoagulation in many centers. Citrate infused in the arterial limb of the CRRT circuit prevents hemofilter thrombosis by chelating calcium, a critical component of the clotting cascade. Calcium chloride infused into the venous line of the system restores normal systemic calcium levels. This approach appears to reduce the risk of hemorrhage and extend hemofilter patency.[23] In addition, citrate can be used for patients with HIT. Serum and ionized calcium levels should be carefully monitored, especially in patients with significant liver dysfunction, and the calcium infusion appropriately adjusted. Citrate is hepatically metabolized into bicarbonate and can cause metabolic alkalosis. In the setting of hepatic failure, citrate accumulation results in elevated serum but low ionized calcium levels, reflecting increased circulating calcium bound to citrate.

Filters

Semipermeable membranes are the basis of all blood purification therapies. The surface area of the membrane depends on the number and length of these fibers. Membrane surface area affects solute clearance and ultrafiltration. Membrane size or surface area varies with the specific model of hemodialyzer or hemofilter. Larger dialysis cartridges are used for patients with a larger surface area or those needing high solute clearances. They allow water and some solutes to pass through the membrane, while cellular components and other solutes remain behind. The water and solutes that pass through the membrane are called the ultrafiltrate. Pore dimensions determine the size selectivity of molecular flux across the membrane, typically pore size membranes are 30,000 Da. Low-flux (< 500 Da) membranes clear small molecules (urea, potassium, and creatinine), but do not clear the larger "middle molecules" that may act as toxins. High-flux membranes (< 20,000 Da) clear middle molecules, such as β_2-microglobulin and perhaps inflammatory cytokines generated by AKI and MOSF. There are 2 types of membranes used in RRT: cellulose and synthetic. Synthetic membranes are biocompatible, high flux, which allow clearance of larger molecules causing less trauma to platelets and white blood cells (WBCs), and are thus primarily used in CRRT. Filters are changed when they become contaminated, clogged, or according to individual hospital protocols.

REPLACEMENT FLUID

RFs are used to increase the amount of convective solute clearance in CVVH by replacing large volumes of ultrafiltrate with fluids that do not contain the solutes targeted for removal. Solute clearance and volume removal are adjusted by altering the ultrafiltration rate and the rate of infusion of RF. They can be replaced before or after the filter depending on individual needs (Figure 99–2). As the filtration fraction (FF), that is, the proportion of plasma flow

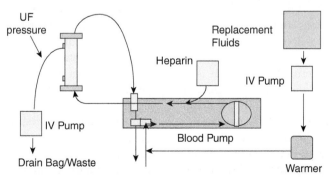

FIGURE 99–2 Early and intensive continuous hemofiltration for severe renal failure after cardiac surgery. (*Reproduced with permission from Bent P, Tan HK, Bellomo R, et al: Early and intensive continuous hemofiltration for severe renal failure after cardiac surgery, Ann Thorac Surg. 2001 Mar;71(3):832-837.*)

that is filtered, increases, the risk of filter thrombosis also rises. Higher rates of ultrafiltration, especially if coupled with low blood flows, predispose to hemofilter thrombosis. Poor filter performance and filter clotting increase sharply at FF greater than 20%. Higher blood flow rates permit greater rates of fluid removal, as hemoconcentration within the filter is limited by the short transit time of blood through the dialysis cartridge. In CVVH, blood flow rates are typically low and ultrafiltration rates are high, which is a significant barrier to effective implementation of these therapies. One approach called predilutional hemofiltration, which is preferred by the authors, involves infusion of RF into the CRRT circuit at a point before the filter, thus lowering the hematocrit through dilution. As a result, a higher ultrafiltration rate may be achieved without compromising filter life. Prefilter RF also dilutes the solute concentration of blood entering the filter and reduces effective clearance. The administration of RF maintains fluid balance and lowers the plasma concentration of solute by dilution. Typical RF rates are 1000 to 2000 mL/h. Rates slower than this are not effective for convective solute removal, but should not exceed one-third of the blood flow rate per hour. There are a number of variable RFs available including normal saline, plasmalyte, or specific commercial products for CVVH with variable electrolyte concentration depending on the clinical condition of the patient as well as the patient's fluid, electrolyte, acid-base, and glucose balance.

COMPLICATIONS OF CVVH

Local bleeding can occur at the vascular access site or might be subcutaneous and not obvious. The access site should be closely monitored for bleeding, hematoma, or ecchymosis. Femoral lines in particular may cause internal bleeding that is not immediately apparent. Monitor the hemoglobin or hematocrit and vital signs closely as they may indicate occult bleeding. Inadvertent disconnection of the CRRT blood circuit could lead to significant blood loss. Modern CRRT machines are equipped with alarms and cutoff switches to minimize this risk. Watch for low access pressure alarms and low return pressure alarms, as they could indicate a

disconnection. Generalized bleeding complications can occur as a side effect of anticoagulation or as a result of critical illness itself. It is vital to monitor the platelet count for thrombocytopenia, coagulation factors, and fibrinogen for signs of disseminated intravascular coagulation (DIC). Care should be taken when priming the tubing as to prevent air bubbles from entering the systemic circulation and causing an air embolism. Hypothermia is another potential complication because of the extracorporeal circulation during CVVH and exposure of RFs to room temperature. Patient's body temperature should be kept above 36°C to maintain adequate hemodynamics and effective hemostasis. Newer CVVH machines have blood warmers integrated into them. Inline fluid and blood warmers are also available so that fluids can be warmed prior to administration. Most CRRT protocols require monitoring of electrolytes and pH every 4 to 6 hours during the first 24 hours of therapy and whenever RFs are changed. CRRT is an invasive process that increases the risk of infection in a patient that is already vulnerable due to renal failure, critical illness, and other invasive lines and procedures. These patients must be monitored closely for signs and symptoms of infection so treatment can be initiated as rapidly as possible. Infections caused by CVVH may be local to the vascular access site or systemic. It is important to remember that when CVVH is in progress fever may be masked due to the cooling effect of extracorporeal circulation. Monitor for other signs of infection such as elevated white blood cell count, increased numbers of immature WBCs, and local symptoms like redness, swelling, and purulent drainage. All connections and vascular access sites must be handled with meticulous aseptic technique to minimize the risk of infection. As patients receiving CVVH will clear renally excreted drugs efficiently, dosing of these drugs should not be reduced for renal function while on CVVH unless clinically indicated. After initiation of CRRT drug levels may need to be drawn to ensure adequate plasma concentrations especially for antibiotics and anticonvulsants. Drips of renally cleared drugs may need to be titrated up while on CVVH and likewise may need to be decreased once CVVH is stopped. Special care must be taken when discontinuing CVVH as certain drugs may build up to toxic levels.

Troubleshooting

Although there are many different types of CVVH machines and each one has its own individual characteristics, we will review some general issues. The access pressure is normally negative; however, excessive negative pressure usually indicates an occlusion somewhere in the access limb of the blood circuit. The complete tubing system should be inspected in search of kinks and stopcocks should be confirmed for proper position. Vascular access should also be evaluated for poor position or swelling at the site. The patient should be positioned properly to minimize flexion near the insertion site and the access port should be aspirated and manually flushed. The return pressure is normally positive and low return pressures could indicate a disconnection at some point, return tubing should be checked for proper connections. Low return pressures can also be encountered when patients are laterally rotated due to orthostatic changes in venous pressure. Alarms that occur due to position changes will usually resolve within a couple of minutes. High return pressures can occur because of occlusions. Filter pressure alarms usually only sound when the filter is clogged or clotted. Initial filter pressures should be measured each time a new filter is placed. Filter pressure usually remains stable throughout therapy. The filter pressure can be trended to help for predict clotting. CVVH machines can detect blood leaks indicating broken filaments in the filter by looking for the presence of blood in the effluent. The sensors will alarm if myoglobin or large amounts of bilirubin are detected in the effluent. A sample should be sent to the laboratory to confirm their presence. The bubble detector is designed to stop the blood pump if air is detected within the line. If it alarms, inspect all tubing carefully for the presence of air bubbles and either reprime or change the filter set. Make sure that all air is cleared from the system during priming, keep all connections tightly joined, and use Luer-lock type connectors. The fluid pump alarms when the bag is empty while the effluent pump alarms when full. Alarms will also sound if a clamp is left closed or a bag is improperly spiked.

REFERENCES

1. Irwin RS, Rippe JM. *Irwin and Rippe's Intensive Care Medicine*. 7th ed. 2012;75:917-931.
2. Martin GS, Mannino DM, Eaton S, Moss M. The epidemiology of sepsis in the United States from 1979 through 2000. *N Engl J Med*. 2003;348:1546.
3. Elixhauser A, Friedman B, Stranges E. *Septicemia in U.S. Hospitals*. Rockville, MD: Agency for Healthcare Research and Quality; 2009. http://www.hcup-us.ahrq.gov/reports/statbriefs/sb122.pdf.
4. Scheel PJ, Liu M, Rabb H. Uremic lung: new insights into a forgotten condition. *Kidney Int*. 2008;74:849-851.
5. Foland JA, Fortenberry JD, Warshaw BL, et al. Fluid overload before continuous hemofiltration and survival in critically ill children: a retrospective analysis. *Crit Care Med*. 2004;32:1771-1776.
6. Goldstein SL, Currier H, Graf Cd, et al. Outcome in children receiving continuous venovenous hemofiltration. *Pediatrics*. 2001;107:1309-1312.
7. Bent P, Tan HK, Bellomo R, et al. Early and intensive continuous hemofiltration for severe renal failure after cardiac surgery. *Ann Thorac Surg*. 2001;71:832-837.
8. Mehta RL, Kellum JA, Shah SV, et al. Acute kidney injury network: report of an initiative to improve outcomes in acute kidney injury. *Crit Care*. 2007;11(2):R31.
9. Coca SG, Peixoto AJ, Garg AX, et al. The prognostic importance of a small acute decrement in kidney function in hospitalized patients: a systematic review and meta-analysis. *Am J Kidney Dis*. 2007;50(5):712-720.
10. Parikh CR, Devarajan P. New biomarkers of acute kidney injury. *Crit Care Med*. 2008;36(suppl 4):S159-S165.
11. Overberger P, Pesacreta M, Palevsky PM, et al. Management of RRT in acute kidney injury: a survey of practitioner prescribing practices. *Clin J Am Soc Nephrol*. 2007;2(4):623-630.
12. Ricci Z, Ronco C, D'Amico G, et al. Practice patterns in the management of acute renal failure in the critically ill patient: an international survey. *Nephrol Dial Transplant*. 2006;21(3):690-696.
13. Uchino S, Kellum JA, Bellomo R, et al. Acute renal failure in critically ill patients: a multinational, multicenter study. *JAMA*. 2005;294(7):813-881.
14. Levy EM, Viscoli CM, Horwitz RI. The effect of acute renal failure on mortality. A cohort analysis. *JAMA*. 1996;275:1489-1494.

15. Chertow GM, Levy EM, Hammermeister KE, et al. Independent association between acute renal failure and mortality following cardiac surgery. *Am J Med.* 1998;104:343-348.

16. Metnitz PG, Krenn CG, Steltzer H, et al. Effect of acute renal failure requiring RRT on outcome in critically ill patients. *Crit Care Med.* 2002;30:2051-2058.

17. Liano F, Junco E, Pascual J, et al. The spectrum of acute renal failure in the intensive care unit compared with that seen in other settings. The Madrid Acute Renal Failure Study Group. *Kidney Int.* 1998;66(suppl):S16-S24.

18. Liano F, Pascual J. Epidemiology of acute renal failure: a prospective, multicenter, community-based study. Madrid Acute Renal Failure Study Group. *Kidney Int.* 1996;50:811-818.

19. Uchino S, Kellum JA, Bellomo R, et al. Acute renal failure in critically ill patients: a multinational, multicenter study. *JAMA.* 2005;294:813-818.

20. Gabrielli A, Layon AJ, Yu M, Civetta JM. *Civetta, Taylor, & Kirby's Manual of Critical Care.* 2012

21. Uchino S, Kellum JA, Bellomo R, et al; Beginning and Ending Supportive Therapy for the Kidney (BEST Kidney) Investigators. Acute renal failure in critically ill patients: a multinational, multicenter study. *JAMA.* 2005;294:813-818.

22. Bellomo R, Cass A, Cole L, et al. Intensity of continuous renal-replacement therapy in critically ill patients. *N Engl J Med.* 2009;361(17):1627-1638.

23. Kutsogiannis DJ, Gibney RT, Stollery D, et al. Regional citrate versus systemic heparin anticoagulation for continuous renal replacement in critically ill patients. *Kidney Int.* 2005;67:2361-2367.

High-Frequency Oscillatory Ventilation

Michael Duff, MD and
Stephen M. Pastores, MD, FACP, FCCP, FCCM

KEY POINTS

1. High-frequency oscillatory ventilation (HFOV) is a form of ventilatory support which delivers very small tidal volumes (1-2 ml per kg) at very high rates (3-15 breaths per second).

2. The major indication for HFOV is for patients with severe acute respiratory distress syndrome (ARDS) whose lungs cannot tolerate high tidal distending pressure.

3. The main determinant of oxygenation during HFOV is the mPaw which is generally initiated at approximately 5 cm H_2O greater than the mPaw noted during conventional ventilation.

4. Carbon dioxide removal during HFOV is directly propportional to the oscillation amplitude and inversely proportional to the oscillation frequency setting.

5. Two recent multicenter randomized trials showed no benefit (OSCAR) and even harm (OSCILLATE) with the use of HFOV in adult patients with ARDS.

INTRODUCTION

High-frequency oscillatory ventilation (HFOV) is a form of ventilatory support that delivers extremely small tidal volumes (V_{Ts}) at very high rates and maintains a relatively constant and higher mean airway pressure (mPaw) than mechanical ventilation. These properties make HFOV an ideal mode of ventilation for lung protection, because it can allow clinicians to operate in a "safe" zone of the volume-pressure curve, avoiding zones of overdistension and derecruitment/atelectasis, provided an optimal mPaw is set and very small V_{Ts} are delivered.

BACKGROUND

HFOV was first described in 1972 and was used to improve oxygenation in neonates with severe respiratory distress syndrome. This was gradually expanded into larger, more mature pediatric patients with severe respiratory failure. In 2001, the Food and Drug Administration approved HFOV devices for use in adult patients with acute respiratory distress syndrome (ARDS) who failed conventional mechanical ventilation (CMV).

PHYSIOLOGY AND MECHANISMS OF GAS EXCHANGE DURING HFOV

Conventional ventilation mimics the respiratory cycle with inspiration and expiration via positive pressure inhalation compared with the negative pressure that drives normal respiration. HFOV is based on several features of nonlaminar flow of gas into and out of a circuit. High-pressure gas flows down the center of the airway, displacing lower pressure gas via coaxial flow and bulk flow. Between cycles and in distal airways, gases mix uniformly so that delivered, oxygen-rich gas saturates available alveoli to maximize the chances of diffusion of oxygen into the bloodstream. This mixing is called pendelluft and essentially accounts for dead space ventilation of any kind, but is especially useful in HFOV. "Exhaled" gases move by previously mentioned bulk and coaxial flows toward the negative pressure generated by the high-velocity "breaths" where they ultimately exit the endotracheal tube into the exhalation circuit. HFOV can be considered to have separated oxygenation and ventilation into 2 separate mechanisms.

Similar to CMV when the respiratory frequency exceeds the time for intrinsic exhalation phase, HFOV delivers breaths that can lead to developing auto–positive end-expiratory pressure (auto-PEEP). This can still occur with very small tidal volumes in HFOV. Whereas auto-PEEP in CMV can be deleterious, the typical small volumes and high rates used in HFOV allow the clinician to avoid auto-PEEP; however, patients with elevated airway resistance are relatively contraindicated for HFOV. The typical maneuver to reduce auto-PEEP is to increase the frequency, which decreases the inspiratory time, and allows for more exhalation and limits breath stacking. Other mechanisms of gas exchange during HFOV include cardiogenic mixing where the contracting heart causes mechanical agitation of gas, especially in lung units surrounding the heart, and molecular diffusion near the alveolar-capillary interface.

INDICATIONS FOR HFOV

HFOV is indicated for patients with severe ARDS whose lungs cannot tolerate high tidal distending pressure. In these patients, HFOV may provide a modality to improve oxygenation and maintain peak airway pressures that are nearly the same as the mean airway pressures. Although the pressure wave at the level of the endotracheal tube has a large gradient, the distending pressures exerted on the alveoli are much closer to the mean airway pressure and the theory suggests that the lung is maintained in a constantly open state. Conversely, the "tidaling" of CMV still exerts a gradient on the distal airways and alveoli. This means that if underrecruited, there

exists the possibility of "atelectrauma" as the lung is opened and closed with each cycle. In the setting of very poor lung compliance, barotrauma is common.

Patient selection begins with moderate to severe ARDS that by strict definition represents patients whose ratio of the partial pressure of oxygen from the arterial blood to the fraction of inspired oxygen (Pao_2:FIo_2) is less than 200, and who require PEEP greater than 10 to 15 cm H_2O to achieve this oxygenation. Patients with plateau pressures greater than 30 cm H_2O and/or mean airway pressures of greater than 24 cm H_2O can also be considered for HFOV. Similarly, patients ventilated by other alternative modes including airway pressure release ventilation (APRV) with P high greater than 35 cm H_2O can be considered. Though not specifically studied, case reports of patients with bronchopleural fistulas have been successfully treated with HFOV.

CONTRAINDICATIONS

HFOV has not been studied in pregnant patients, those with severe chronic obstructive pulmonary disease (COPD), and in patients with hemoptysis or copious thick secretions. Patients with high airway resistance are at increased risk of developing auto-PEEP and should be carefully screened. Pneumothorax is not a contraindication to HFOV, and the clinician must be aware of the possibility that a pneumothorax can occur at any time.

SETUP AND INITIATION OF HFOV

Following patient selection for HFOV, the airway should be suctioned and adequate sedation and analgesia should be provided (Table 100–1). Many patients experience discomfort with the constant insufflation of the lung and vibrations associated with HFOV, and thus may require deeper sedation and occasionally neuromuscular blockade to ensure patient-ventilator synchrony and reduce peripheral oxygen consumption. However, complete cessation of patient respiratory efforts is not recommended and preferably, the patient should be allowed to generate small spontaneous breaths. Once the patient

TABLE 100-1 Initial settings for HFOV.

1. Set initial mPaw at 5 cm H_2O above conventional ventilator mPaw (consider initial alveolar recruiting maneuver with 40 cm H_2O for 40-60 s if severe hypoxemia).
2. Set power to achieve initial ΔP at chest wiggle to mid-thigh or "20+$Paco_2$".
3. Set Hz at 5.
4. Set IT to 33% (may increase to 50% if difficulty with oxygenation; this may further raise carinal pressure an additional 2-4 cm H_2O).
5. If oxygenation worsens, increase mPaw in 3-5 cm H_2O increments Q 30 minutes until maximum setting (approximately 45-55 cm H_2O).
6. If $Paco_2$ worsens (but pH > 7.2), increase ΔP in 10 cm H_2O increments Q 30 minutes up to maximum setting. After maximum ΔP achieved, if necessary, may decrease Hz to minimum of 3 Hz.
7. If severe hypercapnea with pH < 7.2 bag patient, set maximum ΔP, Hz at 3, and try small cuff leak ≈(5 cm H_2O and then compensate bias flow); rule out obstruction in endotracheal tuble with bronchoscopy.
8. If oxygenation improves, gradually wean FiO_2 to 40%, than slowly reduce mPaw 2-3 cm H_2O q 4-6 hours until 22-24 cm H_2O range.
9. When above goal met, switch to PCV (initial settings: peak pressure titrated to achieve delivered TV 6 ml/Kg, Pplat < 30-35 cm H_2O), I:E 1:1 PEEP 12 cm H_2O, rate 20-25, mPaw should be 20 cm H_2O (+/- 2 cm H_2O).

Data from Derdak S. High-frequency oscillatory ventilation for acute respiratory distress syndrome in adult patients, *Crit Care Med.* 2003 Apr;31(4 Suppl):S317-S323.

is stable on HFOV, discontinuation of the paralytic agent should be attempted daily.

Initial bias flow should be set to 35 L/min and may be adjusted according to patient's needs. Inspiratory time is set as a percentage and 33% is recommended as an initial setting. Frequency should be set to 5 Hz, which correlates to a respiratory rate of 300 breaths/min. The main determinant of oxygenation during HFOV is the mPaw, and this is generally initiated at approximately 5 cm H_2O greater than the mPaw noted during conventional ventilation or equal to that of APRV. For severely hypoxemic patients, a recruitment maneuver of 40 cm H_2O for approximately 40 seconds can be considered. The FIO_2 should be set to 1 and then tapered using pulse oximetry to maintain SpO_2 greater than or equal to 88%.

The main determinants of $Paco_2$ removal are the pressure amplitude of oscillation (ΔP) and the frequency (Hz) setting. Increasing the ΔP and

decreasing the frequency reduces the delivered tidal volume and allows $Paco_2$ to rise. The ΔP is usually started at either a value where the chest vibrates down to their midthigh or a value of 20 to 30 cm H_2O above what the patient's $Paco_2$ was on conventional ventilation. For example, if the $Paco_2$ is 60 mm Hg, the ΔP is initiated at 80 cm H_2O. After approximately 30 minutes of HFOV, a repeat blood gas should be analyzed and the power setting should be titrated based on the desired $Paco_2$ level. The chest wall needs to be vibrating; if not, the power setting has to be increased.

TROUBLESHOOTING

On all patients placed on HFOV, it is crucial that oxygen is flowing to the patient. By convention, in the United States oxygen tubing and cylinders are color-coded green. Pressurized air is color-coded yellow, and contains only 20.9% oxygen, the same as room air. Most HFOV ventilators display the amplitude and frequency. While an unexplained rise in amplitude can suggest that the endotracheal tube is becoming obstructed, a sudden decrease in amplitude can suggest pneumothorax. Examining the ventilator tubing can sometimes reveal secretions or hemoptysis. When examining the patient, a decrease in the patient's chest wiggle can suggest pneumothorax, and a prompt chest x-ray should be performed. Although suctioning and bronchoscopy can cause derecruitment, they can be very important in managing the patient on HFOV. Care should be taken to minimize the duration of suctioning and bronchoscopy, and recruitment maneuvers might be considered following any interruption in HFOV.

Routine measures such as obtaining chest x-rays and performing physical examinations are not contraindicated while the patient is on HFOV. Temporarily stopping the piston allows for auscultation of the patient's heart, but stoppage should be minimized. Patients can be moved for imaging studies without stopping HFOV. Daily nursing care remains unaffected. Measures to ensure adequate sedation such as a Bispectral Index Sensor (BIS) monitor should be in place if an infusion of neuromuscular blocking agent is being used as well as routine train-of-four monitoring to minimize the side effects of neuromuscular blockade.

COMPLICATIONS OF HFOV

Complications that may occur during HFOV include hypotension, pneumothorax, and endotracheal tube obstruction. Hypotension occurs occasionally shortly following the switch to HFOV or as mPaw is increased and usually responds to intravenous fluid boluses. A pneumothorax during HFOV may be difficult to detect because of the background noise of the ventilator and the diffuse transmission of airway sounds. However, the loss of chest wiggle that usually occurs on the affected side is an important physical clue to the possibility of a pneumothorax. Obstruction of the endotracheal tube should be considered when there is an abrupt rise in $Paco_2$ during HFOV in an otherwise stable patient. In this circumstance, a suction catheter should be passed immediately to ensure patency of the endotracheal tube; occasionally, bronchoscopy may be required to visually inspect the airway.

WEANING FROM HFOV

Weaning attempts from HFOV usually commences when the patient responds with improved oxygenation and is able to maintain a SpO_2 greater than 90% on a Fio_2 of 0.4. When this occurs, the mPaw is gradually reduced by 2 to 3 cm H_2O every 4 to 6 hours as tolerated as alveolar derecruitment and desaturation may occur if the mPaw is decreased rapidly. As soon as a mPaw of 20 to 24 cm H_2O is achieved while maintaining an Fio_2 of 0.4, the patient can be switched back to a trail of conventional ventilation. The conventional ventilator is usually set to achieve a mPaw of 20 cm H_2O by using pressure control mode with peak pressure set to achieve a delivered tidal volume of 6 to 8 mL/kg of predicted body weight and inspiratory plateau pressure of less than 30 cm H_2O. An arterial blood gas is obtained 20 to 30 minutes after transfer to conventional ventilation to guide further ventilator adjustments.

RECENT STUDIES OF HFOV IN ADULTS

Two large multicenter trials compared HFOV with conventional ventilation in patients with moderate-to-severe ARDS. In the OSCILLATE (Oscillation for ARDS Treated Early), the HFOV strategy with high mean airway pressures was associated with more deaths than the conventional ventilation strategy that used relatively aggressive high PEEP levels (47% vs. 35%) which led to premature termination of the trial. Hemodynamic compromise resulting from the elevated mean airway pressures was thought to be the mechanism accounting for the poor HFOV outcomes. In the OSCAR (High-Frequency Oscillation in ARDS) trial, there was no major difference in the outcome between the HFOV strategy and usual care with conventional mechanical ventilation. In both trials, there was a higher proportion of patients in the HFOV groups who received sedatives and muscle relaxants, which may have also contributed to the poorer outcomes.

SUGGESTED READING

Adhikari NK, Bashir A, Lamontagne F, et al. High-frequency oscillation in adults: a utilization review. *Crit Care Med*. 2011;39(12):2631-2644.

Derdak S. High-frequency oscillatory ventilation for acute respiratory distress syndrome in adult patients. *Crit Care Med*. 2003;31(suppl 4):S317-S323.

Ferguson ND, Cook DJ, Guyatt GH, et al. OSCILLATE Trial Investigators; Canadian Critical Care Trials Group. High-frequency oscillation in early acute respiratory distress syndrome. *N Engl J Med*. 2013;368(9):795-805.

Fort P, Farmer C, Westerman J, et al. High-frequency oscillatory ventilation for adult respiratory distress syndrome—a pilot study. *Crit Care Med*. 1997;25(6):937-947.

Goffi A, Ferguson ND. High-frequency oscillatory ventilation for early acute respiratory distress syndrome in adults. *Curr Opin Crit Care*. 2014;20(1):77-85.

Ip T, Mehta S. The role of high-frequency oscillatory ventilation in the treatment of acute respiratory failure in adults. *Curr Opin Crit Care*. 2012;18:70-79.

Mehta S, Lapinksy SE, Hallett DC, et al. A prospective trial of high frequency oscillatory ventilation in adults with acute respiratory distress syndrome. *Crit Care Med*. 2001;29:1360-1369.

Sud S, Sud M, Friedrich JO, et al. High frequency oscillation in patients with acute lung injury and acute respiratory distress syndrome (ARDS): systematic review and meta-analysis. *BMJ*. 2010;340:c2327.

Young D, Lamb SE, Shah S, et al; OSCAR Study Group. High-frequency oscillation for acute respiratory distress syndrome. *N Engl J Med*. 2013;368(9):806-813.

Intracranial Pressure Monitoring

Nelson Moussazadeh, MD; Philip E. Stieg, PhD, MD and Halinder S. Mangat, MD

OVERVIEW

ICP monitoring is a mainstay of modern neuro-critical care, with a range of devices serving different clinical needs. It is central to the management of severe TBI with suspected intracranial hypertension. In addition, ICP measurement and treatment may also be undertaken in other instances of brain injury associated with intracranial hypertension such as acute subarachnoid hemorrhage, malignant stroke, and meningitis.

The Monro-Kellie hypothesis explains the centrality of ICP to the neurologically ill patient. The rigid cranium limits the volume of its contents; any expansion of the brain, blood, or CSF volume (or addition of orthotopic volume, eg, from neoplasm, abscess, or via inflammation), results an initial compensatory buffering by reduction in CSF and blood volume. If the increase in volume exceeds compensatory mechanisms, elevation in ICP occurs. Pressure elevation presages a volume reduction in tissues in order of compliance and proximity to outlets with large pressure-gradient interfaces. Cerebral herniation including uncal, transtentorial, central, and tonsilar herniation often result in brain stem and vascular compression, respiratory suppression, and irreversible neurologic injury, making malignant intracranial hypertension highly morbid (Figure 101–1).

IVCs remain the gold standard for the measurement of ICP. The procedure of placing an IVC is commonly referred to as ventriculostomy and when combined with a closed drainage system,

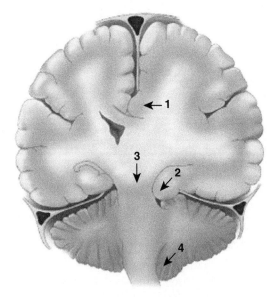

FIGURE 101-1 Schematic drawing of brain herniation patterns. *1.* Subfalcine herniation. The cingulate gyrus shifts across midline under the falx cerebri. *2.* Uncal herniation. The uncus (medial temporal lobe gyrus) shifts medially and compresses the midbrain and cerebral peduncle. *3.* Central transtentorial herniation. The diencephalon and midbrain shift caudally through the tentorial incisura. *4.* Tonsillar herniation. (*Reproduced with permission from Wilkins RH, Rengachary SS: Neurosurgery, 2nd ed. New York: McGraw Hill; 1996.*)

as an external ventricular drain (EVD). The latter combines ICP monitoring with CSF diversion (Figure 101–2). More recently the "transcranial bolt" has also been used as an access to place intraparenchymal probes for direct and continuous measure of ICP (Figure 101–3).

Each technique has distinct advantages and limitations; these notably include the ability to both diagnose and treat intracranial hypertension with an EVD, while posing the occasional technical challenge of cannulating the ventricle and imposing the need for closure to drainage for accurate monitoring. Whereas all monitors furnish instantaneous ICP and allow for derivation of cerebral perfusion pressure (difference between mean arterial pressure [MAP] and ICP), intraparenchymal probes placed using bolts have the added advantage of furnishing continuous data allowing for assessment of trends including ominous Lundberg wave patterns (eg, so-called plateau/A-wave) (Figure 101–4A,B). Bolts

equipped with requisite probes can also measure interstitial brain tissue oxygenation partial pressure ($PbtO_2$), cerebral blood flow, temperature, seizures via intracortical electroencephalography, and brain metabolism via online cerebral microdialysis. When selecting monitoring modalities, the neurointensivist and neurosurgeon should note that TBI and mass lesions may induce deranged CSF flow and pressure gradients resulting in disparate regional parenchymal versus ventricular ICP as well as transient compartmental ICP gradients.

INDICATIONS

Outside of severe TBI, guidelines are not well established for ICP monitoring and its use varies considerably from center to center. ICP monitoring is considered in cases with concern for acute intracranial hypertension resulting from a variety of pathologies causing generalized edema (eg, in the setting of trauma, ischemia anoxia, acute liver failure, diabetic ketoacidosis, venous hypertension, meningitis), mass lesions (traumatic hematoma/contusion, tumor), and hydrocephalus (communicating from, eg, subarachnoid hemorrhage as the most common indication or noncommunicating from a variety of causes). ICP is also commonly monitored in drowning or near-drowning in children. Noncorrectable coagulopathy or antiplatelet use is a contraindication to EVD placement (in addition to scalp infection and intracranial abscess). However, when offered despite this as part of lifesaving maneuvers, particular caution must be exercised during placement.

EVIDENCE FOR ICP MONITORING

ICP monitoring has been best studied in the setting of severe TBI, and is the mainstay in goal-directed treatment. According to the Brain Trauma Foundation guidelines on the basis of Level II evidence, ICP monitoring is indicated for all salvageable severe TBI patients (GCS 3-8 after cardiopulmonary resuscitation) in the setting of an abnormal head computed tomography (CT) (with hematoma, contusion, swelling, herniation, or compressed basal cisterns).

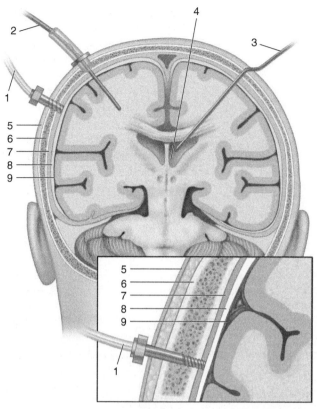

1. Subdural bolt
2. Intraparenchymal monitor
3. External ventricular drain
4. Lateral ventricle
5. Skin
6. Skull
7. Dura mater
8. Subdural space (this is a potential space)
9. Pia-arachnoid

FIGURE 101–2 Compartments for intracranial monitoring. (*Reproduced with permission from Frontera JA:* Decision Making in Neurocritical Care. *New York: Thieme; 2009.*)

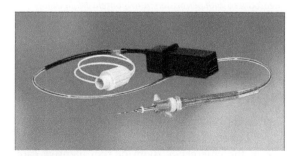

FIGURE 101–3 An intraparenchymal ICP monitor from Integra Life Sciences. (*Permission granted by Integra LifeSciences Corporation, Plainsboro, New Jersey, USA.*)

On the basis of Level III data, invasive ICP monitoring is recommended for patients with severe TBI and a normal CT with 2 or more of age greater than 40, unilateral/bilateral motor posturing, or systolic blood pressure less than 90 mm Hg.

There has been some recent debate regarding the use of ICP monitoring. A study by Chesnut et al, demonstrated that therapy based on ICP monitoring versus serial brain CT imaging had similar outcome benefit. However, this study has several criticisms, the most important being the delay in arrival of patients to the hospital and delay in ICP monitor insertion. Prehospital delay, hypoxia, and

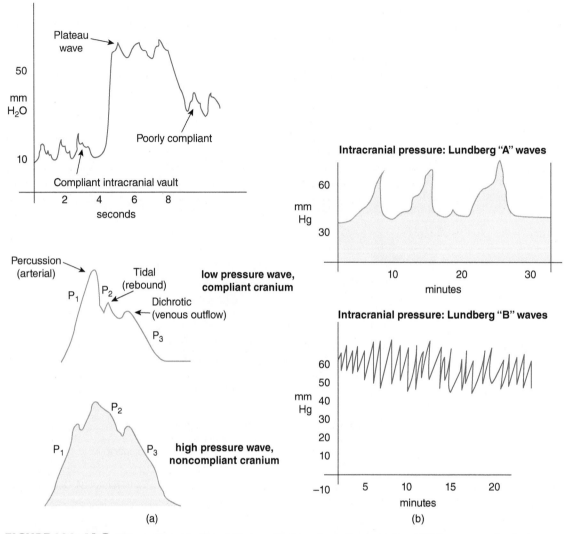

FIGURE 101–4A,B ICP waveforms. In the poorly compliant cranium, elevated rebound (P2) pressures dominate waveform derangement, ultimately leading to transient plateau or Lundberg A-wave hypertension, which CSF and intracranial blood content reduction becomes progressively less (*Reproduced with permission from Frontera JA:* Decision Making in Neurocritical Care. *New York: Thieme; 2009.*)

hypotension have been shown to contribute to worse outcomes in severe TBI patients, and this is an important confounder in the above study. Therefore, the neurosurgical and neurocritical care communities remain circumspect about the significance of these results. Moreover, it has been shown that patients without measurement of ICP have higher mortality and patients who respond to treatment of elevated ICP have improved outcome.

VENTRICULOSTOMY PLACEMENT WITH ICP MONITORING

Ventriculostomy placement and bolt placement can be performed in the operating theater or at the bedside in the emergency room or the intensive care unit (ICU). These procedures should only be performed by qualified and accredited neurosurgeons.

The right frontal approach to cannulation of the lateral ventricle is the neurosurgical workhorse given relative ease of placement in supine patients and avoidance of the nondominant hemisphere; however, this may be modified according to individual circumstances.

In the most typical approach, Kocher point serves as a landmark for a typical safe trajectory. Kocher point lies 10 cm posterior to the glabella and 3 cm lateral to midline and is at the midpupillary line and anterior to the coronal suture. This allows for a nondominant high frontal corticectomy avoiding the superior sagittal sinus medially and precentral gyrus posteriorly.

The patient is positioned supine with head end of the bed elevated with creation of ample working corridors; this is particularly important with intubated patients within constrained ICU rooms. Imaging should be reviewed and displayed. The patient's head should be shaved, cleaned, and the incision site marked using landmarks described earlier.

A procedure time-out should be performed with surgical and nursing staff confirming conformation to standard procedures and availability of necessary equipment. Antibiotics should be administered within 30 minutes of skin incision time, and analgesia/sedation should be used judiciously.

After sterilization and draping the field, skin including tunneling and tack-down sites and the subperiosteal compartment are infiltrated with local anesthetic. An incision is made at Kocher point, anteromedial to posterolateral allowing for incorporation into any future incision, for example, frontotemporal craniotomy. Pericranium is scraped away with the scalpel handle and a self-retaining retractor is placed. Hemostasis should be obtained; while occasional brisk scalp bleeding may pose a challenge without cautery or the full menu of operating room equipment, local pressure, clamps, and suture are usually adequate. The head is firmly held from below the sterile drapes via mandibular grasp by an assistant, and a burr hole is created using a twist drill or an electric drill. A trocar is utilized to create a durotomy and to generate a tunnel for the ventricular catheter. Meticulous hemostasis is ensured to avoid clot formation at catheter inlet at the time of insertion. Bedside burr holes do not allow for

visualization and avoidance of sulci or use of pial cautery, however, in the operating room setting both should be performed.

For a frontal, for example, Kocher point approach, the catheter should be oriented orthogonally to the calvarial surface (the Ghajar Guide may be used to assist in this); as this may frequently be difficult to assess within the confines of a limited incision, the frontal horn and foramen of Monro are typically estimated with a trajectory toward the intersection of a sagittal line from the medical canthus and a coronal line from the external auditory meatus. The ventricular catheter should be passed to a depth of approximately 5 cm from the external calvarial table, with the final 1 cm of that length passed without the rigid catheter stylet, which is removed upon recognition of a trans-ependymal "pop" to avoid blunt vascular or parenchymal injury. Opening pressure should be noted. Should CSF not spontaneously flow, gentle syringe aspiration of any air lock may solve the problem.

Excessive attempts at catheter replacement should be avoided with a low threshold to obtain CT imaging to ensure no shifts in underlying anatomic structures. CT guidance may be used as an adjunct to ventriculostomy placement in difficult cases; neuronavigation is also an option intraoperatively. The free end of the ventricular catheter is subcutaneously tunneled using a trocar available in the placement kit and is then connected to the closed collecting system. The incision is closed, a nonocclusive purse-string suture is placed at the skin exit site, and the catheter is tacked down at several points on the scalp to prevent accidental dislodgement. With a head elevation of 30°, the external auditory meatus lies in approximately the same horizontal plane as the foramen of Monro, allowing its use as a surface landmark for calibrating "zero" isotension. Drainage is continued at a level or rate appropriate to the patient's clinical circumstance.

INTRAPARENCHYMAL ICP MONITOR PLACEMENT

The approach to bolt placement is similar to ventriculostomy placement; the bolt is screwed into place following twist-drill hole creation (ensuring a drill bit of diameter compatible with the available bolt is used). Durotomy is performed, the bolt's sheath is placed, and probes are placed to a suitable depth after requisite calibration/zeroing per the manufacturer's specifications; skin closure is performed around the device margins with meticulous prevention of CSF egress. Many probes allow for tunneling without the use of a bolt (including for intraoperative, postcraniectomy use) for which one should consult the manufacturer's instructions.

DEVICE USE AND MONITORING

CT imaging may be obtained to verify the device placement particularly in the setting of challenging placement or unreliable data or CSF output. ICP monitors are left in place for several days with data monitored continuously, or hourly with EVDs. The routine use of perioperative or prolonged prophylactic systemic antibiotics following ICP monitor introduction remains controversial, with disparate usage patterns. Though ICU-bound comatose patients are at elevated risk for surgical site infection including ventriculitis or cerebritis (see the section on Complications), the literature remains divided with regard to infection rates while potentially creating the risk of multidrug-resistant infections.

Similarly, routine CSF surveillance from EVDs for ventriculitis has been advocated or employed by some centers, though its use remains controversial given the potential for introduction of pathogens upon each instance of instrumenting the system. Prophylactic catheter exchange for infection prevention is not advocated on the basis of studies including one randomized trial performing routine exchange on 103 patients. Others have demonstrated a procedural noninfectious complication rate of 5.6% for EVD placement itself, which likely outweighs any benefit from infection reduction.

COMPLICATIONS AND TROUBLESHOOTING

The primary complications associated with ICP monitor placement are infection, hemorrhage, and malfunction. Ventriculostomy-related infection has

been reported most commonly around 10% of drains placed (2%-25%), or 7.5 to 32 infections per 1000 drain-days, though reported rates depend on the definition used (ie, surveillance data, including the Centers for Disease Control and Prevention [CDC] definition of health care–associated meningitis, are frequently blinded to clinical diagnosis, bacterial culture growth, and treatment ramifications). Associated clinical ventriculomeningitis (a diagnosis made on the basis of CSF cellular and metabolic profile, culture data and clinical parameters including fever, peripheral leukocytosis, and findings of meningismus) is a significant cause of morbidity.

Risk factors for ventriculostomy-related infection include duration of catheterization, catheter irrigation/sampling or replacement, neurosurgical operation, systemic infection, CSF leak, and intraventricular or subarachnoid hemorrhage. Responsible microorganisms most commonly include skin flora (eg, *Staphylococcus aureus* and epidermidis, streptococci, and *Propionibacterium* acnes), and gram-negative bacteria including *Pseudomonas* and *Enterobacteriaceae.* Evidence suggests reduced infection risk with minocycline or clindamycin plus rifampin-impregnated catheters (1.3% vs 9.4% infection and 17.9% vs 36.7% colonization rates), potentially with silver-impregnated ones, and with institution of ICU-based placement bundles and hygiene interventions.

Parenchymal pressure monitors may be associated with a seemingly lower infection rate, though this may be influenced by sampling bias given the ease of CSF access for ventriculostomy surveillance and with few studies culturing device tips in all patients or CSF in all patients. However, retrospective series generally describe clinical infection rates of less than 5% (and mostly < 2%, with higher colonization rates) and either noninferiority or reduced infection risk versus EVD.

While the majority of studies evaluating hemorrhage following invasive ICP device placement do not report radiographic hematoma volume or clinical significance, surgical evacuation of ICP monitor-related hematomas is reported on the order of 0.5% to 3.8%, with one pediatric report describing a 2.7-fold hemorrhage risk reduction with parenchymal monitors versus EVD.

ICP monitors are also subject to technical malfunction. All ICP monitors may provide inaccurate data; in the case of parenchymal sensors this is most often due to insidious zero-drift, which may require replacement (see the section Device Use and Monitoring), or to filament kinking. Zero-drift, occurring on the order of up to 2 mm Hg/8 h in parenchymal monitors (the Integra Camino system is specified to drift up to 2 mm Hg in the first 24 hours and 1 mm Hg/d over the following 5 days), is less of an issue in EVDs as ventriculostomy pressure transducers can be recalibrated to atmospheric pressure. In one large series, some 38% of parenchymal monitors required replacement for drift (Shapiro, $n = 244$). Unlike fiberoptic transducers, ventricular ones can be recalibrated, and rezeroing should be performed each time the reading is in question and when the patient or drain height is altered.

EVDs are additionally susceptible to compromise of CSF drainage. Poor drainage with clinically consistent ICP data (including with a waveform varying appropriately with respiration and head position) may be due to ICP normalization (which can be ruled in via drain-lowering). Alternatively, this may be due to occlusion by blood or brain/ choroidal debris, which can be assessed with visual inspection of EVD tubing and instillation of saline in the distal direction via access ports using sterile technique. Drains also commonly fail due to collapsed lateral ventricle (or ventricles, depending on the degree of compartmentalization) or intraventricular occlusion; CT imaging with particular emphasis on ventricular size/configuration and catheter placement aids in prompt diagnosis and serves as a new baseline prior to replacement should this be required; a nonfunctioning EVD should be promptly removed—regardless of intent to replace— to minimize the risk of infection.

REMOVAL

ICP monitors are removed at the bedside, with the entry point sutured to prevent CSF egress. Removal is dependent on the clinical scenario and the modality of the monitor. For ventricular catheters, necessity is frequently dictated more by the therapeutic need for CSF diversion; in these cases CSF challenge (via drain elevation or clamping) with clinical/ radiographic follow-up is performed prior to drain removal.

SUGGESTED READING

1. Arabi Y, Memish ZA, Balkhy HH, et al. Ventriculostomy-associated infections: incidence and risk factors. *Am J Infect Control.* 2005;33(3):137-143.
2. Brain Trauma Foundation, American Association of Neurological Surgeons, Congress of Neurological Surgeons, et al. Guidelines for the management of severe traumatic brain injury. *J Neurotrauma.* 2007;24(suppl 1):S1-S106.
3. Camacho EF, Boszczowski I, Freire MP, et al. Impact of an educational intervention implanted in a neurological intensive care unit on rates of infection related to external ventricular drains. *PLoS One.* 2013;8(2):e50708.
4. Chesnut RM, Temkin N, Carney N, et al. A trial of intracranial-pressure monitoring in traumatic brain injury. *N Engl J Med.* 2012;367:2471-2481.
5. Eisenberg HM, Frankowski RF, Contant CF, et al. High-dose barbiturate control of elevated intracranial pressure in patients with severe head injury. *J Neurosurg.* 1988;69(1):15-23.
6. Farahvar A, Gerber LM, Chiu YL, et al. Increased mortality in patients with severe traumatic brain injury treated without intracranial pressure monitoring. *J Neurosurg.* 2012;117(4):729-734.
7. Farahvar A, Gerber LM, Chiu YL, et al. Response to intracranial hypertension treatment as a predictor of death in patients with severe traumatic brain injury. *J Neurosurg.* 2011;114:1471-1478.
8. Flint AC, Rao VA, Renda NC, et al. A simple protocol to prevent external ventricular drain infections. *Neurosurgery.* 2013;72(6):993-999.
9. Khan SH, Kureshi IU, Mulgrew T, et al. Comparison of percutaneous ventriculostomies and intraparenchymal monitor: a retrospective evaluation of 156 patients. *Acta Neurochir Suppl.* 1998;71:50-52.
10. Kubilay Z, Amini S, Fauerbach LL, et al. Decreasing ventricular infections through the use of a ventriculostomy placement bundle: experience at a single institution. *J Neurosurg.* 2013;118(3):514-520.
11. Lajcak M, Heidecke V, Haude KH, et al. Infection rates of external ventricular drains are reduced by the use of silver-impregnated catheters. *Acta Neurochir (Wien).* 2013;155(5):875-881.
12. Lozier AP, Sciacca RR, Romagnoli MF, et al. Ventriculostomy-related infections: a critical review of the literature. *Neurosurgery.* 2008;62(suppl 2):688-700.
13. Lundberg N. Continuous recording and control of ventricular fluid pressure in neurosurgical practice. *Acta Psychiatr Scand Suppl.* 1960;36(149):1-193.

14. Narayan RK, Kishore PR, Becker DP, et al. Intracranial pressure: to monitor or not to monitor? A review of our experience with severe head injury. *J Neurosurg*. 1982;56(5):650-659.

15. Ratanalert S, Phuenpathom N, Saeheng S, et al. ICP threshold in CPP management of severe head injury patients. *Surg Neurol*. 2004;61(5):429-434.

16. Shapiro S, Bowman R, Callahan J, et al. The fiberoptic intraparenchymal cerebral pressure monitor in 244 patients. *Surg Neurol*. 1996;45(3):278-282.

17. Srinivasan VM, O'Neill BR, Jho D, et al. The history of external ventricular drainage. *J Neurosurg*. 2014;120(1):228-236.

18. Walti LN, Conen A, Coward J, et al. Characteristics of infections associated with external ventricular drains of cerebrospinal fluid. *J Infect*. 2013;66(5):424-431.

19. Wang X, Dong Y, Qi XQ, et al. Clinical review: efficacy of antimicrobial-impregnated catheters in external ventricular drainage—a systematic review and meta-analysis. *Crit Care*. 2013;17(4):234.

20. Zabramski JM, Whiting D, Darouiche RO, et al. Efficacy of antimicrobial-impregnated external ventricular drain catheters: a prospective, randomized, controlled trial. *J Neurosurg*. 2003;98(4):725-730.

Lumbar Puncture

102

Mai O. Colvin, MD; Ariel L. Shiloh, MD and Lewis A. Eisen, MD

KEY POINTS

1 Lumbar puncture (LP) is essential for the diagnosis of two treatable but potentially fatal conditions, central nervous system (CNS) infection and subarachnoid hemorrhage (SAH) with a negative computed tomography (CT) scan.

2 LP can also be helpful in the differential diagnosis of other conditions including CNS malignancy, pseudotumor cerebri, and demyelinating diseases.

3 Contraindications to LP include skin or soft tissue infection at the puncture site, acute

spinal cord or head trauma, uncorrected severe coagulopathy, and brain shift secondary to a space-occupying lesion (SOL) or diffuse cerebral edema.

4 Ultrasound-guided LPs reduce the risk of a failed or traumatic procedure, the number of needle insertions, and redirections compared to those performed without imaging.

5 Complications from LP include brain herniation, headache, infection, spinal hematoma, and neurologic compromise.

INTRODUCTION

Percutaneous needle LP was first introduced by Quincke in 1891.[1] Since then, LP has become a fundamental method to access cerebrospinal fluid (CSF) in a variety of clinical settings. In the field of critical care, LP is often used to obtain CSF for analysis and to measure the opening pressure of the subarachnoid space. With the advancement of other diagnostic modalities, especially neuroimaging procedures such as CT scans and magnetic resonance imaging (MRI), the numbers of definite indications for LP have been reduced in recent years. However, analysis of CSF remains essential to the diagnosis of two potentially fatal but treatable conditions, which are CNS infections and SAH in patients with a negative CT scan. CSF analysis should always be correlated with history, physical examination findings,

and other diagnostic tests. LP allows clinicians to access CSF in a relatively safe manner in the absence of significant contraindications, although on rare occasions harmful or even serious complications may result. This chapter will review the indications, contraindications, technique, and complications of performing LP in adults.

GENERAL INDICATIONS

The primary indication for LP is to diagnose or exclude bacterial, viral, fungal, and parasitic infections of the CNS. LP is also an indispensable step in the exclusion of SAH when there is a strong clinical suspicion of SAH and brain imaging is nondiagnostic. In addition, CSF analysis and CSF pressure provide clinically valuable information in the diagnoses of many other noninfectious neurologic conditions such as CNS malignancies, pseudotumor cerebri, and demyelinating diseases including multiple sclerosis and Guillain-Barré syndrome.

CNS Infection

Meningitis refers to inflammation of the meninges and could be either infectious or noninfectious. Noninfectious causes of meningitis will not be discussed in this chapter. From 2003 to 2007, the United States had an estimated 4100 cases, including 500 deaths, of bacterial meningitis per year.[2] The annual incidence has declined significantly since the introduction of *Haemophilus influenzae* type b (Hib) and pneumococcal conjugate vaccines. Despite these vaccines, bacterial meningitis continues to be a serious health threat, as both the morbidity and mortality remain high. The two most common pathogens of bacterial meningitis in adults are *Streptococcus pneumoniae* and *Neisseria meningitidis*. Patients with acute bacterial meningitis commonly present with one or more of the following: fever, changes in level of consciousness, nausea or vomiting, headache, and meningeal signs. Thorough physical examinations are certainly important, but the clinical signs and symptoms may be subtle and nonspecific, and should not be used in isolation to rule out potentially life-threatening disease.

Given the high mortality and morbidity of this condition, CSF analysis is often required to diagnose or rule out CNS infection. CSF analysis is the only definitive way to establish the diagnosis and determine the causative pathogen. Therefore, when bacterial meningitis is suspected, LP should be obtained as soon as possible. Early diagnosis with prompt administration of appropriate antibiotics is crucial when managing meningitis. Ideally LP should occur before administration of antibiotics, but it should not delay the antibiotic therapy. While there are contraindications to LP, the decision to forgoing LP should not be undertaken lightly given the seriousness of this condition.

The term encephalitis refers to inflammation of brain parenchyma, most commonly caused by a virus. Viral encephalitis is often characterized by an altered level of consciousness, focal neurologic deficits, seizures, as well as neuropsychiatric symptoms such as psychosis, personality changes, and hallucinations. Clinical manifestations vary depending on the pathogen because different pathogens may affect different areas of the brain. Herpes simplex virus (HSV) 1 is the most common diagnosed pathogen of sporadic viral encephalitis in the western world. In the absence of acyclovir, the mortality for this encephalitis was greater than 70%, and even with acyclovir the 6-month mortality remains high at 14% to 28%.[3-6] Survivors often suffer from serious neurologic sequelae. Other viruses that cause acute encephalitis include other herpes viruses, rabies virus, arboviruses, enteroviruses, and human immunodeficiency virus (HIV). As with bacterial meningitis, when viral encephalitis is suspected, LP should be performed as soon as possible. Polymerase chain reaction (PCR) can detect HSV DNA in CSF rapidly and reliably with sensitivity similar to that of a brain biopsy.[7] Brain imaging such as MRI or CT is often obtained before or after LP to support the diagnosis. When there is high suspicion for HSV encephalitis, initiation of acyclovir treatment should not be delayed. Delays, particularly beyond 48 hours, are associated with poor outcomes.[6,8]

A patient's travel history, geographic location, recreational habits, and arthropod or animal exposure may suggest more unusual pathogens. If a CNS infection is suspected in such patients, CSF analysis should be obtained. In addition, immunocompromised patients may not present with classical signs and symptoms of CNS infections. Therefore, CSF analysis should be obtained when CNS infection is suspected in these patients.

Subarachnoid Hemorrhage

SAH refers to extravasation of blood into the subarachnoid space between the arachnoid membrane and the pia. Although SAH is most commonly caused by trauma, approximately 85% of nontraumatic SAH cases are due to a ruptured cerebral aneurysm.[9] The incidence of spontaneous aneurysmal SAH is approximated to be 27,000 to 30,000 annually in the United States.[10,11] The clinical hallmark of aneurysmal SAH is a sudden, unusually severe headache classically described as the "worst headache of my life." Headache onset is instantaneous, usually within seconds. Additional associated features include a period of unresponsiveness, changes in level of consciousness, nausea or vomiting, pre-retinal subhyaloid hemorrhages, and localized neurologic signs. Nuchal rigidity and low back pain are also commonly seen in patients with SAH, however, these usually take hours to develop after the hemorrhage. If SAH is suspected, noncontrast head CT should be obtained first. Extravasated blood appears hyperdense on CT imaging. The sensitivity of head CT for detecting SAH is highest in the first 6 hours after SAH and declines over time. CT performed in neurologically intact patients has a sensitivity of 93% if the CT is performed within 24 hours of headache onset. The sensitivity declines over time to 58% on day 5.[12,13] Even if the CT is performed within 12 hours after the bleed, about 2% of patients with SAH could have false negatives.[14] Delayed diagnosis of SAH leads to delays in treatment and consequently results in worse overall patient outcomes.[15,16] Therefore, LP should be performed in cases when SAH is suspected despite nondiagnostic CT. LP should not be performed if the CT is diagnostic for SAH or if possible contraindications to LP, such as obstructive hydrocephalus or an intracranial lesion causing mass effect are present. The classic CSF findings of SAH are elevated CSF pressure and xanthochromia, which represents hemoglobin degradation products. Xanthochromia is present when an LP is conducted 12 hours after the onset of bleeding and usually persists for 2 weeks.[17] Although xanthochromia may be confirmed visually, spectrophotometry is a more sensitive method to differentiate xanthochromia and traumatic blood. Xanthochromia may not be apparent if LP is performed early in the disease process, because it takes approximately 4 hours to develop. Angiography should be performed and prompt neurosurgical consult should be requested once the diagnosis of SAH is made.

THERAPEUTICS

LP is both a diagnostic and a therapeutic procedure. LP may be used to access the intrathecal space for drainage of CSF as a treatment for elevated intracranial pressure (ICP), or for injection of contrast dye during neuroimaging studies such as myelogram. LP facilitates the intrathecal administration of medications such as chemotherapy or spinal anesthesia.

CONTRAINDICATIONS

Contraindications to LP include skin or soft tissue infection at the puncture site, acute spinal cord or head trauma, uncorrected severe coagulopathy, and brain shift secondary to a SOL or diffuse cerebral edema. The term "raised ICP" is sometimes used as a contraindication to LP; however, elevated ICP itself does not necessarily incur the risk of herniation after LP, and therefore the term "brain shift" is preferred. Brain shift may end in herniation, and CT should be obtained prior to performing LP in those who are at a higher risk of developing herniation. Determining which adult patients should undergo CT before LP remains somewhat controversial. Physicians should make an attempt to select patients for CT on the basis of clinical findings rather than obtaining routine CT before LP in all patients.[18,19]

Patients with a high likelihood of having intracranial pathology should be evaluated with a CT prior to LP. These include, but are not limited to, an immunocompromised state, history of CNS disease, new-onset seizures, papilledema, abnormal level of consciousness, or focal neurologic deficit.[20-22] CT features that are suggestive of brain shift and unequal pressures between intracranial compartments include obliteration of the ventricles, effacement of sulci, suprachiasmatic, or basilar cisterns, lateral shift of midline structures, and brain herniation.[18,23-25] In addition to these signs, evidence of epidural abscess, ncommunicating hydrocephalus, and large posterior fossa masses preclude an LP.

Other contraindications include coagulopathy. There are no absolute cutoff values that determine when to forgo LP. The decision for emergent LP in such patients should be decided on a case-by-case basis. If time permits and it is clinically feasible, coagulopathy should be corrected before performing LP. In general, an international normalized ratio (INR) of less than 1.4, partial thromboplastin time (PTT) below 50, and a platelet count above 50,000/mm^3 are considered safe parameters. Aberrations can often be corrected with fresh frozen plasma (FFP) and/or platelet transfusions.

PROCEDURE

Anatomy and Physiology

In the average adult, the skull encloses a total volume of 1475 mL, which includes brain parenchyma (~80%), blood (~10%), and CSF (~10%).[26] CSF is produced at a rate of 20 mL/h, for a total of 500 mL/d, by the choroid plexus. CSF is reabsorbed across the arachnoid villi of the superior sagittal sinuses, which act as one-way valves into the venous circulation. Based on the Monro-Kellie hypothesis, the sum of the volumes of brain, CSF, and intracranial blood remains constant. This means that an increase in one will result in a decrease in one or both of the remaining two.[27]

CSF pressure depends on age, body posture, and clinical conditions. The normal CSF pressure in healthy adults in the horizontal position is normally 7 to 15 mm Hg.[28] The spinal cord normally ends at the inferior border of L1 or the superior border of L2. The needle should be inserted into L3/L4 or L4/L5 interspinous spaces. A direct line connecting the two superior iliac crests intersects the midline at the fourth lumbar vertebral body (Figure 102–1) and this allows the clinician to identify L3/L4 and L4/L5 interspinous spaces.

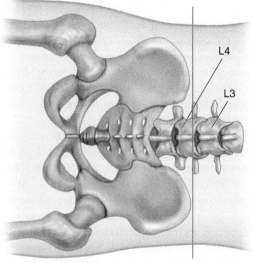

L4

L3

Level of posterior
superior iliac crest

FIGURE 102–1 Anatomy of lumbar spine.

Preparation

Prior to performing an LP, explain the risks and benefits of the procedure to the patient and obtain an informed consent. The operator should wash their hands thoroughly and conduct a time-out at the bedside before starting the procedure. The standard prepackaged LP tray (Figure 102–2) typically includes antiseptic swab sticks, a sterile drape, 1% lidocaine solution, a syringe, needles for anesthetic (27 and 22 gauge), a spinal needle with stylet, a manometer, extension tubing, a 3-way stopcock, four collection tubes, gauze, and bandage. The operator will also need sterile gloves of the appropriate size and a face mask. Before starting the procedure, place the tray where the operator can access it without difficulty. A standard-point Quincke cutting spinal needle is most commonly supplied with the kit, but some physicians prefer to use atraumatic (noncutting) needles such as a Sprotte needle or a Whitacre needle to minimize the risk of post-LP headache (PLPH), also known as post-dural puncture headache (PDPH).

An LP can be performed with the patient in either lateral decubitus or sitting in the upright position. If opening pressure needs to be measured, it is better to position the patient in the lateral decubitus position because it allows for a more accurate measurement. The patient should lie on one side, pull the knees up to the chest, and flex the head toward the knees as much as possible. Placing a pillow under the head helps keep the head in line with the vertebral axis. Ensure that the top shoulder and hip are positioned directly above their bottom counterparts. If LP will be performed while the patient is sitting in the upright position, the patient needs to sit on the side of the bed. The patient should hunch over with the head faced down on a pillow atop a steady bedside table. The arching back will widen the intervertebral spaces. A stool can be used to support the patient's feet as hip flexion in the sitting position optimizes interspinous space width.[29] After positioning the patient, palpate the superior iliac crests again and identify the L3/L4 or L4/L5 interspace. A visual target for the needle insertion site can be made by a skin marker or by making an indentation with gentle pressure using the hub end of a needle sheath or cap of a pen.

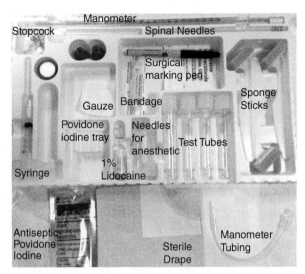

FIGURE 102–2 Prepackaged lumbar puncture tray.

Technique

Clean the patient's back with povidone-iodine. It should be applied in a circular motion while starting at the L3/L4 interspace and moving outward with each motion. Place a sterile drape with an opening over the puncture site on the patient and frame the workspace. Place another sterile drape between the patient's hip and the bed. In adults, LP is normally performed under local anesthesia using 1% lidocaine. Sedation may be necessary to facilitate the procedure for anxious or combative patients. The local anesthesia is injected subcutaneously using a 27-gauge needle, making a wheal. A longer 22-gauge needle is then used to anesthetize the deeper subcutaneous tissues. Aspirate after each advancement of the needle to make sure that the needle is not in a blood vessel. As anesthesia is taking effect, assemble the manometer with a 3-way stopcock and prepare the CSF collection tubes.

A 22-gauge spinal needle is most commonly used in adults. Hold the needle between both the thumbs and index fingers, insert a spinal needle with a stylet in the midline and within the median plane. Staying in the median plane will help avoid damage to the nerve roots. Orient the needle rostrally at a 15° angle as if aiming toward the umbilicus. The bevel of the needle should be parallel to the long axis of the spine, as this will minimize trauma to the dural fibers, which run parallel to the spinal axis. The needle is advanced through the skin, fat, supraspinous ligament, interspinous ligament, ligamentum flavum, epidural space, dura, arachnoid, until it reaches the subarachnoid space (Figure 102–3). Continue advancing the needle with the stylet in place until resistance is felt. A "pop" or reduction in resistance is often felt as the needle passes through ligamentum flavum. Remove the stylet to allow for release of CSF. If no CSF is seen, reinsert the stylet, advance the needle slightly further, and reassess. If bone is encountered, reassess the patient's position and bony landmarks, and ensure the needle is midline. Withdraw the needle into subcutaneous tissue, and reinsert at a slightly modified angle, assessing for the intravertebral space.

Upon confirming the return of CSF, quickly attach a 3-way stopcock to the needle hub using the extension tubing. Ensure to keep the "zero" mark of the manometer at the level of the spinal needle. If the patient is in the lateral decubitus position, ask the patient to relax by slowly extending the neck and legs. Turn the stopcock to allow CSF to flow up the manometer. Opening pressure is measured once the CSF column has leveled out in the manometer. Record the opening pressure and drain the CSF in the manometer into CSF collection tube 1. After removing the manometer, CSF is then serially

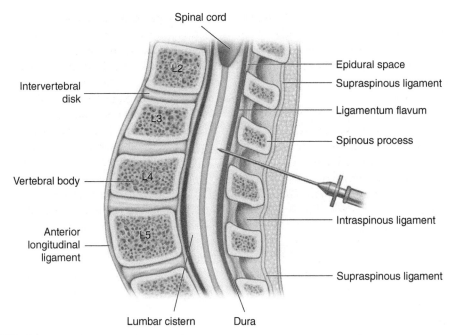

FIGURE 102–3 Midsagittal section of the spinal column with a lumbar puncture needle in place.

collected in sequential tubes. Typically a total of 8 to 15 mL of CSF is removed during a routine LP. More than 15 mL may be removed when special studies are required, such as mycobacteria cultures or cytology. If the opening pressure is elevated, keep the manometer on so that a closing pressure can be measured. When completed, replace the stylet into the needle hub and withdraw the needle. Once the needle is removed, place gauze over the LP site and cover with a bandage. Bed rest after LP is frequently recommended, however, it does not prevent the onset of PDPH regardless of the duration of rest, or the body or head positions of the patient.[30] Similarly, additional fluid intake does not seem to have a preventative effect on the onset of headaches.[30]

Imaging Guidance

Bony landmarks may be difficult to palpate in obese patients as well as patients with generalized edema or scoliosis. LP with imaging guidance may be performed using fluoroscopy or ultrasound. Fluoroscopy-guided LP is performed under real-time continuous x-ray imaging. Fluoroscopy improves success rate, however, it may not be ideal in some situations because it requires a radiologist to perform the procedure, use of radiation, and transportation of potentially critically ill patients.

Imaging guidance may also be provided with ultrasound, which is noninvasive and readily available at the bedside. It is commonly used by critical care physicians for diagnostic evaluation and procedural assistance. In patients with poorly palpable spinal landmarks, ultrasound successfully identified relevant structures in 76% of cases.[31] Ultrasound-guided LPs also reduce the risk of a failed or traumatic procedure, the number of needle insertions, and redirections compared to those performed without imaging.[32]

As the interspaces are small, direct ultrasound guidance can be technically challenging. We will describe a "mark-and-go" technique. An ultrasound-guided LP can be performed with the patient in either lateral decubitus or sitting in the upright position. A linear (high-frequency) probe works well for most patients, allowing for visualization of relatively superficial structures. A curvilinear (low-frequency) probe may be required for patients where deeper visualization is required. In an ultrasound-guided lumbar spinal imaging, the transverse and the longitudinal views are used. The transverse view is obtained by placing the probe perpendicular to the spinal column at the level of the iliac crests. This view is used to determine a midline by identifying the spinous processes. The spinous process appears as a small crescent-shaped hyperechoic (bright) structure with associated posterior hypoechoic (dark) acoustic shadow (Figure 102–4A). Once the spinous process is identified, slide the probe to center the spinous process on the screen. Mark the midline at the midpoint of the probe, both above and below the transducer. Connect these two marks, and this line represents the anatomic midline of the spine. The longitudinal view is acquired next and is used to determine the spinal interspace. This view is obtained by placing the probe parallel to the spinal column. Starting at the superior border of natal cleft, slide the probe in a cephalad direction, while keeping it in the midline, to identify the sacrum and then the spinous processes. The sacrum appears as a continuous hyperechoic band while the spinous process appears as individual hyperechoic crescent-shaped structures (Figure 102–4B). The area between the sacrum and the lowest lumbar spinous process is the L5/S1 intervertebral space. Slide the probe in the cephalad direction, along the spine, to identify L4/L5 and L3/L4 interspinous space. The interspinous

space appears as a hypoechoic gray interspace between the two hyperechoic convexities. The ligamentum flavum appears at the base between the 2 vertebrae. Use the depth indicator to measure the distance between the skin and the ligamentum flavum. This approximates the needle length required to enter the subarachnoid space. Once the L4/L5 interspinous space is identified, center this interspinous space on the screen and mark the midpoint of the probe on both sides of the transducer. Move the probe and connect the two lines. The intersection of this line and the previously identified midline represents the optimal needle insertion site. It is important that patients maintain their body position throughout the ultrasound imaging and the LP so that the relationship between the labeled surface marks and the underlying structures is not altered. Cleanse the skin and perform the remainder of the procedure in the usual fashion as described previously.

COMPLICATIONS

PDPH is one of the most common complications following LP, and the incidence of PDPH varies from 1% to 70%.[33] PDPH is thought to be caused by CSF

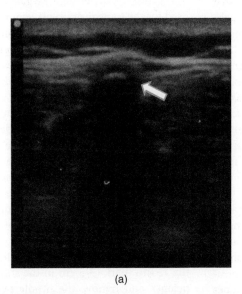
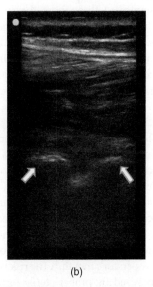

(a)   (b)

FIGURE 102–4 A. Transverse ultrasound view of lumbar spine. Crescent-shaped white line (*arrow*) represents the spinous process. Shadow is cast by the spinous process and this identifies the midline of the spine. **B.** Longitudinal ultrasound view of lumbar spine. Crescent-shaped white lines (*arrows*) represent the spinous processes. The gap between the white lines represents the interspinous space.

leakage into the paraspinous spaces, which decreases the CSF pressure, and results in traction of the meninges and stretching of the pain-sensitive intracerebral veins. Headaches usually start within 24 to 48 hours after the procedure and resolve spontaneously within a few days. PDPH could be mild or disabling, usually exacerbated by an upright position, and relieved in the supine position. The use of smaller-gauge needles and atraumatic needles, stylet reinsertion before withdrawing, and parallel orientation of the bevel to the dural fibers have all been reported to reduce the incidence of PDPH.[34-39] Despite common belief, bed rest and hydration post-LP do not reduce the incidence of PDPH.[30] Most PDPH can be managed by supportive care alone. Epidural blood patch is considered an effective treatment for persistent PDPH associated with a continued CSF leak.[40] Another relatively common complication of LP is back pain, which occurs in about 35% of patients and also resolves spontaneously after several days.[41] Some patients may feel transient electric shock-like pain or dysesthesias during the procedure. The pain is usually transient, but permanent motor and sensory loss can result in very rare cases.[41]

The most serious complication of LP is brain herniation. Removal of CSF via LP usually results in a mild, transient reduction of lumbar CSF pressure that is rapidly communicated throughout the subarachnoid space. In the presence of brain shift, there is a relative pressure gradient with downward displacement of the brain stem and cerebrum. LP will increase this pressure gradient and potentially precipitate brain herniation. Determination of LP as the cause of brain herniation is difficult, and the exact incidence is unknown. Patients with a history of CNS disease, new-onset seizures within 1 week of presentation, papilledema, abnormal level of consciousness, focal neurologic deficit, as well as immunocompromised patients should undergo CT prior to LP.[20-22]

Subarachnoid space infection is a rare complication of LP. Most cases of postdural puncture meningitis are thought to be caused by contamination of the puncture site from the patient's skin flora and aerosolized bacteria from the operator's mouth.[42] The risk of infection can be minimized by proper sterile techniques including hand washing and the use of a face mask.

A small amount of bleeding is relatively common but serious bleeding that results in spinal cord compromise is very rare in the absence of a bleeding risk. If patients experience prolonged back pain or neurologic symptoms such as numbness, weakness, and incontinence after LP, they should be evaluated with a MRI for possible spinal hematoma. Other unlikely complications of LP include extraspinal hematoma, cervical spinal cord infarction, cortical blindness, intraspinal epidermoid tumor, and intervertebral disc herniation.[23,43]

LUMBAR CSF DRAINAGE

A lumbar drain is used for external drainage of CSF, monitoring of CSF flow, and evaluation of ICP. Temporary externalized lumbar catheters are usually used as a treatment of CSF leaks, pressure monitoring, and drainage trials of patients with suspected normal pressure hydrocephalus. More permanent internalized lumboperitoneal shunts are used as the treatment of communicating hydrocephalus or idiopathic intracranial hypertension. Lumbar CSF drainage is also used as a spinal cord protective strategy in thoracic aortic aneurysm repair for patients at high risk of spinal cord ischemic injury.[44] Catheter placement is performed in a similar manner as a standard LP described previously. Instead of a 22-gauge spinal needle, a 14-gauge Tuohy needle is used for the lumbar drain placement. First, approximately 5 mL of sterile saline is injected into a plastic case surrounding the catheter guidewire to lubricate the guidewire. This facilitates threading the guidewire through the catheter. The guidewire is inserted into the open end of the catheter and set it aside. Prepare the area using sterile techniques and local anesthetics as previously described. Appropriate insertion of a Tuohy needle at the L3/4 interspace is confirmed by CSF return. Once the needle is in the subarachnoid space, rotate the needle 90° so that the bevel of the needle points in the cephalad direction. While holding the hub of the needle, the lumbar drain catheter is threaded over the guidewire through the needle. The catheter should advance smoothly. Advance the catheter to approximately the 15-cm mark (3-5 cm in the spinal space is sufficient), and remove the needle over the catheter. Once the needle is removed, carefully remove the guidewire. Thread the catheter tip onto the connector, attach the strain relief device, and snap the connector closed to prevent contamination. Attach a sterile syringe to the connector, aspirate CSF, and confirm correct catheter placement. Secure the catheter to the patient's skin using a sterile dressing. The catheter is then attached to a sterile external lumbar drainage system. CSF is allowed to drain when the lumbar pressure exceeds a previously set threshold. Complications are similar to routine LP and include bleeding, infection, CSF leaks, nerve root irritation, and supratentorial subdural hematoma secondary to CSF overdrainage.

REFERENCES

1. Quincke HI. Ueber hydrocephalus. *Verhandlungen: Deutsche Gesellschaft für Innere Medizin (X).* 1891:321-329.
2. Thigpen MC, Whitney CG, Messonnier NE, et al. Bacterial meningitis in the United States, 1998-2007. *N Engl J Med.* 2011;364(21):2016-2025.
3. Whitley RJ, Gnann JW. Viral encephalitis: familiar infections and emerging pathogens. *Lancet.* 2002;359(9305):507-513.
4. Sköldenberg B, Alestig K, Burman L, et al. Acyclovir versus vidarabine in herpes simplex encephalitis: randomised multicentre study in consecutive Swedish patients. *Lancet.* 1984;324(8405):707-711.
5. Whitley RJ, Alford CA, Hirsch MS, et al. Vidarabine versus acyclovir therapy in herpes simplex encephalitis. *N Engl J Med.* 1986;314(3):144-149.
6. McGrath N, Anderson NE, Croxson MC, Powell KF. Herpes simplex encephalitis treated with acyclovir: diagnosis and long term outcome. *J Neurol Neurosurg Psychiatry.* 1997;63(3):321-326.
7. Lakeman FD, Whitley RJ. Diagnosis of herpes simplex encephalitis: application of polymerase chain reaction to cerebrospinal fluid from brain-biopsied patients and correlation with disease. *J Infect Dis.* 1995;171(4):857-863.
8. Raschilas F, Wolff M, Delatour F, et al. Outcome of and prognostic factors for herpes simplex encephalitis in adult patients: results of a multicenter study. *Clin Infect Dis.* 2002;35(3):254-260.
9. Van Gijn J, Rinkel GJE. Subarachnoid haemorrhage: diagnosis, causes and management. *Brain.* 2001; 124(2):249-278.
10. Schievink WI. Intracranial aneurysms. *N Engl J Med.* 1997;336(1):28-40.
11. Edlow JA, Caplan LR. Avoiding pitfalls in the diagnosis of subarachnoid hemorrhage. *N Eng J Med.* 2000;342(1):29-36.
12. Perry JJ, Stiell IG, Sivilotti ML, et al. Sensitivity of computed tomography performed within six hours of onset of headache for diagnosis of subarachnoid haemorrhage: prospective cohort study. *BMJ.* 2011;343:d4277.
13. Kassell NF, Torner JC, Haley EC Jr, Jane JA, Adams HP, Kongable GL. The International Cooperative Study on the Timing of Aneurysm Surgery: part 1: overall management results. *J Neurosurg.* 1990;73(1):18-36.
14. Van der Wee N, Rinkel GJ, Hasan D, et al. Detection of subarachnoid haemorrhage on early CT: Is lumbar puncture still needed after a negative scan? *J Neurol Neurosurg Psychiatry.* 1995;58(3):357-359.
15. Kassell NF, Kongable GL, Torner JC, et al. Delay in referral of patients with ruptured aneurysms to neurosurgical attention. *Stroke.* 1985;16(4):587-590.
16. Mayer PL, Awad IA, Todor R, et al. Misdiagnosis of symptomatic cerebral aneurysm prevalence and correlation with outcome at four institutions. *Stroke.* 1996;27(9):1558-1563.
17. Vermeulen M, Hasan D, Blijenberg BG, et al. Xanthochromia after subarachnoid haemorrhage needs no revisitation. *J Neurol Neurosurg Psychiatry.* 1989;52(7):826-828.
18. Van Crevel H, Hijdra A, De Gans J. Lumbar puncture and the risk of herniation: When should we first perform CT? *J Neurol.* 2002;249(2):129-137.
19. Gopal AK, Whitehouse JD, Simel DL, Corey GR. Cranial computed tomography before lumbar puncture: a prospective clinical evaluation. *Arch Intern Med.* 1999;159(22);2681.
20. Hasbun R, Abrahams J, Jekel J, et al. Computed tomography of the head before lumbar puncture in adults with suspected meningitis. *N Engl J Med.* 2001;345(24):1727-1733.
21. Tunkel AR, Hartman BJ, Kaplan SL, et al. Practice guidelines for the management of bacterial meningitis. *Clin Infect Dis.* 2004;39(9):1267-1284.
22. Tunkel AR. Approach to the patient with central nervous system infection. In: Mandell GL, Bennett JE, Dolin R, eds. *Principles and Practice of Infectious Diseases.* 7th ed. Philadelphia, PA: Churchill Livingstone Elsevier; 2009:1183.
23. Lawrence RH. The role of lumbar puncture as a diagnostic tool in 2005. *Crit Care Resusc.* 2005;7:213-220.
24. Gower DJ, Baker AL, Bell WO, et al. Contraindications to lumbar puncture as defined by computed cranial tomography. *J Neurol Neurosurg Psychiatry.* 1987;50(8):1071-1074.

25. Holdgate A, Cuthbert K. Perils and pitfalls of lumbar puncture in the emergency department. *Emerg Med (Fremantle).* 2001;13(3):351-358.

26. Oddo M, Le Roux P. What are the etiology, pathogenesis, and pathophysiology of elevated intracranial pressure? In: Deutschman C, Neligan P, eds. *Evidence-Based Practice of Critical Care.* 1st ed. Philadelphia, PA: Elsevier Health Sciences; 2010:399.

27. Mokri, B. The Monro-Kellie hypothesis applications in CSF volume depletion. *Neurology.* 2001;56(12):1746-1748.

28. Albeck MJ, Børgesen SE, Gjerris F, et al. Intracranial pressure and cerebrospinal fluid outflow conductance in healthy subjects. *J Neurosurg.* 1991;74(4):597-600.

29. Fisher A, Lupu L, Gurevitz B, et al. Hip flexion and lumbar puncture: a radiological study. *Anaesthesia.* 2001;56(3):262-266.

30. Arévalo-Rodríguez I, Ciapponi A, Munoz L, et al. Posture and fluids for preventing post-dural puncture headache. *Cochrane Database Syst Rev.* 2013;(7):CD009199.

31. Stiffler KA, Jwayyed S, Wilber ST, Robinson A. The use of ultrasound to identify pertinent landmarks for lumbar puncture. *Am J Emerg Med.* 2007;25(3):331-334.

32. Shaikh F, Brzezinski J, Alexander S, et al. Ultrasound imaging for lumbar punctures and epidural catheterisations: systematic review and meta-analysis. *BMJ.* 2013;346:f1720-f1731.

33. Sudlow C, Warlow C. Posture and fluids for preventing post-dural puncture headache. *Cochrane Database Syst Rev.* 2001;(2):CD001790.

34. Lavi R, Yernitzky D, Rowe JM, et al. Standard vs atraumatic Whitacre needle for diagnostic lumbar puncture: a randomized trial. *Neurology.* 2006;67(8):1492-1494.

35. Thomas SR, Jamieson DRS, Muir KW. Randomised controlled trial of atraumatic versus standard needles for diagnostic lumbar puncture. *BMJ.* 2000;321(7267):986-990.

36. Braune HJ, Huffmann G. A prospective double-blind clinical trial, comparing the sharp Quincke needle (22G) with an "atraumatic" needle (22G) in the induction of post-lumbar puncture headache. *Acta Neurol Scand.* 1992;86(1):50-54.

37. Peterman SB. Postmyelography headache: a review. *Radiology.* 1996;200(3):765-770.

38. Richman JM, Joe EM, Cohen SR, et al. Bevel direction and postdural puncture headache: a meta-analysis. *Neurologist.* 2006;12(4):224-228.

39. Strupp M, Brandt T, Müller A. Incidence of post-lumbar puncture syndrome reduced by reinserting the stylet: a randomized prospective study of 600 patients. *J Neurol.* 1998;245(9):589-592.

40. Van Kooten F, Oedit R, Bakker SL, et al. Epidural blood patch in post dural puncture headache: a randomised, observer-blind, controlled clinical trial. *J Neurol Neurosurg Psychiatry.* 2008;79(5):553-558.

41. Evans RW. Complications of lumbar puncture. *Neurol Clin.* 1998;16(1):83-105.

42. Baer ET. Post-dural puncture bacterial meningitis. *Anesthesiology.* 2006;105(2):381-393.

43. Greenlee JE, Carroll KC. Cerebrospinal fluid in central nervous system infections. In: Scheld WM, Whitley RJ, Marra CM, eds. *Infections of the Central Nervous System.* 3rd ed. Philadelphia, PA: Lippincott Williams & Wilkins; 2004:5-30.

44. Hiratzka LF, Bakris GL, Beckman JA, et al. 2010ACCF/AHA/AATS/ACR/ASA/SCA/SCAI/SIR/STS/SVM guidelines for the diagnosis and management of patients with thoracic aortic disease. *J Am Coll Cardiol.* 2010;55(14):e27-e129.

Temporary Pacemaker Insertion and Management of CV Implantable Electrical Devices in the ICU

103

Michael J. Grushko, MD and Jay N. Gross, MD

KEY POINTS

1 Bradyarrhythmias occur commonly in the intensive care unit (ICU), and most events do not necessitate temporary pacing.

2 Transient bradycardia often occurs in the setting of enhanced vagal tone or other reversible causes.

3 Temporary pacing should be considered when symptoms or hemodynamic compromise develops secondary to the bradyarrhythmia.

4 Transvenous temporary pacing in the ICU setting generally requires intracardiac electrogram (EGM) guidance.

5 Reliable temporary pacing requires adequate sensing and pacing thresholds, stable position of the lead, and secure connections of the pacing system.

6 Permanently implanted pacemakers and implantable cardioverter-defibrillators (ICDs) generally function well in the standard programmed settings, and apparent "anomalous behavior" may be the result of acute rhythm change or electrolyte abnormalities, rather than device malfunction.

TEMPORARY PACEMAKERS IN THE ICU SETTING

Bradyarrhythmias occur commonly in the ICU, and most events do not necessitate temporary pacing. Transient bradycardia often occurs in the setting of enhanced vagal tone due to tracheal irritation, suction, or intubation; abdominal distention; or severe vomiting. Reversible causes such as severe electrolyte or acid-base imbalances should be corrected first whenever possible, as this may obviate the need for pacing or enhance the likelihood that a temporary lead will function appropriately when placed. Isolated sinus pauses, transient extended pauses in atrial fibrillation (AF), and nocturnal bradycardia in patients with obstructive sleep apnea are all common, and generally do not require temporary pacing. Pacing is considered when patients are having symptoms or have developed hemodynamic compromise thought to be secondary to a bradyarrhythmia, or if a rhythm is detected that is associated with a high risk of subsequent malignant bradyarrhythmia (Table 103–1). Recognizing circumstances that portend risk, for example, anterior wall or inferior

TABLE 103–1 Indications for temporary cardiac pacing (based on ACC/AHA guidelines).

Bradycardia associated with acute myocardial infarction
- Asystole
- Sinus bradycardia with symptoms or hypotension not responsive to atropine, typically with inferior infarction
- High-grade AV block (second-degree type II AVB, high-degree AVB, or complete heart block) and/or new bundle branch (especially LBBB) or bifascicular block in patients with anterior/lateral MI with/without hemodynamic insult or syncope
- Ventricular arrhythmia due to bradycardia

Bradycardia not associated with myocardial infarction
- Asystole
- Second-degree type II AVB, high-degree AVB, or complete heart block with hemodynamic insult or syncope
- Severe sinus node dysfunction with recurrent symptomatic long pauses, sinus arrest, or tachy-brady syndrome
- Ventricular arrhythmia due to bradycardia

Support for procedures that may develop bradycardia
- General anesthesia in the setting of 2nd- or 3rd-degree AV block, bifascicular block with a 1st-degree AV block, intermittent AV block
- Cardiac surgery such as ventricular septal defect closure, ostium primum atrial septal defect repair

Overdrive suppression of tachyarrhythmias
- Ventricular tachycardia
- Supraventricular tachycardia

AV, atrioventricular; AVB, atrioventricular block; LBBB, left bundle branch block; MI, myocardial infarction.
Adapted with permission from Gammage MD: Temporary cardiac pacing, *Heart* 2000 Jun;83(6):715-720.

wall myocardial infarction (MI), or preexisting infra-Hisian conduction disease, will help identify patients at high risk for need of temporary pacing.

Transcutaneous Pacing

There are multiple methods for temporary cardiac pacing, including transcutaneous, transvenous, and even transesophageal pacing. In the event of sustained hemodynamic compromise and/or ventricular asystole due to bradyarrhythmia, the most prompt and easiest pacing method is transcutaneous pacing. Current day external defibrillators allow for transcutaneous pacing via the defibrillation pads (Figure 103–1). One should ensure that the pads are applied to dry and intact skin. Ideally, the pads should be positioned in a relative anterior-posterior (AP) location, with the anterior pad placed to the left of the sternum near the point of maximal impulse, and the

posterior pad to the left of the spine and just beneath the scapula. The external generator is set to "pacer" and the rate set based on the acute need. The output is ramped up until reliable capture is obtained, which is usually greater than 40 mA. Due to saturation of the electrocardiogram (ECG) signal from the pacing artifact, myocardial capture may not be clearly evident on the telemetry or ECG. The peripheral pulse can be checked to verify consistent capture. External pacing, despite appropriate technique and multiple adequate pad orientations, achieves consistent capture in only a small majority of patients at best. In addition, it is quite painful to the conscious patient. Hence, it should only be used as a temporizing measure in anticipation of urgent transvenous pacing unless capture is reliable, the patient is deeply sedated or unconscious, and/or when temporary pacing is required for a brief period of time.

Temporary Transvenous Pacing

Like all interventions, the benefits of a temporary transvenous pacemaker (TVP) must be weighed against its risks. Insertion of a temporary pacemaker puts patients at risk for complications related to central venous access, such as bleeding, pneumothorax (level of risk depending on venous access site), thrombosis, line-related sepsis, and cardiac tamponade. Additionally, an unstable temporary pacemaker lead or malfunctioning system has the potential to induce malignant ventricular tachyarrhythmias. Individuals who insert temporary pacemakers should be specifically trained in this area and this procedure should not be equated with other procedures that solely require obtaining central venous access.

Temporary pacemaker leads are most commonly placed via the internal jugular (IJ) or subclavian veins, but when needed, can be placed through the femoral, brachial, or even external jugular veins. When performed at bedside, the right IJ (best with ultrasound guidance) or left subclavian veins are most commonly used as they offer the most direct routes for the shaped balloon-tipped catheters. When fluoroscopy is available (either via portable C-arm or in the interventional laboratory), any of the earlier access sites can be used. In some institutions, the left subclavian is avoided so that this access site is kept available for potential permanent device implantation. Needless to say, strict sterile technique must be adhered to as a pacing wire

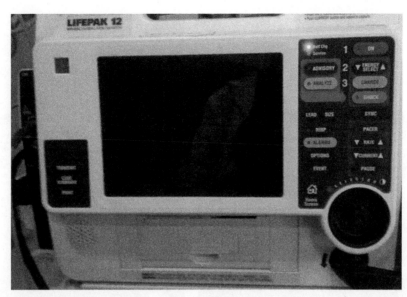

FIGURE 103–1 A typical external defibrillator and transcutaneous pacemaker.

is delivered into the endocardium, which places the patient at risk for bacteremia or endocarditis.

There are various types of temporary pacing leads commercially available. Balloon-tipped leads designed to enhance advancement to the right ventricle are probably the fastest, most accessible, and generally do not require fluoroscopy. These catheters are generally placed via 6-Fr sheaths. Standard multipole electrophysiology (EP) catheters (5 or 6 Fr) or active fixation leads that provide for increased stability can also be used but require fluoroscopy (Figure 103–2). In rare circumstances, when there is a need for very extended temporary pacing, individuals who implant permanent devices have inserted a permanent active fixation lead and connected them to an externalized permanent pacemaker device until the time for permanent implantation.

Methods of Placement

Lead placement can be performed via electrogram (EGM) or fluoroscopic guidance or both. The most practical way to insert a pacing wire is via EGM guidance. The patient is connected to a 12-lead ECG machine, with standard placement of the 4-limb leads (at least). A 12-lead ECG confirming the indication can be obtained (Figure 103–3A). Once the temporary lead is placed into the circulation, the "distal" end

of the pacing lead (marked [−]) is passed to an assistant who connects the electrode to the V1 ECG clip. When connected in this manner, the "V1 lead" on the ECG actually displays the local unipolar intracardiac EGM at the tip of the pacing lead. Of note, care must be taken to cover this connection as this part of the pacemaker wire is no longer sterile. As one advances, the EGM pattern changes from a predominant atrial to a mixed atrial-ventricular signal at the level of the tricuspid valve, and finally when the valve is crossed, a large ventricular EGM is demonstrable. When good contact with the ventricular wall is made, a large localized ST elevation pattern referred to as the "current of injury" is typically seen (Figure 103–3B). The balloon is deflated at this point to allow the lead tip to oppose itself completely to the ventricular myocardium. The most reliable site for temporary pacing is the right ventricular apex. When the lead is positioned in the right ventricular (RV) apex, a paced QRS with a left bundle branch block (LBBB), interior axis pattern will be present (Figure 103–3C). Typically, the RV position is reached between 35 and 45 cm, and if the markers on the lead indicate that significantly more lead is intravascular, it is likely that a large loop is present, which may promote lead instability. When using fluoroscopy, visual guidance makes placement of the lead to the RV apex easier. The position can be confirmed

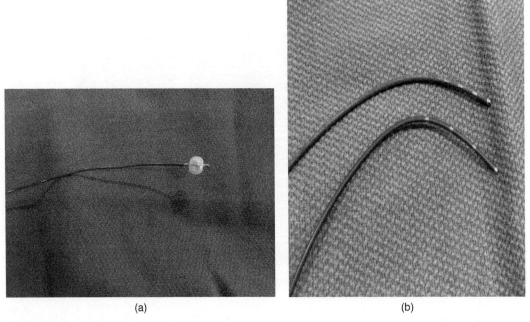

(a)   (b)

FIGURE 103–2 Various examples of temporary transvenous pacing leads. **A.** It shows a standard balloon-tipped catheter with its distal connections. **B.** It shows 2 examples of multipolar-tipped electrophysiology (EP) catheters that can be placed via fluoroscopy.

by AP, right anterior oblique (RAO), and left anterior oblique (LAO) views.

Once the lead is placed in position with a good current of injury, careful assessment of pacing function is required. A normally functioning temporary pacemaker should have a low pacing threshold (typically 1 mA or less) and be capable of sensing spontaneous ventricular activity (preferably 5 mV signals or larger). If there is no underlying rhythm, or if the patient's spontaneous rate is less than the minimal programmable rate of the temporary pacemaker, the sensing threshold cannot be measured.

Once lead stability and functionality is established, suturing the lead at the insertion site in a highly secure manner is critical, as even a minimal displacement of a perfectly placed lead may result in a totally nonfunctioning pacing system. Most operators choose to leave the sheath in place, especially if needed for central venous access (as a sidearm is usually present). In addition, many choose to place a sterile sleeve that is integrated with the introducer around the pacemaker wire, so as to allow for some degree of lead manipulation if a sudden need arises.

Note that the EGM-guided approach is practical only when there is spontaneous ventricular electrical activity. In rare circumstances when there is absolutely no ventricular activity, and fluoroscopy is not immediately available, the only practical option is to advance the lead blindly while pacing in the hope that the lead is advanced to a stable site in the RV and ventricular capture is achieved.

Pacemaker Generators

There are numerous types of temporary pacemaker generators. When a temporary transvenous lead is placed, it is typically connected to a single-chamber generator, though in certain circumstances a temporary transvenous atrial wire can also be placed creating a dual-chamber system. In the cardiothoracic surgical areas, patients may have temporary epicardial wires connected to single- or dual-chamber temporary pulse generators (Figure 103–4). Programming capabilities of these devices vary widely depending on the model type, but all allow for adjustments of pacing rates, outputs, and sensitivities. Most devices also have a capability to deliver rapid antitachycardia

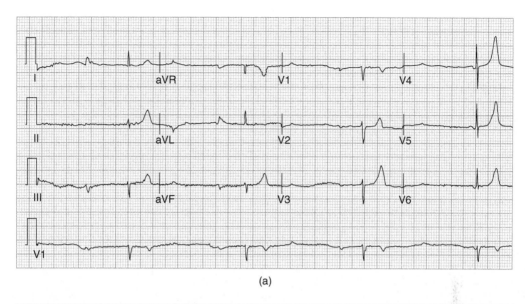

(a)

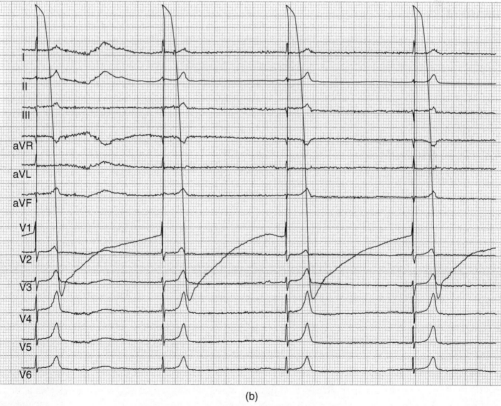

(b)

FIGURE 103–3 A. Electrocardiogram (ECG) with sinus rhythm, complete heart block with a very slow narrow complex escape rhythm. **B.** Lead V1 attached to the temporary distal port displaying a myocardial current of injury, indicating good opposition with the myocardial endocardium. **C.** ECG shows ventricular pacing in a left bundle branch block (LBBB) pattern with negative QRS complexes in the inferior leads and positive QRS complexes in I, L, and augmented voltage right arm (aVR), consistent with right ventricular (RV) apical pacing.

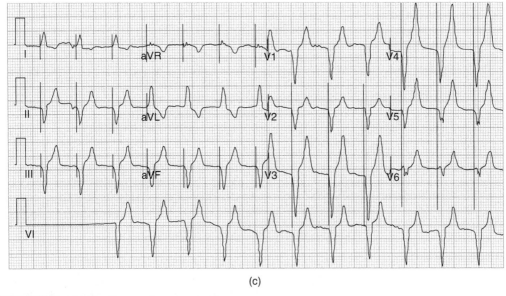

(c)

FIGURE 103–3 (*Continued*)

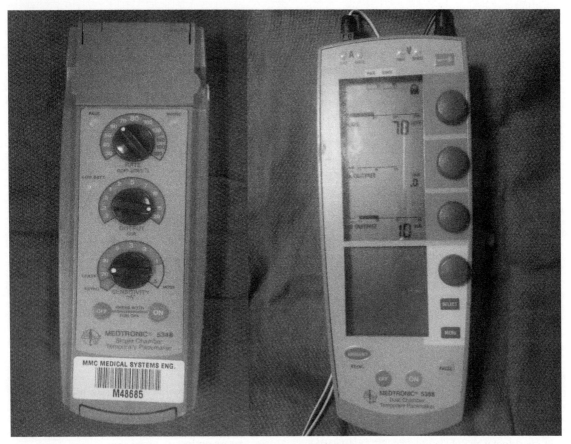

FIGURE 103–4 Typical single- and dual-chamber temporary pacemaker generators.

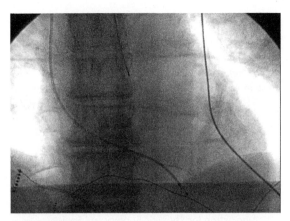

FIGURE 103–5 Chest x-ray (CXR) showing right ventricular (RV) apical lead placement.

pacing, though such activities require the experience of a cardiologist or electrophysiologist.

A chest x-ray should be obtained soon after lead placement to rule out pneumothorax and establish initial radiographic location (Figure 103–5). Should unexplained hypotension or tachycardia ensue any time after placement, a transthoracic echo should be obtained to look for pericardial effusion and/or tamponade from a possible RV perforation. The insertion site should be monitored for bleeding/hematoma. Most importantly, the TVP should be checked at least once daily for both capture threshold and sensitivity, and also after any major movements or transfers. If any changes in device function are noted, a repeat chest x-ray (CXR) should be obtained for evaluation of lead position and a careful check of all connections should be made.

PERMANENT PACEMAKERS IN THE ICU SETTING

Even in the critical care setting, permanent pacemakers usually function normally and special modifications of programmed settings are very infrequently required. Fortunately, most complex mechanical and electrical devices in the critical care unit do not impact on pacemaker function. On occasion, attempts to increase cardiac output by pacing at more rapid rates are pursued, but this usually proves ineffective, as the higher pacing rate is often associated with a concomitant fall in stroke volume. Patients, who develop severe electrolyte or acid-base disturbances, may be at risk for developing pacemaker malfunction. In such circumstances, programming the device to higher pacing outputs and more sensitive settings may offset, at least temporarily, some of these pacing abnormalities.

A basic understanding of pacemaker codes and modes is essential for interpreting pacing patterns seen on ECGs and telemetry. It is important to appreciate that the pacing pattern manifested is a function of both the patient's underlying rhythm and the programmed parameters of the pacemaker. Thus, the absence of any pacemaker activity during regular rhythms most often represents totally normal pacemaker function, and should not trigger any immediate concerns. In order to determine definitively whether function is normal, it is necessary to know the programmed settings of the device. Suspected discrepancies between the programmed settings and pacemaker function should trigger cardiology consultation.

Special Considerations

Cardioversion—In patients with pacemakers or ICDs who are to undergo urgent or planned cardioversion in the ICU setting via external pads, the delivery of direct current energy poses a small risk to both the integrity of the pulse generator and to the lead tip-myocardial interface. The preferred manner is to place the defibrillator pads in an AP orientation near the midline and not overlying the device. In addition, if the device is an ICD, cardiology consultation can be requested to evaluate if cardioversion via the implanted device is appropriate.

Newly implanted cardiac devices—If a hemodynamic monitoring catheter needs to be placed in a patient who has undergone pacemaker or ICD implantation in the previous 6 months, it poses a potential risk for dislodgement. Fluoroscopic guidance is preferred in this setting so as to decrease the risk of unintended lead displacement.

Rate modulation—Many pacemakers are programmed with the rate modulation feature activated. This refers to the ability of the pacemaker to detect the need for an increased heart rate based on the information provided by specialized sensors. The 2 most common forms of rate modulation sensors and associated algorithms are piezoelectric crystal-based accelerometers (ie, equate movement with exertion) or calculated minute ventilation, which is based on transthoracic impedance changes. Infrequently, excessive shaking of the patient or high tidal volume–assisted ventilation may trigger inappropriately elevated pacing rates based on these sensors. In this uncommon circumstance, the rate modulation parameter should be programmed to off.

ICDS IN THE ICU SETTING

Most of the comments described in the pacing section are equally relevant to implantable ICDs, which have analogous pacing capabilities. There are additional considerations that should be kept in mind when dealing with a patient with an active ICD in the ICU setting.

Perhaps the most important consideration is that critically ill patients are frequently tachycardic, either as a physiologic response to their underlying circumstances or resulting from the pharmacologic agents that are being used to support their hemodynamics. This increases the possibility that the ICD patient may receive inappropriate ICD therapies if the heart rate exceeds the detection rate threshold of the device. While many devices have algorithms programmed to try to distinguish ventricular tachycardia (VT) from supraventricular tachycardia (SVT), AF, and sinus tachycardia, none is perfect. The best way to avoid inappropriate shocks is to assure that the tachycardia detection rate is above the patient's heart rate. Since settings vary widely between patients, it is valuable to know the programmed parameters of these devices, so as to avoid the possibility of inappropriate ICD therapies. On occasion, temporary reprogramming to allow for delivery of antitachycardia pacing therapies under the guidance of an electrophysiologist may facilitate minimally invasive and better-controlled treatment of arrhythmias in the critical care setting.

SUGGESTED READING

Ellenbogen KA, Wilkoff BL, Kay GN, Lau C. *Clinical Cardiac Pacing, Defibrillation, and Resynchronization Therapy*. Elsevier-Saunders; 2011.

Epstein AE, DiMarco JP, Ellenbogen KA, et al. ACC/AHA/HRS 2008 guidelines for device-based therapy of cardiac rhythm abnormalities: a report of the American College of Cardiology/American Heart Association Task Force on Practice Guidelines (Writing Committee to Revise the ACC/AHA/NASPE 2002 Guideline Update for Implantation of Cardiac Pacemakers and Antiarrhythmia Devices): developed in collaboration with the American Association for Thoracic Surgery and Society of Thoracic Surgeons. *Circulation*. 2008;117:e350-e408.

Peters RW, Vijayaraman P, Ellenbogen KA. *Cardiac Pacing and ICDs*. 5th ed. Wiley-Blackwell; 2008:35-44.

Tracy CM, Epstein AE, Darbar D, et al. 2012 ACCF/AHA/HRS focused update of the 2008 guidelines for device-based therapy of cardiac rhythm abnormalities: a report of the American College of Cardiology Foundation/American Heart Association Task Force on Practice Guidelines and the Heart Rhythm Society. *Circulation*. 2012;126:1784-1800.

REFERENCES

1. Epstein AE, DiMarco JP, Ellenbogen KA, et al. ACC/AHA/HRS 2008 guidelines for device-based therapy of cardiac rhythm abnormalities: a report of the American College of Cardiology/American Heart Association Task Force on Practice Guidelines (Writing Committee to Revise the ACC/AHA/NASPE 2002 Guideline Update for Implantation of Cardiac Pacemakers and Antiarrhythmia Devices). *Circulation*. 2008;117:e350-e408.

2. Tracy CM, Epstein AE, Darbar D, et al. 2012 ACCF/AHA/HRS focused update of the 2008 guidelines for device-based therapy of cardiac rhythm abnormalities: a report of the American College of Cardiology Foundation/American Heart Association Task Force on Practice Guidelines and the Heart Rhythm Society. *Circulation*. 2012;126:1784-1800.

3. Ellenbogen KA, Wilkoff BL, Kay GN, Lau C. *Clinical Cardiac Pacing, Defibrillation, and Resynchronization Therapy*. Elsevier-Saunders; 2011.

4. Peters RW, Vijayaraman P, Ellenbogen KA. *Cardiac Pacing and ICDs*. 5th ed. Wiley-Blackwell:35-44.

Paracentesis

Claude Killu, MD and Mark Ault, MD

1. Paracentesis is a relatively safe procedure that can be performed in either the inpatient or outpatient setting.

2. Diagnostic paracentesis should be performed on any patient with newly diagnosed ascites or any patient with known ascites that has a change in clinical status.

3. Therapeutic "total paracentesis," the removal of all of the ascites with albumin replacement, is a safe technique for the treatment of symptomatic ascites.

4. Coagulation testing need not be performed and correction of coagulation abnormalities prior to paracentesis is unnecessary.

5. A-2 probe ultrasound technique (low-frequency probe to find an optimal fluid pocket and high-frequency probe to evaluate the abdominal wall for vessels) should be used in all cases.

DEFINITION

Abdominal paracentesis is a procedure in which fluid is removed from the peritoneal cavity with a needle or cannula in patients with ascites. It is a relatively quick and safe procedure and can be done with a minimal amount of equipment as an outpatient procedure or at the bedside for inpatients. Now routinely used as an adjunct to paracentesis, point-of-care ultrasound is a simple procedure that confirms the presence of ascites. Proper analysis of fluid is invaluable in determining the etiology of ascites. The procedure can be done by any trained physician, surgeon, or a midlevel provider. At our institution we have a dedicated team of proceduralists and intensivists experienced in performing paracentesis using exclusively ultrasound guidance.

INDICATIONS

The procedure can be done for therapeutic, diagnostic, or both purposes.

Diagnostic: The procedure helps diagnose.

- The cause of a new-onset ascites or the status of preexisting ascites in patients who are admitted to the hospital for any reason. This is particularly important if there is evidence of infection, hepatic encephalopathy, fever, leukocytosis hypotension, and acute kidney injury.[1]

- Spontaneous bacterial peritonitis where detection at an early stage and expedient initiation of antibiotics can lower mortality. Therefore, the procedure must be performed promptly in virtually all circumstances where a patient with known or newly discovered ascites sustains any change in clinical status. Delays that may occur due to lack of an experienced operator, unfounded concerns for the presence of coagulopathy, or unnecessary administration of blood products prior to paracentesis should be avoided. Analysis of the ascitic fluid may allow not only assessment of the likelihood of spontaneous bacterial peritonitis (SBP) but, with proper collection, identification of a specific microorganism and susceptibility testing to antibiotics guiding treatment in 90% of cases.

- Secondary peritonitis when free fluid is present in peritoneal cavity from rupture or perforation of an abdominal organ. The total protein may be a key differentiating factor in this situation as it is generally low in SBP but may be normal or elevated in secondary causes.

- Malignancy-related ascites (not to be confused with peritoneal carcinomatosis) may be seen with several tumors, including malignancies of the ovary, pancreas, colon, breast, lung, and liver. In addition, the presence of chylous ascites may indicate lymphoma as the cause of the ascites.

- Hemoperitoneum related to trauma, postprocedural or spontaneous intraperitoneal hemorrhage.

Therapeutic: The procedure is usually performed to relieve intra-abdominal pressure causing symptoms of dyspnea, fatigue, early satiety, and/or abdominal discomfort. The amount of fluid a patient can tolerate and the rate of accumulation is highly variable between patients, but will generally establish a predictable pattern in any given patient. Symptoms can be relieved by removal of as little as 1 to 2 L of fluid in a small individual.

CONTRAINDICATION

In general, the diagnostic value of paracentesis outweighs the risks in virtually all circumstances. One of the most frequent concerns in the cirrhotic patient is the potential for bleeding due to coagulopathy and the risks this may pose, yet this concern is largely unfounded. When tested the majority of cirrhotic patients with ascites will be found to have some degree of coagulopathy, but this should preclude paracentesis only in severe cases of disseminated intravascular coagulopathy with overt bleeding or clinically evident primary fibrinolysis. Bleeding from a paracentesis puncture is rare and when it occurs is generally due to injury to a vascular structure which is consistent with the fact that these patients usually have normal coagulation function despite abnormal test results such as the prothrombin time (PT)/international normalized ratio (INR), activated partial thromboplastin time (aPTT), or platelet count. This is partly due to the fact that there is deficiency of both anticoagulants and procoagulants. In fact liver disease can lead to either a hypocoagulable state or a hypercoagulable state. The relative balance or imbalance of these factors is not reflected in conventional tests of coagulation. Clinical evaluation for overt bleeding tends to be a more valuable determinant of bleeding risk than coagulation testing. The inappropriate practice of transfusion of fresh frozen plasma (FFP) and/or platelets' blood product to reverse the coagulopathy before paracentesis is therefore unnecessary and must be discouraged. Routine administration of blood products exposes the patient to a risk of infection and fluid overload and is costly; furthermore, there are no available data to support a threshold or a cutoff value for coagulation parameters beyond which paracentesis should be avoided. It has been shown that approximately 100 to 200 units of FFP would need to be administered prior to paracentesis to prevent transfusion of 2 units of red cells making this practice impractical at best. Grabau and colleagues reported no bleeding complications in series of 1100 patients who underwent large-volume paracenteses without pre- or postprocedure transfusions required despite INRs as high as 8.7 and platelet counts as low as 19,000/mL highlighting the lack of benefit of "corrective" blood product administration in virtually all instances.[2]

COMPLICATIONS

Paracentesis is a safe procedure with a major complication rate of less than 1 in 1000 procedures. Deaths caused by paracentesis are rare but do occur and require meticulous attention to technique. Major complications include procedurally related intraperitoneal bleeding, bowel perforation, and injury to internal organs. The last 2 complications have been virtually eliminated by the adjunctive use of ultrasound. However, until recently hemoperitoneum remained a potentially tragic and unpredictable complication. Recently, this occurrence has largely been attributed to the presence of both normal and abnormal vascular structures buried in the abdominal wall that are generally not palpable, visible, or seen by routine fluid localization with a low-frequency abdominal ultrasound probe. By using in addition, a high-frequency linear probe to specifically evaluate the abdominal wall for the presence and location of these vessels, they may be identified and subsequently avoided (Figures 104–1A, B, and C). In our experience ultrasound assessment both for the optimal location of the fluid and the presence of abdominal wall vessels has nearly eliminated the risk of postprocedural hemoperitoneum and is now considered standard of practice at our institution.[3]

Minor complications are relatively infrequent occurring in 2% to 5% of cases and may include abdominal wall hematoma, leakage from the paracentesis site, the need for more than one attempt to obtain fluid, excessive pain during the procedure, and the inability to completely drain the abdominal cavity. While abdominal wall or rectus sheath hematoma may be extensive, in general these complications can be managed with local measures. Of note, we also track operator injury in the form of needle stick or fluid contact contamination as a complication to emphasize the need for sharp safety and procedural hygiene to our operators.

PRECAUTIONS

Aseptic technique is required when performing this procedure though the need for wide sterile barriers is unnecessary. Caution should be taken especially in patients with massive bowel distension or ileus and in patients with scars indicative of prior abdominal surgeries. Ultrasound should be used in all cases and is invaluable in avoiding these potential anatomic pitfalls. Ultrasound, while essential to the overall safety of the procedure carries its own

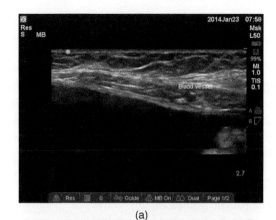

(a)

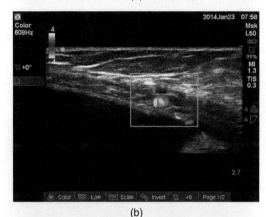

(b)

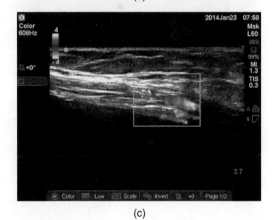

(c)

FIGURE 104–1 A. Cross-sectional ultrasound image of abdomainal wall vessel. **B.** Cross-sect us image abd wall vessel Doppler sig blood flow. **C.** Longitudinal us image of abd wall vessel Doppler sig blood flow.

potential hazards if not applied appropriately. While the learning curve is relatively steep for this application, appropriate training is required to avoid interpretive errors.

PREPARATION AND TECHNIQUE

Patient Positioning

The procedure is usually done with the patient in supine position and the head of the bed flat or slightly elevated. It may be helpful to have the patient tilt slightly to the site of where the entry is planned to allow for pooling and fluid shift.

Sites of Needle Entry and Anatomy

The patient is tilted slightly to the side to allow for fluid shift. The entire abdominal cavity must be scanned with ultrasound using a low-frequency phase array or curvilinear probe to determine the area of "maximum echogenicity" representing the most favorable pocket of fluid. The potential site of entry is then evaluated using a high-frequency linear probe to identify a site within this region devoid of abnormal vasculature. This optimal site of entry is marked on the abdominal wall with an indelible marker (Figures 104–2A, B, and C).

PREPARATION AND EQUIPMENT

An informed consent must be obtained and a formal time-out performed to verify procedure and patient identifier. The following supplies and equipment are needed (Table 104–1):

- Spring-tipped paracentesis drainage kit (Figures 104–3A and B)
- Sterile gloves
- Collection canisters
- Chaux

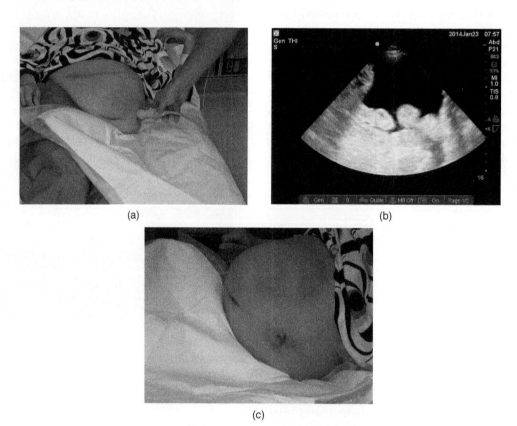

(a)

(b)

(c)

FIGURE 104–2 **A.** Patient is tilted slightly to the side to allow for fluid shift. **B.** Ultrasound using a low-frequency phase array or curvilinear probe to determine the area of "maximum echogenicity". **C.** Optimal site of entry is marked on the abdominal wall with an indelible marker.

TABLE 104–1 Supplies.

- Safe-T-Centesis catheter drainage tray
- 8-Fr catheter drainage device
- Filter needle 19 gauge
- Needle, 25 gauge x 1.5 in
- 10-mL syringe
- 60-mL syringe
- Scalpel
- Universal drainage set
- Collection bag
- ChloroPrep 3-mL applicator
- Drainage tubes
- Gauze pads
- Lidocaine 1% 5 mL
- Fenestrated drape
- Towel
- Bandage

The use of sterile gown, hair cover, or face mask is not required. But the overlying skin is to be prepped in the usual sterile fashion and sterile gloves are used with sterile barriers to create the appropriate sterile field.

PARACENTESIS NEEDLE CHOICE

For local anesthesia the preferred needle is 1.5-in 22- or 25-gauge. In obese patients, a 3.5-in 22-gauge "spinal" needle can be used for diagnostic paracentesis.

Using nonsterile gloves first the skin is sterilized with chlorhexidine. Sterile gloves are then used. If the original X mark has been erased during site preparation, a new mark can be placed with a *sterile*

pen. A sterile drape with a round hole in the middle is placed over the prepped skin and another sterile drape is placed on the side next to the patient to create a wider area. The needle with the syringe to administer lidocaine is inserted intradermally to create a skin wheel. Then the same needle is advanced ideally to the peritoneum providing anesthesia along the needle track. Once the needle enters the peritoneal cavity, fluid is aspirated but this may not be accomplished in obese patients and should not preclude proceeding with the procedure if adequate ultrasound landmarks have been established. At this point the needle is withdrawn and a small skin nick is to be made with a #11 size scalpel at the exact site of needle entry. Attention should be paid to avoid an unnecessarily large skin nick as this will lead to postprocedural leakage and issues with hemostasis. A 6- or 8-Fr catheter over a blunt spring-tipped trocar is then introduced through the skin incision into the peritoneal space with a return of fluid aspirate. When the trocar is at the level of the peritoneum it is helpful to ask the patient to take a deep breath. This tightens the peritoneum and provides countertraction to the trocar making entry into the peritoneal space more comfortable with less rebound. A click of the spring-tip catheter will be appreciated indicating passage of the needle tip past the peritoneum membrane into the peritoneal space. The metal trocar is then held in place and the soft catheter is advanced into the cavity (Figure 104–4A-D). Samples are collected sterilely with the specimens for cell count and chemistries are placed in the clear tubes provided.

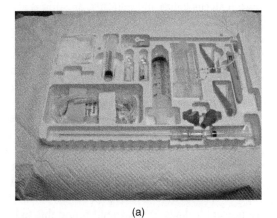

(a)

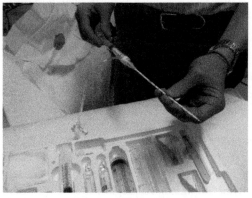

(b)

FIGURE 104–3 A. Spring-tipped paracentesis drainage kit. **B.** Drainage catheter.

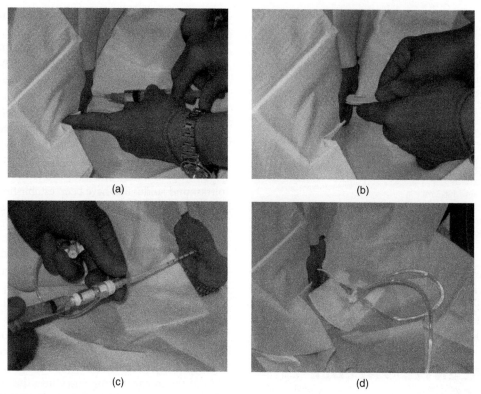

(a) (b) (c) (d)

FIGURE 104–4 A. Needle with the syringe to administer lidocaine is inserted intradermally; the same needle is advanced ideally to the peritoneum. **B.** The needle is withdrawn and a small skin nick is to be made with a #11 size scalpel at the exact site of needle entry. **C.** A 6- or 8-Fr catheter over a blunt spring-tipped trocar is introduced through the skin incision into the peritoneal space with a return of fluid aspirate. **D.** The metal trocar is then held in place and the soft catheter is advanced into the cavity.

Cultures are obtained by inoculating culture bottles directly and if cytology is needed the entire canister is sent to the laboratory to be concentrated. The catheter is then connected to a negative suction bottle or vacuum suction system (Figure 104–5A and B).

As drainage ensues, the bowel and the surrounding omentum may block the flow of the ascitic fluid. Residual ascites may be verified and occasionally the catheter tip itself can then be visualized by placing the ultrasound probe directly adjacent to the catheter insertion site. The stopcock can be opened to release the suction that may have occurred at the catheter tip and the catheter can then be pulled back a few centimeters until flow is restored. In persistent cases it may be worth trying to reposition the patient by further tilting him/her slightly toward the draining site in an attempt to shift the fluid toward the catheter before withdrawing the catheter completely.

When ultrasound examination shows no further fluid to be drained, the 3-way stopcock is turned toward the patient and the catheter is gently pulled out. A sterile gauze and adhesive dressing is applied at the site.

Occasionally, we have noticed a leak from the insertion site after removal of the draining catheter. This, if unrecognized is not serious, but invariably is distressing to the patient and may cause local chemical cellulitis. To address this potential problem, we have been applying a high-viscosity tissue adhesive (Octylseal) or a skin adhesive (Dermabond) to help prevent leakage. This has effectively replaced our prior practice of suturing the puncture site with less skin irritation and no need for suture removal. Multiple references describe the practice of "Z-tracking" to prevent leakage. We have not found this to be an effective option in most patients.

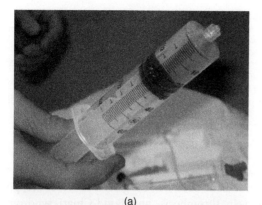

(a)

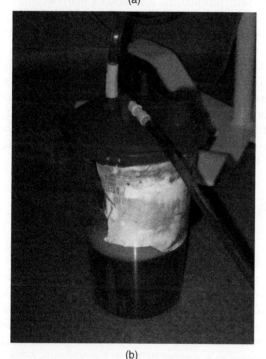

(b)

FIGURE 104-5 A. Samples are collected sterilely and placed in the clear tubes provided. **B.** The catheter is connected to a negative suction bottle or vacuum suction system.

FREQUENCY OF PARACENTESIS AND VOLUME REMOVAL

Removal of 5 L of ascitic fluid in a single session is defined as large-volume paracentesis (LVP) and is considered safe without the need to replace colloids[4] and it used to be considered the safe practical limit to relieve symptoms while preventing hepatorenal syndrome. More recent studies however document the safety of "total paracentesis" where all of the fluid is removed and albumin replacement is given. Standard albumin replacement is performed with 25% albumin administered as 6 to 8 g/L of ascites removed. Occasionally a larger dose of albumin (10 g/L removed) may be given in the setting of baseline renal insufficiency, hypoalbuminemia, or significant edema/anasarca. Additional albumin may also be given postprocedure in the setting of hypotension related to volume shifts. The largest-volume removal reported is 42 L. We have removed 38.8 L without incident.[5]

In our experience, we routinely schedule patients with recurrent ascites refractory to diuretics to return to the clinic at regular intervals that will vary per patient but in general a pattern will be established after 1 to 2 visits. We aim to see them before their ascites interferes with their ability to eat or to exercise in order to prevent muscle breakdown. This has the additional benefit of preventing unwanted emergency department visits for symptom relief and an opportunity for dietary reinforcement.

ANALYSIS OF PERITONEAL FLUID

Clarity and color of the fluid should be noted. The clarity or opacity of the fluid depends largely on the presence and the amount of the neutrophil count or the presence of lipids. The amount of protein, bile, and bilirubin present will determine color. A "benign" fluid sample that has low protein and neutrophil count less than 250/mm³ is usually transparent and slightly yellow-tinged. The presence of bloody or serosanguinous fluid should be noted. A traumatic tap gives a bloody fluid that would clot easily in a nonanticoagulant-containing tube, while a blood-tinged nontraumatic ascitic fluid due to other reasons will not clot. Examples where bloody ascitic fluid may be expected are patients with hepatocellular carcinoma, trauma, and postsurgical and occasionally in peritoneal carcinomatosis. A milky or chylous fluid indicates a high triglyceride concentration and can be seen in advanced stage lymphomas. Bilirubin-stained ascitic fluid occurs in the setting of significant jaundice and appears tea-colored or dark brown. Bile-stained ascites appears greenish and is seen in patients with a bile leak and in patients with hemorrhagic or necrotic pancreatitis.

Only a limited number of diagnostic tests need to be ordered to "profile" the nature of the ascites. A cell count, total protein, and albumin are generally sufficient in most cases and need not be repeated with each paracentesis. The most important test in the symptomatic patient is the cell count and only a few milliliters are needed for evaluation. It is usually agreed that in uncomplicated cirrhosis, the white blood cell (WBC) count will be less than 500/mm^3 and the absolute polymorphonuclear neutrophil (PMN) count should be less than 250/mm^3. A PMN count of greater than 250/mm^3 is considered presumptive evidence of SBP pending culture results but it is important to note that 10% of cases of culture-proven SBP may occur with a PMN count of less than this value. A bloody or serosanguinous ascitic fluid is more difficult to interpret however; using a correction factor subtracting one PMN for each 250 red blood cells (RBCs) may be useful in some scenarios.

Other basic diagnostic tests include Gram stain and culture (aerobic and anaerobic), albumin, total protein, and cytology. More specific tests for diagnosis are triglyceride level in chylous ascites, red blood cell count in trauma and malignancy, bilirubin concentration in bowel perforation, and amylase in pancreatitis (Table 104–2), but need not be ordered routinely.

The serum-to-ascites albumin gradient (SAAG) helps to differentiate etiologies of ascites. The SAAG can be calculated by subtracting the ascitic fluid albumin value from the serum albumin, both measured on the same day. SAAG above 1.1 g/dL suggests the presence of portal hypertension. Etiologies

TABLE 104–3 Diagnostic criteria.

Portal Hypertension (SAAG > 1.1 g/dL)	Nonportal Hypertension (SAAG < 1.1 g/dL)
Cirrhosis • Congestive heart failure • Portal vein thrombosis • Budd-Chiari syndrome	Nephrotic syndrome • Peritoneal tuberculosis • Peritoneal carcinomatosis

SAAG, serum-to-ascites albumin gradient.

of ascites that are associated with portal hypertension include cirrhosis, congestive heart failure, portal vein thrombosis, and Budd-Chiari syndrome. SAAG less than 1.1 g/dL indicates absence of portal hypertension. Examples of causes of ascites without portal hypertension are nephrotic syndrome, peritoneal tuberculosis, and carcinomatosis (Table 104–3). In addition to the ascitic fluid albumin, a total **ascites protein** may be used to assess the risk of SBP with an increased risk associated with levels less than 1 g/dL. It is felt that this level predisposes to SBP because it correlates with complement levels and opsonic activity.

ALBUMIN USE

The use of colloids after a LVP has been debated, but it is generally agreed that paracenteses of 5 L or less would not routinely require albumin replacement. The usual formulation of albumin given in the United States is 25% solution. This provides less volume and less sodium load than the 5% solution. The term postparacentesis circulatory dysfunction (PCD) refers to a state of increased plasma renin activity as a marker of active hypovolemia following LVP and may be responsible for more avid fluid retention and more rapid reaccumulation of ascites. Whether albumin solution administration after LVP has value to correct hypovolemia and improve survival and whether this depends on the amount of fluid removed has been looked at in one study of 105 patients who underwent LVP. These patients were allocated to receive albumin (10 g/L of fluid removed) or no albumin. Those patients who did not receive albumin had an increase in plasma renin activity, developed hemodynamic instability, worsening renal function and hyponatremia.[6] Additionally, albumin replacement has been posited

TABLE 104–2 Ascitic fluid analysis.

Basic Tests	Special Tests
• Cell count and differential • Gram stain, culture, and sensitivity (aerobic, anaerobic) • Albumin • Total protein • Cytology	• Triglyceride level • Red blood cell count • Bilirubin concentration • Amylase

to mitigate fluid extravasation leading to anasarca, and to improve pharmacokinetics of protein-bound medications though data are limited. As noted earlier it is our practice to routinely replace albumin based on volume removed and conditions related to hypovolemia and low oncotic pressure.

In conclusion, paracentesis is a relatively commonly performed procedure that is clearly in the purview of the internist in a variety of settings. It can provide invaluable diagnostic information and significant symptomatic relief. As a benchmark, individuals performing this procedure should maintain records of their procedural activity and be able to document major complication rates approaching 1/1000 procedures. Additionally, it is imperative that the operator be familiar with ultrasound characteristics of the patient with ascites and that ultrasound be used for guidance in all cases.

REFERENCES

1. Runyon BA. In: Feldman M, Friedman LS, Brandt LJ, eds. *Sleisenger and Fordtran's Gastrointestinal and liver disease*. 9th ed. Philadelphia, PA: Saunders Elsevier; 2010:1519.

2. Grabau CM, Crago SF, Hoff LK, et al. Performance standards for therapeutic abdominal paracentesis. *Hepatology*. 2004;40:484.

3. Ault MJ, Rosen BT. Out of sight should not be out of mind: what lurks just beneath the surface of the cirrhotic abdominal wall. *ICU Director*. 2012;3(3):128-129.

4. Runyon BA. Introduction to the revised American Association for the Study of Liver Diseases Practice Guideline management of adult patients with ascites due to cirrhosis 2012. *Hepatology*. 2013;57(4):1651-1653.

5. Ault MJ, Lamba R, Rosen BT. Ultra-large-volume paracentesis: too much of a good thing? *ICU Director*. 2011;2(1-2):12-15.

6. Ginès P, Tito L, Arroyo V, et al. Randomized comparative study of therapeutic paracentesis with and without intravenous albumin in cirrhosis. *Gastroenterology*. 1988;94(6):1493.

Percutaneous Tracheostomy

105

Robert Lee, MD and Mohit Chawla, MD, FCCP

INTRODUCTION

Tracheostomy is defined as creating an artificial airway passage through the neck directly into the trachea. Percutaneous tracheostomy or percutaneous dilatational tracheostomy (PDT) refers to the method of performing tracheostomy using the modified Seldinger (over wire) and dilatational technique. The development of the PDT technique was a natural progression in the era of the rise of minimally invasive approaches. There are, however, notable differences between PDT versus a surgical tracheostomy (ST), in terms of risks and benefits, which will be further discussed in detail. PDT has received wide acceptance by many clinicians, and is now being routinely performed by intensivists, interventional pulmonologists, and surgeons in many countries. It is crucial for those managing patients with tracheostomies to be familiar with PDT in order to provide the best care possible.

HISTORY

Tracheostomy is considered one of the oldest procedures dating back to 3600 BC. The earliest written descriptions are found in Rigveda, a sacred Hindu book, and Babylonian Talmud circa 2000 BC. Percutaneous tracheostomy dates back to 1955, when Sheldon et al used a cutting trocar to place a tracheostomy tube.[1] However, due to the sharp trocar, many deaths occurred. This technique was modified in 1969 when Toye and Weinstein introduced a single tapered dilator with a recessed cutting blade over wire.[2] It was not until 1985, however, when wide acceptance of the percutaneous approach resulted from Ciaglia's new technique of serial dilations over wire in 24 patients.[3] Following this, other techniques came on the horizon including Rapitrach (1989), Griggs (1990), Fantoni, and PercuTwist, which will

be discussed further below. Ciaglia's original multi-dilator method also underwent further refinement leading the Ciaglia Blue Rhino one step dilation technique in 1999, which is undoubtedly considered the most popular approach at this time.[4]

INDICATIONS AND CONTRAINDICATIONS

Indications for PDT are the same as the indications for tracheostomy; however, patient selection is especially important for PDT to minimize potential complications. Unlike ST, the trachea is not directly visualized prior to insertion of the tube during PDT. Only minimal blunt dissection is performed during PDT with rare use of cautery, and therefore, unexpected bleeding can occur during or immediately following the dilatation step.

According to the American Academy of Otolaryngology and Head and Neck Surgery, suggested indications for tracheostomy include the following[5]:

1. Upper airway obstruction
2. Prolonged or expected prolonged intubation
3. Inability of patient to manage secretions (aspiration or excessive bronchopulmonary secretions)
4. Facilitation of ventilation support
5. Inability to intubate
6. Adjunct to manage head and neck surgery
7. Adjunct to manage significant head and neck trauma

In addition, tracheostomy appears to improve the work of breathing and respiratory mechanics.[6-8] In comparison to ST, PDT is an elective procedure typically performed in the intensive care unit (ICU) setting in patients who are already intubated and hemodynamically stable. PDT as an emergent airway management, although possible, is controversial and not universally recommended.[9]

Contraindication for PDT is mostly related to increased risk of bleeding. Although significant bleeding is not common, when it occurs it can be difficult to control.[10,11]

TECHNIQUES

Although several variations in techniques exist for PDT, the basic premise is the same: the trachea is punctured using a hollow needle, guidewire is advanced into the airway, then over the wire, dilatation and eventual placement of the tracheostomy tube is performed. The Fantoni technique is one of the few exceptions that deviates from this basic principle. Bronchoscopic guidance may or may not be used during the procedure depending on the operator's expertise and/or preference.

Ciaglia Blue Rhino Single Dilator

This technique is by far the most widely accepted and practiced approach. When initially introduced by Ciaglia in 1985, multiple separate dilators were used prior to a tracheostomy tube insertion. This multidilation step was consolidated into one single dilator technique in 1999, which simplified the insertion process and reduced the insertion time.[3,4]

Once the entry site is identified by palpation, an incision is made. After minimal dissection, the needle is inserted into the trachea. Bronchoscopic guidance is helpful but not mandatory. Once the wire is inserted into the airway, dilation is made using a punch dilator followed by the single tapered dilator with the subsequent insertion of the tracheostomy tube (Figure 105–1).

Ciaglia Blue Dolphin

This method was designed to prevent significant force exerted from anterior to posterior direction during the single dilator method, which can lead to tracheal ring fracture.[12] Also, an attempt was made to further simplify the tracheostomy insertion by having the dilator and tracheostomy tube loader

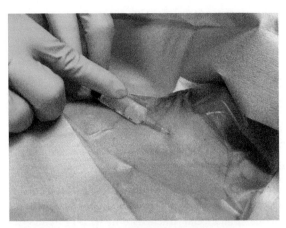

FIGURE 105–1A Local anesthesia (lidocaine and epinephrine mixture) is given at the site of entry.

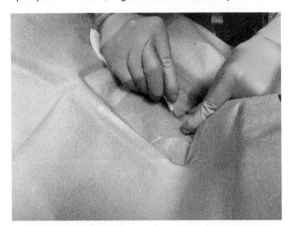

FIGURE 105–1B Incision is made either horizontally or vertically over trachea.

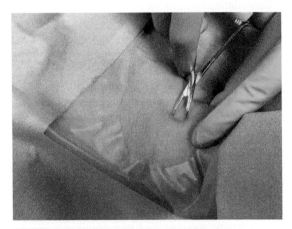

FIGURE 105–1C Minimal blunt dissection is performed (this is considered as an optional step).

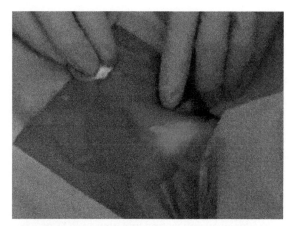

FIGURE 105–1D Bronchoscope light is used to withdraw the endotracheal (ET) tube proximal to the entry point.

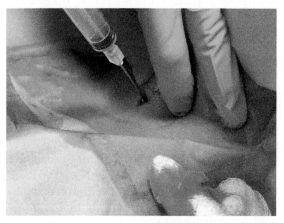

FIGURE 105–1E Introducer needle is inserted into the trachea under direct bronchoscopic visualization.

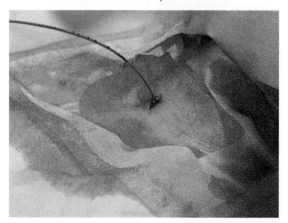

FIGURE 105–1F Wire is passed through the introducer needle.

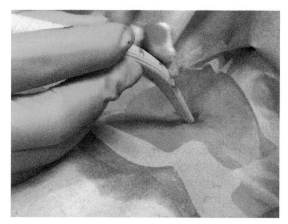

FIGURE 105–1G Dilator is passed over the wire.

connected together. Over the wire, the dilator balloon is inflated causing more radial force rather than the anterior to posterior force. The balloon is then deflated with the advancement of the tracheostomy tube, which is loaded onto the same device connected to the balloon. Therefore, the dilator does not have to be removed first, prior to passing the tracheostomy tube loader over the wire.

Griggs

The Griggs technique uses Griggs forceps, which has grooves to slide over the wire. Using the Griggs forceps, the trachea is dilated and a tracheostomy tube is placed.[13]

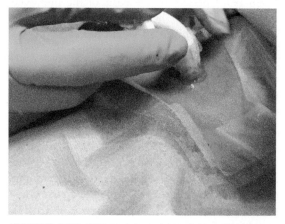

FIGURE 105–1H Tracheostomy tube is passed into the trachea.

Fantoni

The Fantoni technique, also known as retrograde percutaneous translaryngeal tracheostomy, is radically different from other techniques in which the tracheostomy tube is placed from the endoluminal site toward the skin. Once the wire is passed into the trachea percutaneously, it is moved retrograde toward the larynx and attached to a special soft tracheostomy tube. Then the wire is pulled out toward the skin until the tracheostomy tube comes out of the skin. The trachea portion of the trachesotomy tube then needs to be redirected toward the main carina using a rigid bronchoscope.[14]

Percutwist

The Percutwist technique was introduced in 2002, which uses rotational force during dilation using a screw-like dilator that is twisted into the trachea over the wire. The main advantage would be potentially minimizing the chance of tracheal ring fracture, which can occur with techniques using traditional anterior-posterior directional force for dilation.[15]

EVIDENCE

A number of studies comparing PDT to ST have been published. The first meta-analysis published in 1999 by Dulguerov et al, a surgical group in Switzerland, showed increased perioperative complication rate with PDT compared to ST.[16] Of note, ST was divided into older (1960-1985) versus newer (1986-1996) period on the basis of the improved surgical techniques. The difference of perioperative complications between PDT and newer ST period was significant (10% vs 3%). However, this study was widely criticized for including both the observational and randomized trials, and not separating different PDT techniques as different PDT techniques have showed different safety profiles.

The second meta-analysis soon followed in 2000 by Freeman et al in response to the first meta-analysis. This included only prospective randomized trials with the Ciaglia dilatational technique versus ST.[17] Odds ratio (OR) for all operative complications did not show any difference (OR 0.73), but stomal infection (OR 0.02), operative bleeding (OR 0.15), postoperative bleeding (OR 0.39), and all postoperative complications (OR 0.15) seem to favor PDT over surgical tracheostomy. However, the weight of evidence was questioned due to the limited number of patients and studies included in the meta-analysis. There were 5 trials included with a total number of patients being 236 (115 in PDT arm and 121 in ST arm).

The third meta-analysis was published in 2006 by Delaney et al that included 14 randomized trials comparing PDT to ST in critically ill patients, a total of 1212 patients. Pooled estimate of OR did not show any difference between PDT and ST in significant bleeding or mortality. The only significant finding was reduced overall wound infection in PDT of 2.3% compared to 10.7% in ST.[18] The benefit of PDT over ST in surgical site infection was again demonstrated in a trauma population by Park et al in 2013, showing 7% versus 3.4 % that was statistically significant with a P value of 0.04.[19]

As of now, the evidence suggests that PDT has a lower wound infection rate compared to ST, but other complication rates including bleeding and mortality seem comparable.[17-20] Of note, there are other benefits to PDT over ST, which include consumption of less operating room cost and staff resource, less overall cost, and less time it takes to perform the procedure from the time the decision is made to proceed with tracheostomy, given more flexibility in scheduling (28.4 hours compared to 100.4 hours).[17] Because there is no need to transport the patient to the operating room with PDT, it may potentially reduce morbidity associated with the intrahospital transport of critically ill patients.[21]

SPECIAL CONSIDERATION

Bronchoscopic Guidance

It appears intuitive that bronchoscopic guidance would make the PDT procedure safer since it would allow visualization of the needle entry into the airway and prevent posterior wall puncture. Kost et al suggested in his 500 PDT experience that continuous bronchoscopic guidance led to a low complication rate with no incidence of pneumothorax, pneumomediastinum, or paratracheal placement.[22] However, a study published by Dennis et al in 2013, demonstrated a low complication rate in 3162 patients without the use of bronchoscopy, arguing against mandating bronchoscopic guidance for PDT (complication rate of major airway complications and deaths were 0.38% and 0.16%, respectively).[23] The operator's experience is likely a large contributing factor since Kost et al demonstrated a decline in complication rate once the operator performs over 30 PDTs.[22] The decrease in the complication rate occurred even with the percentage of obese and difficult airway patients increasing after the initial 30 patients, suggesting increased comfort level and competency of the operator.

Early Versus Late Tracheostomy

The median tracheostomy timing in United States was reported to be 9 days with interquartile range of 5 to 14 days.[24] The definition of early tracheostomy varied based on the study (ranging from 1 to 8 days). Some of the prior retrospective studies suggested the potential benefits of ICU length of stay and duration of mechanical ventilation. However, 3 main randomized trials showed no such benefits. The only benefit of early tracheostomy seems to be potentially using less sedation, meanwhile showing no evidence in reducing ventilator-associated pneumonia, length of ICU stay, or mortality.[25,26]

Ultrasound Guidance

Ever increasing popularity of using ultrasound has made its way into PDT. By using linear array high-frequency probe, the neck can be examined prior to tracheostomy to reveal aberrant blood vessels in the path of the needle. In obese patients with difficult anatomy, real-time guidance can be used. There is 1 randomized trial that showed an increased success rate of first time puncture when real-time ultrasound is used compared to the traditional landmark method.[27-29] However, no statistically significant finding was noted in complication rate. Additionally, a number of feasibility and case series studies showing the potential benefits of the ultrasound guidance especially in obese patients.[30] Given the unlikelihood of any adverse effect posed by using the real-time ultrasound, it is possible that this will benefit a subgroup of patients with difficult neck anatomy.[27-29]

Operator-Dependent Outcome

One study examined safety and efficiency of PDT performed by physicians trained in either interventional pulmonology or surgery at a tertiary referral center. Of note, all interventional pulmonologists have critical care medicine training background. Almost all procedures were done within 48 hours with no differences in complication rate.[31]

Specific PDT-Related Complications and Death

A specific type of tracheal stenosis was reported termed "corkscrew stenosis" in 11 patients who underwent PDT, which occurred as a result of tracheal ring fracture. Mean time to occur was 13 months (range 1.5-24 months) with 7 requiring tracheal resection.[32] Methods to prevent tracheal ring fracture may be needed to prevent long-term complications like this.

Fatalities that result from PDT arose predominantly from damage to vessels and subsequent bleeding either intraoperatively or up to 22 days after the procedure. Identified factors that led to vessel damage include low placement of tracheostomy below the eighth tracheal ring, prior neck surgery, and radiation therapy. Two fatality cases occurred from loss of airway during the procedure.[10,11]

CONCLUSION

Percutaneous dilatational tracheostomy is a minimally invasive method of placing a tracheostomy tube in intubated patients. It is performed at bedside in the ICU, which reduces cost and resources usually required for a surgical procedure performed in the operating room. It can be safely performed by nonsurgical physicians including interventional pulmonologists and intensivists. Adequate training for the proceduralists, and proper patient selection are crucial in minimizing complications and better outcomes.

REFERENCES

1. Sheldon CH, Pudenz RH, Freshwater DB, Cure BL. A new method for tracheostomy. *J Neurosurg*. 1955;12 (4): 428-431.

2. Toye FJ, Weinstein JD. Clinical experience with percutaneous tracheostomy and cricothyroidotomy in 100 patients. *J Trauma*. 1986;26(11):1034-1040.

3. Ciaglia P, Firsching R, Syniec C. Elective percutaneous dilatational tracheostomy. A new simple bedside procedure; preliminary report. *Chest*. 1985;87(6):715-719.

4. Byhahn C, Lischke V, Halbig S, et al. Ciaglia Blue Rhino: a modified technique of percutaneous dilatational tracheostomy and early results. *Anaesthesist*. 2000;49:202-206.

5. American Academy of Otolaryngology-Head and Neck Surgery (2010). Clinical indicators: tracheostomy. http://www.entnet.org/content/clinical-indicators-tracheostomy.

6. Moscovici da Cruz V, Demarzo SE, Sobrinho JB, et al. Effects of tracheostomy on respiratory mechanics in spontaneously breathing patients. *Eur Respir J*. 2002;20(1):112.

7. Diehl JL, El Atrous S, Touchard D, et al. Changes in the work of breathing induced by tracheostomy in ventilator-dependent patients. *Am J Respir Crit Care Med*. 1999;159(2):383.

8. Davis K, Jr, Campbell RS, Johannigman JA, et al. Changes in respiratory mechanics after tracheostomy. *Arch Surg*. 1999;134(1):59.

9. Davidson SB, Blostein PA, Walsh J, et al. Percutaneous tracheostomy: a new approach to the emergency airway. *J Trauma Acute Care Surg*. 2012;73(2suppl 1):S83-S88.

10. Gilbey P. Fatal complications of percutaneous dilatational tracheostomy. *Am J Otolaryngol*. 2012;33(6):770-773.

11. Simon M, Metschke M, Braune SA, et al. Death after percutaneous dilatational tracheostomy: a systemic review and analysis of risk factors. *Crit Care*. 2013;29;17(5):R258.

12. Gromann TW, Birkelbach O, Hetzer R. Balloon dilatational tracheostomy: initial experience with the Ciaglia Blue Dolphin method. *Anesth Analg*. 2009;108(6):1862-1866.

13. Griggs WM, Worthley LI, Gilligan JE, et al. A simple percutaneous tracheostomy technique. *Surg Gynecol Obstet*. 1990;170:543-545.

14. Fantoni A, Ripamonti D. A nonderivative nonsurgical tracheostomy: the translaryngeal method. *Intensive Care Med*. 1997;23:386-392.

15. Frova G, Quintel M. A simple method for percutaneous tracheostomy controlled rotating dilation. *Intensive Care Med*. 2002;28:299-303.

16. Dulguerov P, Gysin C, Perneger TV, et al. Percutaneous or surgical tracheostomy: a meta-analysis. *Crit Care Med*. 1999;27:1617-1625.

17. Freeman BD, Isabella K, Lin N, Buchman TG. A meta-analysis of prospective trials comparing percutaneous and surgical tracheostomy in critically ill patients. *Chest*. 2000;118:1412-1418.

18. Delaney A, Bagshaw SM, Nalos M. Percutaneous dilatational tracheostomy versus surgical tracheostomy in critically ill patients: a systematic review and meta-analysis. *Crit Care*. 2006;10(2):R55.

19. Park H, Kent J, Joshi M, et al. Percutaneous versus open tracheostomy: comparison of procedures and surgical site infections. *Surg infect (Larchmt)*. 2013;14(1):21-23.

20. Friedman Y, Flides J, Mizock B, et al. Comparison of percutaneous and surgical tracheostomies. *Chest*. 1996;110:480-485.

21. Fanara B, Manzon C, Barbot O, et al. Recommendations for the intra-hospital transport of critically ill patients. *Crit Care*. 2010;14(3):R87.

22. Kost KM. Endoscopic percutaneous dilatational tracheostomy: a prospective evaluation of 500 consecutive cases. *Laryngoscope*. 2005;115(10):1-30.

23. Dennis BM, Eckert MJ, Gunter OL, et al. Safety of bedside percutaneous tracheostomy in the critically ill: evaluation of more than 3,000 procedures. *J Am Coll Surg*. 2013;216(4):858-865.

24. Freeman BD, Morris PE. Tracheostomy practice in adults with acute respiratory failure. *Crit Care Med*. 2012;40(10):2890-2896.

25. Terragni PP, Antonelli M, Fumagalli R, et al. Early vs late tracheotomy for prevention of pneumonia in mechanically ventilated adult ICU patients: a randomized controlled trial. *JAMA*. 2010;303:1483-1489.

26. Trouillet JL, Luyt CE, Guiguet M, et al. Early percutaneous tracheotomy versus prolonged intubation of mechanically ventilated patients after cardiac surgery: a randomized trial. *Ann Intern Med*. 2011;154:373-383.

27. Rudas M, Seppelt I, Herkes R, et al. Traditional landmark versus ultrasound guided tracheal puncture during percutaneous dilatational tracheostomy in adult intensive care patients: a randomized controlled trial. *Crit Care*. 2014;18(4):514.

28. Dinh VA, Farshidoanah S, Lu S, et al. Real-time sonographically guided percutaneous dilatational tracheostomy using a long-axis approach compared to the landmark technique. *J Ultrasound Med*. 2014;33(8):1407-1415.

29. Rudas M, Seppelt I. Safety and efficacy of ultrasonography before and during percutaneous dilatational tracheostomy in adult patients:

a systematic review. *Crit Care Resusc.* 2012;14(4):297-301.

30. Guinot PG, Zogheib E, Petiot S, et al. Ultrasound-guided percutaneous tracheostomy in critically ill obese patients. *Crit Care.* 2012;16(2):R40.

31. Yarmus L, Pandian V, Gilber C, et al. Safety and efficiency of interventional pulmonologists performing percutaneous tracheostomy. *Respiration.* 2012;84(2):123-127.

32. Jacobs JV, Hill DA, Petersen SR, et al. "Corkscrew stenosis": defining and preventing a complication of percutaneous dilatational tracheostomy. *J Thorac Cardiovasc Surg.* 2013;145(3):716-720.

Pericardiocentesis

Martin E. Goldman, MD

INTRODUCTION

The pericardium is a protective double-lined sac that surrounds the heart. The function of the pericardium is to reduce the friction between the heart and surrounding mediastinal structures and also to provide a barrier against spread of infection and malignancies to the heart. Though most cardiac conditions affect the 4 chambers of the heart, its blood supply and/or the conduction system, the surrounding pericardium plays an important role in normal cardiac physiology and disease.

Under certain pathologic conditions, pericardial disease can lead to palpitations, hypotension, and acute cardiac decompensation.[1] Patients presenting with pericardial tamponade accompanied by impending hemodynamic collapse require emergency pericardiocentesis. (An excellent video presentation by Fitch et al in the *N Engl J Med*. should be viewed in conjunction with this review.)[2]

NORMAL ANATOMY AND FUNCTION

The normal pericardium is a double-layered membrane that encases the heart and the origin of the great cardiac vessels. The outer fibrous layer (the parietal pericardium) is attached to the surrounding mediastinal structures: the diaphragm, sternum, and costal cartilages; while the inner serous layer (the visceral pericardium) lies on the surface of the heart and is contiguous with the epicardium.[3] The pericardial lining secretes 15 to 35 mL of serous pericardial fluid (an ultrafiltrate of plasma that contains proteins, electrolytes, and phospholipids) that lubricates the surfaces of the heart to minimize the friction for the contracting heart, and drains through the mediastinal and tracheobronchial lymph nodes.[2] Posteriorly, the pericardium stops at the base of the left atrium so that the posterior wall of the left atrium is not covered by the pericardial space.

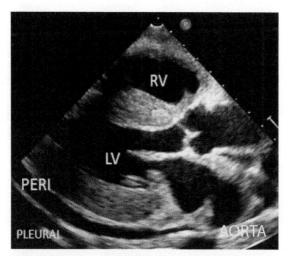

FIGURE 106–1 Small pericardial effusion: parasternal long-axis view, transthoracic echocardiogram; long-axis view of small pericardial effusion. LV, left ventricle; PERI, pericardial effusion; PLEURAL, pleural effusion; RV, right ventricle.

With chronic pericardial fluid that accumulates gradually, pericardial compliance is able to increase to accommodate the slowly accumulating larger volumes. However, because the pericardium is a relatively stiff structure, intrapericardial pressure rises rapidly as intrapericardial volume becomes too large or the volume increases acutely, compressing the cardiac chambers, which could lead to pericardial tamponade.[4]

In suspected pericardial disease, transthoracic echocardiography (TTE) (including 2-dimensional (2D) TTE, M-mode echocardiography, pulse-wave Doppler, and inferior vena cava imaging, collectively 2D TTE) is the first-line imaging technique. 2D TTE can image the size, location, and relative pericardial volume and serve as a guide to therapeutic intervention (pericardiocentesis) (Figure 106–1).[4,5]

PERICARDIAL EFFUSION

Pericardial effusion is the accumulation of greater than 50 mL pericardial fluid within its 2 layers, which can be due to numerous etiologies. Levy found the most common causes of large pericardial effusions were idiopathic (33%), iatrogenic (16%), malignancy (13%), following acute myocardial infarction (MI) (9%), renal failure (uremia, dialysis) (6%), and

collagen vascular disease (6%).[6] Etiologies can vary with institution and referral populations. Pericarditis, a nonspecific inflammation of the pericardium, can be associated with inspiratory chest pain, worse lying than sitting, may be accompanied by a friction rub that may be lost if the effusion is large and may be associated with palpitations and atrial or ventricular arrhythmias.

Pericardial effusion is recognized by echocardiography as an echo-free space between the visceral and the parietal pericardial linings posteriorly in the parasternal long-axis and short-axis views (see Figure 106–1). With M-mode and 2D TTE, a semiquantitative estimate of the pericardial effusion volume can be made by the size and extent of the anterior and posterior echo-free space (if not loculated).[7] A pericardial effusion limited posteriorly, less than 1 cm, is usually less than 250-mL volume (ie, small); greater than 1 cm effusion posteriorly is around 250 to 500 mL (small-moderate); a circumferential, posterior and anterior 1 cm echo-free space is approximately 500 mL (moderate); and if the circumferential echo-free space is greater than 1 cm there is more than 500 mL of effusion (large) (Figure 106–2). A large effusion accompanied by

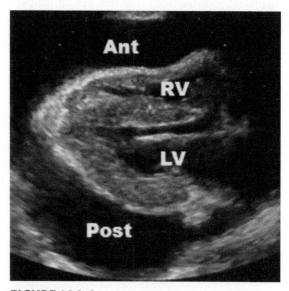

FIGURE 106–2 Large pericardial effusion: parasternal long-axis view. Ant, anterior pericardial effusion; LV, left ventricle; Post, posterior pericardial effusion; RV, right ventricle.

swinging of the heart, may indicate pericardial tamponade and more than 1 L of fluid. Estimation of the fluid volume is relative to cardiac size, which may depend on cardiac chamber enlargement and patient's body surface area. The physiologic consequences of pericardial effusion depend on the effusion volume, rate of fluid accumulation, presence of ventricular hypertrophy, pulmonary hypertension, and the presence or absence of cardiac compression. With increase in effusion size, the fluid extends laterally and once it exceeds 250 to 300 mL, it can appear anteriorly while the patient is in the supine position (Figures 106–2 to 106–5).

Pericardial effusions are usually transudates, seen on 2D TTE as a black nonechogenic (anechoic) space. However, infected or bloody fluid can appear as a hazy-gray rather than clear fluid and should suggest an abnormal exudative content. If not loculated, the pericardial effusion fluid around the heart is dynamic, and shifts with systole and diastole as the heart beats. This is to be distinguished by masses in the pericardial space or postoperative hematomas, which are usually relatively noncompressible.

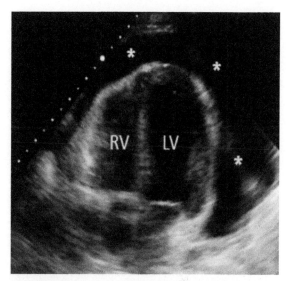

FIGURE 106–4 Pericardial effusion: apical view of large circumferential pericardial effusion. *, pericardial effusion; LV, left ventricle; RV, right ventricle.

Loculated effusions may occur postoperatively in cardiothoracic surgery or due to exudates or inflammatory states following recurrent pericarditis that can occur with infections, viral pericarditis, recurrent rheumatic pericarditis, or in renal disease

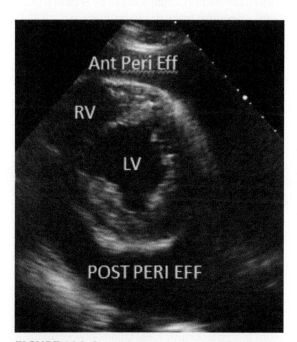

FIGURE 106–3 Pericardial effusion: parasternal short-axis view. Ant Peri Eff, anterior pericardial effusion; LV, left ventricle; POST PERI EFF, posterior pericardial effusion; RV, right ventricle.

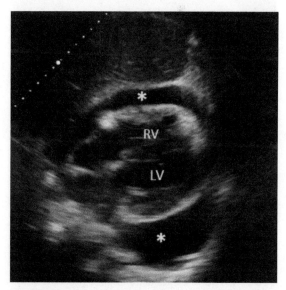

FIGURE 106–5 Pericardial effusion: subxiphoid view, large effusion anterior to right ventricle (RV) and posterior to left ventricle (LV). * pericardial effusion.

(Figure 106–6). Loculated effusions are usually localized, and not circumferential, but may have hemodynamic significance by compression of chambers or vena cava or pulmonary veins. Hematomas appear as immobile, flat or protruding, echodense thickening, usually anteriorly, and may be traumatic or postoperative (common following cardiac surgery where the pericardial space may be violated, uncommon following thoracic or abdominal surgery).

Pericardial fluid should be differentiated from the normal pericardial fat pad that is usually seen anterior to the heart lying within the pericardial sac and has speckled, hyperechoic areas because it is reticulated with echodense fibrous tissue and fatty tissue. The fat pad tissue does not significantly compress with cardiac contraction as free fluid does.

Pleural effusions, which can be easily confused with pericardial effusions, can be distinguished by certain key features. On the parasternal long-axis view, the pericardial reflection usually stops at the atrial-ventricular groove posteriorly, where the left ventricular posterior wall meets the posterior mitral annulus and there is usually no pericardial reflection behind the posterior left atrium; therefore, fluid behind the left atrium and aorta usually represents a pleural effusion (see Figure 106–1). Frequently, atelectatic lung tissue can be seen in the pleural space as well. If there is both a pericardial and pleural effusion, it can be easier to differentiate the 2 spaces. The descending aorta usually lies behind the left atrium and also demarcates the end of the pericardial reflection on the posterior surface of the heart. Fluid, therefore, behind the descending aorta would represent pleural effusion, not pericardial. If the probe is placed far laterally around the chest, the presence of a pleural effusion can be confirmed.

Pericardial effusion can be differentiated from ascites, which can be potentially confusing when imaging from the subxiphoid position. Ascites is usually closer to the liver, separated from heart by the fibrous band of pericardium. With significant ascites, the falciform ligament can be seen as a linear band extending from the liver to the pericardium traversing the black nonechoic ascites.

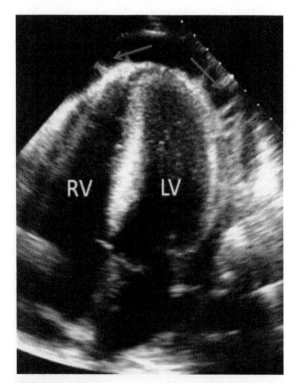

FIGURE 106–6 Pericardial effusion: apical view, with pericardial strands (*arrows*) breaching the pericardial effusion, creating potential loculated pockets. LV, left ventricle; RV, right ventricle.

PERICARDIAL OR CARDIAC TAMPONADE

When fluid accumulates slowly, the parietal pericardium can stretch to accommodate large volumes of fluid. However, if the development and accumulation of the effusion is very rapid or the volume exceeds the capacity of the pericardial space to stretch to contain the volume, increases in intrapericardial pressure begins to impact intracardiac pressure, elevation and equalization of diastolic intracardiac and pericardial pressures, decrease cardiac output, and exaggerated inspiratory decrease in systolic pressure (> 10 mm called pulsus paradox)[4,5] (Figure 106–7).

Circumstances that can lead to pericardial tamponade include all those that cause pericardial effusions including uremic renal failure, hypothyroidism, coronary vessel perforation during percutaneous interventions in the catheterization laboratory, a bleed following cardiac surgery, rupture or dehiscence

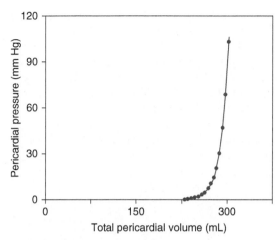

FIGURE 106-7 Pericardial pressure. (*Reproduced with permission from Hoit JP, Rhode EA, Kines H: Pericardial and ventricular pressure,* Circ Res *1960 Nov 1;8(6):1171-1181.*)

following valve surgery or aortic dissection, bleeding into the pericardium from a neoplasm, infection (viral, bacterial, fungal, tubercular), or a marked inflammatory response.[1] One study of 173 patients who underwent pericardiocentesis cited the etiologies as malignant (33%), acute or chronic pericarditis (26%), trauma (12%), uremia (6%), postpericardiotomy (5%), infection (5%), collagen vascular disease (3%), and radiation (2%).[8]

Tamponade following cardiac surgery may be due to bleeding from anticoagulants for prosthetic valves, delayed cessation of antiplatelet drugs, oozing from vascular or aortic anastomoses, or irritation from chest tubes. Loculated effusions may create regions of focal cardiac tamponade that may present with hypotension, but difficult to diagnose unless suspected, especially after cardiac surgery.

Clinically, patients with tamponade may have dyspnea, weakness, tachycardia, and hypotension. On anterior-posterior (AP) x-ray, a large cardiac silhouette, projecting a "water bottle-shaped" heart, in a patient with clear lung fields suggests the presence of a pericardial effusion with at least 250 mL of fluid. An electrocardiogram (ECG) may show signs of pericarditis with sinus tachycardia, and PR depression in leads 2, 3, and aVF. A valuable ECG sign indicative of potential cardiac tamponade is electrical alternans. Computed tomography (CT) and magnetic resonance imaging (MRI) scans

may show incidental large effusions suggestive of tamponade.[5,9-11] If the patient is stable, hemodynamics in the catheterization laboratory will show equilibration of average diastolic pressure across the cardiac chambers produced by the extrinsic pericardial pressure and ventricular interdependence, an inspiratory increase on the right-sided pressures with a concomitant decrease on the left-sided filling pressures—pulsus paradoxus.

Echocardiography is the most expedient modality to diagnose pericardial effusion and confirm the presence of pericardial tamponade. Echocardiography demonstrates circumferential pericardial fluid and compressed cardiac chambers (Figures 106-8). Among echocardiographic signs, the most characteristic is the diastolic right atrial and right ventricular compression. Right atrial collapse may also be seen in patients with hypovolemia who do not have tamponade. With greater compression, the left atrium may also collapse, a more specific finding. The diastolic collapse of the right ventricle usually connotes large enough external pressure to impact stroke volume. Doppler of aortic or pulmonic systolic flow discloses marked respiratory variations: On inspiration, the right ventricle fills at the expense

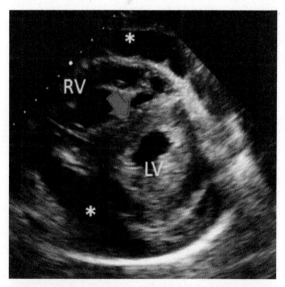

FIGURE 106-8 Ventricular interdependence: 2D echo demonstrating indentation of left ventricular (LV) interventricular septum due to inspiratory increase in right ventricular (RV) pressures.* pericardial effusion

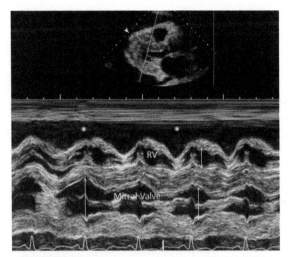

FIGURE 106–9 M-mode echocardiogram demonstrates large anterior pericardial effusion (*), with ventricular interdependence: the right ventricle enlarges with inspiration, while the left ventricle (identified by the mitral valve) becomes smaller and the opposite occurs with expiration.

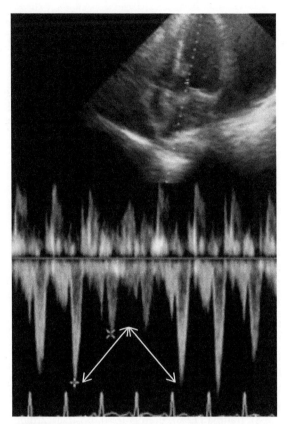

FIGURE 106–10 Transaortic Doppler flow in the left ventricular outflow track, demonstrating higher velocity with expiration and lower with inspiration, creating pulsus paradox (*arrows*).

of the left ventricle, seen as increased peak filling pulsed-wave Doppler velocity; both the ventricular and atrial septa move sharply leftward, reversing on expiration when the left ventricle fills at the expense of the right ventricle (Figure 106–9). A greater than 25% change in peak Doppler flow velocity obtained from the left ventricular outflow track or through the aortic valve, obtained by pulsed Doppler in the apical 4-chamber/5-chamber view or of the pulmonic valve, may connote pericardial tamponade (Figure 106–10). Pulsus paradoxus may also be seen with pulmonary embolism, chronic asthma, chronic obstructive pulmonary disease (COPD) and croup, but may be absent in low cardiac output states. The absence of any cardiac chamber collapse has greater than 90% negative predictive value for cardiac tamponade.[12]

Importantly, pericardial tamponade is a clinical diagnosis based on the presence of tachycardia and hypotension, which can be supported by echo/Doppler findings. Therefore, clinical suspicion of the presence of tamponade or the imminent development of tamponade is extremely important in prevention of acute cardiac collapse. Under certain circumstances, especially with hypertrophy of the left and/or right ventricle and pulmonary hypertension, which may be seen in hypertensive patients with chronic renal failure, who are prone to recurrent pericardial effusion, there may not be the typical findings of tamponade, because the ventricular hypertrophy limits the impact of the external compression on ventricle interdependence.

Management of Acute Cardiac Tamponade

Patients presenting with hypotension and tachycardia in which pericardial pressure from the volume of pericardial effusion causes cardiac compression have cardiac tamponade and require emergency pericardiocentesis that should be performed with echo guidance. The European Society of Cardiology's recent position statement on the triage of patients with potential cardiac tamponade proposed a stepwise scoring system to triage patients requiring

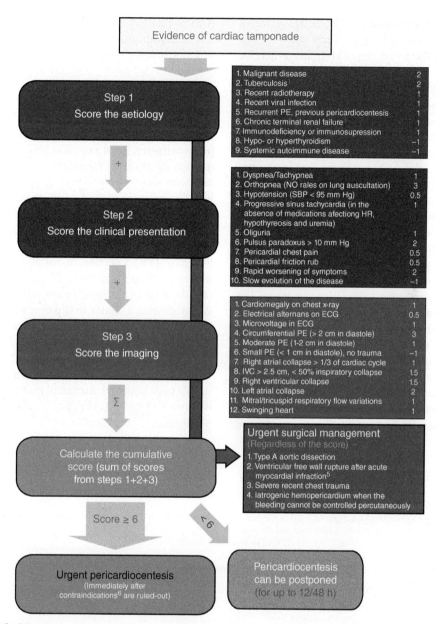

FIGURE 106–11 Triage strategy for urgent management of cardiac tamponade: European Society of Cardiology Working Group on Myocardial and Pericardial Diseases.[14] (*Reproduced with permission form Ristic AD, Imazio M, Adler Y, et al. Triage strategy for urgent management of cardiac tamponade: a position statement of the European Society of Cardiology Working Group on Myocardial and Pericardial Diseases,* Eur Heart J *2014 Sep 7;35(34):2279-2284.*)

pericardiocentesis.[13] The paper incorporates etiology, clinical presentation, and imaging findings (with primary emphasis on echo findings) to determine whether urgent pericardiocentesis, surgical approach, or intervention can be delayed[14] (Figure 106–11).

Pericardial drainage may be performed in the catheterization laboratory with hemodynamic measurement, with sterile technique in which both transthoracic echo and fluoroscopy can be utilized. However, sudden circulatory collapse may mandate the use of pericardiocentesis with imaging where the patient presents, in the emergency ward, ICU, or in the regular ward bed. Surgical drainage may be required if drainage cannot be achieved by percutaneous needle, in the presence of an active intrapericardial bleed, cardiac trauma or laceration, or complicating aortic dissection.

Medical treatment of acute cardiac tamponade can briefly temporize, but even volume infusion may increase intracardiac volume and pressures, thus increasing pericardial pressure and interventricular dependence, exacerbating the hypotension. Mechanical ventilation with positive airway pressure should be avoided in patients with tamponade, because this decreases venous return and may potentiate hypotension.

Pericardiocentesis is the most expedient method to resolve the impending circulatory collapse.[15] The immediate treatment of cardiac tamponade is drainage of the pericardial fluid by either needle pericardiocentesis or surgical pericardial window.

Relative contraindications include suspected effusion due to aortic dissection, traumatic hemopericardium, or myocardial rupture in which the pericardiocentesis may exacerbate the underlying condition that may be temporarily in equilibrium.

Anticoagulation or bleeding dyscrasias are relative contraindications, depending on the acuity of the situation and the severity of bleeding disorder.

PERICARDIOCENTESIS

Medical personnel should be gowned, gloved, and masked. Patients should be sterilely draped and have pulse oximetry, heart rate, and blood pressure continuous monitoring. Emergent intubation or sedation with short-acting hypnotics or anxiolytics may induce more pronounced decompensation.[16]

Materials needed which can be found in prepackaged commercial sets usually include a 21-gauge needle attached to a 5-mL syringe for subcutaneous lidocaine (1%) injection, a scalpel for small skin incision, a 7- to 9-cm 16- to 18-gauge spinal needle or a sheath over the needle catheter, a J-tipped flexible guidewire, a dilator to slip over the guidewire, a 3-way stopcock, a pigtail catheter or dedicated catheter for centesis procedures, several half-filled 10-mL saline syringes, and syringes (20 and 50 mL) for aspiration. An alligator ECG lead can be attached to the needle to monitor for current of injury as the needle is forwarded and hits the epicardium and generates ST elevation ("current of injury") (Table 106–1).

TABLE 106–1 Checklist for pericardiocentesis.

- Lidocaine, 1%, with 10-mL syringe and 25-gauge needle.
- Pericardiocentesis needle: 17-gauge, 12.5-cm (5-in) thin-walled steel needle (usually a spinal needle) for aspiration. It is possible to use 16-gauge and even 14-gauge needles with plastic outer cannulas.
- Syringes: assorted sizes, including 50 mL (2), 30 mL (2), 10 mL (2), and 5 mL (1).
- No. 11 scalpel blade, mounted.
- Sterile conductive monitoring cable with alligator clamps at each end.
- Three-way stopcock.
- Silk suture (5-0) on a cutting needle.
- Straight clamp and needle holder.
- Needles: assorted sizes, including 25 gauge, 1.5 cm (0.59 in) (1); 22 gauge, 2.5 cm (1 in) (2); and 19 gauge, 4 cm (1.5 in) (5), for transferring specimens.
- Drapes.
- Sterile, capped, 15-mL specimen tubes (10).
- Heparin, to lightly heparinize cytologic specimen tubes.
- Specimen tubes, one purple-topped and three red-topped.
- Clean-glass microscope slides.
- Microhematocrit centrifuge tubes with occlusive sealant.
- Ice bucket to hold cytologic specimens.
- Sterile dressing for entry and exit sites.
- Cardiopulmonary resuscitation (CPR) cart.

(Data from Tintinalli JE, Stapczynski JS, Ma OJ, et al: Tintinalli's Emergency Medicine: A Comprehensive Study Guide, 8th edition. New York: McGraw Hill Education, Inc; 2016.)

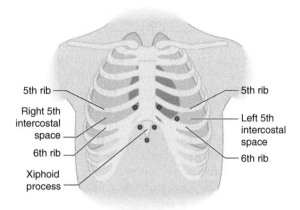

FIGURE 106–12 Potential sites to perform a pericardiocentesis. (*Reproduced with permission from Reichman EF, Simon RR:* Emergency Medicine Procedures, *2nd ed. New York: McGraw-Hill Education; 2013.*)

Before draping and preparing the patient, ECHO imaging should confirm the presence of the effusion, whether the fluid is loculated, the presence of adhesions, the appropriate drainage window, and the approximate angle for needle insertion. Select a window in which the effusion can be clearly visualized, preferably all 4 cardiac chambers (Figure 106–12). The ECHO probe can either be placed in a long sterile plastic sheath with ultrasonic gel at the tip for the probe and used adjacent to the needle in the sterile field or ECHO imaging can also be done at the apex, remote from the needle insertion site at the subxiphoid window or image from the subxiphoid window if the apex window is deemed the safer approach. The echo probe can then be manipulated under the sterile drape, off the sterile field by an experienced echocardiographer physician or sonographer while the pericardiocentesis itself is performed by another experienced physician.

The subxiphoid approach, just underneath the left costal margin, is also the safest for pericardiocentesis performed without ECHO or fluoroscopic guidance, because it avoids the coronary arteries, internal mammary artery, and is extrapleural (Figure 106–12). The alternative apical approach for pericardiocentesis may be closer to the skin surface, but may carry a greater risk of cardiac and pulmonary complications unless the performer is experienced

with this approach. Using sterile technique, the skin should be prepared with a chlorhexidine-based solution and sterilely drape the chest and abdomen with an open window for the procedure location. While monitoring hemodynamically, administer enough anxiolytics and topical pain medicine so the patient is relatively immobile during the procedure to avoid complications such as arrhythmias and cardiac laceration during needle insertion. After topical anesthesia with lidocaine, a small, superficial puncture is made for the spinal needle insertion site with a scalpel blade. The long spinal needle (a 16- to 18-gauge sheathed needle can be used so the metal core can be withdrawn and aspiration injections can be done through the sheath) is slowly advanced at a 30° to 45° angle with its hub depressed so that the point is pointing toward the left shoulder just under the xiphisternum, from the subcostal window. The needle is then advanced slowly, until the piercing of the fibrous pericardium is felt while continuously aspirating (Figure 106–13). Normal pericardial fluid is clear and straw-colored. Aspiration of bloody fluid may be pericardial, pleural, or intracardiac. Once fluid is aspirated back, the sterile clamp can be placed at the skin surface securing the needle and avoiding accidental advancement. By either echo guidance technique, though the tip of the pericardiocentesis needle itself may not be seen, the presence of the needle in the pericardial space is confirmed by "contrast" echo

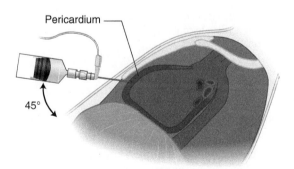

FIGURE 106–13 The subxiphoid approach. The needle is inserted at a 45° angle to the midsagittal plane (**A**) and at a 45° angle to the abdominal wall (**B**). (*Reproduced with permission from Reichman EF, Simon RR:* Emergency Medicine Procedures, *2nd ed. New York: McGraw-Hill Education; 2013.*)

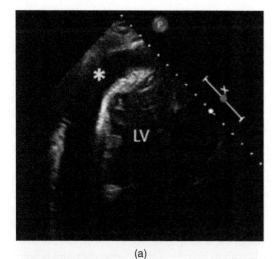

(a)

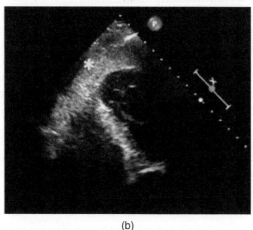

(b)

FIGURE 106–14 A. Apical view of pericardial effusion (*). **B.** Effusion is now opaque following instillation of agitated saline to confirm pericardiocentesis needle position. LV, left ventricle.

created by rapidly injecting either the aspirated fluid or sterile-agitated saline back into the space creates echogenic microbubbles within the pericardial space (Figure 106–14). The microbubbles are easily seen echo-flowing rapidly into the pericardial space, but move slowly in an exudate or bloody effusion. If the needle is not in the pericardial space, microbubbles may be seen injected into a cardiac chamber or may not be seen if injected into a pleural space. Visualizing the microbubbles in the right ventricle or another cardiac chamber requires removal of the needle and very careful monitoring for worsening tamponade if

the cardiac puncture site doesn't self-seal. Repeat the procedure until the needle position is confirmed by the microbubbles.

Once the needle is confirmed to be in appropriate position, a guidewire is then introduced through the needle and a dilator passed over the guidewire to manually drain with 20- or 50-mL syringes, with strict sterile control. Fluid drainage can be followed by ECHO to the point of minimal residual fluid. Because of the steep slope of the intrapericardial pressure-volume curve, aspirating a small volume (50 mL) may be enough to decompress the heart and recover blood pressure and slow the heart rate (Figure 106–7). The source and quality of fluid will determine if a drain should remain in place.

Bloody effusions from iatrogenic cardiac laceration or trauma may require surgical repair. For prolonged drainage, a guidewire passed through the sheath or needle will facilitate the introduction of a pigtail angiographic catheter. However, a drain may occlude, be an irritant, causing arrhythmias and is a potential source of infection. A follow-up TTE should be performed a few hours postpericardiocentesis to ascertain that no further accumulation has occurred.

Loculated effusions may present a problem because a single needle position may only remove fluid from one isolated pocket and those patients may require a pericardial window with lysis of adhesions in the pericardial space.

Pericardiocentesis is usually very safe using ECHO guidance with almost an immediate hemodynamic response of improved blood pressure and slowing of the heart rate.[15,17,18]

Familiarity with the anatomic approaches and contiguous structures will ensure a better outcome.[19] In a large series by the Mayo Clinic, ECHO-guided pericardiocentesis by experienced personnel was safe with a low incidence of minor complications (3.5%) or major complications (1.2%) such as requiring emergency surgery.[20] Cardiac laceration, atrial or ventricular arrhythmias, or vascular injury are very rare complications.

SUMMARY

Pericardial effusions are common, but when they accumulate rapidly or generate enough pressure to impair intracardiac filling, pericardial tamponade can develop. Clinical suspicion, rapid recognition, and confirmation of tamponade by TTE followed by prompt echo-guided pericardiocentesis and drainage of the pericardial fluid can be lifesaving.

REFERENCES

1. Spodick DH. Acute cardiac tamponade. *N Engl J Med*. 2003;349(7):684-690.
2. Fitch MT, Nicks BA, Pariyadath M, McGinnis HD, Manthey DE. Videos in clinical medicine. Emergency pericardiocentesis. *N Engl J Med*. 2012; 366(12):e17.
3. Spodick DH. The pericardium: structure, function, and disease spectrum. *Cardiovasc Clin*. 1976;7(3):1-10.
4. Roy CL, Minor MA, Brookhart MA, Choudhry NK. Does this patient with a pericardial effusion have cardiac tamponade? *JAMA*. 2007;297(16):1810-1818.
5. Klein AL, Abbara S, Agler DA, et al. American Society of Echocardiography clinical recommendations for multimodality cardiovascular imaging of patients with pericardial disease: endorsed by the Society for Cardiovascular Magnetic Resonance and Society of Cardiovascular Computed Tomography. *J Am Soc Echocardiogr*. 2013;26(9):965-1012.e1015.
6. Levy PY, Corey R, Berger P, et al. Etiologic diagnosis of 204 pericardial effusions. *Medicine (Baltimore)*. 2003;82(6):385-391.
7. Weitzman LB, Tinker WP, Kronzon I, Cohen ML, Glassman E, Spencer FC. The incidence and natural history of pericardial effusion after cardiac surgery—an echocardiographic study. *Circulation*. 1984;69(3):506-511.
8. Ben-Horin S, Bank I, Guetta V, Livneh A. Large symptomatic pericardial effusion as the presentation of unrecognized cancer: a study in 173 consecutive patients undergoing pericardiocentesis. *Medicine (Baltimore)*. 2006;85(1):49-53.
9. Cremer PC, Kwon DH. Multimodality imaging of pericardial disease. *Curr Cardiol Rep*. 2015;17(4):24.
10. Ozmen E, Kayadibi Y, Samanci C, et al. Primary pericardial synovial sarcoma in an adolescent patient: magnetic resonance and diffusion-weighted imaging features. *J Pediatr Hematol Oncol*. 2015; 37(4):e230-e233.
11. Groves R, Chan D, Zagurovskaya M, Teague SD. MR imaging evaluation of pericardial constriction. *Magn Reson Imaging Clin N Am*. 2015;23(1):81-87.
12. Merce J, Sagrista-Sauleda J, Permanyer-Miralda G, Evangelista A, Soler-Soler J. Correlation between clinical and Doppler echocardiographic findings in patients with moderate and large pericardial effusion: implications for the diagnosis of cardiac tamponade. *Am Heart J*. 1999;138(4 pt 1):759-764.
13. Velissaris TJ, Tang AT, Millward-Sadler GH, Morgan JM, Tsang GM. Pericardial mesothelioma following mantle field radiotherapy. *J Cardiovasc Surg (Torino)*. 2001;42(3):425-427.
14. Ristic AD, Imazio M, Adler Y, et al. Triage strategy for urgent management of cardiac tamponade: a position statement of the European Society of Cardiology Working Group on Myocardial and Pericardial Diseases. *Eur Heart J*. 2014;35(34):2279-2284.
15. Tsang TS, Barnes ME, Hayes SN, et al. Clinical and echocardiographic characteristics of significant pericardial effusions following cardiothoracic surgery and outcomes of echo-guided pericardiocentesis for management: Mayo Clinic experience, 1979-1998. *Chest*. 1999;116(2):322-331.
16. Ho KM, Mitchell SC. An unusual presentation of cardiac tamponade associated with Epstein-Barr virus infection. *BMJ Case Rep*. 2015;2015.
17. Tsang TS, Seward JB, Barnes ME, et al. Outcomes of primary and secondary treatment of pericardial effusion in patients with malignancy. *Mayo Clin Proc*. 2000;75(3):248-253.
18. Tsang TS, Seward JB. Management of pericardial effusion: safety over novelty. *Am J Cardiol*. 1999;83(4):640.
19. Loukas M, Walters A, Boon JM, Welch TP, Meiring JH, Abrahams PH. Pericardiocentesis: a clinical anatomy review. *Clin Anat*. 2012;25(7):872-881.
20. Tsang TS, Barnes ME, Gersh BJ, Bailey KR, Seward JB. Outcomes of clinically significant idiopathic pericardial effusion requiring intervention. *Am J Cardiol*. 2003;91(6):704-707.

Pulmonary Artery Catheterization

Rafael Alba Yunen, MD and
John M. Oropello, MD, FACP, FCCP, FCCM

KEY POINTS

1. There is a core of accurate and reliable hemodynamic information obtained from the pulmonary artery catheter (PAC) not readily available from any other single device.

2. The most reliable pressure measurements obtained from the PAC are continuous pulmonary artery systolic and diastolic pressures; the least reliable is the pulmonary artery occlusion (or "wedge") pressure.

3. Holding rapid fluid infusions via the introducer and proximal PAC ports and turning off the inflation of sequential

compression devices (SCDs) improves the accuracy of thermodilution cardiac output (CO).

4. Svo_2 does not correlate with CO in critically ill patients; increases in the $P[v-a]co_2$ gradient are inversely proportional to the CO.

5. Information from any hemodynamic monitor must be interpreted in the context of the clinical situation (eg, diagnoses, physical examination, laboratory, radiologic), the treatment goal, and the response to treatment.

The PAC, also called a right heart catheter or named after its creators a Swan-Ganz catheter, was introduced in 1970.[1] Made of flexible plastic (polyvinyl chloride) with an inflatable balloon at the tip, the PAC is directed at the bedside, without the need for fluoroscopy, via a central vein, using the flow of blood through the right heart, into the pulmonary artery, guided by pressure waveforms displayed on the bedside monitor. Harry Swan developed the concept of using a flotation device while observing sailboats and initially planned to use a sail-like device, but a balloon proved to be a safer interface within blood vessels and cardiac chambers. Norman Ganz developed the thermodilution CO capability of the PAC.

Use of the PAC peaked during the 1980s and 1990s, but usage has since trailed off due to its

invasive nature and subsequent randomized controlled studies demonstrating no outcome benefit (ie, reduced mortality, organ failure, length of stay, or costs).[2,3] Despite this, there remains a core of accurate and reliable hemodynamic information, not readily available from any other single device, which can be obtained from the PAC.

The lack of demonstrable improvement in patient outcome when using the PAC is multifactorial. The main factors include reliance on inaccurate data (eg, pulmonary artery occlusion pressure [PAOP]) to guide management; the fact that the PAC is a monitoring technology, not a therapeutic technology; and that the critical illnesses the PAC is used to manage such as septic shock, acute respiratory distress syndrome (ARDS), and multiple organ failure are syndromes that have no specific treatment and outcomes are not directly dependent on hemo-dynamic variables.

This chapter describes standard PAC anatomy, function, indications for insertion, insertion technique, complications, and obtaining reliable data while guiding bedside hemodynamic management.

PAC ANATOMY

A standard triple port VIP 7.5-Fr PAC is described herein. A double-lumen port PAC has identical components, other than lacking the additional infusion lumen.

The PAC insertion length (Figure 107–1) is 110 cm with an outside diameter of 2.3 mm (7.5 Fr). The catheter is yellow color and constructed of polyvinyl chloride extrusions. There are 3 main internal lumens (Figure 107–2): the **distal PA lumen** opens at the catheter tip, the **proximal injectate lumen** (also called the right atrial [RA] or central venous pressure [CVP] lumen) opens at 27 cm proximal to the catheter tip, and an **infusion lumen** opens adjacent to the proximal lumen, at 29 cm. In addition to the 3 main lumens, the tip of the catheter has a small 1.5-mL capacity latex balloon that can be inflated (11-mm diameter) and deflated (7-mm diameter) via an **inflation lumen**. A 3-mL "blood gas" syringe, modified to withdraw a maximum of 1.5 mL of air is connected to the inflation lumen. The inflation lumen has a lock that can prevent unintentional

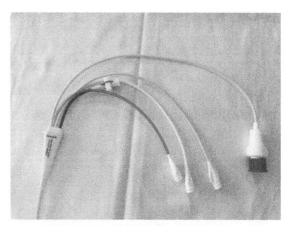

FIGURE 107–2 Close up of PAC ports: yellow tubing (distal PA), blue tubing (proximal injectate), white tubing (proximal infusion), and red tubing (balloon inflation port). The red cap is covering the connection to the thermistor.

balloon inflation or air embolism in the event that both the syringe becomes disconnected and the balloon has a defect (Figure 107–3A and B). The thermistor is located about 4 cm proximal to the PAC tip. At the proximal end of the catheter, a thermistor connector, protected by a red removable cap allows connection to an electrical cable that transmits core body temperature information from the thermistor to the monitor (Figure 107–4).

The introducer kit (see later under PAC Insertion) includes a catheter sheath that is placed over the PAC prior to insertion to allow sterile manipulation of PAC depth after insertion. Some introducers can lock the PAC to prevent migration, in those that do not, a piece of tape is provided to secure the proximal end of the catheter sheath to the PAC that helps resist PAC migration.

PAC FUNCTION

The functional components of the PAC are outlined in Table 107–1. Direct parameters obtained from the PAC are outlined in Table 107–2.

Pressure Data

Pressure information derived from the PAC includes CVP, right ventricular (RV) systolic pressure, RV diastolic pressure, PA systolic and PA diastolic pressure and the PAOP (also called the pulmonary capillary

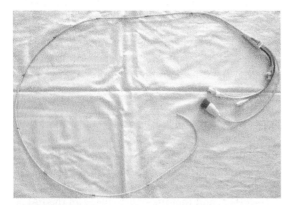

FIGURE 107–1 Standard triple port VIP 7.5-Fr PAC (Edwards Lifesciences, Irvine, CA). The markings indicate the following PAC lengths: each thin band = 10 cm, each thick band = 50 cm, for example, 1 thick + 1 thin band = 60 cm.

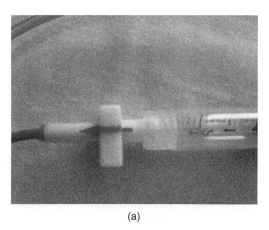
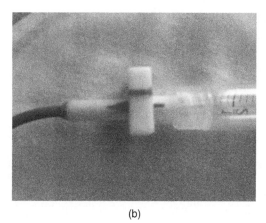

(a)   (b)

FIGURE 107–3 **A.** Inflation port connected to modified blood gas syringe. Note the red markings are in line indicating that the inflation port is open. **B.** The red markings are displaced indicating that the inflation port is locked.

wedge pressure [PCWP] or pulmonary artery wedge pressure [PAWP]). CVP measurement does not require a PAC, only a central venous catheter.

Before the PAC was developed, CVP was recommended as a simple measure of intravascular volume and RV filling or preload. Ventricular preload is the ventricular end-diastolic volume. Either absolute CVP or changes in CVP were proposed to differentiate decreased, normal, or increased intravascular volume or RV preload. However, there is no correlation between CVP and blood volume or cardiac preload in critically ill patients or normal volunteers.[4-6]

CVP does not reflect left ventricular end-diastolic pressure (LVEDP) and the major reason

the PAC was designed was to provide information about left heart function. The PAC was proposed to provide information about the function of the left ventricle (LV) by occluding a segment of the

TABLE 107-1 PAC: functional components.

Component	Function
110-cm length	This length allows passage from the femoral vein to the PA if the neck veins are not accessible
Distal PA lumen	Used to monitor pressure waveforms during PAC insertion and continuous PAP after insertion; PAOP during balloon inflation; true mixed venous blood gas sampling
Proximal RA lumen	CVP/RAP monitoring, fluid bolus for thermodilution CO, infusions
Proximal infusion port (VIP)	Additional infusion port; can perform the functions of the proximal RA lumen port if the RA port becomes occluded
Balloon	Filled via the inflation port during insertion to protect the endocardium from the PAC tip and carry the PAC forward through the right heart; inflated after PAC placement in the PA to determine proper positioning of the PAC; when inflated may provide PAOP
Thermistor	4 cm proximal to the tip; monitors core body temperature; senses temperature change used for thermodilution CO

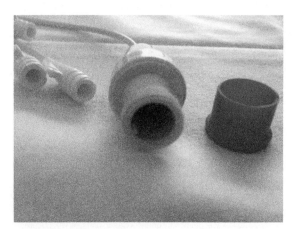

FIGURE 107–4 Red cap removed from the thermistor connection.

CO, cardiac output; CVP, central venous pressure; PA, pulmonary artery; PAC, pulmonary artery catheter; PAOP, pulmonary artery occlusion pressure; RA, right atrial; RAP, right atrial pressure.

TABLE 107-2 PAC: direct measurements.

Direct Data	Accuracy	Comments	Additional Information
CVP/RAP (normal: < 8 mm Hg)	Accurately reflects central venous pressure which is equal to right atrial pressure; RAP = RVEDP in the absence of TR; both CVP and RAP are inaccurate determinants of intravascular volume or RV preload.	This parameter should not be used for hemodynamic clinical decision making.	This parameter does not require a PAC and may be obtained via a central venous catheter. In the PAC the proximal infusion port will be usually located in the SVC, but may also be located within RA or less commonly within the introducer catheter.
RV pressures (systolic/diastolic) 15-30/0-8 mm Hg (normal)	Accurately reflects RV pressures.	Noted during PAC insertion; RV pressures are not present after the distal tip passes into the pulmonary artery.	RV systolic pressure is normally equal to the PA systolic pressure; RV diastolic pressure is normally equal to the mean right atrial pressure.
Pulmonary artery pressures (systolic/diastolic) 15-30/4-12 mm Hg; mean: ≤ 20 mm Hg (normal)	Accurately reflects continuous PA pressures; more accurate than PAP estimated by echocardiography.	Continuously displayed and monitored from the distal port once PAC is in final position in the pulmonary artery.	The true left ventricular end-diastolic pressure is less than the PAD pressure.
PAOP < 12 mm Hg (normal)	The pressure obtained after the PAC balloon is inflated when the tip of the PAC is in the PA. Highly inaccurate, does not reflect LVEDP, LV preload, or intravascular volume.	The most inaccurate parameter derived from the PAC. Interpretation errors, physiologic/pathologic limitations.	The main purpose of balloon inflation should not be to determine a PAOP per se, but to determine that the PAC tip is not located too distally in the PA.
Hemodynamic waveforms	a, c, v waves in RAP tracing; a, v waves in PAOP tracing.	Waveforms are difficult to visualize with standard ICU monitoring equipment.	Waves may be absent in pathologic conditions, eg, large v waves absent with atrial enlargement.
Core body temperature (CBT)	Most accurate measure of CBT.	Measured by a thermistor 4 cm proximal to the PAC tip.	PAC thermistor readings are altered by rapid fluid infusions and sequential compression/decompression devices leading to errors in CO measurement.
Thermodilution cardiac output 3-7 L/min (normal)	Considered the practical "gold standard" for CO measurement; inaccurate in certain situations.	Right heart thermodilution is an indicator dilution method. Under ideal conditions accuracy is within 10%-20% of true CO.	Average 3 measurements; do not measure during rapid fluid infusions, SCD inflation, inaccurate in the presence of tricuspid regurgitation.
True mixed venous blood gases	Most accurate representation of global venous blood; central venous blood gases may sample SVC or IVC blood preferentially and do not reflect true mixed venous blood.	Represent "true" mixed venous blood as the blood is drawn distal to the right ventricle, after the mixing of SVC and IVC blood.	Svo_2 must be interpreted relative to hemoglobin and CO; $Pvco_2$ is a more accurate indicator of flow than Svo_2.

CO, cardiac output; CVP, central venous pressure; ICU, intensive care unit; IVC, inferior vena cava; LV, left ventricular; LVEDP, left ventricular end-diastolic pressure; PA, pulmonary artery; PAC, pulmonary artery catheter; PAD, pulmonary artery diastolic; PAOP, pulmonary artery occlusion pressure; PAP, pulmonary artery pressure; $Pvco_2$, mixed venous carbon dioxide; RA, right atrial; RAP, right atrial pressure; RV, right ventricular; RVEDP, right ventricular end-diastolic pressure; SCD, sequential compression device; Svo_2, hemoglobin saturation of mixed venous blood; SVC, superior vena cava; TR, tricuspid regurgitation.

pulmonary artery via the balloon at the PAC tip, creating a no-flow situation in the vessel, thus the pressure at the PAC tip, the PAOP, would be equal to the pulmonary capillary pressure, pulmonary venous pressure, left atrial pressure, and the LVEDP. In both published research and at the bedside, the PAOP often became equated with LV preload. However, subsequent radionuclide and echocardiography studies have shown that the PAOP does not correlate with LV preload or intravascular volume.[7,8] Pressures do not correlate with volume due to alterations in cardiac compliance induced by positive pressure ventilation, positive end-expiratory pressure (PEEP), intra-abdominal pressure, pulmonary vascular disease, cardiac hypertrophy, ischemia, inopressors, and that the heart functions as a suction pump, that is, diastole is active and can create negative pressures within the chambers.[9] In fact the PAOP may not even reflect the LVEDP due to pathophysiologic factors (eg, mitral valve disease, pulmonary parenchymal and vascular disease) or that PAOP is a very difficult parameter to measure accurately.[8,10] It has also been demonstrated that in stable patients on mechanical ventilation, the PAOP can vary as much as 7 mm Hg in 40% of patients.[11]

The acronym "PCWP" perhaps best describes its role in hemodynamic monitoring: **P**arameter that **C**ommonly gives **W**rong information about the **P**atient. The most reliable pressure measurements provided by the PAC are the PA artery systolic and PA diastolic pressures.

Cardiac Output

PAC CO measurement utilizes the indicator-dilution principle using a thermal load as the indicator, called right heart thermodilution. The thermistor located near the tip of the PAC continuously monitors core body temperature in the PA. There is also an external temperature probe measuring the injectate temperature. To obtain a CO measurement, a thermal load (commonly 10 mL of room temperature fluid [saline or D_5W]) is injected rapidly via the proximal (CVP) infusion port and cools the blood as it travels through the right heart, into the PA and as this cooled blood (indicator) passes the thermistor, the temperature change over time is recorded. The monitor displays the curve of temperature over time and the area under the curve is inversely proportional to the rate of blood flow in the pulmonary artery. These data are converted by the monitor into the CO in liters per minute using the Stewart-Hamilton equation:

$$CO = V_I(T_B - T_I)K_1K_2/\int \Delta T_B(t)dt$$

Where, V_I is the injectate volume, T_B is the blood temperature, T_I is the injectate temperature, K_1 is the injectate density factor, K_2 is a computation constant accounting for the catheter dead space and the heat exchange during transit, and $\int \Delta T_B(t)dt$ is the area under the time-temperature curve.

A single CO measurement is approximately within 30% of the actual CO. When the average of the 3 closest CO measurements are made, accuracy is within 10% to 20% of the actual CO.[12] Average at least 3 similar measurements, for example, within 10% to 15% of the median value discarding those outside this range.[13]

Right heart thermodilution CO is considered the practical gold standard for CO measurement, but there are conditions that can affect the accuracy of thermodilution CO. These include the following:

1. *Tricuspid regurgitation (TR)*. Either falsely low (commonly) or falsely high CO as the regurgitant flow causes changes in the temperature curve due to recirculation or loss of indicator. Echocardiography can assess for TR. If there is significant TR another CO method must be used to determine the CO.

2. Rapid infusion of intravenous (IV) fluids via the introducer port and proximal infusion or VIP port can reduce the thermistor temperature leading to a smaller temperature change and a falsely low CO.

3. *Intermittent SCD*. Not in use at the time the PAC was introduced, but very common today, SCD—used to reduce the incidence of deep venous thrombosis (DVT)—increase the flow of relatively colder blood from the lower extremities when they inflate. If thermodilution CO is performed during inflation of the SCD, the thermistor (reading a lower temperature) will sense a smaller temperature change leading to a falsely low CO determination.[14]

4. *Injectate volume.* If less than the expected (eg, 10 mL) injectate volume is injected, a falsely high CO will occur due to a more rapid than expected temperature change.

5. Respiratory variation can change the temperature of PA blood and alter the CO.

6. Intracardiac left-to-right shunts, for example, ventricular septal defect (VSD).

7. The wrong CO computation constant setting in the monitor. The injectate temperature range and the PAC model determine the computation constant.

Thus holding rapid fluid infusion via the introducer, proximal infusion port, and VIP port of the PAC for at least 30 seconds, turning off the inflation of SCD, and timing the start of injection to the same point of the respiratory cycle, for example, end expiration, improves the accuracy of thermodilution CO. Room temperature injectate is used since ice-cooled injectate does not increase the accuracy[13] and is more burdensome. However, in the setting of hypothermia (low T_B ie, 29°C-30°C) ice-cooled injectate should be used to improve the accuracy by increasing the temperature difference between blood and injectate.

Hemodynamic Waveforms

Hemodynamic waveforms from the PAC consist of "a," "c,", and "v" waves in the right atrial pressure (RAP) tracing and "a" and "v" waves in the PAOP tracing (Figure 107–5). The "a" wave due to atrial contraction occurs after the P wave of the electrocardiogram (ECG). The "c" wave in the RAP waveform is caused by tricuspid valve closure, the "c" wave caused by mitral valve closure is too small to be reflected across the pulmonary vascular bed, and hence the "c" wave is absent from the PAOP waveform. The "v" wave is caused by filling of the atria against a closed atrioventricular valve during ventricular contraction occurs after the ECG T wave. The downslope after an "a" wave is called the "x" descent and similarly for the "v" wave is called the "y" descent (not labeled in Figure 107–5).

Large (cannon) "a" waves may be seen with atrioventricular dissociation. Large "v" waves may be seen with TR or mitral valve regurgitation (MR), decreased ventricular compliance or (in the RAP waveform) with a VSD. Enlarged "v" waves may be absent in TR or MR if the right or left atrium is enlarged. An echocardiogram is more specific and sensitive for the detection of TR and MR. In cardiac tamponade early diastolic compression can lead to a prominent "x" descent. In constrictive pericarditis, late diastolic limitation of ventricular expansion can lead to a prominent "y" descent. However in practice, echocardiography is more sensitive and specific for diagnosis if these conditions are suspected.

In reports about hemodynamic waveforms in patients with these and other cardiac disorders, the waveforms are usually obtained in the cardiac catheterization laboratory or coronary care unit setting using equipment that is more sensitive than that used in the general noncoronary intensive care unit (ICU) setting. It is notable that using standard PACs and recording systems in the general ICU setting, no hemodynamic waveform components can be identified in 52% of PAOP tracings and 20% of RAP tracings.[15] Increased monitor/recorder sensitivity can enhance the detection of waveform components.

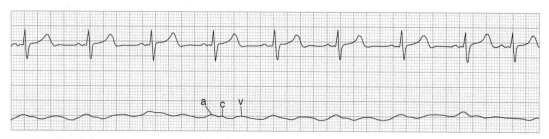

FIGURE 107–5 Right atrial pressure tracing demonstrating "a," "c," and "v" waves relative to cardiac events on the ECG tracing.[15] (*Reproduced with permission from Oropello JM, Leibowitz AB, Geffroy V, et al: Hemodynamic Waveform Detection from Pulmonary Artery Catheters in the ICU, J Intensive Care Med 1999;14(1):46-51.*)

Mixed Venous Blood Gas

Mixed venous oxygen and carbon dioxide levels provide further information about hemodynamics. The most accurate global venous blood gas, the mixed venous blood gas (MVBG), is obtained by drawing PA blood from the distal port of the PAC. The PA is distal to the mixing of superior vena cava (SVC), inferior vena cava (IVC) blood in the RV. The SVC carries blood returning from the head and upper extremities. Due to the relatively high cerebral metabolic rate of oxygen consumption, SVC oxygen levels are normally lower than in the IVC or mixed venous blood. Depending on tip location, a central line may preferentially sample SVC or IVC blood, thus central venous blood gases may differ from true MVBGs.

The normal mixed venous Po_2 (Pvo_2) is 40 mm Hg with a mixed venous hemoglobin-oxygen saturation (Svo_2) of 75%; it is a mixture of venous return from the SVC and IVC. The normal SVC hemoglobin-oxygen saturation ($Ssvco_2$) is 70% and the normal IVC hemoglobin-oxygen saturation ($Sivco_2$) is 80%. The other important component of the MVBG is the mixed venous carbon dioxide level ($Pvco_2$), which normally is within 5 mm Hg higher than the arterial carbon dioxide level obtained on a simultaneous arterial blood gas ($Paco_2$).

Interpretation of Svo_2

Low or decreased Svo_2 levels can result from decreased CO, increased oxygen consumption (vo_2), or anemia. A low Svo_2 value (eg, 40%) does not necessarily mean that the tissues are not getting enough oxygen or that the CO is decreased or inadequate. For example, if the CO is low and the tissues extract more oxygen per unit of blood flow, the Svo_2 will fall, but the tissues may be extracting enough oxygen to meet the metabolic needs. Anemia or increased vo_2 (fever, hypermetabolism) can reduce Svo_2 despite a normal or increased cardiac output.

High or increased Svo_2 levels can result from anatomic systemic left-to-right shunting (arteriovenous [AV] grafts, liver disease) or inability of the cells to utilize oxygen as is commonly seen in sepsis and liver dysfunction as part of the multiple organ failure syndrome—conditions that are the most common in critically ill patients in general medical and surgical ICUs.

Normal Svo_2 levels may not indicate that all is well. Normal Svo_2 may result from the mixing of venous blood returning from both high and low Svo_2 regions, as Svo_2 is a global measure.

From the above information, it should be no surprise that Svo_2 does not correlate with CO in critically ill patients. Further, looking at Svo_2 levels as an indicator of the adequacy of oxygen delivery is similar to looking at the amount of garbage your neighbor throws out to determine if they are getting enough food.

Attempts to increase CO to raise levels of oxygen delivery to arbitrary levels via inotropes or blood transfusions have failed to positively impact patient outcome and may be harmful particularly in older patients.[16-18]

Svo_2 levels should be interpreted with regard to hemoglobin level, CO, vo_2 and lactate level. Lactate levels correlate more closely with the adequacy of tissue oxygen than Svo_2.

Oxygen Content, Delivery, and Consumption

The mixed venous oxygen can be used to calculate oxygen consumption (vo_2), which is the difference in AV oxygen content multiplied by the CO. Table 107–3, contains the formulas for oxygen content (CO_2), delivery (Do_2), and consumption (vo_2).

Fick Cardiac Output

The blood flow to an organ (eg, CO) is equal to the AV difference in the concentration of a substance across the organ multiplied by the release or uptake of that substance by the organ. Using oxygen as the substance and the lung as the organ, CO is equal to the total body oxygen uptake (consumption) as measured by indirect calorimetry divided by the AV oxygen content difference. This is an alternative method to thermodilution indicator-dilution method. The accuracy of Fick-derived CO is limited by considerable inaccuracies in total body oxygen consumption measurement and shunting.

Intracardiac Left-to-Right Shunts

The oxygen levels in the right atrium (RA), RV, and PA are normally similar, for example, Svo_2 approximately 75%. An intracardiac left-to-right shunt, for example, VSD, results in step-up in venous oxygen moving from RA to RV to PA from oxygenated LV blood directly ejected into the RV and pulmonary circulation. This can be assessed by sampling blood

TABLE 107–3 PAC: derived data.

Parameter	Derived From PAC Value	Formula	Limitations
Stroke volume (SV)	CO	CO/HR	
Cardiac index (CI)	CO	CO/BSA	CO is more useful in individual patients. CI is used in research, eg, comparing group data; for individual patients the relationship between CO and BSA is nonlinear; BSA is estimated from height and body weight—this adds additional error to any CO error.
Systemic vascular resistance (SVR) 1100-1500 dynes/s/cm⁻⁵ (normal)	CO, CVP	MAP – CVP × 80/CO (L/min)	SVR is not afterload—CVP used in the SVR calculation is not a determinant of LV afterload; a high SVR does not differentiate between intravascular volume depletion, primary LV dysfunction, or low LV due to a high SVR; it is better to note the CO and the arterial BP for analysis and decision making.
Pulmonary vascular resistance (PVR) 120-450 dynes/s/cm⁻⁵ (normal)	PAP, PAOP, CO	MPAP – PAOP × 80/CO (L/min)	Utilizes the least accurate parameter (PAOP) derived from the PAC; it is better to note the CO and the PAP for analysis and decision making.
Left ventricular stroke work (LVSW) 60-80 g (normal)	CO, PAOP	SV × (MAP – PAOP) × 0.0136	Utilizes the least accurate parameter (PAOP) derived from the PAC; does not answer the question: is it good to do more work or less work? That depends on the clinical picture.
Arterial oxygen content (Cao_2) 19-20 mL/dL (normal)	Not derived from PAC	Hb (g/dL) × 1.34 × SaO_2 + Pao_2 × 0.0031	
Mixed venous oxygen content (Cvo_2) 15 mL/dL (normal)	Distal port blood gas	Hb (g/dL) × 1.34 × Svo_2 + Pvo_2 × 0.0031	
Oxygen delivery (Do_2) 900-1100 mL/min (normal)	CO	Arterial O_2 content × CO (L/min) × 10	No clear target parameters affect outcome; some studies demonstrate worse outcomes with intentional increases in oxygen delivery.
Oxygen consumption (vo_2) 200-250 mL/min (normal)	Svo_2 and CO	Arterial mixed venous O_2 content × CO × 10 (Normal arterial–mixed venous O_2 content difference = 3.5–5.5)	Consumption normally equals demand, but in critical illness, demand may be higher than consumption, this is usually reflected by increased lactate levels.

BSA, body surface area (m²); CO, cardiac output; CVP, central venous pressure; Hb, hemoglobin; HR, heart rate; LV, left ventricle; MAP, mean arterial pressure; MPAP, mean pulmonary artery pressure; PAOP, pulmonary artery occlusion pressure; PAP, pulmonary artery pressure; Pao_2, arterial oxygen; Pvo_2, venous oxygen; SaO_2, arterial oxygen saturation; Svo_2, hemoglobin saturation of mixed venous blood.

gases from the distal port of the PAC as it passes each level.

Interpretation of $Pvco_2$

Although Svo_2 has garnered the most attention to date, $Pvco_2$ levels correlate more closely with blood flow and CO. A consistent finding is the dissociation between venous and arterial Pco_2 (increased P[v-a]co_2 gradient) during reductions in blood flow, that is, decreased CO.[19-21] The normal P[v-a]co_2 gradient is less than or equal to 5. The P[v-a]co_2 gradient is considered to be increased if it is greater than or equal to 7. Increases in the P[v-a]co_2 gradient are inversely proportional to the CO. However, an increased P[v-a]co_2 gradient may also be due to an increased metabolic rate. Hypermetabolic rates are usually associated with a fever. An extreme example is malignant hyperthermia which is associated with very high fever and both a hyperdynamic and hypermetabolic state with increased CO and an increased P[v-a]CO$_2$ gradient.

Derived Parameters

Parameters that are derived from PAC data are outlined in Table 107–3. It is important to understand that systemic vascular resistance (SVR) is not equivalent to LV afterload and the pulmonary vascular resistance (PVR) contains an unreliable parameter in its calculation—the PAOP. A more direct approach is to analyze the arterial blood pressures and the pulmonary artery pressure (PAP) in relation to the CO. See Table 107–3 for additional explanation.

INDICATIONS FOR PAC INSERTION

The decision to insert a PAC should be based on individual clinical assessment where frequent hemodynamic assessments using information obtained from the PAC may allow more effective hemodynamic management. Inability to transport a patient for further diagnostic testing (eg, computed tomography [CT] angiogram) or inadequate echocardiographic windows may influence these decisions as well. The clinical scenarios include the following:

1. Shock (nonhemorrhagic) or hemodynamic instability unresponsive to treatment and when cardiac output determination and trending is deemed valuable.

2. Pulmonary hypertension (PHTN) assessment, trending and treatment in diseases resulting in PHTN (eg, suspected or proven pulmonary embolism, primary or secondary forms of PHTN, severe ARDS).

3. Respiratory failure including severe hypoxemia of undetermined etiology.

PAC INSERTION

The PAC is not utilized as often as in the past. It is especially important to have a physician skilled in PAC insertion be present at the bedside during the insertion when less experienced physicians are involved. The same is true for the nurses in having an experienced nurse skilled in PAC setup and monitoring be available and present.

1. *Introducer insertion.* The first step is obtaining venous access with a large-bore (8.5 Fr) introducer catheter (Figure 107–6). The right internal jugular or left subclavian veins are preferred as these are the least likely to result in kinking of the PAC compared to the left internal jugular or right subclavian vein sites. The femoral vein can be used if the neck veins are not accessible, but it can be more difficult to direct the PAC into proper position. As with any central venous assess, the access site is prepared in sterile fashion with drapes covering the entire patient; venous cannulation, guidewire placement, and confirmation should be done under ultrasound guidance.

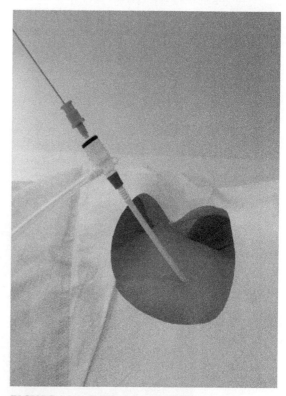

FIGURE 107–6 An 8.5-Fr introducer catheter in the process of insertion into the right jugular vein. The dilator (blue) and guidewire will be removed as the introducer is fully inserted.

2. *Transducer preparation.* The transducers are connected to the monitor via electrical cables and connected to tubing that will be attached to the proximal and distal PAC ports during insertion. Transducers are also connected to a saline flush apparatus.

3. *PAC preparation.* Before insertion of the PAC place the catheter sheath over the PAC and inflate the balloon with 1.5 mL of air via the modified blood gas syringe. Check for symmetric expansion of the balloon and for leaks (Figure 107–7).

    a. Place stopcocks on PAC the distal and proximal ports and then isolate them by using a clamp to pinch the sterile sheets around the proximal catheter while retaining the balloon inflation syringe within the sterile field and hand off the ports to the assistant who connects the transducer tubing to the ports (Figure 107–8). A saline-filled syringe may be connected to the VIP port and that is also flushed. The VIP port is connected to IV fluid after PAC insertion.

    b. The ports are then flushed. The flush should be cleared of any air bubbles. During flushing, the flow out from the distal port should be brisk; if it only trickles, the pressure bag compressing the saline flush is not inflated properly and needs more inflation. The display is checked for waveforms created by shaking the PAC, noting that both the CVP and PAP waveform displays are moving. Place a sterile-gloved finger to occlude the distal port and the distal port waveform should rise on the monitor (Figure 107–9). If the waveforms are not seen, make sure the monitor is set up properly, check the transducer connections, and electrical cables that may need to be reconnected or changed. If the CVP waveform increases when the distal port is occluded, the transducer tubing or the electrical cables are reversed and need to be switched. If the waveforms are small check the scale—if it is set to arterial pressure ranges, for example, 0 to 120 or 0 to 160, the PAC waveforms will appear very small. The scale should be set to 0 to 30 or, if elevated PA pressures are expected or encountered, 0 to 60.

    c. Finally the bed should be leveled with the transducer at the midaxial level and the

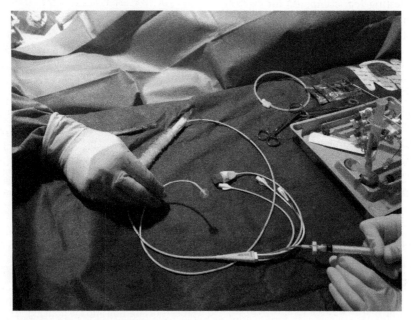

FIGURE 107–7 Prior to insertion via the introducer, the PAC has been passed through the sheath and the balloon has been inflated, testing for air leaks or balloon asymmetry.

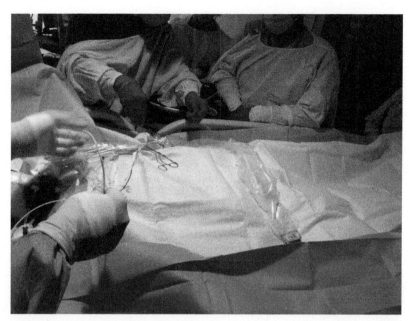

FIGURE 107–8 PAC ports have been handed off to the assistant while retaining the balloon inflation syringe within the sterile field.

transducer zeroed to atmosphere. Then with the PAC connected to the transducer, the distal port is positioned at the midaxillary line and the pressure reading on the monitor should be zero. If not, the level of the bed/transducer should be readjusted.

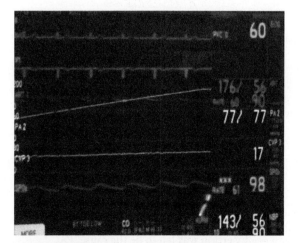

FIGURE 107–9 The PA pressure waveform is increasing when the tip of the PAC (distal PA lumen) is occluded with a gloved finger indicating that the port is properly connected.

4. *PAC insertion.* The ECG is closely observed for arrhythmias during PAC insertion (see 4a later). The PAC is initially inserted until the 15- to 20-cm mark is at the entry of the introducer; this places the balloon tip outside of the introducer, near the SVC or RA level with the nonpulsatile small-amplitude oscillations CVP or RAP waveform displayed on the distal port waveform (Figure 107–10). The normal CVP or RAP is 0 to 8 mm Hg. The balloon is then inflated with 1.5 mL of air and advanced quickly passing the tricuspid valve until the pulsatile RV pressure waveform is obtained, usually at 25 to 30 cm of PAC insertion. The normal systolic/diastolic RV pressure is 15 to 30 or 0 to 8 mm Hg. If the RV pressure waveform is not obtained after insertion to more than 40 cm, the balloon is deflated and the PAC is withdrawn and reinserted as earlier until the RV waveform is obtained. Once the RV pressure waveform is obtained, continue advancing the PAC until a step-up in the diastolic pressure is visible on the waveform, confirming passage across the pulmonic valve and placement into the proximal PA (see Figure 107–10). This usually occurs at

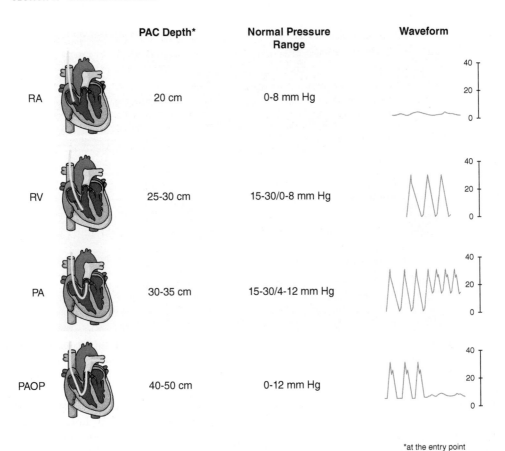

	PAC Depth*	Normal Pressure Range	Waveform
RA	20 cm	0-8 mm Hg	
RV	25-30 cm	15-30/0-8 mm Hg	
PA	30-35 cm	15-30/4-12 mm Hg	
PAOP	40-50 cm	0-12 mm Hg	

*at the entry point of the Introducer

FIGURE 107–10 PAC insertion indicating average insertion length, normal pressures, and hemodynamic waveforms as the PAC is advanced into the PA. (*Adapted from Servier Medical Art, Creative Commons Attribution 3.0 Unported License.*)

35 to 40 cm of insertion, but can be longer, for example, 40 to 60 cm in tall patients and/or with cardiomegaly. A dicrotic notch due to closure of the pulmonic valve may be visible. The normal PA systolic/diastolic pressure is 15 to 30/4 to 12 mm Hg. With further advancement of the PAC into the PA, the pulsatile waveform eventually disappears leaving a nonpulsatile waveform similar to the RAP. This is the PAOP, at the same pressure level as the pulmonary artery diastolic pressure (usually < 12 mm Hg). When the wedge pressure first becomes evident, the balloon at the tip of the catheter should be deflated (see point 5 later).

a. Both atrial and ventricular arrhythmias can occur during passage of the PAC tip through the RA and RV to the PA.

Ventricular are more common. Although inflation of the balloon at the tip of the PAC protects the endocardium from tip irritation, arrhythmias can still occur. These arrhythmias usually resolve as the PAC tip passes into the PA. However, if arrhythmias do not immediately resolve with passage into the PA or if there is difficulty in passing the catheter into the PA, the PAC balloon should be deflated and the PAC immediately removed. Occasionally arrhythmias may persist even after the PAC is removed. After treatment of the arrhythmia, if PAC insertion was felt to be the cause, PAC reinsertion should not be done.

5. *PAC placement.* Once a PA tracing or PAOP is obtained, deflate the balloon and observe

the waveform. If the tracing is in the PA (PA waveform), then after balloon deflation, the PA waveform should remain. If a RV waveform results, the balloon should be reinflated; if the PA tracing is obtained then the PAC should be advanced 1 to 2 cm and the balloon deflated; repeat until a PA tracing remains after balloon deflation. If a PAOP waveform is obtained, deflate the balloon and observe for a PA tracing. If the PAC remains wedged, withdraw the PAC about 1 to 2 cm until a PA tracing is obtained.

6. *PAC fine adjustment.* To ensure that the PAC tip is not further out in the PA than necessary, observe the distal PAC waveform—it should be a PA waveform and not wedged (ie, without a PAOP waveform). If it is wedged, see 5 earlier. If a PA waveform is present, then inflate the balloon to 1 mL (it takes 1 mL to open the balloon, 1.5 mL to fully inflate)—if a PAOP waveform is seen, then deflate the balloon and withdraw about 1 to 2 cm and repeat until the balloon can be filled with the full 1.5 mL of air either without wedging (PA waveform remains)

or a PAOP waveform occurs—with the full 1.5 mL. This will ensure that the tip of the PAC is not too distal. Note that it is safer if the balloon takes the full 1.5 mL remaining in the PA without wedging. Recall that the PAOP is the least reliable number obtained from the PAC, so better to err on the side of a more proximal PAC tip location, as long as it is not in the RV.

7. *PAC postinsertion.* Once the PAC is in proper position with the balloon deflated and displaying a PA waveform via the distal port, the insertion depth at the entry point into the introducer should be noted (eg, 45 cm) and then documented in the procedure note. A chext x-ray (CXR) is obtained to view the course of the PAC and the tip position. Nearly 80% of the time the tip is in the right PA (Figure 107–11), about 20% of the time it is in the left PA. If the tip of the PA catheter is nearer the periphery of the lung, for example, beyond the midclavicular line, the PAC is likely overinserted and needs to be checked (see point 8). In smaller patients, the PAC may wedge at 40 to 42 cm and the PAC may

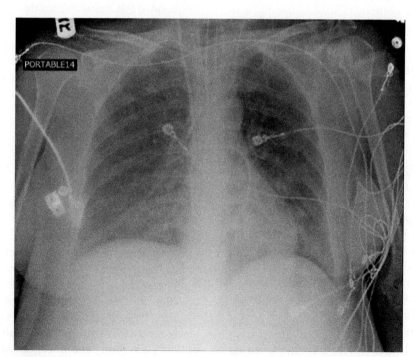

FIGURE 107–11 CXR after insertion of a PAC via the right internal jugular vein. The tip of the PAC is in the right PA.

need to be pulled back into the PA to less than or equal to 40 cm. If this occurs it should be appreciated that the CVP port will lie within the introducer, that is, if the CVP port is at 29 cm and the introducer length is 13 cm and the PAC is inserted to 40 cm (or less), both the VIP and CVP ports will lie within the introducer sheath. This may affect the accuracy of CO measurements.

8. *Post-PAC insertion monitoring.* The PA waveform should be repeatedly assessed by nursing and physician staff, to display a PA waveform and not the wedging (PAOP) or the RV. If a PAOP or an RV waveform is observed, check the insertion depth for migration and adjust the catheter as described in points 5 and 6 earlier. When a PAC is in place, if any atrial or ventricular arrhythmias occur, PAC tip migration should be ruled out as a possible cause by ensuring that the waveforms indicate proper position in the PA (see later).

PAC: SAFETY POINTS

The following are additional points essential to maximize safety when using the PAC.

1. The main principle of balloon deployment is that when **inserting (advancing)** the PAC, the **balloon** should always be **inflated**; when **pulling out (withdrawing)** the PAC, the **balloon** should always be **deflated**. (Except for when you are first inserting the PAC 15 to 20 cm through the introducer—obviously with the balloon deflated.)

2. Usually ventricular (but occasionally atrial) arrhythmias may result from PAC migration or occasionally only from the PAC itself passing through the right heart chambers. If arrhythmias are clearly due to migration and are readily terminated with proper PAC adjustment, then the PAC can remain; however, if they are felt to be due to the PAC, the PAC should be removed.

3. Right bundle branch block (RBBB) may rarely occur with insertion of the PAC. In the setting of left bundle branch block (LBBB) there is

the potential for complete heart block if RBBB occurs during PAC insertion. Therefore, in the presence of a LBBB it is prudent to have a transcutaneous pacemaker immediately accessible when inserting a PAC.

4. Care should be taken to note how much of the PAC has been inserted during PAC placement; no more than 40 cm of PAC should be inserted in attempting to advance the PAC into the RV; the PAC may be coiling in the RA and upon withdrawal, the PAC can wrap around the introducer and become knotted.

5. Multiple attempts at passing the PAC due to difficulty getting into the PA from the RV could result in cardiac perforation and tamponade. It is better to discontinue PAC insertion if things are difficult. Remember, the PAC is an invasive device that is diagnostic, not therapeutic.

6. PACs are heparin coated as this helps prevent thrombosis around the catheter. This bonding also has antimicrobial activity. Patients with heparin-induced thrombocytopenia (HIT) or a history of HIT, should not have a heparin-bonded PAC inserted. There are nonheparin-bonded PACs available for these patients.

7. The PAC balloon is made of latex. In patients with known severe (eg, anaphylactic reactions) latex allergies, a PAC insertion should be avoided unless a PAC with a nonlatex balloon is available via the manufacturer.

COMPLICATIONS

The PAC is an invasive monitor. A task force in 2003 reported the overall deaths due to the PAC to be between 0.02% and 1.5%.[22] Complications can be divided into those resulting from the central venous access versus those resulting from the PAC itself. Complications of central venous access include bleeding, hematoma, arterial puncture, pneumothorax, arrhythmias (from guidewire insertion), air embolism, and hemothorax. Complications of PAC insertion include arrhythmias (greatest risk when the PAC tip is in the RV), RBBB, complete heart block, knotting of the catheter, valvular damage, cardiac perforation, and infection including catheter-related bloodstream infection and endocarditis.

Complications of PAC overinsertion or migration if prolonged and unrecognized, and exacerbated by balloon inflation, include pulmonary infarction and pulmonary artery rupture with hemoptysis and pseudoaneurysm formation.

Complications can be reduced by careful insertion technique, the use of ultrasound for venous access, and only using the PAC when the information is likely to be helpful and for limited time periods—as short as possible, for example, 1 to 3 days.

USING THE PAC TO GUIDE BEDSIDE HEMODYNAMIC MANAGEMENT

Information from any hemodynamic monitor must be interpreted in light of the clinical data (eg, physical examination, ventilator, laboratory, radiologic), the treatment goal and the response to treatment, both hemodynamic and clinical. Hemodynamic data derived from the PAC is not pathognomonic; it is always subject to interpretation.

In the past, Starling curves (the relationship between contractility vs heart muscle stretch) were generated using PAC data comparing stroke volume (SV) on the Y-axis to PAOP on the X-axis. The problem is that PAOP is not an accurate reflection of preload, that is, ventricular cavity dimension or stretch. Subsequent studies have revealed the lack of Starling curves using PAOP versus generating Starling curves using radionuclide or echocardiography-determined preload.[5,23]

The major diagnostic assessments that can be made using PAC data include hyperdynamic circulation, hypodynamic circulation, and pulmonary hypertension. Trends in cardiac output, stroke volume, and PAPs can help to guide hemodynamic interventions.

When using the PAC it is important to use accurate and reliable information:

1. The transducers should be leveled at the midaxillary level and zeroed. No air bubbles should be present within the tubing.

2. The systolic and diastolic PA pressures (PAS and PAD) constitute the reliable pressure data obtained from the PAC. They are more accurate than echocardiography estimates of PA pressure.

The PA pressures are used to assess the presence and degree of PHTN and the changes in PA pressure that occur with changes in condition and treatment. The true LVEDP is less than the PAD with the gap between PAD and LVEDP increasing with PHTN.

3. If the PAC waveform goes from a clear RV tracing to suddenly damped and "wedged" appearing without seeing a PA waveform, suspect a proximal pulmonary embolism—the catheter tip may be lodging in a blood clot.

4. Do not use the CVP or PAOP; they do not reflect ventricular preload or intravascular volume better than flipping a coin.

5. Do not rely on CO measurements if there is evidence of significant TR.

6. Optimize the accuracy of CO measurement by holding rapid fluid infusions via the introducer or PAC for at least 30 seconds, turning off SCDs, and timing the start of injection to the same point of the respiratory cycle.

7. A high CO in the setting of an elevated lactate level rules out heart failure as the etiology and raises the suspicion for a local process, for example, mesenteric ischemia versus a systemic process, for example, septic shock–induced mitochondrial dysfunction. A high CO in the setting of pulmonary edema supports the diagnosis of ARDS rather than heart failure. (The PAOP should not be used to make this differentiation and has in fact been dropped from the current criteria for ARDS diagnosis.)

8. A very low CO on high-dose multiple inotropes should raise the suspicion of dynamic left ventricular outflow tract obstruction due to decreased preload and systemic anterior motion of the mitral valve into the left ventricular outflow tract. Despite an empty left ventricle, the PAOP is usually very high. An echocardiogram should be emergently done to rule this out. The treatment is fluid resuscitation, withdrawal of inotropes, and the use of pure noninotropic alpha agents (ie, phenylephrine) for hypotension.

9. When administering a fluid challenge, repeat the CO immediately after the challenge.

An increase of 15% or more in the SV (or CO if the heart rate [HR] has not increased) constitutes a response to fluid.

10. If removing fluid by diuretic or renal replacement therapy, decreases in the CO ($\geq$ 15%) may indicate the limits of fluid removal.

11. Repeat the CO and SV after starting an inotropic agent to assess the response.

12. Use both the mixed venous oxygen and carbon dioxide. Interpret the Svo_2 in terms of the hemoglobin (Hb) level and CO. An increased $P[v-a]co_2$ gradient (> 7) may signify a low CO unless the patient is hypermetabolic. If the patient is afebrile or only has a low-grade fever, they are not hypermetabolic and the increased $P[v-a]co_2$ gradient is a reflection of lower flow (CO).

13. Use echocardiography to supplement the PAC data that can be interpreted in the light of the direct preload and contractility information provided by echocardiography. Echocardiography can also determine if there is TR and if the CO is accurate.

MODIFIED PACs

We have discussed the standard PAC. Modified PACs include the following:

1. *Continuous cardiac output PAC.* Utilizes a heated coil to increase the temperature of the blood that then passes by a distally located thermistor-generating CO data without the need to inject a bolus of fluid. The CO is not actually continuous in the sense that it is updated every 2 to 3 minutes.

2. *RV ejection fraction PAC.* Estimates RV end-diastolic volume (preload) by measuring the decay in the thermodilution curve gated to the ECG R-R interval. It tends to overestimate the right ventricular end-diastolic volume (RVEDV). Also, accuracy diminishes with rapid or irregular heart rhythm.

3. *Oximetric PAC.* Modified with a fiberoptic bundle to measure continuous Svo_2.

Despite the greater cost of modified PACs, significant clinical advantages over the standard PAC

have not been demonstrated. Finally there are also PACs modified with an RV port to allow simultaneous temporary cardiac pacing and PAC monitoring capability.

REFERENCES

1. Swan HJ, Ganz W, Forrester J, Marcus H, Diamond G, Chonette D. Catheterization of the heart in man with use of a flow-directed balloon-tipped catheter. *N Engl J Med.* 1970;283(9):447-451.

2. Leibowitz AB, Oropello JM. The pulmonary artery catheter in anesthesia practice in 2007: an historical overview with emphasis on the past 6 years. *Semin Cardiothorac Vasc Anesth.* 2007;11(3):162-176.

3. Rajaram SS, Desai NK, Kalra A, et al. Pulmonary artery catheters for adult patients in intensive care. *Cochrane Database Syst Rev.* 2013;2:CD003408.

4. Baek SM, Makabali GG, Bryan-Brown CW, Kusek JM, Shoemaker WC. Plasma expansion in surgical patients with high central venous pressure (CVP); the relationship of blood volume to hematocrit, CVP, pulmonary wedge pressure, and cardiorespiratory changes. *Surgery.* 1975;78(3):304-315.

5. Kumar A, Anel R, Bunnell E, et al. Pulmonary artery occlusion pressure and central venous pressure fail to predict ventricular filling volume, cardiac performance, or the response to volume infusion in normal subjects. *Crit Care Med.* 2004;32(3):691-699.

6. Marik PE, Cavallazzi R. Does the central venous pressure predict fluid responsiveness? An updated meta-analysis and a plea for some common sense. *Crit Care Med.* 2013;41(7):1774-1781.

7. Raper R, Sibbald WJ. Misled by the wedge? The Swan-Ganz catheter and left ventricular preload. *Chest.* 1986;89(3):427-434.

8. Fontes ML, Bellows W, Ngo L, Mangano DT. Assessment of ventricular function in critically ill patients: limitations of pulmonary artery catheterization. Institutions of the McSPI Research Group. *J Cardiothorac Vasc Anesth.* 1999;13(5):521-527.

9. Robinson TF, Factor SM, Sonnenblick EH. The heart as a suction pump. *Sci Am.* 1986;254(6):84-91.

10. Al-Kharrat T, Zarich S, Amoateng-Adjepong Y, Manthous CA. Analysis of observer variability in measurement of pulmonary artery occlusion pressures. *Am J Respir Crit Care Med.* 1999;160(2):415-420.

11. Nemens EJ, Woods SL. Normal fluctuations in pulmonary artery and pulmonary capillary wedge

pressures in acutely ill patients. *Heart Lung*. 1982;11(5):393-398.

12. Critchley LA, Critchley JA. A meta-analysis of studies using bias and precision statistics to compare cardiac output measurement techniques. *J Clin Monit Comput*. 1999;15(2):85-91.

13. Stetz CW, Miller RG, Kelly GE, Raffin TA. Reliability of the thermodilution method in the determination of cardiac output in clinical practice. *Am Rev Respir Dis*. 1982;126(6):1001-1004.

14. Killu K, Oropello JM, Manasia AR, et al. Effect of lower limb compression devices on thermodilution cardiac output measurement. *Crit Care Med*. 2007;35(5):1307-1311.

15. Oropello JM, Leibowitz AB, Geffroy V, Murgolo V, Ezeugwu C, Benjamin B. Hemodynamic waveform detection from pulmonary artery catheters in the ICU. *J Intensive Care Med*. 1999;14(1):46-51.

16. Angus DC, Barnato AE, Bell D, et al. A systematic review and meta-analysis of early goal-directed therapy for septic shock: the ARISE, ProCESS and ProMISe Investigators. *Intensive Care Med*. 2015;41(9):1549-1560.

17. Gattinoni L, Brazzi L, Pelosi P, et al. A trial of goal-oriented hemodynamic therapy in critically ill patients. SvO2 Collaborative Group. *N Engl J Med*. 1995;333(16):1025-1032.

18. Hayes MA, Timmins AC, Yau EH, Palazzo M, Hinds CJ, Watson D. Elevation of systemic oxygen delivery in the treatment of critically ill patients. *N Engl J Med*. 1994;330(24):1717-1722.

19. Cuschieri J, Rivers EP, Donnino MW, et al. Central venous-arterial carbon dioxide difference as an indicator of cardiac index. *Intensive Care Med*. 2005;31(6):818-822.

20. Oropello JM, Manasia A, Hannon E, Leibowitz A, Benjamin E. Continuous fiberoptic arterial and venous blood gas monitoring in hemorrhagic shock. *Chest*. 1996;109(4):1049-1055.

21. Weil MH, Rackow EC, Trevino R, Grundler W, Falk JL, Griffel MI. Difference in acid-base state between venous and arterial blood during cardiopulmonary resuscitation. *N Engl J Med*. 1986;315(3):153-156.

22. American Society of Anesthesiologists Task Force on Pulmonary Artery C. Practice guidelines for pulmonary artery catheterization: an updated report by the American Society of Anesthesiologists Task Force on Pulmonary Artery Catheterization. *Anesthesiology*. 2003;99(4):988-1014.

23. Hansen RM, Viquerat CE, Matthay MA, et al. Poor correlation between pulmonary arterial wedge pressure and left ventricular end-diastolic volume after coronary artery bypass graft surgery. *Anesthesiology*. 1986;64(6):764-770.

Thoracentesis

Satish Kalanjeri, MD and
Stephen M. Pastores, MD, FACP, FCCP, FCCM

KEY POINTS

1 Thoracentesis involves the removal of pleural fluid for diagnostic or therapeutic purposes.

2 The decision to perform thoracentesis should be based on clinical judgment and take into account the perceived safety and utility of the procedure for individual patients.

3 The use of ultrasound to localize the best site for pleural space access is strongly recommended to reduce complications particularly pneumothorax.

4 Caution should be exercised in patients with coagulopathy and those receiving mechanical ventilation.

INTRODUCTION

Pleural effusions occur in 8% to 60% of patients admitted to the intensive care unit (ICU).[1,2] Although majority of these patients are in respiratory failure, pleural effusions may not be the primary cause of the respiratory compromise. This is because pleural effusions are mostly secondary to other conditions, such as pneumonia or malignancy. Often the cause of pleural effusion in ICU patients is presumptive based on the overall clinical picture. For these reasons, the decision to perform a diagnostic or therapeutic thoracentesis is often a judgment call. In a questionnaire-based study in France, only 15% of the intensivists routinely performed thoracentesis in ICU patients with pleural effusions, while 37% of the physicians felt routine thoracentesis would result in a specific diagnosis.[3] Additionally, there are challenges unique to the ICU, such as mechanical ventilation, multiorgan failure, and coagulopathy. This chapter will address the causes of pleural effusions, technique of thoracentesis including sample handling, special considerations in the ICU patient, and the complications of the procedure.

PHYSIOLOGIC EFFECTS OF THORACENTESIS IN THE ICU

In nonventilated patients, regardless of the volume drained, thoracentesis is thought to improve the functional residual capacity (FRC) and total lung capacity (TLC). However, there is no significant improvement in vital capacity (VC), arterial oxygenation, or an improvement in alveolar-arterial (A-a) gradient.[4] In mechanically ventilated patients, the physiologic effects of thoracentesis include a decrease in pleural pressure and ventilator work, and a modest decrease in intrinsic positive end-expiratory pressure (PEEPi), but the A-a gradient, arterial oxygen tension (Pao_2), and lung compliance do not change significantly after drainage of the pleural effusion.[5]

CLINICAL IMPLICATIONS OF PLEURAL EFFUSIONS AND UTILITY OF THORACENTESIS IN THE ICU

Although pleural effusions are rarely the primary reason for respiratory failure in the ICU, because of their physiologic effects, effusions may contribute to the overall morbidity of ICU patients. In a study of 100 ICU patients by Matheson et al, patients with pleural effusions had longer lengths of ICU stay, and spent more days on mechanical ventilation compared to those without effusions.[1] The type of pleural effusion itself seems to have little difference in the clinical outcome. However, Park et al found that patients with transudative effusions needed vasopressor agents more frequently than those with exudative effusions,[6] but there was no difference in terms of length of ICU stay or need for mechanical ventilation. To tap or not is often a question plaguing intensivists, unless faced with a large pleural effusion that automatically warrants a procedure. Fartoukh et al addressed this question in their prospective analysis of 82 thoracentesis procedures in ICU patients.[7] As a result of thoracentesis nearly 10% of patients had an alternative diagnosis for the effusions, and 56% of patients had a change in their management. Such changes included administration of antibiotics, corticosteroids or chemotherapy, insertion of a chest tube, or referral to surgery. Seven patients developed a pneumothorax as a complication of the procedure; majority of the patients were on mechanical ventilation. A meta-analysis by Gollinger et al of pleural fluid drainage in mechanically ventilated patients indicated that thoracentesis resulted in improved oxygenation and lung mechanics, and contributed to change in management, but there was no change in the ICU length of stay or mortality.[8]

ETIOLOGY

Table 108–1 lists the common causes of pleural effusions in the ICU. Congestive heart failure (CHF) and atelectasis are the most common causes of pleural effusions, representing 35% and 22% of all effusions, respectively.[1] Other studies showed parapneumonic effusions (41%-50%) were more

TABLE 108–1 Common causes of pleural effusions in the ICU.

Congestive heart failure
Parapneumonic effusion
Empyema
Atelectasis
Malignancy
Pulmonary embolism
Hepatic hydrothorax
Hypoalbuminemia
Pancreatitis
Hemothorax
Uremia

common than CHF (17%-20%) as cause for the effusions.[6,7] One of the reasons for this disparity is because the cause for effusions is often determined by pleural fluid analysis, and not all patients in the ICU undergo diagnostic studies for effusions. Thus, it is not surprising that these mostly single-center studies demonstrate varying incident rates for the etiologies of pleural effusions. However, there is agreement that the most common cause of a unilateral effusion is infection while CHF is the most frequent cause of bilateral effusions. Light criteria remain the gold standard in classifying effusions as transudates or exudates.[9]

EQUIPMENT AND TECHNIQUE

The first step in a successful and safe thoracentesis procedure is adequate preparation. This begins with confirming the indications for the procedure, review of relevant imaging, and ruling out contraindications. There are no absolute contraindications to the procedure. The relative contraindications are coagulopathy, use of antiplatelet agents and anticoagulants, chest wall cellulitis, and metastasis.

Although several algorithms are available to aid decision making for performing thoracentesis, we do not recommend a rigid approach to ICU patients.

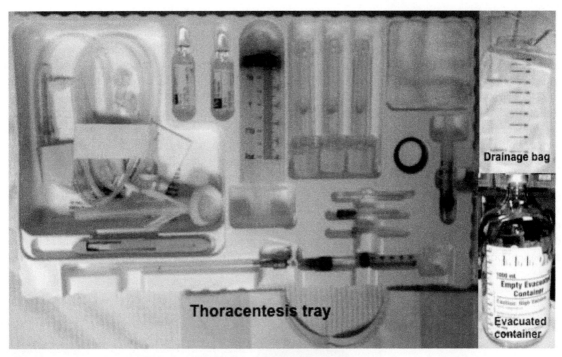

FIGURE 108–1 Thoracentesis tray and drainage bag/bottle (Not to scale).

The decision to perform thoracentesis should be based on clinical judgment, and should take into account the perceived safety and utility of the procedure for individual patients. Informed written consent needs to be obtained from the patient or the health care proxy. Assembling the equipment and paraphernalia is the next step. There are several commercially available kits for thoracentesis that contain the essential equipment. One such kit is shown in Figure 108–1. Table 108–2 lists all the necessary equipment including those contained in readymade kits. It does not matter what type of kit is used for the procedure, since the basic principle of thoracentesis is to access the pleural space with a sharp metallic needle, and once in the pleural space, a flexible nonmetallic catheter is passed into the space either through the access needle or over it.

PROCEDURE

Patient positioning in the ICU can be a challenge. The ideal position for thoracentesis is for the patient to sit up at the edge of the bed leaning forward to rest arms and face on a table such that the back is

TABLE 108–2 Equipment for the procedure.

Portable ultrasound machine
Chlorhexidine 2%/povidone Iodine 1% solution or swabstick
Sterile gloves
Thoracentesis needle/catheter with a 3-way stopcock
16-gauge aspirating needle, 25- and 22-gauge injection needle
10-cc Luer lock syringe
60-cc Luer lock syringe
Scalpel
Collection bag w/ drain tube or evacuated containers
Specimen vials × 3
Sterile towel/drape with fenestration
Lidocaine 1% 5-mL ampule × 2
4 × 4 gauze sponge applicators
Adhesive dressing

accessible for the procedure (Figure 108–2). However, this may not be possible in many patients in the ICU due to mechanical ventilation or other reasons. Access from the infra-axillary area is another approach, with the patient in a semireclined position with the arm to the side (Figure 108–3). We strongly recommend the use of ultrasound to localize the best site for pleural space access. There is clear evidence about favorable safety outcomes and the utility of ultrasound-guided thoracentesis. Mayo et al observed a pneumothorax rate of only 1.3% in their prospective observational study of 211 mechanically ventilated patients (mean PEEP 6.8 cm of water and mean Pao_2/Fio_2 178) who underwent both diagnostic and therapeutic thoracentesis.[10] After appropriate patient positioning, the phased array ultrasound

probe is placed on the chest wall to identify pleural effusion. The criteria for accurate diagnosis of pleural effusion on an ultrasound image are 3-fold—an anechoic/hypoechoic region that represents pleural effusion; identification of anatomic boundaries of this anechoic region: chest wall, diaphragm, and lung tissue that appears like a "fish tail"; and dynamic respiratory movement of the lung surface, diaphragm, or the fluid itself[11] (Figure 108–4). These ultrasound characteristics are meant to minimize the chances of injury to the lung and to prevent subdiaphragmatic insertion of the needle. Presence of debris and floaters (so-called plankton sign) within the anechoic/hypoechoic region are clues to exudative nature of the effusion. In ICUs where portable ultrasonography is unavailable, the classical method

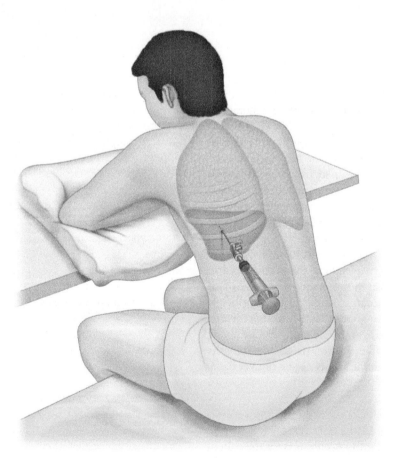

FIGURE 108–2 Patient and needle position—posterior approach. (*Memorial Sloan Kettering Cancer Center © 2014.*)

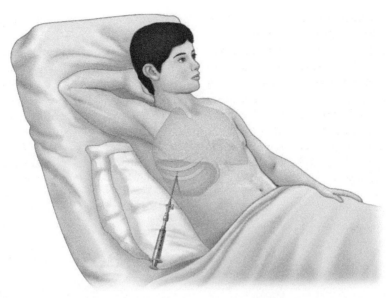

FIGURE 108-3 Patient and needle position—lateral approach. (*Memorial Sloan Kettering Cancer Center © 2014.*)

of choosing a site that has maximum dullness to percussion (usually third-fifth intercostal space in the midaxillary line: "the triangle of safety," or fifth-seventh intercostal space in the posterior scapular line) should be performed. It must be emphasized that this method is fraught with fallacies because a visual identification of effusion is not possible, and chest x-ray (CXR) and percussion findings may not necessarily represent effusion. The point of entry is identified and marked. The point of entry is always "above the rib," that is, along the upper border of a rib in order to avoid neurovascular injury. The neurovascular bundle runs along the lower border of a rib.

The skin is cleaned with 2% chlorhexidine or 1% povidone iodine. If iodine solution is used, it must be allowed to dry on the skin in order to be most effective.[12] A sterile drape with fenestration is then placed over the skin. A 25-gauge needle is used to anesthetize the skin with 1% lidocaine at the intended point of entry. After the skin is anesthetized adequately, the deeper tissues including the pleura are instilled with the local anesthetic using a 22-gauge needle. Negative suction should be performed at all times while entering deeper tissues in order to notice accidental blood vessel injury. Aspiration of free-flowing pleural fluid is indicative of the needle reaching the pleural space—a quick mental note is

made of the direction and depth of the finder needle. The finder needle is withdrawn after adequate analgesia of the deeper tissues including the pleura. If the "catheter over the needle" device is used, a small skin puncture is made with a scalpel. The puncture should be deep enough to traverse the entire thickness of the skin. This step is not necessary with the "catheter within the needle" device. The thoracentesis needle is now prepared for entry into the pleural space—the 60-mL syringe is attached to the distal end of the thoracentesis needle, and care must be taken to align the 3-way stopcock such that pleural fluid flows into the syringe (see Figures 108–2 and 108–3). The thoracentesis needle is then slowly inserted through the skin puncture site, while maintaining negative suction pressure through the syringe. After pleural fluid is aspirated, the needle is further inserted by 2 to 3 mm to ensure the entire bevel of the needle is within the pleural space. The catheter is then slid into the pleural space while maintaining the needle still and in position. Once the catheter is in the pleural space, the needle is withdrawn. Serial pleural manometry may be performed to measure the pleural pressure or pleural elastance (change in pleural pressure/volume removed). Unless this is of diagnostic value or a large-volume thoracentesis is planned, there is no routine indication to perform pleural manometry

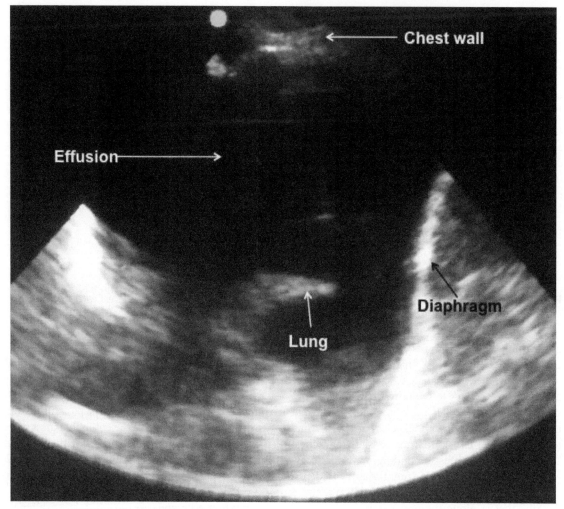

FIGURE 108–4 Ultrasound identification of pleural effusion.

in ICU patients. Patients on mechanical ventilation are at low risk of reexpansion pulmonary edema, and pleural fluid manometry tests may not be useful on mechanical ventilation. A collection tube connected to either a collection bag or vaccutainer bottle is attached to the side port of the 3-way stopcock and the pleural fluid drained. Fluid is drained until one of the following end points is reached:

1. Fluid stops draining despite slightly pulling back the catheter.

2. The patient starts coughing or complains of chest discomfort (nonventilated patients).

3. Pleural fluid manometry indicates a pleural pressure of –20 cm H_2O has been reached, as the risk of reexpansion pulmonary edema is higher with further drop in pleural pressure.[13]

4. About 1- to 1.5-L fluid is drained (although potentially more fluid can be drained if pleural manometry is used).

The catheter is then withdrawn while asking the patient to hum or in the expiratory phase if the patient is on a ventilator. Pressure with gauze is maintained on the skin for a few minutes until there is no pleural fluid or blood seepage from the puncture site.

An adhesive dressing or Band-Aid is placed over the puncture site. We recommend performing a postprocedure CXR to rule out pneumothorax. Although this is not considered a mandatory practice for non-ICU patients, the procedure is riskier in this population and therefore every effort must be made to preempt any complications and take action early. It is a good practice to perform a localized ultrasound immediately after the procedure to look for lung sliding, the absence of which suggests a pneumothorax. However, localized ultrasound for detection of pneumothorax has limitations. Besides pneumothorax may develop hours after the procedure.

Sample Handling

This depends on the local laboratory preferences and guidelines. Ideally at least 50 to 60 mL of pleural fluid should be aspirated for diagnosis. Approximately 30 mL is sent for cytology in a methanol-based solution (CytoLyt bottle) or a plain or heparinized container. If immunocytochemistry is needed, the sample should also be collected in formalin for cellblock. If the sample needs to be sent for flow cytometry, 2 lavender-top bottles (ethylenediaminetetraacetic acid [EDTA]) are used for sample collection. Furthermore, there should no delay in transporting flow cytometry samples to the laboratory in order to prevent cell degradation. Routine biochemical testing (lactate dehydrogenase, cholesterol, glucose, total protein), cell type, and cell count need about 5 mL each and samples are sent in sterile plain or heparinized containers. Microbiological testing requires about 10 mL of the sample. About 2-mL fluid is collected in a heparinized syringe for pH testing. Based on the clinical scenario, tests such as triglyceride and chylomicron levels, amylase, and lipase levels may be sent.

COMPLICATIONS

ICU patients are especially vulnerable to complications because of the critical nature of their illness. Mechanical ventilation and coagulopathy are particularly challenging considerations. Lastly, patient positioning in the ICU can be suboptimal leading to unsuccessful attempts at thoracentesis or complications.

Table 108–3 lists the potential complications of thoracentesis in the ICU. Pneumothorax is the most

TABLE 108-3 Complications of ICU thoracentesis.

Pneumothorax
Bleeding/hemothorax
Hematoma at injection site
Visceral (usually liver or spleen) injury
Soft tissue infection
Pleural infection
Vasovagal episode
Reexpansion pulmonary edema

common complication. Positive pressure ventilation, whether mechanical or noninvasive, renders the patient more susceptible to pneumothorax. The incidence of pneumothorax after thoracentesis while on mechanical ventilation prior to routine ultrasound guidance was 9% to 13%.[14] The use of ultrasound has resulted in a significant reduction in pneumothorax incidence ranging from 1% to 6%.[10] Coagulopathy and bleeding risk from anticoagulant/antiplatelet use have been traditionally considered relative contraindications in the ICU (Table 108–4). Patel et al demonstrated the safety of ultrasound-guided thoracentesis in patients with an international normalized ratio (INR) greater than 3 or a platelet count less than 25,000.[15] Puchalski et al found that the

TABLE 108-4 Key points with thoracentesis.

Coagulopathy is a relative contraindication.
Risk of pneumothorax is higher with mechanical ventilation.
Assemble all equipment, including specimen containers, before the start of procedure.
Ultrasound-guided thoracentesis reduces complications.
Always insert the needle "above the rib" to avoid neurovascular injury.
Thoracentesis generally relieves symptoms, but length of ICU stay and mortality do not improve.
Occasionally chest tube/pigtail catheter insertion may be a safer alternative.

incidence of bleeding with thoracentesis was not any higher even in the presence of multiple bleeding risks such as elevated INR, thrombocytopenia, or use of anticoagulants.[16] However, none of these studies advocating safety of thoracentesis with uncorrected bleeding risks specifically studied ICU patients.[17] Blood products such as fresh frozen plasma and platelet transfusions can be administered to make the procedure safer when coagulopathy is a concern. Use of prophylactic anticoagulation is not considered a contraindication to thoracentesis. However, we recommend holding therapeutic anticoagulation before the procedure, and if this is not feasible inserting a chest tube instead.

Reexpansion pulmonary edema is not a major concern in mechanically ventilated patients as the positive pressure ventilation makes occurrence of reexpansion pulmonary edema unlikely. However, this remains a concern in nonventilated patients or those on noninvasive modes of ventilation. Use of pleural manometry or limiting the amount of fluid drained to 1.5 L reduces the chances of reexpansion pulmonary edema.[13]

CONCLUSIONS

Pleural effusions are rarely the main cause for admission of patients to the ICU. Thoracentesis is a safe procedure, particularly under ultrasound guidance, and has diagnostic utility that helps in management decisions.

REFERENCES

1. Mattison LE, Coppage L, Alderman DF, Herlong JO, Sahn SA. Pleural effusions in the medical ICU: prevalence, causes, and clinical implications. *Chest.* 1997;111(4):1018-1023.
2. Maslove DM, Chen BTM, Wang H, Kuschner WG. The diagnosis and management of pleural effusions in the ICU. *J Intensive Care Med.* 2013;28(1):24-36.
3. Azoulay E, Fartoukh M, Similowski T, et al. Routine exploratory thoracentesis in ICU patients with pleural effusions: results of a French questionnaire study. *J Crit Care.* 2001;16(3):98-101.
4. Brown NE, Zamel N, Aberman A. Changes in pulmonary mechanics and gas exchange following thoracocentesis. *Chest.* 1978;74(5):540-542.
5. Doelken P, Abreu R, Sahn SA, Mayo PH. Effect of thoracentesis on respiratory mechanics and gas exchange in the patient receiving mechanical ventilation. *Chest.* 2006;130(5):1354-1361.
6. Park TY, Lee J, Park YS, et al. Determination of the cause of pleural effusion in ICU patients with thoracentesis. *Korean J Crit Care Med.* 2012;27(4):249-254.
7. Fartoukh M, Azoulay E, Galliot R, et al. Clinically documented pleural effusions in medical ICU patients: how useful Is routine thoracentesis? *Chest.* 2002;121(1):178-184.
8. Goligher EC, Leis JA, Fowler RA, Pinto R, Adhikari NK, Ferguson ND. Utility and safety of draining pleural effusions in mechanically ventilated patients: a systematic review and meta-analysis. *Crit Care.* 2011;15(1):R46.
9. Light RW, Macgregor MI, Luchsinger PC, Ball WC. Pleural effusions: the diagnostic separation of transudates and exudates. *Ann Intern Med.* 1972;77(4):507-513.
10. Mayo PH, Goltz HR, Tafreshi M, Doelken P. Safety of ultrasound-guided thoracentesis in patients receiving mechanical ventilation. *Chest.* 2004;125(3):1059-1062.
11. Mayo PH, Doelken P. Pleural ultrasonography. *Clin Chest Med.* 2006;27(2):215-227.
12. Workman ML. Comparison of blot-drying versus air-drying of povidone-iodine-cleansed skin. *Appl Nurs Res.* 1995;8(1):15-17.
13. Feller-Kopman D, Berkowitz D, Boiselle P, Ernst A. Large-volume thoracentesis and the risk of reexpansion pulmonary edema. *Ann Thorac Surg.* 2007;84(5):1656-1661.
14. Gordon CE, Feller-Kopman D, Balk EM, Smetana GW. Pneumothorax following thoracentesis: a systematic review and meta-analysis. *Arch Intern Med.* 2010;170(4):332-339.
15. McCartney JP, Adams J, Hazard PB. Safety of thoracentesis in mechanically ventilated patients. *Chest.* 1993;103(6):1920-1921.
16. Patel MD, Joshi SD. Abnormal preprocedural international normalized ratio and platelet counts are not associated with increased bleeding complications after ultrasound-guided thoracentesis. *Am J Roentgenol.* 2011;197(1):W164-W168.
17. Puchalski JT, Argento AC, Murphy TE, Araujo KL, Pisani MA. The safety of thoracentesis in patients with uncorrected bleeding risk. *Ann Am Thorac Soc.* 2013;10(4):336-341.

Controversies: Early Tracheotomy

Bradley A. Schiff

INTRODUCTION

Tracheotomy is a common procedure with almost 1 in 4 ICU patients receiving a tracheotomy.[1] While a tracheotomy is a relatively straightforward surgical procedure, the medical complexity of patients requiring tracheotomy, and the debate about its timing and indications, make its utilization complex. Despite its common and widespread use there remains considerable debate in the literature regarding tracheotomies risks, benefits, and indications.

INDICATIONS AND BENEFITS

The indications for tracheotomy have evolved throughout the history of the procedure. With improved understanding of the disease processes affecting the airway, the indications have become more standardized and rigorous in recent years. Today there are numerous indications recognized in the adult population. These indications were defined by the American Academy of Otolaryngology and Head and Neck surgery in the 2010 Clinical Indicators Compendium,[2] and fall into 4 broad categories: to relieve a mechanical obstruction (or potential obstruction), to manage aspiration (and promote improved pulmonary toilet), to provide long-term ventilation (and avoid the complications of long-term translaryngeal intubation), and to promote weaning from the ventilator. The last 2 categories constitute the vast majority of patients included in studies on ET.

Tracheotomy offers a number of potential benefits over endotracheal intubation. Tracheotomy has been shown to decrease the mechanical workload of ventilator-dependent patients,[3,4] and patients with tracheotomies can be placed on and off the ventilator without any significant risk to the patient, potentially facilitating earlier extubation. Tracheotomy improves comfort level when compared with translaryngeal intubation. Patients with tracheotomies have improved tracheal suctioning, oral care, mobility, ability to take oral nutrition and articulate speech,[5,6] and decreased oropharyngeal and laryngeal trauma compared to intubated patients.[7]

RISKS

Different clinicians have different opinions on the risks and timings of tracheotomy. The risk of tracheotomy has decreased over time and varies depending on the skill and experience of the person performing the procedure. In 1833 Trousseau reported a 75% mortality rate for tracheotomy patients, compared with current mortality rates of approximately 1%.[8-10] Today, while tracheotomy is a relatively safe procedure, complications still occur. A recent study looking at 113,653 tracheotomies performed in the United States in 2006 showed a 3.2% complication rate and 0.6% mortality rate.[11] However, the experience and expertize of the physician performing the procedure can greatly impact the risk of tracheotomy. A recent study showed that surgeons performing the fewest tracheotomies demonstrated the highest complication rates, and that intraoperative complication rates varied greatly among practitioners with otolaryngologists having an intraoperative complication rate is 0.39% compared to 3.5% with tracheotomies done by nonotolaryngologists.[12]

TIMING

The optimal timing for a tracheotomy is dependent on the patient and the situation. There is significant controversy regarding the timing of surgery for those patients undergoing an elective tracheotomy after intubation, and it is the timing of tracheotomy in patients undergoing prolonged intubation that is the most debated, and is the focus of this chapter.

Physicians of the 1960s promoted the placement of ET tubes, as high pressure cuffs and rigid endotracheal tubes lead to significant complications rates.[13] With the arrival of the more flexible endotracheal tubes with low-pressure cuffs in the 1970s, combined with the reported high complication rate of tracheotomy, delayed tracheotomy, 3 to 4 weeks after intubation, became the rule. Since the mid-1980s, with the introduction of percutaneous tracheotomy and the decreased complication rates associated with open tracheotomy, there has been a shift toward earlier tracheotomy placement.

The ideal time for tracheotomy in ventilated patients has not been established, despite many studies addressing this topic. The risks of prolonged intubation must be weighed against the benefits of tracheotomy as well as the risks of the procedure.[14] Earlier recommendations suggested that tracheotomy be performed in patients requiring mechanical ventilation for more than 21 days.[6] More recent guidelines advise that translaryngeal intubation be used only for patients requiring fewer than 10 days of artificial ventilation, and that tracheotomy be performed for those requiring artificial ventilation for more than 21 days. The decision is left to the physician for those patients falling between 10 and 21 days.[15] A commonly used method of determining the need and timing of a tracheotomy is the "anticipatory approach." This involves initially stabilizing the patient and treating the primary disease process. If extubation is felt to be possible in the first several days of mechanical ventilation then tracheotomy is not considered necessary. If after a week of translaryngeal intubation the patient is felt (1) likely to benefit from a tracheotomy and (2) likely to require extended intubation (more than 7 additional days), then a tracheotomy should be performed.[13,16] As the clinician's ability to predict the duration of intubation improves, even earlier tracheotomy can be considered. However, despite its widespread use, this approach has yet to be determined to improve the morbidity and mortality of patients requiring prolonged mechanical ventilation.

There are many studies examining the appropriate timing for tracheotomy that typically fall into 3 general categories: (1) nonrandomized retrospective reviews, (2) prospective studies, (3) meta-analysis (of either retrospective reviews or prospective studies). Observational studies retrospectively comparing patients who received a tracheotomy early after intubation with those who received a tracheotomy sometime after intubation are common. However, it is very difficult to extrapolate meaningful conclusions from these observational papers as the patient populations in the 2 groups may be very different, and the difference in management in regards to the timing of tracheotomy may be reflective of differences in perceived outcomes of the patients.

A study by Arabi looked at 531 consecutive nonrandomized patients.[17] They found that the time to tracheotomy was associated with increased duration of ventilation, length of ICU and hospital stay, but not survival. A similar retrospective study by Tong et al, looked at 592 patients, 128 ET patients who received a tracheotomy by day 7, and 464 LT patients who received a tracheotomy after day 7, demonstrating decreased days of mechanical ventilation, length of ICU stay, and length of hospital stays in patients receiving an ET, but no improvement in survival and ventilator-associated pneumonia (VAP).[18]

Shan et al[19] performed a meta-analysis of observational studies comparing ET (< 7 days) with LT (7 or more days) in ICU patients. They combined the data from 6 studies (Armstrong,[20] Arabi,[17] Moller,[21] Flaatten,[22] Zalgi,[23] and Tong[1]) looking at a total of 2037 subjects. They found that the mortality in the early tracheotomy group was significantly lower than the late group at 1 year (26.1% vs 29.8% $P = 0.02$). In addition the duration of mechanical ventilation was shorter in the early group than the late group (mean difference 10.04 days, $P = 0.001$), the ICU stay was shorter in the early tracheotomy group (mean difference 8.8 days, $P < 0.001$), the hospital stay was shorter in the early tracheotomy group (mean 12.18 days, $P < 0.001$), and there was no difference in the incidence of VAP between the 2 groups.

A more recent observational study, looking at tracheotomies in the American College of Surgeon's Trauma Quality Improvement program, used a well-balanced propensity matched cohort of 1154 patients in an attempt to decrease bias and compared early (≤ 8 days) versus late (> 8 days) tracheotomy. They found that ET was associated with fewer mechanical ventilation days (10 vs 16), shorter ICU stay (13 vs 19 days), shorter hospital length of stay (20 vs

27 days), and lower incidence of pneumonia (41.7% vs 52.7%), deep venous thrombosis (DVT) (8.2% vs 14.4%), and decubitus ulcer (4.0% vs 8.9%). Hospital mortality was similar between the 2 groups.[24]

A number of larger observational studies exist, which, like these smaller single-center studies, usually show a benefit for early tracheotomy and contributed to the interest in performing early tracheotomy. A study by Freeman et al[25] looked at the data from 43,916 patients of whom 2473 had tracheotomy. It showed that tracheotomy timing correlated significantly with duration of mechanical ventilation, ICU stay, and hospital stay. A similar study looked at tracheotomy in acute care hospitals in Ontario hospitals.[26] Between 1992 and 2004 10,927 patients received tracheotomy: 3758 received early tracheotomy (≤ 10 days) and 7169 patients received late tracheotomy. Patients receiving early tracheotomy had lower 90 day, 1 year, and study mortality. On multivariate analysis each delay of 1 day was associated with increased mortality. While these observational studies are an excellent starting point, there are a number of reasons why their findings cannot be extrapolated to prospective tracheotomy management. Most important among these is the potential selection biases in determining who received an early versus a late tracheotomy. However, at a minimum, these observational studies promoted the concept that ET might be beneficial, and encouraged larger prospective studies.

A number of prospective studies have been performed comparing early and late tracheotomy. Significant differences in definitions, methodologies, and conclusions exist between studies. A study by Koch et al[27] examined 100 predominately surgical patients in the university hospital in Geiben Germany, prospectively randomized to early (≤ 4 days, average 2.8 days) or late (≥ 6 days, average 8.1 days) tracheotomy. They found no change in mortality between the ET and LT groups, but did find a statistically significant decrease in VAP incidence, duration of mechanical ventilation, ICU and hospital stay in the ET group. A study by Terragni et al[28] in *JAMA* compared ET patients (day 6-8) and LT patients (day 13-15) as part of a randomized control trial across 12 Italian ICUs. Six hundred patients were randomized to early or late tracheotomy after 48 hours: 145/209 ET group patients received tracheotomy and 119/210 LT group patients received tracheotomy. They found a 14% incidence of VAP (measured at 28 days from randomization) in the ET group compared to a 21% incidence in the LT group that approached, but did not reach, statistical significance ($P = 0.07$). The number of ventilator-free days and ICU-free days were statistically significantly decreased in the ET group, but there was no change in hospital stay or mortality between the 2 groups.

Blot et al[29] performed a prospective and randomized study in 2008 evaluating 25 ICUs in France comparing ET (day 4) with prolonged intubation. The study was halted after 2 years because of difficulty accruing patients, and only 123 patients were enlisted in the study. There were no difference in mortality, duration of ventilation, or VAP between the ET and LT group, but there were improvements in patient comfort and late laryngeal symptoms in the ET group. This study was underpowered and fell well short of its recruitment goal partially due to what the authors thought was recruitment bias and therefore it is difficult to draw meaningful conclusions from the study. Trouillet et al[30] performed a prospective randomized controlled study looking at patients after heart surgery at a single French academic hospital expected to need more than 7 days of ventilation. They randomized patients to immediate ET (< day 5) or prolonged intubation with tracheotomy (> day 14). Two hundred sixteen patients were enrolled, 109 in the ET group and 107 in the LT group. There were some differences in the characteristics of the 2 groups with higher rates of heart transplantation, repeat surgery, and renal replacement in the ET group. Only 27% of LT group received tracheotomies. There was no significant difference in ventilation-free days, survival ICU or hospital stay, or rates of VAP between the groups, but more sedation-free days in the ET group with patients in the ET group having more time calm awake or lightly sedated and more days comfortable with easy care, earlier nutrition, and mobilization.

Rumbak et al[31] performed a prospective randomized trial looking at 120 patients in a Florida hospital MICU comparing early percutaneous tracheotomy (48 hours) or delayed tracheotomy (day 14-16). They found that patients in the early group had statistically significant decreased mortality (31.7% vs 61.7%) rates of pneumonia (5% vs

25%), less time in ICU (4.8 vs 16.2 days), and days on mechanical ventilation (7.6 vs. 17.4). This paper has fewer patients than other papers; however, it also stratified patients to the widest difference between ET and LT (< 48 hours vs > 2 weeks).

The TracMan trial[32] is a recent prospective study that was highly anticipated. It was an open multi-centered randomized clinical trial at both university and nonuniversity hospitals in the United Kingdom that identified people within the first 4 days of admission that were likely to require 7 days of ventilator support. ETs were done by day 4 and LTs were done by day 10 or later. Of the people in the LT group over half did not get a tracheotomy (37% were extubated). There was an average of 13.6 days of mechanical ventilation in the ET group versus 15.2 days of mechanical ventilation in the LT group, this approached but did not reach statistical significance ($P = 0.06$). There was no difference in the length of ICU stay and mortality, but less sedation was used in the ET group. This study highlights the limited ability of clinicians to predict which patients would require ventilatory support as over half of the patients in the LT group did not need tracheotomy.

While most of these prospective studies are well designed it is difficult to power a prospective study that would pick up small changes between ET and LT groups. Because of this a number of meta-analysis exists attempting to increase the patient population and the power of the study. A study by Griffiths in 2005[15] looked at 5 studies with 406 participants: the combined studies by Rumbak,[31] Bouderka,[33] Dunham,[34], Rodriguez,[35] and Saffle.[36] They did not find any changes in morality, although the tracheotomy had a slightly lower relative risk (RR), and no change in hospital-acquired pneumonia, (although the tracheotomy had a slighter lower RR). They found that tracheotomy patients had 8.5 fewer days of mechanical ventilation and 15.3 fewer days in the ICU. A recent (2014) meta-analysis by Wang et al[37] looks at all randomized controlled trials regarding early versus late tracheotomy. The analyzed 7 trials (Saffle,[36] Bouderka,[33] Rumbak,[31] Barquist,[38] Blot,[29] Terragni,[28] and Trouillet[30]) encompass 1044 patients. They found no change in mortality (although there again was a lower RR in the ET group) and no change in VAP (although again there was an early with lower RR in the ET group). There

was no appreciable change in length of mechanical ventilation or ICU stay.

DISCUSSION

Despite the numerous studies looking at the timing of tracheotomy no definitive conclusions can be reached. There are a number of potential explanations for the lack of consensus regarding timing of tracheotomy despite numerous papers. First tracheotomy patients are a varied patient population who might require tracheotomy secondary to trauma, general medical issue, respiratory issues both acute (such as pneumonia) and chronic (such as chronic obstructive pulmonary disease [COPD]), and complications from surgery, neurologic injury, etc. It is possible that ET may benefit one type of patient while not benefiting others. Additionally, ET has many different definitions. Some studies compared people who received a tracheotomy within 48 hours versus those who did not receive a tracheotomy until 2 weeks passed, while others compared those earlier than 7 days versus those 7 days or later. It is possible that there are some cutoffs when early tracheotomy may be beneficial, but these were not measured in these studies, or if they were measured then they were underpowered. A comprehensive study would have to randomize people to every day to find ideal timing (and this could vary by disease).

Additionally the decision to perform an ET is based on the clinician's impression that prolonged intubation will be needed while also believing that the patient has a chance of recovery. The studies examining ET are therefore evaluating clinician's ability to determine which patients will need prolonged intubation but have a chance of recovery as much as whether ET is useful. Perhaps in the right patient population early tracheotomy is beneficial, but we are not yet able to accurately determine which patients fit these criteria. A number of studies exist examining clinician's ability to predict ET,[39,40] but as of yet no applicable guidelines exist to determine which patients will need prolonged intubation.

When analyzing the data some studies suggest benefits for ET and some do not. Many studies find a benefit for some aspects of ET (such as increased comfort, or incidence of VAP) but not for others. However, care must be taken when drawing conclusions on some characteristics such as length of mechanical ventilation, ICU stay, and hospital stay as these data may be more indicative of system issues, or of how these patients were managed and triaged, rather than actual medical differences. For example, patients with a tracheotomy may have easier access to step down units or hospice facilities thus decreasing their length of stay. While the data do not find conclusively for or against the use of ET, more of the data suggest benefits for ET and none of the data suggest harm for ET. The meta-analysis did not find a statistically significant benefit in terms of mortality and days of mechanical ventilation, but in both cases the RR of ET was less than that of LT patients.

CONCLUSIONS

Many studies have been written examining the benefits of ET, but as of yet there is no clear consensus on ET. The heterogeneity of the many studies and the patient population receiving tracheotomy makes drawing definitive conclusions difficult. While it cannot be conclusively stated that ET is beneficial there are a number of studies that suggest that it may be (and none that suggest it is harmful). At a minimum more larger and better defined studies are needed before we can say for certain when, and in which patients, ET is conclusively beneficial.

REFERENCES

1. Hsu CL, Chen KY, Chang CH, Jerng JS, Yu CJ, Yang PC. Timing of tracheostomy as a determinant of weaning success in critically ill patients: a retrospective study. *Crit Care*. 2005;9(1):R46-52.
2. Archer SM, Baugh RF, Nelms CR, et al. Tracheotomyeostomy. p. 45. 2000. American Academy of Otolaryngology-Head and Neck Surgery. *2000 Clinical Indicators Compendium*.
3. Diehl JL, El AS, Touchard D, Lemaire F, Brochard L. Changes in the work of breathing induced by tracheotomy in ventilator-dependent patients. *Am J Respir Crit Care Med*. 1999;159(2):383-388.
4. Davis K Jr, Campbell RS, Johannigman JA, Valente JF, Branson RD. Changes in respiratory mechanics after tracheotomyeostomy. *Arch Surg*. 1999;134(1):59-62.
5. Heffner JE. The role of tracheotomy in weaning. *Chest*. 2001;120(suppl 6):S477-S481.
6. Plummer AL, Gracey DR. Consensus conference on artificial airways in patients receiving mechanical ventilation. *Chest*. 1989;96(1):178-180.
7. Heffner JE, Hess D. Tracheostomy management in the chronically ventilated patient. *Clin Chest Med*. 2001;22(1):55-69.
8. Goldenberg D, Ari EG, Golz A, Danino J, Netzer A, Joachims HZ. Tracheotomy complications: a retrospective study of 1130 cases. *Otolaryngol Head Neck Surg*. 2000;123(4):495-500.
9. Borman J, Davidson JT. A history of tracheostomy: si spiritum ducit vivit (Cicero). *Br J Anaesth*. 1963;35:388-390.
10. Heffner JE, Miller KS, Sahn SA. Tracheostomy in the intensive care unit. Part 2: complications. *Chest*. 1986;90(3):430-436.
11. Shah RK, Lander L, Berry JG, Nussenbaum B, Merati A, Roberson DW. Tracheotomy outcomes and complications: a national perspective. *Laryngoscope*. 2012;122(1):25-29.
12. Halum SL, Ting JY, Plowman EK, et al. A multi-institutional analysis of tracheotomy complications. *Laryngoscope*. 2012;122(1):38-45.
13. Heffner JE. Tracheotomy application and timing. *Clin Chest Med*. 2003;24(3):389-398.
14. Esteller-More E, Ibanez J, Matino E, et al. Prognostic factors in laryngotracheal injury following intubation and/or tracheotomy in ICU patients. *Eur Arch Otorhinolaryngol*. 2005;262(11):880-883.
15. Griffiths J, Barber VS, Morgan L, Young JD. Systematic review and meta-analysis of studies of the timing of tracheostomy in adult patients undergoing artificial ventilation. *BMJ*. 2005;330(7502):1243.
16. Heffner JE. Timing tracheotomy: calendar watching or individualization of care? *Chest*. 1998;114(2):361-363.
17. Arabi YM, Alhashemi JA, Tamim HM, et al. The impact of time to tracheostomy on mechanical ventilation duration, length of stay, and mortality in intensive care unit patients. *J Crit Care*. 2009;24(3):435-440.
18. Tong CCL, Kleinberger AJ, Paolino J, Altman KW. Tracheotomy timing and outcomes in the critically ill. *Otolaryngol Head Neck Surg*. 2012;147(1):44-51.
19. Shan L, Hao P, Xu F, Chen YG. Benefits of early tracheotomy: a meta-analysis based on 6 observational studies. *Respir Care*. 2013;58(11):1856-1862.
20. Armstrong PA, McCarthy MC, Peoples JB. Reduced use of resources by early tracheostomy in ventilator-dependent patients with blunt trauma. *Surgery*. 1998;124(4):763-766.

21. Moller MG, Slaikeu JD, Bonelli P, Davis AT, Hoogeboom JE, Bonnell BW. Early tracheostomy versus late tracheostomy in the surgical intensive care unit. *Am J Surg*. 2005;189(3):293-296.

22. Flaatten H, Gjerde S, Heimdal JH, Aardal S. The effect of tracheostomy on outcome in intensive care unit patients. *Acta Anaesthesiol Scand*. 2006;50(1):92-98.

23. Zagli G, Linden M, Spina R, et al. Early tracheostomy in intensive care unit: a retrospective study of 506 cases of video-guided Ciaglia Blue Rhino tracheostomies. *J Trauma*. 2010;68(2):367-372.

24. Alali AS, Scales DC, Fowler RA, et al. Tracheostomy timing in traumatic brain injury: a propensity-matched cohort study. *J Trauma Acute Care Surg*. 2014;76(1):70-76; discussion 76-78.

25. Freeman BD, Borecki IB, Coopersmith CM, Buchman TG. Relationship between tracheostomy timing and duration of mechanical ventilation in critically ill patients. *Crit Care Med*. 2005;33(11):2513-2520.

26. Scales DC, Thiruchelvam D, Kiss A, Redelmeier DA. The effect of tracheostomy timing during critical illness on long-term survival. *Crit Care Med*. 2008;36(9):2547-2557.

27. Koch T, Hecker B, Hecker A, et al. Early tracheostomy decreases ventilation time but has no impact on mortality of intensive care patients: a randomized study. *Langenbecks Arch Surg*. 2012;397(6):1001-1008.

28. Terragni PP, Antonelli M, Fumagalli R, et al. Early vs late tracheotomy for prevention of pneumonia in mechanically ventilated adult ICU patients: a randomized controlled trial. *JAMA*. 2010;303(15):1483-1489.

29. Blot F, Similowski T, Trouillet JL, et al. Early tracheotomy versus prolonged endotracheal intubation in unselected severely ill ICU patients. *Intensive Care Med*. 2008;34(10):1779-1787.

30. Trouillet JL, Luyt CE, Guiguet M, et al. Early percutaneous tracheotomy versus prolonged intubation of mechanically ventilated patients after cardiac surgery: a randomized trial. *Ann Intern Med*. 2011;154(6):373-383.

31. Rumbak MJ, Newton M, Truncale T, Schwartz SW, Adams JW, Hazard PB. A prospective, randomized, study comparing early percutaneous dilational tracheotomy to prolonged translaryngeal intubation (delayed tracheotomy) in critically ill medical patients. *Crit Care Med*. 2004;32(8):1689-1694.

32. Young D, Harrison DA, Cuthbertson BH, Rowan K; TracMan Collaborators. Effect of early vs late tracheostomy placement on survival in patients receiving mechanical ventilation: the TracMan randomized trial. *JAMA*. 2013;309(20):2121-2129.

33. Bouderka MA, Fakhir B, Bouaggad A, Hmamouchi B, Hamoudi D, Harti A. Early tracheostomy versus prolonged endotracheal intubation in severe head injury. *J Trauma*. 2004;57:251-254.

34. Dunham CM, LaMonica C. Prolonged tracheal intubation in the trauma patient. *J Trauma*. 1984;24:120-124.

35. Rodriguez JL, Steinberg SM, Luchetti FA, Gibbons KJ, Taheri PA, Flint LM. Early tracheostomy for primary airway management in the surgical critical care setting. *Surgery*. 1990;108:655-659.

36. Saffle JR, Morris SE, Edelman L. Early tracheostomy does not improve outcome in burn patients. *J Burn Care Rehabil*. 2002;23:431-438.

37. Wang F, Wu Y, Bo L, et al. The timing of tracheotomy in critically ill patients undergoing mechanical ventilation: a systematic review and meta-analysis of randomized controlled trials. *Chest*. 2011 Dec;140(6):1456-1465.

38. Barquist E. A randomized prospective study of early vs late tracheostomy in trauma patients. Proceeding of the American Association for the Surgery of Trauma, 2004. http://www.aast.org/PDF/04absOral.pdf. Accessed May 10, 2005.

39. Veelo DP, Binnekade JM, Buddeke AW, Dongelmans DA, Schultz MJ. Early predictability of the need for tracheotomy after admission to ICU: an observational study. *Acta Anaesthesiol Scand*. 2010;54(9):1083-1088.

40. Papuzinski C, Durante M, Tobar C, Martinez F, Labarca E. Predicting the need of tracheostomy amongst patients admitted to an intensive care unit: a multivariate model. *Am J Otolaryngol*. 2013;34(5):517-522.

Antimicrobial Prophylaxis for Surgery

Jun Makino, MD and
John M. Oropello, MD, FACP, FCCP, FCCM

INTRODUCTION

A surgical site infection (SSI) is an infection related to an operative procedure that occurs at or near the surgical incision within 30 days of the procedure, or within 90 days if prosthetic material is implanted at surgery.[1] SSIs are classified into incisional (superficial/deep) or organ/space infections (Table 110–1A).[1] According to the Centers for Disease Control and Prevention (CDC), prevalence survey in 183 acute care hospitals in the United States, SSIs and pneumonia were the most common health-care-associated infections.[2] Also the National Healthcare Safety Network (NHSN) data for 2006 to 2008 reported the overall SSI rate was 1.9% (16,147 SSIs following 849,659 operative procedures).[3] The aim of antimicrobial prophylaxis is to prevent SSI by reducing the burden of microorganisms at the surgical site during the operative procedure,[4] and ultimately to prevent related morbidity and mortality. Indications for antimicrobial prophylaxis, antibiotic selection, timing, and dosing are reviewed.

Surgical wound infections are historically classified into 4 groups based on the degree of expected microbial contamination during surgery (Table 110–1B).[5] Antimicrobial treatment (vs prophylaxis) is required for dirty procedures or established infections. Antimicrobial prophylaxis is justified for contaminated or most clean-contaminated procedures and in certain clean procedures (eg, prosthetic implants).[6] Also, antimicrobial prophylaxis may be justified for any procedure if the patient has an underlying medical condition associated with a high risk of SSI (Table 110–2).[6]

ANTIMICROBIAL SELECTION, TIMING, DOSING AND DURATION

When antimicrobial prophylaxis is initiated, appropriate antimicrobials should be administered with appropriate timing, dose, and duration to minimize adverse effects, emergence of resistance, and cost.[1]

Antimicrobial agents are selected according to the comparative efficacy for the procedure (eg, *Staphylococcus aureus* and coagulase-negative staphylococci in clean procedures; gram-negative rods and enterococci in abdominal procedures and transplantation of heart, kidney, and liver), the safety

TABLE 110–1A Classification of surgical site infection (SSI).[1]

Type		Description
Incisional SSI	Superficial	Skin and subcutaneous tissue of the incision
	Deep	Deep tissue of the incision (eg, fascial and muscle layers)
Organ/space SSI		Infection involving any part of the body excluding incisional SSIs

Data from Centers for Disease Control. Surgical Site Infection (SSI) Event.

TABLE 110–1B   Wound classification.[5]

Class	Definition	SSI Rate (%)	Microbiology
Clean	An uninfected operative wound in which no inflammation is encountered and the wound is primarily closed.	1.3-2.9	Skin flora; gram-positive cocci
Clean-contaminated	Operative wounds in which a viscus[a] is entered under controlled conditions and without unusual contamination.	2.4-7.7	Gram-negative rods; enterococci
Contaminated	Operative wounds in which the respiratory, alimentary, genital (including reproductive organs), or urinary tracts are entered under controlled conditions and without unusual contamination. Specifically, operations involving the biliary tract, appendix, vagina, and oropharynx are included in this category, provided no evidence of infection or major break in technique is encountered.	6.4-15.2	polymicrobial
Dirty	Old traumatic wounds with retained devitalized tissue and those that involve existing clinical infection or perforated viscera	7.1-40	polymicrobial

[a]Respiratory, alimentary, genital (including reproductive organs), or urinary tracts.
Data from Culver DH, Horan TC, Gaynes RP, et al: Surgical wound infection rates by wound class, operative procedure, and patient risk index. National Nosocomial Infections Surveillance System, *Am J Med* 1991 Sep 16;91(3B):152S-157S.

profile, cost, and the patient's allergic history.[6] There is little evidence that broad-spectrum antimicrobials will lower the rate of SSI compared to narrow-spectrum ones. Therefore, cefazolin is generally chosen for its desirable duration of action, spectrum of activity against organisms commonly encountered in surgery, reasonable safety, and low cost.[1] When patients have known Methicillin-resistant Staphylococcus aures (MRSA) colonization or high risk for MRSA colonization without surveillance data, vancomycin should be considered.[7] However, because vancomycin is less effective for MSSA, cefazolin is sometimes combined with vancomycin to cover both MRSA and Methicillin-sensitive Staphylococcus aureus (MSSA).

TABLE 110–2   Patient-related factors associated with an increased risk for SSI.[6]

- Age (elderly)
- Malnutrition
- Obesity
- Diabetes mellitus
- Tobacco use
- Recent surgical procedure
- Length of preoperative hospitalization
- Colonization with microorganisms
- Receiving immunosuppressants

Data from Bratzler DW1, Dellinger EP, Olsen KM, et al: Clinical practice guidelines for antimicrobial prophylaxis in surgery, *Am J Health Syst Pharm* 2013 Feb 1;70(3):195-283

Also, if the patient is documented or presumed to have IgE-mediated penicillin allergy, cephalosporins and carbapenems should be avoided, and vancomycin, clindamycin, gentamicin, tobramycin, ciprofloxacin, levofloxacin, or aztreonam should be used instead.[6,8] Recommended antimicrobial agents and alternatives for each surgical procedure are listed in Table 110–3.[6]

In order to achieve successful antimicrobial prophylaxis, providing serum and tissue concentrations exceeding the minimum inhibitory concentration at the time of incision and for the duration of the procedure is essential.[9,10]

In the previous studies, patients who received prophylactic antimicrobials 60 to 120 minutes before the initial incision had lower rates of SSI than patients who received prophylaxis outside of this window (Table 110–4).[11,12] Therefore, administration of the first dose of antimicrobials is recommended within 60 minutes before surgical incision.[9,13,14] Vancomycin and fluoroquinolones should begin within 120 minutes before surgical incision because these drugs need more time for infusion. If the duration of the procedure exceeds 2 half-lives of the drug or there is excessive blood loss (> 1500 mL) during the procedure, intraoperative redosing is necessary and the dosing interval will be measured from the time of the initial dosing.[6] Recommended doses and

TABLE 110–3 Recommended antimicrobial agents and alternatives for each surgical procedure.[6]

Type of Procedure	Recommended Agents	Alternative Agents in Patients With β-Lactam Allergy
Cardiac • Coronary artery bypass • Cardiac device insertion • Ventricular assist devices	Cefazolin, cefuroxime	Clindamycin, vancomycin
Thoracic • Lobectomy, pneumonectomy • Lung resection, thoracotomy • Video-assisted thoracoscopic surgery	Cefazolin, ampicillin-sulbactam	Clindamycin, vancomycin
Gastroduodenal • Entry into lumen of GI tract (bariatric, pancreatoduodenectomy) • No entry into gastrointestinal (GI) tract (antireflex, highly selective vagotomy), but high-risk	Cefazolin	Clindamycin or vancomycin + aminoglycoside or aztreonam or fluoroquinolone
Biliary tract • Open procedure • Laparoscopic procedure with high-risk (no indication for low-risk)	Cefazolin, cefoxitin, cefotetan, ceftriaxone, ampicillin-sulbactam	Clindamycin or vancomycin + aminoglycoside or aztreonam or fluoroquinolone, metronidazole + aminoglycoside or fluoroquinolone
Appendectomy • Uncomplicated appendicitis	Cefoxitin, cefotetan, cefazolin + metronidazole	Or vancomycin + aminoglycoside or aztreonam or fluoroquinolone, metronidazole + aminoglycoside or fluoroquinolone
Small intestine • Nonobstructed • Obstructed	Cefazolin Cefazolin + metronidazole, cefoxitin, cefotetan	Clindamycin + aminoglycoside or aztreonam or fluoroquinolone Metronidazole + aminoglycoside or fluoroquinolone
Hernia repair	Cefazolin	Clindamycin, vancomycin
Colorectal	Cefazolin + metronidazole, cefoxitin, cefotetan, ampicillin-sulbactam ceftriaxone + metronidazole, ertapenem	Clindamycin + aminoglycoside or aztreonam or fluoroquinolone, metronidazole + aminoglycoside or fluoroquinolone

Head and neck
• Clean (no indication)
  Clean with placement of prosthesis
• Clean-contaminated cancer
  Other clean-contaminated procedures (except for tonsillectomy, functional endoscopic sinus procedures)
	Cefazolin, cefuroxime
	
	Cefazolin or cefuroxime + metronidazole, ampicillin-sulbactam
		Clindamycin
		
		Clindamycin

Neurosurgery • Elective craniotomy cerebrospinal fluid-shunting procedures, implantation of intrathecal pumps	Cefazolin	Clindamycin, vancomycin

(Continued)

TABLE 110-3 Recommended antimicrobial agents and alternatives for each surgical procedure.[6] (Continued)

Type of Procedure	Recommended Agents	Alternative Agents in Patients With β-Lactam Allergy
Cesarean delivery	Cefazolin	Clindamycin + aminoglycoside
Hysterectomy (vaginal or abdominal)	Cefazolin, cefotetan, cefoxitin, ampicillin-sulbactam	Clindamycin or vancomycin + aminoglycoside or aztreonam or fluoroquinolone, metronidazole + aminoglycoside or fluoroquinolone
Ophthalmic	Topical neomycin-polymyxin B-gramicidin or fourth-generation topical fluoroquinolones (gatifloxacin or moxifloxacin) given as 1 drop every 5-15 min for 5 doses	None
Orthopedic • Clean operation involving hand, knee, or foot without implantation (no indication for antimicrobials) • Spinal procedures with and without instrumentation • Hip fracture repair • Implantation of internal fixation devices (eg, nails, screws, plates, wires) • Total joint replacement	None Cefazolin	None Clindamycin, vancomycin
Urologic • Lower tract instrumentation with risk factors for infection (includes transrectal prostate biopsy) • Clean without entry into urinary tract • Involving implanted prosthesis • Clean with entry into urinary tract • Clean-contaminated	Fluoroquinolone, trimethoprim-sulfamethoxazole, cefazolin Cefazolin (+ a single dose of aminoglycoside for penile prosthesis) Cefazolin ± aminoglycoside, cefazolin ± aztreonam, ampicillin-sulbactam Cefazolin (+ a single dose of aminoglycoside for penile prosthesis) Cefazolin + metronidazole, cefoxitin	Aminoglycoside with or without clindamycin Clindamycin, vancomycin Clindamycin ± aminoglycoside or aztreonam, vancomycin ± aminoglycoside or aztreonam Fluoroquinolone, aminoglycoside with or without clindamycin Fluoroquinolone, aminoglycoside + metronidazole or clindamycin
Vascular	Cefazolin	Clindamycin, vancomycin
Heart, lung, heart-lung transplantation	Cefazolin	Clindamycin, vancomycin
Liver transplantation	Piperacillin-tazobactam, cefotaxime + ampicillin	Clindamycin or vancomycin + aminoglycoside or aztreonam or fluoroquinolone
Pancreas and pancreas-kidney transplantation	Cefazolin, fluconazole for high risk patients	Clindamycin or vancomycin + aminoglycoside or aztreonam or fluoroquinolone
Plastic surgery • Clean with risk factors or clean-contaminated	Cefazolin, ampicillin-sulbactam	Clindamycin, vancomycin

Adapted with permission from Bratzler DW1, Dellinger EP, Olsen KM, et al: Clinical practice guidelines for antimicrobial prophylaxis in surgery, *Am J Health Syst Pharm* 2013 Feb 1;70(3):195-283.

TABLE 110–4 Timing of prophylactic antibiotic administration and subsequent rates of surgical site infections (SSIs).[11,12]

Time of Administration	Percent with SSI	Odds Ratio (95% CI)
Early (2-24 h before incision)	3.8	4.3 (1.8-10.4)
Preoperative (0-2 h before incision)	0.6	1.0 (-)
Perioperative (within 3 h after incision)	1.4	2.1 (0.6-7.4)
Postoperative (> 3 h after incision)	3.3	5.8 (2.4-13.8)

Data from Classen DC, Evans RS, Pestotnik SL, Horn SD, Menlove RL, Burke JP. The timing of prophylactic administration of antibiotics and the risk of surgical-wound infection. *N Eng J Med* 1992;326:281-286; van Kasteren ME, Manniën J, Ott A, et al. Antibiotic prophylaxis and the risk of surgical site infections following total hip arthroplasty: timely administration is the most important factor. Clin Infect Dis 2007; 44:921.

redosing intervals for commonly used antimicrobials are shown in Table 110–5.[6]

Repeat antimicrobial dosing following wound closure is not necessary and may increase antimicrobial resistance.[8,15-16] Also, there is no difference in the rate of SSI with single dose compared with multiple-dose regimens given for less than or more than 24 hours (combined odds ratio 1.04, 95% confidence interval [CI] 0.86-1.25).[15] Therefore, antimicrobial prophylaxis can be stopped within 24 hours after the surgery. There are no data to support the continuation of antimicrobial prophylaxis until all indwelling drains and intravascular catheters are removed.[6]

TABLE 110–5 Recommended doses and redosing intervals for commonly used antimicrobials for surgical prophylaxis.[6]

Antimicrobial	Recommended Doses		Half-Life in Adults with Normal Renal Function (h)	Recommended Redosing Interval (h)
	Adult	Pediatrics		
Ampicillin-sulbactam	3 g (ampicillin 2 g/sulbactam 1 g)	50 mg/kg of the ampicillin component	0.8-1.3	2
Ampicillin	2 g	50 mg/kg	1-1.9	2
Aztreonam	2 g	30 mg/kg	1.3-2.4	4
Cefazolin	2 g (3 g for patients with body weight (BW) > 120 kg)	30 mg/kg	1.2-2.2	4
Cefuroxime	1.5 g	50 mg/kg	1-2	4
Cefotaxime	1 g	50 mg/kg	0.9-1.7	3
Cefoxitin	2 g	40 mg/kg	0.7-1.1	2
Cefotetan	2 g	40 mg/kg	2.8-4.6	6
Ceftriaxone	2 g	50-75 mg/kg	5.4-10.9	NA
Ciprofloxacin	400 mg	10 mg/kg	3-7	NA
Clindamycin	900 mg	10 mg/kg	2-4	6
Ertapenem	1 g	15 mg/kg	3-5	NA

(Continued)

TABLE 110–5 Recommended doses and redosing intervals for commonly used antimicrobials for surgical prophylaxis.[6] (*Continued*)

Antimicrobial	Recommended Doses		Half-Life in Adults with Normal Renal Function (h)	Recommended Redosing Interval (h)
	Adult	Pediatrics		
Fluconazole	400 mg	6 mg/kg	30	NA
Gentamycin	5 mg/kg (dosing weight, single dose)	2.5 mg/kg	2-3	NA
Levofloxacin	500 mg	10 mg/kg	6-8	NA
Metronidazole	500 mg	15 mg/kg	6-8	NA
Moxifloxacin	400 mg	10 mg/kg	8-15	NA
Piperacillin-tazobactam	3.375 g	Infants 2-9 mo: 80 mg/kg of the piperacillin component Children > 9 mo and < 40 kg: 100 mg/kg of the piperacillin component	0.7-1.2	2
Vancomycin	15 mg/kg	15 mg/kg	4-8	NA

Reproduced with permission from Bratzler DW1, Dellinger EP, Olsen KM, et al: Clinical practice guidelines for antimicrobial prophylaxis in surgery, *Am J Health Syst Pharm* 2013 Feb 1;70(3):195-283.

REFERENCES

1. April 2013 CDC/NHSN Protocol Corrections, Clarification, and Additions. http://www.cdc.gov/nhsn/PDFs/pscManual/9pscSSIcurrent.pdf. Accessed March 6, 2015.
2. Magill SS, Edwards JR, Bamberg W, et al. Multistate point-prevalence survey of health care-associated infections. *N Engl J Med.* 2014;370:1198-1208.
3. Yi M, Edwards JR, Horan TC, et al. Improving risk-adjusted measures of surgical site information for the National Healthcare Safety Network. *Infect Control Hosp Epidemiol.* 2011;2(10):970-986.
4. Bratzler DW, Hunt DR. The surgical infection prevention and surgical care improvement projects: national initiatives to improve outcomes for patients having surgery. *Clin Infect Dis.* 2006;43:322.
5. Culver DH, Horan TC, Gaynes RP, et al. Surgical wound infection rates by wound class, operative procedure, and patient risk index. National Nosocomial Infections Surveillance System. *Am J Med.* 1991;91:152S.
6. Bratzler DW, Dellinger EP, Olsen KM, Perl TM, Weinstein RA. Clinical practice guidelines for antimicrobial prophylaxis in surgery. *Am J Health-Syst Pharm.* 2013;70:195-283.
7. Weigelt JA, Lipsky BA, Tabak YP, et al. Surgical site infections: causative pathogens and associated outcomes. *Am J Infect Control.* 2010;38:112.
8. Antimicrobial prophylaxis for surgery. *Treat Guidel Med Lett.* 2012;10:73-78.
9. Bratzler DW, Houck PM, for the Surgical Infection Prevention Guidelines Writers Workgroup. Antimicrobial prophylaxis for surgery: an advisory statement from the national surgical infection prevention project. *Clin Infect Dis.* 2004;38:1706-1715.
10. Galandiuk S, Polk HC, Jr, Jagelman DG, et al. Re-emphasis of priorities in surgical antibiotic prophylaxis. *Surg Gynecol Obstet.* 1989;169:218-222.
11. Classen DC, Evans RS, Pestotnik SL, Horn SD, Menlove RL, Burke JP. The timing of prophylactic administration of antibiotics and the risk of surgical-wound infection. *N Eng J Med.* 1992;326:281-286.
12. van Kasteren ME, Manniën J, Ott A, et al. Antibiotic prophylaxis and the risk of surgical site infections following total hip arthroplasty: timely administration is the most important factor. *Clin Infect Dis.* 2007;44:921.
13. Steinberg JP, Braun BI, Hellinger WC, et al. Timing of antimicrobial prophylaxis and the risk of surgical

site infection: results from the Trial to Reduce Antimicrobial Prophylaxis Errors. *Ann Surg.* 2009;250:10-16.

14. Weber WP, Marti WR, Zwahlen M, et al. The timing of surgical antimicrobial prophylaxis. *Ann Surg.* 2008;247:918-926.

15. McDonald M, Grabsch E, Marshall C, Forbes A. Single-versus multiple-dose antimicrobial prophylaxis for major surgery: a systematic review. *Aust N Z J Surg.* 1998;68:388.

16. Harbarth S, Samore MH, Lichtenberg D, Carmeli Y. Prolonged antibiotic prophylaxis after cardiovascular surgery and its effect on surgical site infections and antimicrobial resistance. *Circulation.* 2000;101:2916.

Units and Conversions

Jun Makino, MD and
John M. Oropello, MD, FACP, FCCP, FCCM

111

INTRODUCTION

The International System of Units (abbreviated SI from the French phrase, Système International d'Unités), or SI, is the standard system of measurement.

Metric Prefixes

Prefix	Symbol	10^n
exa	E	10^{18}
peta	P	10^{15}
tera	T	10^{12}
giga	G	10^9
mega	M	10^6
kilo	k	10^3
hecto	h	10^2
deca	da	10^1
		10^0
deci	d	10^{-1}
centi	c	10^{-2}
milli	m	10^{-3}
micro	μ	10^{-6}
nano	n	10^{-9}
pico	p	10^{-12}
femto	f	10^{-15}
atto	a	10^{-18}

Length

Symbol	Known Quantity	Multiply	Metric Symbol	Known Quantity
in	inches	2.54	cm	centimeters
ft	feet	30	cm	centimeters
ft	feet	0.3	m	meters
yd	yards	0.9	m	meters
—	miles	1.6	km	kilometers

Area

Symbol	Known Quantity	Multiply	Metric Symbol	Known Quantity
sq in	square inches	6.5	cm^2	square centimeters
sq ft	square feet	0.09	m^2	square meters
sq yd	square yard	0.8	m^2	square meters
—	square miles	2.6	km^2	square kilometers

Volume

Symbol	Known Quantity	Multiply	Metric Symbol	Known Quantity
tsp	teaspoons	5	mL	milliliters
tbssp	tablespoons	15	mL	milliliters
fl oz	fluid ounces	30	mL	milliliters
c	cups	0.24	L	liters
pt	US pints	0.47	L	liters
qt	US quarts	0.95	L	liters
gal	US gallons	3.8	L	liters
cu ft	cubic feet	0.03	m³	cubic meters
cu yd	cubic yard	0.76	m³	cubic meters

Mass

Symbol	Known Quantity	Multiply	Metric Symbol	Known Quantity
oz	ounces	28	g	grams
lb	pounds	0.45	kg	kilograms

Pressure or Mechanical Stress

Symbol	Known Quantity	Multiply	Metric Symbol	Known Quantity
cm H_2O[a]	centimeter of water (4°C)	0.01	Pa	Pascal
mm Hg	millimeter of mercury (0°C)	7.5006	kPa	kilopascal
mm Hg	millimeter of mercury (0°C)	1.36	cm H_2O	centimeter of water (4°C)

[a]In clinical practice arterial blood pressure is still measured in mm Hg, cerebrospinal fluid pressure in mm H_2O, and blood gases (P_{CO_2} and P_{O_2}) in mm Hg.

Temperature[a]

Symbol	Known Quantity	Calculation	Metric Symbol	Known Quantity
°F	degree Fahrenheit	([°F] – 32)/1.8	°C	degree Celsius
°C	degree Celsius	[°C] + 273.15	K	Kelvin
°F	degree Fahrenheit	([°F] + 459.67) × 5/9	K	Kelvin

[a]Temperature is normally expressed in degrees Celsius (°C), although the SI base unit for temperature is the Kelvin.

Energy[a]

Symbol	Known Quantity	Multiply	Metric Symbol	Known Quantity
Kcal	kilocalories	4.184	kJ	kilojoules

[a]The kilocalorie (kcal) is still most commonly used to express the energy content of macronutrients, energy expenditure, and energy requirements, although kilojoules (kJ) is the SI unit.

Common Laboratories

Analyte	Specimen	Conventional Unit (Reference Range)	Conversion Factor (Multiply)	SI Unit (Reference Range)
Albumin	Serum	g/dL (3.5-5.0)	10	g/L (35-50)
Alkaline Phosphatase	Serum	U/L (30-120)	0.0167	µkat/L (0.5-2.0)
Alanine aminotransferase (ALT)	Serum	U/L (10-40)	0.0167	µkat/L (0.17-0.68)
Aspartate aminotransferase (AST)	Serum	U/L (10-30)	0.0167	µkat/L (0.17-0.51)
Bicarbonate	Serum	mEq/L (21-28)	1	mmol/L (21-28)
Bilirubin, total	Serum	mg/dL (0.3-1.2)	17.104	µmol/L (5.0-21.0)
Bilirubin, direct	Serum	mg/dL (0.1-0.3)	17.104	µmol/L (1.7-5.1)
Blood urea nitrogen (BUN)	Serum	mg/dL (8-23)	0.357	mmol/L (2.9-8.2)
Carbon dioxide P_{CO_2}	Arterial blood	mmHg (35-45)	0.133	kPa (4.7-5.9)
Oxygen, P_{O_2}	Arterial blood	mmHg (80-100)	0.133	kPa (11-13)
Calcium, total	Serum	mg/dL (8.2-10.2)	0.25	mmol/L (2.05-2.55)
Chloride	Serum, plasma	mEq/L (96-106)	1	mmol/L (96-106)
Cholesterol (total)	Serum, plasma	mg/dL (< 200)	0.0259	mmol/L (< 5.18)
Cortisol	Serum, plasma	µg/dL (5-25)	27.588	nmol/L (140-690)
Creatinine	Serum, plasma	mg/dL (0.6-1.2)	88.4	µmol/L (53-106)
Glutaminyl-transferase (GGT)	Serum	U/L (2-30)	0.0167	µkat/L (0.03-0.51)
Glucose	Serum	mg/dL (70-110)	0.0555	mmol/L (3.9-6.1)
Lactate	Plasma	mg/dL (5.0-15)	0.111	mmol/L (0.6-1.7)
Lactate dehydrogenase (LDH)	Serum	U/L (100-200)	0.0167	µkat/L (1.7-3.4)
Magnesium	Serum	mEq/L (1.3-2.1)	0.5	mmol/L (0.65-1.05)
Phosphorus (inorganic)	Serum	mg/dL (2.3-4.7)	0.323	mmol/L (0.74-1.52)
Potassium	Serum	mEq/L (3.5-5.0)	1	mmol/L (3.5-5.0)
Protein (total)	Serum	g/dL (6.0-8.0)	10	g/L (60-80)
Sodium	Serum	mEq/L (136-142)	1	mmol/L (136-142)
Uric acid	Serum	mg/dL (4.0-8.0)	59.485	µmol/L (240-480)

Medication Dosing During Renal Replacement Therapy

112

Jun Makino, MD and John M. Oropello, MD, FACP, FCCP, FCCM

INTRODUCTION

The aim of drug dosing is to maintain pharmacokinetics (a similar peak, trough, or average steady-state drug concentration) to achieve a desired pharmacodynamic response without adverse side effects.[1] In critically ill patients receiving renal replacement therapy (RRT), however, determining appropriate drug dosing is challenging because pharmacodynamic target attainment is determined by a complex interplay between drug dosing, pharmacokinetic changes within the critically ill patient, and the type of RRT selected (Table 112–1).[2] A stepwise approach for patients with chronic kidney disease and acute kidney injury has been proposed (Table 112–2).[3] For assessment of kidney function, estimation by equation is generally more accurate than measured creatinine clearance, given errors in urine collection.[4] Therefore, the National Kidney Disease Education Program in the United States recommends estimation of the glomerular filtration rate from the Cockcroft and Gault equation for adults: urinary creatinine clearance = (140 – age [years]) × weight (kg) × 0.85 (for female)/serum creatinine (mg/dL) × 72 or the Schwartz equation for children.[5,6]

Table 112–3 contains guidelines by the American College of Physicians for drug dosing in renal failure requiring RRT.[7] There are a variety of RRTs including hemodialysis, continuous RRT, and peritoneal dialysis. When applying these or other guidelines it should be understood that dosing recommendations for one form of RRT usually cannot be applied to other forms of RRT.[8] Dialysis filter type, surface area; the blood, dialysate, and ultrafiltration rates; and interruptions due to circuit clotting influence drug clearance and affect drug dosing.

Drug dosing studies in renal failure have not been conducted in most marketed drugs.[8,9] In addition, the evidence level is weak as most of these studies are small and also the dose of RRT is not uniform. Finally, technological advances in RRT over the last several years have resulted in greater drug clearances; consequently, drug dosing recommendations may be outdated. Therefore, the most effective dosing optimization strategy is to estimate renal function and begin dosing according to the guidelines, followed by closely monitoring drug levels (if possible) or the clinical response, and adjusting the dosing accordingly (Table 112–2).

Table 112–1 Factors to alter pharmacodynamics of critically ill patients.[2]

TABLE 112-1 Factors to alter pharmacodynamics of critically ill patients.[2]

Factors	Pharmacokinetic Change	Response to Change
Fluid overload	Increased volume of distribution	Give a larger loading dose
Increased capillary permeability	Increased volume of distribution	Give a larger loading dose
Hypoalbuminemia	Increased drug availability to exert pharmacologic effect or increased drug elimination	Potential dosage adjustment for highly protein-bound drugs
Augmented renal clearance	Increased drug elimination	More frequent dosing interval
AKI	Decreased drug elimination	Adjust doses on drugs eliminated by the kidney
AKI requiring RRT	Increased drug elimination	Dose adjust as RRT modality chosen
Preserved nonrenal clearance in AKI	Preserved drug elimination in face of AKI in selected drugs	More frequent dosing interval
Increased cardiac output	Increased drug elimination	More frequent dosing interval
Impaired GI motility/reduced GI blood flow	Decreased oral drug absorption	Avoid oral medication

AKI, acute kidney injury; GI, gastrointestinal; RRT, renal replacement therapy.
Reproduced with permission from Scoville BA, Mueller BA: Medication dosing in critically ill patients with acute kidney injury treated with renal replacement therapy, *Am J Kidney Dis*. 2013 Mar;61(3):490-500.

TABLE 112-2 Stepwise approach to adjust drug dosage regimens for patients with CKD and AKI.[3]

Step1	Obtain history and relevant demographic/clinical information	Assess demographic information, past medical history, current clinical, and laboratory data.
Step 2	Estimate GFR	Use most appropriate tools based on age, body size, ethnicity, and concomitant disease status.
Step 3	Review current medications	Is it really necessary or not?
Step 4	Calculate individualized treatment regimen	Calculate dosage regimen based on pharmacokinetic characteristics of the drug and the patient's volume status and eGFR or CLcr.
Step 5	Monitor	Monitor parameters of drug response and toxicity; monitor levels if available/applicable.
Step 6	Revise regimen	Adjust regimen based on step 5.

AKI, acute kidney injury; CKD, chronic kidney disease; CLcr, urinary creatinine clearance; eGFR, estimated glomerular filtration rate; GFR, glomerular filtration rate.
Reproduced with permission from Matzke GR, Aronoff GR, Murray P, et al. Drug dosing consideration in patients with acute and chronic kidney disease—a clinical update from kidney disease: improving global outcomes (KDIGO), *Kidney Int* 2011 Dec;80(11):1122-1137.

TABLE 112-3 Drug dosing in patients treated with RRT.

Drug	Major Excretion Route (percentage of total drug excreted unchanged in the urine for patients with normal renal function)	Dose for Normal Renal Function	Adjustment for Renal Failure GFR > 50	Adjustment for Renal Failure GFR 10-50	Adjustment for Renal Failure GFR < 10	Supplement for Dialysis
Analgesics						
Codeine	Hepatic	30-60 mg q4-6	100% [D]	75% [D]	50% [D]	Intermittent Hemodialysis (IHD): No data PD: No data CRRT: Dose for GFR 10-50 [D]
Fentanyl	Hepatic	Individualized	100% [D]	75% [D]	50% [D]	IHD: Not applicable Peritoneal Dialysis (PD): Not applicable CRRT: Dose for GFR 10-50 [B]
Meperidine	Hepatic	50-100 mg q3-4h	100% [D]	75% [D]	50% [D]	IHD: Avoid PD: Avoid CRRT: Avoid [D]
Methadone	Hepatic	2.5-10 mg q6-8h	100% [D]	100% [D]	50%-75% [D]	IHD: None PD: None CRRT: Dose for GFR: 10-50 [D]
Morphine	Hepatic	20-25 mg q4h	100% [A]	75% [A]	50% [A]	IHD: None PD: None CRRT: Dose for GFR 10-50 [D]
Naloxone	Hepatic	2 mg IV	100% [D]	100% [D]	100% [D]	IHD: Not applicable PD: Not applicable CRRT: Dose for GFR: 10-50 [D]
Acetaminophen	Hepatic	650 mg q4h	q4h [D]	q6h [D]	q8h [D]	IHD: None PD: None CRRT: Dose for GFR: 10-50 [B]
Aspirin	Hepatic	650 mg q4h	q4h [B]	q4-6h [B]	Avoid [B]	IHD: Dose after dialysis PD: None CRRT: Dose for GFR: 10-50 [D]
Antihypertensive and Cardiovascular Agents						
Clonidine	62	0.1-0.6 mg bid	q12h [B]	q12-24h [B]	q24h [B]	IHD: Dose after dialysis [B] PD: Dose for GFR < 10 [B] CRRT: Dose for GFR 10-50 [D]
Methyldopa	25-40	250-500 mg q8	q8h [B]	q8-12h [B]	q12-24h [B]	IHD: Dose after dialysis [D] PD: Dose for GFR < 10 [D] CRRT: Dose for GFR 10-50 [D]
Prazosin	< 5	1-15 mg bid-tid	100% [A]	100% [D]	100% [D]	IHD: None PD: None [D] CRRT: Not applicable

(Continued)

TABLE 112–3 Drug dosing in patients treated with RRT. *(Continued)*

Drug	Major Excretion Route (percentage of total drug excreted unchanged in the urine for patients with normal renal function)	Dose for Normal Renal Function	Adjustment for Renal Failure GFR >50	Adjustment for Renal Failure GFR 10-50	Adjustment for Renal Failure GFR <10	Supplement for Dialysis
Terazosin	20-30	1 mg hs Second dose: 1-20 mg q24h	100% [A]	100% [A]	100% [A]	IHD: None [D] PD: None [D] CRRT: Not applicable
Candesartan	52	16-32 mg q24	100% [A]	100% [A]	100% [A]	IHD: No dose adjustment [A] PD: No dose adjustment [A] CRRT: Dose for GFR 10-50 [D]
Irbesartan	< 5	150-300 mg q24	100% [A]	100% [A]	100% [A]	IHD: No dose adjustment [A] PD: No dose adjustment [D] CRRT: Dose for GFR 10-50 [D]
Losartan	4-10	25-100 mg q24	100% [A]	100% [A]	100% [A]	IHD: None [A] PD: None [A] CRRT: Dose for GFR 10-50 [D]
Valsartan	13	80-320 mg q24h	100% [B]	100% [B]	100% [D]	IHD: None [A] PD: None [D] CRRT: Dose for GFR 10-50 [D]
Benazepril	54	10 mg q24h Second dose: 10-40 mg q12-24h	100% [A]	50%-75% [A]	25%-50% [D]	IHD: None [D] PD: None [D] CRRT: Dose for GFR 10-50 [D]
Captopril	40-50	25-50 mg q8h Second dose: 50-150 mg q8-12h	100% q8-12h [A]	75% q12-18h [A]	50% q24h [A]	IHD: Dose after dialysis [A] PD: Dose for GFR 10-50 [A] CRRT: Dose for GFR 10-50 [D]
Enalapril	88	5-20 mg q12-24h	100% [A]	50%-100% [A]	25% [A]	IHD: Dose after dialysis [A] PD: Dose for GFR < 10 [D] CRRT: Dose for GFR 10-50 [D]
Enalaprilat	88	1.25-5 mg IV over 5 min q6h	100% [A]	50%-100% [A]	25%-50% [D]	IHD: Dose after dialysis [A] PD: Dose for GFR < 10 [D] CRRT: Dose for GFR 10-50 [D]
Lisinopril	88-100	5-10 mg q24h Second dose: 20-40 mg q24h	100% [A]	50%-75% [A]	25%-50% [A]	IHD: Dose after dialysis [A] PD: None [D] CRRT: Dose for GFR 10-50 [D]

Drug		Dose	GFR >50	GFR 10–50	GFR <10	Dialysis
Ramipril	35	2.5 mg q24h Second dose: 5–10 mg q24h	100% [A]	25%–50% [A]	25% [A]	IHD: Dose after dialysis [A] PD: Dose for GFR < 10 [D] CRRT: Dose for GFR 10-50 [D]
Atenolol	85	50–100 mg q24h	50–100 mg q24h [A]	25–50 mg q24h [A]	25 mg q24h [A]	IHD: 25–50 mg after dialysis [A] PD: Dose for GFR < 10 [A] CRRT: Dose for GFR 10-50 [D]
Carvedilol	<2	3.125–6.25 mg q12–24h Second dose: 6.25–25 mg q12–24h	100% [A]	100% [A]	100% [A]	IHD: None [A] PD: None [D] CRRT: Dose for GFR 10-50 [D]
Esmolol	<10	0.5 mg/kg infused over 1 min Second dose: 0.05 mg mg/kg/min for the next 4 min	100% [A]	100% [A]	100% [A]	IHD: None [A] PD: None [A] CRRT: Dose for GFR 10-50 [D]
Labetalol	<5	100 mg bid Second dose: 200–400 mg bid	100% [A]	100% [A]	100% [A]	IHD: None [A] PD: None [A] CRRT: Dose for GFR 10-50 [D]
Metoprolol	8–13	50–400 mg q24h	100% [A]	100% [A]	100% [A]	IHD: None [A] PD: None [A] CRRT: Dose for GFR 10-50 [D]
Nadolol	90	40 mg q24h Second dose: 40–240 mg q24h	q24h [A]	q24–48h [A]	q40–60h [A]	IHD: Dose after dialysis [A] PD: Dose for GFR < 10 [A] CRRT: Dose for GFR 10-50 [D]
Propranolol	<5	80–160 mg bid	100% [A]	100% [A]	100% [A]	IHD: None [A] PD: None [D] CRRT: Dose for GFR 10-50 [D]
Timolol	15	10–30 mg bid	100% [A]	100% [A]	100% [A]	IHD: No dose adjustment [A] PD: No dose adjustment [D] CRRT: Dose for GFR 10-50 [D]
Hydralazine	25	25–50 mg tid	q8h [A]	q8h [A]	q8h [A]	IHD: Dose after dialysis [D] PD: Dose for GFR < 10 [D] CRRT: Dose for GFR 10-50 [D]
Minoxidil	15–20	5–30 mg bid	100% [A]	100% [A]	100% [A]	IHD: Dose after dialysis [D] PD: Dose for GFR < 10 [D] CRRT: Dose for GFR 10-50 [D]

(Continued)

TABLE 112-3 Drug dosing in patients treated with RRT. (*Continued*)

Drug	Major Excretion Route (percentage of total drug excreted unchanged in the urine for patients with normal renal function)	Dose for Normal Renal Function	Adjustment for Renal Failure GFR > 50	Adjustment for Renal Failure GFR 10-50	Adjustment for Renal Failure GFR < 10	Supplement for Dialysis
Nitroprusside	< 10	0.25-8 mcg/kg/min Second dose: by infusion	100% [A]	100% [A]	Avoid [D]	IHD: Avoid [D] PD: Avoid [D] CRRT: Dose for GFR 10-50 [D]
Procainamide	80	500 mg q6-8h	100% q6-8h [A]	50% q8-12h [A]	25% q12-18h [A]	IHD: None CRRT: Dose for GFR 10-50 [D]
Adenosine	< 5	3-6 mg IV bolus	100% [D]	100% [D]	100% [D]	IHD: None PD: None CRRT: Dose for GFR 10-50 [D]
Amiodarone	< 5	800-2000 mg load, then 200-600 mg q24h	100% [A]	100% [A]	100% [A]	IHD None PD: None CRRT: Dose for GFR 10-50 [D]
Bretylium	75	5-30 mg/kg load, then 5-10 mg IV q6h	100% [A]	25%-50% [A]	25% [A]	IHD: None PD: None CRRT: Dose for GFR 10-50 [D]
Disopyramide	35-65	100-200 mg q6h	q8h [A]	q12-24h [A]	q24-48h [A]	IHD: None PD: None CRRT: Dose for GFR 10-50 [D]
Flecainide	43	50-100 mg q12h	100% [A]	50% [A]	50% [A]	IHD: None PD: None CRRT: Dose for GFR 10-50 [D]
Lidocaine	10	50 mg over 2 min, repeat q5 min ×3 Second dose: 1-4 mg/min	100% [D]	100% [D]	100% [D]	IHD: None PD: None CRRT: Dose for GFR 10-50 [B]
Procainamide	59-75	1000-2500 mg q12h	q4h [A]	q6-12h [A]	q8-24h [A]	IHD: Follow levels [A] PD: None [A] CRRT: Dose for GFR 10-50, monitor serum concentration [D]
Propafenone	< 1	150 mg q8h Second dose: 150-300 mg q8h	100% [A]	100% [A]	100% [A]	IHD: None [A] PD: None [A] CRRT: Dose for GFR 10-50 [D]

Quinidine	20	300-600 mg q8-12h	100% [A]	100% [A]	100% [A]	IHD: Dose after dialysis [D] PD: None [D] CRRT: Dose for GFR 10-50, monitor serum concentration [D]
Sotalol	80-90	80 mg q12h Second dose: 120-160 mg q12h	q12h [A]	q24-48h [A]	q48-72h [A]	IHD: Dose after dialysis [D] PD: None [D] CRRT: Dose for GFR 10-50 [D]
Amlodipine	<10	2.5-10 mg q24h	100% [A]	100% [D]	100% [D]	IHD: None [D] PD: None [D] CRRT: Dose for GFR 10-50 [D]
Diltiazem	<5	180-240 mg q24h Second dose: 180-240 mg q24h	100% [A]	100% [A]	100% [A]	IHD: None [A] PD: None [A] CRRT: Dose for GFR 10-50 [D]
Nicardipine	<1	20-40 mg po tid	100% [D]	100% [D]	100% [D]	IHD: None [D] PD: None [D] CRRT: Dose for GFR 10-50 [D]
Nifedipine	<5	10-30 mg q8h	100% [A]	100% [A]	100% [A]	IHD: No dose adjustment [A] PD: No dose adjustment [A] CRRT: Dose for GFR 10-50 [D]
Nimodipine	<10	30 mg q8h	100% [D]	100% [D]	100% [D]	IHD: None PD: None CRRT: Dose for GFR 10-50 [D]
Verapamil	<3	180-480 mg q24h	100% [A]	100% [A]	100% [A]	IHD: None [A] PD: None [A] CRRT: Dose for GFR 10-50 [B]
Digoxin	76-85	1.0-1.5 mg load, then 0.25-0.5 mg q24h	100% q24h [A]	25%-75% q36h [A]	10%-25% q48h [A]	IHD: None PD: None CRRT: Dose for GFR 10-50, monitor serum concentration [D]
Acetazolamide	100	250 mg q6-12h	q6h [A]	q12h [A]	Avoid [A]	IHD: No data PD: No data CRRT: Dose for GFR 10-50 [D]
Furosemide	50-80	20-300 mg q12-24h	100% [A]	100% [A]	100% [A]	IHD: None [A] PD: None [A] CRRT: Not applicable [D]
Hydrochlorothiazide	90	6.25-200 mg q24h	100% [A]	100% [A]	Ineffective [A]	IHD: Not applicable [D] PD: Not applicable [D] CRRT: Not applicable [D]
Metolazone	70	5-20 mg q24h	100% [A]	100% [D]	100% [D]	IHD: None [D] PD: None [D] CRRT: Not applicable [D]

(Continued)

TABLE 112–3 Drug dosing in patients treated with RRT. *(Continued)*

Drug	Major Excretion Route (percentage of total drug excreted unchanged in the urine for patients with normal renal function)	Dose for Normal Renal Function	Adjustment for Renal Failure GFR >50	Adjustment for Renal Failure GFR 10-50	Adjustment for Renal Failure GFR <10	Supplement for Dialysis
Spironolactone	20-30	25 mg tid-qid	q6-12h [D]	q12-24h [D]	Avoid [D]	IHD: Not applicable PD: Not applicable CRRT: Avoid [D]
Dobutamine	<10	2.5 mcg/kg/min	100% [D]	100% [D]	100% [D]	IHD: No data PD: No data CRRT: Dose for GFR 10-50 [D]
Midodrine	75-80	No data	5-10 mg q8h [D]	5-10 mg q8h [D]	No data [D]	IHD: 5 mg q8h PD: No data CRRT: Dose for GFR 10-50 [D]
Milrinone	80-85	15-75 mcg/kg IV load, then 2.5-15 mg po q6h	100% [A]	100% [A]	50%-75% [A]	IHD: No data PD: No data CRRT: Dose for GFR 10-50 [D]
Isosorbide dinitrate	<1	2.5-5 mg 15 min before activity	100% [A]	100% [A]	100% [A]	IHD: None [A] PD: None [D] CRRT: Dose for GFR 10-50 [D]
Isosorbide mononitrate	<5	30-60 mg q24h Second dose: 60-240 mg q24h	100% [D]	100% [D]	100% [D]	IHD: Dose after dialysis [D] PD: None [D] CRRT: Dose for GFR 10-50 [D]
Nitroglycerine	<1	Many routes and methods	100% [D]	100% [D]	100% [D]	IHD: No data PD: No data CRRT: Dose for GFR 10-50 [D]
Antimicrobials						
Amikacin	95	7.5 mg/kg q12h or 15 mg/kg qd	100% q12or 24h [B]	100% q24-72h by levels [B]	100% q48-72h by levels [B]	IHD: 1/2 full dose after dialysis PD: 15-20 mg/L/d CRRT: Dose for GFR 10-50, monitor levels [B]
Gentamycin	95	1.7 mg/kg q8h or 5-7 mg/kg/qd	100% q8-24h [A]	100% q12-48h by levels [A]	100% q48-72h by levels [A]	IHD: 1/2 full dose after dialysis PD: 3-4 mg/L/d CRRT: Dose for GFR 10-50, monitor levels [A]
Kanamycin	50-90	7.5 mg/kg q12h	100% q12 or 24h [D]	100% q24-72h by levels [D]	100% q48-72h by levels [D]	IHD: 1/2 full dose after dialysis PD: 15-20 mg/L/d CRRT: Dose for GFR 10-50, monitor levels [D]

Drug	%	Dose for normal renal function	>50	10-50	<10	Dialysis
Streptomycin	70	1-2 g q6-12h (1.0 g q24h for tuberculosis)	q24h [D]	q24-72h [D]	q72-96h [D]	IHD: 1/2 full dose after dialysis PD: 20-40 mg/L/d CRRT: Dose for GFR 10-50, monitor levels [D]
Tobramycin	95	1.7 mg/kg q8h or 5-7 mg/kg qd	100% q8-24h [A]	100% q24-48h by levels [A]	100% q48-72h by levels [A]	IHD: 1/2 full dose after dialysis PD: 3-4 mg/L/d CRRT: Dose for GFR 10-50, monitor levels [B]
Cefaclor	70	250-500 mg q8	100% [B]	100% [B]	100% [B]	IHD: 250-500 mg after dialysis [B] PD: 250-500 mg q8h CRRT: Not applicable
Cefazolin	75-95	0.25-2 g q6h	100% q8h [A]	100% q12h [A]	50% q24-48h [A]	IHD: 15-20 mg/kg after dialysis PD: 0.5 g q12 CRRT: Doses for GFR 10-50 [D]
Cefepime	85	250-2000 mg q8-12h	100% [A]	50%-100% q24h [A]	25%-50% q24h [A]	IHD: Doses for GFR < 10 PD: Doses for GFR < 10 CRRT: 1-2 g q12h [A]
Cefotaxime	60	1-2 g q6-12h	q6h [A]	q6-12h [A]	q24h or 1/2 dose [A]	IHD: 0.5-2 g after dialysis PD: 1 g/d CRRT: 1 g q12h [B]
Cefotetan	75	1-2 g q12h	100% [A]	1-2 g q24h [A]	1-2 g q48h [A]	IHD: 1 g after dialysis PD: 1 g/d CRRT: Doses for GFR 10-50 [B]
Cefoxitin	80	1-2 g q6-8h	q6-8h [A]	q8-12h [A]	q24-48h [A]	IHD: 1 g after dialysis PD: 1 g/d CRRT: Doses for GFR 10-50 [D]
Ceftazidime	60-85	1-2 g q8h	q8-12h [A]	q12-24h [A]	q24-48h [A]	IHD: 1 g after dialysis PD: 0.5 g/d CRRT: 1-2 g q12 or 2 g load followed by 3 g/d continuous infusion [A]
Ceftriaxone	30-65	0.25-2 g q12-24h	100% [A]	100% [A]	100% [A]	IHD: None PD: 1 g q12 CRRT: Doses for GFR 10-50 [A]
Cefuroxime Axetil	90	250-500 mg q12	100% [A]	100% [A]	100% [A]	IHD: Dose after dialysis PD: None CRRT: Not applicable
Cephalexin	90	250-500 mg q6h	q6-8h [A]	q8-12h [A]	q12-24h [A]	IHD: Dose after dialysis PD: Dose for GFR < 10 CRRT: Not applicable
Azithromycin	6-12	250-500 mg q24h	100% [A]	100% [A]	100% [A]	IHD: None PD: None CRRT: Dose for GFR 10-50 [A]
Clarithromycin	20-30	250-500 mg q12h Second dose: 1 g q24h	100% [D]	50%-100% [D]	50% [D]	IHD: No data, Dose after dialysis PD: None CRRT: Dose for GFR 10-50 [D]

(Continued)

TABLE 112–3 Drug dosing in patients treated with RRT. (Continued)

Drug	Major Excretion Route (percentage of total drug excreted unchanged in the urine for patients with normal renal function)	Dose for Normal Renal Function	Adjustment for Renal Failure GFR > 50	Adjustment for Renal Failure GFR 10-50	Adjustment for Renal Failure GFR <10	Supplement for Dialysis
Erythromycin	15	250-500 mg q6h	100% [A]	100% [A]	100% [A]	IHD: None PD: None CRRT: Dose for GFR 10-50 [D]
Aztreonam	75	500 mg-2 g q8-12h	100% [A]	50% [A]	25% [A]	IHD: 0.5 g after dialysis PD: Dose for GFR < 10 CRRT: 1000 mg q12h [D]
Chloramphenicol	10	12.5 mg/kg q6h	100% [D]	100% [D]	100% [D]	IHD: None PD: None CRRT: Dose for GFR 10-50 [D]
Clindamycin	10	150-450 mg q6h	100% [D]	100% [D]	100% [D]	IHD: None PD: None CRRT: Dose for GFR 10-50 [D]
Dapsone	5-20	50-100 mg q24h (for malaria prophylaxis once weekly)	No data 100% [D]	No data [D]	No data [D]	IHD: No data, None PD: No data, Dose for GFR < 10 CRRT: Dose for GFR 10-50 [D]
Daptomycin	78	4 mg/kg q24h	100% [D]	100% q24-48h [D]	100% q48h [D]	IHD: Dose for GFR < 10 [D] PD: Dose for GFR < 10 [D] CRRT: 8 mg/kg q48h [C]
Ertapenem	38	1 g q24h	100% [D]	100% [D]	50% [D]	IHD: 500 mg qd for GFR < 30, supplemental 150 mg after dialysis if daily dose given less than 6 g before start of dialysis [B] PD: Dose for GFR < 10 [D] CRRT: 100%, no adjustment needed unless GFR < 30 [B]
Imipenem	20-70	0.25-1 g q6h	100% [A]	50% [A]	25% [A]	IHD: Dose after dialysis PD: Dose for GFR < 10 CRRT: 500 mg q6h [A]
Linezolid	30	600 mg q12h	100% [B]	100% [B]	100% [B]	IHD: No dose adjustment [B] PD: No dose adjustment [B] CRRT: 600 mg q12h [A]
Meropenem	65	1-2 g q8h	100% [D]	100% q12h [D]	100% q24h [D]	IHD: Dose after dialysis PD: Dose for GFR < 10 CRRT: 1-2 g q12h [A]
Metronidazole	20	250-500 mg q8-12h	100% [A]	100% [A]	100% [A]	IHD: Dose after dialysis PD: Dose for GFR < 10 CRRT: Dose for GFR 10-50 [B]

Drug		Dose				Dialysis
Nitrofurantoin	30-40	50-100 mg q6h	Avoid < 60 [D]	Avoid [D]	Avoid [D]	IHD: Not applicable PD: Not applicable CRRT: Avoid
Quinupristin/Dalfopristin	Quinupristin 5% Dalfopristin 0%	7.5 mg/kg q8h	100% [B]	100% [B]	100% [B]	IHD: No dose adjustment [D] PD: No dose adjustment [B] CRRT: Dose for GFR 10-50 [C]
Rifaximin	0.023	200 mg pot id	200 mg pot id [D]	100% [D]	100% [D]	IHD: – PD: – CRRT: Has not been studied in renally impaired patients [D]
Sulfamethoxazole	70	1 g q8h	q12h [D]	q18h [D]	q24h [D]	IHD: 1 g after dialysis PD: 1 g/d CRRT: 2.5-5 mg/kg q12h for mild/moderate infections, 10 mg/kg q12 for severe infection [B]
Trimethoprim	60-80	100 mg q12h	q12h [D]	q12h for GFR > 30, q18h for GFR 10-30 [D]	q24h [D]	IHD: Dose after dialysis PD: Dose for GFR < 10 CRRT: 2.5-5 mg/kg q12h for mild/moderate infections, 10 mg/kg q12h for severe infection [D]
Vancomycin	90-100	500 mg-1.25 g q12h	1 g q12-24h [A]	1 g q24-96h [A]	1 g q4-7d [A]	IHD: Dose for GFR < 10 PD: Dose for GFR < 10 CRRT: Dose for GFR 10-50 [A]
Amoxicillin	50-70	250-500 mg q8h	q8h [A]	q8-12h [A]	q24h [A]	IHD: Dose after dialysis PD: 250 mg q12h CRRT: Not applicable
Ampicillin	30-90	250 mg-2 g q6h	q6h [A]	q6-12h [A]	q12-24h [A]	IHD: Dose after dialysis PD: 250 mg q12h CRRT: Dose for GFR 10-50
Nafcillin	35	1-2 g q4-6h	100% [D]	100% [D]	100% [D]	IHD: None PD: None CRRT: Dose for GFR 10-50 [B]
Penicillin G	60-85	0.5-4 million U q4-6h	100% [D]	75% [D]	20%-50% [D]	IHD: Dose after dialysis PD: Dose for GFR < 10 CRRT: Dose for GFR 10-50 [B]
Piperacillin	75-90	3-4 g q6h	q6h [A]	q6-12h [A]	q12h [A]	IHD: 2 g plus 1 g after dialysis PD: Dose for GFR < 10 CRRT: Dose for GFR 10-50 [A]
Piperacillin/Tazobactam	Piperacillin 60%-80% Tazobactam 10%-20%	3.375-4.5 g q6-8h	100% [B]	2.25 g q6-8h [B]	2.25 g q8h [B]	IHD: Dose for GFR < 10, 1.125 g after HD [B] PD: 4.5 g q12h [B] CRRT: 4.5 g q8h
Ciprofloxacin	50-70	500-750 mg (400 mg if IV) q12h	100% [A]	50%-75% [A]	50% [A]	IHD: 250 mg q12h (200 mg if IV) PD: 250 mg q8h (200 mg if IV) CRRT: 400 mg q24h [A]

(Continued)

TABLE 112–3 **Drug dosing in patients treated with RRT.** (*Continued*)

Drug	Major Excretion Route (percentage of total drug excreted unchanged in the urine for patients with normal renal function)	Dose for Normal Renal Function	Adjustment for Renal Failure GFR > 50	Adjustment for Renal Failure GFR 10-50	Adjustment for Renal Failure GFR < 10	Supplement for Dialysis
Gatifloxacin	70-95	400 mg q24h	100% [B]	400 mg initially, then 200 mg q24h [B]	400 mg initially, then 200 mg q24h [B]	IHD: Dose for GFR < 10 [B] PD: Dose for GFR < 10 [B] CRRT: Dose for 30-50 [D]
Levofloxacin	67-87	250-750 mg q24	100% [A]	250-750 mg q24-48h (500-750 mg initial dose) [A]	250-500 mg q48h (500 mg initial dose) [A]	IHD: Dose for GFR < 10 PD: Dose for GFR < 10 CRRT: 500 mg q48h [A]
Moxifloxacin	20	400 mg q24h	100% [B]	100% [B]	100% [B]	IHD: No data [D] PD: No data [D] CRRT: 400 mg q24h [B]
Ofloxacin	68-80	200-400 mg q12h	100% [A]	200-400 mg q24h [A]	200 mg q24h [A]	IHD: 100-200 mg after dialysis PD: Dose for GFR < 10 CRRT: 300 mg q24h [B]
Doxycycline	35-45	100 mg q12h	100% [D]	100% [D]	100% [D]	IHD: None PD: None CRRT: Dose for GFR 10-50 [B]
Minocycline	6-10	100 mg q12h	100% [D]	100% [D]	100% [D]	IHD: None PD: None CRRT: Not applicable
Tetracycline	48-60	250-500 mg bid-qid	q8-12h [D]	q12-24h [D]	q24h [D]	IHD: None PD: None CRRT: Not applicable
Amphotericin B (lipid complex)	< 1	5 mg/kg q24h	q24h [A]	q24h [A]	q24h [A]	IHD: None PD: None CRRT: Dose for GFR 10-50 [A]
Caspofungin	< 2	70 mg initial dose, then 50 mg q24h	No change [B]	No change [B]	No change [B]	IHD: No adjustment necessary [B] PD: No adjustment necessary [B] CRRT: 100% dose [D]
Fluconazole	70	100-400 mg q24h	100% [A]	50% [A]	50% [A]	IHD: 100% after dialysis PD: Dose for GFR < 10 CRRT: 200-400 mg q24h [A]
Flucytosine	90	37.5 mg/kg q6h	q12h [D]	q12-24h [D]	q24-48h [D]	IHD: Dose after dialysis PD: 0.5-1 g/d CRRT: Dose for GFR 10-50 [B]
Itraconazole	35	100 mg q12h	100% [A]	100% [A]	100% [A]	IHD: 100 mg q12-24h (oral only) PD: 100 mg q12-24h (oral only) CRRT: 100% [B]

Drug		Dose				Dialysis
Ketoconazole	13	200-400 mg q24h	100% [D]	100% [D]	100% [D]	IHD: None PD: None CRRT: 100% [D]
Voriconazole	< 2	6 mg/kg IV × 2 doses or 200 mg po q12 Second dose: 4 mg/kg IV or 200 mg po q12h	100% [B]	100% (IV not recommended) [B]	100% (IV not recommended) [D]	IHD: No adjustment necessary [B] PD: No adjustment necessary [D] CRRT: 100% [B]
Ethambutol	75-90	15-25 mg/kg q24h	q24h [A]	q24-36h [A]	q48h	IHD: Dose after dialysis PD: Dose for GFR < 10 CRRT: Dose for GFR 30-50 [D]
Isoniazid	5-30	300 mg q24h	100% [A]	100% [A]	100% [A]	IHD: Dose after dialysis PD: Dose for GFR < 10 CRRT: Dose for GFR 30-50 [D]
Pyrazinamide	1-3	15-30 mg/kg (up to 2.5 g) q24h	100% [A]	100% [A]	50%-100% [A]	IHD: 40 mg/kg 24hr before each 3×/wk dialysis [B] PD: 100% [B] CRRT: Dose for GFR 10-50 [D]
Rifabutin	5-10	300 mg q24h	100% [A]	100% [A]	100% [A]	IHD: None PD: None CRRT: 100% [B]
Rifampin	15-30	600 mg q24h	100% [D]	50%-100% [D]	50%-100% [D]	IHD: None PD: Dose for GFR < 10 CRRT: Dose for GFR 30-50 [B]
Atovaquone	< 1	750-1500 mg q12h	No data; 100% [D]	No data; 100% [D]	No data; 100% [D]	IHD: No data, None PD: No data, None CRRT: Dose for GFR 30-50 [D]
Chloroquine	40	2.5 g (for treatment; 1 g initially, then 0.5 g in 6 h, then 0.5 g daily for 2 d)	100% [D]	100% [D]	50% [D]	IHD: Dose for GFR < 10 PD: Dose for GFR 10-50 CRRT: Dose for GFR 10-50 [D]
Mefloquine	< 1	1250 mg in 2 doses (750 mg initially, then 500 mg 12 h later)	100% [D]	No data; 100% [D]	No data; 100% [D]	IHD: None PD: No data, None CRRT: Dose for GFR 10-50 [D]
Pentamidine	< 5	4 mg/kg q24h	q24h [A]	q24h [A]	q24-36h [A]	IHD: Dose for GFR < 10, 0.75 g after each HD PD: Dose for GFR < 10 CRRT: Dose for GFR 30-50 [D]

(Continued)

TABLE 112–3 Drug dosing in patients treated with RRT. (*Continued*)

Drug	Major Excretion Route (percentage of total drug excreted unchanged in the urine for patients with normal renal function)	Dose for Normal Renal Function	Adjustment for Renal Failure GFR >50	Adjustment for Renal Failure GFR 10-50	Adjustment for Renal Failure GFR <10	Supplement for Dialysis
Primaquine	1	15 mg (base) q24h	No data; 100% [D]	No data; 100% [D]	No data; 100% [D]	IHD: No data, None PD: No data, None CRRT: Dose for GFR 30-50 [D]
Pyrimethamine	15-30	50-75 mg q24h	100% [D]	100% [D]	100% [D]	IHD: None PD: None CRRT: Dose for GFR 30-50 [D]
Acyclovir	40-70	5-10 mg/kg q8h	100% q8 [D]	100% q12-24h [D]	50% q24h [D]	IHD: Dose after dialysis PD: Dose for GFR < 10 CRRT: 5-10 mg/kg q24h [A]
Famciclovir	50-65	500 mg q8h for herpes zoster; 125 mg q12h for genital herpes	100% [D]	q12-24h [D]	50% q24h [D]	IHD: Dose after dialysis PD: No data CRRT: Not applicable, recommend IV ganciclovir
Foscarnet	85	40-60 mg/kg q8h Second dose: to 90 mg/kg q12h	28 mg/kg [A]	15 mg/kg [A]	6 mg/kg [A]	IHD: Dose after dialysis PD: Dose for GFR < 10 CRRT: Cytomegalovirus (CMV) induct; 60 mg q24h; CMV main; 60 mg q48 [B]
Ganciclovir	90-100	5 mg/kg q12h	50% q12-24h [D]	25%-50% q24h [D]	25% 3 wk [D]	IHD: 25% 3×/wk PD: Dose for GFR < 10 CRRT: Induction: 2.5 mg/kg q24h, main: 1.25 mg/kg q24h [B]
Valacyclovir	< 1	500 mg q12h Second dose: to 1000 mg q8h	100% [D]	Full dose q12-24h [D]	0.5 g q24h [D]	IHD: Dose after dialysis PD: Dose for GFR < 10 CRRT: Not applicable, recommend IV form
Valganciclovir	> 90	900 mg bid (induction) 900 mg daily (maintenance)	Induction GFR 40-59; 450 mg bid GFR 25-39; 450 mg qd GFR 10-24 450 mg q2d [A]	Maintenance GFR 40-59; 450 mg qd GFR 25-39 450 mg q2d GFR 10-24 450 mg twice weekly [A]		IHD: Avoid PD: Avoid CRRT: based on GFR

Anticoagulants

Alteplase	No data	60 mg over 1 h, then 20 mg/h for 2 h	100% [D]	100% [D]		IHD: No data [D] PD: No data [D] CRRT: Dose for GFR 10-50 [D]
Dipyridamole	No data	50 mg tid	100% [D]	100% [D]		IHD: None [D] PD: Dose for GFR < 10 [D] CRRT: Not applicable
Heparin	None	75 U/kg load, then 0.5 U/kg/min	100% [A]	100% [A]		IHD: None [A] PD: None [A] CRRT: Dose for GFR 10-50 [D]
Low molecular weight heparin (LMWH)	No data	30-40 mg bid	100% [B]	50% [B]		IHD: Not applicable [D] PD: Dose for GFR < 10 [D] CRRT: 50% and monitor Xa [D]
Streptokinase	None	250,000 U load, then 100,000 U/h	100% [B]	100% [B]		IHD: Not applicable [D] PD: Not applicable [D] CRRT: Dose for GFR 10-50 [D]
Urokinase	No data	4400 U/kg load, then 4400 U/kg qh	100% [B]	100% [B]		IHD: None [D] PD: None [D] CRRT: Dose for GFR 10-50, not available [D]
Warfarin	None	10-15 mg load, then 2-10 mg q24h	100% [A]	100% [A]		IHD: None [B] PD: None [B] CRRT: 100% [D]

Anticonvulsants

Carbamazepine	2-3	200 mg bid Second dose: to 1200 mg q24h	100% [A]	100% [A]	75% [D]	IHD: Dose for FR < 10 give after dialysis [B] PD: Dose for GFR < 10 [D] CRRT: 100% [B]
Clonazepam	< 1	0.5 mg tid	100% [D]	100% [D]		IHD: None [D] PD: No data CRRT: Not applicable
Fosphenytoin	2	15-20 mg PE/kg at 100-150 mg PE/min	100% [B]	100% [B]	100% [B]	IHD: None [A] PD: None [B] CRRT: 100% [B]
Gabapentin	90	300-600 mg tid	400 mg tid [A]	300 mg q12-24h [A]	300 mg qod [A]	IHD: 300 mg load, then 200-300 mg post HD [A] PD: 300 mg qod [D] CRRT: Dose for GFR 10-50 [D]

TABLE 112–3 Drug dosing in patients treated with RRT. (Continued)

Drug	Major Excretion Route (percentage of total drug excreted unchanged in the urine for patients with normal renal function)	Dose for Normal Renal Function	Adjustment for Renal Failure GFR > 50	Adjustment for Renal Failure GFR 10-50	Adjustment for Renal Failure GFR < 10	Supplement for Dialysis
Lamotrigine	10	50 mg q12-24h (initially) 100-500 mg q24h (maintenance)	100% [D]	75% [D]	10 mg qod [A]	IHD: 100 mg after dialysis [A] PD: Dose for GFR < 10 [D] CRRT: Decrease dose by 50% [B]
Levetiracetam	66	500-1500 mg q12h	500-1000 mg q12h [A]	250-750 mg q12h [A]	500-1000 mg q24h [A]	IHD: 250-500 mg after dialysis [B] PD: Dose for GFR < 10 [D] CRRT: 250-750 mg q12h [D]
Oxcarbazepine	30	300-600 mg bid	100% [A]	75%-100% [A]	50% [A]	IHD: Dose for GFR < 10, give after dialysis [D] PD: Dose for GFR < 10 [D] CRRT: Decrease dose by 50%, monitor levels [D]
Phenobarbital	19-31	50-100 mg q8-12h	q8-12h [D]	q8-12h [D]	q12-16h [D]	IHD: Dose before dialysis, 1/2 dose after dialysis [D] PD: 1/2 normal dose [B] CRRT: Normal dose and measure levels [B]
Phenytoin	2	100 mg tid	100% [B]	100% [B]	100% [B]	IHD: None [A] PD: None [B] CRRT: 100% [B]
Topiramate	70-97	200 mg q12h	100% [A]	50% [A]	25% [D]	IHD: Dose for normal renal function after dialysis [D] PD: Dose for GFR 10-50 [D] CRRT: Dose for GFR 10-50 [B]
Valproic acid	< 5	500 mg q24h for 1 wk Second dose: 500-1000 mg q24h	100% [D]	100% [D]	100% [D]	IHD: Dose after dialysis [D] PD: Dose for GFR < 10 [B] CRRT: None [D]
Antihistamines						
Diphenhydramine	2	25 mg tid-qid	100% [D]	100% [D]	100% [D]	IHD: None [D] PD: None [D] CRRT: 100% [D]
Famotidine	65-80	20-40 mg qhs	50%-75% [D]	10%-50% [D]	10% [D]	IHD: Dose after dialysis [A] PD: Dose for GFR < 10 [A] CRRT: Dose for GFR 10-50 [B]
Ranitidine	80	150-300 mg qhs	75% [A]	150 mg q12-24h [A]	75-150 mg q24h [A]	IHD: Dose after dialysis [D] PD: Dose for GFR < 10 [D] CRRT: Dose for GFR 10-50 [D]

Antiparkinson Agents

Drug		Dose	GFR > 50	GFR 10–50	GFR < 10	Dialysis
Carbidopa	30	1 tab tid Second dose: to 6 tabs daily	100% [D]	100% [D]	100% [D]	IHD: No data PD: No data CRRT: Dose for GFR 10-49 [D]
Levodopa	None	250-500 mg bid Second dose: to 8 g q24h	100% [B]	50%-100% [B]	50%-100% [B]	IHD: Dose after dialysis [D] PD: Dose for GFR < 10 [D] CRRT: Dose for GFR 10-50 [D]

Antithyroid Drugs

Drug		Dose	GFR > 50	GFR 10–50	GFR < 10	Dialysis
Methimazole	7	5-20 mg tid	100% [B]	100% [B]	100% [B]	IHD: None [D] PD: None [D] CRRT: Dose for GFR 10-50 [D]
Propylthiouracil	< 10	100 mg tid	100% [A]	100% [A]	100% [A]	IHD: None [D] PD: None [D] CRRT: Dose for GFR 10-50 [D]

Arthritis and Gout Agents

Drug		Dose	GFR > 50	GFR 10–50	GFR < 10	Dialysis
Allopurinol	30	300 mg q24h	75% [B]	50% [B]	25% [B]	IHD: 1/2 dose [B] PD: No data [D] CRRT: Dose for GFR 10-50 [D]
Colchicine	5-17	Acute: 2 mg then 0.5 mg q6h Chronic: 0.5-1 mg q24h	100% [B]	50%-100% [B]	25% [B]	IHD: None [D] PD: Dose for GFR < 10 [D] CRRT: Dose for GFR 10-50 [D]
Diclofenac	< 1	25-75 mg bid	50%-100% [D]	25%-50% [D]	25% [D]	IHD: None [D] PD: None [D] CRRT: Not applicable
Ibuprofen	1	800 mg tid	100% [A]	100% [A]	100% [B]	IHD: None [D] PD: None [D] CRRT: Dose for GFR 10-50 [D]
Indomethacin	30	25-50 mg tid	100% [A]	100% [A]	100% [A]	IHD: None PD: None [D] CRRT: Not applicable
Ketorolac	30-60	30-60 mg load, then 15-30 mg q6h	100% [D]	50% [B]	25%-50% [B]	IHD: None [D] PD: None [D] CRRT: Dose for GFR 10-50 [D]
Naproxen	< 1	500 mg bid	100% [A]	100% [A]	100% [A]	IHD: None [D] PD: None [D] CRRT: Not applicable

(Continued)

TABLE 112–3 Drug dosing in patients treated with RRT. (Continued)

Drug	Major Excretion Route (percentage of total drug excreted unchanged in the urine for patients with normal renal function)	Dose for Normal Renal Function	Adjustment for Renal Failure GFR > 50	Adjustment for Renal Failure GFR 10-50	Adjustment for Renal Failure GFR < 10	Supplement for Dialysis
Bronchodilators						
Albuterol	28	2 inhalations q4-6h	100% [D]	100% [D]	100% [D]	IHD: None [D] PD: None [D] CRRT: 100% [D]
Ipratropium	No data	2 inhalations qid	100% [D]	100% [D]	100% [D]	IHD: None [D] PD: None [D] CRRT: 100% [D]
Salmeterol	< 1	1-2 inhalations bid	100% [D]	100% [D]	100% [D]	IHD: None [D] PD: None [D] CRRT: 100% [D]
Theophylline	< 10	6 mg/kg load, then 9 mg/kg q24h	100% [A]	100% [A]	100% [A]	IHD: 125% during dialysis [B] PD: None [D] CRRT: 100% [D]
Corticosteroids						
Dexamethasone	8	0.75-9 mg q24h	100% [D]	100% [D]	100% [D]	IHD: None [D] PD: None [D] CRRT: 100% [D]
Hydrocortisone	None	20-500 mg q24h	100% [A]	100% [A]	100% [A]	IHD: None [D] PD: None [D] CRRT: 100% [D]
Methylprednisolone	< 10	4-48 mg q24h	100% [A]	100% [A]	100% [A]	IHD: Yes [D] PD: None [D] CRRT: 100% [D]
Prednisone	34	5-60 mg q24h	100% [A]	100% [A]	100% [A]	IHD: Yes [B] PD: None [B] CRRT: 100% [D]
Hypoglycemic Agents						
Glipizide	4.5-7	2.5-15 mg q24h	100% [B]	50% [B]	50% [B]	IHD: None [D] PD: Dose for GFR < 10 [D] CRRT: Not applicable
Glyburide	50	1.25-20 mg q24h	No data	No data	100% [A]	IHD: None PD: None CRRT: Not applicable
Metformin	90-100	500-850 mg bid	50% [B]	25% [B]	Avoid [B]	IHD: Not applicable [D] PD: None [D] CRRT: Not applicable

Drug		Dose	GFR >50	GFR 10–50	GFR <10	
Glipizide	4.5–7	2.5–15 mg q24h	100% [B]	50% [B]	50% [B]	IHD: None [D] PD: Dose for GFR < 10 [D] CRRT: Not applicable
Insulin	None	Variable	100% [A]	75% [A]	50% [A]	IHD: None [A] PD: None [A] CRRT: Dose for GFR 10-50
Hypolipidemic Agents						
Cholestyramine	None	4 g q4–6h	100% [D]	100% [D]	100% [D]	IHD: None [D] PD: None [D] CRRT: 100%[D]
Gemfibrozil	None	600 mg bid	100% [B]	75% [B]	50% [B]	IHD: None [D] PD: Dose for GFR < 10 [D] CRRT: Not applicable
Nicotinic acid	None	1–2 g tid	100% [B]	50% [B]	25% [B]	IHD: None [D] PD: Doses for GFR < 10 [D] CRRT: Dose for GFR 10-50 [D]
Pravastatin	< 10	10–40 mg q24	100% [A]	100% [A]	100% [A]	IHD: None [B] PD: None [B] CRRT: Dose for GFR 10-50 [D]
Simvastatin	< 0.5	5–40 mg q24h	100% [A]	100% [A]	100% [A]	IHD: None [D] PD: None [D] CRRT: Dose for GFR 10-50 [D]
Miscellaneous Drugs						
Metoclopramide	10–22	10–15 mg qid	100% [A]	75% [A]	50% [A]	IHD: None [D] PD: None [D] CRRT: Dose for GFR 10-50 [D]
Ondansetron	< 5	8–10 mg IV q6–12h	100% [A]	100% [A]	100% [A]	IHD: None [B] PD: None [B] CRRT: Dose for GFR 10-50 [D]
Neuromuscular Agents						
Atracurium	None	0.4–0.5 mg/kg load, then 0.08–0.1 mg/kg q15–25 min	100% [D]	100% [D]	100% [D]	IHD: Not applicable [D] PD: Not applicable [D] CRRT: Dose for GFR 10–50 [B]
Etomidate	2	0.2–0.6 mg/kg	100% [D]	100% [D]	100% [D]	IHD: Not applicable [D] PD: Not applicable [D] CRRT: Dose for GFR 10–50 [D]
Fentanyl	6–8	0.002–0.05 mg/kg	100% [D]	100% [D]	100% [D]	IHD: None [D] PD: None [D] CRRT: Dose for GFR 10–50 [B]

(Continued)

TABLE 112–3 Drug dosing in patients treated with RRT. (*Continued*)

Drug	Major Excretion Route (percentage of total drug excreted unchanged in the urine for patients with normal renal function)	Dose for Normal Renal Function	Adjustment for Renal Failure GFR >50	Adjustment for Renal Failure GFR 10-50	Adjustment for Renal Failure GFR <10	Supplement for Dialysis
Ketamine	2-3	1-4.5 mg/kg	100% [D]	100% [D]	100% [D]	IHD: Not applicable [D] PD: Not applicable [D] CRRT: Dose for GFR 10-50 [B]
Pancuronium	30-40	0.04-0.1 mg/kg	100% [A]	50% [B]	Avoid [B]	IHD: Avoid [D] PD: Avoid [D] CRRT: Dose for GFR 10-50 [D]
Propofol	<0.3	2-2.5 mg/kg	100% [B]	100% [B]	100% [B]	IHD: None [D] PD: None [D] CRRT: Dose for GFR 10-50 [B]
Succinylcholine	None	0.3-1.1 mg/kg load, then 0.04-0.07 mg/kg prn	100% [A]	100% [A]	100% [A]	IHD: Not applicable [D] PD: Dose for GFR < 10 [D] CRRT: Dose for GFR 10-50 [D]
Vecuronium	25	0.08-0.1 mg/kg load, then 0.01-0.05 mg/kg q12-15 min	100% [A]	100% [A]	100% [A]	IHD: Not applicable [D] PD: Not applicable [D] CRRT: Dose for GFR 10-50 [D]
Proton-Pump Inhibitors						
Lansoprazole	None	15-60 mg q24h	100% [A]	100% [A]	100% [A]	IHD: None [D] PD: None [D] CRRT: Dose for GFR 10-50 [D]
Omeprazole	Negligible	20-60 mg q24h	100% [A]	100% [A]	100% [A]	IHD: None [B] PD: None [B] CRRT: Dose for GFR 10-50 [D]
Antidepressants						
Bupropion	Hepatic	100 mg q8	100% [D]	100% [D]	100% [D]	IHD: No data [D] PD: Dose for GFR < 10 [D] CRRT: Dose for GFR 10-50 [D]
Trazodone	10-20 (renal)	150-400 mg q24h	100% [B]	100% [B]	100% [B]	IHD: None [D] PD: None [D] CRRT: 100% [D]
Venlafaxine	Hepatic	75-375 mg q24h	75% [B]	50% [B]	50% [B]	IHD: None [D] PD: None [D] CRRT: 100% [D]

Barbiturates

Drug	Metabolism	Normal Dose	GFR >50	GFR 10–50	GFR <10	Supplement
Pentobarbital	Hepatic	30 mg q6-8h	100% [A]	100% [A]	100% [A]	IHD: None [B] PD: None [B] CRRT: Dose for GFR 10-50 [B]
Benzodiazepines						
Lorazepam	Hepatic	1-2 mg q8-12h	100% [A]	100% [A]	100% [A]	IHD: None [B] PD: None [D] CRRT: Dose for GFR 10-50 [B]
Midazolam	Hepatic	Individualized	100% [A]	100% [A]	50% [A]	IHD: Not applicable [D] PD: Not applicable [D] CRRT: Dose for GFR 10-50 [A]
Miscellaneous Sedative Agents						
Buspirone	Hepatic	5 mg q8h	100% [D]	100% [D]	100% [D]	IHD: None [B] PD: Dose for GFR < 10 [D] CRRT: Dose for GFR 10-50 [B]
Haloperidol	Hepatic	1-2 mg q8-12h	100% [D]	100% [D]	100% [D]	IHD: None [D] PD: None [D] CRRT: Dose for GFR 10-50 [D]
Lithium carbonate	Renal	0.9-1.2 g q24h	100% [A]	50%-75% [A]	25%-50% [A]	IHD: Dose after dialysis [B] PD: None [D] CRRT: Dose for GFR 10-50 [A]
Antipyschotic Agents						
Chlorpromazine	Hepatic	300-800 mg q24h	100% [D]	100% [D]	100% [D]	IHD: None [D] PD: Dose for GFR < 10 [D] CRRT: Dose for GFR 10-50 [D]
Promethazine	Hepatic	20-100 mg q24h	100% [D]	100% [D]	100% [D]	IHD: None [D] PD: None [D] CRRT: Not applicable [D]
Selective Serotonin Reuptake Inhibitors (SSRIs)						
Fluoxetine	Hepatic	20 mg q24h	100% [D]	100% [D]	100% [D]	IHD: None [D] PD: None [D] CRRT: Dose for GFR 10-50 [D]
Paroxetine	Hepatic	20-60 mg q24h	100% [A]	50%-75% [B]	50% [B]	IHD: None [D] PD: Dose for GFR < 10 [D] CRRT: Dose for GFR 10-50 [D]

(Continued)

TABLE 112–3 Drug dosing in patients treated with RRT. (Continued)

Drug	Major Excretion Route (percentage of total drug excreted unchanged in the urine for patients with normal renal function)	Dose for Normal Renal Function	Adjustment for Renal Failure GFR > 50	Adjustment for Renal Failure GFR 10-50	Adjustment for Renal Failure GFR < 10	Supplement for Dialysis
Sertraline	Hepatic	50-200 mg q24h	100% [A]	100% [A]	100% [A]	IHD: None [D] PD: None [D] CRRT: Dose for GFR 10-50 [D]
Tricyclic Antidepressants						
Amitriptyline	Hepatic	25 mg q8h	100% [D]	100% [D]	100% [D]	IHD: None [D] PD: None [B] CRRT: Dose for GFR 10-50 [D]
Clomipramine	Hepatic	100-250 mg q24h	100% [D]	100% [D]	100% [D]	IHD: None [D] PD: Dose for GFR < 10 [D] CRRT: Avoid [D]
Desipramine	Hepatic	100-250 mg q24h	100% [D]	100% [D]	100% [D]	IHD: None [D] PD: dose for GFR < 10 [D] CRRT: Avoid [D]
Imipramine	Hepatic	25 mg q8	100% [A]	100% [A]	100% [A]	IHD: None [D] PD: None [A] CRRT: Dose for GFR 10-50 [D]
Nortriptyline	Hepatic	25 mg q6-8h	100% [B]	100% [B]	100% [B]	IHD: None [D] PD: None [D] CRRT: Dose for GFR 10-50 [D]

CRRT, continuous renal replacement therapy; GFR, estimated glomerular filtration rate; IV, intravenous; RRT, renal replacement therapy.

REFERENCES

1. Heintz BH, Matzke GR, Dager WE. Antimicrobial dosing concepts and recommendations for critically ill adult patients receiving continuous renal replacement therapy or intermittent hemodialysis. *Pharmacotherapy.* 2009;29:562-577.
2. Scoville BA, Mueller BA. Medication dosing in critically ill patients with acute kidney injury treated with renal replacement therapy. *Am J Kidney Dis.* 2013;61:490-500.
3. Matzke GR, Aronoff GR, Murray P, et al. Drug dosing consideration in patients with acute and chronic kidney disease—a clinical update from kidney disease: improving global outcomes (KDIGO). *Kidney International.* 2011;80:1122-1137.
4. Levey AS, Stevens LA, Schmid CH, et al. A new equation to estimate glomerular filtration rate. *Ann Intern Med.* 2009;150:604-612.
5. Cockcroft DW, Gault MH. Prediction of creatinine clearance from serum creatinine. *Nephron.* 1976;16:31-41.
6. Anonymous. Health professionals CKD and drug dosing information for providers. Estimation of kidney function for prescription medication dosage in adults. http://nkdep.nih.gov/resources/CKD-drug-dosing.shtml.
7. Aronoff GR, Bennett WM, Berns JS, et al. *Drug Prescription in Renal Failure: Drug Dosing Guidelines for Adults and Children.* Philadelphia, PA: American College of Physicians; 2007.
8. Mueller BA, Smoyer WE. Challenges in developing evidence-based drug dosing guidelines for adults and children receiving renal replacement therapy. *Clin Pharmacol & Therapeutics.* 2009;86:479-482.
9. Janknegt R, Nube M. A simple method for predicting drug clearances during CAPD. *Perit Dial Bull.* 1985;5:254-255.

Drugs in Pregnancy

Natalie Kostelecky, RN, BSN and
Stephen M. Pastores, MD, FACP, FCCP, FCCM

DRUGS IN PREGNANCY

The Food and Drug Administration (FDA) has established 6 categories (A, B, C, D, X, and N) to indicate the potential of a drug to cause birth defects if used during pregnancy.[†] The categories are determined by the reliability of documentation and the risk to benefit ratio. They do not take into account any risks from pharmaceutical agents or their metabolites in breast milk.

Class of Medication	FDA Pregnancy Category Risk	Class of Medication	FDA Pregnancy Category Risk
Analgesics and sedative agents		Amiodarone	D
		Digoxin	C
Acetaminophen	C	Diltiazem	C
Acetylsalicylic acid*	D	Esmolol	C
Fentanyl*	C	Flecainide	C
Hydromorphone*	C	Metoprolol	C
Ibuprofen*	C (first and second trimester); D (third trimester)	*Antimicrobial agents*	
		Penicillins	B
Indomethacin*	C (first and second trimester); D (third trimester)	Cefazolin	B
		Cefepime	B
Ketorolac*	C (first and second trimester); D (third trimester)	Ceftriaxone	B
		Imipenem-cilastatin	C
Meperidine*	C	Meropenem	B
Methadone*	C	Amikacin	D
Morphine*	C	Gentamicin	D
Oxycodone*	C	Tobramycin	D
Oxymorphone*	C	Erythromycin	B
Midazolam	D	Levofloxacin	C
Lorazepam	D	Clarithromycin	C
Propofol	B	Ciprofloxacin	C
Dexmedetomidine	C	Vancomycin	C
Anesthetic agents		Linezolid	C
Halothane	C	Aztreonam	B
Isoflurane	C	Clindamycin	B
Ketamine	N	Metronidazole	B
Lidocaine (local)	B	Trimethoprim-sulfamethoxazole	D
Propofol	B		
Antiarrhythmic agents		Tetracyclines	D
Adenosine	C		

(Continued)

(CONTINUED)

Class of Medication	FDA Pregnancy Category Risk	Class of Medication	FDA Pregnancy Category Risk
Polymyxin B	B	Aminocaproic acid	C
Acyclovir	B	Alteplase	C
Famciclovir	B	Streptokinase	C
Valacyclovir	B	Dabigatran	C
Foscarnet	C	Tinzaparin	B
Ganciclovir	C	Bivalirudin	B
Oseltamivir	C	Desirudin	C
Amantadine	C	Tranexamic acid	B
Rimantadine	C	Clopidogrel	B
Amphotericin B	B	*Anticonvulsant agents*	
Lipid Amphotericin (AmBisome)	B	Phenytoin	D
		Phenobarbital	D
Fluconazole	D	Carbamazepine	D
Ketoconazole	C	Valproic acid	X
Caspofungin	C	Levetiracetam	C
Micafungin	C	Lamotrigine	C
Voriconazole	D	Gabapentin	C
Posaconazole	C	Topiramate	D
Rifampin	C	*Antidepressant, anxiolytic and antipsychotic agents*	
Isoniazid	C	Lorazepam	D
Ethambutol	C	Clonazepam	D
Streptomycin	D	Midazolam	D
Atazanavir	B	Diazepam	D
Didanosine	B	Alprazolam	D
Emtricitabine	B	Aripiprazole	C
Ritonavir	B	Chlordiazepoxide	C
Tenofovir	B	Chlorpromazine	C
Efavirenz	D	Haloperidol	C
Indinavir	C	Olanzapine	C
Lamivudine	C	Quetiapine	C
Lopinavir	C	Risperidone	C
Nevirapine	B	Ziprasidone	C
Zidovudine	C	Bupropion	C
Anticoagulant and antithrombotic agents		Buspirone	B
Unfractionated heparin	C	Zolpidem	C
Warfarin	X	Lithium	D
Enoxaparin	B	*Antihistaminic agents*	
Dalteparin	B	Cetirizine	B
Fondaparinux	B	Chlorpheniramine	B
Rivaroxaban	C	Diphenhydramine	B
Apixaban	B	Fexofenadine	C
Edoxaban	C	Hydroxyzine	C
Argatroban	B	Loratadine	B

(Continued)

(CONTINUED)

Class of Medication	FDA Pregnancy Category Risk	Class of Medication	FDA Pregnancy Category Risk
Meclizine	B	Ranitidine	B
Promethazine	C	Senna	C
Antihypertensive agents		Simethicone	N
Labetalol	C	Sucralfate	B
Nicardipine	C	Ursodiol	B
Esmolol	C	*Respiratory agents*	
Atenolol	D	Acetylcysteine	B
Clonidine	C	Albuterol	C
Methyldopa	B	Budesonide	B
Hydralazine	C	Corticosteroids	C
Sodium nitroprusside	C	Dextromethorphan	C
Captopril	D	Guaifenesin	C
Enalapril	D	Ipratropium	B
Irbesartan	D	Montelukast	B
Candesartan	D	Salmeterol	C
Gastrointestinal agents		Theophylline	C
Cimetidine	B	Zafirlukast	B
Docusate	N	*Urologic agents*	
Famotidine	B	Oxybutynin	B
Lactulose	B	Phenazopyridine	B
Lansoprazole	B	*Vasoconstrictor and Inotropic agents*	
Loperamide	C	Norepinephrine	C
Mesalamine	C	Epinephrine	C
Metoclopramide	B	Phenylephrine	C
Omeprazole	C	Dopamine	C
Ondansetron	B	Vasopressin	C
Opium tincture	B	Dobutamine	B
Pantoprazole	B	Isoproterenol	C
Prochlorperazine	C	Milrinone	C
Promethazine	C		

*All of these agents can be considered category D if used in large doses or for prolonged duration.

Notes:

Category A
Adequate and well-controlled studies have failed to demonstrate a risk to the fetus in the first trimester of pregnancy (and there is no evidence of risk in later trimesters).

Category B
Animal reproduction studies have failed to demonstrate a risk to the fetus and there are no adequate and well-controlled studies in pregnant women.

Category C
Animal reproduction studies have shown an adverse effect on the fetus and there are no adequate and well-controlled studies in humans, but potential benefits may warrant use of the drug in pregnant women despite potential risks.

Category D
There is positive evidence of human fetal risk based on adverse reaction data from investigational or marketing experience or studies in humans, but potential benefits may warrant use of the drug in pregnant women despite potential risks.

Category X
Studies in animals or humans have demonstrated fetal abnormalities and/or there is positive evidence of human fetal risk based on adverse reaction data from investigational or marketing experience, and the risks involved in use of the drug in pregnant women clearly outweigh potential benefits.

Category N
FDA has not classified the drug.
†http://www.gpo.gov/fdsys/pkg/FR-2008-05-29/pdf/E8-11806.pdf

Formulas

Natalie Kostelecky, RN, BSN and
Stephen M. Pastores, MD, FACP, FCCP, FCCM

A. Cardiovascular/Hemodynamics	Equation	Normal Ranges
Systemic systolic blood pressure (SBP)		100-140 mm Hg
Systemic diastolic blood pressure (DBP)		60-90 mm Hg
Pulse pressure (PP)	SBP − DBP	30-50 mm Hg
Mean arterial pressure (MAP)	SBP + (2 × DBP)/3	70-110 mm Hg
Mean pulmonary arterial pressure	[PASP + (2 × DBP)]/3	10-20 mm Hg
Central venous pressure (CVP)		2-6 mm Hg
Pulmonary artery occlusion pressure (PAOP)		4-10 mm Hg
Systemic vascular resistance (SVR)	MAP − RAP/CO × 80	800-1200 dynes s/cm^5
Pulmonary vascular resistance (PVR)	MPAP − PAWP/CO × 80	<250 dynes s/cm^5
Cardiac output (CO)	SV × HR/1000	4.0-8.0 L/min
Cardiac index (CI)	CO/BSA	2.5-4.0 L/min/m^2
Stroke volume (SV)	CO/HR × 1000	60-100 mL/beat
Stroke index (SI)	CI/HR × 1000	33-47 mL/m^2/beat
Left ventricular stroke work index	SVI × (MAP − PAWP) × 0.0136	50-62 g m/m^2/beat
Right ventricular stroke work index	SVI × (MPAP − RAP) × 0.0136	5-10 g m/m^2/beat
Oxygen delivery (DO_2)	CO × CaO_2 × 10	950-1150 mL/min
Oxygen consumption (VO_2)	CO × (CaO_2 − CvO_2) × 10	200-250 mL/min
Arterial oxygen content (CaO_2)	1.39 × SaO_2 × (Hgb) + 0.0031 × PaO_2	17-20 mL/dL
Venous oxygen content (CvO_2)	1.39 × SvO_2 × (Hgb) + 0.0031 × PaO_2	12-15 mL/dL
Arterio-venous oxygen content difference (AVO_2)	CaO_2 − CvO_2	4-6 mL/dL
Oxygen extraction ratio (O_2ER)	CaO_2 − CvO_2/CaO_2 × 100	22%-30%
Coronary artery perfusion	DBP − PAWP	60-80 mm Hg

B. Respiratory	Equation	Normal Ranges
Arterial oxygen tension (PaO_2)		80-100 mm Hg
Arterial oxygen saturation (SaO_2)		95%-100%
Arterial carbon dioxide tension ($PaCO_2$)		35-45 mm Hg
Alveolar gas equation (P_AO_2)	$F_iO_2 (P_{atmos} - P_{H_2O}) - (P_aCO_2 / RQ)$	
Alveolar-arterial oxygen difference (A-a gradient)	$P_AO_2 - PaO_2$	5-25 mm Hg (at $FiO_2 = 0.21$) <150 mm Hg (at $FiO_2 = 1.0$)
Minute ventilation	Respiratory rate × tidal volume	5-6 L/min
Dead space fraction (V_D/V_T)	$Paco_2 - Peco_2/Paco_2$	0.2-0.3
Respiratory system static compliance (C_{st})	$V_T/P_{plat} - PEEP$	60 mL/cm H_2O
Respiratory system dynamic compliance (C_{dyn})	$V_T/PIP - PEEP$	60 mL/cm H_2O
Pulmonary capillary oxygen content (C_cO_2)	$(Hgb \times 1.39 \times 1.0) + (0.0031 \times P_AO_2)$	20.7 ml O_2/dL
Shunt fraction (Q_S/Q_T)	$(Cco_2 - Cao_2)/(Cco_2 - Cvo_2)$	<5%
Oxygen delivery (Do_2)	$Cao_2 \times CO \times 10$	950-1150 mL/min
Oxygen consumption (Vo_2)	$Cao_2 \times Cvo_2 \times CO \times 10$	200-250 mL/min
Carbon dioxide production (Vco_2)		3-4 mL/kg/min

C. Renal, Acid-base, Fluids, and Electrolytes	Equation	Normal Ranges
Anion gap	$[Na^+] - [Cl^-] - [HCO_3^-]$	9-13 mEq/L
Creatinine clearance (CrCl)	Cockcroft-Gault equation (for males) $$\frac{(140-Age) \times (Wt\,in\,kg)}{72 \times Scr}$$ For females = 0.85 × Estimate for males	>100 mL/min
Serum osmolality (S_{osm})	$(2 \times [Na] + [BUN/2.8] + [glucose/18])$	275-295 mOsm/kg
Osmolar gap	Measured serum osmolality – Calculated serum osmolality	0-5 mOsm/kg
Fractional excretion of sodium (F_ENa)	(Urine sodium × Plasma Creatinine)/(Urine Creatinine × Plasma sodium) × 100%	<1% prerenal >1% intrarenal
Total body water (TBW)	Wt (kg) × 0.6 (males) Wt (kg) × 0.5 (females)	
Sodium deficit	TBW × (desired serum Na – Actual serum Na)	
Water deficit	TBW × (Na/140 – 1)	
Henderson-Hasselbalch equation	$pK + log[Hco_3^-]/0.03 \times Paco_2$	

Metabolic acidosis
   Bicarbonate deficit
   Expected $Paco_2$ compensation
	
	 0.5 × Wt (kg) × 24 – Hco_3^-
	 1.5 × Hco_3^- + 8 + 2	

(Continued)

(CONTINUED)

C. Renal, Acid-base, Fluids, and Electrolytes	Equation	Normal Ranges

Respiratory acidosis
  Acute
  Chronic
	$\Delta H^+/\Delta Pa_{CO_2} = 0.8$
	$\Delta H^+/\Delta Pa_{CO_2} = 0.3$	

Respiratory alkalosis
  Acute
  Chronic
	$\Delta H^+/\Delta Pa_{CO_2} = 0.8$
	$\Delta H^+/\Delta Pa_{CO_2} = 0.17$	

D. Nutrition	Equation	Normal Ranges
Ideal body weight (males)	50 kg + 2.3 kg for each inch over 5 ft	
Ideal body weight (females)	45.5 kg + 2.3 kg for each inch over 5 ft	
Body mass index	Weight (kg)/Height (cm)^2	18.5-24.9
Basal energy expenditure (BEE)	$66.5 + (13.75 \times kg) + (5.003 \times cm) - (6.775 \times Age)$ (for males) $655.1 + (9.563 \times kg) + (1.850 \times cm) - (4.676 \times Age)$ (for females)	
Mid-arm muscle circumference (MAC)	Arm circumference (cm) – (0.314 × Tricep skinfold [mm])	
Arm muscle area (mm^2)	(MAC [mm] – [0.314 × TSF]^2)/(4 × 3.14)	
Caloric requirements		Carbohydrate: 3.4 kcal/g Protein: 4.0 kcal/g Fat: 9.1 kcal/g
Protein requirements		1.5-2 g/kg (for most critically ill patients) 1.5-2.5 g/kg (for obese and/or on hemodialysis or renal replacement therapy
Nitrogen balance	Nitrogen consumed – Nitrogen excreted or Protein calories (kcal/day)/25 – Urine nitrogen (g/day) – 5 (g/day)	
Respiratory quotient (RQ)	CO_2 production (mL/min)/O_2 consumption (mL/min) or V_{CO_2}/V_{O_2}	0.8
Maastricht index (MI)	MI = 20.68 – (0.24 × albumin [g/L]) – 19.21 × prealbumin [g/L]) – 1.86 × lymphocytes [10^9/L]) – (0.04 × percentage ideal weight)	Patients with MI > are considered malnourished
Nutritional risk index (NRI)	NRI = (15.9 × plasma albumin [g/dL]) + 41.7 × (present weight/usual weight)	>100: subject is not malnourished 97.5-100: mildly malnourished 83.5 to <97.5: moderately malnourished <83.5: severely malnourished

Algorithms for Resuscitation

Natalie Kostelecky, RN, BSN and
Stephen M. Pastores, MD, FACP, FCCP, FCCM

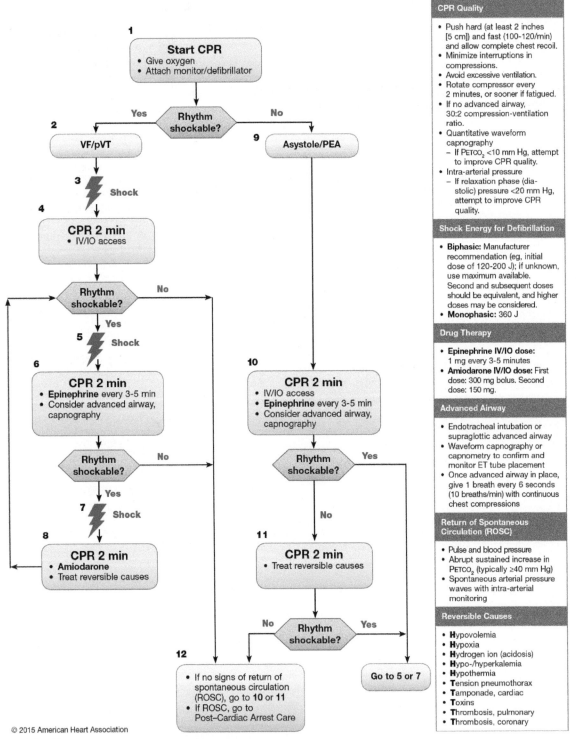

CPR Quality

- Push hard (at least 2 inches [5 cm]) and fast (100-120/min) and allow complete chest recoil.
- Minimize interruptions in compressions.
- Avoid excessive ventilation.
- Rotate compressor every 2 minutes, or sooner if fatigued.
- If no advanced airway, 30:2 compression-ventilation ratio.
- Quantitative waveform capnography
  – If $PETCO_2$ <10 mm Hg, attempt to improve CPR quality.
- Intra-arterial pressure
  – If relaxation phase (diastolic) pressure <20 mm Hg, attempt to improve CPR quality.

Shock Energy for Defibrillation

- **Biphasic:** Manufacturer recommendation (eg, initial dose of 120-200 J); if unknown, use maximum available. Second and subsequent doses should be equivalent, and higher doses may be considered.
- **Monophasic:** 360 J

Drug Therapy

- **Epinephrine IV/IO dose:** 1 mg every 3-5 minutes
- **Amiodarone IV/IO dose:** First dose: 300 mg bolus. Second dose: 150 mg.

Advanced Airway

- Endotracheal intubation or supraglottic advanced airway
- Waveform capnography or capnometry to confirm and monitor ET tube placement
- Once advanced airway in place, give 1 breath every 6 seconds (10 breaths/min) with continuous chest compressions

Return of Spontaneous Circulation (ROSC)

- Pulse and blood pressure
- Abrupt sustained increase in $PETCO_2$ (typically ≥40 mm Hg)
- Spontaneous arterial pressure waves with intra-arterial monitoring

Reversible Causes

- **H**ypovolemia
- **H**ypoxia
- **H**ydrogen ion (acidosis)
- **H**ypo-/hyperkalemia
- **H**ypothermia
- **T**ension pneumothorax
- **T**amponade, cardiac
- **T**oxins
- **T**hrombosis, pulmonary
- **T**hrombosis, coronary

© 2015 American Heart Association

ALGORITHM 1 Adult cardiac arrest. (*Reprinted with Permission 2015 American Heart Association Guidelines for CPR and ECC—Part 7: ACLS © 2015 American Heart Association, Inc.*)

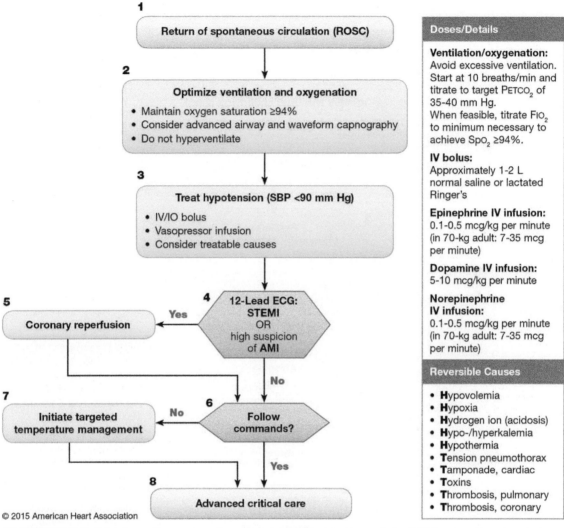

1
Return of spontaneous circulation (ROSC)

2
Optimize ventilation and oxygenation
- Maintain oxygen saturation ≥94%
- Consider advanced airway and waveform capnography
- Do not hyperventilate

3
Treat hypotension (SBP <90 mm Hg)
- IV/IO bolus
- Vasopressor infusion
- Consider treatable causes

4
12-Lead ECG:
STEMI
OR
high suspicion
of AMI

5
Coronary reperfusion ← Yes

No

6
Follow
commands?

7
Initiate targeted
temperature management ← No

Yes

8
Advanced critical care

Doses/Details

Ventilation/oxygenation:
Avoid excessive ventilation.
Start at 10 breaths/min and
titrate to target P_{ETCO_2} of
35-40 mm Hg.
When feasible, titrate F_{IO_2}
to minimum necessary to
achieve S_{pO_2} ≥94%.

IV bolus:
Approximately 1-2 L
normal saline or lactated
Ringer's

Epinephrine IV infusion:
0.1-0.5 mcg/kg per minute
(in 70-kg adult: 7-35 mcg
per minute)

Dopamine IV infusion:
5-10 mcg/kg per minute

**Norepinephrine
IV infusion:**
0.1-0.5 mcg/kg per minute
(in 70-kg adult: 7-35 mcg
per minute)

Reversible Causes

- **H**ypovolemia
- **H**ypoxia
- **H**ydrogen ion (acidosis)
- **H**ypo-/hyperkalemia
- **H**ypothermia
- **T**ension pneumothorax
- **T**amponade, cardiac
- **T**oxins
- **T**hrombosis, pulmonary
- **T**hrombosis, coronary

© 2015 American Heart Association

ALGORITHM 2 Adult immediate post-cardiac arrest care. (*Reprinted with permission 2015 American Heart Association Guidelines for CPR and ECC—Part 8:* Post Cardiac Arrest Care © *2015 American Heart Association, Inc.*)

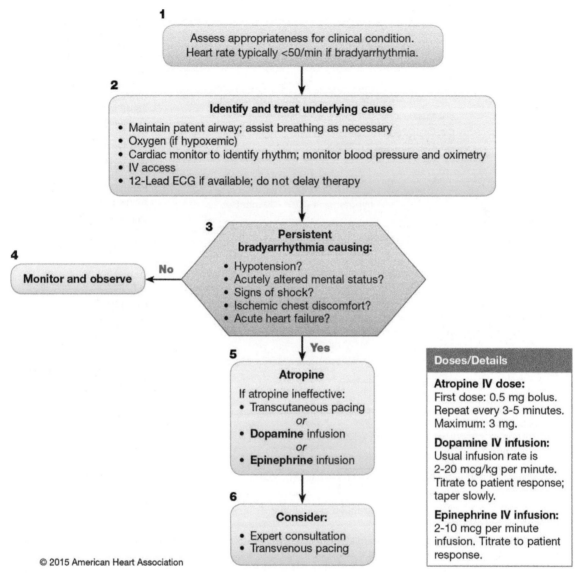

1

Assess appropriateness for clinical condition.
Heart rate typically <50/min if bradyarrhythmia.

2

Identify and treat underlying cause

- Maintain patent airway; assist breathing as necessary
- Oxygen (if hypoxemic)
- Cardiac monitor to identify rhythm; monitor blood pressure and oximetry
- IV access
- 12-Lead ECG if available; do not delay therapy

3

Persistent bradyarrhythmia causing:

- Hypotension?
- Acutely altered mental status?
- Signs of shock?
- Ischemic chest discomfort?
- Acute heart failure?

No →

4

Monitor and observe

Yes

5

Atropine

If atropine ineffective:
- Transcutaneous pacing
  or
- **Dopamine** infusion
  or
- **Epinephrine** infusion

6

Consider:

- Expert consultation
- Transvenous pacing

Doses/Details

Atropine IV dose:
First dose: 0.5 mg bolus.
Repeat every 3-5 minutes.
Maximum: 3 mg.

Dopamine IV infusion:
Usual infusion rate is
2-20 mcg/kg per minute.
Titrate to patient response;
taper slowly.

Epinephrine IV infusion:
2-10 mcg per minute
infusion. Titrate to patient
response.

© 2015 American Heart Association

ALGORITHM 3 Adult bradycardia (with pulse). (*Reprinted with Permission 2015 American Heart Association Guidelines for CPR and ECC—Part 7: ACLS © 2015 American Heart Association, Inc.*)

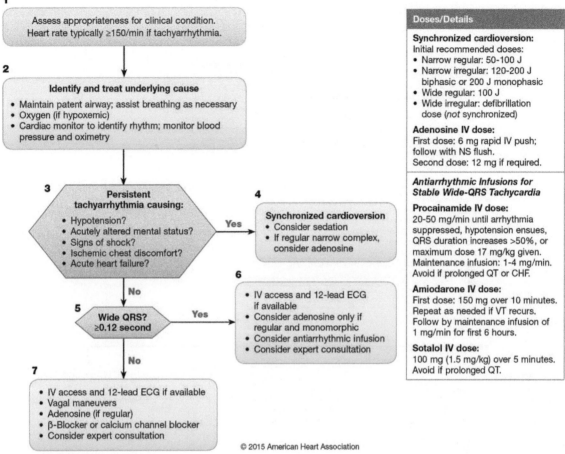

1
Assess appropriateness for clinical condition.
Heart rate typically ≥150/min if tachyarrhythmia.

2
Identify and treat underlying cause
- Maintain patent airway; assist breathing as necessary
- Oxygen (if hypoxemic)
- Cardiac monitor to identify rhythm; monitor blood pressure and oximetry

3
Persistent tachyarrhythmia causing:
- Hypotension?
- Acutely altered mental status?
- Signs of shock?
- Ischemic chest discomfort?
- Acute heart failure?

Yes →

4
Synchronized cardioversion
- Consider sedation
- If regular narrow complex, consider adenosine

No ↓

5
Wide QRS?
≥0.12 second

Yes →

6
- IV access and 12-lead ECG if available
- Consider adenosine only if regular and monomorphic
- Consider antiarrhythmic infusion
- Consider expert consultation

No ↓

7
- IV access and 12-lead ECG if available
- Vagal maneuvers
- Adenosine (if regular)
- β-Blocker or calcium channel blocker
- Consider expert consultation

© 2015 American Heart Association

Doses/Details

Synchronized cardioversion:
Initial recommended doses:
- Narrow regular: 50-100 J
- Narrow irregular: 120-200 J biphasic or 200 J monophasic
- Wide regular: 100 J
- Wide irregular: defibrillation dose (*not* synchronized)

Adenosine IV dose:
First dose: 6 mg rapid IV push; follow with NS flush.
Second dose: 12 mg if required.

Antiarrhythmic Infusions for Stable Wide-QRS Tachycardia

Procainamide IV dose:
20-50 mg/min until arrhythmia suppressed, hypotension ensues, QRS duration increases >50%, or maximum dose 17 mg/kg given. Maintenance infusion: 1-4 mg/min. Avoid if prolonged QT or CHF.

Amiodarone IV dose:
First dose: 150 mg over 10 minutes. Repeat as needed if VT recurs. Follow by maintenance infusion of 1 mg/min for first 6 hours.

Sotalol IV dose:
100 mg (1.5 mg/kg) over 5 minutes. Avoid if prolonged QT.

ALGORITHM 4 Tachycardia (with pulses). (*Reprinted with Permission 2015 American Heart Association Guidelines for CPR and ECC—Part 7: ACLS © 2015 American Heart Association, Inc.*)

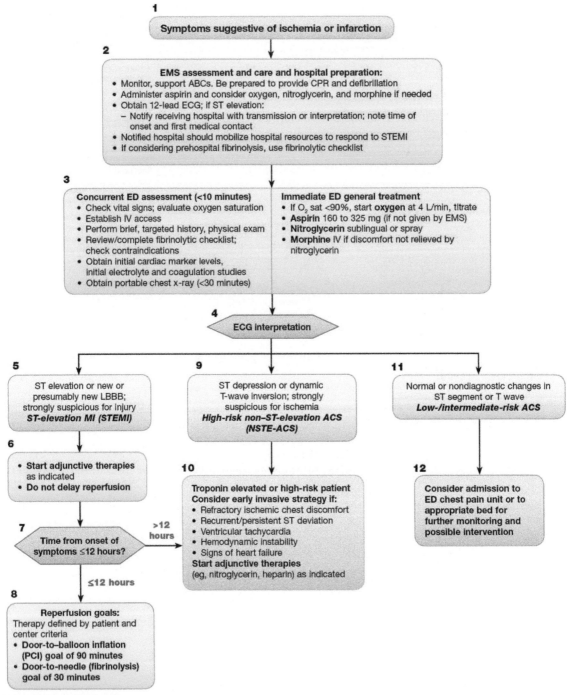

1
Symptoms suggestive of ischemia or infarction

2
EMS assessment and care and hospital preparation:
- Monitor, support ABCs. Be prepared to provide CPR and defibrillation
- Administer aspirin and consider oxygen, nitroglycerin, and morphine if needed
- Obtain 12-lead ECG; if ST elevation:
  – Notify receiving hospital with transmission or interpretation; note time of onset and first medical contact
- Notified hospital should mobilize hospital resources to respond to STEMI
- If considering prehospital fibrinolysis, use fibrinolytic checklist

3
Concurrent ED assessment (<10 minutes)
- Check vital signs; evaluate oxygen saturation
- Establish IV access
- Perform brief, targeted history, physical exam
- Review/complete fibrinolytic checklist; check contraindications
- Obtain initial cardiac marker levels, initial electrolyte and coagulation studies
- Obtain portable chest x-ray (<30 minutes)

Immediate ED general treatment
- If O₂ sat <90%, start **oxygen** at 4 L/min, titrate
- **Aspirin** 160 to 325 mg (if not given by EMS)
- **Nitroglycerin** sublingual or spray
- **Morphine** IV if discomfort not relieved by nitroglycerin

4
ECG interpretation

5
ST elevation or new or presumably new LBBB; strongly suspicious for injury
ST-elevation MI (STEMI)

9
ST depression or dynamic T-wave inversion; strongly suspicious for ischemia
High-risk non–ST-elevation ACS (NSTE-ACS)

11
Normal or nondiagnostic changes in ST segment or T wave
Low-/intermediate-risk ACS

6
- Start adjunctive therapies as indicated
- Do not delay reperfusion

7
Time from onset of symptoms ≤12 hours?

>12 hours

≤12 hours

10
Troponin elevated or high-risk patient
Consider early invasive strategy if:
- Refractory ischemic chest discomfort
- Recurrent/persistent ST deviation
- Ventricular tachycardia
- Hemodynamic instability
- Signs of heart failure
Start adjunctive therapies
(eg, nitroglycerin, heparin) as indicated

12
Consider admission to ED chest pain unit or to appropriate bed for further monitoring and possible intervention

8
Reperfusion goals:
Therapy defined by patient and center criteria
- Door-to–balloon inflation (PCI) goal of 90 minutes
- Door-to-needle (fibrinolysis) goal of 30 minutes

© 2015 American Heart Association

ALGORITHM 5 Acute coronary syndrome. (*Reprinted with permission 2015 American Heart Association Guidelines for CPR and ECC—Part 9: Acute Coronary Syndromes ©2015 American Heart Association, Inc.*)

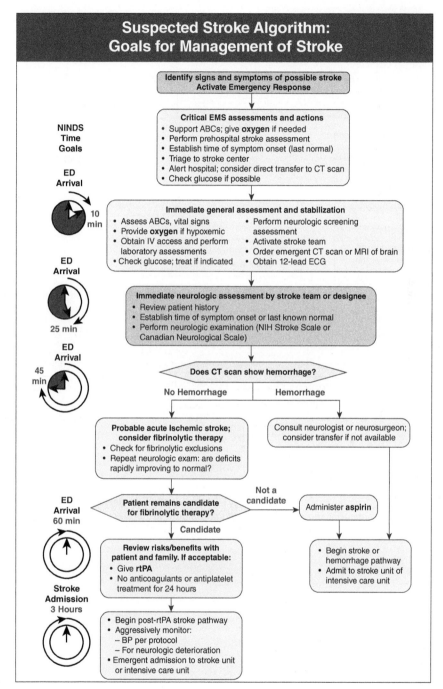

ALGORITHM 6 Algorithm for suspected stroke and goals for management of stroke. (*Reprinted with permission 2015 Handbook of Emergency Cardiovascular Care for Healthcare Providers © 2015 American Heart Association, Inc.*)

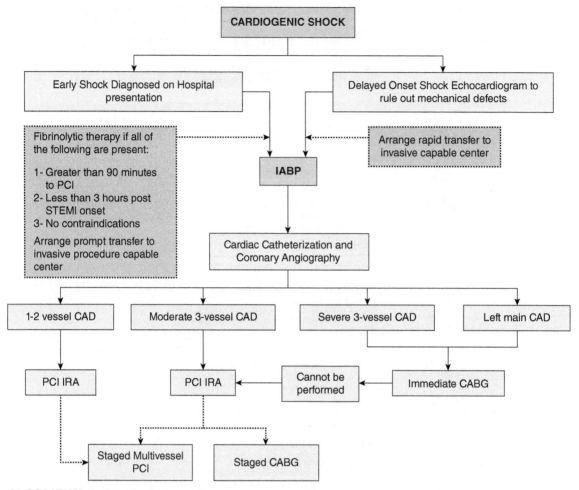

ALGORITHM 7 Algorithm for revascularization strategy in cardiogenic shock. (*Reproduced with permission from Reynolds HR1, Hochman JS: Cardiogenic shock: current concepts and improving outcomes,* Circulation. *2008 Feb 5;117(5):686-697.*)

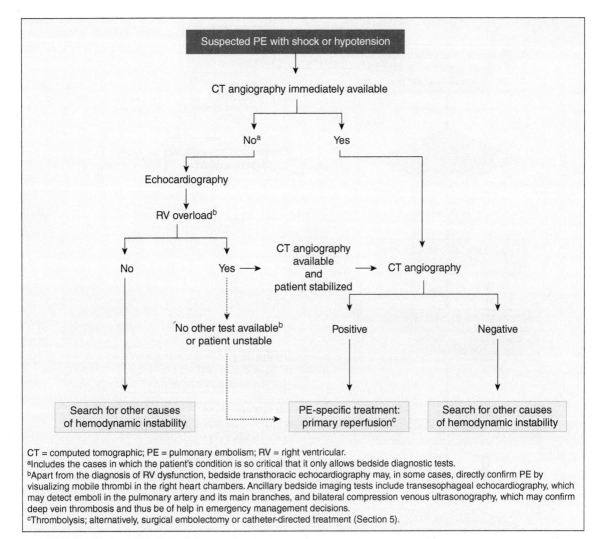

CT = computed tomographic; PE = pulmonary embolism; RV = right ventricular.
[a]Includes the cases in which the patient's condition is so critical that it only allows bedside diagnostic tests.
[b]Apart from the diagnosis of RV dysfunction, bedside transthoracic echocardiography may, in some cases, directly confirm PE by visualizing mobile thrombi in the right heart chambers. Ancillary bedside imaging tests include transesophageal echocardiography, which may detect emboli in the pulmonary artery and its main branches, and bilateral compression venous ultrasonography, which may confirm deep vein thrombosis and thus be of help in emergency management decisions.
[c]Thrombolysis; alternatively, surgical embolectomy or catheter-directed treatment (Section 5).

ALGORITHM 8 Proposed diagnostic algorithm for patients with suspected high-risk PE, ie, presenting with shock or hypotension. (*Reproduced with permission from Konstantinides SV, Torbicki A, Agnelli G, et al: 2014 ESC guidelines on the diagnosis and management of acute pulmonary embolism, Eur Heart J. 2014 Nov 14;35(43):3033-3069.*)

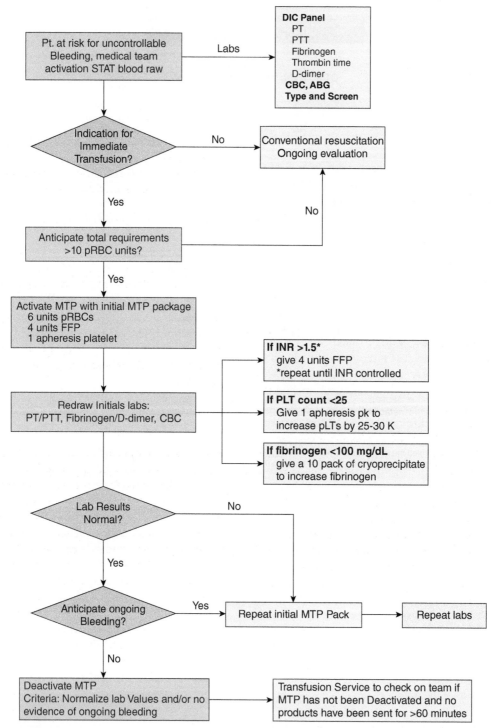

ALGORITHM 9 Algorithm for massive transfusion protocol. (*Adapted with permission from Burtelow M1, Riley E, Druzin M, et al: How we treat: management of life-threatening primary postpartum hemorrhage with a standardized massive transfusion protocol,* Transfusion. *2007 Sep;47(9):1564-1572.*)

Bedside Statistical Tools

John T. Doucette, PhD and Steven Krasnica, MD

INTRODUCTION

A primary goal for clinicians is to evaluate the benefits and harms from the treatment options before them. *Primum non nocere* is a basic principle of ethical practice. "Evidence-based medicine is the conscientious, explicit, and judicious use of the current best evidence in making decisions about the care of individual patients. The practice of evidence-based medicine means integrating the individual clinical expertise with the best available external evidence from systematic review."[1] Since the 1990s, evidence-based medicine (EBM) has been gaining a strong foothold in most disciplines of medicine. In order to practice EBM, however, it is paramount that clinicians are capable of assessing and synthesizing medical literature. Effective physicians comprehend the balance between personal clinical experience and evidence from appropriately conducted research. Clinicians need to proficiently assess the quality of published studies with respect to design, conduct, and analysis, and then to determine the relevance and external validity to their specific patient. Not all evidence is equal, nor does it offer definite clinical plans of care. One needs to understand the basic threats to the validity of studies, namely bias, confounding, and chance. The randomized controlled trial (RCT) and meta-analysis are regarded as the gold standard of EBM. However, RCTs are difficult to perform in critical care medicine.

Critical care medicine is a rapidly evolving discipline that deals with a complex disease spectrum. Sepsis and ARDS, for example, are still poorly understood disease processes with multiple etiologies and phenotypes. Sepsis syndrome may arise from a number of sources all presenting differently in different patients. Consequently, there are many challenges in the conduct of sound clinical research

in this field: critical illness is difficult to precisely define; patient populations may differ drastically with respect to severity of disease, treatment modalities, and other characteristics; subject recruitment may be difficult.

A sound knowledge of fundamental statistics will lay the basis for critical appraisal of the literature, an imperative clinical tool in every practitioner's armamentarium. Statistical tools can be used to describe the performance of diagnostic tests, characterize relationships between clinical decisions and outcomes, and estimate survival probabilities, just to name a few of their many uses. Ultimately, one would like to pair a critical appraisal of evidence with comprehensive clinical judgment at the bedside, where $n = 1$.

STUDY DESIGNS

Perhaps as important as an understanding of the methods of analysis used in clinical studies is an understanding of the various types of study designs, their defining characteristics, and the strengths and weaknesses of each. The most commonly used designs that involve collection and analysis of original data ("primary studies") can be broken into 2 subtypes: experimental or intervention studies and observational studies. Yet another class of studies ("secondary studies") seeks to synthesize information from multiple existing studies of the same research question. For experimental designs, we describe the RCT and other clinical trial designs. For observational studies, we consider cohort studies, case-control studies, cross-sectional studies, case series, and case reports. Finally, we discuss meta-analyses and systematic reviews as types of secondary studies.

EXPERIMENTAL STUDIES

Randomized Controlled Trials

Partly because of its desirable properties, the RCT is widely used in critical care medicine. In this design, patients who meet eligibility criteria are randomly assigned to 1 of 2 or more groups, called the arms of the trial. The groups are often defined by the treatment regimen to be received by the subjects in the group. This is an experimental design, meaning that the investigator actively chooses to give, for example, 1 treatment to 1 group of patients and another to a second group. Thus, the RCT is not suited to research questions where it is not practical or ethical to experimentally assign subjects to the exposure (treatment) of interest.

A key feature of the RCT is the *randomization* of subjects to the arms of the trial. The purpose of this randomization is to create groups of subjects that *tend* to be comparable on other prognostic factors related to outcome, thus ensuring a "fair" comparison. We stress that the groups tend to be comparable, because randomization does not guarantee this. For this reason, it is imperative to compare the subjects in each treatment arm with respect to other factors known to be related to outcome in order to either assure that the groups are similar or to account for any dissimilarities in the analysis of the trial data.

An important issue in the design of an RCT is *blinding* or *masking*. Blinding of a study keeps knowledge of the random treatment assignment of each subject hidden from 1 or more parties. In a so-called double-blind study, both the investigators and the study subjects are thus blinded. The purpose of blinding is to minimize the potential for bias in the study results. Bias can often occur in subtle, unintended ways from well-meaning individuals, and so blinding attempts to remove the potential for many types of bias. For some types of interventions (eg, surgery vs medical management), blinding is not feasible. When this occurs, to the extent possible it is advisable to blind the investigators who assess outcomes. This can be achieved by having outcomes assessed by members of the research team who are not involved in clinical care of the patient or administration of the intervention.

Another important factor, specific to experimental studies, and thus RCTs, is *crossover*, and

related to that, the *intention-to-treat principle*. In some studies, patients who are randomly assigned to 1 treatment group may, at some point during the trial, end up not receiving that treatment and possibly receiving a treatment associated with one of the other arms of the trial. These subjects are said to have crossed over, and the existence of such crossover complicates the analysis of the trial results. The intention-to-treat principle, which is the accepted method of dealing with crossover when it occurs, dictates that data collected from subjects should be analyzed with the group to which the subject was randomized, irrespective of what treatment the subject actually received. Although this may initially seem counterintuitive, this protects the validity of any observed differences between groups. Crossover cannot be assumed to occur at random, and thus to remove crossover subjects from the group to which they were randomly assigned would compromise the randomization, potentially leading to invalid results. Under the intention-to-treat principle, the crossover may dilute the degree of difference between the groups on whatever outcome measure is employed. But the integrity of any observed difference (that is found despite any such dilution) is intact. At the design phase of a trial, if a fair amount of crossover is expected, investigators may be wise to plan for somewhat larger sample sizes to compensate for the dilution of effect sizes due to crossover.

OBSERVATIONAL STUDIES

In observational studies, unlike in studies with an experimental design, the investigator does not decide who has which treatment or exposure but merely observes what happens within each exposure group. As such, extra care must be taken, usually in the analysis, to account for imbalances between the groups on factors related to outcome other than the exposure(s) of interest.

Cohort Studies

In a cohort design, a group of subjects (the "cohort") is identified and followed forward over time to observe the rate of occurrence of the outcome(s) of interest. The cohort is typically divided into 2 or more groups based on exposure to a particular risk factor for the outcome (eg, treatment), with those exposure groups being compared at the end of the study with respect to the outcome rate. Most cohort studies are prospective and proceed as described earlier. Occasionally, if reliable exposure data are available from an earlier time, an investigator can assemble the cohort retrospectively, by determining who had exposure at some specific earlier time and comparing outcomes over the time subsequent to that exposure. These latter studies are alternately referred to as retrospective cohort or historical cohort studies.

Case-Control Studies

In the case-control design, groups of subjects are chosen after the outcome of interest has already occurred. A case group of subjects with a particular disease (or other outcome) are selected, and a comparison group of subjects (the controls) without the disease are chosen. Information about past exposures and risk factors of interest is then collected and compared between the cases and controls. If the exposure data rely on self-report from the study subjects, and if case subjects recall their exposures differently from control subjects, these studies can suffer from a resulting bias known as recall bias. Nonetheless, case-control studies can often be a useful way of addressing a question that needs an observational design.

Cross-Sectional Studies

Another type of observational design is the cross-sectional study. This is sometimes simply called a survey. In a cross-sectional design, no time has passed between the assessment of exposure(s) and outcome(s). Rather, both are assessed or measured at the same point in time. As such, a major limitation of such studies is that the temporal relationship between one factor and the other cannot be established. Cross-sectional designs are often employed for large-scale, population-based surveys to look at the health characteristics of a population.

Case Reports and Case Series

As its name implies, a case report is a description of the characteristics of a single patient. A case series describes a usually small group (series) of patients. These types of studies do not typically involve any data analysis or comparison of subgroups, but merely report on characteristics of interest in the case or series of cases. As such, they are especially useful when something out of the ordinary has occurred that may shed new light on existing knowledge or perhaps even identify a new disease type or syndrome.

SECONDARY STUDIES

In secondary studies, new data are not presented. Rather, existing data from other studies are collected and perhaps reanalyzed to synthesize the body of evidence on a particular topic. All such studies need to consider the possible role of what is known as publication bias, which stems from the belief that studies that find an effect ("positive studies") are more likely to be published than studies that do not ("negative studies"). If this belief is warranted, a synthesis of only published studies will be biased toward finding an effect.

There are 3 main types of secondary studies: review articles, systematic reviews, and meta-analyses. In a review article, the authors identify as many studies as can be found related to a particular research question (and perhaps related topics). They then present in an organized way the key findings of those studies, and draw conclusions based on critical evaluation of the full body of evidence on the question.

Systematic reviews have largely taken the place of the basic review article. In a systematic review, the investigators must spell out the systematic approach used in identifying the research to be included in the review. Typically, a very wide net is cast and a very large number of studies need to be vetted for inclusion or exclusion from the review.

In a meta-analysis, investigators gather all the studies relevant to a particular question in a similar manner as one would do for a systematic review. They then do a new analysis of the combined set of data from those studies, in order to present an overall estimate of the effect of interest that is more precise due to the much larger number of subjects from all studies combined.

Statistical Analysis
Hypothesis Tests

Most clinical studies involve one or more statistical hypothesis tests to address the research question(s) at hand. There are many types of such hypothesis tests. For complex questions or designs, a biostatistician should be consulted, but some of the basic tests used, and issues related to their proper use, are presented here. The types of tests can be grouped as those related to continuous outcomes, categorical or discrete outcomes, and time-to-event (survival) data.

Continuous outcomes—Many of the outcomes we measure are quantitative in nature and lend themselves to inference based on continuous distributions. Many of the tests of this type involve comparing the mean (or other measure of central tendency) of 2 or more populations. When only 2 groups are to be compared, a *t-test for 2 independent samples* is often employed. If a comparison group internal to the study is not available, sometimes the mean of a single group is compared to a known population value using a *one-sample t-test*. If the 2 samples of data to be compared are not from 2 independently selected groups, but are either from the same subjects (paired data) or a comparison group especially selected to match the first group on important characteristics (matched data), then a *paired t-test* is often employed. When more than 2 groups are to be compared to test for equality of means, a method called *analysis of variance* (ANOVA) can be used.

All of these types of *t*-tests and the ANOVA method make an assumption that the data within each population are (approximately) normally distributed. Minor deviations from this assumption can be tolerated, but when this assumption is not realistic, as is often the case, the analyst has 2 options: (1) the data can be transformed in a way that results in a more symmetric distribution (eg, positively skewed data may benefit from a logarithmic transformation) or (2) a *nonparametric* test may be employed instead of the *t*-test or ANOVA. These nonparametric tests, as their name implies, do not make distributional assumptions about the data. They are insensitive to extreme outliers as they make use of the rank ordering of the observations, not their actual values. So, for example, if the 5 oldest patients in a sample were 102, 64, 63, 59, and 56 years of age, in a nonparametric analysis these values would be converted to ranks of 1, 2, 3, 4, and 5 thus diminishing the influence of the extreme value of 102. Examples of nonparametric tests (not an exhaustive list) include the Mann-Whitney U test or the Wilcoxon rank-sum test in

place of the 2-sample *t*-test, the Wilcoxon signed rank test in place of the paired *t*-test, and Friedman's test in place of ANOVA.

Categorical outcomes—When the outcome of interest is a qualitative factor, we say it is a *categorical* variable, meaning that it can only take on a discrete set of possible values. Categorical variables may further be classified as either *nominal* (named categories, such as blood type) or *ordinal* (ordered categories, such as severity of pain if measured as none, mild, moderate, or severe).

Analysis of categorical outcomes often involves using one of a set of tests known collectively as *chi-square tests*. In the *Pearson chi-square test*, 2 or more groups are compared with respect to the proportion exhibiting the outcome. The data are often summarized in a *contingency table or cross-tabulation*, in which subjects are cross-classified by the combination of their exposure group and whether or not they have the outcome. The cross-tabulation presents counts and percentages for each possible combination of the 2 factors, with one factor listed on the rows and the other on the columns. The Pearson chi-square uses a continuous distribution to approximate the behavior of the categorical data; when the number of subjects in 1 or more of the groups (defined by either exposure or outcome) is small, however, the validity of that approximation is questionable, in that case a *Fisher's exact test* should be used instead. Most statistical software is programmed to warn users when use of a Fisher's exact test is preferred. Just as is the case with continuous outcomes, if the groups to be compared are not independently selected but are instead paired or matched, then the method of analysis needs to account for the interdependence within the pairs. In this case, one could use a *McNemar's test* for paired data. The contingency table is set up differently, however, as the unit of observation becomes the matched pairs instead of the individual subjects. Each pair is cross-classified with respect to the outcome for each of the 2 members of the pair.

Time-to-event outcomes (survival analysis)—When the outcome is an event that occurs over time, one is often interested in both whether subjects experience the event and how soon they experience the event. If the event is one for which all subjects can be observed completely with respect to either the fact or the timing of the event, then the methods described earlier can be employed. Many studies, however, follow subjects for the occurrence of an event where, at the end of the study, some subjects have not experienced the event but have been at risk for that event for a period of time. The time to event for such subjects is said to be *censored*, in that we only partially observe it (ie, we know the time is at least as long as the amount of time they were at risk, but do not know how much longer). This arises often in studies where the event of interest is mortality, as such studies will often not be continued until all subjects have died. As such, the analytic methods for dealing with censored time-to-event data are often referred to as *survival analysis*. The survival (or event-free time) experience of 1 or more groups can be estimated using a variety of methods, including the *Kaplan–Meier* or *product-limit* method. This can be illustrated graphically with a Kaplan–Meier curve (actually a step function) that plots study time on the horizontal axis against survival (event-free) probability on the vertical access. The survival experience of 2 or more groups can be compared with various methods, including the *log-rank test*.

P-values—Regardless of the type of statistical test used, a hypothesis test is performed by comparing the observed data to what would be expected to be observed under what is termed the *null hypothesis* which, generally speaking, represents the absence of a difference between groups, or an effect, association, etc. If what was observed would be unlikely under the null hypothesis, then that null hypothesis is rejected in favor of the alternative (eg, that there is a difference or an effect). Specifically, a *test statistic* is calculated (it may be a t statistic, a chi-square statistic, or some other) whose probability distribution under the null hypothesis is known. When "unlikely" values of the test statistic occur, that is, when we reject the null hypothesis. How we define unlikely is determined by the *significance level* of the test, denoted α, which is typically set by convention at 0.05. So, with α = 0.05, if the test statistic falls in the range of values that are the 5% *least* likely to occur, that is, when we reject the null hypothesis. But, in addition to this reject or do not reject dichotomy, our statistical tests produce a measure of the likelihood of our test statistic known as the *P value*. Specifically, the *P* value is the chance of observing a test statistic as large (in absolute value) as the one observed *if* the

null hypothesis were true. Because the test statistic is a function of the observed data, one can think of the *P* value as the chances of observing as great a degree of difference as was observed if, in fact, the populations represented by the groups do not differ at all. One thing that the *P* value is *not*, though it is often misinterpreted as such, is the probability that a conclusion to reject or not reject is due to chance alone.

Measures of Disease Occurrence and Association

The aims of a study often include a desire to quantify the frequency with which, or the rate at which, a disease (or other outcome) occurs and/or the association of 1 or more risk factors with the occurrence of disease. For this, we need to have metrics to describe both disease occurrence and the associations between risk factors and outcomes.

Risks, Rates, and Odds

The proportion of a particular population that develops a particular disease is called the *risk* of disease. The risk is estimated simply as the number with the disease over the total number at risk of the disease. The proportion developing a disease per unit time is called the *rate* of disease. The numerator for the rate is still the same, but the denominator is no longer a count of the at-risk population, but the *person-time* of observation. To calculate person-time, say in years, the number of years that each subject in the at-risk group was followed is summed to get the total person-years for the rate calculation. The line between risks and rates may sometimes be fine, as a risk is often for a fixed period of time, for example, the 5-year risk of cancer recurrence. We do not often think of the *odds* of disease, but we sometimes need to calculate odds for measures of association (described later). If the probability of an outcome is *P*, then the odds of that outcome is $P/(1 - P)$, that is, the chance of it happening divided by the chance of it not happening. Note that if an outcome is rare (*P* close to zero), then the chance of it not happening is close to one, and the odds and the risk are almost the same.

Ratio Measures of Association

If 2 groups are being compared with respect to the occurrence of an outcome, they can be compared with either ratio measures or difference measures. We first consider ratio measures. The *relative risk* is simply the risk in the group of interest divided by the risk in the comparison group. If rates rather than risks are being compared, one may instead compute a *rate ratio*. In the context of survival analysis, the rate of the event in one group divided by the rate in the other is called the *hazard (rate) ratio*. For the case-control study design, risk in each comparison group cannot be observed directly, and we instead calculate an *odds ratio*, defined as the odds of exposure in the cases over the odds of exposure in the controls. If the outcome is rare, one can exploit the fact that odds and risk are almost the same and employ the so-called rare-disease assumption to interpret an odds ratio as an estimate of relative risk. When outcomes are not rare, however, the odds ratio tends to overestimate the relative risk (ie, be further away from a null ratio of one).

Difference Measures of Association

Sometimes the absolute difference in risk or rate between 2 groups is of greater interest than the relative difference. In such cases, a difference measure would be preferred over a ratio measure. The risk difference is simply the risk in one group minus the risk in the other. In clinical studies, where the goal is often to test an experimental treatment to see if it *reduces* risk of an adverse outcome relative to a control treatment, these measures sometimes go by more specific names. The *control event rate* and the *experimental event rate* are simply the rates (or risks) of the outcome in the control group and experimental group, respectively. The difference between these is known as the *absolute risk reduction* (ARR), and is a measure of how much of the event (disease, mortality, etc) could be prevented (or cured) by replacement of the control treatment with the experimental treatment. Another measure of association, related to the ARR and often important in clinical studies, is the *number needed to treat* (NNT). It is defined as NNT = 1/ARR. It is an estimate of how many patients would need to be treated with the experimental treatment in order to prevent 1 adverse outcome (eg, death). So, for example, if a new treatment reduced mortality in a certain patient population from 10% to 4%, the relative risk (of death) would be 0.40 (4%/10%), the ARR would be 6% (10% – 4%), and

NNT = 1/0.06 = 16.67, suggesting that 17 patients would need to be treated to prevent 1 death. The *number needed to harm* is an analogous measure in studies where the groups are being compared with respect to a risk factor or exposure that increases, rather than decreases, the risk of the outcome. It is still calculated as 1 divided by the absolute difference in risk, but has an opposite interpretation because the group with the factor of interest is harmed rather than helped.

Confidence Intervals

Any of the measures mentioned earlier can be estimated from a given set of data. Such an estimate is called a *point estimate*. Because it is based on limited sample data, the point estimate will differ from the actual value it is intended to estimate due to sampling variability. To get a better idea of what the true value of a population parameter may be, one may calculate and present a *confidence interval* (CI) around the point estimate. A CI has a confidence *level* associated with it, denoted $(1 - \alpha)$ and usually expressed as a percent, corresponding to a significance level α for a related hypothesis test. Typically, $\alpha = 0.05$, corresponding to 95% CIs. Even though a CI gives us a better idea of what the true population value is than does the point estimate, any given CI from a single study may or may not contain that true value. But the formulas for calculating 95% CIs are constructed in such a way that, over repeated studies, they will contain the correct value 95% of the time. It is from this that CIs get their name, as we claim 95% *confidence* that the interval will contain the true value.

Diagnostic and Screening Test Performance Measures

Diagnostic and screening tests are used to classify patients with respect to the presence or absence of a disease, syndrome, or other condition. These tests are not always accurate, and their performance is described by various metrics that relate to the correct classification of those with and without disease. To define these measures, consider a population of *N* patients represented in the following "truth table." The columns of the table represent the patients' true presence or absence of disease while the rows represent their test result. In practice, when evaluating

TABLE 116–1 Truth table.

		True Disease Status		
		Disease	**No Disease**	**Total**
Test Result	Positive	a	b	$a+b$
	Negative	c	d	$c+d$
	Total	$a+c$	$b+d$	N

new tests, we may not know with absolute certainty the true disease status of a set of patients, but instead compare a new test to a "gold standard" that is assumed to represent true disease status (Table 116–1).

The *sensitivity* of a test refers to how well it correctly classifies those *with* disease, and is equal to $[a/(a + c)]$, the proportion of those with disease who test positive. The *specificity* of a test refers to how well it correctly classifies those *without* disease, and is equal to $[d/(b + d)]$, the proportion of those without disease who test negative. The *positive predictive value* (PPV) of a test refers to how likely it is that a positive test result indicates the presence of disease, and is equal to $[a/(a + b)]$, the proportion of all those with a positive test result who actually have disease. The *negative predictive value* (NPV) of a test refers to how likely it is that a negative test result indicates the absence of disease, and is equal to $[d/(c + d)]$, the proportion of all those with a negative test result who actually do not have disease.

The sensitivity and specificity of a test are characteristics of the test itself and thus do not change unless something about the test itself is changed (eg, by altering a cutoff for what is considered a positive test result). The PPV and NPV, however, depend not only on how accurate the test is but also on how prevalent the disease is in the population to whom the test is applied. The *prevalence* of a disease is the proportion of the population that has the disease. In our truth table discussed earlier, the prevalence is $[(a + c)/N]$. In particular, if the prevalence is low in the population being tested, a test with fairly high sensitivity and specificity can still have very poor PPV. In such instances, more specific confirmatory tests may be needed in those who initially test positive.

CONCLUSION

The development of comprehensive expertise in statistical methods is beyond the scope of study for most physicians, and only basic methods have been presented here. But the clinician who is equipped with these tools is better prepared to critically appraise the medical literature, where innovations that have the potential to affect clinical practice may appear. The clinical investigator who is equipped with these tools is better prepared to design sound, unbiased studies, and to effectively communicate with coinvestigators (including biostatisticians) in order to make valid inferences from their data. Finally, the physician who can appreciate when the claims of published studies are validly supported by the available data, and when they are not, is better prepared to treat patients in an optimal, evidence-based manner.

REFERENCE

1. Sackett DL, Rosenberg WM, Gray JA, Haynes RB, Richardson WS. Evidence based medicine: what it is and what it isn't. *BMJ.* 1996;312(7023):71-72.

Index

Note: Page numbers followed by f and t indicate figures and tables, respectively.